65828
2 vol.
~~30-~~
20-

VOLUME 28, NO. 1
JANUARY 1985

arthritis and rheumatism

Official Journal of the American Rheumatism Association
Section of the Arthritis Foundation

Arthritis Foundation
Atlanta, Georgia

In osteoarthritis

THE PAIN OF PLEASURE

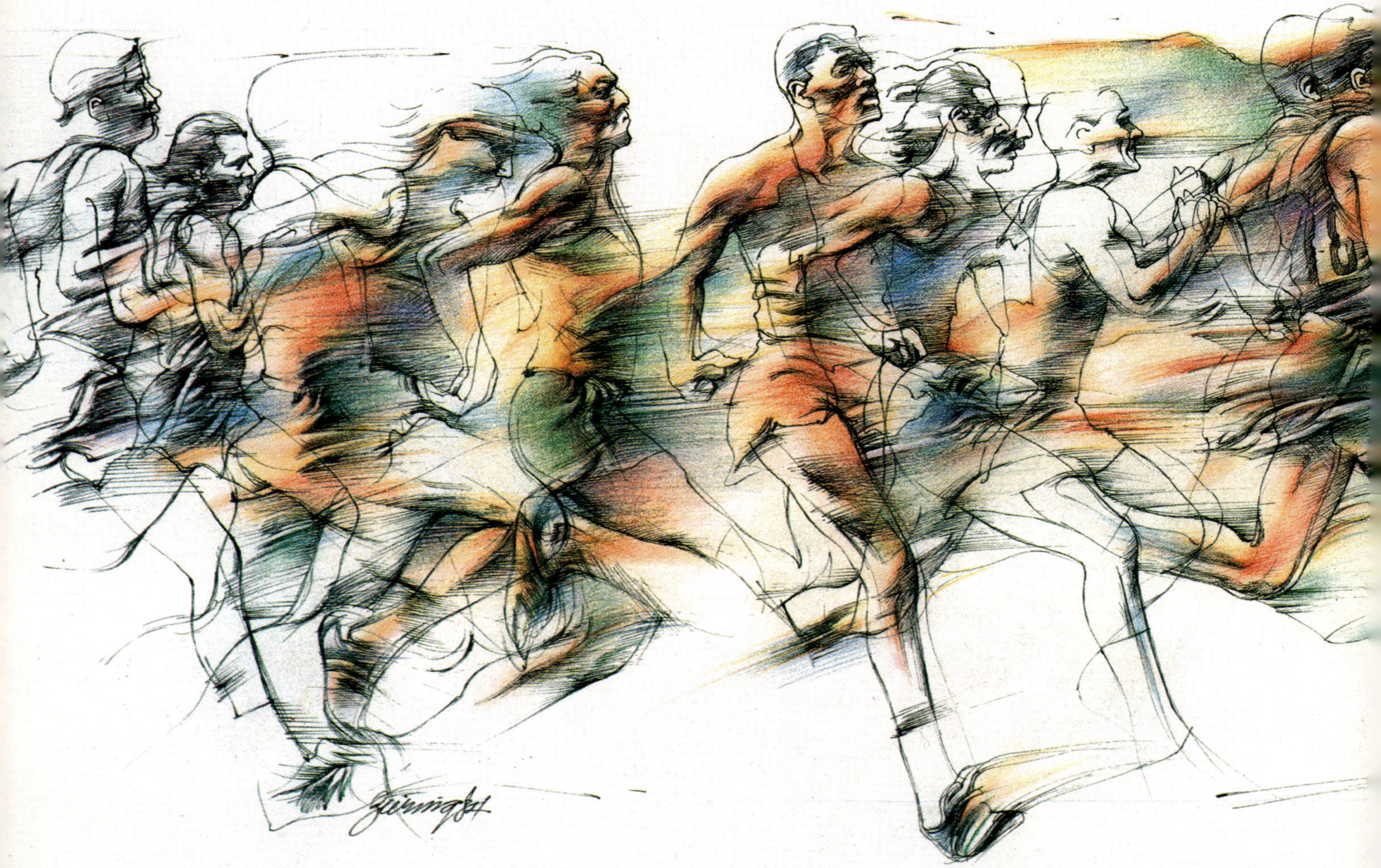

arthritis and rheumatism

Official Journal of the American Rheumatism Association Section of the Arthritis Foundation

VOLUME 28 JANUARY NO. 1

ARA Presidential Address: 1984–2034: The Next Half-Century for American Rheumatology
James R. Klinenberg 1

Characterization of T Cells Bearing HLA–DR Antigens in Rheumatoid Arthritis
Seth H. Pincus, Daniel O. Clegg, and John R. Ward 8

Reproducibility of Multiple-Observer Scoring of Radiologic Abnormalities in the Hands and Wrists of Patients with Rheumatoid Arthritis
John T. Sharp, Gilbert B. Bluhm, Andrew Brook, Anne C. Brower, Mary Corbett, John L. Decker, Harry K. Genant, J. Philip Gofton, Neal Goodman, Arvi Larsen, Martin D. Lidsky, Pekka Pussila, Aaron S. Weinstein, Barbara N. Weissman, and Donald Y. Young 16

Quantitative Histologic Studies on the Pathogenesis of Periarticular Osteoporosis in Rheumatoid Arthritis
Shinichi Shimizu, Shunichi Shiozawa, Kazuko Shiozawa, Shigeaki Imura, and Takuo Fujita 25

Therapeutic Value of Graded Aerobic Exercise Training in Rheumatoid Arthritis
Thomas M. Harkcom, Richard M. Lampman, Barbara Figley Banwell, and C. William Castor 32

Spondylitic Disease Without Radiologic Evidence of Sacroiliitis in Relatives of HLA–B27 Positive Ankylosing Spondylitis Patients
Muhammad A. Khan, Sjef M. van der Linden, Irving Kushner, Hans A. Valkenburg, and Arnold Cats 40

Surface Antigen Specificity of Cold-Reactive IgM Antilymphocyte Antibodies in Systemic Lupus Erythematosus
Akira Yamada, Melody Shaw, and John B. Winfield 44

Effects of L-Canavanine on T Cells May Explain the Induction of Systemic Lupus Erythematosus by Alfalfa
Jorge Alcocer-Varela, Antonio Iglesias, Luis Llorente, and Donato Alarcón-Segovia 52

Lupus Pregnancy. II. Unusual Pattern of Hypocomplementemia and Thrombocytopenia in the Pregnant Patient
Michael D. Lockshin, Peter C. Harpel, Maurice L. Druzin, Carl G. Becker, Renate F. Klein, Rosemarie M. Watson, Keith B. Elkon, and Elizabeth Reinitz 58

The Lupus Anticoagulant: A Disease Marker in Antinuclear Antibody Negative Lupus that is Cross-Reactive with Autoantibodies to Double-Stranded DNA
C. Bernard Colaco and Keith B. Elkon 67

Salmonella Bacteremia in Systemic Lupus Erythematosus: Eight-Year Experience at a Municipal Hospital
Steven Abramson, Sara B. Kramer, Allen Radin, and Robert Holzman 75

The Incidence of Systemic Lupus Erythematosus in Baltimore, Maryland, 1970–1977
Marc C. Hochberg 80

Evolution of Primary Raynaud's Phenomenon (Raynaud's Disease) to Connective Tissue Disease
David D. Gerbracht, Virginia D. Steen, Gayle L. Ziegler, Thomas A. Medsger, Jr., and Gerald P. Rodnan 87

Brief Reports

Beneficial Effect of Intravenous Cyclophosphamide and Oral Prednisone on D-Penicillamine–Associated Bronchiolitis Obliterans
Martinus A. F. J. van de Laar, Cees J. J. Westermann, Sjoerd Sc. Wagenaar, and Huibert J. Dinant 93

Isolation of Echovirus Type 11 from Synovial Fluid in Acute Monocytic Arthritis
Greg Kujala and James H. Newman 98

Systemic Lupus Erythematosus and Common Variable Panhypogammaglobulinemia: A Patient with Absence of Circulating B Cells
Rose Goldstein, Carlos Izaguirre, C. Douglas Smith, Egils Mierins, and Jacob Karsh 100

Ibuprofen May Induce Meningitis in (NZB × NZW)F_1 Mice
Shlomo Berliner, Abraham Weinberger, Yehuda Shoenfeld, Uri Sandbank, Bilha Hazaz, Henry Joshua, Menachem Rosen, and Jack Pinkhas 104

(*Contents continued opposite inside back cover*)

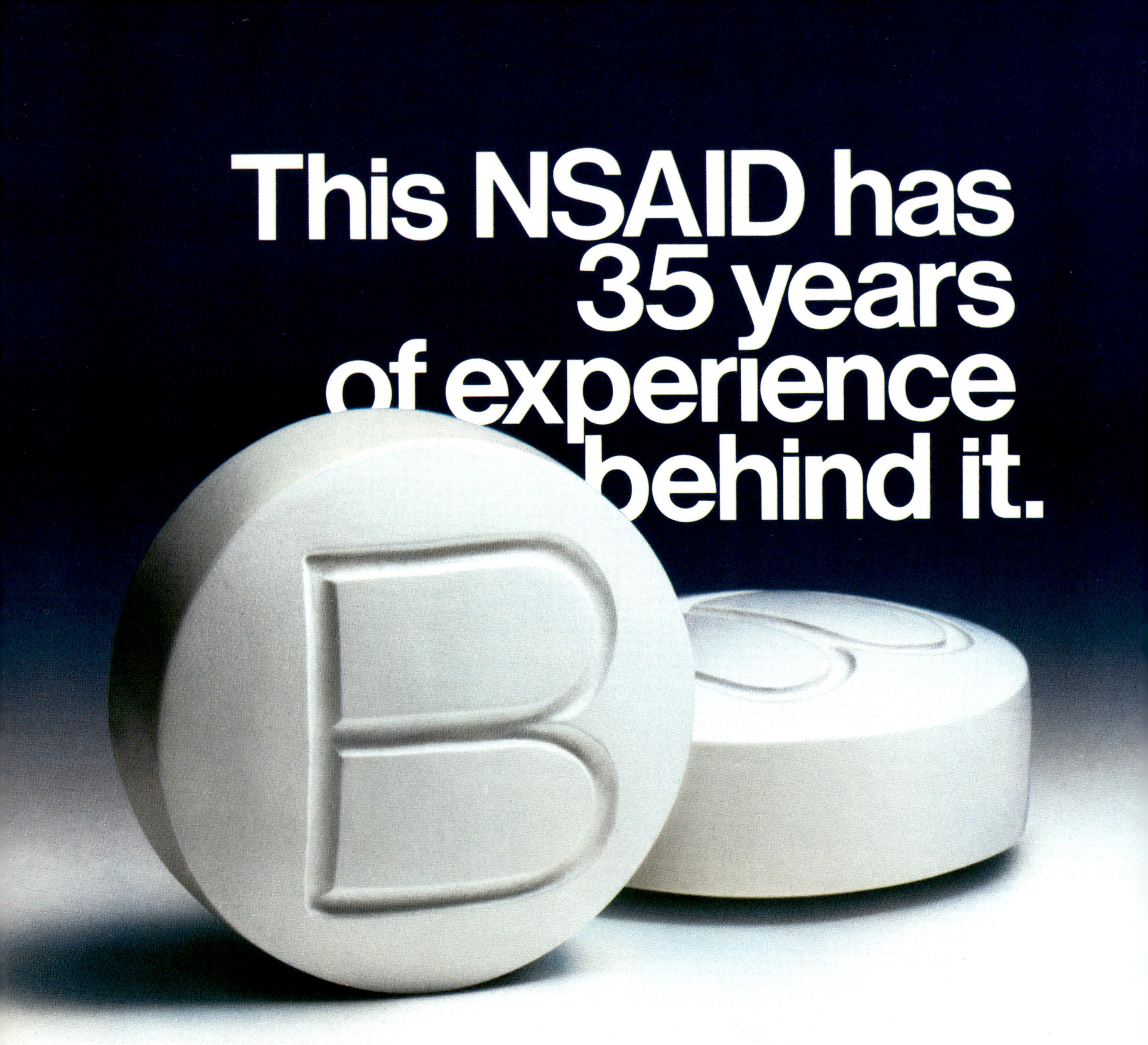
This NSAID has
35 years
of experience
behind it.

Brief Reports (*cont'd*)

Evaluation of an Educational Program for Primary Care Practitioners, on the Management of Osteoarthritis
Jeoffrey K. Stross and Giles G. Bole 108

In Vitro Synthesis of Low Molecular Weight IgM in Rheumatoid Arthritis
D. Neil Jones, Lin Y. Koh, James V. Bertouch, and Peter J. Roberts-Thomson 112

Letters

Pulmonary Hypertension and Chronic Cutaneous Lupus Erythematosus: Association with the Lupus Anticoagulant
Ronald A. Asherson, Stephen H. Morgan, Nigel Harris, Azzudin E. Gharavi, Graham R. V. Hughes, and Ann B. Millar 118

Chondrocytes That Accumulate Proteoglycans and Inorganic Pyrophosphate in the Pathogenesis of Chondrocalcinosis
Koichiro Ishikawa 118

Synovial Fluid Lymphocyte Subpopulations in the Polyarthritis of Immunoblastic Lymphadenopathy
Robert G. Gray 120

INDEX TO ADVERTISERS

Boots Pharmaceuticals
Rufen .... A32 thru A34
Zorprin A9, A10
Bristol-Myers
Bufferin .... Cover 3
Burroughs Wellcome
Imuran .... A46 thru A48
Zyloprim .... A14 thru A16
Classified Ads A48, A49, A61
Geigy Pharmaceuticals
Institutional A23
Glaxo, Inc.
Zantac A39, A40
Eli Lilly & Co.
Nalfon .... A27 thru A30
J. B. Lippincott Co.
Book A31
Merck Sharp & Dohme
Clinoril A17, A18
Dolobid .... A42 thru A44
Flexeril .... A24 thru A26
Indocin SR .... A62 thru A64
Indocin Suppository .... A5 thru A8
Institutional A36, A37
Parke-Davis
Meclomen .... Cover 2, A1, A2
Pfizer Laboratories
Feldene .... A56 Thru A58
Wm. H. Rorer
Ascriptin A/D A19
St. Luke's Medical Center
Conference A55
Syntex Laboratories
Naprosyn .... A11, A12, A50 thru A52
The Upjohn Co.
Motrin .... A20 thru A22
Whitehall Laboratories
Advil A53, 54
WR Medical Electronics Co.
Therabath A13

Advertising Office: Pharmaceutical Media, Inc., 130 Madison Avenue, 6th Floor, New York 10016. Telephone: (212) 685-5010

arthritis and rheumatism

Official Journal of the American Rheumatism Association Section of the Arthritis Foundation

VOLUME 28 FEBRUARY NO. 2

Current Comment: Sex Steroids and the Rheumatic Diseases
Robert G. Lahita 121

Plasma Follicle-Stimulating Hormone, Luteinizing Hormone, and Sex Hormones in Patients with Gout
Enrico Marinello, Giuseppe Riario-Sforza, and Roberto Marcolongo 127

Clinical Characteristics of Fibrositis. II. A "Blinded," Controlled Study Using Standard Psychological Tests
Sharon Clark, Stephen M. Campbell, Mary E. Forehand, Elizabeth A. Tindall, and Robert M. Bennett 132

Juvenile Primary Fibromyalgia Syndrome: A Clinical Study of Thirty-Three Patients and Matched Normal Controls
Muhammad B. Yunus and Alfonse T. Masi 138

HLA Gene Frequencies in Children and Adults with Systemic Onset Juvenile Rheumatoid Arthritis
Marc L. Miller, Stephen Aaron, Jean Jackson, Patricia Fraser, Lloyd Cairns, Susan Hoch, Yves Borel, Martin Larson, and David N. Glass 146

Immunogenetic Studies of Juvenile Dermatomyositis. III. Study of Antibody to Organ-Specific and Nuclear Antigens
Lauren M. Pachman, Jan M. Friedman, Mona L. Maryjowski-Sweeney, Olga Jonnason, Ruta M. Radvany, Gordon C. Sharp, Mike A. Cobb, Norma D. Battles, William E. Crowe, Chester W. Fink, Virgil Hanson, Joseph E. Levinson, Charles H. Spencer, and Donita B. Sullivan 151

The Diagnostic Value of Antihistone Antibodies in Drug-Induced Lupus Erythematosus
Alan Epstein and Peter Barland 158

The Binding of Antihistone Antibodies to *Crithidia Luciliae* Kinetoplasts is Growth Cycle–Dependent
Jau-Shyong Deng, Richard D. Sontheimer, Mary F. Lipscomb, and James N. Gilliam 163

Abnormal Calcium and Magnesium Stores in Erythrocytes and Granulocytes from Patients with Inflammatory Connective Tissue Diseases: Relationship to Inflammatory Activity and Effect of Corticosteroid Therapy
Roger Hällgren, Karin Svenson, Erland Johansson, and Ulf Lindh 169

Immunohistochemical Studies of Interleukin-2 and γ-Interferon in Rheumatoid Arthritis
Gunnar Husby and Ralph C. Williams, Jr. 174

Circulating Natural Killer Cells in Sjögren's Syndrome
Yukinobu Ichikawa, Miyoko Yoshida, Masatoshi Takaya, Mitsuaki Uchiyama, Hiroaki Shimizu, and Shigeru Arimori 182

Soluble Mediators from Mononuclear Cells Increase the Synthesis of Glycosaminoglycan by Dermal Fibroblast Cultures Derived from Normal Subjects and Progressive Systemic Sclerosis Patients
Theresa L. Whiteside, Jennifer G. Worrall, Robert K. Prince, Robert B. Buckingham, and Gerald P. Rodnan 188

Arthroscopy in Septic Arthritis: Lidocaine- and Iodine-Containing Contrast Media are Bacteriostatic
M. A. Dory and M. J. Wautelet 198

Diagnosis-Related Group Regulations: Implications for the Practicing Rheumatologist
Morris Weinberger, Marilyn K. Potts, and Kenneth D. Brandt 204

Brief Reports

Changes in Nongonococcal Septic Arthritis: Drug Abuse and Methicillin-Resistant *Staphylococcus Aureus*
Glorietta Z. Ang-Fonte, Michael B. Rozboril, and George R. Thompson 210

Postgastrectomy Blind Loop Syndrome and the Arthritis–Dermatitis Syndrome
Alice V. Klinkhoff, Howard B. Stein, Otto L. A. Schlappner, and William B. Boyko 214

Bone Crisis of Gaucher's Disease Due to Bone Ischemia: A Case Report
Anne Davidson, Victor Kalff, and Peter F. J. Ryan 218

(*Contents continued opposite inside back cover*)

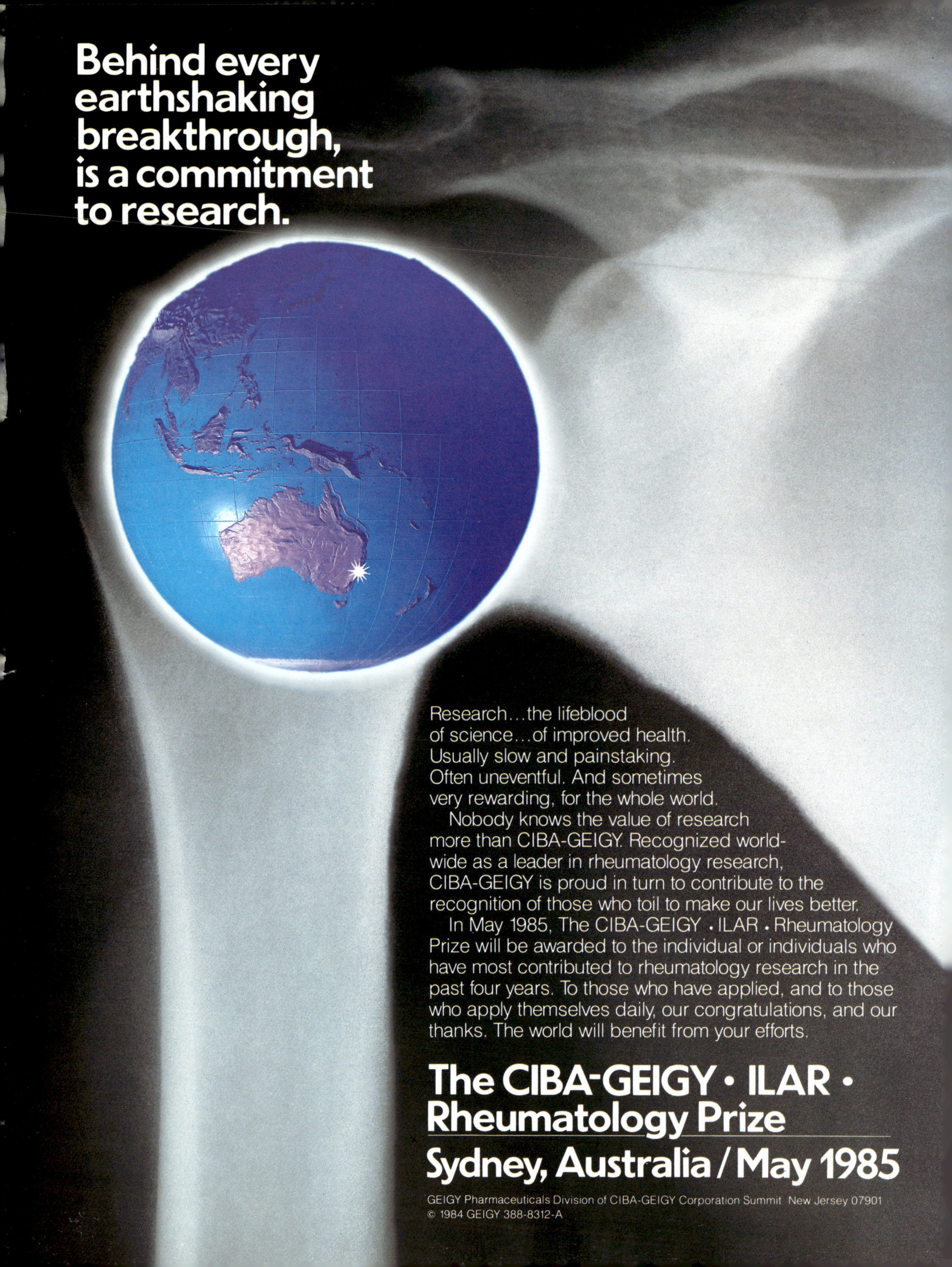
Behind every earthshaking breakthrough, is a commitment to research.
Research…the lifeblood of science…of improved health. Usually slow and painstaking. Often uneventful. And sometimes very rewarding, for the whole world.
Nobody knows the value of research more than CIBA-GEIGY. Recognized worldwide as a leader in rheumatology research, CIBA-GEIGY is proud in turn to contribute to the recognition of those who toil to make our lives better.
In May 1985, The CIBA-GEIGY • ILAR • Rheumatology Prize will be awarded to the individual or individuals who have most contributed to rheumatology research in the past four years. To those who have applied, and to those who apply themselves daily, our congratulations, and our thanks. The world will benefit from your efforts.
The CIBA-GEIGY • ILAR • Rheumatology Prize
Sydney, Australia / May 1985
GEIGY Pharmaceuticals Division of CIBA-GEIGY Corporation Summit New Jersey 07901
© 1984 GEIGY 388-8312-A

Brief Reports (*cont'd*)
Ability to Activate Complement is Not Required for the Detection of Immune Complexes by the Fluid-Phase C1q Binding Assay
Guy P. Fiocco, John S. Davis, IV, and Joseph J. Burge 222
Nucleolar Localization of the PM–Scl Antigen
Ira N. Targoff and Morris Reichlin 226
Multicentric Reticulohistiocytosis: A Cause of Dysphagia with Response to Corticosteroids
Peter J. Zeale, David Miner, Stephen Honig, Marian Waxman, and Harry Bartfield 231
Letters
A Followup Study of Children Exposed to Gold Compounds In Utero
Ulrik Tarp and Hans Graudal 235
HLA–Bw35 and Gold Toxicity in Rheumatoid Arthritis
Graciela S. Alarcón, William J. Koopman, Ronald T. Acton, and Bruce O. Barger 236
Renal Malakoplakia and Systemic Lupus Erythematosus
John Varga 237
Correction of Data on Salicylate and Indomethacin Concentrations in Cartilage
Marshall J. Palmoski and Kenneth D. Brandt 237
Pregnancy and Systemic Sclerosis
Mario Giordano, Gabriele Valentini, Salvatore Lupoli, and Andrea Giordano 237
Reply
Stanley P. Ballou and Irving Kushner 238
Coexistent Rheumatoid Arthritis and Gout
Arthur M. Virshup 238
Epidemiology of Juvenile Arthritis in Rochester, Minnesota
Eric S. Schned 239
Reply
Clement J. Michet 239
Serum C1q Levels in Rheumatoid Arthritis
N. Parhami, C. L. Rosano, and C. Hurwitz 240
ARA Announcements A15

INDEX TO ADVERTISERS

Allergan Pharmaceuticals
Liquifilm Tears A7
Boots Pharmaceuticals
Rufen .... A46 thru A48
Zorprin A11, A12
Bristol-Myers
Bufferin A23
Burroughs Wellcome
Imuran .... A4 thru A6
Zyloprim .... A52 thru A54
Classified Ads A59, A60
Geigy Pharmaceuticals
Institutional .... Cover 3
Glaxo, Inc.
Zantac A35, A36
Lederle Laboratories
Methotrexate A19
Eli Lilly & Co.
Nalfon .... A37 thru A40
Merck Sharp & Dohme
Clinoril A49, A50
Dolobid .... A32 thru A34
Flexeril .... A20 thru A22
Indocin SR .... Cover 2, A1, A2
Indocin Suppository .... A61 thru A64
Institutional A42, A43
Palo Alto Medical Foundation
Symposium A41
Pfizer Laboratories
Corporate A30, A31
Feldene .... A16 thru A18
Norwich Eaton Pharmaceuticals
Didronel A13, A14
Encaprin A44, A45
Wm. H. Rorer
Ascriptin A/D A29
Syntex Laboratories
Naprosyn .... A8 thru A10, A55, A56
The Upjohn Co.
Motrin .... A24 thru A26

Advertising Office: Pharmaceutical Media, Inc., 130 Madison Avenue, 6th Floor, New York 10016. Telephone: (212) 685-5010

arthritis and rheumatism

Official Journal of the American Rheumatism Association Section of the Arthritis Foundation

VOLUME 28 MARCH NO. 3

Autoantibody Specificities of Immune Complexes Sequestered in Articular Cartilage of Patients with Rheumatoid Arthritis and Osteoarthritis
Hugo E. Jasin ... 241

Prognostic Factors in Polymyositis/Dermatomyositis: A Computer-Assisted Analysis of Ninety-Two Cases
Jochanan Benbassat, Dov Gefel, Keren Larholt, Shaul Sukenik, Vladimir Morgenstern, and Avinoam Zlotnick ... 249

Evidence for Intravascular Coagulation in Systemic Onset, But Not Polyarticular, Juvenile Rheumatoid Arthritis
J. Paul Scott, Patricia Gerber, Mona C. Maryjowski, and Lauren M. Pachman ... 256

Subset Specificity of Antilymphocyte Antibodies in Systemic Lupus Erythematosus: Preferential Reactivity with Cells Bearing the T4 and Autologous Erythrocyte Receptor Phenotypes
Akira Yamada, Philip L. Cohen, and John B. Winfield ... 262

Neonatal Lupus Erythematosus Occurring in One Fraternal Twin: Serologic and Immunogenetic Studies
Jeffrey P. Callen, Joseph F. Fowler, Kevin B. Kulick, Gregory Stelzer, and Stephen Z. Smith ... 271

Effects of Long-Term Procainamide Therapy on Immunoglobulin Synthesis
Chia-Li Yu and Morris Ziff ... 276

Patterns of Antihistone Antibody Specificity in Systemic Rheumatic Disease. I. Systemic Lupus Erythematosus, Mixed Connective Tissue Disease, Primary Sicca Syndrome, and Rheumatoid Arthritis with Vasculitis
Robert M. Bernstein, Roderick N. Hobbs, Donald J. Lea, Donald J. Ward, and Graham R. V. Hughes 285

Quantitation of the Sm Nuclear Antigen in Tissues and Activated Lymphocytes
Cinda M. Boyer, Robert A. Eisenberg, and Philip L. Cohen ... 294

Assessing Physician/Patient Perceptions in Rheumatoid Arthritis: A Vital Component in Patient Education
Ilene J. Silvers, Melbourne F. Hovell, Michael H. Weisman, and Mary Rose Mueller ... 300

Double-Blind, Multicenter Controlled Trial Comparing Topical Dimethyl Sulfoxide and Normal Saline for Treatment of Hand Ulcers in Patients with Systemic Sclerosis
H. James Williams, Daniel E. Furst, Stephen L. Dahl, Virginia D. Steen, Carolly Marks, Elaine J. Alpert, Avery M. Henderson, Cecil O. Samuelson, Jr., James N. Dreyfus, Arthur Weinstein, Edmund J. MacLaughlin, Graciela S. Alarcón, Stanley B. Kaplan, Maria Guttadauria, Michael E. Luggen, James C. Reading, Marlene J. Egger, and John R. Ward ... 308

Substrain Heterogeneity in Prostaglandin E_2 Synthesis of Human Dermal Fibroblasts: Differences in Prostaglandin E_2 Synthetic Capacity of Substrains are Not Stimulus-Restricted
Joseph H. Korn ... 315

Kinetics of Extraction of Proteoglycans from Human Cartilage
Lawrence A. Pottenger, June E. Webb, and Nancy B. Lyon ... 323

Radiologic Vignette: Tarsal Coalition
David J. Sartoris and Donald L. Resnick ... 331

Brief Reports

A Subset of Rheumatoid Arthritis Patients with a Pattern of Epstein-Barr Virus Antibodies Similar to That Found in Primary and Secondary Immunodeficiency Diseases
Jacques H. M. Cohen, Thomas L. Vischer, Jocelyn Carquin, and François Blanchard ... 339

Thrombotic Thrombocytopenic Purpura Developing During Pregnancy in a C2-Deficient Patient with a History of Systemic Lupus Erythematosus
R. Dixit, Arthur M. Krieg, and J. P. Atkinson ... 341

Cardiac Involvement in Behçet's Disease
Carolyn A. Bowles, Audrey M. Nelson, Stephen C. Hammill, and J. Desmond O'Duffy ... 345

(Contents continued opposite inside back cover)

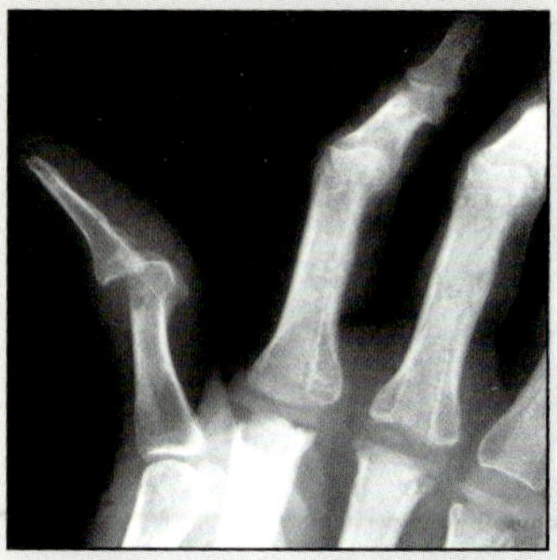
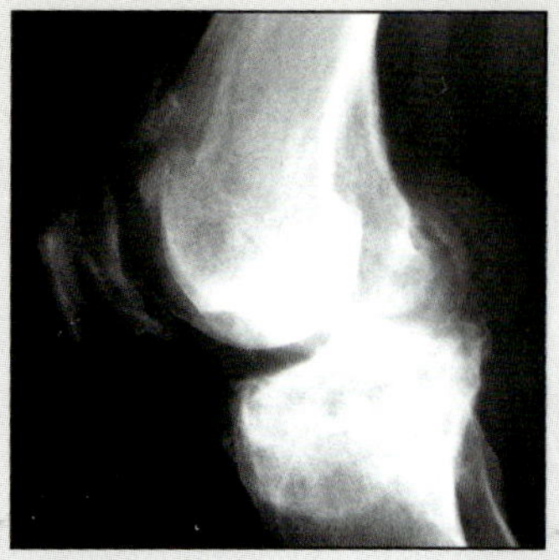
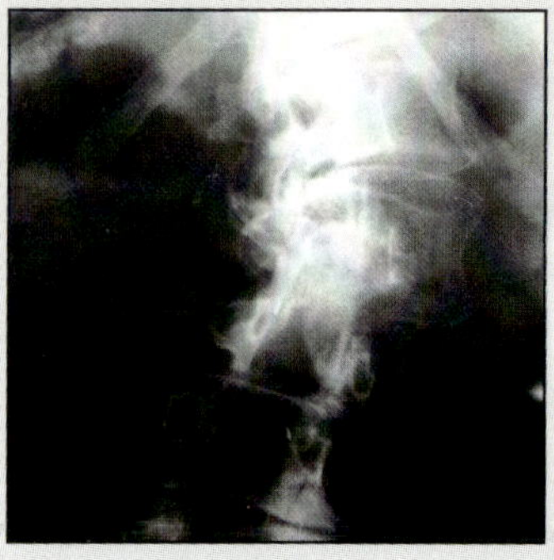
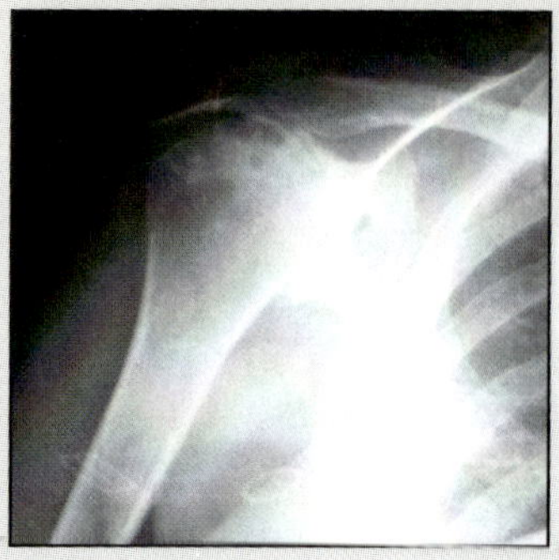

The effects of Sjögren's syndrome don't stop at the joints.

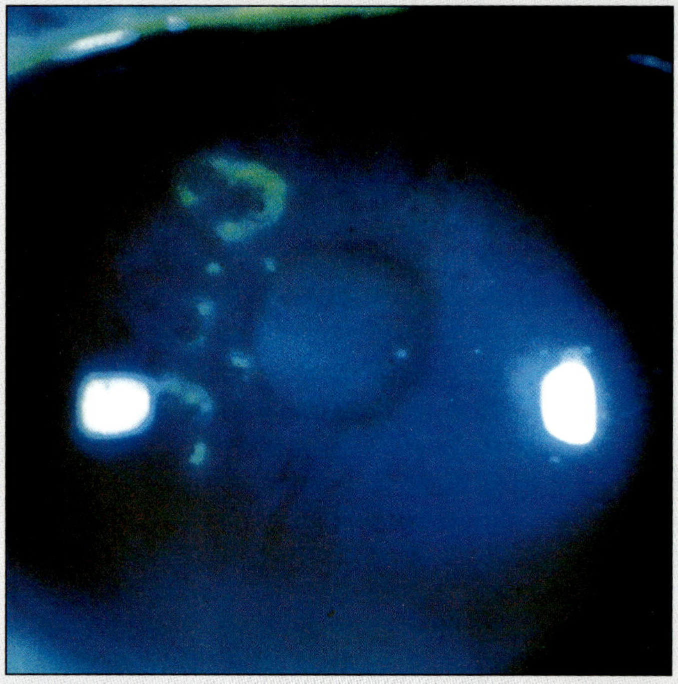

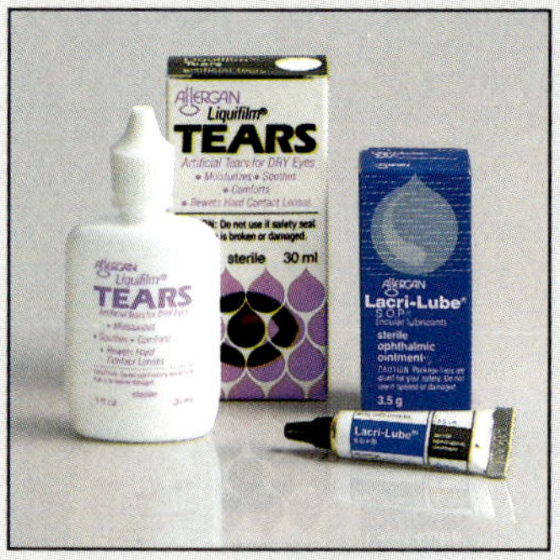

The itchy, scratchy dry eye condition associated with Sjögren's syndrome can result in painful corneal abrasions like the one pictured above.

Liquifilm® Tears artificial tears for day contains time-tested polyvinyl alcohol 1.4% to soothe and lubricate irritated eyes. And Lacri-Lube® S.O.P.® sterile ophthalmic ointment for night helps prevent the ocular dehydration that can result in damaging corneal abrasions.

Liquifilm® Tears for day.

Lacri-Lube® S.O.P.® for night.

ALLERGAN®

Recommended by ophthalmologists for over 20 years.

Allergan Pharmaceuticals, Inc., Irvine, CA 92713

Brief Reports (*cont'd*)

Defective Immune Adherence Receptors (CR1) on Erythrocytes in Autoimmune Diseases: An Association with HLA–Cw3
Yukio Matsumura, Shigeko Inokuma, Tetsuo Hayakawa, and Tomonari Kisaki 349

Response of the Acute-Phase Reactants, C-Reactive Protein and Serum Amyloid A Protein, to Antibiotic Treatment of Whipple's Disease
John I. Reed, Jean D. Sipe, Jeffrey R. Wohlgethan, Wilhelm G. Doos, and Juan J. Canoso 352

Letters

In Vitro IgM and IgM Rheumatoid Factor Production and Response to Remittive Agents in Rheumatoid Arthritis
Graciela S. Alarcón, William J. Koopman, and Ralph E. Schrohenloher 356

Comment on Article by van der Linden et al
Andrei Calin 357

Reply
Sjef M. van der Linden, Arnold Cats, and Hans Valkenburg 358

The CREST Acronym and Some Related Problems
Mario Giordano 359

Digital Angiography for the Diagnosis of Dural Sinus Thrombosis in Behçet's Disease
P. Brissaud, L. Laroche, A. de Gramont, and M. Krulik 359

ARA Announcements A28, A29

INDEX TO ADVERTISERS

Allergan Pharmaceuticals
Liquifilm Tears .... Cover 3
Boots Pharmaceuticals
Rufen .... A6 thru A8
Zorprin A39, A40
Burroughs Wellcome Co.
Imuran .... A52 thru A54
Zyloprim .... A10 thru A12
Classified Ads .... A55 thru A57
Geigy Pharmaceuticals
Institutional A9
Grune & Stratton
Book A19
Lederle Laboratories
Methotrexate A23
Merck Sharp & Dohme
Clinoril A43, A44
Dolobid .... A48 thru A50
Flexeril .... A20 thru A22
Indocin SR .... A58 thru A60
Indocin Suppository .... A30 thru A32
Institutional A4, A5
Parke-Davis
Meclomen .... Cover 2, A1, A2
Pfizer Pharmaceuticals
Corporate A34, A35
Feldene A17, A18, A45, A46
Wm. H. Rorer
Ascriptin A/D A27
Syntex
Naprosyn .... A13, A14, A36 thru A38
The Upjohn Co.
Motrin .... A24 thru A26
Whitehall Laboratories
Advil A15
WR Medical Electronics
Therabath A47

Advertising Office: Pharmaceutical Media, Inc., 130 Madison Avenue, 6th Floor, New York 10016. Telephone: (212) 685-5010

arthritis and rheumatism

Official Journal of the American Rheumatism Association Section of the Arthritis Foundation

VOLUME 28 APRIL NO. 4

Evaluation of Factors Associated with Glucocorticoid-Induced Osteopenia in Patients with Rheumatic Diseases
Thomas R. Dykman, Oscar S. Gluck, William A. Murphy, Theodore J. Hahn, and Bevra H. Hahn 361

The Effect of Glucocorticoids on Bone Mass in Rheumatoid Arthritis Patients: Influence of Menopausal State
Orla Skibsted Als, Anders Gotfredsen, and Claus Christiansen 369

Evaluation of D-Penicillamine in Juvenile Chronic Arthritis: A Double-Blind, Multicenter Study
A. M. Prieur, C. Piussan, P. Manigne, P. Bordigoni, and C. Griscelli 376

Serum C-Reactive Protein in Polymyalgia Rheumatica: A Prospective Serial Study
R. K. Mallya, C. R. K. Hind, H. Berry, and M. B. Pepys. 383

Atrophic Gastritis in Sjögren's Syndrome: Morphologic, Biochemical, and Immunologic Findings
C. P. J. Maury, T. Törnroth, and A-M. Teppo 388

Phagocytosis and Intracellular Killing by Polymorphonuclear Cells from Patients with Rheumatoid Arthritis and Felty's Syndrome
Ferdinand C. Breedveld, Maria T. van den Barselaar, Peter C. J. Leijh, Arnold Cats, and Ralph van Furth 395

Human Rheumatoid Arthritic Cartilage and its Neutral Proteoglycan–Degrading Proteases: The Effects of Antirheumatic Drugs
Johanne Martel-Pelletier, Jean-Marie Cloutier, David S. Howell, and Jean-Pierre Pelletier 405

Cartilage Nucleoside Triphosphate Pyrophosphohydrolase. II. Role in Extracellular Pyrophosphate Generation and Nucleotide Metabolism
Lawrence M. Ryan, Robert L. Wortmann, Barbara Karas, and Daniel J. McCarty, Jr. 413

Cartilage Response to Mechanical Force in High-Density Chondrocyte Cultures
G. P. J. van Kampen, J. P. Veldhuijzen, R. Kuijer, R. J. van de Stadt, and C. A. Schipper 419

A Longitudinal Study of High and Low Avidity Antibodies to Double-Stranded DNA in Systemic Lupus Erythematosus
Hugh McGrath, Jr. and Joseph J. Biundo, Jr. 425

Spontaneous In Vitro Production of Anti-DNA and Anti-RNA by Systemic Lupus Erythematosus and Normal Peripheral Blood Mononuclear Cells
Michael R. Liebling, Curtice Wong, and Jean Radosevich 431

Intraarticular Volume and Clearance in Human Synovial Effusions
Wayne J. Wallis, Peter A. Simkin, Wil B. Nelp, and David M. Foster 441

Government Affairs: FDA Arthritis Advisory Committee Meeting
Harold E. Paulus 450

Brief Reports

Myocarditis in Adult Still's Disease
Ilan Bank, Charles C. Marboe, Rita F. Redberg, and Jerry Jacobs 452

A Persistent Adenovirus Type 1 Infection in Synovial Tissue from an Immunodeficient Patient with Chronic, Rheumatoid-Like Polyarthritis
Kevin J. Fraser, Barry J. Clarris, Kenneth D. Muirden, J. Robert E. Fraser, and Ian Jack 455

Raynaud's Phenomenon of a Single Digit Following Local Intradermal Bleomycin Sulfate Injection
Edwin A. Smith, Frank E. Harper, and E. Carwile LeRoy 459

Concurrent Systemic Lupus Erythematosus and Common Variable Hypogammaglobulinemia
Anthony Stein, Alan Winkelstein, and Amrit Agarwal 462

Bowel Involvement in Systemic Lupus Erythematosus: Crohn's Disease or Lupus Vasculitis?
Dafna D. Gladman, Theodore Ross, Beverley Richardson, and Savita Kulkarni 466

Special Article: Rheumatology Training at Internal Medicine and Family Practice Residency Programs
Don L. Goldenberg, Raphael J. DeHoratius, Stephen R. Kaplan, John Mason, Robert Meenan, Susan G. Perlman, and John B. Winfield 471

(Contents continued opposite inside back cover)

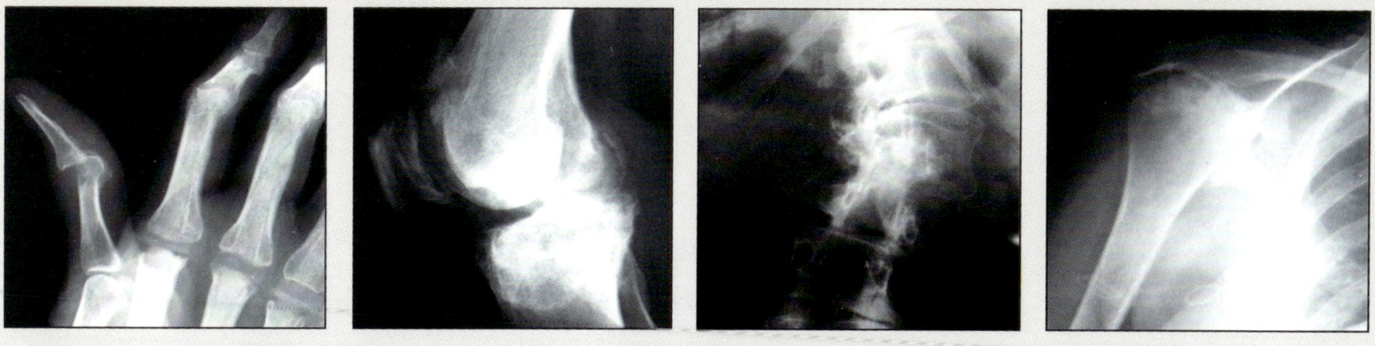

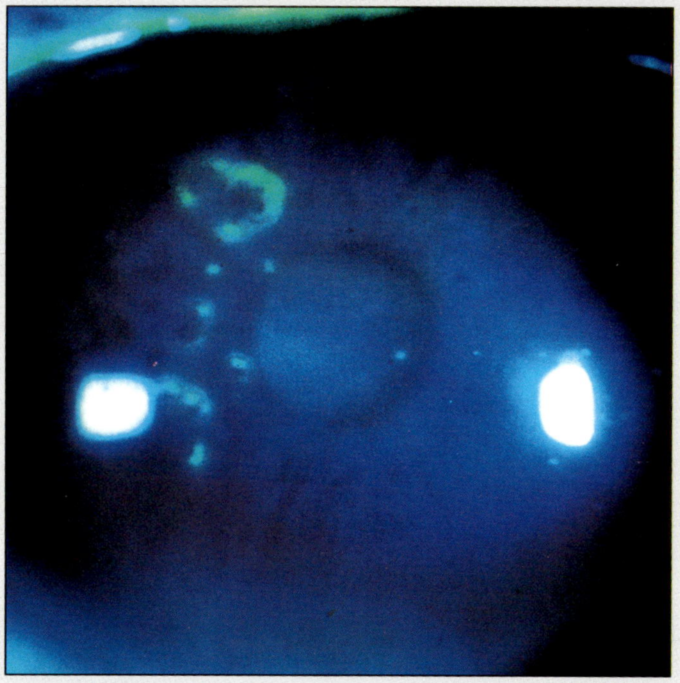

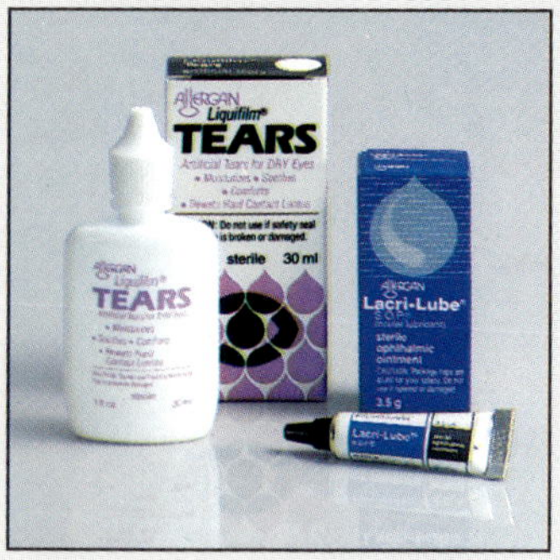
TEARS
Lacri-Lube

Letters

Comment on Article by Faure et al
Barry Lee Myones, Earl D. Silverman, and John J. Miller, III 477

Popliteal Cyst Presenting as an Anterior Tibial Mass
A. Thevenon, P. Hardouin, and B. Duquesnoy 477

Comment on Article by Brenner et al
Stephen Aaron 478

Tender Point Count
Frederick Wolfe 479

Angiotensin Converting Enzyme Inhibitors and Rheumatoid Arthritis
Allen Traficante, Michael A. Catalano, and George E. Ehrlich 480

Book Review 480

ARA Announcements A37

INDEX TO ADVERTISERS

Allergan Pharmaceuticals
Liquifilm Tears . . . . . Cover 3
Boots Pharmaceuticals
Rufen . . . . . A42 thru A44
Zorprin A3, A4
Bristol-Myers
Bufferin A15
Burroughs Wellcome
Imuran . . . . . A6 thru A8
Classified Ads A32, A45, A46
Geigy Pharmaceuticals
Institutional A29
Lederle Laboratories
Symposium A46
Merck Sharp & Dohme
Clinoril A27, A28
Dolobid . . . . . A10 thru A12
Flexeril . . . . . A38 thru A40
Indocin SR . . . . . A34 thru A36
Indocin Suppositories . . . . . Cover 2, A1, A2
Institutional A20, A21
Norwich Eaton Pharmaceuticals
Didronel A13, A14
Pfizer Laboratories
Feldene . . . . . A16 thru A18
Wm. H. Rorer
Ascriptin A/D A33
Seragen, Inc.
ENA Test Kit A9
Syntex Laboratories
Naprosyn . . . . . A22 thru A24
Talcott Laboratories
Parabath A19
The Upjohn Co.
Motrin . . . . . A30 thru A32

Advertising Office: Pharmaceutical Media, Inc., 130 Madison Avenue, 6th Floor, New York 10016. Telephone: (212) 685-5010

arthritis and rheumatism

Official Journal of the American Rheumatism Association Section of the Arthritis Foundation

VOLUME 28 MAY NO. 5

Antibodies to Human T Cell Leukemia Virus are Absent in Patients with Systemic Lupus Erythematosus
Takao Koike, Masaru Kagami, Katsuhiko Takabayashi, Naoki Maruyama, Hisao Tomioka, and Sho Yoshida 481

When Does Rheumatoid Disease Start?
K. Aho, T. Palosuo, V. Raunio, P. Puska, A. Aromaa, and J. T. Salonen 485

Nifedipine and Esophageal Dysfunction in Progressive Systemic Sclerosis: A Controlled Manometric Study
André Kahan, Bruno Bour, Daniel Couturier, Bernard Amor, and Charles J. Menkes 490

Relationship Between Nailfold Capillary Abnormalities and Organ Involvement in Systemic Sclerosis
Michael Lovy, Daryl MacCarter, and James C. Steigerwald 496

Selective Inhibition of Excessive Scleroderma Fibroblast Collagen Production by Lymphokines From Normal Human Mononuclear Cells
Sergio A. Jimenez, William M. McArthur, Reza I. Bashey, and Joel Rosenbloom 502

Synovial Fluid Crystals in Osteoarthritis
Paul A. Gibilisco, H. Ralph Schumacher, Jr., Joseph L. Hollander, and Keith A. Soper 511

Blastomycosis Presenting as Monarticular Arthritis: The Role of Synovial Fluid Cytology
Alfred L. George, Jr., J. Taylor Hays, and Barney S. Graham 516

Induction of Chronic Polyarthritis in Rabbits by Hyperimmunization with *Escherichia Coli*. I. Pathologic and Serologic Features in Two Breeds of Rabbits
Shigehisa Aoki, Koji Ikuta, Tsunemasa Nonogaki, and Yoshitake Ito 522

Etiopathogenesis of the Rheumatoid Arthritis–Like Disease in MRL/l Mice. I. The Histomorphologic Basis of Joint Destruction
Frank X. O'Sullivan, Hans-Georg Fassbender, Steffen Gay, and William J. Koopman 529

The Autologous Mixed Lymphocyte Reaction is Decreased in Freund's Adjuvant–Injected Rats of Arthritis-Susceptible and -Insusceptible Strains
William E. Crowe, Jack R. Battisto, and R. N. Smith 537

Comparative Measurement Efficiency and Sensitivity of Five Health Status Instruments for Arthritis Research
Matthew H. Liang, Martin G. Larson, Karen E. Cullen, and Julie A. Schwartz 542

Proteoglycan Depletion, Rather than Fibrillation, Determines the Effects of Salicylate and Indomethacin on Osteoarthritic Cartilage
Marshall J. Palmoski and Kenneth D. Brandt 548

Role of Synovial Membrane Inflammation in Cartilage Matrix Breakdown in the Pond-Nuki Dog Model of Osteoarthritis
Jean-Pierre Pelletier, Johanne Martel-Pelletier, Latifa Ghandur-Mnaymneh, David S. Howell, and J. Frederick Woessner, Jr. 554

The Specificity of Antibodies to the $F(ab')_2$ Fragment of Human IgG
Ralph Heimer, Lawrence D. Wolfe, and John L. Abruzzo 562

Special Article: Winners of the 1984 Slide Competition
Sidney Block and the Audiovisual Aids Subcommittee of the ARA Education Committee 569

Brief Reports

Systemic Lupus Erythematosus in a Premature Infant
Nancy P. Cummings, Jeffrey Hansen, and J. Roger Hollister 573

Meningococcemia Presenting as Septic Arthritis, Pericarditis, and Tenosynovitis
Michael S. Rosen, Allen R. Myers, and Burton Dickey 576

(Contents continued opposite inside back cover)

Brief Reports (*cont'd*)

Relationship of Autoantibody Expression and HLA Phenotype in Japanese Patients with Connective Tissue Diseases
Masahiko Nishikai and Susumu Sekiguchi 579
Aortic Regurgitation in Giant Cell Arteritis
Alice V. Klinkhoff, Graham D. Reid, and Michael Moscovich 582
Wrist Drop in Progressive Systemic Sclerosis (Scleroderma): Complete Rupture of the Extensor Tendon Mechanism
Lewis H. Rosenbaum, William M. Swartz, Gerald P. Rodnan, and Thomas A. Medsger, Jr. 586
Combination Immunosuppressive Treatment of Steroid-Resistant Dermatomyositis/Polymyositis
Daniel J. Wallace, Allan L. Metzger, and Kathy K. White 590

Letters

Diagnosis of Sjögren's Syndrome
Troy E. Daniels and John P. Whitcher 593
Aortic Arch Syndrome Associated with Anticardiolipin Antibodies and the Lupus Anticoagulant: Comment on Ferrante Paper
Ronald A. Asherson, E. Nigel Harris, Azzudin E. Gharavi, Helen E. Englert, and Graham R. V. Hughes 594
Nephrotic Syndrome Induced by Tiopronin: Association with the HLA–DR3 Antigen
Carlo Salvarani, PierLuigi Macchioni, Fulvia Rossi, Ido Iori, and Giordano Filippi 595
Idiopathic Thrombocytopenic Purpura with High-Titer, Speckled Pattern Antinuclear Antibodies: Possible Marker for Systemic Lupus Erythematosus
H. Daniel Perez, Ernest Katler, and Stephen Embury 596
Autoantibodies During Captopril Treatment
Cees G. M. Kallenberg 597
Systemic Lupus Erythematosus and Down's Syndrome
C. Michael Franklin and Dennis Torretti 598
Low Plasma Renin Activity in Lupus-Prone Mice: A Metabolic Abnormality in MRL/Mp-lpr/lpr Mice?
Ulrich H. Rudofsky, Robert L. Dilwith, Albert M. Magro, and John B. Roths 599
Botticelli and Arthritis
Donato Alarcón-Segovia 600

ARA Announcements A25

INDEX TO ADVERTISERS

Boots Pharmaceuticals
Rufen . . . . *A8 thru A10*
Zorprin A31, A32
Bristol-Myers
Bufferin . . . . Cover 3
Burroughs Wellcome
Imuran . . . . A46 thru A48
Zyloprim A15, A16
Classified Ads A45, A48, A49
Humana/Hollander
Recruitment A49
Lea & Febiger
Medical Tests A19
Lederle Laboratories
Symposium A44
Merck Sharp & Dohme
Clinoril A17, A18, A37, A38
Dolobid . . . . A41 thru A43
Flexeril . . . . A4 thru A6
Indocin SR . . . . A12 thru A14
Indocin Suppositories . . . . A50 thru A52
Institutional A26, A27
Parke-Davis & Co.
Meclomen . . . . Cover 2, A1, A2
Pfizer Laboratories
Feldene . . . . A34 thru A36
Wm. H. Rorer
Ascriptin A/D A7
Seragen, Inc.
ENA Test Kit A11
Syntex Laboratories
Naprosyn . . . . A22 thru A24
University of California
Course A33
The Upjohn Co.
Motrin . . . . A28 thru A30
Whitehall Laboratories
Advil *A20, A21*

Advertising Office: Pharmaceutical Media, Inc., 130 Madison Avenue, 6th Floor, New York 10016. Telephone: (212) 685-5010

arthritis and rheumatism

Official Journal of the American Rheumatism Association Section of the Arthritis Foundation

VOLUME 28 JUNE NO. 6

The Immunoreactivity, Ligand, and Cell Binding Characteristics of Rheumatoid Synovial Fluid Fibronectin
Steven Carsons, Beverly B. Lavietes, Herbert S. Diamond, and Sandra G. Kinney 601

Reduced Joint Count Indices in the Evaluation of Rheumatoid Arthritis
M. J. Egger, D. A. Huth, J. R. Ward, J. C. Reading, and H. J. Williams 613

A Comparison of the Specificity of the 1971 and 1982 American Rheumatism Association Criteria for the Classification of Systemic Lupus Erythematosus
Constance M. Passas, Robert L. Wong, Margaret Peterson, Marcia A. Testa, and Naomi F. Rothfield 620

Relationship Between Circulating Interferon and Anti-Interferon Antibodies and Impaired Natural Killer Cell Activity in Systemic Lupus Erythematosus
Wilmer L. Sibbitt, Jr., Dwayne L. Gibbs, Carol Kenny, Arthur D. Bankhurst, Robert P. Searles, and Kenneth D. Ley 624

Cricopharyngeal Obstruction in Inflammatory Myopathy (Polymyositis/Dermatomyositis): Report of Three Cases and Review of the Literature
Lawrence J. Kagen, Raymond B. Hochman, and Elliot W. Strong 630

Decreased Coronary Reserve in Primary Scleroderma Myocardial Disease
André Kahan, Alain Nitenberg, Jean-M. Foult, Bernard Amor, Charles-J. Menkes, Jean-Y. Devaux, Françoise Blanchet, Jeannine Perennec, Geneviève Lutfalla, and Jean-C. Roucayrol 637

Collagen Synthesis Regulation by the Aminopropeptide of Procollagen I in Normal and Scleroderma Fibroblasts
Jerome S. Perlish, Rupert Timpl, and Raul Fleischmajer 647

Coronary Arteritis in Mice Following the Systemic Injection of Group B *Lactobacillus Casei* Cell Walls in Aqueous Suspension
Thomas J. A. Lehman, Sharyn M. Walker, Vladimir Mahnovski, and Deborah McCurdy 652

Cartilage Surface Charge: A Possible Determinant in Aging and Osteoarthritic Processes
Zahava Laver-Rudich and Michael Silbermann 660

Effectiveness of Cyclosporin Therapy for Behçet's Disease
Robert B. Nussenblatt, Alan G. Palestine, Chi-Chao Chan, Manabu Mochizuki, and Kim Yancey .. 671

Outcomes of Self-Help Education for Patients with Arthritis
Kate Lorig, Deborah Lubeck, R. Guy Kraines, Mitchell Seleznick, and Halsted R. Holman 680

Utilization of Nonsteroidal Antiinflammatory Drugs
Carlene Baum, Dianne L. Kennedy, and Mary B. Forbes 686

Application, to Japanese Patients, of the 1982 American Rheumatism Association Revised Criteria for the Classification of Systemic Lupus Erythematosus
Ryuichi Yokohari and Tokugoro Tsunematsu 693

Brief Reports

Juvenile Progressive Systemic Sclerosis: Clinical and Serologic Findings
María E. Suárez-Almazor, Luis J. Catoggio, José A. Maldonado-Cocco, Rubén Cuttica, and Osvaldo García-Morteo 699

Protective Effect of Poliomyelitis on Psoriatic Arthritis
Steven R. Weiner, Lawrence W. Bassett, and Ronald P. Reichman 703

Allopurinol Hypersensitivity in a Patient with Severe, Chronic, Tophaceous Gout
Ella Webster and Richard S. Panush 707

Oral Gold Therapy in a Patient with Rheumatoid Arthritis and Preexisting Uremia
Winfried Graninger, Gerald Seidl, Josef Kovarik, Wulf Pinggera, and Josef S. Smolen 710

In Appreciation of Nathan J. Zvaifler, MD
Jane Diamond and Irving H. Fox 713

Introducing the New Editor: William J. Koopman, MD
Eng M. Tan 714

(Contents continued opposite inside back cover)

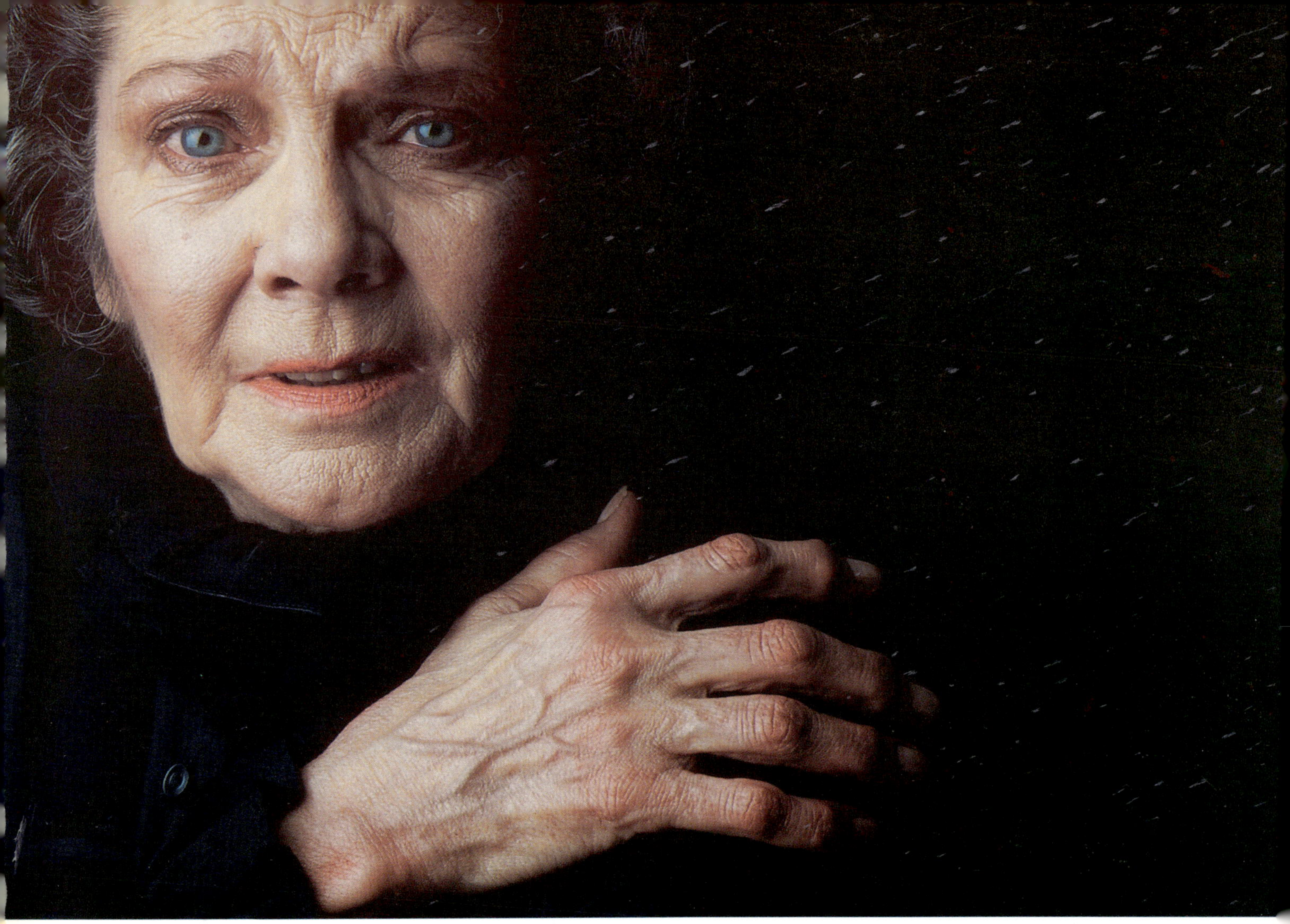

Letters
Evaluation of the 1982 American Rheumatism Association Revised Criteria for the Classification of Systemic Lupus Erythematosus
F. Davatchi, C. Chams, and M. Akbarian 715
Autoantibodies in Argentine Patients with Systemic Sclerosis (Scleroderma)
Luis J. Catoggio, Santiago Rodrigué, Hugo Laborde, Pedro M. Catoggio, and Patricia González Salas 715
Calcium Pyrophosphate Dihydrate Crystal Deposition in Rheumatoid Arthritis
Daniel J. McCarty 717
Reply
Michael Doherty, Paul Dieppe, and Iain Watt 718
Comment on Zea-Mendoza Report
John Varga and Maggie Flinn 719
Book Review 720
ARA Announcements A15

INDEX TO ADVERTISERS

Boots Pharmaceuticals
Rufen .... A38 thru A40
Zorprin A13, A14
Burroughs Wellcome Co.
Imuran .... A4 thru A6
Classified Ads A37, A41
Menley & James Laboratories
Ecotrin .... Cover 3
Merck Sharp & Dohme
Clinoril A17, A18, A35, A36
Dolobid .... A32 thru A34
Flexeril .... A8 thru A10
Indocin SR .... Cover 2, A1, A2
Indocin Suppositories .... A48 thru A50
Institutional A42, A43
Pfizer Laboratories
Feldene .... A26 thru A28
Norwich Eaton Pharmaceuticals
Didronel A23, A24
Rheumatology Diagnostics Laboratory
ANA Profile A7
Wm. H. Rorer
Ascriptin A/D A25
Syntex Laboratories
Naprosyn .... A11, A12, A44 thru A46
The Upjohn Co.
Motrin .... A20 thru A22
WR Medical Electronics Co.
Therabath A16

See additional classified ads on pages A37 and A41

arthritis
and
rheumatism

Official Journal of the American Rheumatism Association Section of the Arthritis Foundation

ARA PRESIDENTIAL ADDRESS

1984–2034: THE NEXT HALF-CENTURY FOR AMERICAN RHEUMATOLOGY

JAMES R. KLINENBERG

It is my special privilege to address you as your President on this occasion of the 50th anniversary of the founding of our Association. Each year the President of this organization has the opportunity to address the membership at the time of the annual meeting, and I am sure that each year the President spends considerable time thinking about an appropriate topic for his Presidential address. Should he take the opportunity to reiterate the concerns of that particular era—whether they be concerns regarding the organization itself or concerns about changes in the practice of medicine—or should it be an opportunity for the President to dwell on past accomplishments of the organization, or raise concerns regarding its directions. Surely, however, each President attempts to take advantage of the unique events of that particular year in order to develop a timely theme for his Presidential address. In that regard, my job was somewhat easier because of the obvious important events of 1984. These include, first and foremost, the 50th anniversary of our organization, but they also include the fact that 1984, the year popularized many years ago by George Orwell in his novel (1), indeed, has finally arrived; and, in addition, especially for those of us living in Los Angeles, 1984 represents the year of the Olympics. Rejecting the latter theme as somewhat overdone and of little direct relevance to rheumatology, I have chosen instead to concentrate on the past 50 years of rheumatology and, as George Orwell attempted to do in his novel, consider projections for rheumatology in the next 50 years to the year 2034—the occasion of our organization's centennial.

It is really somewhat difficult to identify the exact date of birth of the American Rheumatism Association. In May of 1932 the American Committee for the Study and Control of Rheumatic Diseases sponsored a conference on rheumatic diseases at the time of the AMA meeting in New Orleans. This conference was chaired by Dr. Ralph Pemberton of Philadelphia, and the program included distinguished scientists, such as Dr. Philip Hench, Dr. Paul Holbrook, and Dr. Chester Keefer. While this conference caused thoughts to be given to the rheumatic diseases as an important entity and nurtured the subsequent development of our Association, history suggests that its true birth occurred in Cleveland, Ohio on June 11, 1934, at the time of the first annual meeting of the American Association for the Study and Control of Rheumatic Diseases (Figure 1). The President of this organization was Dr. Ernest Irons, who is therefore considered the first President of the American Rheumatism Association. The meeting lasted for 1 day and consisted of 11 papers. Topics reviewed included gout, chronic arthritis in children, focal infection and arthritis in children, the management of atrophic arthritis in relation to the different phases of the disease, arthritis and the influence of vasodilators, and a study of roentgenologic findings in various types of chronic arthritis (Figure 2).

Dr. Irons, in his Presidential address, stated that the purpose of this new Association was "to promulgate a well-rounded concept of the problem of

James R. Klinenberg, MD: Professor and Chairman, Department of Medicine, Cedars-Sinai Medical Center, UCLA School of Medicine, Los Angeles, California: American Rheumatism Association President, 1983–1984.

Address reprint requests to James R. Klinenberg, MD, Department of Medicine, Cedars-Sinai Medical Center, UCLA School of Medicine, Box 48750, Los Angeles, CA 90048.

Submitted for publication August 8, 1984; accepted August 9, 1984.

The

PROCEEDINGS

of

The American Association for the Study and Control of Rheumatic Diseases

FIRST ANNUAL MEETING AND THIRD CONFERENCE HELD AT

Cleveland, June 11, 1934

PRESIDENT .... DR. ERNEST E. IRONS
VICE-PRESIDENT .... DR. RUSSELL L. HADEN
SECRETARY .... DR. LORING T. SWAIM

Figure 1. Program cover of the first meeting of the American Association for the Study and Control of Rheumatic Diseases, June 1934.

arthritis so that rational methods of treatment may be available to the physicians in charge of the many thousands of sufferers from arthritis who must be cared for—not only in larger medical centers but in smaller communities, and in their homes." He suggested that the membership should include "those who have a deep and sincere interest in the study of rheumatic diseases and have made a definite contribution to its literature, or who hold positions of influence in the fields of public health and administration."

I shall not dwell on the history except to note that 3 years later, the American Association for the Study and Control of Rheumatic Diseases became the American Rheumatism Association. The subsequent history of the American Rheumatism Association, including its merger with the Arthritis Foundation, will be fully discussed during the course of this historic meeting, and will be documented in the souvenir booklets which will be available to all the participants in this anniversary celebration. The scientific advances made during the first 50 years of American rheumatology will be discussed and highlighted in the "Landmarks" Symposium.

Considering that "the past is prologue," it is of interest to review some of the key issues brought before this organization by its Presidents in their Presidential addresses. It should be noted that during its first 25 years, the field of rheumatology needed to be established as a real entity, and many of the Presidential addresses dealt with pertinent clinical topics (Table 1). These included such issues as "The Clinical Approach to the Rheumatic Patient," "The Necessity of Certain Criteria for the Diagnosis and

TABLE OF CONTENTS

The New Association and Its Purposes: Introductory Remarks 3
Ernest E. Irons, M. D.

The Rôle of the Reticulo-Endothelial System in the Deposition of Colloidal Dyes and Particulate Matter in Articular Cavities 6
John G. Kuhns, M. D., and H. L. Weatherford, Ph. D.
Discussion: Robert B. Osgood, M. D., and Joseph Kovacs, M. D.

Calcium and Cholesterol Metabolism in Arthritis 14
G. Douglas Taylor, M. D., A. H. Ferguson, M. D., and Maurice Bruger, M. D.

A Study of the Roentgenologic Findings in Various Types of Chronic Arthritis 19
G Douglas Taylor, M. D., A. H. Ferguson, M. D., and Haig Kasabach, M. D.

The Peripheral Blood Circulation in Chronic Arthritis and the Influence of Vasodilators 25
Joseph Kovacs, M. D.
Discussion: Philip S. Hench, M. D., Irving S. Wright, M. D., D. E. Kaufman, M. D., and Joseph Kovacs, M. D.

Nutritional Factors in Chronic Arthritis 34
Frank J. Sladen, M. D., Dwight C. Ensign, M. D., and Clarke M. McColl, M. D.
Discussion: Robert B. Osgood, M. D.

The Influence of Dietetic and Other Factors on the Swelling of Tissues in Arthritis 41
C. W. Scull, Ph. D. and Ralph Pemberton, M. D.
Discussion: A. Almon Fletcher, M. D., Frank J. Sladen, M. D., Ralph Pemberton, M. D., Walter Bauer, M. D., and C. W. Scull, Ph. D.

Focal Infection and Arthritis: A Statistical Study 56
Arthur Steindler, M. D.

The Treatment of Chronic Rheumatoid Arthritis with Streptococcal Vaccine on the Basis of Skin Sensitivity 66
Charles W. Wainwright, M. D.
Discussion: J. Albert Key, M. D., M. H. Dawson, M. D., Russell L. Cecil, M. D., Russell L. Haden, M. D., Joseph L. Miller, M. D., Arthur Steindler, M. D., and Charles W. Wainright, M. D.

The Management of Atrophic Arthritis in Relation to the Different Phases of the Disease 78
W. Paul Holbrook, M. D., and Donald F. Hill, M. D.
Discussion: Robert B. Osgood, M. D., and Ernest E. Irons, M. D.

Chronic Arthritis in Children 88
William T. Green, M. D., and Frank R. Ober, M. D.
Discussion: Robert B. Osgood, M. D.

Gout: Changes in Symptoms and Purin Metabolism Produced by High Fat Diets in Four Gouty Patients 96
L. Maxwell Lockie, M. D., and Roger S. Hubbard, Ph. D.
Discussion: Philip S. Hench, M. D., and Francis C. Hall, M. D.

Figure 2. Papers presented at the first meeting of the American Association for the Study and Control of Rheumatic Diseases, June 1934.

Table 1. American Rheumatism Association Presidential addresses, 1934–1958

Year	President	Title
1934	Ernest Irons	"The New Association and its Purposes"
1936	Russell Haden	"The Clinical Approach to the Rheumatic Patient"
1937	Russell Cecil	"The Necessity of Certain Criteria for the Diagnosis and Cure of Rheumatoid Arthritis"
1938	William Kerr	"Radiculitis Associated with Spinal Arthritis"
1939	Ralph Pemberton	"Considerations Bearing on the Treatment of Arthritics"
1940	Philip Hench	"Palindromic Rheumatism"
1941	Ralph Boots	"Gold Therapy in Rheumatoid Arthritis"
1947	Walter Bauer	"The Challenge of Adolescence"
1951	Otto Steinbrocker	"The Problems of Maturity"
1952	Charles Slocumb	"Relative Cortisone Deficiency Simulating Exacerbation of Arthritis"
1953	Currier McEwen	"Plight of Teaching and Research in Rheumatic Diseases"
1955	Edward W. Boland	"Prednisone and Prednisolone Therapy in Rheumatoid Arthritis: Clinical Evaluations Based on Continuous Observations for Periods of Six to Nine Months"
1958	L. Maxwell Lockie	"A Method to Obtain Data on Arthritic Patients on a Nationwide Scale"

Cure of Rheumatoid Arthritis," "Considerations Bearing on the Treatment of Arthritics," "Palindromic Rheumatism," "Gold Therapy in Rheumatoid Arthritis," "Relative Cortisone Deficiency Simulating Exacerbation of Arthritis," and "A Method To Obtain Data on Arthritic Patients on a Nationwide Scale."

During the second 25 years, the tenor of the Presidential addresses for the American Rheumatism Association became more focal in approach and indicated that rheumatology was more secure in its foundation, and was not considering the questions of "where have we been?" and "where are we going?" (Table 2). Thus, topics such as "Creativity in Arthritis Research," "The Researchers, Practitioners and Teachers of Rheumatology," "The Crusade Against Arthritis: The Role of the American Rheumatism Association," "Some Requirements for the Successful Picture of American Rheumatology," and "Basic Research and Clinical Investigation" all represented a new focus for our organization. Beginning in the late 1960s, the trend toward more futuristic projections began. Evan Calkins talked about "Rheumatology as a Subspecialty: A Comment on its Present Status and Future Paths," Ed Fischel on "The Challenge of Change," John Vaughan on "Taking Steady Aim," and Sid Stillman celebrated "The 40th" 2 years prematurely. Subsequently, John Decker talked about "The Final Common Pathway," Larry Shulman on "Whither or Wither," Gerry Rodnan, in his 1976 address, presented "A Bicentennial Report on the Growth and Development of Rheumatology in the United States," and Dan McCarty continued the trend with "The Future of our Guild: Antidisestablishmentarianism." Gerry Weissmann, last year, very succinctly stated "The Introduction is Over." And indeed, that established for us the theme of the beginning of our next half-century.

Nineteen thirty-four was indeed a banner year! Six days after that first meeting in Cleveland of the American Association for the Study and Control of Rheumatic Diseases, in another midwestern city, Chicago, yours truly made his screaming debut into the real world. I might add parenthetically that other important events of that month in 1934 were the birth of the Dionne quintuplets and the creation of Donald Duck. Although I just made it by 6 days, I therefore have the honor of being the first President of the ARA who was born after its founding. This surely leads to some thoughts about the beginning of a new era and the obvious questions about the directions of rheumatology in the future. George Orwell's predictions regarding 1984, which appear in his novel written in 1949 (1)—35 years ago—have not proved to be totally correct, but surely had certain prophetic qualities. Although we are not living in a state as he described, the development of technology surely has kept pace with his predictions. It might also be stated that in the medical profession at least, his newspeak language may, indeed, have come to pass, since we have clearly entered into the era of DRGs, PPOs, IPAs, HMOs, etc., which all sound very much like newspeak vocabulary.

Dan McCarty began his 1980 Presidential address with a Chinese proverb: "Prediction is difficult, especially when it involves the future." Nevertheless, it seems appropriate as we conclude our 50th year and

Table 2. American Rheumatism Association Presidential addresses, 1960–1983

Year	President	Title
1960	Charles Smyth	"Necrotizing Vasculitis, Mast Cells and Connective Tissue Disease: An Hypothesis"
1961	Edward Hartung	"Creativity in Arthritis Research"
1962	Joseph Hollander	"The Researchers, Practitioners and Teachers of Rheumatology"
1963	Ephraim Engleman	"The Crusade Against Arthritis: The Role of the American Rheumatism Association"
1965	Howard Polley	"Some Requirements for the Successful Picture of American Rheumatology"
1966	Morris Ziff	"Basic Research and Clinical Investigation"
1967	Donald Hill	"Progress for the Patient"
1968	Evan Calkins	"Rheumatology as a Subspecialty: A Comment on Its Present Status and Future Paths"
1969	Edward Fischel	"The Challenge of Change"
1970	Emerson Ward	"Programs of the American Rheumatism Association and Arthritis Foundation"
1971	John Vaughan	"Taking Steady Aim"
1972	J. S. Stillman	"The Fortieth"
1973	John Decker	"The Final Common Pathway"
1974	Thomas Weiss	"Our Continuing Commitment"
1975	Lawrence Shulman	"Whither or Wither"
1976	Gerald Rodnan	"Growth and Development of Rheumatology in the United States: A Bicentennial Report"
1979	Alan Cohen	"Rheumatology 1979: Art, Achievements, and Problems"
1980	Daniel McCarty	"The Future of our Guild: Antidisestablishmentarianism"
1981	Giles Bole	"The American Rheumatism Association: 1990"
1982	J. Claude Bennett	"American Rheumatology: Markings"
1983	Gerald Weissmann	"The Introduction is Over"

enter into a new era, and especially in this year of 1984, that we attempt to make some predictions as to the status of American rheumatology during the next half-century. Unfortunately, most of us will not be here in 2034 when the time capsule is opened, but it is interesting to speculate on the validity of these predictions as tested 50 years from now.

I am indebted to many of you for taking the time to complete the questionnaire which I sent to 150 members of our Association: fellows, practitioners, scientists, academicians, etc. We received 40 completed questionnaires, and the data which I am about to present represent their responses. Of the responders, 24 were under the age of 50, and 16 were 50 or older. Twenty-one considered themselves private practitioners, 15 were basic scientists, and 30 did some type of clinical investigation.

The first question asked was "List the five major scientific breakthroughs relevant to rheumatology which might occur during the next 50 years." As you might expect, the responses were quite variable (Table 3), but they surely suggested certain common themes. First and foremost was an overwhelming sentiment that there would be additional discoveries of relationships between infections and various forms of inflammatory arthritis. This extends beyond the known relationships of so-called reactive arthritides or acute rheumatic fever, or Lyme arthritis, to include the prediction that there would be the elucidation of a specific etiology and pathogenesis for both rheumatoid arthritis and systemic lupus, and that both would ultimately be found to be caused by a virus. Surely this was stimulated by the recent discoveries of Gallo et al (2), of the association of a human leukemia virus with acquired immunodeficiency syndrome (AIDS), and the interesting work suggesting a relationship between a parvovirus and rheumatoid arthritis (3). Based upon this promise was then the suggestion that there would be the development of vaccines for the prevention of both rheumatoid arthritis and systemic lupus, and that with time these diseases would be eradicated. There is a strong feeling in the rheumatologic community today that rheumatoid arthritis and systemic lupus may not exist in the year 2034 because of these scientific advances and appropriate preventative measures.

It was felt that there will be a better understanding of the genetic basis for rheumatic diseases, including rheumatoid arthritis and lupus, and other diseases as well. It is predicted that there will be significant advances in the field of immunogenetics within the

Table 3. Major scientific "breakthroughs" relevant to rheumatology which will occur during the next 50 years

1. Discovery of relationships between infections and various forms of inflammatory arthritis
2. Elucidation of specific etiology and pathogenesis of rheumatoid arthritis (RA) and systemic lupus erythematosus (SLE) (both will be found to be caused by a virus)
3. Development of a vaccine for the prevention of RA and SLE; these diseases will then be eradicated
4. Better understanding of the genetic basis for rheumatic diseases, including RA and SLE
5. Advances in immunogenetics
6. Further understanding of the factors regulating cartilage and bone regeneration

next 50 years, and that this may have significant therapeutic implications. Finally, there was a strong sentiment for the concept that further understanding of the factors regulating cartilage and bone regeneration will offer major breakthroughs in our understanding of osteoarthritis, and may have significant therapeutic implications as well.

The second question was to "List some major clinical advances in rheumatology likely to take place during the next half-century." The more common responses to this question (Table 4) include:

1. The recognition of clinical subsets of rheumatic diseases, such as systemic lupus. While this is already being done to a significant degree, it is predicted that within the next 50 years, lupus may prove to be a series of different diseases—possibly with somewhat different etiologies, but surely with different prognoses and different approaches to therapy.

2. The development of new diagnostic techniques for assessing acute inflammatory arthritis or synovitis, and to allow us to quantitate it better. These might include magnetic resonance imaging, PET scans, advanced techniques in arthroscopy (probably even in small joints), more appropriate use of biopsies, etc.

3. Development of safer and more effective nonsteroidal antiinflammatory drugs, and a much better understanding of how these drugs act and how they should be properly classified. There is also a likelihood that there will be specific classes of drugs with certain major side effects, while other classes of drugs with similar therapeutic benefit may have an entirely different group of side effects. It is further predicted that there will be other explanations for the therapeutic benefit of the antiinflammatory agents and that inhibition of prostaglandin synthetase will represent only one of many modes of action.

4. There will be a greater understanding of the epidemiology of rheumatic diseases, and this may have some beneficial effects regarding prevention.

5. There will be the development of immunotherapy and increased use of genetic engineering for specific treatment of some of the rheumatic diseases.

6. A very important predicted clinical advance in rheumatology will be the development of vaccines to prevent rheumatoid arthritis and systemic lupus, so that these diseases will either become very rare or completely obsolete.

7. There will be major advances in the field of orthopedic surgery, including much better prosthetic joints with the use of entirely different materials and new techniques for seating the prostheses so that there will be no loosening or fracture. During this period of time we will enter into the clinically applicable use of joint transplantation—in some instances, in lieu of the use of artificial joints. The possibility of the bionic arthritic patient is increasingly becoming a reality.

8. Finally, it is suggested that there will be established a role of exercise and diet in the genesis of certain rheumatic diseases, and that appropriate modification of exercise and diet habits will also help in the prevention of rheumatic diseases.

The next question was "What major changes in rheumatologic practice might occur during the next 50 years?" (Table 5). In this regard it was suggested that many existing illnesses will be prevented (such as rheumatoid arthritis and lupus), and others will be cured (such as gout). In their place, however, new illnesses will emerge, such as the emergence of AIDS, during the next 5 years. Most importantly, there will be more emphasis on diseases of the elderly, such as osteoarthritis, and rheumatologic practice will include many more elderly patients (because of the increased life span and, therefore, general aging of the population), as well as the elimination of many of the diseases now seen in rheumatologic practice because of the development of new scientific technologies. Just as in the past 50 years we have seen the disappearance of acute rheumatic fever and the emergence of other rheumatic diseases, so we will see additional changing patterns during the next half-century. It is thought that

Table 4. Major clinical advances in rheumatology during the next 50 years

1. Recognition of clinical subsets of rheumatic diseases (e.g., systemic lupus erythematosus [SLE])
2. Development of new diagnostic techniques for assessing synovitis (e.g., magnetic resonance imaging, position emission tomography scans; advances in arthroscopy; etc.)
3. Development of safer and more effective nonsteroidal antiinflammatory drugs
4. Greater understanding of epidemiology of rheumatic diseases
5. Development of immunotherapy and/or use of genetic engineering for specific disease treatments
6. Development of a "vaccine" to prevent rheumatoid arthritis and SLE
7. Major advances in joint surgery: better prosthetic joints, use of joint transplantation, etc.
8. Establishment of the role of exercise and diet in the genesis of rheumatic disease

there will be more effective therapy for all of the rheumatic diseases and greater emphasis will be placed on prevention, including the use of vaccines, joint protection, genetic engineering, etc.

Rheumatologic practice will entail much more group practice with greater use of a team approach to the rheumatic diseases. It is suggested that there will be a tendency for rheumatology to increasingly merge with general internal medicine, and that most physicians will require fewer specific consultations in the field of rheumatic diseases. It is thought that there will be more scientific rationale for the treatment of rheumatic diseases and, of course, in the next half-century we will enter into an ever-increasing and expanding use of computers in all aspects of the clinical practice of medicine.

The next series of questions had to do with manpower predictions for the next 50 years. Needless to say, there have been many concerns raised about the manpower issue since the GMENAC report (4), and the ARA, along with other professional societies, has given special attention to this issue. All experts seem to agree that it is quite difficult to predict exactly what the manpower needs might be even in the next few years, much less in the next half-century. Therefore, it is not surprising that our colleagues are evenly split regarding available manpower in the next 50 years (Table 6). There is no agreement as to whether there will be more or less practicing rheumatologists per 100,000 population in the next 50 years, and although there is some feeling that the number of research scientists working in the field of rheumatology will be somewhat greater, those numbers are quite soft. There is likewise little agreement as to the number of patient visits to rheumatologists as a percentage of visits to all physicians increasing or decreasing, nor is there any agreement as to the percent of time spent in rheumatology versus primary care medicine. There is, however, overwhelming agreement that the number of hours worked per week by physicians will be less, and that physician income relative to the cost of living will also be less. Finally, it was felt that the number of AHPs per 100,000 population will probably increase during the next 50 years.

Since our organization is made up of a rather heterogeneous group of individuals, including clinicians, basic scientists, clinical investigators, teachers, administrators—most with MDs, some with PhDs, some with both—it has been very hard for the ARA to serve all of its members appropriately. One of the issues over which your officers continually agonize is: How can we better serve our members, including the clinicians and the basic scientists? It seemed appropriate, therefore, to ask "How might we better serve our membership during the next 50 years?" Again, the

Table 5. Major changes in rheumatologic practice in next 50 years

1. Many existing illnesses will be cured or prevented; new illnesses will emerge
2. More emphasis on diseases of the elderly (e.g., osteoarthritis)
3. More effective therapies
4. Greater emphasis on prevention (i.e., use of vaccines, joint protection, etc.)
5. More ambulatory care, less hospital care
6. More group practice, greater use of "team approach"
7. General medicine will merge with rheumatology; less specific consultation on rheumatic diseases
8. Greater use of computers
9. More scientific rationale for treatment of rheumatic disease

Table 6. Predictions as to the state of rheumatologic practice in 2034 (compared with 1984)

	Number of responses		
	More	Less	Same
a) Number of practicing rheumatologists per 100,000 population	17	16	6
b) Number of research scientists working in the field of rheumatology	16	11	12
c) Number of patient visits to rheumatologists (as a percentage of patient visits to physicians)	16	13	15
d) Percent of time spent in rheumatology versus primary care medicine	13	16	10
e) Number of hours worked per week	3	31	11
f) Physician income relative to cost of living	0	33	7
g) Number of arthritis health professionals per 100,000 population	21	11	4

responses were varied, but the overlying theme was to continue to provide a forum for exchange of information and ideas, to provide a broad menu of educational choices so that there is in our program something of interest to everyone, and most importantly, to further the role of our organization as the principal advocate for both practice and research in the field of rheumatic diseases. There was also considerable sentiment for the ARA to become more politically active in speaking for the needs of our members and to be better prepared to deal with government. It was suggested that we should continue to develop our slide collection and that 50 more years would allow it to mature and become a major teaching resource for the rheumatologic community.

It was also predicted that we could enter into new areas of information exchange, largely based on computerization. It was even suggested that our centennial meeting in 2034 may actually consist of a program being conducted in various parts of the country and transmitted by video to individuals' homes, where they can participate in the meeting in an interactive way. It surely may be more efficient, but it doesn't sound like nearly as much fun. One additional innovative suggestion was that the organization might better serve its membership by changing its name.

The replies to the final question, "Any other predictions?" are so varied and interesting that some of them bear repeating. These include: "We will be well into the space age with a variety of new diseases." "There will be more women in rheumatology." "The first major breakthrough will *not* be made by a rheumatologist." "There will be more knowledge by the public that rheumatologists exist." "I will live to see it." "I will be dead in 2034." It was further suggested that the ARA will rent the Rose Bowl for its annual meeting in 2034, with the post-meeting tour being a 10-day trip to Venus at the all-inclusive cost of 120,563 rubles.

Erich Fromm, in his Afterword (1), states that "George Orwell's *1984* is the expression of a mood and it is a warning. The mood that it expresses is that of near despair about the future of man, and the warning is that unless the course of history changes men all over the world will lose their most human qualities, will become soloist automatons and will not even be aware of it." Well, now we are here in 1984 and, in medicine at least, the mood is sometimes that of near despair—not so much about the future of man as the future of medicine. It is reassuring, however, that as we review the predictions of the activities in our field during the next 50 years, they strike a positive note. Despite government intervention, DRGs, prospective reimbursement, PPOs, etc., there is a feeling that scientific advances will be made, the lot of our suffering patients will be improved, and the clinical practice of rheumatology will continue. There is an upbeat note that education will continue to advance, that communications will be enhanced by new technologies, and in fact, one can sense the feeling of excitement about the challenges for the future. We must, however, heed the warning that we might lose our most human qualities which are so necessary to help improve the state of our patients and to further the cause of our sacred profession of medicine.

As we consider that 50 years is really a very short period of time, we can take pride in the great advances made in our discipline and by our Association over this very short period. We must face the next half-century with enthusiasm, vigor, and hope! We have become well established, and now the challenge for the future is ours!

REFERENCES

1. Orwell G: 1984 (with an Afterword by Erich Fromm). New York, Harcourt Brace Jovanovich, Inc., 1949.
2. Gallo RC, Salahuddin SZ, Popovic M, Shearer GM, Kaplan M, Haynes BF, Palker TJ, Redfield R, Oleske J, Safai B, White G, Foster P, Markham PD: Frequent detection and isolation of cytopathic retroviruses (HILV-III) from patients with AIDS and at risk for AIDS. Science 224:500–508, 1984
3. Simpson RW, McGinty L, Simon L, Smith CA, Godzeski CW, Boyd RJ: Association of parvoviruses with rheumatoid arthritis of humans. Science 223:1425–1428, 1984
4. Graduate Medical Education National Advisory Committee: GMENAC Summary Report. US Department of Health and Human Services, Hyattsville, Maryland, 1980

CHARACTERIZATION OF T CELLS BEARING HLA–DR ANTIGENS IN RHEUMATOID ARTHRITIS

SETH H. PINCUS, DANIEL O. CLEGG, and JOHN R. WARD

It has been demonstrated that T cells bearing HLA–DR antigens on their surface are actively involved in an immune response. In diseases of disordered immunoregulation, including rheumatoid arthritis (RA), there are elevated numbers of circulating HLA–DR+ T cells. In this study, we examined the cellular physiology of these T cells in RA patients. Using tritiated thymidine incorporation, we found that, in most patients, HLA–DR+ cells do not account for a significant amount of spontaneous proliferation found in peripheral blood T cells. RNA hybridization studies, using a cloned HLA–DR alpha chain gene probe, indicate that the T cells actively synthesize HLA–DR antigens rather than passively adsorbing them. The cell surface phenotype of the HLA–DR+ T cells was analyzed using double immunofluorescence and a variety of monoclonal antibodies. The expression of T cell differentiation antigens T4, T6, T8, and T10 varied markedly from patient to patient. In some patients, a significant number of cells expressed both T4 and T8 antigens. Most HLA–DR+ cells also express antigens defined by the following antibodies: anti-Tac (the interleukin-2 receptor), J2 (a glycoprotein found on T cell blasts), and ILR-1 (a class II major histocompatibility complex antigen). Activated T cells bearing HLA–DR antigens may play a role in the development of RA. Our data demonstrate that although these cells are not lymphoblasts, they possess a distinct cell surface phenotype.

From the Divisions of Rheumatology and Clinical Immunology, Departments of Medicine, Pediatrics, and Pathology, University of Utah School of Medicine, Salt Lake City, Utah.

Supported by a grant from the Nora Eccles Treadwell Foundation.

Seth H. Pincus, MD; Daniel O. Clegg, MD; John R. Ward, MD.

Address reprint requests to Seth H. Pincus, MD, University of Utah School of Medicine, Salt Lake City, UT 84132.

Submitted for publication February 24, 1984; accepted in revised form August 13, 1984.

The genes within the HLA–D region of the human major histocompatibility complex (MHC) influence diverse aspects of the immune response, including disease susceptibility (1), stimulation of the mixed lymphocyte reaction (2), interactions between T cells and monocytes (3), and the ability to respond to certain antigens (4). Antigens encoded within HLA–D are expressed on a limited number of cell types, including B lymphocytes, monocytes, endothelial cells, and hematopoietic precursors (5). Extremely low levels of HLA–DR antigens are found on the surface of resting T cells, requiring special techniques for their demonstration (6). T cells activated by a variety of stimuli express larger quantities of HLA–DR antigen, which may be detected by less sensitive methods, such as indirect immunofluorescence. In vitro stimulation with mitogens or allogeneic cells results in a five- to tenfold increase in the number of HLA–DR+ T cells in 5 days (7,8). In vivo, following a booster immunization or a bacterial infection, there is a rise in the number of peripheral blood T cells expressing HLA–DR antigens (7). It has been reported that levels of circulating HLA–DR+ T cells are elevated in several diseases involving malfunction of the immune system, including rheumatoid arthritis (RA), systemic lupus erythematosus, and diabetes mellitus (7,9).

A variety of immune abnormalities have been described in RA. Elevated levels of serum immunoglobulins, hyperreactivity of B lymphocytes to pokeweed mitogen, and the presence of autoantibodies are among the defects described in humoral immunity (10). Cellular abnormalities include defective suppressor cell function (11,12) and abnormal ratios of T cells belonging to different subsets defined by monoclonal antibodies (13). The association between RA and the expression of HLA antigen DR4 (1) also suggests that the immune system is involved in RA. In spite of the evidence that has accumulated regarding the immune system in RA, no one has yet identified the immunologic event(s) that initiate or perpetuate the disease process. Nor has it been clearly established that the immune disorders are directly involved in the pathogenesis of the disease.

The finding that activated T cells are present in the peripheral blood and, in higher numbers, in the synovial fluid of patients with RA (7,14) suggests several hypotheses. It is possible that these cells are responding to the antigen that is inciting the disease process and, thus, are intimately involved in the pathogenesis of RA. Alternatively, these cells may be activated by products released during inflammation or other aspects of the disease, in which case their occurrence represents an epiphenomenon. To understand the role of HLA–DR+ T cells in RA, we have begun by exploring the cellular physiology of these cells. In this report we examine the following aspects of HLA–DR bearing T cells: proliferation, synthesis of messenger RNA (mRNA) coding for HLA–DR alpha chains, and expression of other cell surface antigens.

PATIENTS AND METHODS

Antibodies. The production and properties of the monoclonal antibodies used in this study have been described elsewhere. Monoclonal antibodies to T cell antigens T3, T4, T6, T8, and T10 (15,16) were obtained from Ortho Diagnostics (Raritan, NJ). Antibody to the interleukin-2 (IL-2) receptor, anti-Tac (17), was a gift from Thomas Waldmann. ILR-1, which detects a supratypic specificity on the class II major histocompatibility complex antigen SB (18), and J2, which binds to a 26,000 molecular weight glycoprotein found on activated T cells (19), were the gift of Lee Nadler. Three different monoclonal antibodies to monomorphic HLA–DR determinants were used. CA2.06 was obtained from Hugh McDevitt (20), OKIa-1 from Ortho Diagnostics, and rhodamine-conjugated anti-HLA–DR from Becton-Dickinson (Sunnyvale, CA). Fluorescein-conjugated heterologous goat anti-mouse immunoglobulin and goat anti-human IgM were purchased from Cappel Laboratories (Cochranville, PA).

Isolation of T lymphocytes. Heparinized peripheral blood was obtained from patients with definite RA (21) seen in the Rheumatology Division at the University of Utah. Mononuclear cells were separated by centrifugation on a Ficoll-Hypaque density gradient (Pharmacia, Piscataway, NJ). The cells at the interface were harvested and incubated overnight with neuraminidase-treated sheep red blood cells, at 4°C. T cells were separated by centrifugation on Ficoll-Hypaque. The cells in the pellet were resuspended and then centrifuged on another Ficoll-Hypaque gradient. The red cells were removed by lysis with a hypotonic ammonium chloride solution, and the resulting T cells were washed twice with phosphate buffered saline (PBS). The purified T cells were >95% T3+, and ~1% surface immunoglobulin–positive by immunofluorescence. Yields were approximately 10% of the total mononuclear cells isolated on the initial Ficoll-Hypaque gradient.

Cell culture. Purified T cells were cultured at 2×10^5 cells/well in 96-well flat-bottom culture plates (Costar, Cambridge, MA). The media consisted of RPMI 1640 supplemented with 1% autologous serum, 100 units/ml penicillin, 0.03% glutamine, 0.05 mg/ml gentamycin, 0.2 units/ml insulin, 1 m*M* oxaloacetic acid, and 0.5 m*M* sodium pyruvate. Cells were cultured in a 5% CO_2 atmosphere at 37°C. Twelve hours prior to harvest, 1 mCi of ^{3}H-methylthymidine (Amersham Corp., Arlington Heights, IL) was added to each well. All cultures were performed in triplicate.

To eliminate cells expressing HLA–DR antigens, lysis with monoclonal antibody CA2.06 and complement was performed. Hybridoma ascites and neonatal rabbit serum (as a complement source) were titered to obtain maximal specific lysis and a low level of lysis (<10%) in the absence of antibody. The proportion of HLA–DR+ T cells ranged from 8–21%. Ten million T cells were incubated with CA2.06 ascites for 1 hour on ice. The cells were washed and then incubated with the rabbit serum. Efficacy of the lysis was determined by trypan blue dye exclusion viability assessment, and by indirect immunofluorescence with OKIa-1 at 1 and 24 hours following treatment with antibody and complement. Viable cells bearing HLA–DR antigens were not detected after lysis.

RNA hybridization analysis. RNA dot hybridizations were performed according to the protocol of White and Bancroft (22). RNA was extracted from purified T cells, peripheral blood mononuclear cells, and foreskin fibroblasts in primary culture. Cells were lysed in 10 m*M* Tris, pH 7.0, 1 m*M* EDTA, and 1% NP40 (Sigma, St. Louis, MO). Nuclei were pelleted out at 15,000*g* for 2.5 minutes. The supernatant was transferred to an equal volume of 0.15*M* NaCl, 0.015*M* sodium citrate (SSC), and formaldehyde (Sigma) was added to a final concentration of 7%. The mixture was incubated at 60°C for 15 minutes, and then stored at −70°C.

RNA concentration was determined by measuring the absorbance at 260 nm. Twofold serial dilutions of the RNA samples were made in SSC starting with 10 μg/ml, and 100 μl of each dilution was transferred with suction to a 4-mm diameter spot on a nitrocellulose sheet (BA 45) supported on #470 filter paper using a 96-hole minifold apparatus, all from Schleicher and Schuell (Keene, NH). The nitrocellulose sheet was baked at 80°C for 90 minutes in a vacuum oven.

Hybridization was performed at 68°C for 24 hours in 5% sodium dodecyl sulfate (SDS), 100 μg/ml calf thymus DNA, 1 m*M* EDTA, 6× SSC, 1 mg/ml bovine serum albumin (BSA), 1 mg/ml polyvinyl pyrrolidine, 1 mg/ml Ficoll, and 10^7 counts per minute of radiolabeled gene probe. Probes were labeled by nick translation using ^{32}P-dCTP (3,000 Ci/m*M*; New England Nuclear, Boston, MA) to a specific activity of 1–3 × 10^8 cpm/μg of DNA. The hybridized nitrocellulose was washed in 0.1× SSC, 0.1% SDS at 52°C. Autoradiograms were performed using enhancing screens (Cronex; DuPont, Wilmington, DE) for 3 days. The gene probes used for hybridization were: pDRH-7, a clone containing the gene for the alpha chain of HLA–DR inserted in pBR-322 (23); pBR-322; and Ch4-38, which contains the human immunoglobulin mu constant region gene (24).

Immunofluorescence. Prior to use in immunofluorescence assays all reagents were spun in an Airfuge (Beckman, Palo Alto, CA) to remove aggregates. Cells were washed twice in PBS containing 1% BSA and 0.05% sodium azide (polyclonal B cell activator, PBA) and then incubated for 30 minutes at 4°C with a predetermined dilution of the desired monoclonal antibody. After incubation, the cells were washed 3 times with cold PBA and then treated with fluorescein-conjugated goat anti-mouse immunoglobulin. The cells were then washed 3 times in cold PBA. At this point, single indirect immunofluorescence analysis could be performed using a Zeiss Universal microscope. If double immunofluorescence was performed, the cells were incubated in a 1% solution of normal mouse serum in PBA. This procedure bound any free combining sites present on the goat anti-mouse immunoglobulin.

Following a wash in cold PBA, the cells were incubated with rhodamine-conjugated anti-HLA–DR. After the final set of washes, the cells were evaluated for the expression of both fluorescein and rhodamine labels. Both the percent of fluorescein-staining cells costaining with rhodamine, and the fraction of rhodamine-positive cells also bearing fluorescein were determined. Also, to rule out any artifact caused by the double staining, the percent of total cells bearing either the fluorescein or rhodamine label in the double immunofluorescence analysis was compared with the result obtained from a simultaneous single-label experiment. In all cases, results from these simultaneous single- and double-labeling experiments differed by <3%. All determinations were done by counting 100 cells. Data points represent the means of duplicate determinations.

RESULTS

HLA–DR+ T cells and proliferation of peripheral blood T cells from RA patients. It has been reported that peripheral blood T cells from patients with RA have a high level of spontaneous incorporation of radiolabeled thymidine, indicating that at least some of these cells are proliferating more rapidly than in normal individuals (25). To test whether the HLA–DR+ T cells contribute to this proliferation, we compared the uptake of tritiated thymidine in patients' T cells that had been lysed with anti-HLA–DR and complement or were treated with complement alone.

Cells were placed in standard tissue culture conditions and were not stimulated with mitogen, antigen, or heterologous serum components. The efficacy of lysis was assessed by indirect immunofluorescence for HLA–DR+ cells 24 hours later. Viable cell counts were also performed at 24 hours to ensure that the 2 sets of cultures had equal numbers of cells. Proliferative responses were measured on days 3 and 5 and, in one case, on days 1 and 7 as well. The results are shown in Table 1.

In 4 of 5 of the experiments there was a small, and in most cases a statistically nonsignificant ($P > 0.05$), decrease in proliferation in the anti-HLA–DR lysed cell populations. In only 1 experiment (experiment 4) did the HLA–DR+ cell population contribute significantly to the proliferation seen in patient cells. HLA–DR+ T cells may have been proliferating at a higher rate than other T cells, since the number of cells eliminated by anti-DR treatment was small, and there was a decrease in proliferation, albeit not statistically significant. But, clearly, these cells are not the sole source of proliferation in the T cell pool.

T cells synthesize HLA–DR alpha chain mRNA. It has been suggested that since T cells appear to recognize antigen in the context of self-MHC, they have cell surface receptors that might bind MHC gene products, and that the expression of HLA–DR on these T cells might reflect binding of exogenously produced (i.e., by monocytes or by synovial cells) HLA–DR molecules. Using internal labeling with ^{35}S-methionine and immunoprecipitation, we were consistently unable to demonstrate the endogenous produc-

Table 1. Proliferation of T cells lysed with anti-HLA–DR antibody and complement*

	No. days in culture			
	1	3	5	7
Experiment 1				
Total T cells	598 (42)	235 (34)	389 (42)	301 (49)
Lysed T cells	418 (23)	95 (15)	145 (18)	315 (10)
Experiment 2				
Total T cells	NT	805 (375)	495 (124)	NT
Lysed T cells	NT	436 (104)	364 (42)	NT
Experiment 3				
Total T cells	NT	457 (65)	245 (59)	NT
Lysed T cells	NT	394 (29)	232 (53)	NT
Experiment 4				
Total T cells	NT	1,492 (214)	3,022 (488)	NT
Lysed T cells	NT	304 (23)	829 (142)	NT
Experiment 5				
Total T cells	NT	8,841 (798)	7,120 (1,099)	NT
Lysed T cells	NT	8,097 (743)	5,729 (758)	NT

* Total T cells = T cells treated with complement alone; lysed T cells = T cells lysed with monoclonal anti-HLA-DR antibody CA2.06 and complement. Efficacy of lysis was ascertained by indirect immunofluorescence 24 hours after lysis. Values are the amount of tritiated thymidine incorporation (in counts per minute) over 12 hours. Each data point represents the mean (standard error of the mean) of triplicate determinations. NT = not tested.

tion of HLA–DR antigens in peripheral blood T cells either from patients or normal individuals. However, we have used the RNA dot-hybridization technique to demonstrate the presence of RNA having homology to a cloned HLA–DR alpha chain gene probe, pDRH-7. The autoradiogram of this "dot blot" is shown in Figure 1.

RNA was extracted from peripheral blood mononuclear cells of normal individuals, from T cells of normal individuals, and from patient T cells. Serial twofold dilutions of the RNA were made, beginning with 1 μg/dot in the left column. Identical blots were hybridized against 3 different radiolabeled gene probes. Panel A of Figure 1 shows the results with gene probe pDRH-7; panel B with pBR-322, the plasmid that is acting as the carrier for the HLA–DR alpha chain gene. This is a control for nonspecific binding of the radiolabeled DNA to the RNA, as well as for plasmid contamination of the dotted material. Panel C is a measure of B cell contamination, since it is hybridized to a cloned human immunoglobulin mu chain gene, Charon 4-38. The results indicate that in all the cell populations, RNA for HLA–DR alpha chains is being synthesized in roughly equal quantities (panel A). When RNA is obtained from fibroblasts that fail to express HLA–DR antigens on their surface, and blotted against pDRH-7, no hybridization is seen (Figure 2).

Panel B of Figure 1 demonstrates that, although there is some background binding of the plasmid DNA to the RNA samples, the majority of the hybridization seen is specific for the HLA–DR alpha chain gene. Panel C of Figure 1 shows that a low level of B cell contamination can be detected with a cloned mu gene probe. The RNA in rows 1 and 2 was obtained from a cell population containing approximately 10% B lymphocytes, and clear-cut RNA hybridization is seen. Hybridization with the mu chain DNA does not occur with RNA from any other cell preparation. It would thus appear very unlikely that the RNA in the T cell preparations hybridizing with the HLA–DR alpha chain DNA came from contaminating B cells. The

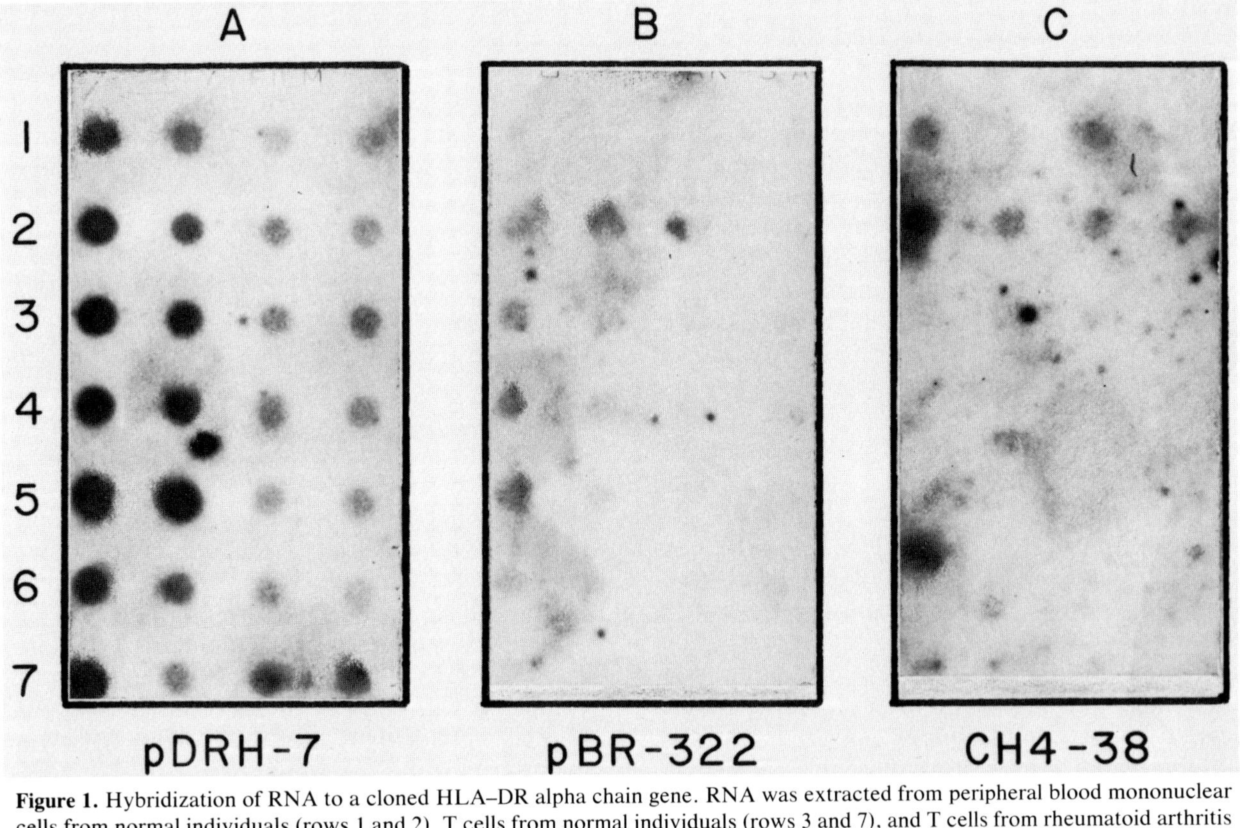

Figure 1. Hybridization of RNA to a cloned HLA–DR alpha chain gene. RNA was extracted from peripheral blood mononuclear cells from normal individuals (rows 1 and 2), T cells from normal individuals (rows 3 and 7), and T cells from rheumatoid arthritis patients (rows 4–6). One microgram of RNA was applied to each dot in the left column of each panel. Serial twofold dilutions were then made toward the right. **A**, Hybridized with pDRH-7, which contains an HLA–DR alpha chain gene inserted into pBR-322. **B**, Hybridized with pBR-322. **C**, Hybridized with the immunoglobulin mu chain probe CH4-38.

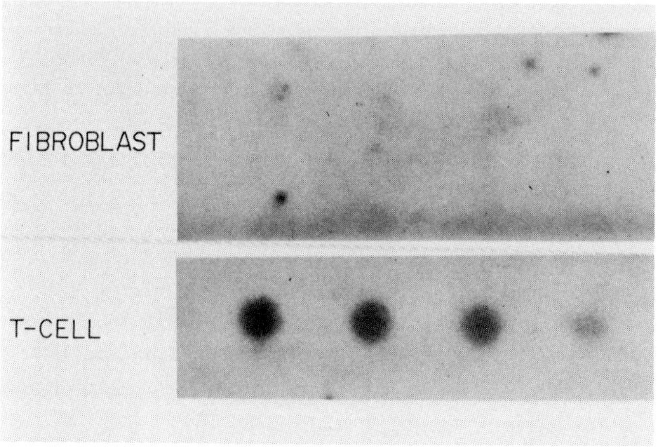

Figure 2. Hybridization of fibroblast and T cell RNA to a cloned HLA–DR alpha chain gene. RNA was extracted from peripheral blood T cells and foreskin fibroblast primary cultures. The blot was prepared as in Figure 1 and hybridized to pDRH-7.

presence of HLA–DR RNA indicates that the HLA–DR antigen expressed on the surface of the T cell is most likely synthesized endogenously. Our failure to detect an HLA–DR protein by immunoprecipitation may have been due to a lack of sensitivity of the assay, since peripheral blood lymphocytes exhibit low levels of protein synthesis.

Cell surface phenotype of HLA–DR+ T cells. The functional status of human T cells has been correlated with the expression of certain cell surface antigens (15,16). We have used double immunofluorescence to study the expression of a number of markers on HLA–DR+ T cells. To rule out artifacts from the system, a variety of control tests were performed (see Patients and Methods), as well as a preliminary experiment using peripheral blood mononuclear cells from a normal individual. In this experiment, cells were successively incubated with anti-T3, fluorescein-labeled goat anti-mouse Ig, and then rhodamine-conjugated anti-HLA-DR. Since, in the peripheral blood, the majority of cells expressing HLA–DR antigens are B lymphocytes and monocytes, there should be little overlap between the T3+ and the HLA–DR+ cell populations. Actually, <3% of HLA–DR+ cells expressed the T3 antigen. The results of double immunofluorescence analyses performed on T cells from 9 patients are shown in Table 2. The data represent the percentage of HLA–DR+ T cells (detected by rhodamine staining) that also express the second antigen (detected by fluorescein staining).

Initial studies evaluating the expression of either T4 or T8 antigens (patients 1–3, sample 1) showed that the total of T4 plus T8 bearing cells greatly exceeded 100%, with a significant majority of the cells being T4+. This suggested that there was a population of HLA–DR+ T cells that expressed both T4 and T8 antigens. Since thymocytes are known to express both antigens, we added a monoclonal antibody that detects a common thymocyte antigen (T6) to see if this marker is also present on a population of HLA–DR+ T cells. The remainder of the studies performed on patients 1–7 demonstrate that there was a variable percentage of T6+ cells (22–100%). Furthermore, the number of T6+ cells approximated the number of cells that were expressing both the T4 and the T8 marker.

The expression of other activation and MHC markers was also studied. The T10 antigen is a structure found on stem cells, thymocytes, null cells, and activated T cells. The majority of HLA–DR+ T cells (42–100%) generally expressed this structure. J2, a 26,000 molecular weight T cell activation antigen, was also frequently expressed on HLA–DR+ T cells (48–88%). A large proportion of the HLA–DR+ T cells have receptors for the lymphokine IL-2 (50–100%), as evidenced by expression of the Tac antigen (which marks the IL-2 receptor). Finally, the coordinate expression of 2 different class II MHC molecules, HLA–DR and SB (which is detected by the monoclonal antibody ILR-1), was examined. In all but 1 case, the majority of HLA–DR+ cells also expressed SB. A similar situation was found when the number of SB+ cells coexpressing HLA–DR was evaluated; in all cases >75% of SB+ cells were also HLA–DR+ (data not shown).

DISCUSSION

Resting T lymphocytes do not normally express HLA–DR in quantities sufficient to allow detection by visual immunofluorescence. But, when they are activated by immunologic stimuli, either in vivo or in vitro, there is a marked increase in the expression of HLA–DR (7,8). An elevated number of HLA–DR+ T cells has been found in the peripheral blood from patients with a variety of conditions of disordered immunoregulation, including RA (7). In our laboratory, we have found that a mean of 16.7% (range 4–33% in 31 samples) of RA patients' T lymphocytes express HLA–DR by visual immunofluorescence, compared with a mean of 2.4% (range 0–7%) seen in normal individuals (Clegg DO, Pincus SH, Ward JR: manuscript in preparation).

In an effort to gain an understanding of how HLA–DR+ T cells may be functioning in RA, we evaluated various aspects of their cellular physiology. Our findings show that: 1) HLA–DR+ T cells do not

Table 2. Cell surface phenotype of HLA–DR-bearing T cells*

	% HLA–DR+ T cells expressing:						
Source	T4	T6	T8	T10	Tac	J2	ILR-1
Patient 1							
Sample 1	100	NT	46	NT	NT	NT	NT
Sample 2	78	22	50	45	NT	NT	NT
Patient 2							
Sample 1	83	NT	50	NT	100	67	100
Sample 2	100	100	100	100	NT	NT	NT
Patient 3							
Sample 1	92	NT	76	NT	67	88	100
Sample 2	82	64	98	72	NT	NT	NT
Patient 4	74	61	66	68	NT	NT	NT
Patient 5	59	40	61	71	NT	NT	NT
Patient 6	66	23	69	42	NT	NT	NT
Patient 7	79	66	82	99	NT	NT	NT
Patient 8	NT	NT	NT	NT	54	48	88
Patient 9	NT	NT	NT	NT	50	60	42

* Cells were incubated with monoclonal antibody to the indicated T cell surface antigen, and then with fluorescein-conjugated goat anti-mouse Ig. The cells were incubated in 1% normal mouse serum and then with rhodamine-conjugated anti-HLA–DR antibody. The results are the percentage of rhodamine-staining cells that also express fluorescein staining. Data points are the mean of duplicate determinations. Replicate samples from the same patient were separated by at least 1 month. NT = not tested.

contribute significantly to the spontaneous proliferation seen in peripheral blood T cells of RA patients; 2) a proportion of these cells bear the T4, T6, and T8 lymphocyte differentiation antigens; and 3) these T cells produce HLA–DR alpha chain RNA. It also appears that characteristics of this cell population, especially expression of cell surface antigens, are variable between patients. With the patients included in this study, we have been unable to detect any correlation between this variability and clinical status. We have ongoing studies to establish whether there is an association between number of HLA–DR+ T cells and clinical status.

The absence of significant proliferation in this T cell population indicates that the HLA–DR+ T cells seen in the peripheral blood of RA patients are not the typical immunoblasts that arise in vitro in response to antigenic challenge. This corresponds with our observation that under light microscopy there is no morphologic difference between T cells in the peripheral blood of patients expressing or lacking HLA–DR (Allred SJ: unpublished observations). Yu et al (7) described 2 types of HLA–DR+ T cells: 1 was a large blastoid cell, and the other was smaller, with a lower level of HLA–DR on its surface. It would appear that the set of cells we are studying in RA patients belongs to the latter group of HLA–DR+ T cells.

It has been clearly demonstrated that T cells recognize antigen within the context of self-MHC antigens (3,26) and, further, that certain T cell populations are capable of passively adsorbing MHC products on their surface (7,27). In experiments demonstrating the endogenous synthesis of HLA–DR antigens by T cells, other investigators have used mitogen- or alloantigen-stimulated T lymphoblasts (i.e., the first type of HLA–DR+ T cell described by Yu et al) as their cell source.

Since the major site of immunologic activity in RA, the synovium, is known to contain large concentrations of non-T cells expressing high levels of HLA–DR antigens (28), it is important to show whether the T cell population we are looking at is adsorbing or synthesizing the HLA–DR antigen expressed on its surface. Because these cells are relatively metabolically inactive, we were unable to directly demonstrate synthesis of HLA–DR. Using the more sensitive technique of DNA-RNA hybridization, we have shown that peripheral blood T cells from patients and from normal individuals contain RNA with homology to a cloned HLA–DR alpha chain gene. The stringency conditions of the hybridization were set so that ≥80% homology between the cloned gene and the RNA was required. With this level of homology, the RNA almost certainly encodes either an HLA–DR alpha chain or another class II MHC molecule.

It is interesting to note that there does not appear to be any significant quantitative difference in alpha chain RNA between T cells from patients or normal individuals, although there is a significant difference in the percentage of the cells expressing HLA–DR antigens, visible by indirect immunofluorescence, in these 2 groups. Extremely sensitive flow cytometry analysis has demonstrated the presence of low levels of HLA–DR on resting peripheral blood T cells (6). Perhaps this quantitative difference in expression of HLA–DR antigens is due to post-transcriptional regulation, rather than due to the amount of RNA actually produced.

Among the most surprising findings of this study was the demonstration that a population of HLA–DR+ T cells express both the T4 and T8 differentiation antigens. It has been assumed that rarely, if ever, will such a doubly marked cell emerge from the thymus, although there have been reports of low numbers of such cells in the peripheral blood of patients with myasthenia gravis (29), as well as in that of normal individuals (30). We have vigorously pursued the possibility that this finding might be due to an experimental artifact or to a cell membrane perturbation that caused the display of HLA–DR or other activation antigens, as has been described by Mittler et al (31). We believe the control studies we performed rule out these possibilities. Since the population of T cells expressing HLA–DR is a small proportion of the total T cells in an RA patient, and the T cells expressing both T4 and T8 antigens is only a proportion of the HLA–DR+ T cells, it is understandable that such a population might be missed when differentiation antigens are assessed on the total population of peripheral lymphocytes in patients (13,14,32).

The finding that the number of cells expressing the thymocyte antigen, T6, approximated the number of cells that were T4+ and T8+ suggests that the double-marked cells also carry thymocyte markers. If such is the case, this cell population may represent cells that are prematurely released from the thymus in response to an immunologic challenge. It has been pointed out that, in RA, the expression of cell markers in the peripheral blood does not mirror that found at the site of inflammation in the joint (32). It is possible that the double-marked population of cells we observed in the peripheral blood was in transit from the thymus to the joint.

The expression of the T cell activation antigens Tac, J2, and T10 on the majority of the HLA–DR+ cells is not unexpected, since HLA–DR itself is considered an activation antigen when it is expressed on T cells (31). However, it does suggest the possibility of immunotherapy with monoclonal antibodies, should this cell population prove to be important in the pathogenesis of RA. It has already been shown that monoclonal antibodies to the Tac antigen can block the activation of lymphocytes to mitogens, soluble antigens, and alloantigens in both proliferative and helper assays (33). Since the Tac antigen is present on the receptor for IL-2, it may be possible to modulate the immune response by blocking the T lymphocyte stimulatory capability of this lymphokine.

It is important to determine whether HLA–DR+ T cells found in the peripheral blood of patients with RA are causally related to the disease process. As a first step, studies of the correlation of levels of HLA–DR+ T cells with RA disease activity, and their changes with treatment, are in progress.

ACKNOWLEDGMENTS

We would like to thank Louise P. Ewing, Clifford J. Stocks, and Sandra J. Allred for expert technical assistance; Charles Auffrey and Phil Leder for their gifts of the cloned genes; Lee Nadler, Hugh McDevitt, and Thomas Waldmann for the monoclonal antibodies; Harry Hill for thoughtful suggestions on the manuscript; and Jana Lawton for word processing.

REFERENCES

1. Ryder LP, Svejgaard A, Daussett J: Genetics of HLA disease association. Annu Rev Genet 15:169–187, 1981
2. Yunis EJ, Amos DB: Three closely linked genetic systems relevant to transplantation. Proc Natl Acad Sci USA 68:3031–3035, 1971
3. Rodey GE, Luehrman LK, Thomas DW: In vitro primary immunization of human peripheral blood lymphocytes to KLH: evidence for HLA-D region restriction. J Immunol 123:2250–2254, 1979
4. Gonwa TA, Peterlin BM, Stobo JD: Human Ir genes: structure and function. Adv Immunol 34:71–96, 1983
5. Torok-Storb B, Nepom GT, Nepom BS, Hanson JA: HLA-DR antigens on lymphoid cells differ from those on myeloid cells. Nature 305:541–543, 1983
6. Mann DL, Sharrow SO: B-cell alloantigens on T-lymphocytes. Transplant Proc 11:1774–1775, 1979
7. Yu DTY, McCune JM, Fu SM, Winchester RJ, Kunkel HG: Two types of Ia-positive T cells: synthesis and exchange of Ia antigens, Proceedings of a Conference on Genetic Control of the Human Immune Response. J Exp Med 152:89s–98s, 1980
8. Charron DJ, Engleman EG, Benike CJ, McDevitt HO: Ia antigens on alloreactive T cells in man detected by monoclonal antibodies: evidence for synthesis of HLA-D/DR molecules of the responder type, Proceedings of a Conference on Genetic Control of the Human Immune Response. J Exp Med 152:127s–136s, 1980
9. Jackson RA, Morris MA, Haynes BF, Eisenbarth GS: Increase in circulating Ia-antigen bearing T cells in type I diabetes mellitus. N Engl J Med 306:785–788, 1982
10. Paget SA, Gibofsky A: Immunopathogenesis of rheumatoid arthritis. Am J Med 67:961–970, 1979
11. Tosato G, Steinberg AD, Blaese RM: Defective EBV-specific suppressor T-cell function in rheumatoid arthritis. N Engl J Med 305:1238–1243, 1981
12. Abdou NI, Lindsley HB, Racela LS, Pascual E, Hassanein KM: Suppressor cell dysfunction and anti-suppressor cell antibody in active early rheumatoid arthritis. J Rheumatol 8:9–18, 1981
13. Veys EM, Hermanns P, Schindler J, King PC, Goldstein G, Symoens J, Wauwe JV: Evaluation of T-cell subsets with monoclonal antibodies in patients with rheumatoid arthritis. J Rheumatol 9:25–29, 1982
14. Burmester GR, Yu DTY, Irani A-M, Kunkel HG, Winchester RJ: Ia+ T cell in synovial fluid and tissues of patients with rheumatoid arthritis. Arthritis Rheum 24: 1370–1376, 1981
15. Reinherz EL, Schlossman SF: The differentiation and function of human T-lymphocytes. Cell 19:821–827, 1980

16. Reinherz EL, Schlossman SF: Regulation of the immune response—inducer and suppressor T-lymphocyte subsets in human beings. N Engl J Med 303:370–373, 1980
17. Leonard WJ, Depper JM, Uchiyama T, Smith KA, Waldmann TA, Greene WC: A monoclonal antibody that appears to recognize the receptor for human T-cell growth factor. Nature 300:267–269, 1982
18. Hurley CK, Shaw S, Nadler L, Schlossman S, Capra JD: The alpha and beta chains of SB and DR antigens are structurally distinct. J Exp Med 156:1557–1563, 1982
19. Hercend T, Nadler LM, Pesando JM, Reinherz EL, Schlossman SF, Ritz J: Expression of a 26,000-dalton glycoprotein on activated human T-cells. Cell Immunol 64:192–199, 1981
20. Charron DJ, McDevitt HO: Analysis of HLA-D region associated molecules with monoclonal antibody. Proc Natl Acad Sci USA 76:6567–6571, 1979
21. Blumberg BS, Bunim JJ, Calkins E, Pirani CL, Zvaifler NJ: ARA nomenclature and classification of arthritis and rheumatism (tentative). Arthritis Rheum 7:93–97, 1964
22. White BA, Bancroft FC: Cytoplasmic dot hybridization: simple analysis of relative mRNA levels in multiple small cell or tissue samples. J Biol Chem 257:8569–8572, 1982
23. Korman AJ, Auffray C, Schamboeck A, Strominger JL: The amino acid sequence and gene organization of the heavy chain of the HLA-DR antigen: homology to immunoglobulins. Proc Natl Acad Sci USA 79:6013–6017, 1982
24. Ravetch JV, Siebenlist U, Korsmeyer S, Waldmann T, Leder P: Structure of the human immunoglobulin mu locus: characterization of embryonic and rearranged J and D genes. Cell 27:583–591, 1981
25. Menard HA, Haim T, Peltier AP: In vitro studies on peripheral blood leukocytes in rheumatoid arthritis. Ann Rheum Dis 33:361–365, 1974
26. Biddison WE, Payne SM, Shearer GM, Shaw S: Human cytotoxic T cell responses to trinitrophenyl hapten and influenza virus: diversity of restriction antigens and specificity of HLA-linked genetic regulation, Proceedings of a Conference on Genetic Control of the Human Immune Response. J Exp Med 152:204s–217s, 1980
27. Nagy Z, Elliott BE, Nabholz M, Krammer PH, Pernis B: Specific binding of alloantigens to T cells activated in the mixed lymphocyte reaction. J Exp Med 143:648–659, 1976
28. Klareskog L, Forsum U, Wingren A, Wigzell H: Relationships between HLA-DR-expressing cells and T-lymphocytes of different subsets in rheumatoid synovial tissue. Scand J Immunol 15:501–507, 1982
29. Berrih S, Gaud C, Bach M-A, LeBrigand H, Binet JP, Bach JF: Evaluation of T-cell subsets in myasthenia gravis using anti-T-cell monoclonal antibodies. Clin Exp Immunol 45:1–8, 1981
30. Robbins DS, Fudenberg HH: Human lymphocyte subpopulations in metastic neoplasia—six years later. N Engl J Med 308:1595–1597, 1983
31. Mittler RS, Rao PE, Talle MA, Look R, Goldstein G: Cell membrane perturbation of resting T cells and thymocytes causes display of activation antigens. J Exp Med 158:99–111, 1983
32. Fox RI, Fong S, Sabharwal N, Carstens S, Kung PC, Vaughan JH: Synovial fluid lymphocytes differ from peripheral blood lymphocytes in patients with rheumatoid arthritis. J Immunol 128:351–354, 1982
33. Depper JM, Leonard WT, Robb RJ, Waldmann TA, Greene WC: Blockade of the interleukin-2 receptor by anti-TAC antibody: inhibition of human lymphocyte activation. J Immunol 131:690–697, 1983

REPRODUCIBILITY OF MULTIPLE-OBSERVER SCORING OF RADIOLOGIC ABNORMALITIES IN THE HANDS AND WRISTS OF PATIENTS WITH RHEUMATOID ARTHRITIS

JOHN T. SHARP, GILBERT B. BLUHM, ANDREW BROOK, ANNE C. BROWER, MARY CORBETT, JOHN L. DECKER, HARRY K. GENANT, J. PHILIP GOFTON, NEAL GOODMAN, ARVI LARSEN, MARTIN D. LIDSKY, PEKKA PUSSILA, AARON S. WEINSTEIN, BARBARA N. WEISSMAN, and DONALD Y. YOUNG

Forty-one coded radiographic films from 16 patients with rheumatoid arthritis were read by 13 observers, using 4 different methods for scoring abnormalities. Although absolute scores differed widely among individual observers, correlation coefficients were greater than 0.850 for approximately 2 of 3 comparisons. When films were ranked, using the median rank of all readers, 72% of individual ranks were within 10% of the median ranks. Among serial films on individual patients, 92% of comparisons between early and late films were interpreted as demonstrating progression of abnormalities when mean standardized scores showed an increase in scores of 15 units or greater. Films with lesser changes were interpreted inconsistently. This study shows good general agreement among readers in scoring radiologic abnormalities of hands and wrists, when applied to a film set showing a broad spectrum of severity, and defines the sensitivity of radiologic detection of disease progression.

Presented at a workshop sponsored by the Joe and Betty Alpert Arthritis Center, Rose Medical Center, Denver, CO, November 28–29, 1983.

Supported by a grant from Eli Lilly Company, Indianapolis, Indiana.

John T. Sharp, MD: Director, Joe and Betty Alpert Arthritis Center, Rose Medical Center, Denver, Colorado; Gilbert B. Bluhm, MD: Coordinator, Clinical Investigation, Rheumatology Research, Henry Ford Hospital, Detroit, Michigan; Andrew Brook, MB: Rheumatologist, Yarralumla, Australia; Anne C. Brower, MD: Department of Radiology, George Washington University Medical Center, Washington, DC; Mary Corbett, MB: Consultant Rheumatologist, Middlesex Hospital, London, England; John L. Decker, MD: Director, Clinical Center, Department of Health and Human Services, NIH, Bethesda, Maryland; Harry K. Genant, MD: Department of Radiology, University of California Medical Center, San Francisco, California; J. Philip Gofton, MD: Rheumatologist, Vancouver, British Columbia, Canada; Neal Goodman, MD: Department of Radiology, St. Anthony Hospital, Denver, Colorado; Arvi Larsen, MD: Spenshults Reumatikersjukhus, Oskarstrom, Sweden; Martin D. Lidsky, MD: Chief, Rheumatology Section, VA Medical Center, Houston, Texas; Pekka Pussila, MD: Department of Radiology, Reumasaation Sairaala, Heinola, Finland; Aaron S. Weinstein, MD: Department of Radiology, University of Cincinnati Medical Center, Cincinnati, Ohio; Barbara N. Weissman, MD: Department of Radiology, Brigham and Women's Hospital, Boston, Massachusetts; Donald Y. Young, PhD: Statistician, ARAMIS Data Bank Network, Stanford University, Palo Alto, California.

Address reprint requests to John T. Sharp, MD, Alpert Arthritis Center, 4567 East Ninth Avenue, Denver, CO 80220.

Submitted for publication February 24, 1984; accepted in revised form July 13, 1984.

Radiologic evaluation has been used by clinicians for many decades to assess the progression of rheumatoid arthritis. A method of staging arthritis which incorporates radiologic abnormalities was adopted by the American Rheumatism Association (ARA) (1). Kellgren and Bier developed a method of grading radiographic changes that was used in epidemiologic studies and a therapeutic trial (2). Several investigators have reported methods of scoring radiologic changes that more fully exploit the advantages of quantitating abnormalities by assessing the changes in multiple joints and expressing the sum of changes as a score (3–6). Radiographic analysis has been used in an increasing proportion of drug trials, particularly in testing agents for disease-modifying activity in trials that extend over a period of 6 months or longer (7–20). Radiologic analysis also has been used as an outcome measure to determine progression of disease and describe the course of illness (21–23).

Radiologic assessment of disease progression is particularly attractive because of the perceived potential of achieving objective measurements. Seemingly, it should be relatively easy to define abnormalities and express the extent of abnormalities by a score. The dates on the films can be hidden or removed, and the sequence can be randomly assigned by a project manager or from random number tables. Multiple interpretations can be obtained by having several readers score the same sets of films, or the reader can compare films representing 2 or more points in time at the same setting, a particularly attractive capability.

Considering that radiographic analysis presents these attractive features, it is somewhat puzzling that radiologic scoring of progression has not been universally adopted in all long-term outcome studies of rheumatoid arthritis, as well as therapeutic trials of agents being tested for their ability to modify the disease. If we ask why there is this failure of acceptance, there are several possible reasons. Perhaps rheumatologists are not convinced of the value of describing disease progression in the individual patient and, as a group, are not committed to studies on drugs that will modify the disease process. Another factor is the influence of drug studies. Pharmaceutical companies have had a major impact on rheumatology during the past 1–2 decades by developing a multiplicity of nonsteroidal antiinflammatory drugs which have short-term benefits, but are not considered to have significant potential for slowing the disease process. Only now that the market is fairly saturated with nonsteroidal antiinflammatory drugs, most of which seem to be relatively interchangeable, have drug companies begun to ask the more profound question of what is required to develop drugs that are capable of slowing or halting the progression of rheumatoid arthritis. Finally, it must be pointed out that methods used in attempting to quantitatively score radiologic abnormalities have not been thoroughly standardized. Relatively few studies have been done on the reproducibility of methods to score radiologic abnormalities (2,4,6,24–26), and the majority of these studies deal with systems for assigning a global grade rather than the more quantitative scoring of multiple joints.

Since lack of clarification of methodologic problems could be a major reason why radiographic evaluation has not yet reached its full potential, a collaborative study to test reproducibility of radiographic analysis of hand and wrist abnormalities in rheumatoid arthritis was organized. Forty-one films from patients with rheumatoid arthritis with different disease durations and in different stages of illness were selected from a film file and read by 13 experienced observers. The results of this study demonstrate the extent to which radiographic scoring is similar among multiple readers, and define the sensitivity of radiologic analysis in detecting progression of rheumatoid arthritis.

MATERIALS AND METHODS

Selection of film readers. Fifteen physicians who were either radiologists with special experience in bone and joint disease or rheumatologists who have experience in radiologic analysis were invited to participate in this study. Seven rheumatologists and 6 radiologists agreed to participate. Two radiologists declined. All of the rheumatologists previously had utilized some method for scoring radiographic changes in clinical studies and 2 radiologists had such experience.

Selection of film set. Films of the hands and wrists were chosen to represent a widely differing extent of radiologic abnormalities, and every film was a part of a film sequence. Sequential films were selected to represent varied differences. Thus, some sets demonstrated minimal, if any, change between sequential films, while others showed extensive progression. The ages of the patients varied, but all were adult and had adult onset of rheumatoid arthritis. The duration of disease was extremely variable. Nine pairs, 15 films from 5 patients with 3 sequential examinations each, and 8 films from 2 patients with 4 sequential examinations each, were chosen. The interval between the first and last films in the sequences varied from 6 weeks to 66 months. Fourteen separate sets of identical films were reproduced from the originals and distributed to each of the collaborating physicians. Dates of films were masked. Individual films were identified as belonging to patients 1–16. Within patient series, the sequence of films was varied so that the letter assignment represented the true sequence of obtaining the films no more often than expected by random chance. In 9 pairs of films, the film labeled "B" was the first film in 4 pairs; the film labeled "A" was the first in 5 pairs. In groups consisting of 3 serial films, the following sequences were represented: B,C,A, once; B,A,C, twice; C,B,A, once; A,C,B, once. In the 2 groups of 4 sequential films, the film order was C,A,D,B in 1 and D,B,C,A in the other. Posteroanterior and oblique views were available for 39 of 41 examinations.

Methods of reading films. Several film readers were chosen because they were known to use different methods for scoring radiographic changes. Four different methods were represented. These included those developed by Genant (6), Gofton and O'Brien (12), Larsen (4,5), and Sharp et al (3). Genant assigned 1 of 5 grades for erosions and joint space narrowing separately to the 10 metacarpophalangeal (MCP) joints and 10 proximal interphalangeal (PIP) joints. These scores were: 0 = normal, 1 = questionable, 2 = minimal, 3 = moderate, 4 = severe. He scored the radionavicular, radioulnar, and ulnar styloid for erosions, but only scored the wrist once for joint space narrowing. Gofton scored 54 joints, including all of the interphalangeal joints, MCP joints, carpometacarpal joints, and 8 areas in each wrist on a 4-point scale: 0 = normal, 1 = minimal, 2 = moderate, and 3 = severe abnormalities. Larsen scored 10 MCP joints, 10 PIP joints, and 4 regions in each wrist, using a standard film set for comparison. Changes were graded as 0 = normal, 1–5 for increasing severity. In this study, each MCP and interphalangeal joint and each wrist region was scored. Sharp scored 54 joints or areas in the 2 hands and wrists, including the proximal and distal interphalangeal joints, MCP joints, carpometacarpal joints, and 8 areas in each wrist, for erosions and joint space narrowing. Erosions were counted individually when they were present as discrete defects in separate areas if the discrete lesions were in the range of 1–4. If an erosion involved half or more of the articulating surface of either bone in a joint, the joint was scored as 5 for destruction. Joint space narrowing was scored as 0 = normal; 1 = focal; 2 = diffuse, but less than 50% narrowing; 3 = more than 50% narrowing; and 4 = ankylosis. Bluhm used the method of Sharp et al for scoring changes, but did not score terminal interphalangeal joints or the pisiform–triquetrum area in the wrist for erosions. He scored each multangular area separately for erosions, rather than together (27). In scoring joint space narrowing, he did not read the terminal interphalangeal joints and scored only 3 carpometacarpal joints, and 4 areas in the wrist.

Those invited to collaborate who had not previously utilized a method of scoring abnormalities (i.e., readers 1, 4, 5, 7, 9, 12, 12, 13, and 15) were instructed by letter and telephone that they were to choose any of the above-described methods with which they were comfortable. They were provided with sets of standard films prepared by one of us (AL), and provided with forms for reading films by any 1 of the 4 methods. It was anticipated that several would choose different methods, but all elected to utilize the method of Sharp et al. Thus, readers 1, 4, 5, 7, 9, 10, 12, 13, and 15 read by the Sharp method. Observers 2, 3, and 6 each used separate methods which they had previously utilized, and observer 8 used the method of Sharp et al, modified by eliminating some of the areas read in the original method.

Statistical methods. The raw data from each investigator were entered into a computer. Total scores were calculated by adding all erosion scores and joint space narrowing for each joint area read. In addition, scores for selected joint groups—for example, all MCP joints and all PIP joints—were computed, and total erosion and joint space narrowing scores were calculated separately when these changes were scored separately. Calculations of Gofton's and Larsen's scores yielded total scores for both hands and wrists, and total scores for specific groups. In addition, a weighted total score was calculated by giving each joint area the higher of either the erosion or joint space narrowing score recorded and adding these high scores for the entire hand and wrist or for specific joint groups.

Statistical analysis was carried out using the Statistical Package for the Social Sciences (28). In addition, the scores for each reader for each film were ranked for the entire set and within sequential sets for individual patients. For example, among pairs, films were ranked 1 or 2; 3 serial films on the same patient were ranked 1, 2, and 3 according to the severity of radiographic findings.

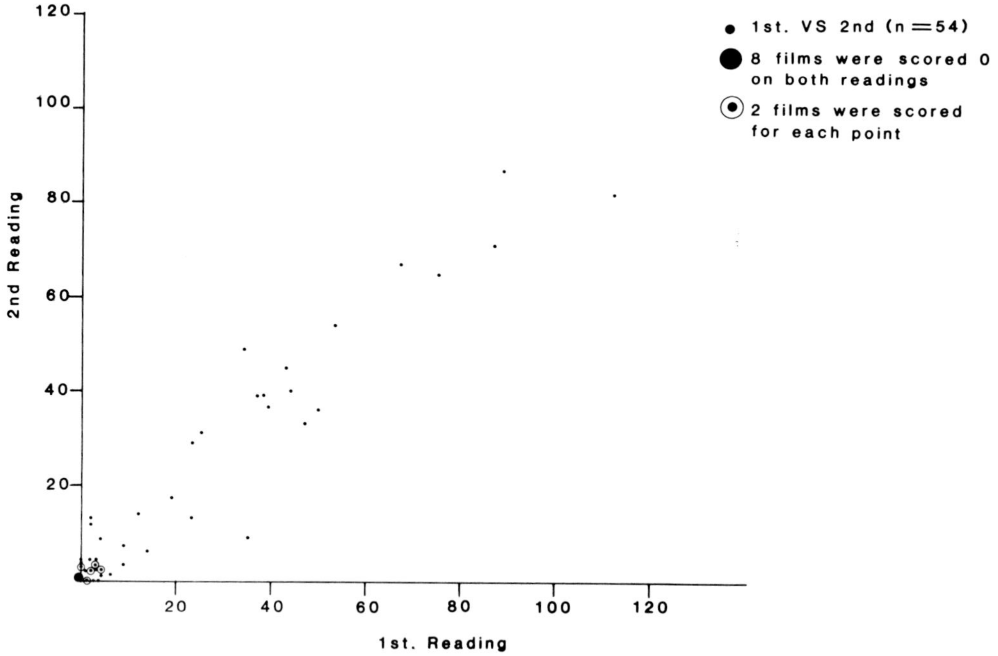

Figure 1. Fifty-four films were read for erosions and joint space narrowing on 2 occasions, 9 or 10 months apart, by 1 observer. Erosion and joint space narrowing scores were added to give total scores. At the time of the second reading, scores of the first reading were not known to the observer and film identity was masked. Film sequence within patient series was varied systematically.

Table 1. Same-observer reproducibility in film reading*

	Second reading			Third reading		
	Total score	Erosion score	Joint space narrowing score	Total score	Erosion score	Joint space narrowing score
First reading (observer 1)						
Total score	0.964 (54)			0.974 (18)		
Erosion score		0.967			0.968	
Joint space narrowing score			0.933			0.962
Second reading (observer 1)						
Total score				0.964 (40)		
Erosion score					0.969	
Joint space narrowing score						0.936
First reading (observer 3)						
Total score	0.915 (19)					

* Values shown are correlation coefficients; numbers in parentheses are the numbers of films read twice.

To facilitate comparison, total scores were standardized between readers by the following formula:

$$\left[\left(\frac{Xi - \bar{X}}{SD}\right) + 2\right] \times 100$$

where Xi is the score for the individual film, $\bar{X}$ is the mean score for all films of the individual reader, and SD is the standard deviation for all scores of the same reader. The value of 2 was added so that all scores were positive, and this was multiplied by 100 to assure a 3-digit scale without decimals.

Observer consistency. Observer consistency was tested by 2 readers. One reader scored 2 overlapping sets of films so that all films in each set were read twice and many were read 3 times. The second reading was carried out 9 or 10 months after the initial reading, and the third reading was done approximately 3 months after the second reading. Dates and names of patients were known to the observer at the time of the first reading, but films were coded for the second and third readings. Films for the second reading were chosen from random numbers generated by a desk-top calculator. Numbers were matched to record numbers in a data bank used to store radiographic and clinical data. Fourteen patients selected had only single films available. Sets of 2 sequential films were available on 17 patients, and sets of 3 sequential films were available on 2 patients. An assistant labeled each film and set, assigning a number for each patient and a letter for each film. The sequence of films was chosen from a table of all possible sequences for the film sets of 3. Among pairs, A and B were assigned to an equal number of first films.

Since the film sets chosen for the collaborative project with 13 observers overlapped to a considerable extent with the second set of films read by observer 1 and did not include any films that had not been read once by observer 1, many films were read a third time.

A second observer read 19 films twice. These 19 films were a subset of the film set distributed to all 13 readers. Films were coded for name and sequence, and sets for individual patients were identified as films belonging to an individual.

RESULTS

Repeated readings of the films by observer 1 were highly consistent (Figure 1). Correlation coefficients for total scores, erosion scores, and joint space narrowing scores for the 3 readings ranged from 0.933 between joint space narrowing scores in the first and second readings to 0.974 between total scores for the first and third readings. Two readings by observer 3 were also highly consistent, with a correlation coefficient of 0.915 (Table 1).

When scores on the same set of films were

Table 2. Individual readers' total scores for 3 illustrative films

Reader	Film 8B	Film 16B	Film 9C
1	20	80	84
2*	29	49	63
3*	0	35	47
4	47	125	104
5	8	47	104
6*	56	110	111
7	60	116	167
8*	23	65	137
9	88	114	181
10	54	166	206
12	0	57	91
13	60	65	151
15	50	89	142

* Different methods (from those of Sharp et al [3]) were used for scoring radiographic changes.

Table 3. Mean scores (all readers)

Reader	n (films)	Erosions	Joint spacing narrowing	Total	Total (weighted)	Metacarpo-phalangeal	Proximal interphalangeal	Wrist
1	41	12.41	16.90	29.32	25.83	9.02	6.73	12.66
2	41	–	–	31.56	–	10.85	10.68	10.02
3	41	–	–	16.88	–	5.41	2.46	8.93
4	41	29.93	26.98	56.90	47.24	14.12	10.68	28.85
5	41	16.98	17.27	34.24	27.17	9.76	5.10	19.27
6	40	30.52	33.08	63.60	42.37	29.07	23.00	11.53
7	41	25.56	47.34	72.90	60.02	18.34	12.78	34.95
8	39	15.62	27.64	43.26	34.51	14.95	11.05	17.26
9	41	29.73	37.12	66.85	51.37	13.63	10.56	37.46
10	41	41.54	41.61	83.15	64.02	19.15	16.29	42.15
12	41	21.54	12.90	34.44	28.49	11.32	5.44	17.59
13	41	45.29	34.24	79.54	60.10	18.46	8.02	51.61
15	41	47.98	33.12	81.10	60.73	25.54	15.41	33.88

tabulated for 13 readers, a great deal of variation was observed. This is illustrated in Tables 2 and 3, which include the individual scores for 3 representative films and mean scores for the entire set of films for each reader. In order to better compare the differences in scores between different readers, standardized scores were calculated as described. Mean standardized scores, ranges, and the coefficient of variation for each film are shown in Table 4.

The coefficient of variation decreased as the total score increased. This reflects the fact that the range and standard deviation of readings were not related to the total score, indicating that the absolute variation was approximately the same for films of all degrees of severity.

In spite of this wide range in individual scores, most of the scores were highly correlated. Correlation coefficients for total scores were ≥0.850 for 50 of the 78 interobserver comparisons, and 31 of 78 were >0.900. Four correlation coefficients were >0.950 (Table 5). Interobserver correlations between joint space narrowing scores and erosion scores were quite similar to correlations between total scores, although slightly lower.

In order to further test the interobserver reproducibility in scoring radiologic changes, the ranks of all 41 films were tabulated for each reader. The median rank for each film was then determined. In those instances in which median ranks tied, the mean of the total scores was utilized as a tie-breaker. After assigning the median rank to each film, the differences between the median rank and the rank assigned by each individual reader were tabulated. The range of differences and the number of individual readers who ranked a given film within 10, 15, or 20% of the median rank are shown in Table 6. Seventy-three percent of the individual readers' ranks were within 10% of the median rank and 91% were within 20%.

Healing of erosions to the extent of filling in a defect and regrowth of cartilage sufficient to be observed as an increase in joint space are considered to be rare events if they occur at all. Taking advantage of this observation, the entire film set was divided into subsets, 1 for each patient. Sequential films were judged to demonstrate progression, remain unchanged, or demonstrate healing by ranking each individual reader's scores for each patient's serial films. This analysis demonstrated that a very high proportion of reader's scores showed progression of disease when the difference between 2 films was large. More divergent interpretations, among serial films whose scores reflected small differences, suggest a limit to the sensitivity of film interpretation. Utilizing the mean standardized scores, differences between sequential films were employed to divide all film comparisons into 4 groups. Ninety-two percent of comparisons in the group with the greatest differences were judged to demonstrate progression of disease, whereas a lesser percent of the comparisons between films with smaller differences in mean scores were read as demonstrating progression (Table 7). Concordance among the readers was very high in judging progression for the group of films with the more progressive disease, but was unimpressive in comparing films showing minimal change.

Comparison of the different methods of scoring films did not disclose any advantage of any of the 4 methods used. Comparison of total scores among individuals using the 4 different methods showed very similar correlation coefficients, and the results of

Table 4. Mean "standardized" scores (all readers)

Film	Mean score*	Range	Coefficient of variation†
13B	82.000	32–128	37.99
15B	82.923	32–122	38.13
11B	102.615	53–132	23.38
5D	107.077	73–147	22.28
5B	111.692	64–150	18.75
1A	122.154	74–187	22.55
7A	122.615	75–182	23.62
7B	126.000	94–182	21.60
1D	125.182	83–202	25.22
13C	102.692	43–138	35.84
13A	111.462	46–146	28.09
5C	126.385	79–160	15.76
11C	130.385	115–151	9.49
5A	129.692	100–181	16.91
3B	129.167	90–162	17.73
3A	134.077	100–167	17.72
11A	141.308	64–200	23.61
8A	148.462	109–192	15.57
8B	159.385	109–235	21.02
2A	152.692	110–235	21.81
12B	178.308	130–215	14.06
4C	190.000	117–287	28.37
4A	188.538	117–302	33.38
4B	202.308	133–293	23.61
4D	208.308	130–314	28.32
2B	210.692	157–283	17.63
14C	210.077	154–261	18.04
6B	214.385	177–256	11.44
12A	219.692	174–262	11.60
15A	269.462	181–327	15.60
14B	277.000	225–371	15.53
10A	265.846	214–312	11.52
10B	295.692	226–352	11.42
16B	279.615	163–359	20.03
16A	309.846	193–394	18.07
9A	327.538	296–351	6.72
14A	348.462	294–421	10.88
6A	351.385	308–380	5.74
9C	369.385	305–427	9.46
6C	404.846	364–463	8.60
9B	412.538	314–566	15.84

* Standardized scores derived by the formula:

$$\left[\left(\frac{Xi - \bar{X}}{SD}\right) + 2\right] \times 100$$

† Coefficient of variation derived by the formula: $\frac{SD}{\bar{X}} \times 100$.

Range of coefficients of variation 5.74–37.99; mean of standard deviations 33.8917.

judging progression of films in sequence suggested that the 4 methods were approximately equally sensitive.

DISCUSSION

This study was undertaken to determine the extent to which scoring of radiologic abnormalities in the hands and wrists of rheumatoid arthritis patients is reproducible. Reproducibility was tested by single observers reading the same films 2 or 3 times without knowing the prior readings and multiple observers reading a standard set of films. Two features in the design of this study were significant in interpreting the results. The film set covered a relatively wide spectrum of disease severity, from films that were considered to show no erosions and no joint space narrowing by some observers, to films that were scored as abnormal in a majority of joints by most observers. Clearly, the results of multiple readers' scoring the film set would have shown less correlation if the range of abnormalities exhibited by the test set had been quite narrow.

The second feature in study design that impacted interpretation was the fact that all films were included within sequences of 2, 3, or 4 films on the same patient. Since there is general agreement that filling in of erosions and recovery toward normal of narrowed joint spaces are rare events, if they occur at all, the interpretation of films in sequences which were scrambled and unknown to the observers was used as an additional means of testing reliability of observations.

With this background information, the results of this study can be interpreted as demonstrating that 1) 2 observers, reading the same films on multiple occasions, were quite consistent in scoring abnormalities, 2) absolute scores of multiple observers, using the same or different methods, were quite divergent, 3) correlation coefficients between total scores of multiple observers were >0.850 in approximately 2 of 3 comparisons, 4) individual observer rankings of films agreed within 10% of the median rank of all observers in 2 of 3 instances, 5) there was agreement on progression of disease in approximately 92% of sequential film comparisons when the difference between the 2 films was >15 units of standardized score, and 6) no statistically significant differences were detected between different methods or different observers (data not shown).

Table 5. Correlation coefficients between readings of multiple observers on the standard set of films*

	n	Range	≥0.850	≥0.900	≥0.950
Total scores	78	0.736–0.956	50	31	4
Erosion scores	55	0.529–0.962	22	12	5
Joint space narrowing scores	55	0.585–0.947	27	12	0

* Correlation coefficients were performed on each reader's scores versus every other reader's scores, using the Statistical Package for Social Sciences program.

Table 6. Readers' differences from median ranks*

Film number	Rank†	Range	Within ± 4 ranks	Within ± 6 ranks	Within ± 8 ranks
13B	1	1–10	12	12	12
15B	2	1–8	12	13	13
11B	3	2–14	9	9	10
5D	4	4–18.5	9	9	11
5B	5	4–15.5	9	11	12
1A	6	2–16.5	9	9	9
7A	7	2–18.5	6	9	11
7B	8	2.5–20	7	10	12
1D	9	4–21	7	8	8
13C	10	2–17	5	7	13
13A	11	2–20.5	3	9	11
5C	12	8–19.5	11	11	13
11C	13	3–20.5	11	11	12
5A	14	7–22	8	10	13
3B	15	7.5–24	5	8	10
3A	16	6–24	7	9	12
11A	17	6–25	7	9	12
8A	18	1.5–21.5	10	10	10
8B	19	1.5–23.5	8	10	11
2A	20	10–25	8	9	12
12B	21	14–27	9	12	13
4C	22	5–32	8	9	10
4A	23	5–33.5	6	7	7
4B	24	18–33	8	11	12
4D	25	14–36	6	11	11
2B	26	18–30.5	11	12	13
14C	27	14–30.5	8	11	12
6B	28	22–29	11	13	13
12A	29	22–30	12	12	13
15A	30	26–35	12	13	13
14B	31	25–38	10	12	13
10A	32	23–34.5	11	12	12
10B	33	30–36	13	13	13
16B	34	21–37	10	11	11
16A	35	24–40	9	11	12
9A	36	33–38	13	13	13
14A	37	34–40	13	13	13
6A	38	35–40	13	13	13
9C	39	32–41	13	13	13
6C	40	38.5–41	13	13	13
9B	41	34–41	13	13	13
Total			385/530 (72.6%)	441/530 (83.2%)	483/530 (91.1%)

* Thirteen readers of each film except for films 1D (11 readers) and 3B (12 readers). Four ranks = within 10% of median; 6 ranks = within 15%; 8 ranks = within 20%.
† Films ranked by median; mean used as tie-breaker.

For part of the analysis, the extent of agreement between multiple observers and the reproducibility of readings by the same observer were described in terms of correlation coefficients. There are no guidelines determining what is an appropriate level when correlation coefficients are used to measure precision of reproducibility as in this study. In general, laboratory tests, based on biochemical reactions that can be measured with great precision, are characterized by correlation coefficients that are >0.950 on repeated testing. Serologic tests which employ titration techniques have greater variability and lower correlation coefficients. Scales obtained from questionnaires used to test psychologic and social functions also have greater variability. Correlation coefficients >0.850, observed in two-thirds of the comparisons of radiographic scores tested here, were an indication of a reasonable similarity of readings, considering the differences in methods and the application of methods used.

The coefficient of variation decreased with increasing severity of involvement. In fact, the extent of variation of readings for each individual film appeared to be independent of the extent of disease. Thus, a given amount of variation represented a smaller proportion of the severity score for films that demonstrated the greatest severity.

The ultimate value in scoring radiographic changes in rheumatoid arthritis is in describing the natural history of the disease, measuring progression to assess the value of clinical variables as prognostic indicators, and testing the ability of treatment to alter the course of the disease. The degree of similarity observed, while generally good after calculating standardized scores, was so low in terms of absolute scores that meaningful comparisons of studies by different observers are probably not possible if only the absolute scores are used. However, the application of a standardized score, derived from a standard film set such as used here, should prove useful in allowing comparisons between different observers.

Determination of progression rates in sequential films resembles the type of analysis appropriate to a therapeutic trial. However, rather than defining the difference between sequential films in terms of a fixed time interval, as is customary in drug trials, sequential films were chosen to represent varying extents of

Table 7. Comparisons among serial films

Range of differences in scores*	Film pairs compared	Change judged as:		
		Progression	Healing	None
−10.9–5	8	47 (46.5%)	46 (45.5%)	8 (7.9%)
5.1–10	2	15 (57.7%)	7 (26.9%)	4 (15.4%)
10.1–15	3	31 (79.5%)	6 (15.4%)	2 (5.1%)
>15	23	274 (91.6%)	14 (4.7%)	11 (3.7%)

* A negative score is a film pair in which the second film had a lower score than the first film, i.e., was judged by that reader as having shown improvement.

progression. This permitted us to test how much progression of disease is detectable by radiologic examination. The results indicated that control subjects would have to have an increase in radiologic abnormality of >15 units of standardized score in order to be reliably characterized as having progressive disease. A change of 15 units of standardized score represents approximately 1% of the maximal score possible. Expressed in terms of actual scores of individual readers, 15 units of standardized score represented from 3 to 9.4 units. An ability to detect a change of this magnitude represents a high degree of sensitivity, considered from this perspective. However, from the standpoint of setting up therapeutic trials, it will be necessary to know what proportion of randomly selected patients have this degree of progression in specific followup intervals and whether standard prognostic features would be helpful in selecting a subset with a higher proportion of patients who have greater progression in shorter intervals.

Although the natural history of radiologic progression in rheumatoid arthritis is not sufficiently well defined at present to resolve this problem, a review of published therapeutic trials and unpublished experience of the authors suggests that an observation interval of 1 year or longer may be necessary in order to establish efficacy, and this estimate is based on inadequate data.

This study establishes the limits of reproducibility of radiologic observations which are necessary to describe progression rates, or, expressed in other terms, the sensitivity of radiologic assessment in detecting progression of disease. By applying these methods to several study populations, it should be possible to obtain more complete information on the natural history of rheumatoid arthritis, which would enable the accurate selection of patient groups for therapeutic trials to give reliable information on modification of disease progression.

REFERENCES

1. Steinbrocker O, Traeger CH, Batterman RC: Therapeutic criteria in rheumatoid arthritis. JAMA 140:659–665, 1949
2. Kellgren JH, Bier F: Radiological signs of rheumatoid arthritis: a study of observer differences in the reading of hand films. Ann Rheum Dis 15:55–60, 1956
3. Sharp JT, Lidsky MD, Collins LC, Moreland J: Methods of scoring the progression of radiologic changes in rheumatoid arthritis. Arthritis Rheum 14:706–720, 1971
4. Larsen A: A radiological method for grading the severity of rheumatoid arthritis. Thesis, University of Helsinki Medical School, Helsinki, Finland
5. Larsen A, Dale K, Eck M: Radiographic evaluation of rheumatoid arthritis and related conditions by standard reference films. Acta Radiol [Diagn] (Stockh) 18:481–491, 1977
6. Genant HK: Methods of assessing radiographic change in rheumatoid arthritis: oral gold therapy in rheumatoid arthritis: auranofin. Am J Med 74:35–47, 1983
7. Cats A: A multicentre controlled trial of the effects of different dosages of gold therapy, followed by a maintenance dosage. Agents Actions 6:355–362, 1976
8. The Cooperating Clinics Committee of the American Rheumatism Association: A controlled trial of cyclophosphamide in rheumatoid arthritis. N Engl J Med 283:883–889, 1970
9. The Cooperating Clinics Committee of the American Rheumatism Association: A controlled trial of gold salt therapy in rheumatoid arthritis. Arthritis Rheum 16:353–358, 1973
10. Empire Rheumatism Council Subcommittee: Multi-centre controlled trial comparing cortisone acetate and acetyl salicylic acid in the long-term treatment of rheumatoid arthritis: results of three years' treatment. Ann Rheum Dis 16:277–289, 1957
11. Gibson T, Huskisson EC, Wojtalewski JA, Scott PJ, Balme HW, Burry HC, Grahame R, Hart FD: Evidence that D-penicillamine alters the course of rheumatoid arthritis. Rheumatol Rehabil 15:211–215, 1976
12. Gofton JP, O'Brien WN: Effects of auranofin on the radiological progression in rheumatoid arthritis. J Rheumatol 9:169–172, 1982
13. Joint Committee of the Medical Research Council and Nuffield Foundation on Clinical Trials of Cortisone, ACTH and Other Therapeutic Measures in Chronic Rheumatic Diseases: A comparison of prednisolone with aspirin or other analgesics in the treatment of rheumatoid arthritis. Ann Rheum Dis 18:173–188, 1959
14. Lidsky MD, Sharp JT, Billings S: Double-blind study of cyclophosphamide in rheumatoid arthritis. Arthritis Rheum 16:148–153, 1973
15. Multicentre Trial Group: Controlled trial of D(-)penicillamine in severe rheumatoid arthritis. Lancet 1:275–280, 1973
16. Research Sub-Committee of the Empire Rheumatism Council: Gold therapy in rheumatoid arthritis. Ann Rheum Dis 19:95–119, 1960
17. Research Sub-Committee of the Empire Rheumatism Council: Gold therapy in rheumatoid arthritis: final report of a multicentre controlled trial. Ann Rheum Dis 20:315–334, 1961
18. Sharp JT, Lidsky MD, Duffy J, Thompson HK Jr, Person BD, Masri AF, Andrianakos AA: Comparison of two dosage schedules of gold salts in the treatment of rheumatoid arthritis: relationship of serum gold levels to

therapeutic response. Arthritis Rheum 20:1179–1187, 1977
19. Sharp JT, Lidsky MD, Duffy J: Clinical responses during gold therapy for rheumatoid arthritis: changes in synovitis, radiologically detectable erosive lesions, serum proteins, and serologic abnormalities. Arthritis Rheum 25:540–549, 1982
20. Sigler JW, Bluhm GB, Duncan H, Sharp JT, Ensign DC, McCrum WR: Gold salts in the treatment of rheumatoid arthritis: a double-blind study. Ann Intern Med 80:21–26, 1974
21. Sharp JT, Calkins E, Cohen AS, Schubart AF, Calabro JJ: Observations on the clinical, chemical and serological manifestations of rheumatoid arthritis, based on the course of 154 cases. Medicine (Baltimore) 43:41–58, 1964
22. Brook A, Fleming A, Corbett M: Relationship of radiological change to clinical outcome in rheumatoid arthritis. Ann Rheum Dis 36:274–275, 1977
23. DeCarvalho A, Graudal H, Jorgensen B: Radiologic evaluation of the progression of rheumatoid arthritis. Acta Radiol [Diagn] (Stockh) 21:115–121, 1980
24. DeCarvalho A: Discriminative power of Larsen's grading system for assessing the course of rheumatoid arthritis. Acta Radiol [Diagn] (Stockh) 22:77–80, 1981
25. Mewa AAM, Pui M, Cockshott WP, Buchanan WW: Observer differences in detecting erosions in radiographs of rheumatoid arthritis. J Rheumatol 10:216–221, 1983
26. Kellgren JH, Lawrence JS: Radiological assessment of rheumatoid arthritis. Ann Rheum Dis 16:485–493, 1957
27. Bluhm GB, Smith DW, Mikulaschek WM: A radiologic method of assessment of bone and joint destruction in rheumatoid arthritis. Henry Ford Hosp Med J 31:152–161, 1983
28. Nie NH, Hull CH, Jenkins JG, Steinbrenner J, Bent DH: SPSS Statistical Package for the Social Sciences. Second edition. New York, McGraw-Hill, 1975

QUANTITATIVE HISTOLOGIC STUDIES ON THE PATHOGENESIS OF PERIARTICULAR OSTEOPOROSIS IN RHEUMATOID ARTHRITIS

SHINICHI SHIMIZU, SHUNICHI SHIOZAWA, KAZUKO SHIOZAWA, SHIGEAKI IMURA, and TAKUO FUJITA

The pathogenesis of periarticular osteopenia in rheumatoid arthritis (RA) was investigated by histomorphometry on juxtaarticular bone removed during joint surgery. Twenty areas from 12 RA patients were compared with 14 areas from 6 osteoarthritis (OA) patients. There was no difference between the 2 groups in the percent of total bone volume. However, increased bone formation was suggested by an increase in the percent of active osteoid surface in RA compared with that in OA. Bone resorption was also increased in RA, as evidenced by increases versus OA in percent total resorptive surface, percent active resorptive surface, and number of osteoclasts. These results demonstrate increased turnover of bone in RA, especially in the resorptive phase of the periarticular trabecular bone. It is proposed that soluble factor(s) synthesized in the contiguous rheumatoid synovium may be transferred to the periarticular bone space, stimulating osteoclasts to resorb bone.

Periarticular osteopenia, also called periarticular osteoporosis, is a common clinical feature in rheumatoid arthritis (RA) (1). Despite its importance, however, few detailed histomorphometric studies have been carried out to elucidate its pathogenesis. There are 3 factors which could possibly contribute to the pathogenesis of periarticular osteopenia: 1) immobilization of the affected joint; 2) increased vascularity around the joint; or 3) local factors derived from adjacent synovial inflammation. The first possibility has not been adequately studied and does not explain the localized osteopenia in juxtaarticular bone. The second possibility, increased vascularity around the joint, has been demonstrated with arteriograms, by Soila and Berglund (2) and Laws et al (3). In a morphologic study, Soila demonstrated changes in periarticular bone in RA and described disintegration with thinning followed by a peculiar distortion of the trabecular bone in the affected joint (4).

Histologic observations by Havdrup et al suggested increased activities of both osteoblasts and osteoclasts in this region (5). Periarticular bone of RA appeared hyperactive by bone scintigraphy (6). Using radioisotope tracer of calcium, Bergmann et al demonstrated increased turnover of bone in the affected joint (7); however, there was no quantitative information reported. Recent development of techniques for preparing undecalcified, thin histologic sections of bone has enabled a quantitative analysis of morphologic changes in the bone (8,9).

Since soluble factor(s) produced by the rheumatoid synovium, such as prostaglandins, may have a direct effect on bone resorption (10–16), it appears important to study the characteristics of rheumatoid osteopenia in relation to the chronic inflammation of RA. The demonstration, by histomorphometric analysis, of increased turnover of bone and, particularly

From the Department of Medicine, Third Division, Kobe University School of Medicine, Kobe, Japan, and the Kakogawa National Hospital, Kakogawa, Japan.

Supported by the North Hyogo Medical and Orthopedic Center and by a Basic Research for Joint Diseases award to S. Shiozawa.

Shinichi Shimizu, MD: Department of Medicine, Kobe University; Shunichi Shiozawa, MD: Lecturer, Department of Medicine, Kobe University; Kazuko Shiozawa, MD: Department of Medicine, Kobe University; Shigeaki Imura, MD: Chief, Department of Orthopedic Surgery, Kakogawa National Hospital; Takuo Fujita, MD: Professor of Medicine, Kobe University.

Address reprint requests to S. Shiozawa, Department of Medicine, Third Division, Kobe University School of Medicine, 7-5-1 Kusunokicho, Chuoku, Kobe 650, Japan.

Submitted for publication December 2, 1983; accepted in revised form June 26, 1984.

increase in osteoclasts in the periarticular trabecular bone of RA patients compared with that of osteoarthritis (OA) patients indicates that synovial inflammation may directly contribute to the pathogenesis of periarticular osteopenia in RA.

PATIENTS AND METHODS

Patients. Twelve patients fulfilling the American Rheumatism Association criteria for definite or classic RA (17), and 6 OA patients as controls, were selected for the study. Their clinical characteristics are shown in Table 1. Patients with RA had a younger mean age, increased erythrocyte sedimentation rate, and a longer duration of disease than those with OA. There was no difference in the sex ratios of the 2 groups. All patients from both groups, except for 2 OA patients, had been treated with a variety of nonsteroidal antiinflammatory agents, and 3 of 12 RA patients were receiving prednisolone, <4 mg/day. There was no significant difference in disease activity between those treated and those not treated with prednisolone, and most of the RA patients had clinically active disease as judged by serologic and joint examination. Most RA patients had radiographic stage 3–4 disease at the time of surgery.

Preparation of bone specimens. Bone specimens adjacent to the articular surface were obtained from the 12 RA and 6 OA patients during total joint replacement surgery. Each specimen was carefully collected from the area of trabecular bone approximately 7 mm below the articular surface, which did not include bone–pannus junction. When possible, we collected more than 2 specimens from some joints at random, in order to minimize the contribution of the difference in weightbearing to the tissue morphology. Specimens were fixed in Millonig's fixative which consisted of 37% (weight/volume) formaldehyde, 0.12*M* monobasic sodium phosphate, 0.11*M* sodium hydroxide, and 0.015*M* sucrose at 4°C for 24 hours. They were dehydrated in graded acetone and embedded in methylmethacrylate. Undecalcified, 5-μm thick sections were cut using a Jung model K microtome (8). Tetracycline labeling was not performed in this study.

Histomorphometric evaluation of bone sections. Tissue sections were stained by a modification of the Masson technique and quantitated by the method of Schenk et al (18). An objective 20× magnification and an integrative eyepiece 10× magnification containing a grid with wave-shaped lines were used. Percent surface was quantitated by counting the number of intersections between grid lines and trabecular bone surface. Volumetric evaluation was done by counting the hit number of points dotted on the eyepiece. The results were expressed in a similar manner as described by Teitelbaum et al (9).

The following histologic parameters were counted: 1) total bone volume (trabecular bones containing both mineralized and nonmineralized bone matrix); 2) total osteoid volume (trabecular bone matrix which was nonmineralized); 3) active osteoid surface (osteoblastic osteoid surface; trabecular bone surface lined by osteoid which was covered by plump, cuboid osteoblasts); 4) inactive osteoid surface (non-osteoblastic osteoid surface; trabecular bone surface lined

Table 1. Characteristics of patients studied

Variable*	Rheumatoid arthritis (n = 12)	Osteoarthritis (n = 6)
Mean age (range)	57 (41–73)	72 (66–82)
M/F (%)	3/9 (25/75)	1/5 (17/83)
Replaced joint, no. (%)		
Knee	10 (84)	4 (67)
Hip	1 (8)	2 (33)
Elbow	1 (8)	0
Mean disease duration, years (range)	13 (6–24)	5 (1–11)
Restriction of ADL, no. (%)		
Mild	2 (17)	3 (50)
Moderate	9 (75)	3 (50)
Severe	1 (8)	0
Radiologic stage, no. (%)		
Stage 3	8 (67)	–
Stage 4	4 (33)	–
ESR, mm/hour, no. (%)		
>30	10 (83)	3 (50)
<30	2 (17)	3 (50)
RA latex test, no. (%)		
–	2 (17)	6 (100)
+	2 (17)	0
>2+	8 (66)	0
Treatment		
Systemic corticosteroids, no. (%)	3 (25)	0
Intraarticular corticosteroids, no. (%)	12 (100)	5 (83)
Nonsteroidal antiinflammatory agents, yes/no (%)	10/2 (83/17)	4/2 (67/33)

* ADL = activities of daily living; ESR = erythrocyte sedimentation rate; RA = rheumatoid arthritis; – = negative, + = positive.

by osteoid which was not covered by active osteoblasts); 5) total osteoid surface (parameters 3 + 4, above); 6) active resorptive surface (osteoclastic resorptive surface; trabecular bone surface containing Howship's lacunae in which osteoclasts were in apposition to the bone surface); 7) inactive resorptive surface (non-osteoclastic resorptive surface; trabecular bone surface containing Howship's lacunae devoid of osteoclasts); 8) total resorptive surface (parameters 6 + 7, above); 9) resting surface (trabecular bone surface exhibiting no histologic evidence of either formation or resorption).

Percent total bone volume and percent total osteoid volume were calculated as follows:

$$\%\ \text{total bone volume} = \frac{N_{mb} + N_{od}}{36 \times F} \times 100$$

$$\%\ \text{total osteoid volume} = \frac{N_{od}}{36 \times F} \times 100$$

where N_{mb} = hit number on mineralized bone; N_{od} = hit number on nonmineralized bone matrix; F = number of fields examined in the eyepiece in which 36 hit points were dotted in a field. The percentage of surface areas of trabecular bone was calculated, in general, as follows:

$$\%\ \text{surface} = \frac{\text{No. for each surface}}{\text{No. for total surface (parameters 5 + 8 + 9)}} \times 100$$

For example, to calculate active osteoid surface, the formula would be as follows:

$$\%\ \text{active osteoid surface} = \frac{\text{No. for active osteoid surface (parameter 3)}}{\text{No. for total surface (parameters 5 + 8 + 9)}} \times 100$$

The number of osteoclasts was counted independently of the above surface countings, and expressed as the absolute number per square millimeter of tissue specimen, as follows:

$$\text{Osteoclasts/mm}^2 = \frac{N_{oc}}{D_f \times F}$$

where N_{oc} = number of osteoclasts in the Howship's lacunae (only osteoclasts with 2 or more nuclei and in contact with the bone surface were counted); D_f = absolute dimensions in a field of eyepiece in a given magnification; F= number of fields examined. One hundred fields per section were usually examined, with a magnification of 200×.

Statistical analysis. Statistical evaluation included the Mann-Whitney rank sum test and Student's *t*-test. When

Table 2. Summary of histomorphometric findings on knee, hip, or elbow joints of rheumatoid arthritis (RA) and osteoarthritis (OA) patients

Variable	RA (12 patients, 20 specimens)	OA (6 patients, 14 specimens)	*P**
% total bone volume			
Median (range)	20.13 (12.25–36.64)	20.19 (12.56–40.36)	
Mean ± SD	21.36 ± 7.44	23.49 ± 10.26	NS
% total osteoid volume			
Median (range)	0.55 (0.03–1.40)	0.39 (0.06–1.92)	
Mean ± SD	0.59 ± 0.39	0.50 ± 0.47	NS
% active osteoid surface			
Median (range)	10.71 (3.19–22.80)	5.72 (0.64–8.69)	
Mean ± SD	12.39 ± 6.36	4.81 ± 3.08	<0.001
% inactive osteoid surface			
Median (range)	15.66 (4.85–37.91)	27.65 (6.12–43.30)	
Mean ± SD	18.34 ± 9.45	23.79 ± 10.93	NS
% total osteoid surface			
Median (range)	31.21 (11.96–48.63)	32.73 (7.87–49.46)	
Mean ± SD	30.73 ± 12.08	28.61 ± 12.99	NS
% active resorptive surface			
Median (range)	2.96 (1.16–6.29)	0.91 (0.36–3.18)	
Mean ± SD	3.21 ± 1.34	1.20 ± 0.90	<0.025
% inactive resorptive surface			
Median (range)	5.29 (2.83–13.87)	2.92 (0.96–7.20)	
Mean ± SD	5.90 ± 2.84	3.35 ± 1.73	<0.01
% total resorptive surface			
Median (range)	8.99 (5.24–16.16)	3.89 (1.32–8.19)	
Mean ± SD	9.11 ± 2.79	4.56 ± 2.22	<0.001
% resting surface			
Median (range)	59.64 (35.21–78.63)	63.92 (48.13–86.25)	
Mean ± SD	60.16 ± 12.55	66.84 ± 13.41	NS
Osteoclasts/mm^2			
Median (range)	0.82 (0.51–1.39)	0.26 (0.09–0.65)	
Mean ± SD	0.84 ± 0.23	0.32 ± 0.17	<0.001

* Calculated by Student's *t*-test or Mann-Whitney rank sum test; NS = not significant.

data from individual patients were presented as an average of several sites examined, statistical significance obtained by applying Student's *t*-test was confirmed using the more critical rank sum method.

RESULTS

All 12 RA patients examined in this study had clinically active disease. Of the 2 RA patients whose synovial tissue was examined, both showed histologic evidence of active disease as well.

Bone specimens adjacent to the articular surface which did not include the bone–pannus junction were observed by quantitative histomorphometry. Macroscopically it appeared that weightbearing sites were more sclerotic and non-weightbearing sites more porotic in the periarticular bone of the RA and OA groups, although the data were not layered nor analyzed by site. Coexistence of sclerotic and porotic areas apparently gave a wide sample variation, even in specimens from the same joint. Accordingly, we collected more than 2 specimens from some randomly-selected joints to minimize the contribution to the tissue morphology of difference in weightbearing.

There was no difference in the percent total bone volume in the 12 RA patients compared with the 6 OA patients, indicating almost equal degrees of osteopenia in the 2 groups (Table 2). In contrast, significant differences were found both in bone formation and resorption. Percent active osteoid surface in RA was 12.39 ± 6.36% (mean ± SD), a significant increase when compared with the percent found in OA (4.81 ± 3.08%, $P < 0.001$). At the same time, in RA there was a decrease (though not significant) in percent of inactive osteoid surface. There was no difference between the 2 groups in the percent total osteoid surface or the percent total osteoid volume.

A significant increase in bone resorption was noted in RA (Table 2). The percent total resorptive surface in RA was 9.11 ± 2.79% (mean ± SD), versus 4.56 ± 2.22% in OA ($P < 0.001$). Percent active resorptive surface was 3.21 ± 1.34% in RA and 1.20 ± 0.90% in OA ($P < 0.025$). The number of osteoclasts in

Table 3. Summary of histomorphometric findings on knee joints of rheumatoid arthritis (RA) and osteoarthritis (OA) patients

Variable	RA (10 patients, 14 specimens)	OA (4 patients, 10 specimens)	P*
% total bone volume			
Median (range)	20.93 (12.25–36.64)	16.29 (12.56–37.81)	
Mean ± SD	23.25 ± 7.99	19.21 ± 8.56	NS
% total osteoid volume			
Median (range)	0.56 (0.03–1.19)	0.46 (0.19–0.80)	
Mean ± SD	0.57 ± 0.32	0.45 ± 0.22	NS
% active osteoid surface			
Median (range)	12.05 (4.42–21.39)	6.32 (1.30–8.69)	
Mean ± SD	12.93 ± 5.96	5.67 ± 2.77	<0.01
% inactive osteoid surface			
Median (range)	20.56 (4.85–37.91)	27.99 (11.85–43.30)	
Mean ± SD	21.59 ± 9.00	26.83 ± 9.53	NS
% total osteoid surface			
Median (range)	37.09 (12.21–48.63)	34.35 (14.48–49.46)	
Mean ± SD	34.52 ± 11.45	32.50 ± 10.68	NS
% active resorptive surface			
Median (range)	2.67 (1.16–5.02)	0.99 (0.36–3.18)	
Mean ± SD	2.67 ± 0.97	1.35 ± 0.99	<0.01
% inactive resorptive surface			
Median (range)	5.67 (3.75–13.87)	2.87 (0.96–7.20)	
Mean ± SD	6.60 ± 2.94	3.28 ± 1.97	<0.01
% total resorptive surface			
Median (range)	8.50 (5.24–16.16)	3.89 (1.32–8.19)	
Mean ± SD	9.27 ± 3.03	4.63 ± 2.52	<0.01
% resting surface			
Median (range)	55.96 (35.21–75.38)	60.81 (48.13–83.33)	
Mean ± SD	56.21 ± 12.13	62.86 ± 11.76	NS
Osteoclasts/mm^2			
Median (range)	0.77 (0.55–1.39)	0.37 (0.09–0.65)	
Mean ± SD	0.80 ± 0.23	0.34 ± 0.17	<0.001

* Calculated by Student's *t*-test or Mann-Whitney rank sum test; NS = not significant.

RA was $0.84 \pm 0.23/mm^2$ (mean ± SD), a significant increase compared with the number found in OA ($0.32 \pm 0.17/mm^2$, $P < 0.001$) (Table 2).

Histomorphometric parameters confined to the knee joint were analyzed separately in order to eliminate the possible effect of difference in joints studied on the evaluation of results (Table 3). There were no significant changes in the statistical results of knees alone when compared with other joints.

The contribution of systemic administration of corticosteroids did not appear to be significant. There was no difference in the percent total resorptive surface in patients who were taking corticosteroids versus those who were not: 8.24 ± 2.05% (mean ± SD) in the former group, 9.68 ± 3.34% in the latter. The number of osteoclasts also did not differ between them: $0.76 \pm 0.21/mm^2$ (mean ± SD) in the patients receiving corticosteroids, $0.81 \pm 0.24/mm^2$ in those not receiving corticosteroids (data not shown).

DISCUSSION

Since it is generally accompanied by little or no synovial inflammation, osteoarthritis serves as an appropriate control in studying the contribution of synovial inflammation to the osteopenia in rheumatoid arthritis. In this study, periarticular trabecular bone of patients with clinically active RA was compared, by histomorphometry, with that of OA patients. There was no difference between RA and OA in the percent total bone volume, suggesting that the contribution of immobilization of the affected joints to the pathogenesis of periarticular osteopenia would be similar in both groups. Older patients are usually expected to have decreased bone volume. However, the mean bone volume was similar in our RA and OA patients, despite the 15-year difference in mean ages. This suggests that an inflammatory factor(s) in RA might have contributed to the periarticular osteopenia.

Bone formation and resorption were both increased in RA. Increased bone formation was suggested by increased active osteoid surface. There was no difference between the 2 groups in total osteoid surface. These results differ from those of Duncan et al, who found inactive osteoid seams to be increased in ribs of patients with RA (19). The systemic trabecular osteopenia found in RA may differ from localized osteopenia in the periarticular trabecular bone.

In studies using tetracycline labeling, histologic parameters of osteoid activity do not always correlate with kinetic findings (20). Since dynamic studies (i.e., fluorochrome labeling) were not performed in this investigation, the findings of increased osteoid based on histologic analysis should be accepted with some reservation. However, it is likely that osteoid activity is increased in RA, especially in the localized area of juxtaarticular bone. It should also be noted that there was no difference in the percent total osteoid surface or percent total osteoid volume between the RA and OA groups. This demonstrates normal mineralization in juxtaarticular bone in RA, suggesting that periarticular osteopenia of the rheumatoid bone observed radiographically is, from a pathogenetic standpoint, "periarticular osteoporosis."

Bone resorption was increased in the periarticular trabecular bone in RA, as measured by a significant increase in total and active resorptive surface. This finding has been supported by comparison of the number of osteoclasts in RA versus that in normal bone. Data available from normal iliac crest bone have indicated the number of osteoclasts to be $0.27 \pm 0.11/mm^2$ (mean ± SD) (21), $0.1/mm^2$ (22), and $0.37/mm^2$ (8). The numbers of osteoclasts in OA periarticular bone in our study were consistent with these numbers in iliac crest bone. The number of osteoclasts found in our RA patients ($0.84 \pm 0.23/mm^2$, mean ± SD) was increased significantly over the number in both OA and normal iliac crest. This indicates active bone resorption, and possibly active bone turnover, in RA periarticular trabecular bone.

Soluble factor(s) synthesized in the rheumatoid synovium may play a role in this process, with the factor(s) being transferred to the periarticular bone and promoting bone resorption by activating osteoclasts. A probable candidate for this would be prostaglandin E, which has been shown to stimulate bone resorption (23). Prostaglandin E, synthesized in rheumatoid synovium (10,11), may be transferred to periarticular bone (24) and may activate osteoclasts by increasing their number (23,25–27). Alternatively, osteoclast activating factor (OAF), produced from lymphocytes interacting with macrophages (28), may participate in this process. Since prostaglandin E is necessary for the production of OAF from lymphocytes, increased prostaglandin E in the rheumatoid synovium may stimulate OAF production (29).

It is important to note that there were no lymphoid cell infiltrations in the periarticular bone in our study. This means that, if OAF is really involved in the osteoporotic process, it could be produced in the rheumatoid synovium and transferred to the periarticular bone space. OAF may act directly on osteoclasts (30) or stimulate prostaglandin E synthesis in the bone. Interaction of lymphocytes with macrophage-type cells plays an important role in many facets of rheumatoid inflammation, such as pannus formation and prostaglandin synthesis (10,11,31).

Contribution of nonsteroidal antiinflammatory agents to the present results appears unlikely, since patients with RA and OA had received similar treatment regimens but showed different results. Although Jee et al showed that in vivo administration of small doses of corticosteroids (<1 mg cortisol/kg/day) increased the number of osteoclasts (32), there is other evidence showing that corticosteroids do not increase bone resorption (32,33). In this study, there was no difference between patients who were and those who were not taking corticosteroids, with regard to bone resorption and number of osteoclasts. This provides further evidence that a contribution of systemic corticosteroids is unlikely.

In summary, histomorphometric analysis in rheumatoid arthritis periarticular trabecular bone demonstrated presence of increased bone resorption through osteoclast activation, suggesting that some soluble factor(s), produced in rheumatoid synovium, may be transferred to the periarticular bone space and stimulate osteoclasts.

ACKNOWLEDGMENTS

We wish to thank Dr. Steven L. Teitelbaum, St. Louis, for his kind instruction on detailed bone histology technique, and Michele A. Bergfeld for technical instruction. We also thank Drs. Ikuo Kobayashi, Chikashi Arita, and Akihiro Oh for supplying tissue and providing continuing support.

REFERENCES

1. Bywaters EGL: The early radiological signs of rheumatoid arthritis. Bull Rheum Dis 11:231–234, 1960
2. Soila P, Berglund K: Angiographic findings in rheumatoid arthritis. Acta Rheum Scand 7:103–106, 1961
3. Laws JW, Lillie JG, Scott JT: Angiographic appearances in rheumatoid arthritis and other disorders. Br J Radiol 36:477–493, 1963
4. Soila P: The causal relations of rheumatoid disintegration of juxta-articular bone trabeculae. Acta Rheum Scand 9:231–236, 1963
5. Havdrup T, Hulth A, Telhag H: The subchondral bone in osteoarthritis and rheumatoid arthritis of the knee: a histological and microradiographical study. Acta Orthop Scand 47:345–350, 1976
6. Desaulniers M, Fuks A, Hawkins D, Lacourciere J, Rosenthall L: Radiotechnetium polyphosphate joint imaging. J Nucl Med 15:417–423, 1974
7. Bergmann P, Mannicourt D, Martin P, Orloff S, Shoutens A: Regional bone calcium turnover rate in rheumatoid arthritis: comparison with the disease activity, Rheumatoid Arthritis. Edited by M Ziff. New York, Raven Press, 1982, pp 303–312
8. Bordier PIIJ, Tunchot S: Quantitative histology of metabolic bone disease, Clinics in Endocrinology and Metabolism (special issue). Vol. 1. Edited by I MacIntyre. Philadelphia, WB Saunders, 1972, pp 197–215
9. Teitelbaum SL, Russell JE, Bone JM, Gilden JJ, Avioli LV: The relationship of biochemical and histometric determinants of uremic bone. Arch Pathol Lab Med 103:228–230, 1979
10. Dayer J-M, Krane SM, Graham R, Russell G, Robinson DR: Production of collagenase and prostaglandins by isolated adherent rheumatoid synovial cells. Proc Natl Acad Sci USA 73:945–949, 1976
11. Shiozawa S, Williams RC Jr, Ziff M: Immunoelectron microscopic demonstration of prostaglandin E in rheumatoid synovium. Arthritis Rheum 25:685–693, 1982
12. Ziff M, Gribetz HJ, Lospalluto J: Effect of leukocyte and synovial membrane extracts on cartilage mucoprotein. J Clin Invest 39:405–412, 1960
13. Wood GC, Pryce-Jones RH, White DD, Nuki G: Chondromucoprotein degrading neutral protease activity in rheumatoid synovial fluid. Ann Rheum Dis 30:73–77, 1971
14. Poole AR, Hembry RM, Dingle JT, Pinder I, Ring EFJ, Cosh J: Secretion and localization of cathepsin D in synovial tissues removed from rheumatoid and traumatized joints: an immunohistochemical study. Arthritis Rheum 19:1295–1307, 1976
15. Dayer J-M, Russell RG, Krane SM: Collagenase production by rheumatoid synovial cells: stimulation by a human lymphocyte factor. Science 195:181–183, 1977
16. Smiley JD, Sachs C, Ziff M: In vitro synthesis of immunoglobulin by rheumatoid synovial membrane. J Clin Invest 47:624–632, 1968
17. Ropes MW, Bennett GA, Cobb S, Jacox R, Jessar RA: 1958 revision of diagnostic criteria for rheumatoid arthritis. Bull Rheum Dis 9:175–176, 1958
18. Shenk RK, Merz WA, Müller J: A quantitative histological study on bone resorption in human cancellous bone. Acta Anat (Basel) 74:44–53, 1969
19. Duncan H, Frost HM, Villanueva AR, Sigler JW: The osteoporosis of rheumatoid arthritis. Arthritis Rheum 8:943–954, 1965
20. Teitelbaum SL, Bates M: Relationships of static and kinetic histomorphometric features of bone. Clin Orthop 146:239–245, 1980
21. Malluche HH, Meyer W, Sherman D, Massry SG: Quantitative bone histology in 84 normal American subjects. Calcif Tissue Int 34:449–455, 1982
22. Johnell O, Wiklund P-E, Hulth A: Osteoclast counting in crista biopsies. Acta Orthop Scand 48:566–571, 1977
23. Klein DC, Raisz LG: Prostaglandins: stimulators of

bone resorption in tissue culture. Endocrinology 86:1436–1440, 1970
24. Robinson DR, Tashjian AH Jr, Levine L: Prostaglandin-stimulated bone resorption by rheumatoid synovia: a possible mechanism for bone destruction in rheumatoid arthritis. J Clin Invest 56:1181–1188, 1975
25. Galasko CSB, Bennett A: Relationship of bone destruction in skeletal metastases to osteoclast activation and prostaglandins. Nature 263:508–510, 1976
26. Santoro MG, Jaffe BM, Simmons DJ: Bone resorption in vitro and in vivo in PGE-treated mice. Proc Soc Exp Biol Med 156:373–377, 1977
27. Schelling SH, Wolfe HJ, Tashjian AH Jr: Role of the osteoclast in prostaglandin E_2-stimulated bone resorption: a correlative morphometric and biochemical analysis. Lab Invest 42:290–295, 1980
28. Horton JE, Oppenheim JJ, Mergenhagen SE, Raisz LG: Macrophage-lymphocyte synergy in the production of osteoclast activating factor. J Immunol 113:1278–1287, 1974
29. Yoneda T, Mundy GR: Prostaglandins are necessary for osteoclast-activating factor production by activated peripheral blood leukocytes. J Exp Med 149:279–283, 1979
30. Raisz LG, Simmons HA, Oppenheim JJ, Mergenhagen SE: Bone resorbing activity in supernatant fluid from cultured human peripheral blood leukocytes. Science 177:793–795, 1972
31. Shiozawa S, Shiozawa K, Fujita T: Morphologic observations in the early phase of the cartilage–pannus junction: light and electron microscopic studies of active cellular pannus. Arthritis Rheum 26:472–478, 1983
32. Jee WSS, Park HZ, Roberts WE, Kenner GH: Corticosteroid and bone. Am J Anat 129:477–480, 1970
33. Raisz LG, Trummel CL, Wener JA, Simmons H: Effect of glucocorticoids on bone resorption in tissue culture. Endocrinology 90:961–967, 1972

THERAPEUTIC VALUE OF GRADED AEROBIC EXERCISE TRAINING IN RHEUMATOID ARTHRITIS

THOMAS M. HARKCOM, RICHARD M. LAMPMAN, BARBARA FIGLEY BANWELL, and C. WILLIAM CASTOR

Women with rheumatoid arthritis performed 1 of 3 low intensity aerobic exercise protocols (15, 25, and 35 minutes) 3 times per week for 12 weeks. A nontraining group served as controls. All exercise groups improved their aerobic capacity, exercise time, and joint counts. Subjects described improvement in activities of daily living and reduced joint pain and fatigue. Exercise duration up to 35 minutes can be therapeutic, and as little as 15 minutes of exercise 3 times/week is sufficient to improve aerobic capacity in rheumatoid arthritis patients with severe limitations.

Recent experimental evidence has indicated that exercise training may be beneficial in rehabilitating patients with chronic diseases including spinal cord lesions (1), cardiovascular disease (2), obesity (3), obstructive lung disease (4), and diabetes mellitus (5). Rheumatoid arthritis (RA) results in muscle wasting, weakness, inactivity, and fatigue with resultant poor aerobic function (6). Exercise therapy in the past has been limited to range of motion and non-stress muscle strengthening coupled with appropriate rest, with the goal of preserving joint movement and strength (7). While this may be appropriate for acute flares of RA, recent studies suggest there may be a role for more vigorous conditioning exercise of a nontraumatizing nature in the long-term management of RA during nonacute or chronic stages (8–12).

Patients with RA have clearly demonstrated a very low level of physical performance ability when measured by aerobic capacity (6,8,9). It has been suggested that regular conditioning exercise can improve aerobic capacity, and improve their functional ability and sense of well-being with no apparent untoward effect on the joint symptoms (6,8–12). In addition, recent animal studies lend support to the theory that exercise is important for joint function. Salter (13) has shown that continuous passive motion favors healing and regeneration of damaged rabbit articular cartilage, and it has also been shown that joint motion with weightbearing is required to maintain normal articular cartilage in dogs (14).

This study was undertaken to evaluate more specifically the amount of exercise necessary to effect significant improvement in exercise tolerance, aerobic capacity, and functional ability without exacerbating joint symptoms. In order to determine appropriate exercise duration, 3 different exercise protocols were devised and a nonexercising group served as controls.

PATIENTS AND METHODS

Twenty women with definite or classic RA (15), American Rheumatism Association functional class II (16), age range 27–68 (mean ± SD, 52 ± 12), were enrolled in the study. Patients independently chose an exercise time slot convenient for them within a 4-hour block of time without knowledge of the protocol to which they would be assigned.

From the Department of Internal Medicine, Rackham Arthritis Research Unit, and the Division of Cardiology, University of Michigan Medical School, Ann Arbor, Michigan.

Supported by USPHS training grant AM 07080.

Thomas M. Harkcom, MD: Rheumatology Fellow; Richard M. Lampman, PhD: Assistant Research Scientist, Division of Cardiology; Barbara Figley Banwell, PT, MA: Program Leader in Physical Therapy, Arthritis Center, University of Michigan; C. William Castor, MD: Professor of Internal Medicine, Rackham Arthritis Research Unit.

Address reprint requests to C. William Castor, MD, University of Michigan Medical School, Rackham Arthritis Research Unit, R-4633 Kresge I, Ann Arbor, MI 48109.

Submitted for publication March 19, 1984; accepted in revised form July 26, 1984.

Table 1. Joint evaluation key

Pain on motion or tenderness on pressure	
0 = none	
1 = minimal (positive response on questioning)	
2 = moderate (spontaneous response elicited)	
3 = severe (withdrawal by patient on examination)	
Swelling	
0 = none	
1 = mild (detectable synovial thickening without loss of bony contours)	
2 = moderate (loss of distinctness of bony contours)	
3 = severe (bulging synovial proliferation with cystic characteristics)	

The 4 different protocols were, in turn, randomly allocated to these time slots. This selection option was deemed necessary in order to facilitate attendance at exercise sessions considering the number of exercise sessions necessary. The control subjects were later informed they would not be attending exercise sessions. This method had the advantage of providing a random assignment of patients to protocols without restricting participation in the study because of scheduling difficulties.

Patients were selected from the large outpatient population followed at this institution and were willing to participate in the program with informed consent. All patients were on stable medical regimens, no major changes in drug therapy occurred during the study, and no intraarticular steroid injections were given. No patients had acute flares of joint symptoms at the time of entry into, nor during, the study. Self-administered questionnaires providing data on education, socioeconomic background, and duration of disease were completed by each subject. Using a modification of the Functional Status Index (FSI) (17), morning stiffness, sleep patterns, self care, ambulation, and activities of daily living were self-assessed by the subjects at baseline and at 2-week intervals during the study. At the end of the training program, subjects were asked to compare their perceptions of changes in fatigue, strength, ability to do housework, participation in social activities, overall mood, amount of joint pain, and tolerance of joint pain. This final inquiry was subsequently referred to as the global assessment. Grip strength, 50-foot walk time, and muscle strength measurement (knee flexors and extensors) using a Cybex II Isokinetic Dynamometer (Lumex Inc., Bay Shore, NY) were tested on all subjects (18). All joint count evaluations were performed by 1 investigator according to the criteria shown in Table 1.

Exercise tolerance tests which followed a standard graded protocol, beginning at 150 kilopond meters (kpm) and advancing by 150 kpm every 3 minutes, using a bicycle ergometer at 50 revolutions per minute (rpm) were performed on all subjects. Aerobic capacities ($\dot{V}O_2$ maximum) were calculated from values obtained using a Parkinson-Cowan Dry Gas Meter for volume determinations, and a Beckman LB-2 carbon dioxide analyzer and an Applied Electro-Chemistry oxygen analyzer for measuring expired CO_2 and O_2 gas composition.

Electrocardiographic rhythms were continuously monitored throughout the test, and heart rate and blood pressure measurements were taken at 1-minute intervals. Exercise was terminated when the subject was unable to maintain cycling cadence to the pace established by the metronome.

In a group setting, the subjects then began their program of bicycle ergometer exercise 3 times/week for 12 weeks, a period previously determined to improve aerobic capacity (19). Each session was supervised by physical education graduate students. The protocols differed in the initial length of total exercise time, the rate of progression, and the final total duration of activity achieved after 6 weeks (15, 25, 35 minutes) and patient groups labeled groups A, B, and C were assigned to the 3 protocols, respectively (Figure 1). The exercise intensity was measured by heart rate, and was maintained for all groups at 70% of the maximal heart rate measured during the baseline exercise tolerance test. The load on the bicycle ergometers was applied at a resistance which achieved and maintained 70% of the maximum heart rate at 50 rpm. Each total daily exercise session was divided into 5 bouts of exercise separated by 1-minute rest periods. Each session was preceded by a warmup and ended with a cool-down period and involved gentle, active, rhythmic range of motion exercises. Control subjects continued their routine daily activities without knowledge of any intervention.

At the end of the 12-week period, repeat exercise tolerance tests for aerobic capacities, joint count, muscle strength testing, walk time, grip strength, and repeat assessments of the FSI were performed exactly as done at baseline. Results were analyzed using the statistical programs of MIDAS for analysis of variance and Student's *t*-test (20).

RESULTS

These subjects, with similar socioeconomic backgrounds and educational levels, showed no differences at entry into the study in age group, duration of disease, aerobic capacity ($\dot{V}O_2$ maximum), exercise

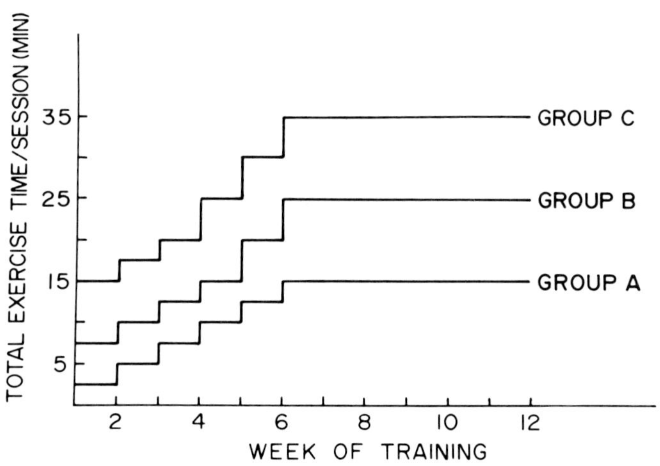

Figure 1. Training scheme. Bicycle ergometer rate at 50 revolutions per minute. Initial training duration, progression, and final training duration are shown. Each session was divided into 5 bouts with 1 minute of rest between bouts.

Table 2. Group means (±SD) for pre- and post-training parameters

	Group A (n = 4)		Group B (n = 3)		Group C (n = 4)		Controls (n = 6)	
	Pre	Post	Pre	Post	Pre	Post	Pre	Post
Age	51.5 ± 3.1		47.3 ± 14.5		44.0 ± 18.3		45.1 ± 19.3	
Duration of disease (years)	12.2 ± 8.7		10.6 ± 5.5		5.6 ± 3.7		8.8 ± 10.1	
Aerobic capacity (ml/kg/minute)	14.6 ± 4.9	21.5 ± 6.5*†	20.3 ± 15.8	22.9 ± 17.9†	21.9 ± 9.0	29.1 ± 17.4†	18.5 ± 7.4	18.6 ± 8.3
Exercise maximum heart rate (beats/minute)	136.5 ± 21.4	151.3 ± 12.3	161.3 ± 44.3	161.3 ± 22.9	162.8 ± 31.3	156.0 ± 30.4	168.2 ± 18.7	162.5 ± 21.4
Exercise pressure rate product (systolic blood pressure × heart rate)/100	252.5 ± 81.7	291.5 ± 36.7	304.7 ± 83.1	318.3 ± 80.4	295.3 ± 56.8	280.5 ± 79.9	278.2 ± 39.4	240.7 ± 97.9
Exercise test time (minutes)	9.0 ± 2.5	12.3 ± 2.5†‡	9.0 ± 8.2	15.0 ± 6.1†	12.5 ± 3.9	14.3 ± 4.4†‡	9.83 ± 2.2	10.1 ± 2.92
Joint count	38.0 ± 21.7	24.0 ± 10.9†	26.0 ± 15.1	10.3 ± 7.0†	32.5 ± 19.4	23.0 ± 10.7†	27.5 ± 7.5	23.0 ± 8.46
Muscle strength (foot pounds)								
Isotonic extension	61.0 ± 17.1	58.5 ± 14.8	86.0 ± 3.5	82.0 ± 6.9	68.0 ± 11.7	61.0 ± 19.6	61.6 ± 13.4	70.6 ± 17.0
Isotonic flexion	35.0 ± 13.4	34.0 ± 6.3	46.6 ± 4.2	45.3 ± 3.1	38.0 ± 9.4	36.0 ± 7.7	35.6 ± 6.8	40.0 ± 10.0
Isometric extension	55.0 ± 13.7	56.0 ± 23.9	72.0 ± 10.4	86.7 ± 9.0*	60.5 ± 15.6	62.5 ± 22.9	63.6 ± 15.7	74.6 ± 13.6
50-foot walk time (seconds)	12.6 ± 3.2	13.5 ± 2.4	12.7 ± 1.5	13.0 ± 1.0	11.4 ± 2.5	12.3 ± 2.1	10.9 ± 1.8	9.55 ± 0.49
Grip strength (mm Hg)	117.8 ± 62.0	102.2 ± 42.2	132.7 ± 88.7	136.0 ± 75.6	101.0 ± 69.0	135.5 ± 45.2	116.35 ± 50.7	133.0 ± 50.3
Functional Status Index								
Self care	3.5 ± 3.1	4.8 ± 3.3	4.0 ± 5.2	5.3 ± 4.9	3.8 ± 3.3	4.7 ± 4.3	4.5 ± 5.3	3.6 ± 5.6
Ambulation	2.8 ± 1.3	4.0 ± 3.5	5.7 ± 3.1	4.7 ± 2.1	4.8 ± 2.2	7.5 ± 4.4	6.0 ± 4.7	5.2 ± 5.1
Activities of daily living	17.0 ± 6.1	14.2 ± 4.2	15.0 ± 14.0	9.7 ± 8.3	16.8 ± 8.3	16.0 ± 13.1	14.8 ± 10.2	14.8 ± 13.8

* $P < 0.05$ compared with baseline.
† $P < 0.01$ for groups A, B, and C combined compared with baseline.
‡ $P < 0.01$ compared with baseline.

maximum heart rates, pressure rate products, exercise test time, joint count, muscle strength, walk time, grip strength, or FSI scores (Table 2). Three patients, 1 from each exercise group, dropped out of the study for personal reasons not related to their disease or the exercise program.

Baseline $\dot{V}O_2$ maximum values were, in general, quite low, reflecting the severely unconditioned state of many of the subjects. Following training, as shown in Figure 2, there was an increase in $\dot{V}O_2$ maximum in all exercise groups compared with controls. While all exercising groups enhanced their aerobic capacities, these improvements only reached statistical significance in group A ($P < 0.05$, Table 2). Exercise tolerance, as measured by time to fatigue during exercise testing, also increased in all 3 exercise groups and was statistically significant for groups A ($P < 0.01$) and C ($P < 0.01$) (Table 2 and Figure 3).

The exercise group (groups A, B, and C combined) showed a significant reduction ($P < 0.01$) in joint counts at the completion of the study (Table 2). Scores for both pain and swelling decreased in the exercising group (Figure 4). The exercising subjects reported a reduction in morning stiffness (Figure 5) and an improvement in sleep patterns (Figure 6) during the study, while no subjective improvements in these parameters were noted by the nonexercising subjects.

Muscle strength, as tested by Cybex II, did not change in any of the groups except isometric extension at 90° in group B ($P < 0.05$) (Table 2 and Figure 7).

Subject assessment of particular aspects of self care, ambulation, and activities of daily living did not change in any general trend. However, in the global assessment of changes in fatigue, exercise tolerance, pain, strength, ability to do household chores, social activity, and overall mood, group A reported the most improvement, a lesser degree of improvement was shown for group B, and little or no change occurred in group C (Figure 8). This coincided with subjective assessments made by each subject as part of the final assessment.

When all exercise subjects were combined into 1 group (n = 11) for statistical purposes, significant improvements were noted on 3 important measures.

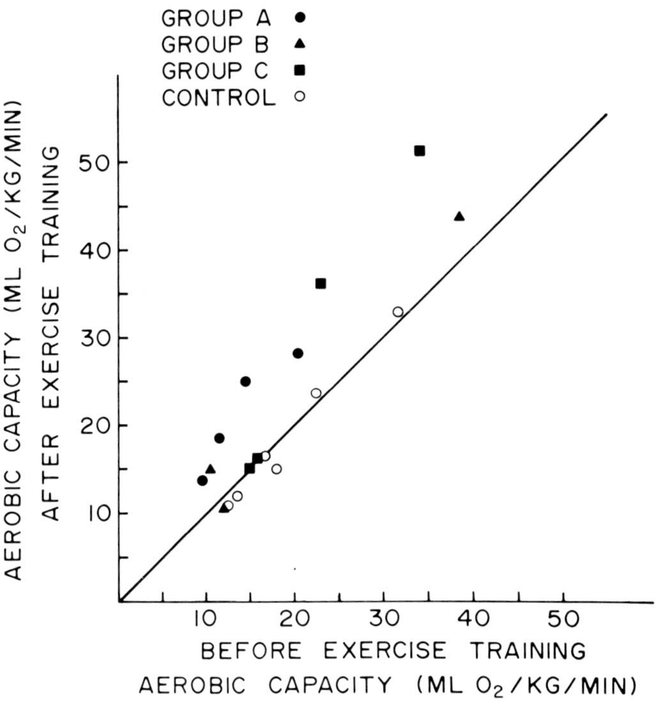

Figure 2. Oxygen uptake (aerobic capacity) for each subject before and after exercise training. $P < 0.05$ for group A.

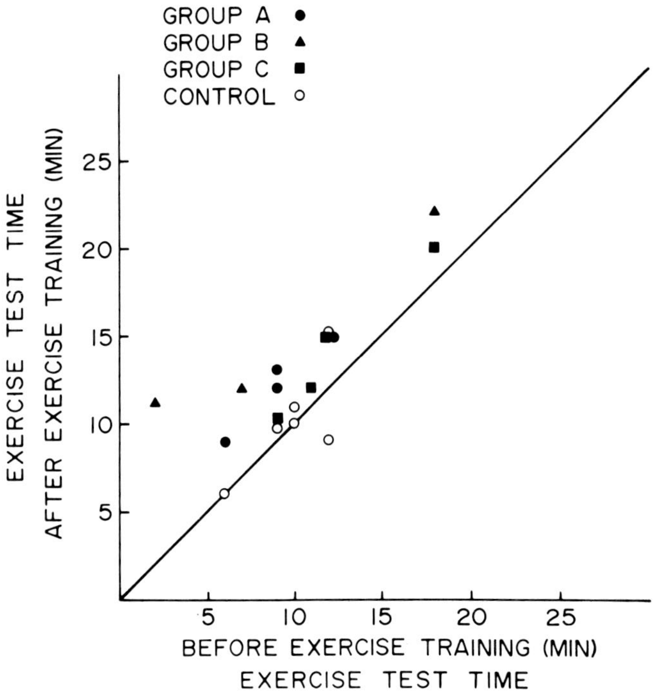

Figure 3. Exercise test time for each subject before and after exercise training. Test was ended when subject became fatigued and could not maintain 50 revolutions per minute. $P < 0.01$ for groups A and C compared with baseline values.

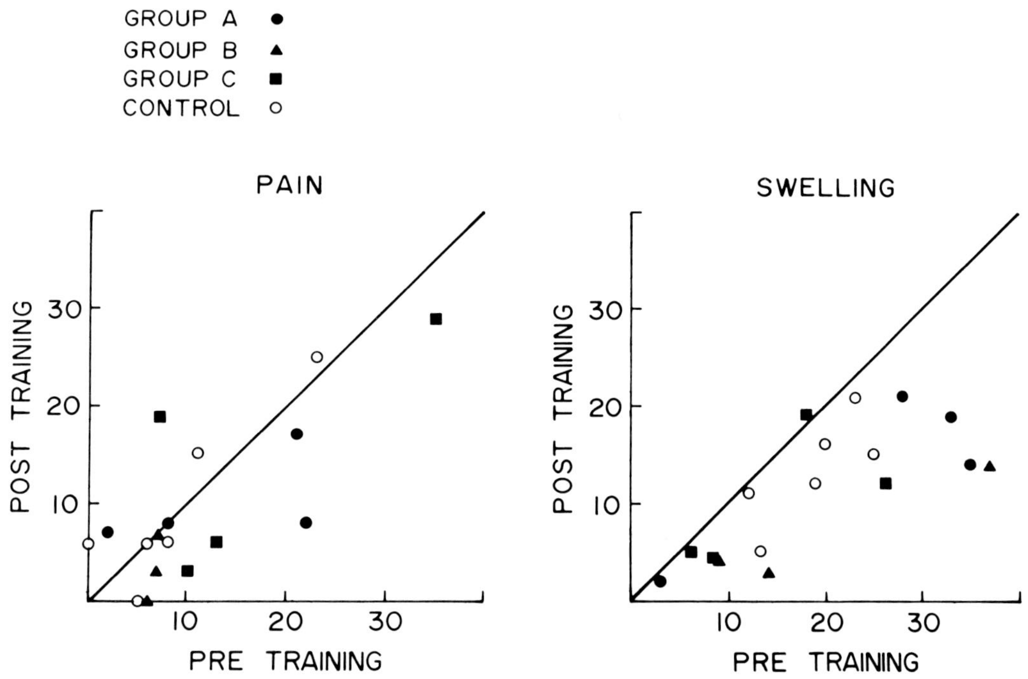

Figure 4. Joint count for each subject, scored for pain and swelling before and after exercise training.

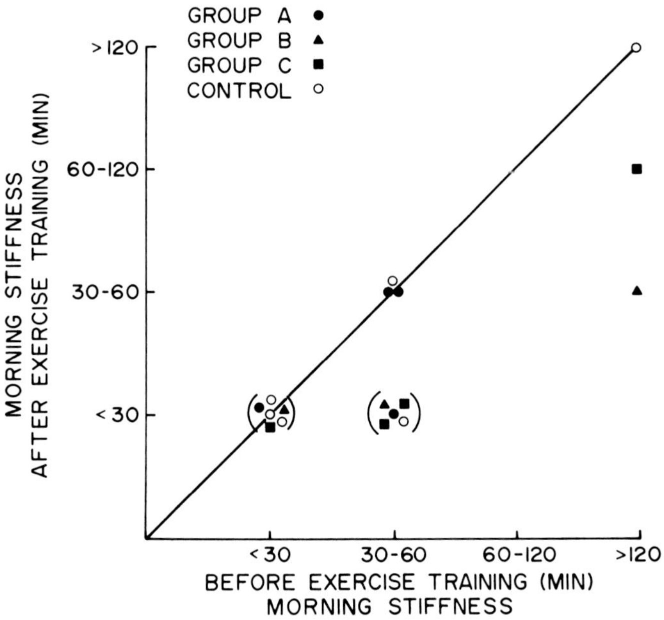

Figure 5. Duration of morning stiffness for each subject. No subject showed an increase in duration of stiffness, and 7 subjects showed a decrease.

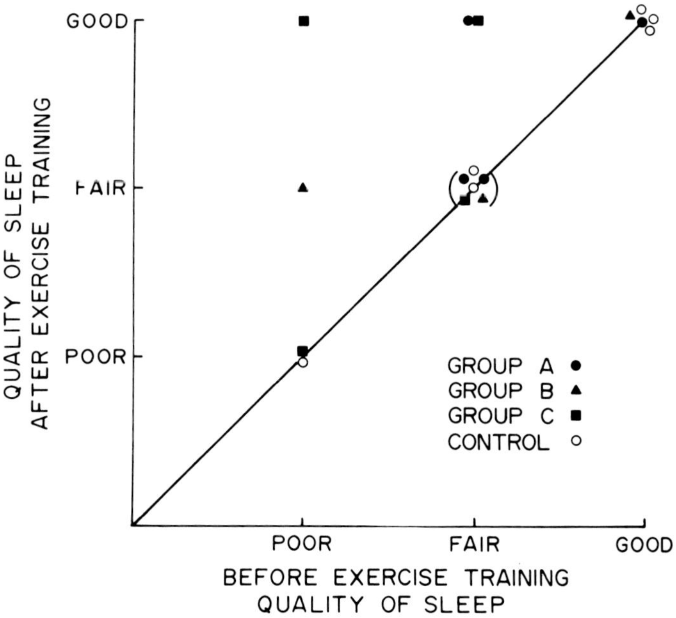

Figure 6. Quality of sleep for each subject. No worsening of sleep pattern was noted during or after training.

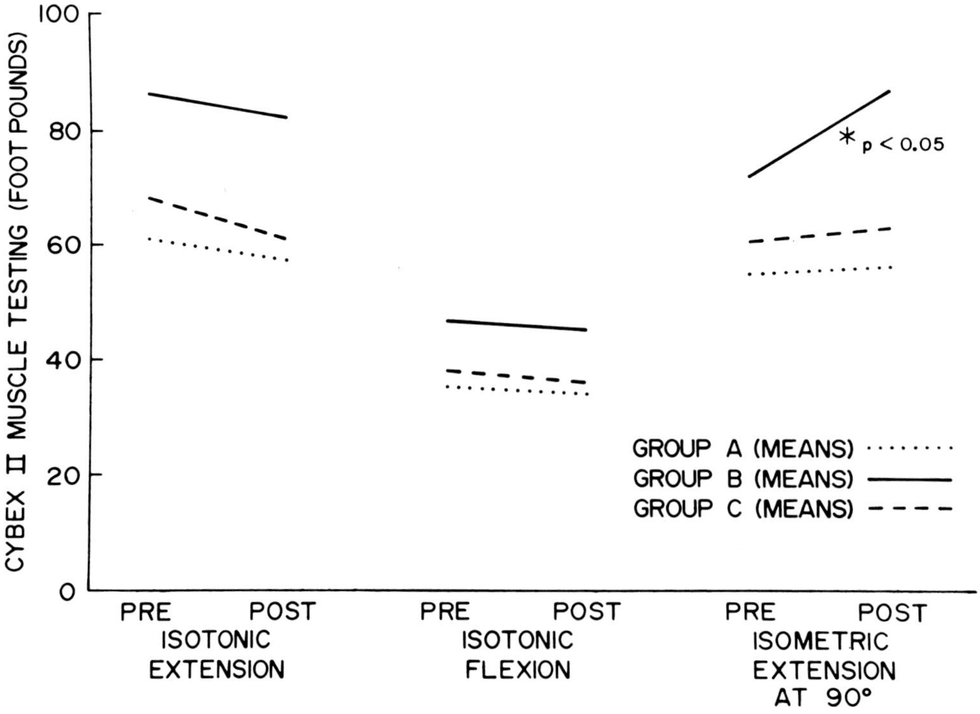

Figure 7. Knee flexors and extensors measured using Cybex II. Group means are shown.

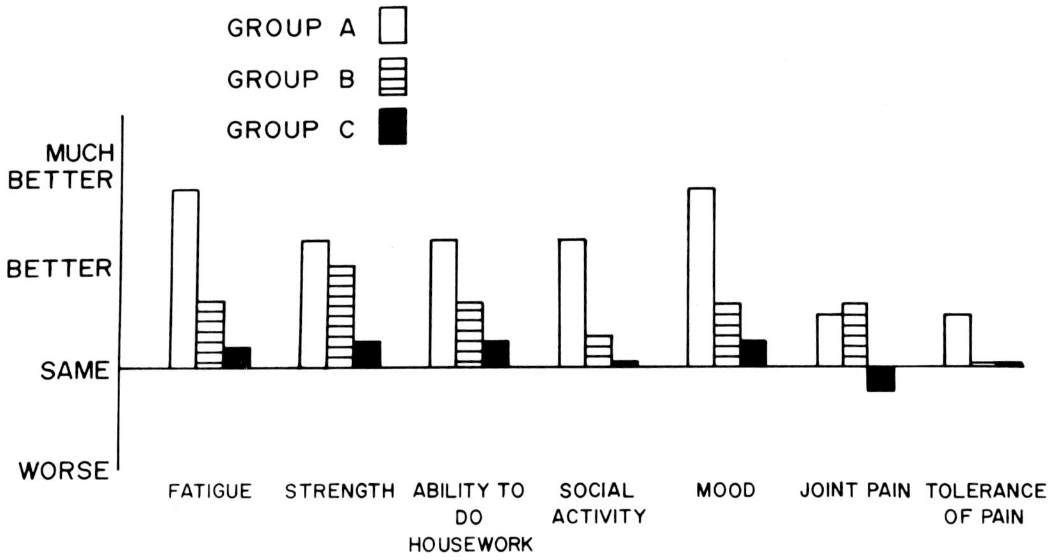

Figure 8. Global assessment by the subjects of changes in categories after completion of exercise training. Numerical assignments made to each level of change. Group means are shown.

Mean joint count decreased from 32.9 to 19.9 ($P < 0.01$); mean aerobic capacity increased from 18.5 to 24.7 ml/kg/minute^{-1} ($P < 0.01$); and mean exercise test time increased from 10.3 to 13.7 minutes ($P < 0.01$). No significant changes were noted for these measures in the control group.

DISCUSSION

In recent years, there has been increasing interest in the role of exercise as a part of various therapeutic programs. Experience with cardiovascular disease has more recently been followed by studies of exercise in chronic obstructive airway disease, diabetes mellitus, and juvenile rheumatoid arthritis (1–5).

Traditionally, and appropriately so, it has been conventional practice to rest inflamed joints and recommend energy conservation to patients with RA. However, it is possible that part of the fatigue and muscle weakness experienced after an acute flare has subsided is because of easily demonstrable poor aerobic capacity, perhaps in association with rheumatoid myositis (21).

This study was designed to evaluate in more specific terms the duration of exercise sufficient to achieve improvements of both an objective and subjective nature, and what duration of exercise might be excessive, causing aggravation of the underlying rheumatic disease. It is recommended that patients with cardiovascular disease exercise for 30 minutes, 3 times/week, at a heart rate of 70–80% of their maximal exercise attainable rates (2). No prior knowledge was available showing whether RA patients require exercise prescriptions similar to those for patients with cardiovascular diseases. Prior studies in RA have not quantified the duration, resistance load, intensity, or progression of exercise, information which is vital to determining a more precise "dosage" of exercise for patients with RA. The exercise protocols devised in this study resulted in increased exercise tolerance and aerobic capacity for all exercising subjects. Our data showed that RA patients initially had low levels of aerobic capacity, which is probably the reason only 15 minutes of exercise per session, the minimum time needed to train normal individuals (19), resulted in significant improvements. It would be expected that continued exercise beyond 12 weeks would cause even greater changes in aerobic capacity and exercise tolerance. The improvements in exercise tolerance were in accordance with improvement in objective scales and subjective comments regarding fatigue and ability to do housework and participate in social activities for longer periods.

In this study the FSI, which was given every 2 weeks and at the end of the study, showed variation in all patients from time to time. Generally, it appeared that the individual tasks evaluated in the index were accomplished without extreme difficulty or had been modified by the subject so that a change in ability to perform these specific tasks was not evident. The difficulty in correlating individual tasks with overall function was noted by Nordemar (10) as well, but changes in our subjects were reflected in more general descriptions, such as in the Global Assessment.

In the final global assessment (Figure 8), the subjects were asked to compare baseline and final self-evaluation of several parameters. Fatigue and general mood were definitely improved and the ability to participate in household and social activities was better for group A and for group B, but with little change for group C. Groups A, B, and C, who exercised 15, 25, and 35 minutes per session, respectively, were able to achieve aerobic, functional, and performance changes without exacerbation of joint discomfort or other symptoms.

The decrease in joint counts in this study was statistically significant for the subjects who exercised, a finding in agreement with those of Beals et al (8) and Ekblom and colleagues (9). The changes in reported pain and/or pain tolerance may be partly responsible for this effect, as well as an overall improvement in the sense of well-being. However, an increase in pain tolerance is not entirely responsible for the decreased counts, as swelling was also noted to be decreased. The role of exercise and its relationship to endogenous opioid peptides such as β endorphins in relief of joint pain remains to be elucidated. This factor may, in part, have influenced these subjective feelings since there is evidence of complex interactions of opioid peptides with exercise training, as well as appetite, thermoregulation, lipolysis, and reproduction (22). An important finding in this study was that all 3 exercise groups tended to have less morning stiffness and maintained or improved their sleep patterns. A concomitant sense of well-being following training may also have caused feelings of improvement, rather than a direct effect on the disease itself. In that our results did show exercise training to be beneficial, further studies need to delineate if this therapy influences synovial fluid and proteoglycan changes and whether it modifies the gelling phenomenon. Changes in pituitary hormones and adrenocortical response to exercise also need to be considered since they may also be responsible for improvements seen in joint count, morning stiffness, and overall enhancement of well-being (23–25).

The lack of improvement in muscle strength probably reflected the methods of training since the program did not involve high intensity isotonic or isometric extension, or flexion exercises that would isolate and specifically train certain muscle groups. Even though the least amount of resistance loading was used in order to avoid exacerbating the joint symptoms, group B still showed an increase in isometric extension at 90°.

A very interesting outcome of this study was the subjective commentary, both solicited and unsolicited, by the participants. In each exercise subject, the responses were uniformly positive, although varied. Comments generally correlated with the global assessment, that fatigue and participation in household, social, and shopping activities improved. The subjects' perceptions of self-image and abilities were better, many being quite surprised at what they could accomplish. The comment was made by several that in spite of control of joint symptoms by medical treatment, their fatigue had not improved until they increased their stamina during the exercise program.

It is apparent from this study that female subjects with nonacute RA in functional class II benefited from regular, supervised aerobic exercise, and this was accomplished without exacerbating joint symptoms. Also of importance is the observation that as little as 15 minutes per session produced improvement in aerobic capacity, exercise tolerance, and sense of well-being. Low intensity aerobic exercise, even at short durations, performed 3 times per week, is beneficial and may be an important adjunct in the long-term treatment of RA.

REFERENCES

1. Hjeltnes N: Oxygen uptake and cardiac output in graded arm exercise in paraplegics with low level spinal lesions. Scand J Rehab Med 9:107–113, 1977
2. Leon G, Blackburn H: Exercise rehabilitation of the coronary heart disease patient. Geriatrics 32:66–76, 1977
3. Foss ML, Lampman RM, Schteingart D: Physical training program for rehabilitation of extremely obese patients. Arch Phys Med Rehabil 57:425–429, 1976
4. Bass H, Whitcomb JF, Forman R: Exercise training: therapy for patients with chronic obstructive pulmonary disease. Chest 57:116–121, 1970
5. Costill DL, Cleary P, Fink WJ, Foster C, Ivy JL, Witzmann F: Training adaptations in skeletal muscles of juvenile diabetics. Diabetes 28:818–822, 1979
6. Beals C, Lampman R, Figley B, Braunstein E, Albers J, Castor C: Oxygen cost of work in rheumatoid arthritis patients (abstract). Clin Res 28:752A, 1980
7. Smith RD, Polley HF: Rest therapy for rheumatoid arthritis. Mayo Clinic Proc 53:141–145, 1978

8. Beals C, Lampman R, Figley B, Shapiro P, Castor C: A case for aerobic conditioning exercise in rheumatoid arthritis (abstract). Clin Res 29:780A, 1981
9. Ekblom B, Lovgren O, Alderin M, Friedstrom M, Satterstrom G: Effect of short-term physical training on patients with rheumatoid arthritis. Scand J Rheumatol 4:80–86, 1975
10. Nordemar R: Physical training in rheumatoid arthritis: a controlled long-term study. Scand J Rheumatol 10:23–30, 1981
11. Ekblom B, Lovgren O, Alderin M, Friedstrom M, Satterstrom G: Effect of short-term physical training on patients with rheumatoid arthritis: a six-month follow-up study. Scand J Rheumatol 4:87–91, 1975
12. Ekblom B: Short- and long-term training in patients with rheumatoid arthritis. Ann Clin Res 34:109–110, 1982
13. Salter RB: Prevention of arthritis through preservation of cartilage. J Can Assoc Radiol 32:5–7, 1981
14. Palmoski MJ, Colyer RA, Brandt KD: Joint motion in the absence of normal loading does not maintain normal articular cartilage. Arthritis Rheum 23:325–334, 1980
15. Ropes MW, Bennett GA, Cobb S, Jacox R, Jessar RA: 1958 revision of diagnostic criteria for rheumatoid arthritis. Bull Rheum Dis 9:175–176, 1958
16. Steinbrocker O, Traeger CH, Batterman RC: Therapeutic criteria in rheumatoid arthritis. JAMA 140:659, 1949
17. Jette AM: Functional Status Index: reliability of a chronic disease evaluation instrument. Arch Phys Med Rehabil 61:395–401, 1980
18. Cybex II Testing Protocol. Lumex Inc., Bay Shore, New York
19. Wasserman K, Whipp B: Exercise physiology in health and disease. Am Rev Respir Dis 112:219–249, 1975
20. Fox DJ, Guire KE: Documentation for MIDAS. Statistical Research Laboratory of the University of Michigan, 1976
21. Halla J, Fallahi S, Oh S, Gay R, Koopman WJ: Rheumatoid myositis (RM): clinical and histological features (abstract). Arthritis Rheum (suppl) 25:S116, 1982
22. Carr DB, Buller BA, Skrinar GS, Arnold MA, Rosenblatt M, Beitins IZ, Martin JB, McArthur JW: Physical conditioning facilitates the exercise-induced secretion of β-endorphin and β-lipotropin in women. N Engl J Med 305:360–362, 1981
23. Cohen JL, May DB, Kim CS, Das B, Austin SM, Ertel NH: Graded exercise induced changes in pituitary hormones (abstract). Clin Res 28:257A, 1980
24. Sharp GO: The role of glucocorticoids in exercise. Med Sci Sports Exerc 7:6–11, 1975
25. Sutton JR, Casey JH: The adrenocortical response to competitive athletics in veteran athletes. J Clin Endocrinol Metab 40:135–138, 1975

SPONDYLITIC DISEASE WITHOUT RADIOLOGIC EVIDENCE OF SACROILIITIS IN RELATIVES OF HLA–B27 POSITIVE ANKYLOSING SPONDYLITIS PATIENTS

MUHAMMAD A. KHAN, SJEF M. VAN DER LINDEN, IRVING KUSHNER, HANS A. VALKENBURG, and ARNOLD CATS

We report 2 independently-conducted family studies of HLA–B27 positive probands with ankylosing spondylitis (AS), both of which support the view that the clinical spectrum of AS is broader than ordinarily assumed, and should include individuals who have symptomatic disease but who do not show radiologic evidence of abnormalities of the sacroiliac joints or the spine. In the Cleveland study of 100 relatives of 30 B27 positive AS probands, 9 relatives did not show radiologic abnormalities of the sacroiliac joints or the spine but had symptoms of chronic inflammatory back pain previously reported to be characteristic of AS. These 9 relatives were all subsequently found to possess B27, in contrast with only 27 of 60 asymptomatic relatives ($P <$ 0.01). In the Leiden study of 101 relatives of 20 randomly chosen B27 positive AS probands, 13 of 86 relatives without radiographic evidence of sacroiliitis reported "thoracic pain and stiffness," as defined in the Rome criteria for AS. Twelve of these 13 symptomatic relatives were B27 positive. In contrast, among the remaining 73 relatives, only 33 were B27 positive ($P < 0.01$). The occurrence of these characteristic spondylitic symptoms in B27 positive, but not B27 negative, relatives of AS probands suggests that the spectrum of the clinical manifestations of AS may include individuals with symptomatic disease, but without radiographic evidence of abnormalities of the sacroiliac joints or the spine. The relatively large number of females we found in this group suggests that women are more likely to manifest this variety of disease than are men.

As in other diseases for which etiology is not clearly defined, the diagnosis of ankylosing spondylitis (AS) is based on clinical and roentgenographic features. Our current concept of the clinical picture of AS is largely based on the manifestations of this condition in patients with florid disease. The first internationally accepted criteria for AS were proposed in Rome in 1961 (1) and were revised 5 years later in New York (2). Radiologic evidence of sacroiliitis is considered to be a sine qua non for the diagnosis of AS according to the New York criteria (2) and, except for rare instances, is required in order for the Rome criteria to be met (1). Although both sets of criteria were originally designed purely for epidemiologic studies, they are widely used in practice for the clinical diagnosis of AS. Most clinicians are reluctant to make the diagnosis in the absence of radiologic changes. We have explored the possibility that the current concept of the spectrum of AS might be too restrictive, and that symptomatic patients with spondylitic disease may not always mani-

Presented in part at the 48th Annual Meeting of the American Rheumatism Association, Minneapolis, MN, June 1984.

From the Department of Medicine, Division of Rheumatology, Case Western Reserve University at Cleveland Metropolitan General Hospital, Cleveland, Ohio, the Department of Rheumatology, University of Leiden, The Netherlands, and the Department of Epidemiology, Erasmus University, Rotterdam, The Netherlands.

Supported in part by the Irma H. Bender Arthritis Research Fund and The Netherlands Prevention Fund.

Muhammad A. Khan, MD: Associate Professor of Medicine, Case Western Reserve University; Sjef M. van der Linden, MD: Department of Rheumatology, University of Leiden (present address: University of Berne, Inselspital, Switzerland); Irving Kushner, MD: Professor of Medicine, Case Western Reserve University; Hans A. Valkenburg, MD: Professor of Epidemiology, Erasmus University; Arnold Cats, MD: Professor of Medicine and Chairman, Department of Rheumatology, University of Leiden.

Address reprint requests to Muhammad A. Khan, MD, Department of Medicine, Cleveland Metropolitan General Hospital, 3395 Scranton Road, Cleveland, OH 44109.

Submitted for publication March 2, 1984; accepted in revised form August 7, 1984.

Table 1. Clinical criteria for "chronic inflammatory back pain"

Onset of back discomfort before the age of 40 years
Insidious onset
Persistence for at least 3 months
Associated with morning stiffness
Improvement with exercise

fest the radiologic abnormalities of the sacroiliac joints. We reviewed our findings from 2 independent studies of relatives of HLA–B27 positive AS probands, conducted in Cleveland, Ohio, and in Leiden, The Netherlands, to determine whether these relatives showed symptoms characteristic of AS.

PATIENTS AND METHODS

In the Cleveland study of the genetics of familial AS (3), we studied 120 relatives of 30 B27 positive unrelated probands (10 females and 20 males; 26 with primary AS and 4 with related spondylarthropathies [SPA]). Probands with a positive family history were preferred. Individuals less than 20 years of age were excluded from the study. HLA typing was done in 100 of the 120 relatives (49 females and 51 males), all of whom had been examined clinically. In all relatives the presence of "chronic inflammatory low back pain" (Table 1) was evaluated, using the criteria of Calin et al (4); inflammatory back pain was considered to be present if the individual fulfilled at least 4 of the 5 criteria. The clinical diagnosis of AS was based on the modified Rome criteria (3,5); a patient was considered to have AS if he or she had at least 2 of the 5 Rome clinical criteria in addition to the radiologic criterion of at least grade 2 bilateral sacroiliitis according to the Atlas of Standard Radiographs (6).

In the Leiden study, first-degree relatives of 20 B27 positive AS probands (1 female and 19 males) were examined for signs and symptoms of AS. Relatives less than 15 years of age were excluded from the study. The probands fulfilled the Rome (1) and the New York (2) criteria for definite AS. The 20 AS probands were randomly chosen from a group of 183 HLA–B27 positive AS patients, as reported earlier (7); 18 had primary AS, 1 had associated psoriasis, and the last proband had associated regional enteritis. Of 116 relatives, 102 were able to take part in the study, which gave a completion rate of 88%. Complete data were not obtained on 1 of the relatives; therefore, this individual is not considered further.

All relatives in the Leiden study were clinically investigated for presence of AS, and chest expansion was measured at the level of the fourth intercostal space. An anteroposterior view of the pelvis was obtained. The pelvic radiographs were read "blindly" twice by 5 observers, and interpretation of the films was done without knowledge of the results of the HLA typing and the clinical examination. The radiographs were scored according to the Atlas of Standard Radiographs (6). The scores of all 10 readings were added and the result was divided by 10 and rounded off to the nearest whole figure (7). Sacroiliitis was considered to be present if at least grade 2 bilateral or grade 3 unilateral changes were observed. All relatives were typed for HLA–B27. The nonradiologic Rome (Table 2) and New York (Table 3) criteria were applied immediately after the physical examination, with the examiner having no knowledge of the radiologic or the HLA typing results. These criteria were also evaluated in 38 B27 negative controls without sacroiliitis, who were drawn from the general population (7,8); all controls were 45 years or older, with a mean age of 55 years.

In both the Cleveland and the Leiden studies, clinical assessment in the probands and relatives was carried out independent of and before the results of HLA typing were known, and the diagnosis was not influenced by the HLA typing result. Statistical analyses were performed using the chi-square method with Yates' correction.

Table 2. Rome clinical criteria for ankylosing spondylitis

Low back pain and stiffness for more than 3 months, not relieved by rest
Pain and stiffness in the thoracic region
Limited motion in the lumbar spine
Limited chest expansion
History or evidence of iritis or its sequelae

Table 3. New York clinical criteria for ankylosing spondylitis

Limitation of motion of the lumbar spine in all 3 planes (anterior flexion, lateral flexion, and extension)
History of pain or the presence of pain at the dorsolumbar junction or in the lumbar spine
Limitation of chest expansion to 1 inch (2.5 cm) or less, measured at the level of the fourth intercostal space

RESULTS

Cleveland study. HLA–B27 was present in 67 of 100 relatives in the Cleveland study (Table 4). There were 31 relatives (15 females and 16 males) affected with AS or related SPA. All were B27 positive; none of the 33 B27 negative relatives was affected. Of the 69 unaffected relatives, 9 had chronic inflammatory back pain. These 9 relatives (4 females and 5 males) did not show roentgenographic evidence of sacroiliitis or spondylitis, had no clinical evidence of peripheral arthritis, and none met 4 of the Rome clinical criteria. When B27 typing was done, all of these 9 individuals were found to be B27 positive. In contrast, only 27 of

Table 4. Prevalence of clinically and radiologically diagnosed ankylosing spondylitis (AS) or spondylarthropathies (SPA) in 100 HLA typed relatives of AS probands (Cleveland study)

	n	HLA–B27 positive	HLA–B27 negative
AS or SPA present	31	31	0
AS or SPA absent	69	36	33

Table 5. Prevalence of "chronic inflammatory back pain" in 69 "unaffected" relatives of ankylosing spondylitis probands (Cleveland study)

	n	HLA–B27 positive*	HLA–B27 negative*
Inflammatory back pain present	9	9	0
Inflammatory back pain absent	60	27	33

* $P < 0.01$, relatives with versus those without inflammatory back pain.

the remaining 60 relatives were B27 positive (Table 5). This difference between the 2 groups in B27 frequency was highly significant ($P < 0.01$). There was no significant difference between the mean ages of the symptomatic and asymptomatic relatives.

Leiden study. HLA–B27 was present in 60 of 101 first-degree relatives (43 males and 58 females) in the Leiden study. Radiologic evidence of sacroiliitis was present in 15 relatives (8 females and 7 males); all were B27 positive (Table 6). Among the remaining 86 relatives without radiologically detectable sacroiliitis, thoracic pain and stiffness were present in 12 females and 1 male (Table 7). B27 was present in 12 of these 13 symptomatic relatives, significantly more common than in those without thoracic pain and stiffness (33 of 73; $P < 0.01$). There was no significant difference in the mean ages of these 2 groups of relatives. All of the 13 relatives with thoracic pain and stiffness had chest expansion greater than 2.5 cm, and in 10 the chest expansion was greater than 5 cm.

DISCUSSION

Most clinicians are reluctant to make the diagnosis of AS in the absence of radiologic changes. However, the results of our 2 independently-conducted family studies of HLA–B27 positive AS probands show an increased prevalence of "chronic inflammatory back pain" in the Cleveland study and "thoracic pain and stiffness" in the Leiden study, among B27 positive relatives without radiologically detectable sacroiliitis. These symptoms, which are characteristic of AS, are not randomly distributed in all relatives; rather, they are virtually limited to the B27 positive relatives, i.e., those at greatest risk of developing AS and related SPA. The association we observed supports the view that these individuals should be regarded as having a spondylitic disorder and that our concept of the spectrum of the clinical manifestations of AS should be broadened.

Roentgenographic evaluation of the sacroiliac joint can be quite difficult because of its anatomic structure (9). Therefore, failure to detect sacroiliitis in films of symptomatic individuals could be suggested as one explanation for our findings. However, we think this explanation is unlikely. When we tested the sensitivity of our process of scoring sacroiliac radiographs, described in Patients and Methods, by mixing the films of 36 sacroiliitis probands with films of relatives and controls, we found that sacroiliitis was never missed (7,10). It is also worth pointing out that some of our patients with clinical evidence of AS but with normal sacroiliac findings on radiographs have been followed for more than 6 years and still do not show radiologic evidence of sacroiliitis.

The major thesis of this study, that arthritis involving the axial skeleton, including the sacroiliac joints, can be present without evidence of erosive disease, should not be surprising. It is recognized that inflammation can occur in joints in the absence of bony erosions. For example, Francois (11) and Shichikawa et al (12) have demonstrated histologic abnormalities of symptomatic sacroiliac joints when pelvic roentgenographs showed absence of sacroiliitis.

The observation that nearly all radiologically normal symptomatic individuals in the Leiden study were females is of interest. This sex distribution is vastly different from the recognized incidence of AS and from the sex incidence in the probands in our 2 studies. It may be explained by the observation that radiologic changes in the sacroiliac joint are less

Table 6. Prevalence of radiologically diagnosed sacroiliitis in 101 HLA typed relatives of ankylosing spondylitis probands (Leiden study)

	n	HLA–B27 positive	HLA–B27 negative
Sacroiliitis present	15	15	0
Sacroiliitis absent	86	45	41

Table 7. Prevalence of "thoracic pain and stiffness" in 86 "unaffected" relatives of ankylosing spondylitis probands (Leiden study)

	n	HLA–B27 positive*	HLA–B27 negative*
Thoracic pain and stiffness present	13	12	1
Thoracic pain and stiffness absent	73	33	40

* $P < 0.01$, relatives with versus those without thoracic pain and stiffness.

marked in affected females than in males. Data supporting this view have been published (7,10,13,14).

The observation that mean ages of symptomatic and asymptomatic relatives in the Leiden study did not differ significantly is of importance, since thoracic pain and stiffness are more common in the older population. For example, among 38 B27 negative population controls, studied in Leiden, who were older than 45 years (mean 55) and did not have sacroiliitis, 7 had thoracic pain and stiffness (18%), compared with only 1 of 41 (2%) younger (mean age 39) B27 negative relatives of AS patients ($P < 0.05$) (unpublished data). This implies that in the older age group, symptoms of thoracic pain and stiffness may also be related to degenerative changes of the vertebral column that occur with aging. However, this implication is still rather speculative and would require further population studies.

In conclusion, these 2 independent family studies of B27 positive AS probands support the view that the clinical spectrum of AS is broader than suggested by the Rome or the New York criteria and probably should include individuals who have symptoms characteristic of AS, but do not have radiologically detectable abnormalities of the sacroiliac joints or the spine. The association between B27 and these symptoms characteristic of AS suggests that individuals with symptomatic disease but normal findings on sacroiliac radiographs should be considered to have spondylitic disease. While radiographically detectable sacroiliitis is very frequent, it is by no means an obligatory manifestation of AS. A history of "chronic inflammatory low back pain" or of "thoracic pain and stiffness" in relatives of AS patients should alert the physician to the possible diagnosis of AS. Since our data are based on family studies, it is not appropriate at this time to extrapolate them to the general population. The prevalence of symptomatic AS without radiographically evident sacroiliitis in the general population is not yet known.

ACKNOWLEDGMENTS

We are grateful to Hermine van der Linden and Evelyn Michalkiewicz for secretarial assistance.

REFERENCES

1. Kellgren JH: Diagnostic criteria for population studies. Bull Rheum Dis 13:291–292, 1962
2. Bennett PH, Burch TA: Population Studies of the Rheumatic Diseases. Amsterdam, Excerpta Medica Foundation, 1968, pp 456–457
3. Hammoudeh M, Khan MA: Genetics of HLA associated disease: ankylosing spondylitis. J Rheumatol 10:301–304, 1983
4. Calin A, Porta J, Fries JF: Clinical history as a screening test for ankylosing spondylitis. JAMA 237:2613–2614, 1977
5. Khan MA, Kushner I, Braun WE: Comparison of clinical features in HLA–B27 positive and negative patients with ankylosing spondylitis. Arthritis Rheum 20:909–912, 1977
6. Kellgren JH, Jeffrey MR: Atlas of standard radiographs in arthritis, Epidemiology of Chronic Rheumatism. Vol. II. Oxford, Blackwell Scientific Publications, 1963, pp 36–40
7. Van der Linden SJ, Valkenburg HA, Cats A: The risk of developing ankylosing spondylitis in HLA–B27 positive individuals: a comparison of relatives of spondylitis patients with the general population. Arthritis Rheum 27:241–249, 1984
8. Van der Linden SJ, Valkenburg HA, Cats A: Evaluation of diagnostic criteria for ankylosing spondylitis: a proposal for modification of the New York criteria. Arthritis Rheum 27:361–368, 1984
9. Grainger RG: Radiological aspects of sacro-iliac arthritis. Proc R Soc Med 50:854–858, 1957
10. Van der Linden SJ: Spondylitis Ankylopoetica: Een Familie en Bevolkingsonderzoek en toetsing van diagnostische Criteria (thesis). Leiden University (The Netherlands), 1982, pp 105–121
11. Francois RJ: Le diagnostic precoce de la spondylarthrite ankylosante bases anatomo-radiologiques. Rhumatologie 35:121–127, 1983
12. Shichikawa K, Tsujimoto M, Nishioka J, Nishibayashi Y, Matsumoto K: Histopathology of early sacroiliitis and enthesitis in ankylosing spondylitis, The First Simmons Center International Symposium on the Spondyloarthropathies. Dallas, TX, May 31–June 2, 1984
13. Khan MA, Kushner I: Diagnosis of ankylosing spondylitis, Progress in Clinical Rheumatology. Edited by AS Cohen. New York, Grune & Stratton, 1984, pp 145–178
14. Van der Linden SJ, Valkenburg H, Cats A: Are women relatively protected from developing ankylosing spondylitis? The First Simmons Center International Symposium on the Spondyloarthropathies. Dallas, TX, May 31–June 2, 1984

SURFACE ANTIGEN SPECIFICITY OF COLD-REACTIVE IgM ANTILYMPHOCYTE ANTIBODIES IN SYSTEMIC LUPUS ERYTHEMATOSUS

AKIRA YAMADA, MELODY SHAW, and JOHN B. WINFIELD

Monoclonal antibodies to known surface antigens on B cells and on resting and activated T cells of various types were used in several approaches to examine the specificity of IgM antilymphocyte antibodies in systemic lupus erythematosus (SLE). Surface determinants that were sought included: T3, T11, Leu-1, Leu-8 (pan-T); T4, T8 (T subset); β_2-microglobulin (β_2m); L243, Leu-10 (DR and DS/DC framework, respectively); anti-Tac (interleukin-2 receptor); 5E9 (transferrin receptor); and 4F2, AA1 (other activation antigens). The first strategy was based on inhibition of rosette formation between mouse monoclonal antibody–coated targets and anti-mouse IgG–coated erythrocytes by SLE sera, either directly at 4°C or after modulation of IgM antilymphocyte antibody–reactive target cell antigen at 37°C. Significant rosette inhibition, defined as >2 standard deviations from the mean value for 10 control sera, was seen only for β_2m (13 of 20 SLE sera were positive; inhibition = 15–58%). Next, relative fluorescence intensity of lymphocyte staining by monoclonal antibodies was assessed by flow microfluorometry after preincubation of cells with SLE serum at 4°C or after modulation of SLE antibody–reactive antigen. Modulation markedly reduced or eliminated SLE antilymphocyte antibody IgM staining. Except for β_2m, neither cold nor warm temperature preincubations altered the relative fluorescence intensity for the known surface antigens. These data confirm anti-β_2m as a common antibody specificity in SLE and suggest that antilymphocyte antibodies in this disorder are not directed to Ia or to certain other defined lymphocyte antigens of functional interest.

A variety of functional effects have been attributed to lymphocyte autoantibodies in systemic lupus erythematosus (SLE). Examples of these include reduced concanavalin A–generated suppressor T cell activity, reduced T cell proliferation to various specific and nonspecific stimuli, inhibition of natural killer cell activity, suppression of antibody-dependent cell-mediated cytotoxicity, inhibition of the generation of alloreactive cytotoxic T cells, and enhancement of B cell immunoglobulin secretion (reviewed in 1). Antilymphocyte antibodies also have been implicated in lymphocyte depletion in vivo in this disorder, especially with respect to T cells and T cell subsets (1). For these reasons, molecular characterization of the determinants on the cell membrane to which different types of SLE antilymphocyte antibodies are directed has been a pressing issue for some time. Despite the considerable effort expended in various laboratories, a remarkable lack of progress has been made in this area. A principle obstacle to the characterization of these determinants is the low avidity and low titer of many of the most interesting antibodies, which greatly limits their utility as probes for immunoprecipitation and analysis of radiolabeled surface molecules. Indeed, with the exception of a single early effort in

From the Division of Rheumatology and Immunology, University of North Carolina at Chapel Hill, School of Medicine, Chapel Hill, North Carolina.

Supported in part by NIH grant R01 AM30863, a Multipurpose Arthritis Center grant, and an Arthritis Foundation Clinical Research Center grant.

Akira Yamada, MD: Fellow in Rheumatology; Melody Shaw, BS: Research Associate; John B. Winfield, MD: Professor of Medicine.

Address reprint requests to John B. Winfield, MD, Division of Rheumatology and Immunology, 932 FLOB, 231H, University of North Carolina at Chapel Hill, School of Medicine, Chapel Hill, NC 27514.

Submitted for publication April 9, 1984; accepted in revised form July 26, 1984.

which the investigators identified a low molecular weight glycoprotein on T cells involved in the allogeneic mixed leukocyte reaction (MLR) (2), this type of approach has been unsuccessful.

The available information has been derived from experimental strategies using antibody absorption or inhibition techniques, such as absorption of SLE serum with purified antigen (3), inhibition of SLE serum cytotoxic activity by precoating target cells with $F(ab')_2$ antibody fragments (4), the lysostrip technique (5), and rosette inhibition using monoclonal antibodies to known antigens (6). The latter method is very sensitive and involves precoating target cells with SLE antilymphocyte antibody, followed by enumeration of rosettes formed between the target cells in the presence of monoclonal antibody of defined specificity and erythrocytes coated with anti-mouse immunoglobulin.

In this investigation, we combined rosette inhibition, indirect immunofluorescence, and flow microfluorometry procedures in a series of experiments to identify SLE serum antibodies directed to 13 surface antigens defined by monoclonal antibodies. We took special advantage of the capacity of SLE IgM antibody–reactive antigen to be modulated by brief incubation of target cells in SLE serum at 37°C.

MATERIALS AND METHODS

Patients and sera. Peripheral blood was obtained from patients with SLE who met the revised American Rheumatism Association diagnostic criteria (7) and from 10 normal subjects. After separation from whole blood, serum was aliquoted and stored at −70°C. Each serum aliquot was heated at 56°C for 30 minutes immediately before use. SLE disease activity was assessed as described previously (8).

Lymphocytes. Normal human peripheral blood mononuclear cells (PBMC) were separated from heparinized venous blood by Ficoll-Hypaque flotation. T cells were obtained by passage of PBMC over nylon wool columns (Fenwall Laboratories, Berkeley, CA) and collecting the nonadherent population, according to the technique of Julius et al (9). Nylon wool–adherent cells, containing enriched numbers of B cells and monocytes, were removed by wringing the nylon wool at cold temperatures. Markers used to assess purity of these enriched cell populations included esterase staining of monocytes and indirect immunofluorescence or complement-dependent cytotoxic reactivity with monoclonal antibodies to Ia, IgM, and pan-T determinants.

Activated T cells were obtained by culturing PBMC for 3 days in tissue culture flasks (Falcon, Oxnard, CA), at a density of 10^6 cells/ml, in RPMI 1640 medium (University of North Carolina Cancer Center, Chapel Hill, NC) containing 1 μg/ml phytohemagglutinin (PHA; Burroughs Wellcome, Research Triangle Park, NC), 2 m*M* glutamine, antibiotics, and 10% fetal calf serum (FCS; Hyclone, Logan, UT) in a humid 5% CO_2, 95% air incubator. Chronic lymphocytic leukemia (CLL) cells were used in certain experiments.

Microcytotoxicity. Two-stage, complement-dependent microcytotoxicity assays using prescreened rabbit complement (C; Pel-Freez Biologicals, Rogers, AR) were performed as previously described (10). Assay temperatures of 15°C were used to detect cold-reactive antibodies, and temperatures of 25°C were used to distinguish warm-reactive anti–T blast antibodies (11). Cytotoxicity, expressed as the percentage of nonviable cells failing to exclude eosin dye, was assessed by inverted phase-contrast microscopy. Cytotoxicity with C alone or with C plus normal serum was <10%.

Special immunologic reagents. Monoclonal antibodies used included the following: L243 (anti-DR framework; American Type Culture Collection, Rockville, MD); anti-Tac (a generous gift from Dr. T. Waldmann, NIH, Bethesda, MD); Leu-1, Leu-8, Leu-10, anti–β_2-microglobulin (anti-β_2m; Becton-Dickinson, Sunnyvale, CA); OKT3, OKT4, OKT8, OKT11 (Ortho Diagnostics, Raritan, NJ); 5E9 (antibody to transferrin receptor; a generous gift from Dr. B. Haynes, Duke University, Durham, NC); AA1 (anti–T blast; a generous gift of Dr. N. Chiorazzi, Rockefeller University, New York, NY); fluorescein isothiocyanate (FITC)–conjugated $F(ab')_2$ goat anti-human IgM; and FITC-rabbit anti-mouse IgG (Cappel Laboratories, Cochranville, PA). Chicken and rabbit anti-human Ia antibodies were gifts of Dr. N Bernard, University of North Carolina, Chapel Hill, NC.

Monoclonal antibody rosettes and rosette inhibition. The monoclonal antibody rosette assay was performed according to the method of Stocker et al (12), using goat anti-mouse IgG–coated bovine red blood cells (BRBC; Biological Products, Winston-Salem, NC) as indicator cells. Two hundred microliters of 50% packed BRBC and 100 μl of affinity-purified goat anti-mouse IgG (800 μg/ml; a gift from Dr. R. Eisenberg, University of North Carolina, Chapel Hill) were mixed, and 200 μl of 2.5 m*M* chromic chloride was added dropwise (13). After incubation of the reaction mixture for 5 minutes at room temperature, anti-IgG–coated BRBC were washed thoroughly and resuspended at 1% in RPMI 1640 supplemented with 10% FCS.

Fifty microliters of a suspension of target lymphocytes (2.5×10^5) was incubated with 50 μl of appropriate dilutions of monoclonal antibody for 30 minutes at 4°C. After washing, target cells were suspended in RPMI 1640, 10% FCS, to a final density of 4×10^6 ml, combined with an equal volume (usually 50 μl) of a 1% suspension of anti-mouse IgG–coated BRBC, and centrifuged for 10 minutes at 200*g* in small tubes (Fisher Scientific, Pittsburgh, PA). After incubation in ice water for 30 minutes, the BRBC/lymphocyte mixture was gently resuspended, stained with Giemsa, and applied to glass microscope slides for microscopy to determine the percentage of rosette-forming cells. At least 200 cells were counted in each assay.

Antibodies to surface determinants recognized by the various monoclonal antibodies were sought in the SLE sera by rosette-inhibition assays. Target lymphocytes (1×10^6) were preincubated with 100 μl of SLE serum or normal serum for 1 hour at 4°C, with frequent agitation. After pelleting and aspiration of serum, the cells were resuspended in the highest dilution of monoclonal antibody giving near-maximal rosette formation, and rosettes were prepared and enumerated as described above. Inhibition was calculated as follows: % inhibition = [(a − b)/b] × 100, where a = % rosettes with normal serum preincubation, and b = % rosettes with SLE serum preincubation.

The major surface antigen(s) on T cells with which cold-reactive SLE antilymphocyte antibodies react can be modulated (i.e., exhibit decreased fluorescence intensity for SLE IgM staining) by brief preincubation of cells in SLE serum at 37°C (14). Therefore, monoclonal antibody rosette inhibition was also examined in experiments where the target cells were preincubated with SLE serum at 37°C for 2 hours prior to rosette assay.

Indirect immunofluorescence and flow cytometry. IgM and IgG antibody binding to T cells in SLE serum was assessed by indirect immunofluorescence at 4°C using FITC-conjugated rabbit $F(ab')_2$ antibodies to human μ or γ chains as the second coat. Appropriate dilutions of mouse monoclonal antibodies and FITC-goat $F(ab')_2$ anti-mouse IgG were used to determine known surface antigens. After staining, cells were kept at 4°C and were examined immediately or were fixed with paraformaldehyde. Analysis of fluorescence intensity (log-integrated green fluorescence) and % positive cells were determined by flow microfluorometry using an Epics V instrument (Coulter Electronics, Hialeah, FL) equipped with argon laser (488 nm), MDADS and EASY 1 computers, and appropriate software. Laser power, photomultiplier tube amplification, and gain settings were calibrated using fluorospheres (Coulter) and kept constant throughout the experimental run on a given lymphocyte preparation. In some experiments, attempts were made to block or modulate known determinants with SLE serum prior to staining with mouse monoclonal antibodies.

RESULTS

In initial experiments, sera from patients with SLE were screened for antibodies to different types of lymphocytes using C-dependent microcytotoxicity and indirect immunofluorescence assays. Of 20 sera with antilymphocyte antibody activity, 13 contained cold-reactive IgM cytotoxic antibodies against resting T cells (mean % ± SD dead cells = 56 ± 24). Sixteen sera were cytotoxic for B cells (mean % ± SD dead cells = 47 ± 23). Relatively warm-reactive IgM antibodies to 3-day PHA-activated T blasts were detected in 7 sera (mean % ± SD dead cells = 55 ± 26) in cytotoxicity assays performed at 25°C. None of these sera gave detectable IgG staining of the different targets. This panel of 20 sera was then used in subsequent experiments to identify IgM antibody reactivity against a series of known cell surface determinants.

Direct rosette inhibition. The monoclonal antibody specificities and the different types of target cells used in rosette-inhibition assays are given in Table 1. Also shown is the mean percent of rosette-forming cells observed in the presence of standard normal AB serum, as well as the variation about this mean when sera from 10 normal individuals were substituted for the standard AB serum in the assay. Figure 1A illustrates the relationship between rosette formation and monoclonal antibody dilution. From preliminary titrations of this sort, a working dilution for each monoclonal antibody was chosen to maximize inhibitability of rosette formation by test sera. Figure 1B shows a typical direct rosette inhibition curve. In this experiment, target cells were preincubated with varying dilutions of rabbit anti-human Ia antiserum before addition of L243, a monoclonal antibody to human Ia.

Thirteen specificities identified by monoclonal

Table 1. Monoclonal antibody specificities and target cells studied

Monoclonal antibody	Specificity (ref.)	Target cell	% rosette-forming cells*	
			Mean	± 2 SD
L243	DR framework (28)	CLL†	73	61–85
Leu-10	DS/DC framework	CLL	52	42–62
$\alpha\beta_2$m	β_2-microglobulin	CLL	71	61–81
OKT4	HLA class II receptor (29)	Resting T	42	34–50
OKT8	HLA class I receptor (30)	Resting T	20	16–24
OKT3	T cell antigen receptor (31)	Resting T	72	60–84
OKT11	E receptor (18)	Resting T	64	52–76
Leu-1	Pan-T	Resting T	53	43–63
Leu-8	Pan-T	Resting T	53	44–62
5E9	Transferrin receptor (32)	T blast	72	61–83
4F2	Activation antigen (33)	T blast	88	63–95
Tac	Interleukin-2 receptor (34)	T blast	63	54–72
AA1	Activation antigen (35)	T blast	30	23–37

* Mean % rosette-forming cells in the presence of standard normal AB serum, and the variation about this mean when substituting 10 normal sera in the rosette inhibition assay (determined as % of total lymphocytes).
† CLL = chronic lymphocytic leukemia.

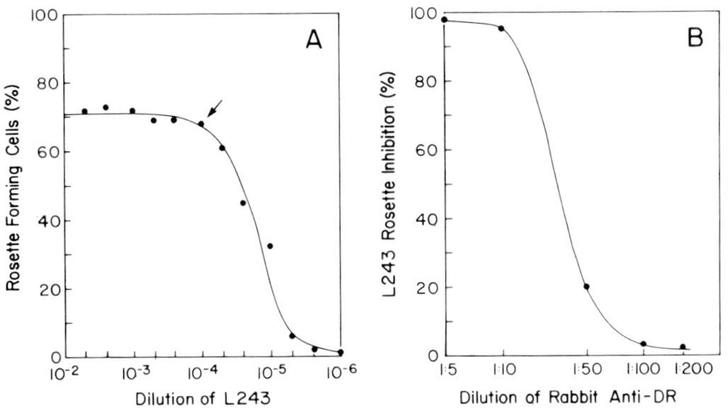

Figure 1. Monoclonal antibody rosette formation and rosette inhibition. **A**, Chronic lymphocytic leukemia (CLL) cells were incubated with various dilutions of L243, a monoclonal anti-DR framework antibody, washed, and then combined with anti-mouse IgG–coated bovine erythrocytes. The **arrow** indicates the dilution of L243 chosen for use in rosette inhibition assays. **B**, A typical rosette inhibition assay. Here the CLL targets were preincubated with rabbit anti-DR framework antiserum prior to addition of L243 and anti-mouse IgG–coated erythrocytes.

antibodies were sought in direct rosette inhibition assays performed at 4°C with the 20 SLE sera (Figure 2). Thirteen of 20 sera inhibited anti-β_2m rosettes (range 15–58%). Rosette inhibition was rarely observed with the other monoclonal antibodies. This was true even when the procedure was modified to allow continuous presence of SLE serum (data not shown). The failure to detect rosette inhibition with L243 rosettes was unexpected since, with this technique, others have identified anti-Ia antibodies directed to the L243 DR framework epitope (6).

To further examine the question of anti-Ia specificities in the SLE sera, an additional series of experiments was performed. First, T cell blasts were used in place of CLL cells as targets in the rosette inhibition assay, but no inhibition was observed (mean % inhibition ± SD = 3 ± 8; % control L243 rosette-forming cells = 14). Second, the anti-Ia rosette assay with CLL targets was modified for use with rabbit anti-DR heteroantiserum by substituting goat anti-rabbit IgG Fc for anti-mouse IgG as the coating for the BRBC indicator cells. In this system, L243 at a 1:1,000 dilution inhibited rosette formation ~40% (85% → 51%), but inhibition by the SLE sera was insignificant (mean ± SD = 1 ± 5%). Third, the presence of anti-Ia antibody was sought in an assay based upon inhibition of C-mediated cytotoxicity using chicken anti-Ia antibody, which does not fix C. Preincubation of nylon wool–purified non-T cells (85% Ia+) with chicken anti-Ia completely prevented killing by L243, but had no effect on cytotoxicity of the SLE sera

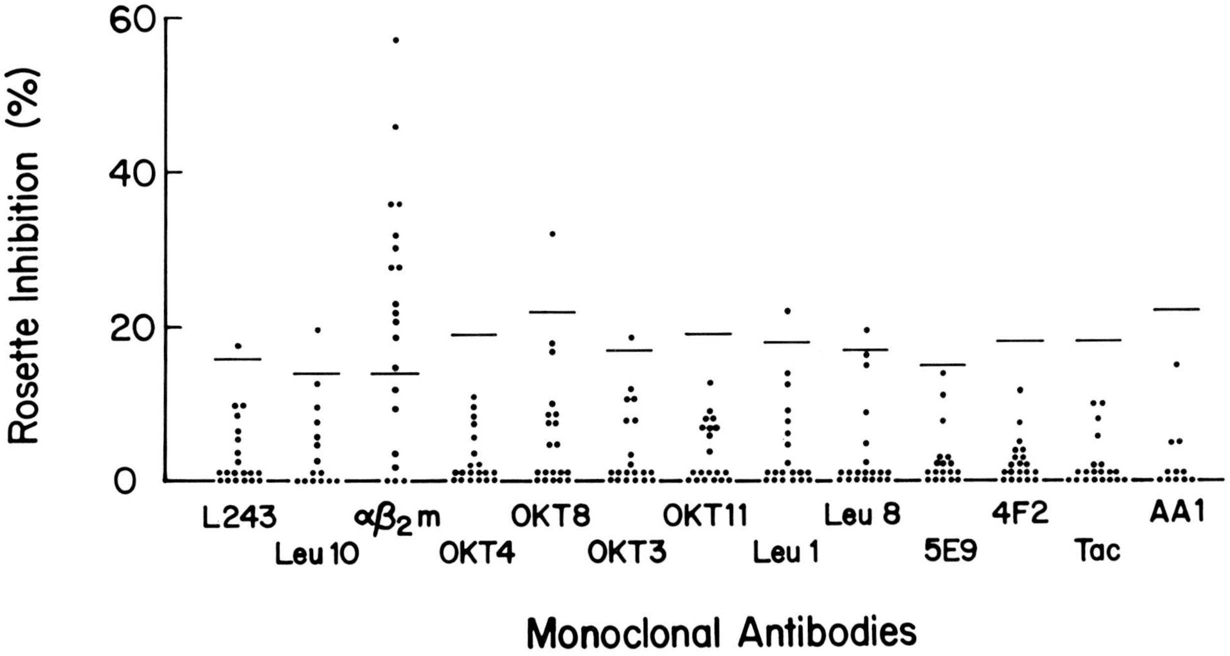

Figure 2. Rosette inhibition by systemic lupus erythematosus (SLE) sera. Target cells were preincubated with SLE serum before performance of the monoclonal antibody rosette assay. Monoclonal antibody specificities and target cells used are shown in Table 1. The horizontal bars represent 2 SD above the mean % inhibition observed with a panel of 10 control sera (within normal limits). With rare exceptions, significant inhibition was found only for β_2-microglobulin (β_2m).

(Table 2). This latter experiment does not exclude the presence of anti-Ia antibodies in SLE sera, but indicates that the predominant anti-B cell specificity is not directed to Ia.

Finally, attempts were made to block indirect immunofluorescent staining by L243 by preincubating T cell blasts with SLE serum at 4°C. Neither the percentage of positively stained cells, nor the relative fluorescence intensity of L243 staining was decreased relative to control preparations preincubated with normal AB serum (data not shown). Inhibition of monoclonal antibody immunofluorescence staining for Tac, OKT3, OKT4, and OKT8 specificities was studied in a similar manner with 10 SLE sera. In no case was monoclonal antibody staining altered by preincubation with the SLE sera.

Modulation studies. In studies to be reported in detail separately (14), it was observed that brief preincubation of lymphocytes with SLE serum at 37°C resulted in loss of IgM-reactive determinant(s) from the cell surface. When cells treated in this manner were incubated at 4°C with a fresh aliquot of the same SLE serum used in the 37°C preincubation, both the percent of IgM+ cells and the relative fluorescence intensity for IgM staining fell sharply. Since SLE IgM antibody-reactive antigen(s) is modulated under these conditions, one would predict that if the IgM antibody were directed to known determinants identified by monoclonal antibodies, these would be modulated as well.

Table 2. Inhibition studies of the cytotoxicity of systemic lupus erythematosus (SLE) sera for peripheral non-T cells, using non--complement-fixing chicken anti-Ia*

	Preincubation of target cells			
SLE serum	None	Normal chicken serum, 1:2	Chicken anti-Ia 1:2	Chicken anti-Ia 1:8
1	90	80	80	ND
2	60	65	65	65
3	60	50	60	50
4	80	80	80	70
5	70	70	65	75
6	50	40	45	35
7	30	ND	ND	35
8	40	50	50	50
9	35	40	45	40
10	80	70	75	70
L243	90	90	<10	<10

* Nylon wool–adherent cell targets were 85% Ia+, 70% sIgM+. Target cells were incubated with indicated dilutions of normal chicken serum or chicken anti-Ia for 30 minutes at 4°C prior to assay. Values expressed as % dead cells, determined in a 2-stage complement-dependent microcytotoxicity assay performed at 15°C. ND = not determined.

This hypothesis was tested with 10 SLE sera for the monoclonal antibody specificities listed in Table 1. Despite a substantial reduction in IgM staining of T cells with 8 of 10 sera following modulation (60 ± 25% IgM+ cells → 26 ± 22%), the percentage of rosettes was unchanged, relative to control values, for all monoclonal antibodies except anti-β_2m. Slight, but significant (>12%) reduction in anti-β_2m rosettes was observed following modulation with 4 of 10 sera. Resting T cells and T cell blasts modulated with SLE serum were also examined by indirect immunofluorescence to detect any subtle change in staining characteristics for the L243, OKT3, OKT4, OKT8, β_2m, and Tac specificities. Anti-β_2m staining was shifted to lower levels of fluorescence intensity by 37°C pretreatment with 7 of 10 sera in the same manner as that observed for SLE IgM (Figure 3). Staining by the other monoclonal antibodies was not altered.

DISCUSSION

This investigation utilized sensitive rosetting and immunofluorescence techniques to define cell surface determinants reactive with IgM antilymphocyte antibodies in SLE. Specificities for epitopes identified by the monoclonal antibodies L243 (DR framework), Leu-10 (DS/DC framework), OKT4, OKT8, OKT3, OKT11 (E receptor), Leu-1, Leu-8, 5E9 (transferrin receptor), 4F2 (activation neoantigen), Tac (interleukin-2 receptor), and AA1 (activation neoantigen) were not demonstrable in direct rosette inhibition assays. Additional evidence against the presence of antibodies to the *molecules* expressing these epitopes was obtained in a series of modulation experiments. Thus, preincubation of target cells with SLE serum at 37°C caused a reduction in cold-reactive IgM staining, but (except for anti-β_2m) did not alter monoclonal antibody rosette formation or relative fluorescence intensity of staining. While it is possible that the known antigens would not be modulated under the conditions used even if specifically bound by SLE antibodies, the dramatic loss of IgM-reactive antigen(s) following modulation indicates that the latter are largely distinct from the molecules recognized by the monoclonal antibodies. It should be emphasized, however, that our approaches to defining the surface antigen specificity of antilymphocyte antibodies in SLE are indirect and subject to certain caveats. For example, the failure of SLE serum to inhibit monoclonal antibody rosette formation could reflect a relative-

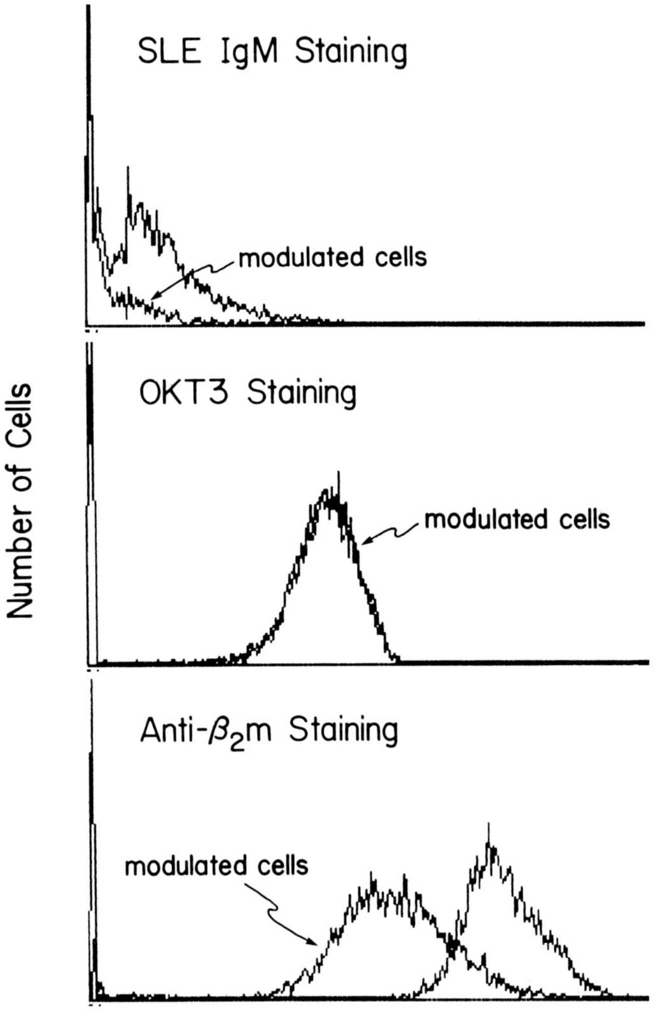

Figure 3. Modulation of systemic lupus erythematosus (SLE) IgM-reactive surface antigen(s) and β_2-microglobulin (β_2m). Nylon wool–purified T cells were modulated by incubation with SLE serum for 2 hours at 37°C. Modulated cells and fresh, untreated T cells were then incubated at 4°C with a fresh aliquot of SLE serum (upper panel), OKT3 (middle panel), or anti-β_2m (lower panel) followed by staining with fluorescein isothiocyanate–conjugated antiimmunoglobulin reagents. Modulation reduced the fluorescence intensity (log-integrated green fluorescence) of SLE IgM and anti-β_2m staining, but did not alter that of OKT3.

ly lower avidity of the autoantibodies. More precise delineation of autoantibody specificities will require immunoprecipitation and immunoblotting procedures.

Each of the experimental approaches identified β_2m as a major specificity of cold-reactive IgM antilymphocyte antibodies in SLE. The data here are consistent with those obtained by previous investigators using different techniques (3,4,15). For example, preincubation of target cells with F(ab')$_2$ fragments of xenoantisera against β_2-microglobulin and heavy chains of HLA–A, B, or C antigens (3), or absorption with purified β_2-microglobulin (4) both inhibit the cytotoxic activity of antilymphocyte antibodies in SLE sera. Antibody to β_2-microglobulin has been found in other diseases, such as Felty's syndrome, as well (16).

The existence of antibodies with Ia specificity is more controversial. In early experiments, F(ab')$_2$ fragments of operationally-specific xenoantisera to HLA–DR antigens reduced the cytotoxicity of SLE sera for B lymphoblastoid cell lines, but not for peripheral lymphocytes (4). The SLE patients had been pregnant, however. More recently, Okudaira et al (6) reported inhibition of anti-DR framework antibody-mediated rosette formation by serum from patients with active SLE. We could not confirm their findings despite our use of the same monoclonal antibody, L243, and both T blasts and CLL cells (~75% Ia+) as targets. Anti-Ia antibodies also were not detected in a series of modulation, indirect immunofluorescence, and inhibition of C-dependent cytotoxicity experiments.

These data may provide some additional insight into conceptualization of the mechanisms by which antilymphocyte antibodies in SLE influence cell function. As an example, there is strong evidence that antilymphocyte antibodies inhibit T cell proliferation to soluble antigen or to allogeneic non-T cells through effects at the level of the responding T cell (2,17). The failure to demonstrate specificities to Ia, Tac, T3, T8, or T4 argues against an inhibitory mechanism involving specific blockade or modulation of, respectively, DR antigens, interleukin-2 receptors, or antigen, or classes I and II molecule-recognition structures. Similarly, the failure of other investigators to inhibit E-rosette formation, and our data against antibodies to the OKT11 epitope suggest that an "off-signal" effect (18) does not occur. It should be emphasized, however, that such arguments represent aids in conceptualization, rather than proofs, since the available data are both limited and indirect. More conclusive answers to questions concerning structure/function relations of antilymphocyte antibodies in SLE will require systematic analyses of the entire array of antibody specificities, using more sophisticated approaches, e.g., cloned cells as targets and human monoclonal antilymphocyte autoantibodies derived from patients.

Given the myriad functional effects attributed to antilymphocyte antibodies in SLE and the range of reactivities seen with cell targets of different types, it is generally assumed that the antibody specificities must reflect this heterogeneity. This presumed diversity contrasts sharply with the unambiguous molecular data in this regard, i.e., β_2m (3,4,15) and a surface determinant cross-reactive with core mononucleosomes (19). Is it possible that cold lymphocytotoxins in this disorder, and in a variety of other disorders, actually are rather limited in specificity in a manner analogous to IgM rheumatoid factor and cold agglutinins? If such were the case, the differential reactivity with various cells and the multiple functional effects might derive from variation in cell density and/or membrane stability of a small number of functionally relevant antigens.

Regardless of the exact antibody specificity, the observation that the predominant antigen(s) with which IgM antibodies react can be easily modulated at physiologic temperatures is of special interest because of the potential for important in vivo effects (20). Shedding of surface antigens in association with antilymphocyte antibody was first postulated by the recovery of allogeneic MLR responsiveness by T cells exposed to MLR-blocking antibodies from SLE serum after short-term culture (2). Further evidence for the existence of circulating complexes of shed surface antigen and antilymphocyte antibody is the demonstration of specific enrichment of antilymphocyte antibody in purified cryoprecipitates from patients with SLE (21,22) and chronic lymphocytic leukemia (23), and the development of antibodies to human lymphocytes in animals immunized with SLE serum cryoproteins (24). Both β_2m and anti-β_2m antibody have been demonstrated in immune complexes isolated from the serum of patients with Felty's syndrome (16).

Although it remains to be determined whether shedding or capping and internalization of antigen is occurring in our experiments, in vivo antigenic modulation has been demonstrated directly in other situations. Thus, treatment of leukemia patients with antibodies to leukemic cells results in the disappearance of reactive membrane antigens (25). Similarly, administration of the monoclonal antibody OKT3 to renal allograft recipients causes a decrease in OKT3+ T cells and the appearance of OKT4+/T3 and OKT8+/T3 cells in peripheral blood followed by re-expression of the OKT3 determinant after overnight incubation in culture (26). Work is in progress to determine whether such phenomena occur spontaneously in SLE, as is perhaps suggested by the observation of Steinberg and colleagues that brightly IgM-staining cells are selectively "lost" in patients with active disease (27). If such proves to be the case, in vivo surface receptor modulation by autoantibodies may be an important mechanism for immune system functional abnormalities in SLE and related disorders.

ACKNOWLEDGMENTS

The technical assistance of Rekha Shah is gratefully acknowledged. We also thank Dr. Philip Cohen for helpful discussions and Cathy Miller-Wells for typing the manuscript.

REFERENCES

1. Winfield JB: Anti-lymphocyte antibodies in SLE: specificity and relationship to abnormal cellular function, Systemic Lupus Erythematosus. Edited by R Lahita. New York, John Wiley & Sons (in press)
2. Wernet P, Kunkel HG: Antibodies to a specific surface antigen on T cells in human sera inhibiting mixed leukocyte culture reactions. J Exp Med 138:1021–1026, 1973
3. Revillard JP, Vincent C, Rivera S: Anti-β_2-microglobulin lymphocytotoxic autoantibodies in systemic lupus erythematosus. J Immunol 122:614–618, 1979
4. Messner RP, DeHoratius R, Ferrone S: Lymphocytotoxic antibodies in systemic lupus erythematosus patients and their relatives: reactivity with the HLA antigenic molecular complex. Arthritis Rheum 23:265–272, 1980
5. Takahashi H, Terasaki PI, Iwaki Y, Nakata S: Identification of surface IgM as the target antigen of cold lymphocytotoxins. Tissue Antigens 16:176–180, 1980
6. Okudaira K, Searles RP, Ceuppens JL, Goodwin JS, Williams RC Jr: Anti-Ia reactivity in sera from patients with systemic lupus erythematosus. J Clin Invest 69:17–24, 1982
7. Tan EM, Cohen AS, Fries JF, Masi AT, McShane DJ, Rothfield NF, Schaller JG, Talal N, Winchester RJ: The 1982 revised criteria for the classification of systemic lupus erythematosus. Arthritis Rheum 25:1271–1277, 1982
8. Winfield JB, Brunner CM, Davis JS IV, O'Brien WM: Assessment of disease activity in systemic lupus erythematosus (abstract). Arthritis Rheum 15:462, 1972
9. Julius MH, Simpson E, Herzenberg LA: A rapid method for isolation of functional thymus-derived murine lymphocytes. Eur J Immunol 3:645–649, 1973
10. Winfield JB, Winchester RJ, Wernet P, Fu SM, Kunkel HG: Nature of cold-reactive antibodies to lymphocyte surface determinants in systemic lupus erythematosus. Arthritis Rheum 18:1–8, 1975
11. Litvin DA, Cohen PL, Winfield JB: Characterization of warm-reactive IgG anti-lymphocyte antibodies in systemic lupus erythematosus: relative specificity for mitogen-activated T cells and their soluble products. J Immunol 130:181–186, 1983
12. Stocker JW, Garotta G, Hausmann B, Trucco M, Cep-

pellini R: Separation of human cells bearing HLA-DR antigens using a monoclonal antibody rosetting method. Tissue Antigens 13:212–222, 1979

13. Goding JW: The chromic chloride method of coupling antigens to erythrocytes: definition of some important parameters. J Immunol Methods 10:61–66, 1976
14. Winfield JB, Shaw M, Yamada A: Modulation of IgM anti-lymphocyte autoantibody-reactive surface antigen in systemic lupus erythematosus. In preparation
15. Ooi BS, Ooi YM, Pesce AJ, Pollak V: Antibodies to β_2 microglobulin in the sera of patients with systemic lupus erythematosus. Immunology 33:535–541, 1977
16. Falus A, Wiik A, Permin H, Brandslund I, Svehag S-E: High serum beta-2-microglobulin levels and circulating immune complexes containing β_2m and anti-β_2m antibodies in Felty's syndrome. Arthritis Rheum 26:721–727, 1983
17. Yamada A, Winfield JB: Inhibition of soluble antigen-induced T cell proliferation by warm-reactive antibodies to activated T cells in systemic lupus erythematosus. J Clin Invest (in press)
18. Palacios R, Martinez-Maza O: Is the E receptor on human T lymphocyte a "negative signal" receptor? J Immunol 129:2479–2485, 1982
19. Rekvig OP, Hannestad K: The specificity of autoantibodies that react with both cell nuclei and plasma membranes: the nuclear antigen is present on core mononucleosomes. J Immunol 123:2673–2681, 1979
20. Chatenoud L, Bach J-F: Antigenic modulation—a major mechanism of antibody action. Immunol Today 5:20–25, 1984
21. Winfield JB, Winchester RJ, Wernet P, Kunkel HG: Specific concentrations of anti-lymphocyte antibodies in the serum cryoprecipitates of patients with systemic lupus erythematosus. Clin Exp Immunol 19:399–406, 1975
22. Zvaifler NJ, Bluestein HG: Lymphocytotoxic antibody activity in cryoprecipitates from serum of patients with SLE. Arthritis Rheum 19:844–850, 1976
23. Day NK, Winfield JB, Gee T, Winchester R, Teshima H, Kunkel HG: Evidence for immune complexes involving anti-lymphocyte antibodies associated with hypocomplementaemia in chronic lymphocytic leukaemia (CLL). Clin Exp Immunol 26:189–195, 1976
24. Klippel JH, Bluestein HG, Zvaifler NJ: Lymphocyte reactivity of antisera to cryoproteins in systemic lupus erythematosus. Clin Immunol Immunopathol 12:52–61, 1979
25. Milier RA, Maloney DG, McKillop J, Levy R: In vivo effects of murine hybridoma monoclonal antibody in a patient with T-cell leukemia. Blood 58:78–86, 1981
26. Chatenoud L, Baudrihaye MF, Kreis H, Goldstein G, Schindler J, Bach J: Human in vivo antigenic modulation induced by the anti-T cell OKT3 monoclonal antibody. Eur J Immunol 12:979–982, 1982
27. Steinberg AD, Klassen LW, Budman DR, Williams GW: Immunofluorescence studies of anti-T cell antibodies and T cells in systemic lupus erythematosus: selective loss of brightly staining T cells in active disease. Arthritis Rheum 22:114–122, 1979
28. Lampson LA, Levy R: Two populations of Ia-like molecules on human B cell line. J Immunol 125:293–299, 1980
29. Biddison WE, Rao PE, Talle MA, Goldstein G, Shaw S: Possible involvement of the OKT4 molecule in T cell recognition of class II HLA antigens: evidence from studies of cytotoxic T lymphocytes specific for SB antigens. J Exp Med 156:1065–1076, 1982
30. Meuer SC, Schlossman SF, Reinherz EL: Clonal analysis of human cytotoxic T lymphocytes: T4+ and T8+ effector T cells recognize products of different major histocompatibility complex regions. Proc Natl Acad Sci USA 79:4395–4399, 1982
31. Reinherz EL, Hussey RE, Schlossman SF: A monoclonal antibody blocking human T cell function. Eur J Immunol 10:758–762, 1980
32. Haynes BF, Hemler M, Cotner T, Mann DL, Eisenbarth GS, Strominger JL, Fauci AS: Characterization of a monoclonal antibody (5E9) that defines a human cell surface antigen of cell activation. J Immunol 127:347–351, 1981
33. Haynes BF, Hemler ME, Mann DL, Eisenbarth GS, Shelhamer J, Mostowski HS, Thomas CA, Strominger JL, Fauci AS: Characterization of a monoclonal antibody (4F2) that binds to human monocytes and to a subset of activated lymphocytes. J Immunol 126:1409–1414, 1981
34. Miyawaki T, Yachie A, Uwadana N, Ohzeki S, Nagaoki T, Taniguchi N: Functional significance of Tac antigen expressed on activated human T lymphocytes: Tac antigen interacts with T cell growth factor in cellular proliferation. J Immunol 129:2474–2478, 1982
35. Chiorazzi N, Bigler R, Hatzfeld J, McCune JM: Distinct human leukocyte activation antigens defined by murine monoclonal antibodies, AA1 and AA2, Human Leukocyte Markers Detected by Monoclonal Antibodies. Edited by A Bernard, L Boumsell. New York, Springer (in press)

EFFECTS OF L-CANAVANINE ON T CELLS MAY EXPLAIN THE INDUCTION OF SYSTEMIC LUPUS ERYTHEMATOSUS BY ALFALFA

JORGE ALCOCER-VARELA, ANTONIO IGLESIAS, LUIS LLORENTE, and DONATO ALARCÓN-SEGOVIA

Alfalfa sprouts can induce systemic lupus erythematosus (SLE) in monkeys. This property of alfalfa sprouts has been attributed to their non-protein amino acid constituent, L-canavanine. Occurrence of autoimmune hemolytic anemia and exacerbation of SLE have been linked to ingestion of alfalfa tablets containing L-canavanine. In this report we show that L-canavanine has dose-related effects in vitro on human immunoregulatory cells, which could explain its lupus-inducing potential. These effects include: 1) diminution of the mitogenic response to both phytohemagglutinin and concanavalin A but not to pokeweed mitogen, as determined in both thymidine incorporation and cell cycle studies, and 2) abrogation of concanavalin A–induced suppressor cell function, which results in increased release of both IgG and DNA binding activity into supernatants by cells from normal subjects and SLE patients. These immunoregulatory effects of L-canavanine may explain the induction or exacerbation of SLE by alfalfa.

A condition similar to systemic lupus erythematosus (SLE) has been observed in monkeys fed alfalfa seeds. The syndrome is characterized by anemia, low serum complement components, antibodies to DNA, and deposition of immunoglobulins and complement in the skin and kidneys (1,2).

L-canavanine sulfate (LCS), a non-protein amino acid constituent of alfalfa sprouts, has been shown to reactivate this syndrome in monkeys; it has therefore been postulated to be the inducer of this primate model of SLE (2). More recently, reactivation of human SLE has been noted in relation to the ingestion of alfalfa tablets (3).

Because several drugs can induce autoantibody formation and an SLE-like disease in a large proportion of treated individuals (4), some by affecting the regulation of the immune response (5,6), we examined the effect of LCS on the in vitro responses of human peripheral blood mononuclear cells (MNC) and found that LCS inhibited the generation of suppressor cells. This suggests that the SLE-like syndrome observed in monkeys and the activation of human SLE by alfalfa both may be explained by interference by LCS with the immunoregulatory role of T cells.

MATERIALS AND METHODS

Cell separation and purification. MNC were obtained from normal adult volunteers (age 23–32) by centrifugation of heparinized venous blood on Ficoll-Hypaque gradients (7). In some experiments we also studied cells from SLE patients who fulfilled the American Rheumatism Association's revised criteria for this disease (8) and were not receiving any treatment.

To obtain T and B cell–enriched populations, MNC were rosetted with sheep erythrocytes (7) and centrifuged on Ficoll-Hypaque cushions. The cells at the interface were harvested, washed, and used as a B cell–enriched population. The pelleted cells were treated with sterile water to rid

From the Department of Immunology and Rheumatology, Instituto Nacional de la Nutrición "Salvador Zubirán," Mexico City, Mexico.

Supported in part by the Fondo para Estudios e Investigaciones Ricardo J. Zevada, Mexico City, Mexico and the Fideicomiso of Fondo Educativo BCH, Mexico City, Mexico.

Jorge Alcocer-Varela, MD; Antonio Iglesias, MD; Luis Llorente, BS; Donato Alarcón-Segovia, MS, MD.

Address reprint requests to Dr. Jorge Alcocer-Varela, Instituto Nacional de la Nutrición "Salvador Zubirán," Vasco de Quiroga No. 15, Delegación Tlalpan, Mexico City, D.F., 14000, Mexico.

Submitted for publication October 25, 1983; accepted in revised form August 13, 1984.

them of erythrocytes, passed over a nylon wool column (7), washed twice with phosphate buffered saline (PBS), and used as a T cell–enriched population.

Purification of T4 and T8 cell subsets was done by negative selection with OKT4 and OKT8 monoclonal antibodies (Ortho Pharmaceuticals, Raritan, NJ) and fresh rabbit serum as a source of complement, as described by Thomas et al (9). Cell viability was controlled by trypan blue dye exclusion, by a technician unaware of the conditions of the experiments.

Mitogen stimulation. All cultures were set up in RPMI 1640 (Gibco, Grand Island, NY) supplemented with 10% heat-inactivated, Ig-free fetal calf serum (FCS; Gibco), 100 units/ml penicillin, 100 μg/ml streptomycin, and 2 m*M* glutamine. This enriched medium is subsequently referred to as culture medium (CM). Cultures were carried out at 37°C in a humidified atmosphere of 5% CO_2 in CM. We dispensed 2×10^5 MNC or T cells to a final volume of 200 μl in flat-bottom microwells. All mitogens were added at concentrations previously determined to be optimal. Concanavalin A (Con A; Sigma, St. Louis, MO) was added to a final concentration of 2 μg/ml, phytohemagglutinin P (PHA; Difco, Detroit, MI) at a final concentration of 2 $\mu g/10^6$ cells, and pokeweed mitogen (PWM; Gibco) at a final concentration of 10 $\mu g/10^6$ cells. We added 0.5 μCi of ^{3}H-thymidine (^{3}HTdR; New England Nuclear, Boston, MA) to some of the cells during the last 18 hours of mitogen stimulation. The remaining cells were fixed with 70% ethanol and kept at 4°C for cytofluorographic analysis.

Concanavalin A–induced suppressor function. MNC (1×10^6 cells/ml) were cultured with or without Con A at a concentration of 12.5 μg/ml for 48 hours at 37°C in plastic tubes (Falcon Labware, Oxnard, CA). LCS (Sigma) was dissolved in minimum essential medium (MEM) and further diluted to the desired concentration in CM. To test the effect of LCS, we added it to both Con A–activated and control cells at the start of the cultures. As another control, Con A was added to the nonactivated cells just before they were harvested. Both Con A–activated and control cells were then washed 3 times with MEM. After treatment with mitomycin C (50 μg/ml), the cells were washed 4 times with MEM and adjusted to a final concentration of 1×10^5 cells in 0.1 ml of CM. The cells were then incubated in 96-well flat-bottom microtiter plates. Fresh autologous MNC (2×10^5) in 0.1 ml of CM and 0.05 ml of PWM were added to each well in a final dilution of 1:100. PWM-stimulated, fresh autologous MNC cultured alone served as controls. Experiments were done in triplicate. Cultures were maintained for 72 hours at 37°C with 5% CO_2 in a humidified incubator. Eighteen hours before harvesting, we added 0.5 μCi of ^{3}H-thymidine to each well. The cells were harvested as previously described (10), using a multiple automated sample harvester. Percent suppression induced by Con A was calculated as follows:

$$\frac{\text{cpm of Con A–treated cocultures + PWM}}{\text{cpm of fresh MNC cultures + PWM}} \times 100$$

Enzyme-linked immunosorbent assay (ELISA) method for IgG measurements. To determine the effect of LCS on IgG production, the same supernatants as in the suppressor cell assays were tested with an ELISA method, described by Ceuppens and Goodwin (11). V-bottom polyvinyl microtiter plates (Dynatech Laboratories, Alexandria, VA) were incubated overnight at 4°C with 100 μl goat anti-human IgG (Accurate Chemicals, Westbury, NY) in a concentration of 1 μg/ml. After washing 4 times with PBS, 100 μl of supernatant, diluted 1:10 in PBS with 5% FCS, was added to the wells. After a 2-hour incubation, the plates were again washed 4 times in PBS. One hundred microliters of alkaline phosphatase–labeled goat anti-human Ig was added to the wells. After a 1-hour incubation, the plates were washed 4 more times with PBS, and 100 μl of freshly prepared substrate was added. After 30 minutes the reaction was stopped by adding 50 μl of 3*N* NaOH. The absorption of each well was measured in a Titertek Multiskan micro-ELISA autoreader at 405 nm, and optical densities were translated to nanograms by plotting from the standard curve.

Effect of LCS on the content of nucleic acids of MNC. Ethidium bromide and propidium iodide staining of MNC was performed as described elsewhere (12). For the analysis of cellular DNA/RNA content with these 2 reagents, we used an FC-200 cytofluorograph (Ortho Diagnostic Instruments, Westwood, MA), interfaced to a 2102 multichannel analyzer (Tektronics, Middleton, WI), also as previously described (12). All studies were done under the same conditions of laser intensity, gain, system pressure, and flow. In most cases, 10,000 cells were analyzed in triplicate.

Concentrations of LCS ranging from 0.1–0.001 mg were added at the start of cultures, and day-to-day determinations of the phases of the cell cycle were made during 6 days of culture with cells under mitogen stimulation. These concentrations of LCS were utilized to cover the possible range of serum concentrations of LCS in monkeys fed 180 mg of LCS/day.

DNA binding assays. Antibodies to double-stranded DNA were studied in culture supernatants by Farr radioimmunoassay as described by Lewkonia et al (13).

RESULTS

Effect of LCS on cell viability. After a 6-day period of culture, there were no significant differences in the viability of MNC cultured with LCS, versus control cells (percent viable cells: control, 89.8 ± 0.6; 100 μg/ml LCS, 90.0 ± 0.7).

Effect of LCS on the response to mitogens. We found a significant diminution of ^{3}HTdR incorporation induced on normal cells by PHA or Con A with LCS at concentrations of $\geq$10 μg/ml (Figure 1a). A more pronounced effect of LCS on the thymidine incorporation induced by these mitogens was noted on MNC from SLE patients (Figure 1b). In contrast, no effect of LCS on cells from either normal subjects or SLE patients was noted on the ^{3}HTdR incorporation induced by PWM (Figure 1). Studies done with 6-hour pulses of ^{3}HTdR to prevent radiation damage to cells gave similar results (data not shown).

Effect of LCS on the cell cycle. Analysis of the DNA/RNA content of cells enables determination of

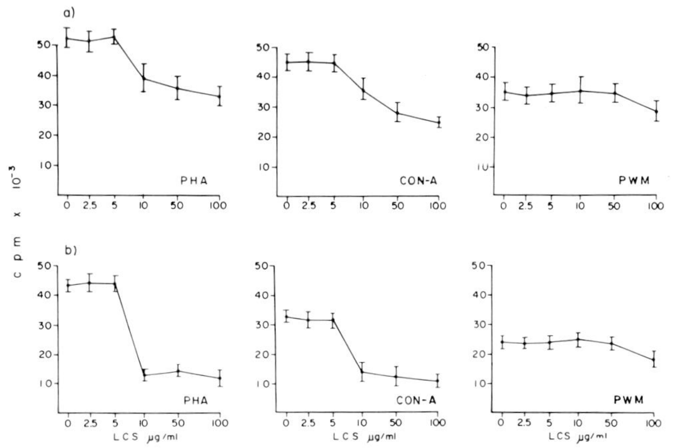

Figure 1. Effect of 5 different concentrations of L-canavanine sulfate (LCS) on the proliferative response of mononuclear cells to phytohemagglutinin (PHA), concanavalin A (Con-A), and pokeweed mitogen (PWM). **a,** Normal cells. **b,** Cells from systemic lupus erythematosus patients. The means ± SE of 7 experiments with each mitogen are shown.

their cell cycle phase (14). The amount of intracellular DNA increases sequentially with progression of the cell cycle from $G_0 + G_1$ (resting) phase to the S and then to the G_2 (pre-mitosis) phase. Incubation with LCS of normal MNC subjected to PHA, Con A, or PWM stimulation caused a significant decrease with PHA and Con A ($P < 0.01$), but not with PWM, in the percentage of MNC that entered into the S and $G_2 + M$ phases of the cell cycle (Table 1). Results of 6-day kinetic studies showing the effect of various concentrations of LCS on the response to PHA and Con A are given in Figure 2. Similar inhibitor effects were noted on separated total T, T4, and T8 subpopulations (Figure 3). However, the decrease was more marked on OKT8 than on OKT4 cells at all 3 doses of LCS, suggesting a preferential effect of LCS on OKT8 cells.

The correlation found between data on thymidine incorporation and cell cycle analysis (r = 0.83) indicates that LCS actually inhibits PHA-induced cell proliferation and is not merely impeding the entrance of thymidine into the cell.

Effect of LCS on Con A–induced suppressor cell function. Mononuclear cells that had been preincubated with Con A were able to suppress the response of fresh autologous MNC to PWM (basal percent suppression: 49.3 ± 3.9, mean ± SEM of 8 different experiments). The addition of LCS at a concentration of 10 μg/ml decreased this suppressor cell function by at least 30% in 5 of 8 experiments (36.3 ± 4.1% suppression). At a 100-μg/ml concentration of LCS, suppressor cell function was decreased in all experiments, albeit modestly in 2 of them (27.7 ± 4.2). The difference was statistically significant at the 0.005 probability level.

To rule out the possibility that LCS was making the fresh PWM-stimulated MNC resistant to suppression, rather than acting on the actual generation of suppression, experiments were done in which we incubated the fresh MNC with LCS. The mean percent suppression in these experiments was similar to that found when no LCS was added (basal, 53.2 ± 1.7; LCS, 51.6 ± 1.6, mean ± SEM) ($P = 0.68$). These findings indicate that LCS interferes with the generation of suppressor cell function upon Con A stimulation.

Effect of LCS on anti-DNA activity in culture supernatants. To determine if the nullifying effect of LCS on Con A–induced suppressor function resulted in increased DNA binding activity in the supernatants of PWM-activated MNC, we tested the supernatants of suppressor cell assays with and without LCS added during their induction phase. These studies were done with MNC from 3 normal subjects and MNC from 3 SLE patients with inactive disease (Table 2). The

Table 1. Effect of L-canavanine sulfate (LCS) on the percentage of cells in each phase of the cell cycle upon mitogen stimulation*

LCS concentration added (μg/ml)	Phase of cell cycle†								
	With PHA			With Con A			With PWM		
	$G_0 + G_1$	S	$G_2 + M$	$G_0 + G_1$	S	$G_2 + M$	$G_0 + G_1$	S	$G_2 + M$
0	59.2 ± 3.0	31.2 ± 2.8	7.3 ± 1.0	65.6 ± 3.7	25.9 ± 2.7	4.2 ± 0.9	72.6 ± 2.8	23.8 ± 3.1	3.1 ± 0.9
2.5	60.3 ± 2.8	27.7 ± 3.5	7.2 ± 1.2	67.2 ± 3.5	26.2 ± 1.9	3.8 ± 0.8	71.5 ± 1.9	22.1 ± 2.6	5.9 ± 0.7
5	62.9 ± 4.2	25.6 ± 3.1	7.1 ± 0.8	71.3 ± 2.5	25.2 ± 3.1	3.0 ± 0.9	76.8 ± 3.1	21.0 ± 1.9	2.9 ± 0.8
10	65.6 ± 2.8	25.6 ± 3.4	6.4 ± 1.0	76.5 ± 2.9	21.7 ± 1.8	3.3 ± 0.5	77.5 ± 2.5	20.4 ± 2.1	3.2 ± 0.4
50	69.6 ± 3.3	23.3 ± 2.7	6.1 ± 0.9	78.1 ± 2.1	18.6 ± 2.8	3.0 ± 0.7	75.4 ± 2.4	22.1 ± 2.0	3.4 ± 0.5
100	81.7 ± 4.0	15.0 ± 3.1	3.1 ± 0.8	84.1 ± 2.5	12.7 ± 2.3	3.1 ± 0.6	74.9 ± 1.7	20.8 ± 2.5	2.5 ± 0.7

* Values shown are mean ± SEM of 6 experiments, after 3 days of culture. PHA = phytohemagglutinin; Con A = concanavalin A; PWM = pokeweed mitogen.
† Determined by DNA content.

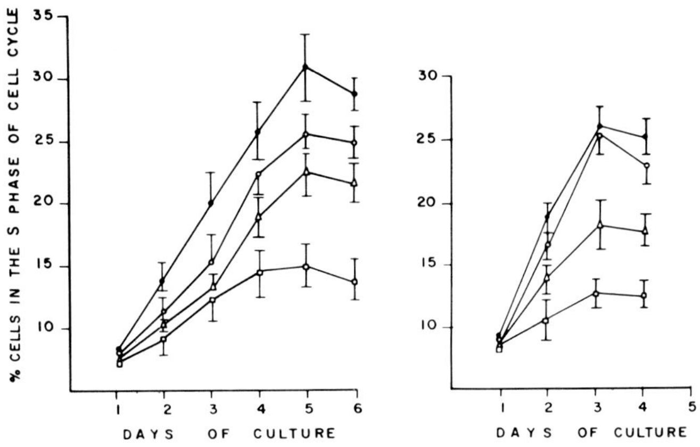

Figure 2. Six-day kinetic studies of the effect of 3 different concentrations of L-canavanine sulfate (LCS) on the percentages of normal cells in the S phase of the cell cycle, with phytohemagglutinin **(left)** and concanavalin A **(right)**. ● = without LCS; ○ = 10 μg/ml of LCS; △ = 50 μg/ml of LCS; □ = 100 μg/ml of LCS.

DNA binding activity found in the supernatants of PWM-stimulated MNC was decreased when they were cocultured with Con A–pretreated cells, but this suppressor effect was abrogated by LCS in a dose-related fashion. This abrogation of suppressor T cell function

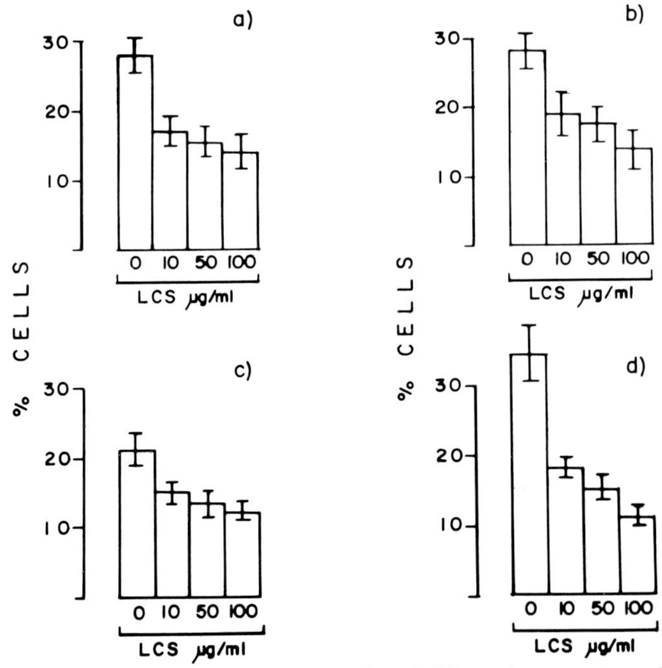

Figure 3. Effect of L-canavanine sulfate (LCS) on the percentage of cells that progress to the S and G_2 + M phases of the cell cycle with phytohemagglutinin stimulation. **a,** Total mononuclear cells. **b,** T cells. **c,** OKT4-enriched cells. **d,** OKT8-enriched cells. Means ± SE of 6 experiments are shown.

Table 2. Effect of L-canavanine added during the induction phase of Con A–induced suppression on the release of DNA binding activity into supernatants of PWM-stimulated normal or SLE mononuclear cells*

Experimental conditions	% binding activity: Normal cells	SLE cells
Suppressor assays		
Without LCS	3.0 ± 1.9	5.5 ± 2.8
With 10 μg/ml LCS	4.4 ± 1.6	13.1 ± 5.9
With 100 μg/ml LCS	6.7 ± 0.7	21.2 ± 5.8
Precultured cells (without Con A)		
Without LCS	6.9 ± 1.4	11.8 ± 1.3
With 10 μg/ml LCS	6.5 ± 1.0	12.3 ± 1.5
With 100 μg/ml LCS	6.8 ± 1.2	11.9 ± 1.2
Control fresh cells (without LCS)		
Without PWM	2.1 ± 0.6	10.4 ± 1.4
With PWM	7.2 ± 2.3	17.8 ± 0.7

* Con A = concanavalin A; PWM = pokeweed mitogen; SLE = systemic lupus erythematosus; LCS = L-canavanine sulfate. Values shown are mean ± SEM of 3 experiments.

on PWM-stimulated B cells was found with both normal and SLE cells but at different levels of DNA binding activity, indicating that further decrease in suppressor T cell control allows for further autoantibody production by polyclonally activated SLE B cells (Table 2).

Effect of LCS on IgG production by B cells from normal subjects and SLE patients. As shown in Table 3, the dose-related effect of LCS on Con A–induced suppression could also be detected by measuring the

Table 3. Effect of L-canavanine added during the induction phase of Con A–induced suppression on the release of IgG into supernatants of PWM-stimulated normal or SLE mononuclear cells*

Experimental conditions	IgG production, ng/ml: Normal cells	SLE cells
Suppressor assays		
Without LCS	735 ± 98	641 ± 106
With 10 μg/ml LCS	918 ± 191	848 ± 171
With 100 μg/ml LCS	1,316 ± 216	1,146 ± 198
Precultured cells (without Con A)		
Without LCS	1,815 ± 196	1,793 ± 148
With 10 μg/ml LCS	1,938 ± 205	2,015 ± 194
With 100 μg/ml LCS	1,748 ± 163	1,976 ± 172
Control fresh cells (without LCS)		
Without PWM	<100	<100
With PWM	2,200 ± 241	1,648 ± 139

* Con A = concanavalin A; PWM = pokeweed mitogen; SLE = systemic lupus erythematosus; LCS = L-canavanine sulfate. Values shown are mean ± SEM of 3 experiments.

release of IgG into the supernatants by PWM-activated B cells.

DISCUSSION

Current concepts of immune regulation in humans postulate a series of T cell circuits on which soluble factors such as lymphokines and thymic hormones act. These T cell circuits have a net regulatory effect on B cells that is mainly determined by the balance of actions of T helper and T suppressor cells (15). Imbalance could result in excessive production of antibodies including autoantibodies. In turn, non-T cells (B cells, monocytes, and perhaps polymorphonuclear leukocytes) activate T lymphocytes in the autologous mixed lymphocyte reaction (16) as well as through soluble mediators (17) and may help regulate them by autoantibodies (18).

Multiple aberrations have been found in spontaneous systemic lupus erythematosus (18), but there is still the unresolved question of whether the primary event is a T cell abnormality leading to the dysregulation or a polyclonal activation of B cells.

Patients who have had drug-related SLE have normal immunoregulatory T cell circuits, whereas patients with long-inactive SLE continue to have detectable abnormalities (19). Several of the main drugs that have been found to be capable of inducing SLE have the property of abrogating the suppressor cell function of normal cells. These include methyldopa (6), diphenylhydantoin (19), procainamide (5,20), and hydralazine (Benveniste P, Llorente L, Alarcón-Segovia D: unpublished observations). Methyldopa causes Coombs'-positive hemolytic anemia more frequently than SLE (21), and it is of interest that the first recognition of the potential for alfalfa to cause autoimmunity was made in a man who developed Coombs'-positive hemolytic anemia (22).

In this study we have shown that LCS causes abrogation of suppressor function in vitro, perhaps by inhibiting the stimulatory effect of Con A, but also possibly by having a preferential effect on the OKT8 (cytotoxic/suppressor) T cell subpopulation.

A dose-response type of effect indicates that this is not due merely to decreased concentrations of mitogen by dilution, but it does not exclude the possibility that LCS counteracts the effect of Con A by acting as a competing ligand. This is unlikely, however, since LCS had an inhibiting effect on both PHA and Con A mitogenic actions.

Studies done on the effect of LCS on autologous mixed lymphocyte reactions and on the production of interleukin-2 excluded the possibility that LCS has an effect on this soluble factor (data not shown). We have also determined that such abrogation of suppressor function leads to increased production of IgG and DNA binding activity by B cells under the effect of PWM. That normal MNC can, when subjected in vitro to mitogenic stimulation, release anti-DNA antibodies into the supernatants has been previously shown by others (20,23,24). The finding of increased IgG in supernatants of B cells subjected to PWM stimulation in the presence of Con A–primed T cells suggests that this DNA binding activity is indeed due to anti-DNA antibodies. The cells from SLE patients readily produced more DNA binding activity than did the normal cells, both upon direct PWM stimulation and when they were subjected to this stimulation after abrogation of Con A suppressor cells by LCS.

The inhibitory effects of LCS on the generation of Con A–induced suppression varied among individual cells. This might help explain why all monkeys fed alfalfa do not develop the disease (1,2). Predisposing factors for the development of drug-related lupus have also been found in either the acetylator phenotype (25), the HLA haplotype (26) or, more likely, both.

Because LCS is an analog of arginine, we conducted studies on the effects of this other amino acid on the cell cycle and found it to have none, thereby indicating the specificity of the effect of LCS (data not shown).

A primate model of human drug-related SLE may be an important tool for research on this disease and its relationship to spontaneously-occurring SLE. More important, however, may be the recognition that some foodstuffs contain substances that can affect immune regulation, and in so doing can elicit autoimmune disease.

There are at least 31 known leguminous plants whose seeds contain L-canavanine (27). Most of them are not usually ingested, at least in America. Whether there may be other LCS-containing plants which, if ingested, might play a role in the development of "spontaneous" SLE in otherwise predisposed individuals is a question that merits further consideration.

REFERENCES

1. Bardana EJ, Malinow MR, Houghton DC, McNulty WP, Wuepper KD, Parker F, Pirofsky B: Diet-induced systemic lupus erythematosus (SLE) in primates. Am J Kidney Dis 1:345–351, 1982
2. Malinow MR, Bardana EJ, Pirofsky B, Craig S: System-

ic lupus erythematosus-like syndrome in monkeys fed alfalfa sprouts: role of a nonprotein amino acid. Science 216:415–417, 1982
3. Roberts JL, Hayashi JA: Exacerbation of SLE associated with alfalfa ingestion (letter). N Engl J Med 308:1361, 1983
4. Alarcón-Segovia D: Drug-induced antinuclear antibodies and lupus syndromes. Drugs 12:69–77, 1976
5. Bluestein HG, Zvaifler NJ, Weisman MH, Shapiro RF: Lymphocyte alteration by procainamide: relation to drug-induced lupus erythematosus syndrome. Lancet 1:816–819, 1979
6. Kirtland HH, Mohler DN, Horwitz DA: Methyldopa inhibition of suppressor-lymphocyte function. N Engl J Med 302:825–832, 1980
7. Laffón A, Alcocer-Varela J, Alarcón-Segovia D: The autologous mixed lymphocyte reaction is not primarily due to xenoantigenic stimulation. Clin Immunol Immunopathol 28:304–308, 1983
8. Tan EM, Cohen AS, Fries JF, Masi AT, McShane DJ, Rothfield NF, Schaller JG, Talal N, Winchester RG: The 1982 revised criteria for the classification of systemic lupus erythematosus. Arthritis Rheum 25:1271–1277, 1982
9. Thomas Y, Sosman J, Irigoyen O, Friedman SM, Kung PC, Goldstein G, Chess L: Functional analysis of human T cell subsets defined by monoclonal antibodies. I. Collaborative T-interactions in the immunoregulation of B cell differentiation. J Immunol 125:2402–2408, 1980
10. Ruíz-Arguelles A, Alarcón-Segovia D, Llorente L, del Giudice-Knipping JA: Heterogeneity of the spontaneously expanded and mitogen-induced generation of suppressor cell function of T cells on B cells in systemic lupus erythematosus. Arthritis Rheum 23:1004–1009, 1980
11. Ceuppens JL, Goodwin JS: Regulation of immunoglobulin production in pokeweed mitogen-stimulated cultures of lymphocytes from young and old adults. J Immunol 128:2429–2434, 1982
12. Alarcón-Segovia D, Llorente L, Fishbein E, Díaz-Jouanen E: Abnormalities in the content of nucleic acids of peripheral blood mononuclear cells from patients with systemic lupus erythematosus: relationship to DNA antibodies. Arthritis Rheum 25:304–317, 1982
13. Lewkonia RM, Barth PT, Hale GM, Hughes GRV: Specificity and clinical relevance of antibodies to double-stranded DNA. Ann Rheum Dis (suppl) 36:114–118, 1977
14. Darzynkiewics Z, Traganos F, Sharpless T, Melamed MR: Cell cycle related changes in nuclear chromatin of stimulated lymphocytes as measured by flow cytometry. Cancer Res 37:4635–4640, 1977
15. Oppenheim JJ, Mizel SB, Meltzer MS: Biological effects of lymphocyte and macrophage derived mitogenic "amplification" factors, Biology of the Lymphokines. Edited by S Cohen, E Pick, JJ Oppenheim. New York, Academic Press, 1978, pp 291–323
16. Kuntz MM, Innes JB, Weksler ME: Lymphocyte transformation induced by autologous cells. IV. Human T lymphocyte proliferation induced by autologous or allogenic non T lymphocytes. J Exp Med 143:1042–1054, 1976
17. Mizel SB: Interleukin 1 and T cell activation. Immunol Rev 63:51–72, 1982
18. Alarcón-Segovia D: Cellular immunity and its regulation in SLE. Clin Rheum Dis 8:63–75, 1982
19. Alarcón-Segovia D, Palacios R: Differences in immunoregulatory T cell circuits between diphenylhydantoin-related and spontaneously occurring systemic lupus erythematosus. Arthritis Rheum 24:1086–1092, 1981
20. Ochi T, Goldings EA, Lipsky PE, Ziff M: Immunomodulatory effect of procainamide in man: inhibition of human suppressor T-cell activity in vitro. J Clin Invest 71:36–45, 1983
21. Worlledge SM, Carstairs KC, Dacie JV: Autoimmune haemolytic anemia associated with α-methyldopa therapy. Lancet 2:135–139, 1966
22. Malinow MR, Bardana EJ Jr, Goodnight SH Jr: Pancytopenia during ingestion of alfalfa seeds (letter). Lancet 1:615, 1981
23. Clough JD, Frank SA, Calabrese LH: Deficiency of T cell mediated regulation of anti-DNA production in systemic lupus erythematosus. Arthritis Rheum 23:24–29, 1980
24. Hoch S, Schur P, Schwaber J: Frequency of anti-DNA antibody producing cells from normals and patients with systemic lupus erythematosus. Clin Immunol Immunopathol 27:28–37, 1983
25. Woosley RL, Drayer DE, Reidenberg MM, Nies AS, Carr K, Oates JA: Effect of acetylator phenotype on the rate at which procainamide induces antinuclear antibodies and the lupus syndrome. N Engl J Med 298:1157–1159, 1978
26. Batchelor JR, Welsh KI, Mansilla Tinoco R, Dollery CT, Hughes GRV, Bernstein R, Ryan P: Hydralazine-induced systemic lupus erythematosus: influence of HLA-DR and sex on susceptibility. Lancet 1:1107–1109, 1980
27. Bell EA: Canavanine in the leguminosae. Biochem J 75:618–620, 1960

LUPUS PREGNANCY

II. Unusual Pattern of Hypocomplementemia and Thrombocytopenia in the Pregnant Patient

MICHAEL D. LOCKSHIN, PETER C. HARPEL, MAURICE L. DRUZIN, CARL G. BECKER, RENATE F. KLEIN, ROSEMARIE M. WATSON, KEITH B. ELKON, and ELIZABETH REINITZ

To explore the causes of complications in pregnant women with systemic lupus erythematosus (SLE), we prospectively evaluated 34 pregnancies in 28 SLE patients, and 2 additional pregnancies in patients with lupus anticoagulant and positive antinuclear antibody, but no other manifestations of SLE. Nineteen pregnancies (55%) were complicated by marked proteinuria, thrombocytopenia, and/or lupus anticoagulant. Hypocomplementemia occurred in 18 pregnancies (52%). Neither thrombocytopenia-anticoagulant nor proteinuria was accompanied by an increase in antibody to double-stranded DNA or by clinical signs of active SLE. Antibody to Ro antigen did not predict fetal death. Both thrombocytopenia and proteinuria appeared abruptly during pregnancy and disappeared quickly after delivery. Fetal death was the result in 7 of 9 (77%) pregnancies in patients with anticoagulant, 6 of 10 (60%) in patients with thrombocytopenia, 6 of 18 (33%) in patients with hypocomplementemia, and 3 of 11 (27%) in patients with proteinuria. Twenty of 29 (68%) children were identified as male. The pathogenesis of hypocomplementemia was evaluated by a new assay, C1s-C1 inhibitor complex, which is thought to measure rate of complement activation by the classical pathway. Most pregnant patients with low CH50 levels and proteinuria had normal levels of C1s-C1 inhibitor complex, whereas nonpregnant patients with equivalent proteinuria and hypocomplementemia had high levels, as did pregnant patients with hypocomplementemia who did not have SLE. Pregnant and nonpregnant hypocomplementemic patients with proteinuria had similar levels of C3 and C4. In pregnant patients with SLE, C1s-C1 inhibitor complex was independent of CH50; in nonpregnant patients a linear relationship between C1s-C1 inhibitor complex and CH50 was seen. We conclude that hypocomplementemia and probably thrombocytopenia (with anticoagulant) occur via different mechanisms in pregnant and nonpregnant patients with SLE.

From The Hospital for Special Surgery, affiliated with The New York Hospital–Cornell University Medical College, New York, The Johns Hopkins University–Good Samaritan Hospital, Baltimore, and The Albert Einstein College of Medicine, New York.

Supported in part by grants from The SLE Foundation, Inc., New York, The Arthritis Foundation Arthritis Clinical Center, NIH (AM 32929 and AM 32845), USPHS (HL-18828: Specialized Center of Research in Thrombosis), and NIH (T32-AM07324).

Michael D. Lockshin, MD; Peter C. Harpel, MD; Maurice L. Druzin, MD; Carl G. Becker, MD; Renate F. Klein, BS; Rosemarie M. Watson, MD; Keith B. Elkon, MB: Rockefeller Brothers Clinical Scholar; Elizabeth Reinitz, MD.

Address reprint requests to Michael D. Lockshin, MD, The Hospital for Special Surgery, 535 East 70th Street, New York, NY 10021.

Submitted for publication January 13, 1984; accepted in revised form July 17, 1984.

In a prospective study of pregnancies in women with systemic lupus erythematosus (SLE), we noted that signs indicating activation of SLE were restricted to proteinuria, thrombocytopenia, and lupus anticoagulant, without other organ system involvement, suggesting that typical lupus exacerbation was not occurring (1). Therefore, in this study we evaluated the pathogenesis of these abnormalities in the pregnant SLE patient and the effect of these abnormalities on fetal outcome.

PATIENTS AND METHODS

Patients. Twenty-eight women with known SLE (2) who did not elect abortion were prospectively evaluated during 34 pregnancies. Twenty of these pregnancies were included in our prior study (1). Of the 28 patients, 2 had first diagnosis of SLE during pregnancy (both with anamnestic evidence for disease duration of more than 2 years); 2 pregnancies in 2 patients with equivocal SLE (positive antinuclear antibody, lupus anticoagulant, and strong family history of rheumatic disease but neither symptoms nor anti-DNA antibody) were also evaluated where indicated in the text. Patients were studied for manifestations of the criteria listed below at least once each trimester, but as frequently as weekly during late pregnancy. For comparisons in the C3, C4, and C1r-C1s-C1 inhibitor studies, pregnant patients with non-SLE rheumatic disease and nonpregnant patients with classic SLE (with CH50 levels equivalent to those of pregnant patients) were selected from the same clinics from which the pregnant patients originated.

Clinical and laboratory evaluations. Serial studies included routine urinalysis, creatinine clearance, 24-hour urine protein, anti-DNA antibody, and CH50. C3, C4, and C1s-C1 inhibitor complex, platelet count, and lupus anticoagulant (identified initially by activated partial thromboplastin time [APTT] >40 seconds and confirmed by coagulation studies including the demonstration that the APTT did not correct when fresh plasma was added) (3) were studied in selected patients. Further clinical evidence included a scoring of SLE activity, obstetric notations of fetal status, and newborn evaluation for congenital defects (especially cardiac arrhythmia by electrocardiogram), Apgar score, weight, and sex.

Laboratory methods. Anti-DNA antibody was measured by the binding assay as previously described (4) or, where indicated, by a millipore filter assay (5). Hemolytic complement was measured by the method of Kent and Fife (6); C3 and C4 protein were measured by nephelometry. C1s-C1 inhibitor (C1s-C1Inh) complex was measured by an enzyme-linked immunosorbent assay previously described (7,8). Antibody to Ro antigen (SS-A) was measured by counterimmunoelectrophoresis using a human spleen antigen (9).

Statistical methods. Two-by-two comparisons were tested by chi-square analysis with Yates' correction. Means

Table 1. Pregnancy outcomes of 30 patients with systemic lupus erythematosus (SLE)*

Patient	Week termination	Sex of child	Live-born	Anti-Ro	CH50 <150 units/ml	APTT >40 seconds	Platelets < 150 × 10^3/mm^3	Protein-uria–hyper-tension	Prior renal disease
1b	6	U	N	ND	0	0	0	0	Y
2b	12	U	N	0	+	+	+	0	N
2c	14	U	N	0	+	+	+	0	N
3	15	U	N	ND	0	+	+	0	N
4b	21	U	N	0	0	+	0	0	N
2a	22	M	N	0	+	+	+	0	N
5	24	F	N	0	+	0	0	+	Y
6	27	M	N	ND	+	0	0	+	Y
7	27	M	Y	0	0	0	0	0	N
8	28	M	Y	0	0	0	0	0	N
29	28	F	Y	0	+	0	+	+	Y
9	29	M	N	0	+	0	+	+	U
4a	30	F	N	0	0	+	+	0	N
10	31	F	Y	0	+	0	0	+	N
11	34	M	Y	0	ND	0	0	+	U
12	35	M	Y	0	0	0	0	0	Y
13	35	M	Y	ND	0	0	0	+	Y
14	36	M	Y	0	+	ND	0	0	N
15	36	M	Y	+	+	0	0	0	N
16a	36	F	Y	0	0	0	+	+	N
27	36	M	Y	+	+	0	0	0	N
17	37	M	Y	0	+	+	+	0	Y
18	38	M	Y	0	+	0	0	+	Y
19	38	M	Y	+	+	0	0	0	N
20	39	M	Y	0	+	0	+	0	Y
21	39	F	Y	ND	0	0	0	+	Y
16b	39	F	Y	0	0	0	0	0	N
1a	40	F	Y	ND	0	0	0	0	Y
1c	40	F	Y	0	0	0	0	0	Y
22	40	F	Y	ND	+	ND	0	0	N
23	42	M	Y	0	+	0	0	0	Y
24	43	M	Y	0	0	0	0	+	Y
25	43	M	Y	0	+	0	0	0	N
26	43	F	Y	0	0	0	0	0	N
29	28	M	N	0	0	0	0	0	N
30	34	M	Y	0	0	0	0	0	N

* Patients 29 and 30 have equivocal SLE. APTT = activated partial thromboplastin time; U = unknown; N = no; ND = not done; 0 = negative or absent; Y = yes; + = positive or present.

Table 2. Mean platelet counts in 4 patients with sustained thrombocytopenia during 6 pregnancies*

Patient	During pregnancy: Determination (no.)	During pregnancy: Platelets/mm^3 × 10^{-3}	More than 1 month after pregnancy: Determinations (no.)	More than 1 month after pregnancy: Platelets/mm^3 × 10^{-3}
2a	1	25	2	203 ± 14
2b	5	93 ± 9	3	145 ± 15
2c	7	91 ± 12	4	130 ± 19
4a	7	143 ± 24	7	219 ± 38
17	16	57 ± 36	9	115 ± 29
28	17	133 ± 41	1	214

* In each pregnancy except 4a, thrombocytopenia was treated with 60–80 mg/day prednisone without recovery of platelet counts. Despite a rapid taper of corticosteroid dose, postpartum platelet count rose, but not always to normal levels.

were tested with Student's *t*-test. Regression analysis was performed with a Visiplot/Visitrend program on an Apple II+ computer.

RESULTS

Pregnancy survival. The 30 women (including the 2 with equivocal disease) carried 36 children. Two patients had 3 pregnancies, and 2 patients had 2. The outcomes of these pregnancies are detailed in Table 1. No recognizable major anatomic congenital anomalies occurred in children that survived or those that died after 20 weeks gestation (anatomic studies on fetuses surviving less than 20 weeks gestation were not satisfactory in any case). Eleven infants (30%) died, 4 during the first 20 weeks gestation and 7 between 21 and 30 weeks (Table 1). All deaths occurred in utero.

Thrombocytopenia and lupus anticoagulant: frequency and fetal outcome. Six pregnant patients had both thrombocytopenia and lupus anticoagulant, 4 had thrombocytopenia alone (3 of the 4 also had preeclampsia), and 3 (2 with equivocal SLE) had anticoagulant alone. Fetal death occurred in 5 of the 6 (83%) pregnancies in patients having both abnormalities, 3 before 20 weeks and 2 after. One patient with preeclampsia and thrombocytopenia miscarried; 2 others were urgently delivered of living children. Only 1 patient with lupus anticoagulant had a normal pregnancy; the other 2 pregnancies resulted in fetal death.

Thrombocytopenia: clinical pattern in pregnant patients. In patients with both thrombocytopenia and anticoagulant, there appeared to be a direct relationship between platelet count and pregnancy (Table 2 and Figure 1). Platelets remained low during pregnancy *despite therapy* and returned to baseline within 3 weeks postpartum. The pregnant patients with thrombocytopenia had a history of prior thrombocytopenia. Two patients studied had abundant megakaryocytes on bone marrow examination; 1 of the 2 studied had antiplatelet antibodies. In only 2 pregnant patients did platelet count fall to less than 50,000/mm^3. In 1 patient, the lowest count was 130,000/mm^3 (Figure 1). None of the 3 live-born children had thrombocytopenia; however, 1 newborn of a mother with normal platelet counts was thrombocytopenic.

Hypocomplementemia (CH50): frequency and fetal outcome. Moderate hypocomplementemia, defined by 150 > CH50 > 50 units/ml, occurred transiently throughout pregnancy in 18 of 27 (66%) pregnancies with antepartum data; CH50 levels in pregnant SLE patients were lower than is usually reported for normal pregnancies (10–17). Complications occurred in 12 of 18 (66%) pregnancies in patients with hypocomplementemia at any time during pregnancy and in 8 of 15 (53%) pregnancies in patients without hypocomplementemia (difference not significant).

Hypocomplementemia (CH50): C3 and C4 pattern. Sera with low CH50 from pregnant patients and from nonpregnant SLE patients were chosen for further evaluation of the complement pathway. Same specimen evaluations demonstrated low normal mean C3 and C4 in both patient groups (Table 3), with linear correlation between C3, C4, and CH50 only in the nonpregnant group (data not shown). Specimens analyzed were primarily from the second trimester, but results were independent of the duration of the pregnancy. In both groups, the C3–C4 pattern suggested classical pathway complement activation. Complement varied independently of anti-DNA antibody; the latter changed little during pregnancy.

Hypocomplementemia (CH50): C1s-C1Inh complex. This test, which is thought to measure the rate of classical complement pathway activation, had normal

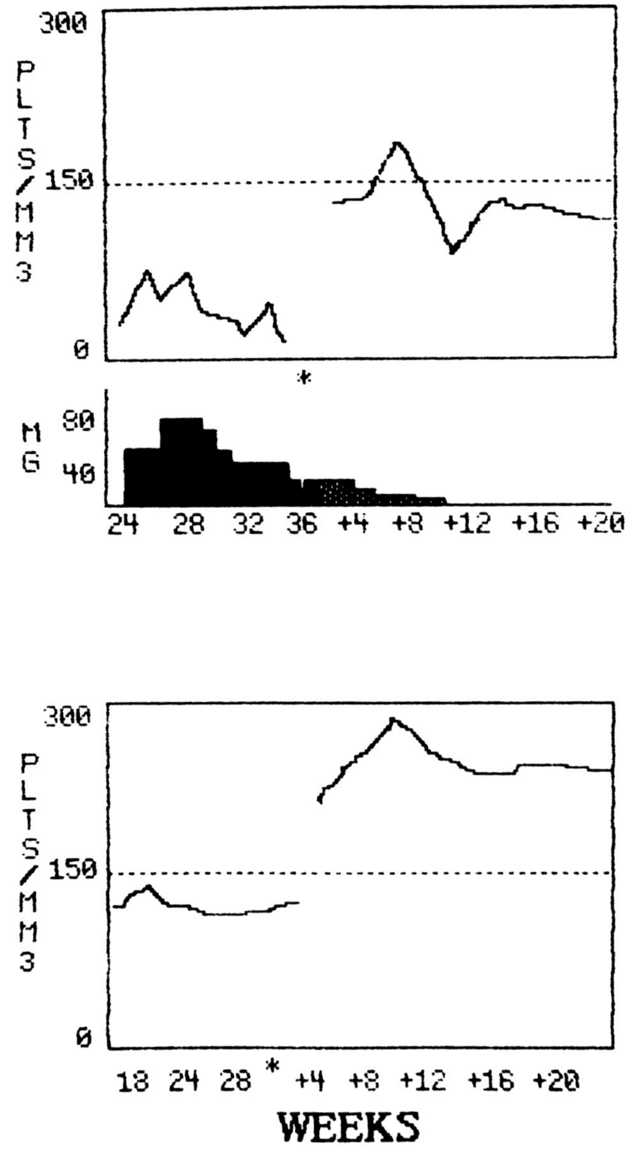

Figure 1. **Top**, Serial platelet counts (PLTS) ($\times 10^{-3}$) in patient 17, noted to be severely thrombocytopenic at 24 weeks gestation (last normal count at week 10). From week 24 on, she received high-dose prednisone therapy (maximum 80 mg/day) without apparent response. At 36 weeks, she received intravenous gamma globulin and delivered by Caesarian section. Despite withdrawal of prednisone therapy, her platelet count remained at a much higher level (although subnormal) for >20 weeks. **Bottom**, Serial platelet counts in patient 4a. Her modest thrombocytopenia first appeared at week 18 (last normal count at week 8). Because the platelet count remained in a "safe" range, she did not receive any corticosteroid therapy, but suffered spontaneous fetal death at 30 weeks, at which time platelet count spontaneously rose to normal levels. (During her second pregnancy her platelet count remained at or above 150,000/mm^3.) Numbers in both panels are weeks ante (no symbol) and post (+) partum. Asterisk indicates time of delivery.

Table 3. C3, C4, CH50, and C1s-C1 inhibitor complex determined on single specimens from pregnant and nonpregnant systemic lupus erythematosus patients with equivalent hypocomplementemia (CH50)

Test	Normal value	12 pregnant patients (mean ± SD)	9 nonpregnant patients (mean ± SD)
CH50, units/ml	≥150	111.6 ± 19.2	102.2 ± 35.9
C3, mg/dl	≥64	84.9 ± 37.2	68.1 ± 7.7
C4, mg/dl	≥10.6	17.5 ± 9.7	11.9 ± 5.2
C1s-C1Inh complex, nmoles/ml*	<12	6.6 ± 7.2	15.3 ± 8.0

* Although the mean values for the C1s-C1 inhibitor complex were abnormal for nonpregnant patients and normal for pregnant patients, none of the differences is statistically significant. There is partial overlap among the patients represented in Tables 3 and 4.

results in hypocomplementemic (CH50) pregnant SLE patients (Tables 3 and 4). Segregating pregnant and nonpregnant SLE patients for both proteinuria and hypocomplementemia demonstrated very high levels of C1s-C1Inh complex in hypocomplementemic proteinuric nonpregnant patients, but in most hypocomplementemic proteinuric pregnant patients levels were normal, despite equivalent levels of C3 and C4 in both groups (Table 4). Four pregnant patients had elevated levels of C1s-C1Inh complex (Figure 2); these patients may have had active SLE. Regression statistics calculated for C1s-C1Inh complex versus CH50 for nonpregnant SLE patients demonstrated strong and highly significant correlation, but for pregnant SLE patients (including the 4 with high levels of C1s-C1Inh complex) no correlation was made (Figure 2).

Nine non-SLE patients, none with proteinuria or abnormal renal function, were also examined. Five (3 with suspected SLE, 1 with discoid LE, 1 with scleroderma) were normocomplementemic and had normal C1s-C1Inh complex (mean 3.3 ± 3.1 nmoles/ml, range 0–4.3). Four (2 with cutaneous vasculitis, 1 with Raynaud's phenomenon, 1 asymptomatic) were hypocomplementemic, and each had abnormal C1s-C1Inh complex (mean 74.5 ± 48.7 nmoles/ml, range 18.8–145). Thus, pregnancy does not prevent abnormal values in this assay. Several of the nonpregnant SLE patients were treated with corticosteroids, as were the 4 SLE pregnant patients with abnormal values (Figure 2). Corticosteroids, therefore, also do not prevent abnormal values in this assay. Since none of the non-SLE patients had evidence of renal disease, clinical nephritis is not required for a positive C1s-C1Inh complex test.

Other phenomena related to fetal survival. *Ro antibody*. Ro antibody was determined in 27 pregnant patients; it was positive in 3, all carrying healthy male infants without heart block. One developed rash and thrombocytopenia within the first week of extrauterine life and was considered to have neonatal SLE. Eight fetal deaths occurred in Ro negative patients.

Fetal sex. Since congenital SLE is predominantly found in women (18,19), we recorded the sex of the newborn, whether living or dead. Twenty of 29 children (68%) (including those of the 2 patients with equivocal SLE) were male; fetal survival was independent of fetal sex after 20 weeks gestation; before 20 weeks (4 pregnancies), sex was unknown. The male predominance of children is statistically significant ($P < 0.05$ in a 2-tailed test). Frequencies of neither thrombocytopenia nor proteinuria were influenced by fetal sex.

Pattern of renal disease. Abrupt proteinuria, usually associated with hypertension and hypocomplementemia but not with edema, occurred in 11 patients and was associated with fetal death in the 3 of 4 cases where onset occurred before 30 weeks gestation. Preexisting known renal disease, hypertension, or proteinuria was present in 6 and absent in 4 pregnant patients with this complication (1 unknown). Conversely, if renal disease was identified prior to pregnancy, the risk of hypertension–proteinuria during pregnancy was 37% (6/16); if kidneys were normal prior to pregnancy the risk was 12% (2/16, $P > 0.2$). Proteinuria, when it occurred during pregnancy, rapidly increased (as high as 17.7 gm/dl), did not respond to corticosteroid therapy, and rapidly decreased after delivery in 9 of 10 patients. Hypocomplementemia was present in 6 of 10 patients with hypertension and proteinuria (1 unknown), but 12 hypocomplementemic patients did not develop renal complications during pregnancy. Significant hematuria and cellular casts did not occur. Other clinical manifestations of active SLE were not present, nor did anti-DNA antibody rise.

Other serologic and clinical manifestations of SLE. Anti-DNA antibody levels were generally low in pregnant patients. Patients with high anti-DNA antibody levels on the first visit had, in general, poorer fetal and maternal outcome, but there was no correlation between DNA antibody and thrombocytopenia–lupus anticoagulant, or between anti-DNA antibody and hypertension–proteinuria. Other clinical manifestations of disease activity were infrequent during pregnancy (1).

DISCUSSION

We previously found that signs of flare during lupus pregnancy appear to be restricted to 2 syndromes: lupus anticoagulant–thrombocytopenia and hypocomplementemia–proteinuria (1). In this study, we specifically asked whether the pathogenesis of these 2 abnormalities occurring in pregnant patients differs from that in nonpregnant patients. The importance of the question is emphasized by the role the abnormalities play in fetal outcome (all but 1 of the fetal deaths were associated with 1 of these abnormali-

Table 4. C1s-C1 inhibitor (C1s-C1Inh) complex in pregnancy complicated by moderate hypocomplementemia (with and without proteinuria)

Patient group: CH50, units/ml	Patient group: Urine protein, gm/dl	Assay*	Pregnant: No.	Pregnant: Mean ± SD	Nonpregnant: No.	Nonpregnant: Mean ± SD
≥150	<0.5	C1s-C1Inh	12	6.2 ± 7.5	7	1.1 ± 2.7
		CH50		210 ± 58		166 ± 34
<150	<0.5	C1s-C1Inh	8	4.3 ± 4.8	6	4.5 ± 9.5
		CH50		117 ± 16		115 ± 9
<150	≥0.5	C1s-C1Inh	9	4.1 ± 5.4	11	22.2 ± 22.2†
		CH50		104 ± 21		102 ± 19

* C1s-C1Inh complex, nmoles/ml; CH50, units/ml. Despite equivalent levels of CH50 and proteinuria, pregnant patients did not demonstrate abnormal levels of C1s-C1 inhibitor complex, while nonpregnant patients did. Patients without proteinuria also had normal levels of C1s-C1 inhibitor complex.
† $T = 2.37$, $P < 0.05$ versus pregnant.

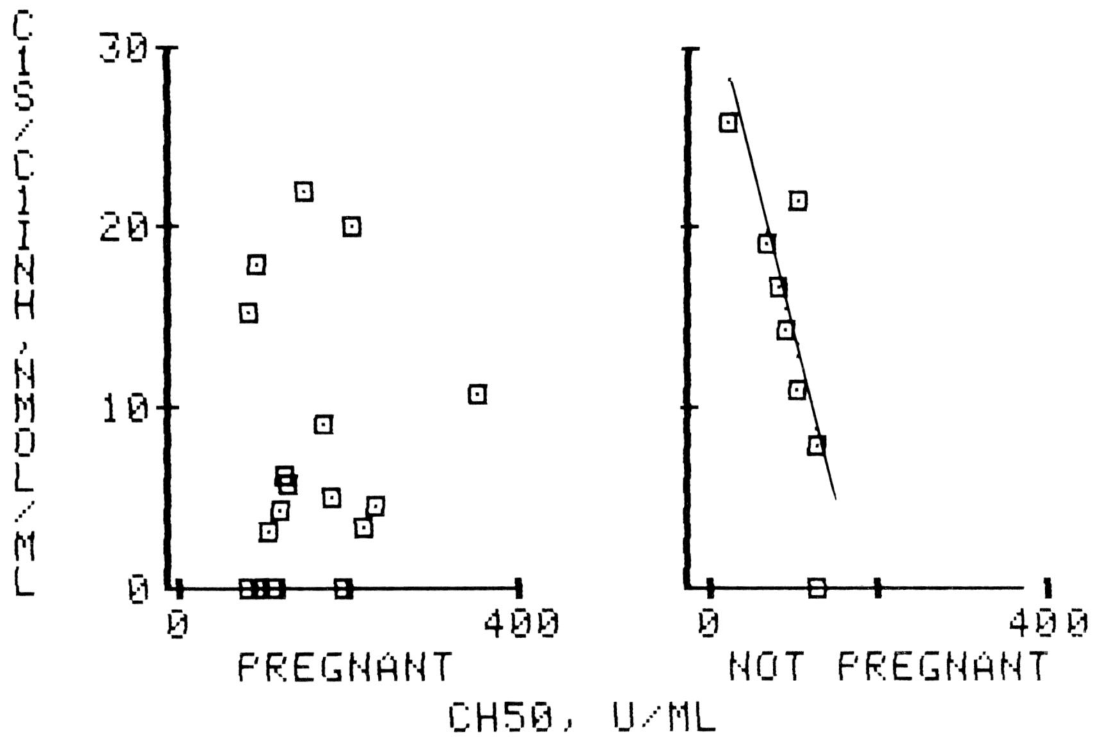

Figure 2. Correlation between C1s-C1 inhibitor (C1s-C1Inh) complex and CH50 in pregnant and nonpregnant systemic lupus erythematosus patients with proteinuria. For pregnant patients no correlation is present, whereas for nonpregnant patients there is close correlation ($P < 0.05$). The 4 abnormal values in pregnant patients (all treated) suggest that neither pregnancy nor corticosteroid therapy can account for negative test results.

ties) and by the need to understand whether these abnormalities occurring in pregnancy should be treated as evidence of active SLE or as pregnancy complications independent of active SLE.

The association of the lupus anticoagulant with fetal death has been noted before (20–25), most frequently as a cause of spontaneous abortion in otherwise healthy women. In the cited patients, mild thrombocytopenia frequently accompanied the anticoagulant, though this was not emphasized. Our experience confirms the prognostic importance of the lupus anticoagulant. Unlike other authors (24), we did not find high-dose corticosteroids uniformly helpful. The mechanism of fetal death in patients with anticoagulant–thrombocytopenia is speculative; placental vasculopathy has been demonstrated in lupus pregnancies, but correlation of specific, clinical SLE-related abnormalities or fetal outcome with placental pathology has not been sought (24,26,27). In our patients with fetal distress or fetal death after 20 weeks, vasculopathy or placental infarction is not the explanation (manuscript in preparation).

The effect of pregnancy on maternal platelet count and APTT, rather than vice versa, has received little attention. In our patients, pregnancy exacerbated preexisting (slight) thrombocytopenia (Figure 1), and remission of thrombocytopenia was prompt following delivery. In normal pregnancies, platelet life-span, measured indirectly, is shortened (28,29). Presumably, increased platelet production prevents the occurrence of clinically apparent thrombocytopenia during normal pregnancy. Recently Miller et al (30) and Gladman et al (31) described 2 patterns of thrombocytopenia in SLE, one a chronic form, which bore no relationship to other signs of clinical SLE activity, the other an acute form, which most frequently appeared during clinical SLE flares. The pattern of thrombocytopenia seen in our pregnant patients matches neither of these forms: it appeared abruptly with pregnancy in the absence of other signs of lupus activity, and it disappeared with the termination of the pregnancy. Although an association between thrombocytopenia and Ro antibody has been noted (32), no such association occurred in our patients.

In patients with hypertension–proteinuria, distinction between pregnancy-induced hypertension (33) and acute lupus glomerulonephritis is both difficult and critical. Although the pathologic pictures of lupus nephritis and pregnancy-induced hypertension differ (34), biopsies could not be done on our patients. We suggest that the abrupt onset, the failure to respond to therapy during pregnancy, the relative absence of formed elements in the urine, and the rapid remission following delivery are more consistent with pregnancy-induced hypertension than with lupus nephritis. Preexisting lupus nephritis predisposing to pregnancy-induced hypertension is probable.

Since hypocomplementemia is typically associated with active immunologically-mediated SLE glomerulonephritis, the occurrence of hypocomplementemia in pregnant patients might suggest that the renal disease seen in pregnancy is active lupus nephritis, not pregnancy-induced hypertension. In a normal pregnancy, complement, measured by C3, C4, CH50, or other assays, usually is supernormal in the third trimester (10–17). In pregnancy-induced hypertension lower mean levels, within the normal range, are seen, but wide scatter of points is typical; many patients have distinctly subnormal values (10–17). In a normal pregnancy, C1 inhibitor is altered only slightly, if at all (13,16), and C3d is increased (35).

The C1s-C1Inh complex assay, which measures classical pathway complement activation, may function as a proxy for classical pathway complement activation rate (6,7,36). In *most* pregnant SLE patients with hypocomplementemia, normal values for C1s-C1Inh complex occurred; in SLE patients with hypocomplementemia and proteinuria who were not pregnant, highly abnormal values occurred. In pregnant patients without SLE, C1s-C1Inh complex levels were high when serum complement levels were low. Thus the normal C1s-C1Inh complex in hypocomplementemic SLE pregnant patients is unusual compared with other hypocomplementemic patients, with or without pregnancy, and with or without nephritis. We therefore believe the pathogenesis of hypocomplementemia in pregnant SLE patients with low levels of C1s-C1Inh complex (but not in those with high levels) differs from that of hypocomplementemia in nonpregnant SLE patients with proteinuria, and we speculate that hypocomplementemia in a subset of pregnant lupus patients is due to decreased complement synthesis rather than to increased activation of the classical pathway. Selective alternate pathway activation is unlikely because of the low C4 levels seen. The eventual identification of complement degradation products will confirm or refute this speculation. However, since C3d levels are increased in a normal pregnancy (35), and since there is considerable controversy regarding measurement of fluid phase (versus cell membrane–associated) complement degradation (37,38), confirmation will prove difficult. Pending this confirmation, we suggest that hypocomplementemia occurring in most pregnant SLE patients does not support the diagnosis of active SLE glomerulonephritis.

The predominance of male births was unexpected. Only 1 prior study presented data on sex ratio of children; it also found male predominance (19 males of 31 births, a ratio similar to ours) (39). The reason for this is not clear, though it is tempting to speculate that female fetuses of SLE patients suffer a selective disadvantage (i.e., die before 20 weeks gestation). The high proportion of newborns with congenital SLE who are girls (18,19) indirectly supports this speculation, if congenital SLE predisposes to fetal death. However, antibody to Ro antigen, which is closely associated with congenital SLE (18,19,40–43), did not explain the in utero deaths in the current series, and the 4 fetuses who had fetal cardiograms recorded, and who subsequently died did not show evidence of congenital heart block.

The findings of this study suggest a reevaluation of our assumptions regarding the pathogenesis of complications of lupus pregnancy. The common assumption that pregnancy complications are manifestations of lupus flare implies that pregnancy induces an increment of (immunologically-defined) lupus activity. Our alternative hypothesis is that pregnancy-related phenomena uncover preexisting, but immunologically stable, SLE-induced organ system damage. The clinical and immunologic differences between pregnant and nonpregnant SLE patients with thrombocytopenia, hypocomplementemia, or abrupt onset of proteinuria support our hypothesis. A third hypothesis, that pregnancy modifies disease expression selectively in different organ systems, currently has no clinical or theoretical support.

The conclusion that pregnancy complications may not be (primarily) immunologically mediated implies that corticosteroid therapy should not be the first treatment, at least for a subset of clinically deteriorating, pregnant SLE patients. Whether a primary induction of remission by corticosteroid therapy should be attempted in all lupus pregnancies, however, is also speculative.

REFERENCES

1. Lockshin MD, Reinitz E, Druzin M, Murrman M, Estes D: Lupus pregnancy. I. Case-control prospective study demonstrating no lupus exacerbation during or after pregnancy. Am J Med 77:893–898, 1984

2. Cohen AS, Reynolds WE, Franklin EC, Kulka JP, Ropes MW, Shulman LE, Wallace SL: Preliminary criteria for the classification of systemic lupus erythematosus. Bull Rheum Dis 21:643–648, 1971
3. Schleider MA, Nachman RL, Jaffe EA, Coleman M: A clinical study of the lupus anticoagulant. Blood 48:499–509, 1976
4. Hughes GRV, Cohen SA, Christian CL: Anti-DNA activity in systemic lupus erythematosus. Ann Rheum Dis 30:259–264, 1971
5. Ginsberg B, Keiser H: A millipore filter assay of antibodies to native DNA in sera of patients with systemic lupus erythematosus. Arthritis Rheum 16:119–207, 1973
6. Kent JF, Fife EH: Precise standardization of reagents for complement fixation. Am J Trop Med Hyg 12:103–116, 1963
7. Harpel PC, Cooper NR: Circulating C1 inactivator-C1s, C1r complexes: quantification by an enzyme-linked differential antibody immunosorbent assay (abstract). Clin Res 30:536A, 1982
8. Inman RD, Harpel PC: C1 inactivator-C1s complexes in inflammatory joint disease. Clin Exp Immunol 53:521–528, 1983
9. Kurata N, Tan EM: Identification of antibodies to nuclear acidic antigens by counterimmunoelectrophoresis. Arthritis Rheum 19:574–580, 1976
10. Johansen KA, Williams JH, Stark JM: Acute-phase C56-forming ability and concentrations of complement components in normotensive and hypertensive pregnancies. Br J Obstet Gynaecol 88:504, 1981
11. Kitzmiller JL, Stoneburner L, Yelenosky PF, Lucas WE: Serum complement in normal pregnancy and pre-eclampsia. Am J Obstet Gynecol 117:312–315, 1973
12. Koslowski JP, Guiguet M, Taquoi G, Jahier J, Feldman JP, Mavel A, Galland JP: Complement (C3 et CH50) et immuno-globulines seriques au cours de la toxemie gravidique. J Gynecol Obstet Biol Reprod (Paris) 7:923–931, 1978
13. Ogston D, Walker J, Campbell DM: C1 inactivator level in pregnancy. Thromb Res 23:453–455, 1981
14. Prall RH, Kantor FS: Serum complement in eclamptogenic toxemia. Am J Obstet Gynecol 95:530–533, 1966
15. Schena FP, Manno C, Selvaggi L, Loverro G, Bettocchi S, Bonomo L: Behaviour of immune complexes and the complement system in normal pregnancy and pre-eclampsia. J Clin Lab Immunol 7:21–36, 1982
16. Tedder RS, Nelson M, Eisen V: Effects of serum complement on normal and pre-eclamptic pregnancy and of oral contraceptives. Br J Exp Pathol 56:389–395, 1975
17. Yang SL, Kleinman AM, Wei PY: Immunologic aspects of term pregnancy toxemia. Am J Obstet Gynecol 122:727–731, 1975
18. Lockshin MD, Gibofsky A, Peebles CL, Gigli I, Fotino M, Hurwitz S: Neonatal lupus erythematosus with heart block: family study of a patient with anti-SS-A and SS-B antibodies. Arthritis Rheum 26:210–213, 1983
19. Lee LA, Weston WL: New findings in neonatal lupus erythematosus. Am J Dis Child 138:233–236, 1984
20. Carreras LO, Machin SJ, Deman R, Defreyn G, Vermylen J, Spitz B, Van Assche A: Arterial thrombosis, intrauterine death and "lupus" anticoagulant: detection of immunoglobulin interfering with prostacyclin formation. Lancet 1:244, 1981
21. Nilsson IM, Astedt B, Hedner U, Berezin D: Intrauterine death and circulating anticoagulant ("antithromboplastin"). Acta Med Scand 197:153–159, 1975
22. Soulier J-P, Boffa M-C: Avortement a repetition, thromboses et anticoagulant circulant anti-thromboplastine. Nouv Presse Med 9:859–864, 1980
23. Firkin BG, Howard MA, Radford N: Possible relationship between lupus inhibitor and recurrent abortion in young women (letter). Lancet 2:366, 1980
24. De Wolf F, Carreras LO, Moerman P, Vermylen J, van Assche A, Renaer M: Decidual vasculopathy and extensive placental infarction in a patient with repeated thromboembolic accidents, recurrent fetal loss and a lupus anticoagulant. Am J Obstet Gynecol 142:829–834, 1982
25. Lubbe WF, Palmer SJ, Butler WS, Liggins GC: Fetal survival after prednisone suppression of maternal lupus-anticoagulant. Lancet 1:1361–1363, 1983
26. Abramowsky CR, Vegas ME, Swinehart G, Byves MT: Decidual vasculopathy of the placenta in lupus erythematosus. N Engl J Med 303:668–672, 1980
27. Abramowsky CR: Lupus erythematosus, the placenta and pregnancy: a natural experiment in immunologically mediated reproductive failure. Prog Clin Biol Res 70:309–320, 1981
28. Fay RA, Hughes AO, Farron NT: Platelets in pregnancy: hyperdestruction in pregnancy. Obstet Gynecol 61:238–240, 1983
29. Horger EO, Keane MWD: Platelet disorders in pregnancy. Clin Obstet Gynecol 22:843–857, 1979
30. Miller MH, Urowitz MB, Gladman DD: The significance of thrombocytopenia in systemic lupus erythematosus. Arthritis Rheum 26:1181–1186, 1983
31. Gladman DD, Urowitz MB, Tozman EC, Glynn MFX: Haemostatic abnormalities in systemic lupus erythematosus. Q J Med 52:424–433, 1983
32. Morley KD, Bernstein RM, Bunn CC, Gharavi AE, Fortin MT, Chipping PM, Hughes GRV: Thrombocytopenia and anti-Ro (letter). Lancet 2:940, 1981
33. Gant NF, Worley RJ: Hypertension in Pregnancy, Concepts and Management. New York, Appleton-Century-Crofts, 1980
34. Spargo BH, Lichtig C, Luger AM, Katz AJ, Lindheimer MD: The renal lesion in pre-eclampsia, Hypertension in Pregnancy. Edited by MD Lindheimer, AJ Katz, FP Zuspan. New York, J Wiley & Sons, 1976, pp 129–138
35. Teisner B, Hau J, Tucker M, Lahood J, Grudzinskas JG: Circulating C3, C4, and C3 split products (C3c and C3d) during normal pregnancy. Am J Reprod Immunol 2:309–311, 1982

36. Hack CE, Eerenberg-Belmer JM, Lim UG, Haverman J, Aalberse RC: Lack of activation of C1, despite circulating immune complexes detected by two C1q methods in patients with rheumatoid arthritis. Arthritis Rheum 27:40–48, 1984
37. Davis AE III, Harrison RA, Lachmann PJ: Physiologic inactivation of fluid phase C3b: isolation and structural analysis of C3c, C3d,g (alpha 2 D), and C3g. J Immunol 132:1960–1966, 1984
38. Medof ME, Lam T, Prince GM, Mold CM: Requirement for human red blood cells in immune complexes and enhancement of binding to spleen cells. J Immunol 130: 1336–1340, 1983
39. Varner MW, Meehan RT, Syrop CH, Strottman MP, Goplerud CP: Pregnancy in patients with systemic lupus erythematosus. Am J Obstet Gynecol 145:1025–1040, 1983
40. Scott JS, Maddison PJ, Taylor PV, Esscher E, Scott O, Skinner RP: Connective tissue disease, antibodies to ribonucleoprotein, and congenital heart block. N Engl J Med 309:209–212, 1983
41. Vetter VL, Rashkind WJ: Congenital complete heart block and connective tissue disease. N Engl J Mcd 309:236–238, 1983
42. Provost TT: Commentary: neonatal lupus erythematosus. Arch Dermatol 19:619–621, 1983
43. Weston WL, Harmon C, Peebles C, Manchester D, Franco HL, Huff JC, Norris DA: A serologic marker for neonatal lupus erythematosus. Br J Dermatol 107:377–382, 1982

THE LUPUS ANTICOAGULANT

A Disease Marker in Antinuclear Antibody Negative Lupus that is Cross-Reactive with Autoantibodies to Double-Stranded DNA

C. BERNARD COLACO and KEITH B. ELKON

The lupus anticoagulant (LA) was demonstrated in 37% of 52 consecutive systemic lupus erythematosus (SLE) patients and patients with lupus-like syndromes, who were referred to our unit. The LA was found to be associated with a biologic false-positive VDRL ($P <$ 0.005), and the apparently paradoxical association of LA with vascular thromboses was confirmed ($P < 0.05$). The presence of LA and a biologic false-positive VDRL defined a group of 7 antinuclear antibody negative patients with characteristic features of recurrent thromboses, spontaneous abortions, neurologic involvement, and renal disease. Further studies on 6 selected sera demonstrated LA in all 6 IgM fractions and in 3 of 6 IgG fractions. Inhibition of LA was shown in 6 of 9 Ig fractions after absorption with double-stranded DNA (dsDNA). Anticardiolipin antibody was shown by immunodiffusion in 3 LA positive IgG fractions from VDRL negative sera. Cardiolipin micelles partially inhibited anti-dsDNA binding of 4 IgG fractions, 3 of which were LA negative. In this report we discuss the overlapping specificities due to cross-reactivity between LA, anticardiolipin, and anti-dsDNA antibodies in human SLE, and we suggest that LA be considered equivalent to the biologic false-positive VDRL as a criterion for the diagnosis of SLE.

The lupus anticoagulant (LA) is an acquired autoantibody that acts as an inhibitor of the prothrombinase complex, thus prolonging in vitro clotting tests for both the intrinsic and extrinsic pathways (1). First described in systemic lupus erythematosus (SLE) in 1952 (2), it has since been shown in other autoimmune, neoplastic, and drug-induced syndromes (3–5). It rarely causes hemorrhage, and then only in association with another clotting factor or platelet deficiency (1,3). No cause is known for the reported associations of LA with vascular thromboses (5–7) and spontaneous abortions (8,9). Several studies have shown the antiphospholipid nature of LA in both IgM and IgG fractions of serum (3,10,11). This may account for its anticoagulant activity and perhaps for the association with a false-positive syphilis test serology (5,12,13).

The possibility that there are cross-reactive antinuclear antibodies (ANA) in SLE sera that account for the biologic false-positive result on VDRL testing was first discussed by Inoue et al (14), who noted the steric resemblance of cardiolipin (CL) to part of the sugar-phosphate backbone of DNA. Soon after, an antibody raised against cardiolipin was shown to bind DNA (15), and later, a monoclonal human IgM with LA activity was observed and used to clearly demonstrate polyspecific binding of the Fabμ (anticoagulant) fragment to several acidic phospholipids (11). Other researchers (16,17) have isolated monoclonal anti–single-stranded DNA (ssDNA) antibodies from lupus mice (MRL/lpr), which may bind a variety of

---

Presented in part at a meeting of the Heberden Society, November 1982.

From the Department of Medicine, Royal Postgraduate Medical School, Hammersmith Hospital, London, United Kingdom.

Supported in part by the Arthritis and Rheumatism Council of Great Britain.

C. Bernard Colaco, MRCP: Research Fellow; Keith B. Elkon, MRCP: Lecturer (present address: Rheumatology Unit, The Hospital for Special Surgery, New York, NY 10021).

Address reprint requests to C. Bernard Colaco, Honorary Lecturer, Department of Immunology, The Middlesex Hospital Medical School, 40–50 Tottenham Street, London W1, United Kingdom.

Submitted for publication October 4, 1983; accepted in revised form July 17, 1984.

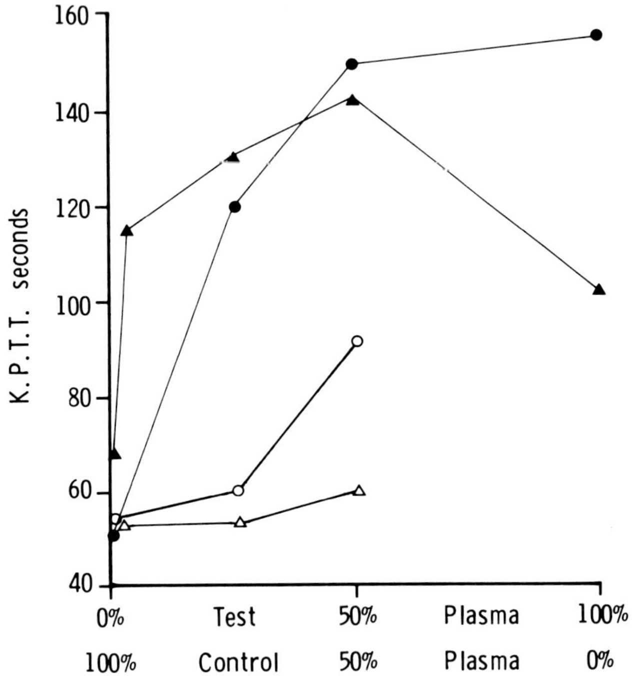

Figure 1. Demonstration of the lupus anticoagulant (LA) in 2 test plasmas and IgM fraction 3 by mixing with dilutions of control plasma and testing with 1:5 diluted phospholipid reagent in the kaolin partial thromboplastin time (KPTT) test. Concentration-dependent anticoagulant effect (●——●). Co-factor deficiency demonstrated (▲——▲), since clotting time in 50% mixture is longer than patients' plasma tested neat. LA effect is dependent on concentration of IgM of fraction 3 (○——○; 1 mg/ml at 50% mixture) compared with pooled normal human IgM (△——△).

polynucleotides and phospholipids. One such antibody also had LA activity.

To assess possible cross-reactivity among these human autoantibodies, we used polyclonal preparations of IgM and IgG, and found that the LA was more frequently IgM and showed that it could be inhibited by double-stranded DNA (dsDNA). Three VDRL negative sera showed IgG anti-CL on immunodiffusion, and CL micelles were able to inhibit IgG anti-DNA activity. The significance of these overlapping cross-reactive phenomena is discussed.

MATERIALS AND METHODS

Patients. We studied 52 patients with SLE and lupus-like diseases (49 women and 3 men), seen consecutively at the Hammersmith Hospital. Forty-one patients satisfied the American Rheumatism Association criteria for SLE (18). The remaining 11 patients had fewer than 4 clinical and laboratory features of SLE, and constituted the group with lupus-like syndromes. Three ANA negative, LA positive patients were identified later, but have been included in the lupus-like syndrome subset.

Screening for LA activity. Platelet-poor plasma was obtained from patients and normal, healthy laboratory staff, by anticoagulation of 9 parts venous blood with 1 part 3.8% sodium citrate and centrifugation at 3,000*g* for 15 minutes.

A commercial kaolin platelet substitute (KPS, a phospholipid extract of bovine brain; Diagen Reagents, Oxon, UK) was reconstituted in distilled water, as recommended for the kaolin partial thromboplastin time (KPTT), at a 1:5 dilution.

For KPTT testing, 100 μl of test plasma was added to 100 μl of KPS. The clotting tube was mixed for exactly 2 minutes in a 37°C water bath. Clotting was initiated by adding 100 μl of 0.025*M* calcium chloride, and the clotting time was recorded.

A mixing test was performed on all test plasma demonstrating a prolonged KPTT, using the 1:5 diluted KPS. Serial dilutions of test plasma in normal control plasma were tested for KPTT after 5 minutes incubation at 37°C. Failure of the 50% control plasma to correct the prolonged KPTT of the test sample to within 10 seconds of normal control values was considered necessary confirmatory evidence for lupus anticoagulant activity. Co-factor deficiency was noted if the addition of normal plasma further prolonged the test plasma KPTT (Figure 1).

All test plasma samples were studied in duplicate on at least 2 separate occasions, and all Ig fractions were tested in duplicate using coded specimens. The effect of dilution was controlled by testing the assay system with phosphate buffered saline (PBS) and normal human Ig, which were used as coded controls.

Separation of immunoglobulin fractions. Six LA positive sera were studied; 3 were VDRL negative, 2 were ANA negative with normal dsDNA binding on Farr assay. Control Ig was prepared from pooled normal sera and from 5 LA negative sera with high anti-dsDNA titers.

Ig fractions were prepared from all test and control sera as previously described (19). In brief, IgG was isolated by ammonium sulfate precipitation and DEAE cellulose chromatography (Whatman Ltd., Kent, UK). IgM was isolated by ammonium sulfate precipitation and Sephacryl S-300 chromatography (Pharmacia, Uppsala, Sweden). Trace amounts of IgG were removed from IgM by passage through a Sepharose 4B protein A column (Pharmacia). All fractions were dialyzed against PBS, pH 7.2, before further use. Purity of the Ig fractions was demonstrated by immunoelectrophoresis and Ouchterlony immunodiffusion. Concentrations of immunoglobulins were measured by Mancini radial immunodiffusion. Test fractions were used at final concentrations of 1 mg/ml of IgM and 10 mg/ml of IgG, unless otherwise stated. For tests requiring pooled human IgG, a commercial Cohn fraction II (Sigma, St. Louis, MO) was used.

Inhibition of LA by dsDNA. Ig samples were tested in the KPTT mixing test pre- and postincubation with native dsDNA (calf thymus nDNA; Sigma) at 20°C for 30 minutes. The final concentration of dsDNA was calculated according to the phosphorus content ($P = 10^0$–10^3 nmoles/liter), and all tests were done at equivalent final concentration of Ig. Keyhole limpet hemocyanin (KLH), at 2 mg/ml, was used as a control inert antigen.

Preparation of cardiolipin micelles. Cardiolipin (diphosphatidylglycerol sodium salt from bovine heart; Sigma), 1 mg in ethanol, was first evaporated under nitrogen and

Table 1. Clinical and laboratory features associated with the lupus anticoagulant (LA)

Feature*	% LA+ (n = 19)	% LA− (n = 33)	χ^2†	*P*‡
Thromboses	26	3	4.3	<0.05
CNS disease	32	18	0.7	NS
Spontaneous abortion	18 (n = 17)	3 (n = 32)	1.5	NS
BFP VDRL	42	3	10.3	<0.005
Thrombocytopenia	37	24	0.4	NS
DNAb >50%	47	52	0.33	NS
DNAb >75%	26	24	0.03	NS

* CNS = central nervous system; BFP VDRL = biologic false-positive VDRL; DNAb = DNA binding (normal <30%).
† With Yates' correction for small numbers.
‡ NS = not significant.

resuspended in 1 ml of buffer (0.15*M* NaCl, 0.02*M* Tris, pH 7.4). Next, it was sonicated for 15 minutes while being cooled on ice. The sonicated suspension was centrifuged at 10,000*g* for 20 minutes at 22°C, and the supernate (cardiolipin micelles) concentration was measured by absorbance at 320 nm.

IgG anti-dsDNA antibody inhibition studies with CL and KPS. Four IgG fractions were used at concentrations adjusted to read in the sensitive range of dsDNA binding on Farr assay (20). One sample was LA positive. Paired samples were tested after 60 minutes incubation with CL micelles (OD 0.15) or with buffer in a 1:1 ratio. Supernates were tested after centrifugation at 3,000*g* for 15 minutes at 22°C. IgG samples were similarly tested after incubation with the commercial phospholipid KPS, at dilutions 1:1, 1:10, and 1:100.

Ig immunodiffusion against CL micelles. Cardiolipin micelles, at several dilutions (OD 0.38–0.09), were tested against Ig fractions by Ouchterlony immunodiffusion in 1% agarose gel in buffer (0.15*M* NaCl, 0.02*M* Tris, pH 7.4). Precipitin lines were stained with Coomassie blue for protein and with Sudan black for phospholipid.

Other testing. The VDRL slide flocculation test was done on all samples using "VDRL Antigen" (cardiolipin 0.03%, cholesterol 0.09%, lecithin 0.2%; Wellcome Reagents Ltd., Kent, UK). Antinuclear activity of sera was tested by indirect immunofluorescence, using rat liver substrate, in 1:20 and 1:100 dilutions to avoid false-negative results due to the prozone phenomenon. Serum dsDNA binding was measured by the Farr assay (20). Examination of sera for extractable nuclear antigen antibodies against Ro, La, Sm, and RNP was performed by counterimmunoelectrophoresis (21).

RESULTS

Of the 52 plasma samples studied, only 4 showed a slightly prolonged prothrombin time or KPTT, using undiluted phospholipid reagents. Six patients had a shortened KPTT, which may reflect a nonspecific increase in Factor VIII levels, but none of these patients had any history of thrombosis. Using the dilute phospholipid, 19 of 52 plasma samples (37%) had LA activity as demonstrated by the mixing test (15 SLE patients and 4 lupus-like syndrome patients). Nine of the 19 LA positive plasma samples (47%) showed co-factor deficiency (Figure 1).

The incidence of selected clinical and laboratory features of the 52 patients is shown in Table 1. LA was significantly associated with thrombosis ($P < 0.05$); 6 patients had experienced a total of 9 thromboses, including 3 cerebral infarcts, 4 deep venous thromboses, and 2 cases of pulmonary embolus. Four of the 49 women studied had experienced 1 or more spontaneous abortions; 3 of these women were LA positive. Thrombocytopenia and neurologic syndromes showed increased frequency, but this was not statistically significant. A highly significant increase in the frequency of biologic false-positive VDRL was found in LA positive patients ($P < 0.005$).

The study helped to define a subset of 7 ANA negative patients with normal dsDNA binding values in the presence of LA and multisystem disease. One serum had antibodies to Ro (SS-A), and 6 of 7 had biologic false-positive VDRL test results. The clinical features common to this subset were arterial and venous thromboses, spontaneous abortions, central nervous system disease, and renal disease as defined by reduced creatinine clearance and/or glomerular disease demonstrated on biopsy (Table 2).

All IgM fractions (from patients 1–6) and 3 IgG fractions (from patients 1–3) demonstrated LA in the mixing test when compared with the effect of pooled normal human IgM and IgG added at equivalent final concentrations (Figure 2). Dilutions of IgM (fraction 3) in the mixing test show that this effect is dependent on antibody concentration (Figure 1).

Clotting times after incubation with dsDNA (P = 10^3 nmoles/liter) were significantly reduced for 5 of 6 IgM fractions and in 1 of the 3 LA positive IgG

Table 2. Lupus anticoagulant positive, antinuclear antibody negative subset of patients, clinical and serologic profile*

	Patient no. (age/sex)						
	1 (30/F)	2 (28/F)	3 (25/F)	4 (52/F)	5 (53/F)	6 (46/M)	7 (36/M)
Thromboses	1	4	5	1	0	1	?
Spontaneous abortion	1	3	NA	2	0	NA	NA
CNS disease	+	–	–	+	+	+	+
Renal disease	–	+	–	+	–	+	+
Rash	+	+	+	+	–	+	+
Arthralgia	+	+	+	+	–	–	–
Raynaud's phenomenon	–	–	–	–	–	+	+
% DNAb	5	11	5	15	7	18	1
ENA	–	Ro (SS-A)	–	–	–	–	–
BFP VDRL	+	+	+	–	+	+	+

* NA = not applicable; CNS = central nervous system; DNAb = DNA binding (normal <30%); ENA = extractable nuclear antigen; BFP VDRL = biologic false-positive VDRL.

fractions. Control samples (before incubation with dsDNA) were tested at equivalent Ig concentrations in PBS without dsDNA (Figures 3A and B). The effect of dsDNA in buffer on control plasma alone showed the contrary nonspecific effect of a slight increase in clotting time.

Incubation of LA positive IgG (fraction 1) with the inert antigen KLH instead of dsDNA, and further controls of Cohn fraction II in PBS or PBS-dsDNA were also found to have no significant effect in the mixing test (Table 3), and dsDNA inhibition of LA in IgG (fraction 1) was found to be linear over the range of dsDNA concentrations equivalent to 10^1–10^3 nmoles of P (Figure 4).

Precipitin lines between cardiolipin and IgG fractions 2–6 and IgM fraction 4 were clearly demonstrated (Figure 5), although sera (samples 3–5) were negative on VDRL testing.

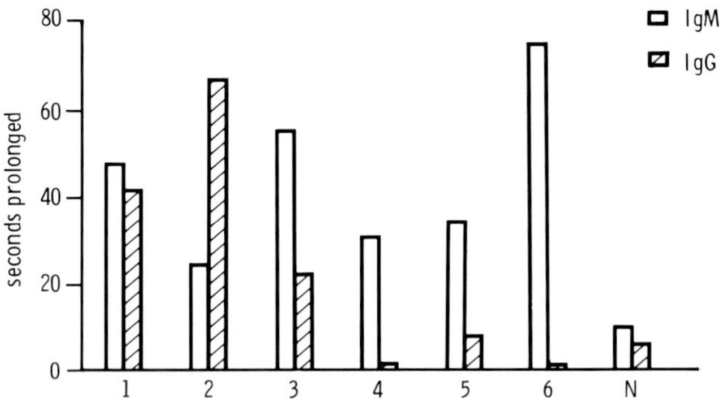

Figure 2. Anticoagulant effect of IgM (from patients 1–6) and IgG (from patients 1–3) fractions from sera (samples 1–6), defined by >10 seconds prolongation of normal control plasma clotting time in a 50% mixing test (kaolin partial thromboplastin time). Pooled normal human Ig (N) was used as a control.

Only IgM fraction 6 was weakly positive on VDRL testing, at the Ig concentrations used. No inhibition was noted after incubation with dsDNA.

Anti-dsDNA binding was inhibited by 10–33% in all 4 IgG samples tested after incubation with pure CL micelles (Table 4). No significant change was noted in samples incubated with the crude phospholipid preparation (KPS) used for the KPTT.

DISCUSSION

The lupus anticoagulant has rarely been the sole cause of serious hemorrhage. On the contrary, several reports have commented on the association of LA with vascular thromboses (5,6), which has been confirmed in this study of 52 consecutive referred patients. The routine screen using neat and 1:5 diluted phospholipid reagent in a standard KPTT and a mixing test has increased the sensitivity of this biologic assay. Without the greater sensitivity of detection, as many as 80% of the positive cases may have otherwise been missed. Assay sensitivity will also vary according to the commercial reagents that are used (22). We could not associate any clinical or laboratory parameter with the absence of co-factor in 9 patients. Co-factor is as yet undefined but has been considered by some to be an immunoglobulin (23) or prothrombin (24).

Early reports had noted an association of LA with false-positive syphilis test serology (12,13,25). Our study shows this association to be strong, occurring in 8 of 19 patients ($P < 0.005$). Four of the 6 patients with thromboses had both LA and a biologic false-positive VDRL. Although the 12% incidence of thrombosis among patients in our study compares with

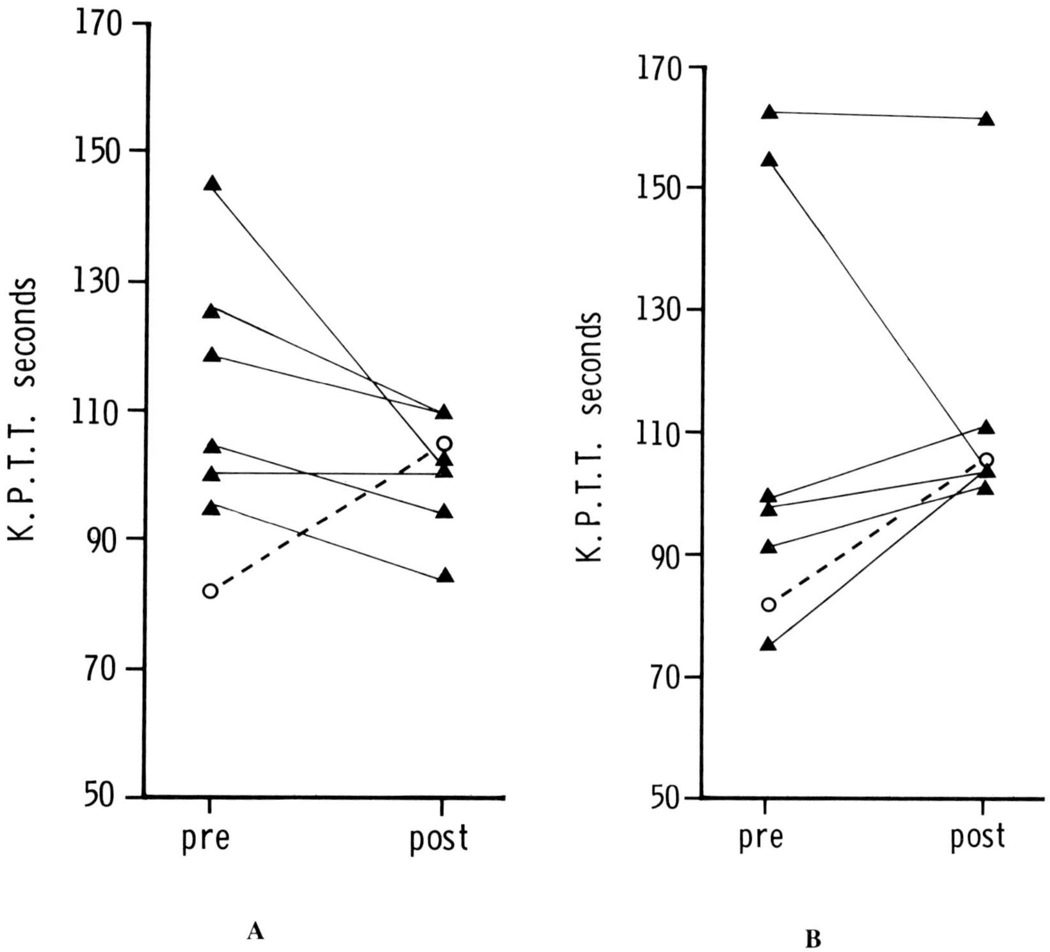

Figure 3. Inhibition of lupus anticoagulant postincubation with double-stranded DNA (dsDNA) (P = 10^3 nmoles) for 30 minutes, as tested by kaolin partial thromboplastin time (KPTT) in a 50% mixing test for **A**, IgM (fractions 1–6) and **B**, IgG (fractions 1–6). Control plasma (○----○) was incubated with dsDNA and phosphate buffered saline (PBS). For samples tested preincubation, PBS without dsDNA was used at equivalent final concentrations of IgM (1 mg/ml) and IgG (10 mg/ml).

that in larger series (26,27), the pathogenesis of thrombosis in SLE is probably multifactorial (28).

Our data did not support any significant association with thrombocytopenia, neurologic disease, or spontaneous abortion. However, when testing revealed 7 ANA negative, LA positive patients, we found that they formed a distinct clinical subset with features of recurrent thromboses, spontaneous abortions, and neurologic disease. Four patients had diminished renal function. One of these 4 patients showed an active diffuse proliferative lupus nephritis with immunoglobulin and C3 deposition in the mesangium and around glomerular capillary loops. These 7 patients' sera had remained ANA negative for periods ranging from 6 months to 2 years, which included episodes of disease flare in 6 patients. Patient 5 showed mild progression of symptoms of transverse myelitis. Her disease resembled that described as lupoid sclerosis by Fulford et al (29).

As a group, our 7 patients differ from the ANA negative group described by Maddison and coworkers (30), whose patients classically showed features of Sjögren's syndrome and photosensitive skin rashes with associated antibodies to Ro (SS-A) and ssDNA. The subset we have defined does share some features with 4 patients described by Firkin et al (9), but we noted more aggressive multisystem disease (Table 2 and Figure 5).

In the second part of the study, we used inhibition assays to define subpopulations of human autoantibodies with overlapping specificities. Of the 6 selected LA positive sera, 3 were VDRL negative, 3 were

Table 3. Specificity of double-stranded DNA (dsDNA) inhibition of IgG (fraction 1) lupus anticoagulant activity in a KPTT mixing test*

	Seconds prolonged		Seconds prolonged
PBS + C	0		
IgG + C	+17	Cohn fraction II + C	+0.5
IgG + dsDNA + C	−2	Cohn fraction II + dsDNA + C	+2
IgG + KLH + C	+15		

* Values are the mean of duplicate experiments. KPTT = kaolin partial thromboplastin time; PBS = phosphate buffered saline; C = control plasma, 50% mixture; KLH = keyhole limpet hemocyanin, an inert control antigen.

VDRL positive, and 2 were ANA negative with normal dsDNA binding values. We confirmed the antibody nature of the LA in all 6 IgM and in 3 of the 6 IgG fractions. Cross-reactive binding of the LA to dsDNA was shown by inhibition in 5 of 6 IgM and 1 of 3 IgG fractions (Figures 3A and B). Interestingly, inhibition of LA by dsDNA was noted in 2 IgM fractions from sera with apparently normal dsDNA binding on Farr assay. This might be explained by the possibility that low-titered IgM anti-dsDNA antibodies were not detected in the sensitive range of the Farr assay, or perhaps the population of cross-reactive anti-dsDNA/antiphospholipid antibodies are of such low affinity that they may not be precipitated in the Farr assay but would still be effectively inhibited by excess antigen in the KPTT.

The VDRL slide flocculation test, however, is likely to be more sensitive for polymeric IgM anti-CL (31), in contrast to our detection of IgG anti-CL by immunodiffusion, which confirmed IgG anti-CL in 5 IgG fractions, 3 of which were from VDRL negative sera (samples 3–5) (Figure 5). Thus anti-CL was shown in serum or IgG fractions of all 6 LA positive sera, but not in the 2 control sera, which were LA negative with high-titered anti-dsDNA. If we accept that LA activity, like the biologic false-positive VDRL, is primarily an IgM response, then this may explain the lack of association of LA with elevated dsDNA binding in whole serum (Table 1), since the latter may be predominantly IgG (32).

To test for cross-reactivity between anti-dsDNA and anti-CL, we selected 4 IgG fractions (1 was LA positive) with high anti-dsDNA activity and demonstrated partial inhibition of binding by prior incubation with cardiolipin in all 4 fractions (Table 4).

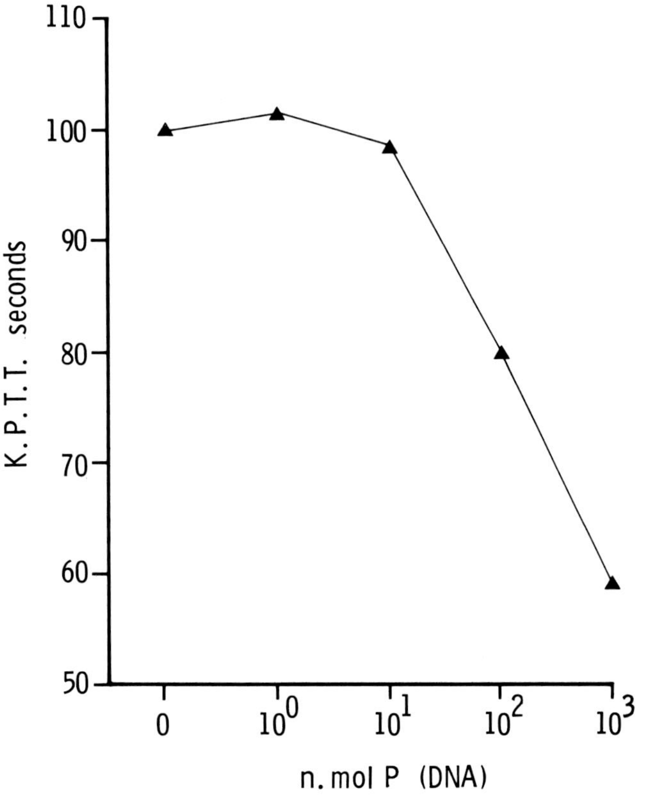

Figure 4. Inhibition of IgG (fraction 1) lupus anticoagulant by incubation with $\log_{10}$ dilutions of double-stranded DNA (P = 10^0–10^3 nmoles) for 30 minutes, as tested by kaolin partial thromboplastin time (KPTT) in a 50% mixing test.

Table 4. Inhibition of IgG anti–double-stranded DNA by incubation with cardiolipin (CL)*

IgG source	% DNA binding Pre CL	Post CL	% inhib.
Patient 7	78	63	19
Patient 1	19	13	31
Patient 8	49	44	10
Patient 9	74	49	33
Control	0	0	–

* % DNA binding measured by the Farr assay (normal <30%); coefficient of variation = ±2%.

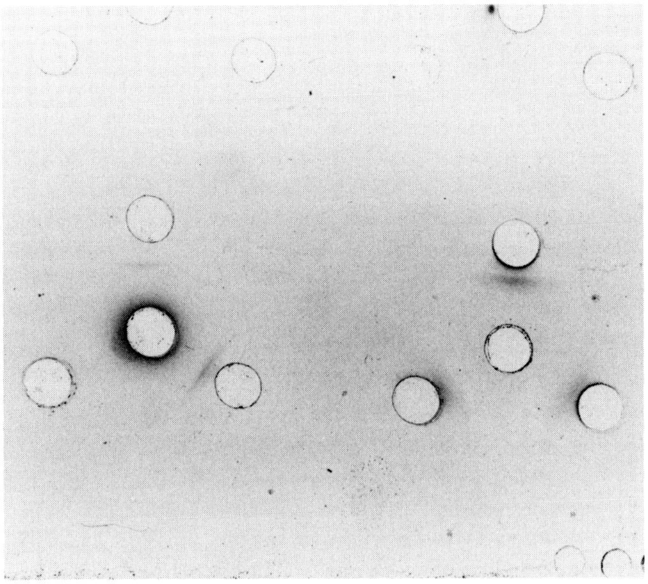

Figure 5. Precipitin lines between IgG fraction 4 and IgG fraction 5 in center wells, and 3 dilutions of cardiolipin micelles (OD 0.09–0.35 at 320 nm) in peripheral wells.

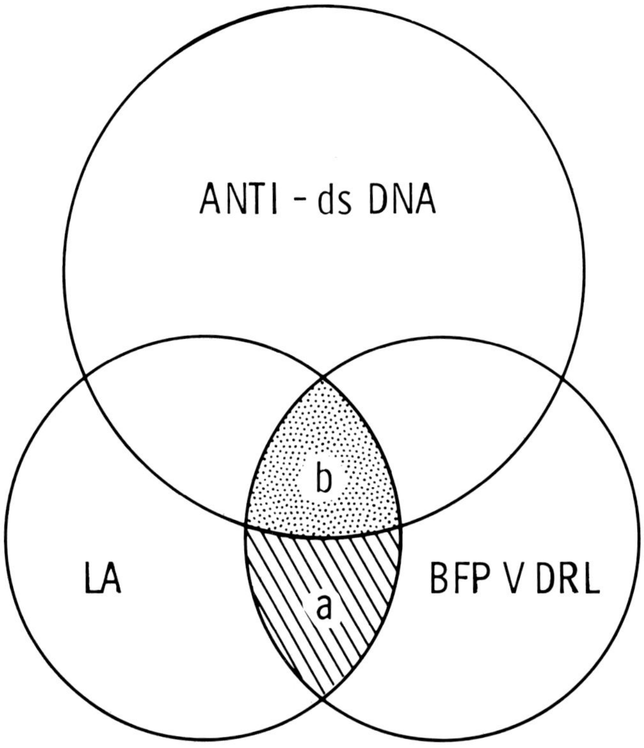

Figure 6. A model for cross-reacting autoantibodies in systemic lupus erythematosus. Anti-dsDNA = antibodies to double-stranded DNA; LA = lupus anticoagulant; BFP VDRL = biologic false-positive VDRL; group a = anti-dsDNA negative (antinuclear antibody negative), LA positive, VDRL positive; group b = anti-dsDNA positive, LA positive, VDRL positive.

These data are similar to those reported on inhibition of anti-ssDNA and anti-dsDNA binding by cardiolipin in a study of 11 SLE sera (33).

Our results suggest that several populations of antibodies with overlapping specificities may occur as part of the polyclonal autoantibody response in human SLE. The ones we have studied can be represented by the model in Figure 6. The biologic false-positive VDRL and LA may be seen mainly as populations of IgM antibodies, often noted on their own as a prodromal feature of SLE.

Why a switch to IgG class antibodies to DNA and other autoantigens appears to herald the full-blown lupus syndrome is as yet unknown. Nevertheless, we have defined a subset of patients who may experience serious disease in the presence of only LA and a biologic false-positive VDRL (group a in Figure 6), and we have demonstrated a group of polyspecific antibodies that bind both phospholipids and dsDNA (group b in Figure 6).

It may be of clinical importance to examine the overlapping specificities of the polyclonal humoral response in human SLE if it delineates pathologic subsets, but one factor contributing to these serologic overlaps may be the presence of an epitope common to phospholipids and various polynucleotides, as has been suggested by recent work on human monoclonal IgM anti-ssDNA antibodies (34).

We have shown that if the lupus anticoagulant is specifically sought, it is commonly found in human SLE. In view of the close association of LA with a biologic false-positive VDRL, we recommend that it be reconsidered as an equivalent criterion to the biologic false-positive VDRL, which has recently been accepted as one of the new diagnostic criteria for SLE (18). Further studies are needed to elucidate the mechanism of action of the LA, but its presence in ANA negative lupus would suggest a potential pathogenetic role.

ACKNOWLEDGMENTS

We are grateful to the patients for their cooperation and to Dr. G. Hughes for helpful advice and permission to study patients under his care. Our thanks to C. Bunn, Dr. V.

Joshi, and Dr. A. Gharavi for technical assistance and to D. L. Mehta and L. K. Bell for typing the manuscript.

REFERENCES

1. Feinstein DI, Rapaport SI: Anticoagulants in systemic lupus erythematosus, Lupus Erythematosus. Second edition. Edited by EL Dubois. Los Angeles, University of Southern California Press, 1974, pp 438–459
2. Conley CL, Hartman RC: A haemorrhagic disorder caused by circulating anticoagulants in patients with disseminated lupus erythematosus. J Clin Invest 31:621–622, 1952
3. Schleider MA, Nachman RL, Jaffe EA, Coleman M: A clinical study of the lupus anticoagulant. Blood 48:499–506, 1976
4. Margolius A Jr, Jackson DP, Ratnoff OD: Circulating anticoagulants: a study of 40 cases and a review of the literature. Medicine (Baltimore) 40:145–202, 1961
5. Mueh JR, Herbst KD, Rapaport SI: Thrombosis in patients with the lupus anticoagulant. Ann Intern Med 92:156–159, 1980
6. Bowie EJW, Thompson JH Jr, Pascuzzi CA, Owen CA Jr: Thrombosis in systemic lupus erythematosus despite circulating anticoagulants. J Lab Clin Med 62:416–430, 1963
7. Angles-Cano E, Sultan Y, Clauvel J: Predisposing factors to thrombosis in systemic lupus erythematosus. J Lab Clin Med 94:312–323, 1979
8. Nilsson IM, Astedt B, Hedner U, Berezin D: Intrauterine death and circulating anticoagulant ("anti-thromboplastin"). Acta Med Scand 197:153–159, 1975
9. Firkin BG, Howard MA, Radford N: Possible relationship between lupus inhibitor and recurrent abortion in young women (letter). Lancet 2:366, 1980
10. Exner T, Rickard KA, Kronenberg H: Studies on phospholipids in the action of a lupus coagulation inhibitor. Pathology 7:319–328, 1975
11. Thiagarajan P, Shapiro SS, De Marco L: Monoclonal immunoglobulin M coagulation inhibitor with phospholipid specificity. J Clin Invest 66:397–405, 1980
12. Laurell AB, Nilsson IM: Hypergammaglobulinaemia, circulating anticoagulant and biologic false positive Wassermann reaction. J Lab Clin Med 49:694–707, 1957
13. Harvey AM, Shulman LE: Systemic lupus erythematosus and the chronic biologic false positive test for syphilis, Lupus Erythematosus. Second edition. Edited by EL Dubois. Los Angeles, University of Southern California Press, 1974, pp 196–205
14. Inoue K, Nojima S, Tomizawa T: The specificity of cardiolipin in the serological reaction. J Biochem 57: 824–826, 1965
15. Guarnieri M, Eisner D: A DNA antigen that reacts with antisera to cardiolipin. Biochem Biophys Res Commun 58:346–349, 1974
16. Lafer EM, Rauch J, Andrzejewski C, Mudd D, Furie B, Schwartz RS, Stollar BD: Polyspecific monoclonal lupus autoantibodies reactive with both polynucleotides and phospholipids. J Exp Med 153:897–909, 1981
17. Rauch J, Schwartz RS: DNA-binding hybridoma antibodies to cardiolipin (abstract). Arthritis Rheum (suppl) 25:S16, 1982
18. Tan EM, Cohen AS, Fries JF, Masi AT, McShane DJ, Rothfield NF, Schaller JG, Talal N, Winchester RJ: The 1982 revised criteria for the classification of systemic lupus erythematosus. Arthritis Rheum 25:1271–1277, 1982
19. Elkon KB, Caeiro F, Gharavi AE, Patel BM, Ferjencik P, Hughes GRV: Radioimmunoassay profile of antiglobulins in connective tissue diseases: elevated level of IgA antiglobulin in systemic sicca syndrome. Clin Exp Immunol 46:547–556, 1981
20. Cohen SA, Hughes GRV, Noel GL, Christian CL: Character of anti-DNA antibodies in systemic lupus erythematosus. Clin Exp Immunol 8:551–561, 1971
21. Bernstein RM, Bunn CC, Hughes GRV: Identification of antibodies to acidic antigens by counterimmunoelectrophoresis. Ann Rheum Dis 41:554–555, 1982
22. Mannucci PM, Canciani MT, Mari D, Meucci P: The varied sensitivity of partial thromboplastin and prothrombin reagents in the demonstration of the lupus-like anticoagulant. Scand J Haematol 22:423–432, 1979
23. Yin ET, Gaston LW: Purification and kinetic studies on a circulatory anticoagulant in a suspected case of lupus erythematosus. Thromb Haemost 14:88–115, 1965
24. Loeliger A: Prothrombin as a co-factor of circulating anticoagulant in systemic lupus erythematosus. Thromb Haemost 3:237–256, 1959
25. Frick PG: Acquired circulating anticoagulants in systemic "collagen disease." Blood 10:691–706, 1955
26. Gladman DD, Urowitz MB: Venous syndromes and pulmonary embolism in systemic lupus erythematosus. Ann Rheum Dis 39:340–343, 1980
27. Estes D, Christian CC: The natural history of systemic lupus erythematosus by prospective analysis. Medicine (Baltimore) 50:85–95, 1971
28. Byrom MA: The clotting defect in SLE, Systemic Lupus Erythematosus. Edited by GRV Hughes. Clin Rheum Dis 8:137–151, 1982
29. Fulford KWM, Catterall RD, Delhanty JJ, Doniach D, Kremer M: A collagen disorder of the nervous system presenting as multiple sclerosis. Brain 95:373–386, 1972
30. Maddison PJ, Mogavero M, Provost TT, Reichlin M: The clinical significance of autoantibodies to a soluble cytoplasmic antigen in systemic lupus erythematosus and other connective tissue diseases. J Rheumatol 6: 189–195, 1979
31. Aho K: Studies of syphilitic antibodies. Br J Vener Dis 44:49–53, 1968
32. Talal N, Pillarisetty R: IgM and IgG antibodies to DNA, RNA and DNA:RNA in systemic lupus erythematosus. Clin Immunol Immunopathol 4:24–31, 1975
33. Koike T, Nagasawa R, Nagata N, Shirai T: Specificity of mouse hybridoma antibodies to DNA. Immunol Lett 4:93–97, 1982
34. Shoenfeld Y, Rauch J, Massicotte H, Datta SK, Andre-Schwartz J, Stollar BD, Schwartz RS: Polyspecificity of monoclonal lupus autoantibodies produced by human–human hybridomas. N Engl J Med 308:414–420, 1983

SALMONELLA BACTEREMIA IN SYSTEMIC LUPUS ERYTHEMATOSUS

Eight-Year Experience at a Municipal Hospital

STEVEN ABRAMSON, SARA B. KRAMER, ALLEN RADIN, and ROBERT HOLZMAN

Non-endemic *Salmonella* bacteremia tends to occur in patients with chronic disease. We reviewed all cases of *Salmonella* infection documented in adults at Bellevue Hospital during the years 1975–1982. Unexpectedly, the most frequent underlying disease found among bacteremic patients was systemic lupus erythematosus (SLE). Patients with SLE accounted for 6 of 30 *Salmonella* bacteremias as compared with 13 of 2,388 non-*Salmonella* gram-negative bacteremias. *Salmonella* was the single most frequent gram-negative isolate from the blood of SLE patients. All lupus patients with *Salmonella* infection were bacteremic. In contrast, isolates from blood represented only 23% of all *Salmonella* infections documented in the non-lupus population. Presentation was characterized by fever (>103°F) and abdominal pain. Four of the 6 patients were hypocomplementemic. All were receiving immunosuppressive therapy. We conclude that SLE patients in a municipal hospital setting are at increased risk for *Salmonella* sepsis. This should be considered when empiric antibiotic therapy is initiated.

It is well recognized that patients with systemic lupus erythematosus (SLE) have an increased susceptibility to infection. This is true even in the absence of renal insufficiency or corticosteroid therapy, and the susceptibility appears to be associated with abnormalities of host defenses (1–10). While the common pyogenic microorganisms are most often implicated in these infections, there have been isolated reports of salmonellosis in patients with SLE (5,6,11–13). Prompted by observation of several cases of *Salmonella* bacteremia among our SLE patients, we reviewed the occurrence of *Salmonella* sepsis at Bellevue Hospital, New York City, from 1975–1982. The majority of these bacteremias occurred in patients with underlying diseases. Unexpectedly, the most common associated illness was SLE, which accounted for 20% of the cases reported. *Salmonella* was the gram-negative organism most frequently isolated from the blood of lupus erythematosus patients during the study period. The clinical features of these patients are examined, with attention to potential factors that may increase the risk of salmonellosis in SLE.

From the Department of Medicine, Divisions of Rheumatology and Infectious Diseases, New York University School of Medicine, New York, New York.

Steven Abramson, MD; Sara B. Kramer, MD; Allen Radin, MD; Robert Holzman, MD.

Address reprint requests to Steven Abramson, MD, Department of Medicine, New York University School of Medicine, 550 First Avenue, New York, NY 10016.

Submitted for publication November 28, 1983; accepted in revised form July 9, 1984.

PATIENTS AND METHODS

At Bellevue Hospital, records of all bacteremias and *Salmonella* isolates from any source are maintained by the Microbiology Department. For the period 1975–1982, all isolates of *Salmonella* from adults (>17 years of age) were reviewed. These represented isolates both from inpatients and from those followed in the outpatient clinics. The charts of patients with *Salmonella* isolated from the blood were examined. Particular attention was given to recent travel to an endemic area, underlying diseases, and concomitant drug therapy. For the same time period (1975–1982), the number of adult patients hospitalized at Bellevue Hospital with sepsis due to any gram-negative organism was determined.

The Rheumatology Division at New York University maintains records on all SLE patients followed at Bellevue Hospital. During the study period, over 120 such patients were followed. The criteria for diagnosis of SLE were those of the American Rheumatism Association (14). Each case of *Salmonella* infection or gram-negative sepsis that occurred in a patient with SLE was ascertained. Patients' charts were reviewed for evidence of lupus disease activity at the time of *Salmonella* bacteremia. Clinical features, including therapy and laboratory values at the time of sepsis, were determined.

RESULTS

***Salmonella* infection in the adult patient population.** During the study period, a total of 30 patients with *Salmonella* sepsis were treated at Bellevue Hospital. As noted in Table 1, most of these patients had a concomitant medical condition. Unexpectedly, the most frequent underlying condition among bacteremic patients was SLE. Diseases of the biliary tract (including silent cholelithiasis) were noted in 5 non-SLE patients. Two of the non-SLE patients had undergone splenectomy, and 2 patients suffered from hematologic malignancy with splenic involvement. One patient had sickle cell anemia. Of the 30 patients, 9 were being treated with corticosteroids, including all 6 with SLE. Only 9 of the 30 patients were in apparent good health; 6 of these 9 had returned within 1 month from regions in which *Salmonella* infection is known to be endemic. These areas were Hong Kong (1 patient), Guyana (1 patient), Haiti (2 patients), Korea (1 patient), and India (1 patient).

During the study period, we identified a total of 112 adult patients with *Salmonella* isolated from any source. Thirty of 112 patients, or 27%, had positive blood cultures, including all 6 patients with SLE. At the time of bacteremia, equal percentages (33%) of the SLE and the non-SLE groups had *Salmonella* isolated from another source. The increased propensity for SLE patients to develop bacteremia when infected with *Salmonella* was statistically significant when

Table 1. Underlying conditions in patients with *Salmonella* bacteremia

Condition	No. of patients*
Systemic lupus erythematosus	6
Cholelithiasis	5
Hemoglobinopathy	3†
Splenectomy	2‡
Hematologic malignancy	2
Diabetic ketoacidosis	1
Intravenous drug abuse	1
Renal failure, receiving dialysis	1
Acquired immune deficiency syndrome	1
Sporadic, healthy	9

* Several patients had more than 1 underlying condition.
† 1 sickle cell anemia, 2 thalassemia minor.
‡ 1 idiopathic thrombocytopenic purpura, 1 post-traumatic.

compared with the non-lupus population (100% versus 23%, $P < 0.001$).

Clinical features of patients with SLE and *Salmonella* bacteremia. All 6 of the SLE patients with *Salmonella* bacteremia occurring during the study period were female. They ranged in age from 18–35. Four of the patients were Hispanic, one was black, and 1 was oriental. None of these patients had recently traveled to an area endemic for *Salmonella* infection. Four of the 6 patients were noted to have bacteremia alone, while 2 also had *Salmonella* recovered from an extravascular site (urine, stool). Two patients with bacteremia had family members with positive stool isolates but without apparent sepsis.

Table 2 reviews the clinical and laboratory features of SLE patients at the time of *Salmonella* sepsis. The patients' temperatures uniformly exceeded 103°F; abdominal pain without diarrhea occurred in 4 cases. With the exception of patient 1, who had increasing arthralgias, the patients were without other symptoms clearly attributable to SLE. Sepsis was strongly suspected in 4 of the patients, leading to the empiric institution of broad-spectrum parenteral antibiotics (an aminoglycoside plus either oxacillin or a cephalosporin). In no case, however, was *Salmonella* bacteremia a consideration at presentation.

Results of the patients' laboratory evaluations were not distinctive. Peripheral leukocyte counts ranged from 5,100–18,300 at the time of sepsis. Only 1 patient (patient 5) had significant azotemia. Despite the stress of acute infection, C3 complement levels were depressed in 4 of the 6 patients.

Outcome for the lupus patients was variable. Patient 5 had a fulminant course, and she succumbed within several days as a result of the adult respiratory distress syndrome and disseminated intravascular coagulation. The 5 remaining patients responded well once specific therapy (i.e., chloramphenicol or ampicillin) was initiated. However, patient 4 has had 2 subsequent recurrences of *Salmonella* bacteremia without an identifiable site of carriage. Patient 6 was successfully treated for *Salmonella* bacteremia but has since been hospitalized for meningococcal sepsis.

Potential predisposing factors to *Salmonella* sepsis were examined in the SLE population. All patients had received corticosteroid therapy, although only patient 5 was receiving >20 mg daily doses of prednisone; 2 patients were also receiving azathioprine at the time of sepsis (Table 2). Three patients had been given broad-spectrum antibiotics for other conditions within 2 weeks of the occurrence of *Salmonella*

Table 2. Clinical and laboratory features of systemic lupus erythematosus (SLE) patients with *Salmonella* bacteremia

Patient	Complaints at presentation	Daily SLE therapy prior to bacteremia	C3, C4 (mg/dl)*	Blood urea nitrogen, serum creatinine (mg/dl)
1	Fever, arthralgias	Prednisone 10 mg, azathioprine 100 mg	140, 27	15, 0.9
2	Fever, abdominal pain	Prednisone 20 mg, azathioprine 75 mg	209, 54	12, 0.9
3	Fever	Prednisone 20 mg	62, 18.5	12, 0.5
4	Fever, abdominal pain	Prednisone 12.5 mg	66, 23	20, 1.1
5	Fever, abdominal pain	Prednisone 60 mg	48, <5	81, 2.6
6	Fever, abdominal pain	Prednisone 12.5 mg	52, 14	17, 0.7

* Normal C3 = 70–175 mg/dl; normal C4 = 16–45 mg/dl.

bacteremia. These conditions included non-*Salmonella* skin abscesses and joint and urinary tract infections. In chronic carriers of *Salmonella*, systemic dissemination has followed antibiotic therapy (15,16). However, we found no evidence to indicate that these patients were chronic carriers. Finally, 4 of the 6 patients were hypocomplementemic. The deficiency of available opsonizing complement components may result in impaired clearance of this organism by tissue macrophages, as has been suggested to be the case in sickle cell anemia (17).

***Salmonella* species isolated in study population.** The *Salmonella* species isolated in the study population are listed in Table 3. The most common isolate was *S enteritidis* serotype enteritidis (10 cases, with 5 in SLE patients), followed by *S typhi* (7 cases, with none in SLE patients). Species identification was not done in 1 case. There was significantly higher frequency of serotype enteritidis in SLE patients compared with that in patients without SLE (5 of 6 versus 5 of 24, $P < 0.05$).

Table 3. *Salmonella* species isolated from blood of patients at Bellevue Hospital, 1975–1982

	Systemic lupus erythematosus patients (%)	Others (%)
S typhi	0	7 (29)
S choleraesuis	1 (17)	0
S enteritidis	5 (83)	17 (71)
Type enteritidis	5	5
typhimurium		5
paratyphi A		2
Heidelberg		1
Newport		1
bareilli		1
muentis		1
Undetermined		1

Since serotype enteritidis was isolated in 5 of the 6 SLE patients, we examined the possibility that patients with lupus might have acquired their *Salmonella* at the hospital's outpatient department. The cases of *Salmonella* in patients with SLE occurred over a 5-year period from 1978–1982, while there was an even distribution throughout the 1975–1982 study period in the non-SLE population. Two of the cases in SLE patients occurred within 2 days of each other, in 1978. One of these cases occurred in a patient who had never attended the Bellevue clinic and had recently arrived from Germany. The other patient had been hospitalized on the pediatric service until 1 month prior to admission, and was originally admitted to an outlying hospital prior to transfer to Bellevue with the *Salmonella* bacteremia. Two other cases occurred in patients who had not previously attended the Bellevue outpatient clinic. Thus, it is unlikely that these cases resulted from a common source.

Gram-negative sepsis in SLE. Review of all gram-negative bacteremia occurring at Bellevue Hospital during the period 1975–1982 revealed 2,418 such episodes. Thirty of these bacteremias were due to *Salmonella* species. Six of the 30 *Salmonella* septicemias (20%) occurred in patients with SLE, in contrast to only 13 of the 2,388 non-*Salmonella* gram-negative

Table 4. Gram-negative bacteremia in systemic lupus erythematosus (SLE) patients and other patients at Bellevue Hospital, 1975–1982

Organism	Number of patients		Percentage with SLE
	SLE	Total hospital	
Salmonella species	6	30	20*
Non-*Salmonella*, gram-negative†	13	2,388	0.54*

* $P < 0.001$.
† Non-*Salmonella* organisms: *Escherichia coli* (5 patients), *Pseudomonas* (2 patients), *Klebsiella* (2 patients), *Enterobacter* (2 patients), *Proteus* (1 patient), *Actinobacter* (1 patient).

bacteremias (0.54%) (Table 4). The greater representation of SLE in the *Salmonella* group as compared with the non-*Salmonella* group was significant ($P < 0.001$).

It was an unexpected finding that *Salmonella* was the most common gram-negative organism isolated from the blood of SLE patients. *Escherichia coli* was the next most common organism, recovered from 5 patients. The remainder of the isolates comprised a variety of enteric organisms as listed in the footnotes to Table 4. None of these other organisms was found in more than 2 patients.

DISCUSSION

We have reviewed all cases of *Salmonella* bacteremia documented among adults at Bellevue Hospital during the period 1975–1982. *Salmonella* bacteremia tended to occur in patients with chronic underlying diseases, as has been previously noted (7,11,18–21). The most common of these illnesses in our population was systemic lupus erythematosus, which accounted for 20% of the cases. *Salmonella* species were, in fact, the most frequent gram-negative isolates from the blood of lupus patients during the study period. Certainly, it must be noted that the patient population served at Bellevue Hospital is generally of low socioeconomic background. Many of the patients are of Hispanic descent, with patients and family members traveling frequently to areas potentially endemic for *Salmonella* infection. The risk of exposure to the *Salmonella* organism in such an inner-city population might therefore be expected to be greater than that of the general population. Nonetheless, our SLE population is unselected and drawn from the same demographic base as are all other Bellevue Hospital patients. The increased risk of *Salmonella* bacteremia in these SLE patients would, therefore, appear to be authentic.

Several distinctive features about *Salmonella* infection in SLE were notable. Most striking was an inability to confine the organism to the extravascular space. Isolates from the blood represented only 23% of all *Salmonella* cultures documented in the non-lupus adult population. This figure is consistent with previous reports that assess the frequency of bacteremia among hospitalized patients with *Salmonella* infection (11). In contrast, all of our lupus patients with *Salmonella* infection treated during the same time period were bacteremic. In 2 illustrative cases, *Salmonella* was isolated from the blood of 2 SLE patients, but from the stool of family members who did not become bacteremic. We believe the data show that SLE patients, when infected with *Salmonella*, are more likely to have bacteremia than those without SLE. Alternatively, it is possible that the SLE patients were in fact at no greater risk of developing *Salmonella* bacteremia than the non-SLE patients, but that the non-SLE patients had transient bacteremias which resolved before they came to medical attention. However, this would seem much less likely.

There are multiple factors that presumably contribute to this dissemination of *Salmonella* infection in lupus patients. First, treatment of SLE directly compromises host defense. All patients in our series were receiving immunosuppressive therapy at the time of bacteremia. This was also true of the SLE patients with *Salmonella* sepsis reported by Lovy (12) and by Cherubin (11). Second, 3 patients had previously been given antibiotic therapy which, as noted earlier, is a recognized risk factor for the dissemination of carried *Salmonella*.

Third, compromised host defense mechanisms characteristic of SLE may have made these patients particularly susceptible to *Salmonella* infection. It is notable that in contrast to more commonly encountered pyogenic organisms, *Salmonella* is an intracellular parasite whose control requires adequate function of the reticuloendothelial system (RES). In experimental animal models, the outcome of *Salmonella* infection is determined by the fate of the organisms that are trapped in the liver and spleen (22). Thus, it is of interest that defective reticuloendothelial function has recently been proposed in SLE.

Frank et al (23) have reported that patients with SLE have decreased clearance of IgG-sensitized ^{51}Cr-labeled erythrocytes. It is suggested that this results from prior occupancy of Fc receptors by circulating immune complexes. Dillon et al (24) have reported that 5 of 70 patients with SLE had peripheral smears consistent with hyposplenism. Three of these patients had ^{99m}technetium-sulfur colloid scans showing no splenic uptake. Hence, potential dysfunction of the RES in lupus patients may leave these patients vulnerable to dissemination of the *Salmonella* organism.

Such a defect in receptor availability may have been compounded by the fact that low levels of the third component of complement (C3) were found in 4 of the 6 SLE patients in this series. Defective alternative pathway function and low levels of C3 have been described previously in patients with sickle cell anemia (17), a disease in which an increased incidence of *Salmonella* infection is well recognized. Consumption of complement occurring in the course of SLE could potentially deplete the serum of C3-opsonizing activity that facilitates the clearance of *Salmonella*.

In summary, our experience with salmonellosis occurring in an inner-city population suggests that such patients with SLE are at increased risk of developing bacteremia. Because of this strong possibility, we suggest that protection against *Salmonella* species should be considered when empiric antibiotic therapy is initiated, particularly in patients who have high fever and abdominal pain.

REFERENCES

1. Perez HD, Andron RI, Goldstein IM: Infection in patients with systemic lupus erythematosus: association with a serum inhibitor of complement-derived chemotactic activity. Arthritis Rheum 22:1326–1333, 1979
2. Staples PJ, Gerding DN, Decker JL, Gordon RS Jr: Incidence of infection in systemic lupus erythematosus. Arthritis Rheum 17:1–10, 1974
3. Jasin HD, Orozco JH, Ziff M: Serum heat-labile opsonins in systemic lupus erythematosus. J Clin Invest 53:343–353, 1974
4. Brandt L, Hedberg H: Impaired phagocytosis by peripheral blood granulocytes in systemic lupus erythematosus. Scand J Haematol 6:348–353, 1969
5. Castelman B, McNeely BU: Case records of the Massachusetts General Hospital. N Engl J Med 278:441–450, 1968
6. Myers AR, Mills JA, Ropes MW: The problem of infection in systemic lupus erythematosus (abstract). Arthritis Rheum 10:300, 1967
7. Cherubin CE, Fodor T, Denmark L, Master D, Fuerst HT, Winter J: The epidemiology of salmonellosis in New York City. Am J Epidemiol 90:285–291, 1969
8. Nived O, Odebeig H, Svensson B: Monocyte in vitro function in systemic lupus erythematosus. III. Bactericidal activity in presence of SLE sera. Scand J Rheumatol (suppl) 31:29–41, 1980
9. Svensson B, Hedberg H: Impaired phagocytosis by macrophages in SLE. Scand J Rheumatol 2:78–80, 1973
10. Svensson BO: Serum factors causing impaired macrophage function in systemic lupus erythematosus. Scand J Immunol 4:145–150, 1975
11. Cherubin CE, Neu HC, Imperato PJ, Harvey RP, Bellen N: Septicemia with non-typhoid salmonella. Medicine (Baltimore) 53:365–376, 1974
12. Lovy MR, Ryan PFS, Hughes GRV: Concurrent systemic lupus erythematosus and salmonellosis. J Rheumatol 8:605–612, 1981
13. Guthaner DF, Stathers GM: Salmonella typhimurium septicemia complicating disseminated lupus erythematosus. Med J Aust 2:1156–1158, 1969
14. Cohen AS, Reynolds WE, Franklin EC, Kulka JP, Ropes MW, Shulman LE, Wallace SL: Preliminary criteria for the classification of systemic lupus erythematosus. Bull Rheum Dis 21:643–648, 1971
15. Rosenthal SC: Exacerbation of salmonella enteritis due to ampicillin. N Engl J Med 280:147–148, 1969
16. Saroglou G, Bisno A: Salmonella bacteremia and gastroenteritis after oral ampicillin therapy for gonorrhea. S Afr Med J 71:964–965, 1978
17. Hand WL, King NL: Serum opsonization of salmonella in sickle cell anemia. Am J Med 64:388–395, 1978
18. Saphra I, Winter JW: Clinical manifestations of salmonellosis in man. N Engl J Med 256:1128–1134, 1957
19. Seligmann E, Saphra I, Wasserman M: Salmonella infections in the USA. J Immunol 54:69–97, 1946
20. Han T, Sokol JR, Netter E: Salmonellosis in disseminated malignant diseases. N Engl J Med 276:1045–1052, 1967
21. Feinfeld DA, Cherubin CE, Carvounis G: An outbreak of salmonella enteritis and septicemia in a population of uremic patients. Arch Intern Med 140:943–945, 1980
22. Kage D, Gill FA, Hook EW: Factors influencing host resistance to salmonella infections: the effects of hemolysis and erythrophagocytosis. S Am J Med Sci 254:205–215, 1967
23. Frank MM, Hamburger MI, Lawley TS: Defective reticuloendothelial system Fc-receptor function in systemic lupus erythematosus. N Engl J Med 300:518–523, 1979
24. Dillon AM, Stein HB, English RA: Splenic atrophy in systemic lupus erythematosus. Ann Intern Med 96:40–43, 1982

THE INCIDENCE OF SYSTEMIC LUPUS ERYTHEMATOSUS IN BALTIMORE, MARYLAND, 1970–1977

MARC C. HOCHBERG

The incidence of systemic lupus erythematosus, based on first hospital discharge diagnosis, in Baltimore, Maryland for the years 1970 through 1977 was determined for individual sex–race groups and the total population. Age-specific incidence rates were consistently highest among black females and lowest among white males: rates for white females exceeded those for black males through age 54, but then declined for ages ≥55. Mean age at diagnosis was significantly lower for black females versus white females (35.5 versus 41.7 years, $P = 0.005$) and for all females versus all males (37.2 versus 44.2 years, $P = 0.012$). There were no temporal trends noted in yearly age-adjusted incidence rates during the 8-year study period. The overall population incidence of systemic lupus erythematosus was 4.6 per 100,000 per year, representing a twofold increase over a comparable study done in New York City 15 years ago.

Previous descriptive epidemiologic studies of systemic lupus erythematosus (SLE) have demonstrated increasing incidence rates from 1.0–7.6 per 100,000 per year during the 20-year period from 1955 to 1974 (1–7). This temporal trend in SLE incidence, however, may in part be artifactual; that is, the increase may be due to 1) increased physician knowledge and recognition of the disease, 2) the development of more sensitive diagnostic tests such as antinuclear antibody (ANA) determinations, and 3) diagnosis of milder cases because of changes in diagnostic criteria. In addition, comparison of previous studies is complicated by methodologic differences, especially in case identification. Studies in New York City (1–3) and Jefferson County, Alabama (2,3) were based on hospital discharge records, while those in Rochester, Minnesota (4) and San Francisco (5) were based on both inpatient and outpatient records. Furthermore, recent studies have not estimated incidence rates by sex–race groups in nonwhites because of the small number of cases (4,5).

Since the ANA test became available in the 1960s and the publication of preliminary criteria for the classification of SLE in 1971 (8), few other major technologic advances have been made which would impact physician diagnosis of SLE. Hence, in a major metropolitan area with 2 university teaching hospitals where knowledge is widely disseminated, one would assume that temporal changes in SLE incidence during the past decade would probably be more real than artifactual. Thus, a population-based study of hospital-diagnosed SLE was done in Baltimore to 1) estimate the average annual age-specific incidence rates by sex–race group; 2) explore potential synergistic interaction between the female sex and the nonwhite race in producing higher incidence rates among nonwhite females; 3) assess possible differences in age at diagnosis between whites and nonwhites; and 4)

From the Rheumatology Division, Department of Medicine, The Johns Hopkins University School of Medicine at the Good Samaritan Hospital, and Department of Epidemiology, The Johns Hopkins University School of Hygiene and Public Health, Baltimore, Maryland.

Supported by grants from the Lupus Foundation of America, the Arthritis Foundation, Maryland Chapter, and The Johns Hopkins Multipurpose Arthritis Center grant 2-P60-AM20558. Dr. Hochberg is the recipient of an Arthritis Investigator Award from the Arthritis Foundation.

Marc C. Hochberg, MD, MPH: Associate Professor of Medicine, Joint Appointment in Epidemiology.

Address reprint requests to Dr. Marc C. Hochberg, c/o Good Samaritan Hospital, 5601 Loch Raven Boulevard, Baltimore, MD 21239.

Submitted for publication March 19, 1984; accepted in revised form August 7, 1984.

examine recent temporal trends in annual age-adjusted incidence rates.

METHODS

The records of 19 Baltimore metropolitan area hospitals, 14 hospitals within the Baltimore city limits, and an additional 5 located in Baltimore County but within the metropolitan area were reviewed for the period 1970 through 1977, and all patients discharged with a diagnosis of SLE (Eighth Revision International Classification of Disease, Code 734.1) (9) were identified. Patient charts were reviewed by a trained research assistant using a predefined protocol to obtain the following information: address at time of discharge including zip code, date of birth, sex, race, date of discharge, marital status, date of diagnosis, number of previous admissions for SLE, and the presence of the American Rheumatism Association (ARA) preliminary criteria for SLE (8). Only the records of Baltimore city residents, with a date of first hospital discharge diagnosis between January 1, 1970 and December 31, 1977, were considered for further analysis.

Based on chart review, cases were required to fulfill at least 4 of the preliminary criteria for SLE to be included in subsequent analyses.

The population data were derived from the 1970 and 1980 United States censuses of the city of Baltimore. Both the 1970 and 1980 censuses reported numbers of persons by age group, sex, and either white or black race. Population denominators for each year of the study were estimated by linear extrapolation using 1970 and 1980 as benchmarks.

Age-specific annual incidence rates of hospital-diagnosed SLE were calculated for each sex–race group per year from 1970 through 1977. Ten-year age groups were used, except for a single group for those below age 15 and one for those age 65 and above. The overall age-adjusted average annual incidence rates for each sex–race group were calculated using the direct method and the total 1980 Baltimore city population as the standard. Standard errors were calculated using the methods of Chiang (10). Time trend analysis of mean age at diagnosis and yearly age-adjusted incidence rates for each sex–race group were conducted using Spearman's rank-order correlation coefficient (R_s) (11). Finally, Rothman's synergy index (12) was determined to evaluate the possible interaction between sex and race as independent risk factors for the development of SLE.

RESULTS

A total of 302 incident cases of SLE were identified among Baltimore city residents discharged during the 8-year study period (Table 1). Black females were most commonly affected, accounting for 63% of cases; females comprised 87% of cases, giving an overall crude sex ratio of 6:1. There was no significant temporal trend in the total number of cases diagnosed per year during the study period ($R_s = -0.44$, $P > 0.05$).

The patterns of the age-specific average annual incidence rates varied between the individual sex–race groups (Table 2 and Figure 1). Incidence rates were lowest among white males, and too few cases were identified during the study period to allow an adequate description of the age distribution except to note that no cases were identified in persons age 24 and under. The overall crude rate among white males was 0.45 per 100,000 per year. Incidence rates among black males showed a unimodal distribution with maximum rates occurring in the 45–54 and 55–64 age groups; the overall crude rate was 2.08 per 100,000 per year. Incidence rates were consistently greater among black males compared with white males in all age groups; the overall crude race ratio for males was 4.6:1 (Table 3).

Age-specific incidence rates among white females showed a bimodal distribution with peaks in the 15–24 and 45–54 age groups; rates declined precipitously above age 55. The overall crude rate was 3.94 per 100,000 per year and the crude rate limited to the 15–54 age groups combined was 6.05 per 100,000 per year. Incidence rates were consistently greater among white females compared with white males; the overall crude sex ratio among whites was 8.8:1 (Table 3).

Age-specific incidence rates for black females showed a unimodal distribution with the maximum rate of 21.6 per 100,000 per year occurring in the 25–34 age group. Incidence rates were higher among black females than any of the other 3 sex–race groups. Comparison of black female with black male rates showed the greatest differences in the 15–34 age groups with an overall crude sex ratio of 5.1:1. Similar comparison of black female rates with white female rates showed variable patterns with age; the overall crude race ratio for females was 2.7:1 (Table 3).

Overall age-adjusted average annual incidence rates were 0.42, 2.50, 3.93, and 11.42 for white males,

Table 1. Number of hospital-diagnosed incident cases of systemic lupus erythematosus by sex–race group and year in Baltimore city residents, 1970–1977*

Year	WM	BM	WF	BF	Total
1970	1	6	10	21	38
1971	0	9	9	28	46
1972	0	4	11	31	46
1973	1	3	8	22	34
1974	1	2	8	17	28
1975	0	3	10	29	42
1976	1	3	7	27	38
1977	3	3	9	15	30
Total	7	33	72	190	302

* WM = white males; BM = black males; WF = white females; BF = black females.

Table 2. Average annual age-specific incidence rates of systemic lupus erythematosus by sex–race group in the city of Baltimore, 1970–1977

	White males		Black males		White females		Black females		Total	
Age group	No.	Rate*	No.	Rate	No.	Rate	No.	Rate	No.	Rate
≤14	0	—	2	0.34	0	—	8	1.45	10	0.53
15–24	0	—	4	1.25	16	5.55	45	12.46	65	5.28
25–34	2	0.87	3	1.56	10	4.73	53	21.57	68	7.69
35–44	2	1.21	6	3.52	12	6.87	34	16.63	54	7.63
45–54	0	—	8	4.97	17	7.23	24	12.95	49	6.22
55–64	2	0.99	6	5.06	9	3.71	15	11.08	32	4.56
≥65	1	0.50	4	4.35	8	2.33	11	8.75	24	3.08
Overall crude rate		0.45		2.08		3.94		10.54		4.40
Overall age-adjusted rate†		0.42		2.50		3.93		11.42		4.62
Standard error		0.16		0.43		0.46		0.83		0.26

* Rates per 100,000 population per year.
† Adjusted to the 1980 Baltimore total population using the direct method.

black males, white females, and black females, respectively (Table 2). Comparison of these age-adjusted rates reflects a marked sex effect and a somewhat less pronounced racial effect (Table 3). To evaluate the possibility of additive interaction or synergism between sex and race as risk factors for high incidence, Rothman's index of interaction was determined (Table 4). The age-adjusted incidence rate for white males was set as the background risk of developing SLE in the absence of either factor, that is, female sex or black race. The calculated values of 1.97 for all age groups and 2.11 for age groups 15–54 (corresponding to reproductive or childbearing years in females) are significantly different from 1.0 and suggest a definite synergistic interaction between female sex and black race.

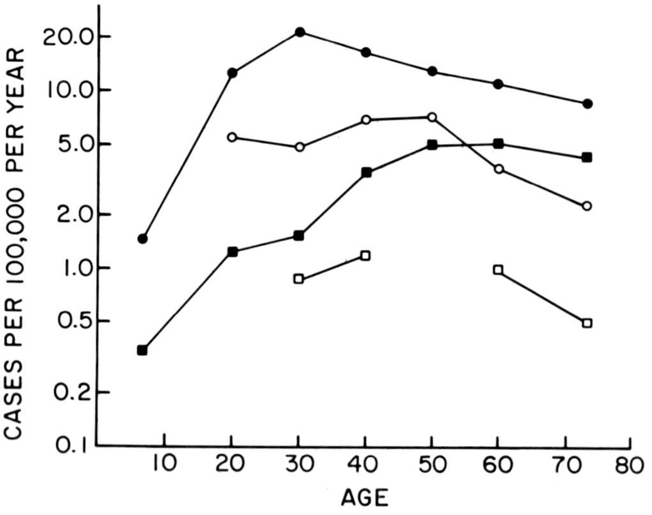

Figure 1. Average annual age-specific incidence rates of systemic lupus erythematosus in Baltimore (city), 1970–1977, for white males (□), black males (■), white females (○), and black females (●). Note that the ordinate axis is a 3-cycle logarithmic scale.

The distribution of age at diagnosis among the sex–race groups is also shown in Table 2. The median age at diagnosis was 36, 46, 42, and 33 years for white males, black males, white females, and black females, respectively. The mean age at diagnosis was significantly younger for black females compared with white females (35.5 ± 15.7 years versus 41.7 ± 17.4 years; $t = -2.79$, $P = 0.005$) and for all females compared with all males (37.2 ± 16.3 years versus 44.2 ± 16.9 years; $t = -2.51$, $P = 0.012$).

There were no significant trends in either the annual age-adjusted incidence rates or the mean age at diagnosis for any of the sex–race groups during the study interval.

DISCUSSION

The incidence of systemic lupus erythematosus in several communities in the United States has been reported previously (1–5), and these studies have been recently reviewed (13). This study represents the largest epidemiologic study of SLE in terms of number

Table 3. Ratios of average annual age-specific incidence rates of systemic lupus erythematosus between sex–race groups

	Female:male		Black:white	
Age group	Black	White	Male	Female
≤14	4.3	–*	–	–
15–24	9.9	–	–	2.2
25–34	13.8	5.4	1.8	4.6
35–44	4.7	5.7	2.9	2.4
45–54	2.6	–	–	1.8
55–64	2.2	3.7	5.1	3.0
≥65	2.0	4.7	8.7	3.7
Overall crude ratio	5.1	8.8	4.6	2.7
Overall age-adjusted ratio	4.6	9.3	5.9	2.9

* No cases present in denominator of ratio.

Table 4. Calculation of Rothman's synergy index (12)*

	Age-adjusted average annual incidence rate†	Relative rate (RR)
All ages‡		
White males	0.42	$1.00 = RR_{00}$
Black males	2.50	$5.95 = RR_{10}$
White females	3.93	$9.36 = RR_{01}$
Black females	11.42	$27.19 = RR_{11}$
Ages 15–54§		
White males	0.46	$1.00 = RR_{00}$
Black males	2.41	$5.24 = RR_{10}$
White females	5.85	$12.72 = RR_{01}$
Black females	15.93	$34.63 = RR_{11}$

* Synergy index $= S = \dfrac{RR_{11} - RR_{00}}{RR_{10} + RR_{01} - 2RR_{00}}$.
† Rates per 100,000 per year.
‡ S = 1.97 (95% confidence intervals: 1.46, 2.66).
§ S = 2.11 (95% confidence intervals: 1.52, 2.93).

of incident cases identified, as well as denominator population, and provides updated information on age-specific average annual incidence rates by sex–race group, as well as new information on differences in mean age at diagnosis between individual sex–race groups and evidence of synergy between the female sex and the black race in producing the highest incidence rates of SLE in black females.

The database used in this study represented patients with SLE who were Baltimore city residents at the time of first hospital diagnosis, who fulfilled 4 or more of the preliminary ARA criteria for SLE, and were discharged from Baltimore area hospitals. Patients with SLE discharged during the study interval who were either first diagnosed before 1970 and/or did not reside in the city of Baltimore were excluded from analyses; they represented an additional 153 cases.

The method of case selection used is similar to that employed by Siegel and Lee (1), who justified their method on the assumptions that patients with SLE would require hospital care because of severity of illness and/or difficulty in diagnosis and would use local facilities for medical care (3). More recent studies in Rochester, Minnesota (4) and San Francisco (5) used both inpatient and outpatient records which were linked through computerized patient registries. Since the assumption of Siegel and Lee relating to the requirement of hospital care for diagnosis is no longer valid, especially in major urban areas with educated internists and rheumatologists, it is likely that the database used in this study is biased due to a systematic underestimation of incident cases of SLE in patients who either have mild disease not requiring hospitalization and/or were diagnosed and managed completely as outpatients during the study period.

In an attempt to quantify the degree of underestimation, the author surveyed the faculty of the Johns Hopkins Rheumatology Division. Of 121 private patients with SLE who were seen during the 12-month period from July 1983 through June 1984 and were under regular followup in our university-based private patient clinic, 11 (9.1%) had never been hospitalized (14). There was a suggestion of racial influence in the proportion of patients never having been hospitalized, 10.7% of 103 whites versus none of 18 blacks, but this is not statistically significant ($P = 0.24$, Fisher's exact 2-tailed test). Whether this underestimation of the number of incident cases applies equally to all 4 sex–race groups in the community is unknown; it is possible that white patients with higher socioeconomic status may seek care earlier in their illness and be more likely to be diagnosed and managed as outpatients by private rheumatologists than blacks with lower socioeconomic status. This is suggested by the private patient data noted above; however, the inaccuracies inherent in attempts to generalize these results to other populations are recognized.

Another potential source of underestimation of incident cases is that patients with SLE might have been discharged with other listed discharge diagnoses. Examples would include other connective tissue disorders such as unspecified collagen vascular disease or mixed connective tissue disease, or glomerulonephritis or lupus nephritis. These reporting errors might be attributable to physician misdiagnosis or coding errors by medical records personnel. Unfortunately, we did not review any such records and are therefore unable to estimate the potential impact on the data presented.

The patterns of the age-specific incidence rates of SLE in Baltimore, based on first hospital discharge diagnosis of SLE, are largely comparable with those patterns noted by Siegel and Lee in New York City and Jefferson County, Alabama (1–3). Among 65 cases in white females identified in the New York City study area, the peak incidence rate of 4.4 per 100,000 per year occurred in the 25–34 year age group, while in the present study, the peak incidence rate of 7.23 per 100,000 per year occurred in the 45–54 year age group. This suggests an increase in the age at diagnosis among white females over the 15-year interval separating these studies. This is supported by an increase in the median age at diagnosis, which rose from 39.7 among

93 cases diagnosed between 1949 and 1968 (3) to 42 among 72 cases in this study. It is important to note, however, the significant decline in incidence rates above age 54 among white females in this study (Table 2 and Figure 1), compatible with the well-recognized sex effect occurring during the reproductive years which is associated with rates varying from 4.73–7.23 per 100,000 per year between ages 15 and 54.

Incidence rates increase 8.5-fold with puberty in black females and reach maximum values in the 25–34 year age group followed by a steady exponential decline. The median age at diagnosis of 33 years in black females is in agreement with that reported by Siegel and Lee in 35 cases diagnosed between 1949 and 1968 (3). The significant difference in mean age at diagnosis between black and white females noted in this study has not been previously reported. Others have noted differences in the racial distribution of patients with late-onset SLE compared with patients with young-onset (15). In this study there was no significant difference in the frequency of diagnosis at or above age 55 among white females compared with black females; 17 (23.6%) of 72 cases versus 26 (13.7%) of 190 cases ($P = 0.08$, Fisher's exact test).

The difference in mean age at diagnosis may, however, be due to bias in case identification if hospitalization for diagnosis of SLE was more likely in younger blacks than whites, especially below age 34, because of differences in medical practice patterns and/or severity of illness. Socioeconomic factors might also be important in this regard; an association of low socioeconomic status with black race and decreased survival in patients with SLE was the reason for an apparent association of black race with decreased survival in a recent multicenter study (16). Thus, if socioeconomic status differed between racial groups, as it would be expected to, differential access to public clinic versus private practitioner care might influence the probability of hospital admission for diagnosis and care of SLE. We took into consideration whether SLE was the primary discharge diagnosis or simply a listed comorbid diagnosis on the medical record. Overall, 36 (11.9%) of the 302 incident cases had SLE listed as a secondary diagnosis; there were no statistically significant differences in the frequency of this parameter between sex–race groups. Despite these possible biases, the difference in age at diagnosis might in fact represent host differences in immune response (17) related to the development of SLE. In any event, this difference is comparable with that noted in mean age at death among black and white females in an 11-year study of mortality from SLE in the United States (18).

Comparison of the age-specific incidence rates between the sex–race groups reveals interesting sex and race ratios (Table 3). Excess female incidence, especially among blacks where adequate numbers of cases occurred, was most striking in the reproductive years through age 34. The importance of endocrine factors related to sex hormones has been repeatedly noted in patients with SLE, with emphasis on their possible role in pathogenesis and expression of disease (19–24). Excess incidence in blacks is less striking but noteworthy and confirms the data of Siegel and Lee (1–3). Increased prevalence (1–3,5) and mortality (13,18,25) among blacks compared with whites with SLE has also been noted. The synergistic interaction of female sex and nonwhite race in producing the highest mortality rates from SLE (18,25), as well as from systemic sclerosis (26) and polymyositis/dermatomyositis (27) in nonwhite females has previously been reported. The present data demonstrate a significant interaction of female sex and black race in producing higher incidence rates in black females not only in the childbearing years, but also throughout the overall age spectrum. Racial differences in sex hormone production and metabolism (28), as well as immune reactivity (17) may interact with the sex factors (20) in ways which remain to be elucidated.

This study found no evidence of temporal trends in either yearly age-adjusted incidence rates among the sex–race groups or mean age at diagnosis. The absence of temporal trends in incidence rates is consistent with our observation of declining mortality rates from SLE (18) in the setting of improvement in survivorship during a time interval which included this study period (29). Furthermore, the absence of secular trends in mean age at diagnosis is consistent with our observation of increasing mean age at death from SLE (18) associated temporally with improved prognosis among SLE patients.

The absence of a temporal increase in hospital-diagnosed SLE incidence rates in this study does not necessarily imply a stability of overall population rates, since increasing numbers of cases may be diagnosed and managed on an outpatient basis. Such data were not obtained in this study, so the possibility of an increase in total SLE cannot be excluded.

The overall population average annual age-adjusted incidence rate, based on first hospital discharge diagnosis of 4.62 per 100,000 per year (95% confidence intervals: 4.10, 5.14) is lower than those reported for Rochester, Minnesota (5.7 per 100,000 per year) (4) and San Francisco (7.6 per 100,000 per year) (5). These studies, as noted above, included both in-hospital and outpatient diagnosed cases in well-defined populations and would be expected to have higher incidence rates since all cases of SLE do not require hospitalization for diagnosis. The overall rate in Baltimore is more than double that of 2.0 per 100,000 per year in New York City (3) and confirms the increase in incidence rates of SLE noted previously. Although this increase may, in large part, be explained by increased physician diagnosis because of doctor and patient awareness and more sensitive laboratory tests, a true increase in incidence cannot be excluded. Nonetheless, SLE can no longer be considered a rare disease, with an incidence in young white females below age 25 and in black females below age 34 which may be comparable to or exceed that of definite rheumatoid arthritis (30). Continued research toward the development of both primary and secondary prevention strategies (31) is clearly warranted.

ACKNOWLEDGMENTS

The author wishes to thank Sheila Brown for abstracting patient records, Katherine vanDyke for assistance in computer programming and data analysis, and Cathay Insley for preparation of the manuscript.

REFERENCES

1. Siegel M, Lee SL: The epidemiology of systemic lupus erythematosus: results of a population study in New York City, Population Studies of the Rheumatic Diseases: Proceedings of the Third International Symposium. Edited by PH Bennett, PHN Wood. New York, Excerpta Medica, 1968, pp 245–255
2. Siegel M, Holley HL, Lee SL: Epidemiologic studies on systemic lupus erythematosus: comparative data for New York City and Jefferson County, Alabama, 1956–1965. Arthritis Rheum 13:802–811, 1970
3. Siegel M, Lee SL: The epidemiology of systemic lupus erythematosus. Semin Arthritis Rheum 3:1–54, 1973
4. Kurland LT, Hauser WA, Ferguson RH, Holley KE: Epidemiologic features of diffuse connective tissue disorders in Rochester, Minn., 1951–1967, with special reference to systemic lupus erythematosus. Mayo Clin Proc 44:649–663, 1969
5. Fessel WJ: Systemic lupus erythematosus in the community: incidence, prevalence, outcome and first symptoms; the high prevalence in black women. Arch Intern Med 134:1027–1035, 1974
6. Svanborg A, Solvell L: Incidence of disseminated lupus erythematosus: follow-up studies indicating increased frequency. JAMA 165:1126–1128, 1957
7. Leonhardt T: Family studies in systemic lupus erythematosus. Acta Med Scand [Suppl] 176(416):1–156, 1964
8. Cohen AS, Reynolds WE, Franklin EC, Kulka JP, Ropes MW, Shulman LE, Wallace SL: Preliminary criteria for the classification of systemic lupus erythematosus. Bull Rheum Dis 21:643–645, 1971
9. US Department of Health, Education and Welfare: Eighth Revision of the International Classification of Disease. Publication No. (PHS) 1693. US Government Printing Office, 1965
10. Chiang CL: Standard error of the age-adjusted death rate, Vital Statistics—Special Report. Selected Studies, No. 9. USDHEW, 1961
11. Snedecor GW, Cochran WG: Statistical Methods. Sixth edition. Ames, The Iowa State University Press, 1967, pp 193–195
12. Rothman KJ: The estimation of synergy or antagonism. Am J Epidemiol 103:506–511, 1976
13. Hochberg MC, Arnett FC: Systemic lupus erythematosus: epidemiology and genetics. Md State Med J 32:524–528, 1983
14. Kosmides VS, Hochberg MC: A data base management system for clinical and epidemiologic studies in systemic lupus erythematosus: design and maintenance, Proceedings of the Eighth Annual Symposium on Computer Applications in Medical Care. Edited by G Cohen. Silver Spring, MD, IEEE Computer Society Press (in press)
15. Ballou SP, Khan MA, Kushner I: Clinical features of systemic lupus erythematosus: differences related to race and age of onset. Arthritis Rheum 25:55–60, 1982
16. Ginzler EM, Diamond HS, Weiner M. Schlesinger M, Fries JF, Wasner C, Medsger TA Jr, Ziegler G, Klippel JH, Hadler NM, Albert DA, Hess EV, Spencer-Green G, Grayzel A, Worth D, Hahn BH, Barnett EV: A multicenter study of outcome in systemic lupus erythematosus. I. Entry variables as predictors of prognosis. Arthritis Rheum 25:601–611, 1982
17. Buckley CE, Dorsey FC: Serum immunoglobulin levels throughout the life span of healthy man. Ann Intern Med 75:673–682, 1971
18. Lopez-Acuna D, Hochberg MC, Gittelsohn AM: Mortality from discoid and systemic lupus erythematosus in the United States, 1968–1978 (abstract). Arthritis Rheum (suppl) 25:S80, 1982
19. Stern R, Fishman J, Brusman H, Kunkel HG: Systemic lupus erythematosus associated with Klinefelter's syndrome. Arthritis Rheum 20:18–22, 1977
20. Masi AT, Kaslow RA: Sex effects in systemic lupus erythematosus: a clue to pathogenesis. Arthritis Rheum 21:480–484, 1978
21. Lahita RG, Bradlow HL, Kunkel HG, Fishman J: Alterations of estrogen metabolism in systemic lupus erythematosus. Arthritis Rheum 22:1195–1198, 1979

22. Lahita RG, Bradlow HL, Kunkel HG, Fishman J: Increased 16 α-hydroxylation of estradiol in systemic lupus erythematosus. J Clin Endocrinol Metab 53:174–178, 1981
23. Lahita RG, Bradlow HL, Fishman J, Kunkel HG: Estrogen metabolism in systemic lupus erythematosus: patients and family members. Arthritis Rheum 25:843–846, 1982
24. Hochberg MC, Kaslow RA: Risk factors for the development of systemic lupus erythematosus: a case-control study (abstract). Clin Res 31:732A, 1983
25. Kaslow RA, Masi AT: Age, sex and race effects on mortality from systemic lupus erythematosus in the United States. Arthritis Rheum 21:473–479, 1978
26. Hochberg MC, Lopez-Acuna D, Gittelsohn AM: Mortality from systemic sclerosis (scleroderma) in the United States, 1969–1979, Proceedings of an International Conference on Progressive Systemic Sclerosis. Edited by GP Rodnan, CM Black. New York, Gower Medical Publishing Co. (in press)
27. Hochberg MC, Lopez-Acuna D, Gittelsohn AM: Mortality from polymyositis and dermatomyositis in the United States, 1968–1978. Arthritis Rheum 26:1465–1471, 1983
28. Hill P, Wynder EL, Helman P, Hickman R, Rona G, Kuno K: Plasma hormone levels in different ethnic populations of women. Cancer Res 36:2297–2301, 1976
29. Hochberg MC: Systemic lupus erythematosus. VIII. Prognosis. Md State Med J 33:114–116, 1984
30. Linos A, Worthington JW, O'Fallon WM, Kurland LT: The epidemiology of rheumatoid arthritis in Rochester, Minnesota: a study of incidence, prevalence, and mortality. Am J Epidemiol 111:87–98, 1980
31. National Arthritis Advisory Board: Proceedings of the Prevention Conference on Arthritis. Washington, DC, US Government Printing Office. In preparation

EVOLUTION OF PRIMARY RAYNAUD'S PHENOMENON (RAYNAUD'S DISEASE) TO CONNECTIVE TISSUE DISEASE

DAVID D. GERBRACHT, VIRGINIA D. STEEN, GAYLE L. ZIEGLER, THOMAS A. MEDSGER, JR., and GERALD P. RODNAN

Eighty-seven patients diagnosed as having primary Raynaud's phenomenon (Raynaud's disease) were reexamined after this symptom had been present for a mean of 8.8 years (range 2.0–34.5). One or more additional clinical feature(s) suggesting an underlying connective tissue disease were found in 12 patients (14%) at first evaluation, and in 23 (26%) by the last evaluation. The most frequent findings were puffy fingers (10 patients), digital tip pitting scars (8 patients), and digital tip ulcerations (6 patients). Distal esophageal hypomotility and/or decreased pulmonary diffusing capacity for carbon monoxide were found in 12 patients. Only 4 individuals (5%) developed clear evidence of a connective tissue disease, and in all cases, the diagnosis was the CREST (calcinosis, Raynaud's phenomenon, esophageal dysmotility, sclerodactyly, telangiectasias) syndrome variant of systemic sclerosis. This condition became obvious 8–17 years after the onset of Raynaud's phenomenon. One or more serologic test values were initially abnormal in 2 of these CREST syndrome patients, as well as in 12 patients who continued to have primary Raynaud's phenomenon at the last evaluation. The combination of puffy fingers, digital pitting scars, and serum anticentromere antibody, all consistent with CREST syndrome, occurred in a small group of patients. None of the 78 patients whose serologic tests were repeated during followup had a change in the serologic profile. These results suggest that only a small proportion of patients with primary Raynaud's phenomenon develop one of the connective tissue diseases during the first decade after onset. When such a disorder does appear, systemic sclerosis with the CREST syndrome variant is the most likely eventual diagnosis.

Raynaud's phenomenon is generally classified as "primary" when no underlying cause or associated condition explaining its presence can be identified (1). This diagnosis is thus made with the realization that some patients may subsequently develop evidence of a connective tissue disease or other disorder with which this circulatory condition is known to be associated, such as systemic sclerosis (scleroderma), systemic lupus erythematosus (SLE), or polymyositis–dermatomyositis (2,3). Our study presents initial and followup information on a group of 87 patients who were initially diagnosed as having primary Raynaud's phenomenon and who had this condition for at least 2 years at the time of their final evaluation. Our objectives were to determine the subsequent frequency of connective tissue disease in these patients, and to identify clinical, laboratory, or serologic findings which might serve to predict this outcome.

PATIENTS AND METHODS

All patients diagnosed as having primary Raynaud's phenomenon by faculty members of the Division of Rheuma-

From the Department of Medicine, Division of Rheumatology and Clinical Immunology, University of Pittsburgh School of Medicine, Pittsburgh, Pennsylvania.

Supported by grants from the National Institutes of Health (FR-00056 and AM-21393); The RGK Foundation, Austin, Texas; and the Arthritis Foundation, Western Pennsylvania Chapter.

David D. Gerbracht, MD: Fellow in Rheumatology; Virginia D. Steen, MD: Assistant Professor of Medicine; Gayle L. Ziegler, RN, BSN: Research Assistant; Thomas A. Medsger, Jr., MD: Associate Professor of Medicine.

Dr. Rodnan is deceased.

Address reprint requests to Virginia D. Steen, MD, Department of Medicine, 985 Scaife Hall, University of Pittsburgh School of Medicine, Pittsburgh, PA 15261.

Submitted for publication March 2, 1984; accepted in revised form June 26, 1984.

tology and Clinical Immunology of the University of Pittsburgh from 1973 through 1981 were identified. This diagnosis was based on history or observation of bilateral, cold-induced blanching and/or cyanosis of the fingers, or fingers and toes. Individuals with historical or physical evidence of arteriosclerosis, thoracic outlet syndrome, pneumatic tool use, or other known causes of Raynaud's phenomenon were excluded, as were those with sufficient additional clinical findings to warrant the diagnosis of one of the connective tissue diseases. All patients had Raynaud's phenomenon for a minimum of 2 years by last evaluation.

Initial evaluation included a detailed history and physical examination, and in most, but not all patients, the following laboratory studies: a complete blood count with platelet count, urinalysis, blood urea nitrogen and serum creatinine concentrations, serum creatine phosphokinase activity, dipstick examination or 24-hour urine collection for protein excretion, a serologic test for syphilis (VDRL or RPR), direct Coombs' test, roentgenograms of the hands and chest, cineesophagram, and pulmonary function tests with diffusing capacity for carbon monoxide (DLco). Serum was also tested for the presence of antinuclear antibody (ANA), anti-ribonucleoprotein antibody (anti-RNP), anti-Sm antibody, anti-DNA, anticentromere antibody (ACA), rheumatoid factor (RF), and concentrations of serum complement components (C3 and C4).

ANA, anti-DNA, and ACA were determined by the indirect immunofluorescence technique using rat liver, the kinetoplast of *Crithidia luciliae*, and the HEp-2 cell line (4), respectively, as substrates. Anti-RNP and anti-Sm antibodies were detected by passive hemagglutination and hemagglutination inhibition techniques, and rheumatoid factor assay was performed by latex agglutination (fixation). The following titers were considered abnormal: ANA $\geq$1:32, anti-RNP $\geq$1:10,000, anti-Sm $\geq$1:10, anti-DNA $\geq$1:10, ACA $\geq$1:40, and RF $\geq$1:80.

Followup evaluation for this study was performed either by return visit or by telephone interview. The former included an interim history and physical examination designed to detect clinical features which might suggest the development of one of the connective tissue diseases. These features consisted of puffy fingers, sclerodactyly, digital pitting scars, digital tip ulcerations, digital telangiectasias, arthralgias, arthritis, pleuritis/pericarditis, photosensitivity, malar rash, and proximal muscle weakness. The definitions used were those published by the Glossary Subcommittee of the American Rheumatism Association (ARA) in the Dictionary of the Rheumatic Diseases (5).

In addition, arthralgia was defined as pain and morning stiffness in multiple peripheral joints without detectable swelling and not accounted for by other conditions, e.g., osteoarthritis. Patients contacted by telephone answered a questionnaire designed to reliably elicit the presence of these features. When possible, we confirmed responses and collected interim data by obtaining similar information and specific physical examination results from the patient's private physician.

Blood was obtained for repeat serologic testing or

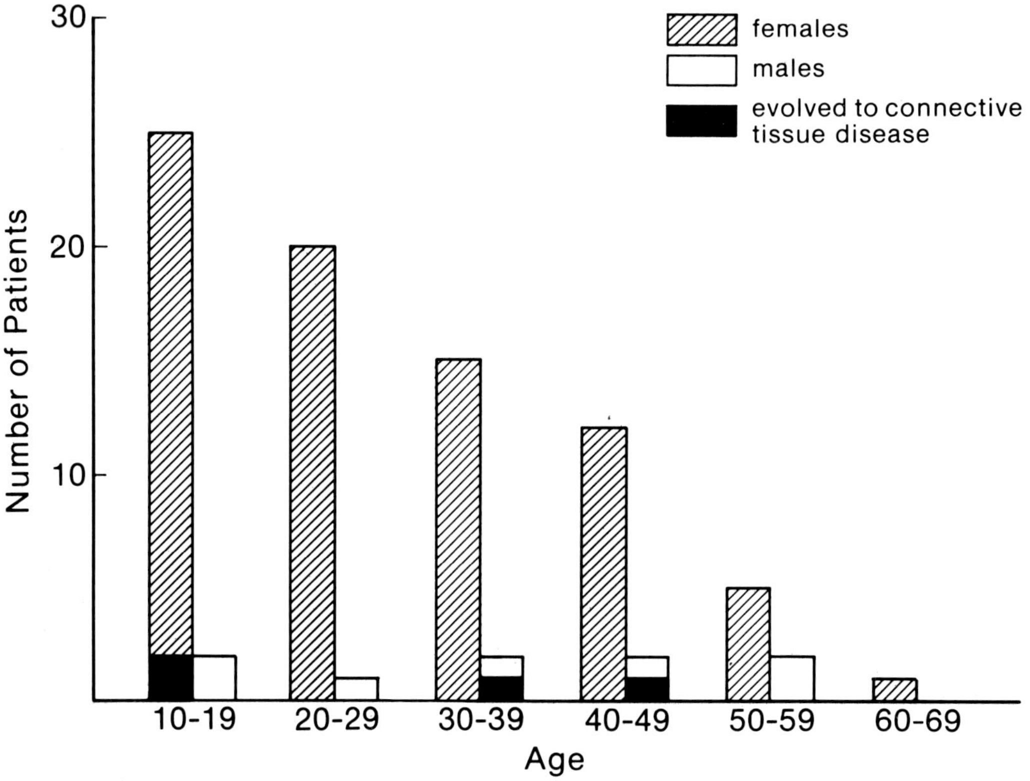

Figure 1. Evolution to connective tissue disease in relation to sex and age at onset of Raynaud's phenomenon.

was mailed from patients unable to return to Pittsburgh. If the patient's serum was found to have an abnormal serologic test result in either the initial (stored frozen) or final (fresh) serum sample, the specific test was repeated simultaneously on both serum samples. In this way, we controlled for any variation in laboratory test technique which might have occurred over time. Additional laboratory studies were ordered only if clinically indicated.

Published preliminary or revised ARA criteria were used for classifying patients as having definite systemic sclerosis, SLE, or definite rheumatoid arthritis at any time during the followup period (6–8). The criteria of Bohan and colleagues were used for the diagnosis of polymyositis–dermatomyositis (9). Patients having only Raynaud's phenomenon and sclerodactyly were considered to have an unclassifiable connective tissue disease most closely resembling the CREST syndrome variant of progressive systemic sclerosis (10).

RESULTS

Ninety-one patients were diagnosed during 1973–1981 as having primary Raynaud's phenomenon. Four patients were excluded, 2 because no followup information was obtainable and 2 because the duration of Raynaud's phenomenon was less than 2 years by last evaluation. Sixty-seven patients were reexamined, and 20 individuals were contacted by telephone.

The final study group thus consisted of 87 individuals, 78 women and 9 men (female:male ratio 8.6:1). The sex and the age at onset of Raynaud's phenomenon according to patient history are shown in Figure 1. The mean age at onset was 30.2 years with a range of 10–61 years. Forty-eight patients (55%) experienced the onset of Raynaud's phenomenon before age 30. Women were younger at onset with a mean age of 28.9, compared with 33.0 years in the men.

These patients had had Raynaud's phenomenon for an average of 5.1 years (median 3.0) at the time of our initial evaluation, with a range of 0.1–34.0 years. Thirty-six patients (41%) were first seen within 2 years (mean 0.8) of the onset of Raynaud's phenomenon symptoms. The total duration of Raynaud's phenomenon from its onset to our final evaluation ranged from 2.0–34.5 years (mean 8.8, median 6.8).

Table 1 lists those individuals who exhibited 1 or more of the clinical features or laboratory abnormalities mentioned above. Initially, 12 patients (14%) were found to have 1 or more clinical findings frequently observed in connective tissue diseases, in addition to Raynaud's phenomenon. This was true of 23 patients (26%) by the time of the final evaluation. Puffy fingers (10 patients), sclerodactyly (4 patients), digital pitting scars (8 patients), digital tip ulcerations (6 patients), arthralgias (5 patients), digital telangiectasias (4 patients), and pleurisy (1 patient) were detected, but no patients had arthritis, malar rash, photosensitivity, or proximal muscle weakness. The mean duration of Raynaud's phenomenon by the last visit was similar in the 23 patients with clinical findings (9.4 years) and the 64 without such findings (8.6 years).

Table 1. Clinical and laboratory abnormalities identified in patients with primary Raynaud's phenomenon (RP)*

Patient	Detected at first visit	Developed during course	Duration of RP at final visit (years)
1	DP, DU, ANA, anti-RNP, DC		5.8
2	PF, DP, ACA, DC		2.8
3	A		15.6
4	DP, ACA	PF	3.5
5	PF, ACA	S, DP, DU, T, A	7.8†
6	A	T	16.3
7	PF		5.8
8	A		13.9
9	PF	DP	4.9
10	DPE, DC		5.5
11	DU	DP	5.1
12	A		6.8
13	ANA, RF	S, DU, DP, T	8.6†
14	DC	DU	13.9
15		P	4.5
16		S	16.8‡
17		S	14.0‡
18		PF, DU	5.8
19		PF	6.6
20		PF	4.9
21		T	32.7
22	ACA	PF	9.1
23		PF	6.8
24	ANA, anti-RNP		5.1
25	ACA, DC		4.9
26	ANA, anti-RNP		5.2
27	ANA		34.5
28	ANA		23.6
29	RF		16.9
30	RF		11.5
31	E		3.9
32	DC		9.5
33	ANA, anti-RNP, DC		8.2
34	DC		5.7
35	DC		4.4
36	DC		9.7
37	DC		29.4

* DP = digital pitting scars; DU = digital tip ulceration; ANA = antinuclear antibodies; RNP = ribonucleoprotein; PF = puffy fingers; ACA = anticentromere antibodies; A = arthralgias; S = sclerodactyly; T = telangiectasias; RF = rheumatoid factor; P = pleurisy; DC = DLco <80% predicted normal; E = esophageal hypomotility.

† Time after the onset of Raynaud's phenomenon that criteria were satisfied for definite systemic sclerosis.

‡ Time after the onset of Raynaud's phenomenon that diagnosis of unclassified connective tissue disease was made.

In 4 of the 23 patients with the above clinical and/or laboratory abnormalities, a connective tissue disease was diagnosed during the followup period. Two individuals (patients 5 and 13) developed sclerodactyly and digital pitting scars and satisfied ARA minor criteria for definite systemic sclerosis (6), 7.8 and 8.6 years, respectively, after the onset of Raynaud's phenomenon. Two others (patients 16 and 17) also developed sclerodactyly after 16.8 and 14.0 years of Raynaud's phenomenon, respectively, but had insufficient additional evidence to satisfy criteria for systemic sclerosis. The latter patients appear to have a disorder most consistent with systemic sclerosis with incomplete CREST syndrome. One of these individuals (patient 5) had a clinical finding (puffy fingers) when first evaluated 4.0 years after the onset of Raynaud's phenomenon, but the other 3 had no clinical findings at the time of the first evaluation.

Distal esophageal hypomotility (2 of 49 patients) and DLco <80% of predicted normal (11 of 43 patients) were the only laboratory abnormalities detected. Interestingly, none of the individuals with these abnormalities had esophageal or pulmonary complaints; all had normal chest roentgenogram results; and none subsequently developed further evidence of a connective tissue disease. Pulmonary fibrosis (0/63) and digital calcinosis (0/50) by roentgenographic examination, urine protein >300 mg in 24 hours (0/39), platelet count $<100,000/mm^3$ (0/42), positive VDRL or RPR (0/50), positive direct Coombs' test (0/29), and elevated serum creatinine phosphokinase activity (0/53) were sought in many patients but not found.

Fourteen patients accounted for 19 abnormal serologic results as defined above (Table 1). ANA was found in 7 (8%) of 84 patients, ACA in 5 of 82 (6%), anti-RNP in 4 of 84 (5%), and RF in 3 of 84 (4%). Anti-DNA and anti-Sm antibodies were not present in any of these patients. Two patients (1 with ANA and RF [patient 13] and 1 with ACA [patient 5]) developed systemic sclerosis with CREST syndrome. Twelve of the 14 remained free of a connective tissue disease after a mean duration of 11.3 years. A significant correlation was found between the occurrence of ACA and puffy fingers ($P < 0.05$) and ACA and digital pitting scars ($P < 0.05$), as well as between the latter physical findings ($P < 0.05$).

Seventy-eight of the original 84 patients with serologic studies had all of these tests repeated. Individual titers of anti-RNP and ACA were identical on repeat testing, while 2 ANA and 2 RF titers had 1–2 tube-dilution differences between the initial and final samples. None of the followup changes in titers in these 4 patients altered the initial designation as normal or abnormal.

DISCUSSION

It is generally thought (11,12), and it is also our own experience, that the majority of patients with Raynaud's phenomenon who develop a connective tissue disease do so within the first 2 years after the onset of this symptom. In this study, we evaluated a large group of patients who were initially diagnosed as having primary Raynaud's phenomenon; patients were evaluated an average of 5.1 years after the onset of symptoms. We were interested in the frequency of evolution to a connective tissue disease in these patients, as well as any clinical, laboratory, or serologic clues at the first visit which might predict such an outcome.

Requirements for the diagnosis of a connective tissue disease vary considerably in the medical literature. We demanded fulfillment of established published ARA criteria (6–9), which, admittedly, is arbitrary. These criteria were promulgated for purposes of classification rather than for early diagnosis and, as shown previously, will exclude some patients believed clinically to have 1 of these conditions. Our 2 study patients who developed sclerodactyly but failed to meet criteria for systemic sclerosis would be considered by many, if not most, observers to have the CREST syndrome variant of this disorder (10,12).

Gifford and Hines (2) performed a medical record review, questionnaire, and reexamination of 377 women and girls with Raynaud's disease seen at the Mayo Clinic during the period 1920–1945. Two hundred eighty had adequate followup (mean 12 years), of whom 10 (3%) developed a clear-cut connective tissue disease. Five patients were considered to have rheumatoid arthritis and 4 had systemic sclerosis of the "acrosclerosis" (CREST syndrome) type; 3 of the latter patients had skin thickening limited to the digits (sclerodactyly alone). One patient developed polyarteritis nodosa.

In a prospective study, Harper et al (3) recorded that 3 (8%) of 39 patients had developed a connective tissue disease after a mean of 2 years followup (7 years mean total duration of Raynaud's phenomenon). None of these 3 patients fully met criteria for 1 of the connective tissue diseases (6–9) and thus their disease was considered "undifferentiated." Based on the descriptions of these patients, we believe that 1 had probable CREST syndrome and the others had features of SLE. Several other studies (13–16) contain important information concerning the evolution of connective tissue disease in patients with Raynaud's phenomenon. However, data from these studies are presented in such a way that the duration of Raynaud's phenomenon prior to the development of these associated conditions cannot be determined.

We have reached similar conclusions regarding the frequency of evolution to a connective tissue disease; 4 (5%) of 87 primary Raynaud's phenomenon patients ultimately developed a connective tissue disease. In contrast, we did not find the diversity of outcomes noted by other authors. All of our 4 patients were considered to have systemic sclerosis with the CREST syndrome (10,17).

Pitted scars and ulcerations of the fingertips are occasionally noted in patients with primary Raynaud's phenomenon (2,3,6,16,18). Their occurrence has been looked upon as concomitant with severe Raynaud's phenomenon rather than an indicator of an underlying disorder (2,16). Three of our 4 patients who developed systemic sclerosis had such scars or ulcerations during followup, but 9 other patients with continued primary Raynaud's phenomenon also had one or both of these findings.

Puffy fingers, which may antedate the development of systemic sclerosis by months or many years (10), were noted in 10 of the 87 patients, only 1 of whom developed systemic sclerosis with the CREST syndrome. Anticentromere antibody has been reported in 49–96% of patients with the CREST syndrome (4,17,19). In our patients, ACA was associated with puffy fingers and with digital pitting scars. This combination of findings may identify a subset of patients destined to develop systemic sclerosis. Thus far, 4 of our 5 patients with ACA have not yet developed systemic sclerosis after 2.8–9.1 years (mean 5.1). More prolonged followup may be required.

Distal esophageal hypomotility and diminished carbon monoxide diffusing capacity have been well-documented as occurring in patients with primary Raynaud's phenomenon (16,18,20). The frequency of these abnormalities in our study was comparable. Although such changes are often found in patients with established connective tissue disease (18,20), none of the 12 patients in this study, with 1 or both of these abnormalities, has yet shown such evolution.

Other authors have noted a low frequency of serum autoantibodies in patients with primary Raynaud's phenomenon (3,17,18,21). In those studies, ANA was present in a total of 23 (26%) of 83 patients (3,21). Our results proved similar; only 17% of patients had autoantibodies. Raynaud's phenomenon and an abnormal serologic test result may coexist for many years before the onset of a connective tissue disease (17). Although 2 of our patients had 1 or more of these abnormal serologic test values prior to the development of systemic sclerosis, 12 others with 1 or more serologic abnormalities did not develop connective tissue disease after a mean followup of 11.3 years. We were surprised to find the serologic profiles of these patients so remarkably constant over time.

We did not perform nailfold capillary microscopy on our patients, although an abnormal capillary pattern has been considered a useful prognostic indicator of the subsequent development of systemic sclerosis (3). In 2 recent studies, a combined total of 3 of 11 patients with "isolated" Raynaud's phenomenon and an abnormal nailfold capillary pattern developed connective tissue disease. However, this transition also occurred in 2 of 72 individuals with Raynaud's phenomenon and a normal capillary pattern (3,22). Prolonged observation and better correlation of capillary microscopy with clinical findings, such as puffy fingers, digital tip lesions, and ACA, are needed to determine the specificity and predictive value of these vascular changes.

We conclude that it is infrequent for patients considered to have primary Raynaud's phenomenon to develop a connective tissue disease during the first decade of their disease. Such transition does occur occasionally, however, and even more time may be required than the 9 years mean duration of Raynaud's phenomenon in this study. Of those who do develop additional findings during the followup period, the clinical features are most commonly those seen in the CREST syndrome variant of progressive systemic sclerosis. Laboratory and serologic abnormalities were nonspecific and, in this study, were not helpful in predicting evolution to connective tissue disease.

REFERENCES

1. Jepson RP: Raynaud's phenomenon—a review of the clinical problem. Ann R Coll Surg Engl 9:35–51, 1951
2. Gifford RW, Hines EA: Raynaud's disease among women and girls. Circulation 16:1012–1021, 1957
3. Harper FE, Maricq HR, Turner RE, Lidman RW,

LeRoy EC: A prospective study of Raynaud's phenomenon and early connective tissue disease. Am J Med 72:883–888, 1982

4. Tan EM, Rodnan GP, Garcia I, Moroi Y, Fritzler MJ, Peebles C: Diversity of antinuclear antibodies in scleroderma: anti-centromere antibody and its relationship to CREST. Arthritis Rheum 23:617–625, 1980
5. Dictionary of the Rheumatic Diseases. Vol. 1: Signs and Symptoms. New York, Contact Associates International, Ltd., 1982
6. Subcommittee for Scleroderma Criteria of the American Rheumatism Association Diagnostic and Therapeutic Criteria Committee: Preliminary criteria for the classification of systemic sclerosis (scleroderma). Arthritis Rheum 23:581–590, 1980
7. Tan EM, Cohen AS, Fries JF, Masi AT, McShane DJ, Rothfield NF, Schaller JG, Talal N, Winchester RJ: The 1982 revised criteria for the classification of systemic lupus erythematosus. Arthritis Rheum 25:1271–1277, 1982
8. Ropes MW, Bennett GA, Cobb S, Jacox R, Jessar RA: 1958 revision of the diagnostic criteria for rheumatoid arthritis. Bull Rheum Dis 9:175–176, 1958
9. Bohan A, Peter JB, Bowman RL, Pearson CM: A computer assisted analysis of 153 patients with polymyositis and dermatomyositis. Medicine (Baltimore) 56:255–286, 1977
10. Rodnan GP: Progressive systemic sclerosis (scleroderma), Arthritis and Allied Conditions. Ninth edition. Edited by DJ McCarty Jr. Philadelphia, Lea & Febiger, 1979, pp 762–809
11. Allen EV, Brown GE: Raynaud's disease: a critical review of minimal requisites for diagnosis. Am J Med Sci 183:187–200, 1932
12. Blain A III, Coller FA, Carver GB: Raynaud's disease—a study of criteria for prognosis. Surgery 29:387–397, 1951
13. De Takats G, Fowler EF: Raynaud's phenomenon. JAMA 179:99–106, 1962
14. Porter JM, Bardana EJ, Baur GM, Wesche DH, Andrasch RH, Rosch J: The clinical significance of Raynaud's syndrome. Surgery 80:756–764, 1976
15. Blunt RJ, Porter JM: Raynaud syndrome. Semin Arthritis Rheum 10:282–308, 1981
16. Velayos EE, Robinson H, Prociuncula FE, Masi AT: Clinical correlation analysis of 137 patients with Raynaud's phenomenon. Am J Med Sci 262:347–356, 1971
17. Fritzler MJ, Kinsella TD, Garbutt E: The CREST syndrome: a distinct serologic entity with anticentromere antibodies. Am J Med 69:520–526, 1980
18. Kallenberg CGM, Wouda AA, The TH: Systemic involvement and immunologic findings in patients with Raynaud's phenomenon. Am J Med 69:675–680, 1980
19. Steen VD, Ziegler GL, Rodnan GP, Medsger TA Jr: Clinical and laboratory associations of anticentromere antibody in patients with progressive systemic sclerosis. Arthritis Rheum 27:125–131, 1984
20. Stevens MB, Hookman P, Siegel CL, Esterly JR, Shulman LE, Hendrik TR: Aperistalsis of the esophagus in patients with connective tissue disorders and Raynaud's phenomenon. N Engl J Med 270:1218–1222, 1964
21. Kallenberg CGM, Pastoor GW, Wouda AA, The TH: Antinuclear antibodies in patients with Raynaud's phenomenon: clinical significance of anticentromere antibodies. Ann Rheum Dis 41:382–387, 1982
22. Spencer-Green G, Hess EV: Prospective analysis of nailfold capillary pattern in Raynaud's phenomenon (abstract). Arthritis Rheum (suppl) 25:S127, 1982

BRIEF REPORT

BENEFICIAL EFFECT OF INTRAVENOUS CYCLOPHOSPHAMIDE AND ORAL PREDNISONE ON D-PENICILLAMINE–ASSOCIATED BRONCHIOLITIS OBLITERANS

MARTINUS A. F. J. VAN DE LAAR, CEES J. J. WESTERMANN, SJOERD SC. WAGENAAR, and HUIBERT J. DINANT

Bronchiolitis obliterans is an infrequent pulmonary complication of rheumatoid disease (1–6). In general, the prognosis is favorable and symptoms subside after prednisone therapy. However, there have been reports of fatalities associated with this condition (1,6,7).

Since the introduction of D-penicillamine as an antirheumatic drug in the early 1970s, a clinically distinct type of bronchiolitis obliterans has been described in several case reports of patients taking D-penicillamine (1,8–13). Geddes et al (1) were the first to suspect a possible relationship between the drug and this type of bronchiolitis obliterans, which is potentially fatal.

We report another case of D-penicillamine–associated bronchiolitis obliterans. Combined immunosuppressive therapy of cyclophosphamide and prednisone altered the downhill clinical course. The probable existence of a distinct histologic picture in D-penicillamine–associated obliterating bronchiolitis is discussed.

Case report. A 32-year-old nonsmoking woman was admitted to our hospital because of progressive dyspnea and nonproductive cough. Her medical history was unremarkable except for a 2-year history of definite rheumatoid arthritis. During the 6 months prior to admission she had been treated with D-penicillamine, 250 mg daily. A gradual improvement of arthritis symptoms had taken place, and she regained full capacity to carry out all activities of daily life.

Four weeks before admission she had minor gynecologic surgery under general anesthesia. Two weeks after this procedure, while riding a bicycle, she experienced acute left-sided chest pain and dyspnea, which forced her to return home on foot. During the following week she became progressively dyspneic and developed a nonproductive cough. Her family physician prescribed amoxycillin, which did not improve her condition.

On admission she was dyspneic and in obvious respiratory distress. The body temperature was 36.8°C, the pulse rate was 96, and the respiration 20. Blood pressure was 120/80 mm Hg. Pulmonary auscultation revealed inspiratory rales with normal expiration. There were no signs of venous thrombosis in the lower extremities.

Erythrocyte sedimentation rate, complete blood count, serum electrolyte, liver, and renal function test, and urinalysis results were normal. Rheumatoid factor titer by sheep cell agglutination was 1:256. The antinuclear factor titer was 1:320. Lupus erythematosus cells were absent. Cryoglobulins and cold agglutinins were not detectable. There were no signs of circulating immune complexes as measured by the C1q binding assay and the leukocyte phagocytosis test. Total hemolytic complement, C3, and C4 complement factors were normal. T lymphocyte proliferation did not occur after stimulation with D-penicillamine; proliferation was normal after stimulation with concanavalin A. Serologic tests for respiratory viral infections showed negative findings. Cultures of sputum,

From the Departments of Rheumatology, Pulmonary Medicine, and Pathology, St. Antonius Hospital, Nieuwegein, The Netherlands.

Martinus A. F. J. van de Laar, MD; Cees J. J. Westermann, MD; Sjoerd Sc. Wagenaar, MD; Huibert J. Dinant, MD.

Address reprint requests to Huibert J. Dinant, MD, Department of Rheumatology, St. Antonius Hospital, Postbus 2500, 3430 EM Nieuwegein, The Netherlands.

Submitted for publication April 25, 1984; accepted in revised form June 26, 1984.

Table 1. Pulmonary function findings in a patient with D-penicillamine–associated bronchiolitis obliterans*

Date	VC	RV	FEV_1	Po_2, mm Hg	Course
12/29/82				73	Admission
1/7/83	1.70		0.90	64	Thoracotomy
1/13/83				52	Start prednisone 60 mg
1/25/83	1.70 (1.70)†	1.57 (1.96)†	0.80 (0.90)†	66	
2/11/83	1.80 (2.30)†		0.85 (0.90)†	67	
2/21/83	2.20		0.79	59	Start cyclophosphamide
3/1/83	2.60		0.85	70	
3/18/83	2.00		0.80	61‡	Respiratory infection
3/31/83				71	
4/27/83	1.60		0.60	59	Respiratory infection
5/19/83	2.30		0.70	60	Discharge
1/30/84	2.40 (2.50)†	(2.20)†	0.65 (0.80)†	69	

* VC = inspiratory vital capacity in liters, measured with a water-sealed spirometer (normal = 3.84); RV = residual volume in liters, measured by the helium dilution technique; FEV_1 = forced expiratory volume in 1 second, in liters, measured with a water-sealed spirometer.
† Values in parentheses were after administration of salbutamol aerosol, 0.2 mg.
‡ With administration of 4 liters of supplemental oxygen/minute by nasal cannula.

urine, and blood were negative. Arterial blood gas analysis revealed a mild hypoxemia and normoventilation (Po_2 73 mm Hg, Pco_2 35 mm Hg, oxygen saturation 95%) (Table 1). An electrocardiogram showed a normal result. Radiographs of the chest showed hyperinflation of the lungs. Pulmonary perfusion scintigraphy revealed multiple subsegmental perfusion defects. Bronchoscopy showed no abnormalities.

Intravenous heparin therapy was started, but was discontinued after 5 days because of progressive dyspnea. At that time, analysis of arterial blood gas, with the patient breathing room air, revealed increasing hypoxemia. Ventilation-perfusion lung scintigraphy showed multiple matched subsegmental defects. Pulmonary angiography using the digital vascular imaging technique showed reduced perfusion of multiple peripheral areas, but no defects suggestive of pulmonary embolism. A graphic registration of the respiration sounds confirmed the auscultatory findings of a mid-inspiratory "squack" suggestive of bronchiolar obstruction (1,11,14) (Figure 1).

On the tenth hospital day, a left anterolateral thoracotomy was performed. Inspection of the left lung revealed no gross abnormalities. During inflation, 2 lung samples measuring 2 × 3 cm each were taken from distant sites. Histologic studies showed a normal aspect of pleural lining and lung parenchyma. There was a concentric bronchiolar process consisting of reparative tissue with predominant fibroblasts and sparsely scattered mononuclear inflammatory cells, with local disruption of the muscularis mucosae and constriction of the bronchiolar lumen (Figure 2). Findings of immunohistochemical studies on fresh-frozen and fixed tissue were negative.

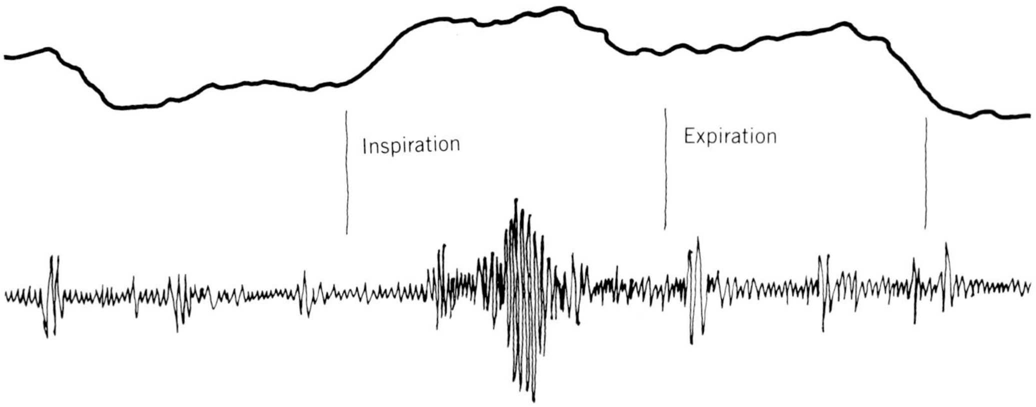

Figure 1. The mid-inspiratory "squack."

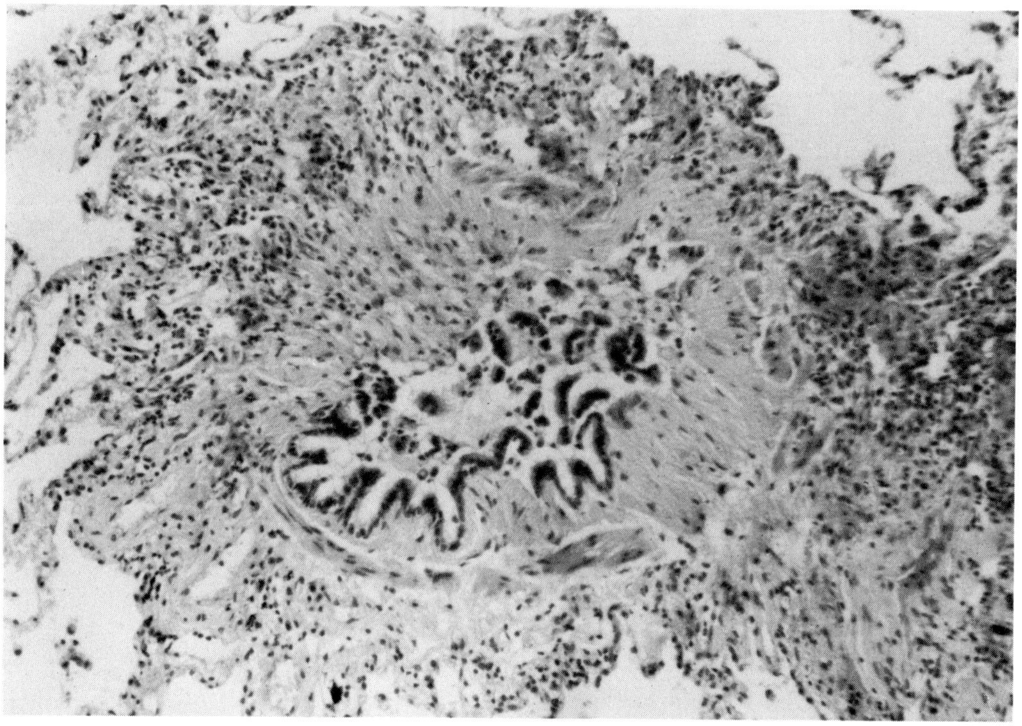

Figure 2. Open lung biopsy showing, by histologic analysis, a concentric bronchiolar process consisting of reparative tissue with fibroblasts and sparsely scattered mononuclear inflammatory cells, local disruption of the muscularis mucosae, and constriction of the bronchiolar lumen.

A diagnosis of bronchiolitis obliterans associated with D-penicillamine treatment for rheumatoid arthritis was made. After discontinuation of D-penicillamine, oral prednisone 60 mg 3 times daily was started. There was temporary improvement of the pulmonary condition, but after 4 weeks, progressive dyspnea and hypoxemia resumed (Table 1). This could not be attributed to respiratory infection. While oral prednisone was continued, a regimen of cyclophosphamide therapy was added. This consisted of an intravenous bolus of 4 mg/kg daily for 6 days, followed by oral cyclophosphamide 2 mg/kg daily in 1 dose.

Ten days after starting this therapy the patient developed lymphopenia (15 lymphocytes/mm^3) and, simultaneously, experienced alleviation of her dyspnea. The improvement of the clinical condition, which was also reflected in improvement of Po_2, was interrupted by respiratory infections with *Hemophilus influenzae* in the fourth and ninth weeks after starting cyclophosphamide therapy. Both infectious episodes resolved with antibiotic therapy. Twelve weeks after starting cyclophosphamide therapy the patient was well enough to return home, taking cyclophosphamide, 125 mg daily, and prednisone, 25 mg daily.

At the time of this writing, 1 year after the onset of pulmonary symptoms and the start of cyclophosphamide therapy, the patient's pulmonary function has stopped declining and remained stable, while her clinical condition has improved (Table 1). Ventilatory function has not improved, but has remained stable in the 8 months following discharge (Table 1). The patient has fully resumed her activities as a homemaker, taking a daily regimen of 100 mg cyclophosphamide and 10 mg prednisone.

Discussion. Although progressive respiratory distress in a nonsmoking patient, with hyperinflation of the chest and mid-inspiratory "squack" on auscultation, is suggestive of bronchiolitis obliterans, the definite diagnosis needs confirmation by open lung biopsy (1,7,15).

Since the early 1970s, when use of D-penicillamine for treatment of rheumatoid arthritis began, 12 cases of bronchiolitis obliterans in patients receiving this drug have been reported. This clinically distinct type of bronchiolitis obliterans is characterized by a rapidly deteriorating course of pulmonary insufficiency. Table 2 shows a summary of information on the 12 previously described patients with this diagnosis.

Table 2. Clinical characteristics of 12 patients with D-penicillamine-associated bronchiolitis obliterans*

Reference	Age/sex	Reason for DP therapy and dosage (mg)	Estimated months of DP therapy before onset of symptoms	Histologic findings	Followup (months)	Therapy	Outcome
1	45/F	RA, 750	12	Bronch. ob.	9	Prednisone	Died
1	50/F	RA, 1,000	6	Bronch. ob.	12	Prednisone	Died
1	36/F	RA, NA	12	ND	24	Prednisone	"Breathless"
11,12	61/F	RA, 750	7	Bronch. ob.	4	Prednisone	Died
11,12	52/F	RA, 500†	3	Bronch. ob.	24	Prednisone	"Ongoing worsening"
10	62/F	RA, NA	12	Bronch. ob.	4	Prednisone + azathioprine	Died
9	42/F	EF, 1,250‡	6	Bronch. ob.	24	Prednisone	"Severe hypoxia"
9	54/F	RA, 750	10	Bronch. ob.	3	Prednisone	"Unchanged"
8	66/F	RA, 900	8	ND	6	Prednisone	"Unchanged"
8	53/F	RA, 600	3	ND	NA	Prednisone	NA
13	63/F	RA, 375	14	Bronch. ob.	5	Prednisone + azathioprine	Died
13	56/F	RA, 375	8	ND	24	Prednisone + azathioprine	"Improved"

* DP = D-penicillamine; RA = rheumatoid arthritis; Bronch. ob. = bronchiolitis obliterans; NA = information not available; ND = not done; EF = eosinophilic fasciitis.
† D-penicillamine discontinued 3 weeks before onset of pulmonary symptoms.
‡ D-penicillamine discontinued 2 weeks before onset of pulmonary symptoms.

Remarkably, all 12 patients were female. Their ages ranged from 36–66. Eleven patients had rheumatoid arthritis. The twelfth actually did not have rheumatoid arthritis but had eosinophilic fasciitis, and is therefore included in the table. The daily dosage of D-penicillamine varied between 375 and 1,250 mg, administered during a period ranging from 3–14 months before the onset of pulmonary symptoms. Pulmonary symptoms started shortly after administration of general anesthetia in 1 patient (13), as in our patient. Yet there is no hard evidence that general anesthetics are capable of triggering D-penicillamine–associated bronchiolitis obliterans.

In 4 patients, no histologic confirmation of the diagnosis was obtained. Five of 8 patients with histologically-confirmed bronchiolitis obliterans died of respiratory failure within 1 year after the onset of pulmonary symptoms. In 2 of the remaining 7 patients, D-penicillamine was discontinued a few weeks before the onset of pulmonary symptoms because of leukopenia (9) or urticaria (11,12). These 2 patients had progressive pulmonary disease at the time their cases were reported. Followup information for periods ranging from 3 months–2 years is available on 4 of the remaining 5 patients. At the time of report, their respiratory conditions varied from severe but stable dyspnea to progressive pulmonary insufficiency; 1 patient improved.

The histologic findings in D-penicillamine–associated bronchiolitis obliterans deserve further consideration. As suggested by Geddes et al (1), we believe the histology of this clinical subtype of bronchiolitis obliterans is distinguishable from bronchiolitis obliterans not associated with D-penicillamine. In the latter, histologic studies usually show obstruction of the bronchiolar lumen by intrabronchiolar polypoid masses of inflammatory tissue (15). In 2 patients with D-penicillamine–associated bronchiolitis obliterans studied by Geddes et al, a concentric, constrictive form of bronchiolar obstruction is described (1), as was seen in the lung biopsy of our patient. The descriptions and pictures of the histologic findings in patients with D-penicillamine–associated bronchiolitis obliterans reported by Epler et al (9), Jansen et al (10), Murphy et al (11), Stein et al (12), and Penny et al (13) are detailed enough to make a distinction between the constrictive and the obstructive forms of bronchiolitis obliterans. In 5 of these 6 patients a constrictive form is described or shown. This almost constant finding supports the view of D-penicillamine as an inductive agent for a distinct clinical as well as histologic subtype of bronchiolitis obliterans.

Direct proof of an etiologic relationship between the drug and this highly aggressive form of bronchiolitis obliterans is lacking and probably difficult to obtain, due to the usually fatal course of the disease, which rules out rechallenging (by purpose or coincidence) to test reproducibility of this complication (16). Supporting evidence of bronchiolitis obliterans being an immunologically-triggered complication of D-penicillamine has not been found, and possibly has not been sought (1,8–13,17–21). In our patient, no signs of autoimmunity could be detected in serologic tests or in immunologic studies of the pulmonary tissue.

Confronted with a progressively dyspneic patient, we decided to add a more aggressive immunosuppressive drug to the regimen of prednisone. Because of its well-known efficacy as an immunosuppressive (regulatory) drug (22) and its ability to be effective quickly, we administered cyclophosphamide as a bolus infusion. The downhill course was arrested soon after the administration of cyclophosphamide, and the patient's pulmonary function has remained stable during the 8 months since discharge. The fact that pulmonary function failed to return to normal is explained by the fibrosis of the bronchioli as seen in the open lung biopsy.

D-penicillamine–associated constrictive bronchiolitis usually occurs within 1 year of beginning the drug and has a rapid evolution. Early detection is imperative. Patients taking D-penicillamine should be instructed to consult a physician as soon as pulmonary symptoms are experienced. We believe symptoms of progressive pulmonary insufficiency in a patient treated with D-penicillamine should lead to cessation of the drug. Auscultation is of great importance because a mid-inspiratory "squack" is suggestive of bronchiolar obstruction. If there is any doubt, intensive diagnostic efforts including open lung biopsy should be made in order to rule out bronchiolitis obliterans. Cyclophosphamide therapy in addition to oral prednisone seems to hold some promise as a treatment for this potentially fatal complication.

REFERENCES

1. Geddes DM, Corrin B, Brewerton DA, Davies RJ, Turner-Warwick M: Progressive airway obliteration in adults and its association with rheumatoid disease. Q J Med 184:427–444, 1977
2. Collins RL, Turner RA, Johnson AM, Whitley NO, Mclean RL: Obstructive pulmonary disease in rheumatoid arthritis. Arthritis Rheum 19:623–628, 1976
3. Cooney TP: Interrelationship of chronic eosinophilic pneumonia bronchiolitis obliterans and rheumatoid disease: a hypothesis. J Clin Pathol 34:129–137, 1981
4. Geddes DM, Webley M, Emerson PA: Airway obstruction in rheumatoid arthritis. Ann Rheum Dis 38:222–225, 1979
5. MacFarlane JD, Dieppe PA, Rigden BG, Clark TJH: Pulmonary and pleural lesions in rheumatoid disease. Br J Dis Chest 72:288–300, 1978
6. Holness L, Tenenbaum J, Cooter NBE, Grossman RF: Fatal bronchiolitis associated with chrysotherapy. Ann Rheum Dis 42:593–596, 1983
7. McCann BG, Hart GJ, Stokes TC, Harrisson BDW: Obliterative brohchiolitis and upper-zone pulmonary consolidation in rheumatoid arthritis. Thorax 38:73–74, 1983
8. Cordier JF, Falconnet M, Moulin J, Brune J, Touraine R: Bronchiolite sévère et polyarthrite rhumatoide rôle très probable de la D-pénicillamine dans deux observations. Lyon Médical 244:113–114, 1980
9. Epler GR, Snider GL, Gaensler EA, Cathcart ES, FitzGerald MX, Carrington CB: Bronchiolitis and bronchitis in connective tissue disease. JAMA 242:528–532, 1979
10. Jansen HM, Elema JD, Hylkema BS, van Leeuwen MA, The TH, van der Mark TW, Shuber HJ: Progressive obliterative bronchiolitis in a patient with rheumatoid arthritis. Eur J Respir Dis [Suppl] 121:43–52, 1982
11. Murphy KC, Atkins CJ, Offer RC, Hogg JC, Stein HB: Obliterative bronchiolitis in two rheumatoid arthritis patients treated with penicillamine. Arthritis Rheum 24:557–560, 1981
12. Stein HB, Patterson AC, Offer RC, Atkins CJ, Teufel A, Robinson HS: Adverse effects of d-penicillamine in rheumatoid arthritis. Ann Intern Med 92:24–29, 1980
13. Penny WJ, Knight RK, Rees AM, Thomas AL, Smith AD: Obliterative bronchiolitis in rheumatoid arthritis. Ann Rheum Dis 41:469–472, 1982
14. Earis J: The inspiratory squack in extrinsic allergic alveolitis and other pulmonary fibrosis. Thorax 37:923–926, 1982
15. Bennington JL: Bronchiolitis obliterans, Surgical Pathology of Non-Neoplastic Lung Disease. Edited by A Katzenstein, F Askin. Philadelphia, WB Saunders, 1982, pp 349–356
16. Meyboom RHB: Penicillamine and the respiratory system, Side Effects of Drugs. Edited by HNG Dukes. Amsterdam, Excerpta Medica, 1980, pp 179–181
17. Brewerton DA: D-penicillamine (letter). Br Med J 273:1507, 1976
18. Lyle WH: D-penicillamine and fatal obliterative bronchiolitis (letter). Br Med J 274:105, 1977
19. Camus PH, Reybet Degat O, Justrabo E, Jeannin L: D-penicillamine induced severe pneumonitis. Chest 81:376–378, 1982
20. Doyle DR, McCurley TL, Sergent JS: Fatal polymyositis in d-penicillamine treated rheumatoid arthritis. Ann Intern Med 98:327–330, 1983
21. Eastmond CJ: Diffuse alveolitis as complication of penicillamine treatment for rheumatoid arthritis. Br Med J 272:1506, 1976
22. Steinberg AD: Immunoregulatory agents, Textbook of Rheumatology. Edited by WN Kelley, ED Harris Jr, S Ruddy, CB Sledge. Philadelphia, WB Saunders, 1981, pp 841–861

BRIEF REPORT

ISOLATION OF ECHOVIRUS TYPE 11 FROM SYNOVIAL FLUID IN ACUTE MONOCYTIC ARTHRITIS

GREG KUJALA and JAMES H. NEWMAN

We describe a patient who had transient, acute synovitis of the knee following a brief diarrheal illness. The case history is noteworthy in regard to the striking monocytosis and low glucose level on synovial fluid analysis, and the unexpected isolation of echovirus type 11 from the synovial fluid. We believe this is the first documented instance of direct echovirus type 11 infection of a joint, causing synovitis.

Case report. A 30-year-old senior medical resident experienced a 24-hour illness characterized by watery diarrhea, sore throat, fever to 38.5°C, sweats, myalgias, and headache. Within 48 hours of symptom onset and 24 hours after the diarrhea had subsided, swelling and pain rapidly developed in the left knee. He had no history of arthritis or of rheumatic symptoms, although he had undergone medial menisectomy and anterior cruciate resection of the left knee 3 years earlier. There were no subsequent knee complaints and he denied recent injury. His remaining medical history was unremarkable.

He was examined by a rheumatologist within 12 hours of the onset of the knee swelling. The general physical examination findings were remarkable only for a temperature of 38°C. He had no rash, lymphadenopathy, ocular, or neurologic signs. Findings in the musculoskeletal system were limited to the left knee. The knee was warm with a moderate effusion. Aspiration produced 60 ml of markedly inflammatory fluid. The white blood cell count was 46,900/mm^3 (85% monocytes, 2% macrophages, 5% polymorphonuclear leukocytes, 8% lymphocytes). The glucose level was 12 mg/dl with a simultaneous serum glucose value of 95 mg/dl. No crystals were identified under compensated, polarizing light microscopy. Repeat synovial analysis 12 hours later confirmed the monocytosis (white blood cell count 32,300/mm^3 with 76% monocytes, 23% lymphocytes, 1% polymorphonuclear leukocytes). Aerobic and anerobic cultures of both specimens failed to grow a pathogen, but aliquots sent to Smith-Kline clinical laboratories grew echovirus type 11. Isolation and identification were performed according to the National Institute of Allergy and Infectious Diseases procedure for using the dried Lim Benyesh-Melnick pools for typing enteroviruses (1), with the following changes: 1) titration of the isolate and the neutralizations were performed in duplicate, and 2) the tissue medium used was Eagle's minimal essential medium with Earl's salts and 2% fetal calf serum. The echovirus 11 grew in both FLOW-4000 cells and rhesus monkey kidney cells, but identification was done with the rhesus monkey kidney cells.

No serologic testing was done. Additional studies included erythrocyte sedimentation rate (Westergren) 14 mm/hour, uric acid 4.6 mg/dl, hemoglobin 14.3, and peripheral white blood cell count 6,900/mm^3 (77% polymorphonuclear leukocytes, 1% bands, 14% lymphocytes, 2% atypical lymphocytes, 5% monocytes).

The patient was given aspirin, 1,300 mg every 6

From the Departments of Medicine and Rheumatology, Wilmington Medical Center, Wilmington, Delaware.

Greg Kujala, MD: Senior Resident, Department of Medicine, Wilmington Medical Center, Wilmington, Delaware (currently, Fellow in Rheumatology, University of Virginia Medical Center, Charlottesville, Virginia); James H. Newman, MD, FACP: Assistant, Section of Rheumatology, Department of Medicine, Wilmington Medical Center, Wilmington, Delaware.

Submitted for publication January 30, 1984; accepted in revised form July 17, 1984.

hours. All symptoms and signs of synovitis resolved within 48 hours of their onset and have not recurred as of 6 months later.

Discussion. Arthritis caused by direct viral infection in the joint space is infrequently documented and presumably unusual. Rubella (2) is the most commonly reported virus recovered from synovial fluid in the United States. Vaccinia (3), varicella (4), herpes simplex, and cytomegalovirus (5) have also been cultured from synovial fluid in acute arthritis. Sanford and Sulkin (6) were the first to report acute arthritis associated with enteroviral infection, specifically, echovirus type 9 cultured from stool only. Blotzer and Myers (7) described a case of polyarthritis associated with echovirus type 9 isolated from the pharynx and rectum. Clinical infection with variola, adenovirus, Epstein-Barr virus, hepatitis B, mumps, influenza A, arboviruses (8), non-B hepatitis virus (9), and coxsackie virus (10) have been associated with arthritis and arthralgias.

Predominant monocytic leukocytosis in synovial effusions in acute (11) or chronic (12) arthritis is relatively rare. Previous reports of mononuclear cells failed to distinguish between monocytes and lymphocytes. Most effusions with mononuclear predominance had leukocyte counts less than 10,000 mm^3. This case is significant because of the patient's monocytosis and high leukocyte count. Blotzer and Myers (7) and Fraser et al (13) provide reviews of synovial fluid leukocyte counts in patients with viral arthritis. Low synovial fluid glucose associated with monocytosis has been reported previously, and we confirm this observation (12).

Acute synovitis is occasionally a sequelum of gastroenteritis. We present the first case of echovirus type 11 cultured from synovial fluid following a self-limited diarrheal illness. The synovial fluid was remarkable for a persistent monocytosis with high leukocyte count and low glucose level. This case suggests that viral infection may be one of the causes of arthritis in some patients with monocytes in their synovial fluid. Such infections may be quite transient.

Acknowledgment. We wish to thank Dr. Gary Haller for his time and assistance in the isolation and thorough identification of the echovirus 11.

REFERENCES

1. Benyesh-Melnick L: Procedure for Using the Dried Lim Benyesh-Melnick Pools for Typing Enteroviruses. Research Resources Branch, National Institute of Allergy and Infectious Diseases, April 1972
2. Weibel RE, Stokes J, Buynak EB, Hilleman MR: Rubella vaccination in adult females. N Engl J Med 280:682–685, 1969
3. Silby HM, Farber R, O'Connell CJ, Ascher J, Marine EJ: Acute monoarticular arthritis after vaccination: report of a case with isolation of vaccinia virus from synovial fluid. Ann Intern Med 62:347–350, 1965
4. Priest JR, Urick JJ, Groth KE, Balfour HH: Varicella arthritis documented by isolation of virus from joint fluid. J Pediatr 93:990–992, 1978
5. Friedman HM, Pincus T, Gibilisco P, Baker D, Glazer JP, Plotkin SA, Schumacher HR: Acute monoarticular arthritis caused by herpes simplex virus and cytomegalovirus. Am J Med 69:241–247, 1980
6. Sanford JP, Sulkin SE: The clinical spectrum of echovirus infection. N Engl J Med 261:1113–1122, 1959
7. Blotzer JW, Myers AR: Echovirus-associated polyarthritis: report of a case with synovial fluid and synovial histologic characterization. Arthritis Rheum 21:978–981, 1978
8. Sauter S, Van H, Utsinger PD: Viral arthritis. Clin Rheum Dis 4:225–240, 1978
9. Fernandez R, McCarty DJ: The arthritis of viral hepatitis. Ann Intern Med 74:207–211, 1971
10. Rahal JJ, Millian SJ, Noriega ER: Coxsackie and adenovirus infection: association with acute febrile juvenile rheumatoid arthritis. JAMA 235:2496–2501, 1976
11. Brawer AE, Cathcart ES: Acute monocytic arthritis. Arthritis Rheum 22:294–300, 1979
12. George D, Hoch S, Cohen E, Kantrowitz F, Weinblatt M: Chronic monocytic arthritis. Arthritis Rheum 26:674–677, 1983
13. Fraser JRE, Cunningham AL, Clarris BJ, Aaskov JG, Leach R: Cytology of synovial effusions in epidemic polyarthritis. Aust NZ J Med 11:168–173, 1981

BRIEF REPORT

SYSTEMIC LUPUS ERYTHEMATOSUS AND COMMON VARIABLE PANHYPOGAMMAGLOBULINEMIA: A PATIENT WITH ABSENCE OF CIRCULATING B CELLS

ROSE GOLDSTEIN, CARLOS IZAGUIRRE, C. DOUGLAS SMITH, EGILS MIERINS, and JACOB KARSH

An association between systemic lupus erythematosus (SLE) and common variable panhypogammaglobulinemia (CVP) has recently been reported (1,2). It is of particular interest that the 2 disorders represent the extremes of B cell dysfunction—SLE characterized by B cell hyperactivity, and CVP by B cell hypoactivity. The results of investigations of the 3 previous cases of SLE and CVP revealed the presence of circulating B cells exhibiting decreased responses to mitogens in all instances (1,2) and to vaccination in 1 case studied for this (2), as well as excessive T cell suppression and subnormal T cell help in the 2 cases studied in vitro (1). We report the fourth case: a patient with an association of SLE and CVP in whom an absence of circulating B cells was the most significant lymphocyte abnormality seen.

Case report. A 61-year-old woman had polyarthralgias and dry eyes since the age of 33. She had had 7 pregnancies—6 ending in spontaneous abortions and 1 in a live birth. SLE was diagnosed formally in 1964 based on the presence of arthritis, Raynaud's phenomenon, alopecia, pleural effusions, and a positive lupus erythematosus cell preparation. Treatment with oral prednisone, 20 mg daily, was initiated. She developed a right corneal ulcer with scarring, secondary to keratoconjunctivitis sicca, which resulted in blindness in the right eye. Left-sided Jacksonian seizures began in 1965, at which time azathioprine was started. In 1966 she developed pancytopenia and a Coombs'-positive hemolytic anemia. Proteinuria was noted in 1969; examination of tissue obtained by renal biopsy revealed focal proliferative glomerulonephritis. Prednisone and azathioprine were discontinued in 1970, when the patient appeared to be in clinical remission. In 1981 corticosteroids were started again because of the development of cerebritis and pneumonitis. Findings at that time included reducible, nonerosive swan-neck deformities of the fingers, a diffusely abnormal result on an electroencephalogram, pulmonary fibrosis, a positive antinuclear antibody test with a titer of 1:20, and a positive lupus band test on sun-exposed, nonlesional skin with IgM, IgG, and C3 staining at the dermal–epidermal junction. In 1981 she developed atrial fibrillation and congestive heart failure. She remained stable taking various doses of oral prednisone, the lowest dosage being 10 mg and 5 mg on alternate days. Her antinuclear antibody test was negative in January 1982. In 1983, she had 2 hospital admissions for pulmonary infiltration compatible with infection or lupus pneumonitis. On each occasion, no microorganism was cultured and the patient recovered quickly with antibiotics and increased doses of corticosteroids.

In August 1983, she was admitted with acute chest and abdominal pain. Her medications were di-

From the Rheumatic Disease Unit, Ottawa General Hospital, University of Ottawa, Ottawa, Ontario, Canada.

Supported by grants from The Arthritis Society of Canada.

Rose Goldstein, MD, CM, FRCP(C): Fellow in Rheumatology, Arthritis Society of Canada; Carlos Izaguirre, MD, PhD: Associate Professor, Department of Medicine; C. Douglas Smith, MD, FRCP(C): Assistant Professor, Department of Medicine; Egils Mierins, MD, FRCP(C): Assistant Professor, Department of Medicine; Jacob Karsh, MD, CM, FRCP(C): Associate Professor, Department of Medicine.

Address reprint requests to Dr. Jacob Karsh, Rheumatic Disease Unit, Ottawa General Hospital, 501 Smyth Road, Ottawa, Ontario, Canada, KlH 8L6.

Submitted for publication April 9, 1984; accepted in revised form July 3, 1984.

goxin, prednisone, furosemide, carbamazepine, and a potassium supplement. She was febrile, with a very tender right upper abdominal quadrant and marked peripheral edema. Abdominal radiographs showed evidence of small bowel obstruction and thickened edematous small bowel walls suggestive of mesenteric ischemia. Blood cultures grew *Morganella morganii*. The provisional diagnoses were lupus mesenteric vasculitis and septicemia, although a mesenteric embolus due to atrial fibrillation could not be discounted. The patient refused surgery and was treated with high-dose intravenous corticosteroids and antibiotics and made a full recovery. Six weeks later, a barium enema revealed a small sessile polyp in the right colon, but no other abnormality. Results of the upper gastrointestinal series were normal. A computerized tomography scan of the abdomen revealed only ascites.

Materials and methods. The frequency distribution of peripheral blood lymphocytes was determined on blood mononuclear cells isolated by density gradient centrifugation on 60% Percoll. T cell subpopulations were identified by direct immunofluorescence with monoclonal antibodies against pan-T cells (OKT11), T helper/inducer cells (OKT4), and T suppressor/cytotoxic cells (OKT8) (Ortho Pharmaceuticals, Raritan, NJ). B cells were identified following staining with fluoresceinated monoclonal antibody to B1 (Coulter Electronics, Hialeah, FL), as well as by staining for the presence of surface IgM, IgA, IgG, and κ and λ light chains (Tago Laboratories, Burlingame, CA).

In vitro immunoglobulin production by peripheral blood lymphocytes of the patient and a control subject was assessed by culturing 1×10^6 lymphocytes, obtained by Ficoll-Hypaque centrifugation of heparinized venous blood, in 1 ml of tissue culture medium consisting of RPMI 1640 (Gibco, Grand Island, NY) supplemented with 10% fetal calf serum and penicillin-streptomycin, in a 5% CO_2 humidified incubator. Lymphocytes were cultured in triplicate in the presence and absence of 1 μg/ml of pokeweed mitogen (PWM; Sigma, St. Louis, MO).

T cell–enriched and B cell–enriched subpopulations of lymphocytes were prepared by rosetting whole lymphocyte preparations with 2-aminoethylisothiuronium–treated sheep red blood cells, followed by centrifugation on Ficoll-Hypaque. T cells were purified from the pellet by hypotonic lysis of the contaminating sheep red cells and provided preparations with >98% T cells, as assessed by re-rosetting. The B cell–enriched preparations usually contained about 50% nonspecific esterase staining cells (monocytes), 30–40% B cells (surface immunoglobulins), and <2% T cells. Autologous and allogeneic mixtures of a 1:1 ratio of T and B cells were established, as well as identical cultures of T and B cell reconstituted populations following irradiation of T cells with 1,000 rads to abrogate suppressor cell activity. Cultures contained a total of 1×10^6 cells.

The presence of pre-formed suppressor cells was evaluated by the method of Waldmann et al (3) by coculturing 0.5×10^6 whole mononuclear cells of the patient and control in the presence of 1 μg/ml of PWM.

All cultures were incubated for 8 days, following which supernatants were harvested and stored at −20°C. Total IgG and IgM in supernatant were measured by enzyme-linked immunosorbent assays developed by Cordis Laboratories (4).

Results. Serum immunoglobulins measured during the acute illness in August 1983 and 5 months later were decreased in the range characteristically seen in CVP: IgG 3.25 gm/liter (normal 5.6–17.7), IgA 0.55 gm/liter (normal 0.85–3.85), and IgM 0.30 gm/liter (normal 0.53–3.75), initially; IgG <2 gm/liter, IgA undetectable, IgM 1.13 gm/liter, 5 months later. Test results for antinuclear antibody (rat liver substrate), rheumatoid factor, and double-stranded DNA antibodies (*Crithidia luciliae*) were negative, and the C3, C4, and CH50 levels were normal. A lupus band test was repeated and found to be positive for IgG and IgM staining at the dermal–epidermal junction.

The total circulating lymphocyte count was mildly decreased (1,001/mm^3, normal 1,120–2,695). Eighty percent of circulating lymphocytes were T cells (800/mm^3). OKT4 (helper/inducer cells) were 638/mm^3 and OKT8 (cytotoxic/suppressor) were 176/mm^3, all at the lower limit of normal, with normal percentage distribution. The ratio of helper to suppressor T cells (OKT4:OKT8) was slightly elevated at 3.6. No cells were found expressing surface immunoglobulins IgM, IgA, IgG, or κ or λ light chains. The number of cells identified by monoclonal antibody to B1, a pan-B cell antigen, was very low (2.8%, absolute 28/mm^3). In contrast, 2 patients with systemic lupus erythematosus but without panhypogammaglobulinemia who were studied at the same time had 36% of circulating lymphocytes B1 marker positive, with normal numbers of cells having polyclonal surface immunoglobulins with both κ and λ light chains.

IgM production by whole mononuclear cells of

Table 1. PWM-induced immunoglobulin production by B cells reconstituted with autologous or allogeneic T cells*

	IgM (ng/ml)	IgG (ng/ml)
Whole mononuclear cells		
Control		
Baseline	504	52
PWM	1,193	1,632
Patient		
Baseline	13	0
PWM	52	0
Bc + Tc	1,343	1,011
Bc + Tc (irr)	1,474	968
Bc + Tp	283	210
Bc + Tp (irr)	2,277	1,973
Bp + Tp	13	0
Bp + Tp (irr)	45	0
Bp + Tc	60	49
Bp + Tc (irr)	31	0

* All experiments performed in the presence of 1 μg/ml pokeweed mitogen (PWM). Results are means of triplicate cultures. Baseline = no PWM; B = B cell–enriched fraction; c = control; T = T cell–enriched fraction; irr = irradiated (1,000 rads); p = patient.

the patient was severely depressed, and IgG production was absent in comparison with normal production by a simultaneously assessed control subject (Table 1). Separation of cells into T and B cell–enriched subpopulations with autologous reconstitution, including T cell irradiation, as well as addition of allogeneic T cells, resulted in no immunoglobulin production by the patient's B cell–enriched fraction. Analysis of this fraction of the patient's cells revealed that 84% stained with the nonspecific esterase and were, therefore, monocytes. In contrast, the patient's T cells supported IgM and IgG production by allogeneic B cells, and the production was markedly enhanced by prior T cell irradiation. The Waldmann-type cell coculture failed to reveal the presence of preformed suppressor cells; the ratio of observed to expected immunoglobulin production was enhanced to 3.6 for IgM and 1.6 for IgG.

Discussion. This patient presents an interesting development of acquired panhypogammaglobulinemia in the course of SLE. Although 3 other similar cases have recently been reported (1,2), this is the first case shown to have an absence of circulating B cells. This finding is surprising in a patient with SLE, which is usually characterized by B cell hyperactivity with increased numbers of circulating B cells, production of multiple autoantibodies, and hypergammaglobulinemia in human and in murine models (5,6). Minor decreases in B cell numbers measured by erythrocyte antibody complement rosettes have been reported rarely in SLE (7). However, our patient did not have agammaglobulinemia, which indicated that B cells were present and functioning outside the circulation.

Traditionally in SLE, B cell hyperactivity is attributed to deficient T suppressor cell numbers and/or function (5). Where measured, however, T cell numbers and T helper to T suppressor ratios frequently have normal values, although the latter can be either increased or decreased (8). The T cell populations in our patient are consistent with those found in SLE.

The results of previous studies of CVP have revealed circulating B cells to be increased (25% of patients), normal (50%), or absent (25%) (3). Associated T cell defects of decreased help and increased suppression have been described (3,9); however, the bulk of current evidence favors a primary B cell defect underlying the loss of immunoglobulin production, with the T cell abnormalities representing secondary epiphenomena. Our patient fits within the immunologic heterogeneity of CVP. Our T cell studies indicate that helper T cell function is adequate, and this is especially evident when suppressor cell activity is abrogated. T cell suppressor function may be increased, as allogeneic immunoglobulin production was markedly augmented following irradiation of the patient's T cells. However, coculture experiments failed to reveal the presence of pre-formed suppressor cells. Overall, the most significant finding in our patient was the absence of B cells and the failure to demonstrate cells capable of differentiation into immunoglobulin-producing cells, even under optimal conditions.

Previous studies reported patients with SLE and CVP who had normal T and B cell numbers, normal concanavalin A–induced suppressor cell activity in 1 patient (2), and excessive T cell suppression and subnormal T cell help in 2 patients studied by similar PWM-stimulated immunoglobulin synthesis assays (1). However, as in our patient, all 3 patients had hyporesponsive B cells, which was considered to be the primary immunologic abnormality (1,2).

Analysis of this and the other cases suggests that the association of SLE and CVP is not related to the duration of SLE. A case has been recently reported where hypogammaglobulinemia coincided with the administration of azathioprine (10); however, in the 3 previously mentioned, 2 had not taken immunosuppressive agents for several years before developing CVP, and the third patient developed CVP prior to administration of azathioprine (1,2). The mechanism of development of acquired panhypogammaglobulinemia in SLE remains poorly understood. Possibilities include coincidence, shared genetic predisposition to the 2 diseases, humoral immunodeficiency associated with malignancy (11), or the development of humoral and cellular immunity against B stem cells or mature B cells analogous to the development of antiplatelet antibodies and thrombocytopenia. There is no evidence in this case to support any of the above possibilities.

Another hypothesis which cannot be ruled out on present evidence is accelerated senescence of B cells after a prolonged period of hyperactivity. Blankwater et al (12) observed an age-related decline in response to *Escherichia coli* lipopolysaccharide, a thymic independent antigen, in New Zealand black (NZB) mice. As in our patient, the abnormality of B cells occurred independently of T cell abnormalities. Accelerated senescence of B cells in the bone marrow and spleen has been observed in the NZB mouse (13). This senescence has been related to cellular and humoral factors that accelerate the maturation of pre-B cells into B cells (14). We are unable to test for such factors in this patient. Two of the 3 previous patients, and the present patient, had significant hemolytic anemia, which is also the most prominent feature of the disease in NZB mice. Thus, these 4 patients may represent a subset of human SLE which closely resembles the disease of NZB mice, including the accelerated senescence of B cells.

Routine screening of immunoglobulins in patients with SLE is warranted, particularly in those with recurrent infections. The awareness of the association between SLE and CVP reported here may lead to the recognition of panhypogammaglobulinemia more often. Further study of B cell development in human and murine SLE will be needed to clarify the pathogenesis of CVP in these patients.

Acknowledgments. We gratefully acknowledge the technical assistance of P. Moffitt and the secretarial assistance of C. Lemay and D. Claude.

REFERENCES

1. Ashman RF, White RH, Weisenhutter C, Canton Y, Lasaron E, Liebling M, Talal N: Panhypogammaglobulinemia in systemic lupus erythematosus: in vitro demonstration of multiple cellular defects. J Allergy Clin Immunol 70:465–473, 1982
2. Sussman GL, Rivera VJ, Kohler PF: Transition from systemic lupus erythematosus to common variable hypogammaglobulinemia. Ann Intern Med 99:32–35, 1983
3. Waldmann TA, Broder S, Blaese RM, Dum M, Blackman M, Stober W: Role of suppressor T cells in pathogenesis of common variable hypogammaglobulinemia. Lancet 2:609–613, 1974
4. Karsh J, Watts CS, Osterland CK: Selective immunoglobulin M deficiency in an adult: assessment of immunoglobulin production by peripheral blood lymphocytes in vitro. Clin Immunol Immunopathol 25:386–394, 1982
5. Blaese RM, Grayson J, Steinberg AD: Increased immunoglobulin-secreting cells in the blood of patients with active systemic lupus erythematosus. Am J Med 69:345–350, 1980
6. Milich DR, Gershwin ME: The pathogenesis of autoimmunity in New Zealand mice. Semin Arthritis Rheum 10:111–146, 1980
7. Glinski W, Gershwin ME, Budman DR, Steinberg AD: Study of lymphocyte subpopulations in normal humans and patients with systemic lupus erythematosus by fractionation of peripheral blood lymphocytes on a discontinuous Ficoll gradient. Clin Exp Immunol 26:228–238, 1976
8. Smolen JS, Chused TM, Leiseron WM, Reeves JP, Alling D, Steinberg AD: Heterogeneity of immunoregulatory T cell subsets in systemic lupus erythematosus—correlation with clinical features. Am J Med 72:783–789, 1982
9. Reinherz EL, Cooper MD, Schlossman SF, Rosen FS: Abnormalities of T cell maturation and regulation in human beings with immunodeficiency disorders. J Clin Invest 68:699–705, 1981
10. Epstein RJ, Ogler RF, Gatenby PA: Lupus erythematosus and panhypogammaglobulinemia (letter). Ann Intern Med 100:162, 1984
11. Smith CK, Cassidy JT, Bole GG: Type I dysgammaglobulinemia, systemic lupus erythematosus and lymphoma. Am J Med 48:113–119, 1970
12. Blankwater M, Levert L, Hijmans W: Age-related decline in antibody responses to E. coli lipopolysaccharide in New Zealand black mice. Immunology 28:847–854, 1975
13. Jyonouchi H, Kincade PW, Landreth KS, Lee G, Good RA, Gershwin ME: Age-dependent deficiency of B lymphocyte lineage precursors in NZB mice. J Exp Med 155:1665–1678, 1982
14. Jyonouchi H, Kincade PW, Good RA, Gershwin ME: B lymphocyte lineage cells in newborn and very young NZB mice: evidence for regulatory disorders affecting B cell formation. J Immunol 131:2219–2225, 1983

BRIEF REPORT

IBUPROFEN MAY INDUCE MENINGITIS IN (NZB × NZW)F_1 MICE

SHLOMO BERLINER, ABRAHAM WEINBERGER, YEHUDA SHOENFELD, URI SANDBANK, BILHA HAZAZ, HENRY JOSHUA, MENACHEM ROSEN, and JACK PINKHAS

Hypersensitivity reactions to ibuprofen, a nonsteroidal antiinflammatory drug, can occur in patients with systemic lupus erythematosus (SLE) (1). A notable feature of the reaction to the drug is the development of aseptic meningitis, not only in SLE patients (1–5), but also in those with mixed connective tissue disease (6). We recently found, by means of a migratory inhibition factor assay, a specific cell-mediated immunity to ibuprofen in SLE patients who had not been previously exposed to this drug (7). The present report deals with the effect of ibuprofen on (New Zealand black × New Zealand white)F_1 ([NZB × NZW]F_1) mice, which spontaneously develop SLE-like disease (8).

MATERIALS AND METHODS

Animals. (NZB × NZW)F_1 mice, from parents obtained from the NIH, were bred in our laboratory. All the animals were kept under laminar flow aseptic conditions in the same room and were observed daily by the same laboratory personnel.

Animal study groups. Twenty female (NZB × NZW)F_1 mice, aged 8 weeks, received daily ibuprofen (30 mg/kg/day) orally (group A). Twenty female (NZB × NZW)F_1 mice, aged 8 weeks, received alcohol and NaOH in their drinking water, and did not receive ibuprofen; they served as controls (group B). Animals in both groups (A and B) lost more than 10 gm of body weight, refused food, and were killed when moribund. Ten female (NZB × NZW)F_1 mice, aged 6 weeks, received ibuprofen (30 mg/kg/day) for 12 weeks and were killed while apparently healthy (group C). Ten female (NZB × NZW)F_1 mice, aged 6 weeks (group D), received only alcohol and NaOH in their drinking water (in equivalent concentrations to that for the previous group but without ibuprofen) and served as controls for group C. These mice were also killed at the age of 12 weeks. Ten female Balb/c mice, aged 6 weeks, received ibuprofen (30 mg/kg/day) orally and were killed at the age of 18 weeks while apparently healthy (group E). Ten female (NZB × NZW)F_1 mice, aged 6 weeks, received ketoprofen (10 mg/kg/day) orally for 5 months and were killed while apparently healthy (group F).

Postmortem examination. Following fixation in formalin, 5 hematoxylin and eosin–stained slides were prepared from each of the following organs of mice from each group: brain and meninges, lungs, liver, spleen, and kidneys.

Ibuprofen. Powdered ibuprofen (Brufen 2-[4-isobutyl phenyl] propionic acid) was kindly donated by the Boots Company Ltd., Nottingham, England. Ibuprofen was dissolved in the drinking water using 95% alcohol (250 cc in 5 liters of distilled water) and 0.1*N* NaOH (10 cc in the above-mentioned 5 liters).

Ketoprofen. Vials with 100 mg ketoprofen and ampules of solvent for ketoprofen were kindly donated

From the Department of Internal Medicine "D," the Rheumatology Unit, the Departments of Pathology, and the Clinical Laboratory, Beilinson Medical Center, Tel Aviv University, Sackler Faculty of Medicine, Petah Tikva, Israel.

Shlomo Berliner, MD: Department of Internal Medicine "D"; Abraham Weinberger, MD: Head, Rheumatology Unit; Yehuda Shoenfeld, MD: Department of Internal Medicine "D"; Uri Sandbank, MD: Head, Department of Pathology; Bilha Hazaz, MSc: Head, Immunopathology Unit; Henry Joshua, MD: Head, Clinical Laboratory; Menachem Rosen, MSc: Head, Animal Laboratory; Jack Pinkhas, MD: Head, Department of Internal Medicine "D."

Address reprint requests to Professor J. Pinkhas, MD, Head, Department of Medicine "D," Beilinson Medical Center, Petah Tikva, 49100, Israel.

Submitted for publication February 4, 1983; accepted in revised form June 11, 1984.

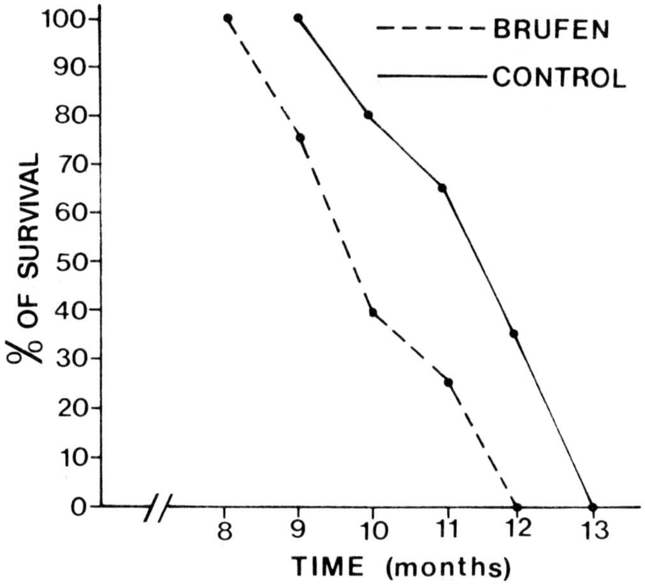

Figure 1. Percentage of survival over time in group A (ibuprofen) and B (control) mice. The difference between the 2 groups at the age of 12 months is statistically significant.

by Specia, Paris, France. The drug was added to the drinking water.

Immunofluorescence studies. Kidney specimens were frozen and stored at −90°C until used. For direct immunofluorescence (IF) staining, unfixed cryocut sections were incubated with fluorescein-conjugated anti-IgG, IgM, and IgA. The sections were examined with an incident light Zeiss microscope. For detecting antinuclear antibodies, a double-stain IF technique was performed. At the first stage, unfixed kidney cryocut sections of normal mice were used as substrate, and were incubated with the mouse serum. At the second stage, these slides were incubated with fluorescein-conjugated anti-mouse IgA, IgM, and IgG.

Statistical analysis. The cumulative proportion of survival was evaluated in groups A and B, and the significance of survival between the 2 groups after 12 months was evaluated, using Fisher's exact test. This test was also used to evaluate statistically significant differences between mice in groups C and D.

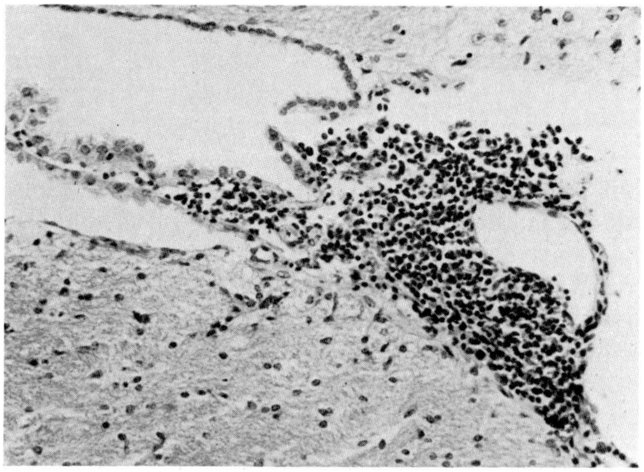

Figure 3. Massive lymphocytic infiltration in the choroid plexus of a mouse from group A (hematoxylin and eosin stained, original magnification × 250).

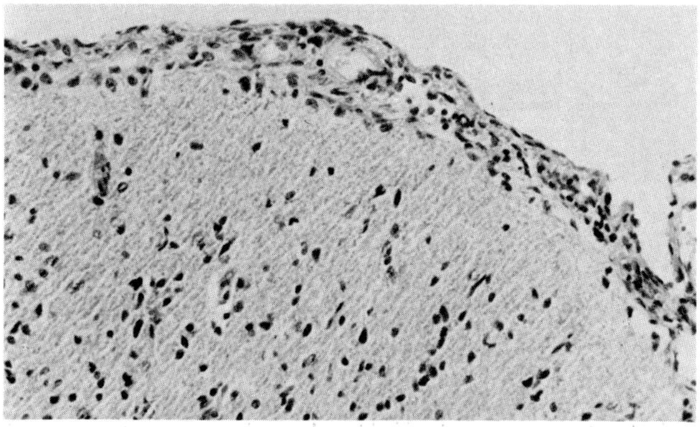

Figure 2. Cerebral cortex of a mouse from group A. The meninges show dense infiltration with lymphocytes and mononuclear cells. Perivascular infiltration is seen (hematoxylin and eosin stained, original magnification × 100).

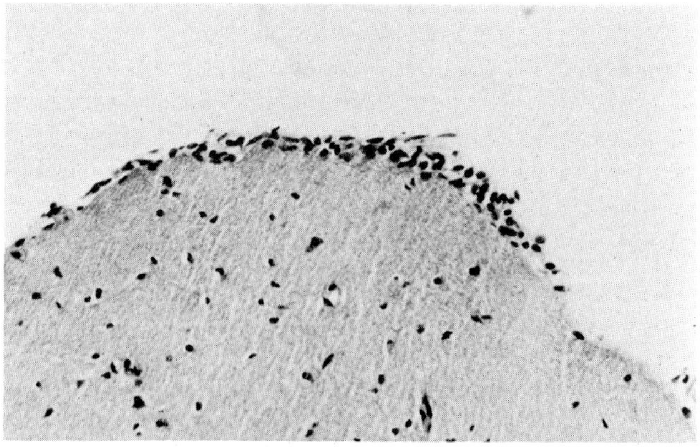

Figure 4. Mild lymphocytic infiltration of meninges in a mouse from group C (hematoxylin and eosin stained, original magnification × 100).

RESULTS

Groups A and B. Survival of the mice in groups A and B is shown in Figure 1. At the age of 12 months, the difference between the 2 groups was slight, although statistically significant ($P = 0.004$). The 10 mice from group A, in whom histopathologic examination was performed, had intensive lymphocytic and mononuclear infiltration in the meninges (Figure 2) and choroid plexus (Figure 3). Other parts of the brain were completely normal, as were the meninges and the choroid plexuses of the 10 control mice (group B) examined. There were no differences between groups A and B in the results of histologic or immunofluorescence examinations of the other organs (kidneys, lungs, liver, or spleen). Similarly, there were no differences in the levels of antinuclear antibodies.

Groups C and D. Mild lymphocytic infiltration was found in all 7 group C animals examined (Figure 4). In 2 of 10 animals from group D, glial nodules were found in the white and the grey matter of the brain, as well as perivascular lymphocytic cuffing of lymphomonocytes. Moderate lymphocytic infiltration of the meninges was noted in these 2 control mice. The choroid plexuses were found to be normal.

Groups E and F. No abnormalities of the brain were found in any of the animals examined from groups E and F.

DISCUSSION

In the present study, meningitis was found in all 17 examined (NZB × NZW)F_1 mice that had received ibuprofen. No brain abnormalities were found in the 10 Balb/c mice that had received ibuprofen or in the 10 (NZB × NZW)F_1 mice that had received ketoprofen.

The meningitis in our animals may have an immune basis since the cellular infiltrate was composed of lymphocytes and mononuclear cells. A similar mechanism was recently reported by Finkelstein et al (9) in several patients with various rheumatic conditions who developed nephropathy after taking fenoprofen, another propionic acid derivative. The meningitis probably develops slowly and is chronic, since we observed a mild lymphomononuclear infiltrate in the young animals, whereas in the older mice it was massive. In addition, this type of infiltrate did not appear in a non-autoimmune strain of mice that received ibuprofen, nor did it appear in the (NZB × NZW)F_1 mice that received ketoprofen, also a propionic acid derivative.

In our study, statistically significant differences between survival of animals in groups A and B were found. This is in contrast to the report of Kelly et al (10), who found no differences in survival between 2 groups of animals, 1 of which had received ibuprofen. The possibility that the different route of drug administration (injection in Kelly's study) accounts for this difference cannot be excluded.

The histologic findings in the 2 control groups of (NZB × NZW)F_1 mice that received only NaOH without ibuprofen are compatible with meningoencephalitis. Although the differences between the numbers of affected animals in groups C and D are statistically significant ($P = 0.002$), the particular histopathologic appearance of meningoencephalitis might be attributed to viral infection.

Infiltrates of lymphocytes and plasma cells were demonstrated recently in the perivascular and subarachnoid spaces of the brain in elderly (NZB × NZW)F_1 mice (11). Evidence of brain injury appearing as macrophages in the parenchyma and perivascular spaces, and myelin degeneration were also observed (11). Chronic stimulation of B cells by infective agents, primary immunoregulatory abnormalities, or both, may underly this infiltration. In the above-mentioned study (11), lymphocyte infiltrates were seen in 39% of 8–12-month-old NZB/NZW mice, in contrast to there being no infiltrates in the 10 mice in our control group B. The reasons for these differences remain unclear.

We conclude that ibuprofen may cause meningitis in (NZB × NZW)F_1 mice, an animal model which reproduces the findings observed in human SLE. This observation should be kept in mind when ibuprofen therapy is considered for SLE patients.

Acknowledgment. We are grateful to Yael Franko of the Head Office of Kupat Holim for performing the statistical analysis.

REFERENCES

1. Ruppert GB, Barth WF: Ibuprofen hypersensitivity in systemic lupus erythematosus. South Med J 74:241–243, 1981
2. Giansinacusa DF, Blumberg S, Kantrowitz FG: Aseptic meningitis associated with ibuprofen (letter). Arch Intern Med 140:1553, 1980
3. Widener HL, Littman BH: Ibuprofen-induced meningitis in systemic lupus erythematosus. JAMA 139:1062–1064, 1978
4. Wasner CK: Ibuprofen, meningitis and systemic lupus erythematosus. J Rheumatol 5:162–164, 1978
5. Samuelson CO, Williamson HJ: Ibuprofen associated aseptic meningitis in systemic lupus erythematosus. West J Med 131:57–59, 1979
6. Bernstein RF: Ibuprofen-related meningitis in mixed

connective tissue disease. Ann Intern Med 92:206–207, 1980
7. Shoenfeld Y, Livni E, Shaklai M, Pinkhas J: Sensitization to ibuprofen in systemic lupus erythematosus. JAMA 244:547–548, 1980
8. Wigley RD: Models of rheumatic disease occurring spontaneously in mice. Semin Arthritis Rheum 7:81–94, 1977
9. Finkelstein A, Fraley DS, Feldman HA, Gandy DR, Bourke E: Fenoprofen nephropathy: lipoid nephrosis and interstitial nephritis: a possible T-lymphocyte disorder. Am J Med 72:81–87, 1982
10. Kelly VE, Izui S, Halushka PV: Effect of ibuprofen, a fatty acid cyclooxygenase inhibitor on murine lupus. Clin Immunol Immunopathol 25:223–231, 1982
11. Rudick RA, Eskin TA: Neuropathological features of lupus-like disorders in autoimmune mice. Ann Neurol 14:325–332, 1983

BRIEF REPORT

EVALUATION OF AN EDUCATIONAL PROGRAM FOR PRIMARY CARE PRACTITIONERS, ON THE MANAGEMENT OF OSTEOARTHRITIS

JEOFFREY K. STROSS and GILES G. BOLE

The quality of health care depends, in part, on the rapidity with which health professionals are willing to adapt to medical innovation and adjust patient care practices in light of new knowledge. By understanding how information is transmitted and under what conditions physicians will accept innovation, we can design educational programs that have a high probability of changing physician behavior.

Primary care physicians practicing in community settings often rely on informal and personal methods of education. Actual experiences in patient care are probably the strongest influences that bring about changes in professional practice. When faced with clinical problems, primary care practitioners commonly turn to colleagues for advice. Previous studies have demonstrated the presence of key individuals in each community who are consulted frequently. These practitioners, referred to as "educationally influential physicians" or EIs, have the ability to change their peers' behavior in a desired manner (1).

This project was based on the hypothesis that EIs can be used to disseminate information to their colleagues about the management of osteoarthritis (OA). Osteoarthritis is the most common disease in humans, with radiologic evidence of the disease found in more than 80% of people over the age of 55 (2). The prevalence rises rapidly with age, with as many as 10% of the population already having radiographic findings by age 25 (3). Over 40 million Americans have radiologically visible OA in the hands or feet, and symptoms of disability have occurred in 5 million (4).

Many physicians have developed pessimistic attitudes about OA because of its frequent downhill course with increasing joint dysfunction and lack of effective treatment. This may not be warranted, because of our growing knowledge about the pathogenesis of the disease process, new treatment approaches, and advances in joint replacement. Since primary care physicians treat most patients with rheumatic diseases, we developed an educational program for these practitioners, on the management of OA. This program was delivered to a small group of physicians identified by their peers as EIs, who then had the responsibility of disseminating the information to their peers. Instructional objectives were defined, a needs assessment carried out, and the educational program was developed. The educational program was self-study in design, utilizing a syllabus and audiovisual aids to minimize faculty teaching time. This report describes the project and our efforts to assess the impact of the educational program on the target population.

Methods. The first step was to identify the project communities. All communities in the state of Michigan were surveyed for the following characteristics: no physician with formal training in rheumatol-

From the University of Michigan Medical School, Ann Arbor.

Supported by Multipurpose Arthritis Center grant 2P 60 AM20557 from the National Institute of Arthritis, Diabetes, Digestive and Kidney Diseases.

Jeoffrey K. Stross, MD: Associate Professor of Internal Medicine and Director, Community Programs Component, University of Michigan Arthritis Center; Giles G. Bole, MD: Professor of Internal Medicine, Director, University of Michigan Arthritis Center, and Physician-in-Charge, Division of Rheumatology, University of Michigan Medical School.

Address reprint requests to Dr. J. Stross, D3211 South Ambulatory Care Building, The University of Michigan Medical Center, Ann Arbor, MI 48109.

Submitted for publication March 6, 1984; accepted in revised form July 9, 1984.

ogy, no ongoing medical educational programs (undergraduate or graduate), at least 15 primary care practitioners in the area, a location at least 25 miles from a referral center, an orthopedic surgeon practicing in the community, and a physical therapy unit in operation at the hospital. Letters were sent to all communities with these characteristics, and 6 communities agreed to participate. Three were randomly selected to be controls, while the other 3 were designated as intervention communities. The EIs were selected using a previously described method (1), and the individual identified in each community was recruited into the project.

The next step was to develop the educational program. Three tasks were identified: defining the instructional goals, performing a needs assessment for the learner group, and developing the instructional materials.

The instructional goals were defined by a group of primary care physicians and rheumatologists. They met to determine what knowledge and skills primary care practitioners should have in order to adequately care for patients with OA. There were 3 major categories identified: diagnosis, management, and referral and education. For each category, instructional objectives relating to knowledge and skills were specified; these are outlined in Table 1. Differences between physicians were minor and were resolved by discussion. No major areas of disagreement were identified, and there was widespread consensus at the end of the session.

After defining the educational objectives, it was necessary to assess the knowledge and skill levels of the EIs and to document the actual practices of primary care physicians in the management of OA. The EIs were asked to complete a written examination prior to the educational program. The questions were derived from the instructional objectives, and 2 questions were developed for each point: 1 for the pre-test and the other for the post-test. The questions were in true/false, multiple choice, or matching format.

The needs assessment included chart audits of all inpatients with a discharge diagnosis of OA. Physical therapy records were reviewed to identify patients not picked up by other methods, and all patients undergoing total hip arthroplasty (THA) for OA were also reviewed. All records were audited against predefined criteria, as were outpatient records in most instances. Data on each patient's history, physical examination, laboratory studies, management, and disposition were collected.

Table 1. Instructional objectives of "educationally influential" physician intervention

I. Diagnosis of osteoarthritis
- A. Knowledge—the learner group, at the completion of the program, must be able to:
  1. Discuss the pathophysiology of osteoarthritis.
  2. Describe the prevalence of osteoarthritis.
  3. Differentiate osteoarthritis from other forms of joint disease.
- B. Skills—the learner group must be able to:
  1. Elicit a history documenting the cardinal features of joint disease.
  2. Perform and record the findings of a joint examination.
  3. Order and interpret laboratory and radiographic studies in patients with osteoarthritis.

II. Management of osteoarthritis
- A. Knowledge—the learner group must be able to describe:
  1. The pharmacology of nonsteroidal antiinflammatory agents.
  2. A comprehensive program for the management of osteoarthritis.
- B. Skills—the learner group must be able to:
  1. Prescribe full-dose aspirin therapy.
  2. Prescribe nonsteroidal antiinflammatory agents.
  3. Instruct a patient in a comprehensive program of management of osteoarthritis.
  4. Perform and interpret an arthrocentesis.

III. Referral and education of patients with osteoarthritis
- A. Knowledge—the learner group must be able to:
  1. Understand the rationale for physical therapy for osteoarthritis.
  2. State the indications for referral for surgical intervention in osteoarthritis.
- B. Skills—the learner group must be able to:
  1. Refer patients to physical therapists and orthopedic surgeons as indicated.

The last step in the development of the educational program was selection of the educational materials. Although this program could be utilized by any physician, it was aimed at a specific group of practitioners identified as EIs. Since these individuals are very busy, a decision was made to develop a self-study program. The 3 components of this program included a basic textbook to serve as a reference source, a syllabus of recent articles, and audiovisual materials. After completion of the pre-test, the educational materials were sent out to each participant, with the areas necessitating further study being highlighted. A post-test was sent 2 months later, after each participant completed the program.

One year after completion of the educational program, the medical records were reaudited using the same criteria. Statistical comparisons were made using chi-square.

Table 2. Pre-program inpatient audit results*

Variable	Control hospitals (n = 44)	Intervention hospitals (n = 41)
Diagnosis		
Osteoarthritis	18	23
Total hip arthroplasty	26	18
Length of stay (days)		
Osteoarthritis	8.4	8.8
Total hip arthroplasty	16.6	17.2
Therapy (osteoarthritis)		
Aspirin	9 (50)	9 (39)
Nonsteroidal antiinflammatory agents	14 (78)	19 (83)
Corticosteroids (systemic)	3 (17)	3 (13)
Corticosteroids (intraarticular)	2 (11)	4 (17)
Physical therapy	15 (83)	20 (87)
Referral	7 (39)	9 (39)
Therapy (total hip arthroplasty)		
Pre-op length of stay (days)	1.5	2.2
Pre-op physical therapy	12 (46)	10 (56)
Post-op narcotics	20 (77)	13 (72)
Post-op physical therapy	26 (100)	18 (100)
Post-op complications	4 (15)	2 (11)

* Numbers in parentheses are percentages.

Results. The average score for the 3 physicians in the pre-test was 58.2%; this improved to 84.1% in the post-test. As a result of this improvement, we felt confident that the participating physicians had the requisite knowledge to disseminate to their peers.

In the pre-intervention period, 85 patients were discharged from the 6 hospitals with a primary discharge diagnosis of OA: 44 in the control and 41 in the intervention hospitals. The male/female distribution and average ages of the patients were similar in the 2 groups. Forty-four of the patients (52%) underwent THA (Table 2). The length of stay and nonoperative management of patients with OA were similar in the control and intervention communities. There were no obvious differences in the management of the THA patients in the 2 groups. A total of 436 outpatient charts were audited: 230 (52.8%) in the control communities and 206 (47.2%) in the intervention communities. There were no significant differences in the therapy received by these groups. Nonsteroidal antiinflammatory agents were the main therapy used (86%), while systemic corticosteroids were rarely used (9%), and intraarticular corticosteroids were given to 15% of outpatients. Physical therapy was recommended in 45% of outpatients, and referral to an orthopedic surgeon or rheumatologist was noted in 18%.

In the post-intervention period, 114 OA patients were discharged from the 6 hospitals: 48 in the control and 66 in the intervention communities (Table 3). The increased number of patients in the intervention communities was seen in operative as well as medically managed cases. While the length of stay was unchanged in THA patients at the control hospitals, there was a 2.0-day reduction in the length of stay of those patients at the intervention hospitals. The only significant changes in therapy for the medically managed patients were increased utilization of intraarticular corticosteroids and decreased use of systemic corticosteroids. In those patients undergoing THA, there was a significant increase in utilization of physical therapy services in the preoperative period, a key point in the educational program. No other significant differences from the pre-intervention period were noted post-intervention. A total of 472 outpatient charts were audited in the post-intervention period: 238 (50.4%) in the control and 234 (49.6%) in the intervention communities. There were no significant changes from the pre-intervention period in the use of systemic medications, physical therapy, or specialty referral. The use of intraarticular corticosteroids increased in the intervention communities from 30 of 206 outpatients (14.6%) to 56 of 234 (23.9%) ($P < 0.05$), while similar changes were not seen in the control communities.

Discussion. Since rheumatologists treat only a small percentage of patients with rheumatic diseases, it is increasingly important to target our educational efforts toward primary care physicians. These individ-

Table 3. Post-program inpatient audit results*

Variable	Control hospitals (n = 48)	Intervention hospitals (n = 66)
Diagnosis		
Osteoarthritis	18	30
Total hip arthroplasty	30	36
Length of stay (days)		
Osteoarthritis	8.6	8.4
Total hip arthroplasty	16.0	15.2
Therapy (osteoarthritis)		
Aspirin	5 (28)	6 (20)
Nonsteroidal antiinflammatory agents	17 (94)	26 (87)
Corticosteroids (systemic)	4 (22)	1 (3)†
Corticosteroids (intraarticular)	2 (11)	12 (40)†
Physical therapy	15 (83)	28 (93)
Referral	6 (33)	9 (30)
Therapy (total hip arthroplasty)		
Pre-op length of stay (days)	1.3	1.6
Pre-op physical therapy	12 (40)	35 (97)†
Post-op narcotics	28 (93)	32 (89)
Post-op physical therapy	30 (100)	36 (100)
Post-op complications	4 (13)	2 (6)

* Numbers in parentheses are percentages.
† $P < 0.05$ versus pre-intervention.

uals often rely on informal methods of communication, so we designed a program to capitalize on this method of information dissemination. A group of physicians, identified by their peers as being educationally influential, were provided with additional knowledge about OA. We then attempted to determine what impact these individuals would have on the behavior of their peers.

While there have not been any dramatic breakthroughs in the management of OA in the past few years, some advances have been made. The preprogram audit demonstrated that nonsteroidal antiinflammatory agents and physical therapy already played an important role in patient management. Our educational efforts were concentrated on 3 therapeutic modalities: the use of intraarticular corticosteroids, the role of physical therapy, and joint replacement.

The post-program audit documents that some changes in behavior occurred. While there were minimal changes in activity in the control hospitals, there was a 60% increase in hospitalizations in the intervention communities, with a doubling of admissions for THA. The indications for THA were examined in each case, and 33 of 36 in the intervention hospitals (92%) were performed because of pain that was unresponsive to a conservative program of pain medication and physical therapy. This suggests that this increase in activity was clinically justified. There was a significant increase in the use of intraarticular corticosteroids in both inpatient and outpatient settings in the intervention communities. It could be argued that this modality may not be clinically indicated, but important diagnostic information can be obtained at the time of arthrocentesis, and intraarticular corticosteroids can provide temporary symptomatic relief.

The major impact of this project was to inform primary care practitioners of the value of joint replacement. The number of procedures doubled in the intervention hospitals, the length of stay decreased by 2.0 days, and preoperative physical therapy was routinely instituted. Since these changes were not seen in the control hospitals and were key features of the educational program, a cause-and-effect relationship is suggested.

One major difference in this project compared with our previous programs using educationally influential physicians was the use of a self-study educational program. In previous studies, we utilized an intensive, academic medical center–based preceptorship. While this approach was successful, it was highly dependent upon scarce resources: an academic center and many hours of faculty time. Consequently, we used a different format in the current study. The change in knowledge was impressive, and the change in behavior of the community practitioners is similar to what has been seen previously (5). These changes are not as dramatically impressive as those seen when a new rheumatologist enters practice (6), but it is very doubtful that there will ever be an adequate supply of rheumatologists to go to communities with populations of less than 25,000.

These data confirm our previous findings concerning the role of EIs in disseminating information to their peers and in influencing their behavior. In those less-populated areas where subspecialty-oriented physicians are unlikely to establish a practice, this approach to educating primary care physicians has utility and value.

REFERENCES

1. Stross JK, Hiss RG, Watts CM, Davis WK, MacDonald R: Continuing education in pulmonary disease for primary care physicians. Am Rev Respir Dis 127:739–746, 1983
2. Kellgren JH, Lawrence JS: Osteoarthrosis and disc degeneration in an urban population. Ann Rheum Dis 17:388–397, 1958
3. Lawrence JS, Bremner JM, Bier F: Osteoarthrosis prevalence in the population and relationship between symptoms and x-ray changes. Ann Rheum Dis 25:1–24, 1966
4. Gordon T: Osteoarthrosis in US adults, Population Studies of the Rheumatic Diseases. Edited by PH Bennett, PHN Wood. New York, Excerpta Medica Foundation, 1968, pp 391–397
5. Stross JK, Bole GG: Evaluation of a continuing education program in rheumatoid arthritis. Arthritis Rheum 23:846–849, 1980
6. Stross JK, Bole GG: The impact of a new rheumatologist on the management of rheumatic disease patients in community hospitals. Arthritis Rheum 26:1033–1036, 1983

BRIEF REPORT

IN VITRO SYNTHESIS OF LOW MOLECULAR WEIGHT IgM IN RHEUMATOID ARTHRITIS

D. NEIL JONES, LIN Y. KOH, JAMES V. BERTOUCH, and PETER J. ROBERTS-THOMSON

Low molecular weight (LMW) IgM, the monomeric subunit of pentameric IgM, has been detected in the sera of patients with a wide variety of rheumatic, infective, and lymphoproliferative diseases but is not found in healthy individuals (1). In seropositive rheumatoid arthritis (RA), serum and synovial fluids contain considerable quantities of the monomeric IgM moiety, and levels of circulating LMW IgM correlate strongly with rheumatoid factor (RF) and with many extraarticular manifestations such as rheumatoid vasculitis (1,2). Furthermore, LMW IgM has been shown to have RF activity (1) (up to 40% of LMW IgM is LMW IgM-RF in some individuals) and can activate the classical complement pathway (3). It is therefore tempting to ascribe an important role for this immunoglobulin in the immunopathogenesis of RA.

The factors concerned in the production of LMW IgM are largely unknown. Four hypotheses have been suggested to explain its presence. First, in vivo breakdown of immune complex–bound pentameric IgM may release monomeric IgM. This could possibly explain the frequent occurrence of LMW IgM in immune complex states (1). Second, a defect during IgM polymerization could result in the liberation of monomeric IgM into the circulation. This is the favored postulate in B cell lymphoproliferative disorders associated with IgM paraproteins (4,5). Third, LMW IgM exists in small quantities as a membrane-bound immunoglobulin on certain B cells, and its release into the circulation could theoretically occur during rapid cell proliferation. However, membrane-bound LMW IgM has different physiochemical properties and low synthetic rates compared with secretory pentameric IgM, and its release into the circulation in quantities comparable with those found is not considered possible (6). Last, the presence of LMW IgM may represent a phylogenetic reversion of the immune response (7), as LMW IgM exists naturally in lower vertebrates (8). This may explain its occurrence in a number of chronic immune-stimulated states such as RA and chronic infective disorders and its close association with RF, which is also frequently found in these conditions (1).

This study explored the second and fourth of these hypotheses. We have documented the active secretion of LMW IgM by pokeweed-stimulated peripheral blood mononuclear cells (PBMC) obtained from RA patients in vitro, but not from healthy control subjects. A correlation was found between the levels of LMW IgM synthesized in vitro and circulating LMW IgM.

From the Department of Clinical Immunology, Flinders Medical Centre, Bedford Park, South Australia.

Supported by a grant from the South Australian Arthritis and Rheumatism Association.

D. Neil Jones: Medical Student and recipient of an Australian Medical Students Association/Lilly Student Research Grant; Lin Y. Koh, BSc: Hospital Scientist; James V. Bertouch, MB BS: recipient of a National Health and Medical Research Council Fellowship; Peter J. Roberts-Thomson, MB BS, DPhil (Oxon): Senior Lecturer and Head, Rheumatology Department.

Address reprint requests to Peter J. Roberts-Thomson, Department of Clinical Immunology, Flinders Medical Centre, Bedford Park, South Australia, 5042.

Submitted for publication August 16, 1983; accepted in revised form July 17, 1984.

PATIENTS AND METHODS

Patients and controls. Seven patients with seropositive, classic RA according to the American Rheumatism Association criteria (9) were studied. Patients 2 and 7 also fulfilled the criteria for Felty's syndrome,

Table 1. Clinical and laboratory data of rheumatoid arthritis patients secreting LMW IgM in vitro*

			Serum					Day 3			Day 7		
Patient	Sex	Age	RF IU/ml	IC units/ml	IgM gm/ liter	% LMW IgM	LMW IgM gm/ liter	IgM μg/ culture†	% LMW IgM	LMW IgM μg/ culture	IgM μg/ culture	% LMW IgM	LMW IgM μg/ culture
1	F	66	1,280	8	1.05	36	0.38	4.59	100	4.59	6.12	100	6.12
2	F	58	>9,999	41	7.7	35	2.7	2.08	94	1.96	2.84	87	2.47
3	M	69	4,000	41	3.24	26	0.84	6.27	89	5.58	6.79	83	5.64
4	F	67	270	4.1	0.64	16	0.10	0.22	51	0.11	2.06	19	0.39
5	M	41	>9,999	>75	5.79	35	2.03	1.39	92	1.29	1.77	87	1.53
6	M	59	1,260	>75	1.48	25	0.37	0.42	51	0.21	0.24	78	0.19
7	F	51	8,810	>75	6.75	26	1.76	4.31	93	4.00	5.26	86	4.52
Normal (n = 5)			<60	<2	0.5–2.2	0	0	0‡	0	0	0.88§	0	0

* LMW IgM = low molecular weight IgM; RF = rheumatoid factor; IC = immune complex.
† Culture = 2×10^6 peripheral blood mononuclear cells.
‡ <0.04 μg IgM/culture.
§ Mean of 5 healthy control subjects.

and patient 1 had diffuse interstitial pulmonary fibrosis. Four of the patients were women, 3 men; their mean age was 59 years (range 41–69) (Table 1). All patients were taking nonsteroidal antiinflammatory drugs, 1 (patient 6) was taking D-penicillamine, 500 mg/day, and patient 1 was taking prednisolone, 10 mg/day. Five healthy laboratory employees (4 males, 1 female; mean age 29 years, range 23–42) were used as controls. Blood was collected by venipuncture, allowed to clot at room temperature, and serum separated by centrifugation and stored at −20°C (−80°C for immune complex determination).

Immunologic investigations. Circulating immune complexes were measured by the fluid-phase C1q binding method and total IgM and rheumatoid factor were determined by rate nephelometry (Beckman, Palo Alto, CA) (1). Nephelometry is a measurement of light scatter caused by antigen–antibody complexes, the degree of scatter being proportional to the amount of immune complex present. To measure rheumatoid factor, a known amount of aggregated human IgG is added to the test serum and the resultant degree of light scatter reflects the quantity of rheumatoid factor present (10).

Quantitation of circulating LMW IgM. Serum LMW IgM was measured as previously described (1). Briefly, 1–2 ml of serum was applied to a 90 × 2.5 cm Sephacryl S300 column (Pharmacia, Uppsala, Sweden). Alternate fractions were collected and assayed for IgM by laser nephelometry using anti-IgM antiserum (Dako Immunoglobulins, Copenhagen, Denmark). An IgM profile was then obtained and the percent LMW IgM was calculated by planimetry from the relative areas of monomeric and pentameric IgM. The absolute quantity of LMW IgM was then calculated from the percent LMW IgM and the total serum IgM values.

Peripheral blood mononuclear cell culture in vitro. Heparinized blood (approximately 40 ml) was collected from patients and controls, diluted 1:1 in phosphate buffered saline (PBS), layered on Ficoll-Hypaque (Pharmacia), and centrifuged at 400*g* for 30 minutes at room temperature. The mononuclear-rich fraction was washed 4 times in PBS (centrifugation at 400*g* for 10 minutes). The cells were then counted and adjusted to a concentration of 1×10^6 cell/ml in RPMI culture medium with 10% fetal calf serum, glutamine, penicillin, and streptomycin (Gibco, Grand Island, NY). Pokeweed mitogen (Sigma, St. Louis, MO) was added at a final concentration of 1 μg/ml to all cultures, but in 2 patients comparative cultures were also incubated without this mitogen. The cell cultures were plated in 2-ml aliquots in Costar 24-well tissue culture dishes and incubated for 3 or 7 days at 37°C (5% CO_2). For 7-day cultures, the medium was changed at day 3. At the completion of culturing, the cell-free supernatants were collected and stored at −20°C.

To confirm active synthesis of IgM, cycloheximide (Sigma) was added to the cultures of 2 patients at day 0 at a final concentration of 10 μg/ml. Viability counts were performed using trypan blue exclusion.

Quantitation of LMW IgM in culture supernatant. For each subject, approximately 20 ml of culture supernatant was concentrated in an Amicon concentrator to a volume of 1 ml and applied to a 90 × 1.6-cm Sephacryl S300 column. Downward filtration was at 20 ml/hour, and 2-ml fractions were collected and assayed for IgM by enzyme-linked immunosorbent assay (ELISA). From the IgM profile obtained, it was possible to calculate the relative percentage of LMW IgM and pentameric IgM.

Enzyme-linked immunosorbent assay for IgM. IgM was measured in culture supernatants and column fractions using a competitive inhibition ELISA as previously described (11). It was previously determined that LMW IgM prepared from a seropositive RA patient by filtration chromatography and affinity chromatography gave an almost identical curve to the pentameric IgM standard, suggesting that the molecular size of the IgM used as the standard did not greatly influence the results (Figure 1).

Radioiodination of purified IgM. A monoclonal IgM rheumatoid factor was purified by repeated cryoprecipitation and filtration chromatography in buffer at pH 4.0, as previously described (12). The purity and pentameric size of the IgM were verified by sodium dodecyl sulfate–polyacrylamide gel electrophoresis. This reagent was then radiolabeled with ^{125}I, using the lactoperoxidase method (13).

Statistical analysis. Variables were compared using rank correlation coefficients.

RESULTS

Circulating LMW IgM was not found in any of the 5 control subjects, and chromatographic analysis of the culture supernatants revealed that all the IgM produced by day 7 of culture was in the pentameric form (Figure 2). In contrast, LMW IgM was found in all 7 serum specimens from the RA patients and contributed from 16 to 36% of the total IgM (Table 1). Furthermore, all pokeweed mitogen–stimulated cell culture supernatants of patients contained LMW IgM, and at day 7, the monomeric IgM contributed from 19 to 100% of the total IgM (Table 1 and Figure 2). In the cultures without pokeweed, insufficient IgM was obtained for chromatographic analysis. Viability counts at the completion of cultures of mitogen-stimulated cells revealed counts ≥87% in all instances. Significant correlations were observed between percent LMW IgM synthesized in vitro at day 7 and percent circulating LMW IgM (r = 0.98, $P < 0.01$) and between circulating LMW IgM and RF (r = 1.0, $P < 0.01$).

Analysis of the RA cell supernatants at day 3 of culture revealed that high levels of LMW IgM were seen in 6 of 7 patients, and LMW IgM continued to be secreted over the next 4 days (Figure 3). In contrast, the levels of pentameric IgM found at day 3 were low and were similar to the levels seen in control cultures (Table 1 and Figure 3).

Addition of cycloheximide to the cultures at day 0 resulted in an almost complete inhibition (>95%) of both pentameric and LMW IgM synthesis at day 3 compared with the control cultures. Viability counts on both sets of cultures were similar (83–90%).

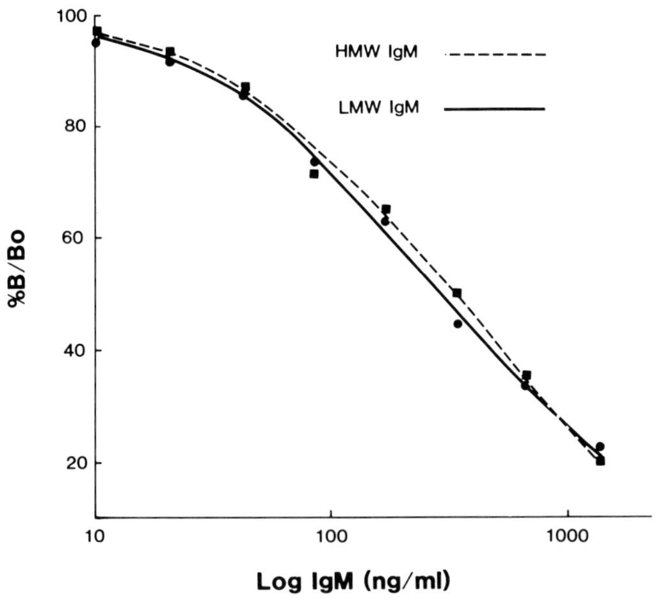

Figure 1. Binding curves for pentameric IgM (HMW IgM) and monomeric IgM (LMW IgM) in competitive inhibition enzyme immunoassay. Ordinate expresses % of conjugate bound (**B**) in relation to sample without IgM (**Bo**), and abscissa reflects the logarithm of IgM concentration (10). HMW IgM was prepared as previously described (10) and LMW IgM was prepared from the serum of a strongly seropositive rheumatoid arthritis patient by Sephacryl S300 chromatography and anti-μ affinity chromatography. The concentration of LMW IgM standard was measured by absorption at 225 nm, by nephelometry, and by the Lowry colorimetric technique. Values did not vary by more than 20% for the 3 methods.

To exclude the possibility that LMW IgM resulted from the breakdown of secreted pentameric IgM during the period of culture, ^{125}I-radiolabeled pentameric IgM was added at day 0 to 2 cultures which were secreting considerable quantities of LMW IgM. At day 4, these culture supernatants were pooled and the ^{125}I column chromatographic profile was compared with the profile of the uncultured ^{125}I-IgM. The profiles were very similar and, in particular, no additional counts were observed in the LMW IgM region after culture, thereby refuting the possibility of spontaneous breakdown of pentameric IgM. Following culture, a new peak which made up to 3% of the total counts was observed eluting at the position of the albumin marker, suggesting some transfer of ^{125}I to fetal calf albumin during the culture period.

DISCUSSION

We have demonstrated that PBMC from seropositive RA patients can be stimulated with pokeweed mitogen to secrete considerable quantities of LMW IgM in vitro. This does not occur with PBMC obtained from healthy controls. Pokeweed stimulation was necessary for the phenomenon to be observed since culture supernatants from unstimulated cells contained insufficient IgM for chromatographic analysis. Cycloheximide, a potent protein synthesis inhibitor, suppressed the phenomenon, illustrating that the production of LMW IgM is dependent on active protein synthesis. Furthermore, our study revealed a significant correlation between percent LMW IgM produced in vitro and percent circulating LMW IgM.

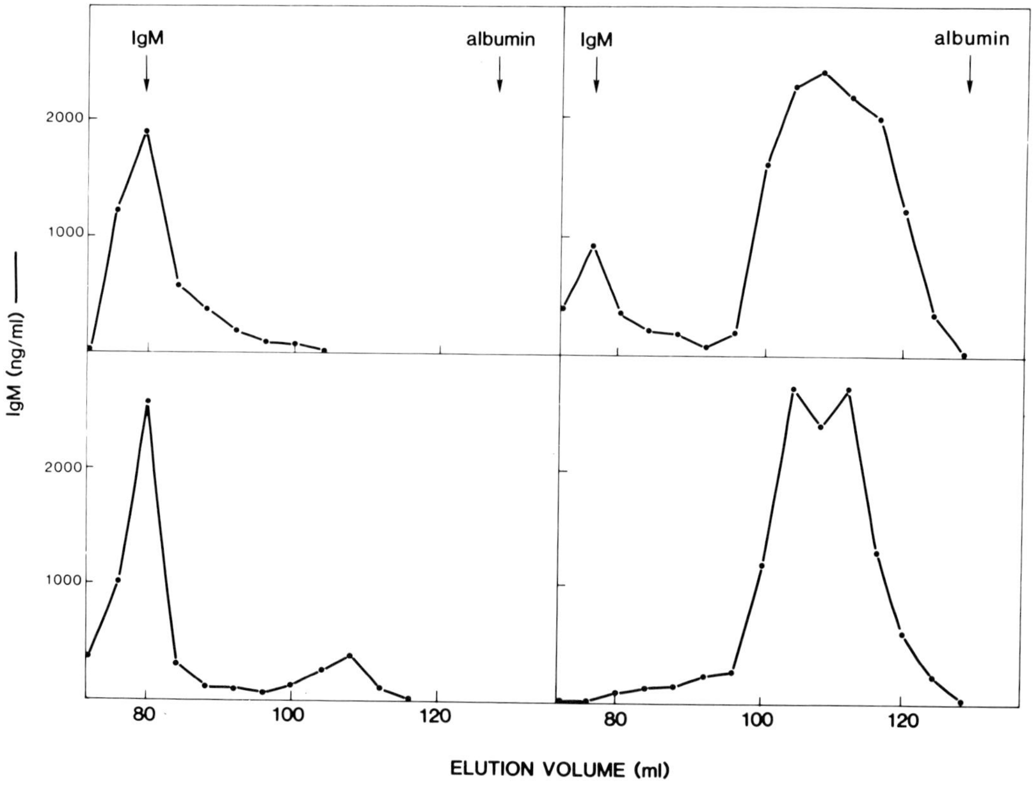

Figure 2. Enzyme-linked immunosorbent assay IgM profiles following column chromatography of cell culture supernatants at day 7. The elution positions of albumin and pentameric IgM are indicated. **Upper left**, Healthy control showing complete absence of monomeric IgM (LMW IgM). **Lower left**, Rheumatoid arthritis patient showing moderate quantities of LMW IgM. **Upper right**, Patient with Felty's syndrome showing large quantities of LMW IgM. **Lower right**, Rheumatoid arthritis patient with pulmonary fibrosis showing large quantities of LMW IgM and no pentameric IgM.

The significance of LMW IgM in RA is unclear. It is found in the serum and synovial fluid in high concentrations, and our previous studies have suggested that a considerable proportion of it possesses RF activity (1). It is an efficient activator of complement (3), and there are indirect data which suggest that it is a nonagglutinating, nonprecipitating antibody with an effective valency of 1 (14). If this is confirmed for LMW IgM in RA, this would suggest that this immunoglobulin could persist in biologic fluids as a small, functionally active immune complex with an antigen:antibody ratio of 1:1. The finding of a close association between LMW IgM and vasculitic complications in a number of studies on RA (2,15) supports an immunopathologic role for LMW IgM.

This study has raised a number of questions related to LMW IgM. The percentage of LMW IgM contribution to the total IgM is greater for that produced by PBMC in vitro than that found in the serum. Whether this reflects an enhancement of the mechanism for LMW IgM production by the mitogen used or whether there is a variation between different origins of IgM production (e.g., bone marrow, spleen, synovium) will need further analysis.

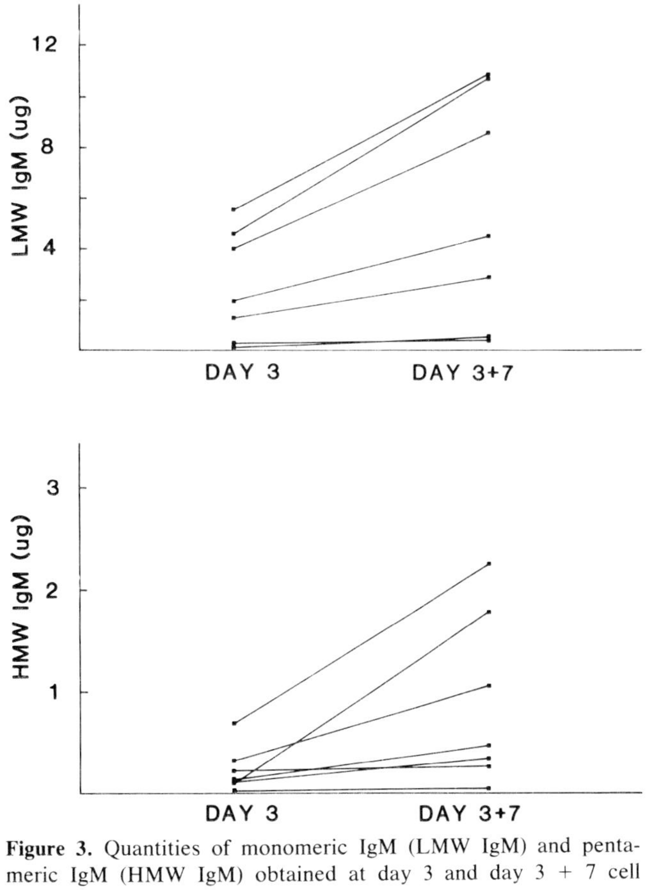

Figure 3. Quantities of monomeric IgM (LMW IgM) and pentameric IgM (HMW IgM) obtained at day 3 and day 3 + 7 cell culture. The lines join values for individual subjects.

The correlation between LMW IgM synthesis in vitro and circulating RF raises questions about the relationship between these 2 entities. Does their presence suggest a closely-related biologic phenomenon, e.g., phylogenetic reversion of the IgM immune response? We would predict from our earlier studies (1) that a proportion of the LMW IgM secreted in vitro will have rheumatoid factor activity, but our initial attempts to demonstrate this have been unsuccessful, probably because of the large dilution that occurs following chromatography of culture supernatants.

The presence of IgM in the early stages (namely, day 3) of culture in the rheumatoid arthritis patients in contrast with its absence at the same time in the control subjects and the predominance of LMW IgM, particularly at day 3, over pentameric IgM raises the possibility of a B cell maturation disorder in RA. Does this suggest that the B cells are already primed and have some IgM polymerizing defect, or are the B cells preprogrammed to secrete LMW IgM? It should be noted, however, that the quantity of IgM produced in culture at day 7 by the rheumatoid PBMC was considerably more than that produced by the controls. This is in contrast to most published studies where, in general, IgM synthesis by rheumatoid PBMC in response to pokeweed mitogen is depressed in comparison with that of normal individuals (16). The explanation of this difference is unclear, but possibly is due to the selection of our rheumatoid arthritis patients. Although they were selected because of their gross serologic abnormalities, 6 of 7 were not taking any specific disease-suppressive medications and some were taking nonsteroidal antiinflammatory drugs infrequently. Further synthetic studies will be required to clarify the difference. Nevertheless, having described the secretion of LMW IgM from RA PBMC in vitro, it is now possible to study many of these questions using this technique. It is hoped that this approach will increase our understanding of the significance of LMW IgM in the rheumatic diseases.

Acknowledgments. We gratefully thank M. Molnar for typing the manuscript and for helpful secretarial assistance and we also thank Dr. S. Neoh for help with the radiolabeling of IgM.

REFERENCES

1. Roberts-Thomson PJ, Wernick RM, Ziff M: Low molecular weight IgM in rheumatoid arthritis and other rheumatic diseases. Arthritis Rheum 24:795–802, 1981
2. Stage DE, Mannik M: 7SγM-globulin in rheumatoid arthritis: evaluation of its clinical significance. Arthritis Rheum 14:440–450, 1971
3. Caldwell JR: Efficient complement fixation by 7SIgM (abstract). Arthritis Rheum 16:537, 1973
4. Carter PM, Hobbs JR: Clinical significance of 7S IgM in monoclonal IgM diseases. Br Med J [Clin Res] 2:260–261, 1971
5. Roberts-Thomson PJ, Jones DN, Koh LY, Neoh SH, Thomas M, Bradley J: Low molecular weight IgM in B cell lymphoproliferative disorders. Aust NZ J Med 14:121–125, 1984
6. Vogler LB: Bone marrow B cell development. Clin Haematol 11:509–529, 1982
7. Solomon A, McLaughlin CL: Biosynthesis of low molecular weight (7S) and high molecular weight (19S) immunoglobulin M. J Clin Invest 49:150–160, 1970
8. Marchalonis J, Edelman GM: Phylogenetic origins of antibody structure. I. Multi-chain structure of immunoglobulins in the South dogfish (Mustelus canis). J Exp Med 122:601–618, 1965
9. Ropes MW, Bennett GA, Cobb S, Jacox R, Jessar RA: 1958 revision of diagnostic criteria for rheumatoid arthritis. Bull Rheum Dis 9:175–176, 1958
10. Roberts-Thomson PJ, Wernick RM, Ziff M: Quantitation of rheumatoid factor by laser nephelometry. Rheumatol Int 2:17–20, 1982
11. Smart IJ, Koh LY: A competitive-inhibition enzyme-immunoassay for the measurement of human IgG, IgA and IgM. J Immunol Methods 60:329–339, 1983
12. Roberts-Thomson PJ: A reappraisal of the monoclonal rheumatoid factor test for circulating immune complexes: a comparison of two monoclonal rheumatoid factor reagents. Clin Exp Immunol 48:52–60, 1982
13. Hesser C, Boesman M, Nordin JH, Isliker H: Effect of chemical and enzymatic radioiodination on in vitro human C1q activities. J Immunol 110:820–828, 1973
14. Chavin SI, Franklin EC: Studies on antigen binding activity of macroglobulin antibody subunits and their enzymatic fragments. J Biol Chem 244:1345–1352, 1969
15. Theofilopoulos AN, Burtonboy G, LoSpalluto JJ, Ziff M: IgG rheumatoid factor and low molecular weight IgM: an association with vasculitis. Arthritis Rheum 17:272–284, 1974
16. Alarcón GS, Koopman WJ, Schrohenloher RE: Differential patterns of in vitro IgM rheumatoid factor synthesis in seronegative and seropositive rheumatoid arthritis. Arthritis Rheum 25:150–155, 1982

LETTERS

Pulmonary hypertension and chronic cutaneous lupus erythematosus: association with the lupus anticoagulant

To the Editor:

Pulmonary hypertension (PH) as a complication of systemic lupus erythematosus (SLE) is uncommon. We have recently reported the association between this condition and the presence of the lupus anticoagulant in 5 of 6 patients (1) and have speculated about whether this antibody, linked to thromboses of various vessels, was in some way connected to the development of PH, possibly by predisposing to microthromboses or "thrombosis-in-situ" in the small pulmonary vessels (2). PH has not, to our knowledge, been previously reported in association with chronic discoid lupus erythematosus (DLE). We wish to report this occurrence in a patient whose sole detectable immunologic abnormalities were the presence of the lupus anticoagulant and high titers of antibodies to cardiolipin (a phospholipid responsible, in part, for the serologic false-positive test for syphilis and also closely linked to the lupus anticoagulant) (3).

The patient, a female, presented in 1977 at age 57, with exertional syncope. These episodes became more frequent, with increasing breathlessness, and 3 years later, the clinical diagnosis of PH was confirmed by right heart catheterization (mean pulmonary artery pressure 64 mm Hg). She was treated with nifedipine, which brought about some improvement.

In 1982 she developed a rash over her sternum and knuckles which had clinical and histologic features of DLE. Simultaneously she developed arthritis in both hands. In the past she had been epileptic, but she had been free of seizures for 10 years and was no longer receiving anticonvulsive therapy. She had been diagnosed as having hypothyroidism 5 years previously and was receiving replacement thyroxine therapy.

By 1983 the pulmonary hypertension symptoms had worsened and her mean pulmonary artery pressure had risen to 85 mm Hg. Pulmonary angiography did not demonstrate embolic disease, and lung function studies suggested mild interstitial disease. However, there was no radiologic evidence of pulmonary fibrosis. Serologic findings (antinuclear antibody, latex fixation, complement, DNA binding, extractable nuclear antigen) were all normal, but there was a false-positive serologic test for syphilis, and the lupus anticoagulant (LA) was found to be present along with high titers of anticardiolipin antibodies (IgG and IgM). The Schirmer's test revealed dryness of the eyes, and salivary gland biopsy demonstrated focal lymphocytic infiltrates consistent with Sjögren's syndrome. She was given anticoagulation treatment and her symptoms improved.

This woman quite clearly had DLE with arthritis and Sjögren's syndrome. Serologically she had no evidence of SLE but, interestingly, she had the triad of false-positive serologic test for syphilis, high-titer anticardiolipin antibodies, and the presence of the LA in the clinical setting of pulmonary hypertension. Neither pulmonary hypertension nor these latter 2 serologic abnormalities has previously been described in DLE, although false-positive serologic tests for syphilis have been documented in 3% of this group of patients (4). Progression of DLE to systemic disease or mixed connective tissue disease was reported to occur in 4 of 62 patients in a recent review (5).

This case represents an important link between PH and the presence of the LA, anticardiolipin antibodies, and a false-positive serologic test for syphilis: these were the only serologic abnormalities demonstrable in this patient.

Ronald A. Asherson, MB, FCP(SA)
Stephen H. Morgan, MB, MRCP
Nigel Harris, MPhil, DM
Azzudin E. Gharavi, MD
Graham R. V. Hughes, MD, MRCP
Royal Postgraduate Medical School
Hammersmith Hospital
Ann B. Millar, MB, MRCP
Royal Free Hospital
London, UK

1. Asherson RA, Mackworth-Young CG, Boey ML, Hull RG, Saunders AE, Gharavi AE, Hughes GRV: Pulmonary hypertension in systemic lupus erythematosus. Br Med J 287:1024–1025, 1983
2. Hughes GRV: Thrombosis, abortion, cerebral disease and the lupus anticoagulant. Br Med J 287:1088–1089, 1983
3. Harris EN, Gharavi AE, Boey ML, Patel BM, Mackworth-Young CG, Loizou S, Hughes GRV: Anticardiolipin antibodies: detection by radioimmunoassay and association with thrombosis in systemic lupus erythematosus. Lancet ii:1211–1214, 1983
4. Prystowsky SD, Herndon JH, Gilliam JN: Chronic cutaneous lupus erythematosus (DLE): a clinical and laboratory investigation of 80 patients. Medicine (Baltimore) 55:183–191, 1975
5. Callen JP: Chronic cutaneous lupus erythematosus. Arch Dermatol 118:412–416, 1982

Chondrocytes that accumulate proteoglycans and inorganic pyrophosphate in the pathogenesis of chondrocalcinosis

To the Editor:

Lust et al have demonstrated that certain cells from patients with hereditary calcium pyrophosphate dihydrate (CPPD) deposition disease produce and accumulate inorganic pyrophosphate (PPi) but barely release it extracellularly (1). Our histologic study seems to confirm their work.

Hyaline cartilage, meniscus, labrum acetabulare, synovium and capsule, or ligamentum flavum obtained by surgery from 9 patients with hereditary or sporadic CPPD deposition disease (2–4) showed characteristic cells in the

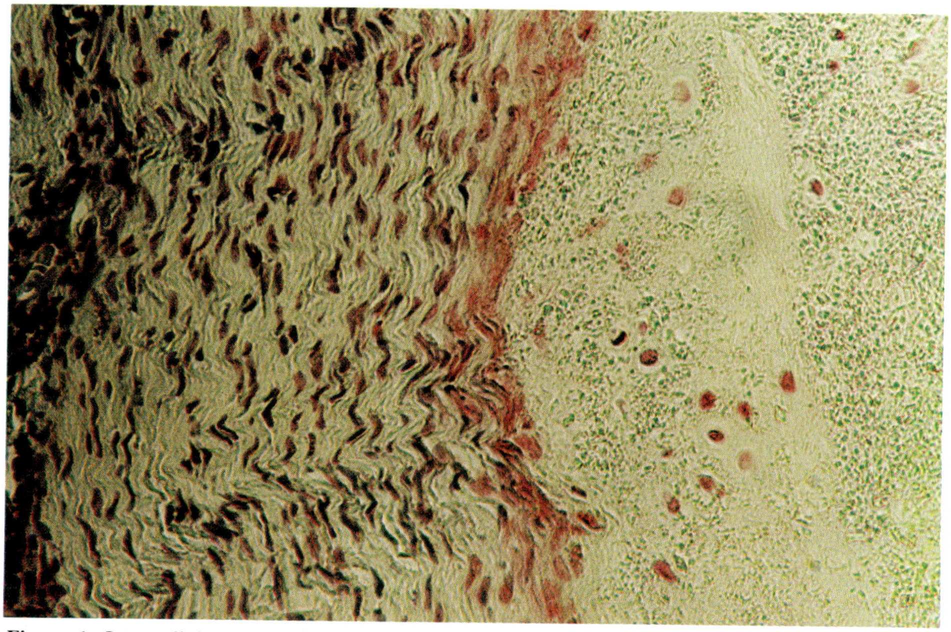

Figure 1. Intracellular proteoglycans shown by staining with Safranin O, fast acid green, and hematoxylin (original magnification × 370).

areas of incipient formation of CPPD crystals. These cells, which were the chondrocytes of hyaline cartilage and the metaplastic chondrocytes in the poorly vascularized regions of other tissues, contained abundant intracellular proteoglycans (PG) as shown by staining with the cationic dye, Safranin O (5).

Most of these cells displayed a reddish coloration and a unique loss of the normal dark staining of the nucleus (Figure 1). Viewed by electron microscopy, these chondrocytes had an abundance of dense material suggestive of PG in the cytoplasm, and a well-developed, rough endoplasmic reticulum. By contrast, light and electron microscopy revealed only a small amount of PG around most cells—a phenomenon reported as "halo" chondrocytes in CPPD-bearing hyaline cartilage (6). These findings suggest that the reddish cells produce and accumulate PG but do not release them extracellularly.

Characteristic changes were evident in the focal crystallization areas of each tissue examined (Figure 1). The reddish-colored cells may originally have been present in this region as ordinary chondrocytes or fibrocytes, subsequently transformed, and left among or pushed aside by the growing crystals. These chondrocytes with the characteristic appearance were scarcely noted around mature deposits of dense aggregates of crystals, and were never present outside the area of formation of CPPD crystals. No similar cell has been described in hydroxyapatite deposition (4,7). The fact that these cells were found constantly, and almost exclusively, in the focal areas of active CPPD crystal formation suggests that they can produce and somehow release enough PPi to cause crystallization.

Crystals were seldom seen adjacent to the apparently viable reddish chondrocytes, whereas the necrotic cells with disrupted cell membrane and decreased staining by Safranin O frequently had crystals around and within them. These findings indicate that not only PG, but probably PPi as well, accumulates in the intact cells and leaks out from the severely degenerated or necrotic cells on disruption of the cell membrane. The debris of cellular components may contribute to crystal nucleation (8). The evident intracellular accumulation of both PG and PPi may indicate that these chondrocytes produce PPi as a by-product of PG synthesis, as has been suggested by Ryan et al (9).

The present study seems to indicate that the mother of crystals is destined to devote herself to her children and to be one with them.

Koichiro Ishikawa, MD
Kumamoto University Medical School
Kumamoto-Shi, Japan

1. Lust G, Faure G, Netter P, Gaucher A, Seegmiller JE: Evidence of a generalized metabolic defect in patients with hereditary chondrocalcinosis: increased inorganic pyrophosphate in cultured fibroblasts and lymphoblasts. Arthritis Rheum 24:1517–1521, 1981
2. Sakaguchi M, Kitagawa T, Ishikawa K, Numata T: Familial pseudogout with destructive arthropathy in Japan (abstract). Arthritis Rheum (suppl) 25:S34, 1982
3. Ogata M, Ishikawa K, Ohira T: Cervical myelopathy in pseudogout. J Bone Joint Surg (in press)
4. Ishikawa K, Heipertz W, Zichner L, Hovy L, Ogata M, Ohira T: Tissue calcification in osteoarthritis: its prevalence, localization, and possible pathogenetic significance. Submitted for publication
5. Ishikawa K: Effect of intra-articular corticosteroid on the meniscus: a histological and histochemical study in rabbit knees. J Bone Joint Surg 63A:120–130, 1981

6. Richardson BC, Chafetz NI, Ferrell LD, Zulman JI, Genant HK: Hereditary chondrocalcinosis in a Mexican-American family. Arthritis Rheum 26:1387–1396, 1983
7. Ishikawa K, Ohira T, Sakata H: Effects of intra-articular injection of halopredone diacetate on the articular cartilage of rabbit knees: a comparison with methylprednisolone acetate. Toxicol Appl Pharmacol (in press)
8. Dieppe P, Calvert P: Crystals and Joint Disease. London, Chapman and Hall, 1983, pp 23–56
9. Ryan LM, Cheung HS, McCarty DJ: Release of pyrophosphate by normal mammalian articular hyaline and fibrocartilage in organ culture. Arthritis Rheum 24:1522–1527, 1981

Synovial fluid lymphocyte subpopulations in the polyarthritis of immunoblastic lymphadenopathy

To the Editor:

Seronegative, inflammatory polyarthritis is an unusual feature of immunoblastic lymphadenopathy (IL) (1–3). Synovianalyses in 2 patients (1,2) showed inflammatory effusions with a polymorphonuclear cell predominance. In a patient with IL and associated polysynovitis, described here, synovial fluid (SF) revealed a marked mononuclear pleocytosis. Lymphocyte subpopulations in the SF were identified by monoclonal antibody testing.

A 45-year-old black man presented in 1981 with a systemic illness ultimately characterized by fever, weight loss, generalized lymphadenopathy, and a polyclonal gammopathy. Findings of peripheral lymph node biopsies were consistent with IL, showing effacement of the normal nodal architecture and a polymorphic infiltration of immunoblasts, plasma cells, and histiocytes. With corticosteroids an initial remission was seen, but adenopathy recurred, waxing and waning with steroid therapy.

In June 1983, at the time of a disease exacerbation, the patient exhibited fever, enlarging adenopathy, and an acute, symmetric, inflammatory polyarthritis involving the metacarpophalangeal, proximal interphalangeal, wrist, elbow, knee, and ankle joints. The following studies gave normal or negative results: complete blood count, urinalysis, serum rheumatoid factor (latex fixation), hepatitis B surface antigen, anti-HA antigen, serum glutamic oxaloacetic transaminase, Monospot test, circulating immune complexes (Raji cell assay), blood cultures, antinuclear antibody, C3, C4, and cryoglobulins. Knee roentgenograms showed no erosions or chondrocalcinosis. Arthrocentesis of the left knee yielded 20 ml of yellow, turbid, poorly viscous fluid with a poor mucin clot, total protein of 5.1 gm/dl, white blood cell count of 20,250 (93% mononuclear, 7% polymorphonuclear), and negative findings on crystal search; bacterial, mycobacterial, and fungal stains and cultures were negative.

Table 1. Lymphocyte subpopulations (% positive cells) identified in the synovial fluid and blood

Monoclonal antibodies reacting to:	Synovial fluid	Blood	Mean normal values, blood (range)
OKT3	80.0	61.0	72.1 (55.5–88.7)
OKT11	73.0	75.0	77.3 (62.9–91.7)
OKT4	75.0	54.0	44.4 (31.2–57.6)
OKT8	8.0	32.0	24.1 (15.0–35.5)
T4:T8 ratio	9.8	1.7	2.0 (0.7–4.0)
B1	4.0	7.0	4.5 (0.0–10.7)

Lymphocytes were separated from heparinized aliquots of blood and SF by density gradient centrifugation. Lymphocyte subpopulations were identified by indirect immunofluoresence after reaction with monoclonal antibodies, and results are shown in Table 1.

Polyarthritis and fever improved with oral indomethacin; corticosteroids were reinstituted shortly thereafter, due to the development of sterile pulmonary lymphoid infiltrates. The patient's disease progressed to a null cell lymphoma, and he died in late 1983.

In contrast to earlier reports of joint fluid analysis in IL polyarthritis, SF lymphocytosis was observed in our patient, possibly reflecting the relatively short time interval between onset of synovitis and arthrocentesis. Peripheral blood T cell numbers and percentages were normal. However, the SF showed a significant increase in the ratio of T helper/inducer to T suppressor/cytotoxic cells. The significance of this finding is unclear. Immunoblastic lymphadenopathy is a disorder in which the primary defect may exist in T cell regulatory function. T helper cells often, but not invariably, have been shown to be the predominant synovial membrane lymphocyte in rheumatoid and other inflammatory arthritides (4,5).

Robert G. Gray, MD
Baystate Medical Center
Springfield, MA

1. Davies PG, Fordham JN: Arthritis and angioimmunoblastic lymphadenopathy. Ann Rheum Dis 42:516–518, 1983
2. Raskin RJ, Tesar JT, Lawless OJ: Polyarthritis in immunoblastic lymphadenopathy. Arthritis Rheum 25:1481–1485, 1982
3. Rothwell RS, Mant MJ, Davis P: Angio-immunoblastic lymphadenopathy associated with polyarthritis. Ann Rheum Dis 39:406–409, 1980
4. Lindblad S, Klareskog L, Hedfors E, Forsum U, Sundström C: Phenotypic characterization of synovial tissue cells in situ in different types of synovitis. Arthritis Rheum 26:1321–1332, 1983
5. Meijer CJLM, deGraaff-Reitsma CB, Lafeber GJM, Cats A: In situ localization of lymphocyte subsets in synovial membranes of patients with rheumatoid arthritis with monoclonal antibodies. J Rheumatol 9:359–365, 1982

arthritis and rheumatism

Official Journal of the American Rheumatism Association Section of the Arthritis Foundation

CURRENT COMMENT

SEX STEROIDS AND THE RHEUMATIC DISEASES

ROBERT G. LAHITA

A new area of research in the rheumatic diseases is the relationship between sex steroids and the morbidity and mortality of these diseases. The majority of rheumatic diseases, or at least those in which immune aberrations are obvious, affect females predominantly. There is no doubt now that sex steroids affect a variety of both normal and pathologic functions, ranging from degree of arthropathy to altered behavior, in both the human and animal models.

Some illnesses, such as systemic lupus erythematosus (SLE), have an impressively higher incidence in females. After puberty, 13 females are affected for each male. The early-age incidence in males of diseases such as gout and Reiter's syndrome suggests that sex steroids are also a major factor in their pathogenesis. The reason for this male or female predominance observed in seemingly unrelated diseases remains a central question today. Could, for example, the pathogenesis and clinical variation of the spondylarthropathies of the female and male be attributed to the effects of sex steroids on host resistance to infection? Could the radiologic picture or other findings in such illnesses reflect this effect?

A current field of interest, called immunoendocrinology, is really the study of the convergence of polypeptide and steroid hormone effects on the immune system. Such studies bear directly on the rheumatic diseases, and the immune system may be only one of several systems affected by these molecules. Moreover, our attempts at understanding the manifestations of most rheumatic diseases from one scientific viewpoint might really be simplistic and lead us to ignore important mechanisms in the pathogenetic process. For example, there is substantial evidence indicating that diseases like SLE, which involve both immune and behavioral abnormalities known to wax or wane with sexual cyclicity, might really be the result of biochemical effects of sex steroids on the lymphoid system and the brain.

Most of the discussion in this review will highlight SLE, since it has been the most thoroughly investigated illness with regard to sex steroid metabolism, though the reader who is familiar with other diseases such as rheumatoid arthritis (RA) and gout might wish to envision similar mechanisms as operative in those illnesses. Hopefully, this discussion will illustrate the point that sex steroid metabolism might contribute to our ultimate understanding of inflammation, the control of autoimmunity, and perhaps mental illness.

The importance of sex has long been recognized in the clinical observation of SLE patients. Females in the childbearing years are generally the most severely affected. Disease severity is often observed by patient and physician to vary with the normal menses (1), the ingestion of conjugated synthetic estrogens used for birth control (2), and during times of great steroid flux, such as pregnancy (3). Although the basic pathogenetic mechanisms during these stages are the subjects of basic investigation in females with the disease, small behavioral changes and rheumatic complaints such as arthralgias and Raynaud's phenomenon are often observed in normal women as well; these often prompt visits to the physician, who must rule out diseases like

From the Rockefeller University, New York, New York.
Robert G. Lahita, MD, PhD.
Address reprint requests to Robert G. Lahita, MD, PhD, The Rockefeller University, 1230 York Avenue, New York, NY 10021.
Submitted for publication July 27, 1984; accepted August 6, 1984.

SLE. There is no question—as patients will admit—that such symptoms can be related to stress, menses, etc., and are perceived by them as hormonal events. In short, these are not random events, but rather physiologic effects that are exaggerated in women.

A clearer understanding of, for example, the genetics of SLE and rheumatoid arthritis (i.e., histocompatibility) might confirm that though these diseases are genetically dissimilar, a common "sexual susceptibility" exists among patients with both diseases. Patients with RA have been thought by many to improve in the presence of estrogens, both natural and synthetic (4), while this is disputed by others (5). The importance of these observations underscores the present interest in the preventive powers of the oral contraceptive on rheumatoid arthritis. In addition, there is solid evidence that genetically-induced hyperestrogenism found in males with Klinefelter's syndrome contributes to the pathology of autoimmune diseases such as SLE (6) and perhaps RA (7,8). No doubt other rheumatologic phenomena will be described in these experiments of nature. Sex chromatin–associated estrogenic metabolites, now being carefully defined, might play a direct role on diverse systems and functions including immunity, brain growth, prostaglandin synthesis, and perhaps even skeletal integrity.

Early work from murine models underscores the importance of "sexual factors." Studies of New Zealand black (NZB) and New Zealand black/New Zealand white (NZB/W) F_1 mice suggested that "femaleness" was important to morbidity and mortality of disease (9), and that alteration of mice either by gonadectomy (10) or therapy with androgens (11) made a significant difference. Various reasons were given for such changes, such as a reduction of tolerance (12), a change in suppressor cell populations (13), and the presence of sex chromatin (14). Despite these data, recent development of hormone-insensitive mice such as the BXSB strain (15) has positioned such phenomena as immunomodulatory, but not essential to pathogenesis. As in this mouse strain, familial male disease has recently been described in humans (16), deemphasizing sex and emphasizing genetic susceptibility. It is, in fact, likely that sex and genetics are 2 of the 3 possible preconditions to the development of SLE. The third precondition may be the presence of or susceptibility to an infectious agent. Though males sporadically develop SLE, sexual abnormalities have been reported in male patients, and whether sex or genetics are important to acquisition of the illness in this sex remains unclear.

Rheumatoid arthritis has only recently come under scrutiny with regard to sexual factors (17), such as the apparent improvement in patients taking oral contraceptives (18,19) and those patients who become pregnant (20), despite the fact that such observations were made over 30 years ago. It has also been apparent for years that sex steroids might influence the course of experimental arthropathy in animals (21) and that such defects, at least in collagen- (22) and streptococcal cell wall–induced arthopathy in rodents (23), were sexually mediated.

Despite all the evidence, the modulating effects of the steroids on immunity remain elusive. The new interest has generated preliminary evidence that androgenic metabolism might be abnormal in female RA patients (Masi AT: personal communication), and new data suggest a direct role for gonadotrophic hormones (24) in the pathogenesis of experimental arthropathy of the rat, emphasizing the importance of the pituitary gland as modifier. Most physicians will undoubtedly concur with all of these findings, citing numerous anecdotal experiences from clinical practice to support the role of pregnancy, stress, or even diet on improvements or exacerbations of disease.

The main thrust of current research into the effects of sex steroids on rheumatic processes and immunologic diseases has been: (a) to understand the role of sex steroids on the immune system, (b) to identify hormonal abnormalities and alterations which might be present in patients with specific rheumatic diseases, and (c) to integrate and identify specific metabolites operative in pathogenesis. As an early example, estrogens were reported to be important as stimulants of immune responsiveness in vitro (25), although such studies involved mitogenic factors such as pokeweed mitogen, without regard to the now known genetic variability of such responses. Recent evidence from studies with mice would suggest that estrogens might act at the level of the thymus gland to secrete immunomodulators which are either inhibitory or excitative to various aspects of the immune system (26). Androgens have a postulated involvement in diverse activities, such as immunosuppression via selection of specific cellular subsets (27) or the induction of specific lymphokines (28). Data suggest that such actions might be wholly dependent on the kind of estrogen or androgen that is active, rather than the amount.

Even though an obvious direction to the study of the effects of sex steroids in the autoimmune diseases would be the detection of receptors on the cells of the lymphoid system, sex steroid receptors have been found only on the thymus (29), with one recent exception in which estrogen receptors were found on OKT8+ T cells (30). This localization of receptors to a specific T cell subset of the suppressor cell variety poses exciting possibilities and awaits further confirmation. The presence or absence of receptors for specific steroids on specific subsets of lymphocytes or other cells of the reticuloendothelial system might change contemporary views about the real importance of these agents.

These exciting possibilities, if confirmed, would make selection and design of active androgenic or estrogenic suppressive agents a reality for the future. Natural androgens like DHEA and synthetic androgens like 19 nortestosterone may offer some interesting possibilities for the future of diseases such as SLE, while non-feminizing estrogens of the cathecol type might be useful in RA.

With the exception of testosterone and 19 nortestosterone in female mice, few androgenic substances have been totally effective in controlling murine lupus in adult animals. Danazol, a 17-substituted anabolic steroid useful in the therapy of angioneurotic edema, has been minimally effective in human lupus (31) and not at all effective in the murine system (32). If data regarding the necessity of thymic interaction are applicable in the mouse, then such manipulation might really be effective only in the neonate or fetus, where thymic tissue is readily available. In addition, more emphasis on the steroid–chromatin interaction is necessary for the observed and predicted effects of such agents to be fully appreciated.

Although there have been many studies on the role of sex steroid metabolism in disease, SLE is the only disease that has been analyzed comprehensively. There are numerous reports of high estrogen levels in both males and females with this disease (33); however, the majority of investigators have not found consistently elevated estradiol levels in males with SLE. Early on, only male patients with Klinefelter's syndrome and SLE were found to have an increase in the hydroxylation of estrone toward the more feminine metabolites, 16 alpha hydroxyestrone and estriol (6). This certainly suggested a role for the X chromosome in the pathogenesis, since such effects were the result of increased levels of estrogen. A series of reports discussing Klinefelter's syndrome and rheumatoid arthritis (7,8) suggested that estrogens might also be operative in RA.

Since Klinefelter patients with SLE had an elevation of feminizing metabolites, a study of males and females with SLE was undertaken (34). Injection of labeled sex steroids into humans in this clinical study revealed that SLE patients of both sexes had elevated levels of 16 alpha hydroxyestrone, while females had the additional elevation of estriol (34). Radiometric studies confirmed this elevation of 16 hydroxylation, along with the persistently observed compensatory decrease in cathecol or 2-hydroxylated estrogens (35). Moreover, study of androgen metabolism in SLE revealed that the oxidation of testosterone at C-17 was increased only in females with active disease (36).

All of these data suggest that there is a fundamental problem with sex steroid metabolism in patients with SLE, and that this problem might be exaggerated in female patients with clinically active disease. There are two ways to attempt to explain these findings: some metabolites of known enzymatic reactions might have unusual potency with regard to immune processes by selectively effecting thymic regulator proteins and either inhibiting or stimulating the immune system (26), or the ratio of estrogen to androgens might be critical, in some unexplained manner, to normal function of the immune system.

The effects of sex steroids on other cell populations have been alluded to above, and as one might expect, the process of inflammation might also be subject to the effects of sex steroids. Though more data on diseases such as gout and polymyalgia rheumatica are needed, the remarkable relationship of age and sex to onset and severity of many of these diseases suggests an important role of sex steroids. Data exist which support the role of sex steroids in the modification of neutrophil activity during normal sexual cycles, including pregnancy (37), and some researchers have suggested that such agents might have a potent role in the mediation of inflammation (38).

Pregnancy is a time of extraordinary shifts in sex steroid metabolism and may provide the investigator with a perfect setting for study. The dramatic alterations in metabolism of steroids normally occurring during pregnancy are probably necessary for the good health of both mother and fetus. As with all normal events, however, the pathologic state might be adversely affected by such shifts with the arrival of new and perhaps dangerous immune complexes (39) and altered T cell function (40,41). Female patients with a predisposition to autoimmune diseases such as RA and SLE might be extremely sensitive to the changes in pregnancy and actually acquire the disease during or after the 9-month gestation period.

SLE has been known to worsen (42) and RA to improve during pregnancy (43) for reasons that elude most investigators. To add to the confusion, there appear to be a substantial number of SLE patients who tolerate the pregnant state rather well, which might indicate that there are separate categories of patients. More intriguing would be the idea that the placenta and the thymus of the fetus might affect the disease of the mother through a series of steroid-dependent reactions which produce specific immunomodulatory thymic or placental hormones.

Some of the most exciting developments in the area of sex steroid involvement in immunity have been the observations with regard to a seemingly unrelated system, the brain. We have known for many years that patients with lupus were subject to behavioral aberrations (44). Emotional stress can and often does result in exacerbations of disease manifestations such as arthralgias and skin rash. Such changes are very provocative and might be the result of the decrease in 2-hydroxylation observed in females with SLE (35). Even right cerebral dominance has been reported in patients with allergies and some forms of autoimmunity (45).

The cathechol estrogens or 2-hydroxylated metabolites are potent neurotransmitters in rodents and may be important mediators of behavior in humans. Shifts in these unusual metabolites are a possible cause of affective disturbance in humans with SLE, although this is speculative and awaits careful analysis. Premenstrual tension, often observed in the normal female, might be exaggerated in SLE patients for this reason, and much of the "central nervous system SLE" or supposed cerebral vasculitis might in fact be related to quantitative changes in the amounts of these estrogens on adrenergic receptor–rich portions of the brain. In addition, further research is necessary to see if such receptors are important to lymphocyte function and the integrity of arterial function in patients with cyclic Raynaud's phenomenon as it relates to stress and disease.

As mentioned, cerebral dominance, learning disabilities, and phenomena such as skeletal abnormalities (kyphoscoliosis) are associated with a higher incidence of immune aberrations. This is not surprising since the migration of neurons in the brain is hormonally mediated during the first few weeks of life in all animals (46). It is plausible that such migration might be altered by varying levels of sex steroids in the fetus as a result of maternal metabolic abnormalities, such as those described above, which are now known to be a part of diseases like SLE. Such changes in neuronal migration have been reported in the NZB autoimmune mouse (47). Alterations of sex steroids in the fetal brain by a variety of mechanisms might account for the apparent changes in behavior and cerebral laterality now observed in patients with autoimmune diseases.

Immunoendocrinology, or the influence of sex steroids on disease, therefore holds great promise for the future of our specialty. The development of new hormonal antiinflammatory agents with fewer side effects is now on the horizon. Monoclonal antibody technology also might afford us a means of studying, isolating, and blocking specific hormone receptors which might be beneficial or detrimental to many disease manifestations. Psychoneurotic conditions, which have heretofore remained elusive, are one area which merits consideration. More important is the role of various sex steroid receptors on the thymus, reticuloendothelial cells, brain, and lymphoid populations of the adult and the developing fetus. They are likely targets of the 16-hydroxylated metabolites and 2-hydroxylated estrogens which are elevated or decreased in various rheumatic diseases.

REFERENCES

1. Rose E, Pillsbury DM: Lupus erythematosus (erythematoides) and ovarian function: observations on a possible relationship with a report of 6 cases. Ann Intern Med 21:1022–1034, 1944
2. Jungers P, Dougados M, Pélissier C, Kuttenn F, Tron F, Lesavre P, Bach J-F: Influence of oral contraceptive therapy on the activity of systemic lupus erythematosus. Arthritis Rheum 25:618–623, 1982
3. Mund A, Swison J, Rothfield N: Effect of pregnancy on the course of SLE. JAMA 183:917–920, 1963
4. Kay CR, Wingrave SJ: Oral contraceptives and rheumatoid arthritis. Lancet 2:1437, 1983
5. Linos A, O'Fallon WM, Worthington JW, Kurland LT: Case-control study of rheumatoid arthritis and prior use of oral contraceptives. Lancet 1:1299–1300, 1983
6. Stern R, Fishman J, Brusman H, Kunkel HG: Systemic lupus erythematosus associated with Klinefelter's syndrome. Arthritis Rheum 20:18–22, 1977
7. MacSween RNM: Reticulum cell sarcoma and rheumatoid arthritis in a patient with XY/XXY/XXXY Klinefel-

ters syndrome and normal intelligence. Lancet 1:460–461, 1965
8. Lamotte M, Labrousse C, Perrault MA, Kleinknecht D, Rozenbaum H: Polyarthrite rheumatoide severe diabete insulino-resistant, syndrome de Klinefelter. Sem Hop Paris 9:525–528, 1965
9. Kelly VA, Winklestein A: Age and sex related glomerulonephritis in New Zealand white mice. Clin Immunol Immunopathol 16:142–150, 1980
10. Roubinian JR, Talal N, Greenspan JS, Goodman JR, Siiteri PK: Effect of castration and sex hormone treatment on survival, anti-nucleic acid antibodies, and glomerulonephritis in NZB/NZW F1 mice. J Exp Med 147:1568–1583, 1978
11. Melez KA, Boegel WA, Steinberg AD: Therapeutic studies in New Zealand mice. VII. Successful androgen treatment of NZB/NZW F_1 females of different ages. Arthritis Rheum 23:41–47, 1980
12. Laskin CA, Taurog JD, Smathers PA, Steinberg AD: Studies of defective tolerance in murine lupus. J Immunol 127:1743–1747, 1981
13. Cooke A, Hutchings P: Sex differences in the regulation of experimentally induced autoantibodies in (NZB × NZW)F1 mice. Immunology 41:819–823, 1980
14. Mazes E, Fuchs S: Linkage between immune response potential to DNA and X chromosome. Nature 249:167–168, 1974
15. Murphy ED, Roths JB: A Y chromosome associated factor in strain BXSB producing accelerated autoimmunity and lymphoproliferation. Arthritis Rheum 22:1188–1194, 1979
16. Lahita RG, Chiorazzi N, Gibofsky A, Winchester RJ, Kunkel HG: Familial systemic lupus erythematosus in males. Arthritis Rheum 26:39–44, 1983
17. Lawrence JS: Rheumatoid arthritis: nature or nurture? Ann Rheum Dis 29:357–379, 1970
18. Blais JA, Demers R: The use of norethynodrel (Enovid) in the treatment of rheumatoid arthritis (preliminary report) (abstract). Arthritis Rheum 5:284, 1962
19. Gilbert M, Rothstain J, Cunningham C, Estrin I, Davedson A, Pincus G: Norethynodrel with mestranol in treatment of RA. JAMA 190:235, 1964
20. Oka M, Vainio U: Effect of pregnancy on the prognosis and serology of RA. Acta Rheum Scand 12:47–52, 1966
21. Mueller MN, Kappas A: Estrogen pharmacology. II. Suppression of experimental immune polyarthritis. Proc Soc Exp Biol Med 117:845–847, 1964
22. Trentham DE, McCune WJ, Susman P, David JR: Autoimmunity to collagen in adjuvant arthritis of rats. J Clin Invest 66:1109–1117, 1980
23. Allen JB, Blatter D, Calandra GB, Wilder RL: Sex hormone effects on the severity of streptococcal cell wall–induced polyarthritis in the rat. Arthritis Rheum 26:560–563, 1983
24. Berczi I, Nagy E, Asa SL, Kovacs K: The influence of pituitary hormones on adjuvant arthritis. Arthritis Rheum 27:682–688, 1984
25. Paavonen T, Andersson LC, Adlercreutz H: Sex hormone regulation of in vitro immune response: estradiol enhances human B cell maturation via inhibition of suppressor T cells in PWM stimulated cultures. J Exp Med 154:1935–1945, 1980
26. Luster MI, Hayes HT, Korach K, Tucker AN, Dean JH, Greenlee WF, Boorman GA: Estrogen suppression is regulated through estrogenic responses in the thymus. J Immunol 133:110–116, 1984
27. Weinstein Y, Berkovich Z: Testosterone effect on bone marrow, thymus and suppressor T cells in the (NZB × NZW)F1 mice: its relevance to autoimmunity. J Immunol 126:998–1002, 1981
28. Dauphinée MJ, Kipper S, Roskos K, Wofsky D, Talal N: Androgen treatment of NZB/W mice enhances IL-2 production (abstract). Arthritis Rheum (suppl) 24:S64, 1981
29. Stimson WH, Hunter IC: Estrogen-induced immunoregulation mediated through the thymus. J Clin Lab Immunol 4:27–33, 1980
30. Cohen JHM, Davel L, Cordier G, Saez S, Revillard JP: Sex steroid receptors in peripheral T cells: absence of androgen receptors and restriction of estrogen receptors to OKT8 positive cells. J Immunol 131:2767–2771, 1983
31. Agnello V, Pariser K, Gell J, Gelfand J, Turksoy RN: Preliminary observations on danazol therapy of systemic lupus erythematosus: effects on DNA antibodies, thrombocytopenia and complement. J Rheumatol 10:682–687, 1983
32. Roubinian JR, Talal N, Greenspan JS, Goodman JR, Nussenzweig V: Danazol's failure to suppress autoimmunity in NZB/NZW F_1 mice. Arthritis Rheum 22:1399–1402, 1979
33. Inman RD: Immunologic sex differences and the female predominance in systemic lupus erythematosus. Arthritis Rheum 21:849–852, 1978
34. Lahita RG, Bradlow L, Fishman J, Kunkel HG: Estrogen metabolism in systemic lupus erythematosus: patients and family members. Arthritis Rheum 25:843–846, 1982
35. Lahita RG, Bradlow HL, Fishman J: Increased 16 alpha hydroxylation of estradiol in systemic lupus erythematosus. J Clin Endocrinol Metab 53:174–178, 1981
36. Lahita RG, Kunkel HG, Bradlow HL: Increased oxidation of testosterone in systemic lupus erythematosus. Arthritis Rheum 26:1517–1521, 1983
37. Cotton DJ, Seligmann B, O'Brien WF, Gallin JI: Selective defect in human neutrophil superoxide anion generation elicited by the chemoattractant n-formylmethionylleucylphenylalanine in pregnancy. J Infect Dis 148:194–199, 1983
38. Buyon JP, Korchak HM, Rutherford LE, Ganguly M, Weissmann G: Female hormones reduce neutrophil responsiveness in vitro. Arthritis Rheum 27:623–630, 1984
39. Masson PL, Delire M, Cambiaso CL: Circulating immune complexes in normal human pregnancy. Nature 266:542–543, 1977

40. Scott JR, Feldbush TL: T- and B-cell distribution in pregnancy. JAMA 239:2769–2772, 1978
41. Tallon DF, Corcoran DJD, O'Dwyer EM, Greally JF: Circulating lymphocyte subpopulations in pregnancy: a longitudinal study. J Immunol 132:1784–1787, 1984
42. Grigor RR, Shervington PC, Hughes GRV, Hawkins DF: Outcome of pregnancy in systemic lupus erythematosus. Proc R Soc Med 70:99–100, 1977
43. Hench PS: The ameliorating effect of pregnancy on chronic atrophic (infectious rheumatoid) arthritis, fibrositis, and interim heat hydrarthrosis. Mayo Clin Proc 13:161–168, 1931
44. Sergent JS, Lockshin MD, Klempner MS, Lipsky BA: Central nervous system disease in systemic lupus erythematosus: therapy and prognosis. Am J Med 58:644–654, 1975
45. Geschwind N, Behan P: Left-handedness: association with immune disease, migraine and developmental learning disorder. Proc Natl Acad Sci USA 74:5097–5100, 1972
46. Kolata GB: Sex hormones and brain development. Science 205:985–987, 1979
47. Sherman GF, Galaburda AM, Geschwind N: Ectopic neurons in the brain of the autoimmune mouse: a neurological model of dyslexia? (abstract). Soc Neuroscience Abstr 9:939, 1983

PLASMA FOLLICLE-STIMULATING HORMONE, LUTEINIZING HORMONE, AND SEX HORMONES IN PATIENTS WITH GOUT

ENRICO MARINELLO, GIUSEPPE RIARIO-SFORZA, and ROBERTO MARCOLONGO

Plasma levels of follicle-stimulating hormone, luteinizing hormone, testosterone, progesterone, 17 beta–estradiol, and cortisol were examined in normal subjects and gout patients under baseline conditions and after clomiphene stimulation. A significant decrease in follicle-stimulating hormone, luteinizing hormone, and 17 beta–estradiol was observed both in male and female gout patients; in the same patients, the plasma testosterone:17 beta–estradiol ratio was found to be significantly higher than in control subjects. The changes observed suggest a possible role played by 17 beta–estradiol in the regulation of purine biosynthesis and uric acid metabolism.

The sex difference in incidence of gout (1) and the rarity of its occurrence in hypogonadal men and premenopausal women (1,2) have led to an interest in the role of sex hormones in this disease.

Plasma uric acid levels are low in children, rise in boys at the time of puberty, and in menopausal women, approach those of adult men (3–5). Nicholls et al (6) observed that plasma uric acid levels fell and urinary uric acid levels rose during estrogen therapy, in a group of transsexual men. Semple et al (7) have shown that there is a significant decrease in serum uric acid concentration which accompanies maximum estradiol levels during pregnancy. However, they did not clearly demonstrate whether the decrease in uric acid is due to the increase in 17 beta–estradiol. In contrast, acute gouty attacks have been observed both in men and women shortly after administration of testosterone (8,9).

At pharmacologic doses, 17 beta–estradiol has shown, in vitro, an antiinflammatory effect on some leukocyte functions (10) and a protective role from the lytic effect of urate crystals on liposomes and lysosomal and plasma membranes of polymorphonuclear leukocytes, in contrast to the disrupting action of testosterone (11,12). While a decreased excretion of 17-ketosteroids was reported in gout patients (13), this finding has not yet been confirmed (14–17). Sŏnka et al (18) claim that urinary DHEA is absent in gout patients, but others have found only a decrease in DHEA (16,17,19,20). Recently, Levinson and Chalker (21) studied the influence of sex hormones on rat liver xanthine oxidase activity, finding an inhibitory effect of estrogen and an increase in enzyme activity following testosterone treatment.

The purpose of this study was to examine the pattern of plasma sex hormones in patients with primary gout. Furthermore, we studied plasma follicle-stimulating hormone (FSH) and luteinizing hormone (LH) behavior in order to assess the physiologic functions of the hypothalamus-hypophysis.

PATIENTS AND METHODS

Seventy-two patients (60 men and 12 postmenopausal women), all with primary metabolic gout, were studied.

From the Institutes of Biochemistry and Rheumatology, University of Siena, Siena, Italy, and the Laboratory of Clinical Chemistry, Hospital of Chieti, Chieti, Italy.

Supported by the CNR (National Research Council) of Italy.

Enrico Marinello, MD: Full Professor of Biochemistry, University of Siena; Giuseppe Riario-Sforza, MD: Director of Clinical Chemistry Laboratory, Hospital of Chieti; Roberto Marcolongo, MD: Full Professor of Rheumatology, University of Siena.

Address reprint requests to Prof. Enrico Marinello, Istituto di Chimica Biologica, Via Pian dei Mantellini, 44, Università Siena, Siena, Italy.

Submitted for publication August 20, 1983; accepted in revised form August 13, 1984.

Table 1. Baseline plasma levels (mean ± SE) of follicle-stimulating hormone (FSH), luteinizing hormone (LH), 17 beta–estradiol, testosterone, progesterone, and cortisol in normal subjects and gout patients

Subjects	FSH (mIU/ml)	LH (mIU/ml)	Testosterone (ng/ml)	17 beta–estradiol (pg/ml)	Cortisol (ng/ml)	Progesterone (pg/ml)	Testosterone: 17 beta–estradiol
Female, normal	112 ± 8.02	78.58 ± 5.57	0.46 ± 0.06	18.25 ± 1.77	110 ± 3.95	305 ± 12.7	25 ± 10
Female, gout	52 ± 8.02*	38.9 ± 5.48*	0.85 ± 0.16	12.45 ± 3.45*	106 ± 3.80	320 ± 14.8	68 ± 30*
Male, normal	11.6 ± 0.92	10.80 ± 0.79	3.9 ± 0.28	44.1 ± 3.80	121 ± 4.2	260 ± 13.9	88 ± 10
Male, gout	7.9 ± 1.05*	7.7 ± 0.48*	4.3 ± 0.29	27.4 ± 1.68*	128.4 ± 4.96	273.0 ± 15.7	190 ± 20*

* $P < 0.01$ versus normal subjects.

The average ages were 43.8 years (range 30–84) for the men and 60 (range 47–80) for the women. The duration of disease ranged from 1–25 years (mean 13 years). All of the patients were hyperuricemic and had no visible tophi. The interval between acute gouty attacks in the patients ranged from 1–3 years. Two weeks before hormone determination, allopurinol administration was suspended, and during this period, all patients were given a free, equilibrated diet, not over 2,500 calories/day (60% sugars, 15% proteins, 25% lipids). No subject was more than 30% overweight. Since all patients were hospitalized 1 week before the experiments, their activities were standardized. The patients were not taking corticosteroids or other medications. Normal controls consisted of 60 subjects (48 men and 12 postmenopausal women) matched for weight and age.

Blood samples, for estimation of plasma uric acid and hormone levels, were obtained at 8:00 AM from fasting subjects at complete rest. Twenty-four–hour urine collections were obtained for basal uric acid and creatinine estimations. Plasma levels of FSH, LH, testosterone, progesterone, 17 beta–estradiol, and cortisol were determined.

Since clomiphene is known to stimulate pituitary gonadotropin secretion, probably through the hypothalamus or higher centers (22), 7 patients with gout and 5 normal subjects were given clomiphene stimulation, using the technique of Rota and Ferlin (23). These subjects were all male volunteers who had no digestive problems, so any absorption variability was excluded. Women were not included in this test, since clomiphene stimulation is effective only in the preovulatory period (22,23). The drug was given orally for 5 days in daily doses of 50 mg. Plasma levels of FSH, LH, 17 beta–estradiol, and testosterone were determined before drug administration and on the third, fifth, seventh, and tenth days after the first clomiphene dose. Plasma and urinary uric acid levels were estimated using an enzymatic spectrophotometric method (24).

All plasma hormones were measured using radioimmunologic techniques. Specifically, FSH and LH, progesterone, testosterone, 17 beta–estradiol, and cortisol were measured according to the methods of Midgley (25,26), De Villa et al (27), Forest et al (28), Doerr (29), and Malvano (30), respectively. The radioimmunoassay method of Doerr (29) measured total plasma 17 beta–estradiol.

Free and bound testosterone levels were determined in 15 gouty males (ages 25–40) and 15 control males (ages 18–42), according to the technique of Forest et al (28).

The following intraassay and interassay coefficients of variance were found: FSH, 5.7–9.5%; LH, 5.5–9.3%; progesterone, 5.2–9.2%; 17 beta–estradiol, 6.8–9.8%; cortisol, 4.5–8.5%; testosterone, 4.3–8.2%. The results were submitted to the following statistical analysis. The relation between plasma levels of hormones and age was studied by the least squares method and by correlation coefficient (r); the same methods were used to study the relation between 17 beta–estradiol levels and the values of plasma and urinary uric acid. Only r values >0.5, corresponding to P values <0.05, were considered significant. The Wilcoxon Mann-Whitney U test, as described by Siegel (31), was used for comparison between groups, to compare the basal plasma levels of hormones in controls and in gout patients; only P values <1% were considered significant.

RESULTS

Plasma values of the hormones examined in controls and gout patients are reported in Table 1. Plasma levels of FSH and LH were significantly lower both in male and female gout patients, compared with controls ($P < 0.01$). Plasma progesterone and cortisol values remained unchanged in male and female gout patients.

The mean plasma 17 beta–estradiol levels in both male and female gout patients were significantly lower in comparison with controls ($P < 0.01$). No significant difference in plasma testosterone levels was found between male gout patients and controls, while a slight but not significant increase was observed in females with gout. Testosterone:17 beta–estradiol ratios were higher both in male and female gout patients than in male and female controls ($P < 0.01$) (Table 1).

No significant variation was observed between male controls and gout patients in the behavior of free and bound testosterone (Table 2). Plasma levels of the

Table 2. Total, bound, and free testosterone (ng/ml, mean ± SE) in 15 male control subjects and 15 males with gout

	Normal subjects	Gout patients
Total testosterone	4.25 ± 0.34	4.60 ± 0.41
Free testosterone	0.95 ± 0.40	0.96 ± 0.68
Bound testosterone	3.30 ± 0.40	3.64 ± 0.51

hormones (FSH, LH, testosterone, and 17 beta–estradiol) were not found to correlate with the patients' age, plasma and urinary uric acid values (values were always lower than 0.5), or disease duration: the *t* values were calculated from linear correlation analysis, and the *P* values thus obtained were always >0.05. A correlation between the FSH:LH ratio and the estradiol levels was also sought. No correlation was found for normal males or females with gout, but in the case of male gout patients, a significant negative correlation was found ($r = -0.352$; $P < 0.05$).

After the clomiphene stimulation test, plasma testosterone levels were sharply and significantly increased both in gouty and normal subjects, and high values were maintained for several days. Plasma FSH, LH, and 17 beta–estradiol concentrations increased progressively in normal subjects after clomiphene administration until, on the tenth day, the FSH and LH returned to baseline values and 17 beta–estradiol decreased significantly. The response was lower in gout patients, although the mean plasma FSH, LH, and 17 beta–estradiol concentrations increased after the third day of clomiphene administration (Figures 1 and 2).

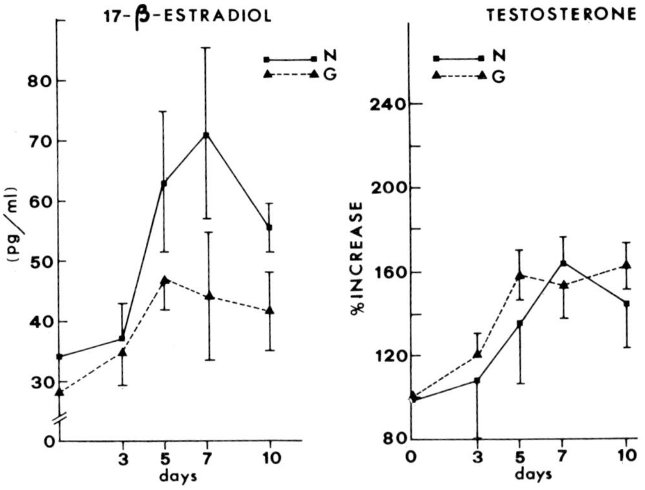

Figure 2. Plasma levels of testosterone and 17 beta–estradiol after clomiphene stimulation in normal subjects (N) and gout patients (G).

DISCUSSION

The finding that gout patients' plasma levels of cortisol and progesterone did not differ from those of the control subjects suggests that alteration of glucocorticoid hormone metabolism is not a significant factor in gout. The similar plasma testosterone levels in patients and controls, at baseline and with the clomiphene test, suggest that testicular endocrine function is normal in this disease.

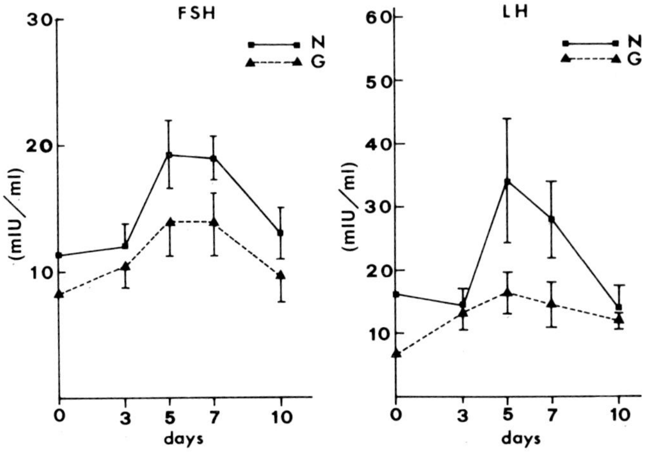

Figure 1. Plasma levels of follicle-stimulating hormone (FSH) and luteinizing hormone (LH) after clomiphene stimulation in normal subjects (N) and gout patients (G).

The lower plasma testosterone values in gout patients reported in a previous study (16) can probably be explained by the small number of patients (23 patients) studied, not all of whom were hyperuricemic. Also, that was a preliminary investigation in which the possible correlation with age was not studied, allopurinol treatment had not been suspended, and diet and activity levels were not standardized. Moreover, statistical analysis of the results was not possible due to the limited number of subjects.

Significantly lower plasma levels of FSH, LH, and 17 beta–estradiol, and a substantially decreased secretion of these hormones after the clomiphene stimulation test, were observed in our gout patients versus controls. The decrease in plasma FSH and LH levels is difficult to explain. It could be genetically determined or caused by some defect in the hypothalamic-pituitary-gonadal axis. However, the latter hypothesis does not provide an adequate explanation for the decrease: even if increased renal excretion cannot be completely excluded, the most reasonable interpretation of this finding is that there is insufficient production of both hormones. Decreased plasma levels of FSH and LH have been observed in obese subjects (32), but our gout patients were not grossly overweight.

The low levels of plasma 17 beta–estradiol may

also have several interpretations, i.e., a decrease of estrogen-binding globulin (33,34) or an increased displacement of estrogens from the binding globulin itself. However, as in FSH and LH, the decreased 17 beta–estradiol secretion after clomiphene stimulation strongly suggests that production of 17 beta–estradiol is deficient. This may be due to changes in the metabolism of this hormone, i.e., to a minor transformation of testosterone to 17 beta–estradiol, as is also indicated by the higher testosterone: 17 beta–estradiol ratio found both in male and female gout patients.

It remains to be determined whether the lower levels of plasma 17 beta–estradiol and the higher testosterone: 17 beta–estradiol ratio can affect purine biosynthesis de novo or uric acid metabolism and, if so, through what mechanism. Hormonal influences are responsible for the differences in plasma uric acid levels due to age and sex which can be correlated with variations in sex steroid hormone levels observed in the different periods of life (35,36). Differences in renal urate clearance as observed by Wolfson et al (13), Scott and Pollard (37), and Nicholls et al (6) seem to be at least partly responsible. However, since no correlation between plasma 17 beta–estradiol and plasma and urinary uric acid values was found in our gout patients, it is likely that 17 beta–estradiol has a more specific effect on the regulation of purine biosynthesis than on uric acid excretion. We must stress that, with the exception of Feigelson's data (38) on the influence of cortisone on purine biosynthesis in rat liver, very few experimental data are available on the regulation of de novo purine biosynthesis in mammals by hormones and, most importantly, by sex hormones.

Recently, Levinson and Chalker (21) found that, in mature rat liver, xanthine oxidase activity (XOA) was 59% greater in males than in females. Pubescence resulted in a twofold increase of XOA in males, which was prevented by prepubertal castration. XOA significantly increased in females after postpubertal castration, prepubertal oophorectomy, or testosterone treatment, while orchiectomy or treatment with 17 beta–estradiol in mature male rats provoked no changes. The hormone-induced changes of XOA have been positively correlated with urinary uric acid excretion.

We emphasize that while our results are statistically significant, they must be confirmed and extended to a larger population; the purpose of the present research is to encourage such further study. We believe a complete study of sex hormone metabolism in gout patients will definitely be useful in furthering understanding of the role of endocrines in the regulation of purine biosynthesis and the pathogenesis of gout.

REFERENCES

1. Wyngaarden JB, Kelley WN: Gout and Hyperuricemia. New York, Grune & Stratton, 1976, pp 21–25
2. McFadzean AJS: A eunuch takes the gout. Br Med J 1:1038–1039, 1965
3. Neel JV: The control of blood uric acid levels—a problem in genetic epidemiology, Population Studies of the Rheumatic Diseases. Edited by PH Bennett, PHN Wood. Amsterdam, Excerpta Medica, 1968, pp 319–335
4. Mikkelsen WM, Dodge NJ, Valkenburg H: The distribution of serum uric acid values in a population unselected as to gout or hyperuricemia. Am J Med 39:242–251, 1965
5. Harkness RA, Nicol AD: Plasma uric acid levels in children. Arch Dis Child 44:773–778, 1969
6. Nicholls A, Snaith ML, Scott JT: Effect of estrogen therapy on plasma and urinary levels of uric acid. Br Med J 1:449–465, 1973
7. Semple PF, Carswell W, Boyle JA: Serial studies of the renal clearance of urate and inulin during pregnancy and after the puerperium in normal women. Clin Sci 47:559–565, 1974
8. Maranon G: Algunos aspectos del problema de la gota. Rev Iber Endocr 4:77–85, 1957
9. Graber-Duvernay J, Graber-Duvernay B: A propos de la goutte aigue feminine. Rhumatologie 9:261–268, 1957
10. Bodel P, Dillard GM, Kaplan SS, Malawista SE: Anti-inflammatory effects of estradiol on human blood leukocytes. J Lab Clin Med 80:373–384, 1972
11. Weissmann G, Rita GA: Molecular basis of gouty inflammation: interaction of monosodium urate crystals with lysosomes and liposomes. Nature 240:167–172, 1972
12. Spilberg I: Current concepts of the mechanism of acute inflammation in gouty arthritis. Arthritis Rheum 18:129–134, 1975
13. Wolfson WQ, Guterman HS, Levine R, Cohn C, Hunt HD, Roseberg EF: Endocrine factors in nucleoprotein metabolism and in gout. J Clin Endocrinol Metab 9:497–501, 1949
14. Butt WR, Marson GW: 17-ketosteroids excretion in gout. Br Med J 2:1023–1024, 1952
15. Casey JH, Hoffman MM, Solomon S: The excretion of urinary dehydroepiandrosterone in gout. Arthritis Rheum 11:444–451, 1968
16. Valentini U, Riario-Sforza G, Marcolongo R, Marinello E: Hormonal aspects of gout patients, Purine Metabolism in Man. Edited by A Rapado, RWE Watts, CHMM De Bruyn. New York, Plenum, 1980, pp 65–71
17. Carcassi A, Lorè F, Manasse G, Macrì P, Pisani M: Gaschromatographic evaluation of urinary 17-ketoster-

oids, etiocholanolone and dehydroepiandrosterone in primary gout and hyperuricemia, Purine Metabolism in Man. Edited by A Rapado, RWE Watts, CHMM De Bruyn. New York, Plenum, 1980, pp 59–63
18. Sŏnka J, Gregorová I, Křižek V: Dehydroepiandrosterone in gout. Lancet 1:671–672, 1964
19. Pittman JA, Starnes WR, Beetham WP, Luketic GC: Dehydroepiandrosterone excretion in gout (abstract). Clin Res 14:66, 1966
20. Sparagana M, Philips G: Dehydroepiandrosterone metabolism in gout. Steroids 19:477–491, 1972
21. Levinson DJ, Chalker D: Rat hepatic xanthine oxidase activity: age and sex specific differences. Arthritis Rheum 23:77–82, 1980
22. Heller CG, Rowley MJ, Heller GV: Clomiphene citrate: a correlation of its effect on sperm concentration and morphology, total gonadotropins, ICSH, estrogen and testosterone excretion, and testicular cytology in normal men. J Clin Endocrinol Metab 29:638–647, 1969
23. Rota G, Ferlin G: Dosaggi radioimmunologici nella pratica clinica: standardizzazione dei parametri operativi. Monografie di Immunologia, Sorin Biomedica, 1979, 5–78
24. Praetorius E, Poulsen H: Enzymatic determination of uric acid, with detailed directions. Scand J Clin Lab Invest 5:273–280, 1953
25. Midgley AR Jr: Radioimmunoassay: a method for human chorionic gonadotropin and human luteinizing hormone. Endocrinology 79:10–18, 1966
26. Midgley AR Jr: Radioimmunoassay for human follicle stimulating hormone. J Clin Endocrinol Metab 27:295–299, 1967
27. De Villa O, Roberts K, Wiest AG, Mikkall G, Flickinger G: A specific radioimmunoassay of plasma progesterone. J Clin Endocrinol Metab 35:458–460, 1972
28. Forest MG, Cathiard AM, Bertrand JA: Total and unbound testosterone levels in the newborn and in normal and hypogonadal children: use of a sensitive radioimmunoassay for testosterone. J Clin Endocrinol Metab 36:1132–1142, 1973
29. Doerr P: Hapten radioimmunoassay of plasma oestradiol. Acta Endocrinol (Copenh) 72:330–334, 1973
30. Malvano R: Recent trends in methodological simplification of steroid radioimmunoassay. Horm Res 9:422–445, 1978
31. Siegel S: Nonparametric Statistics for the Behavioral Sciences. New York, McGraw-Hill, 1956, pp 75–78
32. O'Dea JPK, Wieland RG, Hallberg MC, Llerena LA, Zorn EM, Genuth SM: Effect of dietary weight loss on sex steroid binding, sex steroids, and gonadotropins in obese postmenopausal women. J Lab Clin Med 93:1004–1008, 1979
33. Glass AR, Swerdloff RS, Bray GA, Dahms WT, Atkinson RL: Low serum testosterone and sex-hormone-binding-globulin in massively obese men. J Clin Endocrinol Metab 45:1211–1220, 1977
34. Rosenbaum W, Christy NP, Kelly WG: Electrophoretic evidence for the presence of an estrogen binding globulin in human plasma. J Clin Endocrinol Metab 26:1399–1409, 1966
35. Faiman C, Winter JSD: Gonadotropins and sex hormone patterns in puberty, Control of the Onset of Puberty. Edited by MM Grumbach, GD Grave, FE Meyer. New York, John Wiley and Sons, 1974, pp 39–40
36. Nagai N, Longcope C: Estradiol-17-β and estrone: studies on their binding to rabbit uterine cytosol and their concentration in plasma. Steroids 17:631–647, 1977
37. Scott JT, Pollard AD: Uric acid excretion in the relatives of patients with gout. Ann Rheum Dis 29:397–403, 1970
38. Feigelson P, Feigelson M: Studies on the mechanism of regulation by cortisone of the metabolism of liver purine and ribonucleic acid. J Biol Chem 238:1073–1077, 1963

CLINICAL CHARACTERISTICS OF FIBROSITIS

II. A "Blinded," Controlled Study Using Standard Psychological Tests

SHARON CLARK, STEPHEN M. CAMPBELL, MARY E. FOREHAND,
ELIZABETH A. TINDALL, and ROBERT M. BENNETT

Twenty-two patients with fibrositis and 22 control patients selected from a general medical outpatient population were given 3 standardized psychological questionnaires: the Beck Depression Inventory, the Spielberger State and Trait Anxiety Inventory, and the SCL-90-R. There were no statistically significant differences between fibrositis patients and control patients on any of these tests, a finding at variance with a commonly held belief that patients with fibrositis have an underlying psychological disorder. While psychological factors may be important in some patients with fibrositis, these results indicate that the presence of a psychopathologic condition is not mandatory for the persistence of fibrositis.

The term "fibrositis" has gradually evolved to denote a syndrome of soft tissue rheumatism consisting of diffuse axial musculoskeletal aching, pain, and stiffness, a nonrestorative sleep pattern, and multiple areas of localized soft tissue tenderness (1,2). Fibrositis is a syndrome of clinical symptoms which, individually, are not specific for the diagnosis, and of clinical signs which are subtle and subjective. The use of the term fibrositis for several different syndromes of soft tissue pain (which may or may not be related) has further confused the issue (3,4). There is a common clinical impression that patients with fibrositis tend to have a variety of abnormal psychological behaviors, including depression, somatization, rigidity, and the like. For these reasons many physicians either do not recognize fibrositis as a diagnosis or they consider it a form of psychogenic rheumatism (5,6).

On the other hand, there is increasing evidence that fibrositis is not merely psychogenic in nature. It would be unusual for a primarily psychological disorder to result in a relatively uniform and characteristic constellation of symptoms and signs (2,7). A few studies of the "trigger point" of localized myofascial pain syndromes and of the "tender point" of fibrositis have demonstrated possible histologic and electromyographic abnormalities (8–11), which support a role for a peripheral component of the disease. Despite the common clinical impression of psychological disturbance in fibrositis, there are obviously some patients with fibrositis who have no apparent psychological disorder. Thus, it seems important to determine if psychological disturbances play a major role in fibrositis.

This study was designed to compare the results of standard psychometric tests in patients with and without fibrositis. The patients were selected from a general medical outpatient population, thus reducing bias that might be expected with an inpatient or referral population. Our results do not demonstrate

From the Division of Immunology, Allergy, and Rheumatology, Department of Medicine, and the School of Nursing, Oregon Health Sciences University, Portland, Oregon.

Supported in part by the Oregon Chapter of the Arthritis Foundation, the Tartar Trust Foundation, an Arthritis Foundation Clinical Research Center grant, and grant RR00334 from the GCRC Branch of the Division of Research Resources, NIH.

Sharon Clark, RN, MN, NP: Associate Professor of Nursing; Stephen M. Campbell, MD: Assistant Professor of Medicine; Mary E. Forehand, RN, MN, NP: Research Assistant; Elizabeth A. Tindall, MD: Fellow, OHSU/Providence Medical Center; Robert M. Bennett, MD: Professor of Medicine and Head, Section of Rheumatology.

Submitted for publication August 27, 1982; accepted in revised form August 27, 1984.

any differences between fibrositis and control patients selected in this manner.

PATIENTS AND METHODS

Patient selection. Twenty-two patients with fibrositis and 22 age-, sex-, and race-matched patients without fibrositis were given 3 standardized psychological questionnaires as part of a larger survey of fibrositis. The details of this are reported elsewhere (7). Briefly, 596 patients attending the general medicine and medical subspecialty clinics of the Oregon Health Sciences University completed a brief questionnaire concerning musculoskeletal symptoms and sleep disturbances. On the basis of their answers, 42 of these patients were thought to have possible fibrositis and were asked to return for further evaluation; 27 did so, along with age-, sex-, race-, and clinic-matched patients who did not appear to have possible fibrositis, based on answers to the initial questionnaire.

On the return visit, the patients underwent: 1) an extensive interview concerning a variety of symptoms and other features of their pain syndrome; 2) a physical examination to quantitatively determine tenderness over fibrositic tender points and control nontender points; and 3) 3 standard psychological questionnaires. The examiners were not aware of the results of the first questionnaire or of the results of the other studies done on the return visit.

The diagnosis of definite fibrositis was defined by a constellation of symptoms (7) including diffuse musculoskeletal pain, aching, and stiffness, a nonrestorative sleep pattern, and the development of objective tenderness at dolorimeter pressures of <4 kg/1.54 cm^2 over at least 12 of 17 "tender points" tested. Normal results on the following laboratory tests were required: complete blood count, sedimentation rate, creatine phosphokinase, glutamic oxaloacetic transaminase, antinuclear antibody, rheumatoid factor, and free thyroxine levels. Of the 27 patients with possible fibrositis who returned for further evaluation, 22 fulfilled the criteria for the diagnosis of fibrositis. These 22 were compared with age-, sex-, race-, and clinic-matched patients without fibrositis (Table 1); it is important to note that patients were not excluded from the control group by the presence of musculoskeletal symptoms or sleep disturbances. Thus, the control patients had a certain incidence of musculoskeletal pain and other symptoms; in fact, an inadvertant selection bias, presumably related to those patients who were willing to return for further evaluation, resulted in a higher incidence of musculoskeletal complaints in the control group than in the initial total group of 596 patients.

Table 1. Characteristics of fibrositis and control groups

	Fibrositis group	Control group
Mean age (range)	56.1 (33–67)	56.4 (34–68)
Sex, F/M (number)	16/6	16/6
Race, white/nonwhite (number)	20/2	20/2
% with moderate/severe		
Musculoskeletal pain	100	41
Neck/shoulder pain	91	28
Morning aching	100	32
Morning stiffness	91	23
Waking feeling unrested	100	32
Tired during day	100	41

Psychological testing. Three standardized psychological tests were given in the following order. After a brief instruction period, the patients were left to complete the tests on their own, though an examiner was immediately available for questions. There was no time limit. Patients were encouraged to complete all of the questions on each test. The tests chosen for the study were:

1. Beck Depression Inventory (BDI). The BDI is an inventory of 21 categories (questions) of symptoms and attitudes describing particular manifestations of depression, with each category consisting of a series of 4 self-evaluative statements which are assigned values from 0–3 to indicate the degree of severity. The total score is obtained by adding the scores of the individual symptom categories.

The BDI has been used extensively in the clinical evaluation of depression in psychiatric and medical inpatients and outpatients. It has been shown to be reliable over time and internally consistent, to have impressive concurrent validity with other measures of depression, and construct validity in its use as a criterion measure of depression (12–15).

2. Spielberger State and Trait Anxiety Inventory (STAI). The STAI consists of 40 self-report questions, graded 1 (almost never) to 4 (almost always), measuring A-State, a transitory state of anxiety (questions 1–20), and A-Trait, the tendency one has to respond to situations perceived as threatening with an increase in anxiety state (questions 21–40). This tool was chosen because of its high internal consistency and because it possesses both concurrent and construct validity (16,17). Scores range from 20–80 for both A-State and A-Trait, with the higher scores indicating higher levels of anxiety.

3. SCL-90-R. The SCL-90-R is a multidimensional symptom self-report inventory derived from the Cornell Medical Index and several early versions of the Hopkins Symptom Checklist. It measures 90 items on a 5-point scale of distress from 0 (not at all) to 4 (extremely). The test defines 9 primary symptom dimensions and a global index of distress: Somatization (SOM), distress arising from perceptions of bodily dysfunction, with symptoms and signs demonstrated to have a high prevalence in functional disorders; Obsessive–Compulsive (OC), unremitting and irresistible thoughts, impulses, and actions characteristic of this clinical syndrome; Interpersonal Sensitivity (IS), feelings of personal inadequacy and inferiority, particularly in comparison with others; Depression (DEP), a broad range of the manifestations of clinical depression; Anxiety (ANX), a set of symptoms and signs that are associated clinically with high levels of manifest anxiety; Hostility (HOS), thoughts, feelings, or actions that are characteristics of the negative affect state of anger; Phobic Anxiety (PHOB), persistent, irrational, and disproportionate fear response to a particular person, place, object, or situation; Paranoid Ideation (PAR), paranoid behavior as a disordered mode of thinking; Psychoticism (PSY), a graduated continuum from mild interpersonal aberration to dramatic evidence of psychosis; and the Global Severity Index (GSI), the best single indicator of the current level or depth of psychological distress.

Table 2. Results of Beck Depression Inventory and Spielberger State/Trait Anxiety Inventory*

	Fibrositis group	Control group	*P*
Beck Depression Inventory	10.7 ± 7.3	10.8 ± 5.6	0.960
Spielberger			
State Anxiety	41.9 ± 13.0	45.6 ± 8.5	0.251
Trait Anxiety	39.6 ± 11.4	43.8 ± 8.6	0.162

* Results expressed as mean ± SD.

The SCL-90-R and its predecessors have been subjected to extensive clinical testing. The test is a measure of current psychological symptom status, and not of personality per se. It has excellent test-retest and inter-rater reliability, and has been shown to have criterion and construct validity in a number of medical and psychiatric patient studies. The test appears to be particularly sensitive for detecting the presence of, or changes in, neurotic symptoms in outpatients, and thus would be expected to be particularly valuable in the study of the fairly subtle abnormalities which might occur in outpatients with fibrositis (18–24).

Statistical analysis. Tests were scored using the SPSS 7.2 A and the computer facilities of Portland State University. Tests in which fewer than 82% of the questions were answered were not included in the final analysis; this resulted in the exclusion of 1 fibrositis patient from the BDI, and 1 control patient each from the BDI and STAI. Group differences were analyzed by the 2-tailed *t*-test. Statistical significance was defined as $P < 0.05$. *T*-scores (representing a standardized normal distribution with a mean of 50 and standard deviation of 10) were derived from published data (19).

RESULTS

There was no difference between the 2 groups in the total score for the BDI (Table 2). These results are just above the previously documented cutoff between normal and mildly depressed outpatients (12). There were no statistically significant differences between the 2 groups on individual questions; the fibrositis group complained somewhat more about health concerns.

Similarly, there was no difference between the groups in the total scores for A-State and A-Trait (Table 2). Fibrositis patients complained significantly more frequently of not feeling rested on both A-State and A-Trait but did not differ on any of the other questions.

The fibrositis patients' scores and control patients' scores did not differ significantly on any of the scales of the test or on the GSI (Table 3). All of the mean values fell within 1 standard deviation of published values of normal subjects (19) (Figure 1).

The largest difference between the groups, though not statistically significant, was on the Somatization scale. Closer examination showed that this difference was primarily due to the answers on 2 questions, "headaches" (fibrositis mean 1.8 ± 1.2, control mean 0.9 ± 0.9; $P < 0.01$) and "soreness of your muscles" (fibrositis mean 3.1 ± 0.9, control mean 1.5 ± 1.2; $P < 0.001$), both of which are symptoms possibly associated with fibrositis itself. None of the other responses to questions on this or any other scale differed significantly between groups.

DISCUSSION

Our results fail to demonstrate a difference on standard psychological tests between groups of patients with and without fibrositis who were selected from a general medical clinic population. This suggests that a psychological disturbance is not a necessary component of fibrositis.

The description of fibrositis patients in this study is similar to other recent descriptions of this syndrome (1,2). Although our patients were older than those in previous studies, they otherwise had signs and symptoms similar to those in previously published studies, met the accepted criteria for fibrositis, and by their own evaluation, had moderate to severe pain.

Table 3. Results of SCL-90-R

Scale	Fibrositis group Mean ± SD	Fibrositis group *T*-score*	Control group Mean ± SD	Control group *T*-score*	*P*
Somatization	0.88 ± 0.30	60	0.69 ± 0.44	54	0.078
Obsessive–Compulsive	0.52 ± 0.81	52	0.56 ± 0.55	52	0.843
Interpersonal Sensitivity	0.55 ± 0.25	51	0.59 ± 0.17	52	0.525
Depression	0.60 ± 0.59	55	0.55 ± 0.45	55	0.749
Anxiety	0.53 ± 0.39	54	0.57 ± 0.37	55	0.725
Hostility	0.55 ± 0.32	54	0.49 ± 0.40	52	0.581
Phobic Anxiety	0.12 ± 0.25	52	0.19 ± 0.15	54	0.246
Paranoid Ideation	0.44 ± 0.37	54	0.39 ± 0.40	52	0.669
Psychoticism	0.20 ± 0.05	51	0.23 ± 0.09	54	0.155
Global Severity Index	0.43 ± 0.70	53	0.47 ± 0.79	52	0.859

* Represents mean *T*-score derived from published values for normal populations (19).

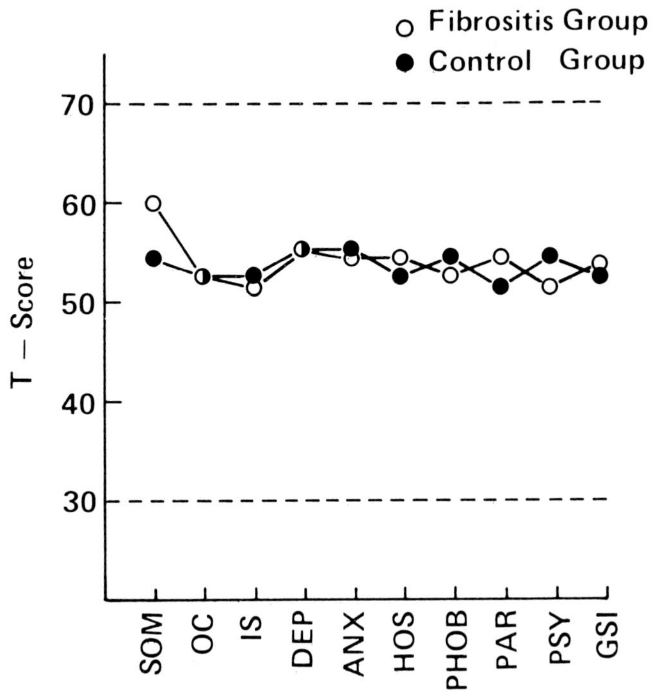

Figure 1. Mean *T*-scores on SCL-90-R scales for fibrositis and control patients. SOM = Somatization; OC = Obsessive–Compulsive; IS = Interpersonal Sensitivity; DEP = Depression; ANX = Anxiety; HOS = Hostility; PHOB = Phobic Anxiety; PAR = Paranoid Ideation; PSY = Psychoticism; GSI = Global Severity Index.

Importantly, they were patients who, despite their pain, had not been referred for rheumatologic evaluation.

The control group of patients did not appear to have artificially elevated results. They did have an increased incidence of musculoskeletal complaints compared with the initial total group, but it would seem unlikely that such bias would produce significant alterations in the results. In any case, a skewed control group would not be compatible with both groups' scores falling well within the published normal ranges.

The psychological tests were appropriate measures for this study. All 3 tests have been documented to be sensitive to the presence of, and changes in, the characteristics they are designed to measure. The 3 tests measure, with some overlap, the psychological characteristics most frequently attributed to fibrositis patients: depression, anxiety, somatization, and obsessive–compulsive behavior. A clinical psychological assessment might have uncovered more instances of psychopathology (25), but the notorious inconsistency of clinical psychological diagnoses (especially when dealing with subtle abnormalities), the lack of quantitative assessments, and the frequent inability to reproduce results limit the usefulness of this method in a comparative study like ours.

Finally, the group size should have been large enough to detect major differences in results of these tests. Except for the Somatization scale on the SCL-90-R, there was no trend to suggest a difference between the 2 groups. Moreover, the group sizes were large enough to detect differences in a number of other variables. Differences small enough to be missed in this study are unlikely to be clinically important.

A number of psychological abnormalities have been attributed to fibrositis patients, particularly somatization, hypochondriasis, hysteria, depression, obsessive–compulsive behavior, and rigidity (26,27). These descriptions have been, in general, based on empiric impressions; quantitative data collected in an organized fashion are scarce. A study in 1942 documented psychological disturbances (hysteria, anxiety, and depression) in 35 of 50 patients with "fibrositis"; however, the evaluations were on clinical grounds only, most of the patients were men, many had evidence of secondary gain, and few had fibrositis by the current definition (28). Moldofsky and colleagues characterized the mood of patients undergoing sleep studies using an objective checklist and found that they tended to be angry–irritable, anxious, and sluggish (29–31). Genoud et al reported that the onset or exacerbation of fibrositis symptoms was temporally related to various life stresses in 15 patients; these stresses ranged from the death of a parent to beginning a low cholesterol diet (32). A comparable control population was not studied.

Payne et al compared the Minnesota Multiphasic Personality Inventory (MMPI) scores of 30 hospitalized fibrositis patients with patients with rheumatoid and other types of chronic polyarthritis (33). Fibrositis patients had elevated scores on 6 of the 10 MMPI scales; on 2 of these scales (Hypochondriasis and Hysteria), scores were in the pathologic range. These results were interpreted as showing that fibrositis patients may be a heterogeneous population with a variety of psychopathologic signs and that these abnormalities are not the result of chronic pain and disability. Ahles et al (34) found similar results in ambulatory fibrositis patients; importantly, though, more than a third were within the normal range. Finally, Wolfe and coworkers (35) administered the MMPI and 4 other psychosocial tests to 78 primary and secondary fibrositis patients and 77 patients with rheumatoid arthritis alone. Fibrositis patients had higher mean scores than rheumatoid arthritis patients on a number of MMPI scales. Analysis of the results classified 28% of fibrositis patients as normal, 35% as somatically concerned, and 37% as psychologically disturbed, compared with 51, 29, and 20%, respectively, for rheumatoid arthritis patients.

The etiology of fibrositis is unknown. The absence of easily demonstrable objective abnormalities has made a primary psychological or somatiform etiology attractive. Our results argue against such a mechanism playing an important role in the perpetuation of fibrositis symptoms in some patients, however. A number of other findings, including the response of the pain to weather fronts, the marked stiffness reminiscent of other rheumatic diseases, the consistent location of the fibrositic tender points, the occasional finding of palpable nodules with electromyographic and histologic abnormalities (8–11), and the disturbance of sleep (29) all suggest a peripheral or, at least, non-psychogenic component of the disease. Despite this, there is a common clinical impression that a number of these patients are psychologically abnormal. We suspect that this may represent variation in patient selection. Longstanding or severe pain and disability may result in the development of emotional abnormalities, for example, the "neurotic triad" of Hypochondriasis, Depression, and Hysteria on MMPI testing of patients with rheumatoid arthritis and other chronic diseases (36–39). Constant uncertainty about the nature or even existence of a disease, or being told by physicians that "there's nothing wrong" or "it's all in your head" could be expected to worsen this problem. There may be a higher incidence of psychopathology in patients with low back pain who fail to respond to conventional therapy than in those who do respond (40–43).

It seems likely that most patients with fibrositis have self-limited disease or learn to live with their pain, and never seek rheumatologic care; those patients who are referred to rheumatologists probably have more severe or chronic disease, have already "made the rounds" of other physicians, or have not responded to therapy, medical or otherwise. This referral group might be expected to have a higher incidence of psychological abnormality. We suggest that this study, by screening a general medical population, selected patients with mild or self-limited disease, while previous studies, using patients hospitalized or referred for rheumatologic care, examined those with more severe disease.

This study must be viewed as being limited in scope. Further work needs to be done using larger numbers of patients and using patients who have not yet sought any medical care for their pain syndrome. We did not study the interaction of stress or recent significant life events with the apparent objective peripheral and central abnormalities associated with fibrositis. Nevertheless, this study does show that not all fibrositis patients can be dismissed as having a psychological abnormality, and indicates that psychopathology is not necessary for the persistence of fibrositis.

ACKNOWLEDGMENTS

We deeply appreciate the superb statistical assistance of Dr. Barbara Stewart and the excellent secretarial assistance of Carol Kleinheksel, Michele Bender, and Pamela Beere-Briggs.

REFERENCES

1. Smythe HA, Moldofsky H: Two contributions to the understanding of the fibrositis syndrome. Bull Rheum Dis 28:928–931, 1978
2. Yunus M, Masi AT, Calabro JJ, Miller KA, Feigenbaum SL: Primary fibromyalgia (fibrositis): clinical study of 50 patients with matched normal controls. Semin Arthritis Rheum 11:151–171, 1981
3. Simons DG: Muscle pain syndromes, part 1. Am J Phys Med 54:289–311, 1975
4. Simons DG: Muscle pain syndromes, part 2. Am J Phys Med 55:15–42, 1976
5. Beetham WP Jr: Diagnosis and management of fibrositis syndrome and psychogenic rheumatism. Med Clin North Am 63:433–439, 1979
6. Weinberger LM: Traumatic fibromyositis: a critical review of an enigmatic concept. West J Med 127:99–103, 1977
7. Campbell SM, Clark S, Tindall EA, Forehand ME, Bennett RM: Clinical characteristics of fibrositis. I. A "blinded," controlled study of symptoms and tender points. Arthritis Rheum 26:817–824, 1983
8. Brendstrup P, Jespersen K, Asboe-Hansen G: Morphological and chemical connective tissue changes in fibrositic muscles. Ann Rheum Dis 16:438–440, 1957
9. Fassbender HG, Wegner K: Morphologie und Pathogenese des Weichteil rheumatismus. Z Rheumaforsch 32:355–374, 1973
10. Yunus M, Kalyanaraman UP, Kalyanaraman K, Masi AT, Berg BC: Microscopic and radioactive bone scan studies in primary fibromyalgia (abstract). Arthritis Rheum (suppl) 25:S146, 1982
11. Simons DG: Electrogenic nature of palpable bands and "jump sign" associated with myofascial trigger points, Advances in Pain Research and Therapy. Vol. 1. Edited

by JJ Bonica, D Albe-Fessard. New York, Raven Press, 1976, pp 913–918
12. Beck AT, Beamesderfer A: Assessment of depression: the depression inventory, Modern Problems in Psychopharmacology. Vol. 7. Edited by P Pichot. Basel, Karger, 1974, pp 151–169
13. Gallagher D, Nies G, Thompson LW: Reliability of the Beck Depression Inventory with older adults. J Consult Clin Psychol 50:152–153, 1982
14. Golin S, Hartz MA: A factor analysis of the Beck Depression Inventory in a mildly depressed population. J Clin Psychol 35:322–325, 1979
15. Hammen CL: Depression in college students: beyond the Beck Depression Inventory. J Consult Clin Psychol 48:126–128, 1980
16. Spielberger CD, Gosuch RL, Lushene RE: STAI Manual. Palo Alto, Consulting Psychologists Press, 1975
17. Morgan W, Horstman DH: Psychometric correlates of pain perception. Percept Mot Skills 47:27–39, 1978
18. Derogatis LR, Lipman RS, Rickels K, Uhlenhuth EH, Covi L: The Hopkins symptom checklist, Modern Problems in Psychopharmacology. Vol. 7. Edited by P Pichot. Basel, Karger, 1974, pp 79–110
19. Derogatis LR: SCL-90-R, Administration, Scoring, and Procedures Manual. Baltimore, LR Derogatis, 1977
20. Derogatis LR, Cleary PA: Confirmation of the dimensional structure of the SCL-90. J Clin Psychol 33:981–989, 1977
21. Evenson RC, Holland RA, Mehta S, Yasin F: Factor analysis of the symptom checklist-90. Psychol Rep 46:695–699, 1980
22. Craig TJ, Abeloff MD: Psychiatric symptomatology among hospitalized cancer patients. Am J Psychiatry 131:1323–1327, 1974
23. Horowitz MJ, Krupnick J, Kaltreider N, Wilner N, Leong A, Marmar C: Initial psychological response to parental death. Arch Gen Psychiatry 38:316–323, 1981
24. Kathol RG, Noyes R, Slymen DJ, Crowe RR, Clancy J, Kerber RE: Propranolol in chronic anxiety disorders. Arch Gen Psychiatry 37:1361–1365, 1980
25. Hamilton M: General problems with psychiatric rating scales (especially for depression), Modern Problems in Psychopharmacology. Vol. 7. Edited by P Pichot. Basel, Karger, 1974, pp 123–138
26. Reynolds MD: Clinical diagnosis of psychogenic rheumatism. West J Med 128:285–290, 1978
27. Smythe HA: Non-articular rheumatism and psychogenic musculoskeletal syndromes, Arthritis and Allied Conditions. Ninth edition. Edited by D J McCarty. Philadelphia, Lea & Febiger, 1979, pp 881–891
28. Ellman E, Savage OA, Witthower E, Rodger TF: Fibrositis—a biographical study of fifty civilian and military cases from the rheumatic unit, St. Stephen's Hospital, and a military hospital. Ann Rheum Dis 3:56–76, 1942
29. Moldofsky H, Scarisbrick P, England RE, Smythe H: Musculoskeletal symptoms and non-REM sleep disturbance in patients with "fibrositis syndrome" and healthy subjects. Psychosom Med 37:341–351, 1975
30. Moldofsky H, Warsh JJ: Plasma tryptophan and musculoskeletal pain in non-articular rheumatism ("fibrositis syndrome"). Pain 5:65–71, 1978
31. Moldofsky H, Lue FA: The relationship of alpha and delta EEG frequencies to pain and mood in "fibrositis" patients treated with chlorpromazine and L-tryptophan. Electroencephalogr Clin Neurophysiol 50:71–80, 1980
32. Genoud P, Gerster JC, Saudan Y: Aspect psychologique du malade souffrant de fibrosite (poly-insertionite). Rev Med Suisse Romande 99:51–56, 1979
33. Payne TC, Leavitt F, Garron DC, Katy RS, Golden HE, Glickman PB, Vanderplate C: Fibrositis and psychologic disturbance. Arthritis Rheum 25:213–217, 1982
34. Ahles TA, Yunus MB, Riley SD, Bradley JM, Masi AT: Psychological studies in primary fibromyalgia syndrome (abstract). Clin Res 31:801A, 1983
35. Wolfe F, Cathey MA, Kleinheksel SM, Amos SP, Hoffmann RG, Young DY, Hawley DJ: Psychological status in primary fibrositis and fibrositis associated with rheumatoid arthritis. J Rheumatol 11:500–506, 1984
36. Zaphiropoulos G, Burry HC: Depression in rheumatoid arthritis. Ann Rheum Dis 33:132–135, 1974
37. Robinson H, Kirk RF Jr, Frye RL: A psychological study of rheumatoid arthritis and selected controls. J Chronic Dis 23:791–801, 1971
38. Polley HF, Swenson WN, Steinhilber R: Personality characteristics of patients with rheumatoid arthritis. Psychosomatics 11:45–49, 1970
39. Rook JC, Pesch RN, Keller ED: Chronic pain and the questionable use of the Minnesota Multiphasic Personality Inventory. Arch Phys Med Rehabil 62:373–375, 1981
40. Crown S: Psychological aspects of low back pain. Rheumatol Rehabil 17:114–124, 1978
41. McCreary C, Turner J, Dawson E: The MMPI as a predictor of response to conservative treatment for low back pain. J Clin Psychol 35:278–284, 1979
42. McCreary CP, Turner J, Dawson E: Emotional disturbance and chronic low back pain. J Clin Psychol 36:709–715, 1980
43. Rosen JC, Frymoyer JW, Clements JH: A further look at validity of the MMPI with low back patients. J Clin Psychol 36:994–1000, 1980

JUVENILE PRIMARY FIBROMYALGIA SYNDROME

A Clinical Study of Thirty-Three Patients and Matched Normal Controls

MUHAMMAD B. YUNUS and ALFONSE T. MASI

Primary fibromyalgia syndrome (PFS) is a common and characteristic rheumatologic condition manifested by diffuse musculoskeletal aches, pains, and stiffness frequently modulated by various factors, e.g., weather, physical activity, sleep quality, and anxiety/stress, and accompanied by discrete tender points at typical soft tissue sites. Although well-recognized in adults, this entity has not been reported separately in juveniles. This study documents PFS in 33 juveniles who presented at age 17 or younger and compares their findings with those in age- and sex-matched normal control subjects. As in adult PFS patients, associated non-musculoskeletal symptoms were common, including fatigue, poor sleep, anxiety/stress, headaches, and paresthesias. Physical examination revealed multiple tender points at characteristic soft tissue sites and no objective evidence of arthritis. Routine laboratory test results were normal or negative. Juvenile PFS is often misdiagnosed. Recognition of this common rheumatologic condition in juveniles is important in order to avoid unwarranted investigations and improper management.

Fibromyalgia syndrome, a form of nonarticular rheumatism manifested by diffuse musculoskeletal aching and tender points at multiple characteristic sites, is now established as a recognizable clinical entity in adults (1–4). We prefer the term primary fibromyalgia syndrome (PFS) rather than "fibrositis" to underscore the absence of an underlying condition (e.g., rheumatoid arthritis, osteoarthritis, trauma, or hypothyroidism) which may also be associated with similar clinical features. This term also indicates lack of inflammation on muscle biopsy (5,6), as well as presence of non-musculoskeletal features (3,7). Although PFS is now well described in adults, this syndrome is not generally recognized among juveniles and has not been separately described in this age group. This report presents detailed results of a clinical study of PFS in 33 juveniles and matched normal controls.

From the Department of Medicine, Division of Rheumatology, University of Illinois College of Medicine at Peoria, Peoria, Illinois.

Supported in part by National Institute of Arthritis, Diabetes, Digestive and Kidney Diseases grant AM-25663.

Muhammad B. Yunus, MD: Assistant Professor of Medicine; Alfonse T. Masi, MD, DrPH: Professor and Head, Department of Medicine.

Address reprint requests to Muhammad B. Yunus, MD, Department of Medicine, University of Illinois College of Medicine at Peoria, P.O. Box 1649, Peoria, IL 61656.

Submitted for publication April 27, 1984; accepted in revised form September 24, 1984.

PATIENTS AND METHODS

Thirty-one patients were white and 2 were black, and all but 2 were females. They had an age range of 9–17 years at presentation (mean 14.7; median 15). The age of the normal controls ranged from 9–19 years (mean 14.5; median 15). Onset age of PFS ranged from 5–17 years (mean 12.3; median 13.5). The presentation and onset ages of patients by subgroups are shown in Table 1. The most frequent age group for both presentation and onset was 13–15 years. All but 1 patient had onset before age 16, and 29 (88%) of the 33 patients presented between ages 13 and 17. The presentation and onset ages of the 2 male patients were 15 and 14, and 14 and 10, respectively.

The mean (± 1 SD) height of patients was 157 ± 11.2 cm and of controls 154.7 ± 9.8 cm, with no significant difference. The mean weight of patients was 45.7 ± 12.1 kg and of controls 39.6 ± 7.0 kg ($P < 0.06$). The mean observed subject/standard height and weight ratios, according to age

Table 1. Distribution of presentation and onset ages in 33 juvenile primary fibromyalgia syndrome patients

Age group (years)	Presentation	Onset
5–6	0 (0%)	4 (12%)
7–9	3 (9%)	5 (15%)
10–12	1 (3%)	4 (12%)
13–15	16 (49%)	19 (58%)
16–17	13 (39%)	1 (3%)
Total 5–17	33 (100%)	33 (100%)

(8), were also calculated for patients and controls, with no significant difference.

All 33 patients were age 17 or younger at presentation, and were seen consecutively by us in ambulatory rheumatology consultation. Older patients with juvenile-onset symptoms were not included. The age limit of 17 at presentation was chosen instead of the suggested pediatric age limit of 20 (9), or onset before age 16 as is the case for juvenile rheumatoid arthritis (10), because many pediatric services include patients until age 17 (which is also the maximum legal age for juveniles). The juvenile presentation age is more reliable than onset age for consistency among centers and for correct diagnosis of juvenile primary fibromyalgia, since time of symptom onset of this condition may not be accurately recalled later in adult years and other conditions at onset, e.g., viral arthralgia or arthritis, cannot be ruled out by recall of symptoms alone.

Data were collected longitudinally by one of us (MBY) according to a standardized protocol which included a physician-administered questionnaire and a physical examination form, as in our previous PFS study (3). All patients had as entry criteria musculoskeletal aching or stiffness for at least 3 months that involved 3 or more areas, as well as at least 4 well-defined tender points (3). None had an underlying condition, including obvious trauma or hypermobility syndrome, to explain their symptoms and signs. None had evidence of synovitis, muscle weakness, or neurologic abnormality. All the usual laboratory test results were normal or negative, including complete blood count, Westergren erythrocyte sedimentation rate, muscle enzymes, serum electrolytes, serum calcium, urinalysis, rheumatoid factor by latex fixation, and roentgenograms of prominently involved sites.

Two female patients had positive antinuclear antibody tests in low titers (both 1:80, speckled pattern) without an underlying cause, including drug or connective tissue disorder, on followup at 15 and 18 months. Test results for serum C3 and C4 and antibodies to native DNA, Sm, and RNP were normal or negative. No patient had clinical hypothyroidism, and thyroid function tests performed on 12 patients had normal results.

Entry criteria did not include strict counting of a required number of minor associated criteria (e.g., fatigue, poor sleep, anxiety) as previously suggested (3). However, clinical diagnosis quite likely involved some consideration of these suggested minor criteria.

Normal controls were chosen from among the friends of patients and were matched for sex, race, and age (±2 years). Six normal controls had musculosketal pain in 1 or more areas for which they did not seek physician consultation.

Tender points were defined as areas of exaggerated tenderness elicited on moderately firm fingertip palpation of specific anatomic sites (3); comparatively less pressure was applied than in adults. Only a response of severe (compared with mild or moderate) pain, physical withdrawal of the local part, characteristic body recoil ("jump sign"), or facial expression of pain qualified as a tender point (3).

Differences between patients and controls and between patient subgroups in proportionate frequencies of dichotomous (yes/no) variables were evaluated using the chi-square test with Yates' correction, as appropriate, or Fisher's exact test. Continuous variables were analyzed by Student's *t*-test or were dichotomized at critical levels and subjected to chi-square or Fisher's exact test, as mentioned above (11).

RESULTS

Frequency of symptoms (Table 2). Diffuse musculoskeletal aching was present in 32 patients (97%); 1 patient consistently complained of stiffness only. Stiffness was present in 79% and subjective soft tissue swelling in 61% of the patients. Non-musculoskeletal symptoms were common, including general fatigue throughout the day in 91%. Although 67% reported not sleeping well, all patients woke up tired in the morning, implicating nonrestorative sleep. Chronic headaches, not due to sinusitis and often related to tension, were reported in 54%, numbness in 36%, and irritable bowel symptoms (altered bowel habits associated with abdominal pain or discomfort) in 27%. Anxiety and depression were self-assessed either by patients and controls or occasionally by their accompanying parent(s); responses were elicited to the questions "do

Table 2. Percent frequency of symptom manifestations in 33 juvenile primary fibromyalgia syndrome (PFS) patients and 33 matched normal controls*

Symptom manifestations	Juvenile PFS patients	Normal controls
Musculoskeletal		
Generalized aches and pains	97	3
Stiffness	79	15
Subjective soft tissue swelling	61	12
Non-musculoskeletal		
Waking up tired	100	48
General fatigue	91	15
Anxiety	70	39
Poor sleep†	67	18
Depression	55	9
Chronic headaches	54	18
Numbness	36	6
Irritable bowel symptoms	27	3

* Differences were significant at $P < 0.005$ or lower, except for anxiety and irritable bowel symptoms, which were significant at $P < 0.05$.

† Indicates negative response to the question "do you sleep well?"

Table 3. Frequency (%) of sites of aches, pains, or stiffness in 33 juvenile primary fibromyalgia syndrome patients*

Site	%	Site	%
Knees	67	Trapezius (upper border)	24
Ankles	42	PIP joints (hands)	24
Elbows	39	Upper lateral thigh	24
Lower back	33	MCP joints	18
Upper/mid-back	30	Fingers	18
Wrists	27	Thighs (diffuse)	15
Cervical spine	27	Feet	12

* PIP = proximal interphalangeal; MCP = metacarpophalangeal.

you regard yourself an anxious or worrying type of person?" and "do you usually feel depressed or low in spirit?" respectively. All symptoms were significantly more frequent among patients than controls.

Sites, duration, and diurnal variation of symptoms. Common sites of aches, pains, or stiffness are shown in Table 3. Aches and pains were symmetric (bilateral in more than 80% of affected sites) in 79% of patients. Total sites of aches and pains among the patients ranged from 4 to 34 (mean 13; median 12), compared with 0 to 5 in the normal controls.

Subjective swelling, when reported (61%), involved 1 to 11 sites (mean 8.1; median 9), commonly in or around knees (45% of patients), followed by metacarpophalangeal (MCP) and proximal interphalangeal (PIP) joints of hands and fingers (18% each), wrists and ankles (15% each). Numbness, when present (36%), was described in 1 to 12 sites (mean 8; median 7), commonly in fingers (52%), hands (24%), and legs (18%).

Duration of aches, pains, or stiffness in patients ranged from 3 to 122 months (mean 30; median 12). Only 1 control subject had aches and pains in 3 or more sites for 3 or more months (but had only 4 tender points). Four controls had pain in 2 anatomic sites each, and another in 1 site. Each PIP or MCP joint area (if specified by the patient), a finger, hand or foot, 1 arm, leg or thigh, cervical spine, upper or mid-back, and lower back were counted as a single site.

Aches and pains were present mostly in the morning in 45%, morning as well as afternoon or evening in 35%, no particular time in 13%, and mostly in the afternoon or evening in 7% of patients. Stiffness was present mostly in the morning in 75%, lasting 10 minutes to all day (mean 107 minutes; median 60), mostly in the morning and afternoon or evening in 12.5%, and at no particular time in 12.5%.

Modulating factors. Factors reported to modulate aches, pains, or stiffness are shown in Table 4. Common aggravating factors were cold and/or humid weather, physical overactivity or inactivity, anxiety/stress, and poor sleep. Commonly, a hot shower or bath, stretching exercises, warm weather, moderate activity, and massage helped alleviate musculoskeletal aching or stiffness.

Physical examination. The patients' mean pulse rate of 76/minute and systolic blood pressure (BP) of 111 were not significantly different from those of the matched controls (75 and 104, respectively). However, the mean diastolic BP of 75 among the patients was significantly greater than that of 65 among the controls ($P < 0.01$), with no correlation between weight and BP in either group. No patient had definite synovitis, including objective joint swelling. However, 1 of the 20 patients complaining of soft tissue swelling also demonstrated mild to moderate diffuse soft tissue swelling of fingers on examination; results of a bone scan in this patient were normal.

The most significant finding among the patients was the presence of multiple tender points (range 5–31; mean 13; median 12). Although 36% of the normal controls had 1 or more tender points, none had more than 4 (range 0 to 4, mean 0.8) ($P < 0.001$). Common sites of tender points are shown in Figure 1. The PIP and MCP joints of the hands were tender in 3 and in 2 patients, respectively. The normal controls had tender points, with significantly less frequency than patients, in the following sites: lateral part of elbows (27%), sternomastoid muscles (18%), medial part of elbows (12%), suboccipital areas (6%), posterior iliac crest (medial aspect), costochondral junctions, and thoracic spine/paraspine (each 3%).

In view of the median presentation age of 15, the 20 patients who presented at age 15 or younger were compared with the 13 patients who presented at ages 16 and 17. No significant difference was found between these 2 groups in any variables except height and weight ($P < 0.05$).

Table 4. Frequency (%) of factors reported to modulate aches, pains, or stiffness in 33 juvenile primary fibromyalgia syndrome patients

Aggravating factors	%	Relieving factors	%
Cold/humid weather	88	Hot shower/bath	85
Physical overactivity	88	Stretching exercises	58
Physical inactivity	64	Warm weather	58
Anxiety/stress	45	Moderate activity	55
Poor sleep*	39	Massage	55
Air conditioning†	18	General rest	27

* Poor sleep defined as "not sleeping well."
† Spontaneous response; not included in protocol questionnaire.

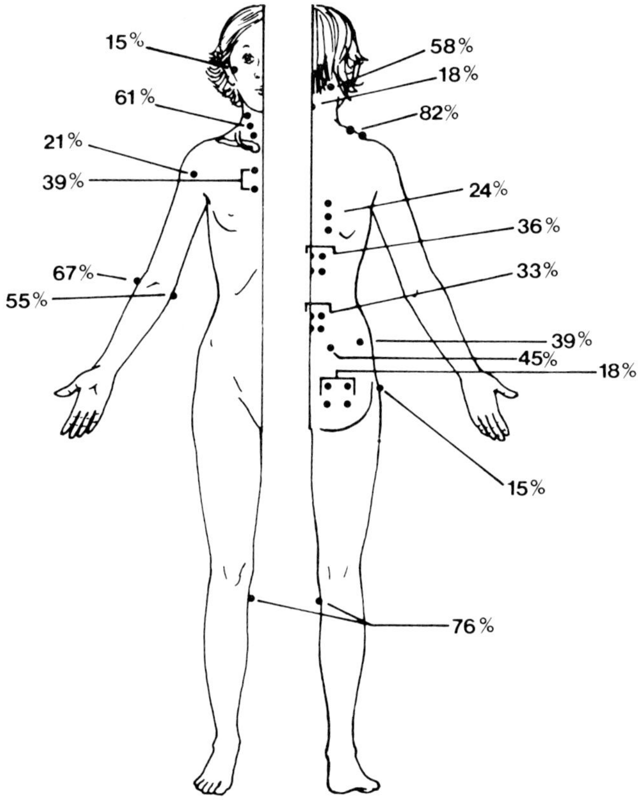

Figure 1. Frequency distribution of common tender points in 33 juvenile primary fibromyalgia syndrome patients; % = percent of positive patients.

Preceding diagnoses and unwarranted investigations. More than half the patients (55%) did not have a definite diagnosis on referral. Referral diagnoses included juvenile rheumatoid arthritis in 8 patients, arthritis in 4, and collagen disease in 1. Only 1 patient had a diagnosis of fibromyalgia ("fibrositis"). Nearly half the patients had 1 or more unwarranted investigation(s), including arthrograms in 4, bone scans in 4, brain scans in 4, myelogram in 1, and spinal tap in 1. Electroencephalograms (EEGs) were performed on 3 patients because of headaches, numbness, or subjective weakness. One patient was treated with oral corticosteroids because of a presumed diagnosis of collagen disease.

Degree of disability, symptom status on followup, and school absenteeism. Information on these features was available in 20 juveniles. At presentation, patients were asked to self-assess their degrees of disability as none, mild, moderate, or severe, considering how much their musculoskeletal symptoms interfered with their normal life activities. All patients reported some disability, graded as mild in 4 (20%), moderate in 12 (60%), and severe in 4 (20%). At presentation, symptoms were graded as mild in 5%, moderate in 45%, and severe in 50%. At followup, after a mean period of 18.8 months (range 4–52; median 14), symptoms had generally improved and were absent in 5%, mild in 55%, moderate in 40%, and severe in none ($P < 0.001$). Juveniles who slept well at the time of referral did better at followup than those who did not ($P < 0.05$). The mean number of days lost from school because of musculoskeletal pain prior to referral was 5.8 ± 8.3, 9.4 ± 9.9, and 13 ± 17.7, in 3, 6, and 12 months, respectively. Followup disability was not assessed.

DISCUSSION

This study, based on 33 juvenile patients and 33 matched normal controls, shows that PFS in juveniles, like that in adults (1–3,7), is a characteristic nonarticular rheumatic syndrome. Both juveniles and adults manifest diffuse musculoskeletal aching and/or stiffness with characteristic modulating factors. Manifestations of a systemic disease, e.g., weight loss, fever, skin rash, and poor appetite, are absent. Physical examination shows no evidence of synovitis, muscle weakness, or neurologic abnormality, but multiple soft tissue tender points are evident at characteristic sites, as was earlier reported in adult PFS patients (3). Symptoms and tender point sites are consistent and reproducible at followup. Routine laboratory test results are normal.

Adult PFS and juvenile PFS are similar conditions, although several differences were noted among the present series of 33 juvenile patients when compared with the 39 adults (age 18 and older) in our previous series (3). Among the juveniles, certain features were more common, i.e., subjective swelling (61% versus 23%; $P < 0.005$), ankle pain (42% versus 15%; $P < 0.05$), and aggravation of pain by overactivity (88% versus 59%; $P < 0.05$), whereas others were less frequent, i.e., low back pain (33% versus 69%; $P < 0.005$), hand pain (33% versus 69%; $P < 0.005$), symptom aggravation by anxiety (45% versus 74%; $P < 0.05$), symptom relief by moderate activity (55% versus 85%; $P < 0.05$), as well as warm/dry weather (58% versus 85%; $P < 0.05$), and tender point at lumbar spine/paraspine area (33% versus 62%; $P < 0.05$). The different frequency of tender points at the suboccipital region is explained by a different (and more sensitive) technique of palpation in our present series (palpation of rectus capitis posterior insertion, rather than below the superior nuchal line). Overall, these relatively few differences between juveniles and adults should be accepted with certain reservations. Subjective perception of symptoms and their reporting may be different and less consistent among the younger juveniles compared with the adults.

PFS, either in adults or juveniles, may be questioned as an entity because no definite physical or laboratory findings are present, or it may be regarded as merely an expression of anxiety or depression. Our psychological studies among adults have shown that only one-third of patients are disturbed psychologically according to the Minnesota Multiphasic Personality Inventory, with high scores on the Depression scale (12,13). Thus, not all PFS patients are unduly anxious or depressed. Psychological studies are not available on juvenile PFS at this time, but our general observations suggest that psychological factors in juveniles are probably similar to adults.

The American Psychiatric Association (APA) guidelines for diagnosis of psychogenic pain include absence of adequate physical findings or pathophysiologic mechanisms for pain (14). In PFS, the tender points on physical examination are usually at specific sites, are consistent, and are reproducible. As in tension headaches, muscle spasm, observed in many patients, probably forms a pathophysiologic basis of PFS. Tension headaches, present in half of our juvenile patients, have specifically been excluded from the APA category of psychogenic pain (14).

Anxiety and stress are important contributory factors for such well-accepted entities as irritable bowel syndrome (IBS) and tension headaches, both of which lack definite physical and laboratory findings and are associated with PFS (3). Conceptually, IBS, PFS, and tension headache syndrome are similar conditions with muscle spasm as a probable pathophysiologic mechanism common to all (15). PFS and IBS have many common and overlapping features (15–17). IBS occurs both in adults and juveniles (17,18). It appears that multiple factors, e.g., constitutional factors, poor sleep, anxiety/stress, subclinical trauma, and poor posture are contributory in PFS. Objective sleep EEG studies have shown disturbed non–rapid eye movement sleep among adult PFS patients (19).

Previous description and prevalence of juvenile PFS. Bates and Grunwaldt described 62 children aged 3–18 years with "trigger areas" among 85 juveniles with myofascial pain caused by a variety of underlying illnesses and injuries (20). These juveniles with nonspecific and heterogeneous myofascial pain are different from our PFS patients, since pain and tender points in these patients were secondary to other conditions, e.g., obvious trauma and infection (20).

Prevalence of juvenile PFS cannot be accurately estimated at this time, but it appears to be common. Over a period of 18 months, from January 1981 to July 1982, we saw 19 new juvenile rheumatoid arthritis (JRA) patients, age 17 years or younger at presentation. We saw 15 new juvenile PFS patients who presented at age 17 years or younger during the same period. However, if adult PFS patients with symptom onset under age 16 are accepted as having juvenile PFS (as is the case in JRA), then the number of juvenile PFS was 24, compared with 22 JRA patients with onset age under 16 years.

Clinical features of juvenile PFS. Several features merit discussion. Subjective swelling of soft tissues may be present in both articular and periarticular locations, leading to a misdiagnosis of arthritis, as was the case in 8 patients. Except in 1 patient, the soft tissue swelling was not objectively seen. However, it is possible that the degree of such swelling is not severe enough to be detected by physical examination. This symptom was not related statistically to anxiety or numbness, but to increased number of pain sites ($P < 0.05$). It was also significantly more common among juveniles who were physically more active ($P < 0.05$). Although a history of definite or obvious trauma was uniformly negative, subclinical trauma or overuse may thus play a role.

Numbness is another feature which did not correlate with anxiety. It may be attributed to altered sensory perception by PFS patients, possibly associated with localized muscle spasm. Neurologic symptoms, including numbness, headaches, and subjective fatigue, are important features of PFS. These symptoms may contribute to unwarranted investigations, e.g., electroencephalograms, brain scans, and myelograms, if the syndrome is unrecognized.

Anxiety and depression were assessed by the patients and occasionally by their parents, as explained earlier. These, as well as other, symptoms which require subjective assessment (e.g., modulating factors of aches and pains) are likely to be less reliable and consistent in juveniles than adults, particularly among the younger children. Further, patients or their parents may report anxiety or stress as rationalization of patients' symptoms. Psychological studies using appropriate tools for children may provide a better evaluation of anxiety, stress, and depression in juvenile PFS.

Poor sleep is an important symptom and is likely to contribute to overall aching (19). Although 67% reported that they do not sleep well, all patients reported fatigue on awakening, implicating nonrestorative sleep (19,21). Morning fatigue may be a more sensitive indicator of nonrestorative sleep than a general statement of not sleeping well. General fatigue during the day is also present in nearly all of the juvenile patients (91%), as in the adults (3).

Our previously demonstrated association of irritable bowel syndrome with PFS was also found in another study (4), and in this juvenile series. Anxiety/stress is likely to be a common associated factor in both PFS and IBS.

Symptoms were significantly more common among the patients than the normal controls. This is in part due to physician selection of PFS symptoms. However, all PFS symptoms, e.g., minor criteria (3,7), were not methodically sought by a physician as entry criteria, although use of clinical judgement in diagnosis is likely to have included some of these symptoms.

Although diffuse soft tissue tenderness may be present in some patients (1,22), localized tenderness at characteristic sites is more usual on physical examination (Figure 1). Distant radiation of pain from site of palpation is rare (22), and thus the term "trigger point" (23) is inappropriate in general, as opposed to the preferred term "tender point." One of our patients presented with pain and tenderness in the temporomandibular joints (TMJ). Fifteen percent had TMJ tenderness in this study. Such tenderness cannot be differentiated from that in TMJ syndrome. However, it is of interest that the most common cause of TMJ syndrome is functional (24). Some PFS patients do have features of this syndrome.

Differential diagnosis. Differentiation of other conditions mimicking juvenile PFS has been fully reviewed elsewhere (25). Juvenile rheumatoid arthritis can be distinguished by objective arthritis and other features (26). Similarly, traumatic arthritis, bursitis, tendinitis, and muscle sprain are differentiated from PFS by history as well as the localized nature of these conditions (in contrast to generalized manifestations in PFS) (25,27). Systemic lupus erythematosus is characterized by its clinical and immunologic features (28). Psychogenic pain is a different entity with bizarre, highly emotional, and highly inconsistent symptoms; patients are tender everywhere, even when touched gently (3). "Growing pains" with musculoskeletal aching in the absence of an abnormal laboratory test result (29,30) might have been confused with juvenile PFS in the past, although tender points were not described in the former. If this term is to be used at all, only patients with nocturnal limb pain (29–31) should be included in this category. Nocturnal pain did not occur predominantly in any of our 33 patients. Some patients with hypermobility of joints have rheumatic symptoms, including myalgia and arthralgia. A diagnosis of hypermobility can be made by the suggested criteria of Beighton and Horan (32). However, patients with hypermobility were excluded from this study. Children with school phobia may have headaches, abdominal pain, and, less commonly, vague body pain, but such symptoms usually occur before school time (33).

Suggested criteria for diagnosis of juvenile PFS. All 33 juveniles in this series and none of the matched normal controls satisfied our previously suggested criteria for PFS (3,7,27). These criteria include generalized musculoskeletal aching at 3 or more sites for 3 or more months in the absence of an underlying condition, e.g., arthritis and obvious trauma. Results of the usual laboratory tests are normal. In addition, 5 or more typical tender points plus 3 of the following 10 features (minor criteria) should be present: 1) chronic anxiety or tension; 2) fatigue; 3) poor sleep; 4) chronic headaches; 5) irritable bowel syndrome; 6) subjective soft tissue swelling; 7) numbness; 8) pain modulation by physical activities; 9) pain modulation by weather factors; and 10) pain modulation by anxiety/stress. Four tender points will also satisfy the criteria, provided a patient has 5 of the above 10 features.

In this study of juveniles, 1 normal control, who had aches and pains at 5 anatomic sites for 4 months, had only 4 tender points and 2 minor criteria, and thus did not satisfy the above criteria. Of the 10 suggested minor criteria, juveniles were significantly different in only 3 (increased frequency of pain aggravation by overactivity and equally decreased frequency of pain relief by moderate activity in juveniles cancelled each other). Frequency distribution of these 3 criteria balanced each other, subjective swelling being more common in juveniles, whereas pain modulation by anxiety and weather is more common in adults. Independently-derived criteria for juvenile PFS, including other control conditions with musculoskeletal aching, e.g., JRA and hypermobility syndrome, will be needed for a future study.

Whether the onset age, or age at presentation, under 17 or 18 years should be accepted as criteria for diagnosis of juvenile PFS is open to discussion. In this study, no significant difference was found between children who presented at age 15 and younger versus those who presented at age 16 and 17. Incidentally, only 1 patient had onset age over age 15 in this study. As explained in Patients and Methods, it may be preferable to classify juvenile patients according to presentation rather than onset age.

Symptoms at followup. Symptoms at followup generally improved among our patients. Optimal management, including a firm diagnosis, reassurance regarding benign nature (compared with juvenile rheumatoid arthritis), management of stress factors if present, moderation of physical activity, physical therapy (heat, stretching exercises), simple, non-addictive analgesics, and a nonsteroidal antiinflammatory agent also contributed to less severe symptoms at followup. Any implication that the pain is "all psychological" should be avoided. Management of juvenile PFS is similar to that of adults (3,7,34), but psychoactive drugs should rarely be used in children. Long-term prognosis of juvenile PFS remains unknown, and needs to be determined in a longitudinal study. From our experience of adult PFS patients with juvenile onset, it appears that symptoms of juvenile PFS may go away in some patients, only to return later in adult life.

In conclusion, juvenile PFS is a common and recognizable condition which should be diagnosed by its own characteristic features and not merely by exclusion of other conditions. Diagnosis of juvenile PFS is important to avoid unwarranted investigations and improper management.

ACKNOWLEDGMENT

We greatly appreciate the technical assistance of Barbara Lundeen in this study.

REFERENCES

1. Tout EF: Fibrositis. J Am Geriatr Soc 16:531–538, 1968
2. Smythe HA: Non-articular rheumatism and psychogenic musculoskeletal syndromes, Arthritis and Allied Conditions. Ninth edition. Edited by DJ McCarty. Philadelphia, Lea & Febiger, 1979, pp 881–891
3. Yunus M, Masi AT, Calabro JJ, Miller KA, Feigenbaum SL: Primary fibromyalgia (fibrositis): clinical study of 50 patients with matched normal controls. Semin Arthritis Rheum 11:151–171, 1981
4. Campbell SM, Clark S, Tindall EA, Forehand ME, Bennett RM: Clinical characteristics of fibrositis. I. A "blinded," controlled study of symptoms and tender points. Arthritis Rheum 26:817–824, 1983
5. Yunus MB, Kalyanraman UP, Kalyanraman K, Masi AT, Berg BC: Microscopic and radioactive bone scan studies in primary fibromyalgia (abstract). Arthritis Rheum (suppl) 25:S146, 1982
6. Kalyanraman UP, Kalyanraman K, Yunus MB, Masi AT: Muscle pathology in primary fibromyalgia syndrome (PFS): a light microscopic, histochemical and ultrastructural study. J Rheumatol 11:808–813, 1984
7. Masi AT, Yunus MB: Primary fibromyalgia syndrome: a commonly unrecognized rheumatologic disorder. Continuing Ed Fam Phys 17:19–32, 1982
8. Tanner JM: Physical growth and development, Textbook of Pediatrics. Edited by JO Forfar, GC Arneil. London, Churchill Livingstone, 1973
9. Council on Child Health, American Academy of Pediatrics: Age limits of pediatrics. Pediatrics 49:463, 1972
10. JRA Criteria Subcommittee of the Diagnostic and Therapeutic Criteria Committee of the American Rheumatism Association: Current proposed revisions of the JRA criteria. Arthritis Rheum (suppl) 20:195–199, 1977
11. Nie NH, Hull CH, Jenkins JG, Steinbrenner K, Bent DH: Statistical Package for the Social Sciences (SPSS). New York, McGraw-Hill, 1975
12. Ahles TA, Yunus MB, Riley SD, Bradley JM, Masi AT: Psychological studies in primary fibromyalgia syndrome (abstract). Clin Res 31:801A, 1983
13. Ahles TA, Yunus MB, Riley SD, Bradley JM, Masi AT: Psychological factors associated with primary fibromyalgia syndrome. Arthritis Rheum 27:637–642, 1984
14. Diagnostic and Statistical Manual of Mental Disorders (DSM III). American Psychiatric Association, 1980, pp 247–249
15. Yunus MB: Primary fibromyalgia syndrome: current concepts. Compr Ther 10:21–28, 1984
16. Yunus MB: Fibromyalgia syndrome: a need for uniform classification (editorial). J Rheumatol 10:841–844, 1983
17. Kirsner JB: The irritable bowel syndrome. Arch Intern Med 141:635–639, 1981
18. Barbero GJ, McKay RJ: Irritable bowel syndrome, Nelson's Textbook of Pediatrics. Edited by RE Behrman, VC Vaughn III. Philadelphia, WB Saunders, 1983, pp 940–941
19. Moldofsky H, Scarisbrick P, England RE, Smythe H: Musculoskeletal symptoms and non-REM sleep disturbance in patients with "fibrositis" syndrome and healthy subjects. Psychosom Med 37:341–351, 1975
20. Bates T, Grunwaldt E: Myofascial pain in childhood. J Pediatr 53:198–209, 1958
21. Moldofsky H, Lue FA: The relationship of alpha and delta EEG frequencies to pain and mood in "fibrositis" patients with chlorpromazine and L-tryptophan. Electroencephalogr Clin Neurophysiol 50:71–80, 1980
22. Yunus MB, Masi AT: A detailed and controlled clinical study of primary fibromyalgia syndrome. In preparation
23. Kraus H: Trigger points. NY State J Med 73:1310–1314, 1973

24. Sheon RP, Moskowitz RW, Goldbert VM: Soft Tissue Rheumatic Pain. Philadelphia, Lea & Febiger, 1982, pp 13–18
25. Yunus MB: Aches and pain: is it juvenile fibromyalgia syndrome? Diagnosis 6:93–102, 1984
26. Calabro JJ, Holgerson WB, Sonpal GM, Khoury MI: Juvenile rheumatoid arthritis: a general review and report of 100 patients observed for 15 years. Semin Arthritis Rheum 5:257–298, 1976
27. Yunus MB: Primary fibromyalgia syndrome: diagnosis and differential diagnosis. IM-Int Med Specialist 4:58–74, 1983
28. Fish AJ, Blau EB, Westberg NG, Burke BA, Vernier RL, Michael AF: Systemic lupus erythematosus within the first two decades of life. Am J Med 62:99–117, 1977
29. Ansell BM: Rheumatic Disorders in Childhood. London, Butterworths, 1980, pp 2–3
30. Øster J, Nielsen A: Growing pains: a clinical investigation of a school population. Acta Paediatr Scand 61:329–334, 1972
31. Calabro JJ, Wachtel AE, Holgerson WB, Repice MM: Growing pains. Postgrad Med 59:66–72, 1976
32. Beighton P, Horan S: Orthopedic aspects of the Ehlers-Danlos syndrome. J Bone Joint Surg 51B:444–453, 1969
33. Gelbert E: Psychosocial Aspects of Pediatric Care. New York, Grune & Stratton, 1978, pp 198–201
34. Yunus MB, Masi AT, Calabro JJ, Shah IK: Primary fibromyalgia. Am Fam Physician 25:115–121, 1982

Erratum

There was an error in Table 2 of an article which appeared in the October 1984 issue of *Arthritis and Rheumatism* (Ahles TA, Yunus MB, Riley SD, Bradley JM, Masi AT: Psychological Factors Associated with Primary Fibromyalgia Syndrome. Arthritis Rheum 27:1101–1106, 1984). The first two values in the table column marked "RA" were listed as 44.8 and 48.3. These values should have been 46.6 and 46.6.

HLA GENE FREQUENCIES IN CHILDREN AND ADULTS WITH SYSTEMIC ONSET JUVENILE RHEUMATOID ARTHRITIS

MARC L. MILLER, STEPHEN AARON, JEAN JACKSON, PATRICIA FRASER, LLOYD CAIRNS, SUSAN HOCH, YVES BOREL, MARTIN LARSON, and DAVID N. GLASS

The HLA genetic region was studied in 51 patients with systemic onset juvenile rheumatoid arthritis: 35 with childhood onset and 16 with adult onset (adult Still's disease). HLA genotypes were established by including family members, 261 of whom were also typed in the study. The most marked difference between patients and controls involved the HLA–DR4 gene, which occurred with a frequency of 0.348 in the childhood onset patients and 0.170 in the controls ($\chi^2 = 8.97$, $P = 0.0028$, adjusted $P = 0.017$). In contrast, the adult onset patients showed a marginal increase in HLA–DR7, but were similar to controls with respect to HLA–DR4. HLA–Bw35 was increased in children with systemic onset disease, in accordance with earlier findings. The results suggest that patients with systemic onset juvenile rheumatoid arthritis have complex HLA associations which are different in childhood onset and adult onset disease.

From the Department of Rheumatology and Immunology, Brigham and Women's Hospital, the Department of Immunology, Children's Hospital Medical Center, the Department of Medicine and Pediatrics, Harvard Medical School, and the Department of Biostatistics, Harvard School of Public Health, Boston, Massachusetts.

Supported by the Easter Seal Society, the Gebbie Foundation, the Leeder Foundation, the Lions Clubs of Massachusetts, the New England Peabody Home for Crippled Children, and by NIH grants AM-30486, CRUAM-05577, and Multipurpose Arthritis Center grant AM-20580.

Marc L. Miller, MD; Stephen Aaron, MD: Fellow of the Canadian Arthritis Society; Jean Jackson, MD; Patricia Fraser, MD; Lloyd Cairns, MD: Fellow of the New Zealand Arthritis Foundation; Susan Hoch, MD; Yves Borel, MD; Martin Larson, ScD; David N. Glass, MD.

Address reprint requests to David N. Glass, MD, Brigham and Women's Hospital, 75 Francis Street, Boston, MA 02115.

Submitted for publication November 14, 1983; accepted in revised form August 24, 1984.

Since the first report of the influence of HLA–B27 in juvenile rheumatoid arthritis (JRA) (1), all clinically distinct forms of JRA have been associated with HLA antigens. Considerable agreement about HLA genetics exists in relation to pauciarticular and polyarticular onset disease (2), but there is less consensus about the HLA antigens associated with systemic onset JRA (2). In an earlier study (3), we reported an increased frequency of HLA–Bw35 in patients with systemic onset disease, but HLA–DR alleles were not examined. An association with HLA–Bw35 has been found in patients with the adult onset form of the disease (adult Still's disease) (4) and in some (5,6), but not all series of patients with onset during childhood (7–11). Most subsets of JRA have stronger associations with HLA–DR, or HLA haplotypes including HLA–DR (2,12), than with HLA–A or B alleles. Accordingly, HLA typing, including typing for HLA–DR, was carried out in patients with systemic onset JRA and their families to ascertain disease-associated genes.

PATIENTS AND METHODS

Patients. Fifty-one white patients (24 female, 27 male) with systemic onset JRA were studied, as were 261 of their relatives. Thirty-five of the probands had disease onset during childhood and 16 as adults (i.e., after their sixteenth birthday). Of the 35 subjects with childhood onset, 16 were reported in an earlier study (3). The patients met the American Rheumatism Association criteria for systemic onset JRA (13). All but 5 had a fever of $\geq$103°F, and all had arthritis at some time in the course of the disease. Forty-two patients had documented evidence of the rash typically associated with the disease. An additional study criterion was the availability and consent of enough family members to establish the possible HLA genotypes.

Probands and family members were typed for HLA–A, B, C, and DR antigens in the Tissue Typing Laboratory of the Department of Rheumatology and Immunology, The Brigham and Women's Hospital, Boston.

Family trees were constructed and haplotype assignments made for each locus when an informative assortment of alleles was demonstrated. If an assignment could not be made for a particular polymorphism, that haplotype was not considered in calculating the gene frequencies for the locus. The denominator used to calculate gene frequencies varied, therefore, with polymorphisms being lower for some than for others.

Control haplotypes. Controls consisted of 398 haplotypes that were established in families with a rheumatic disease proband, but were not inherited by the proband. No haplotype was counted twice, and 1 potential control haplotype that was in recombination with a proband's haplotype was excluded. This method of establishing control gene frequency and control haplotype frequencies using the proband's family has been compared with a method in which haplotype frequencies are derived from families without an affected member. Very comparable results have been obtained between the 2 methods (14). Control gene frequencies for HLA–DR were also compared with HLA–DR data for North American whites from the 8th International Histocompatibility Workshop (15), and no significant differences were found by the application of chi-square statistics (12).

Cells. Peripheral blood mononuclear leukocytes (MNL) were obtained by density gradient centrifugation through Ficoll-Paque (Pharmacia Fine Chemicals, Piscataway, NJ).

HLA–A, B, and C typing. HLA–A, B, and C typing for 39 specificities was carried out by microdroplet complement-dependent cytotoxicity (16). HLA–A, B, and C antisera were kindly supplied by the National Institute for Allergy and Infectious Diseases, NIH, Bethesda.

HLA–DR typing. HLA–DR specificities were typed by complement-dependent cytotoxicity on a nylon-wool B cell–enriched MNL population (17,18). All preparations studied were evaluated by complement-dependent cytotoxicity with a polyvalent rabbit anti-Ia serum kindly supplied by Dr. J. Strominger (Biological Laboratories, Harvard University), and were found to contain 70% Ia-bearing MNL.

The antisera used to type for HLA–DR antigens were either obtained locally or were the gifts of laboratories worldwide. Antisera tested in both the 8th (15) and 9th (19) International Histocompatibility Workshops were included.

Statistical methods. Gene frequencies (counts) for the control series were compared separately with those of childhood onset probands and adult onset probands by chi-square analyses of R × 2 tables (20,21). The number of genes, R, depended on which HLA locus was being considered: A, B, C, or DR. Genes with <5% frequency were pooled with those that could not be serologically defined; the genes so pooled are labeled "other" in the tables.

Each control versus proband comparison yields a chi-square statistic with R − 1 degrees of freedom (df) to test the distribution of genes in the 2 groups, but does not indicate which specific gene frequencies differed. For this we assessed individual contributions to chi-square, each with 1 degree of freedom, computed as the sum in a specific row of $(O - E)^2/E$ for probands and controls. Ignoring the "other" genes, there are R − 1 independent contributions that can be evaluated. This avoids a common problem of correlated tests in HLA analysis (22,23). However, several individual tests were performed, so an adjusted *P* value (P*[R − 1]) was computed for each test to keep the "error rate" at an acceptable level.

The relative risk (RR), or odds ratio, was computed using Woolf's formula (24) for specific genes that had large chi-square contributions.

RESULTS

HLA–A, B, C, and D frequencies are shown in Tables 1, 2, 3, and 4, respectively.

Gene frequencies: childhood onset disease. Analyses of HLA gene frequencies comparing childhood onset probands with controls gave the following results: HLA–A locus $\chi^2 = 5.91$, 6 df, $P = 0.43$; HLA–B locus $\chi^2 = 19.60$, 10 df, $P = 0.033$; HLA–C locus $\chi^2 = 9.40$, 4 df, $P = 0.052$; HLA–DR locus $\chi^2 = 12.45$, 6 df, $P = 0.053$.

The individual genes differing most between probands and controls were HLA–Bw35, HLA–Bw44, and HLA–DR4. The frequency of HLA–Bw44 was 0.235 in probands, compared with 0.128 in controls (RR = 2.09, $\chi^2 = 4.64$, $P = 0.031$, adjusted $P = 0.31$), while the frequency of HLA–Bw35 was 0.191 in probands and 0.093 in controls (RR = 2.30, $\chi^2 = 5.22$, $P = 0.022$, adjusted $P = 0.22$). In the HLA–DR series genes, HLA–DR4 occurred with a frequency of 0.348 in probands and 0.170 in controls (RR = 2.60, $\chi^2 = 8.97$, P = 0.0028, adjusted $P = 0.017$).

Gene frequencies: adult onset diseases. The results for individual HLA loci in adult onset probands versus controls were: HLA–A locus $\chi^2 = 3.68$, 6 df, $P = 0.72$; HLA–B locus $\chi^2 = 16.38$, 10 df, $P = 0.089$; HLA–C locus $\chi^2 = 2.66$, 4 df, $P = 0.62$; HLA–DR locus $\chi^2 = 9.77$, 6 df, $P = 0.14$.

Table 1. HLA–A gene frequencies in patients with childhood onset and adult onset juvenile rheumatoid arthritis and control family members

Gene	Childhood onset (n = 67)	Adult onset (n = 30)	Controls (n = 392)
A1	0.164	0.167	0.153
A2,A28	0.418	0.267	0.301
A3	0.090	0.233	0.135
A9,A23,A24	0.090	0.167	0.143
A10,A25,A26	0.060	0.033	0.087
A11	0.090	0.067	0.066
Other A	0.090	0.067	0.115

Table 2. HLA–B gene frequencies in patients with childhood onset and adult onset juvenile rheumatoid arthritis and control family members

Gene	Childhood onset (n = 68)	Adult onset (n = 30)	Controls (n = 398)
B5 (Bw51,Bw52)	0.015	0.067	0.083
B7	0.132	0.133	0.153
B8	0.118	0.167	0.095
B12 (Bw44)	0.235*	0.067	0.128
B14	0.015	0.200†	0.048
B15 (Bw62)	0.074	0.033	0.050
B17	0.029	0.000	0.073
B18	0.044	0.067	0.058
Bw35	0.191‡	0.100	0.093
Bw40,Bw41 (B41)	0.059	0.067	0.068
Other B	0.088	0.100	0.151

* $\chi^2 = 4.64$, $P = 0.031$, $P^*10 = 0.31$.
† $\chi^2 = 11.07$, $P = 0.0009$, $P^*10 = 0.009$.
‡ $\chi^2 = 5.22$, $P = 0.022$, $P^*10 = 0.22$.

HLA–B14 was found with a frequency of 0.200 in probands and 0.048 in controls (RR = 4.96, χ^2 = 11.07, P = 0.0009, adusted P = 0.009), and the HLA–DR7 gene was present with a frequency of 0.286 in probands and 0.135 in controls (RR = 2.57, χ^2 = 4.08, P = 0.043, adjusted P = 0.26). The HLA–DR4 gene frequency was not increased in the adult onset patients.

DISCUSSION

The increased frequency of the HLA–DR4 gene in children with systemic onset JRA is a new finding which suggests that this disease represents an additional form of arthropathy which can be included with those already associated with this major histocompatibility complex product (rheumatoid arthritis, polyarticular JRA, and psoriatic arthritis) (2). Two other groups of investigators have observed higher levels of HLA–DR4 in children with systemic onset JRA than in control series, but in neither study did the data reach acceptable levels of statistical significance (10,11). Those authors limited their studies to the disease probands, and therefore could not give the data the additional strength of numbers that determination of gene frequencies allows in the present study. Since 6 of our patients are homozygous for HLA–DR4, the family studies permitting calculation of exact gene frequencies are of considerable advantage, especially given that the number of patients available is limited. The increase in HLA–Bw44 may result from its linkage disequilibrium with HLA–DR4 (25).

The increase in the frequency of HLA–DR4 in this series, obtained by comparison with locally defined controls as described above, was based on a control gene frequency of 0.170. This compares with the 0.148 value for the gene frequency of HLA–DR4 found in the 8th International Histocompatibility Workshop (15). In contrast to the children, the adults with systemic onset JRA did not have an increased frequency of HLA–DR4.

The increase in HLA–Bw35 is consistent with the results of earlier studies (3–5), including one study which used some of the same subjects reported here (3). Not all series have shown an increase in HLA–Bw35 antigens, but studies (one in a small series of adults [6] and one in childhood onset patients [9]) have shown an association between HLA–DR5 and systemic onset JRA; HLA–DR5 is in linkage disequilibrium with HLA–Bw35. It is also noteworthy that the HLA–Bw35,Cw4 haplotype, with and without HLA–DR5, is increased in young children with pauciarticular onset JRA (12). The HLA–Bw44,DR5 haplotype, which is also found in early onset pauciarticular JRA (12), was not present in any of the systemic onset patients in this study.

Of the other HLA antigens, HLA–B14 and HLA–DR7 are increased in frequency in patients with

Table 3. HLA–C gene frequencies in patients with childhood onset and adult onset juvenile rheumatoid arthritis and control family members

Gene	Childhood onset (n = 60)	Adult onset (n = 23)	Control (n = 331)
Cw2	0.000	0.043	0.060
Cw3	0.150	0.087	0.097
Cw4	0.200	0.174	0.106
Cw5	0.050	0.000	0.069
Other C	0.600	0.696	0.668

Table 4. HLA–DR gene frequencies in patients with childhood onset and adult onset juvenile rheumatoid arthritis and control family members

Gene	Childhood onset (n = 66)	Adult onset (n = 28)	Controls (n = 364)
DR1	0.106	0.143	0.115
DR2	0.121	0.107	0.154
DR3	0.091	0.071	0.115
DR4	0.348*	0.071	0.170
DR5	0.091	0.214	0.115
DR7	0.136	0.286†	0.135
Other DR	0.106	0.107	0.195

* $\chi^2 = 8.97$, $P = 0.0028$, $P^*6 = 0.017$.
† $\chi^2 = 4.08$, $P = 0.043$, $P^*6 = 0.26$.

the adult onset form of the disease, but not in the childhood onset patients. HLA–B14 has not, to our knowledge, previously been associated with JRA. There is an earlier report of an association between HLA–DR7 and systemic onset childhood JRA, and HLA–DR7 is also associated with psoriatic arthritis (7,26,27). The numbers of adult patients available for study are small, and these associations should be considered as needing further confirmation, as should those in the childhood onset group. This is true particularly since at least two other studies, one from Quebec (4) and the other from England (28), have not found an association with HLA–DR7 in adult onset patients.

As with HLA–DR4, the HLA–DR7 association reported in this series is based on a comparison with locally defined controls. It is noteworthy that the control gene frequency for HLA–DR7 used as the basis for comparing disease and non-disease populations, 0.135, is also very comparable with the 0.126 value obtained for North American whites in the 8th International Histocompatibility Workshop (15).

The HLA genes associated with this group of patients are not unique to systemic onset JRA, having been associated with other arthropathies including other forms of JRA. From this it could be argued that the HLA region effect is limited to the articular features of this illness, and not to its systemic effects. A more complete understanding of this question will evolve when the HLA haplotypes associated with all forms of JRA have been more fully documented. However, it can be concluded, much in agreement with our earlier study (3), that systemic onset JRA is a genetically heterogeneous entity, at least with respect to HLA type, and that this heterogeneity extends to differences between the adult and childhood onset forms of the disease.

ACKNOWLEDGMENTS

The assistance of Agnes Maier in the preparation of this manuscript is gratefully acknowledged. The cooperation of the following physicians in referring patients is very much appreciated: Drs. Ronald Anderson, Arthur Hall, L. Fernandez Herlihy, Michael Kane, Lewis Landsberg, Arthur Morgan, Raymond Partridge, Martin Solomon, Tom Taylor, and Michael Weinblatt.

REFERENCES

1. Rachelfsky G, Terasaki PI, Katz R, Stiehm IR: Increased prevalence of w27 in juvenile rheumatoid arthritis. N Engl J Med 290:892–893, 1974
2. Miller ML, Glass DN: The major histocompatibility complex antigens in rheumatoid arthritis and juvenile arthritis. Bull Rheum Dis 31:21–25, 1981
3. Glass DN, Litvin DA: Heterogeneity of HLA associations in systemic onset juvenile rheumatoid arthritis. Arthritis Rheum 23:796–799, 1980
4. Terkeltaub R, Esdaile JM, Décary F, Harth M, Lister J, Lapointe N: HLA-Bw35 and prognosis in adult Still's disease. Arthritis Rheum 24:1469–1472, 1981
5. Schiavetti L, Galeazzi M, Tuzi T: On the heterogeneity of the HLA association in juvenile rheumatoid arthritis (letter). Arthritis Rheum 24:1216–1217, 1981
6. Hübscher O, Arana RM, Egozcue JM, Silbermins V: Adult onset juvenile rheumatoid arthritis (abstract). Arthritis Rheum (suppl) 25:S23, 1982
7. Statsny P, Fink C: Different HLA D associations in adult and juvenile rheumatoid arthritis. J Clin Invest 63:124–130, 1979
8. Oen K, Petty RE, Schroeder ML: An association between HLA A2 and juvenile rheumatoid arthritis in girls. J Rheumatol 9:916–921, 1982
9. Førre O, Dobloug JH, Høyeraal HM, Thorsby E: HLA antigens in juvenile arthritis: genetic basis for the different subtypes. Arthritis Rheum 26:35–38, 1983
10. Ansell BM, Clemens LE: Chronic arthritis of childhood, Immunogenetics in Rheumatology. Edited by RL Dawkins, FT Chrishansen, PJ Zilko, JA Carrano, M Garlepp, J McCluskey, P Hollingsworth. Amsterdam, Excerpta Medica, 1982, pp 164–166
11. Manners PJ, McCluskey J, Dawkins RL: HLA and complement C4 in chronic arthritis of childhood, Immunogenetics in Rheumatology. Edited by RL Dawkins, FT Chrishansen, PJ Zilko, JA Carrano, M Garlepp, J McCluskey, P Hollingsworth. Amsterdam, Excerpta Medica, 1982, pp 167–171
12. Miller M, Fraser P, Jackson J, Petersen R, Chylack L, Glass D: Inherited predisposition in juvenile rheumatoid arthritis with chronic iridocyclitis. Proc Natl Acad Sci USA 81:3539–3542, 1984
13. Brewer EJ, Bass J, Baum J, Cassidy JT, Fink C, Jacobs J, Hanson V, Levinson JE, Schaller J, Stillman JS: Current proposed revision of JRA criteria. Arthritis Rheum 20:195–199, 1977
14. Raum D, Awdeh Z, Glass D, Kammer G, Khan MA, Coblyn JS, Weinblatt M, Holdsworth D, Strong L, Rossen RD, Brewer E, Yunis E, Alper CA: Extended haplotypes of chromosome 6 in adult rheumatoid arthritis. Arthritis Rheum 27:516–521, 1984
15. Terasaki P, editor: Histocompatibility Testing 1980. Los Angeles, University of California Press, 1980
16. Mittal KK, Mickey MR, Singal ER, Terasaki P: Serotyping for homotransplantation. XVIII. Regimen of microdroplet lymphocyte cytotoxicity test. Transplantation 6:913–927, 1968
17. Lowry R, Goguen J, Carpenter CB, Strom TB, Garovoy

MR: Improved B cell typing for HLA DR using nylon wool column enriched B lymphocyte preparations. Tissue Antigens 14:325–330, 1979
18. Van Rood JJ, van Leuween A, Keuning JJ, van Oud Alblas AB: The serological recognition of human MLC determinants using a modified cytotoxicity technique. Tissue Antigens 5:73–79, 1975
19. Hunter J, Noreen H, Mickelson E, Reinsmoen N: IX International Workshop. ASHI Quarterly 8:5–8, 1984
20. Armitage P: Statistical Methods in Medical Research. New York, Wiley and Sons, 1977, pp 207–211
21. Cavalli-Sforza LL, Bodmer WF: The Genetics of Human Populations. San Francisco, WH Freeman, 1971, pp 828–829
22. Svejgaard A: HLA A antigens and disease: statistical and genetical considerations. Tissue Antigens 4:95–105, 1974
23. Smouse PE, Williams RC: Multivariate analysis of HLA-disease associations. Biometrics 38:757–768, 1982
24. Woolf B: On estimating the relation between blood groups and disease. Ann Hum Genet 19:241–253, 1955
25. Awdeh Z, Raum D, Yunis E, Alper CA: Extended HLA/complement allele haplotypes: evidence for T/t like complex in man. Proc Natl Acad Sci USA 80:250–262, 1982
26. Murray C, Mann DL, Gerber LN, Barth W, Pearlmann S, Decker JL, Nigra TP: Histocompatibility alloantigens in psoriasis and psoriatic arthritis: evidence for the influence of multiple genes in the major histocompatibility complex. J Clin Invest 55:670–675, 1980
27. Armstrong RD, Panayi GS, Welsh KI: Histocompatibility antigens in psoriasis, psoriatic arthropathy and ankylosing spondylitis. Ann Rheum Dis 42:142–146, 1983
28. Elkon KB, Hughes GRV, Bywaters EGL, Ryan PFJ, Inman RD, Bowley NB, James MP, Eady RAJ: Adult onset Still's disease: twenty-year followup and further studies of patients with active disease. Arthritis Rheum 25:647–654, 1982

IMMUNOGENETIC STUDIES OF JUVENILE DERMATOMYOSITIS

III. Study of Antibody to Organ-Specific and Nuclear Antigens

LAUREN M. PACHMAN, JAN M. FRIEDMAN, MONA L. MARYJOWSKI-SWEENEY, OLGA JONNASON, RUTA M. RADVANY, GORDON C. SHARP, MIKE A. COBB, NORMA D. BATTLES, WILLIAM E. CROWE, CHESTER W. FINK, VIRGIL HANSON, JOSEPH E. LEVINSON, CHARLES H. SPENCER, and DONITA B. SULLIVAN

Ninety children with definite juvenile dermatomyositis (JDMS), who had been HLA typed, were tested for the presence of tissue or organ-specific antibodies. Sixty had active disease at the time of study. The mean disease duration was 4 years, and 30 had soft tissue calcifications. The following autoantibodies were sought: thyroid, gastric parietal cells, smooth muscle, striated muscle, microsomes, mitochondria, DNA, extractable nuclear antigen, Sm, PM-1, antinuclear antibody (ANA), and rheumatoid factor. Only the ANA and PM-1 were more frequent in patients than in controls ($P < 0.0002$ and $P < 0.001$, respectively). Higher levels of immune complexes ($P < 0.01$) were found in sera from patients with JDMS than in sera from controls and were correlated with the presence of ANA in patients ($P < 0.01$). Soft tissue calcification was not associated with any autoantibody or HLA antigen, but with disease duration and activity ($P < 0.001$ and $P < 0.05$, respectively). There was no association between the occurrence of any autoantibody and the presence of HLA–B8 or DR3 among the white patients with JDMS. The frequency of autoantibodies in 43 full siblings of children with JDMS was not increased. We conclude that children with JDMS, with or without HLA–B8/DR3, do not show evidence of a generalized nonspecific antibody response to tissue antigens. The significance of the increased antibody to nuclear antigens ANA and PM-1 remains to be determined.

Juvenile dermatomyositis (JDMS) is a multisystem inflammatory disease primarily involving skin and muscle. There is some recent evidence of altered cell-mediated immune function in this disease. Impairment of natural killing activity, but not antibody-dependent cell-mediated cytotoxicity can be demonstrated in peripheral blood leukocytes from JDMS patients (1). We found that frequencies of HLA–B8 and HLA–DR3 were increased in children with JDMS (2,3). A number of other autoimmune diseases are associated with HLA–B8/DR3, and in some of these there is an increase in the occurrence of organ-specific autoantibodies, for example, myasthenia gravis, Graves' disease, and juvenile onset insulin-dependent diabetes (4). Therefore, we have tested our large group of JDMS patients for the presence of antibodies directed toward possible target organs and nuclear antigens.

Supported in part by grants from the National Institutes of Health (AN 21589) and the Illinois Chapter of the Arthritis Foundation.

Lauren M. Pachman, MD: Department of Pediatrics, Northwestern University Medical School and The Children's Memorial Hospital, Chicago, Illinois; Jan M. Friedman, MD: Department of Obstetrics and Gynecology and Pediatrics, University of Texas Health Science Center, Dallas; Mona L. Maryjowski-Sweeney, RN: The Children's Memorial Hospital, Chicago, Illinois; Olga Jonnason, MD: Department of Surgery, University of Illinois, Chicago; Ruta M. Radvany, PhD: Department of Surgery, Northwestern University Medical School; Gordon C. Sharp, MD: Department of Medicine, University of Missouri, Columbia; Mike A. Cobb, MS: The Children's Memorial Hospital; Norma D. Battles, MD: Dallas, Texas; William E. Crowe, MD: Departments of Pediatrics and Medicine, Case Western Reserve University, Cleveland, Ohio; Chester W. Fink, MD: Department of Pediatrics, University of Texas Southwestern Medical School, Dallas; Virgil Hanson, MD: University of Southern California School of Medicine, Los Angeles; Joseph E. Levinson, MD: Departments of Medicine and Pediatrics, Children's Convalescent Pavilion, Cincinnati, Ohio; Charles H. Spencer, MD: Departments of Pediatrics and Rheumatology, Children's Hospital, New Orleans, Louisiana; Donita B. Sullivan, MD: University Hospitals, Ann Arbor, Michigan.

Address reprint requests to Lauren M. Pachman, MD, Division of Immunology/Rheumatology, The Children's Memorial Hospital, 2300 Children's Plaza, Chicago, IL 60614.

Submitted for publication March 19, 1984; accepted in revised form August 13, 1984.

PATIENTS AND METHODS

Patient population. One hundred children with JDMS were enrolled in a multicenter study involving the Pediatric Rheumatology Clinic of the Children's Memorial Hospital (Chicago), the University of Michigan Hospital (Ann Arbor), Los Angeles Children's Hospital, Texas Scottish Rite Hospital (Dallas), and the Children's Hospital Medical Center (Cincinnati). Ninety of these children, including 11 of our original series of 16 (5,6), were considered as having JDMS without evidence of other connective tissue disease according to the strict criteria of Bohan and Peter (7,8). Five children from our original series were excluded, as were 5 others in this study because they had developed features of other connective tissue diseases at various times (4–10 years) following their initial onset of definite juvenile dermatomyositis: e.g., persistent arthritis, Sjögren's syndrome, or scleroderma (5). To qualify for the study, each patient exhibited the typical rash of dermatomyositis and had 3 of 4 of the following additional features: symmetric limb girdle muscle weakness, histologic evidence of myositis demonstrated by muscle biopsy, elevated serum concentration of skeletal muscle enzymes, or electromyographic abnormalities typical of inflammation. Clinical disease activity was determined at the time that the samples were drawn on the basis of muscle weakness/pain and enzyme elevation, in addition to the assessment of cutaneous activity. The age at onset of disease in these patients ranged from 1–21 years, with a mean of 8.0. The mean duration of disease was 4 years. The duration of disease extends from the time of onset to the time that the patients were tested for this study. There were 28 males and 62 females. Sixty-seven of the patients were white, 11 were black, 9 were Latin Americans, 1 was oriental, and 2 were of mixed racial origin.

After obtaining informed consent, interviewing each patient, and reviewing the clinic chart, blood was drawn for serum which was aliquoted and stored at −70°C. At the same time, peripheral blood leukocytes from these subjects were typed for HLA antigens.

Control sera. One hundred five serum samples were obtained in Chicago from blood bank donors, children admitted to the hospital for orthopedic or surgical procedures, health care professionals, and reportedly healthy students entering college. All blood was drawn after informed consent was obtained; the sera were aliquoted and stored at −70°C. These control samples were grouped according to the following age ranges: 0–9 years (39 sera), 10–19 years (41 sera), and 20–29 years (25 sera).

Autoantibody and immune complex studies. All tests except those for antibodies to specific nuclear components were performed in the immunology/rheumatology laboratory of Dr. Pachman at the Children's Memorial Hospital in Chicago. Antibodies to specific nuclear components were assayed in the laboratory of Dr. Gordon Sharp, Columbia, MO.

Immunofluorescence studies. All sera were screened at an initial dilution of 1:20. If positive results were obtained, doubling of dilutions to an endpoint was performed. Antithyroglobulin and antimicrosomal antibodies were studied using monkey thyroid substrate (Zeus Scientific, Raritan, NJ). Fluorescein-conjugated rabbit anti-human IgG (Cappel Laboratories, Cochranville, PA) was used as the indicator serum. Antibody to gastric parietal cells and smooth muscle was measured using rat stomach substrate (Zeus Scientific). Antibody against striated muscle was assayed using both fast and slow muscle from New Zealand white rabbits. The positive control was a serum with known antibody to striated muscle from a patient with myasthenia gravis (kindly provided by BioScience, Van Nuys, CA). Antinuclear antibody (ANA) (9) was initially assessed using human epithelial cells as substrate (Electronucleonics, Bethesda, MD), and confirmed using fresh mouse kidney cells and HEp-2 cells (Immuno Concepts, Sacramento, CA).

Raji cell assay. The Raji cell assay was performed as previously described in detail (10) using both patient and control sera. Internal standards were 3 patients' sera that were known to bind at the low, medium, and high range.

Determination of antibody to specific nuclear components. Extractable nuclear antigen (ENA) preparation, hemagglutination assays for DNA and ENA antibodies, and RNase digestion of ENA-coated tanned red blood cells were performed according to techniques previously detailed (11,12). RNP and Sm antibodies were detected by immunodiffusion (13,14). Antibody to DNA was determined using counterimmunoelectrophoresis (15) and PM-1 (also referred to as PM–Scl) antibody by immunodiffusion as described (16).

HLA typing and data analysis. The patients were typed for HLA–A and HLA–B antigens using a standard 2-stage lymphocyte microcytotoxicity test with NIH sera (17) in the laboratory of one of the authors (OJ). Using sera defining 7 HLA–DR antigens, HLA–DR antigens were determined, in the laboratory of one of the authors (RMR), on peripheral blood B lymphocytes by a minor modification (18) of the microcytotoxicity assay of Terasaki and McClelland (19). These data have previously been reported in detail (2,3).

Family studies. The families of 15 of the Chicago patients were studied intensively. Medical histories with emphasis on immunologic and putative autoimmune diseases were obtained on all first, second, and third-degree relatives. Blood for HLA typing and the serologic studies described above was requested from all parents and siblings of the probands. Thirty parents, 43 full siblings, and 9 half-siblings were tested. None had any history suggestive of JDMS or polymyositis.

Statistical analysis. Correlations between the occurrence of JDMS and various autoantibodies were tested for statistical significance by chi-square analysis, Fisher's exact test, the Mantel-Haenzel test, Welch's approximation of the *t*-test, or by Spearman's rank order coefficient, as appropriate. Differences between groups were considered statistically significant if the probability of observation due to chance alone was <0.05. Data have been grouped for clarity of presentation, but statistics were calculated on ungrouped data.

RESULTS

There was no difference in the frequency of antibody to smooth muscle, thyroglobulin, thyroid microsomes, rheumatoid factor, gastric parietal cells,

Table 1. Autoantibodies in juvenile dermatomyositis patients and control subjects by age group

	Age 0–9		Age 10–19		Age 20–29		Total		
	Patient	Control	Patient	Control	Patient	Control	Patient	Control	*P*
Antithyroid antibody*	0/24†	2/39	2/54	7/41	2/12	0/25	4/90	9/105	NS‡
Antibody to smooth muscle or gastric parietal cells	2/24	2/39	5/54	3/41	0/12	2/25	7/90	7/105	NS
Antimitochondrial	0/24	0/39	1/54	1/41	3/12	0/25	4/90	1/105	NS
Rheumatoid factor	1/23	0/39	0/54	0/41	0/12	0/25	1/89	1/105	NS

* Thyroglobulin or thyroid microsomal.
† Values are no. positive/no. tested.
‡ Not statistically significant using Mantel-Haenszel test.

or mitochondria among JDMS patients and age-matched controls (Table 1). Both control and patient sera bound to rabbit skeletal muscle (21/105 and 20/90, respectively), and in a similar pattern of distribution. However, when antibodies to nuclear components were studied, a highly significant ($P < 0.0002$) increase in ANA positivity was seen among JDMS patients (Table 2). The pattern of ANA at a 1:20 dilution was primarily speckled/granular in the JDMS patients: 17/21 (80%) had this pattern, 1/21 had a rim pattern, and the remaining 3 had both. Of note was that a smaller, but still significantly ($P < 0.05$) increased, number of patients had antibody to PM-1, a calf thymus DNase- and RNase-resistant nuclear antigen (16). Our previous observations (5,20) had suggested than an increase in circulating immune complexes might be present during active disease. In this study, there was a significantly increased ($P < 0.01$) quantity of circulating immune complexes as detected by Raji cell assay among JDMS patients compared with controls (Table 3). No correlations were found between disease activity and either levels of immune complexes or any autoantibody including ANA and PM-1. However, a highly significant association between the level of immune complexes (determined by the Raji assay) and antinuclear antibodies (Table 4) was observed among the JDMS patients ($P < 0.01$).

There was a strong association between the presence of soft tissue calcification and both disease activity ($P < 0.05$, Table 5) and disease duration ($P < 0.001$, Table 6). Soft tissue calcification was not associated with any autoantibody tested, including ANA or PM-1, nor was the presence of immune complexes correlated with calcification.

We had previously found that 25 of the 67 white JDMS patients in the study were positive for the HLA–B8 antigen (2). Nineteen of the 36 white patients tested had HLA–DR3 (3). The frequency of autoantibodies did not differ significantly between the JDMS patients with HLA–B8 or DR3 and those lacking these antigens. Furthermore, there was no association between the presence of soft tissue calcification, disease activity or disease duration, and either HLA antigen among the JDMS patients. Two of these patients had other putative autoimmune diseases: a girl with JDMS, juvenile diabetes mellitus, and recurrent myocarditis

Table 2. Antibody to nuclear antigens in juvenile dermatomyositis patients and control subjects by age group

	Age 0–9		Age 10–19		Age 20–29		Total		
Antibody*	Patient	Control	Patient	Control	Patient	Control	Patient	Control	*P*†
ANA	5/24‡	0/39	14/54	1/40	2/12	2/25	21/90	3/104	<0.0002
DNA	0/19	0/39	1/49	3/39	0/12	0/26	1/80	3/104	NS
ENA	1/19	0/39	1/49	1/39	0/12	0/26	2/80	1/104	NS
RNP	0/22	0/39	0/51	0/40	0/12	0/26	0/85	0/105	NS
Sm	0/21	0/39	0/51	0/40	0/12	0/26	0/84	0/105	NS
PM-1	1/22	0/39	4/51	0/40	1/12	0/26	6/85	0/105	<0.05
Any	6/19	0/30	16/49	5/39	3/12	2/25	25/80	7/94	<0.0005

* ANA = antinuclear antibody; DNA = anti-DNA antibody; ENA = anti–extractable nuclear antigen antibody; RNP = anti-RNP antibody; Sm = anti-Sm antibody; PM-1 = anti–PM-1 antibody; Any = antibody to any nuclear antigen.
† Significance of difference between patients and controls (Mantel-Haenszel test); NS = not significant.
‡ Values are no. positive/no. tested.

Table 3. Circulating immune complexes (μg equivalent of aggregated human IgG) determined by the Raji cell assay*

	n	Mean	SD
Patients	83	162.2	180.5
Controls	103	99.5	120.5

* $t = 2.70$; $P < 0.01$.

(A24,A2,B15,B18,DR3,DR4) and a boy who had rheumatic fever 6 years before he developed JDMS (Aw36,A29,B12).

As reported previously, segregation of HLA haplotypes was normal in unaffected siblings of JDMS patients (2). Studies of 43 full siblings and 30 parents of probands from Chicago did not demonstrate any difference in the incidence of any of the autoantibodies tested when compared with controls. Measurements of immune complexes in sera from family members also fell within normal ranges. Autoimmune disease was identified by taking patient history in 2 siblings and 7 parents of probands with JDMS, but a family history of autoimmune disease was not correlated with the presence of any of the autoantibodies tested in the probands. There was no difference in the frequency of autoimmune disease, autoantibody, or immune complexes measured by Raji cell assay between first-degree relatives of JDMS patients with HLA–B8 or HLA–DR3 and relatives of patients who lacked these antigens.

DISCUSSION

The characteristic clinical presentation of probands with definite juvenile dermatomyositis permits the selection of a relatively homogeneous group of affected children. In the previously reported data from his collaborative study (2,3), we established

Table 4. Association between the presence of immune complexes determined by the Raji assay and antinuclear antibodies in patients with juvenile dermatomyositis

	Antinuclear antibody	
Immune complexes*	Positive	Negative
0–99	4 (24%)†	40 (61%)
100–199	2 (12%)	5 (8%)
200–299	3 (18%)	10 (15%)
300–399	3 (18%)	4 (6%)
400–499	4 (24%)	5 (8%)
≥500	1 (6%)	2 (3%)
Total	17	66

* Microgram equivalent of aggregated human IgG.
† Spearman's rank order correlation coefficient = 0.318 ($P < 0.01$).

Table 5. Association between clinical activity and occurrence of soft tissue calcification in patients with juvenile dermatomyositis*

	Calcification	
Clinical activity	Present	Absent
Definitely active	14 (47%)	20 (34%)
Possibly active	12 (40%)	14 (24%)
Inactive	4 (13%)	25 (42%)
Total	30	59

* Clinical activity based on evidence of proximal muscle weakness, muscle enzyme elevation, and the characteristic rash. Definitely active = present or absent rash, an elevation in serum of muscle-derived enzymes, and definite proximal muscle weakness; possibly active = some muscle weakness, serum levels of muscle-derived enzyme within normal range, present or absent rash; inactive = no physical or laboratory evidence of disease activity. Spearman's rank order correlation = 0.216 ($P < 0.05$).

that the frequency of HLA–B8 and HLA–DR3 is increased in white children with JDMS: for HLA–B8, the relative risk is 2.8 ($P_{corr} < 0.01$), for HLA–DR3, 3.8 ($P_{corr} < 0.01$). These findings suggested that HLA–B8/DR3 (or a gene in tight linkage disequilibrium with HLA–B8/DR3) predisposes to the development of JDMS.

A number of other diseases of complex etiology are associated with HLA–B8/DR3, including dermatitis herpetiformis, celiac disease, myasthenia gravis, Sjögren's syndrome, idiopathic Addison's disease, insulin-dependent diabetes mellitus, and Graves' disease. These diseases all exhibit autoimmune manifestations, including both cellular and humoral dysfunction, raising the speculation that patients bearing the B8/DR3 marker might have a generalized heightened, organ-specific autoimmune response (21,22). Our observation of an increased incidence of HLA–B8/DR3 in JDMS, therefore, raised the possibility that it might be an "autoimmune" disease, and that affected children might exhibit a propensity for developing organ-specific antibody. Support for this hypothesis could be derived from the observation that immunoglobulin and complement components have

Table 6. Association between duration of disease and occurrence of soft tissue calcification in patients with juvenile dermatomyositis*

Disease duration (years)	Calcification	
	Present	Absent
1–4	7 (24%)	44 (73%)
5–9	12 (41%)	11 (18%)
10–14	7 (24%)	3 (5%)
≥15	3 (10%)	2 (3%)
Total	29	60

* Spearman's rank order correlation coefficient = 0.469 ($P < 0.001$).

been identified in the involved small blood vessel wall at the site of muscle damage in patients with JDMS (23,24).

In order to evaluate this hypothesis, we tested sera from a large series of JDMS patients for the presence of antibody directed against various organ and tissue components. Because of the range in age of the subjects and the increased occurrence of autoimmunity with age (25,26), it was necessary to establish frequencies of these autoantibodies in normal individuals of various ages. We found that there was no significant difference between the frequency of reactivity of JDMS and control sera to the organ-specific antigens studied (Table 1). In contrast, when antinuclear antibodies were tested (Table 2), 21/90 JDMS sera were positive compared with only 3/104 controls ($P < 0.0002$). The presence of the positive ANA did not appear to be correlated with the presence of HLA–B8 or DR3 or with disease duration or activity, but was associated with the presence of immune complexes ($P < 0.01$). None of our patients had received β-adrenergic receptor blocking drugs which may be associated with the development of ANA (27). An increased occurrence of ANA positivity among JDMS patients has also been observed by Caspary (28), who found that 9/15 patients were ANA positive in contrast with 0/76 controls and by Sullivan, who found ANA positivity in 8/41 patients with JDMS (29). The sera of adults with polymyositis or dermatomyositis may contain an antinuclear antibody, Jo-1 (30), which has specificity for $tRNA^{His}$ (31) and which appears to occur with increased frequency in those with HLA–DR3 (32).

Immune complexes have been reported in the sera of some children with JDMS (5,18,33). This study provides evidence that they are not correlated with either disease duration or activity, but with the presence of antinuclear antibodies. Previous studies have documented normal levels of complement in JDMS (20), although in polymyositis, low levels have been seen as well (34). We have recently reported increased evidence of complement split products, C3d and C4d, in sera of children with clinically active JDMS, in association with elevated levels of Factor VIII–related antigen, a measure of endothelial cell dysfunction, and fibrinopeptide A, a sensitive measure of intravascular thrombosis (35). This suggests that immune complexes and vascular flow may play a important role in the pathophysiology of JDMS. No correlation of immune complexes was found either with HLA antigens or with soft tissue calcification. Soft tissue calcification seems to be related to disease duration rather than to the presence of any particular antibody in JDMS patients.

In a previous study we did not find an association between HLA antigens and the increased excretion of γ-carboxyglutamic acid (36). There have been no other published reports of HLA antigens and autoantibodies in first-degree relatives of JDMS patients. In an earlier portion of this study, we found no evidence of abnormal segregation of HLA antigens among siblings of patients with JDMS (2). We have now found that even siblings who are HLA–B8/DR3 positive did not have increased frequency of any autoantibody tested.

In several well-established autoimmune diseases, conflicting data have been reported regarding the relationship of the occurrence of specific HLA antigens (usually B8/DR3) and clinical or subclinical evidence of autoimmunity in probands and siblings. In this study, the frequency of overt autoimmune disease in the families of our JDMS patients was not unusually high. Thus, the biologic relationship of HLA–B8/DR3 to the development of autoimmunity in general, or of JDMS in particular, is unclear.

These studies have documented that ANA are positive in 23% of JDMS sera obtained at various time intervals after diagnosis. This is about 8 times greater than expected for children of this age. We have recently reported that sera taken from JDMS patients within 4 months of disease onset have an extraordinarily high frequency of antibody to coxsackie B antigen (37). Of note is that fully 60% of these sera contain an ANA antibody which is coarsely speckled (38), and differs from that seen in polymyositis (39) in that it does not have specificity for $tRNA^{His}$ (31). This observation raises the speculation that the ANA develops in JDMS patients in reaction to an exogenous nucleic acid source, such as a virus. Such viral infection could be related to the pathogenesis of the disease. Further work on this possibility is now in progress.

ACKNOWLEDGMENTS

The authors gratefully acknowledge the superb secretarial assistance of Donna Dickerson and Norma Duarte in the preparation of this manuscript.

REFERENCES

1. Miller ML, Lantner R, Pachman LM: Natural and antibody-dependent cellular cytotoxicity in children with systemic lupus erythematosus and juvenile dermatomyositis. J Rheumatol 10:640–642, 1983

2. Friedman JM, Pachman LM, Maryjowski ML, Radvany RM, Crowe WE, Hanson V, Levinson JE, Spencer CH: Immunogenetic studies of juvenile dermatomyositis: HLA antigen frequencies. Arthritis Rheum 26:214–216, 1983
3. Friedman JM, Pachman LM, Maryjowski ML, Jonasson O, Radvany RM, Battles ND, Crowe WE, Fink CW, Hanson V, Levinson JE, Spencer CH, Sullivan DB: Immunogenetic studies of juvenile dermatomyositis: HLA antigens in patients and their families. Tissue Antigens 21:45–49, 1983
4. Stastny P, Ball EJ, Dry PJ, Nunez G: The human immune response region (HLA-D) and disease susceptibility. Immunol Rev 70:113–153, 1983
5. Pachman LM, Cooke N: Juvenile dermatomyositis: a clinical and immunologic study. J Pediatr 96:226–234, 1980
6. Pachman LM, Jonasson O, Cannon RA, Friedman JM: HLA-B8 in juvenile dermatomyositis. Lancet 2:567–568, 1977
7. Bohan A, Peter JB: Polymyositis and dermatomyositis. N Engl J Med 292:344–347, 1975
8. Bohan A, Peter JB: Polymyositis and dermatomyositis. N Engl J Med 292:403–407, 1975
9. Friou GJ: Clinical application of lupus serum nucleoprotein reaction using the fluorescent antibody technique. J Clin Invest 36:890, 1957
10. Martin CL, Pachman LM: Synovial fluid in seronegative juvenile rheumatoid arthritis: studies of immunoglobulins, complement, and α_2-macroglobulin. Arthritis Rheum 23:1257–1261, 1980
11. Sharp GC, Irvin WS, LaRoque RL, Velez C, Daly V, Kaiser AD, Holman HR: Association of autoantibodies to different nuclear antigens with clinical patterns of rheumatic disease and responsiveness to therapy. J Clin Invest 50:350–359, 1971
12. Sharp GC, Irvin WS, Tan EM, Gould G, Holman HR: Mixed connective tissue disease–an apparently distinct rheumatic disease syndrome associated with a specific antibody to an extractable nuclear antigen (ENA). Am J Med 52:264–272, 1972
13. Norway JD, Tan EM: Differentiations of antinuclear antibodies giving speckled staining patterns in immunofluorescence. Clin Immunol Immunopathol 1:140–154, 1972
14. Sharp GC, Irvin WS, May CM, Holman HR, McDuffie FC, Hess EV, Schmid FR: Association of antibodies to ribonucleoprotein and Sm antigens with mixed connective-tissue disease, systemic lupus erythematosus and other rheumatic diseases. N Engl J Med 295:1149–1154, 1976
15. Kurata N, Tan EM: Identification of antibodies to nuclear acidic antigens by counterimmunoelectrophoresis. Arthritis Rheum 19:574–580, 1976
16. Wolfe JD, Adelstein E, Sharp GC: Antinuclear antibody with distinct specificity for polymyositis. J Clin Invest 59:176–178, 1977
17. National Institute of Arthritis and Infectious Diseases, National Institutes of Health: NIAID Manual of Tissue Typing Techniques, 1976–1977. Bethesda, MD, DHEW #NIH 76-545, 1976
18. Bodner JG, Pickbourne P, Richards S: Ia serology, Histocompatibility Testing. Edited by WF Bodner, JR Batchelor, JG Bodner, H Fertenstein, PS Morris. Munksgaard, Copenhagen, 1977, p 38
19. Terasaki PI, McClelland JD: Microdroplet assay of human serum cytotoxins. Nature 204:998–1000, 1964
20. Pachman LM, Cooke N, Cobb MA: Juvenile dermatomyositis (JDMS): clinical and immunological characterization and evidence of immune complexes (abstract). Clin Res 27:141A, 1979
21. Rose NR, Kong YCM, Sundick RS: The genetic lesions of autoimmunity. Clin Exp Immunol 39:545–550, 1980
22. Aho K: Immunogenetics of rheumatic diseases. Scand J Rheumatol 38:17–23, 1982
23. Whitaker JN, Engel WK: Vascular deposits of immunoglobulin and complement in idiopathic inflammatory myopathy. N Engl J Med 286:330–338, 1972
24. Crowe WE, Bove KE, Levinson JE, Hilton PK: Clinical and pathogenic implications of histopathology in childhood polydermatomyositis. Arthritis Rheum 25:126–139, 1982
25. Andersen I, Andersen P, Graudal H: Smooth-muscle antibodies in rheumatoid arthritis. Acta Pathol Microbiol Immunol [C] Scand 88:131–135, 1980
26. Svec KH, Veit BC: Age-related antinuclear factors: immunologic characteristics and associated clinical aspects. Arthritis Rheum 10:509–516, 1967
27. Booth RJ, Wilson JD, Bullock JY: Beta-adrenergic-receptor blockers and antinuclear antibodies in hypertension. Clin Pharmacol Ther 31:555–558, 1982
28. Caspary EA, Gubbay SS, Stern GM: Circulating antibodies in polymyositis and other muscle-wasting disorders. Lancet 1:941, 1964
29. Sullivan DB, Cassidy JT, Petty RE: Dermatomyositis in the pediatric patient. Arthritis Rheum 20:327–331, 1977
30. Reichlin M, Mattioli M: Description of a serological reaction characteristic of polymyositis. Clin Immunol Immunopathol 5:12–20, 1976
31. Rosa MD, Hendrick JP, Lerner MR, Steitz JA: A mammalian $tRNA^{His}$ containing antigen is recognized by the polymyositis-specific antibody anti-Jo-1. Nucleic Acids Res 11:853–870, 1983
32. Arnett FC, Hirsch TJ, Bias WB, Nishikai M, Reichlin M: The Jo-1 antibody system in myositis: relationships to clinical features and HLA. J Rheumatol 8:925–930, 1981
33. Spencer CH, Jordan SC, Hanson V: Circulating immune complexes in juvenile dermatomyositis (abstract). Arthritis Rheum 23:750, 1980
34. Behan WMH, Barkas T, Behan PO: Detection of immune complexes in polymyositis. Acta Neurol Scand 65:320–334, 1982
35. Pachman LM, Scott JP, Arroyave CM, Maryjowski ML:

Juvenile dermatomyositis (JDMS): activation of coagulation and complement systems (abstract). Clin Res 31:796A, 1983
36. Lian JB, Pachman LM, Gundberg CM, Partridge REH, Maryjowski ML: Gamma-carboxyglutamate excretion and calcinosis in juvenile dermatomyositis. Arthritis Rheum 25:1094–1100, 1982
37. Pachman LM, Christensen ML, Scott JP, Arroyave CM, Friedman JM, Maryjowski ML: Active juvenile dermatomyositis is associated with complement and coagulation activation, and increased titers to antinuclear and coxsackie B viral antigens (abstract). Pediatr Res 18:262a, 1984
38. Pachman LM, Hardin JA, Cobb MA, Arroyave CM: The antinuclear antibody in juvenile dermatomyositis is not Jo-1, suggesting that JDMS and polymyositis are different diseases (abstract). Arthritis Rheum (suppl) 27:S45, 1984

THE DIAGNOSTIC VALUE OF ANTIHISTONE ANTIBODIES IN DRUG-INDUCED LUPUS ERYTHEMATOSUS

ALAN EPSTEIN and PETER BARLAND

This study was undertaken to see whether the presence of antihistone antibodies, measured by indirect immunofluorescence assay, could distinguish between patients who were symptomatic from a drug-induced lupus-like illness (DILE) and asymptomatic patients who had drug-induced antinuclear antibodies (DANA). In this study, 82% of the patients with DILE had antihistone antibodies detectable in their sera, compared with 32% of the patients in the DANA group ($P < 0.01$). When the patients taking procainamide were analyzed separately, it was found that 92% of the patients with DILE had demonstrable antihistone antibodies, contrasted with 33% of the patients in the DANA group ($P < 0.01$). In those patients with antihistone antibodies (DILE versus DANA patients), there were no differences in the mean antibody titers. We conclude that the presence of antihistone antibodies is strong, statistically significant evidence that the symptoms of a given patient are due to drug-induced lupus erythematosus.

It is well known that antinuclear antibodies (ANA) can be detected in the sera of patients with a variety of rheumatic disorders. Moreover, antibodies with different antigenic specificities have been found to characterize specific diseases. Examples of this include the presence of antibodies to native DNA and the Sm antigen in systemic lupus erythematosus (SLE) (1), antibodies to ribonucleoprotein in mixed connective tissue disease (2), and the SS-A and SS-B antibodies in primary Sjögren's syndrome (3).

Convincing evidence that drugs can induce a lupus-like syndrome de novo in individuals not otherwise predisposed to develop it began appearing in the literature in 1953, after the introduction of hydralazine for the treatment of hypertension (4). Prospective studies confirming the ability of a drug to induce a lupus-like syndrome have also been reported for procainamide (5) and isoniazid (6). In addition, many other drugs have been suspected of inducing a lupus-like syndrome (based on small series and case reports, reviewed elsewhere [7]). While a significant percentage of patients taking procainamide (8) or hydralazine (9) develop serum antinuclear antibodies, a relatively small percentage of these patients manifest clinical evidence of a lupus-like illness.

Recently, there has been an increasing awareness of the role of antihistone antibodies as a marker for clinically significant drug-induced lupus erythematosus (10,11). There have not been many studies, however, on antihistone antibodies in the sera of asymptomatic patients with drug-induced antinuclear antibodies (10). We undertook this study to see whether the presence of antihistone antibodies in the sera of patients with ANA secondary to drug treatment could distinguish those patients symptomatic due to a lupus-like illness (DILE) from asymptomatic patients having drug-induced antinuclear antibodies (DANA). The results of such a study might shed some light on the immunopathogenic process involved in drug-induced lupus erythematosus and clarify the diagnostic implications of a positive test result for antihistone antibod-

From the Rheumatology Division, Department of Medicine, Montefiore Medical Center, Albert Einstein College of Medicine, Bronx, New York.

Supported in part by a grant from the New York Chapter of the Arthritis Foundation.

Alan Epstein, MD; Peter Barland, MD.

Address reprint requests to Peter Barland, MD, Montefiore Medical Center, 111 East 210 Street, Bronx, NY 10467.

Submitted for publication October 4, 1983; accepted in revised form September 13, 1984.

ies. We found that although the presence of antihistone antibodies is not absolutely discriminating, their presence remains strong, statistically significant evidence that a patient's symptoms are due to drug-induced lupus erythematosus.

PATIENTS AND METHODS

Patient selection. Clinical information was sought on patients whose sera were sent for antihistone antibody testing to the Immunodiagnostic Laboratory at Montefiore Medical Center during 1981 and 1982. All patients were included in the study except under the following conditions: 1) clinical history was unavailable; 2) the patient had a history of DILE which had resolved at the time the specimen was drawn; 3) the patient had SLE; 4) the routine testing of the specimen for ANA gave negative results.

The clinical data on each patient were thoroughly reviewed by a physician (AE) who was unaware of the results of the antihistone antibody testing. A diagnosis of DILE was made if a patient who was taking a drug known to cause this syndrome manifested 1 or both of the following criteria: 1) arthritis that remitted promptly after discontinuation of the offending drug or that remitted after institution of antiinflammatory therapy without recurrence when the treatment was stopped; 2) pleuritis and/or pericarditis that remitted promptly after discontinuation of the offending drug or that remitted after institution of antiinflammatory therapy without recurrence when the treatment was stopped. The presence of fever, anemia, or thrombocytopenia related to drug administration, though frequently observed, was not considered in making a diagnosis of DILE.

Those patients not fulfilling the criteria for DILE, but who were taking a drug capable of causing DILE and whose test for ANA was positive, were assigned to the DANA group. A small number of patients were excluded from statistical analysis because there was insufficient retrospective data available to make a valid diagnosis. In no instance was a patient's diagnosis changed after the result of the antihistone antibody test was known. Most of the patients ultimately judged not to have DILE did, in fact, have some symptom(s) compatible with this diagnosis. These patients were not completely asymptomatic. Finally, each patient's clinical diagnosis was correlated with the result of the antihistone antibody testing.

Antihistone antibody assay. An indirect immunofluorescent antibody assay technique was used as previously described (11). The assay was based on the ability to extract many nuclear proteins, including histones, from acetone-fixed mouse kidney sections, using 0.1*N* HCl. This treatment does not remove, but may partially denature, the DNA (12). Acid extraction was performed by gently agitating fixed mouse kidney sections in 0.1*N* HCl for 30 minutes at 24°C. The sections were then washed with 0.01*M* phosphate buffered saline (PBS), pH 7.3. Histone reconstitution was performed by incubating the acid-extracted sections in 25 μg/ml histone followed by washing with PBS.

Histones were purchased from Worthington Biochemical Corporation (Freehold, NJ) and were the H-2A fraction. We used this fraction because of its high reactivity with drug-induced lupus sera, as reported by Fritzler and Tan (11). The method of isolation used by Worthington involved sequential extraction and precipitation of calf thymus with ethanol/1.25*N* HCl (4:1 volume:volume) and, later, with 95% ethanol (13). The reconstituted sections were then used as substrates in an indirect ANA assay. Antihistone antibodies were present if the following conditions were satisfied: 1) a greater than twofold fall in the ANA titer after acid extraction of the kidney substrate, and 2) a greater than twofold return of the activity after histone reconstitution.

RESULTS

Eighteen patients met our criteria for the diagnosis of drug-induced lupus erythematosus; 4 patients met both criteria, while the remaining 14 met a single criterion. There were 7 females and 11 males, ranging in age from 7–81 years. The drugs believed to be the causative agents were procainamide in 13 patients, hydralazine in 1, penicillamine in 1, diphenylhydantoin in 1, disopyramide in 1, and ethosuximide in 1 patient. The symptoms, physical findings, and results of routine laboratory investigations of these patients are enumerated in Table 1. Steroids were used in 7 patients.

Twenty-eight patients were diagnosed as having DANA. There were 17 females and 11 males, ranging in age from 36–86 years. The suspected drugs in these patients were procainamide in 12 patients, hydralazine in 10, methyldopa in 1, disopyramide in 1, quinidine in 2, penicillamine in 1, and diphenylhydantoin in 1 patient. These patients either had no symptoms suggestive of lupus erythematosus or had symptoms that were easily explained by another, clearly evident, disease process.

Eight patients were excluded from statistical analysis because there was insufficient retrospective data available to make a valid diagnosis.

When the results of the antihistone antibody testing were examined, we found that 83% of the patients in the drug-induced lupus erythematosus group showed positive results, compared with 32% of the patients in the DANA group ($P < 0.01$). Of the 18 patients in the DANA group who did not have demonstrable antihistone antibodies, 16 had antibodies to an extractable nuclear antigen.

We then tried to find a measurement that would further discriminate between antihistone antibody–positive patients in each group. We examined 2 measurements: 1) the mean of the reciprocal of the log of the antihistone antibody titer in each group, and 2) the amount of reconstitution. There was no statistically significant difference between the 2 groups in either of these measurements (Table 2).

Table 1. Clinical and laboratory features (routine testing) of 18 patients with drug-induced lupus erythematosus*

Clinical feature	n	Laboratory feature	n
Fever	13	Elevated ESR	10
Constitutional symptoms	7	Anemia	7
Arthralgias	9	Leukopenia	0
Arthritis	9	Thrombocytopenia	1
Myalgias	1	Hypergammaglobulinemia	2
Skin rash	2	Positive Coombs' test	3
Malar rash	0	False-positive VDRL	0
Oral ulcers	0	Circulating anticoagulant	1
Alopecia	0		
Pleuropericarditis	13		
Pulmonary infiltrate	1		
Renal involvement	1		
Hepatomegaly	1		
Splenomegaly	1		
Lymphadenopathy	1		
Mononeuritis multiplex	0		

* Not all laboratory tests were available on every patient. ESR = erythrocyte sedimentation rate.

During the course of our study, we became aware of some new observations reported by Portanova et al (14), indicating that the immunofluorescence histone reconstitution assay detects only antihistone antibodies directed against the histone 2A-2B (H-2A–H-2B) fraction. These investigators had also compared the antihistone antibodies found in patients with DILE induced by procainamide with those found in patients with DILE induced by hydralazine. They found that most of their patients with DILE secondary to procainamide treatment developed antibodies to the H-2A–H-2B fraction, detectable by a radioimmunoassay. These same sera were also positive on immunofluorescence assay using total histones for reconstitution. The patients with DILE due to hydralazine treatment did not develop antibodies to the H-2A–H-2B fraction and were negative for antihistone antibodies by immunofluorescence assay. There is no literature on the specificity of the antihistone antibodies induced by other drugs. For these reasons we analyzed separately our patients who were taking procainamide. It was found that of the 13 patients with DILE caused by procainamide, 12 (92%) had demonstrable antihistone antibodies. By contrast, of the 12 procainamide-treated patients in the DANA group, only 4 (33%) had antihistone antibodies ($P < 0.01$ by Fisher's exact test).

DISCUSSION

In a previous study from this laboratory (10), antihistone antibodies were measured in a group of patients with drug-induced lupus erythematosus and in asymptomatic patients with drug-induced antinuclear antibodies, using an indirect immunofluorescence assay and acid-extracted, histone-reconstituted mouse kidney sections as substrate. It was found that 67% of the patients with DILE had antihistone antibodies as the major, or the only, ANA in their sera, but these

Table 2. Results of antihistone antibody (AHA) testing*

	Diagnosis		
	DILE	DANA	P
No. AHA-positive/no. with diagnosis	15/18 (83%)	9/28 (32%)	<0.01
Mean $\frac{1}{\text{log AHA}}$	9.06	7.50	NS
Amount of reconstitution	4.53	5.40	NS

* DILE = drug-induced lupus-like illness; DANA = drug-induced antinuclear antibody. P value calculated using Fisher's exact test. NS = not significant. Amount of reconstitution calculated as:

$$\frac{1}{\text{log AHA after reconstitution}} - \frac{1}{\text{log AHA after extraction}}$$

antibodies were not seen in the sera from patients with DANA.

The present study was undertaken for 2 reasons. First, the original study involved only a small number of patients. Subsequently, we have observed that an occasional patient with DANA has detectable serum antihistone antibodies. Second, the original group of DANA patients was completely asymptomatic, whereas in the present study, most of the DANA patients showed some symptoms that caused us to consider drug-induced lupus erythematosus as a possible explanation. Such patients represent a more important diagnostic group. The present study does not include any of the patients from the original series.

The data from this study show that the majority of patients with drug-induced lupus erythematosus have antihistone antibodies, which is in general agreement with our original study (10) and the study by Fritzler and Tan (11). In this study, 83% of the patients had antihistone antibodies, compared with 67% in the original study and 96% in the series reported by Fritzler and Tan. The present study differs from the original series in that antihistone antibodies were found in the sera of 32% of the patients in the DANA group. This further contrasts with the original series data showing a complete absence of antihistone antibodies in the 12 asymptomatic patients who were tested. Therefore, one can conclude that, although the presence of antihistone antibodies is not absolutely discriminating, as suggested by our original series, it nevertheless remains strong, statistically significant evidence that a given patient's symptoms are due to drug-induced lupus erythematosus.

The studies of Portanova et al (14) indicate that patients with drug-induced lupus erythematosus caused by procainamide develop antibodies to the histone 2A-2B fraction. This histone complex also appears to be the antigenic component reacting in the immunofluorescence assay. We therefore analyzed separately our patients who were taking procainamide. Again, there was a statistically significant, but not absolute, difference in the frequency of antihistone antibodies between the DILE and DANA groups.

The clinical features of these patients were similar to those previously reported (15,16); 2 features deserve special comment. First, the high incidence of pleuropericardial involvement in the DILE patients probably reflects the fact that 13 of the 18 patients in this group were taking procainamide, which has been reported to show a propensity for causing pleuropericarditis (15,17). Second, an elevated erythrocyte sedimentation rate was frequently found in those patients who were ultimately judged as having DILE.

These results, as well as the results of previously reported studies (10,11), indicate that antihistone antibodies account for a large part of the ANA activity in patients with DILE. The antigenic specificity of the ANA activity in patients with DANA remains undefined. Previous studies, using sera from patients with DANA, failed to reveal precipitating antibody activity toward a crude rabbit thymus nuclear extract containing a number of nonhistone nuclear antigens, including Sm, RNP, and La (10). Several observations lead us to believe that the ANA activity in these patients is probably also directed toward a histone component, but that these antibodies differ qualitatively from those found in patients with DILE. Among the patients who were antihistone antibody–positive, there was no significant difference in the mean titers between the 9 patients with DANA and the 15 patients with DILE. These results would argue against a simple quantitative difference between the 2 groups.

A recent study by Portanova et al described a group of patients receiving hydralazine whose ANA activity, by immunofluorescence assay, was lost after acid extraction of the mouse kidney section, but could not be restored by histone reconstitution. When these sera were tested for antihistone antibodies, using a radioimmunoassay, all were positive. The explanation for this discrepancy appeared to be that the immunofluorescence assay, which uses histone-reconstituted nuclei, is selective for antihistone antibodies that react with a mixture of histones 2A and 2B. The low levels of anti–(H-2A–H-2B) activity in the sera of patients taking hydralazine appeared to account for the failure of most, but not all, of the sera to react in the immunofluorescence assay.

It should be noted that the same pattern of reactivity on immunofluorescence assay that Portanova reported for hydralazine-treated patients was also observed in 16 of our 18 DANA patients who were antihistone antibody–negative on immunofluorescence assay. These data could be taken to suggest that many of the patients in the DANA group had antibodies to histone fractions other than the H-2A–H-2B mixture. Preliminary investigations in our laboratory, using an enzyme-linked immunosorbent assay technique to detect antihistone antibodies, have shown that most of our DANA patients do indeed have antihistone antibody titers comparable with those found in the DILE patients. Currently, we are further defining the antigenic specificity of these antibodies.

ACKNOWLEDGMENTS

We gratefully acknowledge the critical advice of Dr. Mark Burns and Dr. Arthur Grayzel, the excellent technical assistance of June Arias, and the expert assistance of Lynne Enoch in the preparation of the manuscript.

REFERENCES

1. Notman DD, Kurata MD, Tan EM: Profiles of antinuclear antibodies in systemic rheumatic diseases. Ann Intern Med 83:464–469, 1975
2. Sharp GC, Irvin WD, Tan EM, Gould RG, Holman HR: Mixed connective tissue disease: an apparently distinct rheumatic disease syndrome associated with specific antibody to an extractable nuclear antigen (ENA). Am J Med 52:148–159, 1972
3. Alspaugh MA, Talal N, Tan EM: Differentiation and characterization of autoantibodies and their antigens in Sjögren's syndrome. Arthritis Rheum 19:216–222, 1976
4. Morrow JD, Schroeder HA, Perry HM Jr: Studies on the control of hypertension by Hyphex. II. Toxic reactions and side effects. Circulation 8:829–839, 1953
5. Fakhro AM, Ritchie RF, Lown B: Lupus-like syndrome induced by procainamide. Am J Cardiol 20:367–373, 1967
6. Rothfield NF, Bierer WF, Garfield JW: Isoniazid induction of antinuclear antibodies: a prospective study. Ann Intern Med 88:650–652, 1978
7. Lee SC, Chase PH: Drug-induced systemic lupus erythematosus: a critical review. Semin Arthritis Rheum 5:83–103, 1975
8. Blomgren SE, Condemi JJ, Bignall MC, Vaughan JH: Antinuclear antibody induced by procainamide: a prospective study. N Engl J Med 281:64–66, 1969
9. Perry HM Jr, Tan EM, Carmody S, Sakamoto A: Relationship of acetyl transferase activity to antinuclear antibodies and toxic symptoms in hypertensive patients treated with hydralazine. J Lab Clin Med 76:114–125, 1970
10. Grossman L, Barland P: Histone reactivity of drug-induced antinuclear antibodies: a comparison of symptomatic and asymptomatic patients. Arthritis Rheum 24:927–931, 1981
11. Fritzler MJ, Tan EM: Antibodies to histones in drug-induced and idiopathic lupus erythematosus. J Clin Invest 62:560–567, 1978
12. Tan EM, Robinson J, Robitaille P: Studies on antibodies to histones by immunofluorescence. Scand J Immunol 5:811–817, 1976
13. Jones EW: Preparative methods for histone fractions from calf thymus. Biochem J 92:55–59, 1964
14. Portanova JP, Rubin RL, Joslin FG, Agnello VD, Tan EM: Reactivity of anti-histone antibodies induced by procainamide and hydralazine. Clin Immunol Immunopathol 25:67–79, 1982
15. Blomgren SE, Condemi JJ, Vaughan JH: Procainamide-induced lupus erythematosus: clinical and laboratory observations. Am J Med 52:338–348, 1976
16. Alarcon-Segovia D, Wakim KG, Worthington JW, Ward LE: Clinical and experimental studies on the hydralazine syndrome and its relationship to systemic lupus erythematosus. Medicine (Baltimore) 46:1–33, 1967
17. Byrd RB, Schanzer B: Pulmonary sequelae in procaine amide induced lupus-like syndrome. Dis Chest 55:170–172, 1969

THE BINDING OF ANTIHISTONE ANTIBODIES TO *CRITHIDIA LUCILIAE* KINETOPLASTS IS GROWTH CYCLE–DEPENDENT

JAU-SHYONG DENG, RICHARD D. SONTHEIMER, MARY F. LIPSCOMB, and JAMES N. GILLIAM

The *Crithidia luciliae* immunofluorescence (CLIF) assay is widely used to test for native DNA (nDNA) antibodies in the diagnosis and management of systemic lupus erythematosus. However, sera from patients with drug-induced lupus erythematosus or rheumatoid arthritis, which should not contain nDNA antibodies, occasionally react with the CL kinetoplast. We examined 36 sera from patients with systemic lupus erythematosus, rheumatoid arthritis, Sjögren's syndrome, and drug-induced lupus erythematosus, who had positive CLIF tests. All 36 sera were also antinuclear antibody–positive with homogeneous and/or peripheral staining patterns on mouse kidney substrates. After hydrochloric acid extraction of the CL smears to remove histone and other nuclear protein antigens, 14 of the 36 sera no longer produced a positive result on the CLIF test. Ten of these 14 sera again gave a positive CLIF result after the hydrochloric acid–extracted *Crithidia* substrate had been reconstituted with purified histone. These studies demonstrated that kinetoplast binding was due to antihistone antibodies in at least 10 of 36 initially CLIF-positive sera. Antihistone antibodies were then purified with a histone-affinity column, and these purified antibodies were reactive with CL kinetoplasts. Thus, the CLIF test is not specific for nDNA antibodies. Additional studies using CL from different days of culture indicated that histone antigen expression in the CL kinetoplast was a function of the life cycle of this organism and is most readily detected 2 days after initiation of culture.

Crithidia luciliae (CL) was introduced by Aarden and associates in 1975 as a substrate for the detection of anti–native DNA antibodies (anti-nDNA) by indirect immunofluorescence (1). The *Crithidia luciliae* immunofluorescence (CLIF) test is currently recognized as being one of the most convenient tests for anti-nDNA, and as such, is used widely in the diagnosis and management of patients with systemic lupus erythematosus (SLE). The CLIF test is simple, reliable, inexpensive, and has been thought to be specific for anti-nDNA (1–11). Results with CLIF tests have been comparable with those obtained from other tests, such as the Farr or millipore filter assays (1,5,6,8–11). However, sera from patients with drug-induced lupus erythematosus (LE), rheumatoid arthritis, or scleroderma occasionally produce a positive result on the CLIF test (1,5,6,8,9).

Recently, data from our laboratory demonstrated that antihistone antibodies purified from sera of patients with drug-induced LE or rheumatoid arthritis could bind to kinetoplasts (12,13). These studies were extended by analyzing additional patients' sera, and it was noted that some sera reacted variably from one batch of *Crithidia* slides to another. Some of this variation was related to the commercial source of the

Presented at the Annual Meeting of the American Federation for Clinical Research, Washington, DC, May 1984.

From the Departments of Dermatology, Internal Medicine, and Pathology, University of Texas Health Science Center at Dallas, Southwestern Medical School, Dallas, Texas.

Supported in part by NIH grants AM00730, AM19101, and AI17363.

Jau-Shyong Deng, MD: Department of Dermatology (current address: Department of Dermatology, University of Pittsburgh School of Medicine, Pittsburgh, PA 15243); Richard D. Sontheimer, MD: Departments of Dermatology and Internal Medicine; Mary F. Lipscomb, MD: Department of Pathology.

Dr. Gilliam is deceased.

Address reprint requests to Richard D. Sontheimer, MD, University of Texas Health Science Center, 5323 Harry Hines Boulevard, Dallas, TX 75235.

Submitted for publication April 23, 1984; accepted in revised form August 13, 1984.

C luciliae substrate. This raised the question of whether growth kinetics of the organism might influence performance in the CLIF test. In this report, evidence is presented which strongly suggests that growth kinetics play an important role in the variability in responses to the CLIF test and are at least partially responsible for the kinetoplast staining by antihistone antibodies.

PATIENTS AND METHODS

Sera. Sera were obtained from patients being evaluated for a wide variety of conditions including connective tissue diseases. All were patients of the Dermatology Outpatient Clinic, the Rheumatology Outpatient Clinic, or the inpatient service of Parkland Memorial Hospital, Dallas, Texas. Over 700 samples were screened for the presence of antinuclear antibodies (ANA) on mouse kidney sections and human HEp-2 cell substrates. Thirty-six were positive for kinetoplast staining with the CLIF test. These 36 samples were included in the subsequent studies, and the patients' diagnoses are listed in Table 1. The diagnoses were made by standard clinical criteria and fulfilled the appropriate American Rheumatism Association criteria for classification (14).

Detection of antinuclear antibodies. ANA were detected by indirect immunofluorescence using 3-μm snap-frozen mouse kidney cryostat sections and human HEp-2 tissue culture cells as previously described (12,13).

Growth kinetics of *Crithidia luciliae*. *C luciliae* was obtained from American Type Culture Collection (Rockville, MD) and inoculated into the recommended culture medium. The cultures were loosely capped, shielded from light, incubated at room temperature for 48–72 hours, and then subcultured at a concentration of 5×10^5 organisms/ml. After subculture, viability determinations were performed daily for 7 days. Viability of the organisms was determined by the percentage of the organisms that were mobile in suspension under the microscope. Organisms from 2-, 4-, and 7-day cultures were harvested, washed in phosphate buffered saline (PBS), and adjusted to a concentration of 20 $\times 10^6$ organisms/ml in PBS. Ten microliters of the suspension was placed on clean glass slides, air-dried, fixed in methanol for 15 minutes at room temperature, kept in a −20°C freezer, and used within 2 months of preparation.

Table 1. Effect of hydrochloric acid extraction on antibody binding to the *Crithidia luciliae* kinetoplast

Diagnosis	Number of patients	Effect of HCl extraction: Positive (group 1)*	Effect of HCl extraction: Negative (group 2)†
Systemic lupus erythematosus	28	22	6
Rheumatoid arthritis	2	0	2
Sjögren's syndrome	2	0	2
Drug-induced lupus erythematosus	4	0	4

* Positive = presence of antibody bound to kinetoplast.
† Negative = absence of antibody bound to kinetoplast.

***Crithidia luciliae* indirect immunofluorescence.** The CLIF assay was performed as described previously (7,12,13). The fluorescein isothiocyanate (FITC)–labeled goat anti-human gamma globulin used had the following characteristics: FITC concentration of 56 μg/ml, protein concentration of 10 mg/ml, and optimal conjugate dilution of 1:20, based on chessboard titrations using the conjugate and 2 reference sera containing ANA of homogeneous and speckled patterns.

Hydrochloric acid extraction of *C luciliae* and mouse kidney sections. *Crithidia* smears and mouse kidney sections were treated with 0.1*N* HCl solution for 30 minutes at room temperature before use. HCl extraction (0.1*N*) has been shown to remove histone and other non-histone nuclear proteins from nuclei without extracting DNA (15,16). After extraction, the slides and smears were rinsed and washed in PBS twice for 10 minutes. The HCl-extracted smears were then separated into 2 groups. One group was reconstituted with purified histone (containing H-2A, H-2B, H-3, and H-4) (Calbiochem-Behring, La Jolla, CA). Both groups were then used as substrates for subsequent indirect immunofluorescence.

Demonstration of antihistone antibodies. Histone antibodies were assayed by indirect immunofluorescence using histone-reconstituted kidney sections and *C luciliae* smears as described previously. The kidney sections and *C luciliae* smears were pretreated as above. The pretreated sections and smears were incubated in a solution containing 25 μg/ml purified histone for 30 minutes at room temperature. The histone-reconstituted sections or smears were washed in PBS and then used as substrates for histone antibodies by indirect immunofluorescence (12,13,15,16).

Detection of anti-nDNA using Farr assay. The anti-nDNA kit (Amersham, Arlington Heights, IL) was used to detect the anti-nDNA. The procedure suggested by the vendor was followed exactly.

Isolation of specific antihistone antibodies. A histone-coated affinity column was used to isolate specific antihistone antibodies as previously described (13). Specific antihistone antibodies were isolated from the sera of 3 patients: 1 with SLE, 1 with rheumatoid arthritis, and 1 with drug-induced LE. Two of these patients have been reported earlier (12,13). The specific antihistone antibodies were used to stain untreated, HCl-extracted, and histone-reconstituted mouse kidney sections and *C luciliae* smears. The presence of immunoglobulin(s) in the eluate was determined by immunoelectrophoresis.

Controls in the indirect immunofluorescence. Normal human sera and sera containing anti-nDNA and antihistone antibodies were used as controls in indirect immunofluorescence. Normal human sera did not stain kinetoplasts, mouse kidney sections, or HEp-2 cells, whether these substrates were treated with HCl only or treated with HCl and reconstituted with histone. The known antihistone antibody–positive sera were used to verify positive staining of histone-reconstituted mouse kidney sections. Anti-nDNA control sera stained untreated, HCl-extracted, or histone-reconstituted mouse kidney sections and *C luciliae* smears. The titers obtained remained within a twofold difference for each of the substrates, regardless of the treatment. The same anti-nDNA control sera were also used to stain the *Crithidia*

Table 2. Relationship between *Crithidia luciliae* and Farr anti–native DNA (anti–nDNA) assay results

	Farr anti-nDNA assay		
Serum group*	>30 units	20–30 units	<20 units
Group 1 (22 patients)	18†	0	4‡
Group 2 (14 patients)	0	4§	10§

* Group 1 = presence of antibody bound to *C luciliae* kinetoplast after HCl extraction; group 2 = absence of antibody bound to *C luciliae* kinetoplast after HCl extraction.
† Titer on untreated *C luciliae* substrate >1:80.
‡ Titer on untreated *C luciliae* substrate <1:40.
§ Titer on untreated *C luciliae* substrate <1:80.

substrates from different stages of growth, and they also gave consistent results.

RESULTS

Histone antibody staining of *C luciliae* kinetoplasts. Over 700 serum samples, each from a different patient, were screened for the presence of ANA and anti-nDNA on mouse kidney sections, human HEp-2 cells, and *C luciliae* smears. Seventy samples gave a homogeneous and/or peripheral nuclear staining pattern on both mouse kidney sections and human HEp-2 cells. Of these 70 samples, 36 were positive for kinetoplast staining on *C luciliae* substrate by indirect immunofluorescence. The 36 serum samples were then tested on *C luciliae* extracted with 0.1*N* HCl. Twenty-two samples remained positive on the HCl-treated *C luciliae* smears. Results of the staining on HCl-extracted *C luciliae* are shown in Table 1. All 22 samples which gave positive staining on HCl-treated *C luciliae* smears (group 1) were from patients with SLE. When histone was added back to the HCl-extracted *C luciliae* smears, these 22 samples remained positive on the histone-reconstituted preparations. Fourteen sera gave negative results on the HCl-extracted *C luciliae* substrate (group 2). Eleven of these 14 sera were positive on histone-reconstituted kidney sections. Ten of these 14 samples also stained the histone-reconstituted HCl-extracted *C luciliae*. Thus, at least 10 of the 36 CLIF-positive samples contained antihistone antibodies, rather than DNA antibodies.

All 36 samples that were positive in the CLIF test were screened for the presence of anti-nDNA using the Farr assay, and results are shown in Table 2. None of the 14 sera in group 2 had significant activity (>30 units) in the Farr assay. This finding suggested that positive kinetoplast staining in the 14 sera in group 2 was not due to anti-nDNA, but to histone or other non-nDNA antibodies.

Histone antibodies were purified from the sera of 3 different patients, 1 with drug-induced LE (patient 1 in Table 3), 1 with rheumatoid arthritis (patient 2 in Table 3), and 1 with SLE (patient 3 in Table 3). Patients 1 and 2 have been described previously (12, 13). The purified histone antibodies were used to stain *C luciliae* smears and mouse kidney sections, and the results are shown in Table 3. The histone antibodies purified from these 3 sera bound to *C luciliae* kinetoplasts, but not HCl-extracted kinetoplasts. They also reacted with kinetoplasts of histone-reconstituted *C luciliae*. However, not all of the *C luciliae* in each smear were positive for kinetoplast staining, as shown

Table 3. Comparison of the antibody binding activity on different substrates of original sera, drop-through fractions from histone-affinity columns, and specific histone antibody fractions*

	Patient 1			Patient 2			Patient 3		
Substrate	Original	Drop-through	Specific antibody	Original	Drop-through	Specific antibody	Original	Drop-through	Specific antibody
Kidney									
Untreated	1,280	640	160	640	160	80	1,280	640	16
HCl-treated	<10	<10	<10	<10	<10	<10	160	160	<2
Histone reconstituted	1,280	160	160	640	<10	80	640	320	16
Crithidia									
Untreated	80	<10	20	40	<10	10	320	160	2
HCl-treated	<10	<10	<10	<10	<10	<10	160	160	<2
Histone reconstituted	10	<10	10	10	<10	10	320	160	1

* Values shown are the reciprocal of the antibody titer on the given substrate. Patient 1 had drug-induced lupus erythematosus and slightly elevated levels of antibody against single-stranded DNA. Patient 2 had rheumatoid arthritis and did not have antibody against single-stranded DNA. Patient 3 had systemic lupus erythematosus; this patient had anti–native DNA based on the Farr assay and also had anti–single-stranded DNA.

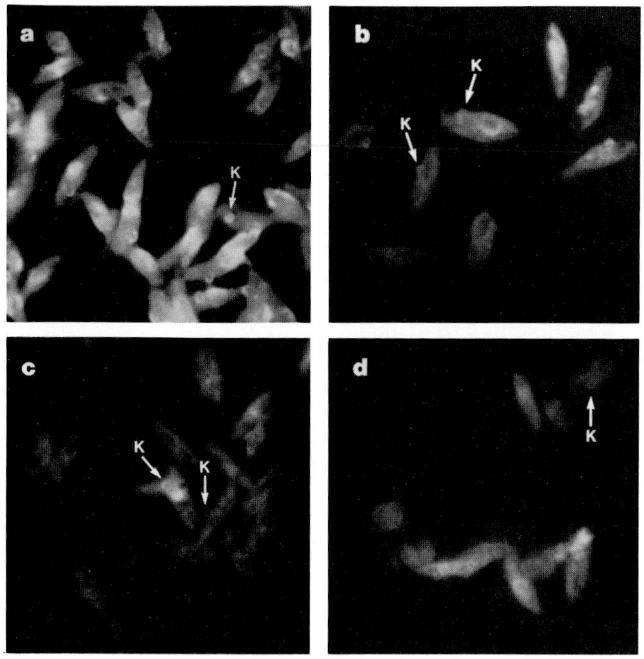

Figure 1. Kinetoplast (**K**) staining in the *Crithidia luciliae* immunofluorescence test. Specific histone antibodies purified from a histone-affinity column were used to stain *C luciliae* at different stages of growth. **a**, Kinetoplast staining on a *C luciliae* smear (2–3-day-old culture) prepared in the standard manner. **b**, Kinetoplast staining on a smear from a 2-day-old culture. **c**, Staining from a 4-day-old culture smear. **d**, Staining from a 7-day-old culture smear. Note the decreasing staining intensity and the decreased number of kinetoplasts stained as the cultures aged. There is background staining of the cytoplasm of the organisms due to Evans blue counterstaining (original magnification × 2,000).

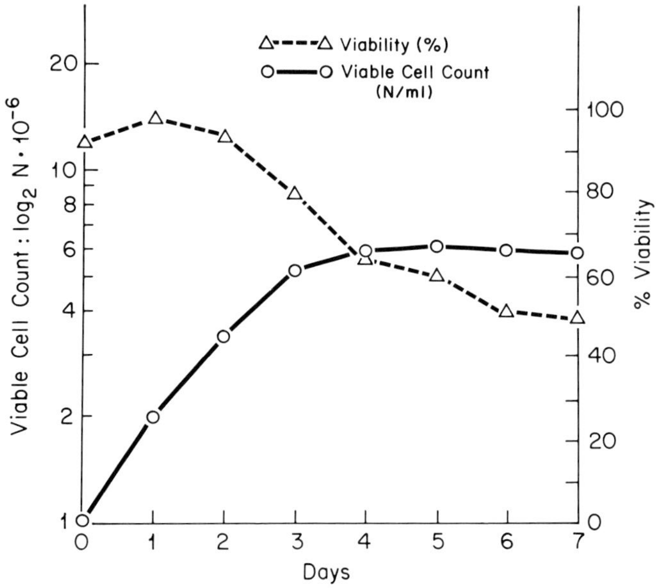

Figure 2. Growth kinetics of *Crithidia luciliae*. *C luciliae* were subcultured from the original stock culture. The viable cell count and the percent viability were determined every 24 hours, without adding new culture medium.

in Figure 1a. The serum from patient 3 contained both histone antibodies and anti-nDNA, and the anti-nDNA was responsible for the staining on the HCl-extracted kidney sections and *C luciliae* smears (Table 3).

Effect of *C luciliae* growth kinetics on kinetoplast staining. In order to evaluate the influence of the growth kinetics of *C luciliae* on the kinetoplast binding by histone antibodies and serum antibodies from patients with different diseases, growth characteristics of *C luciliae* were monitored by quantitating the percentage of viable organisms. Smears from different time points in cultures were prepared. The growth kinetics and the viability of *C luciliae* are shown in Figure 2. Viability began to decrease 48 hours after subculture, while the concentration of viable organisms peaked 4 days after subculture.

Smears from 2, 4, and 7 days of subculture were prepared and used as substrates for the CLIF test, using histone antibodies purified from the 3 sera shown in Table 3. The titers of kinetoplast staining of *C luciliae* by purified histone antibodies are shown in Table 4. In addition to the observed drop in titer, purified histone antibodies stained fewer *C luciliae* kinetoplasts from 4- or 7-day-old culture than from 2-day-old culture (Figure 1b, c, and d). These 2 observations indicated that *C luciliae* lost or decreased histone antigen during its growth in culture as it reached confluency, and the CLIF assay sensitivity decreased when *C luciliae* from older cultures was used as the substrate.

DISCUSSION

Antibodies against nDNA are usually found only in patients with SLE. The methods used to detect the presence of anti-nDNA antibodies include double immunodiffusion, counterimmunoelectrophoresis, Farr assay, millipore filter assay, chromosome spread assay, enzyme-linked immunosorbent assay (ELISA),

Table 4. Effect of *Crithidia luciliae* growth kinetics on the titer of purified histone antibodies staining the kinetoplasts*

2 days	4 days	7 days
8	4	2
8	2	Undiluted
2	Negative	Negative

* Values shown are reciprocal of the antibody titer.

and CLIF assay. These assays differ with regard to sensitivity and specificity. Solid-phase immunoassays (Farr and millipore assays, ELISA) are the most sensitive, but the CLIF test is the easiest to perform and is the least expensive. Thus, the CLIF test is currently used in many clinical laboratories. According to published references (1,5,6,8–11), its results are reliable compared with those from the Farr, millipore filter, and chromosome spread assays. However, there is some controversy about specificity.

Recently, we encountered a patient who had drug-induced LE with high titers of antihistone antibodies (12). This serum had significant reactivity with the kinetoplast of *C luciliae*. Subsequently, we demonstrated that this kinetoplast binding activity was due to antihistone antibodies (13). This observation was compatible with the finding of Aarden et al that some patients with drug-induced LE had antibodies binding to the kinetoplast of *C luciliae* (1). Jonsson and Norberg also suggested that *C luciliae* kinetoplasts might contain nuclear proteins such as histone or histone-like protein in addition to DNA (3).

An important conclusion of this study is that there are 2 (and possibly 3) groups of antibodies that bind to the kinetoplasts of *C luciliae*. These are: anti-nDNA, antihistone antibodies, and, possibly, other unidentified antibodies. Among these 3 groups of antibodies, anti-nDNA antibodies are the most frequent antibodies to demonstrate positive kinetoplast reactivity in the CLIF assay. In our analysis over the past 2 years of over 700 random serum samples, 36 were positive in the CLIF test; 28 of these were from patients with SLE. The reactivity of most of these sera was still positive when histone was extracted from the kinetoplasts. However, there were 10 sera containing antihistone antibodies that also stained the kinetoplasts. These were from patients with SLE, drug-induced LE, rheumatoid arthritis, and Sjögren's syndrome. There were 4 sera that failed to stain the histone-reconstituted *C luciliae* kinetoplasts. These 4 sera might still have had histone antibodies.

As previously shown, procainamide-induced LE is serologically different from LE induced by hydralazine (17,18). Both bind untreated kidney sections, but not HCl-extracted sections. While histone antibodies present in patients with procainamide-induced LE bind to histone-reconstituted kidney sections, sera from hydralazine-induced LE do not. Using the specific histone ELISA, sera from both procainamide and hydralazine-induced LE patients bind histone antigens (18). Another possible explanation for the failure of the 4 sera to stain the histone-reconstituted kinetoplasts is that they contained antibodies other than antihistone antibodies.

The second important conclusion of the present study is that there can be variability in the CLIF test results, independent of changes in disease activity. Our data indicate that the source of *C luciliae* can play an important role in this variability. However, the variability is probably related to the presence of histone antibodies and not to the anti-nDNA antibodies. This possibility was supported when specific antihistone antibodies were used to stain *C luciliae* smears prepared at different times after the initiation of culture. Thus, histone or histone-like proteins are present in the kinetoplasts of *C luciliae* during its rapidly growing stage. By the stationary phase of the culture, the relative concentration of histone or histone-like proteins in kinetoplasts apparently decreases, and the binding of antihistone antibodies to the substrates diminishes. Another possible explanation for the variability in the CLIF test results is that there is also a decrease in DNA in the kinetoplasts. This possibility may not be so important, since 2 sera from SLE patients having high titers of anti-nDNA were used as controls, and their titers did not diminish on *Crithidia* smears prepared at various times of culture.

There is generally good correlation between the results of the Farr and the CLIF assays. The higher the titers observed in the CLIF test, the greater the DNA binding in the Farr assay (8,10,11). None of the sera that failed to stain HCl-extracted *Crithidia* kinetoplasts gave more than 30 units on the Farr assay. All 14 samples had antibody titers of 1:80 or less in the CLIF test. This raises the question of the significance of the CLIF test in terms of antibody titers. We believe, based on our present investigation, that a titer of 1:80 or greater in the CLIF test is more likely to represent a true anti-nDNA. Clearly, clinical information must be considered first and the laboratory data should be used only to verify the clinical impression.

ACKNOWLEDGMENTS

We wish to thank Tuyet Dang for expert technical assistance and Betty Janes for help in preparing the manuscript.

REFERENCES

1. Aarden LA, de Groot ER, Feltkamp TEW: Immunology of DNA. III. Crithidia luciliae, a simple substrate for the determination of anti-dsDNA with the immunofluorescent technique. Ann NY Acad Sci 254:505–515, 1975

2. Stingl G, Meingassner JG, Swelty P, Knapp W: An immunofluorescence procedure for the demonstration of antibodies to native, double-stranded DNA and of circulating DNA-anti-DNA complexes. Clin Immunol Immunopathol 6:131–140, 1976
3. Jonsson J, Norberg R: Effect of enzyme treatment of Crithidia luciliae on the reactivity of its kinetoplast with anti-DNA sera. Scand J Rheumatol 5:221–226, 1976
4. Slater NG, Cameron JS, Lessof MH: The Crithidia luciliae kinetoplast immunofluorescent test in systemic lupus erythematosus. Clin Exp Immunol 25:480–486, 1976
5. Crowe W, Kushner I: An immunofluorescent method using Crithidia luciliae to detect antibodies to double-stranded DNA. Arthritis Rheum 20:811–814, 1977
6. Deegan MJ, Walker SE, Lovell SE: Antibodies to double-stranded DNA: a comparison of the indirect immunofluorescent test using Crithidia luciliae and the DNA-binding assay. Am J Clin Pathol 69:599–604, 1978
7. Sontheimer RD, Gilliam JN: An immunofluorescence assay for double-stranded DNA antibodies using Crithidia luciliae kinetoplast as a double-stranded DNA substrate. J Lab Clin Med 91:550–558, 1978
8. Chubick A, Sontheimer RD, Gilliam JN, Ziff M: An appraisal of tests for native DNA antibodies in connective tissue diseases. Ann Intern Med 89:186–192, 1978
9. Whiteside TL, Dixon JA: Clinical usefulness of the Crithidia luciliae test for antibodies to native DNA. Am J Clin Pathol 72:829–835, 1979
10. Somerfield SD, Roberts MW, Booth RJ: Double-stranded DNA antibodies: a comparison of four methods of detection. J Clin Pathol 34:1032–1035, 1981
11. Graafland HF, Wagner AL: Double stranded DNA antibody quantitation by the Farr assay and indirect immunofluorescent test using Crithidia luciliae. Int J Nucl Med Biol 9:114–117, 1982
12. Steinmetz SF, Deng JS, Rubin RL, Sontheimer RD, Gilliam JN: Reevaluation of the specificity of the Crithidia luciliae kinetoplast as a substrate for detecting antibodies to double-stranded DNA: a case report. J Am Acad Dermatol 11:490–493, 1984
13. Deng JS, Rubin RL, Lipscomb MF, Sontheimer RD, Gilliam JN: Reappraisal of the specificity of the Crithidia luciliae assay for nDNA antibodies: evidence for histone antibody kinetoplast binding. Am J Clin Pathol 82:448–452, 1984
14. Rodnan GP, Schumacher HR, editors: Primer on the Rheumatic Diseases. Eighth edition. Atlanta, Arthritis Foundation, 1983
15. Tan EM, Robinson J, Robitaille P: Studies on antibodies to histone by immunofluorescence. Scand J Immunol 5:811–818, 1976
16. Fritzler MJ, Tan EM: Antibodies to histone in drug-induced and idiopathic lupus erythematosus. J Clin Invest 612:560–567, 1978
17. Tan EM, Portanova JP: The role of histones as nuclear autoantigens in drug-related lupus erythematosus. Arthritis Rheum 24:1064–1069, 1981
18. Portanova JP, Rubin RL, Joslin FG, Agnello VD, Tan EM: Reactivity of antihistone antibodies induced by procainamide and hydralazine. Clin Immunol Immunopathol 25:67–79, 1982

ABNORMAL CALCIUM AND MAGNESIUM STORES IN ERYTHROCYTES AND GRANULOCYTES FROM PATIENTS WITH INFLAMMATORY CONNECTIVE TISSUE DISEASES

Relationship to Inflammatory Activity and Effect of Corticosteroid Therapy

ROGER HÄLLGREN, KARIN SVENSON, ERLAND JOHANSSON, and ULF LINDH

The mass fraction of Ca and Mg in isolated erythrocytes and granulocytes was measured using the nuclear microprobe technique. Conspicuous abnormalities were observed in cells from patients with rheumatoid arthritis and other inflammatory arthritides. Compared with the normal cellular content, total Ca was increased an average of 3 times in erythrocytes and 5 times in granulocytes. Total granulocyte Mg was increased about 3 times, whereas erythrocyte Mg was reduced to as much as 60% of normal. These abnormalities were less prominent or were absent in scleroderma patients, except for levels of granulocyte Ca, which were increased more than 3 times beyond normal in this patient group. A significant positive correlation was found between serum haptoglobin and erythrocyte or granulocyte Ca content among these patients, but not between haptoglobin and erythrocyte or granulocyte Mg values. During corticosteroid treatment, a significant increase in erythrocyte Mg and a significant reduction in erythrocyte Ca were noted, but normalization of these levels was not achieved. Granulocyte Ca was also significantly reduced, while granulocyte Mg remained unaltered. Serum levels of Ca and Mg were within normal ranges and were not influenced by corticosteroid therapy. The results indicate that at least Ca abnormalities in erythrocytes and granulocytes are associated with the intensity of the inflammatory process and that the amounts of Ca and Mg in these cells are influenced by potent antiinflammatory therapy.

During the last 2 decades, there has been a growing awareness that changes in cellular calcium can play an important role in cell injury caused by ischemia (1), biologic toxins (2,3), genetic abnormality (4), or calcium deficiency disease (5). Experimental studies also indicate that the extent of immunologically induced cell injury can be affected by an increase in intracellular calcium (6). A disturbance of the calcium balance could therefore be one of several ways by which the principles of immunologic and inflammatory processes alter cell metabolism and function in chronic inflammatory connective tissue diseases such as rheumatoid arthritis (RA). To test the hypothesis that, in such diseases, there are elevated cellular concentrations of calcium, we measured total cell calcium in erythrocytes and granulocytes isolated from patients with rheumatoid arthritis, scleroderma, and other inflammatory arthritides.

Several other ions exist inside cells, and these may also regulate cell activity. One ion that is particularly important in cell metabolism is Mg^{++}. Since there appears to be a relationship between the concentration ratios of Mg:Ca inside a number of different cells (7), we also measured the cellular levels of magnesium. The possible relationship between abnormal cellular concentrations of calcium and magnesium and the degree of inflammatory activity was explored. Finally, we investigated the effect of potent antiinflammatory drug therapy on the cellular ion content.

From the Department of Internal Medicine, University Hospital, Uppsala and the Gustaf Werner Institute, Department of Physical Biology, Uppsala, Sweden.

Supported by grants from the Swedish Medical Research Council and the Swedish Natural Science Research Council.

Roger Hällgren, MD: Associate Professor of Internal Medicine, University Hospital, Uppsala; Karin Svenson, MD: University Hospital, Uppsala; Erland Johansson, PhD: Gustaf Werner Institute, Uppsala; Ulf Lindh, PhD: Associate Professor of Physical Biology, Gustaf Werner Institute, Uppsala.

Address reprint requests to Roger Hällgren, MD, Section of Rheumatology, Department of Internal Medicine, University Hospital, S-751 85, Uppsala, Sweden.

Submitted for publication February 3, 1984; accepted in revised form August 21, 1984.

PATIENTS AND METHODS

Patients. Blood specimens were collected from 24 inpatients with inflammatory connective tissue diseases: 11 patients had RA, 5 had scleroderma, 3 had ankylosing pelvospondylitis, 3 had psoriatic arthropathy, 1 had Reiter's disease, and 1 had post-infectious arthritis. The RA patients had a mean age of 51 and a mean disease duration of 9 years. The scleroderma patients had a mean age of 55 and a mean disease duration of 6 years. The remaining patients constituted the group with seronegative spondylarthropathies; their mean age was 41, and mean duration of disease was 10 years. The patients with scleroderma were treated with cyclofenil (average 400 mg/day). All other patients had been treated with various nonsteroidal antiinflammatory drugs, which were ceased 3–4 days before blood sampling.

Cellular mass fraction of calcium and magnesium. Venous blood (10 ml) was collected into venoject tubes (Terumo, Tokyo, Japan) containing 0.1 ml of 0.38*M* K_3EDTA as anticoagulant. Erythrocytes and granulocytes were immediately isolated from the blood sample as described elsewhere (8). After washing in sterile phosphate buffered saline, pH 7.3 (SBL, Stockholm, Sweden), the different cell types were resuspended in 1 ml of 0.32*M* sucrose (Analar/BDH, London, UK) that was free of Ca and Mg. Then, 0.5-μl aliquots (equilvalent to approximately 1×10^5 erythrocytes and 0.5×10^4 granulocytes, respectively) were put onto clean Formvar films (Formvar 1595 E; Merck, Darmstadt, West Germany). After cooling to −80°C, the cells were freeze-dried and stored in desiccators at 4°C.

From the blood cell preparations, 10 cells of each type were selected, using light microscopy, prior to microprobe analysis (9). The selected cells were irradiated with a 5-μm beam of 2.5 MeV of protons, using the Van de Graaf accelerator at the Natural Science Research Laboratory, Studsvik, Sweden. Analysis of data was performed as previously described (10). The conversion of x-ray counts to relative amounts was possible by registration of the continuous bremsstrahlung (9,11). The cellular concentrations of Ca and Mg represent median values and are expressed in μg/gm of dry weight.

Blood concentrations of hemoglobin and serum concentrations of haptoglobin, albumin-modified calcium, and magnesium were measured at the Department of Clinical Chemistry, University Hospital, Uppsala, Sweden.

RESULTS

Data on total erythrocyte and granulocyte Ca and Mg obtained from patients and healthy controls showed no sex or age dependency. The serum levels of Ca and Mg were within normal ranges in all patients studied and were not related to the cellular concentrations.

Compared with the controls, all patients with rheumatoid arthritis and those with seronegative spondylarthropathies had increased total Ca in their isolated erythrocytes (Figure 1). In 3 of 5 patients with scleroderma, we noted a modest increase in erythrocyte Ca. A reduction in the Mg content of erythrocytes was obvious in RA patients and was also prominent in those with seronegative spondylarthropathies. There was a tendency toward decreased amounts of erythrocyte Mg in scleroderma patients. Serum haptoglobin was particularly elevated in patients with inflammatory arthritides (Table 1), while a more modest acute-phase reaction was seen in those with scleroderma. There was a significant correlation between haptoglobin and erythrocyte Ca values ($r = 0.54$, $P < 0.01$), but not between levels of haptoglobin and erythrocyte Mg ($P > 0.05$).

Anemia was observed in a number of patients with inflammatory arthritides (Table 1). There was a negative correlation between levels of hemoglobin and erythrocyte Ca ($r = -0.40$, $P < 0.05$) among the patients, and a positive correlation between their hemoglobin and erythrocyte Mg values ($r = 0.47$, $P < 0.05$). No relationship was observed between erythrocyte Ca and Mg content.

The granulocyte content of Ca was considerably elevated in all patients, while a significant increase in granulocyte Mg was noted only in patients with inflammatory arthritides (Figure 2). No correlation was found between granulocyte Ca and Mg levels. The degree of inflammatory activity was linked to levels of granulocyte Ca (Figure 3), but not to levels of granulocyte Mg.

Eight of the patients, 6 with RA and 2 with seronegative spondylarthropathies, were serially studied during treatment with corticosteroids. After 1 week of methylprednisolone treatment (average daily

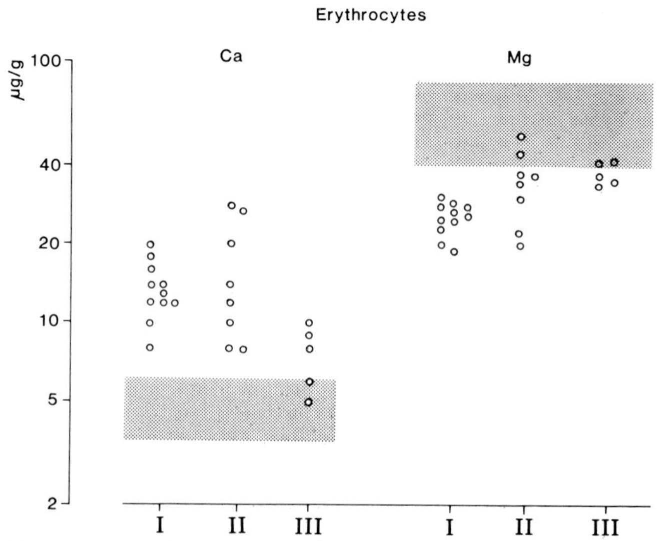

Figure 1. Total Ca and Mg (μg/gm) in erythrocytes isolated from patients with rheumatoid arthritis (I), seronegative spondylarthropathies (II), and scleroderma (III). The shaded areas represent total erythrocyte Ca and Mg in healthy individuals.

Table 1. Laboratory data in 24 patients with chronic inflammatory connective tissue diseases*

Diagnosis (n)	Blood hemoglobin, gm/liter	Serum haptoglobin, gm/liter	Erythrocytes		Granulocytes	
			Ca, μg/gm	Mg, μg/gm	Ca, μg/gm	Mg, μg/gm
Rheumatoid arthritis (11)	115 (88–157)	3.8 (1.7–6.1)	14 (8–20)	25 (19–30)	25 (18–28)	17 (12–22)
Seronegative spondylarthropathies (8)	114 (92–153)	5.2 (3.9–6.0)	16 (8–27)	35 (20–51)	27 (21–34)	13 (8–19)
Scleroderma (5)	141 (130–141)	1.7 (1.5–2.2)	7 (5–9)	38 (34–42)	19 (15–27)	8 (6–10)
Normal controls (15)	113–166†	0.3–2.0†	5 (3.6–6.2)	58 (40–85)	5.6 (4.0–8.6)	5.5 (3.2–8.5)

* Values are the mean values obtained; actual values are shown in parentheses.
† Values are reference ranges. See Patients and Methods.

dose of 20 mg), we observed a significant increase in erythrocyte Mg and a tendency toward a decrease in erythrocyte and granulocyte Ca (Table 2).

After 1 week of steroid treatment only, 100 mg/day of azathioprine was added to the regimen for 3 patients, and 50–100 mg/day of cyclophosphamide was added for 2 other patients, while 3 patients remained on methylprednisolone therapy only. The glucocorticoids were gradually reduced, and after 3 months, the average methylprednisolone dosage was 10 mg/day. At this time, a significant reduction of erythrocyte Ca was noted (Figure 4). Granulocyte Ca was also significantly reduced after 3 months of therapy, while granulocyte Mg remained unchanged (Table 2). The serum levels of Ca and Mg were not altered. During the observation period, the haptoglobin values were reduced from 4.7 ± 0.5 (mean ± SEM) to 2.9 ± 0.4 gm/liter.

Other therapeutic regimens that were tried over a 3-month period in a small number of patients with RA (antiphlogistics were taken alone in 2 patients, in combination with penicillamine in 1 patient, and with chloroquine in a fourth patient) did not influence erythrocyte or granulocyte Ca:Mg ratios or haptoglobin levels (data not shown).

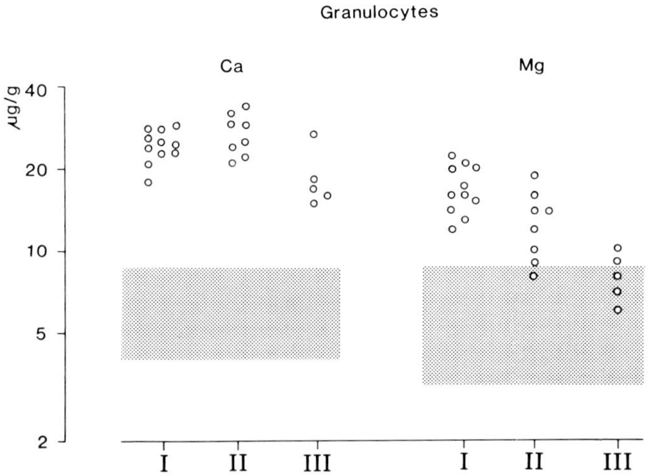

Figure 2. Total Ca and Mg (μg/gm) in granulocytes isolated from patients with rheumatoid arthritis (I), seronegative spondylarthropathies (II), and scleroderma (III). The shaded areas represent total Ca and Mg in granulocytes in healthy individuals.

DISCUSSION

In this study we found a conspicuous accumulation of Ca in erythrocytes and granulocytes isolated from patients with rheumatoid arthritis, other inflammatory arthritides, and scleroderma. The Mg stores were also abnormal—increased in granulocytes but

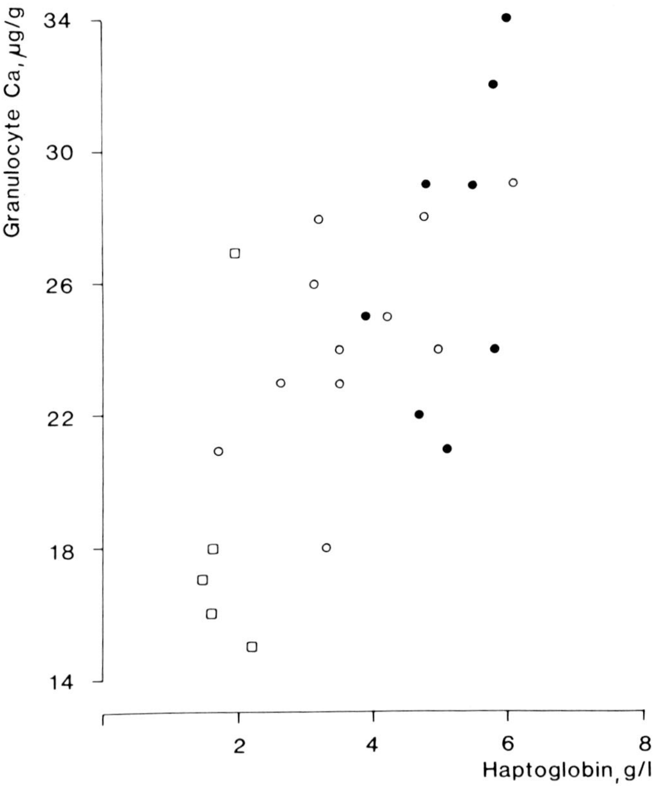

Figure 3. The correlation between granulocyte Ca (μg/gm) and serum haptoglobin (gm/liter) in patients with inflammatory connective tissue diseases (○ = rheumatoid arthritis; ● = seronegative spondylarthropathies; □ = scleroderma). The correlation coefficient was 0.65 ($P < 0.001$), and the equation of the regression line was y = 1.44 × −1.02.

Table 2. The calcium and magnesium content of erythrocytes and granulocytes from 8 patients with inflammatory arthritides, showing the effects of corticosteroid therapy*

	Erythrocytes		Granulocytes	
Time of sampling	Ca (μg/gm)	Mg (μg/gm)	Ca (μg/gm)	Mg (μg/gm)
Before treatment	14.5 ± 2.2	25.8 ± 1.4	27.1 ± 1.3	17.4 ± 1.2
After 1 week of treatment	13.6 ± 1.8	29.1 ± 1.7†	26.1 ± 1.6	17.6 ± 1.3
After 3 months of treatment	10.9 ± 1.6‡	29.6 ± 2.0†	24.3 ± 1.9§	19.0 ± 1.4

* Values represent the mean ± SEM.
† Significant compared with pretreatment values, $P < 0.02$ by Wilcoxon signed rank test.
‡ Significant compared with pretreatment values, $P < 0.01$ by Wilcoxon signed rank test.
§ Significant compared with pretreatment values, $P < 0.05$ by Wilcoxon signed rank test.

reduced in erythrocytes. The mechanisms underlying these alterations are unknown, but the intensity of the inflammatory process seems to be linked to the abnormal Ca balance, since we observed a positive correlation between acute-phase reactants and the erythrocyte and granulocyte content of Ca. Another indirect argument for the hypothesis that inflammatory activity may govern Ca accumulation was provided by the data obtained during corticosteroid therapy, which demonstrated that levels of cellular Ca tended to return toward normal. The Mg levels were not related to the inflammatory activity, but were significantly increased in erythrocytes after administration of corticosteroids.

We have no data on the cellular amount of free Ca or the subcellular localization of Ca in our patients, but at rest, more than 99% of the Ca in nucleated healthy cells is bound to ligands, sequestered in organelles (12–15), or associated with the cell membrane (16). The lack of Ca-binding organelles makes the erythrocytes more dependent on Ca-binding ligands, the most important of which are called calmodulins (17). An increased Ca load to these cells could therefore be compensated for by an increase in the number of Ca-binding sites as a result of enhanced synthesis of the ligand or exposure of new sites for Ca binding. The reduced Mg content in the erythrocytes of our patients might mirror another way by which the cells take care of increased amounts of Ca, namely, by competing with Mg for binding sites on proteins and macromolecules (18). However, the granulocytes could use organelles and granules instead of ligands, allowing for Ca, as well as Mg, accumulation.

A steady-state normally exists between the cytoplasmic free Ca and the bound Ca in the cell. An increase in cytoplasmic Ca over a significant period of time would therefore cause an increase in bound and, hence, total cell Ca. Experimental studies have shown that a number of inflammatory agents (2,6,19–21) relevant to the clinical situations we have studied may all increase cellular Ca, evidently by a change in the permeability of the cell membrane for Ca. Whether in vitro inflammatory stimuli may also change the cellular content of Mg is, at present, unknown. A cellular overload of Ca could also be due to a defect in the mechanism of Ca efflux. This idea could be particularly valid regarding the Mg-deficient erythrocytes observed in inflammatory arthritides, since the Ca efflux in these cells is partly dependent on a Ca-activated MgATPase (22).

At present, it is a matter of speculation as to whether the observed alterations in the balance of Ca

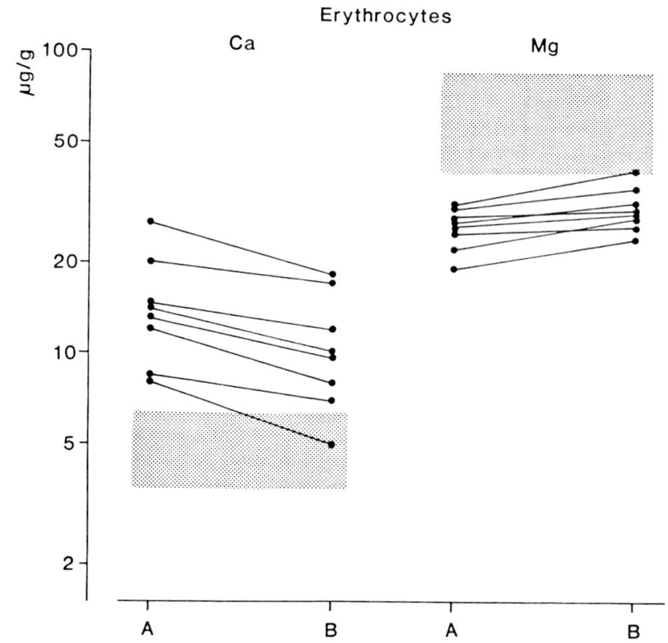

Figure 4. Levels of erythrocyte Ca and Mg (μg/gm) in patients with inflammatory arthritides before (**A**) and after (**B**) 3 months of glucocorticoid therapy. The shaded areas represent the normal erythrocyte content of these cations.

and Mg are primary abnormalities, pathologic changes of the disease process, or perhaps even physiologic changes which check the disease. However, regardless of which proves to be the case, previous in vitro observations indicate that abnormalities of intracellular Ca may have several metabolic consequences (4,23–29) that may influence some of the clinical manifestations of inflammatory connective tissue disease.

REFERENCES

1. Siegel BA, Engel WK, Derrer EC: Localization of technetium-99m diphosphonate in acutely injured muscle: relationship to calcium deposition. Neurology (NY) 27:230–238, 1977
2. Woodin SM: The basis of leucocidin action, The Biological Basis of Medicine. Vol. 2. Edited by EE Bittar. New York, Academic Press, 1968, pp 373–396
3. Okamoto M, Mayer MM: Studies on the mechanism of action of guinea-pig lymphotoxin. II. Increase of calcium uptake rate in LT-damaged target cells. J Immunol 120:279–285, 1978
4. Eaton JW, Skelton TD, Swofford HS, Kolpin CE, Jacob HS: Elevated erythrocyte calcium in sickle cell disease. Nature 246:105–106, 1973
5. Kirby AC, Lindley BD, Picken JR: Calcium content and exchange in frog skeletal muscle. J Physiol (Lond) 253:37–52, 1975
6. Campbell AK, Daw RA, Hallet MB, Luzio JP: Direct measurement of the increase in intracellular free calcium ion concentration in response to the action of complement. Biochem J 194:551–560, 1981
7. Wacker WEC, Williams RJP: Magnesium/calcium balances of biological systems. J Theor Biol 20:65–78, 1968
8. Johansson E, Lindh U, Landström E: The incorporation of selenium and alterations of macro- and trace element levels in individual blood cells following supplementation with sodium selenite and vitamin E: a nuclear microprobe application. Biol Trace Elem Res 5:433–447, 1983
9. Lindh U: Elemental characterization of individual glia and glioma cells in the nuclear microprobe. Nucl Instr Methods 193:343–347, 1982
10. Lindh U: Elemental mapping of tissue sections by means of micro particle-induced x-ray emission spectroscopy and computer graphics. Anal Chim Acta 150:223–244, 1983
11. Uemura YJ, Kuno Y, Koyama H, Yamazaki T, Kienle P: A new way of determining concentrations in PIXE trace element analysis. Nucl Instr Methods 153:573–579, 1978
12. Ashley CC, Campbell AK, editors: Detection and Measurements of Free Ca^{2+} in Cells. Amsterdam, Elsevier/North Holland, 1979
13. Klein RL, Horton CR, Thureson-Klein A: Studies on nuclear amino acid transport and cation content in embryonic myocardium of the chick. Am J Cardiol 25:300–310, 1970
14. Baker PF, Warner AE: Intracellular calcium and cell cleavage in early embryos of xenopus. J Cell Biol 53:579–581, 1972
15. Claret-Berthon B, Claret M, Mazet JL: Fluxes and distribution of calcium in rat liver cells: kinetic analysis and identification of pools. J Physiol (Lond) 272:529–555, 1977
16. Lichtman MA, Weed RI: Divalent cation content of normal and ATP-depleted erythrocytes and erythrocyte membranes. Nouv Rev Fr Hematol 12:799–813, 1972
17. Kretsinger RH: Calcium binding proteins. Annu Rev Biochem 45:239–268, 1976
18. Klee CB, Crouch TH, Richman PO: Calmodulin. Annu Rev Biochem 49:489–515, 1980
19. Campbell AK, editor: Intracellular Calcium: Its Universal Role as a Regulator. New York, John Wiley & Sons, 1983
20. Volsky DJ, Loyter A: Role of Ca^{2+} in virus-induced membrane fusion: Ca^{2+} accumulation and ultrastructural changes induced by Sendai virus in chicken erythrocytes. J Cell Biol 78:465–479, 1978
21. Shearer WT, Atkinson JP, Parker CW: Humoral immunostimulation. VI. Increased calcium uptake by cells treated with antibody and complement. J Immunol 117:973–980, 1976
22. Schatzmann HJ: Active calcium transport and Ca^{2+}-activated ATPase in human red cells. Curr Top Membr Transport 6:125–168, 1975
23. Long C, Mouat B: The influx of calcium ions to human erythrocytes during cold storage. Biochem J 132:559–570, 1973
24. White JG: Effects of an ionophore, A 23187, on the surface morphology of normal erythrocytes. Am J Pathol 77:507–518, 1974
25. Ignarro LJ, George WJ: Mediation of immunologic discharge of lysosomal enzymes from human neutrophils by guanosine 3′,5′-monophosphate. J Exp Med 140:225–238, 1974
26. Becker EL, Showell HJ: The ability of chemotactic factors to induce lysosomal enzyme release. II. The mechanism of release. J Immunol 112:2055–2062, 1974
27. Goldstein IM, Horn JK, Kaplan HB, Weissmann G: Calcium-induced lysozyme secretion from human polymorphonuclear leukocytes. Biochem Biophys Res Commun 60:807–812, 1974
28. Weissmann G, Smolen JE, Korchak HM: Release of inflammatory mediators from stimulated neutrophils. N Engl J Med 303:27–34, 1980
29. Hallet MB, Luzio JP, Campbell AK: Stimulation of Ca^{2+}-dependent chemiluminescence in rat polymorphonuclear leukocytes by polystyrene beads and the nonlytic action of complement. Immunology 44:569–576, 1981

IMMUNOHISTOCHEMICAL STUDIES OF INTERLEUKIN-2 AND γ-INTERFERON IN RHEUMATOID ARTHRITIS

GUNNAR HUSBY and RALPH C. WILLIAMS, JR.

Synovial tissues were studied, using immunofluorescence techniques, for localization of lymphocytic infiltrates and immune reactants, including C3, C5b-9, C9, and Ia antigen. Tissue distribution of interleukin-2 (IL-2) and γ-interferon was also determined, using mouse monoclonal antibodies. IL-2 was found in association with OKT8 and OKT4 T cells, and γ-interferon was noted in association with T cells, B cells, and macrophages. Staining both for IL-2 and for γ-interferon was surprisingly faint in view of the intensity of lymphocytic infiltration.

It is clear from a number of previous studies that rheumatoid arthritis (RA) is associated with many abnormalities of the immune system. Affected patients show serum antibodies, generally referred to as rheumatoid factors, which react with Fc determinants on IgG (1–3). There is considerable evidence for the presence of a number of IgG–IgG and IgM–IgG complexes within serum and synovial fluid, and for activation of the complement system, particularly within prime areas of inflammation such as the rheumatoid synovium and adjacent synovial fluid (4–9). Histologic characteristics of the basic granulomatous lesions of rheumatoid synovitis, as well as those present in extraarticular sites, suggest an active immune reaction with many focal collections of lymphocytes, mononuclear cells, macrophage-like cells, and plasma cells. Currently, very little is known about intercellular communication and precise mechanisms of cell-to-cell interactions within the basic lesions of rheumatoid synovitis.

Recently, considerable attention has been directed toward learning more about messenger/effector molecules, which may regulate and control cell-to-cell interactions in normal or abnormal immune responses in humans. Research has also been conducted on lymphokine products, such as the interferons, interleukin-1 (IL-1), and interleukin 2 (IL-2), since these materials may play a key role in intercellular communication and, therefore, in the modulation of immune reactions. Previous work from this laboratory has indicated that α-interferon may be capable of facilitating humoral immune reactivity by making B cells more responsive to helper cell–derived enhancement (10,11). Studies of interleukin activity and responsiveness, particularly in systemic lupus erythematosus, have indicated a defect or deficiency both in the production of and the response to IL-2 (12).

The present study was directed toward an examination of 2 potentially important lymphokines in RA, γ-interferon and interleukin-2, with particular attention to their cellular source and localization within the lesions of rheumatoid synovitis. The results presented here show that focal collections of cells within the inflamed rheumatoid tissues appeared to show positive immunofluorescence for localization of both γ-interferon and IL-2. However, the extent of

From the Department of Medicine, University of New Mexico School of Medicine, Albuquerque, and the Department of Rheumatology, Tromsø University Hospital, Tromsø, Norway.

Supported in part by grants AMAI-13690 and AMAI-13814 from the U. S. Public Health Service and an Arthritis Foundation Clinical Research Center grant.

Gunnar Husby, MD; Ralph C. Williams, Jr., MD.

Address reprint request to Ralph C. Williams, Jr., MD, Department of Medicine, University of New Mexico, 2211 Lomas Blvd. NE, Albuquerque, NM 87131.

Submitted for publication May 21, 1984; accepted in revised form September 5, 1984.

positive cellular immunofluorescence for both of these lymphokines appeared to be diminished or not as extensive as one would expect in the presence of an apparent florid, aggressive immune reaction such as that seen in active rheumatoid synovitis.

PATIENTS AND METHODS

Synovial tissues from 9 patients with classic or definite rheumatoid arthritis, classified according to the American Rheumatism Association criteria (13), were obtained during synovectomy or joint replacement procedures. Portions of rheumatoid synovial membrane, approximately 0.5 × 1 cm, were dissected free of excess fat and dense connective tissue, snap-frozen in dry ice, and 4μ frozen sections were prepared as previously described (14,15). Normal synovial tissues obtained from 2 patients undergoing operative repair for acute athletic injuries served as controls. Frozen sections were prepared from each tissue, and all histologic sections were stained with hematoxylin and eosin (H & E) to define conventional landmarks and sites of cellular infiltrates.

Immunofluorescence studies. All sections were examined using the reagents shown in Table 1. The degree and anatomic localization of synovial tissue lymphocytic infiltrates were first established by examination of H & E–stained serial sections in conjunction with frozen sections. B cells were identified using affinity-purified fluorescein-conjugated $F(ab')_2$ goat anti-human $F(ab')_2$ as well as with $F(ab')_2$ rabbit anti-human IgM. Synovial tissue T cells and T cell subsets were localized with Ortho OKT3, OKT4, and OKT8 mouse monoclonal reagents followed by goat anti-mouse IgG and, subsequently, with fluorescein-conjugated $F(ab')_2$ rabbit anti-goat IgG or, when simultaneous 2-color immunofluorescence was used, $F(ab')_2$ rabbit anti-mouse IgG conjugated with rhodamine.

Deposition of immune complex material or activated complement components was determined using fluorescein-conjugated rabbit anti-C3. In addition, synovial tissue components containing activation complement neoantigens were identified using fluorescein-conjugated anti–C5b-9 and anti-C9 reagents, kindly furnished by Dr. David Koffler, Hahnemann Medical Center, Philadelphia, PA. Specificity of these reagents has been documented in previous reports by Biesecker et al (16,17). Determinations of the distribution of human Ia antigens within synovial tissues utilized mouse monoclonal reagents (Becton-Dickinson, Sunnyvale, CA) reacting with common framework human Ia antigens.

Cellular and synovial tissue localization of IL-2 was performed using indirect immunofluorescence and a mouse monoclonal anti–IL-2 antibody (18), kindly provided by Dr. S. Gillis, Immunex Corp., Seattle, WA. Specificity of staining for IL-2 was confirmed by absorption of the anti–IL-2 reagent with highly purified gene-cloned human IL-2, kindly furnished by Dr. K. Koths, Cetus Corp., Emeryville, CA.

Gamma interferon was identified within synovial tissues, using a mouse monoclonal anti–γ-interferon antibody (IgG1), kindly furnished by Dr. Charles Burton of Genentech, Palo Alto, CA. Specificity of anti–γ-interferon staining was confirmed by absorption of anti–γ-interferon antibody with gene-cloned γ-interferon, provided by Dr. C. Sevastopoulos, Genentech. Such absorption completely eliminated positive immunofluorescence reactions seen in tissues and confirmed the specificity of the reactions.

Table 1. Immunofluorescence procedures and specific reagents used in identification of various immune reactants within synovial tissues*

Immune reactant	Methods and reagents
B cells	Affinity-purified FITC-conjugated $F(ab')_2$ goat anti-human $F(ab')_2$ Affinity-purified FITC-conjugated $F(ab')_2$ rabbit anti-human IgM
T cells	Mouse monoclonal Ortho OKT3, OKT4, and OKT8 followed by goat anti-mouse IgG and either (a) FITC-conjugated $F(ab')_2$ rabbit anti-goat IgG or (b) Rhodamine-conjugated $F(ab')_2$ rabbit anti-mouse IgG
C3	FITC-conjugated rabbit anti-C3
C5b-9 neoantigen	FITC-conjugated goat anti-human C5b-9
C9	FITC-conjugated rabbit anti-human C9
Ia	Mouse monoclonal anti-Ia followed by goat anti-mouse IgG and either (a) FITC-conjugated rabbit anti-goat IgG or (b) Rhodamine-conjugated rabbit anti-mouse IgG
Interleukin-2	Mouse monoclonal anti–interleukin-2 followed by (a) or (b) above
γ-interferon	Mouse monoclonal anti–γ-interferon followed by (a) or (b) above

* FITC = fluorescein isothiocyanate. FITC-conjugated reagent was used in direct immunofluorescence procedures. Rhodamine-conjugated reagent was used in 2-color immunofluorescence procedures. See Patients and Methods for details.

Controls for the immunofluorescence procedures included mouse monoclonal Ig of the same isotype as the various monoclonal reagents or diluted whole mouse IgG followed by the second labeled reagent. In the case of rabbit or goat antisera, both normal rabbit serum or goat serum followed by conjugate, as well as conjugate for second or third layer alone, served as background controls.

An attempt was made to quantitate γ-interferon in synovial fluids, using a method originally described by Staehelin et al (19). Thirty microliters of monoclonal antibody to γ-interferon (Interferon Sciences, New Brunswick, NJ), at 0.5 μg of mouse γ-globulin per ml, was incubated overnight in flat-bottomed polystyrene plates and in plates washed twice with 5% fetal calf serum (FCS) in 0.01*M* Tris-saline. Serial dilutions of reference gene–cloned γ-interferon (Genentech), using 100 ng/ml to 0.1 ng/ml in 30 μl, were then incubated in plates coated with the original monoclonal anti–γ-interferon. In parallel, 30-μl dilutions of test synovial fluid were studied. After overnight incubation at 4°C, the test plates were washed with Tris-saline/FCS, and 30 μl of a second monoclonal anti–γ-interferon antibody (Genentech) conjugated with horseradish peroxidase at 1 μg/ml was applied, followed by color development and reading in the micro–enzyme-linked immunosorbent assay (ELISA) reader. Addition of known amounts of γ-interferon to synovial

Table 2. Clinical data and synovial tissue immunofluorescence assay results in 9 rheumatoid arthritis (RA) patients and 2 normal controls*

Source (age)	Joint studied	Degree of inflammation	% lymphocytes: B cells	% lymphocytes: T3	MO	% T3 positive: T4	% T3 positive: T8	C3	C5b-9	C9	IL-2	Ia	γ-IFN
RA patient													
1 (61)	Wrist	Severe	15	85	+++	90	10	+	+ (few cells)	+ (few cells)	+	+++	+
2 (71)	Knee	Severe	25	75	++	90	10	+	+	+	+	+++	+
3 (47)	Wrist	Moderate	10	90	++	95	5	+	+	+	+	+++	+
4 (64)	Knee	Moderate	20	80	++	85	15	+	+	+	+	++	+
5 (60)	Knee	Moderate	10	90	+	80	20	+	+	+	+	++	0
6 (57)	Knee	Moderate	10	90	+	90	10	0	0	0	+	++	+
7 (31)	Knee	Mild	20	80	+	95	5	0	0	0	0	+	0
8 (68)	Knee	Mild	5	95	+	80	20	0	0	0	0	+	+
9 (49)	Wrist	Mild	10	90	+	80	20	0	0	0	+	++	+
Normal control													
1 (28)	Knee	Absent	0	0	0	0	0	0	0	0	0	+ (lining cells)	0
2 (26)	Knee	Absent	0	0	0	0	0	0	0	0	0	+ (lining cells)	0

* MO = macrophage; IL-2 = interleukin-2; γ-IFN = γ-interferon. The intensity of immunofluorescence was graded as: absent (0), slight (+), moderate (++), or very strong (+++).

fluids and subsequent quantitation showed that synovial fluid components did not interfere with accurate quantitation.

RESULTS

A summary of our findings on the tissue localization of the various immune reactants studied is given in Table 2. The degree of overall synovial tissue inflammation was arbitrarily graded as mild, moderate, or severe, based on careful assessment of multiple serial H & E–stained sections of each synovial sample. In most cases, lymphocytic infiltrates identified within rheumatoid synovial tissues were predominantly T cells. The extent of synovial tissue macrophage infiltration was identified principally by careful assessment of serial H & E–stained sections and was graded as absent, mild, moderate, or severe (0–3+). T cell subset distribution varied depending on the precise areas examined within the synovium, but in all cases, an overall relative predominance of helper/inducer OKT4 T cells over suppressor/cytotoxic OKT8 T cells was recorded. Similar to observations recorded by several other groups (20–23), T cell infiltrates, particularly those of the OKT4 phenotype, were frequently noted in close anatomic juxtaposition to macrophages staining positively for Ia. Ia antigen–positive cells were identified as B cells, macrophages, activated T cells of both the OKT4 and OKT8 subsets, and as synovial lining cells where, in many sections examined, most of the synovial lining cells were Ia-positive (Figure 1).

Activated complement components identified with anti–C5b-9 neoantigen and anti-C9 were frequently noted within the cytoplasm of phagocytic cells that were concurrently staining positively for Ia. In many portions of rheumatoid synovia, there were small amounts of extracellular granules staining positively for C5b-9 and C9 in parallel with positive anti-Ig immunofluorescence (Figure 2). These changes showed a direct relationship to the degree of histologic evidence of the severity of inflammation within the particular synovial tissue examined.

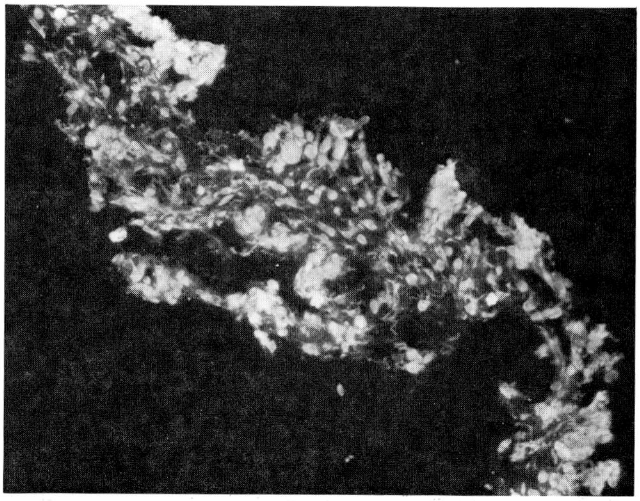

Figure 1. Immunofluorescence demonstration of the localization of Ia antigens on multiple synovial lining cells in tissue from a patient with rheumatoid arthritis (original magnification × 250).

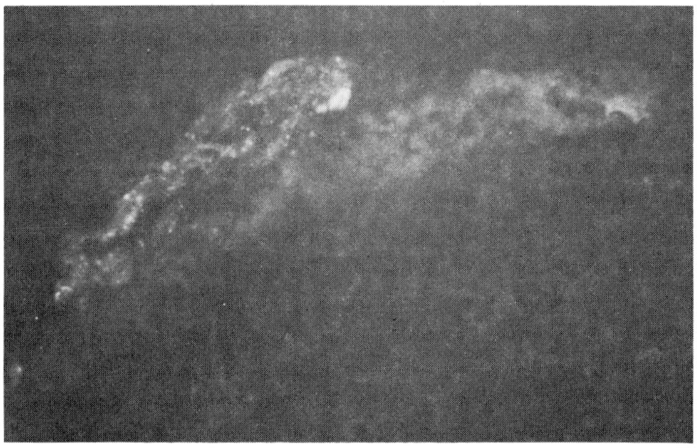

A

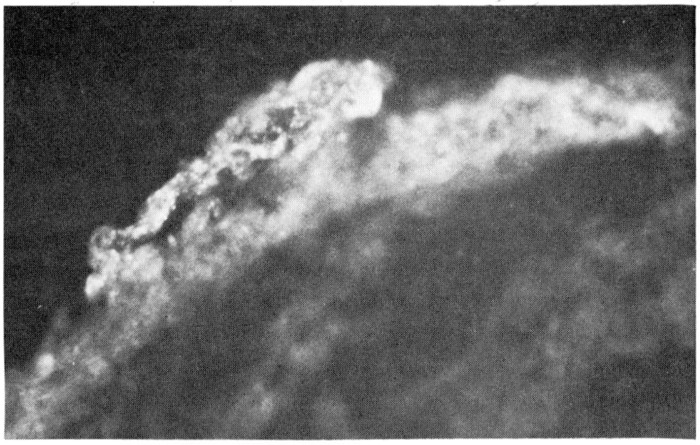

B

Figure 2. Extracellular deposition of C9 (**A**) shown as particulate staining with staining of the connective tissue margin. C9 deposition was present in the same distribution as IgG (**B**) (original magnification × 400).

Despite the apparent intensity of tissue inflammation and lymphocytic infiltration noted in many of the rheumatoid tissues examined, staining for tissue localization of IL-2 was relatively weak and focal compared with the distribution shown by immunofluorescence of other antigens, such as OKT4 or Ia. Specificity of fluorescent staining was confirmed by abolition of T cell membrane reactions after absorption of anti–IL-2 antibody, using cloned IL-2. Double immunofluorescence studies using fluorescein and rhodamine conjugates in parallel sections indicated faint particulate or rim IL-2 membrane localization on OKT4 as well as OKT8 cells. Distinct particulate lymphocyte membrane–bound IL-2 on T cells was identified in 7 of 9 rheumatoid synovial tissues examined. Figure 3 shows examples of these findings. No positive IL-2 membrane or other tissue immunofluorescence was identified in the 2 normal synovial tissues, which were, of course, devoid of lymphocytic infiltrates.

Localization of γ-interferon within rheumatoid synovial tissues was recorded using double immunofluorescence techniques among a number of cell types, including B cells, T cells, and Ia-positive macrophages. Positive identification of γ-interferon was recorded in 7 of 9 RA synovia but was not detected in

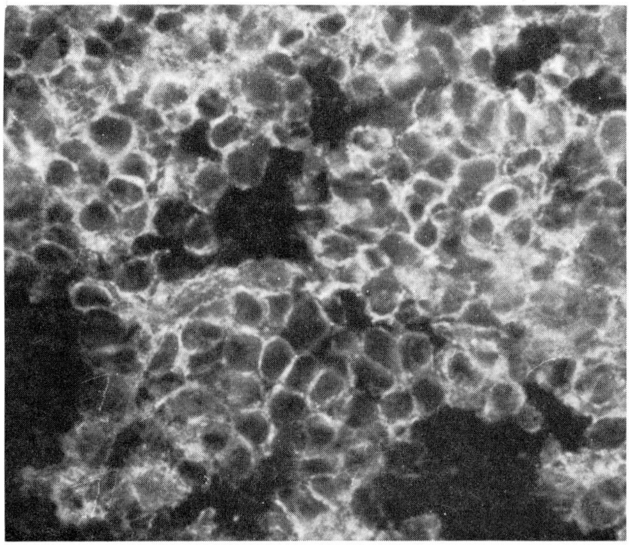

A

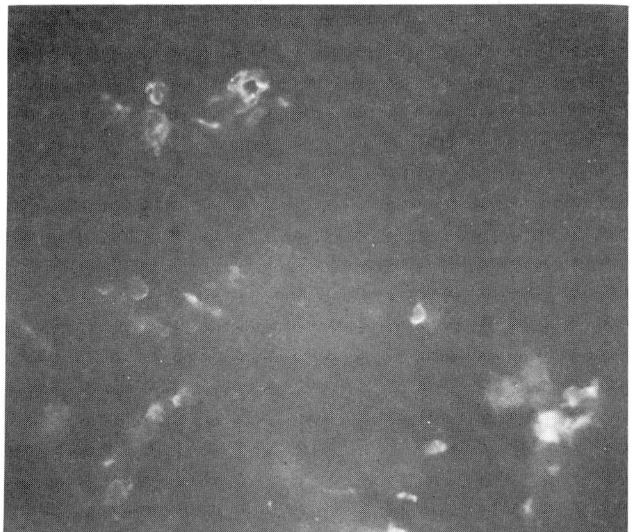

B

Figure 3. A, Indirect immunofluorescence demonstration of T cells infiltrating areas of very active rheumatoid synovitis, stained with OKT3 (original magnification × 400). **B**, Similar field to that shown in **A**, stained with monoclonal antibody specific for interleukin-2. Scattered T cells showing rim membrane or particulate immunofluorescence are seen (original magnification × 250).

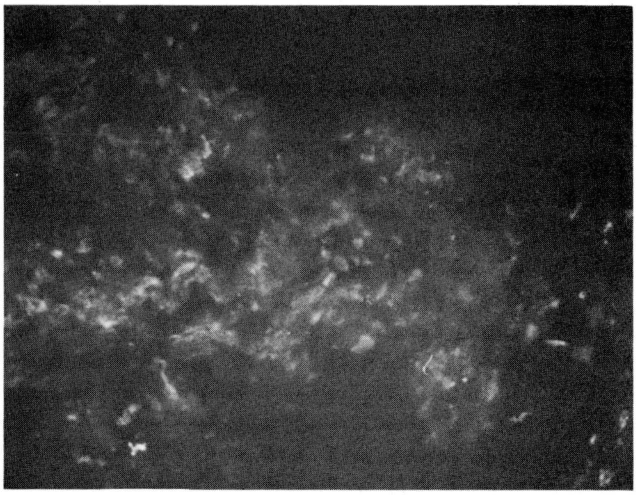

Figure 4. Immunofluorescence demonstration of the localizations of γ-interferon, detected as cytoplasmic and membrane staining among numerous cells infiltrating the rheumatoid synovium. Double immunofluorescence studies indicated γ-interferon associated with T cells, B cells, and macrophage-like cells (original magnification × 250).

normal synovial tissues. An example of rather faint synovial tissue staining for γ-interferon is shown in Figure 4. In general, the cellular localization of γ-interferon was surprisingly sparse compared with the other antigens, such as Ia, OKT4, OKT3, or C5b-9, that were studied in parallel.

Parallel quantitative estimation of γ-interferon, performed using the double monoclonal antibody ELISA method of Staehelin et al (19), showed that only 3 of 9 RA synovial fluids examined contained detectable levels (above 0.1 ng/ml or 3.4 units/ml), using this method (Table 3). No detectable γ-interferon was present in 6 other synovial fluids, including samples from patients with psoriatic arthritis, ankylosing spondylitis, and degenerative arthritis. A single sample from a patient with juvenile rheumatoid arthritis contained detectable γ-interferon.

DISCUSSION

This study provides some direct observations on the immunochemical localization of IL-2 and γ-interferon within the synovial tissues of patients with active rheumatoid arthritis. T cell growth factor, or interleukin-2, has been characterized as an important lymphokine that is necessary for the ongoing growth and nurturing of activated T cells (24–26). There is clear evidence of a marked increment in T cell activation in the rheumatoid synovium, with increased numbers of Ia-positive T cells having been clearly documented both in synovial fluids and tissues of RA patients (27). Recent studies by Young et al (28) have also demonstrated rheumatoid synovial tissue localization of transferrin receptor and epidermal growth factor, possibly also indicative of local tissue activation in some patients. IL-2 is produced by T cells of either the OKT4 or OKT8 phenotype (29–31). Previous studies have shown that the majority of lymphocytes present within the rheumatoid synovium are T cells (14,32), and our own direct immunofluorescence studies during the course of the present work have, by double immunofluorescence, identified IL-2 on the membranes of OKT4 as well as OKT8 synovial T cells.

However, one of the surprising findings of this study was that, within the rheumatoid synovial membranes examined by immunofluorescence, there was relatively sparse evidence for cells either making or having adsorbed membrane IL-2. A priori we had expected to document massive amounts of IL-2 by immunofluorescence localization within all of the rheumatoid tissues examined. Of possible relevance to the apparent scarcity of IL-2–producing cells within the RA synovium are some recent observations by Arya et al (33), indicating a lack of actual expression of the T cell growth factor gene among cells infected with the newly described human T cell leukemia-lymphoma virus (HTLV). In the latter instance, cells transformed by HTLV appear to utilize other mechanisms to regulate control. The relative paucity of cells making IL-2 within rheumatoid synovium may only reflect the fact that a minor cell population within the inflamed synovium is capable of the production and spread of sufficient IL-2 to keep the inflammatory process activated. Kinetic studies comparing actual IL-2 production by rheumatoid synovium versus that of synovial tissues obtained from infected or otherwise activated

Table 3. γ-interferon levels, estimated by immunochemical technique, in synovial fluids from patients with various forms of arthritis

Diagnosis	No. studied	γ-interferon levels ng/ml	γ-interferon levels units/ml
Rheumatoid arthritis	6	<0.1	<3.4
	1	0.2	6.8
	1	0.34	11.5
	1	1.4	47.0
Juvenile rheumatoid arthritis	1	0.2	6.8
Psoriatic arthritis	1	<0.1	<3.4
Ankylosing spondylitis	2	<0.1	<3.4
Degenerative arthritis	3	<0.1	<3.4

patients are necessary before the relative importance of local IL-2 in the rheumatoid inflammatory process can be determined.

Also, it is important to point out that the use of a monoclonal anti–IL-2 antibody and the complete absorption of positive staining using recombinant IL-2 do not rule out the possibility that the anti–IL-2 reagent may, in some instances, be reacting with other cross-reacting determinants. Clearly, T cells from a synovial source in RA patients have been demonstrated to be interleukin-2–dependent when studied as continuous cell lines (34). Moreover, IL-1 activity has been demonstrated in synovial fluids from RA patients (35) and IL-1 provides the stimulus for IL-2 production.

Studies by Rappaport and Dodge (36) have indicated that prostaglandin E (PGE) can inhibit production of IL-2. A number of studies have now clearly documented intense production of PGE by rheumatoid synovium (37,38). As previously stated, precise in vitro data are now required in order to study the actual production of and responsiveness to IL-2 by cells from rheumatoid synovia.

Recent studies by Combe et al (39) and Miyasaka and coworkers (40) have apparently shown a relative deficit in IL-2 production and response by synovial fluid cells, synovial tissues, and peripheral blood lymphocytes from patients with rheumatoid arthritis. These findings would therefore support the results of our immunofluorescence analyses recorded here.

During the course of this study, the presence of γ-interferon was detected in association with a number of cellular phenotypes in rheumatoid synovial tissues. Again, however, the actual intensity of γ-interferon was judged to be low in comparison with conditions noted histologically in the same tissues. The possible relative down-modulation of γ-interferon by rheumatoid synovial tissues may reflect the fact that IL-2 has been shown to control γ-interferon production in several experimental systems (41–43). Studies by Hasler et al (44) also suggest a possible deficiency of γ-interferon production in rheumatoid arthritis and may explain part of the dysregulation of the Epstein-Barr virus response in this disease.

A report by Degre et al (45) has recently provided evidence of γ-interferon in 4 of 10 synovial fluids obtained from RA patients. The results of our quantitation studies of γ-interferon (summarized in Table 3) are similar to those found by this group. It is of interest that we used an immunochemical ELISA technique in our γ-interferon assay, whereas Degre and coworkers used a functional viral inhibition test system. Again, it is clear that there is a need for quantitative studies of γ-interferon production in the peripheral blood as well as the synovial tissues of RA patients. Of considerable interest in the spectrum of questions about the role of γ-interferon in RA are recent observations of Nogueira et al (46), who found defective γ-interferon production in patients with leprosy, a chronic granulomatous disease that, in some ways, is analogous to rheumatoid arthritis. Dissection of the physiologic significance of both IL-2 and γ-interferon will eventually be important in understanding the basic inflammatory process in patients with rheumatoid arthritis.

REFERENCES

1. Franklin EC, Holman HR, Muller-Eberhard HJ, Kunkel HG: An unusual protein component of high molecular weight in the serum of certain patients with rheumatoid arthritis. J Exp Med 105:425–438, 1957
2. Kunkel HG, Franklin EC, Muller-Eberhard HJ: Studies on the isolation and characterization of the "rheumatoid factor." J Clin Invest 38:424–429, 1958
3. Fudenberg HH, Kunkel HG: Specificity of the reaction between rheumatoid factors and gamma globulin. J Exp Med 114:257–278, 1961
4. Kunkel HG, Muller-Eberhard HJ, Fudenberg HH, Holman HR: Gamma globulin complexes in rheumatoid arthritis and certain other conditions. J Clin Invest 40:117–129, 1961
5. Pope RM, Teller DC, Mannik M: The molecular basis of self-association of antibodies to IgG (rheumatoid factors) in rheumatoid arthritis. Proc Natl Acad Sci USA 71:517–521, 1974
6. Winchester RJ, Agnello V, Kunkel HG: Gamma globulin complexes in synovial fluids of patients with rheumatoid arthritis: partial characterization and relationship to lowered complement levels. Clin Exp Immunol 6:689–706, 1970
7. Pekin JT, Zvaifler NJ: Hemolytic complement in synovial fluid. J Clin Invest 43:1372–1382, 1964
8. Zvaifler NJ: Breakdown products of C′3 in human synovial fluids. J Clin Invest 48:1532–1542, 1969
9. Kinsella TD, Baum J, Ziff M: Immunofluorescent demonstration of an IgG B′C complex in synovial lining cells of rheumatoid synovial membrane. Clin Exp Immunol 4:265–271, 1969
10. Rodriguez MA, Prinz WA, Sibbitt WL, Bankhurst AD, Williams RC Jr: α-interferon increases immunoglobulin production in cultured human mononuclear leukocytes. J Immunol 130:1215–1219, 1983
11. Rodriguez MA, Prinz WA, Sibbitt WL, Bankhurst AD, Williams RC Jr: Human alpha-interferon enhances in

vitro synthesis of IgM rheumatoid factor by lymphocytes from normal subjects and rheumatoid arthritis patients. Arthritis Rheum 26:1091–1097, 1983
12. Alcocer-Varela J, Alarcon-Segovia D: Decreased production of and response to interleukin-2 by cultured lymphocytes from patients with systemic lupus erythematosus. J Clin Invest 69:1388–1392, 1982
13. Ropes MW, Bennett GA, Cobb S, Jacox R, Jessar RA: 1958 revision of diagnostic criteria for rheumatoid arthritis. Bull Rheum Dis 9:175–176, 1958
14. Bankhurst AD, Husby G, Williams RC Jr: Predominance of T cells in the lymphocytic infiltrates of synovial tissues in rheumatoid arthritis. Arthritis Rheum 19: 555–562, 1976
15. Husby G, Bankhurst AD, Williams RC Jr: Immunohistochemical localization of prostaglandin E in rheumatoid synovial tissues. Arthritis Rheum 20:785–791, 1977
16. Biesecker G, Katz S, Koffler D: Renal localization of the membrane attack complex in systemic lupus erythematosus nephritis. J Exp Med 154:1779–1794, 1981
17. Biesecker G, Lavin L, Ziskind M, Koffler D: Cutaneous localization of the membrane attack complex in discoid and systemic lupus erythematosus. N Engl J Med 306: 264–270, 1982
18. Steinmann G, Conlon D, Hefeneides S, Gillis S: Serological visualization of interleukin 2. Science 220:1188–1190, 1983
19. Staehelin T, Stahi C, Hobbs DS, Pestka S: A rapid quantitative assay of high sensitivity for human leukocyte interferon with monoclonal antibodies. Methods Enzymol 79:589–595, 1981
20. Klareskog L, Forsum U, Scheynins A, Kabelitz D, Wigzell H: Evidence in support of a self-perpetuating HLA-DR-dependent delayed-type cell reaction in rheumatoid arthritis. Proc Natl Acad Sci USA 79:3632–3636, 1982
21. Duke O, Panayi GS, Janossy G, Poulter LW: An immunohistological analysis of lymphocyte subpopulations and their micro-environment in the synovial membranes of patients with rheumatoid arthritis using monoclonal antibodies. Clin Exp Immunol 49:22–30, 1982
22. Meijer CJLM, de Graaff-Reitsma CB, Lafeber GJM, Cats A: In situ localization of lymphocyte subsets in synovial membranes of patients with rheumatoid arthritis with monoclonal antibodies. J Rheumatol 9:359–365, 1982
23. Klareskog L, Forsum U, Wigren A, Wigzell H: Relationships between HLA-DR-expressing cells and T lymphocytes of different subsets in rheumatoid synovial tissue. Scand J Immunol 15:501–507, 1982
24. Watson J, Mochizuki D: Interleukin 2: a class of T cell growth factors. Immunol Rev 51:257–278, 1980
25. Morgan DA, Ruscetti FW, Gallo R: Selective in vitro growth of T lymphocytes from normal human bone marrows. Science 193:1007–1008, 1976
26. Gillis S, Smith KA: Long term culture of tumour-specific cytotoxic T cells. Nature 268:154–156, 1977
27. Burmester G, Yu D, Irani A, Kunkel H, Winchester R: Ia^+ T cells in synovial fluid and tissues of patients with rheumatoid arthritis. Arthritis Rheum 24:1370–1376, 1981
28. Young CL, Adamson TC III, Vaughan JH, Fox RI: Immunohistologic characterization of synovial membrane lymphocytes in rheumatoid arthritis. Arthritis Rheum 27:32–39, 1984
29. Meuer SC, Hussey RE, Penta AC, Fitzgerald KA, Stadler BM, Schlossman SF, Reinherz EL: Cellular origin of interleukin 2 (IL 2) in man: evidence for stimulus-restricted IL 2 production by $T4^+$ and $T8^+$ T lymphocytes. J Immunol 129:1076–1079, 1982
30. Solbach W, Barth S, Rollinghoff M, Wagner H: Interactions of human T cell subsets during the induction of cytotoxic T lymphocytes: the role of interleukins. Clin Exp Immunol 49:167–175, 1982
31. Luger TA, Smolen JS, Chused TM, Steinberg AD, Oppenheim JJ: Human lymphocytes with either the OKT4 or OKT8 phenotype produce interleukin 2 in culture. J Clin Invest 70:470–473, 1982
32. Van Boxel J, Paget S: Predominantly T cell infiltrate in rheumatoid synovial membranes. N Engl J Med 293: 517–520, 1975
33. Arya SK, Wong-Staal F, Gallo RC: T-cell growth factor gene: lack of expression in human T-cell leukemia-lymphoma virus-infected cells. Science 223:1086–1087, 1984
34. Wilkins JA, Warrington RJ: The generation of interleukin 2 dependent continuous T cell lines from synovial fluid mononuclear cells in rheumatoid arthritis (abstract). Clin Res 30:810A, 1982
35. Fontana A, Hengartner H, Weber E, Fehr K, Grob PJ, Cohen G: Interleukin 1 activity in the synovial fluid of patients with rheumatoid arthritis. Rheumatol Int 2:49–53, 1982
36. Rappaport RS, Dodge GR: Prostaglandin E inhibits the production of human interleukin 2. J Exp Med 155:943–948, 1982
37. Dayer J-M, Krane SM, Russell RGG, Robinson DR: Production of collagenase and prostaglandins by isolated adherent rheumatoid synovial cells. Proc Natl Acad Sci USA 73:945-949, 1976
38. Dayer J-M, Robinson DR, Krane SM: Prostaglandin production by rheumatoid synovial cells: stimulation by a factor from human mononuclear cells. J Exp Med 145:1399–1404, 1977
39. Combe B, Pope RM, Fischbach M, Darnell B, Baron S, Talal N: Interleukin-2 in rheumatoid arthritis: production of and response to IL-2 in rheumatoid synovial fluid, synovial tissue and peripheral blood (abstract). Arthritis Rheum (suppl) 27:S55, 1984
40. Miyasaka N, Nakamura T, Russell IJ, Talal N: Interleu-

kin 2 deficiencies in rheumatoid arthritis and systemic lupus erythematosus. Clin Immunol Immunopathol 31: 109–117, 1984
41. Torres BA, Farrar WL, Johnson HM: Interleukin 2 regulates immune interferon (IFNγ) production by normal and suppressor cell cultures. J Immunol 128:2217–2219, 1982
42. Benjamin WR, Steeg PS, Farrar JJ: Production of immune interferon by an interleukin 2-independent murine T cell line. Proc Natl Acad Sci USA 79:5379–5383, 1982
43. Yamamoto JK, Farrar WL, Johnson HM: Interleukin 2 regulation of mitogen induction of immune interferon (IFNγ) in spleen cells and thymocytes. Cell Immunol 66:333–341, 1982
44. Hasler F, Bluestein HG, Zvaifler NJ, Epstein LB: Analysis of the defects responsible for the impaired regulation of Epstein-Barr virus-induced B cell proliferation by rheumatoid arthritis lymphocytes. I. Diminished gamma interferon production in response to autologous stimulation. J Exp Med 157:173–188, 1983
45. Degre M, Mellbye OJ, Clarke-Jenssen O: Immune interferon in serum and synovial fluid in rheumatoid arthritis and related disorders. Ann Rheum Dis 42:672–676, 1983
46. Nogueira N, Kaplan G, Levy E, Sarno EN, Kushner P, Granelli-Piperno A, Vieira L, Colomer-Gould V, Levis W, Steinman R, Yip YK, Cohn ZA: Defective γ interferon production in leprosy: reversal with antigen and interleukin 2. J Exp Med 158:2165–2170, 1983

CIRCULATING NATURAL KILLER CELLS IN SJÖGREN'S SYNDROME

YUKINOBU ICHIKAWA, MIYOKO YOSHIDA, MASATOSHI TAKAYA, MITSUAKI UCHIYAMA, HIROAKI SHIMIZU, and SHIGERU ARIMORI

Reduced natural killer (NK) cell activity of peripheral blood lymphocytes (PBL) has been reported in a number of diseases including Sjögren's syndrome (SS). In this study, we used 2 monoclonal antibodies directed toward NK cells (anti–Leu-7 and anti–Leu-11) for determining NK cell activity in 29 patients with SS (9 with primary SS and 20 with secondary SS). The NK activity of PBL was simultaneously determined by the ^{51}Cr release method using K562 as target cells. Contrary to previous reports, we did not find reduced NK activity of PBL in our patients compared with sex- and age-matched healthy controls. Although the percentage of Leu-7$^+$ cells was significantly higher in the patients than in the controls ($P < 0.05$), the absolute number of circulating Leu-7$^+$ cells was not different between the groups. The percentage of Leu-11$^+$ cells, however, was not significantly different between the patients and the controls, but the number of circulating Leu-11$^+$ cells was significantly fewer in the patients than in the controls ($P < 0.05$). Between the primary and secondary SS groups, no significant differences were found in NK cell activity or in the percentage of Leu-7$^+$ or Leu-11$^+$ cells. Furthermore, we found a significant correlation of NK activity with the percentage of Leu-11$^+$ cells ($P <$ 0.05) in the controls as well as the SS patients, although a significant correlation was not identified between NK activity and the percentage of Leu-7$^+$ cells. These results are compatible with the known specificities of each monoclonal antibody: the anti–Leu-11 antibody is more specific for functionally active NK cells than is the anti–Leu-7 antibody. The NK activity of PBL, therefore, was proportional to the percentage of NK cells (Leu-11$^+$ cells) and was not impaired in our patients with SS, although the number of circulating NK cells was fewer in the patients than in the healthy controls.

From The Fourth Department of Internal Medicine, School of Medicine, Tokai University, Kanagawa, Japan.

Yukinobu Ichikawa, MD, PhD; Miyoko Yoshida, MT; Masatoshi Takaya, MD, PhD; Mitsuaki Uchiyama, MD; Hiroaki Shimizu, MD; Shigeru Arimori, MD, PhD.

Address reprint requests to Yukinobu Ichikawa, MD, PhD, The Fourth Department of Internal Medicine, School of Medicine, Tokai University, Isehara-shi, Kanagawa-ken, 259-11, Japan.

Submitted for publication April 25, 1984; accepted in revised form September 6, 1984.

Natural killer (NK) cells are defined as spontaneously cytotoxic cells that can lyse certain tumor cell lines in vitro. Attention has been drawn to the NK cells because these cells could be active in the host defense against malignancy and viral infections in vivo (1). Originally, the cells were considered to be null cells which lacked conventional T or B lymphocyte markers (2). The cell lineage of NK cells, however, is still unknown, since some NK cells have been shown to express certain cell surface antigens shared by T lymphocytes or macrophage/monocytes (3,4).

Sjögren's syndrome (SS) is a chronic inflammatory disease characterized by mononuclear cell infiltrations of the exocrine glands, including lacrimal and salivary glands. Although the pathogenesis of this disease is obscure, an autoimmune mechanism has been strongly suggested by a number of observations, including frequent association of this disease with other autoimmune diseases (5), various serologic abnormalities (5), and defects in cellular immunity (6–8). Additionally, the development of lymphoproliferative disorders has been reported to be frequent in patients with SS (9). In this regard, the NK activity of peripheral blood lymphocytes (PBL) has been studied in patients with SS and has been reported to be diminished in these patients (10,11). However, contrasting results have also been reported (12).

Recently, it has become possible to enumerate human NK cells by using monoclonal antibodies directed toward NK cells (13,14). In this study, therefore, we enumerated the NK cells in the peripheral blood of patients with SS by using the 2 monoclonal antibodies, anti–Leu-7 and anti–Leu-11, with simultaneous determination of the NK activity. The anti–Leu-11 antibody has been reported to be more specific for functional NK cells than the anti–Leu-7 antibody (14,15). Contrary to previous reports, neither the activity nor the percentage of NK cells (Leu-11$^+$ cells) was significantly different in our patients compared with sex- and age-matched healthy adult controls. Furthermore, the NK activity of PBLs was proportional to the percentage of NK cells (Leu-11$^+$ cells) in patients with SS, and the functional defects of NK cells were not confirmed in these patients.

PATIENTS AND METHODS

Patients. In this study, there were 29 female patients with SS, 7 of whom had no associated immunologic diseases and 2 of whom had chronic thyroiditis. These latter 9 patients were classified as having primary SS. The remaining 20 patients were classified as having secondary SS in association with rheumatoid arthritis (RA; 4 patients), systemic lupus erythematosus (SLE; 5 patients), progressive systemic sclerosis (PSS; 7 patients), and mixed connective tissue disease (MCTD; 4 patients). One patient with SS secondary to SLE and 2 patients with SS secondary to MCTD also had chronic thyroiditis.

The diagnosis of SS was based on objective evidence of either lacrimal involvement (keratoconjunctivitis sicca), demonstrated by rose bengal staining, or salivary gland involvement, confirmed by secretory sialography or by salivary gland biopsy. SLE, RA, and PSS were diagnosed according to the American Rheumatism Association criteria for each disease (16–18). Patients who had diffuse thyroid enlargement and antithyroid antibodies without hyperthyroidism were diagnosed as having chronic thyroiditis. In our patients, evidence of MCTD was the presence of Raynaud's phenomenon and swollen hands in addition to the presence of high-titer anti-ribonucleoprotein antibody.

At the time of this study, 19 patients were receiving oral prednisolone therapy (average 5.0 ± 2.5 mg/day, range 2.5–12.5). In addition to prednisolone, 2 of these patients were taking nonsteroidal antiinflammatory drugs (NSAID), and 1 was taking D-penicillamine (200 mg/day). Eight patients were taking NSAID alone, and the remaining 2 were taking no medications. There was no significant difference in the mean dosage of prednisolone between the primary and secondary SS groups.

Seventeen healthy women served as normal controls. The mean age of the patients (44.2 ± 10.6, range 26–59) was not significantly different from the mean age of the controls (43.2 ± 13.0, range 23–75) ($P > 0.5$).

Preparation of peripheral blood lymphocytes. Ten milliliters of heparinized peripheral blood was mixed with 1 ml of 5% silica suspension in phosphate buffered saline (PBS; 1/15*M*, pH 7.4) (KAC-2; Nippon Kotai Kenkyu-jo, Gunma, Japan) to deplete phagocytes. After incubation for 60 minutes at 37°C, with intermittent agitation, the mixture was layered on Ficoll-Hypaque gradient (specific gravity 1.077) and centrifuged at 400*g* for 30 minutes. Lymphocytes were washed 3 times with Dulbecco's PBS (0.15*M*, pH 7.6), and the cells were suspended in RPMI 1640 medium supplemented with 25 m*M* HEPES buffer, L-glutamine (300 mg/liter), sodium bicarbonate (2 gm/liter), penicillin (10^5 units/liter), streptomycin (100 mg/liter), and 10% fetal bovine serum (heat-inactivated at 56°C for 30 minutes; Gibco, Grand Island, NY). Then the number of NK cells and the NK activity were simultaneously determined, using freshly separated PBL as described below.

The purity of separated lymphocytes was determined by May-Grünwald–Giemsa staining, and the percentages of contaminating phagocytes, including monocytes and granulocytes, were always <2%.

Determination of the proportion of NK cells. Two commercially available monoclonal antibodies reactive with human NK cells (anti–Leu-7 and anti–Leu-11b) were purchased from Becton-Dickinson, Mountain View, CA. Both antibodies are derived from mouse IgM. The anti–Leu-7 antibody can react with up to 25% of normal PBL (19). Some cells lacking the Leu-7 antigen, however, can mediate a significant proportion of NK activity in PBL. More than 60% of Leu-7$^+$ cells also express a myeloid antigen, OKM1. Additionally, some Leu-7$^+$ cells coexpress T lymphocyte–associated antigen, such as Leu-1 (OKT1), Leu-4 (OKT3), and Leu-2a (OKT8) (15).

The monoclonal antibody, anti–Leu-11, is reported to be reactive with essentially all functional NK cells in PBL, although it is also reactive with neutrophils and basophils (14,15). The antigen identified by the antibody is not expressed on monocytes, eosinophils, resting or mitogen-activated T lymphocytes, or B lymphocytes. Moreover, it has been shown that the most efficient NK activity occurs with the Leu-11$^+$, 7$^-$ subset, although the Leu-11$^-$, 7$^+$ subset mediates weak NK activity. The Leu-11$^+$, 7$^+$ subset has variable NK activity, and the Leu-11$^-$, 7$^-$ cells are not able to mediate NK activity.

The proportion of NK cells was determined by a method similar to that described elsewhere (20). Briefly, 100 μl of PBL (5 × 10^6 cells/ml) was incubated with 5 μl of each monoclonal antibody at 4°C for 30 minutes. After washing with medium, the cells were mixed with fluorescein-conjugated $F(ab')_2$ fragment goat anti-mouse IgM (mu chain–specific; Cappel Laboratories, Cochranville, PA) at a final dilution of 1:50. The cells were further incubated at 4°C and then washed with medium. More than 200 lymphocytes were observed by immunofluorescence microscopy, and the percentages of Leu-7$^+$ and Leu-11$^+$ cells were determined. The PBLs incubated with the fluorescein-conjugated antibody alone were examined in a similar manner, and fluorescence positive cells were always <2%.

Determination of NK cell activity. For the determination of NK cell activity, the standard ^{51}Cr release method using K562, a myelogeneous cell line, as target cells was employed (21). The target cells (1.5×10^6 cells/100 μl in medium) were labeled with 150 μCi of $Na_2{}^{51}CrO_4$ (1 mCi/ml; Daiichi Radioisotope, Tokyo, Japan) for 60 minutes at 37°C. After washing, medium was added to adjust the cells to 1×10^5 cells/ml. Effector cells (PBL) were mixed with 1×10^4 target cells in round-bottom microtiter plates to a final volume of 200 μl (effector:target ratio 25:1 or 40:1). After centrifugation at 800 revolutions per minute for 7 minutes, the mixtures were cultured for 4 hours at 37°C in 5% CO_2–95% air.

One hundred microliters of the supernatant was separated and counted in an automatic well-type gamma counter. Spontaneous release was determined by the incubation of 1×10^4 target cells with medium alone. To determine maximum release, 0.1 ml of the target cell suspension (1×10^4 cells) was mixed with 0.9 ml of distilled water. After incubation for 4 hours at 37°C, 0.5 ml of the supernatant was separated and counted. All cultures were performed in triplicate. The percent cytotoxicity was calculated as follows:

$$\frac{\text{cpm of experimental release} - \text{cpm of spontaneous release}}{\text{cpm of maximum release} - \text{cpm of spontaneous release}} \times 100$$

RESULTS

Percentage of NK cells. Mean lymphocyte counts of peripheral blood were significantly lower in all SS patients (1,330 ± 740/mm^3) than in healthy controls (1,927 ± 757/mm^3) (Table 1). The difference in lymphocyte counts was also significant when each SS group (primary or secondary) was compared with controls. However, no statistically significant difference in lymphocyte counts was demonstrated between the primary and the secondary SS groups ($P > 0.5$).

The percentages of Leu-7$^+$ and Leu-11$^+$ cells were determined simultaneously in the purified PBL (Table 1). The percentage of Leu-7$^+$ cells was significantly higher in all SS patients (12.9 ± 5.3%) than in healthy controls (9.0 ± 3.5%). The percentage of Leu-7$^+$ cells was significantly higher in the secondary SS group (14.1 ± 5.3%) compared with controls.

When the secondary SS patient subgroups were compared with healthy controls, the percentages of Leu-7$^+$ cells were significantly higher in the patients with SS secondary to RA and in those with SS secondary to PSS (Table 2). There was no significant difference between the primary SS group and the controls, or between the primary and secondary SS groups, except for the subgroup of SS patients with RA. When absolute numbers of Leu-7$^+$ cells were considered, no difference was found between the patients (173 ± 122/mm^3) and the controls (171 ± 88/mm^3) ($P > 0.5$). The SS patients with RA, however, had significantly more Leu-7$^+$ cells compared with the healthy controls ($P < 0.01$).

The percentage of Leu-11$^+$ cells, however, was not significantly different between healthy controls (12.4 ± 6.3%) and the total SS patient group (12.5 ± 8.9%). Furthermore, we found no difference in the percentage of Leu-11$^+$ cells when primary and secondary SS groups were compared, except for the patients with RA, who had significantly higher percentages of Leu-11$^+$ cells. The absolute number of Leu-11$^+$ cells, however, was significantly fewer in all patients (148 ± 114/mm^3) than in the controls (217 ± 96/mm^3) ($P < 0.05$). When primary and secondary SS groups were

Table 1. Proportion of natural killer (NK) cells and NK activity in patients with Sjögren's syndrome (SS)*

	Controls (n = 17)	All SS patients (n = 29)	Primary SS (n = 9)	Secondary SS (n = 20)
No. lymphocytes/mm^3	1,927 ± 757	1,330 ± 740†	1,304 ± 507‡	1,341 ± 835‡
% Leu-7$^+$ cells	9.0 ± 3.5 (n = 12)	12.9 ± 5.3‡	10.2 ± 4.4	14.1 ± 5.3§
No. Leu-7$^+$ cells/mm^3	171 ± 88 (n = 12)	173 ± 122	150 ± 113	183 ± 127
% Leu-11$^+$ cells	12.4 ± 6.3	12.5 ± 8.9	10.3 ± 4.5	13.5 ± 10.2
No. Leu-11$^+$ cells/mm^3	217 ± 96	148 ± 114‡	143 ± 88	150 ± 126
NK activity (% cytotoxicity)				
E:T ratio 25:1	37.0 ± 15.8	39.5 ± 21.8	42.9 ± 13.7	38.0 ± 24.7
E:T ratio 40:1	50.1 ± 19.5	51.4 ± 23.3 (n = 28)	55.9 ± 13.0 (n = 8)	49.6 ± 26.4
No. taking prednisolone	–	19	4	15
No. taking NSAID	–	10	3	7

* Percent of NK cells was determined using 2 monoclonal antibodies to human NK cells (anti–Leu-7 and anti–Leu-11); NK activity was measured simultaneously, by ^{51}Cr release, using K562 as target cells. See Patients and Methods for details. E:T = effector:target; NSAID = nonsteroidal antiinflammatory drugs.
† $P < 0.02$ versus controls.
‡ $P < 0.05$ versus controls.
§ $P < 0.01$ versus controls.

Table 2. Proportion of natural killer (NK) cells and NK activity in patients with secondary Sjögren's syndrome (SS)*

	SS–RA (n = 4)	SS–SLE (n = 5)	SS–PSS (n = 7)	SS–MCTD (n = 4)
No. lymphocytes/mm³	1,215 ± 1,078	1,963 ± 1,371	1,177 ± 382†	1,315 ± 411
% Leu-7⁺ cells	16.6 ± 4.8‡	13.6 ± 7.7	14.6 ± 4.1§	11.4 ± 5.1
No. Leu-7⁺ cells/mm³	206 ± 207§	195 ± 155	175 ± 80	161 ± 113
% Leu-11⁺ cells	16.9 ± 3.7¶	16.5 ± 13.2	12.9 ± 12.4	7.3 ± 4.5
No. Leu-11⁺ cells/mm³	199 ± 171	169 ± 134	144 ± 133	89 ± 55#
NK activity (% cytotoxicity)				
E:T ratio 25:1	40.4 ± 21.7	43.2 ± 33.3	35.0 ± 19.9	34.2 ± 32.2
E:T ratio 40:1	52.0 ± 23.0	52.5 ± 34.3	49.1 ± 19.6	44.1 ± 38.4
No. taking prednisolone	2	3	6	4
No. taking NSAID	3	3	1	0

* % of NK cells was determined using 2 monoclonal antibodies to human NK cells (anti–Leu-7 and anti–Leu-11); NK activity was measured simultaneously, by ^{51}Cr release, using K562 as target cells. See Patients and Methods for details. RA = rheumatoid arthritis; SLE = systemic lupus erythematosus; PSS = progressive systemic sclerosis; MCTD = mixed connective tissue disease; E:T = effector:target; NSAID = nonsteroidal antiinflammatory drugs.
† $P < 0.05$ versus controls (see Table 1).
‡ $P < 0.01$ versus controls; $P < 0.05$ versus patients with primary SS (see Table 1).
§ $P < 0.01$ versus controls (see Table 1).
¶ $P < 0.05$ versus patients with primary SS (see Table 1).
# $P < 0.02$ versus controls (see Table 1).

each compared with the controls, no significant difference was identified in the number of Leu-11⁺ cells ($0.05 < P < 0.1$). The patients with MCTD had significantly fewer Leu-11⁺ cells compared with healthy controls ($P < 0.02$). In comparing the primary SS group and the secondary SS subgroups, no significant difference was found in the number of Leu-11⁺ cells.

NK cell activity of PBL. The NK activity of PBL was determined at the time the Leu-7⁺ and Leu-11⁺ cells were enumerated. At the effector:target ratios examined, the NK activity of PBL was not significantly different in SS patients compared with controls ($P > 0.5$) (Tables 1 and 2). Moreover, we found no significant difference in NK activity between the primary and secondary SS groups ($P > 0.5$).

Correlation of NK activity with the proportion of Leu-7⁺ or Leu-11⁺ cells. The correlation of NK activity with the percentage of Leu-7⁺ or Leu-11⁺ cells was analyzed statistically by linear regression. No significant correlation was identified between the NK activity of PBL and the percentage of Leu-7⁺ cells in the SS patients versus controls. We did, however, find a positive correlation of NK activity with the percentage of Leu-11⁺ cells in the 46 subjects studied, healthy controls and SS patients ($y = 20.6 + 1.5x$, $r = 0.58$, $P < 0.05$) (Figure 1). Similar correlations of NK activity with the percentage of Leu-11⁺ cells were also found when the 17 controls ($y = 19.2 + 1.4x$, $r = 0.57$, $P < 0.05$) and the 29 SS patients ($y = 21.4 + 1.5x$, $r = 0.59$, $P < 0.05$) were analyzed separately.

When we analyzed the correlation between the percentage of Leu-11⁺ cells and that of Leu-7⁺ cells, there was a positive correlation between the 2 populations in 41 subjects examined, 29 SS patients and 12 controls ($y = 8.6 + 0.24x$, $r = 0.39$, $P < 0.05$). A similar correlation was identified in the 29 SS patients ($y = 9.2 + 0.3x$, $r = 0.50$, $P < 0.05$), although the correlation was not significant in 12 healthy controls ($y = 7.4 + 0.1x$, $r = 0.20$, $P > 0.05$).

Clinical correlations with NK activity and with the proportion of NK cells. Neither the NK activity nor the percentage of NK cells correlated with erythrocyte

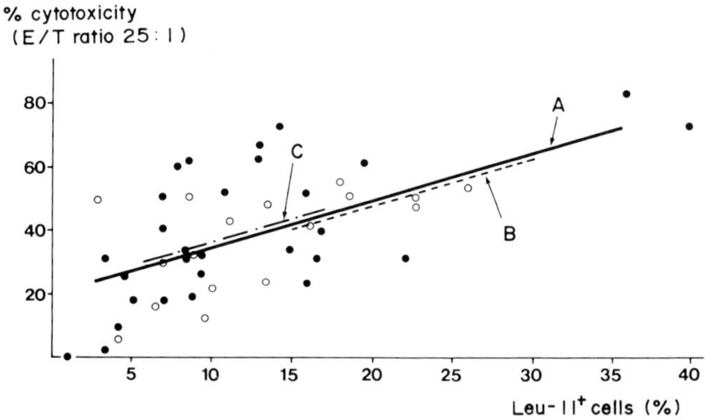

Figure 1. Correlation of natural killer (NK) activity with the percentage of Leu-11⁺ cells, by linear regression analysis. There was a positive correlation in the 46 subjects studied (29 Sjögren's syndrome [SS] patients and 17 normal controls) (**A**; $P < 0.05$). Similar correlations were found when the 17 controls (**B**; $P < 0.05$) and the 29 SS patients (**C**; $P < 0.05$) were analyzed separately. E/T = effector:target; ● = patients with SS; ○ = healthy controls.

sedimentation rates, levels of serum gamma globulin, or serum rheumatoid factor titers in the SS patients. Furthermore, we found no correlations of NK activity or of the percentage of NK cells with history of parotid gland enlargement or with prednisolone therapy at the time of this study.

DISCUSSION

Natural killer cell function has been reported to be abnormal in a number of diseases, such as cancer (22), Chediak-Higashi syndrome (23), and SLE (24). In SLE patients, this abnormality has been thought to be due to serum factors, including circulating immune complexes and antilymphocyte antibodies (25). Additionally, diminished response of NK cells to interferon has been reported in SLE (26).

Reduced NK activity of peripheral blood mononuclear cells has been demonstrated in patients with SS (10,11). The report by Miyasaka et al (11) suggested that multiple causes, including serum factors and the factors derived from macrophages, are involved in the diminished NK activity. Moreover, they have shown that the proportion of NK cells, identified as $OKM1^+$ lymphocytes, was not decreased in their SS patients. Another report has shown that NK activity was not reduced in patients with SS, although interferon-augmented NK activity was significantly depressed in the patients, especially in those with extraglandular disease (12).

Proportional studies of human NK cells have recently become possible because of the availability of monoclonal antibodies directed toward human NK cells (anti–Leu-7 and anti–Leu-11 antibodies) (13,14). One study has shown that there were normal numbers of NK cells, defined by anti–Leu-7 antibody, in PBL of patients with Chediak-Higashi syndrome, but these cells had defective NK function (23). Egan et al (27) reported that the proportion of NK cells, as determined by the $HNK1^+$ antibody, has been found to be variable in patients with SLE, although diminished NK activity was demonstrated. Increased numbers of immature NK cells coexpressing Leu-7 and OKT3 antigens have been suggested as the reason for their results.

In this study, 2 antibodies were used for the determination of NK cells in patients with SS. Contrary to previous reports, we did not find reduced NK activity of PBLs in our SS patients compared with sex- and age-matched healthy controls. Although the percentage of Leu-7^+ cells was significantly higher in patients with SS than in controls, the percentage of Leu-11^+ cells was not different between the 2 groups. When patients with primary SS were compared with those who had secondary SS, neither the NK activity nor the percentage of NK cells (identified by both antibodies) was significantly different. The percentage of NK cells, however, was higher in SS patients with RA compared with either the control group or the group with primary SS.

Peripheral blood lymphocyte counts were significantly lower in the patients compared with the controls. The calculated circulating Leu-11^+ cells, therefore, were significantly fewer in patients than in controls, although the number of Leu-7^+ cells was not different. Furthermore, a similar positive correlation of NK activity with the percentage of Leu-11^+ cells was demonstrated in both the total patient group and the control group. The correlation of NK activity with the percentage of Leu-7^+ cells was not significant, although a positive correlation between the Leu-7^+ and Leu-11^+ cell populations was observed.

These results can be explained from the characteristics of each antibody: the anti–Leu-11 antibody is more specific for functional NK cells than is the anti–Leu-7 antibody (14,15,19). The NK activity, therefore, was proportional to the percentage of NK cells (Leu-11^+ cells) and was not functionally impaired in our SS patients. At present, we do not know the reason for the decreased number of circulating Leu-11^+ cells in the patients. However, this might be due to serum factors, abnormal maturation of NK cells, or local sequestration of NK cells from the circulating pool of NK cells. In this regard, we are attempting to determine the NK cells in exocrine gland tissues of our SS patients. As suggested by previous reports (12,24), the possibility that the patients' NK cells were already activated by stimulation with endogeneous interferon cannot be excluded by our results. Simultaneous determinations of serum interferon and the reactivity of NK cells to interferon in patients with Sjögren's syndrome are required.

REFERENCES

1. Herberman RB, Djeu JY, Kay HD, Ortaldo JR, Riccardi C, Bonnard GD, Holden HT, Fagnani R, Santoni A, Puccetti P: Natural killer cells: characteristics and regulation of activity. Immunol Rev 44:43–70, 1979
2. Herberman RB, Nunn ME, Holden HT, Lavrin DH: Natural cytotoxic reactivity of mouse lymphoid cells against syngeneic and allogeneic tumors. II. Characterization of effector cells. Int J Cancer 16:230–239, 1975
3. Bolhuis RLH, Scuit HRE, Nooyen AM, Ronteltap

CPM: Characterization of natural killer (NK) cells and killer (K) cells in human blood: discrimination between NK and K cell activities. Eur J Immunol 8:731–740, 1978
4. Breard J, Reinherz EL, Kung PC, Goldstein G, Schlossman SF: A monoclonal antibody reactive with human peripheral blood monocytes. J Immunol 124:1943–1948, 1980
5. Bloch KJ, Buchanan WW, Wohl MJ, Bunim JJ: Sjögren's syndrome: a clinical, pathological, and serological study of sixty-two cases. Medicine (Baltimore) 44: 187–231, 1965
6. Leventhal BG, Waldorf DS, Talal N: Impaired lymphocyte transformation and delayed hypersensitivity in Sjögren's syndrome. J Clin Invest 46:1338–1345, 1967
7. Whaley K, Glen ACA, MacSween RNM, Deodhar S, Dick WC, Nuki G, Williamson J, Buchanan WW: Immunological responses in Sjögren's syndrome and rheumatoid arthritis. Clin Exp Immunol 9:721–732, 1971
8. Miyasaka N, Sauvezie B, Pierce DA, Daniels TE, Talal N: Decreased autologous mixed lymphocyte reaction in Sjögren's syndrome. J Clin Invest 66:928–933, 1980
9. Kasan SS, Thomas TL, Moutsopoulos HM, Hoover R, Kimberly RP, Budman DR, Costa J, Decker JL, Chused TM: Increased risk of lymphoma in sicca syndrome. Ann Intern Med 89:888–892, 1978
10. Goto M, Tanimoto K, Chihara T, Horiuchi Y: Natural cell-mediated cytotoxicity in Sjögren's syndrome and rheumatoid arthritis. Arthritis Rheum 24:1377–1382, 1981
11. Miyasaka N, Seaman W, Bakshi A, Sauvezie B, Strand V, Pope R, Talal N: Natural killing activity in Sjögren's syndrome: an analysis of defective mechanisms. Arthritis Rheum 26:954–960, 1983
12. Minato N, Takeda A, Kano S, Takaku F: Studies of the functions of natural killer-interferon system in patients with Sjögren's syndrome. J Clin Invest 69:581–588, 1982
13. Abo T, Balch CM: A differentiation antigen of human NK and K cells identified by a monoclonal antibody (HNK-1). J Immunol 127:1024–1029, 1981
14. Lanier LL, Le AM, Phillips JH, Warner NL, Babcock GF: Subpopulations of human natural killer cells defined by expression of the Leu-7 (HNK-1) and Leu-11 (NK-15) antigens. J Immunol 131:1789–1796, 1983
15. Lanier LL, Engleman EG, Gatenby P, Babcock GF, Warner NL, Herzenberg LA: Correlation of functional properties of human lymphoid cell subsets and surface marker phenotypes using multiparameter analysis and flow cytometry. Immunol Rev 74:143–160, 1983
16. Tan EM, Cohen AS, Fries JF, Masi AT, McShane DJ, Rothfield NF, Schaller JG, Talal N, Winchester RJ: The 1982 revised criteria for the classification of systemic lupus erythematosus. Arthritis Rheum 25:1271–1277, 1982
17. Ropes MW, Bennett GA, Cobb S, Jacox R, Jessar RA: 1958 revision of diagnostic criteria for rheumatoid arthritis. Bull Rheum Dis 9:175–176, 1958
18. Masi AT, Rodnan GP, Medsger TA Jr, Altman RD, D'Angelo WA, Fries JF, LeRoy EC, Kirsner AB, MacKenzie AH, McShane DJ, Myers AR, Sharp GC: Preliminary criteria for the classification of systemic sclerosis (scleroderma). Arthritis Rheum 23:581–590, 1980
19. Abo T, Cooper MD, Balch CM: Characterization of HNK-1^+ (Leu-7) human lymphocytes. I. Two distinct phenotypes of human NK cells with different cytotoxic capability. J Immunol 129:1752–1757, 1982
20. Ichikawa Y, Gonzalez EB, Daniels JC: Suppressor cells of mitogen-induced lymphocyte proliferation in the peripheral blood of patients with common variable hypogammaglobulinemia. Clin Immunol Immunopathol 25: 252–263, 1982
21. Ortaldo JR, Oldham RK, Cannon GC, Herberman RB: Specificity of natural cytotoxic reactivity of normal human lymphocytes against a myeloid leukemia cell line. JNCI 59:77–82, 1977
22. Kadish AS, Doyle AT, Steinhauer EH, Ghossein NA: Natural cytotoxicity and interferon production in human cancer: deficient natural killer activity and normal interferon production in patients with advanced disease. J Immunol 127:1817–1822, 1981
23. Abo T, Roder JC, Abo W, Cooper MD, Balch CM: Natural killer (HNK-1^+) cells in Chediak-Higashi patients are present in normal numbers but are abnormal in function and morphology. J Clin Invest 70:193–197, 1982
24. Goto M, Tanimoto K, Horiuchi Y: Natural cell mediated cytotoxicity in systemic lupus erythematosus: suppression by antilymphocyte antibody. Arthritis Rheum 23: 1274–1281, 1980
25. Herberman RB: Natural killer (NK) cells and their possible roles in resistance against disease. Clin Immunol Rev 1:1–65, 1981
26. Sibbitt WL Jr, Froelich CJ, Bankhurst AD: Abnormal interferon modulation of natural cytotoxicity in systemic lupus erythematosus: relation to suppressive serum factors. Arthritis Rheum 26:1452–1459, 1983
27. Egan ML, Mendelsohn SL, Abo T, Balch CM: Natural killer cells in systemic lupus erythematosus: abnormal numbers and functional immaturity of HNK-1^+ cells. Arthritis Rheum 26:623–629, 1983

SOLUBLE MEDIATORS FROM MONONUCLEAR CELLS INCREASE THE SYNTHESIS OF GLYCOSAMINOGLYCAN BY DERMAL FIBROBLAST CULTURES DERIVED FROM NORMAL SUBJECTS AND PROGRESSIVE SYSTEMIC SCLEROSIS PATIENTS

THERESA L. WHITESIDE, JENNIFER G. WORRALL, ROBERT K. PRINCE, ROBERT B. BUCKINGHAM, and GERALD P. RODNAN

Dermal fibroblast cultures from patients with progressive systemic sclerosis (PSS) synthesize up to 5 times more glycosaminoglycan (GAG) than normal cultures. In an in vitro model of fibroblast-lymphocyte interactions, we show that the supernatants of activated mononuclear cells (MNC) modulate GAG synthesis, as measured by the incorporation of ^{3}H-glucosamine into GAG following incubation of the confluent fibroblast monolayers with active supernatant preparations. GAG accumulation was selectively increased up to 18 times in normal dermal fibroblast cultures. Cell viability was not affected, and ^{3}H-thymidine uptake and cell numbers were depressed in cultures treated with the supernatants. In contrast to normal dermal fibroblast cultures, PSS fibroblasts responded to MNC supernatants by only a 1–2-fold increase in GAG. Supernatants of concanavalin A–activated PSS MNC had higher stimulatory activity than those of normal MNC. Supernatants made with MNC that had been depleted of monocytes on Sephadex G-10 columns were only minimally stimulatory. The GAG-stimulatory supernatants modulated the synthesis, but not the degradation of GAG. Gel filtration on a calibrated Sephadex G-100 column indicated the presence of stimulatory activity in both the 50,000 and 15,000 molecular weight fractions. These activities were trypsin-sensitive, but had different susceptibilities to heat. The active column fractions also contained interleukin-1 activity, as shown in an assay measuring proliferation of mouse thymocytes. Like our factors, interleukin-1 preparations increased GAG in normal and PSS dermal fibroblasts. Products of activated MNC may modulate normal and pathologic processes in human skin.

Presented in part at the 47th Annual Meeting of the American Rheumatism Association, San Antonio, TX, June 1983.

From the Department of Pathology, Division of Clinical Immunopathology, and the Department of Medicine, Division of Rheumatology and Clinical Immunology, University of Pittsburgh School of Medicine, Pittsburgh, Pennsylvania.

Supported by NIH grant AM24019, The Veteran's Administration, and the RGK Foundation, Austin, TX.

Theresa L. Whiteside, PhD: Associate Professor of Pathology, Division of Clinical Immunopathology; Jennifer G. Worrall, MBBS: Fellow in Rheumatology, Divisions of Clinical Immunopathology and Rheumatology and Clinical Immunology, and recipient of the Copeman Travelling Fellowship of The Arthritis and Rheumatism Council of Great Britain; Robert K. Prince, PhD: Research Associate, Division of Rheumatology and Clinical Immunology; Robert B. Buckingham, MD: Clinical Associate Professor of Medicine, Division of Rheumatology and Clinical Immunology.

Dr. Rodnan is deceased.

Address reprint requests to Theresa L. Whiteside, PhD, Room 406, Scaife Hall, University of Pittsburgh School of Medicine, Pittsburgh, PA 15261.

Submitted for publication January 30, 1984; accepted in revised form August 7, 1984.

In progressive systemic sclerosis (PSS, scleroderma), increased accumulation of connective tissue components results in characteristically thickened and indurated skin. Collagen, fibronectin, and glycosaminoglycan (GAG) have all been reported to be present in greater than normal amounts in sclerodermatous skin (1–4). We have demonstrated that dermal fibroblast cultures from patients with PSS accumulate up to fivefold more GAG than do normal cultures and that this accumulation is the result of increased synthesis rather than decreased degradation (5).

PSS skin is often infiltrated with mononuclear cells (MNC) in the early stages of the disease. We have recently shown that these are predominantly T lymphocytes (6). Products of activated T lymphocytes and of monocytes are known to modulate the metabolism of connective tissue cells in culture. Cytokines have been shown to regulate cell growth as well as the synthesis of collagenase-sensitive protein, collagenase, and prostaglandin by human fibroblasts, synovial cells, and chondrocytes in culture (7–11). Through their effects on fibroblast activities in vivo, cytokines may be involved in the processes leading to excessive connective tissue deposition and fibrosis in PSS. In this study, we show that supernatants of mononuclear cells selectively increase the synthesis of GAG by both normal and PSS dermal fibroblasts in culture. We also describe a partial purification and characterization of the factor or factors responsible for this activity.

MATERIALS AND METHODS

Preparation of MNC supernatants. Mononuclear cells from the peripheral blood of normal individuals and patients with PSS were separated on Ficoll-Hypaque gradients, washed, and cultured at 1.5×10^6 MNC/ml of medium 199 (Gibco, Grand Island, NY) supplemented with 0.1% insulin, selenium, transferrin (volume/volume; Collaborative Research, Lexington, MA), 2% fetal calf serum (FCS; Gibco), 20 m*M* HEPES, and 10 μg/ml of gentamicin (Schering, Kenilworth, NJ). Concanavalin A (Con A; Miles Laboratories, Elkhart, IN) was added to the cultures at a concentration of 10–20 μg/ml. Supernatants of the cultures were harvested after 24 hours of incubation at 37°C in a CO_2 incubator, and Con A was inactivated by treatment with 0.1*M* alpha-methyl-D-mannoside (Sigma, St. Louis, MO). In preliminary experiments, control supernatants were generated by incubating medium with MNC without Con A (conditioned medium). To control for possible effects of Con A on fibroblast cultures, Con A was added to medium or conditioned medium and removed by treatment with mannoside. All supernatants were tested on cultured dermal fibroblasts for their effects on connective tissue synthesis.

Fibroblast cultures. Skin biopsy specimens were obtained from the dorsal forearm, midway between the wrist and the elbow, from patients with early, rapidly advancing PSS and from normal volunteers. None of the patients was receiving therapy thought to affect connective tissue metabolism at the time of biopsy, and all were diagnosed as having PSS with diffuse scleroderma in accordance with previously described clinical parameters (12).

Fibroblast cultures were established from explants through subculture of the outgrowing cells and the serial passage as previously described (13). Cultures were studied in the fourth through eighth passage. The cultures to be incubated with MNC supernatants were grown from stock cultures by inoculation of 24-well Falcon plates with 40,000 cells/well on the day the experiment was initiated (day 0). Fibroblast cultures were grown in medium 1066 (Gibco) supplemented with glutamine, proline, HEPES, penicillin, and streptomycin, and 15% pooled human serum. Nutrient medium changes were performed on days 1, 4, and 6. By day 6, all cultures were confluent. To each well, 10 μl of medium containing 4 μCi/ml of D-[1,6-^{3}HN]-glucosamine hydrochloride (New England Nuclear, Boston, MA) was added to label newly-synthesized glycosaminoglycan. Twelve-hour pulses were carried out at the time of the medium change on day 6 and during each of 3 subsequent 24-hour periods without additional medium changes. Ten microliters of ascorbic acid (final concentration 50 μg/ml) was added to each well 2 hours before the addition of labeled glucosamine.

Determination of GAG in fibroblast cultures. GAG measurements were performed as follows. To each well, 100 μl of a solution containing 30 mg/ml of pronase (Calbiochem-Behring, San Diego, CA) in 0.15*M* Tris buffer, pH 8.0 was added. The fibroblasts were rapidly detached and cell numbers were obtained on 0.2 ml of the resultant cell suspension in a Coulter counter. The remaining 0.4 ml of cell suspension was incubated with pronase for 4 hours at 55°C to lyse the fibroblasts. The incubation mixture was centrifuged clear, and aliquots were removed for the measurement of total GAG (from both culture medium and cell layer). Carrier glycosaminoglycan was added to triplicate 100-μl aliquots of each sample, followed by 10 volumes of 0.5% cetylpyridinium chloride (CPC) in 0.002*M* Na_2SO_4.

Reaction tubes were mixed and allowed to stand for 20 minutes at room temperature. The precipitates were collected on Whatman glass fiber filters (Fisher Scientific, Pittsburgh, PA). Individual tubes and filters were washed twice with 0.1% CPC in 0.02*M* NaCl and then washed 4 times with distilled water. They were then placed in liquid scintillation counting vials and dried in an oven at 45°C. Ten ml of toluene-based scintillation fluid was added and counts performed in a Packard liquid scintillation counter.

GAG accumulating in the culture medium was also measured with a modified carbazole technique for uronic acid after isolation of the polymer (14).

Exposure of fibroblast cultures to MNC supernatants. Confluent fibroblast monolayers were incubated with control and active supernatants of MNC (MNC-SN). The supernatants, or soluble factors partially purified from the supernatants, were added, generally at a 1:10 dilution, to triplicate fibroblast cultures at the time of medium change on day 6 and incubated for 72 hours without changing the medium. GAG was measured in the cultures as described above after 12-hour pulses with ^{3}H-glucosamine.

Quantitation of specific GAGs. To distinguish between different species of GAGs produced by the cultured fibroblasts, aliquots of labeled control (no MNC-SN) and experimental cultures (with MNC-SN) were incubated with specific GAG-degrading enzymes. Assays were performed in triplicate. Test samples were placed in reaction tubes, and the following enzymes were added: (a) Hyaluronidase, fungal (*Streptomyces hyaluronlyticus*, Calbiochem-Behring): 0.5 turbidity-reducing units in 0.025 ml of 0.1*M* acetate buffer, pH 5.0, in a total volume of 0.125 ml for 4 hours at 60°C. This enzyme is specific for hyaluronic acid and contains no protease activity at pH 5.0. (b) Chondroitinase AC (Miles Biochemicals, division of Miles Laboratories): 0.1 units in 0.025 ml of 0.4*M* Tris buffer, pH 8.0, in a total volume of 0.125 ml at 37°C overnight. This enzyme degrades hyaluronic acid and chondroitin sulfates A and C (chondroitin 4 and chondroitin 6 sulfates). (c) Chondroitinase ABC (Miles Biochemicals): 0.5 units in 0.025 ml of 0.4*M* Tris buffer, pH 8.0, in a total volume of 0.125 ml at 37°C overnight. This enzyme degrades chondroitin sulfates A, B, and C but has no activity with respect to heparin, heparin sulfate, or keratin sulfate. (d) Pronase: 1.0 mg in 0.1 ml distilled water, added to each reaction tube as a final step for 4 hours at 55°C.

After the pronase step, carrier GAG was added to each tube, and GAG measurements were performed as described above.

Measurements of GAG degradation in fibroblast cultures. The ^{3}H-glucosamine–labeled GAG was prepared by growing normal fibroblasts in ^{3}H-glucosamine–containing medium under standard conditions. The supernatants of confluent cultures were collected, dialyzed extensively against fresh medium, and concentrated. The dialyzed supernatant contained 100,000 counts per minute/ml. It was added to confluent normal fibroblast cultures (44,000 cpm/well) either at the time of addition of the MNC supernatant or for the last 12 hours of incubation with the supernatant. Controls without MNC supernatants and medium controls without fibroblasts were also included. After 24- or 72-hour incubation of fibroblast cultures with MNC supernatant, they were harvested, GAG was precipitated with CPC, and the total radioactive counts in the MNC-supernatant–treated versus untreated cultures were determined.

To ascertain whether excess labeled GAG inhibits ^{3}H-glucosamine uptake by fibroblasts incubated with and without MNC supernatants, we added labeled GAG in the presence and absence of ^{3}H-glucosamine to normal fibroblast cultures incubated with MNC supernatants. Newly-synthesized GAG was estimated by subtracting the CPC-precipitable cpm of cultures containing labeled GAG alone from cpm of cultures incubated with labeled GAG and ^{3}H-glucosamine.

Removal of monocytes from MNC. Adherent cells were removed by passing MNC through a Sephadex G-10 column (15) or by a combination of this method with glass adherence. Monocyte-depleted lymphocytes were tested for the presence of alpha-naphthyl acetate esterase–positive and OKM1-positive cells in acetone-fixed cytocentrifuged preparations. To detect OKM1-positive cells, the avidin-biotin-peroxidase complex (ABC) technique (16) and monoclonal OKM1 reagent (Ortho, Raritan, NJ) were used. To recover monocytes for addition to lymphocyte cultures, cells adherent to glass plates were detached by 20-minute incubation at room temperature and vigorous rinsing with 12 m*M* lidocaine in phosphate buffered saline (PBS), pH 7.4 (17). In some experiments, the isolated adherent cells were irradiated (3,000 rads for 5 minutes) prior to culture with Con A. In addition, MNC depleted of, or enriched with, the adherent cells at a final concentration of 1.5×10^6 cells per ml were incubated with Con A, and the resultant supernatants were tested for GAG stimulatory activity on normal dermal fibroblast cultures as described above.

Preparation of T lymphocyte subpopulations. T lymphocytes were obtained from MNC from normal peripheral blood by "panning" using plastic dishes coated with goat anti-human Ig (18). The isolated T lymphocytes were further fractionated into T4+ and T8+ subpopulations by negative selection using monoclonal antibodies (OKT4 and OKT8; Ortho). T cells treated with OKT8 monoclonal antibody were incubated on plastic plates coated with affinity-purified goat anti-mouse immunoglobulin (18). OKT8+ cells were bound and a nonadherent fraction enriched in T4+ cells was recovered. Similarly, binding of OKT4+ cells to anti-mouse Ig–coated plates yielded a nonadherent fraction enriched in T8+ lymphocytes.

Gel filtration of MNC supernatants on Sephadex G-100. Pooled active supernatants from normal and PSS MNC cultures generated as described above were stored frozen at −70°C. Prior to gel chromatography on Sephadex G-100, the pooled supernatants were concentrated with Aquacide (Calbiochem, San Diego, CA), and 2 milliliters of the concentrate was applied to a 1.5×100 cm column of Sephadex G-100 equilibrated with 0.15*M* PBS at pH 7.2. The column was eluted with PBS, and 2-ml fractions were collected. The column was calibrated using the following markers: bovine serum albumin (BSA, MW 67,000; Sigma); ovalbumin (MW 44,000; Sigma); carbonic anhydrase (MW 29,000; Sigma) and RNase B (MW 14,000; Worthington, Freehold, NJ). The collected fractions were assayed for their protein content and for GAG stimulatory activity on dermal fibroblast cultures.

Interleukin-1 (IL-1) and interleukin-2 (IL-2) activity. IL-1 activity was measured by its capacity to enhance thymocyte proliferation in response to phytohemagglutinin as described (19). Because thymocyte proliferation may also reflect the presence of interleukin-2 (IL-2), supernatant-derived and column-purified fractions were assayed for IL-2 using a standard microassay based on the IL-2–dependent proliferation of a murine T cell line (20). Rabbit IL-1 purified from alveolar and peritoneal macrophages as described by Simon and Willoughby (21) was used as a reference standard. The same preparation of IL-1 was also added to normal and PSS fibroblast cultures in order to study its effect on GAG accumulation.

Characterization of partially-purified GAG stimulatory factor. Aliquots of active fractions from the Sephadex G-100 column were subjected to the following treatments: (a) trypsin digestion (3× crystallized; Worthington) for 30 minutes at 37°C at pH 7.4. Soybean trypsin inhibitor (Sigma) was added to stop the enzymatic reaction; (b) heating at 56°C for 30 minutes and 65°C for 15 minutes; (c) storage at 4°C for 7 days and 37°C for 2 days; (d) dialysis against PBS overnight at 4°C. Control and treated aliquots were assayed for GAG stimulatory activity on normal dermal fibroblasts.

Growth of fibroblasts. Aliquots of unfractionated MNC-SN and of active fractions from the Sephadex G-100 column were investigated for their effect on fibroblast proliferation in both log and confluent cultures. Fibroblasts were seeded into tissue culture plates at a concentration of 20,000 cells per well in the fibroblast culture medium supplemented with 15% human serum. The cells were grown for 24 hours at 37°C in 5% CO_2. Medium was then changed and active or control supernatants or PBS (40 μl/500 μl medium) was added. The cultures were incubated for up to 6 days. Every 24 hours, cells in triplicate wells were pulsed with ^{3}H-thymidine at 1 μCi/well for the last 4 or 12 hours of incubation. In confluent cultures, 12-hour pulses were done at 24-hour intervals during incubation with MNC-SN. The cells were harvested on filter papers, and radioactive counts performed in a liquid scintillation counter. Cell counts were determined in a Coulter counter on additional wells.

Other determinations. Total protein in the partially purified supernatant fractions was measured by the Bio-Rad colorimetric assay using bovine gamma globulin as a standard. Newly-synthesized protein in the fibroblast cultures exposed to MNC supernatants was determined by the incorporation of L-(5-^{3}H) proline into material precipitable with 10% trichloroacetic acid (TCA) in the harvested fibroblast supernatants and trypsinized cell layers. The precipitates were collected on paper filters, washed 3 times with cold

Table 1. The effect of supernatants of concanavalin A–activated normal mononuclear cells on glycosaminoglycan accumulation in normal and progressive systemic sclerosis (PSS) fibroblasts*

	GAG, cpm × $10^{-3}/10^6$ fibroblasts		
	Without MNC supernatant	With MNC supernatant	% increase
Normal lines			
1	92	1,370	1,390
2	44	570	1,198
3	174	702	303
4	113	635	462
Mean ± SD	106 ± 54†	819 ± 371†	
PSS lines			
1	277	776	176
2	485	802	65
3	399	1,055	164
Mean ± SD	387 ± 104‡	877 ± 154‡	

* The supernatants of concanavalin A–activated mononuclear cells (MNC) were diluted 1:10 with complete growth medium and added to confluent fibroblast monolayers at the time of medium change on day 6. Glycosaminoglycan (GAG) content in the cultures was determined following a 12-hour pulse with ^{3}H-glucosamine added 60 hours after the supernatants. Student's paired *t*-test was used to calculate significance.
† $P < 0.001$, with supernatant versus without supernatant.
‡ $P < 0.01$, with supernatant versus without supernatant.

TCA, and radioactive counts performed in a liquid scintillation counter.

RESULTS

The incorporation of ^{3}H-glucosamine into GAG by confluent dermal fibroblast cultures incubated with supernatants of MNC (MNC-SN) was increased in comparison with control cultures incubated with medium alone (Table 1). Control supernatants containing Con A and mannoside had no effect on GAG accumulation in our cultures. Dermal fibroblast cultures exhibited considerable variability in baseline and stimulated GAG synthesis. Nevertheless, the differences in magnitude of response between normal and PSS lines were striking. Following a 72-hour incubation with MNC-SN, the GAG accumulation increased up to fourteenfold in normal dermal fibroblast cultures, but only 1–2-fold in PSS fibroblast cultures. Maximal stimulated synthesis, however, was similar in normal and PSS cultures.

Supernatants of Con A–activated MNC had a significantly greater effect ($P < 0.01$, Student's paired *t*-test) on GAG accumulation than supernatants of unstimulated MNC (data not shown). For example, mean GAG accumulation in 4 normal fibroblast lines was 200 ± 90 cpm × $10^{-3}/10^6$ cells with supernatants of unstimulated MNC, versus 819 ± 371 cpm × $10^{-3}/10^6$ cells with supernatants of Con A–activated MNC. Newly-synthesized cellular protein, as measured by the content of L-(5-^{3}H) proline, did not increase to the same extent (e.g., twofold versus fourteenfold increase in GAG). There was no increase observed in total fibroblast cell numbers, indicating that fibroblast cell division was not appreciably augmented by the MNC-SN in these confluent cultures.

To assure that increases in the labeled precipitable CPC counts observed in cultures incubated with MNC-SN reflected GAG accumulation, we performed sequential hydrolysis of the labeled material with hyaluronidase and chondroitinases AC and ABC in control and experimental cultures. Table 2 shows that hyaluronic acid was the predominant GAG not only in control cultures, as reported by us previously (5), but also in cultures incubated with MNC-SN.

The effect of MNC-SN on hyaluronic acid accumulation in normal dermal fibroblasts was also measured using a colorimetric carbazole technique. We observed a 3.3-fold increase in the uronic acid content of cultures incubated in the active supernatant for 36–72 hours. Using ^{3}H-glucosamine and 12-hour pulses, we measured a sixfold increase in GAG in the same cultures.

To determine the optimal length of fibroblast exposure to the active supernatants, we measured GAG accumulation after 24, 48, 72, and 96 hours of incubation with these supernatants. Data presented in Figure 1 show that a 60–72-hour exposure resulted in maximal enhancement of GAG accumulation by normal dermal fibroblast cultures. In terms of the kinetics of this response, it can be seen in Figure 1 that although increases in GAG accumulation were demonstrable within 24 hours after addition of MNC-SN, the largest differences between control and experimental cultures occurred between 60–72 hours of exposure to these supernatants. Again, PSS fibroblasts exposed to MNC-SNs accumulated only 1–2 times more GAG, in comparison with normal fibroblasts, which accumulated up to 18 times more GAG (data not shown).

It was possible that MNC-SN augmented GAG accumulation by decreasing its degradation, rather than by increasing its synthesis in dermal fibroblast cultures. To test this possibility we prepared tritiated GAG as described in Materials and Methods and added it to normal fibroblast cultures incubated with or without MNC-SN. As shown in Table 3, radioactive

Table 2. Sequential enzymatic hydrolysis of total ^{3}H-glycosaminoglycan (^{3}H-GAG) in dermal fibroblast cultures incubated with and without mononuclear cell (MNC) supernatant*

Enzyme added	Control (without MNC supernatant)	Experimental (with MNC supernatant)		
		1	2	3
^{3}H-GAG				
+ hyaluronidase	54.0 ± 1.9	69.6 ± 0.5	60.6 ± 1.5	64.8 ± 0.4
+ chondroitinase AC	9.5 ± 1.2	7.6 ± 0.3	8.0 ± 1.4	8.7 ± 0.6
+ chondroitinase ABC	12.5 ± 0.1	7.8 ± 0.7	12.9 ± 0.5	8.1 ± 0.6
Residue	24.2 ± 1.5	14.9 ± 0.6	18.8 ± 0.7	18.2 ± 0.1

* Numbers are mean percentages ± SD of hydrolysis of the total labeled GAG. Triplicate cultures were analyzed. The experimental cultures were incubated with 3 different MNC supernatants. Differences between control and experimental cultures were not statistically significant.

counts recoverable by CPC precipitation from the MNC-SN–containing cultures were the same as those from the untreated cultures at all time points up to and including 72 hours after addition of labeled GAG to these cultures. Although degradation almost certainly occurred to some degree in these cultures, all counts were recoverable throughout the experiment. No increased degradation of labeled GAG was measured in experimental cultures. This indicates that the observed increase in GAG is due to increased synthesis in the cultures incubated with MNC supernatants. The addition of excess labeled GAG to normal fibroblasts incubated with MNC supernatants decreased the overall synthesis of GAG, as judged by uptake of ^{3}H-glucosamine in these cultures. However, it did not impair their response to active supernatants (e.g., 8,196 ± 1,264 cpm/well, versus 89,083 ± 7,380 cpm/well in the presence of MNC-SN). Thus, with or without excess GAG present, incorporated radioactive counts in the supernatant-containing cultures were tenfold higher as compared with cultures containing medium alone.

We also determined the effects of increasing dilutions of the supernatants generated with normal MNC on GAG accumulation by human dermal fibroblasts. As shown in Figure 2, a linear relationship existed between concentration of the active supernatants and enhancement of GAG accumulation. The greatest GAG stimulatory activity was seen in the least diluted supernatants, but activity was still present at 1:500 dilution (1 μl of MNC-SN per 500 μl of medium).

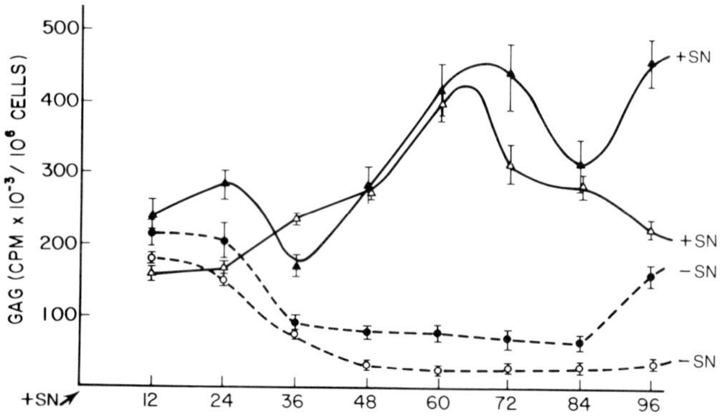

Figure 1. Glycosaminoglycan (GAG) accumulation in 2 normal dermal fibroblast cultures incubated with **(solid lines)** and without **(broken lines)** supernatants (SN) of concanavalin A–activated normal mononuclear cells. The supernatants were diluted 1:10 with complete growth medium and added to the confluent fibroblast monolayers at the time of medium change on day 6. GAG was measured in these cultures using 12-hour pulses with ^{3}H-glucosamine after different exposure times to the supernatants. The data plotted are means ± SD **(vertical bars)** of triplicate cultures. Numbers below the abscissa represent hours of exposure.

Table 3. Effects of mononuclear cell (MNC) supernatant on degradation of labeled glycosaminoglycan (GAG) added to normal dermal fibroblast cultures*

Incubation time with labeled GAG (hours)	cpm × 10^3/well	
	Without MNC supernatant	With MNC supernatant
0–24	16.0 ± 0.1	16.7 ± 0.6
12–24	15.9 ± 0.4	16.7 ± 0.3
0–72	16.4 ± 0.4	17.6 ± 0.9
60–72	15.5 ± 1.1	16.1 ± 0.8
Medium control	16.3 ± 0.2	14.5 ± 0.4

* The tritium-labeled GAG was prepared as described in Materials and Methods and added to confluent fibroblast cultures incubated with or without MNC supernatants. At the end of incubation, radioactive counts of cetylpyridinium chloride–precipitated material were obtained and are expressed as mean ± SD cpm of triplicate wells.

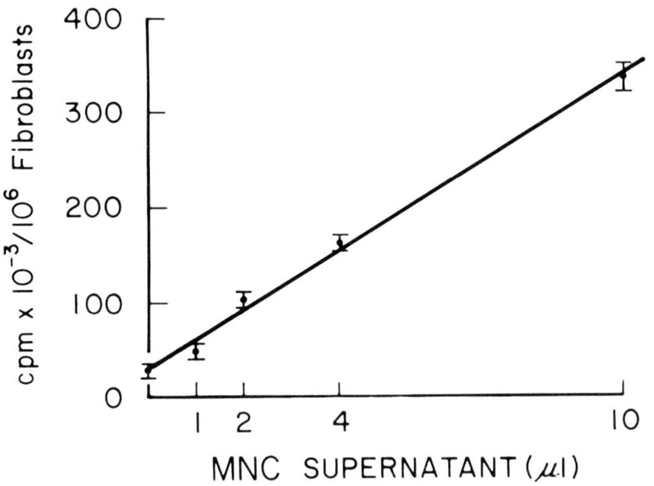

Figure 2. Glycosaminoglycan accumulation in normal fibroblast cultures incubated with increasing dilutions of supernatants from normal mononuclear cells (MNC). Data are presented as means ± SD (**vertical bars**) of quadruplicate cultures from a representative experiment. Fibroblasts were exposed to the supernatant for 72 hours, and ^{3}H-glucosamine was added during the last 12 hours of culture.

Supernatants of both normal and PSS MNC were stimulatory.

MNC used to generate supernatants in all of the above experiments contained 13–14% adherent cells. However, MNC supernatants generated by the cells depleted of monocytes were only minimally stimulatory under the conditions we found to be optimal for demonstrating increases in the GAG content of dermal fibroblasts. In a representative experiment, normal fibroblasts incubated with supernatants of monocyte-containing MNC stimulated GAG accumulation 18.5 times over control, while supernatants prepared with monocyte-depleted MNC gave only a twofold stimulation. The removal of monocytes on a Sephadex G-10 column in this experiment yielded a cell preparation containing <1% monocytes as determined by staining with alpha-naphthyl acetate esterase and by reactivity with OKM1 monoclonal antibody. Nevertheless, this cell preparation incubated with Con A yielded supernatants containing detectable IL-1 activity.

The presence of monocytes appeared to be necessary for the production by MNC of soluble factors modulating GAG accumulation in dermal fibroblast cultures, as well as of IL-1. The addition of adherent cells to monocyte-depleted cultures (the final concentrations of monocytes were 10% and 20%) yielded active supernatants (Table 4). The irradiated (3,000 rads) and non-irradiated adherent cells incubated with Con A yielded supernatants capable of enhancing GAG synthesis up to 16 times (i.e., 4 times as much as unfractionated MNC-SN) in normal dermal fibroblasts (Table 4). When nonadherent cells were added back to the cultures, the GAG stimulatory activity decreased to the levels produced in the unfractionated MNC cultures.

Addition of increasing proportions (10, 25, 50, 75, and 90%) of nonadherent cells to a fixed number of monocytes resulted in supernatants with GAG stimulatory activity comparable with that of unfractionated MNC supernatants. These experiments indicated that adherent cells are themselves capable of releasing the stimulatory activity, that their presence is essential for optimal GAG stimulation by the MNC supernatants, and that nonadherent cells may modulate the production or release of the GAG stimulatory factors.

Isolated T lymphocytes (93% purity and >95% viability) and the subpopulations enriched in T4+ and T8+ cells (>80% and >75% enrichment, respectively, both with >95% viability) were tested for their ability to produce GAG stimulatory activity. T lymphocytes and T lymphocyte subpopulations tested were obtained from different normal individuals, and unfractionated MNC served as positive controls for each individual. Our preparations of T lymphocytes and T4+, as well as T8+ cells, were capable of generating active supernatants containing 70–80% of GAG stimulatory activity present in supernatants of unfractionat-

Table 4. Glycosaminoglycan (GAG) accumulation in normal dermal fibroblast cultures incubated with supernatants made with adherent cell–depleted and –enriched mononuclear cells (MNC) and with purified adherent cells (Mo)*

Exp. no.	Supernatant from 1.5×10^6 cells/ml	GAG cpm $\times 10^{-3}/10^6$ cells
1	Medium control	25 ± 0.5
	MNC	580 ± 45
	MNC − Mo (<1%)	70 ± 4
	MNC + Mo (10%)	451 ± 18
	MNC + Mo (20%)	577 ± 77
2	Medium control	29 ± 1.9
	MNC	103 ± 20
	Mo	467 ± 30
	Mo (irradiated)	439 ± 39
	Mo (irradiated, 10%) + nonadherent cells (90%)	61 ± 2.4

* MNC depleted of adherent cells and adherent cells (Mo) were prepared as described in Materials and Methods. The depleted MNC contained <1% OKM1+ cells. All supernatants were incubated with normal dermal fibroblasts for 72 hours and pulsed with ^{3}H-glucosamine for the last 12 hours of incubation. Data are means ± SD of triplicate cultures from 2 different representative experiments.

ed MNC. It is important to note that all the enriched lymphocyte fractions prepared by panning contained 1–4% monocytes (OKM1+ cells). These results indicated that preparations of T lymphocytes together with a small number (1–4%) of monocytes yield GAG stimulatory activity when activated with Con A in vitro.

In an attempt to characterize the stimulatory factor, active MNC supernatants were concentrated and applied to a calibrated Sephadex G-100 column. The column was eluted with 80 ml of PBS, and the collected fractions were assayed for GAG stimulatory activity on normal dermal fibroblasts. As shown in Figure 3, the stimulatory activity eluted in 2 broad peaks, a major peak of activity at 15,000 MW and a smaller one at 50,000 MW. When tested in the mouse thymocyte proliferative assay for IL-1, combined fractions 29–32 from the 15,000 MW peak contained about tenfold more activity than fractions 17–26 from the higher MW peak (71–105 units/ml versus 7–15 units/ml). Neither of the 2 peaks contained IL-2 as measured in the proliferative assay using a murine T cell line.

The GAG stimulatory factor in the 15,000 MW peak was compared with rabbit IL-1 (purified by affinity chromatography) in terms of effects on cultured dermal fibroblasts. Both were found to enhance GAG synthesis in normal as well as PSS fibroblast cultures (Figure 4). The rabbit IL-1 (pI 5.0) used in this experiment was not purified to homogeneity. Also, an

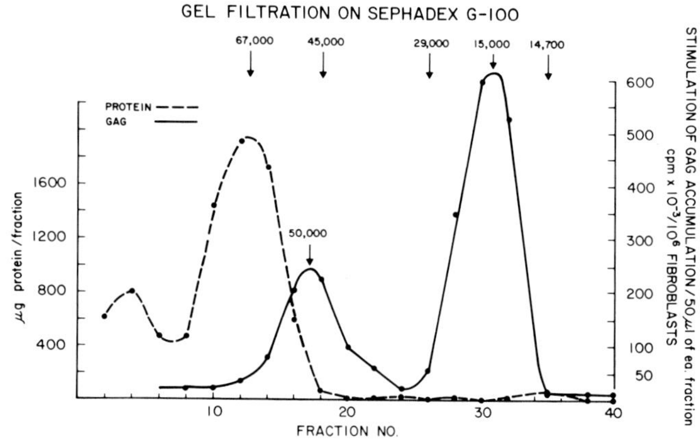

Figure 3. Molecular sieve chromatography of mononuclear cell (MNC) culture supernatants. The supernatants obtained by culturing 1.5×10^6 MNC/ml with concanavalin A for 24 hours were concentrated and applied to a Sephadex G-100 column. Aliquots of the column fractions were added to confluent dermal normal fibroblasts to test their ability to stimulate glycosaminoglycan (GAG) accumulation. The results are means of triplicate determinations. Molecular weight markers were: 67,000, bovine serum albumin; 45,000, ovalbumin; 29,000, carbonic anhydrase; 14,700, RNase B.

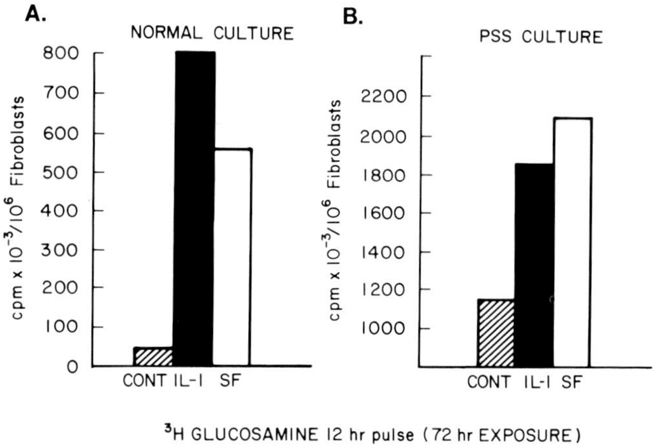

Figure 4. Enhancement of glycosaminoglycan accumulation by a column-purified stimulatory factor (SF; fraction 30, 15,000 MW) and by a preparation of rabbit interleukin-1 (IL-1) in normal (**A**) and progressive systemic sclerosis (PSS) (**B**) dermal fibroblast cultures. Both preparations were added to confluent fibroblasts for 72 hours, and the uptake of ^{3}H-glucosamine was measured during the last 12 hours of the incubation. The data represent means of quadruplicate determinations. An aliquot of phosphate buffered saline was added to control (CONT) cultures.

ultrapure human IL preparation (Genzyme, Boston, MA) did not enhance the GAG accumulation in our system.

Fractions of the 2 peaks obtained by gel filtration on Sephadex G-100 were subjected to dialysis, heat, enzymatic digestion with trypsin, and prolonged storage. The GAG stimulatory activity in the small molecular weight peak was not dialyzable, not sensitive to trypsin, minimally affected by heating at 65°C for 15 minutes (<25% loss of activity), and not affected by storage for 1 week at 4°C. The activity of the 50,000 MW material was also unaffected by trypsin or storage at 4°C. However, heating at 65°C for 15 minutes destroyed it completely.

To determine whether increases in GAG were related to fibroblast proliferation, we measured cell numbers and total ^{3}H-thymidine incorporation in confluent as well as log cultures treated with MNC-SNs. Unfractionated or fractionated supernatants did not alter the growth of fibroblasts in the *confluent* cultures used in cell experiments reported here. No increases in either total fibroblast numbers or in ^{3}H-thymidine uptake (e.g., control 85 ± 10 cpm/cell × 10^3 versus experimental 99 ± 14 cpm/cell × 10^3, means ± SD of quadruplicate wells in a representative experiment, an insignificant difference) were observed in confluent cultures incubated with MNC-SN for 72 hours.

When fibroblast cultures in the *log phase* of growth were incubated with unfractionated MNC-SN or 15,000 MW and 50,000 MW fractions (fractions 32 and 17, respectively) no increases in ^{3}H-thymidine uptake were demonstrable. Rather, MNC-SN consistently caused a depression of ^{3}H-thymidine uptake by normal (Figure 5) as well as PSS fibroblasts (6 different lines were tested with various MNC-SN preparations). MNC-SN also tended to depress cell numbers in log cultures; a small but consistent depression in cell numbers was recorded in 3 different normal dermal fibroblast lines (e.g., Figure 5) and 3 PSS lines. These results indicate that although MNC-SNs may selectively increase GAG synthesis, they do not augment fibroblast proliferation.

DISCUSSION

Our results demonstrate that products of mitogen-activated mononuclear cells modulate accumulation of glycosaminoglycan by normal and PSS fibroblasts in vitro. Increases in GAG following incubation of confluent fibroblast monolayers with supernatants produced by these MNC can be demonstrated by 2 independent techniques (^{3}H-glucosamine uptake into GAG followed by enzymatic degradation to confirm identity of the labeled product, and measurement of total uronic acid content). It appears that the MNC-SNs do not affect the breakdown of GAG in the fibroblast cultures. Rather, the synthesis of GAG is selectively augmented. PSS fibroblasts, which have a high baseline GAG synthesis (5,22), responded less to stimulation by MNC-SNs than normal dermal fibroblasts.

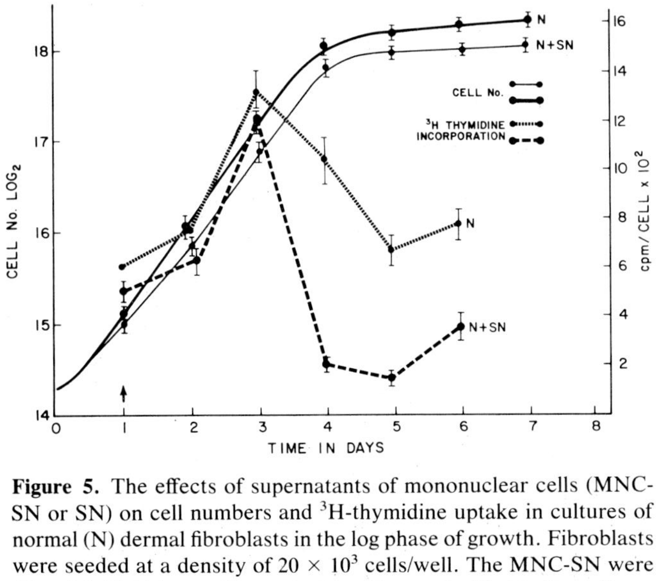

Figure 5. The effects of supernatants of mononuclear cells (MNC-SN or SN) on cell numbers and ^{3}H-thymidine uptake in cultures of normal (N) dermal fibroblasts in the log phase of growth. Fibroblasts were seeded at a density of 20×10^3 cells/well. The MNC-SN were diluted 1:10 with complete growth medium and added to the cultures on day 1. The results of a representative experiment (1 of 6) are shown. The data are means ± SD (**vertical bars**) of triplicate wells.

The factors responsible for the increase of GAG in dermal fibroblasts fractionated into a low molecular weight (15,000) and a high molecular weight (50,000) peak on Sephadex G-100. These stimulatory factors require a long-term incubation (60–72 hours) with target cells to effect optimal GAG stimulation. GAG stimulatory activity is dependent on the presence of adherent cells in the MNC used for the generation of active supernatants. In fact, supernatants of adherent cells alone are capable of stimulating GAG in dermal fibroblasts to a greater extent than unfractionated MNC. Characterization of the 2 peaks of activity in terms of sensitivity to heat and enzymatic digestion by trypsin implies the presence of 2 distinct factors. On the other hand, the chromatography data may be consistent with the existence of a single factor that either aggregates or binds to a carrier molecule.

In view of the fact that interleukin-1 has been recently identified as a GAG stimulatory factor in fibroblasts (23), we considered the possibility that the GAG stimulatory factor(s) may be a monocyte product identical with or related to IL-1. The dependence of GAG stimulatory activity in MNC supernatants on the presence of adherent cells in the cultures further implicates IL-1. Indeed, the low molecular weight peak containing GAG stimulatory activity also had substantial levels of IL-1 activity when tested in the biologic assay for IL-1. Furthermore, we showed that purified rabbit IL-1 is capable of stimulating GAG accumulation in our fibroblast cultures.

Murine and human IL-1 are known to activate collagenase and prostaglandin E_2 production in human synovial cells (24) and fibroblasts (25). There is evidence that human IL-1 does modulate GAG synthesis in foreskin fibroblasts in culture (23), although commercially available ultrapure human IL was not shown to have any GAG stimulatory activity in our experiments. Stringent purification procedures will have to be vigorously applied before the identity of the GAG stimulatory activity and its relation to IL-1 can be ascertained. IL-1, a monokine, may be an important regulator of nonlymphoid cells involved in inflammatory reactions (26). A possible relationship between our GAG stimulatory factor and IL-1 is suggested by our demonstration of GAG stimulatory activity in lymphocyte-depleted cultures of adherent cells. Also, resistance to trypsin in our fractions is reminiscent of IL-1 (27). The fractions containing GAG stimulatory activity are not purified to homogeneity, however, and contaminating proteins may interfere with biochemical characterization.

There are certain differences between our factors and IL-1. Interleukin-1 or lymphocyte activating factor stimulates proliferation in fibroblasts (28). Our MNC-SN or low molecular weight fractions with GAG stimulatory activity did not appreciably augment growth of normal or PSS dermal fibroblasts. In confluent cultures, increases in GAG were never accompanied by an equivalent rise in total newly-synthesized protein (e.g., 13 times more GAG versus 2 times more total protein) or an increase in cell numbers. During the log phase of growth, our active supernatants or fractions did not increase cellular proliferation in relation to untreated controls as judged by cell numbers and/or ^{3}H-thymidine uptake (Figure 5).

It has been reported that soluble mediators mitogenic to cultured fibroblasts are present in supernatants of antigen- or mitogen-activated MNC (29) and of monocyte-enriched, unstimulated MNC (30). In contrast, we could not demonstrate such mitogenic effects; rather, a small, consistent depression in cell numbers was observed in the presence of MNC-SNs in our cultures (Figure 5). Although the nature of this depression is not clear, it may be related to the presence of serum in our cultures or inhibitory substances in the unfractionated or even partially-purified MNC-SN. For example, Korn and coworkers (10) have described a 12,000–20,000 MW factor that is derived from adherent cells and causes prostaglandin-dependent inhibition of dermal fibroblast proliferation. The precise role in tissue fibrosis played by proliferation of fibroblasts is not understood, but it is important to relate changes in connective tissue synthesis to fibroblast replication (31). We have demonstrated that MNC-SNs can selectively increase GAG synthesis without increasing dermal fibroblast replication in vitro. Similar results were obtained by Daireaux et al (32) with human synovial cells in culture.

Connective tissue activating peptides (CTAP), described by Castor and colleagues (33,34), could be related to our GAG stimulatory factors. However, CTAP-I obtained from homogenates of MNC was not active on dermal fibroblasts, and CTAP-III capable of GAG stimulation in these fibroblasts was derived from platelets (34). It is unlikely that platelets contribute to our GAG stimulatory activity, which was present in supernatants generated not only with MNC, but also with purified preparations of cell subsets where contamination with platelets would be negligible. Furthermore, no CTAP-III could be detected by radial immunodiffusion in our preparations.

The local production of GAG stimulatory substances by activated MNC may be responsible for the fibrosis observed in PSS and other diseases characterized by excessive deposition of connective tissue substances. GAG occurs in increased quantity in the skin of patients with PSS (5). Also, fibroblast cultures derived from PSS skin synthesize increased amounts of GAG (5,22). Factors that modulate GAG accumulation in vitro may be of considerable importance in the disease process. Local production, by the MNC infiltrate in PSS skin, of soluble products stimulating and/or inhibiting target connective tissue cells could significantly influence the development of fibrosis. For example, we have evidence that prolonged exposure of normal fibroblasts outgrowing from a skin explant, to active MNC supernatants, results in a propagable change of the fibroblast phenotype in terms of GAG synthesis (35). Since it appears that the MNC supernatants may induce PSS-like behavior in normal dermal fibroblasts, it is most important to identify the responsible factors. Their characterization is necessary for an understanding of the cellular interactions between activated T lymphocytes, monocytes, and dermal fibroblasts, and of the role these interactions play in the pathogenesis of PSS. Studies are in progress to define and further characterize the GAG stimulatory factors.

ACKNOWLEDGMENTS

The authors wish to thank Dr. Philip L. Simon for providing the interleukin-1 preparation and for assaying our samples for interleukin-1 and -2 activities. We are grateful to Dr. C. William Castor for measurement of the CTAP-III content in our preparations.

REFERENCES

1. Buckingham RB, Prince RK, Rodnan GP, Taylor FH: Increased collagen accumulation in dermal fibroblast cultures from patients with progressive systemic sclerosis (scleroderma). J Lab Clin Med 92:5–12, 1978
2. LeRoy EC: Connective tissue synthesis by scleroderma skin fibroblasts in culture. J Exp Med 138:1351–1362, 1972
3. Bashey RI, Perlish JS, Nochumson S, Stephens RS, Fleischmajer R: Connective tissue synthesis by cultured scleroderma fibroblasts. II. Incorporation of ^{3}H glucosamine and synthesis of glycosaminoglycans. Arthritis Rheum 20:879–885, 1977
4. Uitto J, Helin G, Helin P, Lorenzen I: Connective tissue in scleroderma: a biochemical study on the correlation of fractionated glycosaminoglycans and collagen in human skin. Acta Derm Venereol 51:401–406, 1971
5. Buckingham RB, Prince RK, Rodnan GP: Progressive systemic sclerosis (PSS, scleroderma) dermal fibroblasts

synthesize increased amounts of glycosaminoglycan. J Lab Clin Med 101:659–669, 1983
6. Roumm A, Whiteside TL, Medsger TA Jr, Rodnan G: Quantitation and subtyping of lymphocytes in skin of patients with progressive systemic sclerosis (abstract). Arthritis Rheum (suppl) 26:S61, 1983
7. Johnson RL, Ziff M: Lymphokine stimulation of collagen accumulation. J Clin Invest 58:240–252, 1976
8. Whiteside TL, Prince R, Buckingham R, Rodnan G: The effect of lymphokines from normal and PSS lymphocytes on connective tissue synthesis in vitro (abstract). Arthritis Rheum (suppl) 25:S14, 1982
9. Dayer JM, Russell RGG, Krane SM: Collagenase production by rheumatoid synovial cells stimulated by a human lymphocyte factor. Science 195:181–183, 1977
10. Korn JH, Halushka PV, LeRoy EC: Mononuclear cell modulation of connective tissue function: suppression of fibroblast growth by stimulation of endogenous prostaglandin production. J Clin Invest 65:543–544, 1980
11. Herman JH, Nutman TB, Nozoe M, Mowery CS, Dennis MV: Lymphokine-mediated suppression of chondrocyte glycosaminoglycan and protein synthesis. Arthritis Rheum 24:824–834, 1981
12. Rodnan GP, Jablonska S, Medsger TA Jr: Classification and nomenclature of progressive systemic sclerosis (scleroderma). Clin Rheum Dis 5:5–13, 1979
13. Gay RE, Buckingham RB, Prince RK, Gay S, Rodnan GP, Miller EJ: Collagen types synthesized in dermal fibroblast cultures from patients with early progressive systemic sclerosis (scleroderma). Arthritis Rheum 23:190–196, 1980
14. Castor CW, Wright D, Buckingham RB: Effects of rheumatoid sera on fibroblast proliferation and hyaluronic acid synthesis. Arthritis Rheum 11:652–659, 1968
15. Jerrells TR, Dean JH, Richardson GL, Herberman RB: Depletion of monocytes from human peripheral blood mononuclear leukocytes: comparison of the Sephadex G-10 column method with other commonly used techniques. J Immunol Methods 32:11–29, 1980
16. Hsu S, Raine L, Fanger H: Use of avidin-biotin-peroxidase complex (ABC) in immunoperoxidase techniques: a comparison between ABC and unlabeled antibody (PAP) procedures. J Histochem Cytochem 29:557–580, 1981
17. Zanella A, Mantovani A, Mariana M, Silvani C, Peri G, Tedesco F: A modified "low pH" lignocaine method to isolate human monocytes: a comparison with other separation procedures. J Immunol Methods 41:279–288, 1981
18. Wysocki LJ, Sato VL: "Panning" for lymphocytes: a method for cell selection. Proc Natl Acad Sci USA 77:2844–2848, 1978
19. Mizel SB, Oppenheim JJ, Rosenstreich DL: Characterization of lymphocyte-activating factor (LAF) produced by the macrophage cell line P388D1. I. Enhancement of LAF production by activated T lymphocytes. J Immunol 120:1497–1503, 1978
20. Gillis S, Ferm MM, Ou W, Smith KA: T cell growth factor: parameters of production and a quantitative microassay for activity. J Immunol 120:2027–2032, 1978
21. Simon PL, Willoughby WF: Biochemical and biological characterization of rabbit interleukin-1 (IL-1), Lymphokines. Vol. 6. Edited by SB Mizel. New York, Academic Press, 1982, pp 47–63
22. Cabral A, Castor WC: Connective tissue activation. XXVII. The behavior of skin fibroblasts from patients with scleroderma. Arthritis Rheum 26:1362–1369, 1983
23. Postlethwaite AE, Lachman LB, Kang AH: Stimulation of fibroblast hyaluronic acid production by human interleukin 1 (abstract). Arthritis Rheum (suppl) 26:S59, 1983
24. Mizel SB, Dayer JM, Krane SM, Mergenhagen SE: Stimulation of rheumatoid synovial cell collagenase and prostaglandin production by partially purified lymphocyte activating factor (interleukin 1). Proc Natl Acad Sci USA 78:2474–2477, 1981
25. Postlethwaite AE, Lachman LB, Mainardi CL, Kang AH: Interleukin 1 stimulation of collagenase production by cultured fibroblasts. J Exp Med 157:801–806, 1983
26. Lachman LB: Human interleukin 1: purification and properties. Fed Proc 42:2639–2645, 1983
27. Oppenheim JJ, Stadler BM, Siraganian RP, Mage M, Mathieson B: Lymphokines: their role in lymphocyte responses: properties of interleukin I. Fed Proc 41:257–262, 1982
28. Schmidt JA, Mizel SB, Cohen D, Green I: Interleukin 1, a potential regulator of fibroblast proliferation. J Immunol 128:2177–2182, 1982
29. Postlethwaite AE, Kang AH: Induction of fibroblast proliferation by human mononuclear leukocyte-derived proteins. Arthritis Rheum 26:22–27, 1983
30. DeLustro F, Sherer GK, LeRoy EC: Human monocyte stimulation of fibroblast growth by a soluble mediator(s). J. Reticuloendothel Soc 28:519–532, 1980
31. LeRoy EC, Mercurio S, Sherer GK: Replication and phenotypic expression of control and scleroderma fibroblasts: response to growth factors. Proc Natl Acad Sci USA 79:1286–1290, 1982
32. Daireaux M, Penfornis H, Langris M, Bocquet J, Pujol J-C, Belliard R, Loyau G: Effect of a mononuclear cell medium on collagen and glycosaminoglycan production by synovial cells in culture. FEBS Lett 132:93–97, 1981
33. Castor CW: Connective tissue activation. III. Observations on the mechanisms of action of connective tissue activating peptide. J Lab Clin Med 79:285–301, 1972
34. Castor CW, Ritchie JC, Scott ME, Whitney SL: Connective tissue activation. XI. Stimulation of glycosaminoglycan and DNA formation by a platelet factor. Arthritis Rheum 20:859–868, 1977
35. Worrall JG, Whiteside TL, Prince RK, Buckingham RB, Stachura I, Rodnan GP: Persistence of scleroderma-like phenotype in normal fibroblasts following prolonged exposure to soluble mediators from mononuclear cells. Submitted for publication

ARTHROSCOPY IN SEPTIC ARTHRITIS

Lidocaine- and Iodine-Containing Contrast Media are Bacteriostatic

M. A. DORY and M. J. WAUTELET

Puncture of septic foci is usually performed to determine the responsible bacteria. If contrast medium is used instead of saline to rinse the lesion and to withdraw an adequate bacteriologic specimen, the opacification provides valuable information about the extent of the changes. Since lidocaine is usually used as a local anesthetic when patients undergo this procedure, we tested the in vitro antibacterial effects of lidocaine 1%, as well as those of 2 contrast media—meglumine amidotrizoate and metrizamide—on several bacteria. In particular, we looked at the influence of the concentration of inoculum used and the duration of contact before culture. The contrast media did not significantly affect bacterial growth when contact before culture did not exceed 3 hours. In contrast, lidocaine had a significant antibacterial effect, indicating that it should not enter into contact with the bacteriologic specimen.

Puncture of septic lesions does not always provide adequate specimens for bacteriologic examination. In such cases, injection of normal saline is recommended in order to obtain the needed material. If contrast medium is used for this purpose, it can demonstrate the size of the abscess and eventual fistulous tracts, which are often surprisingly extensive. The relation of the septic lesion to the adjacent structures can thus be evaluated more thoroughly. In this paper, we present 4 case reports to illustrate the usefulness of this technique. Since most punctures are performed with the use of lidocaine as a local anesthetic, we have investigated the antibacterial effects of lidocaine and of 2 currently used arthrographic contrast media, on several bacteria. In particular, we examined the variation of bacterial growth with reference to the size of the inoculum and the duration of contact between the drugs and the bacteria before culture.

PATIENTS AND METHODS

Puncture technique. Puncture technique depended on the affected region. If a joint was involved, classic arthrographic technique was used. If an intervertebral disc was affected, a posterolateral approach was used to perform the discography. Other septic lesions were directly punctured under fluoroscopic control and, rarely, under computed tomography (CT) scan control. All punctures were undertaken using 20- or 22-gauge needles. The amount of injected contrast medium varied with the structure to be opacified; however, the injections were always performed very slowly and with minimal pressure.

Depending on the structure to be opacified, dilution of the contrast medium was sometimes necessary in order to reduce the contrast. Lidocaine was always used for this purpose. However, based on previous bacteriologic experiments, we avoided injection of this drug into septic lesions.

Contrast media and lidocaine. Meglumine amidotrizoate (306 mg iodine/ml Angiographine; Schering, Berlin, West Germany) and metrizamide (170 mg iodine/ml Amipaque; Nyegaard, Oslo, Norway), currently used for arthrographic examinations, were tested as contrast media. The antibacterial activity of lidocaine 1% (Xylocaine; Astra, Lakemadel, Sweden) was also investigated. All of these drugs were tested at commonly used concentrations. We also tested a mixture of meglumine amidotrizoate/lidocaine 1% (1:1, volume:volume).

Bacteria. Bacteria studied were *Staphylococcus aureus, Streptococcus viridans* (*milleri*), *Escherichia coli* (4 strains isolated from urine and feces), *Pseudomonas aeru-*

From the Clinique St. Pierre, Ottignies, Belgium.

M. A. Dory, MD: Department of Radiology; M. J. Wautelet, PharmD: Microbiology Laboratory.

Address reprint requests to M. A. Dory, MD, Department of Radiology, Clinique St. Pierre, 1340 Ottignies, Belgium.

Submitted for publication June 11, 1984; accepted in revised form September 20, 1984.

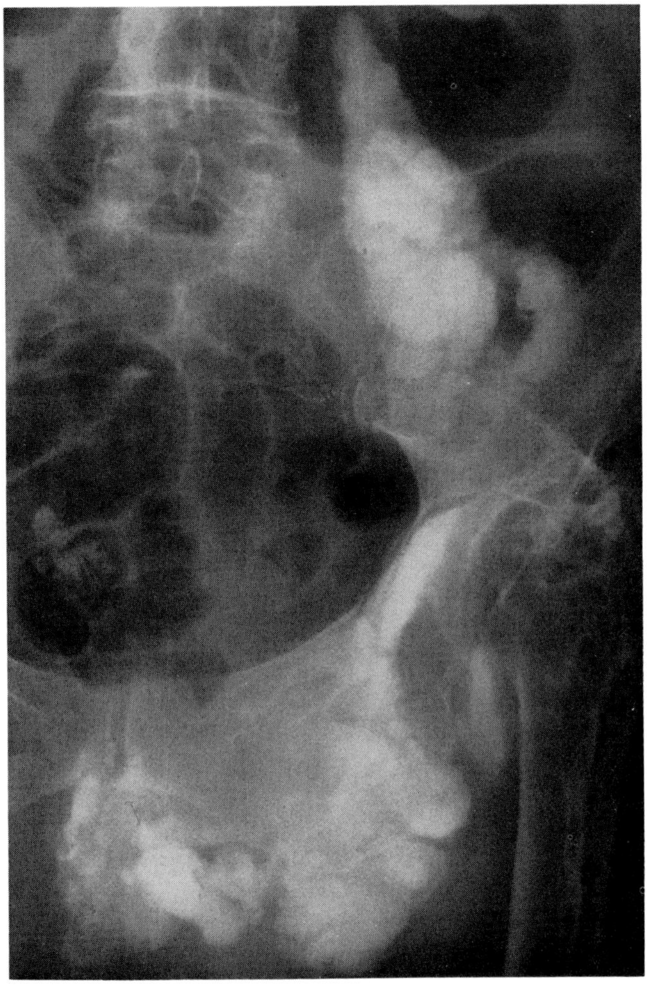

Figure 1. Patient 1. Percutaneous opacification of large prepubic and inguinal abscesses communicating through the hip joint, with another collection spreading high into the psoas muscle.

ginosa, Streptococcus group B (*agalactiae*), and *Mycobacterium tuberculosis*.

Bacteriologic experiments. We used inocula containing 10^8, 10^5, 10^4, and 10^3 bacteria/ml. Except for *M tuberculosis,* 2 colonies of each organism were cultured in 2.5 ml Mueller-Hinton broth or brain heart infusion (BHI) broth and incubated overnight at 35°C. The next morning, each culture was diluted to MacFarland no. 1 standard ($\pm 10^8$ bacteria/ml) with BHI broth, and then diluted to obtain inocula ranging from 10^5–10^3 bacteria/ml. The 4 inocula (10^8, 10^5, 10^4, 10^3 organisms/ml) were then mixed with each contrast medium or lidocaine at a ratio of 1:10 (final bacterial concentration 10^7, 10^4, 10^3, and 10^2 bacteria/ml), allowed to stand at room temperature, and observed at times 0, 30 minutes, 1 hour, 3 hours, 5 hours, and 24 hours. Tubes were covered with aluminum foil to keep out light. For the inocula with 10^8 and 10^5 bacteria/ml, sterile 0.85% NaCl was used as control under the same conditions. At time 0 and at 30 minutes, 1 hour, 3 hours, 5 hours, and 24 hours of incubation, 0.1 ml of each solution was inoculated on the entire surface of BHI-agar plates and incubated overnight at 35°C.

The next morning, results were evaluated as follows: on cultures of inocula containing 10^2–10^4 organisms/ml, the colonies were counted with the naked eye when possible. For the inocula containing $>10^4$ bacteria/ml, the eventual inhibitory effect was evaluated by observing the apparent decrease of the density of the subcultures and the appearance of semiconfluent colonies on the agar plates. If the growth inhibition was already quite pronounced, it was possible to count the colonies.

M tuberculosis drawn from another rich culture was massively inoculated onto Loewenstein medium in the presence of approximately 1 ml meglumine amidotrizoate or 1 ml lidocaine 1%, and incubated 6–8 weeks at 35°C. Growth or lack of growth was thereafter observed.

Patients. *Patient 1.* Patient 1 was a woman who, at the age of 68, developed a septic loosening of a left total hip prosthesis, which subsequently had to be removed. Five years later, she was admitted to the hospital for an inflammatory left inguinal mass. That mass was punctured, and a small

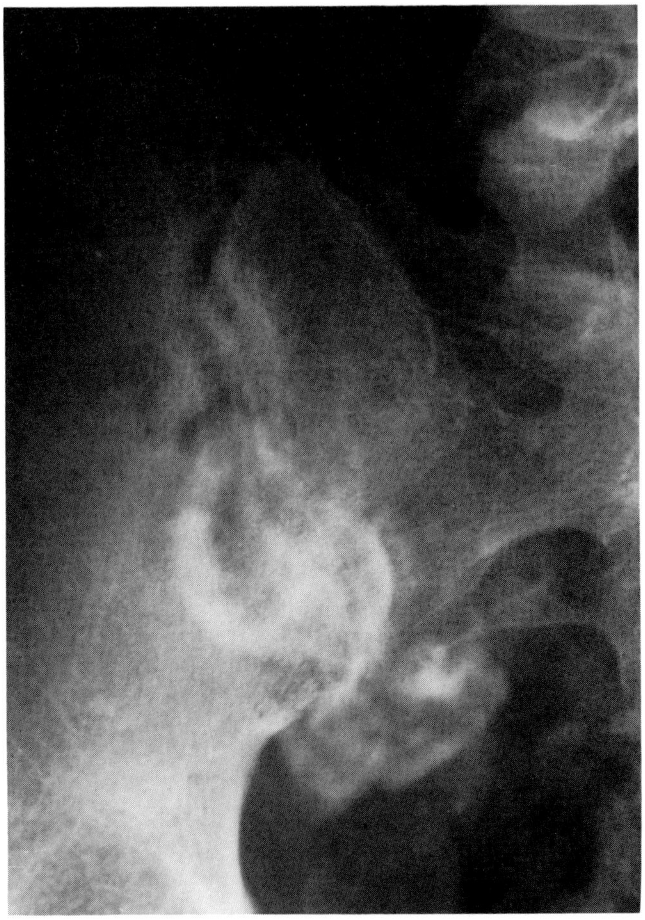

Figure 2. Patient 2. Arthrography of the right sacroiliac joint, anteroposterior view.

amount of green-grey pus was aspirated. Injection of meglumine amidotrizoate demonstrated a large prepubic and inguinal abscess communicating with the hip joint, and another collection located high within the left psoas muscle (Figure 1). Bacteriologic examination of the pus and the reaspirated contrast medium produced negative results; the patient had been receiving antibiotic treatment for a long period of time. Surgical drainage was performed and healing occurred after a few weeks.

Patient 2. Patient 2, a 57-year-old man, presented with arthritis of the right sacroiliac joint. Two previous punctures of the joint had not provided bacteriologic diagnosis. Transiliac puncture of the joint was performed under CT scan control. A 1:1 mixture of meglumine amidotrizoate and lidocaine 1% was injected, and it demonstrated polylobulate collection at the ventral aspect the of the joint (Figures 2 and 3). *M tuberculosis* was isolated by culture of the reaspirated material. Healing occurred after 1 year of specific antibiotic therapy.

Patient 3. Patient 3, a 75-year-old man, had developed right tuberculous trochanteritis at the age of 55. At the time of this admission he was suffering from arthritis of the right hip, of about 2 months duration. No material was withdrawn at articular puncture. Injection of meglumine amidotrizoate demonstrated an abscess which was located at the anterior aspect of the ischium and continued through a posterior fistulous tract to the hip joint (Figure 4). *M tuberculosis* was isolated by culture of the reaspirated contrast medium. The femoral head and neck were removed and the abscess was surgically drained.

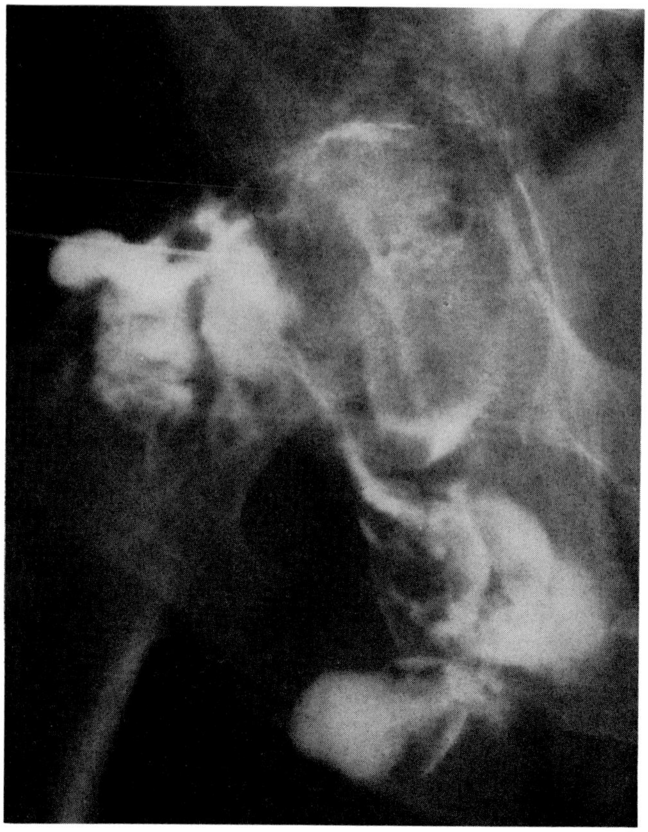

Figure 4. Patient 3. Arthrography of the right hip joint. Abscess located at the ventral aspect of the ischium was also opacified.

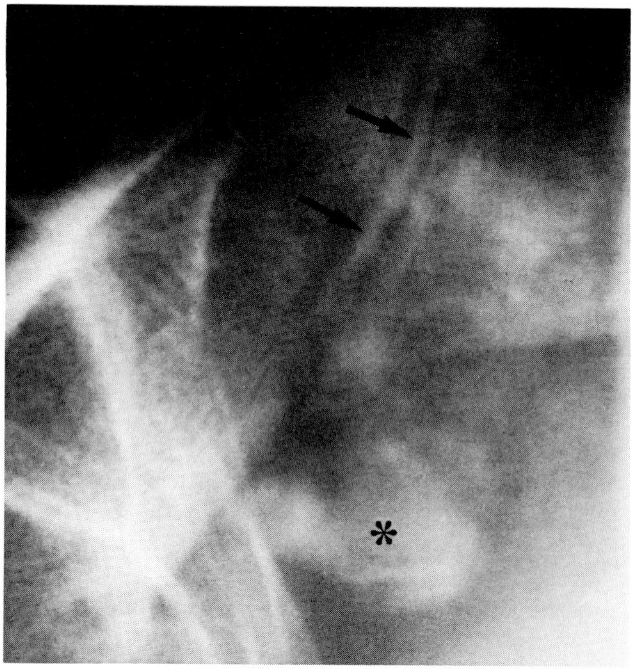

Figure 3. Patient 2. Arthrography of the right sacroiliac joint, craniocaudal view of the opacified area (**arrows**) and the ventral abscess (*).

Patient 4. Patient 4 was a 2-year-old girl who had L5–S1 discitis. Disc puncture by right posterolateral approach was performed, but no material was withdrawn. Injection of metrizamide demonstrated disc destruction and a fistulous tract extending within the left first sacral foramen (Figure 5). *S aureus* was isolated by culture of the reaspirated contrast medium. Antibiotic therapy provided prompt recovery.

RESULTS

Growth inhibition. Table 1 exhibits the maximal growth inhibition observed for each organism. This generally occurred if inoculation was performed after 24-hour contact between the bacteria and the tested drug. However, the tested contrast media did not significantly inhibit bacterial growth if culture was made within 3 hours of incubation; under those conditions the tested bacteria could always be distinguished (Table 2). Lidocaine, however, produced inhibitory effects even in cases of short duration of contact before culture.

Meglumine amidotrizoate and metrizamide. When meglumine amidotrizoate or metrizamide was

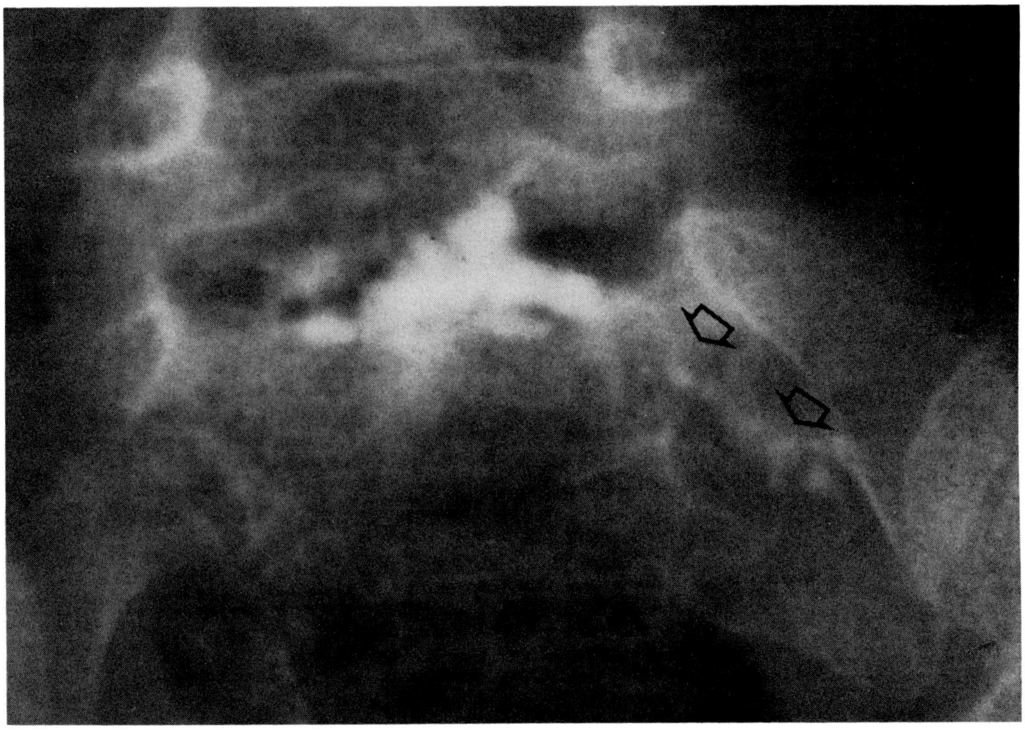

Figure 5. Patient 4. L5–S1 discography showing opacification of a fistulous tract (**arrows**) extending into the first left sacral foramen.

used as contrast medium, no significant growth inhibition of the gram-positive bacteria was observed at the different concentrations tested.

For gram-negative bacteria, metrizamide did not significantly inhibit culture of inocula containing $>10^4$ bacteria/ml. With meglumine amidotrizoate, we observed a partial decrease in the number of the colonies after 5 hours of incubation; growth inhibition was significant but not complete after a 24-hour incubation period. For the inocula containing $<10^4$ bacteria/ml, a significant inhibitory effect of meglumine amidotrizoate was observed on *E coli* and *P aeruginosa* after a 24-hour incubation period. A partial decrease could be observed even after 3 hours of incubation.

The effects of metrizamide on *E coli* were similar to those of meglumine amidotrizoate. However, on *P aeruginosa*, metrizamide produced a reaction

Table 1. Maximal antibacterial effects observed with meglumine amidotrizoate, metrizamide, and lidocaine*

Bacteria	Inoculum size (bacteria/ml)	Meglumine amidotrizoate	Metrizamide	Lidocaine
Gram-positive				
(*Staphylococcus aureus*,	$>10^4$	–	–	–
Streptococcus group B,	$\leq10^4$	–	–	+
Streptococcus viridans)				
Gram-negative				
Escherichia coli	$>10^4$	±	–	+
	$\leq10^4$	+	+	+
Pseudomonas aeruginosa	$>10^4$	±	–	–
	$\leq10^4$	+	–	+

* – = no inhibition; ± = partial inhibition; + = total inhibition (no growth).

Table 2. Antibacterial effects observed with meglumine amidotrizoate, metrizamide, and lidocaine, with ≤3 hours contact before culture*

Bacteria	Inoculum size (bacteria/ml)	Meglumine amidotrizoate	Metrizamide	Lidocaine
Gram-positive				
(*Staphylococcus aureus*,	$>10^4$	–	–	–
Streptococcus group B,	$\leq 10^4$	–	–	±
Streptococcus viridans)				
Gram-negative				
Escherichia coli	$>10^4$	–	–	+
	$\leq 10^4$	±	±	+
Pseudomonas aeruginosa	$>10^4$	–	–	–
	$\leq 10^4$	±	–	+

* – = no inhibition; ± = partial inhibition; + = total inhibition (no growth).

opposite to that seen with meglumine amidotrizoate: the number of the colonies increased with time, showing the ability of some bacteria to multiply when exposed to metrizamide.

Lidocaine. With lidocaine 1%, gram-positive bacteria were not inhibited if the inoculum contained $>10^4$ organisms/ml, but an almost total inhibition was observed after a 24-hour incubation for inocula containing $<10^4$ *S aureus* or *S agalactiae*/ml. Partial inhibition of gram-positive bacteria had already occurred after 3-hour and 5-hour incubations, depending on the size of the inoculum. For *S agalactiae* inoculum containing 10^4 bacteria/ml, the number of colonies decreased steadily from the start of the incubation. Low-concentrated inocula of *S viridans* were not tested.

There was some variation in lidocaine's effects on different gram-negative bacteria. After overnight incubation, the 4 strains of *E coli* were totally inhibited by this drug. Partial inhibition was seen under other conditions, depending on the duration of contact, the initial concentration of the inoculum, and the strain tested. When *P aeruginosa* was used, it was resistant to lidocaine 1% if the inoculum contained $>10^4$ bacteria/ml, but growth inhibition was observed, beginning at 3 hours, for the inoculum at a concentration of 10^4 bacteria/ml. The tests were uninterpretable for the inocula at 10^2 and 10^3 bacteria/ml.

Meglumine amidotrizoate:lidocaine mixture. This solution was tested only on inocula containing $>10^4$ bacteria/ml. It inhibited the strains of *E coli* in proportion to the concentration of lidocaine and was ineffective on the other bacteria.

When *M tuberculosis* was used as the inoculum, the strains grew in the presence of all of the drugs tested.

DISCUSSION

The opacification of septic areas provides valuable information about the size of the lesion, its precise extent, and the eventual presence of adjacent abscesses or fistulous tracts (1,2). This procedure is especially helpful in cases of osteitis or septic arthritis, as in our patients 2 and 3. Detection of an unexpected abscess during arthrography in septic arthritis helps the physician select the most appropriate therapy. This is equally true in spondylodiscitis: opacification of the intervertebral space can provide demonstration of an eventual abscess, particularly one that is spreading into the psoas muscle. In a child presenting with discitis caused by *S aureus* of the L5–S1 space (patient 4), we observed a fistulous tract extending within the first sacral foramen.

During puncture of articular replacements, arthrography has to be performed in order to detect possible loosening. However, positive findings from bacteriologic examination of the aspirated material are quite rare in these cases, even with the use of surgical specimens (3). The injection of contrast medium sometimes allows visualization of fistulous tracts that can extend far from the joint, as in our patient 1. Adequate precautions must be taken so that injection of contrast medium does not disturb bacteriologic isolation of the reaspirated material.

Some researchers have reported an absence of antibacterial effects of meglumine amidotrizoate and metrizamide (4,5); however, in their studies, relatively rich bacterial inocula, containing more than 10^6 bacteria/ml, were used. Kim and Lachman (1) drew our attention to the relation between the concentration of the bacterial inoculum and the antibacterial effects of the contrast media, but they tested only cultures of *S aureus*.

Our experiments do not demonstrate significant effects of the contrast media on gram-positive bacteria, regardless of the concentration of the inoculum. The results regarding gram-negative bacteria are quite different, depending on bacterial concentration. Meglumine amidotrizoate inhibited cultures of *E coli* and *P aeruginosa* to varying degrees, while metrizamide acted only on low-concentrated inocula of *E coli*, ($<10^4$ bacteria/ml). The antibacterial effects of these drugs were altered according to the duration of contact before culture, with the effects being generally insignificant if the specimen was cultured a short time after removal.

Regardless of the duration of the contact, the inhibitory effect of metrizamide on gram-negative bacteria was lower than that of meglumine amidotrizoate. However, we do not believe this justifies the systematic use of this more expansive contrast medium. Rather, it should be reserved for special conditions, e.g., in the case of possible intradural injection.

Inhibitory effects of the contrast media could be due to the release of inorganic iodine in the sample tests. Lang et al (6) demonstrated that samples exposed to sunlight had increased inorganic iodine concentration, whereas room light provoked only slight liberation of this molecule. The influence of duration of contact before culture could be partially due to this phenomenon. During our investigations we covered the test tubes with aluminum foil to prevent light exposure, but this precaution may have been insufficient. The multiplication of *P aeruginosa* observed during incubation in metrizamide was probably due to the capacity of this bacterium to grow easily in aqueous solutions.

Our results with lidocaine were consistent with those previously reported (7,8) for concentrations $>10^4$ bacteria/ml in the inoculum. Gram positive bacteria and *P aeruginosa* were not inhibited, whereas *E coli* were sensitive to this drug, depending on the duration of incubation. Lidocaine did inhibit bacterial growth when the inoculum contained $<10^4$ bacteria/ml. Complete inhibition was observed after 24-hour incubation of some gram-positive bacteria; inhibition began sooner with gram-negative bacteria. Since bacterial concentration within lesions cannot be predicted, lidocaine should not be allowed to enter into contact with the withdrawn specimen.

M tuberculosis seems to be insensitive to all of the tested drugs under the experimental conditions used. These results differ from those of Schmidt and Rosenkranz (7). We may have used much larger concentrations of the inocula. However, our in vitro findings are consistent with our clinical observations. Indeed, we never observed any inhibitory effect of the contrast media or lidocaine on the cultures of samples obtained after opacification of tuberculous lesions. One of us (2) previously reported a case of tuberculous discitis confirmed by bacteriologic examination of the material withdrawn after discography.

Lidocaine must be used very prudently during diagnostic puncture of septic lesions, and it should not come into contact with the lesion. After aspiration of any material, contrast media should be injected to provide adequate demonstration of the extent of the lesion. Thereafter, contrast medium must be reaspirated for bacteriologic examination. Under any circumstance, the specimen should be inoculated as quickly as possible after removal.

ACKNOWLEDGMENTS

We wish to thank Drs. B. Vandermensbrugghe and R. J. Francois for their help during preparation of this paper; C. Godalier, Y. Cordonnier, and A. Genet for technical assistance; M. H. de Crom and D. Gerstmans for secretarial assistance; and C. Georges for the photographic work.

REFERENCES

1. Kim KS, Lachman R: In vitro effects of iodinated contrast media on the growth of Staphylococci. Invest Radiol 17:305–309, 1982
2. Pauls C, Dory M, Lewalle J, Liesenborghs L: Pott's disease: report of a case studied by discography and computerized axial tomography. J Belge Radiol 62:83–86, 1979
3. Postel M: Les complications des prothèses totales de hanche. Rev Chir Orthop (suppl) 61:28–120, 1975
4. Johansen JG, Clausen OG: Antibacterial effects of metrizoate and metrizamide on bacterial growth in vitro. Acta Radiol [Diagn] (Stockh) 18:269–272, 1977
5. Melson GL, McDaniel RC, Southern PM, Staple TW: In vitro effects of iodinated arthrographic contrast media on bacterial growth. Radiology 112:593–595, 1974
6. Lang JH, Lasser EC, Talner LB, Lyon S, Coel M: Inorganic iodide in contrast media. Invest Radiol 9:51–55, 1974
7. Schmidt RM, Rosenkranz HS: Antibacterial activity of local anesthetics: lidocaine and procaine. J Infect Dis 121:597–607, 1970
8. Weinstein MP, Maderazo E, Tilton R, Maggini G, Quintiliani R: Further observations on the antibacterial effects of local anesthetic agents. Curr Therap Res 17:369–374, 1975

DIAGNOSIS-RELATED GROUP REGULATIONS

Implications for the Practicing Rheumatologist

MORRIS WEINBERGER, MARILYN K. POTTS, and KENNETH D. BRANDT

Data from our university hospital on the 2 most common rheumatologic diseases that require hospitalization indicate that total charges for patients admitted with rheumatoid arthritis or systemic lupus erythematosus break down as follows: room, board, and nursing, 55%; tests/procedures, 30%; drugs, 5%; physical and occupational therapy, 5%; and miscellaneous, 5%. Thus, shortening the length of stay would be the most effective mechanism to reduce total charges. We also found marked heterogeneity in the single diagnosis-related group containing rheumatoid arthritis and systemic lupus erythematosus inpatients under 70 years old who had no comorbid conditions. Planners should be sensitive to this as prospective reimbursement is extended beyond Medicare patients.

During the current fiscal year, the federal government will, for each Medicare admission, reimburse hospitals at a prespecified rate based upon the diagnosis-related group (DRG) into which the patient's admitting diagnosis is classified. Psychiatric, rehabilitation, and childrens' hospitals, as well as hospitals in states with alternative diagnosis-based prospective reimbursement systems (i.e., Massachusetts, New York, New Jersey, and Maryland), are exempted. This system is intended to encourage the delivery of cost-effective care. While only Medicare inpatients are currently affected nationally by DRGs, there is every indication that third-party payers will adopt similar pricing systems. For example, Blue Cross/Blue Shield in Arizona, Oklahoma, Kansas, and Cleveland, Ohio are already using modified DRG systems, and Medicaid of Pennsylvania began such a system on July 1, 1984.* Additionally, similar reimbursement programs for physicians' fees for Medicare inpatients are currently being considered (1).

Papers on the development of DRGs (2) and criticism of this system (3–8) appear elsewhere. Our concern is the potential effect of DRGs on practicing rheumatologists. To address this, we have analyzed data on all rheumatoid arthritis (RA) or systemic lupus erythematosus (SLE) patient admissions to the Medicine Services of University Hospital (UH) at Indianapolis during a recent 1-year period.

RA and SLE, the most common rheumatic diseases requiring hospitalization to the UH Medicine Services, provide excellent models for rheumatolo-

From the Regenstrief Institute for Health Care and the Department of Medicine, Indiana University School of Medicine, Indianapolis.

Supported in part by a Multipurpose Arthritis Center grant (AM 20582) from the National Institutes of Health.

Morris Weinberger, PhD: Associate Professor of Medicine, Indiana University School of Medicine; Marilyn K. Potts, MSW: Director, Community Component, Indiana University Multipurpose Arthritis Center; Kenneth D. Brandt, MD: Professor of Medicine and Head, Rheumatology Division, Indiana University School of Medicine and Director, Indiana University Multipurpose Arthritis Center.

Address reprint requests to Morris Weinberger, PhD, Regenstrief Institute for Health Care, 1001 West Tenth Street/5th Floor, Indianapolis, IN 46202.

Submitted for publication April 25, 1984; accepted in revised form August 27, 1984.

* Personal communications: Mr. Joseph Villegas, Director of Professional and Provider Programs, Blue Cross/Blue Shield of Arizona; Mr. Richard Howard, Vice-President for Public Affairs, Blue Cross/Blue Shield of Oklahoma; Mr. Robert Pearcy, Senior Director of Professional and Institutional Affairs, Blue Cross/Blue Shield of Kansas; Mr. Edward Shamrock, Director of Audit and Reimbursement, Blue Cross/Blue Shield, Cleveland, OH; Mr. Richard Lyman, Program Analyst, Bureau of Eligibility, Reimbursement and Coverage, Health Care Financing Administration, Baltimore MD.

gists to study DRGs. These diseases are prevalent: a population survey indicated that 1% of adults have definite RA (9). A retrospective analysis of members of the San Francisco Kaiser Permanente Health Plan, covering 1965–1973, revealed a prevalence rate of SLE of 1/1,960 members; a similar SLE prevalence rate was reported in Minnesota (9). In 1978, average direct medical charges for RA patients living near San Francisco were $2,319 (10). Hospital charges for these patients accounted for 66% of the medical costs, despite the fact that only 26% were hospitalized.

Management of patients with RA and SLE often emphasizes multidisciplinary care. Referral of the RA patient to an occupational therapist (OT) for instruction in energy conservation and joint protection techniques or for provision of adaptive equipment for activities of daily living, and to a physical therapist (PT) for instruction in muscle strengthening and range of motion exercises, is common (11,12). Studies indicate that in the treatment of RA, such care may result in more favorable health outcomes than care by the physician alone (13–16). Under retrospective pricing systems, there had been few financial disincentives for such referrals, since inpatient PT and OT services were generally reimbursed in full. Under DRGs, however, ancillary services, such as PT and OT, are purchased as would be any other item. Therefore, this would encourage such measures as reducing staff and limiting time spent with each patient. Nurses and social workers may be open to similar scrutiny, leading to staff reductions and overburdening of hospital personnel (17). Such changes may affect the nature of interactions between patients and allied health professionals; for example, inpatient education may be sacrificed for a more expedient discharge.

Patients hospitalized with RA and, to a lesser extent, SLE may have a variety of special equipment needs (e.g., aids for self-care and personal hygiene, walkers, canes, wheelchairs). Such equipment may enable patients to perform specific activities and/or reduce stress on affected joints, possibly reducing the likelihood that deformities will develop. Under the DRG reimbursement system, provision of such equipment on an inpatient basis may be decreased.

Finally, clearly defined markers of discharge-readiness for RA and SLE patients are not available. Thus, in non-acute situations, these patients may be discharged before home care instruction is completed or drug therapy is adjusted adequately. Without intensive inpatient instruction, outpatient visits and readmissions may increase.

METHODS

We gathered data on *all* nonsurgical inpatients admitted to UH for RA or SLE between July 1, 1982 and June 30, 1983, who, if classified today, would be assigned to DRG 240 (Connective Tissue Disorder, Age Greater Than 69, and/or Comorbid Condition Present) or DRG 241 (Connective Tissue Disorder, Age Less Than 70, and No Comorbid Condition Present). Thus, it should be emphasized that our analysis is not restricted to Medicare patients.

The 400-bed UH is the only academic referral hospital in Indiana. Over 95% of patients who would be classified in DRG 240 or 241 are admitted to the Rheumatology Service, where a staff rheumatologist is responsible for their care and directs a team composed of a Rheumatology Fellow, house officers, and medical students.

UH's computer provided us with each patient's age, length of stay (LOS), hospital diagnosis (RA or SLE), DRG category (240 or 241), and total charges incurred during the hospitalization. We inflated these charges by approximately 6% annually to estimate 1984 charges. We classified the charges into subcategories, which were then combined into 4

Table 1. Age, length of stay, and 1984 estimated charges for University Hospital inpatients with rheumatoid arthritis (RA) and systemic lupus erythematosus (SLE), by diagnosis-related group (DRG)*

	DRG 240 (Age Greater Than 69 and/or Comorbid Condition Present)		DRG 241 (Age Less Than 70 and No Comorbid Condition Present)	
	RA (n = 26)	SLE (n = 12)	RA (n = 48)	SLE (n = 10)
Age, years	58.50 (13.71)	33.58 (12.60)	52.92 (10.41)	37.20 (15.87)
Length of stay, range, days	2–31	2–19	2–20	3–20
Length of stay, mean, days	9.65 (6.33)	8.58 (5.52)	7.85 (3.52)	9.70 (6.11)
Estimated 1984 charges, dollars	3,646 (2,098)	3,726 (2,277)	3,038 (1,185)	4,124 (2,371)

* Numbers in parentheses = standard deviation; charge estimates are based on 1982–1983 RA and SLE admissions.

Table 2. A comparison of Diagnosis-Related Group (DRG)–based lengths of stay (LOS) and charges and mean LOS and charges found in this study

	DRG 240	DRG 241
DRG-estimated LOS, days	8.6	8.0
University Hospital LOS, days (mean)*	9.3	8.2
1984 DRG base rate for University Hospital†	$4,487	$4,181
University Hospital's DRG rate†	$5,694	$5,360
Mean University Hospital charge*	$3,671	$3,225

* Based on rheumatoid arthritis and systemic lupus erythematosus inpatients at University Hospital between July 1, 1982 and June 30, 1983.
† These are transition rates for 1984. Since 75% of these rates are based on our experience, they apply only to our hospital. The base rate does not include adjustments, such as direct medical education, capital expenditures, and case-mix, while the University Hospital DRG rate includes these adjustments.

broader categories: (a) facility charges (e.g., room, board, nursing); (b) tests/procedures (e.g., radiology, electroencephalograms, clinical pathology, laboratory tests, cardiac studies, and pulmonary function studies); (c) drugs (pharmacy and blood bank); and (d) other services (e.g., occupational therapy, physical therapy, and medical supplies) (18).

T-tests were performed to examine differences between groups for average LOS and total charges; however, we were limited when analyzing differences between individual charge categories (e.g., facilities, tests/procedures). The computer could only provide the total amount spent on a charge item, for example, the total charges for radiographs among all RA patients in DRG 240. This allowed us to compute the mean charge per patient, but not the standard deviation, a statistic necessary to perform *t*-tests. Therefore, we estimated the SD using the coefficient of variation (19), a statistic which assumes that the ratio between the mean and the SD for the total cost is approximately the same as the ratio between the 2 for each category. For example, if the mean charge per hospitalization were actually $4,000, with an SD of $400, the SD would be 10% of the mean. If the average facility charge were $2,000, we would estimate the SD to be ($2,000 × 0.10) = $200. Four separate coefficients of variation were calculated, depending upon the DRG (240 or 241) and the disease (RA or SLE).

RESULTS

Ninety-six patients were analyzed (Table 1). The average age of patients in DRG 240 was 47.2 years, while the mean age of patients in DRG 241 was 50.2 years. This indicates that patients in DRG 240 were classified by comorbid conditions rather than by age. Only 15 patients (15.6%) were 65 years or older, and all had RA. For both DRGs, RA patients were older ($P < 0.001$) than SLE patients, although LOS did not differ. The mean LOSs (9.3 days for DRG 240, 8.2 days for DRG 241) were not significantly different from those established under current federal guidelines (Table 2). The charges for RA patients within

Table 3. Categorization of mean and percent of total estimated 1984 charges for Diagnosis-Related Group 240 (Age Greater Than 69 and/or Comorbid Condition Present), by disease*

	RA (n = 26)	SLE (n = 12)	All patients (n = 38)
Facility			
Room/board/nursing	2,005 (54.99%)	1,794 (48.15%)	1,938 (52.81%)
Other	95 (2.61%)	321 (8.62%)	166 (4.52%)
Subtotal	2,100 (57.60%)	2,115 (56.76%)	2,104 (57.33%)
Tests/procedures			
Radiology/ultrasound	298 (8.17%)	314 (8.43%)	303 (8.26%)
Cardiac studies	97 (2.66%)	45 (1.21%)	81 (2.21%)
Other studies	69 (1.89%)	92 (2.47%)	76 (2.07%)
Clinical pathology laboratory	444 (12.18%)	760 (20.40%)	544 (14.82%)
Anatomic pathology laboratory	12 (0.33%)	39 (1.05%)	20 (0.54%)
Subtotal	920 (25.23%)	1,250 (33.55%)	1,024 (27.90%)
Drugs			
Pharmacy	169 (4.64%)	169 (4.54%)	169 (4.60%)
Blood bank	32 (0.88%)	80 (2.15%)	47 (1.28%)
Subtotal	201 (5.51%)	249 (6.69%)	216 (5.88%)
Other services			
Occupational therapy	132 (3.62%)	0 (0.00%)	90 (2.45%)
Physical therapy	168 (4.61%)	29 (0.78%)	124 (3.38%)
Materials management	91 (2.50%)	68 (1.82%)	84 (2.29%)
Other	34 (0.93%)	15 (0.40%)	28 (0.76%)
Subtotal	425 (11.66%)	112 (3.00%)	326 (8.88%)
Total (dollars)	3,646 (100.00%)	3,726 (100.00%)	3,670 (99.99%)

* RA = rheumatoid arthritis; SLE = systemic lupus erythematosus.

Table 4. Categorization of average and percent of total estimated 1984 charges for Diagnosis-Related Group 241 (Age Less Than 70 and/or No Comorbid Condition Present), by disease*

	RA (n = 48)	SLE (n = 10)	All patients (n = 58)
Facility			
Room/board/nursing	1,664 (54.77%)	2,055 (49.83%)	1,731 (53.67%)
Other	0 (0.00%)	0 (0.00%)	0 (0.00%)
Subtotal	1,664 (54.77%)	2,055 (49.83%)	1,731 (53.67%)
Tests/procedures			
Radiology/ultrasound	348 (11.45%)	569 (13.80%)	386 (11.97%)
Cardiac studies	57 (1.88%)	152 (3.68%)	73 (2.26%)
Other studies	42 (1.38%)	155 (3.76%)	62 (1.92%)
Clinical pathology laboratory	402 (13.23%)	885 (21.46%)	485 (15.04%)
Anatomic pathology laboratory	13 (0.43%)	38 (0.92%)	17 (0.53%)
Subtotal	862 (28.37%)	1,799 (43.62%)	1,023 (31.72%)
Drugs			
Pharmacy	76 (2.50%)	124 (3.01%)	84 (2.60%)
Blood bank	12 (0.40%)	9 (0.22%)	12 (0.37%)
Subtotal	88 (2.90%)	133 (3.23%)	96 (2.98%)
Other services			
Occupational therapy	168 (5.53%)	32 (0.78%)	145 (4.50%)
Physical therapy	160 (5.27%)	38 (0.92%)	139 (4.31%)
Materials management	84 (2.76%)	48 (1.16%)	78 (2.42%)
Other	12 (0.40%)	19 (0.46%)	13 (0.40%)
Subtotal	424 (13.96%)	137 (3.32%)	375 (11.63%)
Total (dollars)	3,038 (100.00%)	4,124 (100.00%)	3,225 (100.00%)

* RA = rheumatoid arthritis; SLE = systemic lupus erythematosus.

DRG 240 were not significantly different from those with SLE ($3,646 and $3,726, respectively). However, within DRG 241, the average charge for SLE patients ($4,124) was higher ($P < 0.001$) than that for RA patients ($3,038).

Table 3 presents the distribution of DRG 240 charges among the 4 previously described categories. The mean estimated 1984 charges for RA and SLE patients who would have been classified in DRG 240 (Connective Tissue Disorder, Age Greater Than 69, and/or Comorbid Condition Present) were $3,646 and $3,726, respectively. Room and board accounted for over half of these amounts (Table 3); laboratory tests and procedures made up approximately 30% of the total. Less than 15% of the total charges was accounted for by the combination of the drugs and other services categories (including PT and OT). The only significant difference between RA and SLE patients in DRG 240 was in the other services category ($t = 4.33$, df = 36, $P < 0.001$), and this was due to the increased use of PT and OT by patients with RA.

Table 4 presents parallel data for DRG 241 (Connective Tissue Disorder, Age Less Than 70, and No Comorbid Condition). Here, however, differences in charges were pronounced. The total estimated 1984 charges for SLE patients (mean $4,124) were significantly higher than for RA patients (mean $3,038; $t = 2.17$, df = 56, $P < 0.05$). As with DRG 240, facility charges accounted for over half of the total, and there were no differences between RA and SLE patients in this area ($t = 1.48$). However, compared with RA patients, SLE patients used more tests/procedures ($t = 5.22$, $P < 0.001$) and drugs ($t = 2.95$, $P < 0.01$), but fewer other services ($t = 4.33$, $P < 0.001$). Additionally, SLE patients had more charges in each subcategory of tests/procedures, as well as in pharmacy (Table 4). RA patients used significantly more OT, PT, and materials management ($P < 0.01$).

Presently, DRG payment rates reflect a combination of local and national charge estimates. During the first year of DRGs, 75% of the rate will be determined by local charges; however, this will be reduced to 50% and 25%, respectively, during the second and third years. In the fourth year, there will be a single national rate paid to all hospitals. Local charges depend on the diagnosis-specific makeup of a hospital's caseload. These rates are then adjusted for medical education, capital expenditures, and bad debts, although such subsidies may be disallowed in the future. Therefore, the 1984 rates for UH are weighted heavily (75%) by our local experiences, and include adjustments specific to UH. Thus, these rates are applicable for our institution only. For RA and SLE, the government estimates the 1984 base rate for all UH medicine admissions to be $4,487 and $4,181, respectively. However, due to adjustments described above, our UH will receive $5,694 for each admission in DRG 240, and $5,360 for each admission in DRG 241.

DISCUSSION

Our results lead to several conclusions. Notably, most admissions for DRG 240 are based on the presence of comorbid conditions rather than the patient's age. Despite this, the only difference in charges is that RA patients used more other services than SLE patients, reflecting the extent of OT and PT that they received (Table 3). This seems to be appropriate.

In contrast, there are large disparities in DRG 241 (Table 4). Since Medicare inpatients are usually at least 65 years old and will therefore be classified predominantly in DRG 240 because of the age criterion, this does not present an immediate problem. However, as prospective reimbursement is extended to non-Medicare patients, planners cannot assume that DRGs which include younger patients with less comorbidity (e.g., DRG 241) will be similar to DRGs designed for older and/or sicker individuals (e.g., DRG 240) with respect to resource allocation. Indeed, our data indicate that, on average, SLE patients accounted for 35.7% more charges than RA patients within DRG 241.

One interesting finding is that DRGs may not present an immediate impact on rheumatologists. Only 15% of inpatients in our study were 65 years or older, the group currently most likely to be affected by DRGs. If UH is representative, hospitals will initially have marginal gains from most inpatients with RA and SLE (Table 2). However, as categories are refined, this gain will be temporary. Also, if allowances for medical education and capital expenditures are eliminated, the picture will be altered dramatically. The rate will also change as national rates are established in 4 years.

Another question concerns the most likely targets for reducing hospital costs. For both DRG 240 and 241, room, board, and nursing account for over half of the expenses, followed by tests/procedures (approximately 30%), drugs (approximately 5%), and other services (10%) (Tables 3 and 4). There are several ways to reduce the room/board/nursing category. One is to lay off nursing staff; however, since this will increase the remaining nurses' workload, this strategy needs to be evaluated in terms of the quality of patient care and the retention of competent nurses.

The strategy with the greatest potential yield is reducing LOS. This will directly affect the facility charge, the largest component of the bill, and will have an indirect impact on the other categories. However, planners must consider the implications upon the quality of patient care and subsequent health outcomes resulting from reduced hospital stays. For example, is it cost-effective to keep a person in the hospital for an additional day to improve his/her medical status if this reduces the risk for rehospitalization? Under retrospective reimbursement, reducing rehospitalization is the most effective way to reduce costs (18); however, under DRGs, hospitals may encourage short-stay, uncomplicated rehospitalizations to remain financially solvent (3).

Physicians may be asked to reduce the number and types of tests and procedures they order. While some laboratory tests and procedures are certainly unnecessary and should be reduced, such a strategy will make only a small dent in total inpatient charges (18).

Hospital pharmacies may alter the medicines they dispense. For example, although aspirin is a widely used, inexpensive treatment for RA, in many individuals it produces dyspepsia, hepatotoxicity, or tinnitus. In such instances, other nonsteroidal antiinflammatory drugs (NSAIDS) may be indicated. Some NSAIDs have the further advantage of requiring fewer doses per day than aspirin, which may improve patient compliance. Since NSAIDs are considerably more expensive than generic aspirin, hospital pharmacies may be encouraged to limit their use under DRGs. Notably, at least 18 states have already deleted, or have considered deleting, NSAIDs from their Medicaid formularies (personal communication: Mr. John McCray, Vice-President for Government Affairs, Arthritis Foundation).

The effect of DRGs on occupational and physical therapists may include increased caseloads and/or staff reductions. If this occurs, therapists may be unable to provide adequate instruction about adaptive equipment and assistive devices, since contact time with each patient would be shortened. OTs and PTs would need to initiate therapy early in the hospital course and use the outpatient setting for followup. It is important to note that in our analysis, combined OT and PT services for RA and SLE patients accounted for less than 10% of the total charge. Therefore, for inpatients with rheumatic disease, OT and PT services may not be the most appropriate target for cost savings. Further, this may lead to patient education being increasingly conducted in outpatient settings. If so, patients who fail to keep their appointments may increase the likelihood of future rehospitalization. Finally, cost-shifting to the outpatient service is only a temporary solution. Future prospective reimbursement systems are likely to encompass all health care services.

How will DRGs affect academic rheumatologists? If university-affiliated hospitals, such as UH, absorb the sickest patients, as may be evidenced by the makeup of DRG 240, national rates will be inappropriate for these institutions. Unless major adjustments are made, there will surely be impending danger.

It must be emphasized that our data should be interpreted cautiously. DRG rates for the first year are dominated by local experiences. Further, DRG 240 at UH consists largely of RA or SLE patients who have comorbid conditions, rather than persons who meet only the age criterion. Therefore, we cannot evaluate whether the current DRG classification system is appropriate for Medicare patients. While the calculations presented are specific to our UH, we strongly urge other hospitals to perform similar analyses and arrive at their own conclusions.

ACKNOWLEDGMENTS

The authors wish to acknowledge the assistance of Dr. Stuart Kleit, Kenneth Beardsley, and Kendra Meetz in the preparation of this manuscript.

REFERENCES

1. Public Law 98-21: Prospective payment for Medicare inpatient hospital services. Amendment passed: March 24, 1983, Federal Register 39752 (September 1, 1983)
2. Vladeck B: Medical hospital payment by diagnosis-related groups. Ann Intern Med 100:576–591, 1984
3. Iglehart JK: Health policy report: New Jersey's experiment with DRG-based hospital reimbursement. N Engl J Med 307:1655–1660, 1982
4. Keith SN: Prospective payment for hospital costs using diagnosis-related groups: will cost inflation be reduced? J Natl Med Assoc 75:609–623, 1983
5. Public Comment of the Committee on Rheumatologic Practice, American Rheumatism Association, to the Health Care Financing Administration. Atlanta, GA, American Rheumatism Association, October 6, 1983
6. Lockshin MD: DRG legislation and rheumatic disease. Submitted for publication
7. Kreitzer SL, Loebner ES, Poveti GC: Severity of illness: the DRGs' missing link. QRB 8:21–34, 1982
8. Bergen SS, Roth AC: Prospective payment and the university hospital. N Engl J Med 310:316–318, 1984
9. Rodnan GP, Schumacher HR, editors: Primer on the Rheumatic Diseases, Atlanta, GA, Arthritis Foundation, 1983, pp 33, 49
10. Meenan RF, Yelin EH, Henke CJ, Curtis DL, Epstein WV: The costs of rheumatoid arthritis: a patient-oriented study of chronic disease costs. Arthritis Rheum 21:827–833, 1978
11. Katz WA: General approach to the management of rheumatic diseases, Rheumatic Diseases: Diagnosis and Management. Philadelphia, JB Lippincott Co., 1979, pp 865–875
12. Melvin JL: Rheumatic Disease: Occupational Therapy and Rehabilitation. Philadelphia, FA Davis Co., 1982
13. Feinberg J, Brandt K: Team management of rheumatoid arthritis patients in functional class I or II: results of a 2-year study. Am J Occup Ther 38:613–620, 1984
14. Katz S, Vignos PJ, Moskowitz RW, Thompson HM, Svec KH: Comprehensive outpatient care in rheumatoid arthritis. JAMA 206:1249–1254, 1968
15. Duff IF, Carpenter JO, Neukom JE: Comprehensive management of patients with rheumatoid arthritis. Arthritis Rheum 17:635–645, 1974
16. Shope JT, Banwell BA, Jette AM, Kulik CL, Edwards NL: Functional status outcome after treatment of rheumatoid arthritis. Clin Rheum Pract 1:243–248, 1983
17. Grimaldi PL, Micheletti JA: Recent Developments in Diagnosis Related Groups: A Practitioner's Guide. Chicago, Pluribus Press, Inc., 1983, pp 208–218
18. Smith DM, Robert SD, Gross TL: Health care costs of medical patients at an urban care center. J Community Health 7:21–32, 1981
19. Colton T: Statistics in Medicine. Boston, Little, Brown & Co., 1974, p 43

BRIEF REPORT

CHANGES IN NONGONOCOCCAL SEPTIC ARTHRITIS: DRUG ABUSE AND METHICILLIN-RESISTANT *STAPHYLOCOCCUS AUREUS*

GLORIETTA Z. ANG-FONTE, MICHAEL B. ROZBORIL, and GEORGE R. THOMPSON

Septic arthritis continues to be a major medical problem for metropolitan hospitals. Previous studies have defined risk factors, joint distribution, and the most common organisms implicated in this condition (1–4). Recently, we became aware of a pattern of septic arthritis that differed significantly from that previously reported. Over a 2-year period, a retrospective analysis of septic arthritis revealed the emergence of a new pattern of antibiotic resistance among the bacteria populating a well-defined subgroup of patients.

Patients and methods. Wayne County General Hospital, a 270-bed general hospital in suburban Detroit, has continuously served indigent citizens of the inner city of Detroit and the population of the surrounding area since the turn of the century. A review of the hospital's records for the 2-year period, January 1, 1981 through December 31, 1982, showed 46 patients with a discharge diagnosis of septic arthritis, excluding all cases of *Neisseria gonorrhea*. These patients' medical records, including their bacteriology laboratory data, were reviewed for inclusion in the study.

Criteria for inclusion were: presentation with an acutely painful, tender, or swollen joint and positive synovial fluid bacterial cultures. Of the 46 medical records reviewed, 28 met our criteria. Of the 18 patients excluded, 6 had positive blood cultures but negative synovial fluid cultures, 10 had negative synovial fluid and blood cultures, and 2 had osteomyelitis on presentation. The records were reviewed with attention to bacteria isolated, joints involved, predisposing factors, and short-term outcome.

Results. During the period of the study, there were 21,442 hospital admissions. Twenty-eight patients met the study criteria, giving an incidence of 1.3 cases per 1,000 hospital admissions. Twenty-two of the 28 patients were male and 6 were female; 19 were black, 8 white, and 1 Hispanic. The age range was 1–56 years, with a mean age of 33.8. Three patients were children (ages 1, 4, and 13).

Table 1 lists the predisposing factors identified, and compares their incidence with those in the 1966–77 series published from this hospital (1). The main predisposing factor in both series was the illicit use of intravenous drugs, which was present in 21 (75%) of the patients in this study. Six of these 21 patients had concomitant extraarticular infections which included septic thrombophlebitis, groin abscess, cellulitis, or pulmonary infections. These infections were caused by the same bacteria as that cultured from the joint. Five had a history of nonpenetrating trauma to the involved joint. In 11 patients, intravenous drug abuse was the only predisposing cause. No patient had evidence of bacterial endocarditis as manifested by embolic phenomena, changing heart murmur, or abnormal cardiac ultrasound findings.

Seven patients had no history of intravenous drug abuse. Three of these patients did have prior arthritis of the involved septic joint, including rheumatoid arthritis, gout, and scleroderma with calcinosis.

From the Rheumatology Section, Department of Medicine, University of Michigan, Ann Arbor, and Wayne County General Hospital, Westland, Michigan.

Glorietta Z. Ang-Fonte, MD; Michael B. Rozboril, MD; George R. Thompson, MD.

Address reprint requests to George R. Thompson, MD, VA Medical Center, 2215 Fuller Rd., Ann Arbor, MI 48105.

Submitted for publication February 27, 1984; accepted in revised form August 21, 1984.

Table 1. Predisposing factors in nongonococcal septic arthritis identified in this study (1981–82) and the previously reported (1966–77) series from the same hospital

	1981–82 (n= 28)	1966–77 (n = 54) (ref. 1)
Intravenous drug abuse (IVDA)	21	19
Extraarticular infection	6	
Local trauma	5	
IVDA alone	11	
Prior arthritis	3	4
Chronic illness	1	13
Immunosuppression	0	0
Preceding trauma	0	14
Other	0	16
None	3	0

None of the patients was immunocompromised by cytotoxic or high-dose steroid drug therapy or malignant disease, though the rheumatoid arthritis patient was receiving 5 mg per day of prednisone. One patient was a chronic alcoholic.

The most frequently involved joint was the knee, with involvement in 15 patients. Three patients each had involvement of the hip or ankle, 2 each the shoulder or elbow; 1 patient each had infection of a wrist, sternoclavicular, sacroiliac, or interphalangeal joint. One patient had both an elbow and a knee involved. The patients with sacroiliac and sternoclavicular joint infections both had histories of intravenous drug abuse.

Thirty-one bacterial isolates were recovered from the 28 patients (Table 2). *Staphylococcus aureus* was the most frequently cultured organism, occurring in 18 patients (64%), and in 7 patients the species isolated was resistant to methicillin. Beta-hemolytic streptococci were recovered from 8 patients (29%). Gram-negative organisms included *Escherichia coli*, *Enterobacter cloacae*, and *Hemophilus influenzae*. *Propionibacterium acnes* was recovered from the synovial fluid of 1 patient.

Table 2. Bacteria cultured from synovial fluid of patients in this study (1981–82) and from the 1966–77 study

	1981–82 (n = 28)	1966–77 (n = 54) (ref. 1)
Staphylococcus aureus	18	19
Methicillin-sensitive	11	19
Methicillin-resistant	7	0
Staphylococcus epidermidis	1	9
Beta-hemolytic streptococci	8	6
Non-beta streptococci	0	2
Gram-negative	3	12
Pseudomonas	0	6
Escherichia coli	1	1
Others	2	5
Propionibacterium acnes	1	0
Other bacteria	0	6

Polymicrobial infections were observed in 2 patients. In 1 patient with rheumatoid arthritis, beta-hemolytic *Streptococcus*, *Staphylococcus epidermidis*, and *P acnes* were all recovered from the wrist joint. In the other patient, both *E coli* and *E cloacae* were grown from right knee synovial fluid. This patient had had urate crystals seen in his joint fluid and for many years also had a metallic foreign body in the soft tissue around the knee.

Twenty-three of the 28 patients studied were treated medically with appropriate intravenous antibiotics and daily needle aspiration of the infected joint. Four of these patients subsequently underwent surgical drainage due to failure to adequately respond to the medical regimen, as manifested by continuing large effusion, high synovial fluid leukocytosis and low glucose, fever, and joint pain. The incriminating organism in 3 of these 4 patients was *S aureus* (2 methicillin-resistant and 1 methicillin-sensitive); it was *E coli* and *E cloacae* combined in the other.

Five patients were treated primarily with surgical drainage in addition to antibiotics, either on admission or shortly thereafter. Three patients had hip involvement (2 were children, ages 4 and 13 years). The other 2 patients were directly admitted to the orthopedic surgical service; they had infections of the knee and ankle, respectively.

The mean duration of hospitalization for those treated medically and surgically was 23.6 days and 29.5 days, respectively, with medians of 28 days and 24 days. Osteomyelitis was diagnosed in 7 patients, 5 in the medically treated and 2 in the surgically treated groups. Criteria for the diagnosis were lucent bone lesions on radiograph, and/or abnormal results on a bone scan.

Two patients died. One was a 30-year-old man with overwhelming sepsis and adult respiratory distress syndrome. The other was a 40-year-old man with rhabdomyolysis, hypertensive crisis, and cardiac arrhythmia. All of the remaining patients were improved when discharged. Seven patients (all intravenous drug abusers) left against medical advice prior to completion of their recommended course of antibiotics. Only 6 patients returned for followup examinations. Five of the 6 were asymptomatic with full range of motion of the affected joint. The sixth patient had had a staphylococcal infection of the glenohumeral joint that had required surgical drainage. That patient had severe limitation of motion of the shoulder.

Discussion. During the period 1966–77, the incidence of nongonococcal septic arthritis was 54 cases out of 156,203 hospital admissions, or 0.34 cases per 1,000 admissions (1). In comparison, in this study we found an incidence of 1.3 cases per 1,000 admissions, or a fourfold increase. The majority of patients were between the ages of 23 and 40 (mean age 33.8). We had only 3 pediatric patients in this series. This is in contrast to Rosenthal's series (2) in which 20 of 71 patients (28%) were under 16 years of age.

The most frequent predisposing cause of septic arthritis was intravenous drug abuse, which occurred in 75% of the patients, compared with an occurrence in 35% (19 of 54 patients) in the 1966–77 series from this hospital (1).

The occurrence of septic arthritis *not* associated with intravenous drug abuse was similar in the 2 studies. While the true prevalence of intravenous drug abuse in the community is unknown, during the period of the present study a marked increase in hospital admissions due to intravenous drug abuse–related disease was observed.

Other studies report a much lower percentage of patients who are intravenous drug abusers. Only 4 of 71 patients (5.6%) were abusers of intravenous drugs in Rosenthal's report (2), and Bayer (4) reported 8 of 21 patients (38%). Seven of Bayer's patients who were drug abusers had involvement of the sternoclavicular joint. That joint, and the sacroiliac, are reported to be frequently involved in drug addicts (4,5). We had 1 patient each (both intravenous drug abusers) with infection of the sternoclavicular and sacroiliac joint.

Staphylococcus aureus is the most common bacterium causing nongonococcal septic arthritis in the adult (1–3). This was true in the 1966–77 series and in our current series. In previously published papers, the *Staphylococcus* isolated was methicillin-sensitive *S aureus*. However, in our drug abuser population a new and not previously reported finding was the recovery of methicillin-resistant *S aureus* from synovial fluid. Thirty-nine percent (7 of 18) of staphylococci isolated were methicillin-resistant. No methicillin resistance was encountered in the 1966–77 series. The occurrence of methicillin-resistant *S aureus* has been previously reported, particularly in the Detroit area (6–8). In those reports the incidence of methicillin-resistant *S aureus* in community-acquired infections rose from 3% in March 1980 to 38% in September 1981 (6).

Gram-negative bacteria were found in 11% (3 of 28) of our patients, compared with 22% (12 of 54 patients) in the 1966–77 series. A higher incidence has been reported in other studies: Goldenberg and Cohen (3) reported 32% (19 of 59), and Rosenthal (2) listed 25% (16 of 63 patients). *Pseudomonas* has been isolated particularly from heroin addicts (4,5). Yet none of our patients had *Pseudomonas*, despite 75% admitting illicit intravenous use of drugs (primarily a mixture of heroin and various adulterants, especially quinine). This is of particular interest since Detroit has had the reputation of leading the nation in the incidence of *Pseudomonas endocarditis* (9).

In view of these bacteriologic findings, in areas where intravenous drug abuse is endemic or methicillin-resistant *S aureus* has been isolated, initial antibiotic therapy while awaiting culture results must include treatment for this bacterium. This may be accomplished with vancomycin, the drug of choice against methicillin-resistant *S aureus*. The aminoglycoside gentamicin, in isolates from our hospital as well as others in Michigan (7,8), also has anti–methicillin-resistant *S aureus* activity, and to achieve cost containment, an initial regimen of nafcillin and gentamicin is satisfactory. For proven methicillin-resistant *S aureus* infections, however, vancomycin is required, and any antibiotic regimen prior to definitive culture results must contain an aminoglycoside for activity against gram-negative bacteria.

The mean duration of hospitalization was not significantly different for patients treated medically versus those treated surgically. Two patients died of nonrelated serious diseases. The remainder were all improved at discharge. Only 6 patients were seen for followup examinations, underscoring the fact that the majority of these patients were not reliable followers of medical advice. It may be speculated, however, that most of them probably did not have recurrences or we would have seen them again at our hospital emergency department, though it is possible that they might have sought care at another hospital.

This study demonstrates 3 important diagnostic and therapeutic considerations for physicians managing patients with suspected septic arthritis. These considerations, which are particularly valid in metropolitan areas with a high prevalence of illicit drug use, are as follows: 1) Septic arthritis is increasing in incidence, as demonstrated by a fourfold increase in admission due to this problem in the 1980s at Wayne County General Hospital. 2) Intravenous drug abuse is now the chief predisposing factor for septic arthritis in our series. 3) Methicillin-resistant *Staphylococcus aureus* has emerged as a frequent and important pathogen for septic arthritis and must be considered in initiating antibiotic therapy.

REFERENCES

1. Manshady B, Thompson GR, Weiss JJ: Septic arthritis in a general hospital 1966–77. J Rheumatol 7:523–530, 1980
2. Rosenthal J, Bole GG, Robinson WD: Acute nongonococcal infectious arthritis: evaluation of risk factors, therapy, and outcome. Arthritis Rheum 23:889–897, 1980
3. Goldenberg DL, Cohen AS: Acute infectious arthritis: a review of patients with non gonococcal joint infections (with emphasis on therapy and prognosis). Am J Med 60:369–377, 1976
4. Bayer AS, Chow AW, Louie JS, Nies KM, Guze LB: Gram-negative bacillary septic arthritis: clinical, radiographic, therapeutic, and prognostic features. Semin Arthritis Rheum 7:123–132, 1977
5. Roca RP, Yoshikawa TT: Primary skeletal infections in heroin users. Clin Orthop 144:238–248, 1979
6. Saravolatz LD, Pohlod DJ, Arking LM: Community-acquired methicillin-resistant Staphylococcus aureus infections: a new source for nosocomial outbreaks. Ann Intern Med 97:325–329, 1982
7. Saravolatz LD, Markowitz N, Arking L, Pohlod D, Fisher E: Methicillin-resistant Staphylococcus aureus: epidemiologic observations during a community-acquired outbreak. Ann Intern Med 96:11–16, 1982
8. Levine DP, Cushing RD, Jui J, Brown WJ: Community-acquired methicillin-resistant Staphylococcus aureus endocarditis in the Detroit Medical Center. Ann Intern Med 97:330–338, 1982
9. Reyes MP, Palutke W, Wylin RF, Lerner AM: Pseudomonas endocarditis in the Detroit Medical Center 1969–1972. Medicine 52:173–194, 1973

BRIEF REPORT

POSTGASTRECTOMY BLIND LOOP SYNDROME AND THE ARTHRITIS–DERMATITIS SYNDROME

ALICE V. KLINKHOFF, HOWARD B. STEIN, OTTO L. A. SCHLAPPNER, and WILLIAM B. BOYKO

The arthritis–dermatitis syndrome is a complication of intestinal bypass surgery in 6–24% of patients. It is related to the overgrowth of bacteria in the excluded segment of the intestine (1–3). Antigenic components of these bacteria probably lead to the formation of immune complexes which then deposit in the target tissues. This theory is partly supported by the occurrence of the arthritis–dermatitis syndrome in 4 patients with a blind loop syndrome not caused by intestinal bypass surgery (4). We report another case of blind loop syndrome resulting from previous gastric surgery.

Case report. A 51-year-old woman complained of pain in the shoulders, lateral epicondyles of the elbows, anterior rib cage, low back, groin, knees, and toes for 6 months. There was no joint swelling, deformity, or morning stiffness. For 2 years she had episodes of pruritic, pustular skin lesions over the shoulders, arms, hands, legs, and feet. These lesions, initially single and subsequently in groups, would begin as vesicles, turn into pustules, umbilicate, become crusted, and heal within 7 days.

From the Departments of Medicine and Pathology, St. Paul's Hospital, and the Divisions of Rheumatology and Dermatology, University of British Columbia, Vancouver, British Columbia, Canada.

Alice V. Klinkhoff, MD: Canadian Arthritis Society Fellow; Howard B. Stein, MD: Clinical Associate Professor of Medicine; Otto L. A. Schlappner, MD: Clinical Associate Professor of Medicine; William B. Boyko, MD: Clinical Assistant Professor of Pathology.

Address reprint requests to Dr. H. B. Stein, 507-1160 Burrard Street, Vancouver, BC, V6Z 2E8, Canada.

Submitted for publication May 21, 1984; accepted in revised form August 13, 1984.

She had several episodes of purplish, tender, swollen nodules on the lower legs and ankles. The skin lesions were accompanied by polyarthralgia, malaise, fever, chills, and sweats. These episodes occurred monthly. An episode of pleurisy had occurred 4 months previously. She had had Raynaud's phenomenon for 2 years.

A subtotal gastrectomy had been performed 10 years previously for a perforated peptic ulcer. For the last 2 years she had diarrhea 3–4 times daily with loose, beige, floating, and foul-smelling stools. She had lost 7 pounds over a 3-month period, and noted easy bruising.

She was thin and had a midline abdominal surgical scar, but no abdominal tenderness or hepatosplenomegaly. Several ecchymoses were present on her extremities but there were no other skin lesions. There was tenosynovitis of the left peroneal tendon with redness, swelling, and tenderness. Muscle strength was normal except for grade 4/5 strength in the neck flexors and quadriceps. The remainder of the physical findings were unremarkable.

The hemoglobin level was 12.7 gm/dl, white blood cell count 7,000/mm^3, platelet count 440,000/mm^3, Westergren erythrocyte sedimentation rate 36 mm/hour, creatinine 1.1 mg/dl, calcium 7.6 mg/dl (normal 8.6–10.3), albumin 3.1 gm/dl (normal 3.3–5.3), alkaline phosphatase 346 units/liter (normal 35–105), and phosphate 2.8 mg/dl (normal 2.5–4.4). Prothrombin time was 27.7 seconds (normal 11–13) and partial thromboplastin time was 47 seconds (normal 25–39), but both corrected to normal following an intramuscular injection of 10 mg of vitamin K. Serum vitamin B_{12} and folate values were normal. Her serum ferritin level was low at 7 ng/ml (normal >20) and carotene was

0.30 μmoles/liter (normal 0.95–3.8). Serum 25-OH vitamin D was markedly reduced at 3 ng/ml (normal >17). A 72-hour fat collection measured 3.8 gm (normal 2.3–7.7). Antinuclear antibody, rheumatoid factor, and cryoglobulins were not detected and C3 and C4 complement levels were normal. Immune complexes measured by C1q binding were 4% (normal <6).

Chest radiograph results were unremarkable. Radiographs of the pelvis and hands showed osteopenia with undisplaced fractures of the left femoral neck and distal phalanx of the right middle finger. A bone scan revealed multiple areas of increased activity involving the ribs, the left femoral head, distal phalanx of the right middle finger, and both feet, consistent with multiple fractures. An upper gastrointestinal series with small bowel follow-through showed a partial gastrectomy and a localized stricture of the efferent loop of the bowel distal to the stoma. Endoscopy revealed a large pouch of small bowel with a very narrow outlet beyond the anastamosis. The mucosa of the afferent loop appeared inflamed. A small bowel biopsy of the afferent loop showed acute and chronic inflammation. Cultures of the small bowel aspirate grew >60,000 coliforms and $>10^5$ lactobacilli. ^{14}C-glycine cholate breath analysis was consistent with bacterial overgrowth at 12% (normal <1%). An iliac crest bone biopsy showed severe osteomalacia with active bone resorption consistent with osteitis fibrosa.

While in the hospital she had an attack of the arthritis–dermatitis syndrome with papulovesicles over the arms, shoulders, and right foot (Figure 1), which resolved over a 4-day period. C3 and C4 complement tests repeated during this episode remained at normal levels; C1q binding was unchanged at 4% and cryoglobulins were absent. Microscopic examination of a skin biopsy showed necrosis of the upper dermis with adjacent vasculitis characterized by endothelial swelling, necrosis, and neutrophilic and mononuclear cell infiltration. Direct immunofluorescence showed deposition of IgM, IgA, and C3 in the vessels of the reticular dermis (Figure 2).

At laparotomy, a stricture was found at the site of the previous Billroth I anastamosis and a second stricture was found in the second part of the duodenum. Between these strictures was a blind loop which was dilated to 10 cm in diameter. The distal bowel was normal. The duodenal stricture was opened and sutured longitudinally and a gastrojejunostomy was performed. When discharged from the hospital, she was prescribed vitamin D, 50,000 IU twice weekly and elemental calcium, 1,500 mg daily.

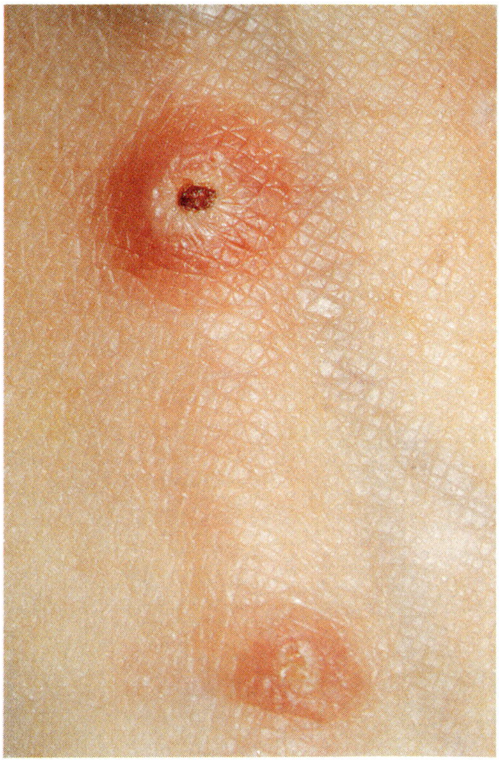

Figure 1. Close-up photograph of the forearm, showing vesiculopustular skin lesions, with crusting apparent on the upper lesion.

Over the subsequent 9 months, there were no further episodes of the arthritis–dermatitis syndrome and no bone pain. She gained 12 pounds. Laboratory data 9 months postoperatively included normal serum calcium, phosphate, and alkaline phosphatase levels.

Discussion. A blind loop syndrome developed in our patient 8 years after a Billroth I gastrectomy. She had malabsorption of carotene, iron, calcium, and vitamins D and K, which resulted in weight loss, osteomalacia with multiple fractures, and bruising. Bacterial overgrowth was proven by the culture of the jejunal aspirate and the elevated ^{14}C-glycine cholate breath analysis. Coincident with the development of this malabsorption syndrome, she experienced episodes of papulovesicular skin lesions, erythema nodosum–like lesions, fever, chills, malaise, Raynaud's phenomenon, polyarthralgia, and tenosynovitis. Biopsy of a fresh skin lesion showed necrosis and vasculitis with immune deposits, although circulating immune complexes were not found by our tests. This picture was similar to that previously described in the arthri-

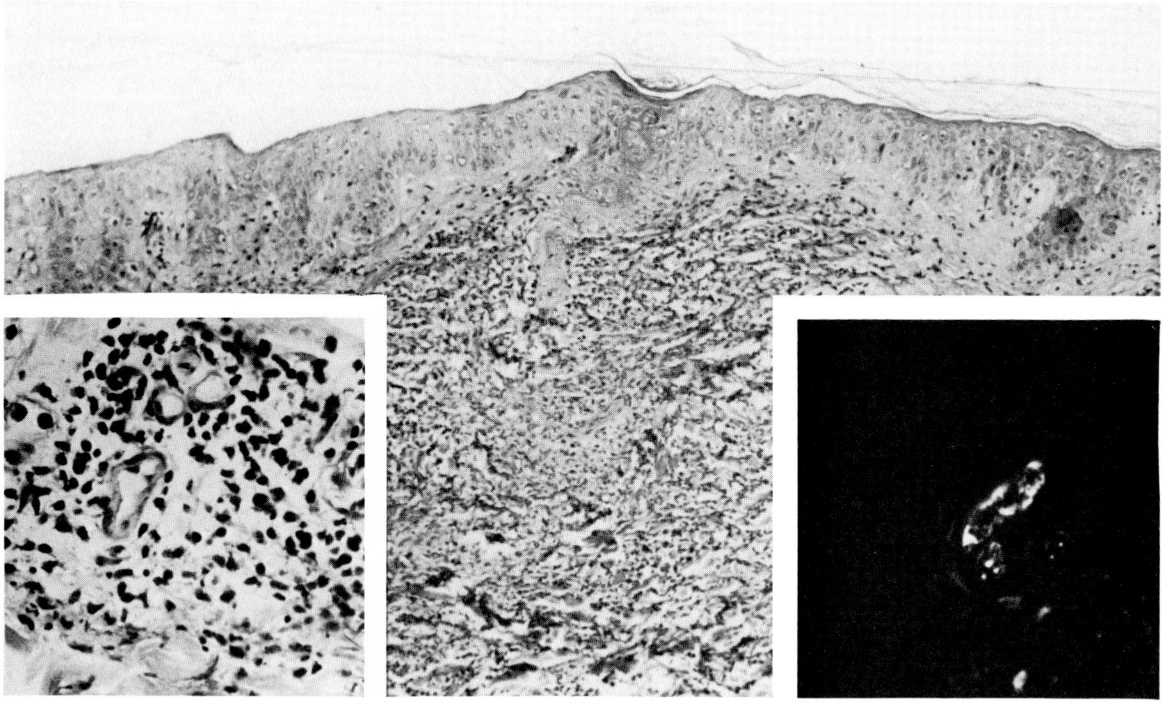

Figure 2. Skin biopsy showing necrosis of papillary and upper reticular dermis (magnification × 100). **Left insert,** Small vessels surrounded by lymphocytes, and intact and degenerating neutrophils (magnification × 400). **Right insert,** Direct immunofluorescent preparation demonstrating coarse granular deposition of IgM in dermal vessels. Vascular IgA and C3 deposition is also present.

tis–dermatitis syndrome associated with intestinal bypass surgery (1–4).

An association between the intestinal bypass procedure and arthritis was first recognized by Payne, who reported polyarthritis and tenosynovitis in 32% of jejunocolostomy patients (1). The incidence of this complication has been diminished to 6–24% by the modification of the procedure to jejunoileostomy (5–9). The syndrome consists of recurrent episodes of arthralgia, nondeforming polyarthritis, tenosynovitis, and cutaneous vasculitis. Skin lesions are typically vesiculopustular or erythema nodosum–like. Paresthesias and Raynaud's phenomenon are common. Antibiotics such as tetracycline or clindamycin can sometimes improve symptoms of the syndrome. In resistant cases, prednisone may be necessary (10). Surgical reconstitution of normal bowel anatomy is curative (11,12).

This syndrome appears to be caused by the overgrowth of bowel bacteria in the blind loop created by the intestinal bypass. Bacterial antigens may then enter the circulation, leading to the formation of antibodies and immune complexes. Such complexes, containing IgG, IgA, IgM, and complement, have been detected during episodes of arthritis (13,14). The finding of antibodies to *Escherichia coli* and *Bacterioides fragilis* in the cryoglobulins of these patients further supports the role of intestinal bacteria in this syndrome (15).

The presence of the syndrome in association with bacterial overgrowth in the bowel and its disappearance with the eradication of the bacterial overgrowth and the finding of immune deposits in skin lesions in our patient partially supports this theory. However, we did not find immune complexes, cryoglobulins, or complement abnormalities in the circulation of our patient during an active phase of the syndrome.

The intestinal bypass arthritis–dermatitis syndrome has recently been described in 4 patients who did not have bowel bypass (4). Two patients, both with previous partial gastrectomy, developed diarrhea followed by cutaneous pustules, arthritis, arthralgia, and fever. Skin biopsy specimens showed features consistent with the intestinal bypass arthritis–dermatitis syndrome, including the deposition of IgG and C3 in the upper dermis. Two other patients in the same series, 1 with Crohn's disease and the other with ulcerative colitis, had episodic fever, arthralgia, and papulovesicular skin lesions, pathologically indistinguishable from those seen complicating bypass surgery. The skin lesions and arthralgia responded to prednisone.

The finding of the arthritis–dermatitis syndrome in patients with a blind loop syndrome not caused by intestinal bypass surgery supports the notion that the bacterial overgrowth is the initiating event. Blind loop syndrome occurring after gastrectomy and with inflammatory bowel disease has now been associated with the arthritis–dermatitis syndrome. It is unclear why this syndrome has escaped notice in these patients in the past. It may be that the quantities of bacteria which inhabit the small bowel after intestinal bypass are greater than after gastrectomy, or that different organisms are involved. Furthermore, the liver disease which complicates obesity and the intestinal bypass procedure may impair the clearance of immune complexes by the reticuloendothelial system.

Acknowledgment. The authors wish to thank Ruth Minchington for typing the manuscript.

REFERENCES

1. Payne JH, DeWind LT, Commons RR: Metabolic observations in patients with jejunocolic shunts. Am J Surg 106:273–289, 1963
2. Shagrin JW, Frame B, Duncan H: Polyarthritis in obese patients with intestinal bypass. Ann Intern Med 75:377–380, 1971
3. Mir-Madjlessi SH, Mackenzie AH, Winkelman EI: Articular complications in obesity patients after jejunocolic bypass. Cleve Clin Q 41:119–125, 1974
4. Jorizzo JL, Apisarnthanarax P, Subrt P, Hebert AA, Henry JC, Raimer SS, Dinehart SM, Reinarz JA: Bowel-bypass syndrome without bowel bypass. Arch Intern Med 143:457–461, 1983
5. Buchanan RF, Willkens RF: Arthritis after jejunoileostomy. Arthritis Rheum 15:644–645, 1972
6. Fernandez-Herlihy L: Arthritis after jejunoileostomy for intractable obesity. J Rheumatol 4:135–138, 1977
7. Campbell JM, Hunt TK, Karam JH, Forsham PH: Jejunoileal bypass as a treatment for morbid obesity. Arch Intern Med 137:602–610, 1977
8. Drenick EJ, Ament ME, Finegold SM, Passaro E Jr: Bypass enteropathy: an inflammatory process in the excluded segment with systemic complications. Am J Clin Nutr 30:76–89, 1977
9. Hallberg D, Backman L, Espmark S: Surgical treatment of obesity. Prog Surg 14:46–83, 1975
10. Stein HB, Schlappner OLA, Boyko W, Gourlay RH, Reeve CE: The intestinal bypass arthritis-dermatitis syndrome. Arthritis Rheum 24:684–690, 1981
11. Drenick EJ, Ament ME, Finegold SM, Corrodi P, Passaro E: Bypass enteropathy: intestinal and systemic manifestations following small bowel by-pass. JAMA 236:269–272, 1976
12. Leff RD, Aldo-Benson MA, Madure JA: The effect of revision of the intestinal bypass on post-intestinal bypass arthritis. Arthritis Rheum 26:678–681, 1983
13. Utsinger PD, Farber N, Shapiro RF, Ely PH, McLaughlin GE, Weisner KB: Clinical and immunologic study of the post-intestinal bypass arthritis–dermatitis syndrome (abstract). Arthritis Rheum 21:599, 1978
14. Rose E, Espinoza LR, Osterland CK: Intestinal bypass arthritis: association with circulating immune complexes and HLA B27. J Rheumatol 4:129–134, 1977
15. Wands JR, LaMont JT, Mann E, Isselbacher KJ: Arthritis associated with intestinal bypass procedure for morbid obesity: complement activation and characterization of circulating cryoproteins. N Engl J Med 294:121–124, 1976

BRIEF REPORT

BONE CRISIS OF GAUCHER'S DISEASE DUE TO BONE ISCHEMIA: A CASE REPORT

ANNE DAVIDSON, VICTOR KALFF, and PETER F. J. RYAN

Adult-onset, or type 1, Gaucher's disease is an autosomal disorder, characterized by deficiency of a lysosomal enzyme, β-glucocerebrosidase. This results in the accumulation of a glycolipid, glucosylceramide, in distinctive "foam" cells which are seen in the bone marrow, reticuloendothelial tissue, and other organs (1). Infiltration of the bone marrow with resulting bone resorption and destruction has been well described previously (2,3); however, the pathogenesis of bone crisis in this disease still remains a subject of conjecture. The use of bone scanning may aid in elucidating this problem. We present a case of bone crisis in Gaucher's disease involving the pelvis, in which an extensive cold area became hot on serial bone scanning, suggesting that the lesion was due to ischemia. We also comment on the possible mechanism of this complication.

Case report. A previously well, 19-year-old white man was found to have Gaucher's disease when his bone marrow was examined in August 1981 following presentation with recurrent epistaxis and thrombocytopenia. Leukocyte β-glucocerebrosidase levels were less than 10% of normal, and screening of the family resulted in the diagnosis of Gaucher's disease in an asymptomatic brother aged 21.

Because of persistent thrombocytopenia (platelets 36×10^9/liter), splenectomy was performed in December 1981. The spleen weight was 4,700 gm and tissues from the liver, spleen, and a splenic hilar node biopsy revealed infiltration with Gaucher cells.

He remained well until April 1982 when he presented with a 3-week history of pain in the right hip, associated with fever and anorexia. On admission he looked unwell, was febrile (temperature 38.5°C), and walked with a pronounced right-sided limp.

Examination revealed right hip irritability with pain on passive movement in all directions. Laboratory investigations revealed leukocytosis of 14.4×10^9/liter, thrombocytosis of 672×10^9/liter, and an erythrocyte sedimentation rate (ESR) of 47 mm/hour (Westergren). Results of a hip radiograph were normal, and bone scan results using ^{99m}Tc phosphate were normal. Four days following admission, an arthrotomy was performed at which time a large right hip "honey-like" effusion was found. The effusion contained no inflammatory cells and no organisms were cultured. Synovial biopsy showed no inflammation and no evidence of infiltration by Gaucher cells, and synovial vessels appeared normal on light microscopy. He was started on flucloxacillin therapy, 500 mg every 6 hours, was discharged after 9 days, but was readmitted 8 days later with persistent fever. A repeat bone scan showed an area of increased uptake in the right hip, which was attributed to his recent surgery. His temperature returned to normal in 2 days with conservative measures.

He remained well until February 1983 when he was readmitted with pain in the left iliac crest and the left hip, fever, and anorexia. His temperature was 37.8°C. In addition, new findings of 2 finger-breadths of hepatomegaly and several spider nevi over the chest

From the Departments of Rheumatology and Nuclear Medicine, Alfred Hospital, Prahran, Victoria, Australia.

Anne Davidson, MBBS: Fellow in Rheumatology; Victor Kalff, MBBS, FRACP: Nuclear Medicine Department; Peter F. J. Ryan, MBBS, FRACP: Head, Rheumatology Unit.

Address reprint requests to Dr. P. F. J. Ryan, Department of Medicine, Monash Medical School, Alfred Hospital, Prahran, 3181, Victoria, Australia.

Submitted for publication March 12, 1984; accepted in revised form August 13, 1984.

were documented. Hemoglobin level was 13.3 gm/dl, white cell count 15.8 × 10^9/liter, platelet count 370 × 10^9/liter, and ESR 29 mm/hour. Results of a pelvic radiograph were again normal. A bone scan revealed multiple cold areas in the left wing of the ileum, left superior pubic ramus, and superior aspect of the left sacroiliac joint. He was treated with traction and antiinflammatory agents and his condition normalized after 5 days. A repeat bone scan 17 days later showed markedly increased uptake of tracer which corresponded to the cold areas on the previous scan (Figures 1 and 2). Three months after discharge, hemostatic and platelet function tests were performed on the patient and his affected nonsplenectomized sibling. These test results were normal except that in the splenectomized patient, circulating platelet aggregates were demonstrated to be present by comparing the platelet counts of platelet-rich plasma of blood collected simultaneously in buffered EDTA and buffered EDTA formalin (circulating platelet aggregate ratio = 0.40; normal range 0.8–1.1).

Discussion. The main clinical manifestations of type 1 Gaucher's disease are related to infiltration of the liver, spleen, and bone marrow by lipid-laden cells. Hypersplenism and thrombocytopenia are common, and mild anemia and leukopenia may occur (1). Bone marrow infiltration may lead to vertebral compression fractures, pathologic fracture of long bones, or aseptic necrosis, particularly of the femoral heads (2,3).

The sites involved have invariably been at the metaphyseal plate of long bones of children or growing adolescents and reports have noted involvement of femur, tibia, ribs, and clavicle (2–4). The metaphyseal plate in children and adolescents, which is also characteristically the site of acute hematogenous osteomyelitis (5), has a unique blood supply consisting of non-

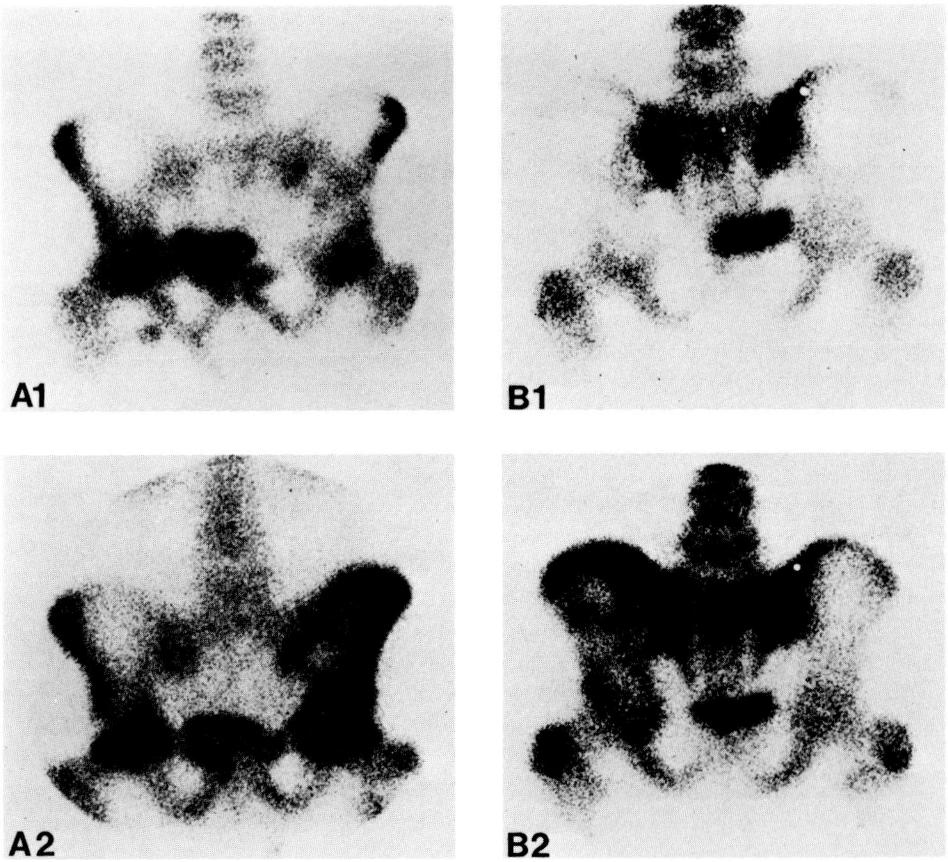

Figure 1. ^{99m}Tc diphosphonate scans showing views of pelvis. On presentation, the bone scans of the pelvis shown in the anterior (**A1**) and posterior (**B1**) projections demonstrate multiple subtle, but definite, areas of decreased uptake over the sacroiliac crest, acetabulum, and superior pubic ramus of the left hemi-pelvis. Corresponding views taken 17 days later (**A2**, **B2**) demonstrate that these abnormal regions now show markedly increased uptake.

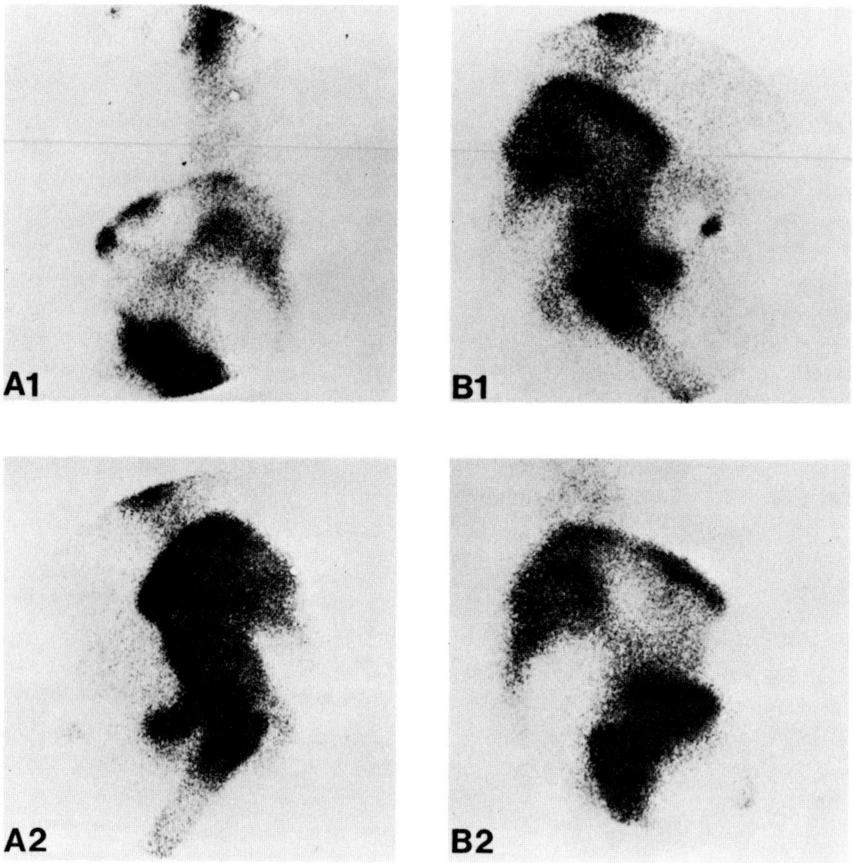

Figure 2. The bone scans of the left and right lateral projections at presentation (**A1, B1**) and 17 days later (**A2, B2**).

anastomosing arteriolar loops enclosed by rigid bony walls, which drain into a pool of venous sinusoids with a sluggish blood flow. The epiphyseal bone is also supplied by vascular loops but in contradistinction to the metaphyseal vessels, these anastamose freely with each other. In growing bone, there is no communication between the epiphyseal and metaphyseal blood supply (6). Thus, the metaphyseal bone is particularly prone to infarction if the nonanastomosing arcades of vessels are compromised by increased intraosseous tension resulting from infiltrating Gaucher cells, local edema, or subperiosteal hemorrhage. Although bone crisis involving the pelvis has not previously been reported, flat and irregular bones such as the pelvis also have metaphyseal equivalent locations with comparable vascular arcades bordering epiphyseal growth plates or articular cartilage (6,7) (Figure 3).

Clinically, bone crisis of Gaucher's disease resembles that of sickle cell disease, which is thought to be related to focal areas of bone ischemia or infarction secondary to thrombosis of small vessels by

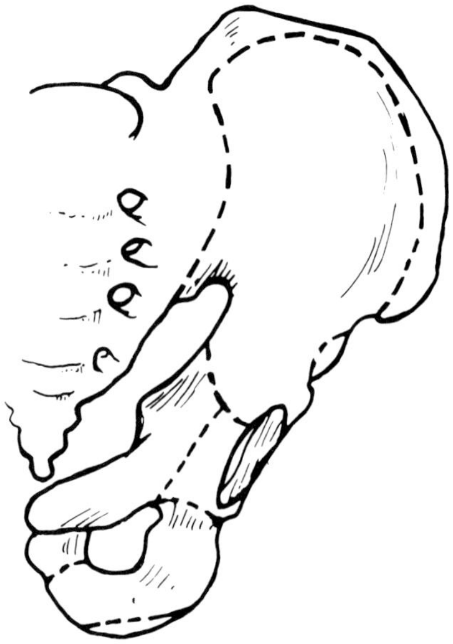

Figure 3. Left hemi-pelvis. The metaphyseal-equivalent sites are indicated by broken lines (adapted from Nixon, ref. 7 and descriptions by Brookes, ref. 6). Note the excellent correspondence between these sites and the observed scan abnormalities.

sickled cells (8). However, unlike sickle cell disease, bone marrow scintigraphy, using ^{99m}Tc-labeled sulfur colloid, appears to have little utility in Gaucher's disease. In sickle cell disease, there is active bone marrow expansion, and thus, increased uptake of the radiopharmaceutical. Bone marrow infarction can therefore be readily diagnosed by the appearance of areas of diminished uptake in the regions of expanded bone marrow. However, in Gaucher's disease, there is marrow replacement with characteristic cells which do not take up sulfur colloid and, therefore, there is little or no uptake of the radiopharmaceutical (9). This would therefore make bone marrow infarction difficult or impossible to discern using this method.

The use of bone scanning in bone crisis of Gaucher's disease has only been reported on 2 previous occasions. In 1 patient, an area of decreased uptake corresponded to the site of bone pain but no followup scans were performed (9). In the second patient, scans revealed a persistent cold area in the tibial plateau corresponding to the site of symptoms. This patient also had a hemorrhagic bursitis of the knee, suggestive of subperiosteal hemorrhage. There was no change in the cold area over a period of 16 months (9). In our patient, serial bone scanning suggested local ischemia involving pelvic metaphyseal equivalent sites followed by reactive bone formation 17 days later.

The first episode of bone crisis described in our patient occurred 4 months following splenectomy. The effect of splenectomy on the onset or progression of bone lesions in Gaucher's disease has been a subject of considerable discussion in the literature, with some authors suggesting an increased incidence of bone lesions in splenectomized patients (2,3,4,10). Silverstein and Kelly (3) postulate that removal of the spleen could divert large numbers of Gaucher cells to the bone marrow and other reticuloendothelial tissue. In this context, rapidly advancing hepatomegaly has been reported following splenectomy (11), a finding also noted in our patient. The effect of postsplenectomy thrombocytosis and the presence of increased numbers of platelet aggregates, as seen in our patient, has not been investigated.

We have reported a case of bone crisis in Gaucher's disease that involved metaphyseal-equivalent sites of the pelvis in which bone scanning was suggestive of an ischemic lesion. We postulated that the unique blood supply of the growing metaphysis made this area susceptible to ischemic insult and accounted for the age distribution of this complication. Differentiation of bone crisis from osteomyelitis, which also occurs in these patients, is difficult but may be aided by the use of serial bone marrow scanning as in sickle cell disease. Whether bone involvement is accelerated by splenectomy is still a subject of conjecture, but it may be possible to delay bony complications in Gaucher's disease with the use of anti-platelet agents. Further investigation of this area is warranted.

REFERENCES

1. Brady RO, Barranger JA: Glucosyl ceramide lipidosis, Gaucher's Disease, The Metabolic Basis of Inherited Disease. Fifth edition. Edited by JB Stanbury, JB Wyngaarden, DS Fredrickson. New York, McGraw-Hill, 1983, pp 842–856
2. Amstutz HC, Carey EJ: Skeletal manifestations and treatment of Gaucher's disease: review of twenty cases. J Bone Joint Surg 48A:670–701, 1966
3. Silverstein MN, Kelly PJ: Osteoarticular manifestations of Gaucher's disease. Am J Med Sci 253:569–576, 1967
4. Yossipovitch ZH, Herman G, Makin M: Aseptic osteomyelitis in Gaucher's disease. Isr J Med Sci 1:531–536, 1965
5. Welt S, Rosenthal N, Oppenheimer BS: Gaucher's splenomegaly with reference to skeletal changes. JAMA 92:637–649, 1929
6. Brookes M: Blood Vessels in Bone Marrow, Vascular Patterns: The Blood Supply of Bone, An Approach to Bone Biology. London, Butterworths, 1971, pp 74–81
7. Nixon GW: Hematogenous osteomyelitis of metaphyseal-equivalent locations. AJR 130:123–129, 1978
8. Espinosa LR, Spilberg I, Osterland CK: Joint manifestations of sickle cell disease. Medicine (Baltimore) 53:295–305, 1974
9. Cheng TH, Holman BL: Radionuclide assessment of Gaucher's disease. J Nucl Med 19:1333–1336, 1978
10. Gelford G, Bienenstock H: Hemorrhagic bursitis and bone crises in chronic adult Gaucher's disease. Arthritis Rheum 25:1369–1373, 1982
11. Matoth Y, Fried K: Chronic Gaucher's disease: clinical observations on 34 patients. Isr J Med Sci 1:521–530, 1965

BRIEF REPORT

ABILITY TO ACTIVATE COMPLEMENT IS NOT REQUIRED FOR THE DETECTION OF IMMUNE COMPLEXES BY THE FLUID-PHASE C1q BINDING ASSAY

GUY P. FIOCCO, JOHN S. DAVIS, IV, and JOSEPH J. BURGE

Complement (C) activation by immune complexes (IC) is known to have an important role in the pathogenesis of tissue inflammation. Therefore, among the assays that detect circulating IC, those which distinguish C-activating complexes are accorded greater clinical significance. The modified fluid-phase ^{125}I-C1q binding assay (C1q-BA) (1) is one such assay that has come into general use. Since its introduction, however, questions have arisen as to why endogenous C1q does not block detection of putative C1q-binding IC, and why the C1q-BA does not always correlate with other serologic markers of C activation. We present direct evidence that IC need not be capable of binding to C1q or of activating the C system under physiologic conditions in order to be detected in the C1q-BA. Furthermore, we show that it is the presence of polyethylene glycol (PEG) that induces the binding of ^{125}I-C1q (in the C1q-BA) to these otherwise non–C-activating IC.

PATIENTS AND METHODS

Patients. The patients were diagnosed as having systemic lupus erythematosus according to the 1982 American Rheumatism Association revised criteria (2). Patients were selected randomly from those known to have a positive result on the C1q-BA. Normal human serum was obtained from volunteer donors. All sera were stored at $-70°C$ and were thawed only once.

Reagents and the C1q-BA. The fluid-phase C1q binding assay was performed as described by Zubler et al (1). Aliquots of ^{125}I-C1q, which had been stored at $-70°C$, were freshly thawed and dialyzed against veronal buffered saline (5 m*M* barbital, pH 7.5, containing 0.15*M* NaCl) immediately before use. Aggregated human IgG (AHG) was prepared from Cohn fraction II by heating at a concentration of 10 mg/ml in phosphate buffered saline, pH 7.4, for 20 minutes at 63°C. This material was then centrifuged at 500*g* for 30 minutes. The upper three-fourths of the supernatant was used. Reduction and alkylation of AHG was accomplished by incubation with 0.1*M* dithiothreitol for 60 minutes and then with 0.033*M* N-ethylmaleamide for 10 minutes at room temperature. The material was then dialyzed against phosphate buffered saline.

In the following experiments, we used the conventional method of expressing input of AHG or reduced and alkylated AHG as the pre–heat aggregation quantity of IgG, even though only a small proportion of the total IgG is actually in aggregated form. Our method of heat aggregation routinely results in $<15\%$ aggregation (data not shown) and, furthermore, involves the subsequent isolation of only the *soluble* (at 500*g*) fraction of the aggregates. Thus, our reported input levels of aggregates may differ from those reported by other researchers.

Complement fixation assay. The ability of AHG or reduced and alkylated AHG (R & A–AHG) to consume complement was tested by first establishing

From the University of Virginia Medical Center, Department of Medicine, Division of Rheumatology, Charlottesville, Virginia.

Supported by grants AM31311 and AM11766 from the National Institutes of Health.

Guy P. Fiocco, MD: Rheumatology Fellow; John S. Davis, IV, MD: Professor; Joseph J. Burge, MD: Assistant Professor.

Address reprint requests to Joseph J. Burge, MD, University of Virginia Medical Center, Box 412, Charlottesville, VA 22908.

Submitted for publication April 23, 1984; accepted in revised form July 17, 1984.

the dilution of normal serum that resulted in 50% lysis of sheep red blood cells in a CH50 assay. The CH50 assay was performed according to the method of Kabat and Mayer (3), but was modified into a microassay, using 100 μl of diluted serum and 100 μl of sensitized sheep red blood cells (1×10^8 cells/ml). Fifty microliters of this dilution of normal serum was incubated with serial dilutions of AHG or R & A–AHG for 15 minutes at 37°C. The mixture was then incubated with the sheep red blood cells for 45 minutes at 37°C, and the resultant hemolytic activity was determined by spectrophotometric measurement of hemoglobin release. No loss of hemolytic activity was detected, using up to 2,500 μg/ml of R & A–AHG. Complete depletion of hemolytic activity was observed using as little as 20 μg/ml of AHG.

Sucrose density gradients. Linear isokinetic gradients were prepared from 60/10% (weight/volume) sucrose in borate buffer, pH 8.2. When PEG was used, it was added to the borate buffer, to a final concentration of 2.5%, prior to the addition of the sucrose. ^{125}I-C1q (100 μl) was preincubated with either AHG (100 μl of 10 mg/ml), R & A–AHG, normal human serum, or patient serum, and 0.2*M* EDTA (200 μl) for 30 minutes at 4°C prior to layering it on top of the gradient. Ultracentrifugation was performed with an SW-50 rotor and a Sorval ultracentrifuge at 100,000*g* for 18 hours. Fractions (0.5 ml) were collected and counted in a Beckman gamma counter.

RESULTS

Detection of AHG versus R & A–AHG in the C1q-BA. To test our hypothesis that C activation is not necessary for IC detection in the C1q-BA, we used AHG and R & A–AHG in the standard fluid-phase C1q-BA. We first established that reduction and alkylation of the AHG completely destroyed the ability of these model IC to consume complement (see C fixation assay above). Moreover, although the R & A–AHG were totally incapable of activating C, they were easily detected in the C1q-BA (Figure 1). Compared with the unreduced AHG, the R & A–AHG showed only a 30% reduction in detection in the assay.

C1q binding detected by sucrose gradient ultracentrifugation. Figure 2 shows the binding of AHG or R & A–AHG to ^{125}I-C1q as detected by sucrose density ultracentrifugation in the absence or presence of PEG. One thousand micrograms of AHG or R & A–AHG was added to ^{125}I-C1q, layered on top of the sucrose density gradient, and centrifuged (100,000*g*) at 4°C. Fractions (0.5 ml) of the gradient were collected and counted for ^{125}I radioactivity. A shift in the position of the ^{125}I-C1q (compared with its position in a control gradient run separately) toward the bottom (denser) area of the gradient was interpreted as having been due to binding. Note that in the presence of PEG, sedimentation of the ^{125}I-C1q control changed.

Figure 2A shows that in the absence of PEG, AHG causes a shift in position of the ^{125}I-C1q, whereas the R & A–AHG shows little direct binding of C1q. However, Figure 2B shows that the inclusion of PEG in the gradient induces binding of C1q to the R & A–AHG and a shift in position of the ^{125}I curve, as indicated by the cross-hatched area. The AHG bound C1q as before. These results are representative of 3 identical experiments that were performed on separate occasions.

We next chose sera from 6 lupus patients known to have a positive result on the C1q binding assay and used these sera in the ultracentrifuge binding experiments as above. Figure 3 shows the results of these experiments, using 2 representative sera. When ^{125}I-C1q was added to these sera and subjected to ultracentrifugation, there was no increased binding of C1q in the patients' sera compared with that of normal serum in the absence of PEG (Figure 3A). In the presence of PEG (Figure 3B), the reference position of sedimentation of the ^{125}I-C1q in the normal serum control changed, as expected, because of the added PEG density. The important point, however, is

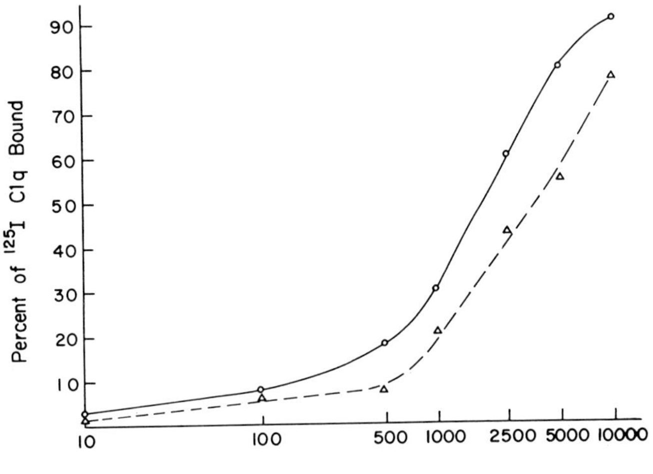

Figure 1. Binding of ^{125}I-C1q to aggregated human IgG (AHG) (○——○) or reduced and alkylated AHG (R + A AHG) (△----△) in the standard C1q binding assay.

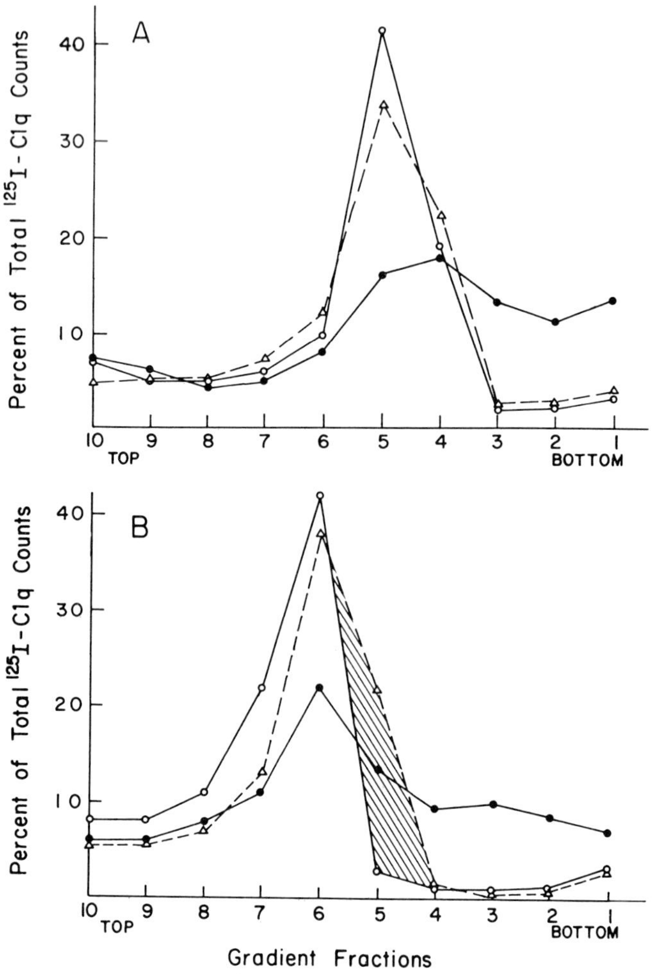

Figure 2. Binding of aggregated human IgG (AHG) (●——●) or reduced and alkylated AHG (△----△) to ^{125}I-C1q in sucrose density gradients in the absence (**A**) and presence (**B**) of polyethylene glycol. The sedimentation of ^{125}I-C1q alone (○——○) is shown for comparison.

that for both patients' sera, a shift to higher densities in the ^{125}I-C1q curve occurred relative to the normal serum control curve, indicating C1q binding. The fact that PEG induced a bipartate curve in the case of patient 1 and a homogenous shift in position of the curve in the case of patient 2 may relate to differences in the immune complex–like material present in each serum, since 4 other patients' sera that were tested also exhibited such variation (data not shown). Thus, while these patients had high levels of apparent IC material detected by the fluid-phase C1q-BA, there was no evidence of direct binding of ^{125}I-C1q, using the sucrose density gradient measurement, unless PEG was introduced.

Preincubation with unlabeled C1q of AHG versus R & A–AHG. We next tested the effects of preincubation with unlabeled C1q on the subsequent detection of AHG and of R & A–AHG in the C1q-BA. One would predict that if an IC could bind C1q under physiologic conditions, then this C1q would block subsequent detection of the IC in the C1q-BA. Indeed, we observed that the incubation of AHG (500 μg/ml) with equimolar amounts of unlabeled C1q decreased

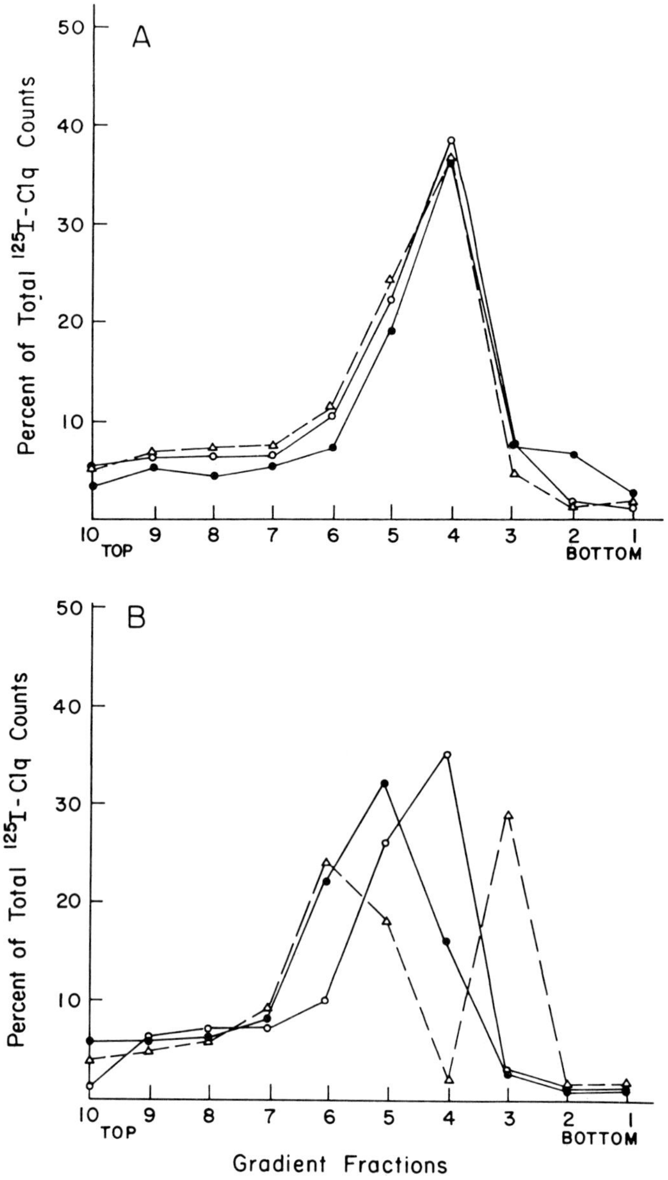

Figure 3. Binding of endogenous serum immune complexes to ^{125}I-C1q in sucrose density gradients in the absence (**A**) and presence (**B**) of polyethylene glycol. The change in sedimentation of ^{125}I-C1q from the position of the normal human serum control (●——●) is shown for patient 1 (△----△) and patient 2 (○——○).

its detection in the C1q-BA by 60% compared with preincubation with buffer alone. However, identical preincubation of R & A–AHG with the C1q did not affect its detection in the assay.

DISCUSSION

Several observations by other researchers suggest that the fluid-phase C1q-BA may not be specific for those IC which activate C, i.e., (a) PEG enchances the binding of ^{125}I-C1q as well as endogenous serum C1q to AHG-coated tubes (4); (b) the fluid-phase C1q-BA does not correlate with the solid-phase C1q-BA (5); (c) addition of PEG into the solid-phase C1q-BA increases the number of positive results (4); (d) PEG is known to artificially induce protein–protein association and, hence, might induce C1q to bind artifactually to certain materials (6); and (e) C1q-BA results do not always correlate with serologic markers of in vivo C activation (7).

However, this evidence is indirect, and these observations might be explained by the following: (a) PEG may not induce all proteins to associate, but rather may enhance molecular interactions with low affinity constants; (b) the interactions between ICs and the C system in vivo are quite complex and may not be fully reflected by serologic testing; (c) not all positive C1q-BA results represent the presence of circulating IC, i.e., many non-IC materials are known to cause false-positive test results. For example, Hack et al (7) recently reported that, although the majority of their rheumatoid arthritis patients had positive fluid-phase C1q-BA results, only a small number showed evidence of C1 activation products generated in vivo or in vitro. They concluded that "measurement of CIC [circulating immune complexes] by means of C1q [solid- or fluid-phase C1q-BA] does not mean that these CIC activate C1" (7). However, only their rheumatoid factor–positive patients had significantly elevated C1q-BA results or C activation. Rheumatoid factor is known to induce an in vitro false-positive result in the C1q-BA (7,8). Thus, their observations were, in all likelihood, based on false-positive C1q-BA results, which would not be expected to relate directly to in vivo events.

In this study, we used 3 different approaches to demonstrate *directly* that C fixation is not required for IC detection by the fluid-phase C1q-BA. First, we showed that R & A–AHG (model immune complexes) which were incapable of activating C in a CH50 assay were nonetheless easily detectable in the C1q-BA. Second, using a direct method of identifying C1q binding that is independent of the C1q-BA, i.e., sucrose density ultracentrifugation, we have demonstrated that neither R & A–AHG nor patient serum known to give positive results in the C1q-BA was capable of directly binding ^{125}I-C1q unless PEG was added. Third, the addition of unlabeled C1q to C-fixing AHG inhibited the subsequent detection of AHG in the C1q-BA; however, similar preincubation of R & A–AHG had no such effect. Thus, the C1q-BA does not distinguish the complexes that activate complement from those that do not.

REFERENCES

1. Zubler RH, Lange G, Lambert PH, Miescher PA: Detection of immune complexes in unheated sera by a modified ^{125}I-C1q binding test: effect of heating on the binding of C1q to immune complexes and application of the test to systemic lupus erythematosus. J Immunol 116:232–235, 1976
2. Tan EM, Cohen AS, Fries JF, Masi AT, McShane DJ, Rothfield NF, Schaller JG, Talal N, Winchester RJ: The 1982 revised criteria for the classification of systemic lupus erythematosus. Arthritis Rheum 25:1271–1277, 1982
3. Kabat EA, Mayer MM: Experimental Immunochemistry. Second edition. Springfield, Illinois, Charles C. Thomas, 1961, pp 135–139
4. Hack CE, Eerenberg-Belmer AJM, Hannema AJ, Out TA, Aalberse RC: Polyethylene glycol enhances the binding of C1q to circulating immune complexes. J Immunol Methods 44:211–221, 1981
5. Abrass CK, Nies KM, Louie JS, Border WA, Glassock RJ: Correlation and predictive accuracy of circulating immune complexes with disease activity in patients with systemic lupus erythematosus. Arthritis Rheum 23:273–282, 1980
6. Creighton DW, Lambert PH, Miescher PA: Detection of antibodies and soluble antigen-antibody complexes by precipitation with polyethylene glycol. J Immunol 111:1219–1227, 1973
7. Hack CE, Eerenberg-Belmer AJM, Lim UG, Haverman J, Aalberse RC: Lack of activation of C1, despite circulating immune complexes detected by two C1q methods, in patients with rheumatoid arthritis. Arthritis Rheum 27:40–48, 1984
8. Zilberfarb JL, Davis JS IV, Andrews BA: Enhancement of C1q binding by IgM rheumatoid factor (abstract). Arthritis Rheum (suppl) 25:S73, 1982

BRIEF REPORT

NUCLEOLAR LOCALIZATION OF THE PM–Scl ANTIGEN

IRA N. TARGOFF and MORRIS REICHLIN

Precipitating antibodies to antigens in calf thymus extract (CTE) can be detected by immunodiffusion in the sera of 60% of patients with polymyositis (PM) and dermatomyositis (DM) (1). The specificity of these antibodies can be determined by identity reactions in Ouchterlony experiments with reference sera, and such analysis indicates that they are directed at a heterogeneous group of antigens (2). The frequency with which these different antigenic specificities were seen was recently determined in a large group of patients who satisfied the criteria for PM and DM (including overlap patients) (1). The 3 most common specificities encountered were Jo-1 (seen in 18%, predominantly in patients with PM) (2), nuclear RNP (nRNP; 12%, predominantly in overlap syndrome), and PM–Scl (formerly PM-1, seen in 8%) (3).

Anti-PM–Scl has been reported to occur in patients with PM, DM, and polymyositis– or dermatomyositis–scleroderma overlap (PM/S), and a higher frequency of PM/S is seen in patients who have PM–Scl antibody than in the PM population as a whole. Antibody to Ku is also associated with PM/S (4), but Ku is antigenically independent from PM–Scl by immunodiffusion (1). Anti-PM–Scl is occasionally found in patients who have scleroderma without apparent myositis (5), but has not been reported in other connective tissue diseases. The antigen is trypsin-sensitive and RNase- and DNase-resistant (3), but has not yet been completely purified or characterized. Although it can be demonstrated in nuclear extracts (3), its subcellular localization has not been reported. The sera of all our patients with this precipitin produced nucleolar staining by indirect immunofluorescence (IIF) on HEp-2 cells (1). We now report evidence supporting a nucleolar localization of the PM–Scl antigen, using IIF with specifically purified antibody and extraction from isolated nucleoli.

MATERIALS AND METHODS

Serum Lx, from a patient with PM/S, is the prototype reference serum used in our laboratory for identifying the PM–Scl specificity. Two lines are formed on immunodiffusion of this serum with CTE (whole CTE prepared as described in reference 2), the minor second line found, thus far, only in sera with anti-PM–Scl. The major line showed immunologic identity with PM–Scl reference sera used in other laboratories (1).

Preparation of specific antibody. A 3:1 saline extract of calf thymus (approximately 10 mg/ml protein) was fractionated by ammonium sulfate between 30 and 50% saturation, and then dialyzed against $0.01M$ $NaPO_4$, pH 7.0. This was applied to a similarly equilibrated diethylaminoethyl ion exchange column,

From the Department of Medicine, University of Oklahoma Health Sciences Center, Oklahoma City, Oklahoma.

Supported by National Institutes of Health grant AM 32214.

Ira N. Targoff, MD: Associate Investigator, Veterans Administration Medical Center, and Assistant Professor of Research, Department of Medicine, University of Oklahoma Health Sciences Center, Oklahoma Medical Research Foundation, Oklahoma City, Oklahoma; Morris Reichlin, MD: Professor of Medicine, Chief, Combined Immunology Section, Department of Medicine, University of Oklahoma Health Sciences Center, and Head, Arthritis and Immunology Program, Oklahoma Medical Research Foundation, Oklahoma City, Oklahoma.

Address reprint requests to Ira N. Targoff, MD, Arthritis and Immunology Program, Oklahoma Medical Research Foundation, 825 NE 13th Street, Oklahoma City, OK 73104.

Submitted for publication January 3, 1984; accepted in revised form July 9, 1984.

and PM–Scl activity (as detected by counterimmunoelectrophoresis) was eluted with an NaCl gradient between 0.05*M* and 0.2*M* ionic strength. Concentrated pooled active fractions (at approximately 50 mg/ml protein) and whole Lx serum were clarified by centrifugation and mixed 1:1 and 2:1 by volume, and sodium azide was added. These mixtures were incubated at 37°C for 1 hour, and then at 4°C for 96 hours. Precipitates formed and were separated by centrifugation (3,000 revolutions per minute in an IEC PR-J centrifuge) and washed 3 times in phosphate buffered saline (PBS), the final wash having an optical density at 280 nm of <0.015. The washed precipitates were resuspended in 1 ml of 1*M* acetic acid and kept at 4°C overnight. Undissolved material was removed by centrifugation (3,000 rpm), and the supernatant was dialyzed against PBS. The sediment was resuspended in 4*M* guanidine and kept at 4°C overnight. After centrifugation, this supernatant was also dialyzed against PBS.

Preparation of nucleolar extract. Rat liver nuclei were prepared by a procedure similar to that used by Widnell and Tata (6). Perfused liver was homogenized in 0.32*M* sucrose, 3 m*M* $MgCl_2$; nuclei were sedimented at 700*g* for 10 minutes, resuspended in 2.4*M* sucrose, 1 m*M* $MgCl_2$, and ultracentrifuged at 50,000*g* for 1 hour. Nucleoli were isolated from these nuclei by the procedure of Busch and Daskal (7), by resuspending the nuclei in 0.34*M* sucrose, 0.05 m*M* $MgCl_2$ for sonication (Branson Sonifier), which was continued until most nuclei were lysed (usually about 45 seconds) with the sample in ice water. The sonicate was underlayered with 0.88*M* sucrose, 0.05 m*M* $MgCl_2$ and centrifuged for 20 minutes at 2,000*g*. The pellet was resuspended in PBS overnight. The supernatant was nucleoli-poor nuclear extract. Microscopic examination with methylene blue stain revealed almost all nucleoli, with rare intact nuclei. This procedure was also applied to calf liver nuclei isolated by repeated low-speed centrifugations, including washes with 0.5% Triton X-100.

Other procedures. Indirect immunofluorescence was performed using mouse cryostat sections and prefixed slides of HEp-2 tissue culture cells (Anti-

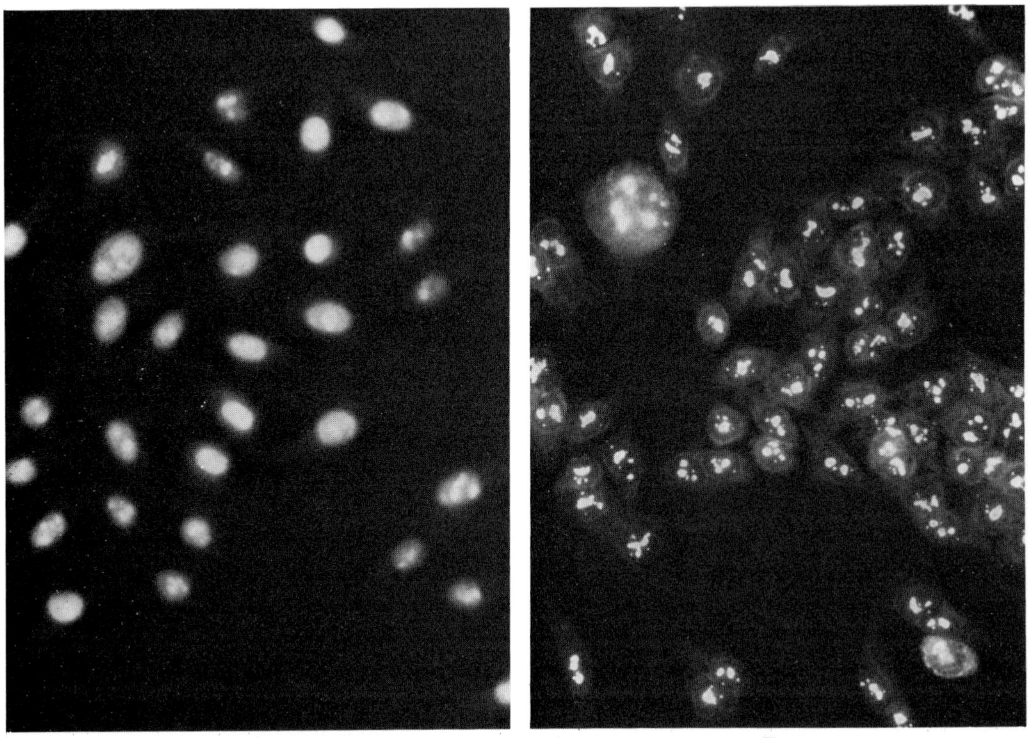

A B

Figure 1. Indirect immunofluorescence of whole Lx serum (**A**) versus purified antibody (**B**), showing that the nucleolar staining seen with whole serum is the result of precipitating antibody, which is identified by immunodiffusion as anti-PM–Scl. The nuclear staining is due to a different antibody, either a nonprecipitating or insoluble system.

bodies, Inc., Davis, CA) as substrates. Lx serum, normal serum, positive controls (another serum without anti-PM–Scl, known to give a nucleolar pattern, and a serum with anti-nRNP, known to give a nuclear pattern), and the acid and guanidine redissolved precipitates (specific antibody I [SAI] and specific antibody II [SAII]) were tested on both substrates.

Ouchterlony immunodiffusion was performed in 0.6% agarose gel in PBS with sodium azide, and 1.6% polyethelene glycol 6,000 (8).

RESULTS

Both SAI and SAII had precipitating anti-PM–Scl activity on immunodiffusion, showing the major precipitin line in a reaction of identity with whole serum (although the second line could not be seen at the concentration tested). SAI had 0.3 mg/ml as immunoglobulin, and SAII had 0.45 mg/ml by using the optical density of the whole preparation.

IIF with normal human serum (1:20) and human Cohn fraction II (1 mg/ml) was negative on both mouse liver and HEp-2 cell substrates, while strongly positive reactions were obtained with the positive controls. On mouse liver substrate, Lx serum showed a 2+ nucleolar pattern of IIF at 1:20 dilution, the SAI gave a weak nucleolar pattern, and the undiluted SAII gave a strongly positive nucleolar pattern. On HEp-2 cells, Lx serum gave a bright, 4+ nucleolar pattern at 1:20 dilution which disappeared at 1:100 dilution (Figure 1). A background speckled nuclear fluorescence, which persisted weakly at 1:100 dilution, was also present. SAI showed bright nucleolar fluorescence on HEp-2 cells, both undiluted and diluted 1:5 (0.06 mg/ml), and there was no background nuclear fluorescence. SAII gave a similar pattern that still had a trace of activity at 1:25 dilution. There was 12.5 mg/ml immunoglobulin G in Lx serum, and thus the 1:20 dilution had 0.62 mg/ml. At least tenfold more activity per mg of protein is present in the redissolved precipitates.

The rat liver nucleolar extract had to be concentrated in different runs, from 1.5 to 8 mg/ml protein,

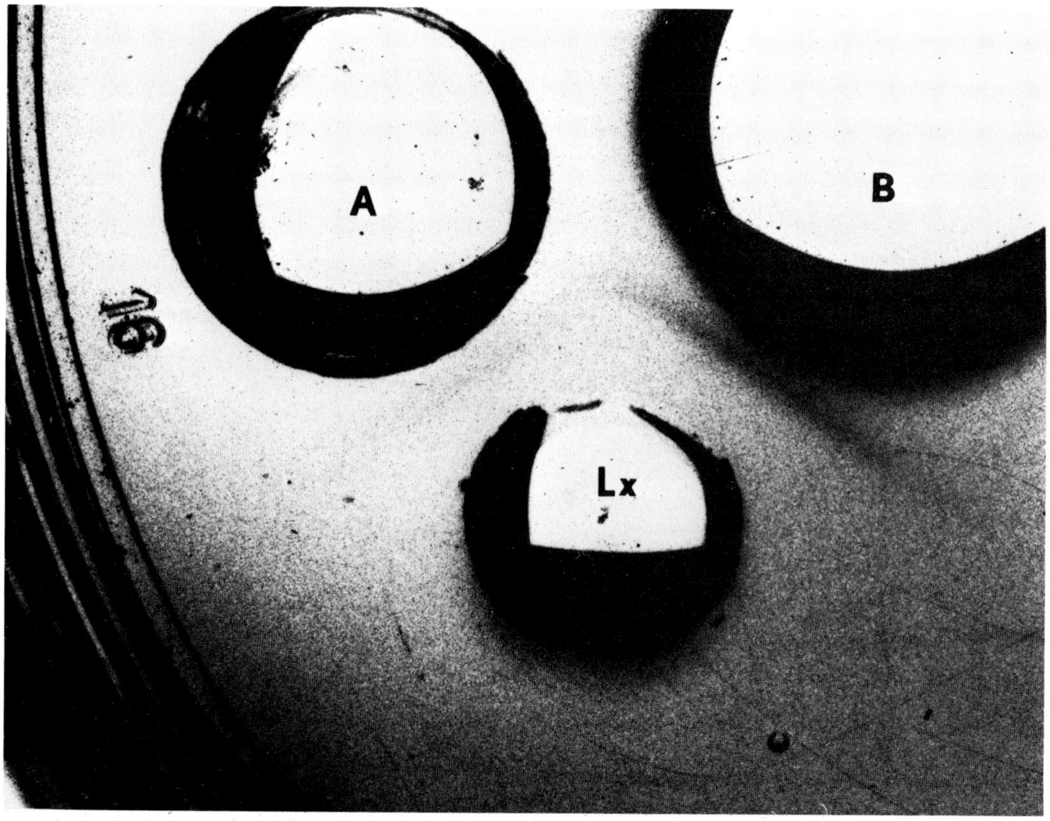

Figure 2. Anti-PM-Scl containing serum (well Lx) forms a precipitin line with the calf liver nucleolar extract (well B), which fuses with the line formed with whole calf thymus extract (well A). Under these conditions, only 1 line was seen with both extracts.

before it reacted with Lx serum on immunodiffusion. A single line was seen; it was antigenically identical to the major precipitin line with CTE, and similar in appearance (Figure 2). Rat liver and nucleoli–poor nuclear extract could not be demonstrated to have PM–Scl antigen by immunodiffusion, at comparable concentrations. The nucleolar extract was 10–50-fold enriched for the PM–Scl antigen over whole extract, which required 80 mg/ml protein to react with Lx serum. Similar results were obtained with calf liver nucleoli, which were at least tenfold enriched over whole cell extract and twofold enriched over nuclei. While the nucleoli preparation contained nRNP and a trace of Jo antigens, these were not at all enriched over nuclei.

DISCUSSION

The evidence presented here shows that specific antibody from washed immune precipitate is enriched in nucleolar reactivity, and supports a nucleolar localization for the PM–Scl antigen. In addition, the recovery of the precipitating antigen from isolated nucleoli, with much more activity per milligram protein than whole extract, confirms this. These findings do not rule out the possibility that the molecule is also present in other parts of the cell. The ribosomal RNP antigen, for example, was found to be present in both the nucleolus and the cytoplasmic ribosomes (9,10). However, specific antibody to PM–Scl stained only the nucleolus on IIF, with both substrates used. Even the nuclear staining seen with whole serum had disappeared, and neither whole serum nor specific antibody had ever stained cytoplasm. Lx serum did not react in immunodiffusion with a preparation of cytoplasmic ribosomes (unpublished observation).

After dialysis of CTE to 1*M* acetic acid or 4*M* guanidine, the PM–Scl antigenic activity of the CTE was decreased or destroyed. Thus, these solutions would be expected to release specific antibody from the immune precipitate. Specific antibody was studied on HEp-2 cells in addition to conventional substrates such as mouse liver, because antibodies to nucleoli can be more sensitively detected by HEp-2 cells that have larger nucleoli (11).

The nucleolar pattern of immunofluorescence has been reported in a number of autoimmune diseases, including systemic lupus erythematosus, DM and PM, and Sjögren's syndrome. However, it is most frequently found in progressive systemic sclerosis (PSS), where an incidence of 43% of 76 patients was recently reported (5). There is some heterogeneity among the antinucleolar antibodies in myositis, since some of our myositis patients have a high titer of antinucleolar antibody by IIF, but do not have precipitating PM–Scl. There appears to be some heterogeneity among the antinucleolar antibodies found in PSS as well, since 3 distinct patterns of nucleolar IIF staining on HEp-2 cells have recently been described (5).

The nature of the nucleolar antigens in PSS has been studied. Pinnas et al (12) reported a trypsin-resistant antigen extracted from calf thymus nucleoli that contained a 4–6S RNA. This antigen formed a precipitate on immunodiffusion, in 18 of 26 patients who had antinucleolar antibodies by IIF. Sixteen of those 18 patients had scleroderma, CREST syndrome (calcinosis, Raynaud's phenomenon, esophageal dysmotility, sclerodactyly, and telangiectasias), or Raynaud's phenomenon. A similar trypsin-resistant, phenol-resistant 4–7S RNA antigen that reacted on immunodiffusion with 16 of 16 patients with antinucleolar antibodies was described by Miyawaki and Ritchie (13). Recently, Reddy et al (14) studied the antinucleolar antibodies of 24 patients with PSS, by Pansorbin immunoprecipitation of extracts of ^{32}P-labeled cells, as originally described by Lerner and Steitz (15). None of these sera precipitated phenol-extracted or proteinase K–treated RNAs, and none contained antibodies reacting directly with U3RNP, the small ribonucleoprotein particle characteristic of nucleoli. However, 8 of the 24 sera reacted with large particles, presumed to be preribosomal particles, that contained U3RNP. In addition, 1 of the 24 sera ("To") reacted with a nucleolar 7–2 ribonucleoprotein and a cytoplasmic 8–2 ribonucleoprotein. Another such serum, Th, from a patient with systemic lupus erythematosus, has also been described (16). In a study by Matter et al (17), no nucleolar RNAs were precipitated by 19 sera with a nucleolar pattern of IIF, using a similar immunoprecipitation technique (although one, which also had nuclear IIF, precipitated Sm RNAs).

Thus, the spectrum of nucleolar antigens that have been previously described includes: 1) the ribosomal RNP antigens; 2) the small RNA antigen that does not require protein (not detected by Pansorbin immunoprecipitation); 3) the protein-dependent antigen on large preribosomal particles; and 4) the Th ("To") antigen. It has not been directly demonstrated that all of these are independent antigens, but PM–Scl is clearly different from all of them. It is trypsin-sensitive, does not stain cytoplasm, is non-identical with ribosomal RNP (provided by Dr. Hajime Yamagata), and in Pansorbin immunoprecipitation, performed in Dr. J. A. Steitz's laboratory (Steitz JA, Black D, Rieder R: personal communication), did not precipitate any of the recognized RNAs, including U3, 5.0S, 5.8S, 7–2, or 8–2. Although other precipitating antibodies may have been confused with PM-1 in the past (1,8), PM–Scl has now been established as a unique precipitating system, distinct from other recognized precipitating specificities including Sm, nRNP, SS-A (Ro), SS-B (La), Mi, Ku, and Jo-1 (1). Therefore, PM–Scl may be added to the list of nucleolar antigens as a clearly defined independent specificity.

The purification of PM–Scl has thus far proved difficult, but it will be necessary in order to develop more sensitive tests for the detection of anti-PM–Scl antibody and to further explore its etiologic, pathogenic, and clinical significance. It was possible in this study to achieve a substantial purification by extracting isolated nucleoli, rather than whole tissue or nuclei, and this may make subsequent physicochemical separation procedures more successful.

REFERENCES

1. Reichlin M, Maddison PJ, Targoff I, Bunch T, Arnett F, Sharp G, Treadwell E, Tan EM: Antibodies to a nuclear/nucleolar antigen in patients with polymyositis–overlap syndromes. J Clin Immunol 4:40–44, 1984
2. Nishikai M, Reichlin M: Heterogeneity of precipitating antibodies in polymyositis: characterization of the Jo-1 antibody system. Arthritis Rheum 23:881–888, 1980
3. Wolfe JF, Adelstein E, Sharp GC: Antinuclear antibody with distinct specificity for polymyositis. J Clin Invest 59:176–178, 1977
4. Mimori T, Akizuki M, Yamagata H, Inada S, Homma M: Characterization of a high molecular weight acidic nuclear protein recognized by autoantibodies in sera from patients with polymyositis-scleroderma overlap. J Clin Invest 68:611–620, 1981
5. Bernstein RM, Steigerwald JC, Tan EM: Association of antinuclear and antinucleolar antibodies in progressive systemic sclerosis. Clin Exp Immunol 48:43–51, 1982
6. Widnell CC, Tata JR: A procedure for the isolation of enzymatically active rat liver nuclei. Biochem J 92:313–317, 1964
7. Busch H, Daskal Y: Methods for isolation of nuclei and nucleoli, Methods in Cell Biology. Vol. XVI. Edited by DM Prescott. New York, Academic Press, 1977, pp 1–43
8. Treadwell EL, Takano M, Alspaugh MA, Harmon D, Kobel J, Gray J, Sharp GC: Distinction of PM-1 from three new antigens associated with rheumatic disease (abstract). Arthritis Rheum (suppl) 24:S94, 1981
9. Miyawaki S, Kohmoto K, Kurata N, Ofuji T: Identification and characterization of two new soluble nuclear antigens reactive with sera of patients with connective tissue diseases. Arthritis Rheum 21:803–810, 1978
10. Miyachi K, Tan EM: Antibodies reacting with ribosomal ribonucleoprotein in connective tissue diseases. Arthritis Rheum 22:87–93, 1979
11. Tan EM, Rodnan GP, Garcia I, Moroi Y, Fritzler JM, Peebles C: Diversity of antinuclear antibodies in PSS: anti-centromere antibody and its relationship to CREST syndrome. Arthritis Rheum 23:617–625, 1980
12. Pinnas JL, Northway JD, Tan EM: Antinucleolar antibodies in human sera. J Immunol 111:996–1004, 1973
13. Miyawaki S, Ritchie RF: Nucleolar antigen specific for antinucleolar antibody in the sera of patients with systemic rheumatic diseases. Arthritis Rheum 16:726–736, 1973
14. Reddy R, Tan EM, Henning D, Nohga K, Busch H: Detection of nucleolar 7-2 ribonucleoprotein and a cytoplasmic 8-2 ribonucleoprotein with autoantibodies from patients with scleroderma. J Biol Chem 258:1383–1386, 1983
15. Lerner MR, Steitz JA: Antibodies to small nuclear RNA's complexed with proteins are produced by patients with systemic lupus erythematosus. Proc Natl Acad Sci USA 76:5495–5499, 1979
16. Hashimoto C, Steitz JA: Sequential association of nucleolar 7-2 RNA with two different autoantigens. J Biol Chem 458:1379–1382, 1983
17. Matter L, Schopfer K, Wilhelm JA, Nyffenegger T, Parisot RF, DeRobertis EM: Molecular characterization of ribonucleoprotein antigens bound by antinuclear antibodies: a diagnostic evaluation. Arthritis Rheum 25:1278–1283, 1982

BRIEF REPORT

MULTICENTRIC RETICULOHISTIOCYTOSIS: A CAUSE OF DYSPHAGIA WITH RESPONSE TO CORTICOSTEROIDS

PETER J. ZEALE, DAVID MINER, STEPHEN HONIG, MARIAN WAXMAN, and HARRY BARTFIELD

Multicentric reticulohistiocytosis (MR) is a rare disorder characterized by the widespread infiltration of tissue with lipid-laden histiocytes (1). The most disabling feature is polyarthritis, which ultimately may result in joint destruction. Patient response to corticosteroids has been inconsistent and difficult to distinguish from naturally occurring spontaneous remission. We describe a patient with MR whose articular and extraarticular symptoms responded dramatically to corticosteroids on 2 separate occasions.

Case report. A 38-year-old black woman was first admitted to St. Vincent's Hospital and Medical Center in January 1983, because of progressive weakness and pain in the right hand associated with decreased function over several months. Several weeks prior to admission, she noted the onset of pain and stiffness in her knees, shoulders, and proximal interphalangeal (PIP) joints of both hands. Several days before admission, she began to experience dysphagia. There was no history of fever, skin rash, Raynaud's phenomenon, alopecia, visual disturbances, or subcutaneous nodules. She had no history of arthritis, and the family history was noncontributory.

Physical examination revealed a thin, 38-year-old black woman in no acute distress. Vital signs were normal except for a rectal temperature of 100°F. Abnormal findings were limited to the joints. She had diffuse swelling, warmth, and tenderness of the metacarpophalangeal (MCP) joints and the PIP joints of both hands (the right greater than the left). There was markedly diminished range of motion of the PIP joints bilaterally, and the extension of the elbows was also limited. No skin nodules were present.

Her hemoglobin value was 11.3 gm, hematocrit 35.6%, and the white blood cell count was 7,300 cells/mm^3. The erythrocyte sedimentation rate ranged from 25–43 mm/hour during her hospitalization. Roentgenographic studies of her chest and hands showed normal results, as did the barium esophagram. The bone scan revealed increased uptake of the radioisotope in the hands, wrists, elbows, sternoclavicular joints, ankles, and knees, bilaterally. Tests for rheumatoid factor and antinuclear antibodies gave negative results. An electromyogram of the muscles of both upper extremities was interpreted as being consistent with bilateral carpal tunnel syndrome.

The patient was discharged with a presumptive diagnosis of reflex sympathetic dystrophy of the hands in association with an undifferentiated connective tissue disease. She was treated with prednisone, 30 mg twice a day, with prompt and dramatic relief of all symptoms. Hand strength and range of motion returned to normal. Her dysphagia, the etiology of which remained uncertain, fully resolved.

She continued to improve over the ensuing 3 months, while the dosage of prednisone was gradually tapered. However, upon discontinuation of her corticosteroid therapy, the dysphagia and arthritis recurred. Aspirin was prescribed but did not alleviate her symptoms. She noted an outbreak of painless nodules over her face and the dorsum of her hands,

From the Departments of Medicine and Pathology, St. Vincent's Hospital and Medical Center, New York, New York.

Peter J. Zeale, MD; David Miner, MD; Stephen Honig, MD, FACP; Marian Waxman, MD; Harry Bartfield, MD.

Address reprint requests to Stephen Honig, MD, FACP, St. Vincent's Hospital and Medical Center, 153 West 11th Street, New York, NY 10011.

Submitted for publication January 17, 1984; accepted in revised form August 21, 1984.

and she was readmitted to the hospital, approximately 4 months after her first admission, for further evaluation.

Examination at the time of readmission revealed numerous firm, yellow-brown nodules, ranging in size from 1.5 cm to about 5 cm, involving the skin of the nose, nasolabial folds, hands, and elbow areas, bilaterally. There was swelling, warmth, and tenderness of the MCP, PIP, and distal interphalangeal joints, bilaterally. There was extensive synovial thickening and limited ability to extend her fingers. Hand grip strength was markedly diminished.

Barium esophagram again showed normal results as did a manometric study of the esophagus. However, upper endoscopy revealed a 2-cm nodule on the posterior wall of the hypopharynx, and below this area, several 2–3-mm nodules were seen. Biopsies of the skin nodules from the right elbow area, including the fascia, were performed, followed by a biopsy of the pharyngeal nodule.

The biopsy samples revealed nodular aggregates and diffuse collections of large histiocytic cells, situated in the dermis and subcutaneous fat (Figure 1). The cells were characterized by abundant cytoplasm, which was either finely granular and pinkish-glassy or pale and foamy (Figure 2). The nuclei were round and vesicular.

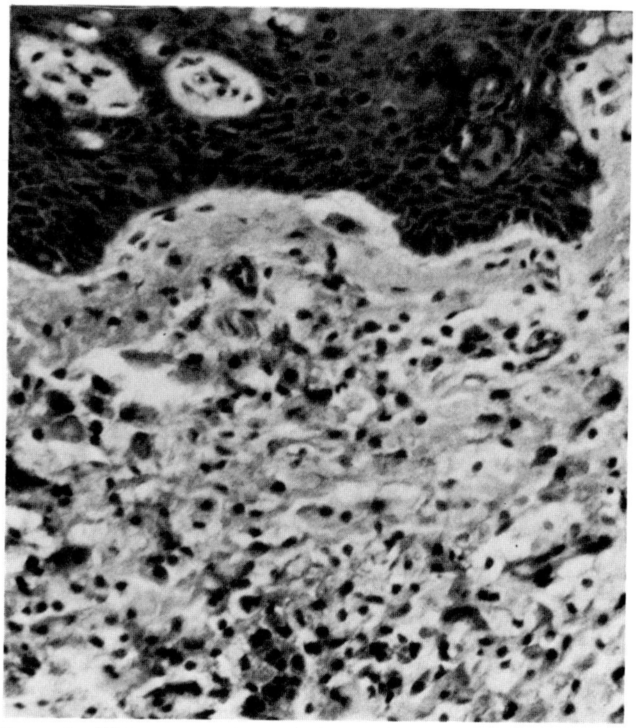

Figure 2. High-power view of the multinucleated reticulohistiocytes with abundant pink-glassy cytoplasm (hematoxylin and eosin stained, magnification × 40).

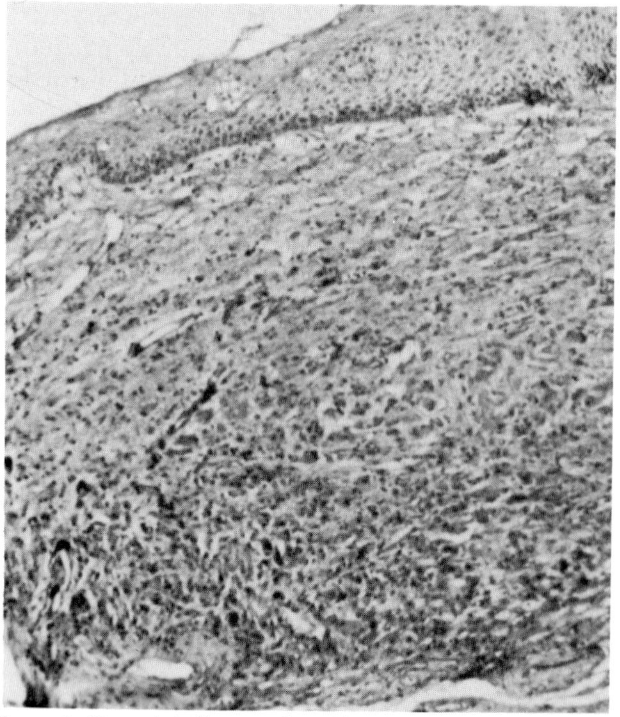

Figure 1. Dermal infiltrate of multinucleated reticulohistiocytes (hematoxylin and eosin stained, magnification × 100).

Although the infiltrate was principally mononuclear, rare multinucleate histiocytic giant cells were also readily identified (Figure 3). The cytoplasm of the histiocytes stained strongly with periodic acid–Schiff reagent stain, which remained resistant to prior digestion with diastase. Identical histiocytic infiltrates were found in the biopsy sample of the right elbow fascia and in the specimen of the nodule from the posterior pharyngeal wall (Figure 4).

The patient was again started on a regimen of prednisone, 30 mg twice daily. Within days, her hand grip strength returned to normal, and her dysphagia resolved. Over the ensuing weeks, the nodules on her hands and face began to regress, and many of them have subsequently disappeared. As of July 1983, the patient exhibited no evidence of arthritis or skin nodules, while being maintained with prednisone treatment of 10 mg/day.

Discussion. Multicentric reticulohistiocytosis is a rare disorder of unknown cause, manifested clinically by polyarthritis, mucocutaneous nodules, and a variety of systemic symptoms (1). Because of the

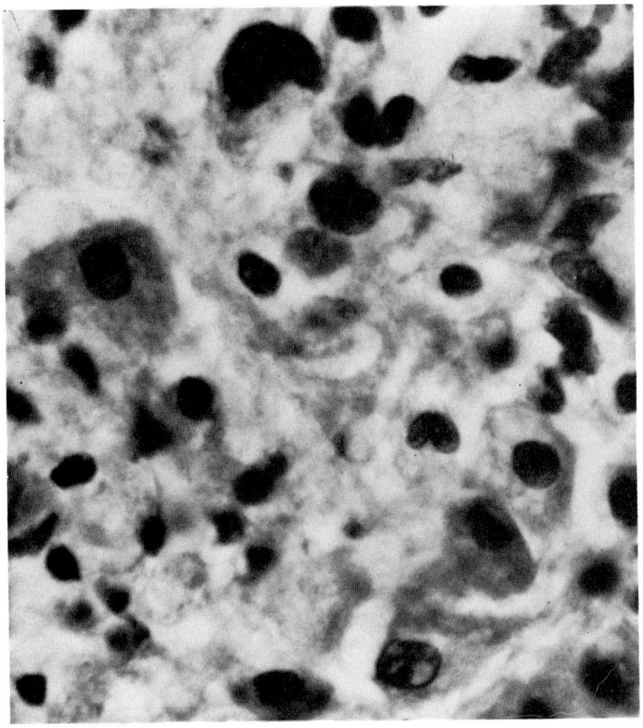

Figure 3. Multinucleate histiocytes with foamy cytoplasm (center) (hematoxylin and eosin stained, magnification × 400).

rarity of the disease, it remains a difficult diagnostic and therapeutic problem for the rheumatologist. Early in the disease course it is frequently misdiagnosed, since the examination and radiographs may suggest such entities as gout, rheumatoid arthritis, or psoriatic arthritis (2). The nodules typically appear months to years after the onset of polyarthritis, frequently raising the diagnostic possibility of sarcoidosis or even leprosy (3). The definite diagnosis of MR requires a biopsy of skin nodules or synovium, which reveals the typical nodular aggregates of histiocytes with multinucleated cells showing a ground-glass or foamy cytoplasm (4).

The clinical presentation and histologic findings in our patient are classic for a diagnosis of MR. The unusual and interesting aspects of this case are twofold: 1) the patient experienced dysphagia that was caused by a pharyngeal nodule; and 2) the patient responded dramatically to corticosteroid therapy on 2 separate occasions.

Mucosal nodular infiltrates are commonly seen in MR. Barrow and Holubar (1) found them in 52% of their 33 patients, mostly involving the lips, buccal mucosa, nasal septum, tongue, and gingiva. Warin et al (5) reported the finding of typical MR nodules in the larynx of 1 of their patients. We do not know of any reports citing the presence of a dysphagia-causing hypopharyngeal nodule as one of the presenting symptoms in MR. We are confident in attributing our patient's dysphagia to the presence of the nodule, in light of the negative results of the barium swallow and upper endoscopy and motility studies.

Of additional interest is this patient's dramatic response to corticosteroid therapy on 2 separate occasions. Because of the rarity of the disease and its obscure etiology, there has been no consistent approach to therapy. Response to therapy has been difficult to assess because of the highly variable nature of the disease. Various modalities have been used in treating this disease, including salicylates, corticosteroids, adrenocorticotropic hormone, hydroxychloroquine, nitrogen mustard, cyclophosphamide, azathioprine, chlorambucil, as well as low-fat diets, all of which have shown variable response (1,2,4,6–8).

Our patient demonstrated a marked response, in that all symptoms—arthritis, dysphagia, and the presence of skin nodules—resolved with steroid therapy. We believe that her response was not part of the natural remission one may see in this disorder, because her second disease flare and remission subse-

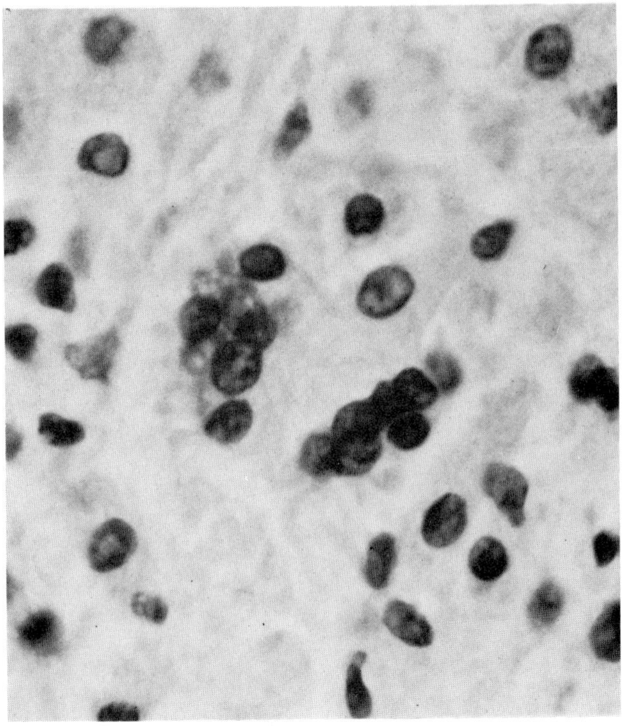

Figure 4. Diffuse mucosal infiltrate of multinucleated reticulohistiocytes in the pharyngeal biopsy specimen (hematoxylin and eosin stained, magnification × 400).

quent to a second course of therapy were so temporally related to the use of steroids.

We have presented a case of MR with distinctive articular and extraarticular symptoms that responded to corticosteroid therapy on 2 separate occasions. The patient presently remains asymptomatic on tapering doses of steroids.

REFERENCES

1. Barrow MV, Holubar K: Muticentric reticulohistiocytosis: a review of 33 patients. Medicine (Baltimore) 48:287–305, 1969
2. Gold RH, Metzger AL, Mirra JM, Weinberger HJ, Killibrew K: Multicentric reticulohistiocytosis (lipoid dermato-arthritis): an erosive polyarthritis with distinctive clinical, roentgenographic and pathologic features. AJR 124:610–624, 1975
3. Flam M, Ryan S, Mak-Poy GL, Jacobs KF, Nelder KH: Multicentric reticulohistiocytosis: report of a case with atypical features and electron microscopic study of skin lesions. Am J Med 52:841–848, 1972
4. Davies NEJ, Roenigk HH, Hawk WA, O'Duffy JD: Multicentric reticulohistiocytosis: a report of a case with histochemical studies. Arch Dermatol 97:543–547, 1968
5. Warin RP, Evans CD, Hewitt M, Taylor AL, Price CHG, Middlemiss JH: Reticulohistiocytosis (lipoid dermato-arthritis). Br Med J 1:1387–1391, 1957
6. Krey PR, Comerford FR, Cohen AS: Multicentric reticulohistiocytosis: fine structural analysis of the synovium and synovial fluid cells. Arthritis Rheum 17:615–633, 1974
7. Hanauer LB: Reticulohistiocytosis: remission after cyclophosphamide therapy. Arthritis Rheum 15:636–640, 1972
8. Taylor DR: Multicentric reticulohistiocytosis. Arch Dermatol 113:330–332, 1977

LETTERS

A followup study of children exposed to gold compounds in utero

To the Editor:

Drug teratogenicity is a problem that must be considered when planning therapy for female rheumatoid arthritis (RA) patients who are fertile (1). In experimental studies, gold has been demonstrated to be present in oocytes and in hepatocytes of the fetus (ref. 2 and Møller-Madsen B: personal communication). In doses exceeding those used in therapy by a factor ≥25, gold has been found to have dose-related teratogenic and embryotoxic effects in rats and rabbits (3–6). Few reports are available regarding possible effects of gold on the human fetus, and none of the published studies has dealt with possible long-term consequences. A study published in Japanese reported 2 cases of hip anomalies occurring in the offspring of 69 women who had been treated with gold during part of or throughout pregnancy (7). In the English literature, there are 3 case reports describing the outcome of pregnancies in women treated with gold. One child was healthy (1). Another child had severe malformations and died 5 days after birth (8). In a third woman the pregnancy was terminated because of gold exposure. No obvious abnormality was found, but gold was demonstrated in the liver and kidney of the fetus (9).

It is unlikely that treatment with gold or equivalent drugs would be considered for RA patients who are known to be pregnant. If pregnancy occurs during gold treatment, it is common practice to stop therapy. Contraception practice has been advocated as a prerequisite of gold therapy in fertile women, and the possibility of induced abortion may be considered in women who have received the drug while pregnant.

Among the patients examined and followed in our clinic during the years 1965–83, 107 women aged 15–45 years were treated for varying periods with gold sodium thiosulfate (GSTS) or gold sodium thiomalate (GSTM). Eight pregnancies occurred in 7 women during treatment. Gold treatment was stopped when the pregnancy was discovered. Abortion was not advised. Detailed and reliable information was also obtained on 2 additional women who had become pregnant during gold treatment before being admitted to the clinic.

We studied the course and outcome of these 10 pregnancies. Two women wanted induced abortion for personal reasons. One woman gave birth at full term to a stillborn girl (weight 4,500 gm, length 54 cm) after an otherwise uncomplicated pregnancy. The child had been dead for approximately 20 hours. The gold therapy had been started 6 weeks prior to conception and had continued through the first 5 weeks of pregnancy at a dosage of 20 mg of GSTM weekly. At autopsy of the infant, no anomalies were found. The cause of death was a tight knot of the umbilical cord.

Six women, with 7 pregnancies, gave birth to live infants. The 7 children received several followup examinations: they were examined immediately after birth by a midwife and a physician, several times during the first years by public health nurses, and at the ages of 5 weeks, 5, 10, and 15 months, 2, 3, 4, 5, and 6 years by family doctors. In addition to the histories given by the parents, information was obtained from the records of lying-in hospitals, public health nurses, and family doctors.

The doses of gold given during the mothers' pregnancies are shown in Table 1. The mean total dose of pure gold given during pregnancy was 67.8 mg. The mean exposure period was 5.7 weeks. In some patients the doses were low because the gold tended to produce side effects. During the pregnancy 3 patients had taken 0.5–1 gm acetylsalicylic acid daily. One patient had taken 100 mg indomethacin daily for a short period; another had taken 1,200 mg ibuprofen and 100 mg ketoprofen daily. Two patients did not take drugs other than gold. None had been exposed to infection, radiographs, or excessive amounts of alcohol. Four smoked 4–10 cigarettes daily. One patient had a slightly depressed estriol level during the last months of pregnancy, and 1 had slight hypertension and proteinuria during the last weeks.

One woman delivered 4 weeks before term, the others at term. The births were normal. The mean weight at birth was 3,200 gm (range 2,600–3,900), the mean length 50.9 cm (range 48–53). No malformations occurred, and there were no problems during the neonatal period.

The mean age of the children when their records were reviewed was 7.4 years (range 0.8–15.9). Their somatic

Table 1. Amounts of gold given and duration of exposure

Patient	Duration of gold therapy (weeks)	Weeks of pregnancy exposed to gold	Dose of gold (mg)*	Total amount of pure gold given during pregnancy (mg)
1	23	8	GSTS 50/week	148.0
2	88	6	GSTS 50/week	92.5
3	25	6	GSTM 10–20/week	27.5
4	200	2	GSTM 20/4 weeks	10.0
5	13	9	GSTS 50/week	166.5
6	121	6	GSTM 10/2 weeks	15.0
7	3	3	GSTM 10/week	15.0

* GSTS = gold sodium thiosulfate, 37% gold; GSTM = gold sodium thiomalate, 50% gold.

development, as estimated by length and weight attained curves, was normal. Their psychomotor and intellectual development was assessed to be normal, based on the presence of key indicators of development and present achievement. No behavioral disorders were reported. The physical examinations did not reveal any malformations, and the children appeared physically and psychologically healthy.

No teratogenic, embryotoxic, or long-term adverse effects of gold have been demonstrated in this study. We believe the study method used was appropriate. An evaluation of the statistical risk of malformations possibly caused by gold, D-penicillamine, and other antirheumatic drugs will, however, require a very comprehensive study. A central recording of pregnancies in women with RA might contribute to a final answer.

Ulrik Tarp, MD
Hans Graudal, MD
University of Aarhus
Orthopedic Hospital
Aarhus, Denmark

1. Cohen DL, Orzel J, Taylor A: Infants of mothers receiving gold therapy (letter). Arthritis Rheum 24:104–105, 1981
2. Møller-Madsen B, Danscher G: Transplacental transport of gold in rats exposed to sodium aurothiomalate. Exp Mol Pathol 39:327–331, 1983
3. Kidston ME, Beck F, Lloyd JB: The teratogenic effects of myochrysine injection in rats. J Anat 108:590–591, 1971
4. Szabo KT, Guerriero FJ, Kang YJ: The effects of gold-containing compounds on pregnant rats and their fetuses. Vet Pathol [Suppl] 15:89–96, 1978
5. Szabo KT, DiFebbo ME, Phelan DG: The effects of gold-containing compounds on pregnant rabbits and their fetuses. Vet Pathol [Suppl] 15:97–102, 1978
6. Eiseman JL, Alvares AP: Heme metabolism in the fetoplacental unit and neonatal livers during lactation: effect of gold sodium thiomalate. J Pharmacol Exp Ther 214:250–256, 1980
7. Miyamoto T, Miyaji S, Horiochi Y, Hara M, Ishihara K: Gold therapy in bronchial asthma: special emphasis upon blood levels of gold and its teratogenicity. Nippon Naika Gakkai Zaashi 63:1190–1197, 1970
8. Rogers JG, Anderson RM, Chow CW, Gillam GL, Markman L: Possible teratogenic effects of gold. Aust Paediatr J 16:194–195, 1980
9. Rocker I, Henderson WJ: Transfer of gold from mother to fetus (letter). Lancet ii:1246, 1976

HLA–Bw35 and gold toxicity in rheumatoid arthritis

To the Editor:

We previously reported the frequency distribution of DR antigens in a group of 148 white rheumatoid arthritis (RA) patients undergoing chrysotherapy, and its relation to the occurrence of toxicity in general and renal toxicity in particular (1). The analysis of our data at that time failed to demonstrate a relationship between any HLA–A, B, or C specificity and gold toxicity; thus, our report focused on the DR associations. A recent report from Germany, however, describing an association between Bw35 and mucocutaneous lesions in gold-treated RA patients (2), prompted us to reevaluate our previously unpublished data on this set of patients.

Table 1. Selected HLA antigens in rheumatoid arthritis patients undergoing chrysotherapy

HLA antigen	Patients not exhibiting side effects (n = 105), % (A)	Patients exhibiting side effects, %: Renal (n = 12) (B)	Muco-cutaneous (n = 25) (C)	P*: A vs. B	A vs. C
A1	14.3	16.6	20.0	NS	NS
B8	19.0	8.3	16.0	NS	NS
Bw35	9.5	16.6	8.0	NS	NS
DR3	9.5	33.3	16.0	<0.05	NS

* NS = not significant.

From a total of 143 patients on whom we had complete HLA–A, B, C, and DR data, there were 39 toxic reactions in 38 patients (25 mucocutaneous, 12 renal, and 2 miscellaneous). As shown in Table 1, Bw35 was present with similar frequency in patients who exhibited no side effects, compared with those who exhibited either renal or mucocutaneous side effects. Furthermore, the association of DR3 with renal toxicity does not necessarily imply the presence of the HLA–A1, B8, DR3 haplotype, as reported by Nüsslein et al (2), and previously reported by Bardin et al (3). In fact, only 2 of our 4 patients who had renal toxicity and the DR3 antigen exhibited this haplotype.

It will be of interest to obtain information from other investigators who have conducted research in this field (3–6), concerning this reported association of mucocutaneous toxicity with Bw35 as found by Nüsslein and colleagues. As in the case of the DR3 association with gold toxicity, where the relative risk may not be as high as originally reported (4), the relative risk for Bw35 may not be as high as reported by the German group, but may indeed be increased. Clearly, additional data are required in order to resolve this issue.

Graciela S. Alarcón, MD, MPH
William J. Koopman, MD
Ronald T. Acton, PhD
Bruce O. Barger, PhD
University of Alabama in Birmingham
Birmingham, AL

1. Barger BO, Acton RT, Koopman WJ, Alarcón GS: DR antigens and gold toxicity in white rheumatoid arthritis patients. Arthritis Rheum 27:601–605, 1984
2. Nüsslein HG, Jahn H, Lösch G, Guggenmoos-Holzmann I, Leibold W, Kalden JR: Association of HLA–Bw35 with mucocutaneous lesions in rheumatoid arthritis patients undergoing sodium aurothiomalate therapy. Arthritis Rheum 27:833–836, 1984

3. Bardin T, Dryll A, Debeyre N, Ryckewaert A, Legrand L, Marcelli A, Darsset J: HLA system and side effects of gold salts and D-penicillamine treatment of rheumatoid arthritis. Ann Rheum Dis 41:599–601, 1982
4. Panayi GS, Wooley PH, Batchelor JR: Genetic basis of rheumatoid disease: HLA antigens, disease manifestations, and toxic reactions to drugs. Br Med J 2:1326–1328, 1978
5. Gran JT, Husby G, Thorsby E: HLA DR antigens and gold toxicity. Ann Rheum Dis 42:63–66, 1983
6. Bensen WG, Moore N, Tugwell P, D'Souza M, Singal DP: HLA antigens and toxic reactions to sodium aurothiomalate in patients with rheumatoid arthritis. J Rheumatol 11:358–361, 1984

Renal malakoplakia and systemic lupus erythematosus

To the Editor:

I read with interest the article by Wener et al which describes a patient with systemic lupus erythematosus (SLE) and renal malakoplakia (Wener MH, Ramsey PG, Hill HR, Striker L, Mannik M: Renal malakoplakia in a patient with systemic lupus erythematosus. Arthritis Rheum 27:704–707, 1984). In the article, the authors state: "We are not aware of previous reports of renal malakoplakia associated with SLE."

Mitchell reported a similar patient seen at the Mayo Clinic (Mitchell JC: Malacoplakia: an unusual but potentially preventable complication of recurrent urinary tract infections in patients with systemic lupus erythematosus. Med Grand Rounds 2:57–66, 1983). The patient was a 30-year-old woman with the diagnosis of SLE, who had a course marked by clinical flares of disease activity associated with urinary symptoms. Flares were treated with increased doses of prednisone; associated bacteriuria was attributed to recurrent urinary tract infections not thought to contribute significantly to the course of her underlying disease. It is noteworthy that 4 years after the diagnosis of SLE was made, her serologic markers became normal; nonetheless, episodes of fever, malaise, and dysuria recurred and were treated with increased doses of prednisone, as well as empirically selected antibiotics.

Once the diagnosis of renal malakoplakia was made (by renal biopsy demonstrating dense calcific granules of Michaelis-Gutmann bodies), the significance of persistent bacteriuria became apparent, and appropriate antibiotic therapy and partial nephrectomy led to stabilization of renal function and eradication of the infection; prednisone was discontinued.

John Varga, MD
Boston University Medical Center
Boston, MA

Correction of data on salicylate and indomethacin concentrations in cartilage

To the Editor:

We wish to correct an error in a paper we recently had published in *Arthritis and Rheumatism* (Palmoski MJ, Brandt KD: Effects of salicylate and indomethacin on glycosaminoglycan and prostaglandin E_2 synthesis in intact canine knee cartilage ex vivo. Arthritis Rheum 27:398–403, 1984). In that paper we reported that the concentrations of salicylate and of indomethacin in cartilage were lower than those in the culture medium, and we concluded that neither drug diffused freely into the cartilage.

Since the paper was published we have recognized that our calculations of the molar concentrations of the drugs in the cartilage were incorrect. In actuality, when the concentration of salicylate in the culture medium was $10^{-3}M$, its concentration in cartilage from habitually unloaded sites of the femoral condyles was $6.7 \times 10^{-2}M$. When the concentration of indomethacin in the culture medium was $4 \times 10^{-6}M$, its concentration in cartilage from unloaded sites was $5.6 \times 10^{-6}M$. Thus, the concentration of indomethacin in unloaded cartilage was essentially the same as that in the incubation medium, while the concentration of salicylate in the cartilage was somewhat greater than that in the medium, suggesting that some type of binding of salicylate may have occurred in the tissue.

As we stated in our paper, the concentration of both drugs in cartilage from unloaded regions of the articular surface was at least 50% greater than that in cartilage from habitually loaded sites. Our data, both in the above-mentioned paper and in a previous report (Palmoski MJ, Brandt KD: Relationship between matrix proteoglycan content and the effects of salicylate and indomethacin on articular cartilage. Arthritis Rheum 26:528–531, 1983), indicate that the suppressive effects of salicylate and indomethacin on glycosaminoglycan biosynthesis in vitro are greater in articular cartilage from habitually unloaded sites than in cartilage from loaded areas, and that this is associated with a greater uptake of drug in the unloaded areas, presumably due to their relatively lower proteoglycan content.

Marshall J. Palmoski, PhD
Kenneth D. Brandt, MD
Indiana University School of Medicine
Indianapolis, IN

Pregnancy and systemic sclerosis

To the Editor:

In their interesting paper, Ballou et al report on patients they have seen and review previously reported cases of pregnancy and systemic sclerosis (Ballou SP, Morley JJ, Kushner I: Pregnancy and systemic sclerosis. Arthritis Rheum 27:295–298, 1984). We have retrospectively analyzed 86 married women with progressive systemic sclerosis (PSS). Six of the 86 patients, and 4 of 86 healthy married women used as controls, had no pregnancies. The remaining 80 PSS patients had a total of 299 pregnancies. Fifty of those pregnancies were interrupted by spontaneous abortion. The 82 control women had 332 pregnancies, 32 of which were interrupted by spontaneous abortion. The percentage of abortion in PSS patients was found to be statistically different from that of controls ($\chi^2 = 6.36$; $P < 0.05$).

It is not easy to establish the exact time of onset of PSS. Nonetheless, our 86 PSS patients could be subdivided into 3 subgroups according to their age range at disease onset. In the first subgroup (n = 24) the disease began before age 30; in the second (n = 22) it began between the ages of 30 and 39; in the third (n = 40) it began after age 40. The percentage of abortions was not statistically different among the 3 subgroups. It is noteworthy that among the 24 women in the first group, only 3 had no pregnancies. The remaining 21 had 68 pregnancies, of which 16 were interrupted by abortion.

These data suggest that abortions occur more frequently in women with PSS. This would appear to be the case even before the PSS is diagnosed. In contrast to Ballou's finding that pregnancy is uncommon in PSS, only 6 of 86 patients in our series had no pregnancy. The finding of a lower total number of pregnancies in our PSS women (n = 299) as compared with controls (n = 332) might be related to psychological or other factors, i.e., localized scleroderma of genital areas (Stenever MA, Ng ABP: Scleroderma of the uterine cervix. Am J Obstet Gynecol 107:965–966, 1970), as opposed to decreased fertility in women with PSS.

Mario Giordano, MD
Gabriele Valentini, MD
Salvatore Lupoli, MD
Andrea Giordano, MD
University of Naples
Naples, Italy

Reply

To The Editor:

The data of Giordano et al, indicating an increased frequency of spontaneous abortion in pregnant patients with progressive systemic sclerosis (scleroderma), are of particular interest in view of the large number of patients reported. In addition, the evidence suggesting that abortions may be more frequent even prior to onset of clinically evident disease is especially intriguing, and may imply subclinical abnormalities in these patients prior to recognized disease onset.

A second point made by the authors is that married women who develop scleroderma do not have diminished fertility. While this may well be the case, we cannot tell from this letter whether the patients' fertility was manifested prior to or after the onset of scleroderma. We fear the possibility still exists that there is diminished fertility after the onset of scleroderma.

Finally, it is unfortunate that Dr. Giordano and colleagues did not provide information regarding the course of pregnancy in the scleroderma patients. Although our review as well as several other reports suggest that maternal complications are frequent in patients with established scleroderma, this conclusion is far from firm.

Stanley P. Ballou, MD
Irving Kushner, MD
Case Western Reserve University
Cleveland Metropolitan General Hospital
Cleveland, OH

Coexistent rheumatoid arthritis and gout

To the Editor:

I am writing regarding the article by Agudelo et al (Agudelo CA, Turner RA, Panetti M, Pisko E: Does hyperuricemia protect from rheumatoid inflammation? A clinical study. Arthritis Rheum 27:443–448, 1984).

The hypothesis assumed and investigated by those authors is that the low concurrence of two common rheumatic conditions, gout and rheumatoid arthritis (RA), is due to a protective effect in gout, preventing the development of rheumatoid arthritis. An equally attractive and logical explanation that may be operative in part is that patients were protected from developing gout by the fact that traditionally—until perhaps 10 years ago—nearly all, if not all, of these patients were taking high-dose salicylates, which had a significant uricosuric effect.

During my training as a rheumatology fellow, the dictum that rheumatoid arthritis patients did not develop gout was frequently hammered into my calvarium, and indeed during that 2-year fellowship I saw no patients with both diseases. However, at the time that I started in clinical practice, Motrin appeared on the pharmacologic scene and was followed by the multiple other nonsteroidal antiinflammatory drugs which have been marketed since then. These other agents are much more attractive to the patients because of the fewer number of pills that they must swallow less often, and to the physician because they insure greater patient compliance. Accordingly, in my own practice I see that aspirin now is used by only a minority of my patients with RA. In the last 10 years, I have also seen several patients with concurrent rheumatoid arthritis and gout. Perhaps there is a relationship between these two phenomena.

Arthur M. Virshup, MD
West Palm Beach, FL

Epidemiology of juvenile arthritis in Rochester, Minnesota

To the Editor:

Towner et al (1) recently reported higher prevalence and incidence rates of juvenile arthritis (JA) in Rochester, Minnesota than those previously reported. The higher incidence rate was apparently due to a higher proportion of pauciarticular disease (74% of the total number) compared with previous studies. The impression of the authors was that the pauciarticular form of disease was clinically mild with few nonarticular manifestations. For example, only 4% of the patients had iridocyclitis.

The authors suggested that higher rates of mild pauciarticular disease were observed because the study was community based, whereas previous studies were university hospital or clinic based. They speculated further that the mild pauciarticular disease may represent 1 or more JA subtypes with distinct etiologies.

A possible etiologic agent in at least a proportion of the pauciarticular forms of JA in Rochester is the Lyme disease spirochete. Patients with Lyme disease may meet the 1977 revised American Rheumatism Association criteria for JA (2), especially if the erythema chronicum migrans rash doesn't occur (as is the case in up to 25% of patients [3]) or if it is overlooked or misidentified (4). Lyme disease is being reported with increasing frequency in Minnesota (5,6), including in and around Olmsted County. Several patients have had onset of the disease in the 1970s (4), overlapping the ascertainment time of Towner's study.

Several observations by Towner et al are consistent with the possibility that Lyme disease contributes to the increased rates of JA in Rochester. First, the frequent pattern of pauciarthritis (including one-third of patients with monarthritis) matches the most common pattern of arthritis in Lyme disease (3). Second, the low incidence of eye inflammation in this series could reflect the existence of a form of arthritis, such as Lyme disease, not susceptible to eye involvement. Third, 16 of 49 patients had symptom-free intervals of at least 3 months. Attacks of arthritis in Lyme disease are often separated by symptom-free intervals of weeks to months (3). Fourth, the sex ratio was approximately equal (9 males and 11 females) among children whose age at onset was between 5 and 15 and whose arthritis was of at least 3 months duration. The ratio of males to females was 1:11 when age at onset was <5. It is possible that the inclusion of cases of Lyme disease in the older age group of JA patients might account for the near equalization of incidence rates among males and females.

It is unclear whether Lyme disease has emerged as a truly new disease or has simply been recently recognized (3). In any event, there are few cases with known onset prior to the 1970s in Connecticut (7) or in the upper midwest (5,6,8). It would be of interest to learn whether the incidence of pauciarticular forms of JA in Rochester increased in the 1970s compared with the 1960s. If so, it might lend further support to the notion that Lyme disease is part of the "JA" population in Rochester and could partially account for the unusually high rates of JA seen there.

Eric S. Schned, MD
Park Nicollet Medical Center
Minneapolis, MN

1. Towner SR, Michet CJ Jr, O'Fallon WM, Nelson AM: The epidemiology of juvenile arthritis in Rochester, Minnesota 1960–1979. Arthritis Rheum 26:1208–1213, 1983
2. Brewer EJ Jr, Bass J, Baum J, Cassidy JT, Fink C, Jacobs J, Hanson V, Levinson JE, Schaller J, Stillman JS: Current proposed revision of JRA criteria. Arthritis Rheum 20:195–199, 1977
3. Steere AC, Malawista SE, Hardin JA, Ruddy S, Askenase PW, Andiman WA: Erythema chronicum migrans and Lyme arthritis: the enlarging clinical spectrum. Ann Intern Med 86:685–698, 1977
4. Schned ES: Lyme disease as an etiology of "unexplained" recurrent monoarthritis. Minn Med 65:325–328, 1984
5. Williams DN, Vance JC, Hedberg C, Foley C, Osterhold M: Lyme disease and erythema chronicum migrans in Minnesota. Minn Med 65:217–220, 1982
6. Lyme disease: an emerging public health problem. Minnesota Department of Health, Disease Control Newsletter 11:21–28, 1984
7. Steere AC, Malawista SE: Cases of Lyme disease in the United States: locations correlated with distribution of Ixodes dammini. Ann Intern Med 91:730–733, 1979
8. Dryer RF, Goellner PG, Carney AS: Lyme arthritis in Wisconsin. JAMA 241:498–499, 1979

Reply

To the Editor:

Dr. Schned raises the important issue of Lyme disease as an etiology for some cases of pauciarticular juvenile arthritis in endemic areas. In our study, we observed no significant difference in the overall incidence rates of pauciarticular arthritis for the years 1960–69 versus 1970–79. This was also true for the specific age group 5–15 years. Among the patients in this age group, there was a slight preponderance of children with onset of disease between the months of March–October, the high-risk period for Lyme disease. Eighty-one percent of the 1960s cases and 70% of the 1970s cases began during this 8-month period. Because the numbers are small, however, it is likely that this observation can be attributed entirely to chance. None of the children developed neurologic or cardiac manifestations suggestive of Lyme disease.

We would agree that Lyme disease should be seriously considered as an etiologic agent in some cases of juvenile arthritis in endemic areas. Seroepidemiologic studies of juvenile arthritis may eventually elucidate the magnitude of its contribution.

Clement J. Michet, MD, MPH
Mayo Clinic
Rochester, MN

Serum C1q levels in rheumatoid arthritis

To the Editor:

We read with great interest the article by Ochi et al (1) on serum C1q levels as a prognostic guide to articular erosions in patients with rheumatoid arthritis (RA).

We agree with their statement that serum C1q levels are elevated in patients with active RA; we have previously reported such increases in RA uncomplicated by vasculitis (2–5). These increases were not found in patients with other arthritides such as systemic lupus erythematosus, gout, Paget's disease, ankylosing spondylitis, psoriatic arthritis, and lymphomas. Levels of C1q return to normal or subnormal levels in those RA patients whose disease results in vasculitis.

In addition, we have shown that the increased levels of C1q found in patients with active RA are not accompanied by increased levels of C1r and C1s, indicating that active RA is characterized by an approximately fivefold increase in C1q unbound to C1r and C1s (5). These findings may have pathogenic significance in RA, since the unbound collagen-like stem region has specific physiologic properties. It is to this region that $C1r_2$-$C1s_2$ and fibronectin bind (6,7). Furthermore, there are specific receptor sites for this region on subsets of B lymphocytes, macrophages, neutrophils, and null cells (8).

We cannot agree with the correlation, suggested by Ochi et al (1), between the extent of initial elevation of serum C1q level and the extent of later articular erosion. In our experience with 65 patients who had RA in various classes and stages, elevated levels of C1q did not correlate with any specific tissue damage, including articular erosion. Contrary to their findings that C1q serum levels in clinically "burned out" RA returned to normal values, levels of C1q in our patients remain high in "burned out" cases, even after 20 years duration of the disease, except in those cases that result in vasculitis or rheumatoid nodulosis, where levels of C1q do return to normal or subnormal values. It may be of interest to note that in 1 case of subacute RA in remission, C1q levels returned to normal values and then doubled about a month before the patient's disease flared. This finding suggests that levels of C1q may correlate with the activity of the disease.

We also question the serum C1q values reported by Ochi et al (1), since we have shown that assays of serum levels of C1q by single radial immunodiffusion are inaccurate if there is not compensation for the nonspecific effects of serum proteins on the size of the C1q–anti-C1q precipitin ring (5). Unless the standard curves are prepared in C1q-depleted serum, the immunodiffusion assay will yield values 2–3-fold too high (5).

N. Parhami, MD, FACP
C. L. Rosano, MS
C. Hurwitz, PhD
VA Medical Center
Albany, NY

1. Ochi T, Yonemasu K, Iwase R, Sasaki T, Tsuyama I, Ono K: Serum C1q levels as a prognostic guide to articular erosions in patients with rheumatoid arthritis. Arthritis Rheum 27:883–887, 1984
2. Rosano CL, Hurwitz C: Separation of hydroxyproline-containing protein from C1q (a subcomponent of complement) in serum. Clin Chem 23:1335–1337, 1977
3. Rosano CL, Parhami N, Hurwitz C: The clinical significance of protein-bound hydroxyproline fractions in sera of patients with adult rheumatoid arthritis. J Rheumatol 6:656–663, 1979
4. Rosano CL, Parhami N, Hurwitz C: Determination of C1q in human sera. J Lab Clin Med 94:593–599, 1979
5. Rosano CL, Parhami N, Hurwitz C: Serum levels of C1 subunits in rheumatoid arthritis. J Lab Clin Med 103:313–321, 1984
6. Bing DH, Almeda S, Isliker H, Lahav J, Hynes RO: Fibronectin binds to the C1q component of complement. Proc Natl Acad Sci USA 79:4198–4201, 1982
7. Pearlstein E, Sorvillo J, Gigli I: The interaction of human plasma fibronectin with a subunit of the first component of complement, C1q. J Immunol 128:2036–2039, 1982
8. Ross GD: Structure and function of membrane complement receptors: summary. Fed Proc 14:3089–3093, 1982

arthritis and rheumatism
Official Journal of the American Rheumatism Association Section of the Arthritis Foundation

AUTOANTIBODY SPECIFICITIES OF IMMUNE COMPLEXES SEQUESTERED IN ARTICULAR CARTILAGE OF PATIENTS WITH RHEUMATOID ARTHRITIS AND OSTEOARTHRITIS

HUGO E. JASIN

To define autoantibody specificities of immune complexes sequestered in articular cartilage of patients with rheumatoid arthritis and osteoarthritis, extracts were obtained from articular cartilage specimens from 16 patients with rheumatoid arthritis, 11 patients with osteoarthritis, and 6 normal controls. Radioimmunoassays of the extracts revealed that rheumatoid cartilage contained 37 times more IgM and 14 times more IgG than did normal cartilage extracts. In addition, osteoarthritic cartilage contained 3 times more IgM and IgG than the normal tissues. IgM rheumatoid factor was found in 13 of 16 rheumatoid cartilage extracts but in none of 11 osteoarthritic or 6 normal control extracts. IgG rheumatoid factor was detected in 4 of 7 seropositive rheumatoid but in none of 5 osteoarthritic cartilage extracts. More than 60% of the rheumatoid cartilage extracts were positive for native and denatured collagen II antibodies. Surprisingly, 50% of the osteoarthritic specimens also contained significant titers of collagen antibodies. Similar results were obtained with osteoarthritic menisci extracts. These findings indicate that the immune complexes sequestered in rheumatoid cartilage contain autoantibodies that are probably synthesized locally by cells infiltrating the inflamed synovium. If immune complexes trapped in cartilage play an important role in cartilage damage, our findings would provide a possible pathogenic mechanism that explains the self-perpetuating and chronic nature of cartilage degradation in rheumatoid arthritis and osteoarthritis.

From the Harold C. Simmons Arthritis Research Center and the Department of Internal Medicine, University of Texas Health Science Center at Dallas, Southwestern Medical School, Dallas, Texas.

Supported by USPHS grants AM-16209 and AM-09989.

Hugo E. Jasin, MD: Professor of Internal Medicine, University of Texas Health Science Center at Dallas, Texas.

Address reprint requests to Dr. Hugo E. Jasin, Department of Internal Medicine, UTHSCD, 5323 Harry Hines Boulevard, Dallas, TX 75235.

Submitted for publication June 19, 1984; accepted in revised form October 1, 1984.

Arthritis and Rheumatism, Vol. 28, No. 3 (March 1985)

The pathophysiologic mechanisms operative in articular cartilage damage in rheumatoid arthritis (RA) are not completely understood. However, the pathologic changes observed in advanced disease indicate that most of the cartilage erosive lesions are associated with the invasion of the articular and deep areas of cartilage by pannus originating from the inflamed synovium (1,2). Although the conditions that initiate and facilitate pannus invasion are unknown, previous work in our laboratory suggested that sequestered immune complexes commonly found in the superficial areas of rheumatoid cartilage (3) may play a role in the destructive process by inducing pannus invasion (4) or by activation of the resident mononuclear phagocytes within this granulation tissue (5,6). Rheumatoid synovial fluids frequently contain large amounts of immunoglobulin with autoantibody specificities, synthesized in part by plasma cells infiltrating the subsynovial membrane (7,8). Thus, it was of particular interest to define the possible autoantibody specificities of immune complexes sequestered in articular cartilage. Our findings indicate that rheumatoid factor (RF) and/or collagen antibodies are found in the majority of cartilage tissue specimens obtained from joints of patients with advanced RA. Surprisingly, more than 50% of specimens from patients with osteoarthritis (OA) also contained collagen antibodies. These findings may provide an explanation for the self-perpetuating and chronic nature of RA and OA.

MATERIALS AND METHODS

Materials. Fresh cartilage specimens from the hip and knee joints of 16 patients with RA and 11 patients with OA undergoing total joint replacement were obtained during surgical procedures from several hospitals in the Dallas metropolitan area. Diagnoses were confirmed by histologic examination of cartilage and synovium. Normal cartilage specimens from the knee joints of 6 organ donors over age 40 were obtained within 24 hours of the donor's death.

Cartilage slices grossly free of synovium or pannus were washed free of blood and synovial fluid with Hanks' balanced salt solution (HBSS) and stored at −70°C until used. Small sections were fixed in buffered formalin for routine histologic examination. Synovial fluids obtained from patients with RA and OA were centrifuged at 2,500 revolutions per minute for 10 minutes. The cell-free fluids were stored at −70°C until assayed.

Bovine type II collagen was purified according to the method of Trelstad et al (9) from articular cartilage slices of 1-year-old cows slaughtered 1–2 hours previously. Chick type II collagen was purchased from Genzyme Corporation, Boston, MA. Bovine type I collagen was obtained commercially (Sigma, St. Louis, MO) and repurified by 2 cycles of salt precipitation and diethylaminoethyl cellulose chromatography. Analytic polyacrylamide gel electrophoresis of the bovine collagens showed no evidence of contamination by proteoglycans. Human IgG was purified from Cohn fraction II by diethylaminoethyl cellulose chromatography (10).

Extraction of immune complexes. Approximately 0.5-gm cartilage slices from each specimen were thawed, weighed, and minced with a scalpel blade into 1 × 1-mm pieces. The minced cartilage was suspended in 40 ml phosphate buffered saline (PBS), pH 7.2, 0.02% Na azide and washed at 4°C, with continuous tumbling for 5 days. PBS washes were changed twice daily. At the end of 5 days, the tissues were resuspended in 40 ml of 0.1*M* NaH_2PO_4, 0.15*M* NaCl, pH 5.3, and washed for several hours at 37°C with continuous tumbling. The washed tissues were then transferred to 12 × 75-mm polystyrene tubes (Falcon Labware, Oxnard, CA) and washed overnight with 1.5 ml of PBS, pH 5.3, at 37°C. The tubes were centrifuged at 1,000 rpm for 10 minutes, and the supernatants were collected (PBS wash). The pelleted tissues were resuspended in 1.5 ml PBS, pH 5.3, containing 1 mg/ml testicular hyaluronidase (Sigma) and then further incubated for 18 hours at 37°C. The tissues were pelleted by centrifugation and the supernatants (hyaluronidase extracts) collected. The tissues were washed 6 times with 4 ml HBSS and incubated for 10–15 hours at 37°C with HBSS containing purified bacterial collagenase, 400 units/ml (Worthington Biochemical Corp., Freehold, NJ).

Collagenase digestion was terminated when at least two-thirds of the cartilage mince had been digested. The remaining tissues were pelleted by centrifugation, and the supernatants (collagenase extracts) were collected. To inhibit collagenase activity, Na_2EDTA and newborn calf serum (NBCS) were added to the PBS washes, hyaluronidase, and collagenase extracts to final concentrations of 0.01*M* and 10%, respectively. These were dialyzed at 4°C against several changes of PBS–0.01*M* EDTA and stored at −70°C until assayed.

Radioimmunoassays. The tissue extracts, synovial fluids, and sera were assayed for IgG, IgM, human serum albumin (HSA), IgM rheumatoid factor (IgM-RF), and IgG and IgM anti-native and denatured types I and II collagen antibodies by solid-phase radioimmunoassay.

Selected collagenase supernatants were assayed for IgG rheumatoid factor (IgG-RF) (11). The general technique used for IgG and IgM-RF measurements has been previously described by us (12). Briefly, affinity-purified rabbit anti-IgG or anti-IgM (10 μg/ml) or human IgG aggregates (50 μg/ml) were coated onto polyvinyl chloride round-bottom microtiter wells (Dynatech Laboratories, Alexandria, VA) for 4 hours. Between steps, the wells were washed twice with PBS and twice with PBS–10% NBCS. The extracts were assayed undiluted for IgM-RF. The synovial fluids and sera were diluted 1:1,000 for IgM-RF, 1:10,000 for IgG and IgM, and 1:40,000 for HSA. The assays were developed with affinity-purified ^{125}I-F(ab')$_2$ rabbit anti-human IgG or anti-IgM. For the IgG antibody assays, the diluting and washing buffers contained 0.05*M* dithiothreitol to avoid possible artifacts created by the presence of IgM-RF in the samples to be tested. All samples were tested in duplicate.

Standard curves for IgG, IgM, and HSA were constructed for each determination, using 7 dilutions of stock solutions in triplicate ranging from 10–5,000 ng/ml. The results for IgM-RF were expressed as ng of F(ab')$_2$ anti-IgM bound per well. Since binding of ^{125}I–anti-IgM varied somewhat between different preparations and decreased slowly with storage, the results for each assay were normalized by the use of curves constructed for every determination, with 5 standard seropositive rheumatoid sera of low, medium, and high IgM-RF titers and 2 normal sera. Samples binding more than 2.5 ng of anti-IgM per well were considered positive (mean + 2 SD).

Radioimmunoassays for collagen antibodies were performed by a modification of the method of Clague et al (13). Solutions of native and heat-denatured (56°C for 30 minutes) types I and II collagen in PBS (50 μg/ml) were added to polyvinyl chloride round-bottom microtiter wells for 4 hours. Control wells incubated with PBS alone were used for each sample tested. Between steps, the wells were washed as described above. Synovial fluids and sera were diluted 1:200 in PBS-NBCS; the extracts were assayed undiluted. For the IgG antibody assays, the diluting and washing solutions contained dithiothreitol as described above. All samples were tested in duplicate. Seven standard rheumatoid synovial fluids positive for collagen antibodies were included for every determination. The assays were developed with affinity-purified ^{125}I-F(ab')$_2$ rabbit anti-human IgM or IgG containing 1–2 μg/ml and $\sim 10^6$ counts per minute/ml.

The results are expressed as ng of anti-IgM or anti-IgG bound per well. Samples binding ≥0.8 ng per well (mean + 2 SD) were considered positive. The collagen antibody assays were validated by testing 13 normal and 30 rheumatoid sera, as well as 17 rheumatoid, 8 inflammatory, and 13 osteoarthritic synovial fluids. The results shown in Table 1 are similar to values previously published (14,15). Absorption of RF by the addition of excess aggregated human IgG to cartilage extracts containing IgM-RF and type II collagen antibodies did not alter the collagen antibody titers that were present in the original samples (results not shown).

Table 1. Collagen antibodies in sera and synovial fluids

		Type II collagen antibodies (% positive)	
	n	Native	Denatured
Sera			
Rheumatoid arthritis	30	13	30
Control	13	0	0
Synovial fluids			
Rheumatoid arthritis	17	53	71
Inflammatory*	8	12	12
Osteoarthritis	13	0	0

* This group included 3 patients with gout, 1 with Reiter's syndrome, 1 with psoriatic arthritis, 1 with ankylosing spondylitis, and 2 with palindromic rheumatism.

Table 3. Immunoglobulin:albumin ratios in cartilage extracts and synovial fluids*

		Ratios†			
	n	IgM:HSA ± SEM		IgG:HSA ± SEM	
RA extracts	16	0.65 ± 0.4	(20.3)	2.1 ± 0.05	(11.1)
RA synovial fluids	15	0.032 ± 0.03		0.19 ± 0.03	
OA extracts	11	0.25 ± 0.1	(65.0)	2.1 ± 0.9	(26.3)
OA synovial fluids	9	0.004 ± 0.0007		0.08 ± 0.01	
Control extracts	6	0.026 ± 0.005		0.20 ± 0.02	

* HSA = human serum albumin; RA = rheumatoid arthritis; OA = osteoarthritis.
† Numbers in parentheses represent relative enrichment of Ig in cartilage extracts compared with synovial fluids.

RESULTS

The amounts of IgM and IgG measured in the collagenase extracts of the 3 groups of articular cartilage specimens are shown in Table 2. It is noteworthy that the rheumatoid cartilage extracts contained 14 and 37 times more IgG and IgM, respectively, than did the normal cartilage extracts, confirming the qualitative findings previously obtained in our laboratory by immunofluorescence ultraviolet microscopy (3). Moreover, there was evidence of increased IgM and IgG content in the OA specimens, which contained 3 times more IgG and IgM than the normal control tissues. Hyaluronidase extraction of the tissues prior to collagenase treatment yielded small amounts of Ig comparable with those found in the PBS washes (results not shown). However, collagenase digestion resulted in a 3–5-fold increase in Ig release, suggesting that a major part of the immune complexes were trapped by the collagen fiber meshwork (16).

Despite the exhaustive washing procedure to which the tissues had been subjected, it was still possible that the Ig extracted may have represented contaminating molecules that originated in the synovial fluids diffusing into the cartilage from the joint cavity. For this reason, HSA levels were measured in the collagenase extracts as a marker of synovial fluid protein contamination, and for comparison, in a group of 15 RA and 9 OA synovial fluids. The IgM:HSA and IgG:HSA ratios obtained are shown in Table 3. The relative Ig concentrations in rheumatoid synovial fluids approached the values found in sera in previous tests by other investigators (17). Comparison of the ratios measured in rheumatoid cartilage extracts indicated that there was an 11–20-fold relative enrichment of Ig with respect to synovial fluids. Similar measurements carried out with the OA extracts and synovial fluids yielded even higher relative Ig enrichments of 26-fold for IgG and 65-fold for IgM. The ratios found in the normal cartilage extracts were identical to the expected ratios in normal sera derived for the normal values for Ig and HSA. Normal synovial fluids were not available for comparison.

Table 2. Immunoglobulins in collagenase extracts of articular cartilage (ng/gm of tissue, mean ± SEM)

Cartilage extracts	n	IgM	IgG
Rheumatoid arthritis	16	3,575 ± 1,596	11,380 ± 3,423
Osteoarthritis	11	287 ± 95	2,602 ± 666
Normal control	6	97 ± 17	821 ± 111

The collagenase extracts were tested by radioimmunoassay for the presence of IgM-RF (Figure 1). Thirteen of the 16 RA supernatants showed variable amounts of IgM-RF, whereas no IgM-RF was detectable in the 6 normal and 11 OA specimens. Two of the 3 negative rheumatoid cartilage extracts were from seronegative patients (serum was not available from the third). Seven collagenase extracts from seropositive rheumatoid cartilage specimens and 5 from control OA tissues were assayed for IgG-RF. Four of the 7 rheumatoid extracts contained variable amounts of IgG-RF ranging from 122–1,710 ng/gm of tissue. None of 5 control extracts had detectable IgG-RF (<28 ng/gm of tissue) (Figure 2).

The PBS washes and hyaluronidase and collagenase extracts were assayed for the presence of IgM and IgG antibodies against native and denatured type II collagen (Table 4). Of the 27 extracts assayed, only 2 rheumatoid PBS washes showed the presence of small concentrations of collagen antibodies. Hyaluronidase treatment released small amounts of anti–denatured collagen antibodies from the rheumatoid tissues. However, collagenase digestion resulted in the release of

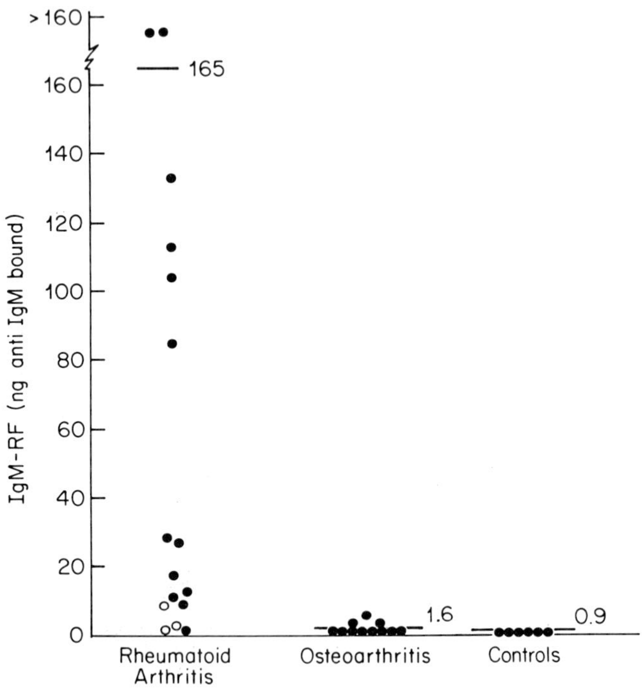

Figure 1. IgM rheumatoid factor (IgM-RF) in collagenase extracts of rheumatoid and osteoarthritic cartilage. Open circles represent extracts from seronegative patients. Numbers are the mean values for each group.

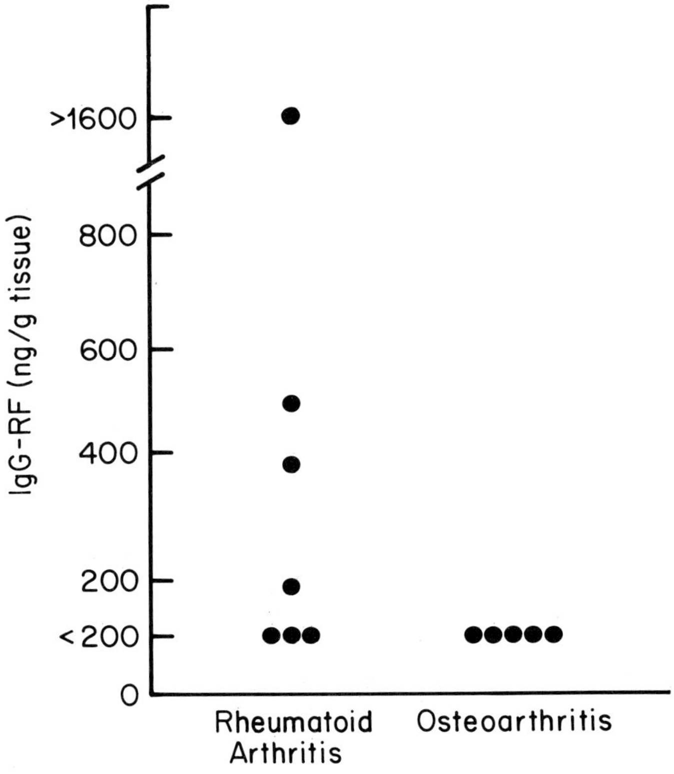

Figure 2. IgG rheumatoid factor (IgG-RF) in collagenase extracts of rheumatoid and osteoarthritic cartilage.

native and denatured anticollagen antibodies in more than 60% of the rheumatoid and 50% of the osteoarthritic tissues. None of the 6 normal tissue extracts contained detectable levels of anticollagen antibodies. The individual values for the IgM and IgG antibodies are shown in Figures 3 and 4. As a group, the collagen antibody titers found in the OA extracts were lower than those found in the rheumatoid digests. However, the Ig concentrations in the latter were several times higher than in the osteoarthritic specimens (Table 2), which suggests that the Ig extracted from OA cartilage was relatively enriched for collagen antibodies. The mean values for all extracts assayed are shown in Table 5.

To investigate the species specificities of the antibodies extracted, the samples were also tested with chick type II collagen. The fact that all positive extracts for bovine collagen were also positive for the chick protein and vice versa suggests wide cross-reactivity between chick and bovine collagen. Comparison of the results obtained with native and heat-denatured collagens also indicated the presence of heterogeneous antibody subpopulations with wide specificities and cross-reactivities. As noted previously by others (15), in sera and synovial fluids, the majority of the cartilage extracts contained antibodies that reacted with both native and denatured molecules. Similar data were obtained when the extracts were assayed for the presence of antibodies against bovine type I collagen (Table 5). Most extracts exhibiting reactivity against type II collagen also contained antibodies against type I collagen. However, the extracts containing antibodies against type I collagen tended to react mainly with the native molecule, whereas little difference in reactivity was detected between native and denatured type II collagen.

Collagenase extracts from menisci of 4 osteoar-

Table 4. IgM and IgG antibodies to native and denatured type II collagen in rheumatoid and osteoarthritic cartilage extracts*

	Extracts					
	PBS		Hyaluronidase		Collagenase	
	N	D	N	D	N	D
Rheumatoid arthritis	2/16	2/16	2/16	8/16	9/16	10/16
Osteoarthritis	0/11	0/11	0/11	2/11	5/11	6/11

* PBS = phosphate buffered saline; N = native collagen; D = denatured collagen. Values expressed as number positive/total.

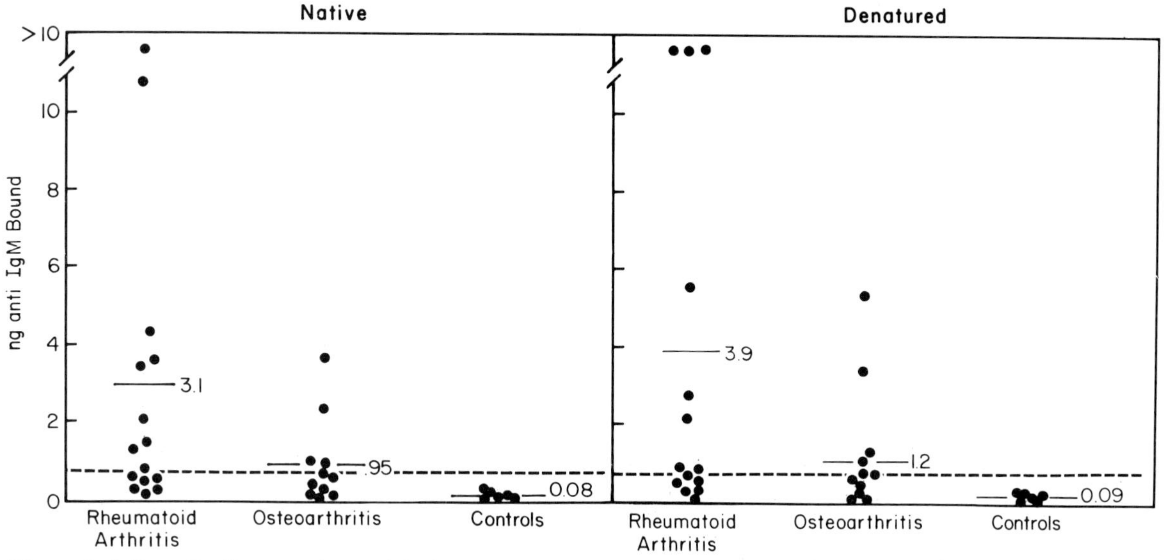

Figure 3. IgM antibodies to native and denatured type II collagen in collagenase extracts of rheumatoid, osteoarthritic, and normal cartilage. Values above the broken line are considered positive. Numbers are the mean values for each group.

thritic and 9 normal trauma patients were also tested for autoantibodies. None of the 13 extracts contained detectable RF. All 4 osteoarthritic extracts contained anticollagen antibodies, with average titers of 2.3 ng for IgG anti–native and 1.3 ng for IgG anti–denatured type II collagen. The specimens obtained from the trauma patients were uniformly negative.

DISCUSSION

A variety of immunologic mechanisms have been clearly implicated in the pathogenesis of RA (18). The rheumatoid synovial membrane contains large numbers of inflammatory cells, among them plasma cells, which synthesize and secrete immunoglobulins and autoantibodies in amounts comparable in magnitude with those synthesized and secreted by spleen and lymph node cells (7). Thus, it is reasonable to assume that the composition of immune complexes found in rheumatoid cartilage (3) may reflect the antibody specificities commonly found in synovial fluids. Although the pathogenic significance of the immune complexes sequestered in rheumatoid articu-

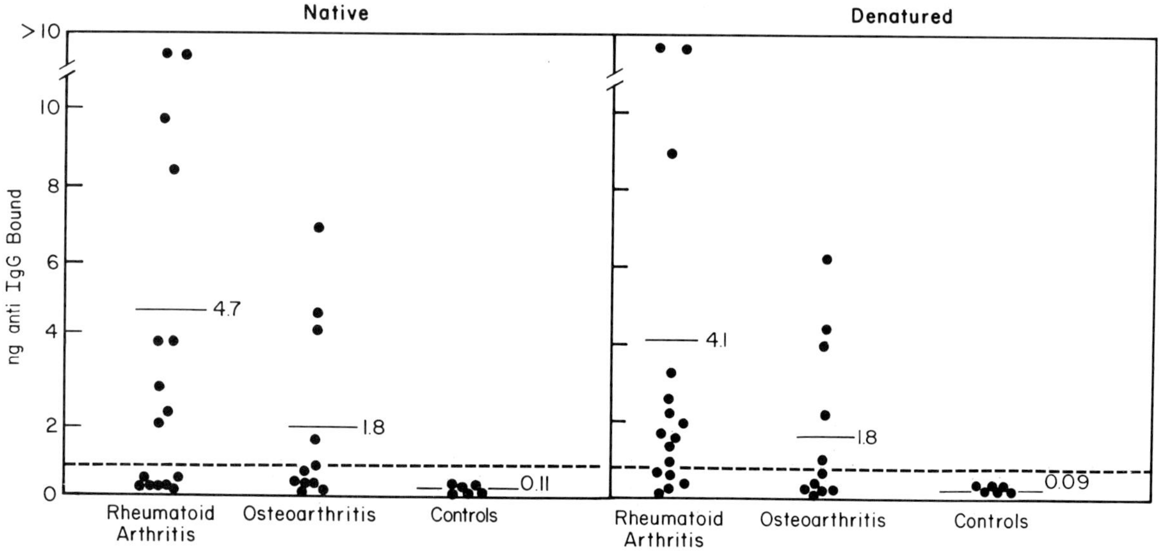

Figure 4. IgG antibodies to native and denatured type II collagen in collagenase extracts of rheumatoid, osteoarthritic, and normal cartilage. Values above the broken line are considered positive. Numbers are the mean values for each group.

Table 5. Collagen antibodies extracted from rheumatoid and osteoarthritic articular cartilage*

	Type II collagen antibodies				Type I collagen antibodies			
Tissue extracts	Native, IgM	Native, IgG	Denatured, IgM	Denatured, IgG	Native, IgM	Native, IgG	Denatured, IgM	Denatured, IgG
Rheumatoid arthritis	3.1 ± 1.3	4.7 ± 1.7	3.9 ± 1.4	4.1 ± 1.5	4.0 ± 2.0	2.2 ± 0.8	1.9 ± 1.2	1.2 ± 0.6
Osteoarthritis	0.95 ± 0.3	1.8 ± 0.6	1.2 ± 0.4	1.8 ± 0.5	2.2 ± 0.8	1.9 ± 0.6	1.1 ± 0.4	0.8 ± 0.3

* Values expressed as ng of anti-Ig bound, mean ± SEM.

lar cartilage is not known, previous studies in our laboratory have suggested that they may play a role in the generation of invasive pannus (4) and in irreversible cartilage matrix degradation (5,6). For these reasons, it was considered important to investigate the possible autoantibody specificities of Ig trapped in cartilage. The presence of autoantibodies sequestered in avascular joint collagenous tissues would provide an explanation for the self-perpetuating and chronic destructive features that are the hallmark of RA.

Our studies confirm and extend previous qualitative observations made in our laboratory, showing that immune complexes trapped within joint collagenous tissues were found in the majority of patients with RA (3). Exhaustive washing of finely minced cartilage specimens was carried out to ensure that the immunoglobulins released by collagenase digestion represented sequestered immune complexes and not merely loosely bound immunoglobulins derived from synovial fluid bathing the tissues. Several findings indicated that this was the case. Increasing the cartilage permeability for large molecules by hyaluronidase digestion to facilitate diffusion did not significantly increase the Ig released, whereas collagenase digestion resulted in a 3–5-fold increase in Ig in the extracts. Moreover, simultaneous measurements of HSA as a marker of synovial fluid contamination confirmed these findings.

Comparison of Ig:HSA ratios between RA and OA extracts and synovial fluids indicated that there was an 11–65-fold enrichment of Ig in the tissue digests. In addition, rheumatoid cartilage extracts contained 14–37 times more IgG and IgM than did normal cartilage. Finally, the presence of collagen antibodies in osteoarthritic cartilage and its absence in synovial fluids indicated that the immunoglobulins extracted from cartilage were part of immune complexes sequestered within the collagen meshwork or bound to matrix macromolecules.

Of interest was our finding that osteoarthritic tissue released significantly more Ig than did tissues from normal controls. We had previously reported that more than 30% of "primary" osteoarthritis joint collagenous tissues contained immune complexes detectable by immunofluorescence microscopy (19). The significance of those findings was not readily apparent at that time. The presence of trapped Ig coupled with the frequent detection of collagen antibodies in the osteoarthritic cartilage extracts suggests that immune complex deposition may be a common feature in this disease.

IgM-RF was detected by radioimmunoassay in 13 of 16 rheumatoid cartilage specimens and in none of 11 osteoarthritic and 6 normal cartilage extracts. Of the 3 negative rheumatoid extracts, 2 were from seronegative patients, and serum was not available from the third. IgG-RF was also found in 4 of the 7 seropositive rheumatoid specimens tested. It is likely that the failure to detect this autoantibody more frequently was due, in part, to the much lower sensitivity of the assay which requires pepsin digestion of each sample (11). Thus, the immune complexes trapped in rheumatoid cartilage probably reflect the specificities present in synovial fluid over a period of time. However, trapping of these autoantibodies within the tissues would also depend on their capacity to form large and relatively insoluble immune complexes once they penetrate the tissues (16). It is possible that the relative avidities of RF in synovial fluids may differ from those of RF molecules trapped in cartilage. Studies on this issue are currently in progress.

Trapped collagen antibodies were found in more than 60% of rheumatoid cartilage specimens extracted. The incidence of positive extracts approached that found for rheumatoid synovial fluids. Unfortunately, it was not possible to obtain fluids from the patients prior to surgery, so a side-by-side comparison of the quantitative and qualitative properties of the collagen antibodies in both compartments could not be carried out. The presence of collagen antibodies in 50% of the osteoarthritic cartilage extracts was an unexpected finding. Inflammatory synovitis and pannus formation do not constitute a prominent feature in osteoarthritis. However, our previous studies (19) showed that immune complexes were frequently detected in the group of osteoarthritic patients with "primary" disease, which may show a prominent inflammatory component (20,21) associated with evidence of severe cartilage deterioration (21,22). It is likely that the incidence of positive extracts may reflect a minimum estimate of the actual occurrence of autoantibodies, since the enzymatic digestion steps involved in extraction may have destroyed part of the antibody reactivities. Moreover, solid-phase radioimmunoassays tend to detect only high avidity antibodies.

Analysis of the specificity of the extracted antibodies suggested wide interspecies cross-reactivity and the presence of antibody populations reacting both with native and denatured types I and II collagen. This pattern has been noticed previously by other investigators, in sera and synovial fluids obtained from patients with rheumatoid arthritis (14,15). Absorption studies are in progress to establish if the cross-reactions observed represent distinct antibodies to different epitopes present in the native and denatured molecules. It is likely that only a restricted subpopulation of antibodies with distinct specificity to native type II collagen may have pathogenic significance. In the rodent model of collagen-induced arthritis, for instance, the disease develops only after immunization with native type II collagen (23–25).

The presence of trapped collagen antibodies in osteoarthritic cartilage and menisci extracts associated with increased total immunoglobulins within these tissues indicates that sequestration of immune complexes in cartilage is not a phenomenon seen exclusively in rheumatoid arthritis. Indeed, cellular and humoral immunity to collagen has been detected with variable frequency in many diseases where chronic connective tissue injury and collagen degradation constitute a prominent feature (15,26–28). The suggestion that the emergence of collagen antibodies may be secondary to collagen degradation does not exclude the possibility that one or more of the antibody subpopulations may play a prominent role in the facilitation of tissue injury and in the maintenance of chronic and progressive cartilage damage. There is persuasive evidence derived from clinical observations and animal investigations to support this hypothesis. In patients with relapsing polychondritis, collagen antibody titers are detected almost exclusively in patients with active, untreated disease (28,29). In the experimental model of collagen-induced arthritis in rodents, it has been shown recently that the disease can be passively transferred with serum concentrates obtained from animals immunized against native type II collagen (30,31). In addition, the infused collagen antibodies localized in the superficial areas of articular cartilage (32), which is the same anatomic localization found in the human counterpart (3). The facilitating role of these antibodies in the induction of chronic polyarthritis is clearly illustrated by recent investigations carried out by Taurog et al (33), who have shown that passive transfer of adjuvant arthritis in the rat by immune spleen cells is facilitated, and the severity of the arthritis significantly enhanced, by previous injection of the recipients with sera containing collagen antibodies.

The possible pathogenic role of collagen antibodies in a relatively noninflammatory disease such as osteoarthritis is more difficult to surmise. Although there are no studies dealing with possible interactions of these antibodies with chondrocytes, Maoz et al (34) demonstrated that antibodies against a collagen-like synthetic peptide and antisera against rat tail collagen had a specific cytotoxic activity against rat embryo fibroblasts, suggesting the presence of collagen-like molecules on the fibroblast membrane. Moreover, in the collagen-induced arthritis in rats, widespread cartilage chondrocyte degeneration is apparent in the early stages of the disease (35). It is therefore possible that collagen antibodies may play a pathogenic role in osteoarthritis by interacting directly with the chondrocyte, inducing functional alterations and cell death. This hypothesis should be easily amenable to experimental verification.

The present studies do not add evidence that would permit us to assign an unequivocal pathogenic role to the immune complexes trapped in cartilage. However, their availability and the delineation of their autoantibody specificities will allow us to investigate further their pathophysiologic significance. The present findings provide a possible pathogenic mechanism to explain the self-perpetuating and chronic nature of rheumatoid arthritis and osteoarthritis.

ACKNOWLEDGMENTS

I am grateful to Dr. Morris Ziff and to Dale Edelbaum for measurements of IgG rheumatoid factor in the cartilage extracts, to Ellis Lightfoot for expert technical help, and to Debbie McInnis for excellent secretarial assistance.

REFERENCES

1. Ball J: Pathological aspects of rheumatoid arthritis, Early Synovectomy in Rheumatoid Arthritis. Edited by W Hijmans, WD Paul, H Herschel. Amsterdam, Excerpta Medica, 1969, p 23

2. Gardner DL: The Pathology of Rheumatoid Arthritis. Baltimore, Williams & Wilkins, 1982, p 27
3. Cooke TD, Hurd ER, Jasin HE, Bienenstock J, Ziff M: Identification of immunoglobulins and complement in rheumatoid articular collagenous tissues. Arthritis Rheum 18:541–551, 1975
4. Jasin HE, Cooke TD: The inflammatory role of immune complexes in joint collagenous tissues. Clin Exp Immunol 33:416–424, 1978
5. Jasin HE, Dingle JT: Human mononuclear cell factors mediate cartilage matrix degradation through chondrocyte activation. J Clin Invest 68:571–581, 1981
6. Jasin HE: Factors controlling articular cartilage degradation by activation of chondrocytes, Advances in Inflammation Research. Vol. 5. Edited by G Weissmann. New York, Raven Press, 1983, pp 87–105
7. Smiley JD, Sachs C, Ziff M: In vitro synthesis of immunoglobulin by rheumatoid synovial membrane. J Clin Invest 47:624–632, 1968
8. Sliwinsky AS, Zvaifler NJ: In vivo synthesis of IgG by the rheumatoid synovium. J Lab Clin Med 76:304–310, 1970
9. Trelstad RL, Kang AH, Toole BP, Gross J: Collagen heterogeneity. J Biol Chem 247:6469–6473, 1973
10. LoSpalluto J, Chegoriansky J, Lewis A, Ziff M: Chromatographic properties of gamma globulin: behavior of serum gamma macroglobulins. J Clin Invest 39:473–480, 1960
11. Wernick R, LoSpalluto JJ, Fink CW, Ziff M: Serum IgG and IgM rheumatoid factors by solid phase radioimmunoassay: a comparison between adult and juvenile rheumatoid arthritis. Arthritis Rheum 24:1501–1511, 1981
12. Olsen N, Ziff M, Jasin HE: In vitro synthesis of immunoglobulins and IgM-rheumatoid factor by blood mononuclear cells of patients with rheumatoid arthritis. Rheumatol Int 2:59–66, 1982
13. Clague RB, Brown RA, Weiss JB, Holt PJL: Solid-phase radioimmunoassay for the detection of antibodies to collagen. J Immunol Methods 27:31–41, 1979
14. Steffen C: Collagen as an autoantigen in rheumatoid arthritis, Studies in Joint Disease. Edited by A Maroudas, EJ Holborow. Turnbridge Wells, UK, Pitman Medical Publishing Co., 1981, p 201
15. Stuart JM, Huffstutter EH, Townes AS, Kang AH: Incidence and specificity of antibodies to types I, II, III, IV, and V collagen in rheumatoid arthritis and other rheumatic diseases as measured by ^{125}I-radioimmunoassay. Arthritis Rheum 26:832–840, 1983
16. Jasin HE: Mechanism of trapping of immune complexes in joint collagenous tissues. Clin Exp Immunol 22:473–485, 1975
17. Cecere F, Lessard J, McDuffy S, Pope RM: Evidence for the local production and utilization of immune reactants in rheumatoid arthritis. Arthritis Rheum 25:1307–1315, 1982
18. Zvaifler NJ: The immunopathology of joint inflammation in rheumatoid arthritis. Adv Immunol 16:265–336, 1973
19. Cooke TDV, Richer S, Hurd E, Jasin HE: Localization of antigen-antibody complexes in intraarticular collagenous tissues. Ann NY Acad Sci 256:10–24, 1975
20. Ehrlich GE: Osteoarthritis beginning with inflammation. JAMA 232:157–159, 1975
21. Huskisson EC, Dieppe PA, Tucker AK, Cannell LB: Another look at osteoarthritis. Ann Rheum Dis 38:423–428, 1979
22. Kellgren JH, Moore R: Generalized osteoarthritis and Heberden's nodes. Br Med J i:181–184, 1952
23. Trentham DE, Townes AS, Kang AH: Autoimmunity to type II collagen: an experimental model of arthritis. J Exp Med 146:857–869, 1977
24. Courtenay JS, Dallman MJ, Dayan AD, Martin A, Mosedale B: Immunization against heterologous type II collagen induces arthritis in mice. Nature 283:666–668, 1980
25. Wooley PH, Luthra HS, Stuart JM, David CS: Type II collagen-induced arthritis in mice. I. Major histocompatibility complex (I region) linkage and antibody correlates. J Exp Med 154:688–700, 1981
26. Gioud M, Meghlaoui A, Costa O, Mouier JC: Antibodies to native type I and II collagens detected by an enzyme linked immunosorbent assay (ELISA) in rheumatoid arthritis and systemic lupus erythematosus. Coll Relat Res 2:557–560, 1982
27. Stuart JM, Postlethwaite AE, Kang AH: Evidence for cell-mediated immunity to collagen in progressive systemic sclerosis. J Lab Clin Med 88:601–607, 1976
28. Foidart JM, Shigeto S, Martin GR, Zizic TM, Barnett EV, Lawley TJ, Katz SI: Antibodies to type II collagen in relapsing polychondritis. N Engl J Med 299:1203–1207, 1978
29. Ebringer R, Rook G, Swana GT, Botazzo GF, Doniach D: Autoantibodies to cartilage type II collagen in relapsing polychondritis and other rheumatic diseases. Ann Rheum Dis 40:473–479, 1981
30. Stuart JM, Cremer MA, Townes AS, Kang AH: Type II collagen-induced arthritis in rats: passive transfer with serum and evidence that IgG anticollagen antibodies can cause arthritis. J Exp Med 155:1–7, 1982
31. Stuart JM, Dixon FJ: Serum transfer of collagen-induced arthritis in mice. J Exp Med 158:378–392, 1983
32. Stuart JM, Tomoda K, Yoo TJ, Townes AS, Kang AH: Serum transfer of collagen-induced arthritis. II. Identification and localization of autoantibody to type II collagen in donor and recipient rats. Arthritis Rheum 26:1237–1244, 1983
33. Taurog JD, Kerwar SS, McReynolds RA, Mahowald ML: Striking synergy between passively transferred collagen-induced and adjuvant-induced arthritis in rats (abstract). Arthritis Rheum (suppl) 27:S23, 1984
34. Maoz A, Dym H, Fuchs S, Sela M: Cytotoxic activity of antibodies to a collagen-like synthetic polytripeptide on cells in tissue culture. Eur J Immunol 3:839–842, 1973
35. DeSimone DP, Parsons DB, Johnson KE, Jacobs RP: Type II collagen–induced arthritis: a morphologic and biochemical study of articular cartilage. Arthritis Rheum 26:1245–1258, 1983

PROGNOSTIC FACTORS IN POLYMYOSITIS/DERMATOMYOSITIS

A Computer-Assisted Analysis of Ninety-Two Cases

JOCHANAN BENBASSAT, DOV GEFEL, KEREN LARHOLT, SHAUL SUKENIK, VLADIMIR MORGENSTERN, and AVINOAM ZLOTNICK

An effort was made to identify all patients with polymyositis/dermatomyositis (PM/DM) admitted to hospitals in Israel from 1956–1976. The diagnosis of PM/DM was retrospectively reviewed in 92 (46 definite, 26 probable, and 20 possible) cases. The most common complaints and physical findings in the course of the disease were muscle weakness (86 patients), rash (53 patients), arthritis or arthralgia (39 patients), and dysphagia (35 patients). Elevated serum aldolase levels were found in 64% of the patients for whom data were available; 92% had abnormal electromyogram results, and 60.9% had muscle histopathology consistent with PM/DM. Malignancy was diagnosed in 13 patients. Malignancy, ischemic heart disease, and pulmonary complications were the most common causes of death. The actuarial survival curve was heterogeneous, with an accelerated mortality during the first year after diagnosis and a slower mortality during the following 7 years. Independent unfavorable prognostic signs were: failure to induce remission, leukocytosis, fever, older age, a shorter disease history, and dysphagia.

From the Department of Medicine and the Medical Computing Unit, Hadassah University Hospital, Jerusalem; and the Department of Medicine and Medical Computing Unit, Soroka Medical Center, Beer Sheva, Israel.

Jochanan Benbassat, MD: Department of Medicine, Hadassah University Hospital; Dov Gefel, MD: Department of Medicine, Hadassah University Hospital; Keren Larholt, BA: Medical Computing Unit, Soroka Medical Center; Shaul Sukenik, MD: Department of Medicine, Soroka Medical Center; Vladimir Morgenstern: Medical Computing Unit, Hadassah University Hospital; Avinoam Zlotnick, MSc, MD: Department of Medicine, Hadassah University Hospital.

Address reprint requests to J. Benbassat, MD, Department of Medicine, Hadassah University Hospital, Mt. Scopus, PO Box 24035, Jerusalem, 91240, Israel.

Submitted for publication August 29, 1983; accepted in revised form September 7, 1984.

There are several studies of survival in polymyositis/dermatomyositis (PM/DM) (1–5). Mortality in this disorder has been reported to be between 13.7% (6) and 50% (7) within an unspecified length of follow-up period. Associated autoimmune disease (4,8) and malignancy (4,6,8), the length and severity of the illness (5,8), age (2,4), and childhood onset of polymyositis (9) have been reported to be predictive of a reduced length of survival. On the other hand, Bohan et al (6) reported favorable survival statistics for all groups of patients with PM/DM, with the exception of those with associated malignancy, and there were no deaths among the patients with childhood DM reported by Sullivan et al (10).

The differences in the reported mortality in PM/DM, and the conflicting conclusions on the prognostic significance of the various manifestations of the disease could be because of limited interpretation of followup data. We know of only one study (3) of the actuarial survival of patients with PM/DM. This report is a retrospective computer-assisted analysis of all the hospital records we were able to collect, between 1956 and 1976, of PM/DM patients in Israel. An attempt is made to determine the effect of the various manifestations of PM/DM on the actuarial survival of the patients in order to identify factors of possible prognostic significance.

METHODS

The archives of the general hospitals in Israel, all of which maintain medical research indexing systems, were searched for patients discharged between 1956 and 1976 with diagnoses of polymyositis, dermatomyositis, or myositis. Each chart was evaluated according to the criteria of Bohan et al (6): (a) symmetric muscle weakness; (b) typical histologic findings on muscle biopsy; (c) increased levels of muscle enzymes in the serum; (d) compatible electromyographic (EMG) findings; and (e) characteristic dermatologic manifestations. Patients suspected of having muscular dystrophy, endocrinopathy, alcoholism, muscle infections, or evidence of a central or peripheral nervous system disease were excluded from the study.

One hundred sixty charts were reviewed, and 92 cases partially or completely fulfilled the diagnostic criteria. PM/DM was considered definite in 46 patients who presented at least 4 manifestations, probable in 26 patients with 3, and possible in 20 patients with 2 of the 5 manifestations. There were 30 known deaths with 16 autopsies. Classification by diagnostic category (group I: primary idiopathic polymyositis [PM]; group II: primary idiopathic dermatomyositis [DM]; group III: polymyositis with malignancy [PM/DM–Mal]; group IV: polymyositis of childhood onset [PM/DM–Child]; group V: overlap syndromes [PM/DM–Os]) was according to the criteria of Bohan et al (6). PM/DM–Child was defined as PM/DM in a subject age 18 or less.

The available clinical, laboratory, and followup data were compiled according to a predesignated format, and a digital computer was used for their analysis. Followup information was limited to that found in the patients' hospital and outpatient department records. In December 1980, information on additional deaths was obtained from the Ministry for Internal Affairs, which keeps a central registry of vital records. The large number of attending physicians and the heterogeneity of the clinical departments involved precluded standardization of the assessment of muscle strength and dysphagia. Therefore, muscle weakness and dysphagia were assumed to have been present whenever recorded as such in the patients' charts. Remission was defined as an increase in muscle strength, or 2 or more of the following: disappearance of skin rash, normalization of muscle enzyme levels in serum, and normalization in EMG tracings.

Survival functions were processed by the biomedical computer program P series of the University of California Press, 1979 (BMDP 79). The Berkson and Gage (11) option was selected for actuarial survivorship curves. The differences between curves were tested by the analogs of nonparametric rank tests provided by the program, the Breslow and Mantel-Cox tests (12,13). Both statistics are asymptotically distributed as chi-square. The Breslow test gives greater weight to early observations and is less sensitive to late events which occur when few study patients remain alive (12,14). Independent risk factors were identified by stepwise logistic regression using the BMDP-81 statistical software of the University of California.

RESULTS

Incidence. Data on the age-adjusted annual incidence rates of PM/DM in Israel derived from the patients in this series have been presented elsewhere (15). Briefly, there were 2.18 new cases annually per 1,000,000 population. The age distribution was heterogeneous, with modes in the second and seventh decades and with a relatively low incidence among subjects in their twenties. The male:female ratio among patients <60 years old was 0.14–0.57, while that among patients ≥ 60 was 1.10–1.50. DeVere and Bradley (4) have also found the female preponderance to be restricted to patients aged 55 or less.

Clinical features. Patients with childhood polymyositis comprised 21.7% of our series. Another 31.5% were classified as having primary idiopathic dermatomyositis, and 19.6% had primary idiopathic polymyositis. The remaining patients had overlap syndromes (13.0%) and polymyositis with malignancy (14.1%). The time interval from first manifestation of the disease to diagnosis was 1 year or less in 69 patients, the average for the whole series being 13.0 months. Patients with PM/DM–Mal, PM/DM–Child, and PM/DM–Os presented with nonsignificantly shorter disease histories than did those with PM or DM.

Skin rash was the most common presenting complaint in DM and PM/DM–Mal, muscle weakness in PM and PM/DM–Child, and arthralgia in PM/DM–Os. The most common complaints throughout the duration of the disease were muscle weakness (93.5%), muscle pain (46.7%), rash (57.6%), and arthralgia (42.4%). By definition, skin rash characterized DM and was never present in PM. It was observed in 76.9% of the patients with PM/DM–Mal, in half of those with PM/DM–Child, and in one-third of the patients with PM/DM–Os. Dysphagia was reported by 38.0% of the patients and it was nonsignificantly more common in PM/DM–Mal and PM/DM–Child. Temperature above 38°C was found in 21.7%, while hepatomegaly, splenomegaly, and lymphadenopathy were found in 31.5, 20.7, and 10.9% of the patients, respectively.

Laboratory findings. The EMG results were abnormal in 72 (92.3%) of the 78 patients examined. There were no differences in the frequency of EMG disturbances among the various diagnostic categories. Muscle biopsies were interpreted as compatible with polymyositis in 60.9% of the 80 cases that had available data. Abnormal histologic findings were seen in 85% of the muscle biopsies in PM/DM–Child, but only in 30.8% of those in PM/DM–Mal ($P < 0.05$).

Serum aspartate aminotransferase (AST), creatine phosphokinase (CPK), aldolase (ALD), and lactic dehydrogenase (LDH) exceeded twice the upper level of normal in 39 of 83 (47.0%), 33 of 66 (50.0%, 29 of 45 (64.4%), and 34 of 59 (57.6%) cases with available data, respectively. The highest incidence of muscle enzyme abnormalities was observed in PM/DM–Child.

The levels of AST, CPK, ALD, and LDH correlated significantly ($P < 0.005$) with one another, although product-moment correlations were generally low (0.290–0.495).

Rheumatoid factor was found in the sera of 6 patients with PM/DM–Os and in 1 patient with PM. Rheumatoid arthritis was diagnosed in 6 of the patients with PM/DM–Os, scleroderma was diagnosed in 4, and Sjögren's syndrome in 2. Antinuclear antibodies (ANA) were found in the sera of 23.6% of the 55 patients with available data and were evenly distributed among the various diagnostic categories. In most cases the ANA titers were not recorded in the patients' charts. White blood cell counts exceeded 10,000/μl in 12 (15.6%) of the 77 patients with available data. There were no marked abnormalities in red blood cell counts or in liver functions. Blood urea nitrogen (BUN) levels exceeded 50 mg/dl in 11.9%, and proteinuria was found in 14.5% of the patients.

Cardiac and electrocardiographic abnormalities. Electrocardiogram (EKG) results were available for 73 patients. EKG abnormalities, including nonspecific ST-T changes, supraventricular arrhythmias, Q waves, and conduction disorders, were detected at the time of diagnosis in 23 patients (31.5%). In 11 of these 23 patients, the EKG abnormalities could be accounted for by an associated hypertensive (4 patients), ischemic (5 patients), or pulmonary (2 patients) heart disease. In the 4 patients with hypertensive heart disease, arterial hypertension preceded the diagnosis of PM/DM by 2, 3, 5, and 10 years. In 5 patients, ischemic and/or hypertensive heart disease was thought to be the primary cause of death.

The abnormalities on the EKGs of the remaining 12 patients were paroxysmal atrial tachycardia (3 patients), ST-T changes (6 patients), and conduction disturbances (3 patients). None of the 16 autopsies revealed edema, lymphocytic infiltration, necrosis, or other inflammatory myocardial changes which have been described in PM/DM (16). However, the amount of effort invested in the search for such changes in the patients is unknown.

Pulmonary manifestations. Twelve patients had lung involvement, and in 8 of these 12, pulmonary disease was thought to be the primary cause of death. Interstitial lung disease (17) was diagnosed in 2 patients and was confirmed at autopsy in 1. Pulmonary emboli were the suspected cause of sudden death in 3 patients, and this was confirmed at autopsy in 1. The most common pulmonary involvement was pneumonia. It was found at autopsy in 7 patients and was the main cause of death in 4 of them. The extent to which aspiration contributed to the development of pneumonia was not recorded.

Polymyositis with malignancy. Thirteen patients (14.1%; 3 with PM, 10 with DM) had malignancies, including Hodgkin's lymphoma, angiosarcoma, and carcinoma of the bronchus, stomach, colon, breast, ovary, and prostate. Malignant tumors were found in 6 (18%) of the 34 male patients in this series and in 7 (12%) of the 58 female patients. The diagnoses of PM/DM and malignancy were made simultaneously at

Table 1. Recorded primary causes of death in 30 patients with polymyositis/dermatomyositis, by diagnostic category*

	PM (n = 18)	DM (n = 29)	PM/DM–Mal (n = 13)	PM/DM–Child (n = 20)	PM/DM–Os (n = 12)	Total (n = 92)
Uncontrolled activity		2		1		3 (10.0%)
Pulmonary		4	2	2		8 (26.7%)
Cardiac		4			1	5 (16.7%)
Cerebrovascular		1				1 (3.3%)
Malignancy			5			5 (16.7%)
Uremia	1		2			3 (10.0%)
Not given	2	1	1		1	5 (16.7%)
All causes	3	12	10	3	2	30 (100%)
Total mortality in diagnostic category (%)	16.6	41.4	76.9	15.0	16.6	32.6
Length of followup (person years)	22.5	79.2	22.7	26.2	10.7	161.3
Mortality per person years followup (×100)	13.3	15.2	44.0	11.5	18.6	18.6

* PM = polymyositis; DM = dermatomyositis; Mal = malignancy; Child = childhood onset; Os = overlap syndromes.

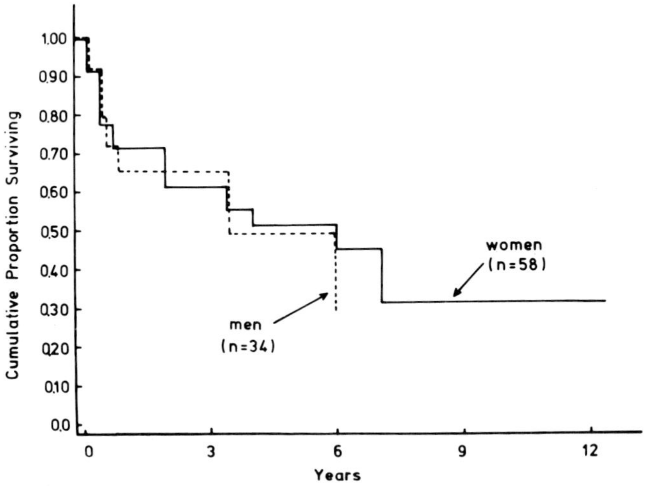

Figure 1. Actuarial survival since diagnosis of 92 patients with polymyositis/dermatomyositis, by sex. After 6 years followup, only 1 man and 7 women remained in the study.

presentation in 8 patients. In 2 patients, the malignant neoplasm was detected 1 month and 8 months prior to diagnosis of PM/DM. In the remaining 3 patients, the diagnosis of PM/DM preceded that of malignancy by 6, 18, and 24 months. The frequency of malignancy increased with age. Malignant tumors were found in 1 (3%) of the 34 patients aged 40 years or less, 5 (16%) of the 32 patients aged 41–59, and in 7 (27%) of the 26 patients aged 60 or more.

Survival and factors of possible prognostic significance. Malignancy, ischemic heart disease, and pulmonary complications were the most common causes of the 30 known deaths. Three patients died of uremia and 3 died from uncontrolled activity of PM/DM (Table 1). Actuarial survival depicted a heterogeneous curve, which revealed an accelerated mortality the first year after diagnosis and a slower mortality over the following 7 years. There were no

Table 2. Factors affecting actuarial survival of 92 patients since diagnosis of polymyositis/dermatomyositis

	Cumulative proportion surviving after (months)			*P*	
Variable*	9	36	72	Breslow test	Mantel-Cox test
Sex					
Men (34)	0.72	0.66	0.30	0.8323	0.8802
Women (58)	0.75	0.61	0.46		
Interval from first manifestation to diagnosis					
<7 months (53)	0.65	0.49	0.27	0.0308	0.0082
>7 months (37)	0.88	0.82	0.63		
Diagnostic category					
PM (18)	1.00	0.56	0.28	0.3362	0.2874
DM (29)	0.67	0.66	0.50		
PM/DM–Mal (13)	0.62	0.44	0.22		
PM/DM–Child (20)	0.86	0.75	–		
PM/DM–Os (12)	0.72	0.72	–		
Age at diagnosis (years)					
<20 (23)	0.88	0.78		0.0855	0.0304
21–60 (46)	0.79	0.64	0.51		
>61 (23)	0.55	0.49	0.17		
Temperature (°C)					
<38 (72)	0.86	0.74	0.49	0.0006	0.0001
>38 (20)	0.36	0.24	0.24		
Remission achieved					
Yes (57)	0.85	0.78	0.59	0.0000	0.0000
No (17)	0.34	0.26	–		
White blood cells					
<10,000/μl (65)	0.78	0.68	0.50	0.0003	0.0000
>10,000/μl (12)	0.39	–	–		
Dysphagia					
No (57)	0.84	0.81	0.51	0.0072	0.0066
Yes (35)	0.60	0.36	0.28		
Rash					
Yes (53)	0.64	0.54	0.43	0.0341	0.1482
No (39)	0.92	0.77	0.36		

* Figures in parentheses indicate the number of patients with available data. See Table 1 for diagnostic category abbreviation definitions.

Table 3. Stepwise logistic regression analysis of the effect of variables on actuarial survival of 92 patients with polymyositis/dermatomyositis diagnosed in Israel between 1956 and 1976

Step no.	Variable entered	Entered as	Improvement		Global	
			χ^2	P	χ^2	P
1	Clinical remission	Yes/no	12.674	0.000	15.307	0.000
2	Leukocyte count	Number	9.687	0.002	30.138	0.000
3	Temperature	°C	9.108	0.003	39.754	0.000
4	Age	Years	9.063	0.003	45.620	0.000
5	Time since first manifestation	Months	3.857	0.050	45.942	0.000
6	Dysphagia	Yes/no	3.117	0.077	50.484	0.000

differences in length of survival time for male and female patients (Figure 1).

Patients with PM/DM–Mal had a higher mortality rate than those in the remaining diagnostic categories (Table 1). The mortality of patients with PM/DM–Mal was 44.0 per 100 person years of followup, but it was only 11.5–18.6 in the remaining diagnostic categories. There were no significant differences in actuarial survival among the various diagnostic categories, probably because of the small numbers of patients (Table 2).

A shorter disease history, rash, dysphagia, temperature above 38°C, older age, leukocyte counts exceeding 10,000/μl at diagnosis, and failure to induce a clinical remission were associated with a significantly reduced actuarial survival (Table 2). BUN levels >30 mg/dl, proteinuria, and elevated serum aldolase levels were associated with a nonsignificantly shorter actuarial survival. Stepwise logistic regression revealed that failure to induce a clinical remission, leukocyte counts of $\geq$10,000/μl at diagnosis, temperature above 38°C at diagnosis, and older age were independent risk factors. A shorter disease history and dysphagia contributed to mortality with borderline significance (Table 3).

Stepwise logistic regression using entry variables only (i.e., excluding clinical remission) showed that white blood count, temperature, and age remained independent significant risk indicators (P = 0.004, 0.002, and 0.011, respectively). Repeated analysis after excluding 12 patients with pulmonary involvement identified only white blood cell count (P = 0.001) and age (P = 0.005) as independent risk factors. Temperature contributed to mortality with borderline significance (P = 0.07).

Survival was not affected by the presence of arthritis or arthralgia, abnormal histologic findings on muscle biopsy, increased levels of 1 or more of the remaining muscle enzymes, erythrocyte sedimentation rate, abnormalities revealed in the EMG tracing, hemoglobin level, presence of Raynaud's phenomenon, antinuclear antibodies in the serum, blood pressure at diagnosis, abnormalities shown in the EKG, splenomegaly, or degree of certainty in the diagnosis.

DISCUSSION

The presented data should be interpreted with caution. They are based on a retrospective study of a relatively small number of patients seen over a long period of time at a large number of institutions. The degree of evaluation varied, and evaluations of serum levels of muscle enzymes, EMG, and biopsies were missing in many cases; hence the relatively high proportion of probable and possible cases of PM/DM in the series. However, our study was unique in employing a stepwise logistic regression, which combined multivariate analytic techniques and actuarial

Table 4. Mortality in published series of patients with polymyositis/dermatomyositis

Reference	Number of patients at risk	Surveyed time interval	Mortality %
O'Leary and Waisman (7)	40	1925–1938	50.0
Sheard (19)	25	1927–1947	52.0
Wedgewood et al (9)*	26	Not given	40.0
Pearson (20)	48	Not given	25.0
Logan et al (2)	63	1950–1963	41.1
Winkelman et al (8)	289	Not given	27.6
Medsger et al (3)	124	1947–1968	35.0
Sullivan et al (10)*	18	1960–1969	0.0
Riddoch and Morgan-Hughes (5)	20	1960–1970	40.0
DeVere and Bradley (4)	118	1954–1974	27.9
Bohan et al (6)	153	1956–1971	13.7
Carpenter et al (21)†	62	1947–1971	45.1
Henriksson and Sandstedt (18)	107	Not given	23.0
This series	92	1956–1976	32.0

* Including cases of polymyositis/dermatomyositis of childhood only.
† Including cases of polymyositis and dermatomyositis only.

Table 5. Prognostic factors in published series of patients with polymyositis/dermatomyositis (PM/DM)*

Reference	Number of cases	Unfavorable prognostic signs	Signs with no prognostic significance
Riddoch and Morgan-Hughes (5)	20	Prolonged disease history, low serum CPK levels	
Winkelman et al (8)	289	Raynaud's phenomenon, severity of activity, malignancy, scleroderma, pharyngeal and chest muscle weakness	Skin rash, "routine" test results, sex, duration of disease, age
Logan et al (2)	63	Older age, "fulminating" type of PM/DM	
DeVere and Bradley (4)	118	Prolonged duration prior to Rx, overlap syndrome, malignancy, older age	Severity of activity, ESR
Medsger et al (3)	124	Older age, degree of muscle weakness, dysphagia, pneumonitis	Sex, skin rash, ESR, EMG abnormalities, hematocrit, abnormal muscle histopathology
Bohan et al (6)	153	Malignancy, older age, prolonged duration prior to Rx	Severity of activity, scleroderma, Raynaud's phenomenon
Carpenter et al (21)	62	Dysphagia, severe proximal muscle weakness	Corticosteroid Rx, degree of inflammation on muscle biopsy
Henriksson and Sandstedt (18)	107	Older age, prolonged duration prior to Rx, cardiac manifestations, malignancy, no response to Rx	
This series	92	Independent risk factors: Older age; Fever; Leukocytosis; Failure to induce remission. Comorbid factors: Malignancy; Skin rash; Dysphagia; Shorter disease history	Arthritis, ESR, abnormal muscle histopathology, EMG abnormalities, Raynaud's phenomenon, hemoglobin level, blood pressure, EKG abnormalities, splenomegaly, sex, ANF, level of muscle enzymes

*CPK = creatine phosphokinase; Rx = treatment; ESR = erythrocyte sedimentation rate; EMG = electromyogram; EKG = electrocardiogram; ANF = antinuclear factor.

survival rates. Using these methods, failure to induce remission, leukocytosis of 10,000/μl or more, temperature above 38°C, and older age, and to a lesser degree, a shorter history and dysphagia, were identified as independent risk factors for mortality. Pneumonia was the main reason fever was identified as a risk. After exclusion of the remission variable and of pneumonia patients, the significant risk indicators identified were white blood cell count and age.

Our findings are similar to those in other series with regard to the overall proportion of patients with PM/DM who died during followup (2–5,8,9) (Table 4), main causes of death (3–6,8,18) (Table 1), and shape of the actuarial survival curve (3) (Figure 1). Similarly to other series of patients with PM/DM, older age (2,4,6), dysphagia (3,8), and acute progressive onset of the disease (2,8) with fever and leukocytosis predicted poorer survival. Surprisingly, malignancy, which has been reported to be associated with reduced survival in PM/DM (4,6,8,18), was not independently found to affect survival in our subjects (Table 5).

We could not confirm that the overlap syndromes (4,8), a prolonged disease history (5,6), the degree of elevation of serum CPK (5), cardiac manifestations (18), or Raynaud's phenomenon (8) had any effect on survival. In agreement with other studies, sex (3,6,8), sedimentation rate (3,4), hemoglobin level (3), and EMG abnormalities (3) had no prognostic significance. Additional parameters which did not affect survival were arthritis, splenomegaly, high blood pressure levels at diagnosis, antinuclear antibodies in the serum, or abnormal histologic findings on muscle biopsy (Table 5).

REFERENCES

1. Rose AL, Walton JN: Polymyositis: a survey of 89 cases with particular reference to treatment and prognosis. Brain 89:747–768, 1966
2. Logan RL, Bandera JM, Mikkelsen WM, Duff IF: Polymyositis: a clinical study. Ann Intern Med 65:996–1007, 1966
3. Medsger TA, Robinson H, Masi AT: Factors affecting survivorship in polymyositis: a life table study of 124 patients. Arthritis Rheum 14:249–258, 1971
4. DeVere R, Bradley WG: Polymyositis: its presentation, morbidity and mortality. Brain 98:637–648, 1975
5. Riddoch D, Morgan-Hughes JA: Prognosis in adult polymyositis. J Neurol Sci 26:71–80, 1975
6. Bohan A, Peter JB, Bowman RL, Pearson CM: A computer assisted analysis of 153 patients with polymyositis-dermatomyositis. Medicine (Baltimore) 56:255–286, 1977
7. O'Leary PA, Waisman M: Dermatomyositis: a study of 40 cases. Arch Dermatol Syphilol 41:1001–1009, 1940
8. Winkelman RK, Mulder DW, Lambert EH, Howard EH, Diessner RG: Course of dermatomyositis and polymyositis: comparison of untreated and cortisone treated patients. Mayo Clin Proc 43:545–556, 1968
9. Wedgewood RJP, Cook CD, Cohen J: Dermatomyositis: report of 26 cases in children with discussion of endocrine therapy. Pediatrics 12:447–466, 1953
10. Sullivan DB, Cassidy JT, Petty RE, Burt A: Prognosis in childhood dermatomyositis. J Pediatr 80:555–562, 1972
11. Berkson J, Gage RP: Calculation of survival rates for cancer. Mayo Clin Proc 25:270–296 1950
12. Breslow NE: Analysis of survival data under the proportional hazard model. Intern Stat Rev 43:45–52, 1975
13. Mantel N: Evaluation of survival data and two new rank order statistics arising in its consideration. Cancer Chemother Rep 50:163–170, 1966
14. Peto R, Pike MC, Armitage P, Breslow NE, Cox DR, Howard SV, Mantel N, McPherson K, Peto J, Smith PG: Design and analysis of randomized clinical trials requiring prolonged clinical observation of each patient. Br J Cancer 35:1–27, 1977
15. Benbassat J, Gefel D, Zlotnick A: Epidemiology of polymyositis-dermatomyositis in Israel (1960-1976). Isr J Med Sci 16:197–200, 1980
16. Denbow CE, Lie JT, Tancredi RG, Bunch TW: Cardiac involvement in polymyositis: a clinicopathologic study of 20 autopsied patients. Arthritis Rheum 22:1088–1092, 1979
17. Schwartz MI, Matthay RA, Sahn SA, Stanford RE, Marmostein BL, Steinhorn DJ: Interstitial lung disease in polymyositis-dermatomyositis: analysis of six cases and a review of the literature. Medicine (Baltimore) 55:89–112, 1976
18. Henriksson KG, Sandstedt P: Polymyositis: treatment and prognosis: a study of 107 patients. Acta Neurol Scand 65:280–300, 1982
19. Sheard C: Dermatomyositis. Arch Intern Med 88:640–653, 1951
20. Pearson CM: Patterns of polymyositis and their responses to treatment. Ann Intern Med 59:827–838, 1963
21. Carpenter JR, Bunch TW, Engel AG, O'Brien PC: Survival in polymyositis: corticosteroids and risk factors. J Rheumatol 4:207–214, 1977

EVIDENCE FOR INTRAVASCULAR COAGULATION IN SYSTEMIC ONSET, BUT NOT POLYARTICULAR, JUVENILE RHEUMATOID ARTHRITIS

J. PAUL SCOTT, PATRICIA GERBER, MONA C. MARYJOWSKI, and LAUREN M. PACHMAN

After observing a child with systemic onset juvenile rheumatoid arthritis (S-JRA) who developed purpura fulminans in association with disseminated intravascular coagulation, with subsequent gangrene and autoamputation, we undertook a prospective study of coagulation parameters in children with JRA. Ten consecutive children with S-JRA, 10 children with rheumatoid factor–negative, polyarticular juvenile rheumatoid arthritis (P-JRA), and 10 age- and sex-matched controls were studied. Routine coagulation screening tests were performed, as were tests for plasma fibrinopeptide A (a sensitive measure of intravascular thrombin generation), factor VIII–related antigen (an endothelial cell protein), and platelet factor 4 (a platelet-secreted protein). Our studies suggest that activation of intravascular coagulation is common in systemic onset JRA, but not in rheumatoid factor–negative, polyarticular disease. The coagulopathy may cause severe morbidity. In addition, marked elevations of plasma factor VIII–related antigen suggest perturbation of endothelial cells and vascular involvement in S-JRA, but not in P-JRA. Normal ranges of platelet factor 4 indicate that intravascular platelet consumption does not occur in either type of JRA, despite the thrombocytosis common in both.

From Northwestern University Medical School, Chicago, Illinois.

Supported in part by grants from the Marlene Apfelbaum Memorial Foundation and the Boothroyd Foundation.

J. Paul Scott, MD: Assistant Professor of Pediatrics, Division of Hematology, Northwestern University Medical School; Patricia Gerber, MD: Raleigh, North Carolina; Mona C. Maryjowski, RN: Nurse Clinician, Division of Immunology/Rheumatology, Northwestern University Medical School; Lauren M. Pachman, MD: Professor of Pediatrics, Division of Immunology/Rheumatology, Northwestern University Medical School.

Address reprint requests to John Paul Scott, MD, Division of Hematology, Children's Memorial Hospital, 2300 Children's Plaza, Chicago, IL 60614.

Submitted for publication March 6, 1984; accepted in revised form September 13, 1984.

Juvenile rheumatoid arthritis (JRA) is a chronic illness of unknown etiology, which can present with at least 3 patterns of onset: systemic, polyarticular (more than 5 joints involved), and pauciarticular (4 or fewer joints) (1). To what degree these patterns represent a single disease entity or diseases with different pathophysiology is unclear, since there may be evolution of one disease onset pattern into another (i.e., systemic or pauciarticular forms of the disease may develop into the polyarticular form). We observed a child in whom fulminant disseminated intravascular coagulation (DIC) developed when an upper respiratory infection became superimposed upon active systemic onset JRA, with subsequent disastrous consequences: gangrene and autoamputation of several fingers, the forefoot, and the tip of her nose. The association of thrombocytosis with JRA has been described previously (2–4). We speculated that the thrombocytosis could reflect a state of compensated intravascular coagulation, in view of the thrombocytosis seen in some chronic inflammatory diseases (5). These studies describe coagulation abnormalities found in children with systemic onset JRA (S-JRA) and contrast them with findings in children with rheumatoid factor–negative, polyarticular JRA (P-JRA).

PATIENTS AND METHODS

Patients with a diagnosis of systemic or polyarticular onset (rheumatoid factor–negative) juvenile rheumatoid arthritis, according to the 1983 American Rheumatism Association nomenclature and classification (6), who were enrolled in the Rheumatology/Immunology Clinic of the Children's Memorial Hospital were studied during the period March 1982 through May 1983. Ten consecutive children with systemic onset JRA were matched with 10 children of similar age and sex with polyarticular JRA and 10 normal age- and sex-matched controls during the period of study.

Disease activity was graded clinically, with overlapping criteria for systemic and polyarticular manifestations. A rating of 0 indicated inactive disease in both. For S-JRA, 1+ indicated minimal activity characterized by lymphadenopathy, hepatosplenomegaly of <2 cm, and could also include the 1+ criteria for P-JRA: a loss of 5° in range of motion, with or without pain or morning stiffness of <1 hour. A 2+ rating in S-JRA indicated hepatosplenomegaly (>2 cm below the costal margins), fevers that occurred as either low-grade or occasional spikes, and/or intermittent rash. These could be accompanied by the symptoms found for moderately active polyarticular disease. Polyarticular activity rated as 2+ indicated morning stiffness >1 hour, development of new joint involvement or persistent pain, decreased range of motion (loss of 10°), and evidence of local inflammation (heat and swelling). For systemic JRA, 3+ activity designated a child with daily spiking fevers, evanescent rash, and generalized activation of the reticuloendothelial system. These findings could be accompanied by pericardial disease. P-JRA patients with 3+ activity had morning stiffness >2 hours, joint effusions, >10° loss of range of motion in any joint, and the appearance of new joint involvement. It was recognized that no patient could fulfill all criteria at each level, but the presence of 2 or more of the signs/symptoms aided in assessing activity. The basic clinical and laboratory data of the patients with S-JRA and P-JRA are presented in Table 1.

After informed consent was obtained from parents, blood for coagulation studies was drawn from a freely flowing antecubital vein by a 2-syringe technique using a 21-gauge butterfly needle. Routine clotting studies (prothrombin time [PT], activated partial thromboplastin time [PTT], fibrinogen, and fibrin degradation products) and factor VIII coagulant assays (VIII:C) were performed as previously described (7). Factor VIII–related antigen (VIIIR:Ag) was measured by immunoelectrophoresis using rabbit antisera (8,9). Fibrinopeptide A (FPA) was measured by radioimmunoassay using a commercially available kit (Mallinkrodt Industries, St. Louis, MO) according to the method of Nossel et al (10). Platelet factor 4 (PF-4) was measured by radioimmunoassay using a kit (Abbott Laboratories, North Chicago, IL) as described by Levine and Krentz (11). Plasma samples for FPA and PF-4 measurements were anticoagulated with the specific anticoagulant supplied by the manufacturer. Routine clotting studies were performed immediately. Samples for PF-4 and FPA were stored at −70°C for less than 1 month.

RESULTS

There were no clinical findings suggestive of a coagulopathy in any of the patients with P-JRA. One patient with S-JRA developed acrocyanosis and poor peripheral perfusion in association with high, spiking fevers, hepatosplenomegaly, and a skin rash at the presentation of her illness. She was prescribed a regimen of aspirin, 100 mg/kg/day. Initial laboratory studies showed a platelet count of 123,000/mm^3 which fell to 47,000/mm^3, accompanied by a PT of 21 seconds (normal 11.0–14.5), PTT >150 seconds (normal 30–45), fibrinogen 37 mg/dl (normal 150–400), and fibrin degradation products (FDP) >40 μg/ml (normal <10).

Table 1. Clinical and laboratory data on patients with systemic onset juvenile rheumatoid arthritis (S-JRA) and rheumatoid factor–negative, polyarticular juvenile rheumatoid arthritis (P-JRA)*

	S-JRA	P-JRA
n	10	10
Age (years)	9.9 ± 4.5	11.1 ± 4.5
Disease duration	2.0 ± 4.0	5.5 ± 4.4
(range)	(<1 month–14 years)	(1.4–12 years)
Males/females	4/6	4/6
Disease activity score	2.9 ± 0.3	2.1 ± 0.8
ESR (mm/hour)	52 ± 12	24 ± 13
Platelet count ($\times 10^3$/mm^3)	408 ± 188	467 ± 125
Therapy (no. receiving)		
ASA alone	7	2
Hydroxychloroquine + NSAID	3	0
ASA + remittive agent	0	2
NSAID + remittive agent	0	4
Prednisone	0	2

* Data on age, disease duration, disease activity score, ESR, and platelet count are mean ± SD. See text for explanation of disease activity scoring. ESR = erythrocyte sedimentation rate; ASA = aspirin; NSAID = nonsteroidal antiinflammatory drug. NSAIDs include ASA, tolmentin, naproxen. Remittive agent = penicillamine.

The symptoms of hypoperfusion and the coagulopathy improved markedly after institution of corticosteroid therapy and heparin, 10 units/kg/hour, by continuous infusion.

Mild thrombocytosis, as previously noted, was common in both groups of children with JRA (Table 1). Thrombocytopenia was found in only 1 patient (described above) who had clinical and laboratory findings compatible with acute disseminated intravascular coagulation. Serum glutamic pyruvic transaminase (SGPT) was measured in each of the S-JRA patients. Six of 10 had normal levels, and 4 had mildly elevated levels (<200 IU). The serum albumin was normal or mildly decreased in each of the patients with S-JRA (mean 2.8 gm/dl, range 2.1–3.5). Review of daily aspirin doses and serum levels in the 9 S-JRA patients receiving therapy with aspirin showed that 7 were receiving standard doses (101 ± 13 mg/kg/day, mean ± SD) with satisfactory levels (16.2 ± 7.2 mg/dl, mean ± SD). No patient had a serum aspirin level >27 mg/dl, and 1 patient had a very low level of 4.3 mg/dl with a daily dose of 37 mg/kg. Information on SGPT, aspirin doses and levels, and summaries of the abnormal coagulation findings for each patient with S-JRA are presented in Table 2.

In Table 3, the results of the coagulation studies performed on the S-JRA and P-JRA patients and normal controls are shown. The prothrombin time was generally normal in each group, but the PTT was frequently prolonged (5 of 10 patients) in the S-JRA group. The cause for this prolongation is unclear. Fibrinogen concentrations were also frequently elevated in the S-JRA group (5 of 10 patients) and were normal in all patients with P-JRA. Levels of FDP were increased in 5 patients with S-JRA and normal in all patients with P-JRA. Plasma levels of factor VIII clotting activity and factor VIIIR:Ag were normal in patients with P-JRA; in contrast, both VIIIC and VIIIR:Ag were significantly increased in patients with S-JRA. The increase in factor VIIIR:Ag was much greater than that in VIII:C; the ratio of VIII:C to VIIIR:Ag for S-JRA patients was 0.77 ± 0.6 (mean ± SD), in contrast to a ratio of 1.4 ± 0.4 for patients with P-JRA and 1.2 ± 0.7 for the normal controls (P = 0.07). Marked elevations of plasma FPA were common in S-JRA; only 1 patient with S-JRA had a normal plasma FPA level. Mildly increased plasma FPA concentrations were also common in P-JRA. Concentrations of the platelet release protein, PF-4, were similar in all groups and usually within normal limits.

DISCUSSION

We have observed 2 cases of acute disseminated intravascular coagulation in association with systemic JRA. In 1 patient, purpura fulminans developed, with subsequent gangrene and autoamputation of several fingers, the forefoot, and tip of the nose. In the second, the child presented with classic S-JRA and was begun on a regimen of aspirin. One week later the clinical findings of decreased peripheral perfusion with

Table 2. Summary data on 10 patients with systemic onset juvenile rheumatoid arthritis*

Patient	SGPT (normal 3–36 IU)	Serum albumin (normal 3–4.5 gm/dl)	ASA dose (mg/kg/day)	Serum ASA level (mg/dl)	Coagulation abnormalities
1	12	2.8	0		↑ PTT, ↑ FPA
2	30	2.4	110	18	↑ PT, ↑ Fib, ↑ VIIIR:Ag, ↑ FPA
3	24	3.4	77	20	↓ Plts, ↑ PT, ↑ PTT, ↑ FDP, ↑ VIIIR:Ag, ↑ FPA
4	162	3.5	37	4.3	↑ Fib, ↑ FDP, ↑ VIIIR:Ag, ↑ FPA
5	26	2.3	103	14	↑ PTT, ↑ Fib, ↑ VIIIR:Ag, ↑ FPA
6	154	2.6	120	8.5	↑ FDP, ↑ VIIIR:Ag, ↑ FPA
7	5	2.1	100	18	↑ PTT, ↑ Fib, ↑ FPA
8	54	2.8	104	24	↑ PT, ↑ PTT, ↑ FDP, ↑ VIIIR:Ag, ↑ FPA
9	3	2.7	93	12	↑ Fib, ↑ FDP, ↑ VIIIR:Ag, ↑ FPA
10	222	3.4	42	27	↑ VIIIR:Ag
Mean ± SD	69.2 ± 79	2.8 ± 0.5	87 ± 30	16 ± 7	

* All studies on patients 4, 5, 6, 7, 9, and 10 were performed within 2 months of diagnosis. SGPT = serum glutamic pyruvic transaminase; ASA = aspirin; PTT = partial thromboplastin time; FPA = fibrinopeptide A; PT = prothrombin time; Fib = fibrinogen; VIIIR:Ag = factor VIII–related antigen; Plts = platelets; FDP = fibrin degradation product.

Table 3. Results of coagulation studies performed on patients with systemic onset juvenile rheumatoid arthritis (S-JRA), patients with rheumatoid factor–negative, polyarticular juvenile rheumatoid arthritis (P-JRA), and normal children as controls. Data are presented as mean ± 1 SD*

	PT (seconds)	PTT (seconds)	Fibrinogen (mg/dl)	FDP (μg/ml)	VIII:C (units/dl)	VIIIR:Ag (units/dl)	FPA (ng/ml)	PF-4 (ng/ml)
Normal values	11–14.50	30–45	150–400	<10	50–150	50–150	<2.5	<11.0
S-JRA	14.0 ± 1.5	47.5 ± 11†	415 ± 187†	15 ± 14	242 ± 122†	406 ± 250†	9.7 ± 0.4†	7.7 ± 2.8
P-JRA	12.2 ± 0.5	40.3 ± 6.5	286 ± 55	<10	113 ± 29	83 ± 25	3.7 ± 2.5‡	8.5 ± 5.5
Control	12.3 ± 0.8	37.3 ± 4.3	217 ± 38	<10	121 ± 53	118 ± 72	1.9 ± 0.5	6.0 ± 3.3

* VIII:C = factor VIII clotting activity; PF-4 = platelet factor 4. See footnote to Table 2 for definitions of other abbreviations.
† $P < 0.01$ versus controls.
‡ $P < 0.05$ versus controls.

cool, cyanotic fingers and toes, in association with laboratory findings suggestive of disseminated intravascular coagulation, prompted us to institute therapy with systemic corticosteroids and heparin. Aspirin therapy was continued and she showed a rapid clinical and laboratory improvement.

Coagulopathy in association with systemic onset JRA was described by Pinedo et al (12), who described a 15-year-old boy with systemic JRA who developed evidence of DIC and hepatitis while receiving aspirin. When aspirin was discontinued, the symptoms resolved, but evidence of hepatic dysfunction and coagulopathy recurred upon reintroduction of aspirin. Sbarbaro and Bennett (13) described a similar case in a 17-year-old female with systemic onset JRA. Silverman and colleagues (14) recently reported 7 cases of consumption coagulopathy in systemic JRA. They noted an association between this coagulopathy and hypoalbuminemia. They speculated that disordered coagulation may be a result of reduced endothelial cell prostacyclin synthesis caused by high levels of unbound nonsteroidal antiinflammatory medication.

Our studies of children with S-JRA suggest that activation of the coagulation system is common in S-JRA. These studies were performed when disease was very active (mean activity score = 2.9), and 6 patients were studied during the first 2 months after onset. The most frequent findings on routine testing were prolongation of the PTT (5 of 10 patients), elevation of fibrinogen concentration (5 of 10 patients), and elevated FDP (5 of 10 patients). Fibrinopeptide A is a sensitive measure of intravascular thrombin generation because it is the initial peptide cleaved from fibrinogen by thrombin and has a very short half-life in the circulation (15). Nine of the 10 patients with S-JRA demonstrated elevated plasma FPA concentrations, with the mean value approximately 4 times the upper limit of normal. The association of elevated plasma FPA and elevated serum FDP suggests that both thrombin and plasmin are being generated in S-JRA, with subsequent derangement of the host hemostatic mechanism. The FPA values were also elevated in 6 of 10 patients with P-JRA. The mechanism for this is unclear. We speculate that generation of FPA in P-JRA is caused by local inflammation and thrombin generation in areas of acute arthritis. We were unable to demonstrate a correlation between disease activity and plasma FPA in patients with P-JRA.

Studies of the factor VIII molecular complex were undertaken because we hypothesized that vasculitis may be the underlying pathophysiologic mechanism in S-JRA. Factor VIIIR:Ag is a glycoprotein synthesized in endothelial cells and megakaryocyte (16–18); it normally circulates in association with the factor VIII coagulant protein in a 1:1 ratio (19). Factor VIII levels in our P-JRA patients were normal, although the ratio of VIII:C to VIIIR:Ag was slightly greater than 1.0. In S-JRA, the ratio of VIII:C to VIIIR:Ag was 0.77, with 6 of 10 patients having ratios <0.6. These findings suggest that perturbation of endothelial cells, with subsequent release of factor VIIIR:Ag, occurs in S-JRA. An alternative hypothesis is that the generation of thrombin and plasmin may cause limited proteolysis of the factor VIIIR:Ag. Factor VIIIR:Ag was measured by immunoelectrophoresis, and limited proteolysis could expose more antigenic determinants, resulting in an artifactual elevation in factor VIIIR:Ag concentrations.

When one compares the findings of our study with those obtained from studies of other vasculitic disorders, certain similarities stand out. In systemic lupus erythematosus (SLE), elevations of plasma fibrinopeptide A concentrations are common (10). Factor VIII is also found in increased concentrations (20), and this elevation is thought to be related to endothelial damage, with consequent release of VIIIR:Ag. Endothelial damage resulting from vasculitis in SLE may predispose to thrombus formation. In scleroderma and Raynaud's phenomenon (21), marked elevations of factor VIII von Willebrand factor have also been reported. In Kawasaki disease, a childhood arteritis, evidence of activation of coagulation and increased factor VIII activity has been reported (22).

These reports are in agreement with our findings of increased FPA levels and markedly increased factor VIIIR:Ag concentrations in S-JRA. Common to the disorders of SLE, scleroderma, and Kawasaki disease are endothelial damage and a predisposition to intravascular thrombosis. The similar findings in S-JRA suggest that S-JRA is a vasculitis. Further investigations of other endothelial cell proteins and the histologic characteristics of S-JRA are warranted. In addition, the pathophysiologic mechanism of the coagulopathy seen in S-JRA is unknown. If a vasculitis is demonstrated, studies of prostaglandin metabolism, plasma coagulation inhibitors, and generation of plasminogen activator would be of interest.

The role of aspirin and hepatic dysfunction remains unclear. As depicted in Table 2, there was no clear-cut relationship between the coagulopathy we found in S-JRA and elevated SGPT levels. Seven of 10 patients had mildly decreased serum albumin concentrations, but no patients were clinically edematous or jaundiced, and 3 patients with normal serum albumin levels (patients 3, 4, and 10) had evidence of altered coagulation parameters. The 3 patients with the lowest serum albumin concentrations each had elevated plasma fibrinogen concentrations; therefore, a simple failure of hepatic protein synthesis does not explain the coagulopathy we observed. The dosage and serum level of aspirin were within usual therapeutic ranges in the majority of patients. The amount of aspirin circulating unbound in these patients, and how it interferes with the normal hemostatic mechanism, will need to be addressed in future studies.

We measured platelet factor 4 to determine whether the thrombocytosis of JRA was associated with widespread platelet activation. In other disease states, elevated plasma concentrations of platelet release proteins have been used as a means to distinguish between intravascular and extravascular platelet consumption (23,24). The mean values for PF-4 were similar in our S-JRA and P-JRA patients. For both groups, mean PF-4 concentrations were within normal limits. Occasional patients in both groups showed mild increases in PF-4, but no consistent pattern was noted. From these data, we conclude that evidence of platelet activation, as measured by plasma PF-4 levels, is lacking in JRA, despite the thrombocytosis.

In conclusion, our findings suggest that activation of intravascular coagulation is common in systemic onset juvenile rheumatoid arthritis, but not in polyarticular disease. This activation may be manifested clinically by a thrombotic event and in the laboratory by abnormal coagulation screening test results. Fibrinopeptide A assays indicate that intravascular thrombin generation is common in S-JRA. Studies of the factor VIII molecular complex suggest that perturbations of endothelial cell function, compatible with a vasculitis, may occur in S-JRA, but not in P-JRA. Our study of a platelet release protein did not indicate widespread platelet activation in either S-JRA or P-JRA. The mechanism of the thrombocytosis found in juvenile rheumatoid arthritis remains unclear, but our studies do support the concept of vasculitis as the underlying pathophysiologic alteration in systemic onset JRA.

REFERENCES

1. Brewer EJ, Giannini EH, Person DA: Juvenile Rheumatoid Arthritis. Philadelphia, WB Saunders, 1982, p 73
2. Endresen GKM, Hayerael HM, Kass E: Platelet count and disease activity in juvenile rheumatoid arthritis. Scand J Rheumatol 6:237–240, 1977
3. Balogh ZF, Katalin M, Falus A, Baszosky S: Serologic abnormalities in juvenile chronic arthritis: a review of 46 cases. Ann Rheum Dis 39:139–134, 1980
4. Hutchinson RA, Davis P, Jayson MIV: Thrombocytosis in rheumatoid arthritis. Ann Rheum Dis 35:138–142, 1976
5. Wintrobe MM: Clinical Hematology. Eighth edition. Philadelphia, Lea & Febiger, 1981, pp 1113–1132
6. Decker JL and the Glossary Subcommittee of the ARA Committee on Rheumatologic Practice: American Rheumatism Association nomenclature and classification of arthritis and rheumatism (1983). Arthritis Rheum 26: 1029–1032, 1983
7. Scott JP, Morgan ER: Coagulopathy of disseminated neuroblastoma. J Pediatr 103:219–222, 1983
8. Laurell CB: Quantitative estimation of proteins by electrophoresis in agarose gels containing antibodies. Anal Biochem 15:45–52, 1966
9. Zimmerman TS, Ratnoff OD, Powell AE: Immunologic differentiation of classic hemophilia (factor VIII deficiency) and von Willebrand's disease. J Clin Invest 50:244–252, 1971
10. Nossel HL, Yudelman I, Canfield RE, Butler VP,

Spanondis K, Wilner GD, Qureshi GD: Measurement of fibrinopeptide A in human blood. J Clin Invest 54:43–53, 1974
11. Levine SP, Krentz LS: Development of a radioimmunoassay for human platelet factor 4. Thromb Res 11:673–678, 1977
12. Pinedo AM, Van de Putte LBA, Loeliger EA: Salicylate-induced consumption coagulopathy. Ann Rheum Dis 32:66–68, 1973
13. Sbarbaro JA, Bennett RM: Aspirin hepatotoxicity and disseminated intravascular coagulation. Ann Intern Med 86:183–185, 1977
14. Silverman ED, Miller JJ, Bernstein B, Shafari T: Consumption coagulopathy associated with systemic juvenile rheumatoid arthritis. J Pediatr 103:872–876, 1983
15. Nossel HL: Radioimmunoassay of the fibrinopeptides in relation to intravascular coagulation. N Engl J Med 293:428–432, 1976
16. Jaffe EA: Endothelial cells and the biology of factor VIII. N Engl J Med 296:377–383, 1977
17. Hoyer LW, de los Santos RP, Hoyer JR: Anti-hemophilic factor antigen: localization in endothelial cells by immunofluorescent microscopy. J Clin Invest 52:2737–2744, 1973
18. Sixma JJ, Kater L, Bouma BN, Schmitz du Moulin F, DeGraaf S, Tuit S: Immunofluorescent localization of factor VIII-related antigen, fibrinogen and several other plasma proteins in hemostatic plugs in humans. J Lab Clin Med 87:112–119, 1976
19. Hoyer LW: The factor VIII complex: structure and function. Blood 58:1–13, 1981
20. Angles-Cano E, Sultan Y, Clauvel JP: Predisposing factors to thrombosis in systemic lupus erythematosus: possible relation to endothelial cell damage. J Lab Clin Med 94:312–323, 1979
21. Kaheleh MB, Osborn I, LeRoy EC: Increased factor VIII/von Willebrand factor antigen and von Willebrand factor activity in scleroderma and Raynaud's phenomenon. Ann Intern Med 94:482–484, 1981
22. Burns JC, Glode MP, Clarke SH, Hathaway WE: Evidence for activation of coagulation in Kawasaki syndrome (abstract). Pediatr Res 17:135A, 1983
23. White GC, Maroux A: Platelet factor 4 levels in patients with coronary artery disease. J Lab Clin Med 97:369–378, 1981
24. Han P, Turpie AGC, Genton E: Plasma B-thromboglobulin: differentiation between intravascular and extravascular platelet destruction. Blood 54:1192–1196, 1979

SUBSET SPECIFICITY OF ANTILYMPHOCYTE ANTIBODIES IN SYSTEMIC LUPUS ERYTHEMATOSUS

Preferential Reactivity with Cells Bearing the T4 and Autologous Erythrocyte Receptor Phenotypes

AKIRA YAMADA, PHILIP L. COHEN, and JOHN B. WINFIELD

The relative specificity of systemic lupus erythematosus antilymphocyte antibodies for T cell subsets bearing the OKT4, OKT8, or autologous erythrocyte rosette (A-RFC) markers was examined in complement-dependent microcytotoxicity assays and by indirect immunofluorescence. Target cells included normal OKT4+ or OKT8+ T cell clones established from mitogen-activated blasts, resting or phytohemagglutinin-activated peripheral T cells highly enriched for OKT4+ cells or OKT8+ cells, and A-RFC+ and A-RFC− populations. In the majority of sera, cytotoxicity for T4+ cells was greater than that for T8+ cells regardless of cellular activation status. Overall cytotoxicity was considerably higher for activated cells, however, especially when warm assay temperatures were used. A-RFC+ targets were more reactive than nonrosetting T cells, and this was associated with strikingly higher relative fluorescence intensity of IgM staining. Despite these consistent differences in relative cytotoxicity or staining, antibody titers against all cell types were strongly correlated in individual sera. Absorption experiments failed to demonstrate distinct antibody specificities for T4+ and A-RFC+ cells. These data suggest that the major determinant of cytotoxic reactivity may be a single or limited number of surface antigens common to all T cells. Superimposed on this dominant system(s) is a special reactivity with certain distinct subsets and with activated T cells generally.

From the Division of Rheumatology and Immunology, University of North Carolina at Chapel Hill, School of Medicine, Chapel Hill, North Carolina.

Supported in part by NIH grant R01 AM-30863, the UNC Multipurpose Arthritis Center, and an Arthritis Foundation Clinical Research Center grant.

Akira Yamada, MD: Fellow in Rheumatology; Philip L. Cohen, MD: Associate Professor of Medicine; John B. Winfield, MD: Professor of Medicine.

Address reprint requests to John B. Winfield, MD, Division of Rheumatology and Immunology, 932 FLOB 231H, University of North Carolina at Chapel Hill, School of Medicine, Chapel Hill, NC 27514.

Submitted for publication July 9, 1984; accepted in revised form September 25, 1984.

Many T cell functional abnormalities are recognized in systemic lupus erythematosus (SLE). For certain of these, a causative role for antilymphocyte autoantibodies has been suggested (reviewed in 1). Examples include: reduced suppressor T cell activity (2,3), impaired T cell proliferation to various stimuli (4–6), decreased production of cytotoxic T cells (7), and enhanced immunoglobulin secretion by B cells (8).

Associated with T cell dysfunction is an absolute reduction of circulating T cells and variation in the relative proportions or numbers of different T cell subpopulations. The nature of T cell subset abnormalities in SLE is complex, however, with disparate data from different laboratories: decreased Tγ cells (9–11), decreased OKT5+/T8+ or Leu-2a (cytotoxic/suppressor) cells (12–15), decreased OKT4+ (helper/inducer) cells (14,16), low or high Leu-3a/Leu-2a (helper/suppressor) ratio depending on the type of clinical manifestations (14), and decreased T cells which form spontaneous rosettes with autologous erythrocytes (A-RFC) (17).

Some evidence suggests that cold-reactive IgM lymphocytotoxic antibodies have distinct specificities for discrete, functionally relevant subsets. This initially was suggested by the demonstration that a T cell subset staining brightly with serum IgM was markedly depleted in patients with active SLE (18). More recently, antibodies to T8+ cytotoxic/suppressor cells

(15,19), T4+ suppressor inducer cells (14,15), and A-RFC+ suppressor effector cells (20) have been identified. Correlation of antibody specificity in patient plasma with subset ratio of patient lymphocytes and their suppressor functional capacity in vitro further suggests that antilymphocyte antibodies may contribute directly to immunoregulatory abnormalities in this disorder (15).

A firm consensus has not been achieved in this important area, however, and for this reason, the specificity of lymphocytotoxic antibodies for T4+, T8+, A-RFC+, and A-RFC− T cells was reexamined in the present investigation. Targets included subsets purified from normal resting and mitogen-activated T cells and from T cell clones. Special efforts were made to define the relationship of antibody titer and antibody thermal amplitude to complement (C)–dependent cytotoxicity for these various types of T cells. In addition, relative surface membrane antigen density of the different subsets, a determinant of cytotoxic antibody reactivity, was assessed by indirect immunofluorescence and flow cytometry.

MATERIALS AND METHODS

Patients and serum. Peripheral blood was obtained from patients with SLE who met the American Rheumatism Association revised diagnostic criteria (21). After separation from whole blood, serum was aliquoted and stored at −70°C. Each serum aliquot was heated at 56°C for 30 minutes immediately before use.

Lymphocytes. Normal human peripheral blood mononuclear cells (PBMC) were separated from heparinized venous blood by Ficoll-Hypaque flotation. T cells were obtained as the nonadherent population after passage of PBMC over nylon-wool columns (Fenwall Laboratories, Berkeley, CA) according to the technique of Julius et al (22). Activated T cells were obtained by culturing PBMC for 3 days with 1 μg/ml phytohemagglutinin (PHA; Burroughs Wellcome, Research Triangle Park, NC) in tissue culture flasks (Falcon, Oxnard, CA) at a density of 10^6 cells/ml in RPMI 1640 medium (UNC Cancer Center, Chapel Hill, NC) containing 2 m*M* glutamine, antibiotics, and 10% fetal calf serum (Hyclone, Logan, UT) in a humid 5% CO_2, 95% air incubator. Both resting and activated T cells were >95% OKT11+ as determined by complement-dependent cytotoxicity assays or indirect immunofluorescence.

Isolation of T cell subsets. Purified T4+ and T8+ cells were prepared using negative selection monoclonal antibody rosetting procedures as described by Stocker et al (23). Two hundred microliters of 50% packed bovine red blood cells (BRBC; Biological Products, Winston-Salem, NC) and 100 μl of affinity-purified goat anti-mouse IgG (800 μg/ml; a gift from Dr. R. Eisenberg, University of North Carolina, Chapel Hill, NC) were mixed, followed by dropwise addition of 200 μl of 2.5 m*M* chromic chloride (24). After incubation of the reaction mixture for 5 minutes at room temperature, anti-IgG–coated BRBC were washed thoroughly and resuspended to 1% in RPMI 1640 supplemented with 10% fetal calf serum. Five million resting or activated T cells were incubated with 100 μl of appropriate dilutions of OKT4 or OKT8 monoclonal antibody (Ortho Diagnostics, Raritan, NJ) for 30 minutes at 4°C. After washing, the T cells were suspended in RPMI 1640–10% fetal calf serum, to a final density of 4×10^6/ml, combined with an equal volume of a 1% suspension of anti-mouse IgG–coated BRBC, and centrifuged for 10 minutes at 200*g* in 16 × 100-mm tubes (Falcon).

After incubation at 4°C for 20 minutes, the BRBC/lymphocyte mixture was layered over Ficoll-Hypaque and centrifuged. Interface cells were >95% T11+ and, depending on the monoclonal antibody used for rosetting, either >80% T4+ (<5% T8+) or >80% T8+ (<5% T4+). In certain experiments, T cell subsets were prepared by OKT4 or OKT8 plus complement as described by Morimoto et al (15). The subsets were 80–90% pure by this technique. Subsets were also isolated by positive selection using Leu-2a and Leu-3a reagents (Becton-Dickinson, Sunnyvale, CA). Rosette-forming cells were collected in the pellet, and after lysis of erythrocytes with 0.83% ammonium chloride, consisted of >95% pure populations.

A-RFC+ and A-RFC− subsets were isolated from concanavalin A (Con A)–activated T cells. Plastic adherent cells (3×10^5) treated with mitomycin C (Sigma, St. Louis, MO) were mixed with nylon-wool–purified T cells (4×10^6) and cultured with 40 μg Con A (Pharmacia, Piscataway, NJ) in a final volume of 4 ml of medium as described above. After 3 days of culture, Con A–activated cells (2×10^6 in 200 μl) were combined with 200 μl fetal calf serum and 500 μl 2.5% autologous erythrocytes. This mixture was incubated at 37°C for 15 minutes, centrifuged at 150*g* for 5 minutes, and kept at 4°C for 2 hours. Rosetting (A-RFC+) and nonrosetting (A-RFC−) cells were then separated by centrifugation over Ficoll-Hypaque. A-RFC− cells collected at the interface contained <2% A-RFC+ cells. The pellet consisted of >80% A-RFC+ cells.

T cell clones. Clones of PHA-activated cells were established by limiting dilution in suspension culture. Briefly, T cells were isolated by sheep erythrocyte rosetting, and seeded at 0, 0.25, 0.5, 1.0, and 5.0 cells per well in round-bottom tissue culture plates (Costar 3799) in 200 μl of medium containing PHA (2 μg/ml), 20% interleukin-2 (IL-2; Electronucleonics Laboratories, Silver Spring, MD), and ~5×10^4 irradiated (4,000R) autologous PBMC.

After 7 days of incubation at 37°C as described above, medium, IL-2, and feeder cells were replaced. Seven days later, positive wells were scored by inverted phase-contrast microscopy, and cells were transferred to 96-well flat-bottom tissue culture plates (Falcon 3072; Becton-Dickinson, Oxnard, CA). Clones were fed with medium and IL-2 every 3 days thereafter. Fresh, irradiated autologous PBMC were added weekly. Approximately 16% of cells seeded at a density of 0.5 per well gave rise to clones, which were expanded using 24-well flat-bottom plates (Costar 3524). Before use as targets in C-dependent cytotoxicity assays, cloned T cells were centrifuged on Ficoll-Hypaque to remove cellular debris.

Microcytotoxicity. Two-stage, C-dependent microcytotoxicity assays using prescreened rabbit C (Pel-Freez

Table 1. Surface phenotype of target cells

	Percentage of cells positive for surface marker									
	Unfractionated†		Purified‡						Clones§	
Surface marker*	Resting T	Activated T	Resting T4+	Resting T8+	Activated T4+	Activated T8+	A-RFC+ T	A-RFC− T	T4+ clone	T8+ clone
T11	>95	>95	>95	>95	>95	>95	>95	>95	100	100
T4	~60	~60	80–95	<5	80–90	<5	~80	~60	100	0
T8	~30	~30	<5	80–90	<5	80–90	~20	~30	0	100
A-RFC	<5	~20					>80	<2		

* A-RFC = autologous rosette-forming cells.
† Resting T cells were isolated from fresh peripheral blood mononuclear cells as the nylon-wool nonadherent fraction. Activated T cells were phytohemagglutinin (PHA)–activated for 3 days.
‡ T4+ and T8+ subsets were purified from resting or PHA-activated T cells by negative selection monoclonal antibody rosetting procedures using OKT4 or OKT8 reagents. A-RFC+ and A-RFC− cells were prepared from cultures that were stimulated with concanavalin A for 3 days.
§ T4 and T8 clones were established from PHA-stimulated T cell blasts by limiting dilution.

Biologicals, Rogers, AR) were performed as previously described, to quantitate antilymphocyte antibody activity in the SLE sera (25). Assay temperatures of 15°C were used to detect cold-reactive antibodies; temperatures of 25°C were used to distinguish warm-reactive anti–T blast antibodies (6,26). Cytotoxicity, expressed as the percentage of nonviable cells failing to exclude eosin dye, was assessed by inverted phase-contrast microscopy. Cytotoxicity with C alone or C plus normal serum was <10%.

Each SLE serum was examined in separate assays against resting or activated T cell subsets from at least 3 different normal subjects. Titer was determined by testing of serial twofold dilutions (endpoint = 30% killing), and is expressed as 1/log$_2$. In comparisons of relative cytotoxicity of SLE sera for different subsets, a dilution was chosen on the descending part of the curve in order to maximize differences. Preferential killing of one subset versus another was always greatest at lower dilutions, i.e., differences in relative cytotoxicity became less at higher dilutions.

Indirect immunofluorescence and flow cytometry. IgM and IgG antibody binding to T cells in SLE serum was assessed by indirect immunofluorescence at 4°C using fluorescein isothiocyanate (FITC)–conjugated rabbit F(ab')$_2$ antibodies to human μ or γ chains as the second coat. Appropriate dilutions of mouse monoclonal antibodies and FITC-goat F(ab')$_2$ anti-mouse IgG were used to determine known surface antigens. After staining, cells were kept at 4°C and either examined immediately or fixed with paraformaldehyde. Analysis of fluorescence intensity and percent positive cells was determined by flow microfluorometry using an Epics V instrument (Coulter Electronics, Hialeah, FL) equipped with argon laser (488 nm), MDADS and EASY 1 computers, and appropriate software. Laser power, photomultiplier tube amplification, and gain settings were calibrated using fluorospheres (Coulter), and kept constant throughout the experimental run on a given lymphocyte preparation.

Absorption techniques. SLE sera were exhaustively absorbed at 4°C with purified resting T4+ or T8+ cells (40 μl volume per ~2×10^6 cells, repeated 5 times). Completeness of absorption was confirmed by absence of C-dependent cytotoxicity against the absorbing cell type.

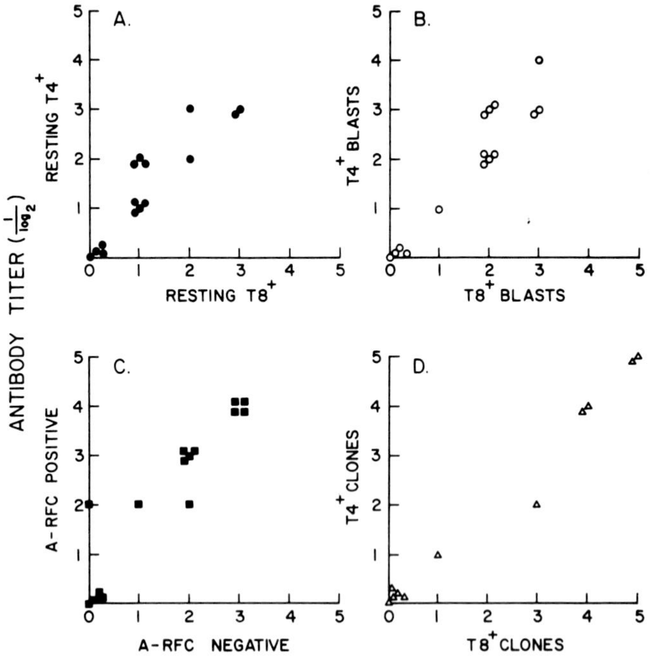

Figure 1. Relationship of complement-dependent cytotoxic antibody titers in systemic lupus erythematosus sera against phenotypically distinct T cell targets. Comparisons include: resting T4 versus resting T8 (**A**), phytohemagglutinin-activated T4 versus activated T8 (**B**), autologous rosette-forming cell (A-RFC)+ versus A-RFC− (**C**), and T4 clones versus T8 clones (**D**). In each case, a highly significant linear relationship is evident.

Table 2. Cytotoxicity (at 15°C) of systemic lupus erythematosus sera for different lymphocyte subsets (n = 15)*

	Resting T cells		T blasts			
	T4+	T8+	T4+	T8+	A-RFC+	A-RFC−
Titer (1/log$_2$)†	1.5 ± 1.0	1.1 ± 1.0	2.2 ± 1.5	1.9 ± 1.2	2.3 ± 1.6	1.5 ± 1.3
Maximum (%)‡	62 ± 26	51 ± 21	65 ± 29	56 ± 26	73 ± 26	57 ± 27
Preferential (%)§	62 ± 26	51 ± 21	59 ± 26	46 ± 23	67 ± 25	48 ± 21
Δ (%)¶	12 ± 8		14 ± 15		19 ± 11	
Ratio	T4/T8 = 1.2 ± 0.2		T4/T8 = 1.3 ± 0.4		+/− = 1.5 ± 0.3	

* Values are mean ± SD. A-RFC = autologous rosette-forming cells.
† Endpoint = 30% dead cells.
‡ Maximum cytotoxicity of a given patient serum.
§ Cytotoxicity of neat serum or dilution of serum where difference in relative killing of one subset versus another, e.g., T4+ versus T8+ or A-RFC+ versus A-RFC−, was greatest.
¶ Difference in relative killing of target subsets, i.e., T4 killing minus T8 killing and A-RFC+ killing minus A-RFC− killing.

Statistical analysis. Statistical analysis of data, which included Pearson product moment correlation coefficients and paired *t*-tests, was performed by Dr. Sandra Stinnett, Biometrics Consulting Laboratory, UNC Department of Biostatistics.

RESULTS

The surface phenotype and purity of the different types of lymphocytes studied as targets are shown in Table 1. Although the magnitude of overall cold-reactive lymphocytotoxicity varied in individual patient sera, antibody titer for one subset correlated highly with that for other subsets, regardless of activation status (Figure 1). Correlation coefficients were in the range of 0.89–0.96 in each case ($P < 0.001$). When cytotoxicity titers for resting subsets were compared with titers for PHA-activated subsets, a similar, strongly positive correlation was observed, although the latter were relatively more reactive (r = 0.86). These data indicate that reactivity of T cells to cytotoxic antibodies in SLE serum at cold assay temperatures is determined primarily by the presence of surface antigen(s) widely shared by T4+, T8+, A-RFC+, and A-RFC− subsets. In addition, the relationship of cytotoxicity for resting T cells to that for activated T cells suggests that a common antigen–antibody system(s) is operant here.

Preferential cytotoxicity for T4+ and A-RFC+ targets. Superimposed on this major antigen–antibody system(s) common to multiple phenotypically distinct subsets and to resting and activated T cells was a consistent preferential cytotoxicity for T4+ and A-RFC+ targets. As illustrated in Table 2 and Figure 2, 13 of 15 patient sera were more cytotoxic for resting T4+ than for T8+ cells (mean ± SD difference in relative killing of the group of 15 sera = 12 ± 8%; T4/T8 killing ratio = 1.2 ± 0.2). This difference, while small, was highly significant ($P = 0.0001$). Greater cytotoxicity for T4+ cells also was observed when PHA-activated T cells were used as targets: the difference in relative killing between T4+ and T8+ was 14 ± 15%; T4/T8 killing ratio was 1.3 ± 0.4 ($P = 0.004$). Fourteen of 15 sera exhibited preferential cytotoxicity for A-RFC+ targets relative to A-RFC− targets. As shown in Table 2, mean cytotoxicity for A-RFC+ cells

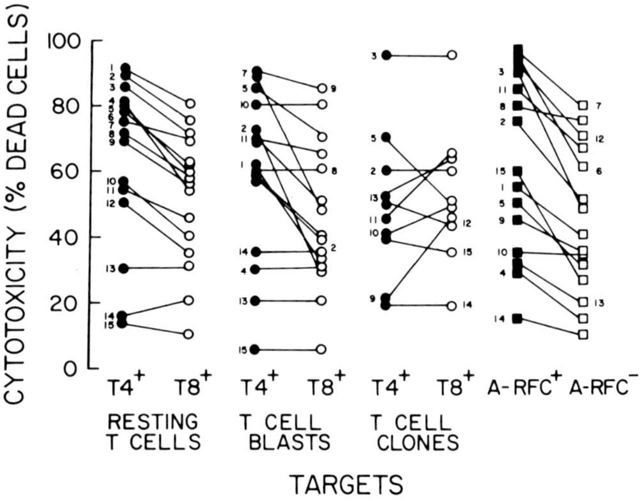

Figure 2. Preferential killing of T4+ cells and autologous rosette-forming cells (A-RFC) by systemic lupus erythematosus sera. Values represent the maximum difference in cytotoxic antibody reactivity of the different subsets observed with a given serum or dilution thereof. Individual patient sera are identified by numbers 1–15.

was 19% higher than for A-RFC− cells (P = 0.001). A-RFC+/A-RFC− killing ratio for the group of sera was 1.5 ± 0.3.

In order to exclude an effect of the method of isolating the T4+ and T8+ cells on the relative cytotoxic activity in SLE sera, subsets were purified by positive selection rosetting and by monoclonal antibody plus complement. Six sera were examined for cytotoxicity against Leu-2a+ (T8+) and Leu-3a+ (T4+) T cells isolated by positive selection. Each serum exhibited greater killing for Leu-3a+ resting T cell targets (mean ± SD percent killing of Leu-3a+ cells = 83 ± 14%; killing of Leu-2a+ cells = 44 ± 13%; Leu-3a/Leu-2a killing ratio = 1.9). Five of 6 sera also were more cytotoxic for PHA-activated Leu-3a+ cells (66 ± 30% versus 51 ± 26%), although the Leu-3a/Leu-2a killing ratio was less (=1.3). Similar data were obtained in experiments comparing the cytotoxicity of SLE sera for subsets isolated by negative selection rosetting (T4/T8 killing ratio = 1.2 ± 0.2) with that for residual cells after treatment with monoclonal antibody plus complement (T4/T8 killing ratio = 1.2 ± 0.3).

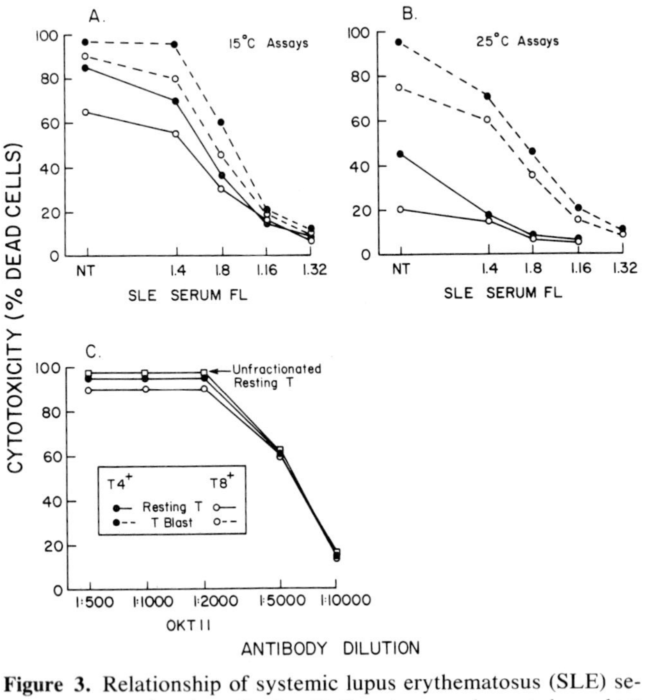

Figure 3. Relationship of systemic lupus erythematosus (SLE) serum or monoclonal antibody dilution to complement-dependent cytotoxicity for different types of targets. Both T4+ and T8+ blasts are more reactive than resting T4+ and T8+ cells, a difference especially apparent at warm (25°C) assay temperatures (**A** and **B**). Reactivity of resting T4 and T8 cells with the pan-T cell monoclonal antibody OKT11 is similar (**C**). NT = neat serum

Three sera with preferential cytotoxicity for the T4+ and A-RFC+ subsets were absorbed with T4+ cells, T8+ cells, or A-RFC− cells. T8+ cells absorbed all cytotoxic activity against T4+ cells, and vice versa. Absorption with A-RFC− cells eliminated cytotoxicity for both A-RFC− and A-RFC+ targets. These findings suggest that the preferential cytotoxicity for T4+ and A-RFC+ targets may not involve antibodies to subset-specific surface determinants.

Each of the purified subsets consisted of >95% T cells (Table 1), indicating that preferential killing of T4+ and A-RFC+ targets was not due to artifactual inclusion of non-T cells or nonlymphoid cells in the T8+ and A-RFC− preparations. Nor were the T4+ and A-RFC+ subsets inherently more susceptible to complement-mediated lysis. Thus, unfractionated T cells and T4+ and T8+ subsets were lysed to the same extent by dilutions of OKT11, a pan-T monoclonal antibody (Figure 3C). Similar results were obtained in comparisons of PHA-activated T4+ and T8+ cells and of A-RFC+ and A-RFC− cells (data not shown).

Increased cytotoxicity for activated T cells. Cytotoxicity of SLE sera for mitogen-activated T cells was greater than that for resting T cells (Figures 3A and B and Figure 4). As shown, this difference was especially striking in assays performed at warm (25°C) tempera-

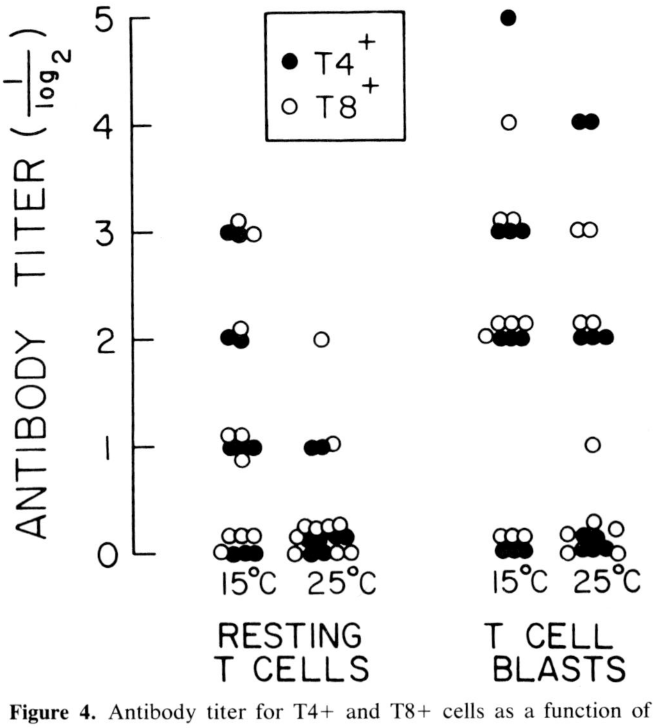

Figure 4. Antibody titer for T4+ and T8+ cells as a function of complement-dependent cytotoxicity assay temperatures.

tures. Indeed, at 25°C, maximum cytotoxicity for resting T4+ and T8+ cells was only 21 ± 20% and 17 ± 18%, respectively, which contrasted with values of 51 ± 31% for activated T4+ cells and 46 ± 31% killing for activated T8+ cells ($P < 0.001$). Using 25°C assay temperatures, however, the preferential killing of T4+ cells, whether resting or activated, was <5% for each serum. For the resting T cell targets, this low differential killing undoubtedly reflects the generally low lymphocytotoxicity at 25°C. But with activated T cell targets, the loss of preferential cytotoxicity for T4+ cells suggests that increased expression of a surface antigen(s) shared by both subsets, possibly a neoantigen, may play the predominant role in determining cytotoxic reactivity.

T cell clones. Ten sera were examined for cytotoxic antibody against a T4+ clone (LC-5) and a T8+ clone (LC-3) established from a single normal lymphocyte donor. Individual serum antibody titers against these clones were similar (Figure 1), as was the group mean cytotoxicity at the serum dilution exhibiting greatest differential cytotoxicity (T8+ clone mean ± SD percent killing = 52 ± 19%; T4+ clone killing = 48 ± 21%) ($P = 0.19$).

Four of 10 sera were preferentially cytotoxic for the T8+ clone, 3 were preferentially cytotoxic for the T4+ clone, and the remaining 3 were equally cytotoxic for both clones (Figure 2). For each of the 4 sera showing slightly greater killing for the T8+ clone,

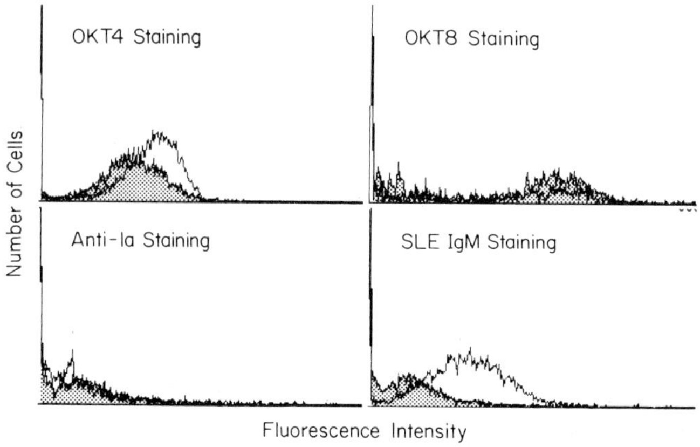

Figure 5. Relative fluorescence intensity of monoclonal antibody and systemic lupus erythematosus (SLE) IgM antilymphocyte antibody staining with autologous rosette-forming cell (A-RFC)+ and A-RFC− cells. Purified A-RFC+ and A-RFC− lymphocytes were studied by indirect immunofluorescence and flow cytometry using an EPICS V instrument. Histograms of fluorescence intensity of A-RFC− targets are shaded; A-RFC+ histograms are clear. As illustrated on the lower right for a representative SLE serum, SLE IgM staining was more intense with A-RFC+ cells.

however, cytotoxicity for both resting and PHA-activated peripheral T cells was greater for the T4+ subset. This apparent paradox presumably is due to heterogeneity within the clones with respect to cell cycle phase, i.e., reactivity of the SLE sera with shared antigen(s) expressed differentially at different stages of activation obscured the minor degree of preferential cytotoxicity seen with resting or PHA-stimulated T4+ cells.

Surface antigen density of T cell subsets. One of the factors which might contribute to increased cytotoxic reactivity of a given subset to SLE antibodies is greater surface membrane density of target antigen. This question was examined by comparing the different targets with respect to the relative fluorescence intensity of staining for SLE IgM or monoclonal antibodies to known surface determinants. In comparisons of T4+ and T8+ cells, little difference in intensity of staining was observed with OKT3, OKT11, and anti–β_2-microglobulin, and with 10 SLE sera. A higher proportion of cells staining more brightly with OKT4+ was evident in the A-RFC+ population, but staining with anti-Ia, OKT3, OKT8, OKT11, and anti–β_2-microglobulin was identical in the A-RFC+ and A-RFC− subsets. Of special interest, however, was the increased intensity of SLE IgM staining with A-RFC+ targets, observed with each of 6 different patient sera (Figure 5). Similar comparisons were performed with resting and PHA-activated T cells (Figure 6). Both monoclonal antibody (OKT4, OKT8, OKT3, OKT11, anti–β_2-microglobulin) and SLE IgM staining were more intense with activated cells.

To determine directly whether higher surface antigen density was associated with increased susceptibility to lysis by a given concentration of antibody, twofold dilutions of several monoclonal antibodies were examined in C-dependent cytotoxicity assays against the different targets. As predicted from the fluorescence intensity data, little difference in cytotoxicity titer was observed when OKT11 and anti–β_2-microglobulin were tested with T4+ versus T8+ and A-RFC+ versus A-RFC− subsets. With PHA-activated T cell targets, however, both of these monoclonal antibodies exhibited a titer which was 2 tubes higher than that seen with resting T cells.

DISCUSSION

The present data indicate that the major determinant of C-dependent lymphocytotoxic activity in SLE sera against different T cell subsets is a common antigen–antibody system or systems, shared by all T cells. Superimposed on this dominant system(s) is a special reactivity with certain distinct subsets and with activated T cells. These 2 principal observations should provide the basis for precise delineation of a variety of complex antibody–lymphocyte interactions in this and other disorders.

Several lines of evidence support the presence of a predominant system common to most T cells. The overall cytotoxicity of a given SLE serum was similar for purified, phenotypically distinct T cells of different types. While preferential killing of one subset versus another was frequently observed and was highly significant, differences in relative killing were minor. Second, regression analyses established strong positive correlation of cytotoxic antibody titer for the various subsets. Third, reciprocal absorptions of serum with cells of one subset removed all cytotoxic antibody for other subsets.

Although the exact identity of the surface antigen(s) in this widely shared antigen–antibody system remains to be defined, it is possible that β_2-microglobulin is a significant component. Four different groups of researchers have identified antibody to β_2-microglobulin in SLE sera (27–30). For example, in recent studies in our laboratory, anti–β_2-microglobulin was the only demonstrable specificity in rosette inhibition and modulation experiments using monoclonal antibodies to 13 known surface antigens, including T4 and T8 (30). Such observations raise the possibility that this antigen–antibody system common to all lymphocytes may involve a single or limited number of surface determinants. Further work will be required in order to resolve this question.

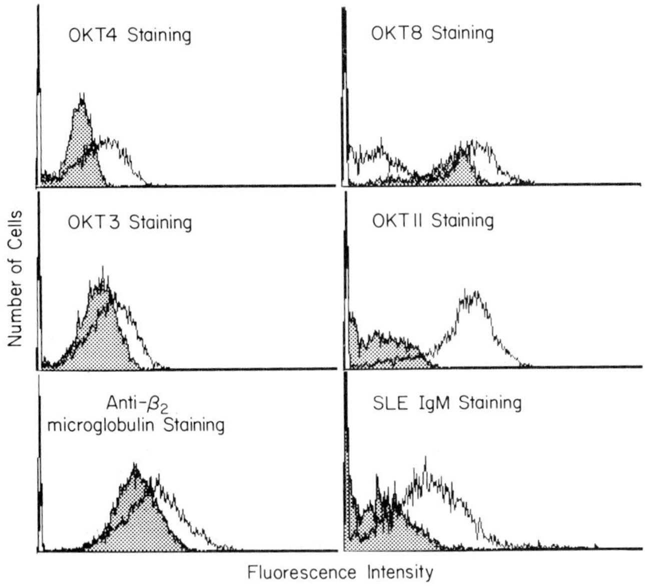

Figure 6. Relative fluorescence intensity of monoclonal antibody and systemic lupus erythematosus (SLE) IgM antilymphocyte antibody staining for resting and phytohemagglutinin-activated T cells. Methods were as described in Figure 5. Resting cell histograms are shaded. In each case, activated T cells exhibited a relatively higher fluorescence intensity of staining than resting T cells.

In addition to antibodies directed to shared T cell antigen(s), the majority of sera exhibited increased killing of mitogen-activated T cells and T cell subsets expressing the T4 and autologous erythrocyte receptor phenotypes. There are several possible explanations for such preferential cytotoxicity. The first is based on the presence of additional antibody directed to membrane antigens expressed on one type of lymphocyte and not on another. Previous data consistent with this concept have been obtained using many different approaches, and have led to the currently prevailing idea that SLE sera contain a panoply of discrete antibody specificities for T cells, activated T cells, B cells, monocytes, natural killer cells, and a variety of T cell subsets (reviewed in 1). Although absorption data, e.g., B cells versus T cells (25) and resting T cells versus activated T cells (6,26), argue convincingly for the existence of cell type–specific antibodies in SLE sera, at least in certain cases, it remains to be established that preferential cytotoxicity for T4+ or A-RFC+ targets is due to subset-specific antibodies. Our limited data on this question would suggest that antibodies to truly distinct determinants on these 2 populations may not exist in SLE sera.

A second explanation for preferential cytotoxicity is that T4+ and A-RFC+ cells are inherently more "lysable" than T8+ and A-RFC− cells. This is not supported by the present data, which showed equal killing of the different subsets by OKT11, a pan-T monoclonal antibody.

Variation in surface antigen density has not generally been considered to be a mechanism by which different types of lymphocytes might be lysed preferentially by SLE antibodies. It is well-recognized that percent cytotoxicity, hemagglutination titer, and degree of hemolysis are all functions of target cell: antibody ratio. Decreased (insufficient) surface antigen density may limit cytotoxic reactivity to a given serum; conversely, sufficient or relatively increased target antigen density enables effective or enhanced cell killing by the same concentration of antibody.

This phenomenon undoubtedly is operant in our observation of increased lysis of activated T cells, relative to resting T cells, by monoclonal antibodies to certain T cell antigens which exhibit increased expression on activated cells. Such a mechanism also may underly the increased reactivity with SLE sera of A-RFC+ and PHA-activated T cells, although antibodies specific for activation neoantigens appear to contribute substantially in the latter case, especially at warm assay temperatures (6,26).

Previous data from other laboratories suggest that preferential killing of OKT8+ cells predominates in SLE when sera are preselected for T cell cytotoxicity of >20% at a dilution of 1:5 (15,19). Our data are conflicting on this point, showing instead a consistent, slightly increased cytotoxicity for T4+ cells. Differences in technique for purifying the T cell subsets, or in preparation and handling of SLE serum samples, do not seem sufficient to explain the discrepant results. Thus, assays using T4+ and T8+ cells purified by monoclonal antibody plus complement gave results identical to those using subsets prepared by positive or negative selection monoclonal antibody rosetting procedures.

Virtually all of the 15 unselected patient sera exhibited increased cytotoxicity for T4+ and A-RFC+ targets. While it is difficult to generalize from such a small patient group, particularly in the absence of serial observations, the consistency of the selective reactivity of these 2 subsets is striking. Furthermore, since antilymphocyte antibodies appear to be fundamentally involved in lymphopenia (31) and in a variety of in vitro lymphocyte functional abnormalities in SLE (1), subset-selective interactions of this type may be of significance in vivo. Of particular interest here is the potential relationship of our findings to recent reports of T4+ (14,16) and A-RFC+ (17,20) subset depletion, and to T suppressor abnormalities in SLE. The latter may involve reduction and/or dysfunction of both T4+ suppressor inducer cells (12,15) and A-RFC+ suppressor effector cells (17,20).

It should be emphasized, however, that the present investigation was not directed to T cell subpopulation abnormalities in the patients studied. Several laboratories, including our own, have demonstrated a disproportionate reduction in $T\gamma$ cells and T8+/Leu-2a+ cells in patients with active SLE (9–15). Furthermore, the preferential cytotoxicity of our patient sera for T4+ cells in vitro does not necessarily imply that a similar situation occurs in vivo. For example, it is possible that antibodies more active against T8+ cells are absorbed from plasma in vivo, in a fashion analogous to that shown previously for high-avidity anti-DNA antibodies in this disorder (32); as a consequence, in vitro assays may detect "leftover" antibodies primarily, e.g., antibodies relatively less cytotoxic for T8+ cells or low-avidity anti-DNA antibodies. Serial observations and additional correlative studies will be required in order to provide answers to these interesting questions.

ACKNOWLEDGMENTS

The technical assistance of Rekha Shah and Melody Shaw is gratefully acknowledged. We also thank Linda Tillman for typing the manuscript.

REFERENCES

1. Winfield JB: Anti-lymphocyte antibodies in SLE: specificity and relationship to abnormal cellular function, Systemic Lupus Erythematosus. Edited by R Lahita. New York, John Wiley & Sons (in press)
2. Sakane T, Steinberg AD, Reeves JP, Green I: Studies of immune functions of patients with systemic lupus erythematosus: complement-dependent immunoglobulin M anti-thymus-derived cell antibodies preferentially inactivate suppressor cells. J Clin Invest 63:954–965, 1979
3. Sakane T, Steinberg AD, Reeves JP, Green I: Studies of immune functions of patients with systemic lupus erythematosus: T-cell subsets and antibodies to T-cell subsets. J Clin Invest 64:1260–1269, 1979
4. Wernet P, Kunkel HG: Antibodies to a specific surface antigen on T cells in human sera inhibiting mixed leukocyte culture reactions. J Exp Med 138:1021–1026, 1973
5. Williams RC Jr, Lies RB, Messner RP: Inhibition of mixed leukocyte culture responses by serum and γ-globulin fractions from certain patients with connective tissue disorders. Arthritis Rheum 16:597–605, 1973
6. Yamada A, Winfield JB: Inhibition of soluble antigen-induced T cell proliferation by warm-reactive antibodies to activated T cells in systemic lupus erythematosus. J Clin Invest (in press)
7. Huber C, Pfister R, Stingl G: Complement-dependent lymphocytotoxic antibodies (CLA) in systemic lupus erythematosus preferentially inhibit the generation of allo-reactive cytotoxic T cells in secondary CML. Clin Exp Immunol 50:525–533, 1982
8. Takeuchi T, Abe T, Kiyotaki M, Toguchi T, Koide J, Morimoto C, Homma M: In vitro immune response of SLE lymphocytes: the mechanism involved in B-cell activation. Scand J Immunol 16:369–377, 1982
9. Fauci AS, Steinberg AD, Haynes BF, Whalen G: Immunoregulatory aberrations in systemic lupus erythematosus. J Immunol 121:1473–1479, 1978
10. Hamilton ME, Winfield JB: T_γ cells in systemic lupus erythematosus: variation with disease activity. Arthritis Rheum 22:1–6, 1979
11. DeHoratius RJ, Tung KSK, Pincus T: Reduced T-

lymphocyte subsets in systemic lupus erythematosus: effects of immune complexes and lymphocytotoxic antibodies. Clin Immunol Immunopathol 17:245–256, 1980
12. Sakane T, Kotani H, Takada S, Murakawa Y, Ueda Y: A defect in the suppressor circuits among OKT4+ cell populations in patients with systemic lupus erythematosus occurs independently of a defect in the OKT8+ suppressor T cell function. J Immunol 131:753–761, 1983
13. Morimoto C, Reinherz EL, Schlossman SF, Schur PH, Mills JA, Steinberg AD: Alterations in immunoregulatory T cell subsets in active systemic lupus erythematosus. J Clin Invest 66:1171–1174, 1980
14. Smolen JS, Chused TM, Leiserson WM, Reeves JP, Alling D, Steinberg AD: Heterogeneity of immunoregulatory T-cell subsets in systemic lupus erythematosus: correlation with clinical features. Am J Med 72:783–790, 1982
15. Morimoto C, Reinherz EL, Distaso JA, Steinberg AD, Schlossman SF: Relationship between systemic lupus erythematosus T cell subsets, anti-T cell antibodies, and T cell functions. J Clin Invest 73:689–700, 1984
16. Bakke AL, Kirkland PA, Kitridou RC, Quismorio FP Jr, Rea T, Ehresmann GR, Horwitz DA: T lymphocyte subsets in systemic lupus erythematosus: correlations with corticosteroid therapy and disease activity. Arthritis Rheum 26:745–750, 1983
17. Takada S, Ueda Y, Murakawa Y, Suzuki N, Sakane T: Functional heterogeneities among concanavalin A-activated OKT4+ and OKT8+ cells by using autologous erythrocyte rosette technique. J Clin Invest 72:2060–2071, 1983
18. Steinberg AD, Klassen LW, Budman DR, Williams GW: Immunofluorescence studies of anti-T cell antibodies and T cells in systemic lupus erythematosus: selective loss of brightly staining T cells in active disease. Arthritis Rheum 22:114–122, 1979
19. Morimoto C, Reinherz EL, Abe T, Homma M, Schlossman SF: Characteristics of anti-T-cell antibodies in systemic lupus erythematosus: evidence for selective reactivity with normal suppressor cells defined by monoclonal antibodies. Clin Immunol Immunopathol 16:474–484, 1980
20. Kumagai S, Steinberg AD, Green I: Immune responses to hapten-modified self and their regulation in normal individuals and patients with SLE. J Immunol 127:1643–1652, 1981
21. Tan EM, Cohen AS, Fries JF, Masi AT, McShane DJ, Rothfield NF, Schaller JG, Talal N, Winchester RJ: The 1982 revised criteria for the classification of systemic lupus erythematosus. Arthritis Rheum 25:1271–1277, 1982
22. Julius MH, Simpson E, Herzenberg LA: A rapid method for isolation of functional thymus-derived murine lymphocytes. Eur J Immunol 3:645–649, 1973
23. Stocker JW, Garotta G, Hausmann B, Trucco M, Ceppellini R: Separation of human cells bearing HLA-DR antigens using a monoclonal antibody rosetting method. Tissue Antigens 13:212–222, 1979
24. Goding JW: The chromic chloride method of coupling antigens to erythrocytes: definition of some important parameters. J Immunol Methods 10:61–66, 1976
25. Winfield JB, Winchester RJ, Wernet P, Fu SM, Kunkel HG: Nature of cold-reactive antibodies to lymphocyte surface determinants in systemic lupus erythematosus. Arthritis Rheum 18:1–8, 1975
26. Litvin DA, Cohen PL, Winfield JB: Characterization of warm-reactive IgG anti-lymphocyte antibodies in systemic lupus erythematosus: relative specificity for mitogen-activated T cells and their soluble products. J Immunol 130:181–186, 1983
27. Revillard JP, Vincent C, Rivera S: Anti-β_2-microglobulin lymphocytotoxic autoantibodies in systemic lupus erythematosus. J Immunol 122:614–618, 1979
28. Messner RP, DeHoratius R, Ferrone S: Lymphocytotoxic antibodies in systemic lupus erythematosus patients and their relatives: reactivity with the HLA antigenic molecular complex. Arthritis Rheum 23:265–272, 1980
29. Ooi BS, Ooi YM, Pesce AJ, Pollak V: Antibodies to β_2 microglobulin in the sera of patients with systemic lupus erythematosus. Immunology 33:535–541, 1977
30. Yamada A, Shaw M, Winfield JB: Surface antigen specificity of cold-reactive IgM antilymphocyte antibodies in systemic lupus erythematosus. Arthritis Rheum 28:44–51, 1985
31. Winfield JB, Winchester RJ, Kunkel HG: Association of cold-reactive antilymphocyte antibodies with lymphopenia in systemic lupus erythematosus. Arthritis Rheum 18:587–594, 1975
32. Winfield JB, Faiferman I, Koffler D: Avidity of anti-DNA antibodies in serum and IgG glomerular eluates from patients with systemic lupus erythematosus: association of high avidity anti-native DNA antibody with glomerulonephritis. J Clin Invest 59:90–96, 1977

NEOPNATAL LUPUS ERYTHEMATOSUS OCCURRING IN ONE FRATERNAL TWIN

Serologic and Immunogenetic Studies

JEFFREY P. CALLEN, JOSEPH F. FOWLER, KEVIN B. KULICK, GREGORY STELZER, and STEPHEN Z. SMITH

Neonatal lupus erythematosus (LE) is a syndrome that is manifested by LE skin lesions and/or congenital heart block, occurring in infants at, or shortly after, birth. The syndrome is believed to be caused by transplacental passage of an IgG antibody, usually the anti-Ro (SS-A) antibody, from the mother to the infant. Although the mother may have a connective tissue disease or may be healthy, the common characteristic is the presence of maternal circulating anti-Ro antibody. It has been believed that the HLA determinants demonstrated in children who have neonatal LE were not a factor in the expression of the syndrome. We report the occurrence of neonatal LE, manifested by photosensitivity and discoid LE skin lesions, in one fraternal twin. HLA studies of this affected twin demonstrated the presence of DR3. Anti-Ro antibody was present in the mother, but was not present in either child at 4 months post-delivery. HLA determinants may be involved in the expression of disease in neonates who have been exposed to the anti-Ro antibody. Furthermore, the presence of circulating antibodies in the unaffected twin causes us to question the assumption that the anti-Ro antibody is the causative factor for the occurrence of tissue injury in children with neonatal LE.

Presented in part at the 48th Annual Meeting of the American Rheumatism Association, Minneapolis, MN, June 1984.

From the Department of Medicine, Division of Dermatology, University of Louisville, Kentucky; the Department of Medicine and Dermatology, State University of New York at Buffalo, VA Medical Center, Buffalo, New York; and the Histocompatibility Laboratory, Jewish Hospital, University of Louisville, Department of Microbiology and Immunology, Louisville, Kentucky.

Supported in part by the Ralph Hockstetter Medical Research Advance in honor of Dr. Henry C. and Mrs. Bertha H. Buswell and by a grant from the Lupus Foundation of Kentuckiana.

Jeffrey P. Callen, MD: Department of Medicine, Division of Dermatology, University of Louisville; Joseph F. Fowler, MD: Department of Medicine, Division of Dermatology, University of Louisville; Kevin B. Kulick, MD: Department of Medicine and Dermatology, State University of New York at Buffalo, VA Medical Center, Buffalo; Gregory Stelzer, PhD: Director, Histocompatibility Laboratory, Jewish Hospital, University of Louisville, Department of Microbiology and Immunology, Louisville; Stephen Z. Smith, MD: Department of Medicine, Division of Dermatology, University of Louisville.

Address reprint requests to Jeffrey P. Callen, MD, 310 East Broadway, Louisville, KY 40202.

Submitted for publication March 27, 1984; accepted in revised form September 13, 1984.

Since the discovery of the anti-Ro antibody system (SS-A), interest in neonatal lupus erythematosus (LE) has been rekindled (1–4). Passive transfer of this IgG antibody from the mother has been strongly linked with the occurrence of cutaneous LE lesions in neonates, as well as with the occurrence of complete congenital heart block (1,5,6). However, not all children of mothers who have anti-Ro antibody develop symptoms or signs of cutaneous or cardiac disease (7). This report describes the serologic and immunogenetic findings in dizygotic twins of a mother with anti-Ro antibodies, in whom the disease expression was discordant. Differences in HLA determinants may explain the discordant disease expression we observed.

PATIENTS AND METHODS

Patients. Medical histories and physical examinations were obtained from all members of the family of the patient with neonatal lupus erythematosus (propositus). Blood was collected from the twins, the mother, and the father. Specimens were collected from the children and the mother at 3 and 4 months post-delivery. Two types of specimens were collected, 1 for HLA and T cell studies and 1 for serologic studies. The blood collected for serologic studies was allowed to clot, and the serum was then separated and frozen. Prior to all serologic studies, the sera were heated at 56°C for 30 minutes to destroy complement.

Serology. Antinuclear antibodies (ANA) were detected by direct immunofluorescence according to the method of Coons (8). Sera drawn at 3 months were tested using the HEp-2 cell line. Sera drawn at 4 months were tested by one of us (KBK), and were screened at a dilution of 1:20 on mouse liver substrate using commercially prepared goat anti-human immunoglobulin (Kallestadt). Sera that were positive at 1:20 dilution were then serially diluted, and the greatest dilution demonstrating detectable immunofluorescence was recorded.

Precipitating antibodies against soluble nuclear and cytoplasmic antigens were detected through the use of gel double-immunodiffusion in Ouchterlony plates containing 0.6% agarose. The source of antigen was calf thymus and human spleen extract, prepared as previously described (9). The identity of the precipitin was determined with monospecific antisera. Antibodies to native DNA (nDNA) were detected with indirect immunofluorescence using *Crithidia luciliae* substrate (10). Antibodies to single-stranded DNA (ssDNA) were detected using a modified Farr assay with ^{125}I-ssDNA, as previously described (11).

HLA–A, B, C, and DR alloantigens. Peripheral blood lymphocytes were typed for HLA–A, B, C, and DR antigens. The T and B cells were separated using a modified nylon wool technique. HLA typings were performed by the standard 2-stage microcytotoxicity test procedure, using an extended antigen/antibody and complement incubations for B cell typings. Sera for the tissue typing were obtained primarily from commercially available typing trays and the National Institutes of Health (12,13).

Patient 1, MYW, propositus. This 3-month-old black female was the second of fraternal twins from an otherwise uncomplicated pregnancy and low forceps delivery. Shortly after birth, the child developed an eruption on the face and scalp; there was erythema and slight scaling. The initial differential diagnosis included transient neonatal pustular melanosis and traumatic injury from the forceps. The eruption failed to resolve. By 2½ months, the eruption was worsening and had spread to the trunk, arms, and legs.

Physical examination revealed multiple atrophic, confluent patches with moderate scar formation on the temple (Figure 1). There were erythematous, "owl-eye" type mask lesions on the face surrounding the eyes. Discoid erythematous lesions with slight scale, erythema, and telangiectasias were present on the shoulders, chest, arms, legs, and vulvar area. The eruption was worse in areas that had been exposed to the sun. On repeat questioning, the parents noted that the rash had worsened after exposure to the sun.

Results of her electrocardiogram were normal, as were the complete blood count and multiphasic analysis of her serum. A 3-mm punch biopsy specimen was taken from a lesion on the temple. Analysis of the sample revealed an atrophic epidermis with a perivascular and periappendageal round-cell infiltrate. Basal cell vacuolopathy was present, and lymphocytes were also present at the dermal–epidermal junction. Immunofluorescence analysis of the biopsy sample was not done.

Followup evaluation at 4 months post-delivery revealed a cessation of new lesions, but by 7 months, the disease was in a regressive phase. At the time of the last followup, residual pigmentary abnormalities and scarring still remained.

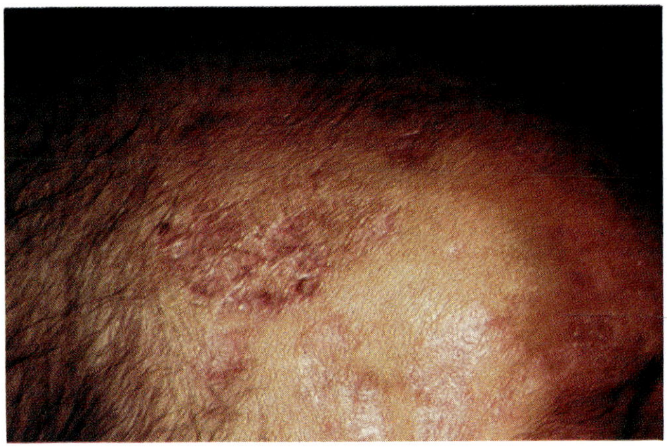

Figure 1. The temple area of a 3-month-old child, showing erythematous discoid lesions with atrophy and early scarring. The child's fraternal twin showed no clinical evidence of disease.

Patient 2, MW, twin sibling. The sister of MYW was born first, also by forceps delivery. She did not develop any skin lesions nor was any photosensitivity noted. Results of her electrocardiogram and complete blood count were normal. At 7 months of age, no disease had been found.

Patient 3, DW, mother. The mother of MYW and MW was a 28-year-old black woman who had been healthy her entire life, had not had any skin diseases, arthralgias, or arthritis, nor had she ever demonstrated photosensitivity. The twins were a product of her second pregnancy. Her first pregnancy was normal and resulted in a healthy male child with no evidence of cardiac or cutaneous disease.

RESULTS

Neonatal lupus erythematosus was manifested in only 1 of the twins, and no evidence of LE was seen in any of the other family members (Figure 2). By 4 months of age, the LE lesions had begun to become quiescent, and no new lesions were appearing. Photosensitivity was present only in the propositus despite the presence of ANA in the other twin and the presence of anti-Ro in the mother. Neither congenital heart block nor any conduction defect was found in any of the family members examined.

Serologic studies. The results of the serologic studies are summarized in Table 1. When the twins were 3 months of age, the family members were tested for ANA only, using the HEp-2 cell line; the twins and their mother showed positive results. The propositus demonstrated a speckled pattern with a titer of 1:1,280, while the mother and the unaffected twin demonstrated speckled patterns at a titer of 1:160. At the age of 4 months, the serologic findings in the twins were altered; no cytoplasmic or nuclear antibodies

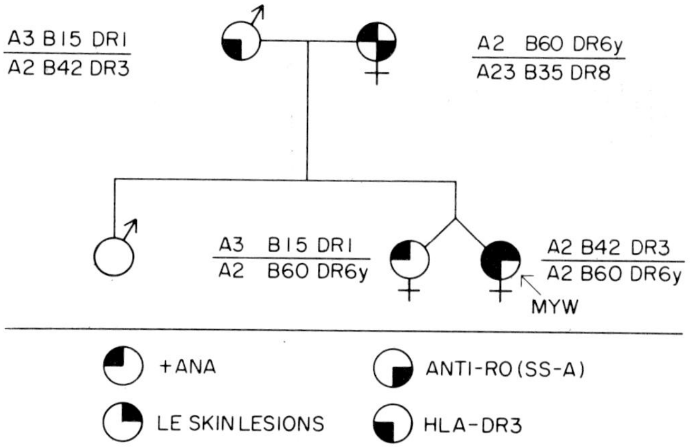

Figure 2. Clinical, serologic, and genetic findings in the family of a child with neonatal lupus erythematosus (LE). +ANA = antinuclear antibody–positive.

were demonstrated in the serum of either infant. The mother's serum was ANA-negative on mouse liver substrate, but was positive for anti-Ro (SS-A) antibody. The mother's serum was negative for anti-La (SS-B), anti-ssDNA, and anti-nDNA.

Histocompatibility typing. The HLA antigens found in the family members tested are shown in Figure 2. None of the family members possessed HLA–B8. The mother did not demonstrate either the DR2 or DR3 locus. The affected infant was DR3-positive, whereas the unaffected infant was DR3-negative.

DISCUSSION

McCuistion and Schoch (14) are credited with the first report of neonatal lupus erythematosus. In their report, the authors suggested that an agent that was capable of crossing the placenta was responsible for the development of LE in the infant. Although the mother of their patient was then in good health, 11 months later she developed systemic lupus erythematosus (SLE). Neonatal LE has since been reported in approximately 38 patients (15–30). Only 5 patients reported as having the cutaneous lesions of neonatal LE were males. About half of the mothers of these 38 infants had one of a variety of connective tissue diseases (LE, rheumatoid arthritis, Sjögren's syndrome); the other mothers were normal. The cutaneous lesions of neonatal lupus are transient and are generally considered to be benign. However, the other common manifestation of neonatal LE, congenital heart block, may result in permanent disease or even death.

The role of transplacental transmission of a factor responsible for the development of neonatal LE was postulated in McCuistion and Schoch's report (14). However, in 1966, Beck et al (31) reported the transplacental passage of 7.0S gamma globulin, the antinuclear antibody, from 3 mothers with SLE. The infants were studied serologically, but failed to manifest any disease associated with LE. Beck et al showed that the antibody transfer was through the placenta, and ANA were not found in the colostrum, milk, or amniotic fluid. The investigators monitored the ANA titers in these infants and found that the titers fell, showing a half-life of about 20 days.

In 1981, Miyagawa et al (25) demonstrated that transplacental transmission of anti-Ro antibodies (SS-A) and anti-La antibodies (SS-B) can occur. These authors described 2 children (born to 1 mother) who both developed an annular LE eruption. Subsequently, Weston et al (4), Franco et al (2), and Kephart et al (3) have analyzed cases of neonatal LE and have shown a definite relationship between the occurrence of skin lesions and the presence of the anti-Ro antibody. Similar data have been reported for patients with congenital heart block (32).

Genetic studies of patients with neonatal LE have been performed in only a few cases. Lee et al (5) recently reported that DR3 was present in the mothers of patients with neonatal LE, but they failed to demonstrate a genetic (HLA) predisposition for disease development in affected infants versus their unaffected siblings. Similarly, Lockshin et al (7) found that their patient with neonatal LE and congenital heart block had neither the B8 nor DR3 antigen, yet the affected sibling did. HLA studies in patients with LE have shown significant correlations of DR3 with subacute cutaneous lupus erythematosus and of DR3 with the presence of anti-Ro (SS-A) (33).

Table 1. Serologic studies of a patient with neonatal lupus erythematosus (LE), her healthy fraternal twin, and their mother*

	Mother	Infant with neonatal LE	Healthy twin sibling
ANA			
Twins age 3 months	1:160 (sp)	1:1,280 (sp)	1:160 (sp)
Twins age 4 months	–	–	–
Anti-Ro (SS-A)	+	–	–
Anti-La (SS-B)	–	–	–
Anti-ssDNA	–	–	NT
Anti-nDNA	–	–	–

* Sera were tested only for antinuclear antibodies (ANA) at 3 months post-delivery, using the HEp-2 cell line (normal <1:40). At 4 months post-delivery, sera were again tested for ANA, using mouse liver substrate (normal <1:10); the remaining serologic studies were performed at this time. sp = speckled pattern; – = negative; + = positive; ssDNA = single-stranded DNA; NT = not tested; nDNA = native DNA.

The clinical characteristics of the skin lesions of neonatal LE generally fall into 1 of 2 types, either discoid lupus erythematosus (DLE) lesions, or subacute cutaneous lupus erythematosus (SCLE) lesions. Our patient demonstrated scarring, atrophy, telangiectasias, and pigmentary changes consistent with DLE. Her lesions occurred more prominently on the head and neck but were also present on unexposed skin surfaces. Most of the patients reported in the literature have demonstrated DLE lesions similar to those of our patient, but there have also been reports of annular erythema typical of SCLE. The lesions may be present at birth or may occur shortly after birth. Resolution of the process begins by 3–4 months of age, and by 6 months, it is uncommon for the infant to develop new lesions or to demonstrate photosensitivity.

Exacerbation by sunlight was present in our patient, but similar photosensitivity did not occur in any other family member. Others have reported photoexacerbation in the infant as well as in the mother. Weston et al (4) noted that the neonatal DLE lesions occurring in 4 of their 6 patients were sun-induced. They did not challenge the other patients. Similarly, Lane and Watson (30) noted photosensitivity in 2 of the 3 patients they described.

The mother of our patient was healthy, even though she possessed the anti-Ro (SS-A) antibody. Anti-Ro has been correlated with the presence of SCLE, arthritis, SLE, Sjögren's syndrome, and cutaneous vasculitis (1). Controversy still exists over whether anti-Ro has a specific clinical correlation or prognostic implication in SLE patients (1,34). Also, it is not known whether the presence of this antibody in an otherwise healthy individual, such as our patient's mother, portends a poor prognosis. Weston et al (4) described 4 mothers of neonatal LE patients who were clinically normal, but serologically positive, and in followup, none had developed symptoms or signs of connective tissue disease. Moreover, the disease that occurred in the 4 other mothers was not progressive. However, the followup period was short, ranging from 1–6 years.

Our patient was seen at age 3 months and demonstrated ANA on tests using HEp-2 cells, but at the same time, her twin sister showed ANA, though in a low titer. Sera for anti-Ro and anti-La testing were not drawn until 4 months of age, at which time the results were negative in both infants. The mother's serum was positive for ANA in tests using the HEp-2 cell line, but negative when tested on mouse liver substrate. However, tests for anti-Ro were positive. The negative results of tests for the anti-Ro antibody in the infants' sera can be explained by the timing of the blood sampling.

In the family we describe here, HLA–DR3 was present in the affected infant and in the father. It is likely that the twins were both exposed to anti-Ro (SS-A), particularly in view of the presence of ANA in the sera initially tested. It may be that our patient's susceptibility to neonatal LE was genetically determined by the presence of DR3. Three possible explanations for disease susceptibility in this case are: 1) photosensitivity, which has been associated with the presence of DR3 and anti-Ro antibodies; 2) a different response of the skin to sun exposure in DR3-positive individuals; or 3) a different clearance of antibody in the affected, DR3-positive child. An interesting postulate is that the presence of both DR3 and anti-Ro may have been necessary for disease expression in this family, since only the affected infant possessed both of these characteristics. Furthermore, the unaffected sibling had antinuclear antibodies and, presumably, circulating anti-Ro antibody but developed no clinical evidence of disease.

Although it has been suggested that the common characteristic among patients with neonatal LE is the presence of anti-Ro, this observation raises questions regarding the pathogenesis of the disease. The anti-Ro antibody cannot be the sole factor involved in the occurrence of tissue injury in neonatal LE patients.

We have described fraternal twins with discordant disease expression of neonatal LE. Their mother was healthy, but possessed anti-Ro antibodies. HLA differences demonstrated in the twins may help explain this discordant disease expression, particularly since DR3 was present in the affected twin only.

REFERENCES

1. Provost TT: Commentary: neonatal lupus erythematosus. Arch Dermatol 119:619–622, 1983
2. Franco HL, Weston WL, Peebles C, Forstot L, Phanuphak P: Autoantibodies directed against sicca syndrome antigens in neonatal lupus syndrome. J Am Acad Dermatol 4:67–72, 1981
3. Kephart DC, Hood AF, Provost TT: Neonatal lupus erythematosus: new serologic findings. J Invest Dermatol 77:331–333, 1981
4. Weston WL, Harmon C, Peebles C, Manchester D,

Franco HL, Huff JC, Norris DA: A serologic marker for neonatal lupus erythematosus. Br J Dermatol 107:377–382, 1982
5. Lee LA, Bias WB, Arnett FC, Huff JC, Norris DA, Harmon C, Provost TT, Weston WL: Immunogenetics of the neonatal lupus syndrome. Ann Intern Med 99:592–593, 1983
6. Scott JS, Maddison PJ, Taylor PV, Esscher E, Scott O, Skinner P: Connective tissue disease, antibodies to ribonucleprotein, and congenital heart block. N Engl J Med 309:209–212, 1983
7. Lockshin MD, Gibofsky A, Peebles CL, Gigli I, Fotino M, Hurwitz S: Neonatal lupus erythematosus with heart block: family study of a patient with anti–SS-A and SS-B antibodies. Arthritis Rheum 26:210–213, 1983
8. Coons AM: Fluorescent antibody methods. Gen Cytochem Methods 1:399–422, 1958
9. Clark GM, Reichlin M, Tomasi TB: Characterization of a soluble cytoplasmic antigen reactive with sera from patients with systemic lupus erythematosus. J Immunol 102:117–122, 1968
10. Aarden LA, DeGroot ER, Feltkamp TE: Immunology of DNA. III. Crithidia luciliae, a simple substrate for the determination of anti-dsDNA with the immunofluorescence technique. Ann NY Acad Sci 254:505–515, 1975
11. Kulick KB, Provost TT, Reichlin M: Antibodies to single-stranded DNA in patients with discoid lupus erythematosus. Arthritis Rheum 25:639–646, 1982
12. Eighth International Workshop on Histocompatibility Testing. Los Angeles, UCLA Press, 1980
13. Ayoub G, Terasaki PI: Improved Dr typing of cadaver donor by lymphocyte incubation. Tissue Antigens 18: 289–293, 1981
14. McCuistion CH, Schoch ER Jr: Possible discoid lupus erythematosus in newborn infant. Arch Dermatol Syphilol 70:781–785, 1954
15. Epstein HC, Litt JZ: Discoid lupus erythematosus in a newborn infant. N Engl J Med 265:1106–1107, 1961
16. Jackson R: Discoid lupus in a newborn infant of a mother with lupus erythematosus. Pediatrics 33:425–430, 1964
17. Reed WB, May SB, Tuffanelli D: Discoid lupus erythematosus in a newborn. Arch Dermatol 96:64–66, 1967
18. Soltani K, Pacernick LJ, Lorincz AL: Lupus erythematosus-like lesions in newborn infants. Arch Dermatol 110:435–437, 1974
19. Vonderheid EC, Koblenzer PJ, Ming PML, Burgoon CF Jr: Neonatal lupus erythematosus: report of four cases with review of the literature. Arch Dermatol 112:698–705, 1976
20. Nice CM: Congenital disseminated lupus erythematosus. AJR 88:585–587, 1962
21. Levy SB, Goldsmith LA, Morohashi M, Hashimoto K: Tubuloreticular inclusions in neonatal lupus erythematosus. JAMA 235:2743–2744, 1976
22. Winkler RB, Nora AH, Nora JJ: Familial congenital complete heart block and maternal systemic lupus erythematosus. Circulation 56:1103–1107, 1977
23. Draznin TH, Esterly NB, Furey NL, DeBofsky H: Neonatal lupus erythematosus. J Am Acad Dermatol 1:437–442, 1979
24. Wallach D, Meyer O, Desbois JC: Lupus erythemateux neo-natal. Ann Dermatol Venereol 109:829–830, 1982
25. Miyagawa S, Kitamura W, Yoshioka J, Sakamoto K: Placental transfer of anticytoplasmic antibodies in annular erythema of newborns. Arch Dermatol 117:569–572, 1981
26. Lecha V, Herrero C, Bordas X, Lecha M, Mascaro JM, Gelpi C, Rodriguez JL: Lupus erythemateux neo-natal. Ann Dermatol Venereol 109:779–780, 1982
27. McCue CM, Mantakas ME, Tinglestad JB, Ruddy S: Congenital heart block in newborns of mothers with connective tissue disease. Circulation 56:82–90, 1977
28. Bremers HH, Golitz LE, Weston WL, Hays WG: Neonatal lupus erythematosus. Cutis 24:287–290, 1979
29. Brustein D, Rodriquez JM, Minkin W, Rabhan NB: Familial lupus erythematosus. JAMA 238:2294–2296, 1977
30. Lane AT, Watson RM: Neonatal lupus erythematosus. Am J Dis Child 138:663–666, 1984
31. Beck JS, Oakley CL, Rowell NR: Transplacental passage of antinuclear antibody (studies in infants of mothers with SLE). Arch Dermatol 93:656–662, 1966
32. Lee LA, Reed BR, Harmon C, Wolfe R, Wiggins J, Peebles C, Weston WL: Autoantibodies to SS-A/Ro in congenital heart block (abstract). Arthritis Rheum (suppl) 26:S24, 1983
33. Sontheimer RD, Stastny P, Gilliam JN: Human histocompatibility antigen associations in subacute cutaneous lupus erythematosus. J Clin Invest 67:312–316, 1981
34. Dillon CF, Jones JV, Reichlin M: Antibody to Ro in a population of patients with systemic lupus erythematosus: distribution, clinical and serological associations. J Rheumatol 10:380–386, 1983

EFFECTS OF LONG-TERM PROCAINAMIDE THERAPY ON IMMUNOGLOBULIN SYNTHESIS

CHIA-LI YU and MORRIS ZIFF

Procainamide is a potent inducer of autoantibodies. In order to evaluate the immunologic effects of this drug in vivo, 23 cardiac disease patients who had received procainamide for at least 6 months and an equal number of matched cardiac disease control subjects were studied, and percentage of circulating T cell subsets, concanavalin A–induced suppressor cell activity, and pokeweed mitogen–stimulated generation of immunoglobulin-secreting cells was quantitated. There was no significant difference between patient and control groups in the percentage of T cell subsets defined by OKT4 and OKT8 monoclonal antibodies or in concanavalin A–induced suppressor cell activity. The numbers of pokeweed mitogen–induced immunoglobulin-secreting cells were markedly decreased in the patient group, as measured by the protein A–augmented reverse hemolytic plaque assay (3,000 ± 644, mean ± SEM in patients versus 10,826 ± 1,529, mean ± SEM in control subjects, *P* < 0.005). Removal of the adherent cell fraction did not improve the hyporesponsiveness. When B and T cell fractions of 6 patients were mixed with normal T and B cell fractions, all of the patients demonstrated diminished B cell responses, and one-half also had diminished T cell responses. Addition of patient adherent cells to a co-culture of normal B cells with deficient patient T cells restored plaque formation to normal levels, suggesting that the T cell defect was correctable by a macrophage-derived factor. The data obtained suggest that procainamide exerts an immunosuppressive action on both B and T cell function in patients receiving this drug.

A number of drugs with differing chemical structures have been implicated in the induction of lupus erythematosus (LE) (1–7). Among these, procainamide (PA) is the most potent inducer of antinuclear antibody (ANA) (1,3,6). Prospective studies have revealed that this drug produces positive ANA tests in 50–83% of patients receiving long-term therapy (8–11). In addition to ANA, a spectrum of serologic and hematologic changes has been observed (1,2,4,12–18). The most common mechanism proposed to explain the development of autoantibodies in drug-induced LE is a drug–nucleoprotein interaction believed to enchance the autoimmunogenicity of nuclear components (2,19–22). However, this mechanism does not explain the occurrence of autoantibodies to non-nuclear antigens in this condition. Genetic factors (1,11,13,23–25) and the pharmacologic properties of the drug (26,27) appear to have important roles in the pathogenesis of the autoimmunity. Recently, evidence has shown that PA may interfere with the regulation of the immune system, either directly (14,28–31) or indirectly (2,32).

In this report, the effects of PA on immunoregulatory function have been studied in a group of patients with cardiac arrhythmias who had received PA for a

From the Harold C. Simmons Arthritis Research Center and the Department of Internal Medicine, University of Texas Health Science Center, Southwestern Medical School, Dallas, Texas.

Supported by grants AM-09989 and AM-18505 from the NIADDK and an Arthritis Clinical Research Center grant from the Arthritis Foundation.

Chia-Li Yu, MD: Fellow in Internal Medicine; Morris Ziff, PhD, MD: Ashbel Smith Professor of Internal Medicine, Director, Harold C. Simmons Arthritis Research Center.

Address reprint requests to Morris Ziff, PhD, MD, Harold C. Simmons Arthritis Research Center, Department of Internal Medicine, University of Texas Health Science Center at Dallas, Southwestern Medical School, 5323 Harry Hines Boulevard, Dallas TX 75235.

Submitted for publication March 16, 1984; accepted in revised form September 4, 1984.

minimum of 6 months. To evaluate the effects of this drug on immunoregulatory function in these patients, the percentage of T cell subsets in the blood, concanavalin A (Con A)–induced suppressor cell activity, and pokeweed mitogen–induced generation of immunoglobulin-secreting cells (PWM-ISC) have been examined.

PATIENTS AND METHODS

Patients. Twenty-three patients with coronary or hypertensive cardiovascular disease who had taken procainamide for at least 6 months were studied. Seventeen were men and 6 were women. As controls, simultaneous measurements were made in age-, sex-, and race-matched patients with coronary or hypertensive cardiovascular disease not receiving PA. Patients who were receiving hydralazine or other drugs known to induce lupus erythematosus were excluded. Five patients and 3 control subjects were receiving propranolol at the time of study. In the control patients, the daily dose of propranolol was approximately the same (80–140 mg/day) as in PA-treated patients.

The average age of the patients was 59.4 ± 6.5 years (range 47–69) and that of the controls was 59.0 ± 5.6 years (range 51–68). Male to female ratio was 3:1. The mean daily PA dose was 2.91 ± 1.0 gm and the mean duration of therapy was 2.5 years (range 6 months–11 years). Eleven of 22 patients tested had positive antinuclear antibody tests. All reactions were homogenous in pattern (33). This was combined with a speckled pattern in 2 patients and a peripheral pattern in 1. Two patients had drug-induced lupus erythematosus. None of the controls had a positive ANA test. Cold-reactive antilymphocyte antibody was not detected in the patient sera using normal peripheral blood mononuclear cells (PBMC) as targets.

Culture conditions. All cell suspensions were cultured in RPMI 1640 (Gibco, Grand Island, NY) supplemented with penicillin (100 units/ml), streptomycin (100 μg/ml), L-glutamine (0.3 mg/ml) (Microbiological Associates, Walkersville, MD), HEPES buffer (10 mmoles/ml, Gibco), and 15% heat-inactivated fetal bovine serum (Gibco) at 37°C in 5% CO_2, 95% air, for varying periods of time.

Cell preparation. Peripheral blood mononuclear cells were obtained by Ficoll-Hypaque (specific gravity 1.077; Gallard-Schlesinger, NY) density gradient centrifugation. To remove adherent cells (AC), the PBMC were incubated in glass petri dishes at 37°C in 5% CO_2 for 1 hour. The nonadherent cells (NC) were collected and the same procedure repeated once. The AC were harvested with a rubber policeman. More than 98% of the AC were nonspecific esterase–positive. These cells were used in the macrophage add-back study.

In order to obtain T and B cell–enriched populations, NC were further rosetted with neuraminidase-treated sheep red blood cells followed by centrifugation over density gradient cushions. The interphase cells were harvested, washed twice with Hanks' balanced salt solution (HBSS), and suspended in culture medium as the B cell–enriched population. The pellets were hemolyzed with cold ammonium chloride solution, washed, and suspended in culture medium as the T cell–enriched population. The purity of both B and T cell–enriched populations was approximately 90% in each case, as indicated by membrane immunoglobulin and OKT3 fluorescent antibody staining, respectively. In B cell–enriched populations, about 3–5% nonspecific esterase–positive cells were present.

Detection of T cell subsets. Commercially available mouse monoclonal antibodies, OKT3, OKT4, and OKT8 (Ortho Pharmaceutical Corp., Raritan, NJ), were used to define the human peripheral T cell subsets. OKT3 identifies human peripheral T lymphocytes, OKT4 identifies human helper/inducer, and OKT8 identifies cytotoxic/suppressor T cell subsets. The indirect immunofluorescence antibody method was used in 9 experiments. Briefly, 1×10^6/0.2 ml T cells were mixed with 5 μl of reconstituted mouse monoclonal antibody in an ice water bath, with occasional agitation for 30 minutes. After washing twice with 0.2% sodium azide in HBSS, the cells, suspended in a 100-μl volume of HBSS, were stained with 100 μl of a 1:40 dilution of fluorescein-conjugated goat anti-mouse immunoglobulin (Cappel Laboratories, West Chester, PA) and analyzed in a Becton-Dickinson III cell sorter (Becton-Dickinson, Sunnyvale, CA).

Protein A–augmented reverse hemolytic plaque assay (RHPA). To count the immunoglobulin-secreting cells, an RHPA was employed utilizing *Staphylococcus aureus* protein A–coated sheep red blood cells (SPA-SRBC) as indicator cells (34). The lymphocytes to be tested and the SPA-SRBC were suspended in agarose on microscopic slides. After an initial 1-hour incubation at 37°C, the slides were placed on Jerne racks and floated in a developing polyvalent rabbit anti-human immunoglobulin antiserum (Cappel). After another 1-hour incubation, the slides were floated in a 1:20 dilution of absorbed guinea pig serum (Cappel). After a final 1-hour incubation at 37°C, the resulting hemolytic plaques were counted using a stereomicroscope. Data were corrected by subtracting the number of ISC/10^6 responding cells in unstimulated cultures.

Con A–induced suppressor cell activity. Nonspecific suppressor cell activity was evaluated by a 2-stage method as described by Ochi et al (30). Briefly, 5×10^6/ml unseparated PBMC were stimulated with concanavalin A (Pharmacia Fine Chemicals, Uppsala, Sweden) at a final concentration of 30 μg/ml and cultured at 37°C in 5% CO_2 in petri dishes, with continuous shaking for 48 hours. As a control, Con A was added to the nonactivated control cells just before harvest. After induction, the whole population was harvested and intensively washed with 0.06*M* α-methyl-D-mannoside (Sigma, St. Louis, MO) in HBSS. The cells obtained were then added to PWM-stimulated cultures of freshly prepared PBMC from normal individuals. Suppressor and effector cells were co-cultured in U-bottomed microtiter wells in the presence of 10 μg/ml of PWM (Gibco) for 7 days. The total number of cells cultured per microwell was kept constant (1×10^5/well) while the proportion of the suppressor to effector cells was varied (0:4, 1:3, 2:2, 3:1, and 4:0). At the end of the incubation, cells from triplicate samples were pooled and the number of ISC generated at the various suppressor:effector ratios counted. The percent suppression was calculated according to the formula:

$$\%\ \text{suppression} = \left(1 - \frac{\text{ISC observed}}{\text{ISC predicted}}\right) \times 100$$

The predicted number of ISC was the sum of the values obtained by multiplying the number of ISC generated when each population of cells was cultured alone at a concentration of 1×10^6/ml by the fraction of the number of cells in the co-culture made up by that population.

PWM responsiveness of PBMC and NC. PWM responsiveness was quantitated by measuring PWM-induced ISC. To do this, 0.6 ml of PBMC or NC (5×10^5/ml) was cultured in 5-ml polystyrene tubes (Falcon Labware, Oxnard, CA) in the presence of 10 μg/ml PWM for 7 days. ISC were quantitated by the RHPA. In order to exclude the possibility of a change in kinetics in the patient group, 3 kinetic studies were done in which the ISC were measured

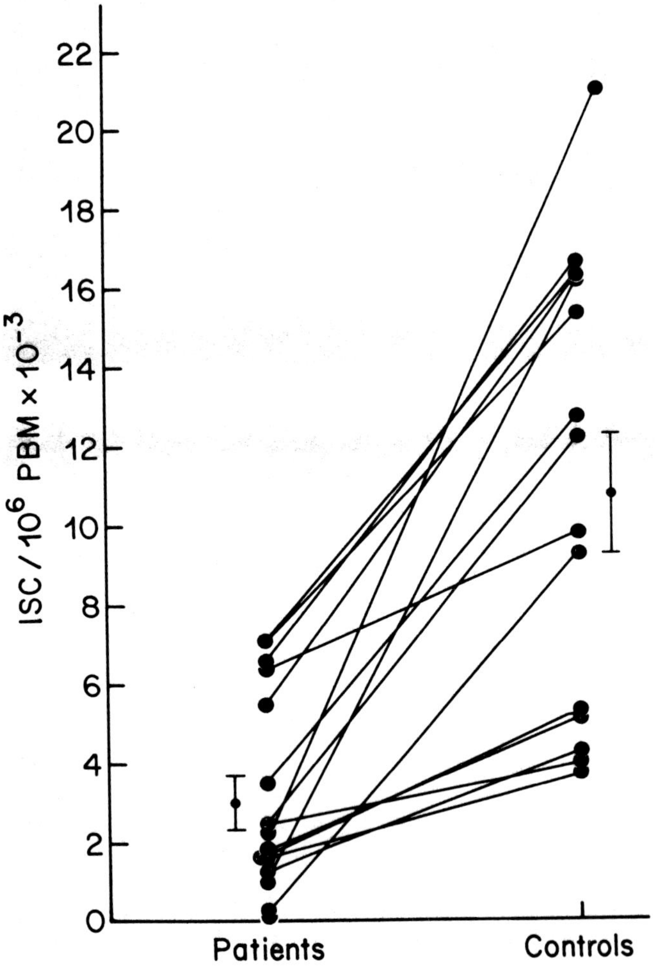

Figure 1. Comparison of pokeweed mitogen–induced generation of immunoglobulin-secreting cells (PWM-ISC) in patients and controls. Each line represents a paired experiment in which patient and matched control were studied simultaneously. ISC were assayed on day 7 after stimulation with PWM, 10 μg/ml. Brackets indicate mean ± SEM. The response is clearly decreased in the patient group compared with the control group ($P < 0.005$ by Student's t-test; $P < 0.005$ by 2-tailed paired t-test). PBM = peripheral blood mononuclear cells.

Table 1. Spontaneous and pokeweed mitogen (PWM)–induced immunoglobulin-secreting cells (ISC) in patients and control subjects

	ISC/10^6 peripheral blood mononuclear cells		
	Patients (n = 14)	Controls (n = 14)	*P*
Spontaneous	750 ± 174*	728 ± 195	NS†
PWM-induced	3,000 ± 644	10,826 ± 1,529	<0.005
Δ ISC‡	2,513 ± 596	10,118 ± 1,553	<0.005

* Values are mean ± SEM.
† Not statistically significant by Student's t-test.
‡ Δ ISC = PWM-induced ISC minus spontaneous ISC.

every other day until day 11. In addition, spontaneous ISC were measured between 18 and 24 hours after the blood drawing to determine the level of spontaneous activation in patients and controls.

Effect of addition of normal cells to patient cells. B or T cell–enriched populations from 6 patients were mixed in polystyrene tubes with normal T or B cells, in various ratios. The number of B cells was kept constant at 0.25×10^6/ml and the T cells were added to the tubes to establish T:B ratios varying from 0.5:1 to 4:1. PWM-ISC were assayed after 7 days of co-culture. At the same time, parallel cultures were set up using T cells previously treated with 25 μg/ml mitomycin C (Sigma) at 37°C for 45 minutes to abrogate suppressor cell activity. The pretreated T cells were intensively washed and cultured with B cells as above.

RESULTS

Percentage of T cell subsets defined by monoclonal antibody reagents. There was no significant difference in the percent of OKT4 or OKT8 cells, or in the OKT4:OKT8 ratio between the patient group (1.73 ± 0.33, mean ± SEM) and the control group (2.09 ± 0.21, mean ± SEM).

Con A–induced suppressor cell activity. Con A–activated suppressor cell activity directed against the generation of PWM-ISC in cultures of freshly prepared normal PBMC was quantitated at suppressor:effector cell ratios of 3:1, 1:1, and 1:3. Maximum suppression was observed at the 1:1 ratio. At this ratio, percent suppression was 80.2 ± 2.9 in the patient group and 69.6 ± 0.3 in the control group. These values did not differ significantly.

Kinetics of PWM-induced ISC response. A kinetic study of the PWM-ISC response was done to establish the optimum time to measure the ISC in the cultures. In 3 experiments with PBMC, ISC were measured every other day until day 11. In both patients and controls, maximum numbers of ISC were observed on the seventh day of culture.

PWM-ISC were then measured in patients and

controls in pairs. The cultures from the patient and his or her matched control were performed simultaneously in all cases. ISC were assayed on the seventh day of culture. Marked hyporesponsiveness to PWM stimulation was noted in the patient group relative to the control group, as shown in Figure 1 and Table 1. It can be seen in Figure 1 that in all matched pairs, the patient value was smaller than the control value and, as shown in Table 1, the difference between the mean values in the patients and controls was highly statistically significant ($P < 0.005$). Furthermore, 9 of the 14 control measurements were above the upper range of the patient values. The hyporesponsiveness was not different in the ANA-positive and ANA-negative patients.

PWM-induced and spontaneous ISC in patients and controls. Since polyclonal B cell activation has been reported in SLE (34,35), spontaneous ISC were determined between 18 and 24 hours after blood drawing in the absence of antigenic or mitogenic stimulation. No evidence of increase in spontaneous ISC was noted in the patient group, including the 2 patients with PA-induced lupus erythematosus (Table 1).

Mixing experiments. Six mixing experiments were carried out in which patient B or T cells were co-cultured for 7 days with normal T or B cells in the presence of 10 μg/ml PWM. The T:B cell ratio varied between 0.5 and 4. In a parallel series of experiments, T cells were pretreated with mitomycin C to abrogate the activity of the suppressor population before mixing with the B cells (30,34,36). It was observed that in 3 of the 6 patients, diminished generation of PWM-ISC was associated with decreased function of both B and T cells; in the other 3 patients, this was associated with decreased B cell function alone (Table 2). Thus, all of the 6 patients examined had a B cell defect and one-half also exhibited a T cell defect. Figure 2 shows the findings in a patient in whom both T cells and B cells exhibited deficient responses. Figure 3 shows the

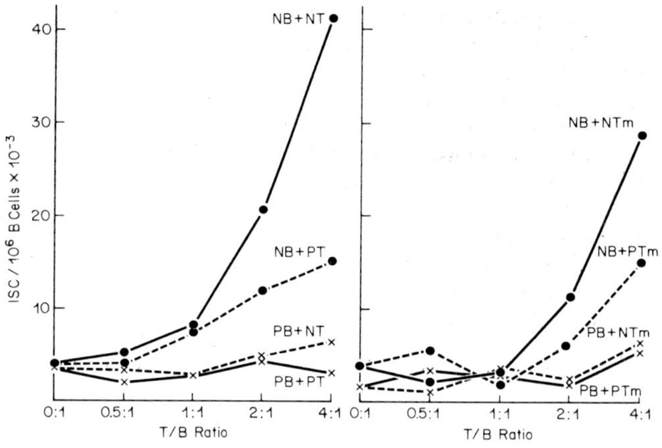

Figure 2. Pattern of deficient B and T cell responses to pokeweed mitogen (PWM) stimulation in a long-term procainamide (PA)–treated patient. NB = normal B cells; NT = normal T cells; PB = patient B cells; PT = patient T cells. The patient was a 66-year-old white man who had received 3 gm PA daily for 5 years without developing antinuclear antibody. In the co-culture study, both B and T cells were defective (**left**). After mitomycin-C treatment of the T cells either from the normal donor (NTm) or the patient (PTm), no distinct increase occurred in PWM-induced immunoglobulin-secreting cells (ISC) above that observed with untreated T cells (**right**).

Table 2. Pokeweed mitogen–induced immunoglobulin-secreting cells (PWM-ISC) in mixtures of patient and control cells

Mixing experiment	PWM-ISC (ISC/10^6 unseparated peripheral blood mononuclear cells) Patients	Controls	PWM-ISC after co-culture (ISC/10^6 B cells)* Normal B + Normal T (a)	Patient B + Patient T (b)	Patient B + Normal T (c)	Normal B + Patient T (d)	Deficient† population
1	3,250	24,450	30,600	4,400	6,000	39,200	B
2	7,400	18,000	50,000	13,600	18,200	49,000	B
3	3,500	12,700	32,180	3,600	5,800	34,000	B
4‡	650	12,500	41,200	3,200	6,400	15,200	B, T
5‡	2,250	12,200	38,400	3,200	10,200	14,600	B, T
6	3,500	15,500	40,400	6,000	11,200	14,000	B, T

* B cells (7.5×10^4), either patient or normal (cardiac disease control), were co-cultured with 3×10^5 T cells, either patient or normal (cardiac disease control) in the presence of 10 μg/ml PWM for 7 days. About 3–5% of nonspecific esterase–positive cells were contained in the B cell population.

† A deficient B cell response was indicated by a decreased value in column c compared with column a; deficient T cell function was indicated by a decreased value in column d compared with column a.

‡ Experiments 4 and 5 utilized the same patient with different controls.

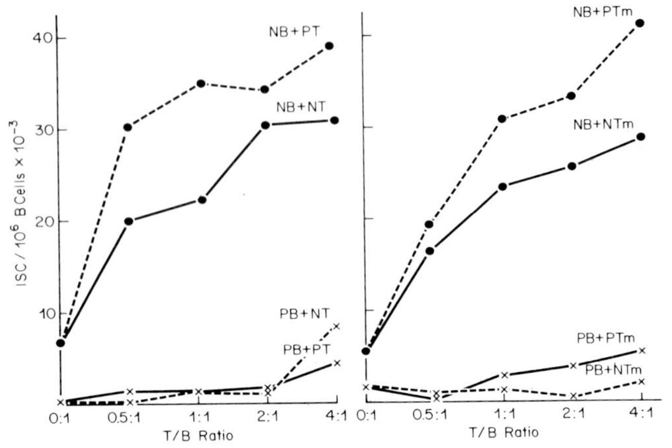

Figure 3. Pattern of deficiency of the B cell response alone to pokeweed mitogen in a long-term procainamide–treated patient. This 50-year-old black female patient received 3 gm of procainamide daily for approximately 1 year and then developed fever, arthralgias, myalgias, pericarditis, and a high antinuclear antibody titer (1:2,560, homogenous pattern). The patient B cell response was deficient, while the T cell response was intact (**left**). Mitomycin-C treatment of the T cells did not increase the number of PWM-induced immunoglobulin-secreting cells (**right**). See legend to Figure 2 for definitions.

findings in a patient in whom only the B cells were deficient. Mitomycin-C pretreatment of the patient T cells had no effect on the generation of PWM-ISC in either type of patient, indicating that the reduced ISC responses were not due to the proliferation of a suppressor T cell (36).

Table 2 summarizes the results of the 6 experiments in which patient B or T cells were mixed with normal T or B cells. In all cases, the number of ISC generated by PWM stimulation of mixtures of patient T and B cells was less than that of the simultaneously assayed normal B plus normal T cells. In all cases, the patient B cell response was also decreased, even in the presence of normal T cells. In experiments 4, 5, and 6, mixtures of patient T cells with normal B cells yielded decreased responses. Moreover, since experiments 4 and 5 utilized the same patient with different controls, it would appear that the defects in B and T cells observed were not dependent on the source of the normal cells.

Role of macrophages in procainamide-induced hyporesponsiveness. Activated macrophages may exert suppressive activity (37). To examine the possibility that the decreased PWM-ISC response observed in the patient group might be due to a macrophage-induced suppression, we compared PWM-ISC generation before and after removal of the glass-adherent cell fraction in 8 experiments. It was observed that the generation of PWM-ISC was decreased in 7 of 8 patients following removal of the adherent cells in the patient group, and less consistent change was noted in the control group (Figure 4). It would appear from this that the decreased PWM-ISC generation noted in the patient group was not due to an abnormal suppressor activity on the part of the adherent cell fraction. Moreover, the patient PWM response appeared to be more dependent on the presence of an adherent cell fraction than was the normal response.

Using isolated B and T cell fractions, additional

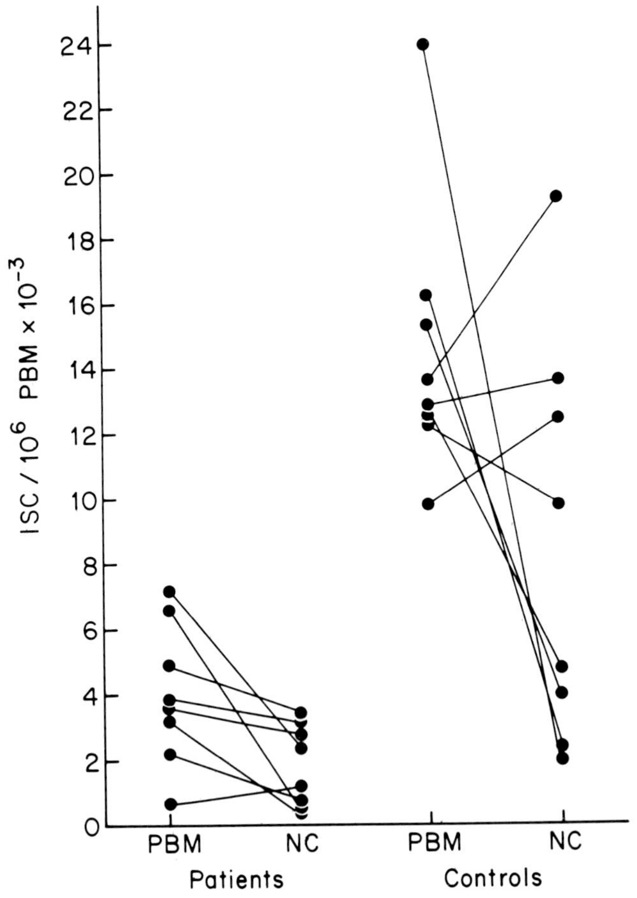

Figure 4. Role of adherent cells in pokeweed mitogen–induced immunoglobulin-secreting cell (ISC) generation. Nonadherent cells (NC) were collected after removing adherent cells by twice incubating peripheral blood mononuclear cells (PBM) in glass petri dishes at 37°C in 5% CO_2 for 1 hour each time. The lines connect measurements before and after removing the adherent cells. The fall in response in the patient group following removal of adherent cells indicates that the macrophage fraction was not exerting a suppressor effect and that the patient response was more dependent on the macrophage than was the control response.

Table 3. Pokeweed mitogen–induced immunoglobulin-secreting cells (PWM-ISC) in B cell and T cell mixtures supplemented with increasing numbers of adherent cells*

Cell combination	ISC/10^6 B cells	Cell combination	ISC/10^6 B cells
PB + PT		PB + NT	
+5% NAC	12,800	+5% NAC	13,200
+10% NAC	18,000	+10% NAC	13,200
+20% NAC	12,800	+20% NAC	12,400
+30% NAC	14,400	+30% NAC	17,600
+0% PAC	11,600	+0% PAC	14,400
+5% PAC	13,200	+5% PAC	14,800
+10% PAC	18,400	+10% PAC	15,200
+20% PAC	18,800	+20% PAC	12,400
+30% PAC	22,000	+30% PAC	14,000
NB + NT		NB + PT	
+0% PAC	83,200	+0% PAC	14,400
+5% PAC	72,800	+5% PAC	15,200
+10% PAC	66,400	+10% PAC	26,000
+20% PAC	79,600	+20% PAC	52,800
+30% PAC	62,800	+30% PAC	74,400

* B cells (0.25 × 10^6/ml) were mixed with 1 × 10^6/ml T cells in the presence of increasing numbers of syngeneic or allogeneic adherent cells. The same normal (control) and the same patient cells were used throughout the experiment. PB = patient B cells; PT = patient T cells; NT = normal T cells; NB = normal B cells; NAC = normal donor adherent cells; PAC = patient adherent cells.

experiments were carried out to determine whether the deficient B and T cell functions noted in the patient group were associated with an abnormality of macrophage function. In some of these experiments, patient B cells were mixed with either normal or patient T cells (in a ratio of 1:4) and then supplemented with increasing numbers of normal or patient adherent cells. In other experiments, normal B cells were mixed with either normal or patient T cells and similarly supplemented with adherent cells. As expected, no increase in PWM-ISC was noted following addition of normal adherent cells (NAC) to co-cultures of patient B cells with either patient or normal T cells (Table 3), indicating that the B cell deficiency in the patient was not remedied by normal macrophages. Neither was there a decrease in ISC when patient adherent cells (PAC) were added to mixtures of patient B cells with patient or normal T cells or normal B cells with normal T cells, indicating that the patient macrophages did not manifest suppressor activity. Finally, it is of particular interest that the addition of PAC to cultures of normal B cells with patient T cells progressively increased the number of ISC, indicating that the deficient T cell function of the patient group could be restored by increased numbers of adherent cells.

DISCUSSION

Because of the capability of PA to induce a spectrum of autoantibodies in treated patients, including antihistone antibody (2,12,19,38), anti–single-stranded DNA (2,6), antilymphocyte antibody (6,14,31), and rheumatoid factor (2,6,12,13,15), it appears likely that this drug has the capacity to interfere with normal immunoregulatory control mechanisms. There is evidence both in vivo (28) and in vitro (14,30,31) to indicate that PA interferes with such mechanisms. In this investigation, experiments have been carried out to further explore the effect of PA on immunoregulation in patients receiving long-term PA therapy, by measuring the separate functions of their T lymphocytes, B lymphocytes, and macrophages in PWM-stimulated cultures. The subjects were cardiac disease patients who had received PA for at least 6 months. Simultaneous paired control measurements were made in age-, race-, and sex-matched cardiac disease patients, hospitalized on the same wards or attending the same outpatient clinics, who had not received PA.

In preliminary experiments, it was found that there were no significant differences between patients and controls in the percentage of circulating T4 and T8 cells or in the suppressor activity of Con A–stimulated PBMC acting on PWM-induced generation of ISC in cultures of normal PBMC. However, when comparisons were made of the numbers of ISC generated in PWM-stimulated cultures of PBMC of PA-treated patients and untreated controls, the numbers of ISC generated in the PA-treated group were observed to be highly significantly decreased.

In experiments in which isolated populations of normal or patient T cells were mixed with normal or patient B cells and stimulated in culture with PWM, all 6 patients tested had a reduced ISC response to PWM in the presence of normal T cells, indicating that the PA-treated patient B cell function was deficient. Three of the 6 patients also manifested defective T cell function when their T cells were cultured with normal B cells. That the diminished PWM responsiveness was not attributable to an inhibitory action of macrophages was demonstrated in experiments in which removal of adherent cells from PBMC resulted in a fall rather than a rise in PWM-stimulated ISC. Also, addition of normal or patient adherent cells to PWM-stimulated cultures of patient B cells with normal T cells failed to increase the response, indicating that the decreased B cell response was not attributable to deficient macrophage function. With regard to the diminished T cell function, which was observed in 3 of 6 patients tested, it is of interest that this was corrected by addition of syngeneic patient adherent cells to cultures of normal B cells with patient T cells, indicating that the T cell defect, when it occurred, could be corrected by increased numbers of macrophages. The basis for this effect of macrophages on the defective T cells is not clear at the present time. However, it suggests that the T cell defect in PA-treated patients may be rectified by macrophages or a macrophage-derived factor.

The observed deficiency of B cell function in the PA-treated patients is similar to that reported in active idiopathic SLE in humans (39–42) and in aged New Zealand black mice (43). Although the decreased B cell function in patients with active SLE has been variously attributed to defective differentiation of the B cell population (42), combined B cell and helper T cell functional defects (39) and combined B cell and suppressor T cell functional defects (44) have been reported in this disease. Bluestein et al (14,31) found that 65% of patients with PA-induced LE and 20% of the long-term PA-treated patients had cold-reactive serum antilymphocyte antibody and proposed that PA might react with lymphocyte membranes to provide a neoantigen which could stimulate the formation of antilymphocyte antibody.

In experiments not discussed in this report, we did not detect antilymphocyte antibodies in this group of patients. With regard to a membrane effect, however, it is possible that PA, like the local anesthetic group of compounds of which it is an analog (45), may react with the cell membranes of B cells and T cells to provide either a membrane-stabilizing effect or an actual immunosuppressive effect, leading to the observed inhibition of mitogen-induced lymphocyte transformation. It is of interest that 2 other drugs known to stimulate positive ANA reactions, penicillamine and chlorpromazine, have been shown to inhibit mitogen-induced proliferation in vitro. Penicillamine is known to inhibit the response of helper T cells in culture (46); and it has been observed that chlorpromazine inhibits lymphocyte responsiveness to mitogens (47,48).

Two other reports have appeared in which the action of PA on immunoregulatory function has been investigated. One report from this laboratory by Ochi et al (30) has described an in vitro inhibition by PA of suppressor T cells, leading to the generation of increased numbers of ISC. This in vitro finding is in contrast with the present observation, in vivo, of diminished B cell function and in some patients also diminished T helper cell function. With respect to the findings of Ochi et al, it is perhaps to be expected that the action of a potential membranotropic agent, like PA, on the lymphocyte response would vary with the conditions of the drug-lymphocyte interaction. This report describes a long-term in vivo effect of PA while that of Ochi and colleagues described a local action on PBMC in culture. It is noteworthy that both reports observed an inhibitory effect on lymphocyte function.

In a report by Miller and Salem (28), increased cumulative IgG secretion was observed in PWM-stimulated cultures of PBMC from ANA positive PA-treated patients. This finding differs from our observation of consistently decreased PWM-induced ISC generation in similar cultures. Although only 50% of our patients were ANA positive, there appeared to be no difference between ANA positive and ANA negative patients in our observations. It should be noted that Miller and Salem measured IgG secretion, while we asssayed ISC of all immunoglobulin classes. It is, moreover, possible that measurement of plaque formation on the seventh day, as performed in our experiments, may provide information different from that obtained by Miller and Salem, measuring cumulative IgG secretion. Perhaps the most significant reason for the difference in results between the 2 studies, however, lies in the difference in the PWM responses in the control subjects in the 2 studies. The response to PWM stimulation in the control group of Miller and Salem appears inappropriately low (stimulation index [SI] = 3.3) in comparison with that of our control subjects (SI = 14.9), with that of Ginsburg et al (SI = 10.4) (34), and with that of Olsen et al (SI = 8.4) (49) in similar cultures.

The following hypotheses have been proposed regarding the autoimmune potential of PA: 1) it interacts with nucleoprotein to form a neoantigen (2,19–22); 2) it acts as an adjuvant for polyclonal activation of autoantibody producing clones (7); 3) it reactivates a latent virus (2,32); and 4) it interferes with immunoregulation (14,28–31). Our finding of the induction of PWM-ISC hyporesponsiveness is in accordance with similar findings with other autoimmunity-inducing drugs in vitro (46–48,50,51). Moreover, it resembles the diminished responsiveness to mitogen observed in patients with active idiopathic SLE (34). The defects in B and T cell function observed by us in long-term PA–treated patients may result from the ability of this drug to inhibit membrane depolarization by a mechanism similar to that observed in the cardiac conduction system (45). This effect, which may be related to the local anesthetic action of its analog, procaine, may endow PA with the capacity to suppress the function of immunocompetent cells.

ACKNOWLEDGMENT

The authors are grateful to Debbie McInnis for her excellent help in typing this manuscript.

REFERENCES

1. Alarcón-Segovia D: Drug-induced lupus syndromes. Mayo Clin Proc 44:664–681, 1969
2. Blomgren SE, Condemi JJ, Vaughan JH: Procainamide-induced lupus erythematosus: clinical and laboratory observations. Am J Med 52:338–348, 1972
3. Siegel M, Lee SL, Peress NS: The epidemiology of drug-induced systemic lupus erythematosus. Arthritis Rheum 10:407–415, 1967
4. Rutherford BD: Procainamide-induced systemic lupus erythematosus. NZ Med J 68:235–240, 1968
5. Lee SL, Chase PH: Drug-induced systemic lupus erythematosus: a critical review. Semin Arthritis Rheum 5:83–103, 1975
6. Weinstein A: Progress in Clinical Immunology. Vol. IV. Edited by RS Schwartz. New York, Grune & Stratton, 1980, pp 1–21
7. Schoen RT, Trentham DE: Drug-induced lupus: an adjuvant disease? Am J Med 71:5–8, 1981
8. Blomgren SE, Condemi JJ, Bignall MC, Vaughan JH: Antinuclear antibody induced by procainamide: a prospective study. N Engl J Med 281:64–66, 1969
9. Molina J, Dubois EL, Bilitch M, Bland SL, Friou GJ: Procainamide-induced serological changes in asymptomatic patients. Arthritis Rheum 12:608–614, 1969
10. Hope RR, Bates LA: The frequency of procainamide-induced systemic lupus erythematosus. Med J Aust 2:298–303, 1972
11. Henningsen NC, Cederberg A, Hanson A, Johansson BW: Effects of long-term treatment with procainamide: a prospective study with special regard to ANF and SLE in fast and slow acetylators. Acta Med Scand 198:475–482, 1975
12. Fakhro AM, Ritchie RF, Lown B: Lupus-like syndrome induced by procainamide. Am J Cardiol 20:367–373, 1967
13. Lappat EJ, Cawein MJ: A familial study of procainamide-induced systemic lupus erythematosus: a question of pharmacogenetic polymorphism. Am J Med 45:846–852, 1968
14. Bluestein HG, Zvaifler NJ, Weisman MH, Shapiro RF: Lymphocyte alteration by procainamide: relation to drug-induced lupus erythematosus syndrome. Lancet 2:816–819, 1979
15. Sheldon PJHS, Williams WR: Procainamide-induced systemic lupus erythematosus. Ann Rheum Dis 29:236–243, 1970
16. Utsinger PD, Zvaifler NJ, Bluestein HG: Hypocomplementemia in procainamide-associated systemic lupus erythematosus (letter). Ann Intern Med 84:293, 1976
17. Weinstein J: Hypocomplementemia in hydralazine-associated systemic lupus erythematosus. Am J Med 65:553–556, 1978
18. McLain DA, Hahn BH: Cryoglobulin in the procainamide-induced lupus syndrome. Arthritis Rheum 22:305–307, 1979
19. Tan EM, Portanova JP: The role of histones as nuclear autoantigens in drug-related lupus erythematosus. Arthritis Rheum 24:1064–1069, 1981
20. Eldredge NT, Robertson WVB, Miller JG III: The interaction of lupus-inducing drugs with deoxyribonucleic acid. Clin Immunol Immunopathol 3:263–271, 1974
21. Gold EF, Ben-Efraim S, Faivisewitz A, Steiner Z, Klajman A: Experimental studies on the mechanism of induction of anti-nuclear antibodies by procainamide. Clin Immunol Immunopathol 7:176–186, 1977
22. Dubroff LM, Reid RJ Jr: Hydralazine-pyrimidine interactions may explain hydralazine-induced lupus erythematosus. Science 208:404–406, 1980
23. Tannen RH, Weber WW: Antinuclear antibodies related to acetylator phenotype in mice. J Pharmacol Exp Ther 213:485–490, 1980
24. Davies DM, Beedie MA, Rawlins MD: Antinuclear antibodies during procainamide treatment and drug acetylation. Br Med J 3:682–684, 1975
25. Woosley RL, Drayer DE, Reidenberg MM, Nies AS, Carr K, Oates JA: Effect of acetylator phenotype on the rate at which procainamide induces antinuclear antibodies and the lupus syndrome. N Engl J Med 298:1157–1159, 1978
26. Uetrecht JP, Freeman RW, Woosley RL: The implications of procainamide metabolism to its induction of lupus. Arthritis Rheum 24:994–1003, 1981
27. Kluger J, Drayer DE, Reidenberg MM, Lahita R: Acetylprocainamide therapy in patients with previous procainamide-induced lupus syndrome. Ann Intern Med 95:18–23, 1981
28. Miller KB, Salem D: Immune regulatory abnormalities produced by procainamide. Am J Med 73:487–492, 1982
29. Tannen RH, Cunningham-Rundless S: Inhibition of Con A mitogenesis by serum from procainamide-treated patients and patients with systemic lupus erythematosus. Immunol Commun 11:33–45, 1982
30. Ochi T, Goldings EA, Lipsky PE, Ziff M: Immunomodulatory effect of procainamide in man: inhibition of human suppressor T cell activity in vitro. J Clin Invest 71:36–45, 1983
31. Bluestein HG, Redelman D, Zvaifler NJ: Procainamide-lymphocyte reactions: a possible explanation for drug-induced autoimmunity. Arthritis Rheum 24:1019–1023, 1981
32. Lerner RA, Dixon FJ, Crocker BP, Delvillano BC, Jensen FC, Kennel S, McConahey PJ: Schering Sympo-

sium on Immunopathology. Adv Biosci 12:356–360, 1974
33. Klajman A, Camin-Belsky N, Kimchi A, Ben-Efraim S: Occurrence, immunoglobulin pattern and specificity of antinuclear antibodies in sera of procainamide treated patients. Clin Exp Immunol 7:641–649, 1970
34. Ginsburg WW, Finkelman FD, Lipsky PE: Circulating and pokeweed mitogen-induced immunoglobulin-secreting cells in systemic lupus erythematosus. Clin Exp Immunol 35:76–88, 1979
35. Jasin HE, Ziff M: Immunoglobulin synthesis by peripheral blood cells in systemic lupus erythematosus. Arthritis Rheum 18:219–228, 1975
36. Lipsky PE, Ginsburg WW, Finkelman FD, Ziff M: Control of human B lymphocyte responsiveness: enhanced suppressor T cell activity after in vitro incubation. J Immunol 120:902–910, 1978
37. Laughter AH, Twomey JJ: Suppression of lymphoproliferation by high concentrations of normal human mononuclear leukocytes. J Immunol 119:173–179, 1977
38. Fritzler MJ, Tan EM: Antibodies to histones in drug-induced and idiopathic lupus erythematosus. J Clin Invest 62:560–567, 1978
39. Okudaida K, Tanimoto K, Nakamura T, Horiuchi Y: Spontaneously enhanced in vitro immunoglobulin synthesis by B cells in systemic lupus erythematosus. Clin Immunol Immunopathol 16:267–278, 1980
40. Nies KM, Stevens RH, Louie JS: Impaired immunoglobulin M synthesis by peripheral blood lymphocytes in systemic lupus erythematosus: a primary B cell defect. Clin Immunol Immunopathol 19:118–130, 1981
41. Pelton BK, Denman AM: Defective B cell function in systemic lupus erythematosus. Clin Exp Immunol 48:513–518, 1982
42. Bobrove AM, Miller P: Depressed in vitro B-lymphocyte differentiation in systemic lupus erythematosus. Arthritis Rheum 20:1326–1333, 1977
43. Primi D, Hammarström L, Smith CI: Genetic control of lymphocyte suppression. I. Lack of suppression in aged NZB mice is due to a B cell defect. J Immunol 121:2241–2243, 1978
44. Nishinarita S, Takizawa I, Hiria H, Morita K, Amaki I: Suppressor T cell dysfunction and depressed immunoglobulin production by B cells in vitro in patients with SLE. J Rheumatol 8:19–30, 1981
45. Seeman P: The membrane actions of anesthetics and tranquilizers. Pharmacol Rev 24:583–655, 1972
46. Lipsky PE, Ziff M: The effect of D-penicillamine on mitogen-induced human lymphocyte proliferation: synergistic inhibition by D-penicillamine and copper salts. J Immunol 120:1006–1013, 1978
47. Ferguson RM, Schmidtke JR, Simmons RL: Inhibition of mitogen-induced lymphocyte transformation by local anesthetics. J Immunol 116:627–634, 1976
48. Canoso RT, Yunis EJ: Immunogenetic markers in chronic schizophrenic males treated with long-term chlorpromazine therapy (abstract). Clin Res 28:341A, 1980
49. Olsen N, Ziff M, Jasin HE: In vitro synthesis of immunoglobulins and IgM-rheumatoid factor by blood mononuclear cells of patients with rheumatoid arthritis. Rheumatol Int 2:59–66, 1982
50. Pugh S, Pelton B, Raftery EB, Denman AM: Abnormal lymphocyte function is secondary to drug-induced autoimmunity. Ann Rheum Dis 35:344–348, 1976
51. Kirtland HH III, Mohler DN, Horwitz DA: Methyldopa inhibition of suppressor lymphocyte function: a proposed cause of autoimmune hemolytic anemia. N Engl J Med 302:825–832, 1980

PATTERNS OF ANTIHISTONE ANTIBODY SPECIFICITY IN SYSTEMIC RHEUMATIC DISEASE

I. Systemic Lupus Erythematosus, Mixed Connective Tissue Disease, Primary Sicca Syndrome, and Rheumatoid Arthritis with Vasculitis

ROBERT M. BERNSTEIN, RODERICK N. HOBBS, DONALD J. LEA, DONALD J. WARD, and GRAHAM R. V. HUGHES

A new fluorimetric assay was used to measure the relative amounts of antibodies to individual nuclear histones in sera from 102 patients with systemic lupus erythematosus (SLE), mixed connective tissue disease, primary sicca syndrome, and rheumatoid arthritis with vasculitis. In SLE sera, the predominant responses were to histones H-1, H-2B, and H-3, with marked elevations of binding to H-1 and H-2B in one-third of the patients, and to H-3 in one-fourth; antibodies of both the IgG and IgM classes were also detected. In a few SLE sera, the pattern of histone response differed or was restricted to 1 immunoglobulin class. In mixed connective tissue disease, only 2 of 9 sera showed elevated histone binding activity, the response being predominantly to H-3 in 1 patient and to H-1 and H-2B in the other. Binding to H-2B was also prominent in 2 of 3 patients with primary sicca syndrome. The highest antihistone reactivity and the most heterogeneous response patterns were observed in patients who had rheumatoid arthritis with vasculitis; 6 of 8 of those sera had elevated histone reactivity. In SLE, the highest histone binding results were found among patients with a history of photosensitivity. Histones are closely associated with DNA in the nucleosome, and we speculate that antihistone antibodies could arise as a result of damage to DNA, induced by drugs or irradiation.

From the Rheumatology Unit, Hammersmith Hospital, London, and the Rheumatology Department, Robert Jones and Agnes Hunt Orthopaedic Hospital, Oswestry, Shropshire, England.

Robert M. Bernstein, MA, MD, MRCP: Hammersmith Hospital; Roderick N. Hobbs, PhD: Robert Jones and Agnes Hunt Orthopaedic Hospital; Donald J. Lea, PhD: Robert Jones and Agnes Hunt Orthopaedic Hospital; Donald J. Ward MB, FRCP: Robert Jones and Agnes Hunt Orthopaedic Hospital; Graham R. V. Hughes, MD, FRCP: Hammersmith Hospital.

Address reprint requests to Dr. R. M. Bernstein, Rheumatism Research Unit, Manchester Royal Infirmary, Oxford Road, Manchester M13 9WL, England.

Submitted for publication September 14, 1983; accepted in revised form September 13, 1984.

Autoantibodies reactive with cellular components are a characteristic finding in systemic rheumatic disease. Among the antigens best characterized are DNA and the histones. The histones are a group of similar, small, highly conserved nuclear proteins (1) that bind to DNA by virtue of their many basic residues. They can be prepared in high purity as 5 distinct molecular fractions: H-1, H-2A, H-2B, H-3, and H-4.

The presence of antihistone antibodies has been reported in idiopathic and drug-induced systemic lupus erythematosus (SLE) (2–5), rheumatoid arthritis (RA) (5,6), and other conditions (7), and they are thought to be responsible for the lupus erythematosus cell phenomenon. We have developed a solid-phase fluorimetric assay for the measurement of antihistone antibodies, using highly-purified histone fractions (8). In this paper we report the diverse patterns of antihistone reactivity seen in different connective tissue diseases, emphasizing the predominant response to histones H-1, H-2B, and H-3 in SLE.

PATIENTS AND METHODS

Patients. We studied 82 patients with SLE fulfilling the American Rheumatism Association classification criteria (9), 9 patients with mixed connective tissue disease (MCTD) defined by the presence of anti-RNP antibody and high-titer speckled antinuclear antibody (ANA) in the absence of antibodies to Sm and with normal DNA binding (10), and 8 patients who had RA with vasculitis, presenting as cutaneous purpura and ulceration in 6 and mononeuritis multiplex in 5. Also studied were 3 patients who had primary sicca syndrome with keratoconjunctivitis sicca and salivary gland lymphoid follicles observed on lip biopsy; all 3 had rheumatoid factor and precipitating antibodies to Ro, and 2 had anti-La. Eight healthy controls were studied. Sera were stored at −20°C and examined with the investigator having no knowledge of the diagnosis.

Antihistone antibody assay. Purified individual histones were prepared using standard methods (11) and further purified by Biogel P-100. Histones H-1 and H-3 were from pig thymus; H-2A, H-2B, and H-4 were from calf thymus (Figure 1). In addition, whole calf thymus histones (Sigma, St. Louis, MO) were used in a screening study comparing the overall antihistone response with clinical features and HLA antigens. The assay buffer contained 3.02 gm/liter boric acid, 1.87 gm/liter disodium tetraborate ($Na_2B_4O_7 \cdot 10H_2O$), and 100 m*M* sodium chloride. Tween 20 (0.1%) was added to make up Tween buffer, a solution that minimizes nonspecific protein binding (12). The fluorescein-labeled sheep antisera to whole human IgG and IgM (Wellcome Reagents Ltd.) had fluorescein/protein molar ratios of about 3.5.

The assay was performed as described in detail previously (8). Polystyrene enzyme immunoassay cuvettes (Gilford, Oberlin, OH) were coated with tyrosine–glutamic acid copolymer with an average molecular weight of 66,000 (TGA; Miles-Yeda Ltd., Rehovot, Israel) by adding 100 μl of a 100-μg/ml solution in borate buffered saline to the cuvette bottom and tapping gently to ensure complete coverage. Cuvettes were sealed with Parafilm M (American Can Co., Greenwich, CT), left overnight at 20°C, and washed thoroughly with distilled water.

Individual histones were coated onto the prepared surfaces by overnight incubation of 100-μl volumes of histone (50 μg/ml) in borate buffered saline. Unbound protein was washed away quickly with buffer. Duplicate samples of 5% serum in Tween buffer were added to the cuvettes and left overnight at 20°C. Cuvettes were washed 3 times with Tween buffer, and a 100-μl solution containing a mixture of 1 volume fluorescein-labeled antiserum, 3 volumes normal sheep serum, and 56 volumes Tween buffer was added.

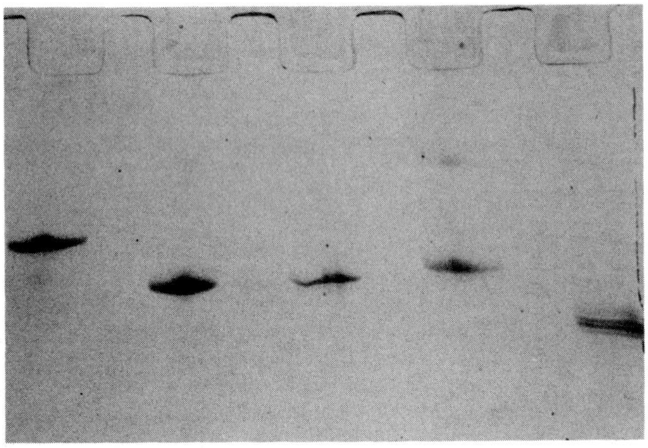

Figure 1. Purified histones used in the fluorimetric assay, displayed on a 6*M* urea/15% polyacrylamide gel. Left to right: H-1, H-2A, H-2B, H-3 (with a trace of dimer), and H-4 (showing the mono-, di-, tri-, and tetra-acetylated forms).

After incubation for 5 hours and then washing 3 times with Tween buffer, bound conjugate was released from the cuvette surface by addition of 750 μl of 0.2% sodium dodecyl sulfate (SDS) in 0.1*M* NaOH. The fluorescence of this solution was measured in a Locarte fluorimeter (13), using an SDS–NaOH solution blank. The fluorimeter was adjusted to read 1.000 with a 200-fold dilution of the mixture containing labeled antiserum in the SDS–NaOH solution. All binding values were the mean of estimations made in duplicate. An upper limit of normal was set arbitrarily at 2 standard deviations above the mean of the values for healthy controls.

Antibodies to DNA and soluble cellular antigens. Antibody to double-stranded DNA was measured by the Farr assay (14). Antibodies to acidic soluble cellular antigens were detected by counterimmunoelectrophoresis using extracts of rabbit thymus and human spleen (15).

HLA typing and clinical correlation in SLE. HLA–A, B, C, and DR antigens were determined in 64 SLE patients, and in all 12 patients with MCTD or primary sicca syndrome, by a microcytotoxicity assay (16) using antisera standardized against sera of the 8th Histocompatibility Workshop (17). Medical records of 64 SLE patients were reviewed retrospectively, and the following individual features were recorded: discoid lupus, facial rash, photosensitivity (light-induced rash or flare of lupus activity), alopecia, mouth ulcers, livedo reticularis, Raynaud's phenomenon, digital ischemia or vasculitis, arthritis, myositis, tendinitis, pleurisy, pericarditis, dyspnea, abnormal pulmonary function test results, proteinuria (>0.5 gm in 24 hours), urine granular or red cell casts, renal biopsy findings, hypertension, noninfective fever, sicca syndrome (dryness on Schirmer's test, with wetting <5 mm in 5 minutes, and/or salivary lymphoid follicles on lip biopsy), seizures, psychosis, depression, thrombosis, stroke, abortion, splenomegaly, lymphadenopathy, raised IgG, low IgA, low C3, low C4, anemia (<10 gm/dl), leukopenia ($<4.0 \times 10^9$/liter), lymphopenia, thrombocytopenia ($<100 \times 10^9$/liter on 2 occasions unrelated to therapy), steroid therapy, cytotoxic therapy, antimalarial therapy, Coombs' test result, rheumatoid factor, lupus anticoagulant, biologic false-positive test result for syphilis, and antibodies to nuclei DNA, Sm, RNP, Ro, La, SL, proliferating cell nuclear antigen, ribosomal RNP, and PL-4 (18).

For the purposes of this analysis, whole histone binding results were defined as normal (<0.1 fluorimeter units), moderately elevated (0.1–0.2), or high (>0.2), and the results were compared with the presence or absence of clinical features and HLA antigens by chi-square tests with 2 degrees of freedom (df). The 1 statistically significant correlation obtained was then examined further by Student's *t*-test using the binding results for each of the purified histones.

RESULTS

Controls. In the absence of serum, very little fluorescent conjugate was bound to the histone-TGA–

Table 1. Fluorimeter readings of 8 healthy control sera and comparison with 13 systemic lupus erythematosus (SLE) sera selected for results just above the arbitrary normal range

	Purified histones				
	H-1	H-2A	H-2B	H-3	H-4
Normal sera					
1	0.111	0.096	0.078	0.098	0.083
2	0.105	0.078	0.069	0.085	0.084
3	0.094	0.091	0.073	0.099	0.094
4	0.082	0.068	0.053	0.106	0.063
5	0.091	0.087	0.062	0.086	0.080
6	0.108	0.100	0.075	0.111	0.096
7	0.085	0.058	0.065	0.069	0.062
8	0.092	0.060	0.086	0.107	0.076
No serum	0.012	0.009	0.016	0.015	0.008
Mean of 8 normal sera	0.096	0.080	0.070	0.095	0.080
SD	0.010	0.015	0.010	0.013	0.012
Mean + 2 SD (arbitrary upper end of normal range)	0.116	0.110	0.090	0.121	0.104
Mean of 13 SLE sera	0.131	0.095	0.134	0.123	0.114
SD	0.031	0.029	0.031	0.035	0.028

coated cuvettes, and fluorimeter readings were about 0.01. Readings for 8 normal sera averaged approximately 0.08 for individual histone fractions (Table 1), suggesting that low levels of antihistone antibodies are a normal finding, although the possibility of some nonspecific Fc binding of IgG is not excluded.

SLE patients. Figure 2 shows SLE sera binding values >2 standard deviations above the mean values

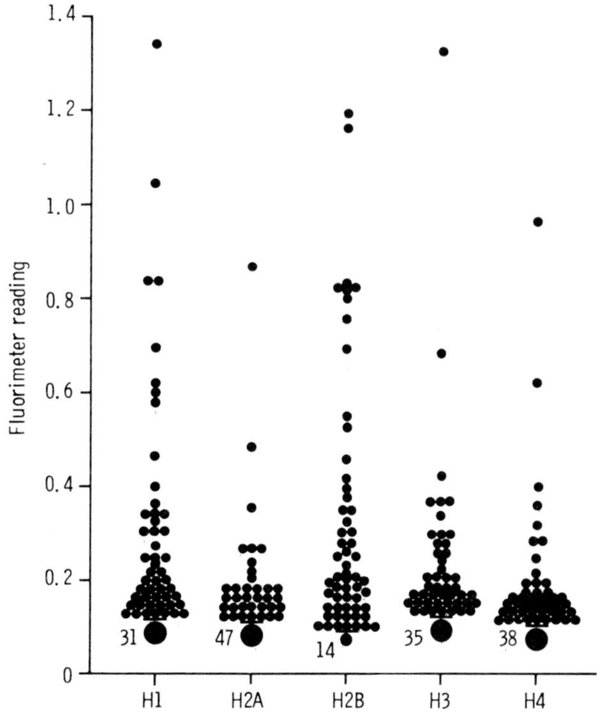

Figure 2. Binding values to the 5 individual histones in sera from 82 patients with systemic lupus erythematosus. Elevated values were defined as >2 standard deviations above the mean values of 8 normal sera.

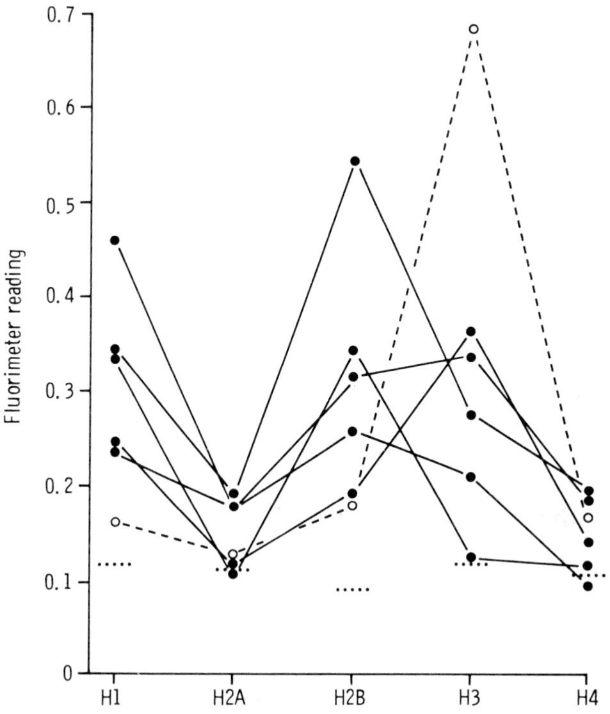

Figure 3. Typical binding patterns to the 5 individual histones in 6 systemic lupus erythematosus sera, showing greatest reactivity with histones H-1, H-2B, and H-3. One serum (○— —○) is unusual in that it shows mainly H-3 reactivity.

of the normal sera, for each of the individual histones. Binding to H-1 was elevated in 51 (62%), to H-2A in 35 (43%), to H-2B in 68 (83%), to H-3 in 47 (57%), and to H-4 in 44 (54%) of the 82 SLE sera tested. Although many SLE sera gave results only slightly above the normal range, a more marked elevation (>0.2 fluorimeter units) of binding to H-1 and H-2B was seen in about 32% of sera, to H-3 in 24% of sera, and to H-2A and H-4 in 10%.

Typical patterns of binding to the 5 individual histones are shown in Figure 3. In almost all cases, binding to histones H-1, H-2B, and H-3 was greater than binding to H-2A or H-4. As shown in Table 1, this pattern of reactivity was apparent even in SLE sera showing only modest binding (0.1–0.2 units), in contrast with the normal sera, where H-2B binding was lowest. A few SLE sera showed a more restricted pattern of binding to just 1 or 2 histones, such as to H-1 and H-2B or only H-3. Histone H-4 appeared to be least immunogenic, and antibodies to H-4 were predominant in only 1 patient.

MCTD patients. In keeping with the restricted nature of the antinuclear antibody response implicit in the serologic definition of MCTD (10), histone binding was normal in 7 of 9 MCTD sera tested. However, binding was elevated in 2 patients (Figure 4). The predominant response was to H-3 in 1 patient with photosensitive rash, alopecia, and Raynaud's phenomenon, and to H-1 and H-2B in a patient with Raynaud's phenomenon, depression, telangiectasia, and active ulcerative colitis. The latter patient was receiving therapy with salazopyrine, a drug capable of inducing ANA. All patients with normal histone binding activity had severe Raynaud's phenomenon, 2 had myositis and sicca syndrome, 1 had erosive arthritis and telangiectasias, and 2 had recurrent pleuritic pain controlled by low-dose prednisone.

Primary sicca syndrome patients. Histone binding was elevated in 2 of the 3 sera from patients with primary sicca syndrome. In 1 serum the response was to H-1 and H-2B; in the other it was to all histones except H-2A, with strikingly high binding to H-2B (Figure 4).

RA patients with vasculitis. Histone binding values were greatly elevated in 6 of the 8 sera from patients who had RA with vasculitis. The binding pattern was much more heterogeneous than in SLE, and very high binding to H-2A and H-4 was observed in this group (Figure 5). Titers of IgM rheumatoid factor were high in all cases, ranging from 160–1,280,

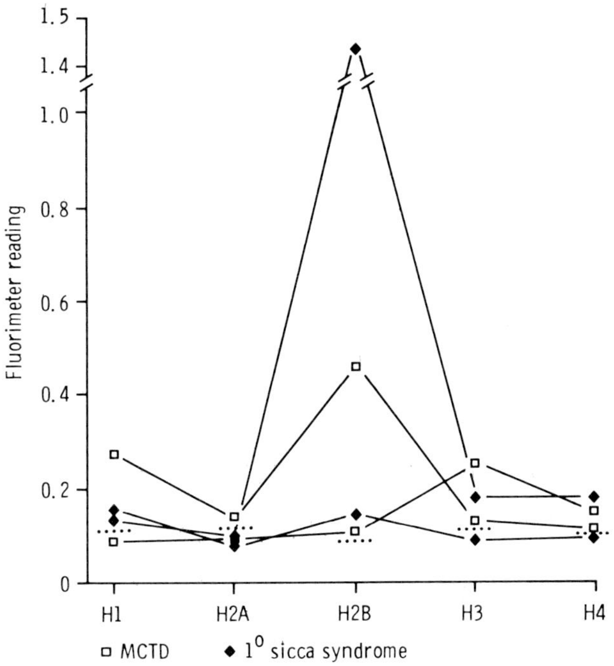

Figure 4. Histone reactivity patterns of sera from 2 patients with mixed connective tissue disease (MCTD) and 2 with primary sicca syndrome. Seven additional MCTD sera and 1 serum from a patient with primary sicca syndrome gave normal results.

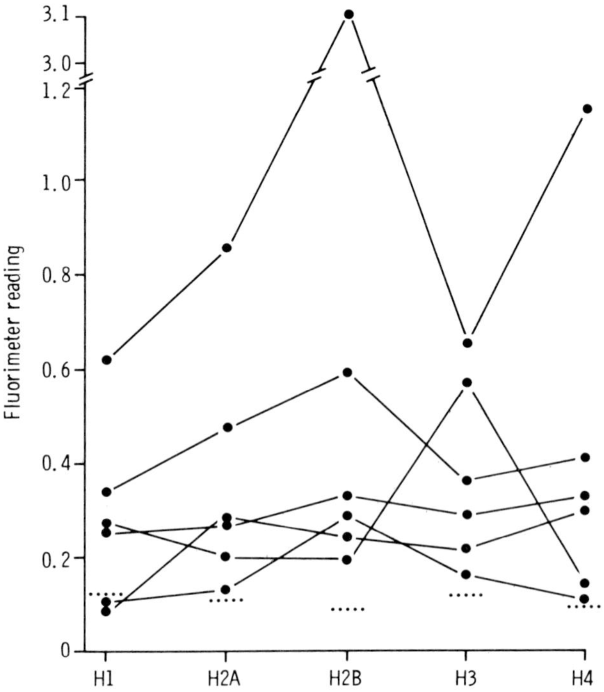

Figure 5. Heterogeneous histone binding patterns of sera from 6 patients with rheumatoid vasculitis. Two additional sera showed normal binding.

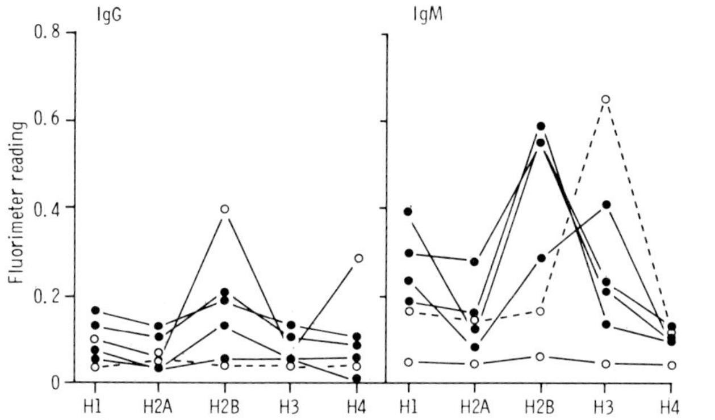

Figure 6. IgG and IgM binding patterns of sera from 6 systemic lupus erythematosus patients. ○— —○ is the same H-3–reactive serum shown in Figure 3. IgM reactivity predominates in 5 sera, and IgG reactivity in 1 (○——○).

but there was no correlation with the level, pattern, or immunoglobulin class of histone binding.

IgG and IgM antihistone responses. Eleven sera with high binding values were selected for separate examination of the IgG and IgM responses. In SLE (Figure 6), histone-binding antibodies were predominantly of the IgM class in 4 of 6 sera tested, and exclusively IgM in the 1 serum showing mainly anti–H-3 specificity. Only the sixth serum with predominantly anti–H-2B and anti–H-4 reactivity contained mainly IgG antibodies. In rheumatoid vasculitis, a greater proportion of the antibodies were of the IgG class. Only 1 of these sera showed clearly different patterns of histone reactivity when the IgG and IgM responses were compared (Figure 7).

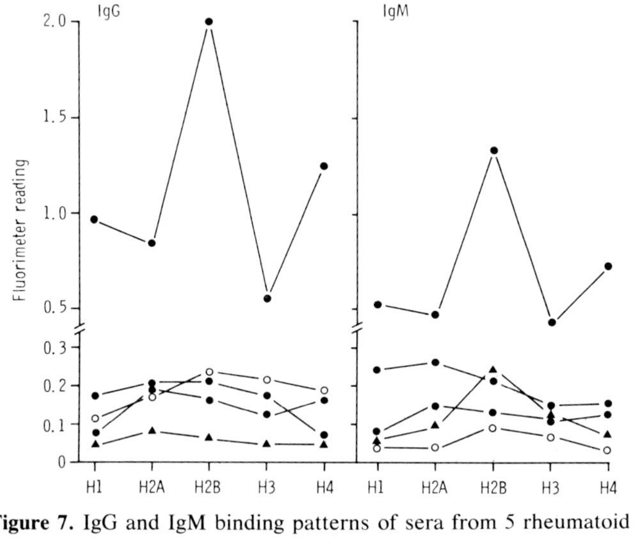

Figure 7. IgG and IgM binding patterns of sera from 5 rheumatoid vasculitis patients. The pattern of binding differed in 1 serum (▲——▲). IgG binding predominated in the highest binding serum, and in one other (○——○).

Table 2. Histone binding values in 60 systemic lupus erythematosus patients, by history of photosensitivity

Histone	History of photosensitivity		No history of photosensitivity		P (Student's t-test)
	Mean	SD	Mean	SD	
H-1	0.241	0.189	0.138	0.068	<0.005
H-2A	0.135	0.084	0.088	0.033	<0.005
H-2B	0.289	0.279	0.137	0.073	<0.005
H-3	0.161	0.078	0.128	0.072	<0.05
H-4	0.143	0.111	0.101	0.035	<0.05

Clinical-serologic correlation in SLE. In SLE sera, elevated binding to total histones showed no correlation with clinical features, HLA antigens, abnormal laboratory findings, or other autoantibodies,

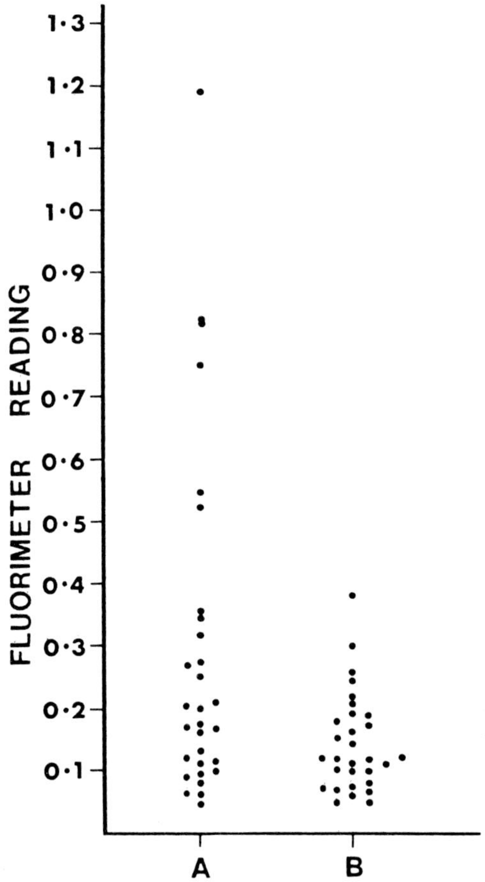

Figure 8. Histone H-2B binding values in systemic lupus erythematosus patients, according to the presence (**A**) or absence (**B**) of a history of photosensitivity.

except for a possible association with a history of photosensitivity (χ^2 = 9.2, 2 df, P = 0.01), but even this was not significant when corrected for the number of chi-square tests carried out. Nevertheless, the relationship between photosensitivity and elevated binding values for the individual histones was apparent on analysis by Student's *t*-test (Table 2). This relation is illustrated in Figure 8, which shows H-2B binding; all 6 patients with highest histone binding had histories of photosensitivity. Among the patients included in the clinical review, these 6 showed the highest binding to all histones, and an additional 2 patients had particularly high H-1 binding. All 8 patients were among the 30 with a history of photosensitivity, although this was not particularly severe or recent at the time blood was drawn for the study.

DISCUSSION

The pattern or relative magnitude of the immune response to the 5 histone proteins described in this study shows differences between SLE and the other rheumatic conditions examined. Further patterns are emerging among the antihistone antibodies induced by drugs (ref. 19 and Hobbs RN, Lea DJ, Bernstein RM: manuscript in preparation).

In SLE, the predominant responses were usually to H-1, H-2B, and H-3, but not to H-2A or H-4. Only 1 of the 82 SLE sera showed markedly elevated binding to a single histone (H-3), and this patient was unusual in that features of SLE were newly developing after a long prodrome of idiopathic thrombocytopenic purpura. In a serial study of patients with SLE (8), we found that the pattern of histone reactivity remains stable, although absolute levels may fluctuate with disease activity. Using the immunoblot technique, Hardin and Thomas (20) found antihistone antibodies in 11 of 24 SLE sera, with anti–H-1 and anti–H-2B predominant in most cases. We found above-normal levels of binding to 1 or more histones in 83% of the SLE patients tested, and marked elevations in 32% (as is readily apparent in Figure 2). This is in keeping with previous findings on antihistone antibodies in 30–60% of SLE sera (2,5,20,21).

Although overlap syndromes abound, the concept of MCTD remains controversial. The condition was originally defined by the presence of anti-RNP antibodies in the absence of other types of ANA (10,22), yet 2 of our 9 MCTD patients had elevated histone binding, and 2 others had antibody to the cellular antigen Ro (SS-A). Thus, it would appear unwise to adhere too rigidly to the serologic definition of MCTD, both because additional anticellular antibody specificities may be defined in these sera and because anti-RNP–negative overlap syndromes can be so clinically similar (22,23).

Although the highest binding values were found in serum from patients with rheumatoid vasculitis, these measurements are complicated by the possibility of rheumatoid factors binding either to the specific IgG antihistone antibody or to histones directly. A subset of rheumatoid factors does cross-react with histones (6). However, using the present assay, we demonstrated cross-reactivity only when rheumatoid factors were isolated from serum (24), and ANA-negative, rheumatoid factor–positive RA sera showed normal antihistone reactivity (8).

In normal sera, the low level of immunoglobulin binding measured in our assay may represent true antihistone antibody or nonspecific binding. The presence of autoantibodies in normal serum is well-documented for ANA (25), rheumatoid factor (26), antimitochondrial antibodies (27), and immune complexes (28). In SLE, many results were clustered just above the normal range, which we defined as 2 standard deviations above the mean of healthy control values. These slightly elevated values could reflect the elevated immunoglobulin levels often found in SLE, but as evidence against that possibility, histone binding was mostly normal in MCTD, where serum IgG is also often elevated. That the higher binding values measured in the patients' sera represent specific antibodies is supported first by the finding of various patterns of histone reactivity, and second by the restriction of antibody class in some cases.

Several assays for the detection of antihistone antibodies in SLE have been described, including (a) immunofluorescence after reconstitution of acid-extracted tissue sections with purified histones (2–4), (b) solid-phase radioimmunoassays (5,19,29), (c) enzyme-linked immunosorbent assays (ELISA) using a solid phase of polystyrene (21,30) or glass (31), and (d) immunoblot techniques (20). These methods have given conflicting results. For example, by an ELISA method (31), antibodies were found to be restricted to H-1 and H-2B in some cases, whereas by radioimmunoassay (5), little antibody to these histones was detected.

The fluorimetric assay developed for our studies is simple, specific, and sensitive, and gives results that are in substantial agreement with the findings of the 2 most recent reports (20,21). Specificity is ensured by the use of well-defined, highly-purified histones, while sensitivity is enhanced by the increased amount of histone antigen bound to the solid phase via the TGA copolymer (8). Although antibody binds nonspecifically to naked TGA, this binding is greatly diminished when the TGA is saturated with histones; indeed, normal sera show lower reactivity with histone-TGA than with naked TGA (8). In the absence of TGA, the sensitivity of the assay is lower, but the patterns of histone reactivity are unchanged.

There is one interesting exception. As shown in Figure 9, reactivity of antibody with histone H-4 was sometimes undetectable when H-4 was adsorbed directly onto the polystyrene. This observation suggests that antigenic sites on H-4 are restricted to the hydrophobic C-terminal region that is probably hidden when the protein binds directly to plastic. H-4 is known to undergo major conformational changes on binding to DNA or other histones (32,33), and TGA may have a similar effect on the conformation of H-4, which could be important to its recognition by antibody. To analyze in detail the antigenic site on this histone, we have predicted likely epitopes from the amino acid sequence and synthesized the relevant polypeptides to test with antibody.

The diverse patterns of antihistone reactivity described in this report may reflect differences in the underlying ability of each patient to mount an immune response to the histones. However, other factors such as differences in clearance and degradation cannot be ignored. A similar differential responsiveness to the closely-related Sm and RNP antigens appears to have a racial basis, in that the anti-Sm specificity is nearly 10 times more common in black and Chinese patients than in white patients (18). There are now several examples of autoantibody specificities involving more than 1 component of a nucleoprotein particle: antibodies are found simultaneously to DNA and several histones in the nucleosome, to high molecular weight RNA and 3 proteins in the ribosome (18), to the Ro and La antigens (which, together, form complexes with hyRNAs), and to several proteins in the soluble (U) RNP particles (34). It seems possible that, in each case, the immune response develops against the particle as a whole. In patients with SLE, MCTD, and primary sicca syndrome, antibodies to the different types of particle occur separately more often than together. The antinuclear response in all these related conditions is not merely polyclonal, but highly selective, and quite possibly, antigen-driven (18).

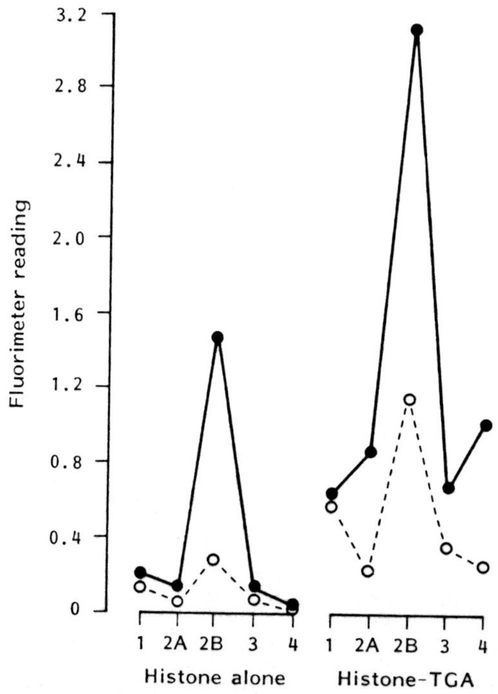

Figure 9. Immunoglobulin binding to tubes coated with purified histones in the absence (left) or presence (right) of the tyrosine-glutamic acid (TGA) copolymer. Two examples are shown.

The highest antihistone reactivity in SLE was found among patients with photosensitivity. Light therapy with psoralens and ultraviolet A irradiation damages DNA and may lead to ANA (but not anti-native DNA) production (35). Therapy with hydralazine (a drug that binds to DNA) induces antibodies directed against histones (16,36) and poly(ADP-ribose) (37), but rarely against DNA. In SLE, the most common antihistone response is to H-1 and H-2B (20,21, and this report). Both these histones lie in exposed positions on the nucleosome, again suggesting that the whole particle is the immunogen. In experimental studies the immunogenicity of histones is greatly enhanced by the addition of nucleic acid (38), and the soluble cellular Jo-1 and La antigens can interact with viral RNA (39). We would speculate that DNA acts as an immunologic carrier to which T lymphocytes are normally tolerant; damage to DNA by drugs or ultraviolet irradiation (40) could lead to a breakdown of tolerance, enabling anti-hapten responses to develop against DNA-associated molecules such as histones.

ACKNOWLEDGMENTS

We are indebted to Dr. G. H. Goodwin for the kind gift of highly-purified histones. We thank Dr. J. R. Batchelor and A. Dodi for the HLA determinations, C. C. Bunn for the DNA binding measurements, and Dr. Evelyn Hess for helpful discussions.

REFERENCES

1. Isenberg I: Histones. Annu Rev Biochem 48:159–191, 1979
2. Tan EM, Robinson J, Robitaille P: Studies of antibodies to histones by immunofluorescence. Scand J Immunol 5:811–818, 1976
3. Fritzler MJ, Tan EM: Antibodies to histones in drug-induced and idiopathic lupus erythematosus. J Clin Invest 62:560–567, 1978
4. Grossman L, Barland P: Histone reactivity of drug-induced antinuclear antibodies: a comparison of symptomatic and asymptomatic patients. Arthritis Rheum 24:927–931, 1981
5. Rubin RL, Joslin FG, Tan EM: A solid-phase radioimmunoassay for anti-histone antibodies in human sera: comparison with an immunofluorescence assay. Scand J Immunol 15:63–70, 1982
6. Aitcheson CT, Peebles C, Joslin F, Tan EM: Characteristics of antinuclear antibodies in rheumatoid arthritis: reactivity of rheumatoid factor with a histone-dependent nuclear antigen. Arthritis Rheum 23:528–538, 1980
7. Kubokawa T, Ishikawa H: Antibody to histone commonly observed in pemphigus and connective tissue disease. Arch Dermatol Res 273:149–152, 1982
8. Hobbs RN, Lea DJ, Ward DJ: fluorimetric assay for human antibodies to all the histones. J Immunol Methods 65:235–243, 1983
9. Tan EM, Cohen AS, Fries JF, Masi AT, McShane DJ, Rothfield NF, Schaller JG, Talal N, Winchester RJ: The 1982 revised criteria for the classification of systemic lupus erythematosus. Arthritis Rheum 25:1271–1277, 1982
10. Tan EM: Autoantibodies to nuclear antigens: their immunobiology and medicine. Adv Immunol 33:167–240, 1982
11. Johns EW: The isolation and purification of histones, Methods in Cell Biology. Edited by G Stein, J Stein, LJ Kleinsmith. London, Academic Press, 1977, pp 183–203
12. Smith JA, Hurrell JGR, Leach SJ: Elimination of non-specific adsorption of serum proteins by Sepharose-bound antigens. Anal Biochem 87:299–305, 1978
13. Lea DJ, Ward DJ: Estimation of IgM rheumatoid factors by fluorimetry. Ann Rheum Dis 37:247–251, 1978
14. Pincus T, Schur PH, Rose JA, Decker JL, Talal N: Measurement of serum DNA binding activity in SLE. N Engl J Med 281:701–705, 1969
15. Bernstein RM, Bunn CC, Hughes GRV: Identification of antibodies to acidic antigens by counterimmunoelectrophoresis. Ann Rheum Dis 41:554–555, 1982
16. Compston DHS, Batchelor JR, McDonald WI: B-lymphocyte alloantigens associated with multiple sclerosis. Lancet 2:1261–1265, 1976
17. Terasaki P, editor: Histocompatibility Testing 1980. Los Angeles, University of California Press, 1980
18. Bernstein RM, Bunn CC, Hughes GRV, Francoeur AM, Mathews MB: Cellular protein and RNA antigens in autoimmune disease. Mol Biol Med (in press)
19. Portanova JP, Rubin RL, Joslin FG, Agnello VD, Tan EM: Reactivity of anti-histone antibodies induced by procainamide and hydralazine. Clin Immunol Immunopathol 25:67–79, 1982
20. Hardin JA, Thomas JO: Antibodies to histones in systemic lupus erythematosus: localization of prominent autoantigens on histones H1 and H2B. Proc Natl Acad Sci USA 80:7410–7414, 1983
21. Costa O, Monier JC: Detection of antibodies to histones in human systemic lupus erythematosus and in murine lupus-like syndromes using micro-ELISA. Ann Immunol (Paris) 134:365–376, 1983
22. Alarcon-Segovia D: Mixed connective tissue disease: a decade of growing pains. J Rheumatol 8:535–540, 1981
23. Bernstein RM, Morgan SH, Chapman J, Bunn CC, Mathews MB, Turner-Warwick M, Hughes GRV: Anti-Jo-1 antibody: a marker for myositis with interstitial lung disease. Br Med J 289:151–152, 1984
24. Hobbs RN, Lea DJ, Phua KK, Johnson PM: Binding of isolated rheumatoid factors to histone proteins and basic polycations. Ann Rheum Dis 42:435–438, 1983
25. Lowenstein MB, Rothfield NF: Family study of systemic lupus erythematosus: analysis of the clinical history, skin immunofluorescence, and serologic parameters. Arthritis Rheum 20:1293–1303, 1977
26. Bartfield H: Distribution of rheumatoid factor activity in non-rheumatoid states. Ann NY Acad Sci 168:30–38, 1969
27. Baum H, Palmer C: Significance of anti-mitochondrial antibodies. Lancet 2:1411–1412, 1981
28. Contreras CE, Orozco A, Sanchez P, Ortega G, Bianco NE: Physiological aspects of circulating immune complexes in the normal population. Clin Exp Immunol 48:693–699, 1982
29. Blankstein LA, Stollar BD, Levy SB: Immunochemical distinction among histones and their variants in a solid-phase radioimmunoassay. Anal Biochem 104:168–172, 1980
30. Romac J, Bouley JP, Van Regenmortel MHV: Enzyme-linked immunosorbent assay in the study of histone antigens and nucleosome structure. Anal Biochem 113: 366–371, 1981
31. Aitkaci A, Monier JC, Mamelle N: Enzyme-linked immunosorbent assay for antihistone antibodies and their presence in systemic lupus erythematosus sera. J Immunol Methods 44:311–322, 1981
32. Lewis PN: Fluorescently labelled histones as probes of nucleosome structure: preparation and general properties of methionine-labelled histone H4. Eur J Biochem 99:315–322, 1979
33. Burch JBE, Martinson HG: Iodination of nucleosomes at low ionic strength: conformational changes in H4 and

stabilisation by H1. Nucleic Acids Res 9:4367–4385, 1981

34. Petterson I, Hinterberger M, Mimori T, Gottlieb E, Steitz JA: The structure of mammalian small nuclear ribonucleoproteins: identification of multiple protein components reactive with anti-(U1) RNP and anti-Sm autoantibodies. J Biol Chem 259:5907–5914, 1984
35. Kubba R, Steck WD, Clough JD: Antinuclear antibodies and PUVA photochemotherapy. Arch Dermatol 117:474–477, 1981
36. Portanova JP, Rubin RL, Joslin FG, Bernstein RM, Tan EM, Agnello VD: Antihistone antibodies induced by pronestyl and hydralazine (abstract). Arthritis Rheum (suppl) 24:S110, 1981
37. Clayton AL, Bernstein RM, Tavassoli M, Shall S, Bunn CC, Hughes GRV, Chantler SM: Measurement of antibody to poly(adenosine diphosphate-ribose): its diagnostic value in systemic lupus erythematosus. Clin Exp Immunol 56:263–271, 1984
38. Stollar BD, Ward M: Rabbit antibodies to histone fractions as specific reagents for preparative and comparative studies. J Biol Chem 245:1261–1266, 1970
39. Mathews MB, Bernstein RM: Myositis autoantibody inhibits histidyl-tRNA synthetase: a model for autoimmunity. Nature 304:177–179, 1983
40. Emerit I, Michelson AM: Mechanism of photosensitivity in systemic lupus erythematosus patients. Proc Natl Acad Sci USA 78:2537–2540, 1981

QUANTITATION OF THE Sm NUCLEAR ANTIGEN IN TISSUES AND ACTIVATED LYMPHOCYTES

CINDA M. BOYER, ROBERT A. EISENBERG, and PHILIP L. COHEN

Anti-Sm antibodies are specific for the diagnosis of systemic lupus erythematosus both in humans and in mice. Because the autoantibody response to this nuclear ribonucleoprotein particle is probably antigen driven, we have quantitated the Sm antigen in cells and tissues, using a highly sensitive and specific enzyme-linked immunosorbent assay. The Sm content of several in vitro cell lines was determined to be approximately 1 pg of Sm/cell. We found that murine spleen cells stimulated in vitro with either T cell or B cell mitogens contained up to 10 times more Sm than did unstimulated cells and that they also released increased amounts of Sm. In a survey of organs from several mouse strains, we found that lymphoid tissues had the largest amounts of Sm and that the Sm content of a particular tissue correlated with its DNA content. Increased amounts of Sm in and around activated lymphocytes, as found in systemic lupus erythematosus, may provide a source of antigen for the induction of the anti-Sm autoantibody.

From the Division of Rheumatology–Immunology, Department of Medicine, the Department of Microbiology–Immunology, and the Department of Hospital Laboratories, University of North Carolina School of Medicine, Chapel Hill, North Carolina.

Supported by grants from the National Institutes of Health (AM-26574 and AM-30701), the North Carolina Board of Science and Technology, University of North Carolina Research Council, the Kroc Foundation, and an Arthritis Foundation Clinical Research Center grant.

Cinda M. Boyer, PhD: Department of Hospital Laboratories, North Carolina Memorial Hospital, University of North Carolina, Chapel Hill (present address: Box 3010, Division of Immunology, Duke University Medical Center, Durham, NC 27710); Robert A. Eisenberg, MD: Division of Rheumatology–Immunology, Department of Medicine and the Department of Microbiology–Immunology, University of North Carolina, Chapel Hill, and Senior Investigator of the Arthritis Foundation; Philip L. Cohen, MD: Division of Rheumatology–Immunology, Department of Medicine and the Department of Microbiology–Immunology, University of North Carolina, Chapel Hill, and Senior Investigator of the Arthritis Foundation.

Address reprint requests to Robert A. Eisenberg, MD, Division of Rheumatology–Immunology, Department of Medicine, University of North Carolina School of Medicine, 932 FLOB 231H, Chapel Hill, NC 27514.

Submitted for publication July 17, 1984; accepted September 14, 1984.

Antibodies to the nuclear ribonucleoprotein antigen, Sm, are found in the sera of approximately 25% of patients with systemic lupus erythematosus (SLE) (1). The MRL/Mp-lpr/lpr mouse strain, which develops an SLE-like autoimmune disease, shows a similar frequency of anti-Sm antibodies (2). It is not known why anti-Sm antibodies are produced specifically in SLE, or why only a minority of patients produce this specificity. One possible factor in the induction of anti-Sm antibodies is the Sm antigen itself. Results of investigations from a variety of laboratories have characterized this antigen as a ribonucleoprotein particle. The ribonucleic acid moiety is composed of the U1, U2, U4, U5, and U6 small nuclear RNAs (3). The polypeptide(s), which contains the antigenic determinants, has been more difficult to characterize precisely (4–6). Recent evidence obtained, using Sm translated in a cell-free system, demonstrated that anti-Sm recognizes 8 different polypeptides ranging in molecular weight from 9,000–32,000 (7). The Sm protein–RNA complex may play a role in the processing of messenger RNA in normal cellular metabolism (8,9).

Previous work has shown that the distribution of the Sm antigen varies throughout the cell cycle (10). In addition, immunofluorescence analysis has suggested that activation of lymphocytes increases the intracellular content of Sm (11). In the present study, using a sensitive enzyme-linked immunosorbent assay (ELISA) to quantitate the Sm antigen, we have found that mitogen-stimulated lymphocytes contain and release increased amounts of Sm. In addition, we have defined the Sm content of various murine tissues and compared that with the cellular DNA content. Enhanced expression of the Sm antigen may occur in activated lymphocytes in SLE and thus contribute to the induction of anti-Sm antibodies in this disease.

MATERIALS AND METHODS

Animals. MRL/Mp-+/+ and MRL/Mp-lpr/lpr mice were obtained from our breeding colony. CBA mice were purchased from Dr. G. Haughton, University of North Carolina, Chapel Hill.

Cell lines. HEp-2 (human epidermal carcinoma cells), MRC (human embryonic lung fibroblasts), and McCoy (mouse carcinoma cells) cultures were purchased from Flow Laboratories, McLean, VA. P3HR1 (human lymphoblastoid cells) were obtained from the Tissue Culture Facility, University of North Carolina Cancer Center.

Preparation of cell and tissue lysates. Mice were killed by cervical dislocation, and the tissues were removed. Lymphoid organs were teased with a needle to obtain single cell suspensions. Cells were counted and viability determined by trypan blue exclusion. Supernatants and cell lysates from cultured lymphoid cells were prepared by centrifuging microtiter plate cultures, removing an aliquot of the supernatant, washing the cells, and resuspending the cell pellet in lysing buffer (0.2*M*, pH 8.3, borate buffered saline [BBS] plus 1% Nonidet P40, and the following protease inhibitors [Sigma, St. Louis, MO]: 0.5 m*M* phenylmethylsulfonyl fluoride, 10 m*M* ethylenediamine tetraacetic acid, 10 m*M* benzamidine, 1 m*M* o-phenanthrolene, and 50 m*M* ε-aminocaproic acid). For preparation of tissue lysates, tissue was weighed and pressed through stainless steel wire mesh into lysing buffer. Culture supernatants and cell and tissue lysates were stored at −20°C until testing.

Purification of Sm antigen and affinity columns. Sm antigen was prepared as described in detail elsewhere (6). Briefly, lyophilized acetone powder of rabbit thymus (Pel-Freez, Rogers, AR) was extracted in the cold with phosphate buffered saline in the presence of protease inhibitors. The phosphate buffer extract was digested with RNase and DNase. Sm antigen was differentially salted out between 35% and 60% saturated ammonium sulfate, and further purified by an affinity column containing anti-Sm antibodies. The purified Sm antigen contained immunoreactive polypeptides of 15,000 and 17,000 molecular weight (6) and was used as a standard for the Sm antigen ELISA assay. For construction of standard curves, the antigen was assumed to have an extinction coefficient at 280 nm of 10 for a 1% solution.

For use in antibody purification, affinity columns containing Sm antigen or SS-B antigen were prepared by coupling the 60% pellet (Sm antigen) or 80% pellet (SS-B antigen), obtained from the purification procedure described above, to CNBr-activated Sepharose (Pharmacia Fine Chemicals, Piscataway, NJ).

Preparation of antibody and enzyme reagents. Serum from an SLE patient (RM), containing antibody to Sm, RNP, SS-A, and SS-B defined by standard reference antisera, was purified on an affinity column containing Sm antigen. After the anti-Sm serum was bound to the column, the column was washed extensively with BBS containing protease inhibitors followed by the same buffer, plus 1*M* NaCl and 0.01% Nonidet P40. The column was eluted with 0.5*M* glycine, pH 2.5; the eluate was neutralized, concentrated by ultrafiltration, and dialyzed against BBS. The eluted material contained strong anti-Sm activity and weak anti–SS-B activity by immunodiffusion, and was further absorbed on an affinity column containing SS-B antigen. The unbound fraction contained only anti-Sm activity by immunodiffusion. The affinity-purified anti-Sm was pepsin-digested, and Fc fragments were removed with goat anti-human Fc coupled to CNBr-activated Sepharose (Pharmacia). The resulting $F(ab')_2$ fragments were biotinylated with biotinyl-N-hydroxysuccinimide ester (12). Avidin and alkaline phosphatase (Sigma) were conjugated with 0.1% glutaraldehyde.

Anti-Sm Fab fragments were purified from the sera of 2 SLE patients (RM and AW). IgG obtained by DEAE chromatography was digested with papain, and Fab fragments were isolated by sequential passage through DE52, G150, and affinity columns containing protein A and goat anti-human Fc coupled to CNBr-activated Sepharose (Pharmacia).

ELISA assay. Polyvinylchloride microtiter plates (Dynatech Laboratories, Alexandria, VA) were coated with 1 μg/ml of affinity-purified anti-Sm $F(ab')_2$ fragments in BBS containing protease inhibitors, for 5 hours at room temperature. Plates were washed 5 times with BBS and nonspecifically coated with BBS containing protease inhibitors, 0.4% Tween 80 (Sigma), and 0.5% bovine serum albumin (Fraction V; Miles Laboratories, Elkart, IN) for 1 hour at 4°C. Wells were aspirated, test samples added in a 100-μl volume, and plates were incubated overnight at 4°C. After 5 washes with BBS, biotinylated anti-Sm $F(ab')_2$ fragments were added, and the plates were incubated for 3 hours at 4°C. Plates were washed 5 times with BBS, avidin-conjugated alkaline phosphatase was added, and plates were incubated for 3 hours at 4°C. Following 5 washes with BBS, the substrate disodium paranitrophenylphosphate (Sigma) was added at 1 mg/ml in 0.01*M* diethanolamine buffer, pH 9.8. Plates were incubated at room temperature in a humidified changer.

Absorbance at 405 nm was measured several times with a micro-ELISA autoreader (Dynatech). The amount of Sm antigen in unknown samples was determined by referring average OD_{405} ELISA readings to a standard curve constructed with affinity-purified Sm antigen. The detection limit of the ELISA assay was approximately 0.1–1 ng of Sm protein. Reactivity of Sm antigen in the assay was completely inhibitable by anti-Sm Fab fragments purified from the sera of 2 SLE patients (RM and AW).

Lymphocyte blastogenesis. Mouse spleen cells were placed in round-bottom sterile microtiter plates (Costar, Cambridge, MA) at 5×10^6 cells/ml, in 0.2 ml complete RPMI 1640 (UNC Cancer Center, Chapel Hill, NC) supplemented with 5% heat-inactivated fetal calf serum (Gibco, Grand Island, NY), 2 m*M* glutamine, 15 m*M* HEPES, 100

Table 1. Detection of Sm antigen in nucleated cell lysates

Cell line	OD_{405}* 10[5] cells	10[4] cells	10[3] cells	pg of Sm/cell†
McCoy	1.429	0.307	0.020	0.83
HEp-2	0.802	0.445	0.071	1.53
MRC	0.778	0.425	0.051	1.45
P3HR1	0.802	0.283	0.030	0.75

* Average of duplicate samples. The SEM for all duplicates averaged <10% of the mean value. Average OD_{405} for lysing buffer was −0.003.

† Average OD_{405} values for 10^4 cells were referred to a standard curve constructed with affinity-purified Sm antigen.

units/ml penicillin, and 100 μg/ml streptomycin. Spleen cells were cultured with or without the mitogens phytohemagglutinin (PHA; Burroughs Wellcome, Greenville, NC) at 1 μg/ml, concanavalin A (Con A; Pharmacia) at 2 μg/ml, or lipopolysaccharide (LPS 055:B5; Difco, Detroit, MI) at 100 μg/ml. Cultures were incubated at 37°C in a humidified 5% CO_2 atmosphere for specified periods and then labeled with 1 μCi ^{3}H-thymidine (ICN Pharmaceuticals, Irvine, CA) for 8 hours. In kinetics experiments, cultures were labeled for 2 hours. Cultures were harvested onto filter discs with an automatic Mash II harvester (MA Bioproducts, Walkersville, MD). The discs were dried, placed in vials with scintillation fluid (National Diagnostics, Somerville, NJ), and counted in a liquid scintillation counter (Beckman LS200).

Colorimetric DNA assay. DNA was determined by the diphenylamine reaction as described by Burton (13). Briefly, calf thymus DNA standard (Sigma) and unknown samples in 0.5*N* $HClO_4$ were mixed with diphenylamine reagent containing acetaldehyde. Samples were incubated at 30°C for 16–20 hours, and absorbance at 600 nm was determined using a spectrophotometer. The amount of DNA in unknown samples was determined by referring OD_{600} readings to the calf thymus DNA.

RESULTS

Release of Sm antigen from nucleated cells. In preliminary experiments, various methods of cell disruption, including freezing, sonicating, and detergent treatment, were evaluated for releasing Sm antigen from cells. We found that the optimal procedure was 1 freeze–thaw cycle in BBS containing 1% Nonidet P40. Using this method, several tissue culture cell lines were assayed for Sm antigen. Sm antigen activity was detectable in cell lysates derived from 10^5, 10^4, and 10^3 cells, but not in lysing buffer (Table 1). Sm content varied from 0.8–1.5 pg of Sm/cell for the cell lines tested.

Sm antigen and DNA in lysates of murine tissues. Weighed tissue samples from various organs of 3 mouse strains were evaluated for Sm content by ELISA. OD readings were referred to a standard curve constructed with affinity-purified Sm antigen. Tissue Sm content for 2 mice of each strain is shown in Figure 1. Lymph node, spleen, and thymus contained relatively large amounts of Sm antigen, whereas brain, heart, and muscle contained small amounts of Sm. Intermediate values were obtained for liver, kidney, and lung tissue. The content of DNA, determined by the diphenylamine technique, was positively correlated with tissue Sm content ($r = 0.79$, $P < 0.01$, by linear regression).

Sm antigen in T cell mitogen–stimulated normal mouse spleen cells. CBA mouse spleen cells were cultured with or without mitogens, and ^{3}H-thymidine incorporation was assayed at 72 hours in quadruplicate cultures. PHA-stimulated and Con A–stimulated cultures incorporated 17–18 times as much labeled thymidine as did unstimulated cells (Table 2). Cell lysates and supernatants from cohort cultures were tested in the Sm ELISA assay. After 72 hours in culture, lysates from unstimulated cells contained an average of 32 ng

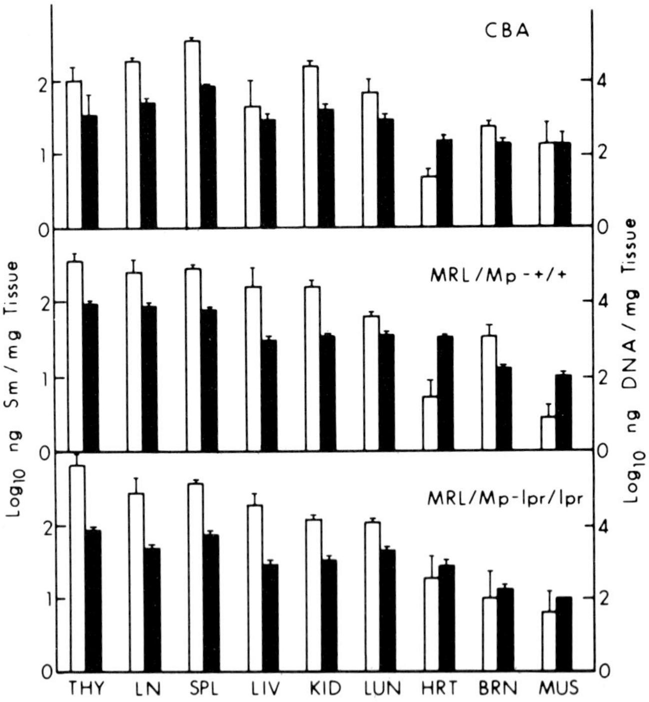

Figure 1. Sm and DNA content of murine tissues. Tissue lysates were assayed for Sm by enzyme-linked immunosorbent assay (open bars) and for DNA by diphenylamine (closed bars). Determinations were made for 2 mice for each of the 3 strains, except that only 1 DNA determination was obtained for MRL/Mp-lpr/lpr muscle. Data are expressed as average $\log_{10}$ ng/mg tissue (wet weight) ± SEM. THY = thymus; LN = lymph node; SPL = spleen; LIV = liver; KID = kidney; LUN = lung; HRT = heart; BRN = brain; MUS = muscle.

Table 2. Sm antigen in mitogen-stimulated mouse spleen cells*

	^{3}H-thymidine incorporation (cpm)	Cell lysates (ng of Sm/well)	Culture supernatants (ng of Sm/well)
Cells alone	4,371 ± 331	32 ± 7	12 ± 1
Cells + PHA	73,490 ± 1,196	276 ± 28	44 ± 1
Cells + Con A	79,860 ± 1,757	314 ± 24	42 ± 6

* Values represent the average of quadruplicate cultures ± SEM. PHA = phytohemagglutinin; Con A = concanavalin A.

of Sm/well (or 0.03 pg/cell added at the initiation of culture) and 12 ng of Sm/well in the supernatant. Cells cultured for 72 hours with PHA or Con A, however, contained tenfold more Sm in the cell lysates and 3.5-fold more in the supernatants (Table 2).

Kinetics of increase in Sm antigen expression in lectin-stimulated normal mouse spleen cells. CBA spleen cells were cultured with or without Con A, and quadruplicate cultures were assayed for ^{3}H-thymidine incorporation and Sm content by ELISA. In Con A–stimulated cultures, proliferation peaked at 48 hours, with 40 times more thymidine incorporation than in unstimulated cultures, and decreased at later time points (Figure 2). Maximal Sm antigen expression also occurred at 48 hours, with 7 times more Sm antigen in mitogen-stimulated cultures than in unstimulated cultures.

Sm antigen in LPS-stimulated normal mouse spleen cells. To determine if activated B cells could produce an increase in Sm, LPS, a mitogen selective for bone marrow–derived lymphocytes, was used to

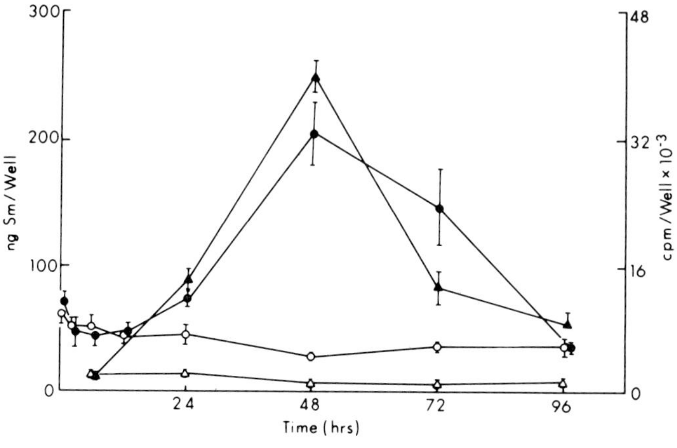

Figure 2. Kinetics of Sm antigen expression in cell lysates of concanavalin A–stimulated mouse spleen cells. Sm antigen activity in cell lysates of quadruplicate cultures was determined by enzyme-linked immunosorbent assay. ○——○ = unstimulated cells; ●——● = cells + concanavalin A; △——△ = ^{3}H-thymidine incorporation by unstimulated cells; ▲——▲ = ^{3}H-thymidine incorporation by cells + concanavalin A; bars = standard error.

Table 3. Sm antigen expression in cell lysates of LPS-stimulated mouse spleen cells*

	Time		
	0	24 hours	48 hours
Cells alone			
cpm/well	NT	3,576 ± 112	3,947 ± 240
ng of Sm/well	219 ± 78	122 ± 26	67 ± 17
Cells + LPS			
cpm/well	NT	32,995 ± 489	29,505 ± 814
ng of Sm/well	168 ± 28	341 ± 99	146 ± 9

* LPS = lipopolysaccharide; NT = not tested. Values represent the average of quadruplicate cultures ± SEM.

stimulate CBA spleen cells. ^{3}H-thymidine incorporation was tenfold higher in stimulated cultures at 24 and 48 hours. Sm antigen content was threefold higher in stimulated cultures at 24 hours, and twice as high at 48 hours (Table 3).

DISCUSSION

We have quantitated the Sm nuclear antigen in a variety of cell sources, using a highly sensitive micro-ELISA assay. In a survey of lysates of tissues from 3 different strains of mice, we have found the highest Sm content in lymphoid organs, such as thymus, lymph node, and spleen. These same tissues also had a high DNA content per mg of wet tissue. Overall, there was a strong correlation of amounts of DNA with amounts of Sm in all the tissues tested. This is consistent with the largely nuclear localization of the Sm antigen as has been demonstrated in immunofluorescence studies (10). We found an increase in Sm expression following mitogenic stimulation of T and B lymphocytes in vitro. Our results are consistent with those obtained by Jonsson and Norberg, who quantitated cellular Sm levels by indirect immunofluorescence (11). The enhanced Sm expression we observed paralleled the increased DNA synthesis, as evidenced by tritiated thymidine uptake. However, since mitogenic stimulation also results in increased RNA and protein synthesis in vitro (14), it cannot be assumed that Sm expression is directly related to DNA synthesis. In fact, others have proposed that small nuclear ribonucleoprotein particles are important in the processing of messenger RNA (8,9,15).

Although the assay's specificity for the Sm antigen was confirmed by inhibition with anti-Sm Fab fragments, it cannot distinguish the individual Sm antigen from that contained in nuclear ribonucleoprotein (nRNP) (16). Earlier work has shown that the nRNP particle cannot be purified free of the Sm antigenic determinant, while more recent biochemical studies have indicated that the Sm polypeptides are mostly a subset of those associated with nRNP (6). Since both forms of the Sm antigenic determinant are precipitable by anti-Sm antibodies, it would be expected that our assay would, likewise, detect them both.

The role of Sm and nRNP antigens in the induction of autoantibodies is unknown. One possibility is that autoantibodies to nuclear constituents may be induced by a cross-reacting, unrelated foreign antigen. However, this seems unlikely, since antibodies to such a wide variety of nuclear constituents are found in several autoimmune diseases. The clinical correlation of the presence of anti-Sm antibodies with anti-RNP antibodies (17) is an indication that the Sm antigen itself plays a role in the induction of anti-Sm antibodies. Since the Sm and nRNP antigens are found together on a single particle, the coexistence of their autoantibodies suggests that this particle plays a role in immunization. Similarly, the recent observation that several anti-Sm sera contain antibodies specific for each of the 8 separate polypeptide chains found in Sm translated in vitro from K562 cell messenger RNA, is also consistent with the Sm ribonucleoprotein particle's being immunogenic (7), since it is unlikely that a non–antigen-dependent mechanism would lead to the simultaneous generation of so many anti-Sm specificities.

It is possible that generalized lymphoid activation, which is a prominent feature of SLE (18), results in enhanced expression of the Sm nuclear antigen, as suggested by our in vitro results, and thereby favors the production of autoantibodies to this particular specificity. Alternatively, the Sm antigen may be expressed in a different form of SLE. For example, Mathews and Bernstein (19) have suggested that the Jo-1 autoantigen, autoantibodies to which are specific for polymyositis, might be made immunogenic by complexing it with RNA from a possible etiologic virus. Further work quantitating and characterizing the Sm antigen in mice and in humans with SLE might elucidate the mechanism of anti-Sm antibody formation in SLE and its relationship to underlying immunoregulatory abnormalities.

ACKNOWLEDGMENT

The authors would like to thank Dr. James D. Folds for encouraging this research as part of Dr. Boyer's postdoctoral training in clinical immunology in the Department of Hospital Laboratories at North Carolina Memorial Hospital, University of North Carolina, Chapel Hill.

REFERENCES

1. Notman DD, Kurata N, Tan E: Profiles of antinuclear antibodies in systemic rheumatic diseases. Ann Intern Med 83:464–469, 1975
2. Eisenberg RA, Tan EM, Dixon FJ: Presence of anti-Sm reactivity in autoimmune mouse strains. J Exp Med 147:582–587, 1978
3. Lerner MR, Steitz JA: Antibodies to small nuclear RNAs complexed with proteins are produced by patients with systemic lupus erythematosus. Proc Natl Acad Sci USA 76:5495–5499, 1979
4. Takano M, Golden SS, Sharp GC, Agris PF: Molecular relationships between two nuclear antigens, ribonucleoprotein and Sm: purification of active antigens and their biochemical characterization. Biochemistry 20:5929–5936, 1981
5. Billings PB, Allen RW, Jensen FC, Hoch SO: Anti-RNP monoclonal antibodies derived from a mouse strain with lupus-like autoimmunity. J Immunol 128:1176–1180, 1982
6. Eisenberg RA, Klapper DG, Cohen PL: The polypeptide structure of the Sm and RNP nuclear antigens. Mol Immunol 20:187–195, 1983
7. Fisher DE, Conner GE, Reeves WH, Blobel G, Kunkel HG: Synthesis and assembly of human small nuclear ribonucleproteins generated by cell-free translation. Proc Natl Acad Sci USA 80:6356–6360, 1983
8. Lerner MR, Boyle JA, Mount SM, Wolin SL, Steitz JA: Are snRNPs involved in splicing? Nature 283:220–224, 1980
9. Rogers J, Wall R: A mechanism for RNA splicing. Proc Natl Acad Sci USA 77:1877–1879, 1980
10. Deng JS, Takasaki Y, Tan EM: Nonhistone nuclear antigens reactive with autoantibodies: immunofluorescent studies of distribution in synchronized cells. J Cell Biol 91:654–660, 1981
11. Jonsson J, Norberg R: Some functional properties of the RNP nucleoplasmic antigen. Scand J Immunol 12:119–127, 1980
12. Bayer EA, Skutelsky E, Wilchek M: The avidin-biotin complex in affinity cytochemistry, Methods in Enzymology. Vol. 62. Edited by DB McCormick, LD Wright. New York, Academic Press, 1979, pp 308–315
13. Burton K: A study of the conditions and mechanism of the diphenylamine reaction for the colorimetric estimation of deoxyribonucleic acid. Biochem J 62:315–323, 1956
14. Takasaki Y, Deng J-S, Tan EM: A nuclear antigen associated with cell proliferation and blast transformation: its distribution in synchronized cells. J Exp Med 154:1899–1909, 1981
15. Hinterberger M, Pettersson I, Steitz JA: Isolation of small nuclear ribonucleoproteins containing U1, U2, U4, U5, and U6 RNAs. J Biol Chem 258:2604–2613, 1983
16. Mattioli M, Reichlin M: Physical association of two

nuclear antigens and mutual occurrence of their antibodies: the relationship of the Sm and RNA protein (Mo) systems in SLE sera. J Immunol 110:1318–1324, 1973
17. Sharp GC, Irvin WS, May CM, Holman HR, McDuffie FC, Hess EV, Schmid FR: Association of antibodies to ribonucleoprotein and Sm antigens with mixed connective-tissue disease, systemic lupus erythematosus and other rheumatic diseases. N Engl J Med 295:1149–1154, 1976
18. Ropes MW: Systemic Lupus Erythematosus. Cambridge, MA, Harvard University Press, 1976, pp 48–49
19. Mathews MB, Bernstein RM: Myositis autoantibody inhibits histidyl-tRNA synthetase: a model for autoimmunity. Nature 304:177–179, 1983

ASSESSING PHYSICIAN/PATIENT PERCEPTIONS IN RHEUMATOID ARTHRITIS

A Vital Component in Patient Education

ILENE J. SILVERS, MELBOURNE F. HOVELL, MICHAEL H. WEISMAN, and MARY ROSE MUELLER

Patient education surveys were completed by 101 patients with rheumatoid arthritis and by 28 rheumatologists to assess and compare patients' reports with physicians' perceptions of patients' needs regarding content, provider, and education program delivery methods. Both groups agreed on the importance of patients' education about arthritis, especially on the topics of medication, physician/patient communication, quackery, and maintaining ambulation. A higher proportion of physicians reported that patient education was needed in psychosocial areas, activities of daily living, sexual concerns, and community resources. Patients sought more education in disease process, diagnostic procedures, and nutrition. Patients rated pharmacists and nutritionists significantly more important as educational sources than did physicians. Both groups reported individual patient/practitioner meetings as the preferred delivery method. Physicians reported group education to be valuable for some psychosocial topics; patients disagreed significantly. Despite considerable consensus, disagreements were evident in the psychosocial area and in the role of allied health professionals. Clarification, understanding, and resolution of these differences should be sought before implementing patient education programs.

Patient education is accepted as a valid component in management of rheumatoid arthritis (RA) (1–4). Traditionally, the identification of health education needs for chronic diseases has been made by providers whose generalizations have often been based on casual clinical observations, individual case studies, stereotypical attitudes toward patients, or by arbitrary decree (5). These practices may result in erratic or poorly structured programs. Little information is available to permit a more empiric decision-making process for planning patient education programs in the management of chronic disease (6,7).

Patients with RA represent a prototype for long-term disease management because of their changing functional status and the need for their cooperation in the treatment regimen. It has become recognized that components in the treatment program may exacerbate or create psychosocial problems (7). It seems reasonable, therefore, to expect that RA education protocols should be based on a systematic assessment of patients' needs. Results of patient/provider surveys attempting to determine educational content, treatment components, or overall beliefs about arthritis have been reported (8–10). However, these studies examined a heterogeneous patient population as well

From the Graduate School of Public Health, San Diego State University, and the Department of Medicine, Division of Rheumatology, University of California School of Medicine, San Diego, California.

Supported by grant AM-07062-07 from the National Institutes of Health Rheumatic Disease Training Program, an Arthritis Foundation Clinical Research Center grant, and the UCSD Clinical Research Center, NIH grant RR-00827.

Ilene J. Silvers, MPH: Health Education Specialist, San Diego Area Arthritis Foundation and Adjunct Faculty Member, Division of Health Promotion, Graduate School of Public Health, San Diego State University; Melbourne F. Hovell, PhD, MPH: Associate Professor and Head, Division of Health Promotion, Graduate School of Public Health, San Diego State University; Michael H. Weisman, MD: Associate Professor of Medicine, Department of Medicine, Division of Rheumatology, UCSD Medical Center; Mary Rose Mueller, FNP: Clinical Nurse, Department of Medicine, Division of Rheumatology, UCSD Medical Center.

Address reprint requests to Michael H. Weisman, MD, University of California School of Medicine, H-811G, 225 W. Dickinson Street, San Diego, CA 92103.

Submitted for publication March 27, 1983; accepted in revised form October 3, 1984.

as a mixed sample of health care providers. Given the unique differences between RA and other rheumatic diseases, it was determined that a more homogeneous study of RA patients and rheumatologists was needed.

There exists a body of theoretical and practical information recommending physician/patient negotiation of medical treatment goals toward increasing patient satisfaction, compliance, and treatment outcome (11–17). Another reasonable approach involves a dual perspective needs assessment to establish goals for effective medical and educational services. This approach permits the development of more personalized and comprehensive education programs by providing information useful in determining priorities, focusing the scope and content, and setting mutually determined goals (18).

This study was undertaken to determine the scope and content of RA education through (a) the self-expressed needs of RA patients, and (b) rheumatologists' perceptions of RA patients' educational needs. Identifying the priorities set by both may permit development of educational interventions that are flexible yet specific to patients' needs and compatible with the complexities of the treatment regimen. Exploration of the differences between patient and physician perspectives may provide insights into that relationship, permit more cooperation, and alert planners to postpone educational services until disagreements are resolved.

METHODS

Participants. *Patient selection.* The patient sample was derived from University of California/San Diego (UCSD) Medical Center's computerized active patient data file. All of the 185 ambulatory patients with RA diagnosed by staff rheumatologists were surveyed. Included were patients seen in rheumatology clinics of the University and VA Medical Centers and private patients of faculty physicians.

Patient respondent profile. Of 101 patients (55%) who returned the survey, 55 were women, 44 were men, and 2 did not indicate. All were being treated by 1 of the responding physicians. Forty patients had VA providers, 42 were private patients of faculty rheumatologists, and 19 were seen by rheumatology fellows in the UCSD Arthritis Clinic. Patients' ages ranged from 24–79 years (mean 58.2). There was a range of 1–49 years (mean 14.2) since first diagnosis of RA. Patients were predominantly white (87%) and were English-speaking (91%). The median level of education was high school. Ten patients reported completing less than high school; 45 reported completing more than high school. Most patients reported incomes from $10,000–$15,000. Fifteen patients reported incomes under $5,000; 11 patients reported incomes over $35,000.

Age, sex, and source of patients were factors considered to determine whether respondents appeared to represent a different population from nonrespondents. Both groups had a mean age of 58 years. Women comprised 55% of the respondents and 61% of the nonrespondents; men comprised 45% of the respondents and 39% of the nonrespondents. Approximately the same proportions (63%, 53%, 44%) of respondents were obtained from each of the patient settings relative to each group's eligible pool of patients. Thus, no substantial differences in respondents and nonrespondents were apparent.

Physician selection. Physicians were chosen from those designated as rheumatology specialists on the approved referral list from the San Diego and Imperial County Arthritis Foundation. Sixteen physicians represented major teaching institutions including the University of California, Scripps Clinic and Research Foundation, Kaiser-Permanente Medical Plan, VA Medical Center, and Naval Regional Medical Center. Another 16 physicians were in community private practice. In addition, all 6 fellows from the Division of Rheumatology at UCSD Medical Center were queried. Thirty-six physicians were men, 2 were women, and all were white.

Physician respondent profile. The 28 physicians who responded (74%) reported an average of 9.7 years in practice. At least 10 (36%) were known to have 1 or more of their patients among those who responded. The percentage of clinical practice time spent in rheumatology ranged from 10–100% with an average of 67%. Twenty-six respondents were men; 2 were women. No significant differences between the respondents and nonrespondents were noted.

Survey procedures. *Patient survey: design and content.* Questions were personalized to ask, "how important would this be to you?" Respondents simply checked 1 of 4 categories from extremely important (scale 3) to not at all important (scale 0), or 3 categories including always, sometimes, never. Some questions only required a yes or no answer. A subset of sixth-grade students verified an elementary school readability level after standard readability formulas were determined to be inappropriate for this instrument.

Patients were questioned on 51 variables which included RA education experience, desire for information, importance of various topics in RA education, and the importance of 8 allied health professionals for providing arthritis education. Furthermore, patients were asked to rate the importance of 5 communication channels by which they might receive arthritis information. Then they were asked to indicate the preferred method of receiving topic-specific education pertinent to RA.

Patient survey: administrative procedures. The survey was mailed to 185 patients. Ten patients were predominately Spanish-speaking; 4 Spanish language surveys were returned. The cover letter explained that the purpose of the survey was to identify needs, concerns, and feelings prior to establishment of an educational program. Patients were guaranteed anonymity and confidentiality. Reminder follow-up phone calls were made after 3 weeks to solicit questionnaires not yet received. Two months after initial mailing, analyses were initiated for the 101 responses.

Physician survey: design and content. The physician survey was directed to rheumatologists. The design followed the same format as the patients' survey. Several of the questions were mirror images, which facilitated comparison of physicians' and patients' views on the same issues. Some language modification was necessary in order to assess the physicians' perceptions of the needs of the RA patients. The physicians' questionnaire also inquired about the type of group education believed to be suited best to the community and to their respective practices.

Physician survey: administrative procedures. A cover letter to physicians explained the origin and purpose of the survey, i.e., "to better plan and facilitate a comprehensive, structured, community-based patient education program." It also guaranteed individual confidentiality and provided for strictly voluntary participation. An adjunct to the cover letter was a personal note from one of the authors (MHW). Within 2 weeks, one-half of the 38 physicians had responded. Subsequently, the physicians from whom no response had been received were called. A total of 28 (74%) responded.

Statistical analysis. Descriptive statistical analyses were performed on each survey. Frequency distributions and proportions were reported for all questions. Chi-square analyses were employed for categorical data that examined associations between patients' and physicians' judgments concerning health education. Because of selective failure to answer some individual questions, the sample size for analyses varied. However, for most questions, no more than 6 answers were missing.

RESULTS

Patients. *General need: RA education.* To assess the general need for an education program, patients were asked 3 questions: 1) "Have you ever taken part in an arthritis education program?" 2) "How much do you know about RA?" 3) "Would you like to learn more?" Seventy-six percent had never participated in an arthritis education program. On a scale of 0–3 (0 = nothing, 3 = a lot), 42% reported knowing a lot, 33% reported knowing a moderate amount, 24% reported knowing a little, and 1 patient reported knowing nothing. Ninety-two percent indicated that they wished to learn more.

Allied health professionals in RA education. Patients were asked to rate the importance of allied health professionals (nonphysician) in facilitating arthritis education. While most patients (49–75%) reported that all the professionals were extremely or very important, those professionals receiving the highest proportion (69–75%) of patients rating them as extremely or very important were: physical therapist, pharmacist, occupational therapist, and nutritionist. Rated very important by smaller proportions (49–60%) were: nurse, trained group leader, Arthritis Foundation representative, and social worker.

Topics for RA education. Patients rated the importance of 18 possible topics for RA education. All content areas were considered extremely or very important by a strong minority (44%) to a large majority (95%) of patients. The 3 topics for which training was reported to be extremely or very important by the highest proportion of patients (91–95%) were interpersonal communication between physician and patient, medication, and disease process.

Nine other topics also received high proportions (72–82%) of patient responses rating them very or extremely important. They included: recognizing quackery, maintaining ambulation, nutrition, diagnostic procedures, special pain relief, surgical procedures, cooperative disease management, prescribed exercises, and stress reduction, rest and relaxation.

Still important, but receiving only about 65% of responses, were energy conservation, weight management, and psychosocial needs. The patient population was roughly divided (44–55%) concerning the need for training in activities of daily living, sexual concerns, and community resources.

Arthritis education channels. For general information regarding arthritis, patients were asked to rate the importance of 5 possible communication channels. A clear majority reported individual meetings with health practitioners (80%), printed material (73%), and media programming (63%) as extremely or very important. A simple majority indicated that planned education groups (55%) and self-care or support groups (58%) were somewhat to not important.

Channel preference for RA concerns. Patients were asked to choose 1 of 4 channels for education on selected RA topics. The largest proportion (35–59%) favored individual meetings with a health practitioner for most content areas. The next highest proportion reported printed materials as their choice for receiving information on nutrition (48%), medication (37%), and stress reduction, rest and relaxation (26%). Smaller proportions indicated that planned group sessions may be acceptable for learning about stress reduction, rest and relaxation (31%), occupational therapy (29%), physical therapy (26%), and relating to family and friends (26%). It is particularly noteworthy that an important minority of patients responded to "none" of the channels for the following areas: sexual concerns (31%), relating to family and friends (23%), dealing with emotions and feelings (19%), and stress reduction, rest and relaxation (13%).

Physicians. *Present RA education practice.* To determine rheumatologists' perceptions of the need for an RA education program, physicians were asked if they thought that structured patient education would be beneficial in the management of RA; 100% responded "yes." Furthermore, 75% indicated that they did not currently have such a program.

Perception of patients' wishes. Each physician estimated what percentage of his/her patients wanted to know more about RA. Estimates ranged from 5–100%, with an average of 70%. Seventy-one percent thought that 60% or more of their patients wanted additional arthritis education.

Importance of nonphysician allied health professionals. Regarding the importance of nonphysician allied health professionals in providing arthritis education, physical therapists (85%) and occupational therapists (79%) received the largest proportions of extremely or very important ratings by physicians. Education provided by trained group leaders (68%), Arthritis Foundation representatives (65%), and nurses (63%) was reported to be very important by the majority of physicians. On the contrary, the following 3 professionals were considered to be less important (ratings of somewhat or not at all important) by the majority of physicians: pharmacist (61%), social worker (64%), and nutritionist (86%).

Topics for RA education. Physicians were asked to respond to the importance of 18 possible topics for an RA education program. While more than 60% of physicians rated 13 of the 18 topics as extremely or very important, it is noteworthy to examine the extremes. The 4 topics receiving the greatest proportion of physicians rating them as extremely or very important were: interpersonal communication between physician and patient (100%), psychosocial needs (100%), medication (96%), and activities of daily living (93%). A clear majority of physicians (68–89%) rated 9 topics as very important: maintaining ambulation, recognizing quackery, rest and relaxation, sexual concerns, special pain relief, prescribed exercises, community resources, cooperative disease management, and surgical procedures.

Approximately one-half of the physicians reported energy conservation (59%), disease process (56%), and weight management (46%) as very or extremely important. Receiving the lowest ratings were diagnostic procedures and nutritional issues; 61% and 78% of physicians, respectively, rated them as somewhat or not at all important.

Arthritis education channels. To determine what they believed to be the most effective communication channels for delivering RA education, physicians were asked to rate the importance of 5 different channels. Individual meetings with a health practitioner and planned group sessions were both reported to be extremely or very important by approximately 85% of physicians. Printed material received a clear majority with 64%. Physicians were roughly divided over the importance of media programming (57%) and arthritis support or self-care groups (50%).

Channel preference for RA concerns. When physicians were asked to select 1 of 4 communication channels to deliver specific RA education topics, the majority (46–86%) reported individual meetings with a health practitioner as the preferred method for 6 of the 10 topics: interpersonal communication between patient and physician, physical therapy, occupational therapy, diagnostic procedures, sexual concerns, and medication. Planned group sessions were preferred for patients' psychosocial concerns, including dealing with emotions and feelings (54%), stress reduction, rest and relaxation (82%), and patients' relations with family and friends (86%). Nutrition was reported as best presented through planned groups (36%) or printed materials (25%). Printed materials were reported as a secondary choice for education concerning medication by 29% of physicians.

Format and facilitators of RA education groups. Ninety-three percent of physicians responded affirmatively (yes/no scale) to offering structured self-help group programs conducted by trained lay leaders. When asked which of 2 programs (a trained volunteer–conducted self-help course for lower fees compared with an allied health personnel–conducted course which might require higher fees) was most in line with their practices and patients' needs, 75% of physicians preferred a course facilitated by trained volunteers, 18% preferred the allied health professional conducted course, and 7% were undecided.

Patient/physician comparison. In order to compare the expressed needs and desires of patients with the perceptions of physicians who are responsible for the delivery of their health care, the results of several mirror questions were analyzed.

Allied health professionals. Figure 1 compares the physicians' and patients' ratings, as extremely or very important, for each of 8 allied health professionals (nonphysician) concerning their roles in RA education. Patient/physician reported preferences were unremarkable for most of the professionals considered. Significant differences between physicians' and patients' responses ($P \leq 0.001$, $\chi^2[1]$) were demonstrated for the importance of the pharmacist and nutritionist. Seventy-three percent of patients rated the pharmacist

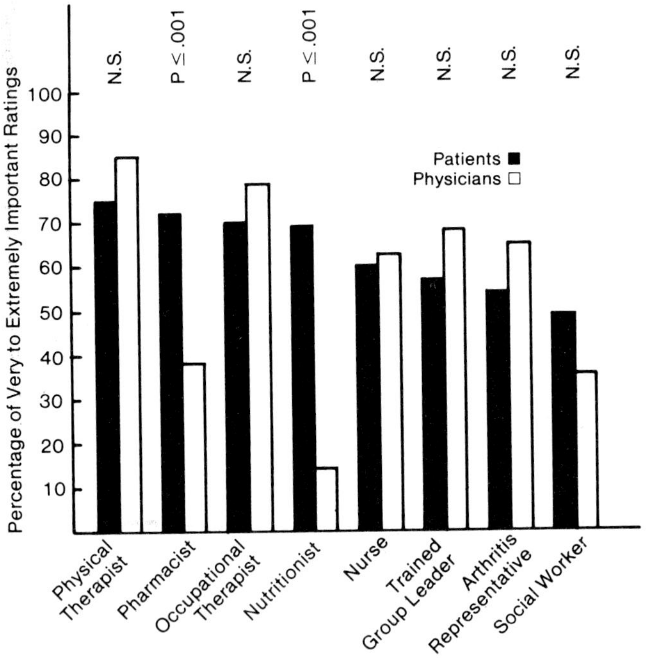

Figure 1. Percentages of patients' and physicians' ratings reported as extremely important (scale 3) to very important (scale 2) for nonphysician health professionals involved in education of arthritis patients. NS = not significant.

as extremely or very important, compared with only 39% of physicians. Similar results occurred with nutritionists, with 69% of patients reporting them as important, while only 14% of physicians judged them as extremely or very important. It is also noteworthy that the social worker was reported as important by less than 50% of both physicians and patients.

Topics. For the majority of the topics, there was little difference between the proportion of physicians and patients who rated a given topic as very to extremely important. The 2 groups differed significantly ($P \leq 0.015$, $\chi^2[1]$) however, on 7 topics (Figure 2). The 4 topics which received high proportions of physicians' ratings (72–100%) in contrast to patients' ratings (44–64%) were psychosocial needs, activities of daily living, sexual concerns, and community resources. The reverse was found for the topics of disease process, diagnostic procedures, and nutrition, with a high proportion of patients (81–91%) rating these as extremely or very important, compared with a smaller proportion of physicians (21–55%).

Channels for delivery of arthritis education. Both patients (78%) and physicians (86%) agreed that the individual meeting between patient and practitioner was the most important communication channel. Physicians (85%), however, also rated as extremely or very important the planned education group, in contrast to patients' responses (45%), a difference which proved to be statistically significant ($P \leq 0.002$, $\chi^2[1]$).

Channel/content distribution. When physicians and patients were compared regarding their preferences for delivery of specific topics, the greatest differences occurred in those areas commonly considered to be psychosocial ($P \leq 0.01$), $\chi^2[1]$). They included the issues of stress reduction, relaxation and rest; relations with family and friends; sexual concerns; and dealing with emotions and feelings. Physicians (36–86%), unlike patients, (13–31%) indicated that those psychosocial issues were best dealt with through group sessions, except for sexual concerns where 50% of physicians indicated that individual meetings were the best method of delivery; group sessions were selected as the next best method by 36%.

Another important difference ($P \leq 0.05$, $\chi^2[1]$) existed in the way patients and physicians responded to "none" of the proposed channels. Physicians' responses indicated that all psychosocial issues should be dealt with through some channel, whereas a minority of patients (13–31%) responded "none."

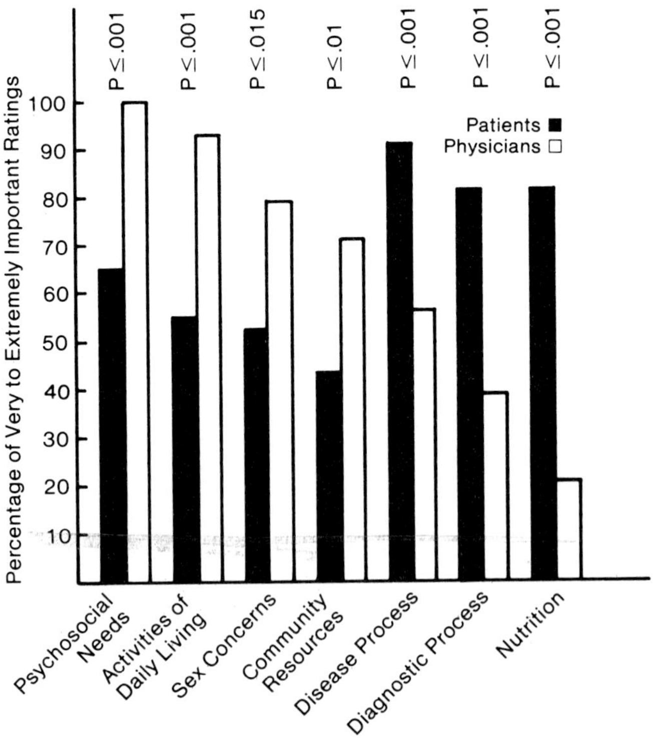

Figure 2. Percentages comparing significant patients' and physicians' ratings reported as extremely important (scale 3) to very important (scale 2) for various topics in arthritis patient education where group differences were significant.

DISCUSSION

This study sought to obtain the expressed educational needs of arthritis patients and the perceptions of those needs by the rheumatologist-providers. In so doing, we had a dual perspective in defining the scope, content, and method of delivery of an educational program and also in discovering a mechanism for exploring differences in opinion—a start in the process of eliminating barriers to optimal disease management.

Health surveys have been accepted as a valid and effective method of gathering self-reported data on particular target groups (19). Although based on self report and subject to reporting error, this survey provided a relatively quick and inexpensive way to assess and describe overall physician/patient perspectives for RA education. The responses represented a broad group of urban, predominantly white patients with RA, who are treated by private physicians or in rheumatic disease teaching clinics. The rheumatologists practiced in either private or institutional settings. Although in this study a person-to-person analysis was not possible, we think these samples were highly interactive and reflective of one another. Therefore, results may generally apply to similar patient/physician groups, which very likely represent the majority of RA patients and their physicians in urban settings. Generalizations to special groups, such as non–English-speaking, minority, short-term disease duration, or severely disabled patients, should be made with caution.

Based on their history of health education, their expressed desires, and the importance assigned to most topics, patients and physicians reported a substantial need for health education. This corresponds to the findings of other studies which document that over 80% of RA patients seek more information (11,20). Despite considerable agreement, few physicians (<25%) reported offering educational services in their current practices.

The data derived from patients' responses to content suggested that most patients were seeking greater knowledge in the pathophysiology and therapeutic processes in RA, more training and information in areas which could impact their treatment regimen, and better communication and cooperation with their physicians. Rheumatologists' reported content preferences suggested that RA patients needed more information in the personal, community, or psychosocial areas, in addition to training which might enhance the treatment regimen and improve physician/patient relationships. Pathophysiology, diagnostic procedures, and nutrition were rated important by the fewest physicians. Thus, rheumatologists seemed to reflect the views of Mazzuca who, following an extensive review of chronic disease education and treatment regimens, reported that less emphasis should be placed on pathophysiology and more on behavioral change which might impact the treatment regimen (21).

We are uncertain why in this study significantly fewer patients than physicians reported the need for patient training in the psychosocial areas; this appears to be inconsistent with recent studies which demonstrate widespread sociomedical effects of RA (22–24). However, other observations have also demonstrated that arthritis patients are less concerned about topics of sexuality, family relationships, and activities of daily living (9,11). Some investigators have noted that psychosocial stability in RA patients is a complex process, evolving and fluctuating, and often depending upon such variables as premorbid intrapsychic adjustment, stage in the life cycle, age, intelligence, education, socioeconomic level, disease duration, severity of disease, and functional limitation (4,25–27). While it would be ideal to characterize or select a subgroup of patients or a particular time when educational interventions and ancillary support services in psychosocial areas would be optimal, this study is limited in that it did not control for such variables as disease duration or functional classification.

Physicians' responses may have reflected their awareness of the overall deleterious effects of RA on patients' social relationships, marriage and family life, leisure activities, and most frequently, on vocational and economic situations (22,23). In addition, this particular patient sample represented older patients (mean 58 years) with a long disease duration (mean 14 years). It may be that many of these patients have already altered their expectations and learned to adjust to their physical and functional status (23,25). Without further testing, however, we cannot be sure what mechanisms occurred that accounted for fewer patients reporting a need for training in the psychosocial areas. Thus, some unique coping mechanisms might have been present or the disinterest may have reflected an avoidance of sensitive issues.

Furthermore, it is possible that a health education approach may not be appropriate in addressing an individual's psychosocial needs. Patients may be less interested in the general issues of how RA affects psychosocial health than in seeking specific help for their own problems. Nonetheless, it may be prudent to reassess psychosocial needs periodically in order to avoid omitting behavioral service needs that may arise during the course of RA management.

It is noteworthy that physicians, unlike patients, selected group programs as particularly valuable for dealing with patients' psychosocial concerns. We are not certain of the reasons for this finding; however, it has been suggested by Rogers et al that many physicians avoid direct contact with sensitive psychosocial areas for fear of uncovering problems which they may be ill-prepared to address (26).

Two inconsistencies in physicians' responses warrant further examination. While over 95% of physicians reported the topics of medication and patients' psychosocial needs as highly important for patient education, the 2 allied health professionals who might have been expected to deliver educational services concerning medication and psychosocial needs—the pharmacist and the social worker—were rated as very important by a minority of physicians (<40%). Physicians may be unaware of the extent to which their patients already interact with pharmacists in seeking counsel on drug side effects or drug–drug interactions. Furthermore, they may not recognize the expanded clinical and patient education training that pharmacists receive (28).

Other researchers have found that social workers are underutilized by rheumatologists (22,29). The reasons for this are largely unknown, although we might speculate that social workers are utilized predominantly in acute care hospital settings for discharge planning and public assistance functions. Perhaps the role of the social worker with respect to ambulatory RA patients should be expanded, consistent with the modern-day utilization of social service workers for counseling in the community setting (30). It may also be important to resolve the discrepancy between patients' and physicians' perceptions of the importance of pharmacists and nutritionists. As suggested by Meenan et al, the underutilization of trained and skilled allied health professionals may reflect a practice habit or bias that warrants change (22).

In developing educational interventions, caution should be exercised when content or process is selected without clear evidence of its effect on outcome. For example, although in our study patients sought more information on disease process, at least 1 other study of RA patients concluded that overemphasis on disease process and joint protection may have been responsible for increased patient self-perception of pain and disability in the treatment group (3).

While it may be convenient to draw broad generalizations regarding content priorities, it is also important to examine topics reported by smaller proportions of patients. For example, a failure to examine why sexuality and community resources were judged to be important by a minority of patients may lead to erroneously denying vital information to a significant proportion (<49%) of the population who believed these issues were important.

Finally, although both patients and physicians reported physician/patient interpersonal communications as a high priority for patient education, little work has been directed toward increasing patients' interpersonal communication skills (12). Perhaps a reason for this has been demonstrated in a parallel situation dealing with physician/patient communication concerning the issue of "informed consent." In that setting traditional medical decision-making involves the medical bias that treatments range from superior to inferior, with physicians exercising the best judgment. Physicians may see little to be gained by giving the patient a choice (31). In rheumatoid arthritis, this traditional model may be particularly inappropriate because many physician-preferred and most useful treatments may be toxic, expensive, or lack definitive proof of effectiveness. Thus, choosing between alternate treatments may be an important venture requiring skillful communication between the physician and the informed, educated patient.

Most communication studies have focused on health care professionals rather than on patients, and these efforts have been fraught with problems of limited evaluation of the teaching methods, imperfect research methodologies, and failure to evaluate in terms of patient health–related outcomes (32). Thus, investigators in rheumatology might seek to collaborate with communication and behavioral medicine investigators to expand this important research area, which might significantly alter the management of chronic disease.

Results of this study suggest that group programs must be cautiously planned, implemented, and evaluated since the data confirm that perceptions of providers do not necessarily reflect or agree with the expressed group needs of RA patients. Education by groups (versus individual) may be important to a smaller number of patients (<45%), but resolution of the differences in opinion between patients and physicians on the importance of topics and on the potentially influential roles of nonphysician allied health professionals in patient education is a necessary prerequisite. Future studies will be necessary to help us understand the disagreements and resolve the issues concerning the relative importance of content, service providers, and delivery methods for RA education.

ACKNOWLEDGMENTS

The authors gratefully acknowledge the technical assistance of G. Paul Schragg, the encouragement and support of Jeannie Swindle and Dr. Nathan J. Zvaifler, and the expert secretarial assistance of Lisa Russell and Kathy Russell.

REFERENCES

1. Vignos PJ, Parker WT, Thompson HM: Evolution of a clinic education program for patients with rheumatoid arthritis. J Rheumatol 3:155–165, 1976
2. Kaye RL, Hammond AH: Understanding rheumatoid arthritis: evaluation of a patient education program. JAMA 239:2466–2467, 1978
3. Parker J, Singsen B, Hewett J, Moeschberger M, Walker S, Hazelwood S, Hall P: Patient education for rheumatoid arthritis: short-term positive and adverse consequences (abstract). Arthritis Rheum (suppl) 25:S38, 1982
4. Kaplan S, Kozin F: A controlled study of group counseling in rheumatoid arthritis. J Rheumatol 8:91–99, 1981
5. Green LW, Lewis FM, Levine DM: Balancing statistical data and clinician judgements in the diagnosis of patient educational needs. J Community Health 6:79–91, 1980
6. Green LW, Kreuter MH, Deeds SG, Partridge KB: Health Education Planning: A Diagnostic Approach. Palo Alto, CA, Mayfield Publishing Co., 1980
7. Udelman HD, Udelman DL: Emotions and rheumatologic disorders. Am J Psychother 35:576–587, 1981
8. Wade KJ, Brown S, Wasner CK: Rheumatoid arthritis patient education: a consensus on main topics (abstract). Arthritis Rheum (suppl) 25:S86, 1982
9. Potts M, Weinberger M, Brandt K: Views of patients and providers regarding the importance of various aspects of an arthritis treatment program. J Rheumatol 11:71–75, 1984
10. Lorig K, Cox T, Cuevas Y, Guykraines R, Britton M: Converging and diverging beliefs about arthritis: Caucasian patients, Spanish speaking patients, and physicians. J Rheumatol 11:76–79, 1984
11. Knudson K, Spiegel T, Furst D: Outpatient educational program for rheumatoid arthritis patients. Patient Counsel Health Educ 3:77–82, 1981
12. Roter DL: Patient participation in the patient-provider interaction: the effects of patient question asking on the quality of interaction, satisfaction, and compliance. Health Educ Monogr 5:281–315, 1977
13. Frances V, Korsch BM, Morris MJ: Gaps in doctor-patient communication: patients' response to medical advice. N Engl J Med 280:535–540, 1969
14. Brody DS: The patient's role in clinical decision-making. Ann Intern Med 93:718–722, 1980
15. DiMatteo MR, DiNicola DD: Achieving Patient Compliance: The Psychology of the Medical Practitioner's Role. New York, Pergamon Press, 1982
16. Eraker SA, Kirscht JP, Becker MH: Understanding and improving patient compliance. Ann Intern Med 100:258–268, 1984
17. Zisook S, Gammon E: Medical noncompliance. Int J Psychiatry Med 10:291–303, 1981
18. Kosecoff J, Fink A: Needs assessment: selecting goals for a clinical program. Drug Intell Clin Pharm 15:986–989, 1981
19. Aday LA, Sellers C, Andersen RM: Potentials of local health surveys: a state of the art summary. Am J Public Health 71:835–840, 1981
20. Sweezey R, Rudd E, Robinson H: Public education in rheumatic diseases. J Rheumatol 1:343–347, 1974
21. Mazzuca SA: Does patient education in chronic disease have therapeutic value? J Chronic Dis 35:521–529, 1982
22. Meenan RF, Yelin EH, Nevitt M, Epstein WV: The impact of chronic disease: a sociomedical profile of rheumatoid arthritis. Arthritis Rheum 24:544–549, 1981
23. Deyo RA, Inui TS, Leininger J, Overman S: Physical and psychosocial function in rheumatoid arthritis: clinical use of a self-administered health status instrument. Arch Intern Med 142:879–882, 1982
24. Kramer JS, Yelin EH, Epstein WV: Social and economic impacts of four musculoskeletal conditions: a study using national community-based data. Arthritis Rheum 26:901–907, 1983
25. Zeitlin DJ: Psychological issues in the management of rheumatoid arthritis. Psychosomatics 18:7–14, 1977
26. Rogers MP, Liang MH, Partridge AJ: Psychological care of adults with rheumatoid arthritis. Ann Intern Med 96:344–348, 1982
27. Earle JR, Perricone PJ, Moultsby DM, Perricone N, Turner RA, Davis J: Psychosocial adjustment of rheumatoid arthritis patients from two alternative treatment settings. J Rheumatol 6:80–87, 1979
28. McGhan WF, Stimmel GL, Hall TG, Gilman TM: A comparison of pharmacists and physicians on the quality of prescribing for ambulatory hypertensive patients. Med Care 21:435–444, 1983
29. Yelin EH, Feshbach DM, Meenan RF, Epstein WV: Social problems, services and policy for persons with chronic disease: the case of rheumatoid arthritis. Soc Sci Med 13C:13–20, 1979
30. Erfling JL: The role of the social worker in the rehabilitation of rheumatic disease patients, Rehabilitation Management of Rheumatic Conditions. Edited by GC Ehrlich. Baltimore, Williams & Wilkins, 1980, pp 170–188
31. Lidz CW, Meisel A, Osterweis M, Holden JL, Marx JH, Munetz MR: Barriers to informed consent. Ann Intern Med 99:539–543, 1983
32. Strecher V: Improving physician-patient interaction: a review. Patient Counsel Health Educ 4:129–135, 1983

DOUBLE-BLIND, MULTICENTER CONTROLLED TRIAL COMPARING TOPICAL DIMETHYL SULFOXIDE AND NORMAL SALINE FOR TREATMENT OF HAND ULCERS IN PATIENTS WITH SYSTEMIC SCLEROSIS

H. JAMES WILLIAMS, DANIEL E. FURST, STEPHEN L. DAHL, VIRGINIA D. STEEN, CAROLLY MARKS, ELAINE J. ALPERT, AVERY M. HENDERSON, CECIL O. SAMUELSON, JR., JAMES N. DREYFUS, ARTHUR WEINSTEIN, EDMUND J. MACLAUGHLIN, GRACIELA S. ALARCÓN, STANLEY B. KAPLAN, MARIA GUTTADAURIA, MICHAEL E. LUGGEN, JAMES C. READING, MARLENE J. EGGER, and JOHN R. WARD

A prospective, randomized, double-blind trial compared topical therapy with 0.85% normal saline, 2% dimethyl sulfoxide (DMSO), and 70% DMSO for treatment of digital ulcers in 84 patients with systemic sclerosis. There were no statistically significant differences among the 3 treatment groups in the improvement in the total number of open ulcers, total surface area of open ulcers, average surface area per open ulcer, number of infected ulcers, number of inflamed ulcers, or patient pain assessment. While some patients improved during the study, improvement could not be attributed to a specific treatment. Over one-quarter of the patients treated with 70% DMSO were withdrawn for significant skin toxicity.

From the Cooperative Systematic Studies of Rheumatic Diseases Program, University of Utah School of Medicine, Salt Lake City.

Supported by NIAMDD contract no. 6-2218 and Public Health Service research grants no. RR-64, RR-68, and FR-56 from the Division of Research Resources.

H. James Williams, MD: Department of Internal Medicine, University of Utah School of Medicine; Daniel E. Furst, MD: Division of Rheumatology, University of California, Los Angeles; Stephen L. Dahl, PharmD: Department of Internal Medicine, University of Utah School of Medicine; Virginia D. Steen, MD: School of Medicine, University of Pittsburgh; Carolly Marks, RN: Division of Arthritis, Harborview Medical Center, Seattle; Elaine J. Alpert, MD: Arthritis Section, Boston University Medical Center; Avery M. Henderson, PhD, MPH: Division of Rheumatic and Genetic Diseases, Duke University Medical Center, Durham, North Carolina; Cecil O. Samuelson, Jr., MD: Division of Rheumatology, University of Utah School of Medicine; James N. Dreyfus, MD: Arthritis Research Unit, University of Michigan, Ann Arbor; Arthur Weinstein, MD: Division of Rheumatic Diseases, University of Connecticut, Farmington; Edmund J. MacLaughlin, MD: University of Missouri–Columbia; Graciela S. Alarcón, MD: Division of Clinical Immunology and Rheumatology, University of Alabama in Birmingham; Stanley B. Kaplan, MD: Department of Medicine, University of Tennessee, Memphis; Maria Guttadauria, MD: Department of Medicine, State University of New York, Downstate Medical Center, Brooklyn; Michael E. Luggen, MD: Division of Immunology, University of Cincinnati; James C. Reading, PhD: Department of Family and Community Medicine, University of Utah School of Medicine; Marlene J. Egger, PhD: Department of Family and Community Medicine, University of Utah School of Medicine; John R. Ward, MD: Department of Internal Medicine, University of Utah School of Medicine.

Address reprint requests to H. James Williams, MD, Cooperative Systematic Studies of Rheumatic Diseases, University of Utah Medical Center, 50 North Medical Drive, Salt Lake City, UT 84132.

Submitted for publication May 29, 1984; accepted in revised form October 1, 1984.

Dimethyl sulfoxide (DMSO) is a highly polar organic solvent which was introduced for clinical studies in 1963. Because long-term toxicity studies with DMSO showed changes in the refractive index of the lens of some species of treated animals, the Food and Drug Administration severely restricted clinical testing (1). Limited clinical testing was subsequently permitted in 1968. Ocular toxicity in humans has not been described, but efficacy remains controversial (2). While DMSO has been recommended for the treatment of many conditions, controlled data have been lacking.

Patients with scleroderma (systemic sclerosis) are known to develop painful cutaneous ulcerations, particularly on the fingertips and on the dorsum of the proximal interphalangeal and metacarpophalangeal joints (3–5). These ulcers can also occur on the skin overlying the olecranon, the malleolus, and calcaneus. The ulcerations may become secondarily infected and are difficult to treat. Treatment is nonspecific and measures include protection, immobilization, and appropriate antibiotics for local infection (6).

Scherbel et al (7) reported that topical DMSO improved skin pliability in 19 patients with systemic sclerosis and ischemic ulcers. They concluded that no resistant ischemic ulcers had been encountered since the immersion technique had been substituted for topical application. More recently, a small controlled study has shown accelerated healing of scleroderma ulcers in 6 of 9 patients (personal communication: Research Industries Corp., Salt Lake City, UT). In contrast, Tuffanelli (8) failed to demonstrate any benefit in the management of scleroderma, and others have questioned the efficacy of DMSO in the treatment of skin ulcers (9).

Because of persistent controversy about the efficacy of DMSO, the 13 clinics participating in the Cooperative Systematic Studies of Rheumatic Diseases (CSSRD) Program* undertook a 3-month, double-blind, controlled study comparing 0.85% normal saline (NS), 2% DMSO, and 70% DMSO, using the immersion technique in the treatment of digital skin ulcers in patients with systemic sclerosis.

PATIENTS AND METHODS

Cooperating clinics. The CSSRD was funded under a National Institute of Arthritis, Metabolism, and Digestive Diseases contract in 1976, with the Coordinating Center (CC) at the University of Utah in Salt Lake City. The protocol was developed at the CC with the assistance and approval of the member clinics and under the direction and guidance of an Advisory Committee. Data, collected at each clinic and sent to the CC, were monitored for completeness and adherence to the protocol. Analysis was performed at the CC.

Patients. Eighty-four consenting patients 18 years of age or older, with definite systemic sclerosis by American Rheumatism Association preliminary criteria (10) and with skin ulcers of the hands and/or fingers of at least 3 weeks duration were accepted into the trial. One or more ulcers had to be at least 4 mm^2 in surface area or have a diameter of 2 mm. Because the origin of digital ulcers is not readily discernible and the significance of the differences between pressure and ischemia is not known, no effort was made to separate ulcers as ischemia- or pressure-induced. However, ulcers must not have resulted primarily from cutaneous calcinosis.

Patients were permitted a stable background regimen of nonsteroidal antiinflammatory medication, corticosteroids, penicillamine, analgesics, vasodilators, or antihypertensive medication. All patients stated they had not used DMSO in the 3 months preceding the trial. Patients with localized or chemically-induced scleroderma-like conditions were excluded, as were patients with rapidly progressive disease, severe pulmonary or renal involvement, uncontrolled hypertension, or infection of the hand other than that related to the skin ulcers. Pregnancy and concomitant therapy with another experimental drug were also reasons for exclusion.

Treatment plan. Patients were randomly assigned within each clinic to 1 of the 3 treatment groups: normal saline, 2% DMSO, or 70% DMSO. Each patient in this 12-week study was instructed to treat only the more severely involved hand, with a thrice-daily soaking in a small polyethylene bag filled with the study solution at room temperature. The hand and wrist were immersed for 15 minutes during each treatment. The polyethylene bag was held in place by an elastic wrist band. After completion of the soaking, the treated hand was air-dried and the used solution was discarded. Containers for all 3 solutions were physically indistinguishable.

Clinical assessment. The global severity of each patient's systemic sclerosis was assessed by the opinion of the evaluating physician on a scale of mild, moderate, or severe. Each patient was evaluated for treatment compliance and therapy was evaluated for efficacy and adverse effects, at baseline, 2, 4, 8, and 12 weeks by the same observer. Every attempt was made to perform the evaluation at the same time of day on each visit.

The clinical description of the skin ulcers on both the treated and untreated hands included: (a) total number of ulcers, (b) number of open ulcers, defined as ulcers that had not epithelialized, (c) location of ulcers, (d) size of each ulcer in millimeters in 2 directions with 1 measurement being the longest axis and the second measurement perpendicular to that axis, (e) presence or absence of infection for each ulcer, and (f) presence or absence of cellulitis (inflammation) around each ulcer. Each observer determined the amount of redness, blistering, or sloughing of the skin of each hand. Without questioning the patient, the observer also determined the amount of characteristic breath odor, which was graded as 1 = none, 2 = mild (barely noticeable), 3 = moderate (noticeable but not offensive), and 4 = severe (offensive).

At each visit, the patient was asked to assess pain from the skin ulcers, using both an analog scale (11) and a scale of none, mild, moderate, severe, or very severe. Compliance with the treatment protocol was determined by direct query and by review of a daily diary recording each treatment. Patients were also questioned to determine if they were applying the study solution properly.

A urinalysis, complete blood count including differential cell count and platelet count, Westergren erythrocyte

* The participating clinics and clinic directors are: Boston University, Robert F. Meenan, MD; Duke University, Richard P. Polisson, MD; University of Alabama in Birmingham, Graciela S. Alarcón, MD; University of California, Los Angeles, Harold E. Paulus, MD; University of Cincinnati, Michael E. Luggen, MD; University of Connecticut, Farmington, Arthur Weinstein, MD; University of Michigan, Ann Arbor, William Mikkelsen, MD; University of Missouri–Columbia, Gordon C. Sharp, MD; State University of New York, Downstate Medical Center, Brooklyn, David Kaplan, MD; University of Pittsburgh, Virginia D. Steen, MD; University of Tennessee, Memphis, Stanley B. Kaplan, MD; University of Utah, Salt Lake City, Cecil O. Samuelson, Jr., MD; University of Washington, Seattle, Robert F. Willkens, MD.

Table 1. Characteristics of patients at entry, by treatment group

Variable*	Normal saline (n = 31)	2% DMSO (n = 25)	70% DMSO (n = 28)
Mean age	45	47	48
Male/female	9/22	6/19	7/21
Race			
White	24	20	25
Other	7	5	3
Scleroderma severity			
Mild	6	4	8
Moderate	19	14	12
Severe	6	7	7
Mean duration of scleroderma (months)	113	111	134

* $P > 0.18$ for all variables.

sedimentation rate, and blood chemistry survey were done at entry into and at completion of the study. An ophthalmologic evaluation including slit lamp examination was performed by an ophthalmologist at the beginning and end of the trial.

Statistical analysis. Quantitative data not having a Gaussian distribution were analyzed by the Kruskal-Wallis test using the difference between the first and last visits utilizing median values rather than mean values. Mantel-Haenszel chi-square tests were used to analyze discrete variables with a restricted number of values. One-way analysis of variance was also performed to verify the nonparametric results.

To control for possible differences at entry among treatment groups, efficacy analyses were repeated using an analysis of covariance (ANCOVA). Since the treatments had a natural ordering, the Jonckheere-Terpstra test (12) was used to test the alternative of increasing or decreasing effect with dose.

RESULTS

Patient population. Each of the clinics enrolled 2–17 patients. Statistical testing by the ANCOVA procedure did not detect any significant bias introduced by the use of patients from multiple clinics. Thirty-one patients received NS, 25 were assigned to receive 2% DMSO, and 28 used 70% DMSO. There were no significant differences among the treatment groups at the beginning of the trial in age, sex, race, or in severity or duration of systemic sclerosis (Table 1). Fifty-five patients completed the study: 22 in the NS group, 19 in the 2% DMSO group, and 14 in the 70% DMSO group. Patients in these groups were also comparable in the variables mentioned above and in number and severity of open digital ulcers at entry (Table 2). The proportions of patients taking corticosteroids, penicillamine, and vasodilators were similar in these groups.

Efficacy. Open ulcers were evaluated, since epithelialized ulcers were difficult to distinguish from scars. Efficacy, evaluated by a change in the open ulcer variables between the beginning and end of 12 weeks of immersion therapy, was determined for all 3 treatment groups (Table 3). While the total number of open ulcers remained unchanged for the 3 groups, the total surface area of the open ulcers decreased by a mean of 15 mm^2 and the averge surface area per ulcer was diminished by at least 3 mm^2. However, these changes in surface area were similar in all 3 groups and no significant differences were noted among the groups. Likewise, the number of infected and inflamed ulcers was unchanged for all 3 treatment groups.

Patient assessment of ulcer pain, utilizing the continuous analog scale, suggested improvement with 70% DMSO but varied widely among the patients using this treatment. Ranges are displayed in Table 3; standard deviations were 31.3, 42.7, and 29.3 for NS, 2% DMSO, and 70% DMSO, respectively. The improvement did not achieve statistical significance. This was confirmed by pain assessment on the categorical scale, where no major differences were noted.

Because all 3 treatment groups demonstrated improvement in total surface area of open ulcers and in average surface area per ulcer, evaluations of the untreated hand were also analyzed for the efficacy variables (Table 3). On the untreated hands, the total surface area of open ulcers improved slightly in all 3 groups but was less than one-third the improvement seen in the treated hands. The changes in average surface area per ulcer in the untreated hands were

Table 2. Median values at entry for open ulcers on treated hand of patients completing trial, by treatment group*

Variable	Normal saline	2% DMSO	70% DMSO
Total number of ulcers	2 (0–7)	3 (1–8)	4 (1–6)
Total surface area ulcers (mm^2)	32 (0–116)	39 (6–75)	44 (16–180)
Average surface area per ulcer (mm^2)	12 (0–39)	10 (2–70)	14 (4–180)
No. of infected ulcers	0 (0–4)	0 (0–2)	0 (0–1)
No. of inflamed ulcers	0 (0–3)	0 (0–2)	0 (0–1)

* Values in parentheses are ranges. $P > 0.21$ for all variables.

Table 3. Median changes in efficacy variables for open ulcers on treated and untreated hands between initiation and completion of the trial, by treatment group*

Variable	Normal saline		2% DMSO		70% DMSO	
	Treated†	Untreated‡	Treated	Untreated	Treated	Untreated
Total number ulcers	0 (−7–7)	1 (−8–6)	1 (−6–5)	0 (−8–2)	1 (−2–4)	0 (−2–3)
Total surface area ulcers (mm²)	15 (−36–107)	2 (−51–76)	18 (−307–70)	6 (−273–50)	15 (0–130)	3 (−12–25)
Average surface area/ulcer (mm²)	4 (−57–34)	−3 (−34–38)	3 (−71–70)	2 (−68–30)	4 (−8–130)	0 (−19–15)
No. of infected ulcers	0 (−2–2)	0 (−1–1)	0 (−4–2)	0 (−4–2)	0 (0–1)	0 (−2–2)
No. of inflamed ulcers	0 (−1–2)	0 (0–2)	0 (−1–2)	0 (0–2)	0 (−1–1)	0 (−1–1)
Patient pain assessment, analog (mm)	−1 (−48–80)	0 (−40–83)	6 (−91–86)	1 (−90–55)	20 (−16–77)	−10 (−69–50)
Patient pain assessment, categorical (score 1–5)	0 (−2–3)	0 (−1–3)	0 (−3–3)	0 (−3–2)	1 (−1–2)	−1 (−2–1)

* Ranges given in parentheses; improvement indicated by a positive value.
† $P > 0.21$ for all comparisons among groups for treated hands.
‡ $P > 0.19$ for all comparisons among groups for untreated hands.

variable and inconsistent among the 3 groups of patients. Changes in the total number of open ulcers and the number of ulcers that were infected or inflamed were similar in treated and untreated hands. Patients treated with 70% DMSO experienced worsening of pain in the untreated hand (analog scale worsening of 10 mm), while the treated hand seemed to improve (analog scale improvement of 20 mm). Less striking differences were seen in the 2% DMSO group. These differences were also seen on the categorical pain scale for the 70% DMSO group.

In an effort to determine if a subset of patients experienced greater benefit from any of the treatments, all patients who completed the trial were evaluated for 50% reduction in the total number of open ulcers and for 50% reduction in the total surface area of all open ulcers of the treated hand (Table 4). These arbitrary definitions were used to detect meaningful change in ulcer healing among the groups. Approximately 40% of patients in each treatment group experienced a decrease of at least 50% in the number of open ulcers. Similarly, half of the patients in the NS and 2% DMSO groups had a reduction in total surface area of ulcers by at least 50%, compared with 40% of the patients using 70% DMSO. These differences were not statistically significant. Thus, the 3 treatments were similar with respect to efficacy when analyzed for these degrees of ulcer healing.

Adverse reactions. A review of laboratory variables and ophthalmologic findings showed no significant changes within each group or among the groups between the start and end of the trial.

During the 12-week study, 29 patients were withdrawn (Table 5). Nine patients were withdrawn because of severe skin reactions including cracking, blistering, sloughing, and burning (Figure 1). Eight of these patients were using 70% DMSO; they constituted 29% of all the patients receiving that concentration of DMSO. One patient treated with 2% DMSO and none using NS had severe skin reactions. Three patients using NS withdrew from the study for lack of response, while no patients using either concentration of DMSO withdrew for this reason. Lack of patient cooperation resulted in withdrawal of 12 patients and protocol violations led to withdrawal of 5 patients, but patients in these 2 categories were divided equally among all 3 treatment groups.

Patients using DMSO frequently develop a distinctive odor to their breath. The presence of this odor was 4 times more frequent in patients using 70% DMSO than in those in the other 2 groups (Table 6). Odor was graded on a scale of 1 to 4, and scores were

Table 4. Percentage of patients with 50% improvement of selected measurements for treated hands, by treatment group

	Normal saline	2% DMSO	70% DMSO	P*
% with 50% of open ulcers improved	38	38	43	0.932
% with 50% reduction in total surface area of open ulcers	50	50	39	0.670

* By Mantel-Haenszel chi-square test.

Table 5. Reason for withdrawal, by treatment group

	Normal saline (n = 31)	2% DMSO (n = 25)	70% DMSO (n = 28)
Skin reactions	0	1	8
Lack of response	3	0	0
Lack of cooperation	4	4	4
Protocol violation	2	1	2
Total	9	6	14

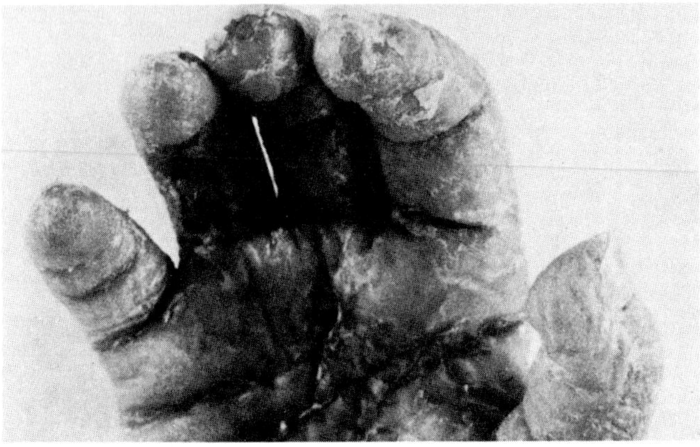

Figure 1. Typical skin reaction from 70% DMSO, resulting in patient's withdrawal from the study.

obtained by summing the severity grade for each of the 5 clinic visits. Patients with breath odor while using 70% DMSO had higher individual scores as well as higher maximum scores. All 3 treatment groups had some patients with detectable breath odor.

DISCUSSION

The use of DMSO has been controversial (2,13). We have limited the current report to a trial of DMSO in the treatment of digital ulcers in patients with systemic sclerosis. A 70% DMSO concentration was chosen because it is most frequently recommended and used (9). A second group was treated with 2% DMSO because though it is believed to possess little potential benefit (14), it causes a characteristic breath odor in some patients, which prevented the unblinding of patients or physicians. This strategy was partially successful. All 3 treatment groups had some patients with breath odor, but this effect was more frequent and more noticeable in patients receiving 70% DMSO. However, more than one-third of the patients using 70% DMSO never developed the characteristic odor. While the presence of a strong characteristic odor had the potential to unblind subjects and observers, there was enough odor in other treatment groups to confound the participants.

It has been suggested that double-blind trials for DMSO are impossible (15). While perfect blinding may not be possible, the proportions of false-positive and false-negative reports of breath odor suggest that double-blind procedures were at least partially successful. Significant skin reactions with 70% DMSO also could lead to "unmasking" of the participants.

In 1967 Scherbel et al (7) reported using various concentrations of DMSO in an open study of patients with systemic sclerosis. The DMSO was initially applied by painting and subsequently, in resistant patients, by immersion. Six of 12 patients receiving topical treatment experienced healing of their skin ulcers in 1–3 weeks and 3 additional patients reported healing by 6 weeks. Two of the 3 patients with refractory symptoms were treated by immersion with resolution of the ulcers in 1 week. Thereafter, all patients were treated by immersion, with no resistant ulcers encountered.

In a subsequent open-label study, Scherbel (16) described 22 patients with cutaneous ulcers and systemic sclerosis. These patients treated 1 extremity by the immersion technique with 46% DMSO. After 3 months of therapy, 73% of ulcers on the treated extremity had healed, compared with 17% of the ulcers on the untreated extremity. In contrast, Tuffanelli (8) treated 24 systemic sclerosis patients with 90% DMSO applied topically. On treated hands, 6 of 16 ulcerations healed, while 4 new ulcers developed. On the untreated hands, 5 of 15 ulcers healed and 3 new ulcerations occurred.

In the current study, treatment by immersion therapy failed to demonstrate significant differences between 2% DMSO and 70% DMSO or between either

Table 6. Presence and amount of characteristic breath odor by treatment group, for patients finishing or withdrawing from study

Variable	Efficacy group: Normal saline	2% DMSO	70% DMSO	Withdrawal group: Normal saline	2% DMSO	70% DMSO
No. of patients	22	19	14	9	6	14
Patients with any odor	3 (14%)	3 (16%)	9 (64%)*†	0	1 (17%)	8 (58%)*
Maximum individual severity‡	2	3	4	1	2	4
Average odor score§	5.2	5.4	7.4	–	–	–
Patients with odor at last visit	0	0	5	0	1	7

* $P < 0.007$, 70% DMSO versus normal saline.
† $P = 0.013$, 70% DMSO versus 2% DMSO.
‡ Scale 1–4 (see Patients and Methods).
§ Minimum score = 5, maximum score = 20 (see Patients and Methods).

concentration of DMSO and normal saline. The number of open ulcers did not appreciably improve for any specific group. While the total surface area of ulcer involvement decreased, this improvement was seen in all 3 groups. The untreated hands improved to a lesser degree. Perhaps the daily soaking of the hand with ulcerations resulted in faster improvement, irrespective of the solution used. Patients using the higher concentration of DMSO reported greater pain relief but the differences were not statistically significant.

Although the differences between treatment groups appeared small in our study, power calculations do not exclude the probability of Type II error. Thus, in the best case, the final sample size in this study provided approximately 90% power to detect a difference of 72 percentage points in improvement in the number of infected open ulcers between any 2 treatment groups, given the observed standard deviations. Alternatively, 212 patients per group would have been required to detect a 30 percentage point difference between the high and low treatment groups with 90% power. These calculations assume an overall 5% significance level for all possible pairs of treatment group comparisons. For the other ulcer variables, lower power was available.

Therefore, an effect of DMSO could conceivably have been missed by this study, although there is no evidence of such an effect in the data. Two factors contribute to the marked reduction in statistical power. First, observed standard deviations were much larger than expected. Second, the actual dropout rate was higher than the anticipated dropout rate of 20% per group. The actual dropout rates were 29%, 24%, and 50% for the NS, 2%, DMSO, and 70% DMSO groups, respectively.

The DMSO used in our study was not benign. Twenty-nine percent of the patients receiving 70% DMSO were withdrawn for severe skin reactions. Even 1 patient receiving 2% DMSO developed urticaria during therapy. No other toxicity was manifested in this 3-month trial.

Our results fail to confirm that DMSO is effective in enhancing the rate of healing of digital ulcers in systemic sclerosis patients. Since 70% DMSO can lead to significant skin blistering and peeling, care should be exercised when it is used.

ACKNOWLEDGMENTS

The direction, advice, and supervision given by the Advisory Committee were greatly appreciated. Members of the Advisory Committee during the period of this study were: Kenneth D. Brandt, MD, Indiana University Medical School, Indianapolis; Byron W. Brown, PhD, Stanford College of Medicine, Palo Alto, CA; Doyt L. Conn, MD, Mayo Clinic, Rochester, MN; John G. Harter, MD, Food and Drug Administration, Rockville, MD; Marc C. Hochberg, MD, Good Samaritan Hospital, Baltimore; Stephen R. Kaplan, MD, Roger Williams Hospital, Providence, RI; James R. Klinenberg, MD, Cedars Sinai Medical Center, Los Angeles; Mary Betty Stevens, MD, Johns Hopkins University, Baltimore; Alexander S. Townes, MD, VA Medical Center, Memphis; and Robert B. Zurier, MD, University of Pennsylvania, Philadelphia. Harold E. Paulus, MD, University of California, Los Angeles was the Participating Clinic director on the Advisory Committee. The assistance of the staff at the Coordinating Center was most valuable. Specific important contributions were made by Miki L. Coleman, MS, applied biostatistician; Gerald Wise, data manager; and Wanda L. Moore, administrative assistant. Treatment solutions were supplied by Research Industries Corporation.

REFERENCES

1. Dimethyl sulfoxide (DMSO) preparations: termination of clinical testing and investigational use. Federal Register 30:14639, 1965
2. Harter JG: The status of dimethyl sulfoxide from the perspective of the Food and Drug Administration. Ann NY Acad Sci 411:1–5, 1983
3. Tuffanelli DL, Winkelmann RK: Systemic scleroderma: a clinical study of 727 cases. Arch Dermatol 84:359–371, 1961
4. Herman BE, Fischl R, Frankel A, Herman P: Successful skin graft in patient with generalized scleroderma. JAMA 182:578–579, 1962
5. Rodnan GP: Progressive systemic sclerosis: clinical features and pathogenesis of cutaneous involvement (scleroderma). Clin Rheum Dis 5:49–79, 1979
6. Rodnan GP: Progressive systemic sclerosis (scleroderma), Arthritis and Allied Conditions. Ninth edition. Edited by DJ McCarty, Jr. Philadelphia, Lea & Febiger, 1979, pp 762–809
7. Scherbel AL, McCormack LJ, Layle JK: Further observations on the effect of dimethyl sulfoxide in patients with generalized scleroderma (progressive systemic sclerosis). Ann NY Acad Sci 141:613–629, 1967
8. Tuffanelli DL: A clinical trial with dimethyl sulfoxide in scleroderma. Arch Dermatol 93:724–725, 1966
9. Fleischmajer R: Methodology and techniques in the evaluation of dimethyl sulfoxide for connective tissue disorders (discussion paper). Ann NY Acad Sci 243:393–394, 1975
10. Subcommittee for Scleroderma Criteria of the American Rheumatism Association Diagnostic and Therapeutic Criteria Committee: Preliminary criteria for the classification of systemic sclerosis (scleroderma). Arthritis Rheum 23:581–590, 1980
11. Huskisson EC: Assessment for clinical trials. Clin Rheum Dis 2:37–49, 1976

12. Hollander M, Wolfe DA: Nonparametric Statistical Methods. New York, John Wiley & Sons, 1973, p 120
13. Jimenez RAH, Willkens RF: Dimethyl sulfoxide: a perspective of its use in rheumatic diseases. J Lab Clin Med 100:489–500, 1982
14. Brown JH: Clinical experience with DMSO in acute musculoskeletal conditions comparing a noncontrolled series with a controlled double blind study. Ann NY Acad Sci 141:496–505, 1967
15. Kantor TG: Design of therapeutic trials for dimethyl sulfoxide. Ann NY Acad Sci 243:390, 1975
16. Scherbel AL: The effect of percutaneous dimethyl sulfoxide on cutaneous manifestations of systemic sclerosis. Ann NY Acad Sci 411:120–130, 1983

SUBSTRAIN HETEROGENEITY IN PROSTAGLANDIN E_2 SYNTHESIS OF HUMAN DERMAL FIBROBLASTS

Differences in Prostaglandin E_2 Synthetic Capacity of Substrains Are Not Stimulus-Restricted

JOSEPH H. KORN

We examined prostaglandin E_2 (PGE_2) biosynthetic heterogeneity in fibroblast substrains and possible mechanisms that might mediate this heterogeneity. PGE_2 synthesis of fibroblast substrains, in response to phytohemagglutinin-stimulated mononuclear cell supernates, ranged from 9.0 ± 1.0 ng/ml to 79.3 ± 7.4 ng/ml (mean ± SD). The phenotypic behavior of individual substrains was stable. Substrains were also heterogeneous in PGE_2 response to phorbol myristate acetate, and displayed stability in this phenotype as well. Substrains which were high responders to mononuclear cell supernate also ranked high in response to phorbol myristate acetate. Similar heterogeneity was observed in response to purified interleukin-1. Arachidonic acid added exogenously did not raise interleukin-1 responsiveness of low-producer substrains to that of high producers, suggesting that differences in PGE_2 synthesis among substrains did not reflect differences in substrate availability or phospholipase activity. Supernates of high- and low-responder phenotype substrains, when added to cells of the reciprocal strain or to unrelated fibroblasts, did not affect the pattern of PGE_2 synthesis. The concordance of substrain responsiveness to mononuclear cell supernate and phorbol myristate acetate suggests that heterogeneity among substrains in PGE_2 synthesis is related to the ability to produce PGE_2 rather than to the ability to respond to a given mediator. In addition, differences in PGE_2 synthesis among substrains do not appear to result from release of regulatory autokines.

From the Division of Rheumatic Diseases, Veterans Administration Medical Center, University of Connecticut School of Medicine, Newington, Connecticut.

Supported by grants from the VA Medical Research Service, NIH (AM-32343), and Arthritis Foundation and NIH Arthritis Center grants.

Joseph H. Korn, MD: Associate Professor of Medicine.

Address reprint requests to Dr. Joseph H. Korn, Research Building #5, VA Medical Center, Newington, CT 06111.

Submitted for publication July 20, 1984; accepted in revised form September 25, 1984.

Cytokines released by lymphocytes and monocytes have been shown to play a critical role in modulating fibroblast metabolism. Recent studies have shown that a monokine closely related to, if not identical with, interleukin-1 (IL-1) regulates fibroblast proliferation, prostaglandin E_2 (PGE_2) synthesis, and release of the enzyme collagenase (1–6). Release of interleukin-1 at sites of inflammation might thus be responsible, at least in part, for fibroproliferative, vasoregulatory, and degradative events at the site of inflammatory lesions. The extent to which such events occur might depend not only on the degree of immunologic activation and amount of mediator release, but also on the responsiveness of the target connective tissue cell population.

We have recently demonstrated that exposure of fibroblasts to mononuclear cell products for several weeks results in subsequent hyperresponsiveness in the fibroblasts' PGE_2 synthetic response to IL-1–containing mononuclear cell supernates (7). Furthermore, this hyperresponsiveness persists in vitro for more than 4 months and for 20 cell generations after the original exposure to mononuclear cell products (7). This in vitro experimental observation parallels the finding in rheumatoid synovial cells; these cells are hyperresponsive to mononuclear cell–derived mediators and maintain this phenotypic expression in vitro after removal from the inflammatory in vivo environment (8).

One explanation for the induction of permanent phenotypic alterations in cells following in vitro or in vivo exposure to mononuclear cell–derived mediators is an alteration in the normal heterogeneity of connective tissue cells, leading to an overgrowth of populations that produce more PGE_2 in response to IL-1. Such alteration could be the result of differences among subpopulations in their response to growth mediators released by lymphocytes and monocytes. We have, in fact, shown that substrains of normal human dermal fibroblasts derived from a single parent culture are heterogeneous in the extent to which mononuclear cell factors affect their growth (9). This heterogeneity is largely explained by differences in PGE_2 synthesis among the substrains; supernates of mononuclear cells inhibited proliferation of fibroblast substrains in proportion to the stimulation of PGE_2 synthesis, an effect that was reversed with indomethacin.

This study examines PGE_2 synthesis of human foreskin fibroblast substrains isolated by limiting dilution cloning from a single parent line. These substrains are demonstrated to be heterogeneous in their PGE_2 synthetic response to mononuclear cell supernates (MC-SN) and to maintain the pattern of responses as a stable phenotype. Two possible mechanisms for heterogeneity in MC-SN–stimulated PGE_2 synthesis are explored: 1) differences in ability of various substrains to interact with MC-SN, and 2) production by different substrains of an autokine that either augments or inhibits response to exogenous mediators.

MATERIALS AND METHODS

Cell culture. Fibroblast cultures were derived from human neonatal foreskin as described previously (7). Substrains were isolated from a primary culture by limiting dilution cloning (9). Cloning efficiency was improved by supplementing culture media with pooled fibroblast–conditioned medium (FCM) (medium removed from 3-day confluent foreskin fibroblast cultures). Fibroblasts were cultured in basal Eagle's medium (BME) supplemented with 25 m*M* HEPES buffer, 100 units/ml penicillin, 100 μg/ml streptomycin, and 2 m*M* L-glutamine and containing 10% fetal bovine serum (FBS). All substrains were fed weekly from the same pool of conditioned medium.

Fibroblast cloning. Four weeks after initiation, a confluent primary culture was harvested by brief 0.25% trypsin–0.02*M* EDTA exposure. Cells were washed and resuspended in BME containing 20% FBS. A final cell concentration of approximately 35 cells/10 ml was achieved by serial dilution of fibroblasts starting at a cell concentration of $5–10 \times 10^5$ cells/ml (determined by cell counts using a hemacytometer chamber). Cell concentrations were verified and adjusted as necessary at intermediate concentrations. The final cell suspension (35 cells/10 ml) was added in 100-μl aliquots to 4 replicate 96-well culture dishes (35 cells/100 wells), and the volume of each well was brought to 200 μl with BME–20% FBS–25% FCM. Wells were examined to assure that no more than a single fibroblast per well was present; in more than half the wells no fibroblasts were visible.

Confluent wells were expanded into 24-well culture dishes in the same culture medium and then into 60-mm culture dishes over 4–7 weeks. Once confluent in 60-mm dishes, substrains were fed twice weekly with BME–10% FBS, harvested at confluence, and passaged serially (every 7–10 days) in 100-mm culture dishes. (The term "substrain" is used throughout this paper since the clonal origin of the substrains has not been definitively demonstrated.) No substrain showed evidence of in vitro transformation. All showed density-dependent growth inhibition and normal senescence, with first slowing and then cessation of proliferation after approximately 15 subpassages (following initial attainment of mass culture).

Cloning efficiency. The parent strains, GL and DW, derived from different foreskins, were each seeded initially into 4 96-well plates (approximately 35 cells/plate). Substrain growth was apparent in microwells within 10–14 days. Cloning efficiency was 20% for strain GL (30 positive wells) and 28% for strain DW (40 positive wells). Fourteen substrains were expanded in culture and used for assay of PGE_2 synthesis (5 GL substrains, 9 DW substrains). Other substrains were used for unrelated experiments or were lost due to poor growth or contamination. Substrains were identically fed and passaged; all were tested simultaneously at the same subpassage. The parent line was similarly maintained and tested.

Mononuclear cell cultures. Human peripheral blood mononuclear cells were obtained and cultured as previously described (4). Briefly, 10^6 MC/ml were cultured in the presence of 2.5 μg/ml phytohemagglutinin (PHA) for 72 hours. Culture supernates were harvested by centrifugation, rendered cell-free by passage through a 0.40μ filter, pooled, and frozen (−20°C). A single pool of MC supernates was used for all experiments. We have previously shown that PGE_2 stimulatory activity in these supernates elutes principally with an M_r of 12,000–20,000 (3) and is probably identical to IL-1 (1).

Test cultures. PGE_2 synthesis was assessed in cultures of untreated fibroblasts and fibroblasts treated with 3-day supernates of PHA-stimulated MC cultures as described previously (7), except that all data in the present paper refer to fibroblast cultures incubated for 24 hours rather than 48 hours. Preliminary experiments demonstrated that PGE_2 synthesis in the substrains was near maximal at 24 hours, as shown previously for parent strains (3), and that relative synthesis of PGE_2 among substrains was the same at 24 hours and 48 hours.

Briefly, 1×10^4 fibroblasts were seeded in replicate wells of 96-well culture dishes in RPMI 1640–10% FBS. To each well was added 0%, 2.5%, 10%, or 25% (final concentration) MC-SN. Cells were cultured for 24 hours and the culture media harvested and frozen (−20°C) for PGE_2 assay. PHA alone, at the concentration present in test MC-SN, did not significantly stimulate PGE_2 synthesis. Proliferation was measured simultaneously by ^{3}H-thymidine incorporation (3).

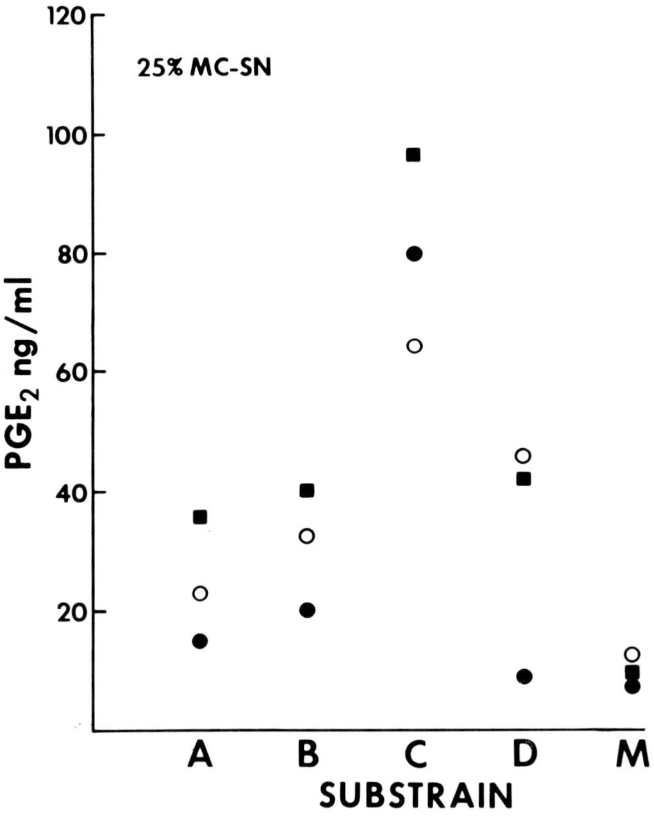

Figure 1. Stimulation of prostaglandin E_2 (PGE_2) synthesis in GL substrains by 25% mononuclear supernates (MC-SN). Substrains were tested 2 weeks (■), 11 weeks (○), and 24 weeks (●) after initial confluence in mass culture (60–100-mm dishes) was achieved. Each point represents the mean of duplicate assays.

Incorporation of ^{3}H-leucine into trichloroacetic acid–precipitable protein was used as an index of protein synthesis.

Interleukin-1, purified by affinity chromatography, was obtained from Genzyme (Cambridge, MA). Phorbol myristate acetate (PMA; Sigma, St. Louis, MO) diluted in culture medium was added at concentrations of 0.01–5 μM. Arachidonic acid (Sigma) was diluted in 100 μl ethanol and used in final concentrations of 20 μM and 100 μM (final ethanol concentration <0.2%). Ethanol, at the concentrations used, did not affect fibroblast PGE_2 synthesis. Both PMA and arachidonic acid were present throughout the 24-hour test culture period.

Radioimmunoassay for PGE_2. Radioimmunoassay for PGE_2 was performed as described previously (7). A monoclonal antibody to PGE (generously supplied by Dr. Ned Lally, University of Pennsylvania) was used. The antibody showed a 1.5% cross-reaction with $PGF_2\alpha$ and PG-6-keto-$F_1\alpha$. These are the other major prostaglandin metabolites present in culture media of MC-SN–treated fibroblast cultures as determined by thin-layer chromatography (unpublished observations).

Reagents. Culture media and supplements were obtained from Gibco (Grand Island, NY), serum from Sterile Systems (Logan, UT), and culture dishes from Costar (Bellco Glass, Vineland, NJ). Radiolabeled thymidine and PGE were obtained from New England Nuclear (Boston, MA), phytohemagglutinin was obtained from Burroughs Wellcome (Research Triangle Park, NC), and PGE_2, $PGF_2\alpha$, and PG-6-keto-$F_1\alpha$ were courtesy of Mr. Paul Coughlin (Upjohn Co., Kalamazoo, MI).

RESULTS

MC-SN–stimulated PGE_2 synthesis. MC-SN–stimulated PGE_2 synthesis of 5 substrains is depicted in Figure 1. The 5 substrains of strain GL were tested at 3 time-points over a period of 6 months. Baseline PGE_2 synthesis was not significantly different among the substrains and ranged from 1–3 ng/ml/10^4 cells. Although each strain increased PGE_2 synthesis in response to mononuclear cell supernate, the magnitude of response was heterogeneous (Figure 1). Substrain M was poorly responsive, with a PGE_2 synthesis of 9.0 ± 1.1 ng/ml (mean ± SE). Substrain C was a high responder, with a mean PGE_2 synthesis of 79.3 ± 7.4 ng/ml. Substrains A, B, and D demonstrated mean PGE_2 synthesis of 24.0 ± 5.4, 29.8 ± 4.8, and 31.7 ± 9.5 ng/ml, respectively, in the 3 assays. Mean PGE_2 synthesis of the parent strain, tested for comparison at the same 3 time-points, was 18.4 ± 4.3 ng/ml. PGE_2 of substrain C was significantly greater than that of each of the other 4 substrains and of the parent line ($P <$ 0.05, Student's paired t-test). The pattern of response among substrains was the same when lower concentrations of MC-SN (2.5% and 10%) were used (see below).

One mechanism that would account for differences in PGE_2 synthesis among the substrains might be differences in plating efficiency and/or cellular proliferation. Fibroblast substrains were assayed simultaneously for ^{3}H-thymidine incorporation (as an index of cell number) and for PGE_2 synthesis in the presence of MC-SN (Table 1). PGE_2 synthesis corre-

Table 1. Relationship between cellular proliferation and prostaglandin E_2 (PGE_2) synthesis in fibroblast substrains*

Substrain	PGE_2, ng/ml	^{3}H-thymidine, cpm
A	36.5 ± 4.7	1,780 ± 470
B	39.4 ± 5.0	2,824 ± 403
C	95.2 ± 1.2	2,687 ± 287
D	41.6 ± 8.4	1,212 ± 304
M	8.6 ± 1.0	1,980 ± 77

* ^{3}H-thymidine incorporation and PGE synthesis were assessed in the presence of 25% mononuclear cell supernates. Fibroblasts were cultured simultaneously for determination of PGE and proliferation in replicate wells; all substrains were assayed at the same time. Values are mean ± SD.

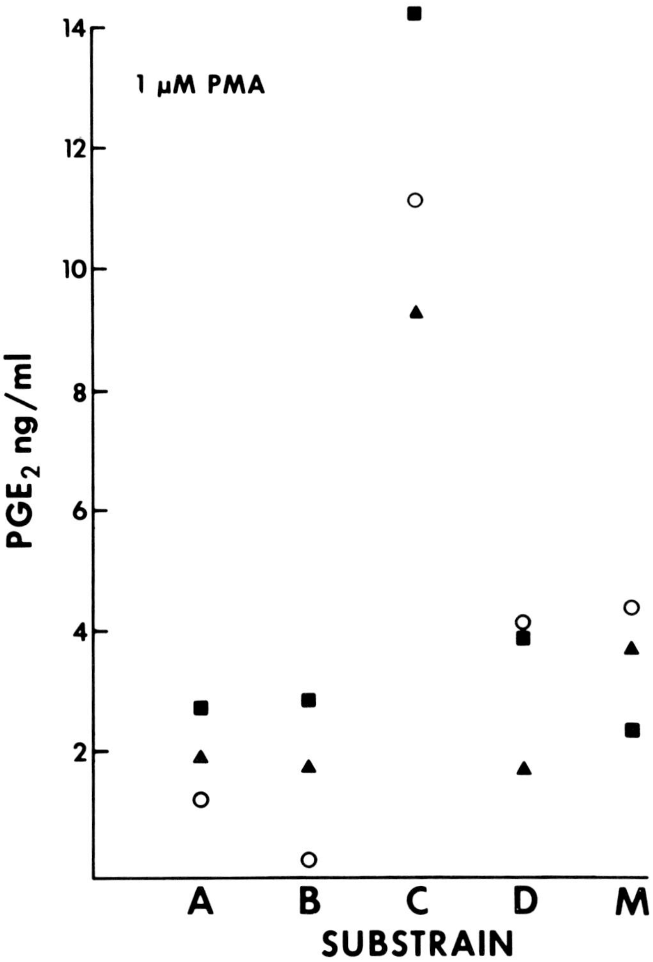

Figure 2. Stimulation of prostaglandin E_2 (PGE_2) synthesis in GL substrains by 1 μM phorbol myristate acetate (PMA). Substrains were tested at 11 weeks (○), 20 weeks (▲), and 24 weeks (●) after initial confluence in mass culture. Each point represents the mean of duplicate assays.

lated poorly with ^{3}H-thymidine incorporation ($r = 0.42$, $P > 0.3$). The high PGE_2 synthesis of substrain C and the low PGE_2 synthesis of substrain M did not appear to merely reflect the relative number of viable cells.

PMA-stimulated PGE_2 synthesis. To attempt to distinguish whether the differences observed among substrains in MC-SN–stimulated PGE_2 synthesis reflected primary differences in the responsiveness to MC-SN or differences in the inherent capacity to produce PGE_2, the PGE_2 synthetic response to PMA was investigated. In response to 1 μM PMA, the parent line showed mean PGE_2 synthesis of 2.7 ± 0.15 ng/ml of PGE_2, a 240% increase compared with baseline levels. PMA was thus a considerably less potent stimulus for PGE synthesis than was MC-supernate.

Table 2. Responses of fibroblast substrains to varying concentrations of mononuclear cell supernate (MC-SN)*

Sub-strain	Prostaglandin E_2, ng/ml 0% MC-SN	2.5% MC-SN	10% MC-SN	25% MC-SN
A	1.4 ± 0.2	15.8 ± 3.4	26.2 ± 16.2	24.0 ± 5.4
B	1.1 ± 0.3	24.6 ± 7.0	23.3 ± 5.5	29.8 ± 4.8
C	3.2 ± 0.8	70.0 ± 1.1	96.9 ± 13.6	79.3 ± 7.4
D	1.1 ± 0.3	12.2 ± 0.6	39.1 ± 5.4	44.5 ± 1.2
M	1.1 ± 0.3	14 ± 4.4	29.2 ± 16.5	9.0 ± 1.1

*All substrains were tested simultaneously under identical culture conditions. Each value represents the mean ± SEM of 2–3 separate experiments.

The responses of the 5 substrains to PMA (tested at the same time) are depicted in Figure 2. The mean PGE_2 synthesis for substrain C was 11.5 ± 1.2 ng/ml, a level which was 3–8-fold greater than that in the other substrains. At each of the time-points tested, substrain C synthesized considerably more PGE_2 than did any of the other substrains ($P < 0.05$ for each substrain comparison). Furthermore, PGE_2 synthesis for the 5 substrains in response to MC-SN stimulation correlated highly with PGE_2 synthesis in response to PMA stimulation ($r = 0.89$, $P < 0.02$, Pearson's test).

We examined whether the differences in PGE_2 synthesis shown in Figures 1 and 2 were due to differences in the dose-response curves of the substrains (i.e., the maximal PGE_2 synthesis of each substrain might be the same, but the threshold concentration of mediator that is needed to achieve this maximum might be different). In fact, substrain C PGE_2 synthesis exceeded that for the other substrains at MC-supernate concentrations of 2.5–25% and PMA concentrations of 0.01–5 μM (Tables 2 and 3). Furthermore, although there were differences among substrains in the concentration of mediator needed for maximal stimulation, response of the substrains generally plateaued at 10% MC-SN and 0.5–1.0 μM PMA. It

Table 3. Responses of fibroblast substrains to varying concentrations of phorbol myristate acetate (PMA)*

Sub-strain	Prostaglandin E_2, ng/ml 0 μM PMA	0.01 μM PMA	0.5 μM PMA	1 μM PMA	5 μM PMA
A	1.1 ± 0.4	1.1 ± 0.2	2.4 ± 0.1	2.5 ± 0.1	3.8 ± 0.7
B	1.0 ± 0.4	0.1 ± 0.0	2.3 ± 0.4	1.7 ± 0.6	1.4 ± 0.9
C	3.9 ± 0.9	10.9 ± 3.8	17.5 ± 5.6	11.6 ± 1.2	9.0 ± 2.0
D	1.1 ± 0.2	6.8 ± 0.7	2.7 ± 0.4	3.3 ± 0.6	5.6 ± 2.0
M	1.2 ± 0.2	4.1 ± 1.1	3.2 ± 0.7	3.6 ± 0.5	2.8 ± 0.5

* All substrains were tested simultaneously under identical culture conditions. Each value represents the mean ± SEM of 2–3 separate experiments.

Table 4. Failure of fibroblast substrain supernatants to transfer cell phenotype*

Substrain	Grown in	Prostaglandin E_2, ng/ml 0% MC-SN	10% MC-SN	25% MC-SN	^{3}H-thymidine, cpm	C:M†
Experiment 1						
C	M	1.6 ± 0.2	43.8 ± 3.6	56.8 ± 5.9		
M	C	2.4 ± 0.1	15.0 ± 0.4	21.8 ± 1.1		
Experiment 2						
C	M	1.5 ± 0.0	38.4 ± 4.8	47.8 ± 4.0		
M	C	1.6 ± 0.0	9.7 ± 0.2	8.6 ± 0.1		
Proliferation studies						
C	–‡				2,300 ± 93	0.31
M	–‡				7,511 ± 1,400	
C	M				1,365 ± 106	0.26
M	C				5,208 ± 93	

* Fibroblasts of substrains M and C were cultured for 2 weeks in 50% spent medium of the reciprocal strain. Following this period of culture, the substrains were tested for proliferation and stimulated prostaglandin E_2 synthesis. Values are mean ± SD. MC-SN = mononuclear cell supernate.
† Ratio of substrain C cpm to substrain M cpm.
‡ Grown in normal culture medium.

is thus unlikely that still greater mediator concentrations would raise PGE_2 synthesis of all substrains to the levels achieved by substrain C.

Effect of substrain supernates on PGE synthesis. We investigated the possibility that the differences in responses among these substrains might be the result of the release of some regulatory mediator by a substrain that influenced its phenotypic expression in response to a stimulus. Fibroblasts from GL substrain C (Figures 1 and 2) were cultured for 2 weeks in the presence of 50% (volume/volume) conditioned culture medium from substrain M. Conversely, fibroblasts from substrain M were similarly cultured in conditioned media from substrain C. Following this culture period, both strains were tested for PGE_2 synthesis in response to MC-SN (Table 4).

In each of 2 "cross-culture" experiments, substrain C synthesized considerably greater amounts of PGE_2 than did substrain M. The high-responder phenotype (substrain C, Figure 1) and low-responder phenotype (substrain M) were thus unaffected by prior incubation in the culture medium of the reciprocal substrain. The relative proliferative capacities of the 2 substrains were similarly unaffected by prior incubation in culture medium of the reciprocal strain (Table 4).

Table 5. Lack of prostaglandin E_2 (PGE_2) modulatory activity in supernates of fibroblast substrains

Addition to culture substrain supernate*	Mononuclear cell supernate	PGE_2, ng/ml (mean ± SD)
0	0	2.1 ± 0.01
10% C	–	2.3 ± 0.01
10% M	–	2.2 ± 0
–	10%	10.5 ± 0.0
10% C	10%	11.2 ± 0.6
20% C	10%	11.4 ± 1.0
10% M	10%	11.3 ± 0.3
20% M	10%	11.6 ± 0.4

* Supernates of substrain C or M were added to cultures of an unrelated fibroblast strain.

Culture media of substrains C and M were also tested for direct effects of PGE_2 synthesis of foreskin fibroblasts of an unrelated strain (Table 5). Addition of 10% substrain C supernate to unrelated fibroblasts did not directly stimulate fibroblast PGE_2 synthesis. Furthermore, in the presence of 10% MC-SN, 10% or 20% substrain C supernate did not further augment PGE_2 synthesis. Conversely, supernate of substrain M did not inhibit the PGE_2 synthetic response of unrelated fibroblasts. Thus, the PGE_2 responder phenotype of substrains was not transmissible by products elaborated and released by those substrains.

Stimulation of PGE_2 synthesis by IL-1 and arachidonic acid. Differences in PGE_2 synthesis among fibroblast substrains that were not transmissible could have been due to differences in substrate availability (e.g., availability of membrane phospholipid). We therefore examined whether addition of arachidonic acid to IL-1–stimulated cultures would increase IL-1–stimulated PGE_2 synthesis by low PGE_2 producers to levels achieved by high-producing substrains. Table 6 presents data for 4 substrains of parent strain DW. Two substrains, A and D, were consistent high pro-

Table 6. Effect of interleukin-1 (IL-1) and arachidonic acid (AA) on prostaglandin E_2 (PGE_2) synthesis of fibroblast substrains*

	PGE_2, ng/ml				^{3}H-leucine incorporation, cpm × 10^{-2}/culture†			
Addition to culture	Substrain A	Substrain D	Substrain G	Substrain J	Substrain A	Substrain D	Substrain G	Substrain J
0‡	2.9 ± 1.0	2.3 ± 0.3	1.5 ± 0.3	1.5 ± 0.2				
MC-SN, 10%‡	32.2 ± 5.7	38.1 ± 14.7	13.9 ± 4.8	13.4 ± 2.3				
0	2.0 ± 0.5	1.5 ± 0.1	1.1 ± 0.2	1.4 ± 0.1				
IL-1, 1:300	7.8 ± 1.9	7.2 ± 2.2	3.3 ± 0.3	3.8 ± 0.1				
IL-1, 1:100	11.8 ± 3.8	10.5 ± 1.2	3.7 ± 1.5	3.4 ± 0.2				
IL-1, 1:30	8.9 ± 1.8	6.6 ± 0.4	2.4 ± 0.1	2.3 ± 0.1				
IL-1 (1:100) + AA, 10 μM	25.7 ± 4.6	20.9 ± 1.7	5.7 ± 1.9	3.7 ± 0.8				
IL-1 (1:100) + AA, 30 μM	33.6 ± 0.4	28.2 ± 1.3	5.3 ± 0.9	15.2 ± 4.0				
AA, 10 μM	1.9 ± 0.1	2.0 ± 0.2	1.2 ± 0.0	1.6 ± 0.2				
AA, 30 μM	8.3 ± 1.4	3.3 ± 0.0	1.7 ± 0.2	3.4 ± 1.5				
MC-SN, 10%	35.9 ± 4.7	58.2 ± 15.2	8.2 ± 0.4	9.9 ± 0.1				
0					3.7 ± 0.4	4.3 ± 1.3	3.0 ± 1.2	4.4 ± 0.9

* Except for the first 2 rows, values are mean ± SD. MC-SN = mononuclear cell supernate.
† Parallel cultures to those used for measuring PGE_2 synthesis were pulsed overnight with 1 μCi/well of ^{3}H-leucine. Trichoroacetic acid–precipitable protein was washed, collected, and counted. Results represent mean ± SD of quadruplicate samples.
‡ Mean ± SEM responses of the substrains in 5 separate experiments.

ducers in response to MC-SN, while G and J were low producers; in 5 experiments, mean PGE_2 production for substrains A and D was more than twice that of G and J (n = 5; $P < 0.01$ A versus G, $P < 0.025$ A versus J, $P < 0.05$ D versus G, $P < 0.06$ D versus J, by Student's paired t-test).

Substrains A and D, high producers in response to MC-supernate, were also better responders to purified IL-1, with peak PGE_2 production approximately 3 times that of substrains G and J. The poorer responses of substrains G and J were not the result of impaired viability or metabolic activity. Incorporation of ^{3}H-leucine into trichloroacetic acid–precipitable protein was similar in the 4 cell substrains (Table 6).

Addition of arachidonic acid, 10 μM and 30 μM, to IL-1 augmented PGE_2 production of all the substrains but failed to raise PGE_2 synthesis of substrains G and J to the levels of substrains A and D. Arachidonic acid alone at the concentrations used was a weak stimulator of PGE_2 synthesis; only substrain A showed an appreciable response. Arachidonic acid appeared to act synergistically with IL-1, particularly with substrains A and D, rather than additively. If arachidonic acid can act by presenting available substrate for PGE_2 synthesis, the data would suggest that differences among substrains in IL-1–stimulated PGE_2 synthesis are not due solely to substrate availability.

DISCUSSION

It has been demonstrated previously that fibroblast clones derived from a single source differ in their proliferative capacity, age of senescence, and production of collagen and collagenase (10–13). Fibroblast subpopulations also show small differences in baseline PGE_2 synthesis, differences which are, however, enough to influence relative proliferative capacity (14). In this study, we have demonstrated that fibroblast substrains derived from a single parent strain differ in their PGE_2 synthetic responses to 2 unrelated stimuli of PGE_2 synthesis, IL-1–containing mononuclear cell supernates and phorbol myristate acetate. The substrains isolated displayed a PGE phenotype that was stable over multiple cell generations and months in culture.

There are several possible explanations for differences in PGE_2 synthesis among substrains. One possibility is that the substrains differ in their general level of cellular activation. In this study, PGE_2 synthesis did not correlate with proliferative capacity of the substrains or with protein synthesis. In addition, PGE_2 synthesis in substrains does not correlate with levels of synthesis of collagenase or the procoagulant protein, tissue factor (15).

A second possibility is that substrains differ in their interaction with a given stimulus (e.g., number of receptors), that is, the differences are stimulus-restricted. The concordance of substrain responses to MC-SN and PMA would suggest that, if this is the case, these substrains have similar degrees of interaction with 2 chemically unrelated stimuli.

A third possibility is that substrains release autokines that regulate gene expression. Our results would suggest that if such a regulatory substance is produced, it is not released into the culture medium in a stable form or at a high enough concentration to alter the phenotype of other fibroblast populations.

Finally, it is possible that substrains differ in their inherent capacity to produce PGE_2, possibly as a result of differences in the levels of substrate (arachidonic acid) or enzyme (phospholipase, cyclooxygenase) available. Arachidonic acid, added exogenously, failed to bring IL-1–stimulated PGE_2 synthesis of the substrains to equal levels. This would suggest that the substrains differed at a point distal to arachidonate in the metabolic pathway.

However, it is not clear that exogenous arachidonic acid stimulates PGE_2 synthesis by directly forming part of the arachidonic acid pool available to the cell. Recent data suggest that exogenous arachidonic acid is rapidly incorporated into membrane phospholipid without an increase in the levels of free arachidonic acid (16,17). Heterogeneity in substrain response to exogenous arachidonic acid may still, therefore, be a result of differences in phospholipase activity or other mechanisms that govern free arachidonic acid levels. We have not yet been able to study rates of arachidonic acid incorporation into and release from membrane phospholipid in these substrains.

It has been recently shown, in murine peritoneal macrophages, that the rate-limiting step for PGE_2 synthesis is an enzyme in the endoplasmic reticulum, i.e., distal to arachidonic acid (18). Consistent with this observation are the findings of Rodan et al, who isolated osteosarcoma lines with different PGE_2 synthetic capacity (19). In these lines, the content of the enzyme cyclooxygenase, measured by radioimmunoassay, correlated with the amount of PGE synthesized; lines that produced no PGE_2 lacked this enzyme which converts arachidonic acid to the PGE_2 precursor, PGG_2 (19). Whether cells which do not contain the enzyme are constitutionally unable to make it or are unresponsive to stimuli that might induce the enzyme is unknown.

The extent to which the isolated substrains are reflective of the population mix in the original parent strain is unknown. Only the high-producing substrain differed markedly from the parent strain in its PGE_2 synthetic profile. This would suggest that this and other high-producing substrains form a relatively small portion of the parent population. Population heterogeneity may, however, become more significant where connective tissue cell proliferation takes place. In such settings, the potential exists for an alteration in the normal population phenotype as a result of differential proliferation of subpopulations in response to lymphocyte-, monocyte-, platelet-, and serum-derived growth factors. The change in the clonal distribution of connective tissue cell populations could be responsible for the permanent changes in population phenotype seen in vivo in inflammatory disease and in vitro in experimental settings.

ACKNOWLEDGMENTS

The expert technical assistance of Daria Torres, Elaine Downie, and Mark Dobrzanski is gratefully acknowledged.

REFERENCES

1. Schmidt JA, Mizel SB, Cohen D, Green I: Interleukin 1, a potential regulator of fibroblast proliferation. J Immunol 128:2177–2181, 1982
2. Postlethwaite AE, Kang AH: Induction of fibroblast proliferation by human mononuclear leukocyte–derived proteins. Arthritis Rheum 26:22–27, 1983
3. Korn JH, Halushka PV, LeRoy EC: Mononuclear cell modulation of connective tissue function: suppression of fibroblast growth by stimulation of endogenous prostaglandin production. J Clin Invest 65:543–554, 1980
4. Dayer JM, Robinson DR, Krane SM: Prostaglandin production by rheumatoid synovial cells: stimulation by a factor from human mononuclear cells. J Exp Med 145:1399–1404, 1977
5. Dayer JM, Russell RGG, Krane SM: Collagenase production by rheumatoid synovial cells: stimulation by a human lymphocyte factor. Science 195:181–183, 1977
6. Postlethwaite AE, Lachman LB, Mainardi CL, Kang AH: Interleukin 1 stimulation of collagenase production by cultured fibroblasts. J Exp Med 157:801–806, 1983
7. Korn JH: Fibroblast PGE_2 synthesis: persistence of an abnormal phenotype after short term exposure to mononuclear cell products. J Clin Invest 71:1240–1246, 1983
8. McGuire MKB, Meats JE, Russell RG: Cell-cell interactions in the rheumatoid joint. Agents Actions 10:486–490, 1980
9. Korn JH, Torres D, Downie E: Clonal heterogeneity in the fibroblast response to mononuclear cell derived mediators. Arthritis Rheum 27:174–179, 1984
10. Smith JR, Hayflick L: Variation in the life-span of clones derived from human diploid cell strains. J Cell Biol 62:48–53, 1984
11. Botstein GR, Sherer GK, LeRoy EC: Fibroblast selection in scleroderma: an alternative model of fibrosis. Arthritis Rheum 25:189–195, 1982
12. Brinckerhoff CE, Nagel JE: Collagenase production by cloned populations of rabbit synovial fibroblasts. Coll Relat Res 5:433–444, 1981
13. Bordin S, Page RC, Narayanan AS: C1q receptors on cultured human gingival fibroblasts: analysis of binding properties. Science 223:171–173, 1984

14. Ko SD, Page RC, Narayanan AS: Fibroblast heterogeneity and prostaglandin regulation of subpopulations. Proc Natl Acad Sci USA 74:3429–3432, 1977
15. Korn JH, Brinckerhoff CE, Edwards RL: Fibroblast responses to mononuclear cell-derived mediators: fibroblast substrains are differentially activated for different metabolic products (abstract). Arthritis Rheum (suppl) 27:S37, 1984
16. Robinson DR, Hamer P, Pichiarello D: Regulation of prostaglandin synthesis: evidence for a new mechanism (abstract). Arthritis Rheum (suppl) 27:S28, 1984
17. Hunter SA, Burstein S, Sedar C: Stimulation of prostaglandin synthesis in WI-38 human lung fibroblasts following inhibition of phospholipid acylation by p-hydroxy-mercuribenzoate. Biochim Biophys Acta 793:202–212, 1984
18. Darte V, Beaufay H: Subcellular localization of the PGE_2 synthesis activity in mouse resident peritoneal macrophages. J Exp Med 159:89–102, 1984
19. Rodan SB, Wesolowski G, Rodan G: Prostaglandin synthesis in osteoblastic and non-osteoblastic osteosarcoma cell lines (abstract). Calcif Tissue Int 34:14, 1982

KINETICS OF EXTRACTION OF PROTEOGLYCANS FROM HUMAN CARTILAGE

LAWRENCE A. POTTENGER, JUNE E. WEBB, and NANCY B. LYON

Fifty-one uniformly sliced human patellar cartilage specimens were extracted with physiologic buffer containing inhibitors. Galactosamine-rich proteoglycans were more easily extracted than glucosamine-rich proteoglycans. Extraction occurred in 2 phases. There was a large proteoglycan extraction during the first 30 minutes, followed by a steady loss proportional to the square root of time. The amount of proteoglycans extracted during phase 1 was approximately half that of phase 2. Extraction of proteoglycans varied with age, structural integrity, and cartilage thickness. Intact osteoarthritic cartilage had normal proteoglycan extraction.

Many of the biomechanical characteristics of cartilage result from interactions between proteoglycans and collagen. Proteoglycans are trapped in a compressed state within the fine type II collagen mesh (1). An external force upon the cartilage causes extrusion of water with further compression until a new equilibrium is achieved. Removal of the force leads to imbibition of water and resumption of the original shape (2). For this system to work effectively, the proteoglycans must be rigidly immobilized within the cartilage. Escape of proteoglycans from the surface would lead to loss of ability to withstand compression; movement of proteoglycans within the cartilage would distort its shape.

In osteoarthritis and other conditions in which the cartilage mesh is disrupted, there are decreased concentrations of proteoglycans in areas of disruption (3,4). The reduced concentrations may be due to chondrocyte necrosis with concomitant decrease in proteoglycan synthesis (5), degradation of proteoglycans by enzymes secreted by either chondrocytes (6) or inflammatory cells in synovial fluid (7), or inability of a fragmented collagen mesh to prevent leakage of proteoglycans from the surface (8). The present investigation was stimulated by the final possibility.

Many aspects of the proteoglycan entrapment within cartilage remain poorly understood. A portion of the core protein of some proteoglycans have a region which is capable of binding hyaluronic acid (9,10) and "link" proteins (11,12). High molecular weight proteoglycan aggregates, which are formed when many proteoglycans bind to one long hyaluronic acid chain, appear to be too large to migrate through the fine collagen mesh present in cartilage (13,14). Many proteoglycans, however, are not capable of binding hyaluronic acid, yet still appear to be trapped within the cartilage (13).

We recently presented data concerning extraction of proteoglycans with a buffer of physiologic pH and ionic strength from bovine nasal cartilage slices of varying thicknesses (14). The extraction occurred in 2 phases. There was a rapid loss of proteoglycans occurring in less than 30 minutes followed by a prolonged, slower phase which was approximately proportional to the square root of time. As much as 65% of the proteoglycans could be extracted from 20μ cartilage slices using buffer alone.

From the Department of Orthopaedic Surgery and the Department of Pathology, University of Chicago, School of Medicine, Chicago, Illinois.

Supported by NIH grant AM-32538.

Lawrence A. Pottenger, MD, PhD: Associate Professor of Surgery and Pathology; June E. Webb, BA: Research Assistant; Nancy B. Lyon, AB: Graduate Student, Department of Pathology.

Address reprint requests to Lawrence A. Pottenger, MD, PhD, The University of Chicago, Department of Orthopaedic Surgery, 5841 South Maryland Avenue, Box #102, Chicago, IL 60637.

Submitted for publication June 21, 1984; accepted in revised form September 25, 1984.

In this report, the extractability of proteoglycans from 51 specimens of human patellar cartilage was studied. Physiologic buffer with inhibitors was found to extract approximately 40% of the total cartilage uronic acid from 20μ sections of all cartilage types, although the amount varied with age and condition of the cartilage. The kinetics of extraction was similar to that seen with bovine nasal cartilage.

MATERIALS AND METHODS

Human patellar cartilage specimens were obtained from 3 different sources: 7 specimens were obtained during amputation for sarcomas not affecting the knee joint, 4 specimens were removed from osteoarthritic knees during total joint replacement, and 40 specimens were harvested from 30 individuals at autopsy within 24 hours of death. In addition, cartilage samples were taken from the femoral condyles of the 4 osteoarthritic joints and from 6 autopsy specimens. These specimens were either used immediately or stored at -20°C for analysis within 3 weeks.

All specimens were analyzed for surface disruption using the India ink staining method of Meachim (15). Samples that had no evidence of surface disruption were designated grade 1, and those with disruption affecting only the tangential layer of the cartilage were called grade 2. Areas where the tangential layer was completely missing with partial disruption of the radial zone were designated grade 3. Different grades of cartilage from the same patella were collected and analyzed separately. Grossly fibrillated cartilage was not studied because it could not be accurately sliced to specific thicknesses.

Variation in proteoglycan extractability by slice thickness. Slices from the same cartilage were prepared in 3 different thicknesses. Fresh cartilage was immediately sectioned with a vibratome (14) at 100μ and 500μ; frozen cartilage was sectioned at 20μ with a cryostat. During the cutting process, care was taken not to expose the slices to any liquid which might prematurely extract proteoglycans. In each case, the slices were taken from full-thickness pieces of cartilage. They were cut perpendicular to the surface and parallel to the longitudinal axis of the patella. These particular slice thicknesses were selected because they have successive fivefold increases in surface area and the smallest size, 20μ, is slightly smaller than 25–70μ, which is the reported thickness of fibrillated cartilage (16).

Samples of slices (0.2 gm) were extracted with 15 volumes of buffer at physiologic pH and ionic strength, containing inhibitors of proteolysis (0.05 phosphate, pH 7.4, with 100 m*M* NaCl, 10 m*M* EDTA, 5 m*M* benzamidine HCl, 100 m*M* 6-aminohexanoic acid, 1 m*M* phenylmethylsulfonyl fluoride, and 10 m*M* N-ethylmaleimide). Buffer ionic strength was verified with a conductance meter. The samples were rotated on a multipurpose rotator (Model 150 V, Scientific Industries) for 30 minutes. The buffer was then carefully decanted and the slices were rinsed with an additional 10 volumes and resuspended in another 15 volumes of buffer. Extraction with buffer was continued for 7 days, with changes of buffer and rinsing on days 1, 2, 4, and 7. The sections were then extracted with 2*M* guanidine-HCl (GdnHCl) for 2 days followed by 4*M* GdnHCl for 2 days, and finally, the extracted cartilage was solubilized by digestion with papain (17). Cartilage samples were kept at 4°C throughout the entire extraction process. Extracts and digests were analyzed for uronic acid (18), glucosamine, and galactosamine (19).

Variation of proteoglycan extractability with age and cartilage grade. Twenty-micron cryostat sections of 51 cartilage specimens were prepared and extracted as previously described, except that the GdnHCl extractions were omitted. In most cases, 0.2-gm samples of each cartilage were analyzed in triplicate. The relative percentages of proteoglycan aggregates and non-aggregated monomers of some extracts were assessed by Sepharose CL-2B gel filtration (14).

Because of the long extraction periods, interpretation of the results of these studies was dependent on the absence of in vitro autolysis. The use of inhibitors has been shown to prevent autolysis (20). Two additional experiments were performed to insure that significant autolysis was not occurring. A cartilage sample was extracted with buffer for 5 minutes. Half of the sample was then immediately placed on a Sepharose CL-2B column while the other half was stored at 4°C for 48 hours and then placed on the column. The 2-column elution patterns were indistinguishable.

The second experiment was designed to determine whether autolysis, which did not occur in 4*M* GdnHCl, was occurring in physiologic ionic strength buffer. For 2 days, 0.2 gm of cartilage, sliced at 20μ, was extracted with buffer containing inhibitors. Then, without removing the original extract, dry GdnHCl was added to a final concentration of 4*M* and extraction was continued for another 2 days. Simultaneously, a 0.2-gm sample from the same cartilage was extracted for 4 days with 4*M* GdnHCl. Both extracts were then dialyzed against 9 volumes of buffer to induce aggregation and applied to Sepharose CL-2B columns. Their column elution patterns were also indistinguishable, indicating that the original buffer extraction did not alter the molecular weight or degree of aggregation of the proteoglycans.

RESULTS

Table 1 shows the extraction patterns of uronic acid, galactosamine, and glucosamine from a patellar autopsy specimen of a 39-year-old man. Amounts extracted are expressed as percentages of the total amount present. The extraction pattern of galactosamine tended to parallel that of uronic acid; both are components of chondroitin sulfate. Glucosamine, a component of keratan sulfate, tended to resist extraction with buffer alone. As slice thickness increased, this disparity between the amount of galactosamine and glucosamine extracted with buffer increased.

Also with increasing slice thickness, greater amounts of all constituents remained within the cartilage after extraction with 4*M* GdnHCl. The percentages of glucosamine remaining in the extracted carti-

Table 1. Sequential extraction of proteoglycans (variation with slice thickness)*

	Uronic acid (%)	Galactosamine (%)	Glucosamine (%)	Galactosamine/glucosamine†
20μ slices				
Buffer	25.8	31.3	17.4	1.38
2*M* GdnHCl	27.4	27.2	26.6	0.68
4*M* GdnHCl	22.1	19.6	33.3	0.39
Residual	24.7	22.1	22.9	0.63
100μ slices				
Buffer	10.8	12.3	4.4	2.21
2*M* GdnHCl	19.3	23.2	19.3	0.95
4*M* GdnHCl	38.4	34.7	50.0	0.55
Residual	31.5	29.8	26.3	0.90
500μ slices				
Buffer	6.9	6.6	2.0	2.64
2*M* GdnHCl	10.0	15.7	7.5	1.69
4*M* GdnHCl	40.2	35.9	54.7	0.53
Residual	42.9	41.7	35.8	0.94

* Cartilage slices from a 39-year-old man were first extracted for 7 days with buffer, then for 2 days with each guanidine-HCl (GdnHCl) concentration. Unextractable constituents (residual) were analyzed after papain solubilization of the extracted cartilage.
† Ratios were determined from amounts extracted, not from percentages.

lage were generally less than the percentages of uronic acid and galactosamine remaining. This was due to increased extraction of glucosamine with 4*M* GdnHCl compared with extraction of galactosamine and uronic acid. Similar results were obtained when other cartilage specimens were analyzed in the same way.

Figure 1 shows the cumulative buffer extraction of uronic acid, galactosamine, and glucosamine from the same cartilage specimen over a 7-day period. Extraction of all components appeared to occur in 2 phases. There was an immediate loss of proteoglycans from the slices that occurred in less than 30 minutes, followed by a slower loss that was roughly proportional to the square root of time. The percentage extracted during the first 30 minutes was approximately half the percentage extracted over the next 7

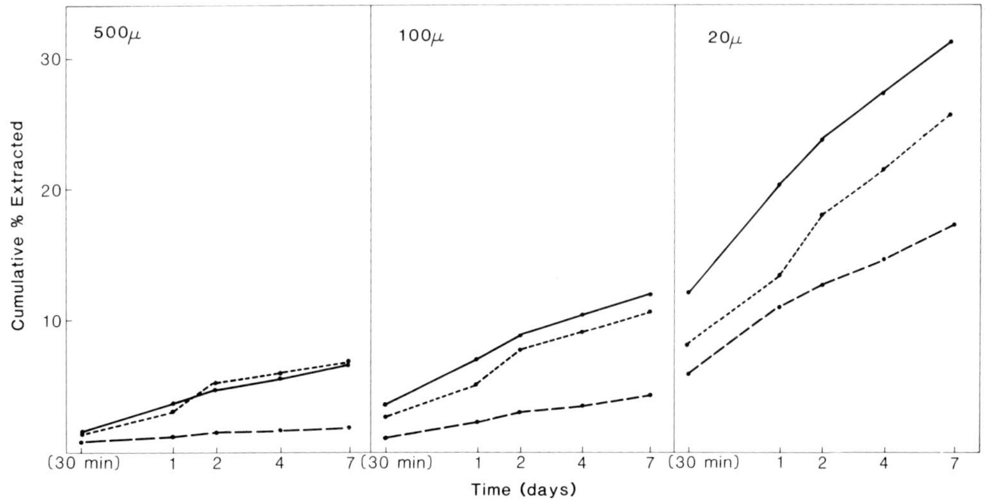

Figure 1. Extraction of galactosamine (——), uronic acid (- -), and glucosamine (- - -) from human cartilage with buffer of physiologic ionic strength and pH. A patellar autopsy specimen from a 39-year-old man was sliced at 500μ and 100μ with a vibratome and at 20μ with a cryostat. Cumulative extractions are expressed as percentages of total cartilage content of each particular constituent. X axis is a square root scale.

days. With decreasing slice thickness, buffer extraction of proteoglycans increased, but the increase was much less than the fivefold difference in surface area between the groups. Thus, the loss of proteoglycans per surface area was much less in the 20μ sections than in the 500μ sections. This indicated that slicing cartilage at 20μ was not causing a fundamental change in the ability of the cartilage collagen mesh to retain proteoglycans. Therefore, for the remaining studies 20μ sections were used because they yielded greater amounts of proteoglycans for analysis.

Table 2 gives the cumulative buffer extraction of uronic acid separated according to tissue source. Samples from osteoarthritic joints were taken from areas free of fibrillation. Although there was a large variation within each group as demonstrated by the large standard deviation, there was no significant difference among the groups in the mean amount of uronic acid extracted. The average standard deviation for triplicate studies of the 7-day extraction of 34 specimens was 1.4%, indicating that the large standard deviation seen within each group was not due to variation in analysis of individual cartilage samples. Data from specimens of condylar cartilage were not included in subsequent analyses.

Figure 2 shows the percentage of total cartilage uronic acid extracted in 7 days using buffer alone, in relation to the age of the individual from which the sample was taken. Immature cartilage tended to lose greater amounts of proteoglycans. There was a large variation within each age group. In spite of this, the linear regression of mature cartilage showed little variation with age.

The percentage of uronic acid extracted with buffer in 7 days correlated with the percentage extracted in 30 minutes (Figure 3). Again, the amount of uronic acid extracted in 30 minutes was approximately half the amount extracted during the next 7 days, regardless of the total amount extracted.

Skeletally immature grade 1 cartilage (no surface disruption) lost much greater amounts of uronic acid in both phases of extraction than did skeletally mature grade 1 cartilage (Table 3). The skeletally immature cartilage consisted of both articular cartilage and underlying cartilage which would have eventually undergone endochondral ossification (21). It is possible that the underlying cartilage was responsible for the different extraction pattern.

Table 2. Buffer extraction of uronic acid from 20μ cartilage slices, according to tissue source

Cartilage source	30-minute (% ± SD)	7-day (% ± SD)
Amputation (n = 7)	13.9 ± 4.3	44.0 ± 3.9
Autopsy (n = 36)	13.1 ± 3.0	40.3 ± 7.2
Osteoarthritis (n = 4)	14.2 ± 2.2	45.5 ± 8.6
Condyle (n = 10)	13.2 ± 1.5	43.8 ± 4.2

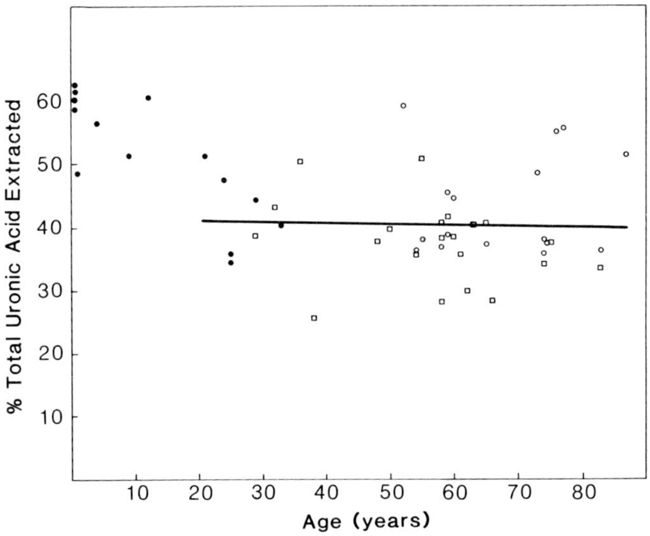

Figure 2. Percentage of total cartilage uronic acid extracted in 7 days with buffer according to the age of the individual from which the cartilage was obtained. The linear regression line is for specimens from skeletally mature individuals only. ● = grade 1 cartilage; □ = grade 2 cartilage; ○ = grade 3 cartilage.

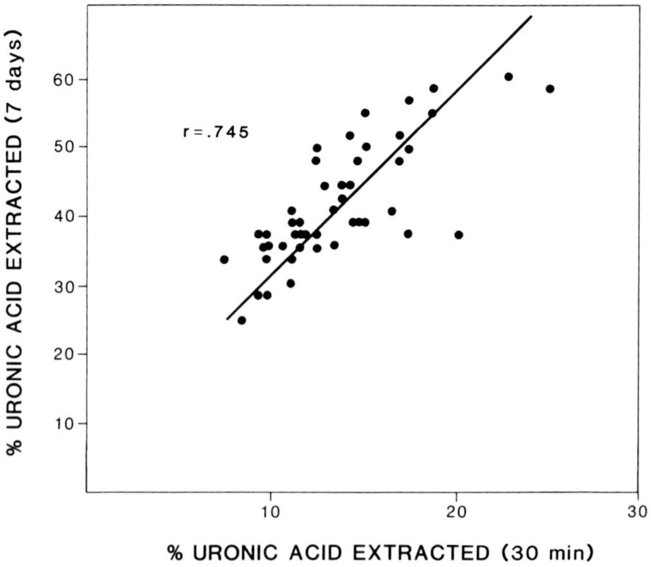

Figure 3. Correlation between percentage of the total cartilage uronic acid which was extracted from 20μ slices with buffer in 30 minutes and the percentage extracted over 7 days. Solid line = linear regression.

Table 3. Variation, with age and condition of cartilage, of extraction of uronic acid from 20μ slices

	Grade	30-minute (% ± SEM)	7-day (% ± SEM)
Skeletally immature	1 (n = 8)	22.5 ± 1.51	57.6 ± 1.6
Skeletally mature	1 (n = 6)	12.2 ± 0.7	42.2 ± 2.6
	2 (n = 21)	12.3 ± 0.7	37.7 ± 1.4
	3 (n = 16)	13.2 ± 0.8	43.4 ± 2.0

Extraction of skeletally mature cartilage showed little variation with cartilage grade (Table 3). Grades 1 and 3 cartilage lost similar amounts of uronic acid in 7 days while grade 2 lost a slightly, but significantly, lesser amount. None of the cartilage from subjects over 33 years old was grade 1, so the differences between grade 1 and grade 2 extraction patterns may be due to changes with age. Analysis of grade 2 and grade 3 extraction patterns within the same age range (52–83 years) showed a significant increase of extraction from grade 3 cartilage, which occurred mainly during the second phase (Figure 4). It should be emphasized that grossly fibrillated cartilage was not studied because it could not be accurately cut to 20μ. Grade 3 cartilage was softer and tended to fragment during the extraction process, while grades 1 and 2 maintained their size and shape throughout.

Figure 5 shows typical Sepharose CL-2B analyses of the buffer extracts of skeletally immature and skeletally mature cartilage. In all specimens analyzed, extraction of skeletally immature cartilage yielded a much greater proportion of aggregates. Regardless of the donor's age, the ratio of aggregates to monomers increased as the extraction progressed. Many adult samples showed very few aggregated proteoglycans in the buffer extracts in spite of the fact that over 40% of their total cartilage uronic acid had been extracted.

For purposes of quantitation, Sepharose CL-2B elution patterns were divided into 4 equal segments. Proteolgycans eluting with K_{av} 0–0.25 were considered aggregates. Those eluting with K_{av} 0.25–0.5 were considered large monomers and those eluting between 0.5–0.75 were small monomers. Few, if any, proteoglycans eluted after K_{av} 0.75. Since cartilage samples yielded different amounts of each category of proteoglycans, it was difficult to compare the kinetics of extraction between cartilage samples unless the amounts extracted at different times were compared with the total amount of each type of proteoglycan extracted during the 7-day period (Figure 6). The extraction patterns of all proteoglycan types were approximately linear with respect to the square root of time, but their rates of extraction varied greatly. Proteolgycan monomers were extracted more rapidly than aggregates. The kinetics of extraction of small monomers had a curve indicative of depletion of the diffusable molecules, with less than the predicted amount being extracted as the extraction progressed.

DISCUSSION

Cartilage proteoglycans consist of keratan sulfate and chondroitin sulfate chains covalently attached to a linear core protein (22,23). At one end of the core protein of aggregating proteoglycans, there is a hyaluronic acid binding site which is free of glycosaminoglycan chains. Immediately adjacent to this site is a region containing mainly keratan sulfate chains, while

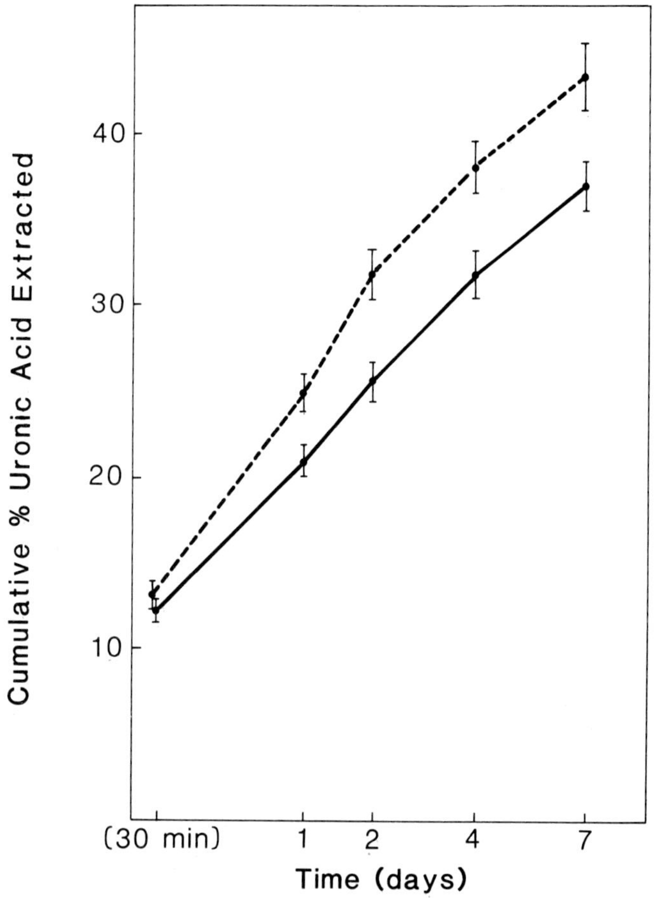

Figure 4. Cumulative buffer extraction of uronic acid from grade 2 (——) and grade 3 (– – –) cartilage. Lines represent the combined extraction data on 14 grade 2 specimens and 16 grade 3 specimens from individuals between 52 and 83 years of age. Error bars are SEM. X axis is a square root scale.

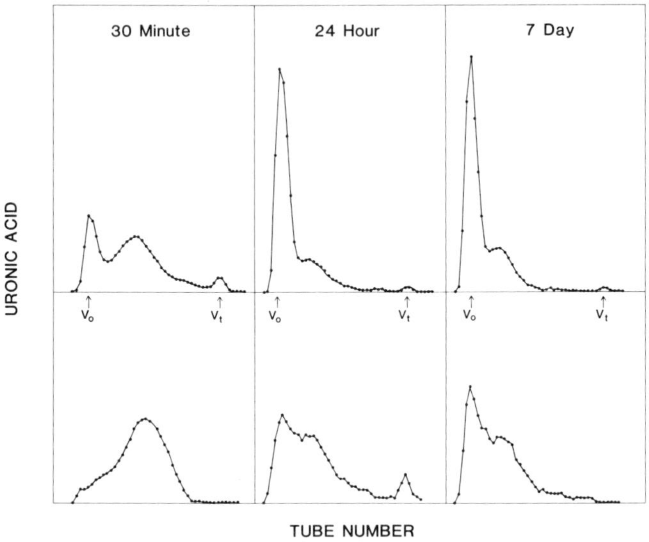

Figure 5. Sepharose CL-2B gel filtration patterns of proteoglycans extracted from 20μ human cartilage sections with buffer alone. The upper panels are from cartilage of a 3-month-old; the lower panels are from grade 2 cartilage of a 52-year-old. For comparison, the curves have been drawn with the same areas: uronic acid extracted in the first 30 minutes (30 Minute); between 30 minutes and 24 hours (24 Hour); between 24 hours and 7 days (7 Day). V_0 = void volume; V_t = total volume.

the remaining molecule contains the majority of chondroitin sulfate chains (24).

Cartilage also contains proteoglycans incapable of binding hyaluronic acid, at least some of which are probably in vivo degradation products of previously aggregating proteoglycans (25). Organ culture experiments of rabbit articular cartilage suggest that proteoglycan degradation is initiated by limited proteolysis of the core protein to yield a non-aggregating proteoglycan only slightly smaller than the original proteoglycan (26). Because many of the keratan sulfate chains are close to the hyaluronic acid binding site, released non-aggregating proteoglycans would be expected to be relatively enriched with respect to chondroitin sulfate.

In this study, the most easily extracted proteoglycans, which contained a high concentration of non-aggregated proteoglycans, had high galactosamine:glucosamine ratios indicating a high proportion of chondroitin sulfate. Similar findings have been previously described (25,27,28). Fragments of proteoglycans remaining attached to the hyaluronic acid chain after limited proteolysis, although relatively small in size, would be resistant to extraction with physiologic buffer because of their aggregation with hyaluronic acid. Under conditions which dissociate attachment to hyaluronic acid, such as 4*M* GdnHCl, these small molecules should be efficiently extracted, as was shown in these experiments. That is, the greatest percentages of glucosamine were extracted with 4*M* GdnHCl, and the percentages of glucosamine that remained within the extracted cartilage after 4*M* GdnHCl extraction were similar to those of galactosamine and uronic acid.

Recent studies have demonstrated that the composition of proteoglycans within articular cartilage varies with depth from the surface (29,30). With increasing depth, average proteoglycan monomer size decreases and the percentage of keratan sulfate and protein increases. We chose to study full-thickness cartilage slices for two reasons. First, it would be technically difficult to compare the extraction of proteoglycans from grade 3 samples where an unknown depth had already been abraded. Second, the experiments were designed to simulate fibrillation, which is longitudinal cleft formation that exposes almost the entire depth of the cartilage.

In spite of the large variation in extraction percentages, all of the samples displayed the same biphasic extraction pattern. The first phase of extraction probably represented loss of proteoglycans close to the newly-cut surface. The relatively large percent-

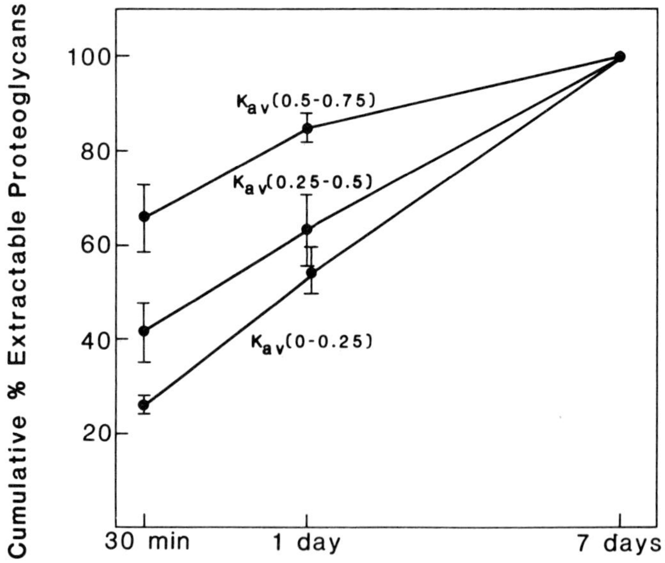

Figure 6. Buffer extraction of individual proteoglycan types. Four different cartilage specimens of 20μ thickness from skeletally mature individuals were extracted with buffer in the usual manner. Extracts were analyzed by Sepharose CL-2B gel filtration as in Figure 5 and the percentages of aggregates (K_{av} 0–0.25), large monomers (K_{av} 0.25–0.5), and small monomers (K_{av} 0.5–0.75) were determined. X axis is a square root scale.

age of small and large monomers extracted during the first phase suggests that non-aggregated proteoglycans are capable of migration within intact cartilage, while movement of aggregates is probably very limited. In previous studies, extraction of aggregates from bovine nasal cartilage was found to be directly proportional to the surface area, suggesting that they were shed from the surface without internal movement (14).

The second phase of extraction exhibited kinetics typical of a diffusional process (31). The entire cumulative extraction and the extraction of individual proteoglycan types was approximately proportional to the square root of time, although different types eluted from the cartilage at different rates. The decision to extract with buffer for 7 days was arbitrary. From the kinetics, one can predict that longer extraction would yield progressively lesser amounts. Some of the 20μ samples lost less than the predicted amount between the fourth and seventh days, which suggested that the amount of extractable proteoglycans had been depleted.

For all samples studied, the amount extracted in phase 1 was approximately half that of phase 2. This was true regardless of slice thickness. Both phases therefore appear to be related to the surface area exposed during slicing. The fact that thicker sections lost greater amounts of proteoglycans per surface area than thinner sections indicated that thicker sections are rapidly extracted to a greater depth. Our bovine nasal cartilage studies showed that this was due to a loss of non-aggregated proteoglycans from a depth of cartilage which was greater than the entire thickness of thinner sections (14).

Earlier studies indicated that extraction of cartilage with 0.15*M* NaCl yielded only non-aggregating proteoglycans (25,27). With the use of proteinase inhibitors, the percentage of extracted aggregates greatly increased (20). Also, the early investigators extracted large pieces of cartilage, so the surface area available for loss of aggregates was relatively small compared with the depth from which non-aggregated proteoglycans could be extracted.

Experiments outlined in Materials and Methods demonstrated that at 4°C there is no significant proteoglycan degradation during extraction with buffer of physiologic ionic strength and pH, containing inhibitors of proteolysis. In addition, sequential low ionic strength extraction followed by 4*M* GdnHCl does not yield greater amounts of non-aggregated proteoglycans than immediate 4*M* GdnHCl extraction. Furthermore, the kinetics of extraction were indicative of a diffusional process rather than a degradative process, and the percentage of aggregates increased with the time of extraction, which is the opposite of what would be expected if the extraction was the result of continuing autolysis.

Because they yielded large numbers of proteoglycans yet were technically easy to handle, 20μ cartilage slices were used to screen specimens. Slices thinner than 20μ tended to fall apart making it difficult to separate small fragments from the extract, and the amount of fragmentation tended to vary among specimens so that their surface areas were no longer comparable. Even at 20μ, some grade 3 samples had a tendency to fragment, which may account for their increased susceptibility to proteoglycan extraction. This fragmentation may represent an in vitro change similar to in vivo fibrillation. Whether fragmentation results in disruption of the integrity of the entire collagen mesh or merely increased surface area would be difficult to determine.

The present studies show that, even without additional fragmentation, 20μ sections of adult articular cartilage, on the average, lose almost half of their proteoglycans when extracted with buffer at physiologic ionic strength and pH. There is a variation in proteoglycan extractability which cannot be explained by the current studies even when cartilage grade is taken into account. This variation remains the subject of continuing research.

Fibrillated osteoarthritic cartilage has been shown to yield a high percentage of proteoglycans when extracted with low ionic strength solutions (32). In this study, extraction of 20μ cartilage sections from nonfibrillated areas of 4 osteoarthritic knees did not demonstrate significantly increased extractability compared with cartilage from normal knees. Several investigators have recently analyzed proteoglycans of intact cartilage specimens from osteoarthritic knees (33,34). They found no difference between intact osteoarthritic cartilage and normal cartilage with regard to percentage water content, proteoglycan concentration, percentage of proteoglycans capable of aggregating, and proteoglycan monomer size. Their results suggest that in intact osteoarthritic cartilage there is no predisposition toward proteoglycan loss due to alteration in the composition of the proteoglycans; our results suggest that there is no predisposing weakness of the collagen mesh. Loss of proteolgycans as a result of mechanical disruption of the collagen mesh probably plays a very important role in the pathogenesis of osteoarthritis, although chondrocyte necrosis and enzymatic degradation in areas of fibrillation are probably also important.

REFERENCES

1. Maroudas A: Balance between swelling pressure and collagen tension in normal and degenerate cartilages. Nature 260:808–809, 1976
2. Kempson GE: Mechanical properties of articular cartilage, Adult Articular Cartilage. Second edition. Edited by MAR Freeman. Kent, England, Pitman Medical Publishing, 1979, pp 333–414
3. Venn M, Maroudas A: Chemical composition and swelling of normal and osteoarthrotic femoral head cartilage. I. Chemical composition. Ann Rheum Dis 36:121–129, 1977
4. Sweet MBE, Thonar EJ-MA, Immelman AR, Solomon L: Biochemical changes in progressive osteoarthrosis. Ann Rheum Dis 36:387–398, 1977
5. Weiss C: Normal and osteoarthritic articular cartilage. Orthop Clin North Am 10:175–189, 1979
6. Sapolsky AI, Malemud CJ, Norby DP, Moskowitz RW, Matsuta K, Howell DS: Neutral proteinases from articular chondrocytes in culture. Biochim Biophys Acta 658:138–147, 1981
7. Janoff A, Feinstein G, Malemud CJ, Elias JM: Degradation of cartilage proteoglycan by human leukocyte granule neutral proteases—a model of joint injury. J Clin Invest 57:615–624, 1976
8. Freeman MAR: The fatigue of cartilage in the pathogenesis of osteoarthritis. Acta Orthop Scand 46:323–328, 1975
9. Hardingham TE, Muir H: The specific interaction of hyaluronic acid with cartilage proteoglycans. Biochim Biophys Acta 279:401–405, 1972
10. Hascall VC, Heinegard D: Aggregation of cartilage proteoglycan. I. The role of hyaluronic acid. J Biol Chem 249:4232–4241, 1974
11. Hascall VC, Sajdera SW: Proteinpolysaccharide complex from bovine nasal cartilage: the function of glycoprotein in the formation of aggregates. J Biol Chem 244:2384–2396, 1969
12. Tang L-H, Rosenberg L, Reiner A, Poole AR: Proteoglycans from bovine nasal cartilage: properties of a soluble form of link protein. J Biol Chem 254:10523–10531, 1979
13. Pottenger LA, Lyon NB, Hecht JD, Neustadt PM, Robinson RA: Influence of cartilage particle size and proteoglycan aggregation on immobilization of proteoglycans. J Biol Chem 257:11479–11485, 1982
14. Pottenger LA, Lyon NB, Webb JE: Proteoglycan extraction of sized cartilage particles. Arch Biochem Biophys 227:440–447, 1983
15. Meachim G: Light microscopy of India ink preparations of fibrillated cartilage. Ann Rheum Dis 31:457–464, 1972
16. Minns RJ, Steven FS, Hardinge K: Osteoarthrotic articular cartilage lesions of the femoral head observed in the scanning electron microscope. J Pathol 122:63–70, 1977
17. Paulsson M, Heinegard D: Matrix proteins bound to associatively prepared proteoglycans from bovine cartilage. Biochem J 183:539–545, 1979
18. Bitter T, Muir HM: A modified uronic acid carbozole reaction. Anal Biochem 4:330–334, 1962
19. Wagner WD: A more sensitive assay discriminating galactosamine and glucosamine in mixtures. Anal Biochem 94:394–396, 1979
20. Pearson JP, Mason RM: The stability of bovine nasal cartilage proteoglycans during isolation and storage. Biochim Biophys Acta 498:176–188, 1977
21. Walmsley R: The development of the patella. J Anat 74:360–368, 1940
22. Mathews MB, Lozaityte I: Sodium chondroitin sulfate protein complexes of cartilage. I. Molecular weight and shape. Arch Biochem Biophys 74:158–174, 1958
23. Hascall VC, Sajdera SW: Physical properties and polydispersity of proteoglycans from bovine nasal cartilage. J Biol Chem 245:4920–4930, 1970
24. Heinegard D, Axelsson I: Distribution of keratan sulfate in cartilage proteoglycans. J Biol Chem 252:1971–1979, 1977
25. Hardingham TE, Ewins RJF, Muir H: Cartilage proteoglycans—structure and heterogeneity of the protein core and the effects of specific protein modifications on the binding of hyaluronate. Biochem J 157:127–143, 1976
26. Sandy JD, Brown HLG, Lowther DA: Degradation of proteoglycan in articular cartilage. Biochim Biophys Acta 543:536–544, 1978
27. Hardingham TE, Muir H: Hyaluronic acid in cartilage and proteoglycan aggregation. Biochem J 139:565–581, 1974
28. Mayes RW, Mason RM, Griffin DC: The composition of cartilage proteoglycans: an investigation using high- and low-ionic-strength extraction procedures. Biochem J 131:541–553, 1973
29. Franzen A, Inerot S, Hejderu SD, Heinegard D: Variations in the composition of bovine hip articular cartilage with distances from the articular surface. Biochem J 195:535–543, 1981
30. Bayliss MT, Venn M, Maroudas A, Ali SY: Structure of proteoglycans from different layers of human articular cartilage. Biochem J 209:387–400, 1983
31. Crank J: The Mathematics of Diffusion. Oxford, Clarendon Press, 1975, p 11
32. Brandt KD: Enhanced extractability of articular cartilage proteoglycans in osteoarthrosis. Biochem J 143: 475–478, 1974
33. Brocklehurst R, Bayliss MT, Maroudas A, Coysh HL, Obst D, Freeman MAR, Revell PA, Ali SY: The composition of normal and osteoarthritic articular cartilage from human knee joints. J Bone Joint Surg 66A:95–106, 1984
34. Santer V, White RJ, Roughley PJ: Proteoglycans from normal and degenerate cartilage of the adult human tibial plateau. Arthritis Rheum 24:691–700, 1981

RADIOLOGIC VIGNETTE

TARSAL COALITION

DAVID J. SARTORIS and DONALD L. RESNICK

Tarsal coalition, or fusion, refers to the union of 2 or more tarsal bones into a single structure, with consequent absence of normal relative motion between them (1,2). The connection may be fibrous (syndesmosis), cartilaginous (synchondrosis), or osseous (synostosis) (1,3). Congenital cases are thought to arise from altered differentiation and impaired segmentation of primordial mesenchyme, resulting in failure of joint formation (3,4). Incorporation of accessory ossicles into tarsal articulations has also been proposed as an etiology (5,6). Acquired causes include trauma, previous surgery, infection, osteoarthritis, and rheumatoid arthritis (1,3). Paleopathologic remains have documented the occurrence of this condition as early as 900–950 AD (7,8). This vignette describes the epidemiologic, clinical, radiographic, and scintigraphic features of the various forms of tarsal coalition.

Epidemiology

The overall prevalence of tarsal coalition in the general population is approximately 1% (6,9). In some instances, particularly those with multiple tarsal fusions, a familial tendency has been noted (3,8). Autosomal dominant inheritance with variable penetrance has been proposed, based on a 39% incidence among first-degree relatives of 31 affected individuals in 1 study (8). Tarsal coalitions may be isolated phenomena or may be associated with congenital malformation syndromes, including hereditary symphalangism, Apert's acrocephalosyndactyly, and the hand–foot–uterus syndrome (3,10,11). Many cases of peroneal spastic flatfoot are accompanied by tarsal fusions, although the former finding may also be caused by a previous fracture, osteoarthritis, tuberculosis, juvenile chronic arthritis, or other conditions (12–15).

Clinical manifestations

Signs and symptoms of tarsal coalition generally develop during the second or third decade of life (3,16). This delayed presentation of a congenital problem has been attributed to the conversion of fibrous or cartilaginous union to osseous fusion, the former being rarely symptomatic (2,3). Typically, vague foot pain exaggerated by vigorous use or prolonged standing is noted, often beginning after minor trauma or unusual activity (1,17). Physical examination reveals intermittent or constant peroneal muscular spasm, restricted subtalar joint mobility, pes planus, and valgus positioning of the foot (1,3). Concomitant spasm of the tibialis anterior may, however, result in varus deformity, and pes cavus has also been observed (1,3). Tarsal coalition may present as an incidental radiographic finding in an asymptomatic individual (3).

Radiographic classification

Solitary tarsal coalitions are categorized according to the bones that are united (1,3). Calcaneonavicular fusions are slightly more common than talocalcaneal fusions, whereas talonavicular and calcaneocuboid involvement occur far less frequently (3,9).

From the Radiology Service, Veterans Administration Medical Center, San Diego, California.

David J. Sartoris, MD; Donald L. Resnick, MD.

Address reprint requests to Donald L. Resnick, MD, Radiology Service, VA Medical Center, 3350 La Jolla Village Drive, San Diego, CA 92161.

Submitted for publication August 16, 1984; accepted in revised form September 4, 1984.

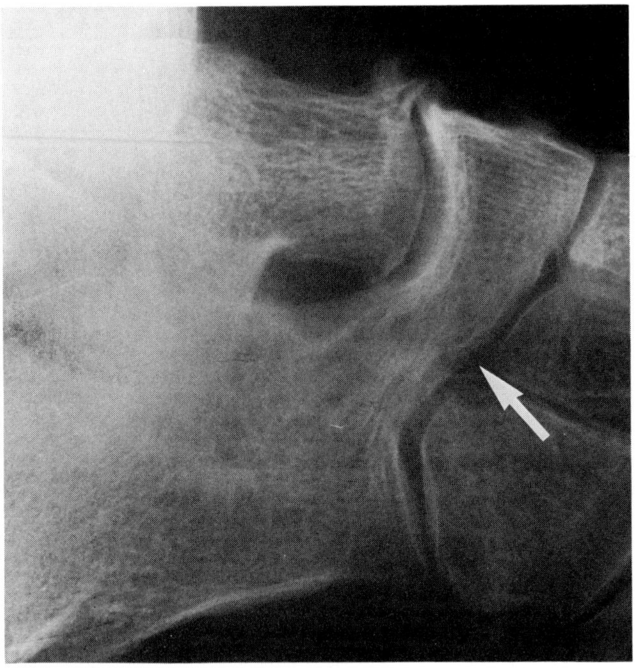

Figure 1. Oblique view demonstrating osseous fusion between the calcaneus and navicular (**arrow**). Secondary degenerative changes are present in the talonavicular articulation.

Coalitions involving multiple bones or unusual sites are characteristically associated with other congenital abnormalities (3). In general, radiographic findings in tarsal fusion can be classified as either primary (direct or indirect visualization of the fibrous, cartilaginous, or osseous bridge) or secondary (adaptive alterations in the affected or adjacent bones and articulations) in type.

Calcaneonavicular coalition. Normally, an articulation does not exist between the calcaneus and the navicular (3). In cases of bony coalition, which generally occurs in children between the ages of 8 and 12 (2,3), routine frontal and lateral radiographs may fail to demonstrate the site of union between these structures, although a 45° medial-oblique view of the foot establishes the diagnosis (Figure 1) (1,3). Close approximation of the adjacent calcaneal and navicular cortices, particularly in association with bone sclerosis or irregularity, suggests fibrous or cartilaginous fusion (1,3). Secondary radiographic signs are less pronounced than those accompanying talocalcaneal coalition, and include hypoplasia of the talar head (1,3) (Table 1). Clinical manifestations are also less severe; spastic flatfoot may be evident, although the condition is commonly asymptomatic. This coalition may predispose to ankle sprain (3,18). Fracture of an osseous calcaneonavicular bridge has also been reported (6).

Talocalcaneal coalition. Fusion of the talus and the calcaneus occurs most commonly at the level of the sustentaculum tali and involves the middle facets of the anterior subtalar joint. Rarely are the anterior facets or posterior subtalar joint affected (3,17). Talocalcaneal coalition is seen more frequently in males and occurs bilaterally in up to 25% of patients (3,17). Ossification occurs between the ages of 12 and 16 (2). Osseous coalitions may be overlooked on standard frontal and lateral radiographs, or even simulated in normal feet (3,19). Plain film radiography, utilizing oblique or axial (Harris-Beath views) projections (Figure 2), and conventional tomography are more diagnostic (1,3). Close apposition, eburnation, or sclerosis of adjacent articular surfaces implies fibrous or cartilaginous union (3). The latter may be confirmed by contrast arthrography of the talocalcaneonavicular joint, during which failure of normal opacification of the fused posterior portion of the articular cavity is noted (Figure 3) (3,20).

The numerous secondary radiographic signs of talocalcaneal coalition are summarized in Table 1. Subtalar rigidity leads to dorsal subluxation of the navicular, resulting in periosteal elevation and reactive bone formation at the attachment of the talonavicular ligament (1,17). An osseous outgrowth, or "beak," is formed at the dorsal aspect of the talar head adjacent to the talonavicular articulation (Figure 4). Less constantly, a similar excrescence develops on the proximal–dorsal surface of the navicular (1,3). These findings, best recognized in the lateral projection, are also observed in diffuse idiopathic skeletal hyperostosis, acromegaly, rheumatoid arthritis, and other conditions with altered motion of the talonavicular joint (1,3).

Table 1. Secondary radiographic signs of tarsal coalition

Calcaneonavicular
Hypoplasia of head of talus
Talocalcaneal
Osseous excrescence at dorsal aspect of talus
Narrowing of posterior talocalcaneal joint space
Broadening or rounding of lateral process of talus
Ball-and-socket tibiotalar articulation
Failure of visualization of middle facets of anterior subtalar joint
Concave undersurface of talar neck with asymmetry of talocalcaneonavicular joint

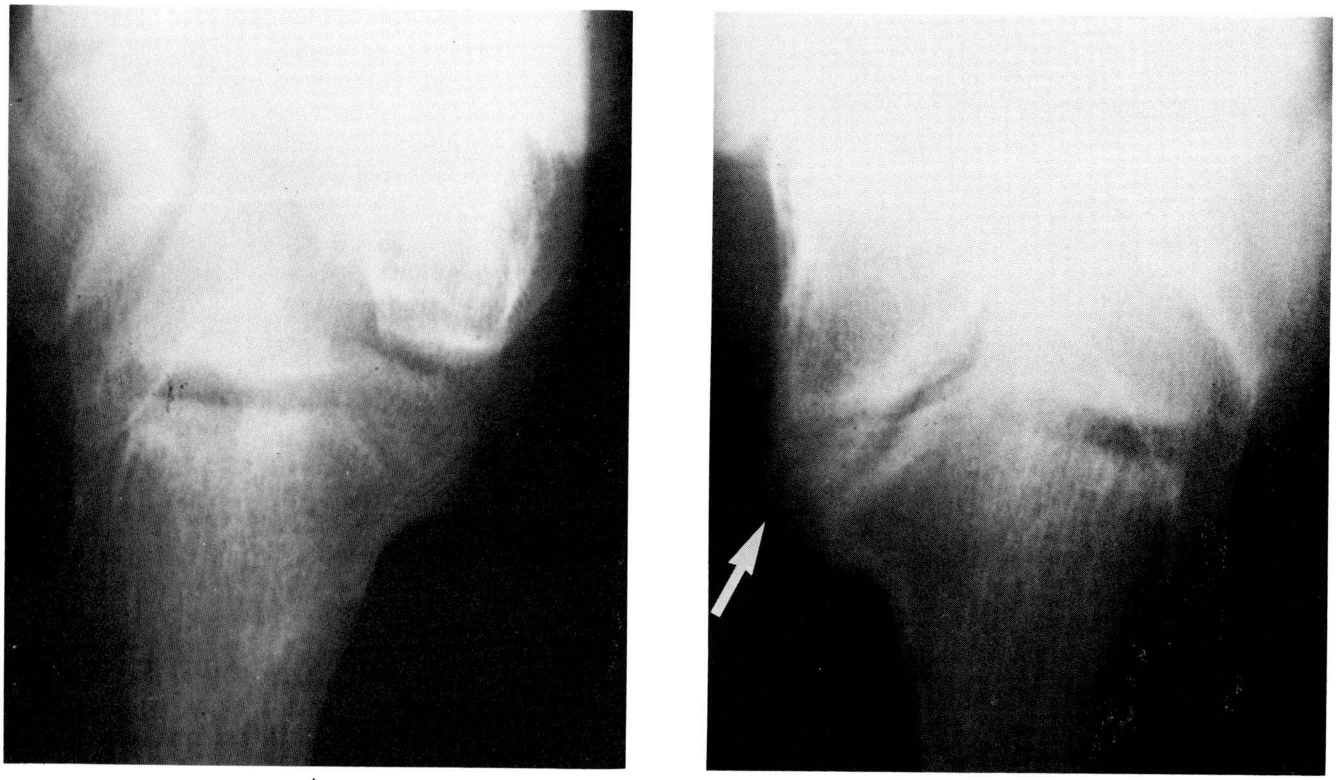

A B

Figure 2. Axial (Harris-Beath) views at the level of the sustentaculum tali. **A**, Normal side. **B**, Osseous talocalcaneal coalition (**arrow**).

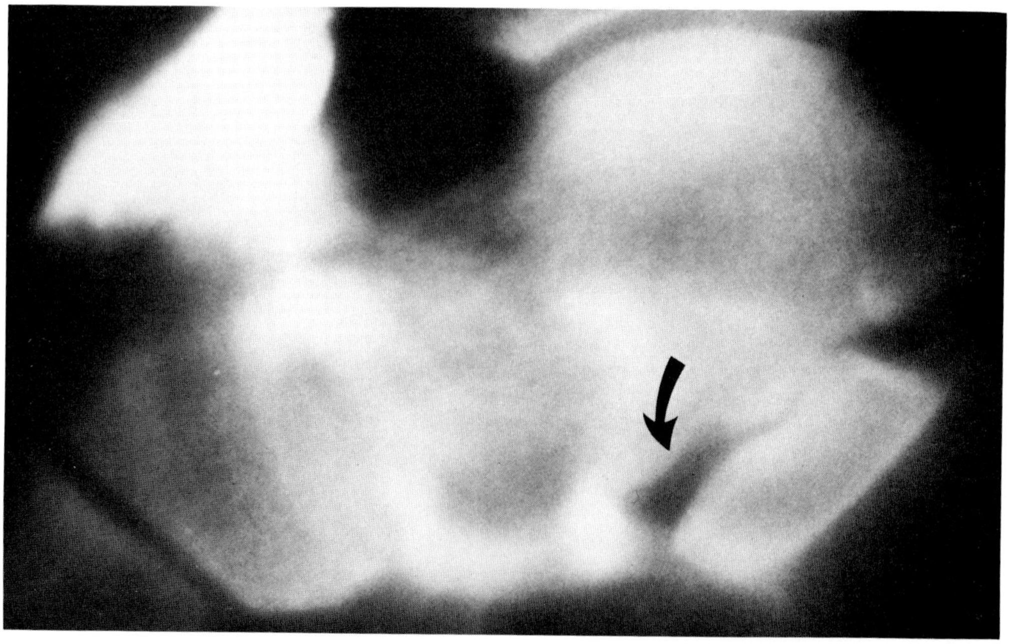

Figure 3. Tomogram (lateral view) following contrast injection of talocalcaneonavicular joint revealing absence of opacification posteriorly in region of sustentaculum tali, due to nonosseous talocalcaneal coalition (**arrow**).

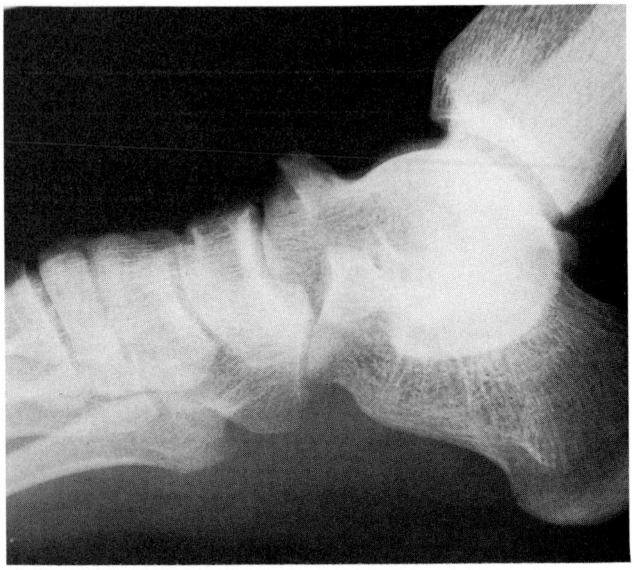

Figure 4. Radiograph (lateral view) showing prominent osseous excrescence arising from dorsal aspect of talar head. Obliteration of articular interval between talus and calcaneus also suggests coalition.

However, they are readily distinguished from osteophyte formation related to osteoarthritis of the ankle or midfoot, and should not be mistaken for excrescences which may develop normally at the insertion of the capsule of the ankle joint in the talar neck (3,21).

At its typical site, talocalcaneal coalition may lead to eversion of the calcaneus, or premature degenerative arthritis of the posterior subtalar articulation (3). Either of these phenomena results in apparent narrowing of the posterior subtalar joint space, a secondary radiographic sign seen in as many as 60% of patients (3,17). Valgus angulation of the calcaneus resulting from talocalcaneal fusion leads to broadening, or rounding of the lateral process of the talus in approximately 50% of patients (1,3,17). Furthermore, in the presence of a talocalcaneal coalition, the functions of inversion and eversion which are normally performed by the subtalar articulations are assumed by the tibiotalar joint (3,22). This phenomenon converts the normally mesa-shaped superior talar joint surface to a rounded convexity which articulates with a correspondingly concave distal tibia, a finding that is termed the "ball-and-socket" ankle joint (Figure 5) (3,22).

The middle facets of the anterior subtalar joint are normally seen in tangent on a properly-positioned lateral radiograph of the foot (Figure 6). Failure to visualize this articulation is a helpful ancillary sign of talocalcaneal coalition, although technical error may result in false-positive diagnoses (3,17). Comparison radiographs of the uninvolved foot may be useful in detecting talocalcaneonavicular joint asymmetry and associated concavity of the plantar aspect of the talar neck (3,17). The reliability of these signs depends upon comparable positioning on the 2 sides of the body (3,17).

Talonavicular coalition. Conventional radiographs, particularly the lateral view, are usually adequate for the diagnosis of this uncommon variety of tarsal fusion (Figure 7) (1,3). Osseous bridging occurs between the ages of 3 and 5 years, and may be asymptomatic or associated with peroneal spasm (1,2). Abnormalities of the fifth digit of the hand may occur concomitantly, and both autosomal dominant and recessive inheritance patterns have been observed (10,23).

Calcaneocuboid coalition. This extremely rare entity is readily diagnosed in its osseous form by routine radiography (1,3). Calcaneocuboid fusion may be asymptomatic, coexistent with peroneal spasm, bilateral, or associated with other congenital anomalies (1,3).

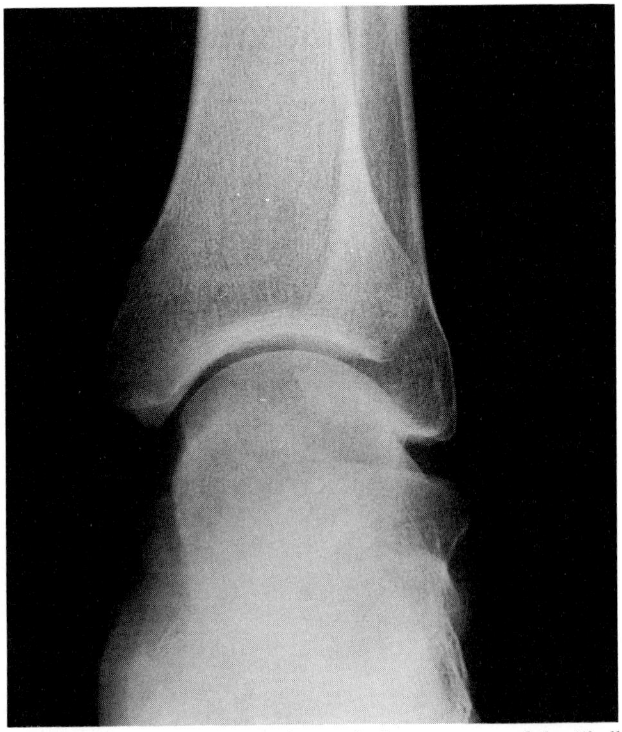

Figure 5. Frontal view illustrating typical appearance of the "ball-and-socket" ankle joint.

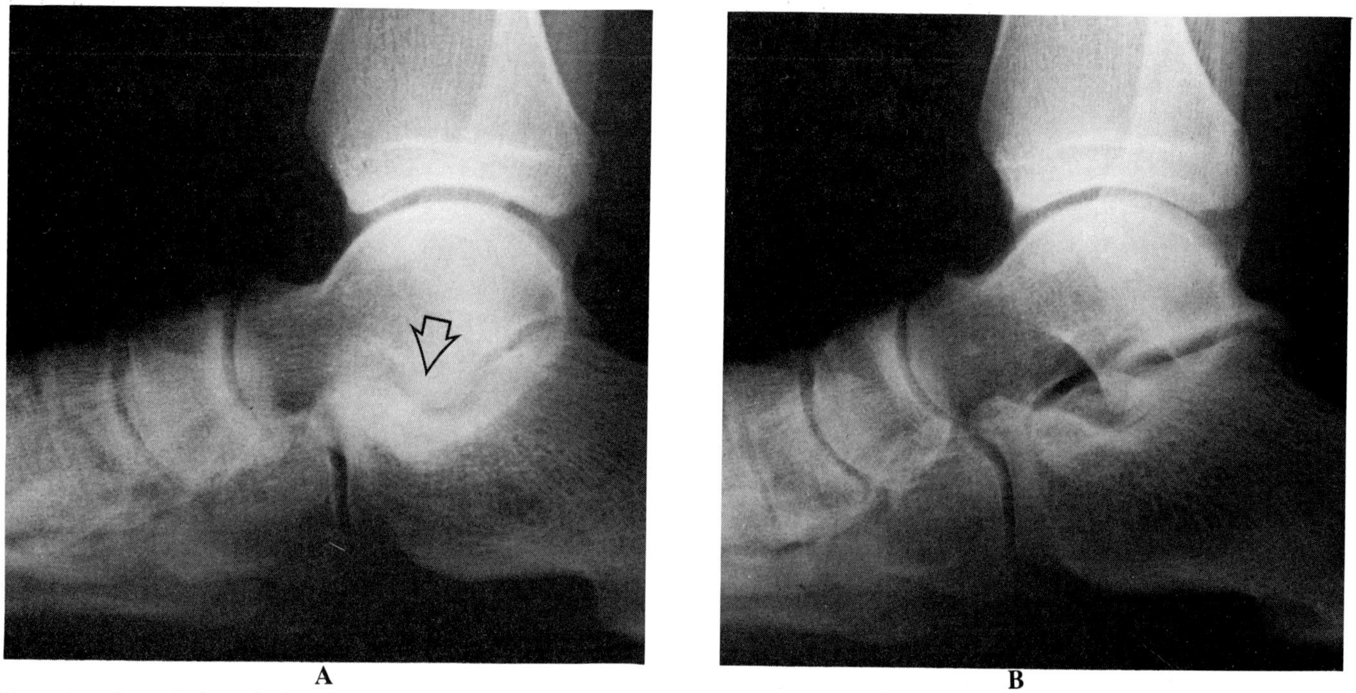

A B

Figure 6. A, Lateral view of talocalcaneal coalition showing obscuration of middle facets of anterior subtalar joint (**arrowhead**), with associated narrowing of the posterior subtalar articulation. **B**, Lateral view of normal foot, for comparison.

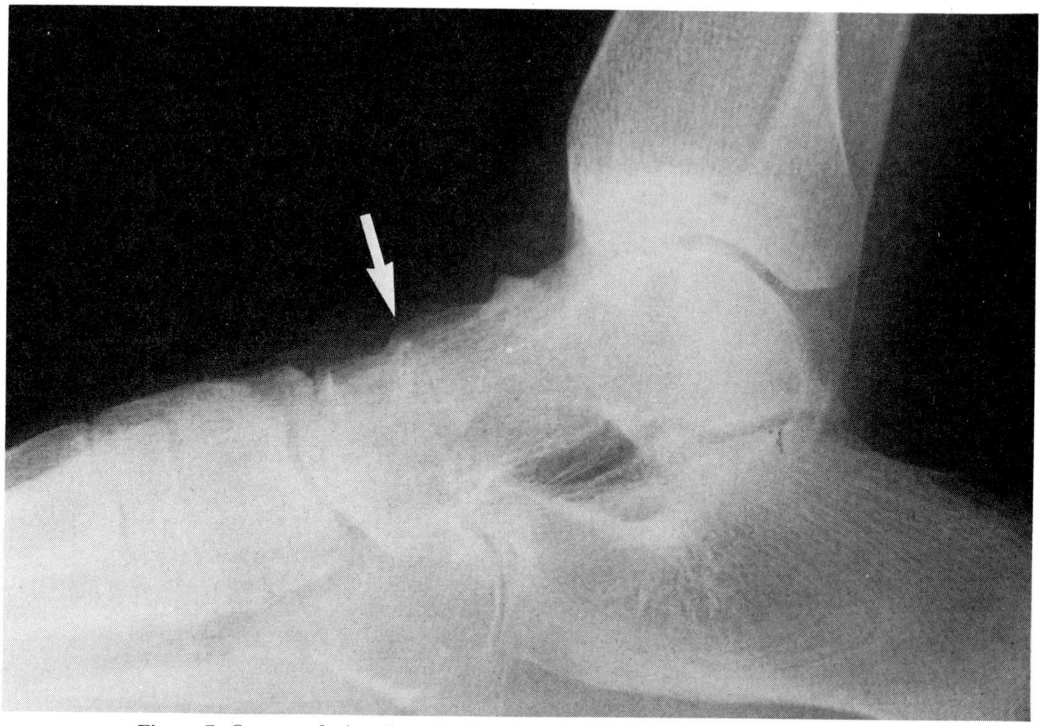

Figure 7. Osseous fusion (lateral view) between the talus and navicular (**arrow**).

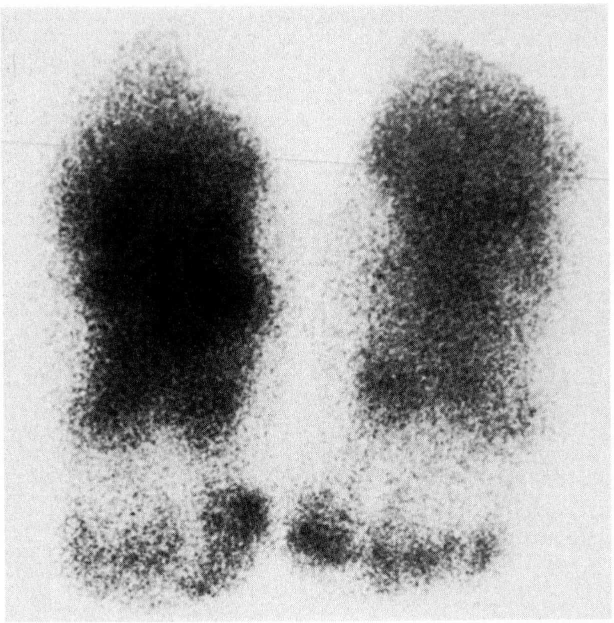

Figure 8. Skeletal scintigram of both feet (frontal view) revealing augmented radionuclide accumulation in the tarsal region of the right foot.

Miscellaneous coalitions. Sporadic case reports of isolated naviculocuneiform and cubonavicular coalition exist (24,25).

Newer imaging modalities

Recently, skeletal scintigraphy using ^{99m}Tc-methylene diphosphonate has been found to be useful as a noninvasive screening procedure for subtalar coalition (16,26). Positive findings include augmented radionuclide accumulation in the region of the subtalar joint, as well as in the dorsal aspect of the talus or talonavicular joint (Figures 8 and 9) (16,26). The former probably results from accentuated stress on articular surfaces adjacent to the site of fusion, whereas the latter is probably secondary to the same mechanism that produces dorsal talar and navicular excrescences (26).

High-resolution computed tomography has recently been shown to be an extremely valuable technique in the identification and characterization of talocalcaneal coalitions (Figure 10) (16,27). Its advantages include noninvasiveness, precise evaluation of adjacent osseous and soft tissue structures, potential for demonstration of associated abnormalities, and an ability to simultaneously image the opposite foot (16).

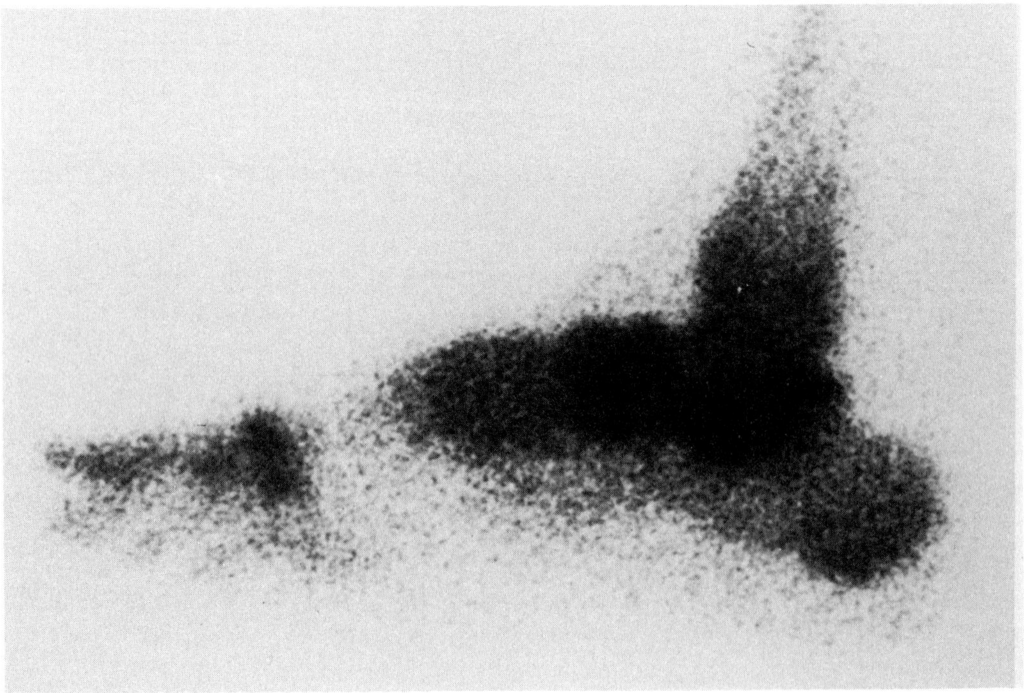

Figure 9. Lateral image of right foot (shown in Figure 8) localizes the increased activity to the subtalar and talonavicular joint areas.

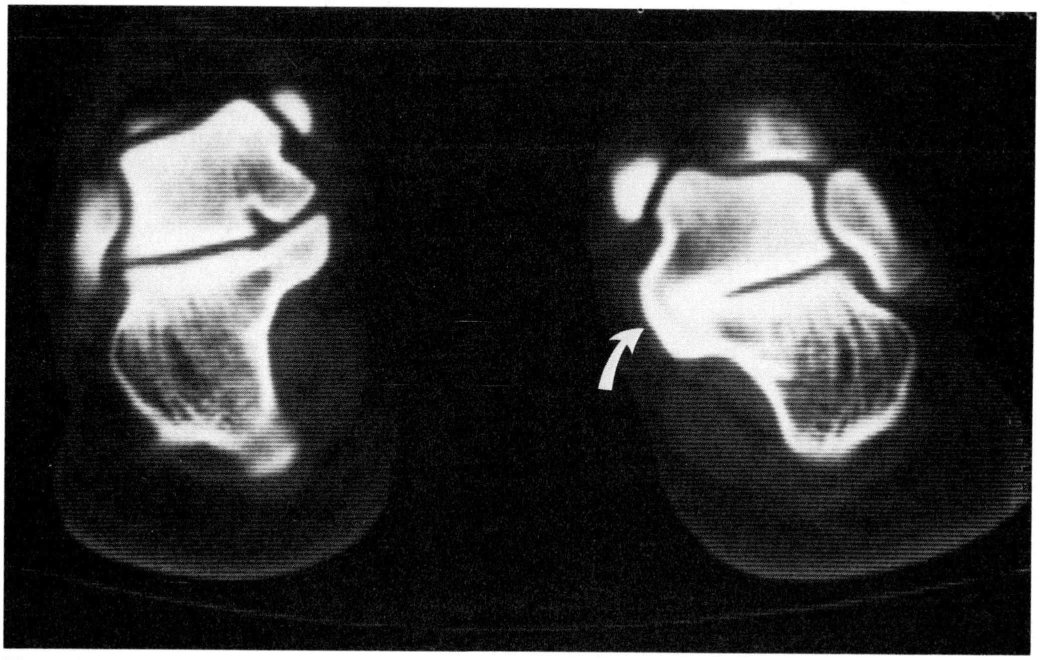

Figure 10. Computed tomographic image at the level of sustentacula tali demonstrating osseous bridging of the middle facets of the anterior subtalar joint on the right (**arrow**). The normal appearance of this articulation is seen in the left foot.

Acknowledgment. Special thanks are extended to Geri Hubble for typing the manuscript.

REFERENCES

1. Conway JJ, Cowell HR: Tarsal coalition: clinical significance and roentgenographic demonstration. Radiology 92:799–811, 1969
2. Cowell HR, Elener V: Rigid painful flatfoot secondary to tarsal coalition. Clin Orthop 177:54–60, 1983
3. Resnick D: Additional congenital or heritable anomalies and syndromes, Diagnosis of Bone and Joint Disorders with Emphasis on Articular Abnormalities. Edited by D Resnick, G Niwayama. Philadelphia, WB Saunders Co., 1981, pp 2559–2565
4. Wheeler R, Guevera A, Bleck EE: Tarsal coalitions: review of the literature and case report of bilateral dual calcaneonavicular and talocalcaneal coalitions. Clin Orthop 156:175–177, 1981
5. Galinski AW, Crovo RT, Ditmars JJ Jr: Os trigonum as a cause of tarsal coalition. J Am Podiatry Assoc 69:191–196, 1979
6. Richards RR, Evans JG, McGoey PF: Fracture of a calcaneonavicular bar: a complication of tarsal coalition: a case report. Clin Orthop 185:220–221, 1984
7. Heiple KG, Lovejoy CO: The antiquity of tarsal coalition: bilateral deformity in a pre-Columbian Indian skeleton. J Bone Joint Surg 51A:979–983, 1969
8. Leonard MA: The inheritance of tarsal coalition and its relationship to spastic flatfoot. J Bone Joint Surg 56B:520–526, 1974
9. Stormont DM, Peterson HA: The relative incidence of tarsal coalition. Clin Orthop 181:28–36, 1983
10. Challis J: Hereditary transmission of talonavicular coalition in association with anomaly of the little finger. J Bone Joint Surg 56A:1273–1276, 1974
11. Geelhoed GW, Neel JV, Davidson RT: Symphalangism and tarsal coalitions: a hereditary syndrome: a report on two families. J Bone Joint Surg 51B:278–289, 1969
12. James EA: Tarsal coalitions and peroneal spastic flatfoot. Austral Radiol 14:80–83, 1970
13. Cowell HR: Talocalcaneal coalition and new causes of peroneal spastic flatfoot. Clin Orthop 85:16–22, 1972
14. Jayakumar S, Cowell HR: Rigid flatfoot. Clin Orthop 122:77–84, 1977
15. Kendrick JI: Tarsal coalitions. Clin Orthop 85:62–63, 1972
16. Deutsch AL, Resnick D, Campbell G: Computed tomography and bone scintigraphy in the evaluation of tarsal coalition. Radiology 144:137–140, 1982
17. Beckly DE, Anderson PW, Pedegana LR: The radiology of the subtalar joint with special reference to talocalcaneal coalition. Clin Radiol 26:333–341, 1975

18. Snyder RB, Libscomb AB, Johnston RK: The relationship of tarsal coalitions to ankle sprains in athletes. Am J Sports Med 9:313–317, 1981
19. Shaffer HA Jr, Harrison RB: Tarsal pseudo-coalition–a positional artifact. J Can Assoc Radiol 31:236–237, 1980
20. Kaye JJ, Ghelman B, Schneider R: Talocalcaneonavicular joint arthrography for sustentacular-talar tarsal coalitions. Radiology 115:730–731, 1975
21. Keats TE, Harrison RB: Hypertrophy of the talar beak. Skeletal Radiol 4:37–39, 1979
22. Channon GM, Brotherton BJ: The ball-and-socket ankle joint. J Bone Joint Surg 61B:85–89, 1979
23. Zeide MS, Wiesel SW, Terry RL: Talonavicular coalition. Clin Orthop 126:225–227, 1977
24. Gregersen HN: Naviculocuneiform coalition. J Bone Joint Surg 59A:128–130, 1977
25. Cavallaro DC, Hadden HR: An unusual case of tarsal coalition: a cuboid navicular synostosis. J Am Podiatry Assoc 68:71–75, 1978
26. Goldman AB, Pavlov H, Schneider R: Radionuclide bone scanning in subtalar coalitions: differential considerations. AJR 138:427–432, 1982
27. Azouz EM: Tarsal pseudo-coalition (letter). J Can Assoc Radiol 33:105, 1982

BRIEF REPORT

A SUBSET OF RHEUMATOID ARTHRITIS PATIENTS WITH A PATTERN OF EPSTEIN-BARR VIRUS ANTIBODIES SIMILAR TO THAT FOUND IN PRIMARY AND SECONDARY IMMUNODEFICIENCY DISEASES

JACQUES H. M. COHEN, THOMAS L. VISCHER, JOCELYN CARQUIN, and FRANÇOIS BLANCHARD

Alspaugh and Tan (1) first observed that patients with rheumatoid arthritis (RA) had antibodies against a peculiar Epstein-Barr virus (EBV)–induced antigen which they called RANA (RA-associated nuclear antigen). In further studies, several groups reported that patients with RA had higher titers of antibodies against the viral capsid antigen (VCA) when compared with controls (2–4). These results, however, were not confirmed by others (5–7). Similarly, some authors found increased titers of antibodies against the Epstein-Barr nuclear antigen (EBNA) in patients with RA (2,3), but others did not (6,7).

In the course of a multicenter study on HLA antigens in rheumatoid arthritis (8), sera were tested for their titers of VCA and EBNA antibodies. These titers were then compared with those found in a control group of healthy persons with similar characteristics.

Patients and methods. Sera were obtained from 151 patients with definite or classic, adult-onset rheumatoid arthritis of at least 5 years duration. The patients were participating in the Swiss Collaborative Study on HLA antigens; a previously published paper outlines the details of this study (8). The control sera were from 88 healthy adults participating in a study on HLA-linked susceptibility factors in childhood leukemia (9); the subjects were the parents of children with leukemia. Age and sex distributions were similar in the patient and control groups.

Antibodies to VCA were determined by a double antibody immunofluorescence technique on P3HR1 cells as described by Henle and Henle, using fluorescein-conjugated antibodies against human IgM and general immunoglobulin (10). The antibodies to EBNA were determined with the anticomplement immunofluorescence technique of Reedman and Klein (11). The details of both methods have been previously described (12). Three sera were excluded from this study due to the presence of antinuclear antibodies, which interfered with the reading of the anti-EBV immunofluorescence. They were detected by their positivity on an EBV-negative T lymphoma (JM cell line). All sera from patients with RA were absorbed on glutaraldehyde-insolubilized pooled IgG for 18 hours at 4°C to remove rheumatoid factor, and then cleared by ultracentrifugation at 40,000*g* for 2 hours. This absorption rendered 84% of the sera latex-negative when tested at a 1:40 dilution (Latex slide test; Behring, Marburg, FRG); it did not modify the EBV antibody titers of control sera.

Results. The VCA and EBNA antibody titers are given in Table 1. The RA patients had significantly higher anti-VCA titers and lower anti-EBNA titers than the controls. Biparametric analysis of the titers in both groups revealed a subpopulation of 21 patients in the RA group (14%) who had anti-VCA titers ≥1:1,280 and anti-EBNA titers ≤1:40; no member of the control group had such a pattern ($P < 0.004$, Fisher's

From the Immunology Laboratory, University Hospital Center, University of Reims, France, and the Division of Rheumatology, Geneva University Medical School, Geneva, Switzerland.

Supported by grants from the Swiss Federal Department of Public Health and the Swiss National Fund for Scientific Research.

Jacques H. M. Cohen, MD: University of Reims; Thomas L. Vischer, MD: Geneva University Medical School; Jocelyn Carquin, BScPharm: University of Reims; François Blanchard, MD: University of Reims.

Address reprint requests to T. L. Vischer, MD, Division of Rheumatology, Hôpital Cantonal Universitaire, CH-1211, Geneva 4, Switzerland.

Submitted for publication June 11, 1984; accepted in revised form October 11, 1984.

Table 1. Titers of antibodies to viral capsid antigen (VCA) and Epstein-Barr nuclear antigen (EBNA) in rheumatoid arthritis (RA) patients and control subjects

	Anti-VCA*	Anti-EBNA*
Control sera (n = 88)	6.06 ± 1.65	4.34 ± 2.15
Sera from all RA patients (n = 151)	6.38 ± 2.14†	3.73 ± 1.95‡
Sera from RA patients without the subpopulation defined by an anti-EBNA titer ≤1:40 and an anti-VCA titer ≥1:1,280 (n = 130)	5.96 ± 1.96§	4.02 ± 1.80§

* Values shown are mean ± SD, $\log_2 \times 10^{-1}$ of titer.
† $\chi^2 = 13.5$, $P < 0.00024$ (nonparametric median test).
‡ $\chi^2 = 9.05$, $P < 0.0026$ (nonparametric median test).
§ $\chi^2 = 3.03$, $P > 0.08$ (nonparametric median test).

exact probability test). When this subpopulation of 21 RA sera was removed from the RA group, the mean titers were similar in the 2 groups.

Discussion. After primary infection by EBV, both EBNA and VCA antibodies usually remain at a detectable level in the serum for the rest of the subject's lifetime. In the general population, the range of the titers of antibodies to each antigen is wide, but for a given subject, the titers are related to each other. High anti-VCA titers in association with very low anti-EBNA titers are rare among normal subjects but frequent in patients with primary and secondary immunodeficiencies (13–15). The 21 RA patients with this pattern of EBV antibodies did not differ from the other RA patients with regard to age, sex, duration of disease, or treatment. The group with the peculiar EBV serology pattern had slightly higher titers of rheumatoid factors (mean ± SD, $\log_2 \times 10^{-1}$ of the titer: 4.8 ± 2.4 versus 4.2 ± 2.3; $P = 0.371$) and significantly raised erythrocyte sedimentation rates (47.9 ± 29.6 versus 32.3 ± 27.7; $P = 0.036$, separate variance estimate). Thus, this group seems to have had more active disease at the time of study than the other RA patients.

Some of the discrepancies in EBV serology found in published studies of RA patient series could be explained by the inclusion of various proportions of patients with this immunodeficiency pattern of EBV serology.

Acknowledgments. We thank the participants in the Swiss Collaborative Study on HLA–DR Antigens in Rheumatoid Arthritis for their cooperation and P. Schilling-Doriot for typing the manuscript.

REFERENCES

1. Alspaugh MA, Tan EM: Serum antibody in rheumatoid arthritis reactive with a cell-associated antigen. Arthritis Rheum 19:711–719, 1976
2. Ferrel PB, Aitcheson CT, Pearson GR, Tan EM: Seroepidemiological study of relationships between Epstein-Barr virus and rheumatoid arthritis. J Clin Invest 67:681–687, 1981
3. Alspaugh MA, Henle G, Lennette ET, Henle W: Elevated levels of antibodies to Epstein-Barr virus antigens in sera and synovial fluids of patients with rheumatoid arthritis. J Clin Invest 67:1134–1140, 1981
4. Venables PJW, Roffe LM, Erhardt CC, Maini RN, Edwards JMB, Porter AD: Titers of antibodies to RANA in rheumatoid arthritis and normal sera: relationship to Epstein-Barr virus infection. Arthritis Rheum 24:1459–1464, 1981
5. Catalano MA, Carson DA, Slovin SF, Richman DD, Vaughan JH: Antibodies to Epstein-Barr virus-determined antigens in normal subjects and in patients with seropositive rheumatoid arthritis. Proc Natl Acad Sci USA 76:5825–5828, 1979
6. Silverman SL, Schumacher HR: Antibodies to Epstein-Barr viral antigens in early rheumatoid arthritis. Arthritis Rheum 24:1465–1468, 1981
7. Slovin SF, Luberski TT, Carson DA, Catalano MA, Reitz EM, Vaughan JH: Antibodies to Epstein-Barr virus associated antigens in Pima Indians with and without rheumatoid arthritis. Rheumatol Int 3:65–68, 1983
8. Vischer TL: HLA-DR antigens in rheumatoid arthritis: a Swiss collaborative study. Rheumatol Int 1:111–113, 1981
9. Cohen JHM, Vischer TL, Carquin J, Blanchard F, Von Fliedner VE, Jeannet M: HLA-DR antigens and the antibody response against Epstein-Barr virus. Tissue Antigens 23:156–162, 1984
10. Henle W, Henle G: Immunofluorescence in cells derived from Burkitt's lymphoma. J Bacteriol 91:1248–1256, 1966
11. Reedman BM, Klein G: Cellular localisation of an Epstein-Barr virus (EBV) associated complement fixing antigen in producer and non-producer lymphoblastoid cell lines. Int J Cancer 11:499–520, 1973
12. Cohen JHM, Lenoir GM: Epstein-Barr virus and rheumatoid arthritis: are rheumatoid arthritis associated nuclear antigen and Epstein-Barr virus nuclear antigen different? Biomedicine 36:246–249, 1982
13. Henle W, Henle G: Epstein-Barr virus-specific serology in immunologically compromised individuals. Cancer Res 41:4222–4225, 1981
14. Cheeseman SH, Henle W, Rubin RH, Tolkoff-Rubin NE, Cosimi B, Cantell K, Winkle S, Herrin JT, Black PH, Russell PS, Hirsch MS: Epstein-Barr virus infection in renal transplant recipients. Ann Intern Med 93:39–42, 1980
15. Sakamoto K, Freed HJ, Purtilo DT: Antibody responses to Epstein-Barr virus in families with the x-linked lymphoproliferative syndrome. J Immunol 125:921–925, 1980

BRIEF REPORT

THROMBOTIC THROMBOCYTOPENIC PURPURA DEVELOPING DURING PREGNANCY IN A C2-DEFICIENT PATIENT WITH A HISTORY OF SYSTEMIC LUPUS ERYTHEMATOSUS

R. DIXIT, ARTHUR M. KRIEG, and J. P. ATKINSON

Thrombotic thrombocytopenic purpura (TTP) is an uncommon syndrome characterized by the clinical pentad of fever, microangiopathic hemolytic anemia (MAHA), thrombocytopenia, neurologic symptoms, and renal abnormalities. The occasional occurrence of TTP during pregnancy, and also its occurrence in association with systemic lupus erythematosus (SLE), have been reported (1). Whereas TTP has not been described in patients with hereditary deficiencies of complement, the association between homozygous C2 deficiency and SLE is well-recognized (2). We describe here a patient with C2 deficiency and SLE who developed thrombocytopenia, MAHA, seizures, and renal abnormalities during the first trimester of pregnancy. Corticosteroid therapy did not alter her clinical status, but there was a prompt response to termination of pregnancy.

Case report. The clinical and family history of this 31-year-old white woman have been previously described (3,4). At age 5 she developed discoid lupus erythematosus. She also had a history of photosensitivity and recurrent oral ulcerations. She was otherwise well until age 20 (1972), when she developed fever, a maculopapular erythematous skin rash involving the face and arms, petechiae, scleral icterus, thrombocytopenia (platelet count 2,000/mm^3), Coombs-positive hemolytic anemia (hematocrit 11%, reticulocytes 27%), renal involvement (serum creatinine 1.3 mg/100 ml, creatinine clearance 20–30 ml/minute, 24-hour urine protein 3.6 gm, urine sediment that showed 30–50 erythrocytes/high power field, and a few granular casts), retinal hemorrhages and cytoid bodies, and an acute psychosis which did not appear to be associated with her steroid treatment. There was no evidence of disseminated intravascular coagulation. Anti-DNA antibodies were positive at 27% (normal <17%), but antinuclear antibody (ANA) was negative (titer <1:10).

Clinically, the skin lesion was judged to be typical of SLE. The biopsy showed compatible pathology, and immunofluorescent staining was positive for IgG only. Total hemolytic complement activity was undetectable. Further investigation revealed functional and antigenic absence of C2, with normal levels of the other complement components. A diagnosis of C2 deficiency and SLE was made, and the patient was treated with steroids and azathioprine. Following a protracted hospital course, she went into a sustained remission.

For the next 10 years she was asymptomatic. Examination at least twice yearly showed normal peripheral blood counts and normal renal function and urine sediment. Prednisone was tapered over a 2-year period to 10 mg 3 times per week. This dosage was continued until the present admission. Azathioprine was reduced over a 2-year period prior to admission and discontinued in June 1980. Until the fall of 1980 she had practiced contraception using mechanical barriers. She had never used oral agents. She had a

From the Howard Hughes Medical Institute Laboratories and the Department of Medicine, Division of Rheumatology, Washington University School of Medicine, St. Louis, Missouri.

R. Dixit, MD: Fellow, Division of Rheumatology, Washington University School of Medicine; Arthur M. Krieg, MD: Medical Resident, Department of Internal Medicine, University of Minnesota; J. P. Atkinson, MD: Professor of Medicine, Division of Rheumatology, Washington University School of Medicine.

Address reprint requests to Dr. John P. Atkinson, Division of Rheumatology, Washington University School of Medicine, 660 S. Euclid, Box 8045, St. Louis, MO 63110.

Submitted for publication June 11, 1984; accepted in revised form September 5, 1984.

spontaneous abortion at 7 weeks gestation in May 1981. No clinical abnormalities were noted during this pregnancy or in the period following the abortion. She had a normal complete blood count and platelet count in July 1981.

In December 1981, when she was 11 weeks pregnant, the patient presented to her physician, following a brief episode of epistaxis. Outpatient evaluation revealed a hematocrit value of 26% and platelet count of 19,000/mm^3. On admission to the hospital she had no complaints. Physical examination demonstrated normal vital signs, lower extremity petechiae, normal neurologic findings, and an appropriately enlarged uterus for gestational age.

Laboratory findings on admission were: white blood cells 11,600/mm^3 with a normal differential count, hemoglobin 9.9 gm/100 ml, hematocrit 29.5%, reticulocytes 20%, platelet count 12,000/mm^3, lactate dehydrogenase 950 IU/liter, indirect bilirubin 2.0 mg/100 ml, and erythrocyte sedimentation rate 28 mm/hour. The peripheral smear showed numerous fragmented red cells, nucleated red cells, and polychromasia. Renal function and urinalysis results fluctuated during the early part of her hospital stay. Urinalysis revealed 1+–3+ protein, 1–3 granular casts/high power field, and 10–50 red cells/high power field. Creatinine clearance was 52–103 ml/minute, with a serum creatinine of 0.7–1.2 mg/100 ml, and 24-hour urine protein of 393–754 mg. ANA, anti-DNA antibodies, Raji cell assay, prothrombin/partial thromboplastin time, C3, C4, factor B, fibrinogen (275 mg/100 ml), cryoglobulins, VDRL, sucrose hemolysis, and direct and indirect Coombs' tests all showed results that were negative or within normal limits. Total hemolytic complement and C2 activity were again undetectable. A highly sensitive quantitative assay (5) for red cell–bound C3d and immunoglobulin demonstrated extremely low-normal levels of C3d and low-normal levels of immunoglobulin.

A review of the patient's 1972 hospitalization record revealed that anti-DNA antibodies were positive 1 of the 6 times they were evaluated. The Coombs' tests for Ig and C3 were negative on 6 determinations and weakly positive for only IgG on 1 occasion. The peripheral smear demonstrated extensive red cell fragmentation. Bone marrow aspiration showed erythroid hyperplasia with adequate megakaryocytes. Since thrombocytopenia, neurologic symptoms, and renal abnormalities were also present during the 1972 admission, the similarity in presentation and possible response to steroids during that admission prompted us to initiate treatment with prednisone. She received oral prednisone (50 mg/twice a day) for 5 days. This was followed by 4 days of intravenous pulse methylprednisolone therapy (500 mg/twice a day), and then 3 days of oral prednisone (50 mg/twice a day). There was no improvement in her hematologic status. During this 12-day period the platelet count remained unchanged and 6 units of saline-washed red blood cells was required to maintain the hematocrit above 23%. The peripheral smear showed increasing red cell fragmentation.

Because of the temporal association of her disease process with pregnancy and the ineffectiveness of steroid therapy in reversing the life-threatening thrombocytopenia, the pregnancy was terminated by suction curettage. The patient received 10 units of platelets and 2 units of saline-washed red blood cells prior to the procedure. There were no complications. Approximately 4 hours later, however, she suffered the first of 2 witnessed grand mal seizures which occurred about 2 hours apart. The results of computerized tomography of the head, serum electrolyte testing, and lumbar puncture (performed after transfusion of another 10 units of platelets) were unremarkable. One and a half hours after transfusion, the platelet count was 100,000/mm^3. She was treated with diphenylhydantoin and there were no further seizures. In the 24 hours following the procedure, her hematocrit fell from 36% to 23%, the peripheral smear showed increased red blood cell fragmentation, and the platelet count decreased to 28,000/mm^3. Subsequently, her platelet count progressively increased, and the peripheral smear demonstrated fewer fragmented red cells.

By the eighth postoperative day, the platelet count was >100,000/mm^3, and all laboratory indicators of hemolysis had resolved. Throughout the rest of the hospital course there was no deterioration in renal status and no laboratory evidence of disseminated intravascular coagulation. She was discharged on a regimen of 50 mg of prednisone twice daily, which was tapered over 6 weeks to 5 mg 3 times per week. Over the subsequent 18 months, she has been asymptomatic, with normal blood and platelet counts and normal renal function.

A stored sample of the patient's serum was recently evaluated for the presence of anti-Ro (SS-A) antibodies, which have been demonstrated to have an increased prevalence (75%; 9 of 12 patients) in the sera of C2-deficient SLE patients (6). The serum was found to contain anti-Ro (SS-A) antibodies.

The presence of high levels of unusually large plasma factor VIII:von Willebrand factor multimers that decreased during periods of relapse has been reported in 4 patients with chronic relapsing TTP, which is a rare subset of TTP (7). This patient's plasma, collected following remission of disease activity, did not reveal abnormal multimer distribution.

Histologic examination of the products of conception for evidence of TTP was unfruitful since the specimen was devoid of maternal tissue (1).

Discussion. This patient with C2 deficiency and discoid lupus erythematosus in early childhood had 2 similar disease episodes separated by 10 asymptomatic years. MAHA, severe thrombocytopenia, relatively mild and reversible renal disease, and neurologic symptoms characterized these 2 illnesses. Diagnostic possibilities include both SLE and TTP, either alone or in combination.

The classic diagnostic pentad of TTP consists of fever, MAHA, thrombocytopenia, neurologic symptoms, and renal abnormalities (1). With the exception of fever, which was present only during the first hospitalization, the patient demonstrated the remaining criteria. Fever has been reported to be absent in 40% of patients with TTP (8). The lack of evidence of an antibody- and/or complement-mediated hemolytic anemia and thrombocytopenia also favors a diagnosis of TTP over SLE. A tissue biopsy may have contributed further evidence toward establishing the diagnosis of TTP, but was not performed. However, since biopsies frequently produce negative results, TTP often has to be considered on clinical grounds exclusively, and lack of histologic evidence in an otherwise compatible setting is not considered decisive in excluding the diagnosis (9).

Diagnostic certainty in this patient, however, is confounded by the fact that she satisfies at least 7 of the 11 1982 revised criteria for the classification of SLE (10) and has C2 deficiency, which is associated with the occurrence of an SLE-like disease (2,6). Indeed, several features manifested by this patient, i.e., the presence of photosensitive skin involvement, mild renal disease, low or insignificant titers of anti-native DNA and antinuclear antibodies, and the presence of anti-Ro (SS-A) antibodies, are features that characterize C2 deficiency patients with SLE-like disease (2,6).

The other possibility to be considered is that the patient may have both SLE and TTP. TTP has been described in association with SLE (1,9,11). It has also been reported to occur during pregnancy, with a few patients having been successfully treated by plasma exchange or plasma infusion (1). There has been, however, no report of TTP occurring in a patient with C2 deficiency.

It is impossible to be certain whether our patient had SLE, TTP, or perhaps both syndromes. While the neurologic and renal manifestations of SLE and TTP can be indistinguishable, there are often hematologic differences. Thrombocytopenia in SLE is usually immune-mediated (12), while that occurring in TTP is not (8,9). The remarkable improvement in platelet count following transfusion and the lack of any response in the platelet count to high doses of prednisone argue against an immune-mediated thrombocytopenia in this patient (13).

There are also differences in the red cell hemolysis seen in SLE and TTP. MAHA is characteristic of TTP, and occurs rarely in SLE in the setting of diffuse vasculitis or severe hypertension (9,14). Clinically significant hemolysis in SLE is usually immune-mediated and associated with a positive result on the Coombs' test (12). Indeed, even when Coombs-negative immune hemolytic anemias have been examined, abnormally large numbers of IgG molecules have been shown to be present on the red cells of almost all patients, albeit in quantities below the sensitivity of the standard Coombs' assay (15). Using a highly sensitive radiolabeled anti-antiglobulin method (5), this patient's red cells were found to have surface IgG, IgA, and IgM levels in the low-normal range. (Her red cells had been fortuitously tested for C3d in 1979. At that time she had a lower value than any of several hundred normal donors [5], and when this assay was repeated during her illness in 1981, the value was even lower.) These data strongly suggest that this patient's red cell destruction was not antibody- and/or complement-mediated.

The 1982 episode appears to have been provoked by pregnancy. There was an exacerbation in the first trimester after a 10-year disease-free period, and a prompt response after termination of pregnancy.

In summary, this case illustrates the diagnostic dilemma that may be encountered in attempting to distinguish between SLE and TTP, documents that TTP or a TTP-like syndrome may accompany C2 deficiency, and suggests that pregnancy may be a potential initiating factor in some patients with TTP.

Acknowledgments. The authors thank Dr. H. Chaplin, Washington University, for measuring red blood cell–bound C3d and immunoglobulins and for his helpful comments; Dr. Gordon Sharp, University of Missouri and Dr. Morris Reichlin, Oklahoma Medical Research Foundation, for performing the antinuclear antibody profile; Drs. Alex Denes, Washington University, and Robert Schwartz, Tufts University Medical School, for their evaluation of the patient's hematologic status; Dr. J. Moake, Boston University, for determination of her plasma factor VIII:von Willebrand factor multimer distribution; and Dr. K. Osterland, McGill University, for his review of the patient's initial hospitalization and continued interest in her case.

REFERENCES

1. Bukowski RM: Thrombotic thrombocytopenic purpura: a review. Prog Hemost Thromb 6:287–337, 1982
2. Agnello V: Complement deficiency states. Medicine (Baltimore) 57:1–20, 1978
3. Osterland CK, Espinoza L, Parker LP, Schur PH: Inherited C2 deficiency and systemic lupus erythematosus: studies on a family. Ann Intern Med 82:323–328, 1975
4. Wahl R, Meo T, Shreffler D, Miller W, Atkinson JP, Schultz J, Osterland CK: C2 deficiency and a lupus erythematosus-like illness: family reevaluation. Ann Intern Med 90:717–718, 1979
5. Chaplin H, Nasongkla M, Monroe MC: Quantitation of red blood cell-bound C3d in normal subjects and random hospitalized patients. Br J Haematol 48:69–78, 1981
6. Provost TT, Arnett FC, Reichlin M: Homozygous C2 deficiency, lupus erythematosus, and anti-Ro (SSA) antibodies. Arthritis Rheum 26:1279–1282, 1983
7. Moake JL, Rudy CK, Troll JH, Weinstein MJ, Colannino NM, Azocar J, Seder RH, Hong SL, Deykin D: Unusually large plasma factor VIII: von Willebrand factor multimers in chronic relapsing thrombotic thrombocytopenic purpura. N Engl J Med 307:1432–1435, 1982
8. Ridolfi RL, Bell WR: Thrombotic thrombocytopenic purpura: report of 25 cases and review of the literature. Medicine (Baltimore) 60:413–428, 1981
9. Byrnes JJ: Thrombotic thrombocytopenic purpura. Med Clin North Am 64:131–157, 1980
10. Tan EM, Cohen AS, Fries JF, Masi AT, McShane DJ, Rothfield NF, Schaller JG, Talal N, Winchester RJ: The 1982 revised criteria for the classification of systemic lupus erythematosus. Arthritis Rheum 25:1271–1277, 1982
11. Cecere FA, Yoshinoya S, Pope RM: Fatal thrombotic thrombocytopenic purpura in a patient with systemic lupus erythematosus: relationship to circulating immune complexes. Arthritis Rheum 24:550–553, 1981
12. Budman DR, Steinberg AA: Hematologic aspects of systemic lupus erythematosus: current concepts. Ann Intern Med 86:220–229, 1977
13. Wintrobe MM: Clinical Hematology. Eighth edition. Philadelphia, Lea & Febiger, 1981, pp 1092–1103
14. Gatenby PA, Smith H, Kirwan P, Lauer CS: Systemic lupus erythematosus and thrombotic thrombocytopenic purpura: a case report and review of relationship. J Rheumatol 8:504–508, 1981
15. Gilliland BC: Coombs-negative immune hemolytic anemia. Semin Hematol 13:267–275, 1976

BRIEF REPORT

CARDIAC INVOLVEMENT IN BEHÇET'S DISEASE

CAROLYN A. BOWLES, AUDREY M. NELSON, STEPHEN C. HAMMILL, and J. DESMOND O'DUFFY

The classic features of Behçet's disease are recurrent oral and genital aphthous ulcers with uveitis (1). Additional features include cutaneous vasculitis, synovitis, meningoencephalitis, and gastrointestinal ulcers (1). Major vessel lesions with phlebitis, arteritis, and aneurysm formation also have been reported (2–6) and can present as ischemic extremities (2), massive hemoptysis (3), caval occlusions (4,5), or aortic aneurysms (6). Various cardiac abnormalities also have been described (7) but are rare and seldom recognized antemortem. We describe a young woman with Behçet's disease who suffered a myocardial infarction and left ventricular dysfunction that were believed to be due to coronary arteritis and myocarditis.

Case report. In July 1981, a 22-year-old woman was hospitalized after a 6-week history of fever, recurrent oral and genital ulcers, and buttock papules. Two weeks before admission, while febrile, she experienced episodes of anterior chest pain and numbness of the left arm. Her local physician noted aphthous oral and genital ulcers. The leukocyte count was 12,400/mm^3, hemoglobin 12.5 gm/dl, and Westergren erythrocyte sedimentation rate (ESR) 100 mm/hour. Results of microbiologic and radiologic studies for fever of unknown origin were negative, and treatment with antibiotics and salicylates was ineffective.

On examination, the blood pressure was 100/70 mm Hg without a paradoxical pulse. Her pulse rate was 120/minute, respirations 18/minute, and oral temperature 39°C. Multiple aphthous ulcers were present on the inferior surface of her tongue, buccal mucosa, and lips. A 3 × 3-cm ulcer was present on the right labium majus, and a 1 × 1-cm ulcer was present on the left labium majus. Several superficial ulcers were noted on the vaginal and cervical mucosae. A grade 2/6 short systolic flow murmur was heard at the left sternal border, and a systolic bruit was heard in the epigastrium. Results of ophthalmologic examination with slit lamp biomicroscopy were normal.

Laboratory studies revealed a leukocyte count of 16,000/mm^3 with 75% polymorphonuclear leukocytes, hemoglobin 11.2 gm/dl, platelet count 362,000/mm^3, creatine kinase 33 units/liter, and ESR 107 mm/hour. Results of the following studies were also normal: urinalysis, chest roentgenogram, serology for syphilis and hepatitis B antigen, monospot test, antinuclear antibody, total hemolytic complement, test for cryoglobulins, aspartate transaminase, alkaline phosphatase, bilirubin, lactic dehydrogenase, and creatinine. Results of viral, bacterial, and fungal cultures of the oral and genital ulcers were negative. Dark-field examination of the ulcers gave negative results. A biopsy specimen of an oral ulcer showed nonspecific inflammation and no evidence of immunoglobulin or complement deposition by indirect immunofluorescence. Findings of proctoscopy and roentgenography of the colon and terminal ileum were normal. Aneurysms were not seen on ultrasound study of the upper abdomen. An electrocardiographic (EKG) evaluation showed no abnormalities (Figure 1A). The prothrombin time, partial thromboplastin time, and thrombin time were normal, as was the antithrombin III level. The protamine gel test result was positive; plasma

From the Division of Rheumatology and Internal Medicine and the Division of Cardiovascular Diseases and Internal Medicine, Mayo Clinic and Mayo Foundation, Rochester, Minnesota.

Carolyn A. Bowles, MD; Audrey M. Nelson, MD; Stephen C. Hammill, MD; J. Desmond O'Duffy, MBBCh.

Address reprint requests to C. A. Bowles, MD, Division of Rheumatology and Internal Medicine, Mayo Clinic, 200 First Street SW, Rochester, MN 55905.

Submitted for publication July 3, 1984; accepted in revised form November 14, 1984.

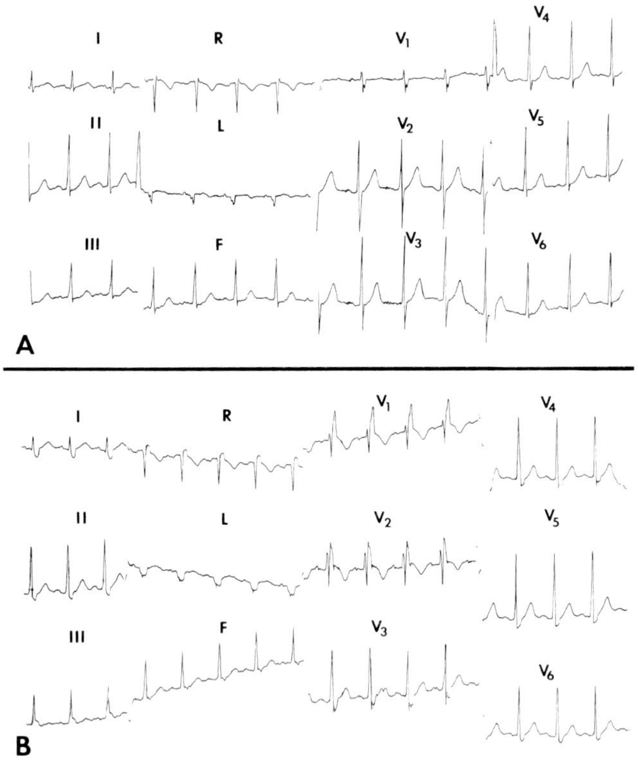

Figure 1. A, Normal electrocardiogram reading, on admission to the hospital. **B,** Electrocardiogram reading after myocardial infarction, demonstrating right bundle-branch block.

fibrinogen was 611 mg/dl (normal 190–365), factor V 154% (normal 50–150), factor VIII 233% (normal 55–145), and the fibrin split products level was 5 μg/ml (normal $\leq$3).

A diagnosis of incomplete Behçet's disease was made. Salicylates did not reduce the fever, but indomethacin, 100 mg/day, led to its prompt disappearance. Five days after admission, the patient experienced left anterior chest pressure. An EKG revealed frequent unifocal, premature ventricular complexes and a new right bundle-branch block (RBBB) (Figure 1B). The axis remained normal. The creatine kinase (CK) level increased to 103 units/liter (normal 15–57), with 22% myocardial band. Serial CK levels returned to 9 and 11 units/liter. A technetium pyrophosphate scan showed focal increased uptake in the interventricular septum, a finding compatible with an acute subendocardial infarction (Figure 2). The patient was considered to have had an acute myocardial infarction. A 2-dimensional echocardiogram showed global decrease in left ventricular function, an estimated left ventricular ejection fraction of 37% (normal >50) (8), and akinesis of the interventricular septal wall. There was no pericardial effusion shown on echocardiogram. The left ventricular end-diastolic dimension was 57 mm (upper limit of normal range) by M-mode echocardiography. These abnormalities were interpreted as being consistent with a dilated cardiomyopathy.

Nine days after admission, she had a recurrence of fever, chills, and oral ulcers while receiving indomethacin therapy (150 mg/day). Sterile pustules and superficial phlebitis were noted at each venipuncture and intravenous catheter site. Chest pain recurred, and an EKG showed a persistent RBBB. Coronary angiography showed a focal dilatation of the left anterior descending coronary artery at the origin of the first septal perforating coronary artery (Figure 3).

The first septal perforating coronary artery was completely occluded, while the remaining coronary arteries were normal. Ergonovine and nitroglycerin administration did not affect the coronary artery findings. A left ventriculogram showed moderate dilatation with generalized hypokinesis and dyskinesis of the basal-septal segment. The calculated ejection fraction was not considered reliable because of the pronounced ventricular ectopy.

For presumed coronary arteritis with probable myocarditis, prednisone, 60 mg daily, was begun, and she had no further chest pain while in the hospital. When released, she was receiving prednisone and hydroxychloroquine. Two weeks later, bigeminy and trigeminy developed and disopyramide, 150 mg 4 times a day, was added to her regimen.

At the 3-month followup examination, she reported no recent oral or genital lesions, but chest pain had recurred when the dosage of prednisone was reduced below 15 mg/day. An EKG still showed RBBB. Two-dimensional echocardiography showed normal left ventricular size and function, with an ejection fraction of 55%. The left ventricular end-diastolic dimension was 50 mm by M-mode echocardiography. Levels of plasma fibrinogen, factor VIII, and factor V were normal. The protamine gel test result was negative, and the value for fibrin split products was 0 μg/ml. Her leukocyte count was 13,500/mm^3, and the ESR was 12 mm/hour.

During the next 1½ years, she had recurrent, mild episodes of oral and genital ulcers and continued with the hydroxychloroquine therapy, 200 mg/day, prednisone, 10–12.5 mg/day, and disopyramide. In April 1983, she developed pericarditis associated with a flare of oral and genital ulcers. Transfer factor therapy was begun, but she died suddenly. An autopsy was not performed.

Discussion. This patient had recurrent aphthous oral and genital ulcers, with cutaneous pustules and hypersensitivity at venipuncture sites. In addition, she had fever, coronary artery occlusion with myocardial

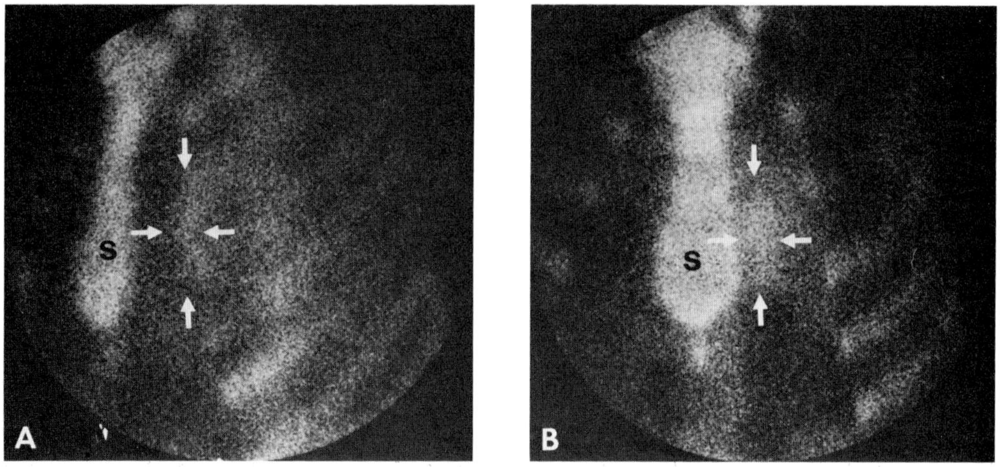

Figure 2. Left anterior oblique (**A**) and anterior (**B**) views of the technetium pyrophosphate infarction scan. Focal uptake is localized to the interventricular septum (**arrows**), a finding consistent with acute myocardial infarction. S = sternum.

infarction, left ventricular myocardial dysfunction, ventricular ectopy, and coagulation abnormalities. We believe that all of these abnormalities were due to Behçet's disease. An atherosclerotic etiology for her heart disease would seem unlikely because of her age, the absence of physical findings of atherosclerosis on examination, and the absence of any other atherosclerotic lesions on angiogram. She also had a negative family history for atherosclerosis, and she had normal serum cholesterol and triglyceride levels. Corticosteroid therapy provided prompt resolution of her symptoms, reversal of the lowered ejection fraction, and normalization of her sedimentation rate and coagulation abnormalities.

Few cardiac abnormalities have been noted in patients with Behçet's disease. When present, cardiac involvement has rarely been a serious clinical problem. Isolated instances of pericarditis (9,10), myocarditis (3,9,11), coronary artery aneurysm or occlusion (7,12), electrocardiographic disturbance (13), and aortic insufficiency (14) have been reported in this disease. We could find only 2 other reported cases of coronary artery occlusion and diminished left ventricular function documented by angiographic and echocardiographic methods, but in 1 case, the hepatitis B surface antigen test was positive (12,15). Coronary artery aneurysm and thrombotic coronary occlusion have been associated with vasculitis in other connective tissue disorders, for example, systemic lupus erythematosus and periarteritis nodosa.

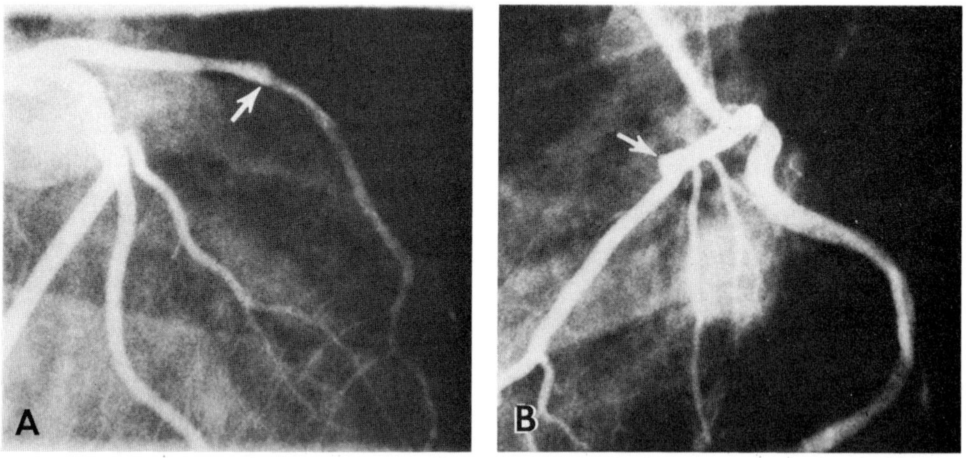

Figure 3. Right anterior oblique (**A**) and left anterior oblique (**B**) views of the left anterior descending and circumflex coronary arteries during coronary angiography. A focal dilatation of the left anterior descending coronary artery at the origin of the first septal perforating coronary artery is present (**arrows**) with complete occlusion of the septal artery. The remaining coronary arteries are normal.

In our patient, the coronary artery occlusion that was presumed to be due to vasculitis may have been promoted by clotting abnormalities. Thrombotic arterial occlusion has been reported in the pulmonary and peripheral arteries of patients with Behçet's disease (2,3). In these instances, the arterial walls contained inflammatory infiltrates, with either polymorphonuclear leukocytes or plasma cells and lymphocytes (2,3).

Numerous coagulation abnormalities have been reported in Behçet's disease, including defective fibrinolysis with prolongation of the euglobulin lysis time and increased levels of fibrinogen and factor VIII activity (16). Our patient had elevated levels of fibrinogen, factor VIII, and fibrin split products—findings compatible with a low-grade, chronic disseminated intravascular coagulation. Whether these coagulation abnormalities contributed to the coronary artery occlusion remains speculative.

The left ventricular dysfunction in our patient may have been due to myocarditis, small vessel vasculitis, or both. Myocardial abnormalities have been reported in Behçet's disease (3,9,11). Occasionally, patients present with clinical evidence of myocardial dysfunctions (9,11). Inflammatory infiltrates in the myocardium also have been noted in autopsy reports of patients with Behçet's disease (11). In these patients, the myocardium contained foci of granulocytes, lymphocytes, and histiocytes compatible with chronic myocarditis.

Agents that have been used in the treatment of Behçet's disease include corticosteroids, colchicine, fresh blood or plasma, transfer factor, fibrinolytic agents, and immunosuppressive drugs. The emergent nature of our patient's coronary artery and myocardial involvement appeared to justify corticosteroid therapy. Because the cytotoxic agent chlorambucil, which has been effective in preventing recurrences of uveitis and meningoencephalitis (17), requires several weeks of treatment before benefit is seen, it was not used. In retrospect, chlorambucil probably should have been prescribed, since the corticosteroid therapy proved only temporarily palliative.

REFERENCES

1. O'Duffy JD: Behçet's disease, Textbook of Rheumatology. Vol. 2. Edited by WN Kelley, ED Harris Jr, S Ruddy, CB Sledge. Philadelphia, WB Saunders, 1980, pp 1197–1202
2. Enoch BA, Castillo-Olivares JL, Khoo TCL, Grainger RG, Henry L: Major vascular complications in Behçet's syndrome. Postgrad Med J 44:453–459, 1968
3. Davies JD: Behçet's syndrome with haemoptysis and pulmonary lesions. J Pathol 109:351–356, 1973
4. Chajek T, Fainaru M: Behçet's disease: report of 41 cases and a review of the literature. Medicine (Baltimore) 54:179–196, 1975
5. Kansu E, Özer FL, Akalin E, Guler Y, Zileli T, Tanman E, Kaplaman E, Müftüoğlu E: Behçet's syndrome with obstruction of the venae cavae: a report of seven cases. Q J Med 162:151–168, 1972
6. Hills EA: Behçet's syndrome with aortic aneurysms. Br Med J 4:152–154, 1967
7. Shimizu T, Ehrlich GE, Inaba G, Hayashi K: Behçet disease (Behçet syndrome). Semin Arthritis Rheum 8:223–260, 1979
8. Quinones MA, Waggoner AD, Reduto LA, Nelson JG, Young JB, Winters WL Jr, Ribeiro LG, Miller RR: A new, simplified and accurate method for determining ejection fraction with two-dimensional echocardiography. Circulation 64:744–753, 1981
9. Lewis PD: Behçet's disease and carditis. Br Med J 1:1026–1027, 1964
10. Scarlett JA, Kistner ML, Yang LC: Behçet's syndrome: report of a case associated with pericardial effusion and cryoglobulinemia treated with indomethacin. Am J Med 66:146–148, 1979
11. Higashihara M, Mori M, Takeuchi A, Ogita T, Miyamoto T, Okimoto T: Myocarditis in Behçet's disease—a case report and review of the literature. J Rheumatol 9:630–633, 1982
12. Kaseda S, Koiwaya Y, Tajimi T, Mitsutake A, Kanaide H, Takeshita A, Kikuchi Y, Nakamura M, Mayumi H, Komori M, Tokunaga K: Huge false aneurysm due to rupture of the right coronary artery in Behçet's syndrome. Am Heart J 103:569–571, 1982
13. Stucchi C, Vollenweider A: Maladie de Behçet et manifestations atypiques. Ophthalmologica 135:573–578, 1958
14. Comess KA, Zibelli LR, Gordon D, Fredrickson SR: Acute, severe, aortic regurgitation in Behçet's syndrome. Ann Intern Med 99:639–640, 1983
15. Schiff S, Moffatt R, Mandel WJ, Rubin SA: Acute myocardial infarction and recurrent ventricular arrhythmias in Behçet's syndrome. Am Heart J 103:438–440, 1982
16. Chajek T, Aronowski E, Izak G: Decreased fibrinolysis in Behçet's disease. Thromb Diath Haemorrh 29:610–618, 1973
17. O'Duffy JD, Robertson DM, Goldstein NP: Chlorambucil in the treatment of uveitis and meningoencephalitis of Behçet's disease. Am J Med 76:75–84, 1984

BRIEF REPORT

DEFECTIVE IMMUNE ADHERENCE RECEPTORS (CR1) ON ERYTHROCYTES IN AUTOIMMUNE DISEASES: AN ASSOCIATION WITH HLA–Cw3

YUKIO MATSUMURA, SHIGEKO INOKUMA, TETSUO HAYAKAWA, and TOMONARI KISAKI

A possible role of erythrocyte immune adherence receptor (C3b receptor, CR1) in removal of circulating immune complexes has been postulated. Miyakawa and coworkers (1) reported that defective CR1 on erythrocytes was observed in the majority of the patients with systemic lupus erythematosus (SLE) but in only 5% of normal subjects. The defect was suspected to be genetically determined because it was not affected by disease activity or the amount of circulating immune complexes, but stayed unchanged during the course of the disease even after years in remission induced by steroid therapy. It was also found frequently in consanguineous relatives of the patients with defective CR1, even when they had no symptoms or serologic disorders related to any autoimmune diseases.

We investigated a correlation between CR1 abnormality and the major histocompatibility antigens, HLA–A, B, C, and DR, and we noticed in a preliminary study that most patients with SLE who had defective CR1 also had HLA–Cw3, although the frequency of HLA–Cw3 among a Japanese population has been reported to be 46.5% (2).

This study provides evidence for the association of defective CR1 with HLA–Cw3 tested in 73 subjects: 38 patients with autoimmune diseases and 35 of their consanguineous relatives.

Patients and methods. Patients with autoimmune diseases treated in our division of allergy and immunology from 1979 through 1981 were tested for erythrocyte CR1 by immunoadherence as described (1). Twenty-one patients in the defective CR1 group, including 10 with SLE, were typed for HLA. Seventeen patients with normal CR1, including 9 with SLE, were also HLA typed. These patients served as controls. Thirty-five consanguineous relatives of 14 patients from 11 families were also tested for CR1 and HLA.

HLA–C typing was performed using a standard 2-stage microlymphocytotoxicity assay.

The prevalence of HLA–Cw3 was compared among those with defective CR1 and those with normal CR1, according to 4 different groups: 19 patients with SLE; 38 patients with autoimmune disease; 35 consanguineous relatives of 14 patients from 11 families; and 49 members of the 11 families, including the propositi. Statistical analysis was performed using the chi-square test. In cases where the numbers were too small for the chi-square test, Fisher's exact test was used.

Results. Defective CR1 was found in 38% of the patients with SLE, and in approximately 33% of the patients with other autoimmune diseases, such as Sjögren's syndrome, rheumatoid arthritis, and polymyositis/dermatomyositis, and in 10% of patients with progressive systemic sclerosis (Table 1). However, the defect was not observed in 10 patients with Behçet's disease.

A comparison of the prevalence of HLA–Cw3 among those with defective CR1 and the control

Presented at the 5th International Congress of Immunology, Kyoto, Japan, August 1983.

From the Matsumura Clinic and Research Institute for Asthma and Immunological Diseases, Tokyo, and the Division of Allergy and Immunology, Tokyo Metropolitan Komagome Hospital, Tokyo, Japan.

Yukio Matsumura, MD; Shigeko Inokuma, MD; Tetsuo Hayakawa, MD; Tomonari Kisaki, MD.

Address reprint requests to Y. Matsumura, MD, Matsumura Clinic and Research Institute for Asthma and Immunological Diseases, 5-52-2 Higashi-nippori, Arakawa-ku, Tokyo 116, Japan.

Submitted for publication February 8, 1984; accepted in revised form September 20, 1984.

Table 1. Prevalence of defective CR1 in patients with autoimmune diseases

	No. with defective CR1/ no. tested	%
Systemic lupus erythematosus	15/39	38.4
Sjögren's syndrome	11/31	35.4
Rheumatoid arthritis	4/13	30.7
Polymyositis/dermatomyositis	2/6	33.3
Progressive systemic sclerosis	1/10	10.0
Mixed connective tissue disease	0/2	0

subjects with normal CR1 is shown in Table 2. In all 4 groups, HLA–Cw3 was found with unusually high frequency, 71–80%, in those with defective CR1, while it was found with less frequency, 24–35%, in the controls with normal CR1. This difference was statistically significant in each group.

The overall prevalence of HLA–Cw3 in the subjects with defective CR1 was 23 of 32 (71.9%), which was significantly higher than in those subjects with normal CR1 (12 of 41; 29.3%) ($P < 0.001$).

HLA–Cw3, however, did not always coexist with defective CR1. This was true even in the family studies (Figure 1).

Discussion. Although the possible masking of CR1 on erythrocytes by circulating immune complexes has been noted (3,4), defective CR1 found in SLE patients was suspected to be inborn, and not acquired, because it stayed unchanged even after the disease was in remission induced by steroid therapy, although circulating immune complexes were shown to be decreased. Defective CR1 was found frequently in relatives who did not have circulating immune complexes or symptoms of autoimmune diseases (1).

In this study, circulating immune complexes were measured by a radioimmunoassay (5), at the same time as CR1. There were no significant differences in mean immune complex levels between those with defective CR1 and those with normal CR1.

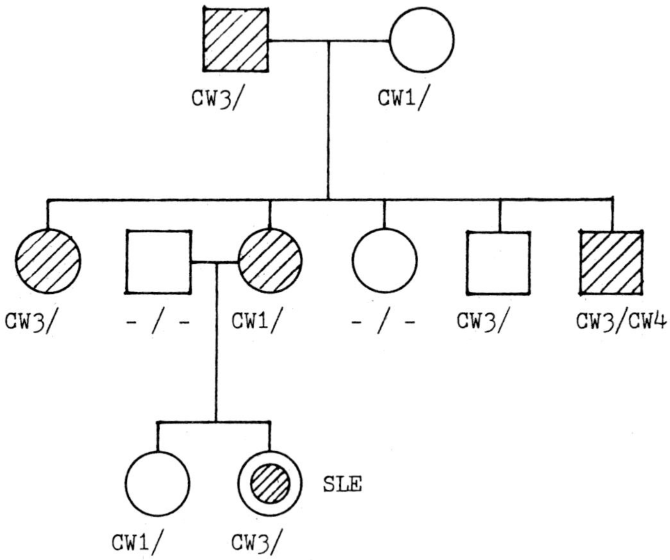

Figure 1. A pedigree of a family, suggesting the association of defective CR1 with HLA–Cw3. All consanguineous relatives within third degree of a patient with systemic lupus erythematosus were tested for CR1 and HLA–C. Shaded symbols indicate defective CR1, and open symbols indicate normal CR1. □ = male; ○ = female; - / - = HLA–Cw1 through HLA–Cw8 were not detected.

Wilson and coworkers (6), counting the number of receptor sites per erythrocyte, divided CR1 into 3 groups—a high, an intermediate, and a low phenotype group—which were suspected to be inherited in an autosomal codominant manner according to their pedigree analyses.

In a preliminary study, we noticed a high frequency of HLA–Cw3 in the SLE patients with defec-

Table 2. Comparison of the prevalence of HLA–Cw3 between those with defective CR1 and those with normal CR1, in different groups

	Defective CR1 (%)	Normal CR1 (%)	χ^2 test	Fisher's exact test*
Systemic lupus erythematosus	8/10 (80.0)	3/9 (33.3)		$P = 0.05$
All autoimmune diseases	15/21 (71.4)	6/17 (35.3)	$P < 0.01$	
Family members except propositi†	8/11 (72.7)	6/24 (25.0)		$P = 0.01$
Family members including propositi	15/20 (75.0)	7/29 (24.1)	$P < 0.001$	
Total tested	23/32 (71.9)	12/41 (29.3)	$P < 0.001$	

* Fisher's exact test was used when numbers tested were too small for chi-square analysis.
† Thirty-five relatives of 14 patients from 11 families were tested.

tive CR1. In order to confirm the association, we compared the prevalence of HLA-Cw3 in those with defective CR1 and matched controls with normal CR1, in separate populations. The patients with autoimmune diseases and their family members were chosen for the study because defective CR1 was frequently found in these populations. A normal population was not tested because those with defective CR1 were found in numbers too small to allow for the analysis of the frequency of HLA–Cw3. In all groups tested, HLA–Cw3 was found at an unusually high frequency in those with defective CR1, significantly higher than in those with normal CR1.

The results of the present study strongly suggest that defective CR1 is genetically determined and associated with HLA–Cw3. HLA–Cw3, however, did not always coexist with defective CR1, even in the family studies. It might not be the HLA–Cw3 gene itself, but closely linked genes that would influence the development of defective CR1. It might also be possible that in our study some of those with HLA–Cw3 were judged to have normal CR1 by the immune adherence test, although they had partially decreased numbers of CR1, which Wilson and coworkers (6) classified as intermediate phenotype.

Further studies are needed to clarify the roles of defective CR1 in the etiology of autoimmune diseases.

Acknowledgments. The authors thank Drs. M. Mayumi, F. Tsuda, and M. Shimizu for their useful discussions and help in the measurement of CR1.

REFERENCES

1. Miyakawa Y, Yamada A, Kosaka K, Tsuda F, Mayumi M: Defective immune-adherence (C3b) receptor on erythrocytes from patients with systemic lupus erythematosus. Lancet 2:493–497, 1981
2. Baur MP, Danilovs JA: Population analysis of HLA-A, B, C, DR, and other genetic markers, Histocompatibility Testing 1980. Edited by PI Terasaki. Los Angeles, UCLA Tissue Typing Laboratory, 1980, pp 955–998
3. Iida K, Mornaghi R, Nussenzweig V: Complement receptor (CR1) deficiency in erythrocytes from patients with systemic lupus erythematosus. J Exp Med 155:1427–1438, 1982
4. Inada Y, Kamiyama M, Kanemitsu T, Hyman CL, Clark WS: Studies on immune adherence (C3b) receptor activity of human erythrocytes: relationship between receptor activity and presence of immune complexes in serum. Clin Exp Immunol 50:189–197, 1982
5. Tsuda F, Miyakawa Y, Mayumi M: Application of human erythrocytes to a radioimmune assay of immune complexes in serum. Immunology 37:681–688, 1979
6. Wilson JG, Wong WW, Schur PH, Fearon DT: Mode of inheritance of decreased C3b receptors on erythrocytes of patients with systemic lupus erythematosus. N Engl J Med 307:981–986, 1982

BRIEF REPORT

RESPONSE OF THE ACUTE-PHASE REACTANTS, C-REACTIVE PROTEIN AND SERUM AMYLOID A PROTEIN, TO ANTIBIOTIC TREATMENT OF WHIPPLE'S DISEASE

JOHN I. REED, JEAN D. SIPE, JEFFREY R. WOHLGETHAN, WILHELM G. DOOS, and JUAN J. CANOSO

Whipple's disease is a chronic systemic illness that, to varying degrees, affects the gastrointestinal tract, the joints, heart, lungs, muscles, and the brain (1). An infectious etiology is suggested by the constant presence of intracellular bacillary bodies in involved tissues, as well as by the success of antibiotic therapy, but the results of bacterial cultures have been inconclusive (2). In order to study the effect of antibiotics on the course of Whipple's disease, we prospectively evaluated the response of the acute-phase reactants, C-reactive protein (CRP) and serum amyloid A protein (SAA), to treatment with penicillin. Upon initiation of treatment, the Jarisch-Herxheimer reaction occurred; serum levels of CRP and SAA rose abruptly, then returned to pretreatment values within several days. The serum CRP and SAA levels fell virtually to normal within 2 weeks, while clinical symptoms and signs resolved slowly over a period of 6 months.

Case report. A 57-year-old white man was first admitted to the Boston Veterans Administration Medical Center on September 16, 1982 for evaluation of arthritis, abdominal pain, lymphadenopathy, and weight loss. Since 1976, he had had monthly attacks of acute arthritis predominantly affecting the wrists, knees, ankles, and the metacarpophalangeal and metatarsophalangeal joints. The attacks involved 1 or more of these joints, and resolved spontaneously, in 1–3 days, without residual symptoms.

Aching low back pain radiating to the left buttock and trochanteric area began in 1979. Treatment with nonsteroidal antiinflammatory agents gave him moderate relief. Also during this period, he had bouts of epigastric and right upper quadrant pain exacerbated by breathing and coughing, lasting from a few minutes to a few days. He became anorectic and lost 18 kg during the 3 years prior to his admission. He also noted generalized weakness; hypersomnia, sleeping 14–16 hours a day; and impotence, with infrequent morning erections.

Physical examination revealed a thin, debilitated man. His weight was 52 kg, oral temperature 36.8°C, and blood pressure 104/68 mm Hg. Multiple firm, discrete lymph nodes ranging from 1–3 cm in diameter were palpable in the cervical, axillary, epitrochlear, and inguinal regions, bilaterally. A grade I/VI systolic ejection murmur was audible at the lower left sternal border. The lungs were clear. The liver spanned 16 cm and was of normal consistency. The spleen was not palpable. Findings of peripheral joint examination were entirely within normal limits. However, there was limited motion of the lumbar spine, with only 3 cm lengthening in flexion (normal range 4.6–8.1 cm, average 6.9 cm) (3). Neurologic examination showed normal responses.

Laboratory studies showed the following values: hematocrit 34.9%, white blood cell count 8,600/

From the Medical and Laboratory Services, Boston VA Medical Center; the Thorndike Memorial Laboratory, Boston City Hospital; and the Boston University School of Medicine, Arthritis Center, Boston, Massachusetts.

Supported by the Veterans Administration and by grants from the USPHS, the NIADDK (AM-04599 and AM-07014), an NIH Multipurpose Arthritis Center grant (AM-20613), and an Arthritis Foundation Clinical Research Center grant.

John I. Reed, MD: Former Arthritis Fellow; Jean D. Sipe, PhD: Associate Research Professor of Medicine and Biochemistry; Jeffrey R. Wohlgethan, MD: Assistant Professor of Medicine; Wilhelm G. Doos, MD: Assistant Professor of Pathology; Juan J. Canoso, MD: Associate Professor of Medicine.

Address reprint requests to Juan J. Canoso, MD, Rheumatology, Room D10-93, Boston VA Medical Center, 150 South Huntington Avenue, Boston, MA 02130.

Submitted for publication July 2, 1984; accepted in revised form September 25, 1984.

mm^3 (72% polymorphonuclear leukocytes, 6% bands, 15% lymphocytes, 2% monocytes, and 3% eosinophils), and platelet count 433,000/mm^3. Westergren erythrocyte sedimentation rate (ESR) was 77 mm/hour. Total serum protein was 7.2 gm/dl, with 3 gm/dl of albumin. Radiographs of the chest and an upper gastrointestinal series with small bowel follow-through were unremarkable. A radiograph of the pelvis revealed definite left-sided sacroiliitis. Results of urinalysis and D-xylose test were normal, and several qualitative determinations of stool fat were negative.

Tests for antinuclear antibodies, HLA–B27 antigen, latex fixation, and a serologic test for the agent of Lyme disease (performed at the Centers for Disease Control, Atlanta, GA) were negative. Intradermal tuberculin and mumps tests were nonreactive, but there was a response to the *Candida* antigen. Serum IgG was 2,260 mg/dl (normal 700–1,500), IgA was 539 mg/dl (normal 55–350), and IgM was 243 mg/dl (normal 50–265). Lymphocyte studies were performed on November 29, 1982 and revealed absolute lymphopenia of 500/mm^3, and a normal T4/T8 ratio of 1.41.

Specimens obtained from biopsies of cervical and axillary nodes revealed heavy infiltration of the tissue by diastase-resistant, periodic acid–Schiff (PAS)–positive macrophages, suggesting the diagnosis of Whipple's disease. Electron microscopic demonstration of intra- and extracellular exogenous bodies interpreted as bacilli confirmed the diagnosis. Occasional PAS-positive macrophages were present in the lamina propria on jejunal biopsy. Acid-fast stains and cultures for mycobacteria were negative.

Central nervous system evaluation included an electroencephalogram and computerized tomography, which showed normal results. Analysis of fluid obtained by lumbar puncture revealed 8 erythrocytes/mm^3 and 6 leukocytes/mm^3 (1 polymorphonuclear and 5 mononuclear) in the fourth tube, and normal glucose and protein concentrations. Serum T4, T3 resin uptake, thyroid-stimulating hormone, and testosterone levels were normal, thus decreasing the likelihood that hypothalamic involvement was the cause of the patient's impotence.

Treatment with penicillin was elected, and high doses (20 million units per 24 hours, intravenously) were used initially because of the suspicion of subclinical cerebral involvement.

Materials and methods. Serum amyloid A protein was measured in a competitive binding assay using ^{125}I-amyloid A fibril protein for binding to the wells of flexible microtitration plates coated with anti–amyloid A antibodies (4). Aliquots of test serum were heated at 60°C for 1 hour prior to the addition of the radioimmunoassay buffer. SAA was measured in triplicate wells and expressed in terms of amyloid A equivalents (μg/ml). With this assay, normal values of SSA are <1 μg/ml.

C-reactive protein was measured by rate nephelometry using the Beckman kit for CRP and the Beckman ICS Analyzer II nephelometer (Beckman Instruments, Brea, CA). Normal values are those values that are less than the threshold concentration for the method, which is 6 μg/ml.

Results. Prior to treatment there were moderate elevations of SAA and CRP, along with a high ESR and thrombocytosis (Figure 1). Intravenous penicillin treatment was begun at 9:00 AM on December 1, 1983, day 0. Approximately 12 hours later, the patient developed a frontal headache and had a shaking chill. His temperature rose to 39.6°C, and his blood pressure dropped to 82/48 mm Hg. Penicillin was discontinued. Blood and urine cultures obtained during the febrile episode were negative.

On day 1, fever and hypotension had resolved, but there was a sharp increase in CRP level and a lesser elevation of SAA concentration, along with a further rise in the ESR. Penicillin treatment was resumed at progressively increasing doses on the morning of day 2. That evening there was an episode of pleuritic-like pain in the right upper quadrant, which subsided following a single dose of indomethacin, 25 mg. By day 3, CRP and SAA returned to pretreatment levels, but 2 weeks later, the ESR was still above the day 0 value. Full doses of penicillin were again reached on day 5. By day 14, CRP and SAA levels were normal, but both transiently increased between day 26 and day 30, without change in the clinical condition.

Intravenous penicillin was discontinued on day 30, and treatment with penicillin V, 500 mg 4 times a day, plus probenecid, 500 mg 3 times a day, was begun, to be continued indefinitely. By this time, strength, appetite, and joint pain were beginning to improve. Over the ensuing 6 months the peripheral arthritis, adenopathy, and hypersomnia completely resolved, though the mild buttock pain persisted.

Fifteen months after initiation of therapy, the patient felt well, and his weight was 65.9 kg. At that time, results of a physical examination were normal, including range of motion of the lumbar spine, which had increased to 5 cm lengthening in flexion; all laboratory values were normal as well. Impotence, however, had persisted.

Discussion. This patient's illness exemplifies the

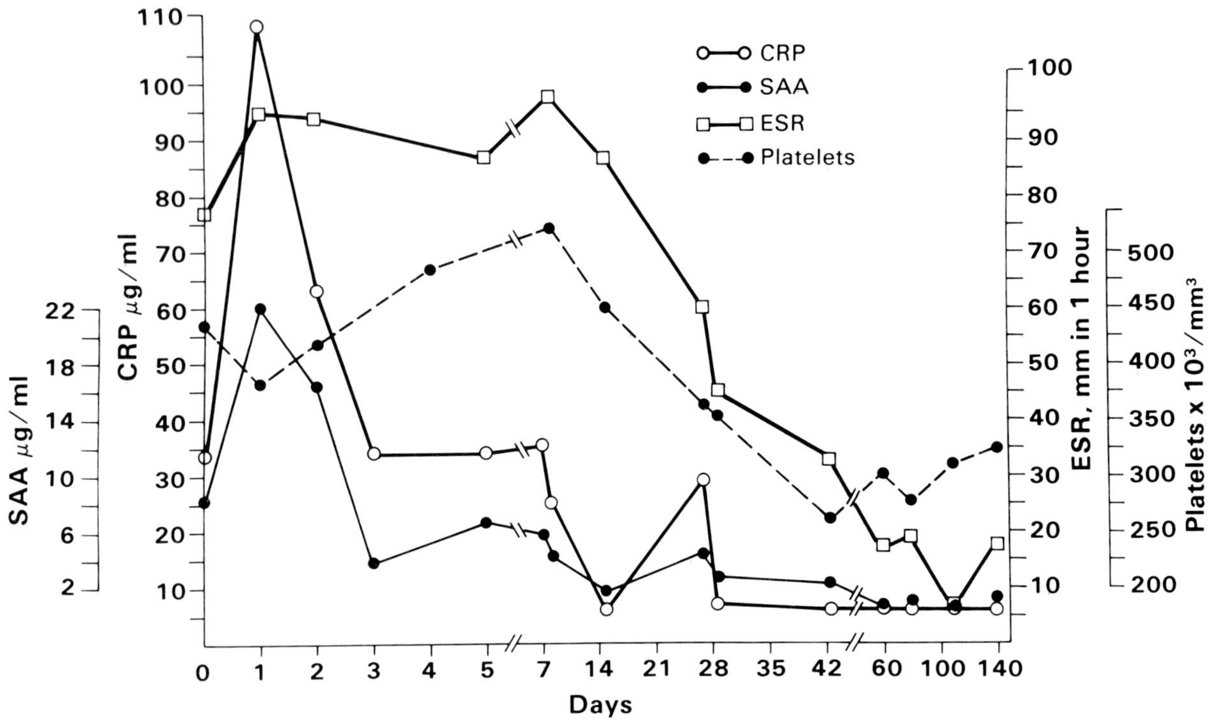

Figure 1. Serum levels of the acute-phase reactants, C-reactive protein (CRP) and serum amyloid A protein (SAA), along with erythrocyte sedimentation rate (ESR) and platelet count in a patient with Whipple's disease. Intravenous penicillin treatment was begun on day 0; oral penicillin was substituted on day 30.

protean nature of Whipple's disease, in which departures from the classic description are commonplace. His initial presentation with palindromic rheumatism was followed, years later, by weight loss, generalized lymphadenopathy, hypersomnia, and impotence, along with early spondylitis. Although evidence of intestinal involvement was lacking, the diagnosis of Whipple's disease was established based on findings from light and electron microscopic studies of the lymph node biopsy specimen, the negative cultures for mycobacteria, and the absence of serologic evidence of definable infectious disease. Since we could not rule out brain involvement, we chose treatment with high-dose, intravenous penicillin that presumably would reach bactericidal levels within the central nervous system (5). The response was gratifying; even spinal motion improved, as has been reported in another case (6). Fifteen months later, our patient was in remission while receiving long-term penicillin therapy.

CRP has long been used as a marker of activity in inflammatory and infectious diseases. SAA is a newly recognized acute-phase reactant (7); it was originally identified as the serum counterpart of amyloid A protein (AA protein), the major constituent of tissue deposits in secondary amyloidosis (8,9). We are not aware of any studies of SAA in Whipple's disease. Farr et al (10) reported on a patient whose CRP levels were persistently elevated and whose disease resisted treatment; SAA levels were presumably elevated as well, since that patient developed amyloidosis, proven immunologically to be of the AA type.

SAA and CRP are inducible proteins (11) with extremely short plasma half-lives in experimental animals: 80–90 minutes for SAA in the mouse (12), and about 5 hours for CRP in the rabbit (13). In contrast, those constitutive proteins such as fibrinogen, haptoglobin, and other serum alpha globulins, which contribute most significantly to elevation of the ESR, have half-lives of at least 3–5 days (14). It is not surprising, then, that in our patient, CRP and SAA levels decreased early in the course of treatment, while his ESR returned to normal more slowly.

The patient's platelet count was elevated, and declined in parallel with the ESR. In Whipple's disease thrombocytosis is common (15). It has been attributed to chronic inflammation, with a possible contribution from hyposplenism (16).

Our patient became febrile and hypotensive several hours after beginning penicillin treatment. Pleuritic chest pain followed reinstitution of therapy after a brief cessation. We believe these developments constitute a Jarisch-Herxheimer reaction.

The pathogenesis of this syndrome is obscure. Proposed mechanisms include release of bacterial endotoxin (17), unidentified pyrogens (18), immune complex disease with activation of the complement system (19), and depletion of endogenous opioids (20).

In Whipple's disease, the Jarisch-Herxheimer reaction has rarely been reported. One patient (21) had temperature of 40°C with shaking chills and incontinence of urine and stool on the day following initiation of oral penicillin. The fever continued for several days, and the ESR rose to 85 mm/hour. Another patient (22) had temperature of 39.7°C 16 hours after intramuscular injection of procaine penicillin and streptomycin. A third patient (23) had shaking chills, temperature of 40°C, and abdominal and pleuritic pain following initiation of parenteral penicillin and ampicillin treatment.

It is unclear whether Jarisch-Herxheimer reactions are truly rare in this condition or if they are just not reported. We speculate that serial determinations of SAA and CRP would identify subclinical reactions, providing an early indication of response to antibiotics.

Measurement of acute-phase reactants before and after treatment may be useful in the evaluation and management of suspected Whipple's disease, particularly in the recognition of the obscure late flares which are not unusual after discontinuation of "successful" treatment.

REFERENCES

1. Bayless TM, Knox DL: Whipple's disease: a multisystem infection. N Engl J Med 296:290–291, 1979
2. Keren DF: Whipple's disease: a review emphasizing immunology and microbiology. CRC Crit Rev Clin Lab Sci 14:75–108, 1981
3. Wright V, Moll JMH: Seronegative Polyarthritis. Amsterdam, Elsevier/North Holland, 1976, p 151
4. Sipe JD, Ignaczak TF, Pollock PS, Glenner GG: Amyloid fibril protein AA: purification and properties of the antigenically related serum component as determined by solid phase radioimmunoassay. J Immunol 116:1151–1156, 1976
5. Lowhagen G-B, Brorson J-E, Kaijser B: Penicillin concentrations in cerebrospinal fluid after intramuscular, intravenous, and oral administration to syphilitic patients. Acta Derm Venereol (Stockh) 63:53–57, 1983
6. Bowman C, Dieppe P, Gettas L: Remission of pseudospondylitis with treatment of Whipple's disease. Br J Rheumatol 22:181–182, 1983
7. Rosenthal CJ, Franklin EC: Variation with age and disease of an amyloid A protein-related serum component. J Clin Invest 55:746–753, 1975
8. Levin M, Pras M, Franklin EC: Immunologic studies of the major nonimmunoglobulin protein of amyloid. I. Identification and partial characterization of a related serum component. J Exp Med 138:373–380, 1973
9. Linke RP, Sipe JD, Pollack PS, Ignaczak TF, Glenner GG: Isolation of a low molecular weight serum component antigenically related to an amyloid fibril protein of unknown origin. Proc Natl Acad Sci USA 72:1473–1476, 1975
10. Farr M, Hollywell CA, Walton KW, Morris C, Scott DL, Bacon PA: Amyloidosis in Whipple's arthritis. J R Soc Med 76:963–965, 1983
11. Kushner I: The phenomenon of the acute phase response. Ann NY Acad Sci 389:39–48, 1982
12. Hoffman JS, Benditt EP: Plasma clearance kinetics of the amyloid-related high density lipoprotein apoprotein, serum amyloid protein (apoSAA), in the mouse: evidence for rapid apoSAA clearance. J Clin Invest 71:926–934, 1983
13. Chelladurai M, MacIntyre SS, Kushner I: In vivo studies of serum C-reactive protein turnover in rabbits. J Clin Invest 71:604–610, 1983
14. Koj A: Acute phase reactants, Structure and Function of Plasma Proteins. Vol. I. Edited by AC Allison. New York, Plenum Press, 1974, pp 73–131
15. Nuzum CT, Sandler RS, Paulk HT: Thrombocytosis in Whipple's disease. Gastroenterology 80:1465–1467, 1981
16. Corazza GR, Frisoni M, Millette S, Vaira D, Gasbarrini G: Mechanisms of thrombocytosis in Whipple's disease (letter). Gastroenterology 82:165, 1982
17. Bryceson ADM: Clinical pathology of the Jarisch-Herxheimer reaction: J Infect Dis 133:696–704, 1976
18. Young EJ, Weingarten NM, Baughn RE, Duncan WC: Studies on the pathogenesis of the Jarisch-Herxheimer reaction: development of an animal model and evidence against a role for classical endotoxin. J Infect Dis 146:606–615, 1983
19. Editorial: The Jarisch-Herxheimer reaction. Lancet 1:340–341, 1977
20. Teklu B, Habte-Michael A, Warrell DA, White NJ, Wright DJM: Meptazinol diminishes the Jarisch-Herxheimer reaction of relapsing fever. Lancet 1:835–839, 1983
21. Trier JS, Phelps PC, Eidelman S, Rubin CE: Whipple's disease: light and electron microscopic correlation of jejunal mucosal histology with antibiotic treatment and clinical status. Gastroenterology 48:684–707, 1965
22. Pastor BM, Geerken RG: Whipple's disease presenting as pleuropericarditis. Am J Med 55:827–831, 1973
23. Vellar ID, Niall JF, Davis NA, Hope R: Whipple's disease: a report of two cases. Med J Aust 1:661–663, 1974

LETTERS

In vitro IgM and IgM rheumatoid factor production and response to remittive agents in rheumatoid arthritis

To the Editor:

We have been interested in the relationship between in vitro patterns of IgM and IgM rheumatoid factor (IgM-RF) production in patients with rheumatoid arthritis (RA), and the response to remittive agents. Our previous studies, carried out on a cross-sectional sample of our RA patients, failed to show any significant relationship between the quantity of IgM-RF or IgM produced and the remittive agents the patients were receiving at the time of the study (1,2). Nonetheless, in vivo data have shown that serum immunoglobulin levels, including RF titers, are reduced during treatment with gold salts (GS) (3,4). Therefore, it was of interest to perform a prospective in vitro study of IgM and IgM-RF production in a group of patients undergoing chrysotherapy.

Eleven patients with seropositive classic or definite RA (5) undergoing a 1-gm loading dose of GS (Myochrysine: 7 patients, Solganal: 4 patients) were studied. Peripheral blood was obtained at the initiation (T_0) and at the completion (T_1) of the GS loading dose (mean interval: 22 weeks). Peripheral blood mononuclear leukocytes (MNL) were prepared by Ficoll-Hypaque density centrifugation, cultured for 7 days in the presence and absence of the polyclonal B cell activator pokeweed mitogen (PWM), and the culture supernatants were assayed for total IgM and IgM-RF using methods previously described in detail (6).

Each patient was examined by one of us (GSA) at T_0 and T_1, and clinical activity was assessed using both duration of morning stiffness and number of swollen and tender joints (modified Ritchie Index [7]). If a patient had at least a two-thirds reduction in both indices of disease activity at T_1, he or she was considered a responder to GS therapy.

The results of these studies are summarized in Table 1. Spontaneous in vitro production of IgM-RF was observed at T_0 in only 4 of 11 of the gold-treated patients. These patients were equally divided between those who responded and those who did not respond to GS. MNL from each of these individuals spontaneously synthesized less RF at T_1 than at T_0. Although the numbers were too few to permit definite conclusions regarding the true effect of chrysotherapy on spontaneous in vitro IgM-RF production, it is noteworthy that RF production by 11 RA control patients on stable therapeutic regimens did not differ between T_0 and T_1 (data not shown). Spontaneous in vitro production of IgM was observed for each of the gold-treated patients at T_0, but did not demonstrate significant changes at T_1. Results with the RA control patients on stable therapeutic regimens were comparable.

In contrast with spontaneous in vitro synthesis, MNL from most (10 of 11) of the gold-treated patients exhibited in vitro IgM-RF production when stimulated with PWM at T_0 (mean $\pm$ SD = 50 ± 57 ng/10^6 cells). A significant decrease in RF synthesis was observed at T_1 (14.5 ± 10.0; $P < 0.05$). This decrease was apparent for all patients, whether responders or nonresponders. Similarly, PWM-stimulated in vitro IgM production was less at T_1 than at T_0 ($P < 0.01$), regardless of response to therapy. Significant changes in PWM-stimulated in vitro IgM-RF and IgM production were not observed for the RA control group on stable therapeutic regimens.

Table 1. Spontaneous and pokeweed mitogen (PWM)–induced IgM and IgM rheumatoid factor (IgM-RF) production in relation to clinical response, in rheumatoid arthritis patients undergoing chrysotherapy, at initiation (time 0) and completion (time 1) of loading dose

	IgM (ng/10^6 cells)				IgM-RF (ng/10^6 cells)*			
	Spontaneous		PWM-induced		Spontaneous		PWM-induced	
	Time 0	Time 1	Time 0	Time 1	Time 0	Time 1	Time 0	Time 1
Responder patients								
1	42	140	1,200	500	10	<10	16	11
2	306	232	4,300	535	28	<10	61	11
3	330	94	1,400	380	42	<10	42	18
4	171	78	3,800	150	<10	<10	80	<10
5	222	240	2,450	725	<10	<10	29	<10
6	54	156	390	742	<10	<10	14	<10
7	42	15	1,000	580	<10	<10	43	37
Nonresponder patients								
8	42	83	1,255	875	<10	<10	16	11
9	142	79	1,500	850	<10	<10	61	11
10	360	138	5,000	2,000	93	<10	<10	<10
11	414	96	4,750	1,050	208	17	218	31

* Sensitivity of the assay: ≥ 10 ng/10^6 cells.

Our results suggest that spontaneous in vitro production of IgM-RF by peripheral blood MNL is not a useful indicator of response to chrysotherapy, as suggested by Olsen et al (8), for 2 reasons. First, many RA patients (64% in the present series) do not demonstrate significant in vitro IgM-RF production in the absence of PWM stimulation. Second, decreases in spontaneous in vitro RF production were observed regardless of response to therapy, although the number of patients studied was too small to permit statistical analysis. Decreases in PWM-induced in vitro IgM and IgM-RF production by peripheral blood MNL following GS therapy occurred with most of our patients, but were comparable in patients who showed clinical improvement and those who did not.

Graciela S. Alarcón, MD, MPH
William J. Koopman, MD
Ralph E. Schrohenloher, PhD
University of Alabama in Birmingham
Birmingham, AL

1. Koopman WJ, Schrohenloher RE: Enhanced in vitro synthesis of IgM rheumatoid factor in rheumatoid arthritis. Arthritis Rheum 23:985–992, 1980
2. Alarcón GS, Koopman WJ, Schrohenloher RE: Differential patterns of in vitro IgM rheumatoid factor synthesis in seronegative and seropositive rheumatoid arthritis. Arthritis Rheum 25:150–155, 1982
3. Gotlieb NL, Kiem IM, Penneys NS, Schultz DR: The influence of chrysotherapy on serum protein and immunoglobulin levels, rheumatoid factor and antiepithelial antibody titers. J Lab Clin Med 86:962–972, 1975
4. Lorber A, Simon T, Leeb J, Peter A, Wilcox S: Chrysotherapy: suppression of immunoglobulin synthesis. Arthritis Rheum 21:785–791, 1978
5. Ropes MW, Bennett GA, Cobb S, Jacox R, Jessar RA: 1958 revision of diagnostic criteria for rheumatoid arthritis. Bull Rheum Dis 9:175–176, 1958
6. Koopman WJ, Schrohenloher RE: In vitro synthesis of IgM rheumatoid factor by lymphocytes from healthy adults. J Immunol 125:934–939, 1980
7. Ritchie DM, Boyle JA, McInnes JM, Jasani MK, Dalakos TG, Grieveson P, Buchanan WW: Clinical studies with an articular index for the assessment of joint tenderness in patients with rheumatoid arthritis. Q J Med 37:393–406, 1968
8. Olsen N, Ziff M, Jasin HE: Spontaneous synthesis of IgM rheumatoid factor by blood mononuclear cells from patients with rheumatoid arthritis: effect of treatment with gold salts or D-penicillamine. J Rheumatol 11:17–21, 1984

Comment on article by van der Linden et al

To the Editor:

Van der Linden and colleagues (1) have proposed a modification of the New York criteria (2) for the diagnosis of ankylosing spondylitis. They elected to substitute a modified form of the Rome pain criterion (3) for that used in the New York counterpart.

We have long favored a more simple approach, the use of symptomatic sacroiliitis as the key determining factor (4). Although the modification by van der Linden et al includes the symptoms that we described in 1977 (5), it remains unclear why they wish to continue to include measurement of spinal and chest mobility. Criteria should be simple, reproducible, and readily definable. The New York criteria that depend on measurements are none of these. By contrast, the proposed criteria for Reiter's syndrome are indeed simple (6). They require the occurrence of an episode of arthritis lasting for at least 1 month, in conjunction with urethritis or cervicitis (6).

Whatever approach is used—straightforward as with ours (4), or more tortuous as in the New York (2) and Rome (3) reports—all criteria demand certain exclusions, such as brucellosis, tuberculosis, metastatic disease, and other entities that can result in sacroiliac disease and pain. In the final analysis, the diagnosis must depend on the subjective reading of the pelvic radiograph, and however much modification of criteria is applied, this reading will remain a subjective phenomenon, though the sine qua non for diagnosis.

Broadly, there are 3 main reasons criteria are needed. The first is to allow comparison of different patient groups, the second is to help the clinician reach a diagnosis, and the third is to provide investigators with a clue as to whether the putative "trigger" has been pulled in a genetically susceptible individual. Regarding the first reason, it is imperative to define the entry variables used, given that there are numerous additional demographic and clinical features that define the patient population. With regard to the second, a patient with sacroiliitis and back pain should be treated, regardless of whether the spine moves to a "normal" or lesser extent. Clearly, in terms of the last, evidence of bilateral sacroiliitis is sufficient to define the endpoint.

Too much time can be spent analyzing, reanalyzing, defining, and redefining criteria.

Andrei Calin, MD, MRCP
Royal National Hospital for Rheumatic Diseases
Bath, UK

1. Van der Linden S, Valkenburg HA, Cats A: Evaluation of diagnostic criteria for ankylosing spondylitis: a proposal for modification of the New York criteria. Arthritis Rheum 27:361–368, 1984
2. Bennett PH, Burch TA: Population Studies of the Rheumatic Diseases. Amsterdam, Excerpta Medica Foundation, 1968, pp 456–457
3. Kellgren JH, Jeffrey MR, Ball J: The Epidemiology of Chronic Rheumatism. Vol. 1. Oxford, Blackwell Scientific Publications, 1963, pp 326–327
4. Calin A: Ankylosing spondylitis, Textbook of Rheumatology. Edited by WN Kelley, ED Harris Jr, S Ruddy, CB Sledge. Philadelphia, WB Saunders, 1981, pp 1017–1032
5. Calin A, Porta J, Fries JF, Schurman DJ: Clinical history as a

screening test for ankylosing spondylitis. JAMA 237:2613–2614, 1977
6. Willkens RF, Arnett FC, Bitter T, Calin A, Fisher L, Ford DK, Good AE, Masi AT: Reiter's syndrome: evaluation of preliminary criteria for definite disease. Arthritis Rheum 24:844–849, 1981

Reply

To the Editor:

Dr. Calin correctly stresses that criteria may serve several purposes. As we stated in our article (1), they permit comparison between groups of patients at different centers and help in defining and diagnosing a disease. Besides that, criteria can be used to further understanding of the natural history of a condition, aid in its treatment, estimate its prognosis, and help to establish subtypes of disease. Finally, they are indispensable in epidemiologic investigation (2).

The New York criteria for ankylosing spondylitis (AS) were developed for use in population studies; they were proposed in 1966 by a committee of experts on the basis of clinical experience, as was usual at the time (2). It became customary to evaluate criteria with a challenge set of data (3), reflecting the development of a more scientific methodology. The study by Moll and Wright (4) and our study (1) justify *modification* of the New York criteria to accomplish what the criteria were initially aimed to do.

Dr. Calin criticizes the New York criteria. Using these criteria, he and Fries reported a 20% prevalence of AS in HLA–B27 positive individuals (5). He especially criticizes the use of measurements of spinal and chest mobility, which are not "simple, reproducible, and readily definable." Not everyone would agree with this statement. A recent textbook (2) states: "The New York criteria share the objectivity and simplicity of the earlier (Rome) prototype. . . The definition of what constitutes normal, and as such abnormal, lumbar spine motion has troubled some investigators. In assessment of this parameter, the use of carefully graded and measured quantitation of spinal motion proved no more effective than qualitative evaluation. . ."

We would agree with Calin that specifications of internal criteria, e.g., how the measurements should be done and what will be considered to be abnormal, will improve reproducibility by reducing intra- and interobserver variation, once these specifications have been widely accepted (3). In our paper, we did indicate how the measurements were done (1).

Applying the (modified) New York criteria or defining AS as "symptomatic sacroiliitis" will not solve the problem of observer variation in the radiologic interpretation of sacroiliac joint findings, which might contribute largely to the existing discrepancies in the reported prevalence rates of AS in HLA–B27 positive individuals (6). Investigators' reading of reference sets of pelvic films might be expected to improve the validity of radiologic diagnosis of sacroiliitis.

We do not agree with Calin's remark that radiologic evidence of bilateral sacroiliitis is sufficient to define whether the putative "trigger" has been pulled in a genetically susceptible individual. Sacroiliitis is clearly a heterogeneous condition; at the open population level, sacroiliitis is mostly HLA–B27 *negative*, and clinical evidence of AS was not observed in B27 negative individuals (7). In our family study on the prevalence of AS, some HLA–B27 positive AS relatives with radiologic sacroiliitis were fully asymptomatic (7). Pain may also be absent in classic AS (8). Therefore, defining AS as symptomatic sacroiliitis does not seem to be supported by the findings.

We found the New York criteria of "limitation of the lumbar spine" and "limitation of chest expansion" to reflect a longer duration of disease better than they help in early diagnosis of AS (unpublished observations). The clinical history screening test, as proposed by Calin et al (9), although only showing moderately positive findings in our epidemiologic study (7), might be more useful for the detection of early AS in clinical practice. However, this screening test was developed from data obtained from 42 *known* AS patients, and the predictive value of a positive result was only 6–14% (9,10). The merits of this test for AS must still be assessed in patients with early AS, and the specificity has yet to be evaluated in an open population study. Additional effort to complete these types of investigation is needed.

Sjef M. van der Linden, MD
University of Bern
Bern, Switzerland
Arnold Cats, MD
University of Leiden
Leiden, The Netherlands
Hans A. Valkenburg, MD
Erasmus University
Rotterdam, The Netherlands

1. Van der Linden S, Valkenburg HA, Cats A: Evaluation of diagnostic criteria for ankylosing spondylitis: a proposal for modification of the New York criteria. Arthritis Rheum 27:361–368, 1984
2. Willkens RF: Criteria, Spondylarthropathies. Edited by A Calin. New York, Grune & Stratton, 1984, pp 9–19
3. Feinstein AR: Clinical Biostatistics. XLVI. What are the criteria for criteria? Clin Pharmacol Ther 28:108–116, 1979
4. Moll JMH, Wright V: New York clinical criteria for ankylosing spondylitis. Ann Rheum Dis 32:354–363, 1973
5. Calin A, Fries JF: Striking prevalence of ankylosing spondylitis in "healthy" W27 positive males and females: a controlled study. N Engl J Med 293:835–839, 1975
6. Hollingsworth PH, Cheah PS, Dawkins RL, Owen ET, Calin A, Wood PHN: Observer variation in grading sacroiliac radiographs in HLA-B27 positive individuals. J Rheumatol 10:247–254, 1983
7. Van der Linden SM, Valkenburg HA, de Jongh BM, Cats A: The risk of developing ankylosing spondylitis in HLA–B27 positive individuals: a comparison of relatives of spondylitis

patients with the general population. Arthritis Rheum 27:241–249, 1984
8. Hochberg MC, Bornstein DG, Arnett FC: The absence of back pain in classical ankylosing spondylitis. Johns Hopkins Med J 143:181–183, 1978
9. Calin A, Porta J, Fries JF, Schurman DJ: Clinical history as a screening test for ankylosing spondylitis. JAMA 237:2613–2614, 1977
10. Calin A, Kaye B, Sternberg M, Ansell B, Chan M: The prevalence and nature of back pain in an industrial complex. Spine 5:201–205, 1980

The CREST acronym and some related problems

To the Editor:

Tramposch et al, in their interesting paper (1), used terminology which calls for comment. The authors made an admirable effort to report the clinical facts very accurately. Therefore, in their Table 2, they pointed out in detail that among patients 1–4 there were 2 with CRST, 1 with CREST, and 1 with CRS. Among the other 7 patients there were 3 with CREST, 3 with REST, and 1 with CRST. Thus, of the 5 features that are expressed by the acronym CREST (calcinosis, Raynaud's phenomenon, esophageal dysmotility, sclerodactyly, telangiectasias), only 2 were present in all 11 patients, namely, Raynaud's phenomenon (R) and sclerodactyly (S). If the presence of only 2 features (R and S) is sufficient basis for a diagnosis of CREST syndrome, one could infer that only these are essential to the diagnosis.

Furthermore, in Table 2, progressive systemic sclerosis (PSS) patients 5–11 are labeled as having PSS (+ CREST) or PSS (+ REST) or PSS (+ CRST). Although some authors use more detailed PSS classifications (2–4), most specialists in scleroderma basically divide PSS patient groups according to those with CREST and those with diffuse scleroderma. According to this classification, in CREST patients, skin sclerosis is limited to hands, forearms distal to the elbow, and/or face (5). These CREST patients are often anticentromere antibody (ACA)–positive and usually have a better prognosis. However, in patients with diffuse scleroderma, skin sclerosis also involves the trunk; these patients usually are ACA-negative and have a worse prognosis.

What is crucial in this discussion is that most patients with diffuse scleroderma also have features R, E, and T, and that a significant percentage of these also have feature C. Therefore, if we consider only the 5 features expressed with the CREST acronym, it is evident that only feature S clearly distinguishes between CREST patients and non-CREST patients. The other features are substantially the same in both subgroups.

Such are the clinical facts. Therefore, when it is said that CREST syndrome is a variant of PSS with a better prognosis (and often associated with ACA positivity), this actually means that patients with limited skin sclerosis represent this variant. Also, Steen et al (5), in the same issue of *Arthritis and Rheumatism* as the Tramposch article, wrote that "calcinosis and telangiectasia were not required for the diagnosis of CREST syndrome." They did require that "skin involvement be limited to the distal portions of the extremities and/or face, and that tendon friction rubs be absent."

An accurate analysis of the clinical data (as they appear in the Tramposch article, for example) thus points out that the concept of the CREST syndrome may be confusing. The acronym is useful to depict a constellation of diagnostic criteria which, in most cases of PSS, make diagnosis definite. Nevertheless, if one considers CREST to be a nosologic entity, uncertainties might arise.

Mario Giordano, MD
University of Naples
Naples, Italy

1. Tramposch HD, Smith CD, Senecal J-L, Rothfield N: A long-term longitudinal study of anticentromere antibodies. Arthritis Rheum 27:121–124, 1984
2. Giordano M, Ara M, Capelli L, Tirri G, Vatti M: Vorschlag zu einer neuen Klassifizierung und Nomenklatur der progredienten generalisierten Sklerodermie (PGS). Verh Dtsch Ges Rheumatol 6:379–382, 1980
3. Giordano M: Classification of progressive systemic sclerosis, International Conference on PSS (Scleroderma). Austin, TX, October 20–23, 1981
4. Catoggio LJ, Skinner RP, Maddison PJ: Frequency and clinical significance of anticentromere and anti-Scl-70 antibodies in an English connective tissue disease population. Rheumatol Int 3:19–21, 1983
5. Steen VD, Ziegler GL, Rodnan GP, Medsger TA Jr: Clinical and laboratory associations of anticentromere antibody in patients with progressive systemic sclerosis. Arthritis Rheum 27:125–131, 1984

Digital angiography for the diagnosis of dural sinus thrombosis in Behçet's disease

To the Editor:

In the July 1984 issue of *Arthritis and Rheumatism*, Bank and Weart (1) reported a case of dural sinus thrombosis (DST) in Behçet's disease. DST is a rare complication in this disease, and diagnosis was made using conventional angiography.

We report here another case which supports the observation, stated by Modic et al (2), that digital intravenous subtraction angiography (DSA) could be the procedure of choice for detecting DST.

In 1982, a 29-year-old Algerian man was diagnosed as having Behçet's disease with recurrent aphthous stomatitis, genital ulcers, and bilateral uveitis. He had received no therapy for his disease until he was hospitalized in 1983 for

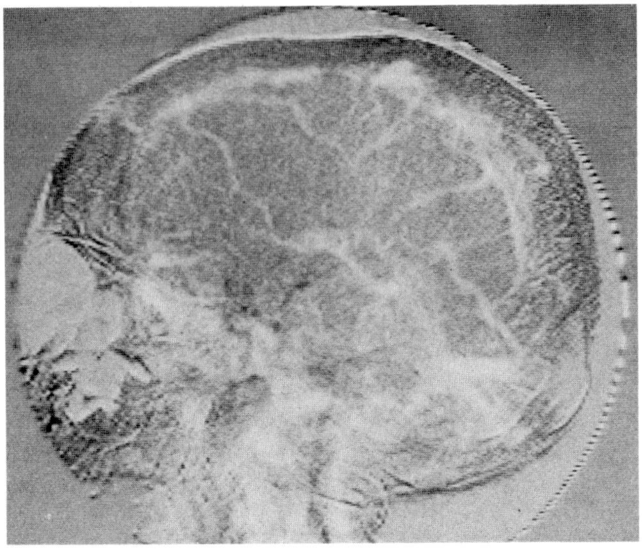

Figure 1. Digital intravenous subtraction angiogram, revealing a superior sagittal sinus thrombosis.

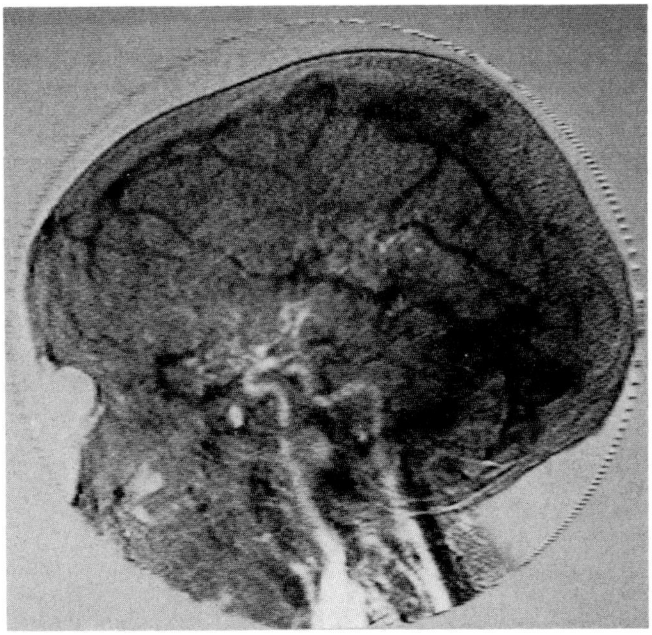

Figure 2. Digital intravenous subtraction angiogram, 2 months after initiation of therapy, showing incomplete recanalization of the superior sagittal sinus.

severe bitemporal headache and visual loss. The ophthalmologic examination found bilateral retinal vasculitis without papilledema. Computerized tomographic scan of the head produced normal results, but digital intravenous subtraction angiography revealed a superior sagittal sinus thrombosis (Figure 1). The patient was then treated with prednisone, 1 mg/kg/day, and chlorambucil, 0.2 mg/kg/day, for 2 months. The headache disappeared, signs of retinal vasculitis regressed, and a second digital angiography showed an incomplete recanalization of the superior sagittal sinus (Figure 2).

Bank and Weart found 9 cases in the literature (including their patient) of DST with Behçet's disease; however, they omitted a case reported by Feuilhade et al (3).

Our patient appears to represent the eleventh documented case of DST with Behçet's disease. The exact frequency of this complication is not known; it should be sought in patients with symptoms of increased intracranial pressure or severe headache. Digital intravenous subtraction angiography, which is less invasive and safer than conventional angiography (2), should be performed initially, whereas conventional selective angiography remains useful when DSA is not diagnostic. Another advantage of DSA is that it can easily be repeated, giving further information on possible recanalization of thrombosis, as occurred in our patient.

P. Brissaud, MD
L. Laroche, MD
A. de Gramont, MD
M. Krulik, MD
Hôpital Saint-Antoine
Paris, France

1. Bank I, Weart C: Dural sinus thrombosis in Behçet's disease. Arthritis Rheum 27:816–818, 1984
2. Modic MT, Weinstein MA, Chilcote WA, Pavlicek W, Duchesneau P-M, Furlan AJ, Little JR: Digital subtraction angiography of the intracranial vascular system. AJR 138:299–306, 1982
3. Feuilhade C, Touboul JL, Wechsler B, Guillard A: Thrombophlébite cérébrale au cours de la maladie de Behçet (letter). Nouv Presse Méd 11:3351, 1982

A&R's Birmingham Editorial Office to Begin Receiving New Manuscripts April 1

Dr. William J. Koopman will officially succeed Dr. Nathan J. Zvaifler as Editor of *Arthritis and Rheumatism* on July 1, 1985. As of April 1, 1985, Dr. Koopman's office will begin reviewing new manuscripts submitted for consideration. Any manuscripts submitted after that date should be sent to: William J. Koopman, MD, Editor, *Arthritis and Rheumatism*, University of Alabama at Birmingham, PO Box 55657, Birmingham, AL 35255-5657. All followup correspondence regarding manuscripts that were submitted to Dr. Zvaifler before April 1 should continue to be directed to San Diego.

arthritis and rheumatism

Official Journal of the American Rheumatism Association Section of the Arthritis Foundation

EVALUATION OF FACTORS ASSOCIATED WITH GLUCOCORTICOID-INDUCED OSTEOPENIA IN PATIENTS WITH RHEUMATIC DISEASES

THOMAS R. DYKMAN, OSCAR S. GLUCK, WILLIAM A. MURPHY, THEODORE J. HAHN, and BEVRA H. HAHN

In 161 ambulatory rheumatic disease patients receiving long-term prednisone therapy, diaphyseal mass (DM) and metaphyseal mass (MM) of the forearm were measured by single photon absorptiometry, and bone radiographs were reviewed when available. Multivariate analysis of treatment and patient characteristics demonstrated that glucocorticoid-induced osteopenia (defined as an elevated DM:MM ratio) and bone fractures occurred with similar frequency in patients of each sex, in whites and blacks, in patients with various rheumatic diseases, and in patients receiving different regimens of prednisone therapy. However, large cumulative doses of prednisone were associated with elevated DM:MM ratios as well as with bone fractures, and menopause or age ≥50 years (males or females) was associated with bone fractures. We conclude that long-term therapy with various prednisone regimens results in glucocorticoid-induced osteopenia and fractures. This affect is cumulative, occurs in all patient groups, and results in more bone fractures in certain groups.

It has long been recognized that long-term administration of oral glucocorticoids can result in a significant loss of bone mass (1–3). The degree of loss is more severe in areas of the skeleton with a high content of trabecular bone, such as vertebrae and ribs. It is less striking in the diaphyses of long bones, which consist primarily of compact cortical bone (4–6).

We have previously used single photon absorptiometry to measure appendicular bone mineral mass in normal individuals and rheumatic disease patients (7–10). Measurements at diaphyseal and metaphyseal sites of the radius demonstrate a constant relationship between bone mineral mass at the diaphyseal site and that at the metaphyseal site, both in normal individuals and in most patients with conditions associated with osteopenia (for example, idiopathic osteoporosis). However, in osteopenia associated with glucocorticoid therapy, there is a greater loss of metaphyseal mass (MM) than diaphyseal mass (DM), and the DM:MM ratio increases (7–10). A combination of factors may account for this observation. First, the metaphyseal site contains a higher proportion of trabecular bone (>25%) than the diaphyseal site (~5%) (11). Second, the metaphyseal site has a greater surface area than the diaphyseal site, and endosteal resorption of cortical bone may be more easily measured at the metaphyseal site.

Since measurement of DM:MM ratios provides a simple, inexpensive, and rapid method of identifying patients with glucocorticoid-induced osteopenia, we have measured these ratios in 161 patients with various rheumatic diseases treated with long-term glucocorticoid therapy. This report evaluates whether different glucocorticoid treatment regimens and patient characteristics are associated with glucocorticoid-induced osteopenia and bone fractures.

From the Department of Medicine and the Mallinckrodt Institute of Radiology, Washington University School of Medicine, St. Louis, Missouri, and the Department of Medicine, UCLA School of Medicine and Wadsworth VA Hospital, Los Angeles, California.

Supported in part by NIH training grant AM-07279-06.

Thomas R. Dykman, MD; Oscar S. Gluck, MD; William A. Murphy, MD; Theodore J. Hahn, MD; Bevra H. Hahn, MD.

Address reprint requests to Bevra H. Hahn, MD, Department of Medicine, UCLA School of Medicine, Center for Health Sciences, 10833 Le Conte Avenue, Los Angeles, CA 90024.

Submitted for publication June 26, 1984; accepted in revised form October 26, 1984.

PATIENTS AND METHODS

Patient selection. All ambulatory patients attending rheumatology clinics at Washington University between July 1979 and December 1980 were screened by review of written medical records. Any ambulatory patients who met the following criteria were invited to participate in the study: 1) at least 6 weeks of daily or alternate-day prednisone therapy; 2) no prior therapy with sodium fluoride, supplemental calcium, or vitamin D in doses exceeding the minimal daily requirement of 400 IU/day; 3) no evidence of significant renal dysfunction (creatinine >1.5 mg/dl); 4) no clinical or chemical evidence of intestinal malabsorption, liver disease, or primary hyperparathyroidism.

Of 366 patients who met these criteria, 205 refused to participate and were not further evaluated. In the 161 who consented, the following information was obtained:

1. Historical information. Sex, age, race, diagnosis, and prednisone dosage were recorded in every patient. Cumulative dose of prednisone for each patient was also calculated from review of the written medical record and/or personal interview, by adding daily doses over the entire length of therapy. Functional class was assigned based upon the patient's activities at the time of study (12). Dieticians estimated calcium intake by review of food consumption during the 8 weeks before testing.

2. Radiographic studies. Single photon absorptiometry of the radius, as described by Cameron et al (13), was performed in all 161 patients. This method utilizes a monochromatic beam from a ^{125}I source. The forearm is wrapped in a tissue-equivalent material to maintain constant thickness and is transversely scanned. The arm was carefully positioned so that the photon beam passed in a perpendicular path to the long axis of the radius. Two sites of the radius of the nondominant arm were scanned: a metaphyseal site 3 cm proximal to the distal end of the radius, and a diaphyseal site at a distance one-third the total length of the radius from its distal end.

Results of 3 scans at each site were averaged, and the bone mineral mass (gm/cm^2) was calculated. In our laboratory, the coefficient of variation was ±3% at the diaphyseal site and ±3–5% at the metaphyseal site (7). The DM:MM ratio was then calculated for each patient. This method has 2 advantages. First, it is known that although the DM and MM may decrease with age, the loss of bone mineral occurs in parallel so that the DM:MM ratio remains constant regardless of age, sex, or race (7,8). Second, because glucocorticoid therapy is associated with a disproportionate loss of MM, elevation of the DM:MM ratio would identify patients with glucocorticoid-induced osteopenia (7,8).

In the 161 patients, all available radiographs taken 2 years before or at the time of study were also reviewed, and the presence of bone fractures was recorded. Radiographs of both vertebral and extravertebral sites were available on 93 patients.

Statistical methods. Analysis of data was performed with assistance from the Division of Biostatistics at Washington University. Chi-square testing of contingency tables with Yates' correction and Student's *t*-tests were performed as noted. A multiple linear regression model was used for analysis of treatment and patient characteristics and DM:MM ratios. Adequacy of this model is represented by F = 4.28, P = 0.0001. Multiple logistic regression was utilized for analysis of treatment and patient characteristics and fractures. The adequacy of this model is represented by the goodness of fit χ^2 = 80.0, P = 0.24.

RESULTS

Patient characteristics. Characteristics of the 161 rheumatic disease patients studied are shown in Table 1. Fifty percent were ≥50 years old. The majority of patients were females (82%), 56% of whom were postmenopausal. Sixty-one percent of the patients were white and all remaining patients were black. The 2 most frequent disease categories were rheumatoid arthritis (53%) and systemic lupus erythematosus (33%). The remaining 22 patients (14%) included 4 patients with scleroderma or its variants, 4 with polymyositis/dermatomyositis, 4 with undefined or mixed connective tissue disease, 4 with Reiter's syndrome, 2 with juvenile rheumatoid arthritis, and 1 patient each with polyarteritis nodosa, Behçet's syndrome, ankylosing spondylitis, and psoriatic arthritis. Functional classification by Steinbrocker's criteria (12) revealed that 41% of these patients were in functional class I, 55% were in class II, and 4% were in class III. (The low percentage in class III is not surprising since only patients who were ambulatory were included in the study.) Drug therapies were recorded in 120 patients who had medical records that were complete enough to enable an assessment of drugs taken in the previous 2 years. Many patients took nonsteroidal antiinflammatory agents (51%) or aspirin (24%). Cytotoxic agents or estrogens were used infrequently.

Glucocorticoid therapy. The mean dosage of prednisone taken by the 161 patients at the time of absorptiometry was 15.6 ± 1.1 mg/day (mean ± SEM), with a range of 1–80 mg/day. Thirty-two patients (20%) were receiving alternate-day rather than daily therapy. Duration of therapy ranged from 42–9,275 days, with a mean ± SEM of 1,473 ± 116 days, approximately 4 years. Cumulative dose of prednisone was 16.0 ± 1.3 gm (mean ± SEM), with a range of 0.2–118.5 gm.

Absorptiometry. In a healthy St. Louis population including all ages above 18 years, the DM:MM ratio remains constant and has a value of 1.37 ± 0.12 (mean ± SD) (7). In this study, any DM:MM values that were more than 2 standard deviations above this normal mean (i.e., ≥1.62) were defined as elevated. Sixty-one of 161 patients receiving prednisone (38%)

Table 1. Characteristics of patients with normal or elevated diaphyseal mass:metaphyseal mass (DM:MM) ratios

Characteristic*	All patients (%)	DM:MM ratio Normal (%)	DM:MM ratio Elevated (%)	P†
Sex				
Female	133/161 (82)	79/100 (79)	54/61 (88)	NS
Male	28/161 (18)	21/100 (21)	7/61 (12)	
Age				
≥50	81/161 (50)	50/100 (50)	30/61 (49)	NS
<50	80/161 (50)	50/100 (50)	31/61 (51)	
Menopausal status (females)				
Postmenopause	69/123 (56)	37/71 (52)	32/52 (61)	NS
Premenopause	54/123 (44)	34/71 (48)	20/52 (39)	
Race				
White	98/161 (61)	59/100 (59)	39/61 (63)	NS
Black	63/161 (39)	41/100 (41)	22/61 (37)	
Rheumatic disease				
RA	86/161 (53)	55/100 (55)	31/61 (51)	NS
SLE	53/161 (33)	34/100 (34)	19/61 (31)	
Other	22/161 (14)	11/100 (11)	11/61 (18)	
Functional class‡				
I	63/153 (41)	41/92 (45)	22/61 (36)	NS
II	84/153 (55)	48/92 (52)	36/61 (59)	
III	6/153 (4)	3/92 (3)	3/61 (5)	
Therapy‡				
NSAID	61/120 (51)	37/67 (55)	24/53 (45)	NS
Aspirin	29/120 (24)	16/67 (24)	13/53 (25)	NS
Cytotoxic drugs	9/120 (8)	3/67 (4)	6/53 (9)	NS
Estrogen	5/120 (4)	2/67 (3)	3/53 (6)	NS

* RA = rheumatoid arthritis; SLE = systemic lupus erythematosus; NSAID = nonsteroidal antiinflammatory drugs.
† Probability by chi-square analysis, between patients with normal and those with elevated DM:MM ratios. NS = not significant.
‡ Information not available on every patient.

had elevated ratios characteristic of glucocorticoid-induced osteopenia.

Demographic characteristics including sex, age, menopausal status, race, disease category, functional class, and nonglucocorticoid therapies were not significantly different in patients with normal DM:MM ratios versus those with elevated ratios (Table 1). Weekly calcium ingestion was also not significantly different in the 2 groups: patients with elevated DM:MM ratios ingested 5.26 ± 0.56 gm/week (mean ± SEM) of calcium, versus 4.51 ± 0.50 gm/week in patients with normal ratios. Since demographic characteristics were not significantly different in patients with normal and elevated DM:MM ratios, these characteristics probably did not account for the greater loss of bone mineral mass in patients with elevated DM:MM ratios.

Bone fractures. Radiographs of both vertebral and extravertebral sites were available for review in 93 of the 161 patients who had absorptiometry. To evaluate whether review of radiographs in only some patients would potentially increase the observed number of fractures, demographic parameters were compared in the 93 patients who had radiographs versus the 68 patients who did not. There was no significant difference in sex, age, race, disease category, mean daily dose of prednisone, or cumulative dose (data not shown). However, functional class was significantly better in patients with radiographs (1.57 ± 0.05, mean ± SEM) than in those without (1.76 ± 0.08), (t = 2.01, $P < 0.05$). This may have led to a finding of fewer fractures in patients who had radiographs.

Twenty-eight of the 93 patients with radiographs (30%) had bone fractures (Table 2). Fractures were found significantly more often in patients with elevated DM:MM ratios (42%) than in patients with normal ratios (19%). When fractures were analyzed by site of occurrence, 17 patients (18%) had vertebral

Table 2. Bone fractures and diaphyseal mass:metaphyseal mass (DM:MM) ratio in 93 rheumatic disease patients with radiographs and absorptiometry

	No. (%) of patients with fracture
All patients	28/93 (30)
Elevated DM:MM ratio	19/45 (42)*
Normal DM:MM ratio	9/48 (19)*

* $P < 0.05$, chi-square analysis.

fractures and 17 had extravertebral fractures (data not shown). Sites of extravertebral fractures included feet and hands (6 patients), humerus (4 patients), ribs (4 patients), tibia (2 patients), and femoral neck (1 patient). Elevated DM:MM ratios were found in 11 of the 17 patients with vertebral fractures (65%) and in 12 of the 17 patients with extravertebral fractures (71%).

Association of previous glucocorticoid therapy with elevated DM:MM ratios and fractures. Patients receiving different doses of prednisone at the time of absorptiometry had similar frequencies of elevated DM:MM ratios and fractures (Table 3). However, since doses taken by patients at the time of absorptiometry may not reflect dosages taken previously, the 32 patients receiving ≤5 mg prednisone/day were carefully evaluated. Review of medical records disclosed that 10 of these patients had consistently taken ≤5 mg prednisone/day in the past. Three of these 10 (30%) had elevated DM:MM ratios (data not shown). Patients receiving alternate-day therapy at any dose were also evaluated. They did not have better DM:MM ratios; 11 of 32 (34%) had elevated ratios (data not shown).

High cumulative doses of prednisone were associated with a significant increase in the frequency of elevated DM:MM ratios. This trend was found, by multivariate analysis, to be independent of patient age; elevated DM:MM ratios were not more common in patients ≥50 years of age than in those <50 years. High cumulative doses were also associated with elevated DM:MM ratios in various subgroups versus the patient group as a whole (data not shown), including females ($P = 0.0003$), males ($P = 0.05$), patients with rheumatoid arthritis ($P = 0.01$), and patients with systemic lupus erythematosus ($P = 0.0005$). Fractures were also found significantly more often in patients with high cumulative doses of prednisone.

Elevated DM:MM ratios and bone fractures. When patients were analyzed by sex, age, menopausal status, race, disease category, and functional class, no significant differences in the frequency of elevated DM:MM ratios were found (Table 4). However, age ≥50 years and menopause were each associated with a significant increase in fractures. Increases in fractures in patients age ≥50 were similar in men and women (data not shown); 5 of 11 men ≥50 years old (45%) and 14 of 38 women ≥50 years old (37%) had fractures.

Among patients age ≥50, 13 of the 19 with fractures (68%) had elevated DM:MM ratios. Among postmenopausal females, 10 of the 15 with fractures (67%) had elevated ratios. Therefore, evidence for glucocorticoid-induced osteopenia was found in two-thirds or more of the patients age ≥50 who had fractures and in two-thirds or more of the postmenopausal females with fractures. No significant differences in number of fractures were detected in female patients versus male, whites versus blacks, or patients with different rheumatic diseases.

DISCUSSION

Using photon absorption techniques and bone radiographs, we examined glucocorticoid-induced osteopenia in ambulatory rheumatic disease patients

Table 3. Association of previous prednisone therapy with elevated diaphyseal mass:metaphyseal mass (DM:MM) ratios and with fractures

	Patients with elevated DM:MM ratio (%)	P*	Patients with fracture (%)	P*
Daily dose				
≤5 mg	11/32 (34)		6/19 (32)	
6–20 mg	42/105 (40)	NS	18/58 (31)	NS
>20 mg	8/24 (33)		4/16 (25)	
Cumulative dose				
<10 gm	18/77 (23)		10/45 (22)	
10–30 gm	25/61 (40)	<0.005	10/33 (33)	<0.05
>30 gm	18/23 (78)		8/15 (53)	

* By multiple regression analysis. NS = not significant.

Table 4. Elevated diaphyseal mass:metaphyseal mass (DM:MM) ratios and fractures, by patient subgroup*

	Patients with elevated DM:MM ratio (%)	*P*†	Patients with fracture (%)	*P*†
Sex				
Male	7/28 (25)	NS	5/14 (36)	NS
Female	54/133 (41)		23/79 (29)	
Age				
<50	31/80 (39)	NS	9/44 (20)	<0.05
≥50	30/81 (37)		19/49 (39)	
Menopausal status				
Premenopause	20/53 (37)	NS	7/36 (19)	<0.05
Postmenopause	31/69 (45)		15/40 (38)	
Race				
White	39/98 (40)	NS	21/63 (33)	NS
Black	22/63 (35)		7/30 (23)	
Rheumatic disease				
RA	31/86 (36)	NS	15/44 (34)	NS
SLE	19/53 (37)		9/34 (26)	
Other	11/22 (50)		4/15 (26)	
Functional class				
I	22/63 (35)	NS	8/44 (18)	NS
II	36/84 (42)		18/47 (38)	
III	3/6 (50)		2/2 (100)	

* RA = rheumatoid arthritis; SLE = systemic lupus erythematosus.
† By multiple regression analysis. NS = not significant.

receiving long-term prednisone therapy. Since patients with a history of osteopenia or fracture may have preferentially enrolled in this study, some selection bias may have occurred. Furthermore, since radiographs of only two-thirds of the patients were reviewed, further bias may have occurred, so the observed incidence of fractures may be artificially high. The rates of vertebral and extravertebral fractures we found (18% each) were slightly higher than those reported in other unselected populations (7–17%). However, our goal in performing this study was to evaluate whether certain glucocorticoid regimens or patient characteristics are associated with glucocorticoid-induced osteopenia and bone fractures. Therefore, although some selection bias was possible, comparisons of treatment and patient characteristics within the study population should remain valid.

Among patients with rheumatoid arthritis, vertebral fractures have been reported in 8–17% of those receiving glucocorticoid therapy (2,3,14). The only other large series of rheumatic disease patients studied is a recent preliminary report of 309 patients attending an outpatient clinic in Salt Lake City; approximately 80% of the patients in this series had rheumatoid arthritis. Vertebral fractures were found in 15% of patients receiving glucocorticoids, compared with 7% of patients not receiving glucocorticoids (15). Although these series are not directly comparable due to differences in patient diagnoses, functional class, and duration of therapy, the occurrence of vertebral fractures in 18% of our patients is not inconsistent with these reports. It is of interest that extravertebral fractures and vertebral fractures were found with the same frequency in our patients. In our experience, extravertebral fractures may be a significant source of morbidity.

Our decision to use DM:MM ratios was based largely on our previous experience showing a characteristic elevation of DM:MM ratios in patients receiving long-term glucocorticoid therapy (7–10). Although a single preliminary report did not find this relationship (16), a recent publication has used this methodology and identified elevated DM:MM ratios in asthma patients receiving long-term glucocorticoid therapy (17). Other investigators have measured vertebral as well as forearm bone mineral mass using photon absorptiometry in individuals with Cushing's syndrome. In 17 patients with iatrogenic and idiopathic Cushing's syndrome, a much greater loss of bone mineral mass was found at vertebral sites than at proximal or distal forearm sites (6).

Although measurements at either proximal or distal forearm sites may not be as sensitive in detecting loss of vertebral bone mineral as measurements at vertebral sites, our study provides evidence that measurement at 2 appendicular sites and calculation of the DM:MM ratio may identify many patients who have loss of bone mass at vertebral sites. Elevated DM:MM ratios were found in approximately two-thirds of the patients with vertebral fractures in our study. Elevated DM:MM ratios were also found in a similar number of patients with extravertebral fractures.

The inability of DM:MM ratios to identify all patients with bone fractures in this study may reflect the many factors which contribute to bone fractures in patients receiving glucocorticoid therapy. In addition to loss of bone mass induced by glucocorticoid therapy, inactivity due to poor functional class, age, and menopause may contribute to low bone mass and fracture (3,14). In this study, patients with elevated DM:MM ratios had significantly more fractures (42%) than patients with normal DM:MM ratios (19%). Although our study supports an association between elevated DM:MM ratios and bone fractures, we do not believe a single measurement of DM:MM ratio can be used to predict risk for fracture in an individual patient.

Multivariate analysis of DM:MM ratios and previous glucocorticoid therapy in this study demonstrated that the cumulative dose of prednisone is the most important factor which determines glucocorticoid-induced osteopenia. Patients who had taken a cumulative dose of >30 gm of prednisone had the highest incidence of fractures (53%) and elevated DM:MM ratios (78%). Several previous reports have also emphasized the association between cumulative glucorticoid dose and radiographic osteopenia or bone fracture (15,18). Two studies of rheumatic disease patients, however, did not emphasize this relationship (3,14). Cumulative dosage in both of these latter studies was <10 gm, and duration of therapy may not have been long enough to produce a significant increase in radiographic osteopenia or fractures. Correlations between elevated DM:MM ratios and large cumulative dose of glucocorticoids were present in various patient subgroups in our study, including those with rheumatoid arthritis, those with systemic lupus erythematosus, males, and females.

Although previous investigators have suggested that therapy with low daily doses of glucocorticoids is not associated with glucocorticoid-induced osteopenia (3,19), our earlier (10) and present results demonstrate that some patients receiving daily low-dose therapy, as well as patients on alternate-day regimens, may have elevated DM:MM ratios. Bone mineral loss during glucocorticoid therapy is due to decreased bone formation and increased bone resorption (9,20,21). Glucocorticoids inhibit intestinal calcium absorption and inhibit osteoblast differentiation and osteoblast synthesis of collagen and noncollagen protein. Although oral doses of prednisone >10 mg are usually required to inhibit intestinal calcium absorption (22), we have found some patients receiving ≤10 mg/day who have decreased intestinal calcium absorption (unpublished observations). Furthermore, the dose of prednisone that inhibits bone formation has not been determined, and low daily or alternate-day doses could possibly inhibit bone formation in some individuals. Overall, we believe our data suggest that long-term therapy at any dose may produce glucocorticoid-induced osteopenia.

Analysis of patient characteristics demonstrated that the frequency of elevated DM:MM ratios was similar in different patient groups. Comparisons by sex, race, functional class, and various disease categories disclosed no significant differences. These findings suggest that the risk for development of glucocorticoid-induced osteopenia (elevation of DM:MM ratio) is similar in all patient groups. However, fractures were significantly increased in patients age ≥50 years (males or females) and in postmenopausal females. One explanation for the higher number of fractures in these elderly patients would be that preexisting low bone mass secondary to age or postmenopausal status results in an increased risk of fracture. However, elevated DM:MM ratios were found in two-thirds or more of the patients who were ≥50 years old or were postmenopausal females with fractures. Therefore, evidence for glucocorticoid-induced osteopenia was common in these patients, and glucocorticoid-induced

Table 5. Patient and treatment characteristics associated with elevated diaphyseal mass:metaphyseal mass ratios and/or bone fracture

Definite association	Probable association	No association
Cumulative prednisone dose	Functional class	Sex (excluding menopause)
Age ≥50 years (male and female)		Race
		Disease category
Menopause		Current prednisone regimen

bone loss superimposed on low bone mass may have increased bone fractures.

One previous study has demonstrated that radiographic evidence of osteopenia of the vertebral spine is more common in women ≥50 years old receiving glucocorticoids (3). A recent study has also demonstrated that glucocorticoid therapy increases the risk of hip fractures in postmenopausal women (23). Although males have a greater bone mass than females at all ages, other series have also noted that men as well as women develop fractures during glucocorticoid therapy (15,17,24).

No previous studies have evaluated fracture rates in blacks versus whites receiving glucocorticoid therapy. Although blacks have a greater bone mass throughout life than whites, we did not find a significant difference in fracture rates between these 2 races. Fractures were found more often in patients with worsening functional class (class I, 18%; class II, 38%; class III, 100%); these differences, however, were not significant. Since most of our patients (96%) were in functional class I or II, we cannot exclude the possibility that in a more disabled population of rheumatic disease patients, low bone mineral mass due to immobilization could increase fractures.

In summary, certain treatment and patient characteristics are associated with elevated DM:MM ratios and/or bone fractures in ambulatory rheumatic disease patients receiving long-term glucocorticoid therapy (Table 5). Large cumulative doses of prednisone are associated with elevated DM:MM ratios and fractures. Age ≥50 years or postmenopausal state is associated with fractures, and many of these elderly patients with fractures have evidence of glucocorticoid-induced osteopenia (elevation of DM:MM ratio). Although worsening functional class is not associated with a significant increase in fractures, based upon previous reports (1,2) and trends found in this study, functional class may be a significant factor. Finally, elevated DM:MM ratios and fractures occur with similar frequency in males and females, in whites and blacks, in patients with different rheumatic diseases, and in those on different regimens of prednisone.

These findings using DM:MM ratios suggest that long-term glucocorticoid therapy in various regimens may result in glucocorticoid-induced osteopenia. This effect is cumulative, occurs in all patient groups, and results in more fractures in patients ≥50 years of age, postmenopausal females, and patients receiving large cumulative doses.

REFERENCES

1. Curtiss PH, Clark WS, Herndon CH: Vertebral fractures resulting from prolonged cortisone and corticotrophin therapy. JAMA 156:467–469, 1954
2. Badley BWD, Ansell BM: Fractures in Still's disease. Ann Rheum Dis 19:135–142, 1960
3. Saville PD, Kharmosh O: Osteoporosis of rheumatoid arthritis: influence of age, sex and corticosteroids. Arthritis Rheum 10:423–430, 1967
4. Sussman ML, Copelman B: The roentgenologic appearance of the bones in Cushing's syndrome. Radiology 39:288–292, 1942
5. Howland WJ, Pugh DG, Sprague RG: Roentgenologic changes in the skeletal system in Cushing's syndrome. Radiology 71:69–78, 1968
6. Seeman E, Wahner HW, Offord KP, Kumar R, Johnson WJ, Riggs BL: Differential effects of endocrine dysfunction on the axial and the appendicular skeleton. J Clin Invest 69:1302–1309, 1982
7. Hahn TJ, Boisseau VC, Avioli LV: Effect of chronic corticosteroid administration on diaphyseal and metaphyseal bone mass. J Clin Endocrinol Metab 39:274–282, 1974
8. Hahn TJ, Hahn BH: Osteopenia in patients with rheumatic diseases: principles of diagnosis and therapy. Semin Arthritis Rheum 6:165–188, 1976
9. Hahn TJ, Halstead LR, Teitelbaum SL, Hahn BH: Altered mineral metabolism in glucocorticoid-induced osteopenia: effect of 25-hydroxyvitamin D administration. J Clin Invest 64:655–665, 1979
10. Gluck OS, Murphy WA, Hahn TJ, Hahn B: Bone loss in adults receiving alternate day glucocorticoid therapy: a comparison with daily therapy. Arthritis Rheum 24:892–898, 1981
11. Wahner HW, Riggs BL, Beabout JW: Diagnosis of osteoporosis: usefulness of photon absorptiometry at the radius. J Nucl Med 18:432–437, 1977
12. Steinbrocker O, Traeger CH, Batterman RC: Therapeutic criteria in rheumatoid arthritis. JAMA 140:659–667, 1949
13. Cameron JR, Mazess RB, Sorenson JA: Precision and accuracy of bone mineral determination by direct photon absorptiometry. Invest Radiol 3:141–150, 1968
14. McConkey B, Fraser GM, Bligh AS: Osteoporosis and purpura in rheumatoid disease: prevalence and relation to treatment with corticosteroids. Q J Med 124:419–427, 1962
15. Clegg DO, Egger MJ, Ward JR: Osteoporotic vertebral compression fractures in rheumatologic patients treated with prednisone (abstract). Arthritis Rheum (suppl) 26:S47, 1983
16. Mueller MN: Effects of corticosteroids on bone mineral

in rheumatoid arthritis and asthma (abstract). AJR 126:1300, 1976
17. Adinoff AD, Hollister JR: Steroid-induced fractures and bone loss in patients with asthma. N Engl J Med 309:265–268, 1983
18. Reifenstein EC Jr: Symposium on adrenal corticoid therapy: control of corticoid-induced protein depletion and osteoporosis by anabolic steroid therapy. Metabolism 78:78–88, 1958
19. Klinefelter HF, Winkenwerder WL, Bledsoe T: Single daily dose prednisone therapy. JAMA 241:2721–2723, 1979
20. Caniggia A, Nuti R, Lore F, Vattimo A: Pathophysiology of the adverse effects of glucoactive corticosteroids on calcium metabolism in man. J Steroid Biochem 15:153–161, 1981
21. Raisz LG: Effect of corticosteroids on calcium metabolism. Prog Biochem Pharmacol 17:212–219, 1980
22. Klein RG, Arnaud SB, Gallagher JC, DeLuca HF, Riggs BL: Intestinal calcium absorption in exogenous hypercortisonism: role of 25-hydroxyvitamin D and corticosteroid dose. J Clin Invest 60:253–259, 1977
23. Paganini-Hill A, Ross RK, Gerkins VR, Henderson BE, Arthur M, Mack TH: Menopausal estrogen therapy and hip fractures. Ann Intern Med 95:28–31, 1981
24. Seeman E, Melton LJ, O'Fallon WM, Riggs BL: Risk factors for spinal osteoporosis in men. Am J Med 75:997–1003, 1984

THE EFFECT OF GLUCOCORTICOIDS ON BONE MASS IN RHEUMATOID ARTHRITIS PATIENTS

Influence of Menopausal State

ORLA SKIBSTED ALS, ANDERS GOTFREDSEN, and CLAUS CHRISTIANSEN

We studied 97 patients with definite or classic rheumatoid arthritis (RA). Fifty-four patients (19 premenopausal women, 25 postmenopausal women, and 10 men) had been treated with low-dose glucocorticoids for at least 12 months (mean dose <10 mg/day). The remaining 43 patients (15 premenopausal women, 17 postmenopausal women, and 11 men) had been treated with penicillamine, and served as a patient control group. The distal forearm bone mineral content (BMC) was measured in all patients by single photon absorptiometry using ^{125}I, and the total body bone mineral (TBBM) was measured in 61 patients by dual photon absorptiometry using ^{153}Gd. Compared with normal controls, both treatment groups had significantly decreased BMC and TBBM ($0.01 < P < 0.001$). When the patients were stratified according to pre- and postmenopausal state, we found significantly lower BMC and TBBM values in the premenopausal glucocorticoid-treated women than in penicillamine-treated women. However, no differences in BMC and TBBM values were found in the corresponding postmenopausal groups. In the premenopausal women treated with glucocorticoids, the duration of treatment and cumulative dose correlated with BMC. No such correlations were found in the postmenopausal women. We conclude that 1) RA is associated with loss of bone mass, 2) systemic glucocorticoid treatment further aggravates the bone loss, 3) in postmenopausal RA patients, the bone loss resulting from menopause and from the disease itself is not accelerated by low-dose glucocorticoids, and 4) in premenopausal RA patients, however, the bone mass is significantly affected by glucocorticoid treatment. We therefore suggest that these factors be considered when prescribing glucocorticoids, in order to minimize the bone loss.

Rheumatoid arthritis (RA) is associated with the development of both generalized and periarticular osteoporosis (1–10). It is uncertain whether the loss of bone mass is primarily dependent on disease activity, duration of RA, or the type of drug treatment given. Some investigators have found a significant correlation between the degree of functional impairment and the amount of the reduction of bone mineral (1,8,11,12), and it is widely accepted that the duration of RA is a determinant in the degree of the loss of bone mass (5,10,12).

There is substantial evidence indicating that glucocorticoids induce osteoporosis in patients receiving treatment for RA (1–3,10,13–16, and Nagant de Deuxchaisnes C: personal communication) and for other diseases (16–19). Nevertheless, it is still unclear to what extent the dosage or the duration of treatment is related to the degree of bone loss.

Furthermore, the reduction in bone mineral occurring in the female population with the onset of menopause (20,21) necessitates differentiation between pre- and postmenopausal RA patients, when interpreting data on glucocorticoid-induced osteo-

From the Department of Clinical Chemistry, Glostrup Hospital, University of Copenhagen, Glostrup, Denmark.

Supported by grants from the Danish Rheumatism Association, the Ferdinand and Ellen Hindsgauls Fund, the Fund of September 28, 1972, the Einar Willumsens Memorial Award, and the Dagmar Marshall Fund.

Orla Skibsted Als, MD; Anders Gotfredsen, MD; Claus Christiansen, MD.

Address reprint requests to Orla Skibsted Als, MD, Department of Clinical Chemistry, Glostrup Hospital, DK-2600, Glostrup, Denmark.

Submitted for publication May 21, 1984; accepted in revised form September 27, 1984.

penia. Those investigators who have made this distinction have found that there was no effect on bone in premenopausal women receiving glucocorticoids for RA, but that there was a pronounced loss of bone mass in men and postmenopausal women receiving this treatment (1,14, and Nagant de Deuxchaisnes C: personal communication).

In order to investigate the impact of glucocorticoids on bone mass, especially as a function of the menopausal condition, we measured the state of bone mineralization in 97 patients with RA who were receiving either glucocorticoids plus nonsteroidal antiinflammatory drugs (NSAID) or penicillamine plus NSAID.

PATIENTS AND METHODS

All patients entering this study fulfilled the American Rheumatism Association criteria for classic or definite RA (22). None of the patients had any other diseases known to interfere with calcium metabolism nor was any of them receiving any medication (other than glucocorticoids or female hormones) known to interfere with calcium metabolism. The 97 patients (76 women and 21 men) comprised a consecutive series of patients attending the rheumatic disease outpatient clinic of Glostrup Hospital. All had been receiving continuous medical treatment for at least 6 months.

The patients were assigned to 1 of 2 groups according to the treatment given; 1 group was receiving glucocorticoids plus NSAID (n = 54), and the other was receiving penicillamine plus NSAID (n = 43). The 2 treatment groups were further divided into subgroups according to sex and menopausal state. Table 1 shows the relevant clinical data of all patients, by subgroup.

In order to assess the disease activity of each patient, we estimated the functional class according to the criteria of Steinbrocker et al (23). Normal values for the bone mineral variables measured were obtained from the following groups of healthy subjects: group 1 consisted of 358 subjects (129 men with a mean age [±SD] of 46.1 ± 16.5, and 229 women with a mean age [±SD] of 46.0 ± 16.6) in whom we measured the distal forearm bone mineral content (BMC); there were 67 subjects in group 2 (30 men having a mean age [±SD] of 46.4 ± 15.1, and 37 women with a mean age [±SD] of 44.2 ± 12.2) in whom we measured the total body bone mineral (TBBM). All participants were thoroughly informed about the purpose and consequences of the study, and all gave their written consent (Helsinki Declaration II). Approval was obtained from the local and the national ethical committees.

Measurement of bone mineral content. The BMC of the distal forearm was measured according to the method of Christiansen et al (24), by single photon absorptiometry using a 30 mCi ^{125}I radiation source emitting photons at 27.5 keV. The subject's forearm was immersed in a water bath so as to obtain a constant thickness of soft tissue/soft tissue equivalent. Six scans were made on each forearm, beginning at the site where the radius and ulna are 0.8 cm apart, and moving proximally and rectilinearly, perpendicular to the long axis of the arm (distance between scans = 0.4 cm). To correct for the influence of fat in the subcutaneous tissue, special computer algorithms were used (25). BMC is expressed in arbitrary units (dimension = mass per unit length) and is calculated as the mean of all scans on both arms, i.e., 12. This method has been shown to have a long-term reproducibility of 1.2% in normal subjects (26).

Measurement of total body bone mineral. The TBBM was measured by dual photon absorptiometry using a whole body scanner developed at our laboratory (27). The source of radiation is 1 Ci of ^{153}Gd having principal photon peaks at 44 and 100 keV. During the 90-minute scanning procedure, the subject was placed in a supine position on the scan-table, with the radiation source under the table and the detector above. The subject was scanned in a rectilinear pattern with a transverse scan speed of 1 cm/second and longitudinal steps of 2.5 cm. Data were recorded in 0.5-second intervals, yielding lines of 150 measuring points and a total of about 11,000 pixels. TBBM is expressed in units (gm/cm^2). The reproducibility of the TBBM measurement has been shown to be 2.4%, and the accuracy 1.5% (27,28). The total amount of absorbed radiation in one scan procedure is 50 μGy, or 5 mrads, per unit of body area.

The BMC was measured in all RA patients. The TBBM was measured in 61 patients (5 men receiving penicillamine treatment, 9 men receiving glucocorticoids, 11 women receiving penicillamine, and 36 women receiving glucocorticoids).

Table 1. Clinical data on 97 rheumatoid arthritis (RA) patients, by treatment group and subgroup

Treatment group/subgroup (n)	Mean age, years (range)	Mean disease duration, years (range)	Mean treatment duration, years (range)	Mean daily dose, mg (range)	Mean functional class (range)
Corticosteroid-treated RA patients (54)					
Men (10)	56.7 (40–73)	15.6 (5–30)	10.2 (1–21)	7.9 (2–10)	2.2 (1–3)
Women with RA onset before menopause (19)	46.2 (23–67)	15.1 (2–47)	8.4 (1–24)	7.6 (1–19)	2.6 (2–4)
Women with RA onset after menopause (25)	67.6 (55–82)	14.5 (2–46)	5.6 (1–26)	8.3 (3–21)	2.4 (1–4)
Penicillamine-treated RA patients (43)					
Men (11)	53.8 (30–73)	9.8 (2–35)	1.8 (1–4)	485 (375–600)	1.7 (1–3)
Women with RA onset before menopause (15)	39.7 (24–50)	8.9 (2–37)	1.8 (1–5)	462 (250–750)	1.6 (1–3)
Women with RA onset after menopause (17)	58.7 (50–68)	13.4 (2–30)	2.9 (1–6)	471 (250–750)	1.9 (1–3)

Analysis of data. The Student's *t*-test for unpaired data, and single and multiple linear regression analyses were used in the statistical evaluation of the data (29). Since TBBM and BMC are functions of sex and age, the values were calculated as percentages relative to the normal mean values in the corresponding sex and age groups.

RESULTS

Because our patients were consecutively entered in the study, we achieved a degree of randomness. Thus, the 2 treatment groups (those receiving glucocorticoids and those receiving penicillamine) were not comparable for age or duration of disease (Table 1). The glucocorticoid-treated group had a higher mean age and longer mean duration of disease than did the penicillamine-treated group. Linear regression analyses within the subgroups showed no significant correlation between age and BMC or between disease duration and BMC.

When the TBBM values for the RA patients were compared with values obtained from normal subjects (Figure 1A), the following pattern emerged. The penicillamine-treated male patients showed a tendency toward decreased TBBM, although this decrease was not significant. The glucocorticoid-treated male patients had TBBM values significantly lower than those of the normal subjects and of the penicillamine-treated male patients ($P < 0.001$ and $P < 0.01$, respectively). The TBBM values in the female patients were significantly lower than normal values in both the penicillamine-treated and the glucocorticoid-treated groups ($P < 0.01$ and $P < 0.001$, respectively). The glucocorticoid-treated female patients showed a (nonsignificant) tendency toward lower TBBM values compared with the penicillamine-treated female patients. Compared with normal subjects, both the glucocorticoid- and the penicillamine-treated male and female patients had significantly decreased BMC ($0.01 < P < 0.001$) (Figure 1B). Both male and female glucocorticoid-treated patients showed a tendency toward lower BMC values than the penicillamine-treated patients; again, the difference was not significant. However, when the statistical analyses were performed using absolute values instead of values expressed as percent of age-matched normal, there was a significant difference in BMC between glucocorticoid-treated and penicillamine-treated women ($P < 0.01$).

When the female RA patients were stratified into 2 groups according to menopausal state at the time of onset of RA, we found the relationships demonstrated in Figure 2. In premenopausal RA patients, both

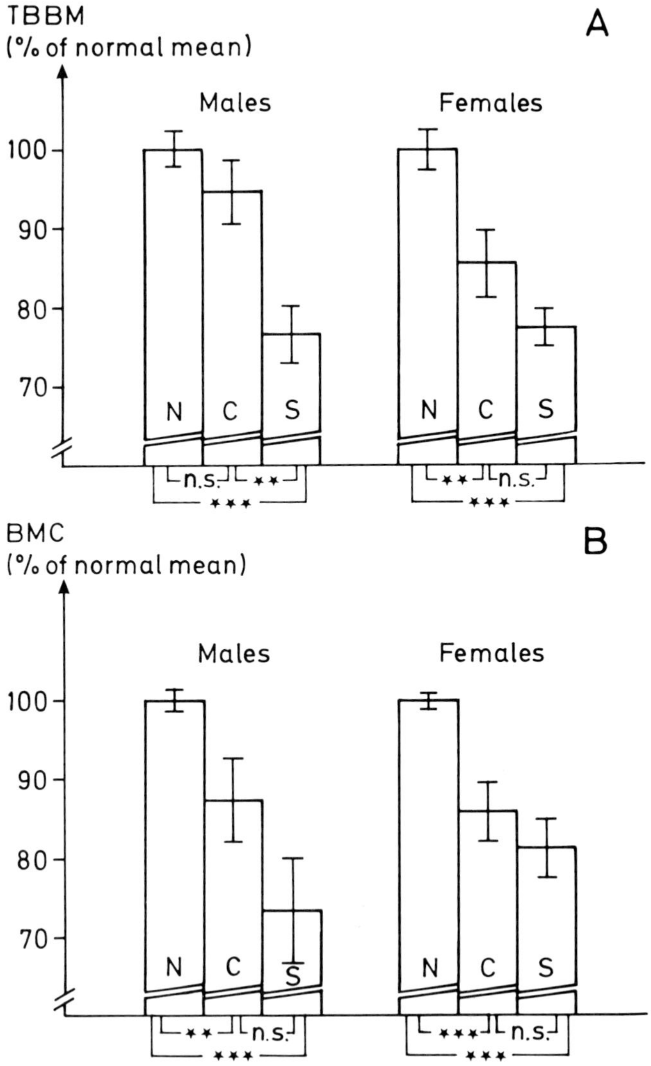

Figure 1. A, Total body bone mineral (TBBM), and **B,** distal forearm bone mineral content (BMC) in healthy subjects (N), penicillamine-treated rheumatoid arthritis (RA) patients (C), and glucocorticoid-treated RA patients (S). BMC and TBBM are given as percentage of normal values for an age- and sex-matched population. Bars indicate the mean ± SEM; ns = not significant; $^{**}P < 0.01$; $^{***}P < 0.001$.

BMC and TBBM were significantly lower in the glucocorticoid-treated group ($P < 0.01$ and $P < 0.05$, respectively). In postmenopausal patients, however, there was no significant difference in the effect of either of the 2 treatments on the 2 densitometric variables.

Figure 3 shows the pooled regression analysis of BMC versus TBBM in all patients in whom both the TBBM and the BMC were measured (n = 61). The correlation coefficient was highly significant (r =

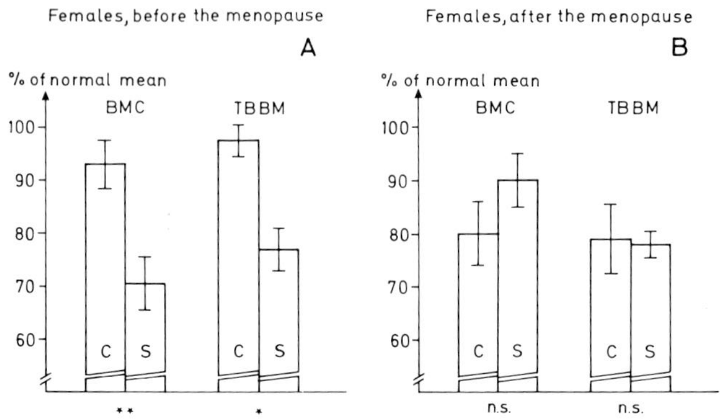

Figure 2. Total body bone mineral (TBBM) and distal forearm bone mineral content (BMC) in penicillamine-treated female rheumatoid arthritis (RA) patients (C) and in glucocorticoid-treated female RA patients (S), with disease onset before **(A)** and after **(B)** menopause. BMC and TBBM are given as percentage of normal values for an age- and sex-matched population. Bars indicate the mean ± SEM; $**P < 0.01$; $*P < 0.05$; ns = not significant.

0.89), and the standard error of estimate (SEE) was 9.6%. When linear regressions were performed in the separate subgroups, r values, slopes, and intercepts were virtually identical.

Table 2 shows the partial coefficients of correlation as well as the results of a stepwise multiple regression analysis of BMC, as the dependent variable, versus duration of RA, functional class, duration

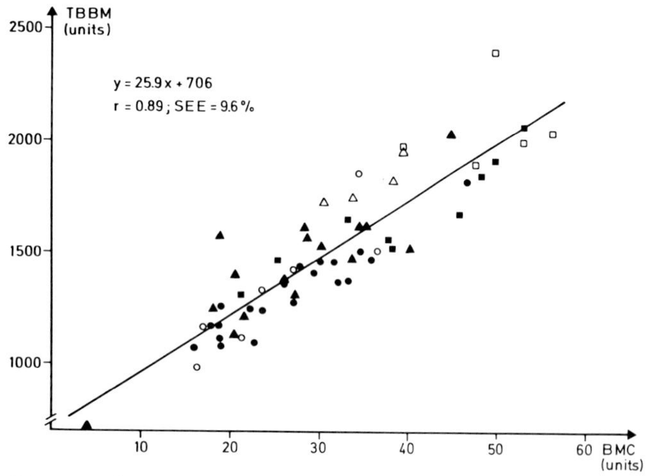

Figure 3. Correlation between distal forearm bone mineral content (BMC) and total body bone mineral (TBBM) in 61 patients with rheumatoid arthritis (RA). Penicillamine-treated patients: men (□); women with RA onset before menopause (△); women with RA onset after menopause (○). Glucocorticoid-treated patients: men (■); women with RA onset before menopause (▲); women with RA onset after menopause (●). SEE = standard error of estimate. BMC values are given as arbitrary units (dimension = mass per unit length) and TBBM values are given as absolute units (gm/cm^2).

of glucocorticoid treatment, and the cumulative dose of glucocorticoids, in the 3 subgroups of glucocorticoid-treated patients. In women with premenopausal onset of RA, only the duration of treatment and dose given before menopause were used in the calculations. From the data shown in Table 2, it can be seen that most predictor variables were found to be irrelevant in women with postmenopausal onset of RA and in men. Only the partial coefficient of correlation of the cumulative glucocorticoid dose versus BMC reached significance in the male group.

In the group of women who had premenopausal onset of RA, the partial correlations between each of the 4 independent variables and BMC were significant, except for duration of RA. The multiple regression expressions were also significant at all levels, except in the case of disease duration. Moreover, the coefficients of correlation increased when the variables were included in the order shown in Table 2; with all 4 independent variables, the coefficient of correlation was 0.74. This means that more than 50% (R^2) of the variation of BMC could be explained by the contribution of the 4 independent variables. The partial coefficient of correlation of premenopausal cumulative glucocorticoid dose versus BMC, 0.62, deteriorated when the total glucocorticoid dose (pre- + postmenopause) was used instead (0.46), although it remained statistically significant.

Figure 4 shows the regression between premenopausal duration of glucocorticoid treatment and BMC in women with onset of RA before menopause. The rate of decline in BMC was 2.55% per year of glucocorticoid treatment. Figure 4 includes 8 premenopausal penicillamine-treated women who were selected in order to match the functional class of the glucocorticoid-treated premenopausal patients as closely as this population sample permits (glucocorticoid-treated women 2.6, 8 penicillamine-treated women 2.1, mean BMC ± SD). The intercept of the regression line (83.5 ± 8.08%) was comparable with the BMC level maintained by penicillamine-treated premenopausal women with RA (92.1 ± 18.91%).

DISCUSSION

The patients were entered consecutively into the study to obtain the closest possible representative random sample. The glucocorticoid-treated group and the penicillamine-treated group were therefore not comparable for age, duration of RA, or functional class. However, comparability for age and duration of RA proved to be immaterial since neither of these 2

Table 2. Multiple regression analysis of % bone mineral content versus 4 independent variables in glucocorticoid-treated rheumatoid arthritis (RA) patients

	Women with premenopausal onset of RA (n = 19)			Women with postmenopausal onset of RA (n = 25)			Men (n=10)		
Independent variable	Partial coefficient of correlation	R^2 of multiple regression	SEE of multiple regression (%)	Partial coefficient of correlation	R^2 of multiple regression	SEE of multiple regression (%)	Partial coefficient of correlation	R^2 of multiple regression	SEE of multiple regression (%)
Duration of RA, years	−0.3866*	0.1495*	30.4	−0.2378*	0.0566*	28.0	0.1277*	0.0163*	29.0
Functional class, 1–4	−0.6229†	0.4468‡	25.3	0.2496*	0.1813*	26.6	0.0355*	0.0210*	31.0
Duration of glucocorticoid treatment, years§	−0.4513¶	0.5095‡	24.6	−0.1773*	0.1238*	26.7	−0.3996*	0.5210*	23.3
Cumulative glucocorticoid dose, mg§	−0.6208†	0.5518‡	24.3	−0.1952*	0.2413*	26.9	−0.6732‡	0.7207*	19.5

* Not significant.
† $P < 0.01$.
‡ $P < 0.05$.
§ For men and postmenopausal women, values used in analyses were the total duration of treatment and total cumulative dose; for premenopausal women, only the duration of treatment and cumulative dose before menopause were used.
¶ $P = 0.0534$.

variables was found to correlate significantly with BMC. We have shown elsewhere that the decline in BMC resulting from duration of RA, if any, is seen within the first 3 years (30). Furthermore, the relative contribution of each of the 4 variables (disease duration, functional class, duration of glucocorticoid treatment, and glucocorticoid dose) was evaluated in the multiple correlation analysis.

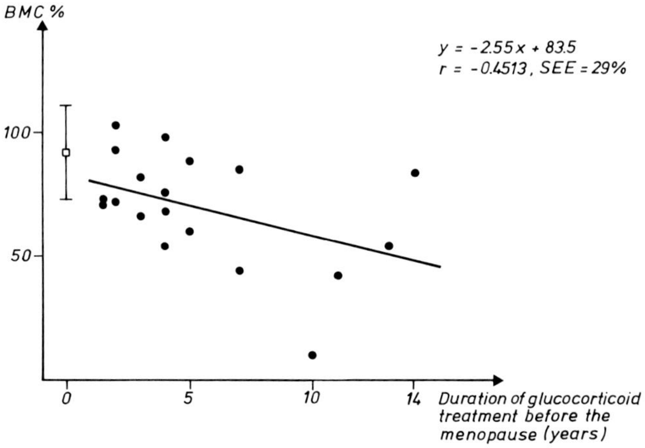

Figure 4. Relationship between duration of glucocorticoid treatment before menopause and distal forearm bone mineral content (BMC) in 19 women with onset of rheumatoid arthritis (RA) before menopause. BMC is expressed as percentage of mean normal value for an age-matched population. The open square and bars (□ ± SD) represent the mean BMC of 8 penicillamine-treated women with premenopausal onset of RA, matched with the glucocorticoid-treated women according to functional class.

It has been proposed that, since the bone loss resulting from RA is both generalized and periarticular, the only accurate means of evaluating RA-associated osteoporosis is to measure the total skeletal mineralization (10). The TBBM and BMC measurements are 2 different methods of assessing skeletal mineralization. They usually correlate well, and the slope and intercept of the regression line tend to be identical in healthy controls and in patients having a variety of calcium metabolic disorders (31–34), ranging from patients with very osteoporotic bones (including RA patients) (31,34) to patients with only subtle changes in skeletal mineralization (32). The pooled regression analysis of BMC versus TBBM in the patients in our study (Figure 3) replicates and confirms this relationship. Furthermore, the regression lines were identical in the separate groups. We have also clearly shown that the patterns of the BMC and the TBBM changes were virtually identical (Figure 1), displaying significant trends toward reduced mineralization in all RA patients. These trends become further accentuated on addition of glucocorticoids to the treatment regimen.

The role of glucocorticoids in calcium metabolism and their interaction with estrogens are not entirely clear. They have been shown to decrease intestinal absorption of calcium (17,35,36), although detrimental changes in serum concentrations of $1,25(OH)_2D$ and immunoreactive parathyroid hormone have not occurred (36,37). The catabolic and proteolytic action of glucocorticoids certainly account for part of their osteopenic effect. Finally, some investigators have found a positive relationship between urinary cortisol excretion and bone loss in oophorectomized women (38,39), and reduced levels of androstenedione, estrone, and testosterone in glucocorticoid-treated postmenopausal women (40). These findings may indicate that exogenously supplied glucocorticoids suppress adrenocorticotropic activity, thereby leading to a lowered production of dehydroepiandrosterone, androstenedione, estrone, and estradiol. This would therefore cause women treated with glucocorticoids after menopause to lose calcium at a fast rate; an appreciably more powerful action of glucocorticoids on bone mass would be expected in postmenopausal than in premenopausal women, in whom the estrogen level is high. Indeed, some results obtained in other series favor this theory (1,14, and Nagant de Deuxchaisnes C: personal communication). Our results contradict this.

The premenopausal glucocorticoid-treated patients had significantly reduced bone mass (as evidenced by measurements of BMC and TBBM) compared with both the healthy control group and the group of penicillamine-treated patients (Figure 2A). The postmenopausal glucocorticoid-treated patients, although osteopenic when compared with healthy controls, showed no greater reduction of bone mass than the penicillamine-treated patients (Figure 2B). The validity of our results is further accentuated by our having found significant correlations between BMC versus duration of glucocorticoid treatment and between BMC and cumulative glucocorticoid dose in premenopausal RA patients, but no correlations between these variables and BMC in postmenopausal patients (Figure 4 and Table 2).

It is interesting that the 8 premenopausal women who were selected from the penicillamine-treated group to match by functional class the glucocorticoid-treated premenopausal patients, had a mean value close to the intercept of the regression line for duration of glucocorticoid treatment versus BMC (Figure 4). This indicates that the lower bone mass in premenopausal glucocorticoid-treated RA patients, compared with those treated with penicillamine, was not due to differences in the degree of functional impairment, but was largely a result of the glucocorticoid treatment itself. The loss of bone was 2.55% per year, indicating that after 10 years of glucocorticoid treatment, about 25% of bone would be lost. If premenopausal non–glucocorticoid-treated RA patients have, on average, 90% of normal BMC, 10 years of glucocorticoid treatment is expected to reduce the bone mass to about 65% of normal values.

Therefore, on the basis of our data, care should be exercised when prescribing glucocorticoids for the treatment of RA in premenopausal women. In the case of postmenopausal women with RA, we have found that the BMC is much less affected by this type of treatment. The mean daily dose given in the premenopausal group (7.6 mg/day) is regarded as safe; however, the dosages ranged from 2–19 mg/day. The highly significant correlation between cumulative dose and BMC in this group of patients further emphasizes the necessity of keeping dosages low.

Theories about the pathophysiologic role of glucocorticoid hormones in the development of osteoporosis are conjectural. Our findings lend little support to the concept that inhibition of dehydroepiandrosterone and its metabolites is the critical factor in the osteoporosis of RA. In addition to the bone loss that accompanies both aging and the onset of menopause, premenopausal women who have RA are at increased risk of developing more severe osteoporosis as a result of 1) the disease process itself, 2) physical inactivity, 3) disease duration, and 4) the duration and cumulative dose of glucocorticoid treatment. It should also be recognized that the disease processes and pathophysiologic mechanisms in premenopausal women may be entirely different from those in postmenopausal women.

ACKNOWLEDGMENT

We thank Dr. C. Hellesen, Chief, Department of Rheumatology and Rehabilitation, Glostrup Hospital, for permission to study his patients.

REFERENCES

1. Saville PD, Kharmosh O: Osteoporosis of rheumatoid arthritis: influence of age, sex and corticosteroids. Arthritis Rheum 10:423–430, 1967
2. O'Brien WM, Samuels BM, Jasani MK, Anderson JA, Boyle JA, Buchanan WW: The role of corticosteroids in causing osteoporosis in rheumatoid arthritis (abstract). Arthritis Rheum 11:501, 1968
3. Bjelle AO, Nilsson BE: Osteoporosis in rheumatoid arthritis. Calcif Tissue Res 5:327–332, 1970
4. Duncan H: Osteoporosis in rheumatoid arthritis and corticosteroid induced osteoporosis. Orthop Clin North Am 3:571–583, 1972
5. Kennedy AC, Smith DA, Buchanan WW, Anderson JB, Jasani MK: Bone loss in patients with rheumatoid arthritis. Scand J Rheumatol 4:73–79, 1975
6. Kennedy AC, Smith DA, Anton HC, Buchanan WW: Generalised and localised bone loss in patients with rheumatoid arthritis. Scand J Rheumatol 4:209–215, 1975
7. Kennedy AC, Lindsay R: Bone involvement in rheumatoid arthritis. Clin Rheum Dis 3:403–420, 1977
8. Oka M, Rekonen A, Kuikka J, Anttinen J: Bone mineral

density in rheumatoid arthritis measured by the gamma transmission method. Scand J Rheumatol 4:28–32, 1975
9. Hahn TJ, Hahn BH: Osteopenia in patients with rheumatic diseases: principles of diagnosis and therapy. Semin Arthritis Rheum 6:165–188, 1976
10. Reid DM, Kennedy NSJ, Smith MA, Tothill P, Nuki G: Total body calcium in rheumatoid arthritis: effects of disease activity and corticosteroid treatment. Br Med J 285:330–332, 1982
11. Virtama P, Helelä T, Kalliomäki JL: Osteoporosis in rheumatoid arthritis: a follow-up study. Acta Rheum Scand 14:276–284, 1968
12. Mueller MN: Effects of corticosteroids on bone mineral in rheumatoid arthritis and asthma (abstract). AJR 126:1300, 1976
13. Mueller MN, Jurist JM: Skeletal status in rheumatoid arthritis: a preliminary report. Arthritis Rheum 16:66–70, 1973
14. Zanzi I, Roginsky MS, Ellis KJ, Blau S, Cohn SH: Skeletal mass in rheumatoid arthritis: a comparison with forearm bone mineral content (abstract). AJR 126:1305–1306, 1976
15. Hahn BH, Dykman T, Lewis-Stevens D, Haralson K, Murphy W, Hahn TJ: Incidence of bone fracture in rheumatic disease patients treated with and without glucocorticoids (abstract). Clin Res 29:782A, 1981
16. Hahn TJ, Boisseau VC, Avioli LV: Effect of chronic corticosteroid administration on diaphyseal and metaphyseal bone mass. J Clin Endocrinol Metab 39:274–282, 1974
17. Gallagher JC, Aaron J, Horsman A, Wilkinson R, Nordin BEC: Corticosteroid osteoporosis. Clin Endocrinol Metab 2:355–368, 1973
18. Deding Å, Tougaard L, Krogh-Jensen M, Rødbro P: Bone changes during prednisone treatment. Acta Med Scand 202:253–255, 1977
19. Adinoff AD, Hollister JR: Steroid-induced fractures and bone loss in patients with asthma. N Engl J Med 309:265–268, 1983
20. Smith DM, Khairi MRA, Norton J, Johnston CC Jr: Age and activity effects on rate of bone mineral loss. J Clin Invest 58:716–721, 1976
21. Christiansen C, Christensen MS, Transbøl I: Bone mass in postmenopausal women after withdrawal of oestrogen/gestagen replacement therapy. Lancet i:459–461, 1981
22. Ropes MW, Bennett GA, Cobb S, Jacox R, Jessar RA: Diagnostic criteria for rheumatoid arthritis—1958 revision. Ann Rheum Dis 18:49–53, 1959
23. Steinbrocker O, Traeger CH, Batterman RC: Therapeutic criteria in rheumatoid arthritis. JAMA 140:659–662, 1949
24. Christiansen C, Rødbro P, Jensen H: Bone mineral content in the forearm measured by photon absorptiometry: principles and reliability. Scand J Clin Lab Invest 35:323–330, 1975
25. Rickers H, Balslev I, Foltved H, Rødbro P: Bone mineral content before and after intestinal bypass operation in obese patients. Acta Med Scand 209:203–207, 1981
26. Christiansen C, Rødbro P: Long-term reproducibility of bone mineral content measurements. Scand J Clin Lab Invest 37:321–323, 1977
27. Gotfredsen A, Borg J, Christiansen C, Mazess RB: Total body bone mineral in vivo by dual photon absorptiometry. I. Measurement procedures. Clin Physiol 4: 343–355, 1984
28. Gotfredsen A, Borg J, Christiansen C, Mazess RB: Total body bone mineral in vivo by dual photon absorptiometry. II. Accuracy. Clin Physiol 4:357–362, 1984
29. Armitage P: Statistical Methods in Medical Research. Oxford, Blackwell Scientific Publications, 1971
30. Als OS, Gotfredsen A, Riis BJ, Christiansen C: Are disease duration and degree of functional impairment determinants of bone loss in rheumatoid arthritis? Ann Rheum Dis (in press)
31. Als OS, Gotfredsen A, Christiansen C: Relationship between local and total bone mineral in patients with rheumatoid arthritis and normal subjects. Clin Rheumatol 2:265–271, 1983
32. Tjellesen L, Gotfredsen A, Borg J, Christiansen C: Relationship between local and total body bone mineral in epileptic patients and normal subjects. Clin Physiol 3:359–364, 1983
33. Nilas L, Gotfredsen A, Christiansen C: The relationship between local and total bone mineral content after gastric surgery. Scand J Gastroenterol 19:591–595, 1984
34. Gotfredsen A, Als OS, Tjellesen L, Nilas L, Borg J, Christiansen C: Clinical applicability of in vivo estimation of total body bone mineral by dual photon absorptiometry: measurement on normals and osteopenic patients. J Comput Assist Tomogr 7:558–559, 1983
35. Wajchenberg BL, Periera VA, Kieffer J, Ursic S: Effect of dexamethasone on calcium metabolism and ^{47}Ca kinetics in normal subjects. Acta Endocrinol (Copenh) 61:173–192, 1962
36. Hahn TJ, Halstead LR, Baran DT: Effects of short term glucocorticoid administration on intestinal calcium absorption and circulating vitamin D metabolite concentration in man. J Clin Endocrinol Metab 52:111–115, 1981
37. Seeman E, Kumar R, Hunder GG, Scott M, Heath H III, Riggs BL: Production, degradation, and circulating levels of 1,25-dihydroxyvitamin D in health and in chronic glucocorticoid excess. J Clin Invest 66:664–669, 1980
38. Lindsay R, Hart DM, Manolagas S, Anderson DC, Coutts JRT, Maclean A: Sex steroids in pathogenesis and prevention of postmenopausal osteoporosis, Osteoporosis II. Edited by US Barzel. New York, Grune & Stratton, 1979, pp 161–181
39. Manolagas SC, Anderson DC, Lindsay R: Adrenal steroids and the development of osteoporosis in oophorectomized women. Lancet ii:597–600, 1979
40. Crilly RG, Horsman A, Marshall DH, Nordin BEC: Postmenopausal and corticosteroid-induced osteoporosis. Front Horm Res 5:53–75, 1978

EVALUATION OF D-PENICILLAMINE IN JUVENILE CHRONIC ARTHRITIS

A Double-Blind, Multicenter Study

A. M. PRIEUR, C. PIUSSAN, P. MANIGNE, P. BORDIGONI, and C. GRISCELLI

Seventy-four children with juvenile chronic arthritis were entered into a 6-month, multicenter, comparative double-blind study of the efficacy of D-penicillamine versus placebo. The results were evaluated in 70 patients, 55 of whom completed 6 months of the study. Improvement was observed in the total number of stiff joints, total number of painful joints, and total severity index measuring joint pain. There was also a significant reduction in the concurrent use of nonsteroidal antiinflammatory drugs. D-penicillamine was well-tolerated in all but 2 patients. Some children in the placebo group exhibited definite improvement; however, relapses that were observed were mainly in that group. These results confirm the efficacy of D-pencillamine for the treatment of joint involvement in juvenile chronic arthritis.

Juvenile chronic arthritis (JCA) is a heterogeneous disease which is not usually associated with the presence of IgM rheumatoid factor. Three types of onset have been described (1–3). The principal complication of this disease is the occurrence of progressive joint involvement. The systemic onset form can develop into chronic polyarthritis without systemic symptoms. The polyarticular onset form has an unpredictable course and can lead to severe polyarthritis. In some children who have the pauciarticular onset variety, the disease can progress insidiously to polyarthritis. This latter situation occurs especially in girls, with or without the presence of antinuclear antibodies in the serum.

Slow-acting antirheumatic drugs (SAARD) such as D-penicillamine (DP) have been used for patients who have JCA with progressive joint involvement (4–7). The outcome of this disease is unpredictable, however, and in many patients, unexpected spontaneous improvement occurs. We therefore decided to conduct a double-blind multicenter study of the effect of DP versus that of placebo.

PATIENTS AND METHODS

The study was approved by the Comité d'Ethique Médicale de l'INSERM. All JCA patients who were admitted to the study met previously established diagnostic criteria (1). Criteria for exclusion were the following: persistence of systemic extraarticular symptoms, mainly spiking fever, during the previous 6 months; arthritic involvement of <4 joints; use of nonsteroidal antiinflammatory drugs (NSAID) not authorized for pediatric use in France; systemic corticosteroid therapy >0.5 mg/kg/day of prednisone or the equivalent; use of SAARD during the previous 3 months; any modification of treatment, including physiotherapy, during the past month; presence of renal, blood, or hepatic disorders during the previous 6 months; and history of penicillin allergy. The presence of at least 2 of the following inflammation criteria was necessary for admission to the study: erythrocyte sedimentation rate (ESR) >25 mm/hour, serum fibrinogen >400 mg/dl, and elevation (>2 SD) of IgG, IgA, or IgM.

From the French Immunology and Pediatric Rheumatology Group, Hôpital des Enfants Malades, Paris, France.

Supported by Caisse Nationale de l'Assurance Maladie des Travailleurs Salariés.

A. M. Prieur, MD: Senior Researcher, Hôpital des Enfants Malades, Paris; C. Piussan, MD: Professor of Pediatrics, Centre Hospitalo-Universitaire, Amiens, France; P. Manigne, MD: Assistant of Pediatrics, Hôpital des Enfants Malades, Paris; P. Bordigoni, MD: Assistant of Pediatrics, Hôpital d'Enfants, Vandoeuvre les Nancy, France; C. Griscelli, MD: Professor of Pediatrics, Hôpital des Enfants Malades, Paris, France.

Address reprint requests to Anne Marie Prieur, MD, INSERM U 132, Hôpital des Enfants Malades, 149 rue de Sèvres, 75730 Paris Cedex 15, France.

Submitted for publication November 14, 1983; accepted in revised form October 19, 1984.

Arthritis and Rheumatism, Vol. 28, No. 4 (April 1985)

The trial regimen was as follows: scored 50-mg tablets of DP and identical placebo tablets were prepared by Bayer Pharma (Puteaux, France). Patients were randomly assigned to the DP or the control group. They were grouped according to weight by increments of 5 kg (10–15 kg, 15–20 kg, 20–25 kg, etc.), and a minimum dose of 5 mg/kg/day during the first 2 months and 10 mg/kg/day during the next 4 months was administered. Throughout the trial, 10 mg/kg/day of pyridoxine hydrochloride was given concomitantly, and physiotherapy was continued. A sealed envelope containing information on the patient's treatment was available in case of emergency.

Seventy-four patients (51 girls and 23 boys) with a mean age of 9 years (range 3–18) were included in the study. Informed consent was obtained from parents or guardians. The children were followed either as outpatients or in 1 of 3 specialized centers: Villa Richelieu, La Rochelle, France (P. Labeaumont, MD, P. Michel, MD), Centre Helio Marin, Roscoff, France (M. Jehanne, MD, J. M. Ledeunff, MD), or Chateau des Cotes, Jouy en Josas, France (M. C. Toumieux, MD).

The group included 35 patients with polyarticular onset JCA (4 with rheumatoid factor [RF], 2 with antinuclear antibodies [ANA], and 2 with both RF and ANA). Fourteen had pauciarticular onset disease (8 were ANA-positive, of whom 2 had uveitis) which was polyarticular at the time of the study. Twenty-five had systemic onset disease but had been free of extraarticular systemic symptoms for a minimum of 6 months.

Patients were assessed monthly as follows: 1) Physical examination was performed and general findings including height, weight, and temperature were noted. 2) Functional class according to the Steinbrocker criteria (8) was recorded. 3) The duration (minutes) of morning stiffness was assessed. 4) Each joint was evaluated individually except the cervical spine, carpal joints of each hand, and tarsal joints of each foot, each of which was considered 1 joint. Each joint was rated for the intensity of pain (0 = painless, 1 = pain on motion, 2 = pain on motion and spontaneous pain), of inflammation (0–3, with 1 point each allocated for swelling, heat, and redness), and of stiffness (by adding the results in degrees obtained by the measurement of each sector of motion of the joint tested with a goniometer and establishing a percentage of motion compared with normal joints, as previously described [9]). Intensity of stiffness was graded from 0–10 for each joint, with 1 point given per 10% loss of total normal motion. This assessment led to the evaluation of total painful joints, total inflamed joints, and total stiff joints and to the development of the sum of the severity ratings of pain, inflammation, and stiffness. 5) Average daily consumption of NSAID and/or prednisone was recorded. 6) The laboratory data including the measurement of ESR, fibrinogen level, and immunoglobulin levels (radial immunodiffusion) were recorded. 7) Adverse effects were recorded by monthly clinical evaluation (skin, mucosa, gastrointestinal, respiratory, and visceral examination), weekly verification of proteinuria, monthly laboratory investigation (complete blood count, platelets, hepatic transaminase), and determination of RF and ANA every 3 months. Ophthalmologic examination was performed at the start and the end of the study. 8) Before breaking of the code at the end of the 6-month trial, patients and/or parents were asked if they believed the drug had helped them, and the physician's overall evaluation was recorded. 9) Patients were considered

Table 1. Distribution of types of disease onset in juvenile chronic arthritis patients studied*

Group (n)	Systemic onset	Poly-articular onset	Pauci-articular onset
D-penicillamine (38)	16	15	7
Placebo (36)	9	20	7
Total (74)	25	35	14

* No significant difference in distribution between D-penicillamine and placebo groups (chi-square test).

Table 2. JCA patient characteristics, by treatment group, at the beginning of the study*

Characteristic	D-penicillamine	Placebo
Females/males	27/11	24/12
Age (years)	8.2 ± 3.9	9.8 ± 3.9
JCA duration (years)	3.1 ± 2.3	4.2 ± 3.3
No. of inflamed joints	10.5 ± 6.5	13.9 ± 19.1
Morning stiffness (minutes)	51.1 ± 36.9	46 ± 29.5
ESR (minutes/hour)	50.6 ± 28.8†	38.5 ± 22.2†
Previous SAARD (no. receiving)		
Gold salts	4	3
Pyrithoxine	1‡	2‡
Levamisole	0	1‡
Chlorambucil	3‡	1
NSAID (no. receiving)		
Aspirin	31	28
Propionic acid derivatives	4	3
Prednisone		
No. receiving	7	10
Dosage (mg/kg/day)	0.38 ± 0.62	0.25 ± 0.62

* Except where otherwise noted, values are mean ± SD. JCA = juvenile chronic arthritis; ESR = erythrocyte sedimentation rate; SAARD = slow-acting antirheumatic drugs; NSAID = nonsteroidal antiinflammatory drugs.
† Significant difference ($P < 0.05$, Student's t-test).
‡ Two children had previously received 2 SAARD.

Table 3. Reasons for dropout during the study

	D-penicillamine group (no. patients)	Placebo group (no. patients)
Lost to followup	4	4
Misdiagnosed	0	2
Primary tuberculosis*	0	2
Relapse		
Polyarticular	0	2
Systemic	1	2
Side effect	2†	0

* Purified protein derivative skin test gave a positive result during the trial.
† Thrombocytopenia, mucocutaneous symptoms.

Table 4. General assessment of patients, beginning and end of the trial

	D-penicillamine group (n = 38)	Placebo group (n = 32)
No. in functional class 3–4		
Initial	9	6
Final	4	6
No. with general symptoms*		
Initial	14	4
Final	9	5
No. in remission at final assessment	7	4

* Low-grade fever, lymphadenopathy, hepatosplenomegaly.

to be in remission when they had no articular symptoms and a normal sedimentation rate. 10) If parents agreed, 15 mg/kg/day DP was given to patients who did not respond well enough to a 10 mg/kg daily dose.

Criteria for removal of patients from the trial were worsening of the disease, the occurrence of severe intercurrent illness, the appearance of side effects, or noncompliance by the patient.

Statistical analysis of the data was performed by the chi-square test, Student's *t*-test, and the Wilcoxon test.

RESULTS

Patients. As shown in Table 1, there was no significant difference between the DP-treated group and the placebo-treated group in terms of distribution among systemic, polyarticular, and pauciarticular onset disease. The main characteristics of the patients at the beginning of the study are shown in Table 2. There were no significant differences between the DP group and the placebo group except for ESR values, which were higher in the DP group. Twenty percent of the patients had previously received SAARD. Most of the children were receiving aspirin treatment. Seventeen patients were receiving prednisone, but in relatively low doses.

Reasons for dropout during the study are shown in Table 3. Twelve children did not complete the study. Eight were noncompliant or lost to followup. Two girls had been included in the study with a disease meeting the criteria of seropositive JCA, for 1 and 5 years, respectively. These 2 girls were previously free of any biologic features of other connective tissue disease. During the study, while receiving placebo, 1 developed characteristic laboratory manifestations of mixed connective tissue disease with the appearance of antibodies to RNP, and the second developed proteinuria and characteristic histologic renal features associated with the appearance of anti-DNA antibodies and a decrease in the hemolytic complement level, indicating a subsequent course of systemic lupus erythematosus. Primary tuberculosis was detected in 2 other children, which required breaking the code in order to avoid the addition of antibiotics, which could have interfered with DP treatment and might have augmented the risk of drug-induced lupus.

Effect of therapy on clinical symptoms. The results were analyzed in 70 children, including the 8 who were lost to followup. Seven patients were withdrawn from the trial because of relapse or side effects (Table 3). Four patients in the placebo group exhibited a relapse between the second and the third months of treatment, and a fifth patient had a systemic flare while receiving DP. Two severe side effects led to the withdrawal of DP: 1 girl who had previously experienced cytopenia during chlorambucil therapy developed reversible thrombocytopenia (75,000/mm^3) while receiving 5 mg/kg/day of DP, and a male patient developed a cutaneous rash and mouth ulceration in the fifth month of treatment. Fifty-five patients (31 in the DP group and 24 in the placebo group) completed the entire study.

Table 5. Effects of therapy on articular symptoms*

Symptom	D-penicillamine group (n = 38) Initial	D-penicillamine group (n = 38) Final	Placebo group (n = 32) Initial	Placebo group (n = 32) Final	P†
Morning stiffness (minutes)	47.5 ± 36.2	26.8 ± 38.7	48.2 ± 32.5	37.2 ± 43.8	<0.06
No. of painful joints	6.3 ± 5.5	3.3 ± 3.8	7.6 ± 5.3	5.5 ± 5.5	<0.04
No. of inflamed joints	5.2 ± 5.2	2.5 ± 3.4	2.6 ± 2.7	1.7 ± 2.1	<0.2
No. of stiff joints	11.7 ± 9.0	8.5 ± 7.9	10.6 ± 7.5	11.1 ± 9.2	<0.01
Sum of severity of pain	7.2 ± 5.8	3.6 ± 4.2	8.3 ± 6.6	6.5 ± 6.3	<0.01
Sum of severity of inflammation	5.8 ± 5.5	2.7 ± 4.1	3.3 ± 3.5	2.0 ± 2.7	<0.08
Sum of severity of stiffness	17.1 ± 14.8	14.5 ± 13.3	16.7 ± 13.6	17.0 ± 13.1	<0.2

* Values are mean ± SD.
† By Wilcoxon test; $P < 0.05$ considered significant.

Table 6. Patients' daily consumption of antiinflammatory drugs*

	D-penicillamine group (n = 38)		Placebo group (n = 32)		
	Initial	Final	Initial	Final	*P*†
Aspirin (mg/kg/day)	81 ± 21	69 ± 26	71 ± 22	76 ± 17	<0.05
Prednisone (mg/kg/day)	0.17 ± 0.16	0.17 ± 0.20	0.15 ± 0.08	0.07 ± 0.06	<0.20

* Values are mean ± SD.
† By Wilcoxon test; $P < 0.05$ considered significant.

As shown in Table 4, overall functional improvement was observed only in the DP group: 5 of 9 children who were in functional class 3–4 at the beginning of the study were in class 1–2 at the end of the study. The general symptoms were initially different in the DP and placebo groups and could not be compared objectively.

The duration of morning stiffness was reduced, though not significantly, in the group receiving DP. Significant improvement was observed in the total number of stiff joints and the total number of painful joints. The sum of severity of pain was markedly decreased in the treated group (Table 5). Seven children in the DP group (1 with systemic onset, 3 with polyarticular onset, and 3 with pauciarticular onset) and 4 in the placebo group (all with pauciarticular onset) were in remission at the end of the 6-month study (Table 4).

In the DP group, the daily consumption of aspirin was significantly reduced. Prednisone dosage was not significantly reduced in either group (Table 6). One child receiving DP developed a relapse of uveitis, and prednisone therapy was increased to 0.2 mg/kg/day.

Effects of therapy on laboratory results. ESR was lower at the end of the study than at the beginning in both the DP and the placebo groups. While more pronounced in the DP group, however, the difference was not significant (Wilcoxon test). No difference between the beginning and the end of the study was observed in fibrinogen levels or in the levels of IgG, IgA, or IgM (Table 7). The RF titer was unaffected in 4 patients who completed the entire study (2 in the DP group and 2 in the placebo group). Modifications in ANA titers were similar in the 2 groups (Table 8). During the study, ANA became positive in 5 patients, 2 in the DP group and 3 in the placebo group. Further evaluation of these antibodies did not show any specificity against DNA or soluble antigens.

Adverse effects. Adverse effects were observed in 19 patients (Table 9). In 2, both receiving DP, these effects were severe enough to necessitate stopping the trial (see above). In 10 patients receiving DP and 7 receiving placebo, effects were generally mild and disappeared without withdrawal of the drug. In 10 patients (6 in the DP group and 4 in the placebo group), vomiting and abdominal pain were recorded. In 4 (3 in the DP group and 1 in the placebo group), transient rashes were observed. Two children receiving DP developed measles but experienced a definite improvement in their JCA for 3 and 5 weeks, respectively. One boy in the placebo group developed mumps. Although he had no immediate marked change in his rheumatic symptoms, he had significant articular and overall improvement during the study. Laboratory results showed no drug-related modifications except in 1 girl who developed thrombocytopenia.

Assessments by patients and/or parents and by physicians. At the end of the trial, the patients' and/or parents' and physicians' assessments favored the DP treatment (Table 10). When results with 10 mg/kg/day

Table 7. Laboratory findings in patients studied*

	D-penicillamine group (n = 38)		Placebo group (n = 32)	
	Initial	Final	Initial	Final
ESR (mm/hour)	49 ± 32	31 ± 26	41 ± 26	33 ± 23
Fibrinogen (mg/dl)	472 ± 217	432 ± 138	517 ± 138	460 ± 116
IgG (mg/liter)	1,774 ± 493	1,632 ± 580	2,010 ± 335	1,920 ± 615
IgA (mg/liter)	279 ± 207	270 ± 141	238 ± 174	230 ± 195
IgM (mg/liter)	213 ± 140	201 ± 98	170 ± 69	182 ± 69

* Values are mean ± SD. No significant difference between initial value and final value for any parameter studied. ESR = erythrocyte sedimentation rate.

Table 8. Antinuclear antibody titers

	D-penicillamine group (n = 38)	Placebo group (n = 32)
No. increased	1	1
No. became positive	2	3
No. unchanged	4	2
No. reduced	1	2

of DP were not sufficiently satisfactory, parents were asked if they would agree to having their child try 15 mg/kg/day. This was administered to 6 patients. After 6 months, complete failure of the increased dosage was observed in 2. In 4, definite clinical improvement was observed based on reduced duration of morning stiffness and on articular involvement, although sedimentation rate decreased only in 2.

Ten patients in the placebo group who showed persistence of active disease were subsequently treated with DP using the same protocol as was used in the DP study group. No therapeutic effects were observed in 5 patients after 6–18 months (mean 10.4 months). Three of these patients had polyarticular onset disease (1 with RF, 1 with both RF and ANA) and 2 had pauciarticular onset disease (both with ANA). Five other patients exhibited a marked clinical improvement. They had received DP for 1–3.5 years (mean 2.5 years). Sedimentation rate remained elevated in 3. Of these 5 patients, 3 had systemic onset disease and 2 had polyarticular onset disease without any biologic autoimmune features.

DISCUSSION

Slow-acting antirheumatic drugs are indicated for the treatment of juvenile chronic arthritis, and open studies appear to show that these second-line agents induce beneficial effects (4–6). However, except for the rare patients in whom IgM rheumatoid factor is present, spontaneous improvement is not uncommon, and within 10 years of followup a significant proportion of patients regain normal joint function without these drugs (10). Thus, investigators must carefully consider the indications before prescribing the long-term use of drugs which do not have immediate spectacular effects and are not devoid of side effects.

Table 9. Number of patients experiencing adverse effects

Location or type of effect	D-penicillamine group (n = 38)	Placebo group (n = 32)
Gastrointestinal tract	6	4
Rash	3	1
Dysgeusia	0	1
Viral infection	2	1
Thrombocytopenia	1	0

Table 10. Patients' and/or parents' and physicians' assessments of the usefulness of the drug taken*

	No assessment recorded	Reported useful	Reported useless, relapse, or side effects
Patients and/or parents (no.)			
DP	7	22	9
Placebo	7	12	13
Physicians (no.)			
DP	2	21	15
Placebo	1	10	21

* For both patient and/or parent assessment and physician assessment, $0.05 < P < 0.02$, D-penicillamine (DP) versus placebo.

For this reason, we designed a 6-month, double-blind cooperative study on the efficacy of D-penicillamine versus placebo. Although the duration of our study may seem short compared with others (4–6), we considered it more ethical to break the code after a 6-month evaluation in order to avoid depriving some children with JCA of SAARD, even if they were receiving background antiinflammatory drugs. Study patients were selected based on their joint disease and included children with chronic polyarthritis following a systemic onset, patients with polyarthritis (either seropositive or seronegative), and patients with pauciarticular onset in whom the disease eventually involved more than 4 joints.

The effect of DP on clinical symptoms was assessed using several clinical parameters. Improvement in general functional status was observed only in the treated group, with a significant number of patients moving from class 3–4 to class 1–2. Among the crippled patients included in class 3–4, only 2, who were nearly unable to walk, were in class 4. One, in the DP group, had a severe knee flexion contracture due to patella luxation and another, in the placebo group, had severe stiffness of the ankles and hips. The overall functional improvement observed in the treated group was not biased by physiotherapy, which was performed in both groups under the same conditions.

Improvement was also marked when evaluated on the basis of the reduction in duration of morning stiffness in the DP group. Detailed joint evaluation was analyzed using a methodology similar to that proposed by the American Rheumatology Collaborative Study Group (11), i.e., by counting and grading the severity of joint involvement. However our procedure was slightly different since we evaluated 3 different criteria separately, as described in Patients and Methods. Although some of our criteria, such as spontaneous pain or cutaneous redness, could be of little importance in children, our method of assessment seemed to facilitate evaluation by several observers, and despite some difference from the methods of other investigators (11,12), it provided a simple and rapid tool for joint examination in this study.

The main effects observed on the articular parameters were a significant decrease in pain and a reduction in the total number of stiff joints. The lack of a significant reduction in joint inflammation could be due to several factors: (a) our method of evaluation, which did not give enough weight to swelling, an important symptom of joint inflammation in children; (b) the duration of our trial, which was only 6 months and was even less for the 15 patients who did not complete the entire study; (c) the dosage of DP, which was not above 10 mg/kg/day. In this regard, it should be noted that 4 of 6 patients who received a subsequent course of 15 mg/kg/day of DP showed definite clinical improvement.

These results confirm those of previous open studies on the clinical efficacy of DP in JCA (5,6). However, in those reports, results were given as an overall evaluation of the disease activity and were not based on evaluation of precise modification of various joint symptoms, as in the present report. Although accurate assessment methods can be biased by many factors, such as the age of the child, the time of day, and the observer, these methods should be used for future drug studies and be adapted according to the experience of various observers (11,12).

Results of laboratory tests of inflammation did not significantly change in our study. Although ESR more clearly appeared to decrease in the DP group, this difference was not significant by the Wilcoxon test. The reduction of RF titers is an important biologic parameter of the effect of DP in adults (13). No conclusion on this could be drawn from our study, however, since only 2 patients in the DP group were seropositive.

The daily consumption of aspirin was significantly reduced in the DP group (Table 6), indicating less need for the use of rapidly-acting agents in these patients. This therapeutic parameter can be interpreted as indicating the efficacy of DP.

Adverse effects were systematically recorded at each visit. In 2 patients, they were severe enough to break the code, revealing that the patients were receiving DP. The patients' conditions returned to normal after withdrawal of the drug. In the other cases, adverse effects were mild and disappeared rapidly without modification of the protocol. When the code was broken, it appeared that these effects were not due to DP, since they occurred in both groups. Side effects are an important problem in adult patients receiving DP (14). In children, side effects seem to be less frequent, and they often occur only after 1–2 years of therapy (5).

It is interesting to analyze the improvement observed in the placebo group. In fact, these patients were not receiving strict placebo treatment since they were also taking NSAID. Furthermore, they were under close medical surveillance with monthly evaluations, and the effect of the medical attention itself must be taken into consideration. Among the 24 patients receiving placebo who completed the entire study, 4 of 7 with pauciarticular onset disease had complete remission, with no arthritis and normal ESR. This observation raises the question of the indication of SAARD for each type of disease onset, particularly for pauciarticular onset. The number of children studied in our trial is too small to warrant objective conclusions about this. However, this question certainly merits consideration in a larger number of patients and suggests the need for further cooperative studies using the maximum possible number of patients from each clinical subgroup. Heterogeneity in JCA remains an important stumbling block in the assessment of drug effectiveness.

ACKNOWLEGMENTS

The authors are grateful to P. Reinert, MD, F. de Gouyon, MD, J. M. Lefur, MD, and J. M. Garnier, MD for providing some of the patients' data. We also thank J. Goujart, MD and M. Prieur, MD for their expert advice in statistical analysis and Véronique Beauvais for skillful secretarial assistance.

REFERENCES

1. Brewer EJ Jr, Bass J, Baum J, Cassidy JT, Fink C, Jacobs J, Hanson V, Levinson JE, Schaller J, Stillman JS: Current proposed revision of JRA criteria. Arthritis Rheum 20:195–199, 1977
2. Ansell BM: Chronic arthritis in childhood. Ann Rheum Dis 37:107–120, 1978
3. Mozziconacci P, Hayem F: Formes cliniques des polyarthrites de l'enfant. Bull Mem Soc Med Hop Paris 118:763–771, 1967
4. Brewer EJ Jr, Giannini EH, Barkley E: Gold therapy in the management of juvenile rheumatoid arthritis. Arthritis Rheum 23:404–411, 1980
5. Ansell BM, Hall MA: Penicillamine in chronic arthritis of childhood. J Rheumatol (suppl) 8:112–115, 1981
6. Shairer H, Stoeber E: Long term follow-up of 235 cases of juvenile rheumatoid arthritis treated with D penicillamine, Penicillamine Research in Rheumatoid Disease. Edited by E Munthe. Oslo, Fabritius and Sonner, 1976, pp 279–281
7. Giannini EH, Brewer EJ, Person DA: Auranofin in the treatment of juvenile rheumatoid arthritis. J Pediatr 102:138–141, 1983
8. Steinbrocker O, Traeger CH, Batterman RC: Therapeutic criteria in rheumatoid arthritis. JAMA 140:659–662, 1949
9. Schwab P: Representation graphique simplifiée de l'évolution de la fonction articulaire. Ann Pediatr (Paris) 30:611–612, 1983
10. Calabro JJ, Holgerson WB, Sonpal GM, Khoury MI: Juvenile rheumatoid arthritis: a general review and report of 100 patients observed for 15 years. Semin Arthritis Rheum 5:257–298, 1977
11. Brewer EJ Jr, Giannini EH: Standard methodology for Segment I, II, and III Pediatric Rheumatology Collaborative Study Group studies. I. Design. J Rheumatol 9:109–113, 1982
12. Kvien TK, Høyeraal HM, Sandstad B: Assessment methods of disease activity in juvenile rheumatoid arthritis—evaluated in a prenisolone/placebo double-blind study. J Rheumatol 9:696–702, 1982
13. Wernick R, Merryman P, Jaffe I, Ziff M: IgG and IgM rheumatoid factors in rheumatoid arthritis: quantitative response to penicillamine therapy and relationship to disease activity. Arthritis Rheum 26:593–598, 1983
14. Munthe E, Kåss E: Penicillamine in rheumatic diseases: a prospective study of tolerance and efficacy. J Rheumatol (suppl) 8:107–111, 1981

SERUM C-REACTIVE PROTEIN IN POLYMYALGIA RHEUMATICA

A Prospective Serial Study

R. K. MALLYA, C. R. K. HIND, H. BERRY, and M. B. PEPYS

A prospective serial study of 13 well-documented, previously untreated cases of polymyalgia rheumatica was undertaken in order to assess the behavior of the nonspecific indices of disease activity, erythrocyte sedimentation rate and serum C-reactive protein (CRP) concentration, during induction of disease remission by prednisolone therapy. The clinical manifestations of all patients responded rapidly and completely to steroids, and the serum CRP value, which was raised in all patients at presentation, fell to normal at a rate which precisely reflected the clinical improvement. The erythrocyte sedimentation rate also fell, but did so much more slowly than the CRP concentration and, in half the patients, was still not normal after 14 days. These results indicate that assay of serum CRP provides a precise means of objectively assessing the course of polymyalgia rheumatica during initial therapy with steroids, and suggest that routine measurements of CRP may make a useful contribution to the management of the disease.

From the Department of Rheumatology, King's College Hospital, London, and the MRC Acute Phase Protein Research Group, Immunological Medicine Unit, Department of Medicine, Royal Postgraduate Medical School, London, United Kingdom.

Supported in part by Medical Research Council Programme grant G979/51 to Professor Pepys. Dr. Hind is a Medical Research Council Training Fellow.

R. K. Mallya, MB, MRCP: Senior Registrar in Rheumatology, Department of Rheumatology, King's College Hospital (current address: Department of Rheumatology, Guy's Hospital, St. Thomas's Street, London, SE1); C. R. K. Hind, BSc (Hons), MB, MRCP: Research Fellow and Honorary Senior Registrar, MRC Acute Phase Protein Research Group, Immunological Medicine Unit, Department of Medicine, Royal Postgraduate Medical School; H. Berry, DM, MRCP: Consultant Rheumatologist, Department of Rheumatology, King's College Hospital; M. B. Pepys, MD, PhD, FRCP: Professor of Immunological Medicine, MRC Acute Phase Protein Research Group, Immunological Medicine Unit, Department of Medicine, Royal Postgraduate Medical School.

Address reprint requests to Prof. M. B. Pepys, Department of Medicine, Royal Postgraduate Medical School, Hammersmith Hospital, Du Cane Road, London W12 0HS, England.

Submitted for publication June 13, 1984; accepted in revised form October 3, 1984.

Polymyalgia rheumatica (PMR) is a common disorder of the elderly, characterized by symmetric pain and stiffness affecting the proximal muscles of the limbs and torso (1,2). Giant cell arteritis (temporal arteritis), with its associated high risk of eye involvement, may occur in association with PMR, the incidence having been shown to be between 6% (3) and 50% (4), but it also occurs without PMR. The etiology and pathogenesis of these syndromes are not known, although, together with the clinical findings, serologic abnormalities indicative of active inflammation are almost always present. These abnormalities include an elevated erythrocyte sedimentation rate (ESR) in most, but not all, cases (5,6) and increased concentrations of various acute-phase plasma proteins (7,8) and of liver enzymes such as alkaline phosphatase and γ-glutamyl transferase (9). These nonspecific abnormalities provide diagnostic evidence; the ESR has been widely used for this purpose and for monitoring the patient's response to therapy. Treatment with oral prednisolone is effective in all cases, and progress is usually very rapid, provided a sufficient dose is given (10). In patients with temporal arteritis, this form of prompt intervention is mandatory in order to minimize the risk of loss of sight.

Although previous studies have established the correlation at presentation between disease activity and objective indices such as ESR and serum C-reactive protein (CRP) (7,8), and have demonstrated normalization once clinical remission has been induced, the relative rates of response of these variables during induction of remission have not previously been precisely monitored. We report here a prospective serial study in which patients with PMR were evaluated clinically in detail, and their levels of ESR, serum CRP, and hepatic enzymes were monitored at frequent intervals after starting prednisolone therapy. Our results indicate that serum CRP responds much more rapidly than the ESR and, furthermore, it returns to normal by day 7–14 in almost all cases. This information provides a framework for using the CRP measurement on a real-time basis in the objective assessment and management of PMR.

PATIENTS AND METHODS

Thirteen patients (12 women and 1 man) with a mean age of 67 years (range 58–82), who presented to the rheumatology clinics at King's College and Lewisham Hospitals during a 6-month period, were included in the study. The diagnosis of PMR was made on the basis of established criteria (7,11), including the complaint of severe proximal upper limb stiffness and pain lasting for an hour or more each morning. The mean duration of symptoms at presentation was 9.3 months (range 6–18 months), and none of the patients had received any medication before the diagnosis was made. Two patients who also had pain and tenderness over the temporal artery, which was associated with blurring of vision, underwent temporal artery biopsy; the sample from only 1 of these patients showed giant cell arteritis. It was not considered justifiable or necessary to perform biopsies on the remaining patients who had typical PMR.

Patients who had PMR without proven temporal arteritis were given prednisolone at a dosage of 15 mg/day for 1 week and 10 mg/day for the second week. The dosage was subsequently reduced by 1 mg/day/week to reach the lowest dosage capable of maintaining clinical remission. Patients with temporal arteritis were given prednisolone at a dosage of 60 mg/day for 1 week and 50 mg/day for the second week. Subsequently, the dosage was reduced by 5 mg/day/week until the lowest dosage able to maintain clinical remission was achieved. All these patients remained in complete clinical remission for at least the next 12 months.

All patients were assessed clinically on days 0 (initial presentation), 3, 7, and 14 by the same observer (RKM). Samples of venous blood were obtained at the time of clinical assessment and were drawn at approximately the same time each day to minimize the possibility of diurnal variation in the ESR (12). The duration (in minutes) of muscle stiffness (MS) was recorded. The pain scale (PS) was represented by a 10-cm horizontal visual analog scale (13). The ESR was measured by the Westergren method (14). Hemoglobin, alkaline phosphatase, and γ-glutamyl transferase were estimated by standard laboratory methods, and CRP was measured by electroimmunoassay as previously described (15). The coefficient of variation of CRP values was <10% both between and within assays, and the lower limit of sensitivity of the test was 0.1 mg/dl. For healthy subjects, the serum CRP concentration is <0.3 mg/dl in 90% of the subjects and <1.0 mg/dl in 99% (16).

The statistical significance of correlations between the ESR values and MS or PS was calculated using linear regression analysis, and the significance of correlations between CRP levels and MS or PS was determined using Spearman's rank correlation coefficient. Student's *t*-test was used to analyze the significance of differences in hemoglobin concentration obtained over time.

RESULTS

At presentation to the clinic, and before initiation of steroid therapy, both the CRP concentration and the ESR were elevated in all patients. Prednisolone caused a rapid improvement in symptoms, which was closely paralleled by a fall in the CRP value in all patients (Figure 1), so that the CRP level was normal in 11 of 13 patients by day 7, and in 12 of 13 patients by

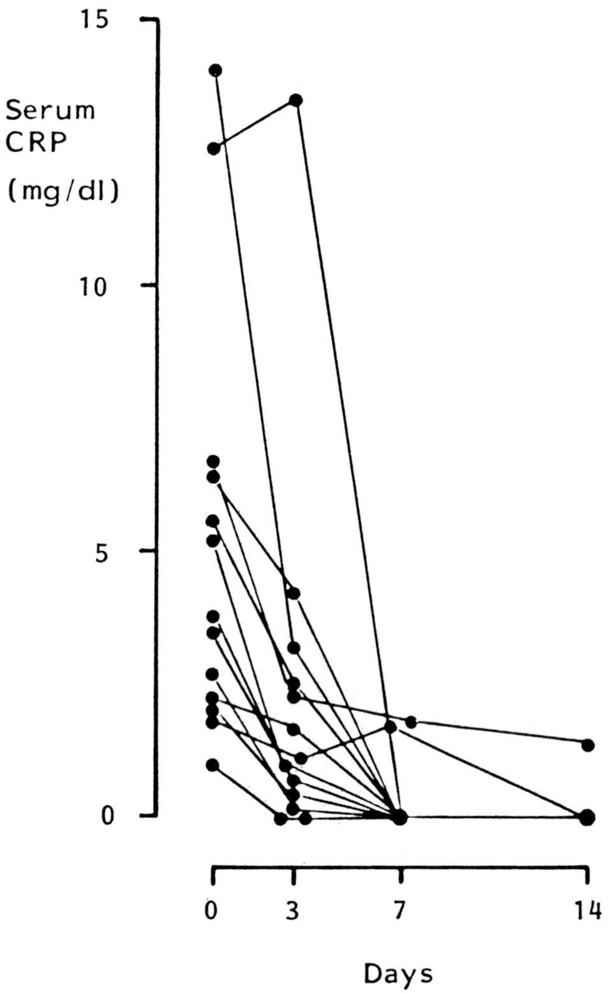

Figure 1. Effect of steroid therapy on serum C-reactive protein (CRP) concentration in 13 patients with polymyalgia rheumatica.

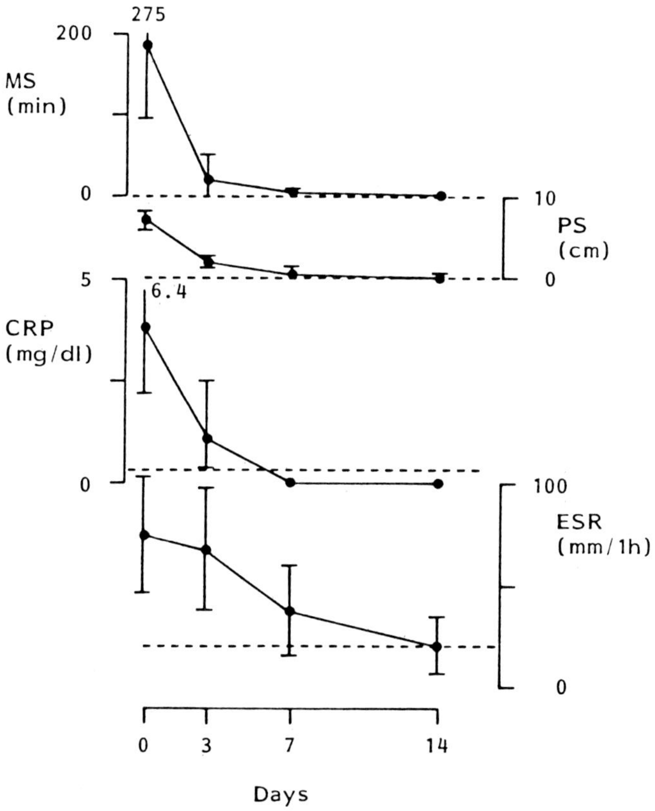

Figure 2. Response to steroid therapy of subjective and objective indices of disease activity in polymyalgia rheumatica. For muscle stiffness (MS), the pain scale (PS), and the erythrocyte sedimentation rate (ESR), each point represents the mean ± SD; for C-reactive protein (CRP), each point represents the median and interquartile range.

Table 1. Correlation between subjective and objective indices of disease activity during steroid treatment of polymyalgia rheumatica*

	Day 0	3	7	14
CRP with MS				
r_s	0.8109	0.7197	0.6329	0.9000
P	<0.01	<0.01	<0.02	<0.02
ESR with MS				
r	0.5287	0.3922	0.5010	0.2301
P	<0.05	NS	<0.05	NS
CRP with PS				
r_s	0.8230	0.4132	0.4263	0.6592
P	<0.01	NS	NS	<0.02
ESR with PS				
r	0.7041	0.2583	0.1601	0.1880
P	<0.01	NS	NS	NS

* CRP = C-reactive protein; MS = muscle stiffness; r_s = Spearman's correlation coefficient; ESR = erythrocyte sedimentation rate; r = linear correlation coefficient; NS = not significant; PS = pain scale. See Patients and Methods for details.

day 14. In marked contrast, the ESR responded much more slowly (Figure 2). The different response rates of these 2 nonspecific indices of disease activity were reflected by significantly higher correlation coefficients between the CRP level and the subjective clinical variables than those between the ESR and these variables (Table 1).

The serum concentrations of hepatic enzymes, alkaline phosphatase, and γ-glutamyl transferase, were elevated in a proportion of patients, presumably reflecting the systemic nature of the disease in these individuals. All patients with a high γ-glutamyl transferase concentration (7 of 13) also had elevated levels of alkaline phosphatase. Two other patients presented with high levels of alkaline phosphatase, but without abnormal γ-glutamyl transferase levels. The levels of these enzymes fell during induction of remission but did so more slowly than the CRP or even the ESR, and they did not correlate closely with the clinical manifestations (data not shown).

Since there were only 2 patients with temporal arteritis in this series, it was not possible to conduct any statistical analysis; however, there seemed to be no difference in the quality of these patients' symptomatic or objective responses to prednisolone. Similarly, there was no difference in response between patients with raised levels of hepatic enzymes and those without.

A further, interesting, feature of PMR observed in this study was that, although there was, overall, no significant anemia at presentation (hemoglobin 11.97 ± 1.17 gm/dl, mean ± SD), the hemoglobin concentration rose steadily over the first 14 days of treatment (12.23 ± 1.19 gm/dl on day 3, 13.00 ± 1.23 gm/dl on day 7, and 13.31 ± 0.93 gm/dl on day 14). The value obtained on day 14 was significantly higher than that obtained at presentation ($P < 0.005$).

DISCUSSION

The CRP is the classic acute-phase plasma protein which is produced by hepatocytes in response to most forms of tissue injury, inflammation, or infection (17). Its concentration in serum increases rapidly, from trace amounts in healthy subjects to levels which closely reflect the extent and activity of underlying disease. With spontaneous or therapeutically induced remission, the serum CRP value falls equally as quickly, with a half-life of 5–8 hours. Measurement of serum CRP has been well established as a sensitive means of objectively assessing disease activity (18).

In contrast, the ESR depends on the plasma concentration of fibrinogen, immunoglobulin, and some acute-phase globulins, all of which have half-lives of days or weeks, as well as on the number, size, and conformation of the erythrocytes (19). Therefore, the ESR generally responds more slowly to exacerbation and to remission of disease activity than does CRP.

Measurements of CRP, other acute-phase proteins, and of ESR in patients with PMR have been reported previously (7,8). However, in one report (7), although many patients were studied, many of them were tested more than once, the number of tests per patient varied, and yet all the results were pooled together for analysis. Furthermore, only some of the individuals were studied serially during progress of their disease. In the other study (8), only semiquantitative and relatively insensitive assays for CRP were used. For these reasons, information may have been obscured; nonetheless, a clear correlation of CRP and ESR with each other and with disease activity was observed.

Although we investigated a smaller number of patients, our study was prospective, each individual was very carefully assessed clinically with respect to the major symptoms of muscle stiffness and pain, and ESR and CRP levels were measured over the period when clinical changes were occurring most rapidly in response to introduction of steroid therapy. Our results show clearly that a fall in CRP value occurred rapidly, closely paralleling the improvement in symptoms, and did so more quickly and over a greater incremental range than did the ESR. The serum CRP concentration was restored to normal by steroid therapy at the same time the symptoms were abolished. In contrast, although the ESR fell, it remained above normal in many patients.

It is interesting to compare these results with those obtained from monitoring the behavior of serum CRP in other inflammatory diseases of unknown etiology, particularly as it relates to treatment with steroids and other antiinflammatory or immunosuppressive drugs. For example, in systemic vasculitis (including polyarteritis nodosa, microscopic polyarteritis, and Wegener's granulomatosis), treatment with both cyclophosphamide and steroids seems to be required to induce remission and control the disease. However, when this is achieved, the CRP level falls rapidly to normal and remains there as long as remission is maintained (20,21). Also during this phase, there is no extension of lesions or deterioration of organ function. In rheumatoid arthritis, however, in which the serum CRP concentration closely reflects clinical and radiologic assessment of disease activity, it is rare for the CRP value to fall within the normal range—even during clinical remission and even while receiving steroid treatment (22,23). This may be because the dosage required to completely abolish disease activity is so high that an unacceptable incidence of side effects occurs, and such steroid dosages are therefore rarely given.

The therapeutic response to steroids in PMR patients is known to be rapid and dramatic, so much so that initiation of steroid therapy is sometimes used as a diagnostic test (11). Nevertheless, an objective test for disease activity remains important for proper management of the PMR patient, and not simply as a means of independently confirming the diagnostic impression of clinical improvement. Individuals differ in their subjective response to and reporting of symptoms such as muscle pain and stiffness, and the patient's assessment of these conditions may be complicated by the euphoric effect of steroids. Our results demonstrate that the behavior of serum CRP, unlike that of the ESR, reflects precisely and concurrently the classic response to steroid treatment. Furthermore, for all patients whose CRP decreased to within the range of normal, their disease remained in remission, with minimal steroid dosage, for the next 12 months.

REFERENCES

1. Barber HS: Myalgic syndrome with constitutional effects: polymyalgia rheumatica. Ann Rheum Dis 16:230–237, 1957
2. Calamia KT, Hunder GG: Clinical manifestations of giant cell (temporal) arteritis. Clin Rheum Dis 6:389–403, 1980
3. Hunder GG, Allen GL: The relationship between polymyalgia rheumatica and temporal arteritis. Geriatrics 28:134–142, 1973
4. Malmvall BE, Bengtsson BA: Giant cell arteritis: clinical features and involvement of different organs. Scand J Rheumatol 7:154–158, 1978
5. Healey LA, Wilske KR: Manifestations of giant cell arteritis. Med Clin North Am 61:261–270, 1977
6. Ellis ME, Ralston S: The ESR in the diagnosis and management of the polymyalgia rheumatica/giant cell arteritis syndrome. Ann Rheum Dis 42:168–170, 1983
7. Park JR, Jones JG, Hazleman BL: Relationship of the erythrocyte sedimentation rate to acute phase proteins in polymyalgia rheumatica and giant cell arteritis. Ann Rheum Dis 40:493–495, 1981

8. Eshaghian J, Goeken JA: C-reactive protein in giant cell (cranial, temporal) arteritis. Ophthalmology 87:1160–1166, 1980
9. Dickson ER, Maldonado JE, Sheps SG, Cain JA: Systemic giant-cell arteritis with polymyalgia rheumatica: reversible abnormalities of liver function. JAMA 224:1496–1498, 1973
10. Huston KA, Hunder GG, Lie JT, Kennedy RH, Elveback LR: Temporal arteritis: a 25-year epidemiologic, clinical and pathologic study. Ann Intern Med 88:162–167, 1978
11. Hunder GG, Hazleman BL: Giant cell arteritis and polymyalgia rheumatica, Textbook of Rheumatology. Vol. 2. Edited by WN Kelley, ED Harris Jr, S Ruddy, CB Sledge. Philadelphia, WB Saunders, 1981, pp 1189–1196
12. Mallya RK, Berry H, Mace BEW, de Beer FC, Pepys MB: Diurnal variation of erythrocyte sedimentation rate related to feeding. Lancet i:389–390, 1982
13. Berry H, Huskisson EC: Treatment of rheumatoid arthritis. Clin Trials J 9:13–15, 1972
14. International Committee for Standardisation in Haematology: Reference method for the erythrocyte sedimentation rate (ESR) test on human blood. Br J Haematol 23:671–673, 1973
15. Fagan EA, Dyck RF, Maton PN, Hodgson HJF, Chadwick VS, Petrie A, Pepys MB: Serum levels of C-reactive protein in Crohn's disease and ulcerative colitis. Eur J Clin Invest 12:351–359, 1982
16. Shine B, de Beer FC, Pepys MB: Solid phase radioimmunoassays for C-reactive protein. Clin Chim Acta 117:13–23, 1981
17. Pepys MB: C-reactive protein fifty years on. Lancet i:653–657, 1981
18. Pepys MB, Baltz ML: Acute phase proteins with special reference to C-reactive protein and related proteins (pentaxins) and serum amyloid A protein. Adv Immunol 34:141–212, 1983
19. Pepys MB: Acute phase phenomena, The Science and Practice of Clinical Medicine: Rheumatology and Immunology. Edited by AS Cohen. New York, Grune & Stratton, 1979, pp 85–89
20. Hind CRK, Winearls CG, Lockwood CM, Rees AJ, Pepys MB: Objective monitoring of activity in Wegener's granulomatosis by measurement of serum C-reactive protein concentration. Clin Nephrol 21:341–345, 1984
21. Hind CRK, Savage CO, Winearls CG, Pepys MB: Objective monitoring of disease activity in polyarteritis by measurement of serum C-reactive protein concentration. Br Med J 288:1027–1030, 1984
22. Amos RS, Constable TJ, Crockson RA, Crockson AP, McConkey B: Rheumatoid arthritis: relation of serum C-reactive protein and erythrocyte sedimentation rates to radiographic changes. Br Med J 1:195–197, 1977
23. Mallya RK, de Beer FC, Berry H, Hamilton EDB, Mace DEW, Pepys MB: Correlation of clinical parameters of disease activity in rheumatoid arthritis with serum concentration of C-reactive protein and erythrocyte sedimentation rate. J Rheumatol 9:224–228, 1982

ATROPHIC GASTRITIS IN SJÖGREN'S SYNDROME

Morphologic, Biochemical, and Immunologic Findings

C. P. J. MAURY, T. TÖRNROTH, and A-M. TEPPO

Gastric studies were carried out in 16 patients with well-documented Sjögren's syndrome (SS), 43 matched rheumatic disease patients without SS, and 7 patients with chronic atrophic gastritis not associated with SS. Chronic atrophic gastritis was a much more common finding in the SS patients than in the rheumatic disease control patients. Significant hypopepsinogenemia was present in 11 of 16 SS patients. In 6 patients this was combined with hypergastrinemia, a combination highly specific for chronic atrophic gastritis. The lowest pepsinogen levels were seen in patients with primary SS associated with high levels of SS-B antibody. On a histologic and biochemical basis, it was not possible to distinguish the gastric findings in primary SS from those in secondary SS, nor to distinguish chronic atrophic gastritis associated with SS from that not associated with SS. We conclude that chronic atrophic gastritis is a prominent feature in SS and that the severity of the gastritis appears to correlate with some serologic parameters of SS.

Sjögren's syndrome (SS) is a systemic autoimmune disease in which destructive inflammatory cell infiltration of the lacrimal and salivary glands gives rise to the characteristic sicca component (1). Systemic manifestations include vasculitis, renal tubular acidosis, thyroiditis, interstitial pulmonary fibrosis, and myositis (1–5). Gastric studies in SS have revealed deranged acid secretion (6,7), hypopepsinogenemia (8), autoantibodies to parietal cells (7,9), and inflammatory cell infiltration in gastric mucosa (7,10,11). It is not known, however, to what extent the gastric findings are specific for SS, nor if there is any correlation between the degree of gastritis and serologic parameters of the disease.

Since recent studies have revealed immunologic and genetic differences between primary and secondary SS (12–14), a comparison of the gastric findings in these 2 forms of the disease was of interest. We therefore performed gastroscopic, morphologic, biochemical, and serologic studies in patients with primary and secondary SS, and report our findings here.

PATIENTS AND METHODS

Patients. Sixteen female SS patients, with a mean age of 58 years (range 35–72), were studied prospectively. Eight patients had primary SS (sicca complex without other associated connective tissue/autoimmune disease) and 8 had secondary SS. The associated diseases in the latter patients were rheumatoid arthritis (3 patients), primary biliary cirrhosis and arthritis (2 patients), systemic lupus erythematosus (1 patient), mixed connective tissue disease (1 patient), and unclassified polyarthritis (1 patient). Sicca complex features found in the patients and major medications taken are shown in Table 1.

All SS patients had normal serum creatinine levels; 1 had renal tubular acidosis. Endoscopic examination was performed on all patients. Nausea and epigastric pain were common symptoms. Six of the SS patients had complained of prolonged dyspepsia.

Forty-three female rheumatic disease patients with-

From the Fourth Department of Medicine, University of Helsinki, Helsinki, Finland.

Supported by the Sigrid Juselius Foundation, Helsinki, Finland.

C. P. J. Maury, MD: Senior Lecturer in Medicine; T. Törnroth, MD: Senior Lecturer in Pathology; A-M. Teppo, MSc: Clinical Chemist.

Address reprint requests to Dr. C. P. J. Maury, Fourth Department of Medicine, University of Helsinki, Unioninkatu 38, SF-00170 Helsinki, Finland.

Submitted for publication December 12, 1983; accepted in revised form October 23, 1984.

Table 1. Sicca complex features and major medications taken by 8 female patients with primary Sjögren's syndrome (SS) and 8 female patients with secondary SS*

		Lacrimal gland findings			Salivary gland findings			
Patient	Age	Xerophthalmia	Schirmer's test	Rose bengal stain	Xerostomia	Minor salivary gland biopsy	Sialography	Major medication
Primary SS								
1	35	+	+	+	+	+	NS	Ibuprofen
2	42	+	+	+	+	NS	+	–
3	59	+	+	+	+	+	NS	Aspirin
4	60	+	+	+	+	+	NS	–
5	68	+	+	+	+	+	NS	–
6	68	+	+	+	+	+	+	Methylprednisolone
7	69	+	+	+	+	NS	NS	–
8	72	+	+	+	+	+	+	Ibuprofen
Secondary SS								
9	35	+	+	+	+	+	+	Prednisone
10	38	+	–	NS	+	NS	+	Prednisone
11	50	+	+	+	+	+	+	Ibuprofen
12	60	+	+	NS	+	NS	NS	Gold
13	61	+	+	+	+	+	+	Prednisone
14	66	+	+	+	+	+	NS	Prednisone
15	67	+	+	NS	+	NS	NS	Prednisone
16	70	+	NS	NS	+	+	+	Prednisone

* + = positive finding; – = negative finding; NS = not studied.

out any signs or symptoms of SS (30 with rheumatoid arthritis, 5 with systemic lupus erythematosus, 5 with polymyalgia rheumatica, and 3 with systemic sclerosis), with a mean age of 61 years (range 29–77), all receiving some form of antirheumatic medication (gold/steroids/nonsteroidal antiinflammatory drugs), served as the matched control group. All were undergoing upper gastrointestinal endoscopy because of various epigastric complaints. Seven female patients, with a mean age of 54 years (range 30–68), with chronic atrophic gastritis but no SS were also included in the study. All control patients had normal renal function. Informed consent was obtained from all subjects undergoing endoscopy.

Histology. One to four mucosal biopsy specimens were taken at random from the corpus of the stomach for morphologic and biochemical studies. For histologic examination, the specimens were fixed in 10% neutral buffered formaldehyde and embedded in paraffin. Sections were stained with hematoxylin and eosin and alcian blue–periodic acid–Schiff and assessed blindly.

Specimens were classified according to common criteria for gastritis (15,16), with special attention to inflammatory cell infiltration, atrophy of gland layer, and metaplasia. "Inflammatory epithelial destruction" was recorded when there was infiltration of the foveolar area, including surface and crypt epithelium, by neutrophilic granulocytes, i.e., alterations reflecting an acute inflammatory component. Each morphologic parameter was graded in severity from + (mild, slight) to +++ (severe, abundant). The findings in the corpus biopsies from individual patients were usually similar; if there were inter-biopsy differences, the classification was based on the most representative specimens.

Carbohydrate analysis. For glycoconjugate analysis, the biopsy specimens were homogenized in water and analyzed for monosaccharides by gas-liquid chromatography as described previously (17–19) and for protein as described by Hartree (20). A Perkin-Elmer Model 900 gas chromatograph, with hydrogen flame ionization detectors and nitrogen as carried gas, was used. Columns (2 m × 3 mm) were packed with 2.2% SE-30 Gas Chrom Q.

Biochemical and immunologic assays. Serum pepsinogen I was measured by radioimmunoassay (21,22). Serum β_2-microglobulin was assayed by the Phadebas β-2-micro Test (Pharmacia, Uppsala, Sweden) as previously described (23). Antibodies to SS-A were measured by double immunodiffusion in 0.6% agarose gel using saline-soluble extract (24) from acetone powder or rabbit thymus (Pel-Freez Biologicals, Rogers, AR) as antigen. The specificity of the precipitin lines was confirmed with reference sera obtained from Dr. Eng Tan (Scripps Clinic and Research Foundation, La Jolla, CA). Antibodies to SS-B were assayed by enzyme immunoassay (25). Other assays were carried out by commonly used laboratory methods.

Statistical analysis. Chi-square test and linear regression analysis using the least squares method were used in the statistical calculations.

Table 2. Morphologic features of gastritis in Sjögren's syndrome (SS) patients (based on endoscopic mucosal biopsies from the corpus of the stomach)

		Chronic atrophic gastritis		
Patients (n)	Superficial gastritis	Mild	Moderate	Severe
Primary SS (8)	1	3	2	2
Secondary SS (8)	2	3	1	2
Total (16)	3	6	3	4

Table 3. Summary of morphologic changes in gastric mucosa of patients with Sjögren's syndrome (SS)

Finding	Primary SS (n = 8)	Secondary SS (n = 8)	All SS patients (n = 16)
Inflammatory epithelial destruction			8 (50%)
Mild	–	1	
Moderate	3	3	
Severe	–	1	
Round cell infiltration, foveolar area			12 (75%)
Slight	3	1	
Moderate	2	4	
Abundant	1	1	
Round cell infiltration, gland layer and muscularis mucosae			15 (94%)
Slight	1	2	
Moderate	4	3	
Abundant	3	2	
Atrophy of gland layer			13 (81%)
Mild	3	3	
Moderate	2	1	
Severe	2	2	
Metaplasia, intestinal			7 (44%)
Mild	1	3	
Moderate	2	1	
Metaplasia, pseudopyloric			6 (38%)
Mild	3	1	
Moderate	1	1	
Amyloidosis	–	1	1 (6%)

RESULTS

Histologic findings. Thirteen of the 16 patients with SS (81%) had chronic atrophic gastritis, compared with 15 of the 43 age-, sex-, and medication-matched rheumatic disease controls (35%) ($P < 0.01$). The morphologic findings in the endoscopic gastric corpus biopsy specimens from the SS patients are summarized in Tables 2 and 3. Four SS patients, 2 with primary and 2 with secondary SS, had severe atrophic gastritis. Seven of the 8 patients with primary SS had atrophic gastritis.

Histologically it was not possible to distinguish the gastric findings in the primary SS patients from those in the secondary SS patients, nor to distinguish chronic atrophic gastritis associated with SS from that not associated with SS. Typical gastric mucosal findings in the SS patients are shown in Figures 1–3. No obvious correlations were observed between the degree of gastrointestinal symptoms and the endoscopic or histologic findings.

Mucosal glycoconjugate patterns. The composition of monosaccharides of the mucosal glycoconjugates was similar in the primary SS and the secondary SS patients (Table 4). This pattern was also similar to that found in the patients with atropic gastritis not associated with SS.

Laboratory features of chronic gastritis in SS patients. Hypopepsinogenemia was found in 11 of 16

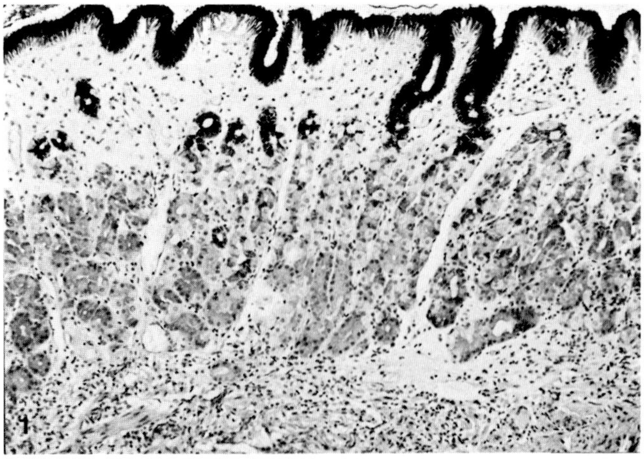

Figure 1. Biopsy specimen from a patient with Sjögren's syndrome, showing mild atrophy of mainly the deep part of the gland layer, with slight infiltration of round cells (alcian blue–periodic acid–Schiff stained, original magnification × 115).

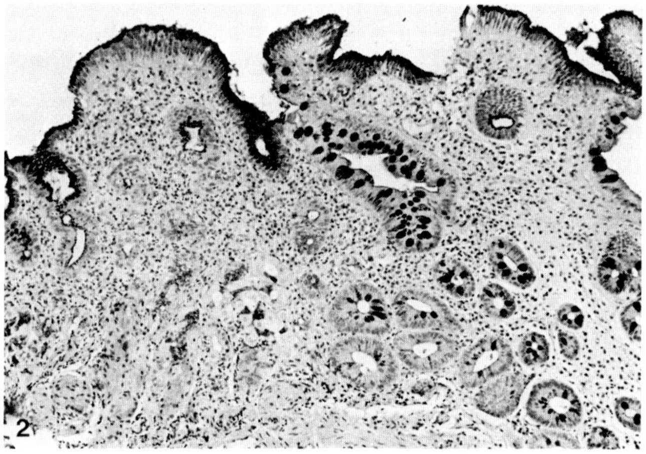

Figure 2. Biopsy specimen from a patient with Sjögren's syndrome, showing moderate atrophic gastritis, with moderate intestinal metaplasia (goblet cells stained dark) and moderate inflammatory cellular infiltration (alcian blue–periodic acid–Schiff stained, original magnification × 115).

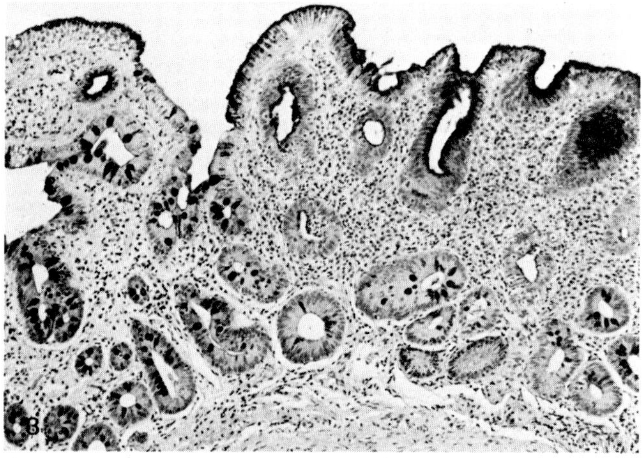

Figure 3. Biopsy specimen from a patient with Sjögren's syndrome, showing severe atrophy, with complete loss of body glands, severe intestinal metaplasia, and moderate inflammatory cellular infiltration (alcian blue–periodic acid–Schiff stained, original magnification × 115).

patients with SS (69%) (Table 5). In 6 patients this was combined with elevated serum gastrin (>100 pmoles/liter), a combination highly specific for atrophic gastritis (26). Only 2 patients had parietal cell antibodies (1 with atrophic gastritis, 1 without); none had intrinsic factor antibodies. No patient had overt pernicious anemia. Seven of the patients had hemoglobin values <12.0 mg/dl (range 9.7–11.5); 6 of them had secondary SS.

Serum pepsinogen I and gastric mucosal morphology. Figure 4 illustrates the relationship between serum pepsinogen I levels and gastric mucosal histology. As shown, all patients with moderate and severe atrophic gastritis had hypopepsinogenemia.

Serologic profiles of SS patients. High erythrocyte sedimentation rate, high immunoglobulin and β_2-microglobulin levels, low C4 level, and rheumatoid factor positivity were characteristic findings in the patients (Table 6). Three of the 5 patients with high SS-B antibody levels (1.55, 0.74, and 0.73 absorbance units, respectively) had primary SS; they were the same patients who had the lowest serum pepsinogen levels (6, 7, and 3 μg/liter, respectively). Three of the patients had antibodies against the nuclear antigen SS-A.

Serum pepsinogen I levels correlated positively with serum vitamin B_{12} levels (r = 0.59, $P < 0.05$) and negatively with erythrocyte sedimentation rate (r = −0.54, $P < 0.05$). Serum pepsinogen tended to correlate negatively with serum β_2-microglobulin (r = −0.40, not significant) and IgA (r = −0.37, not significant).

DISCUSSION

A previous study from this laboratory showed that in SS the type of lymphocytic infiltrations in the gastric mucosa corresponds to that in the salivary glands (11). Moreover, serum β_2-microglobulin levels, which correlate with the degree of lymphocytic infiltration in the salivary glands (27), also correlate negatively with serum pepsinogen I (8) and, hence, with the degree of chronic gastritis (28–30).

Table 4. Monosaccharide composition of mucosal glycoconjugates in patients with primary Sjögren's syndrome (SS), patients with secondary SS, and patients with atrophic gastritis without SS*

Patient group (n)	Mannose	Galactose	N-acetylgalactosamine	N-acetylglucosamine	Sialic acid
Primary SS (8)	6.1 ± 2.4	9.6 ± 6.1	10.4 ± 5.2	11.6 ± 4.4	1.5 ± 0.7
Secondary SS (8)	5.2 ± 1.5	8.6 ± 3.3	11.7 ± 3.1	12.1 ± 2.2	1.6 ± 0.3
Atrophic gastritis without SS (7)	5.4 ± 1.6	9.9 ± 4.7	12.2 ± 4.8	11.5 ± 4.8	2.3 ± 1.5

* Values represent the relative amount of monosaccharide/protein and are mean ± SD. Differences between the patient groups were not significant for any of the values (Student's *t*-test).

Table 5. Laboratory features of chronic gastritis in Sjögren's syndrome (SS) patients

Parameter	Primary SS (n = 8)	Secondary SS (n = 8)	All SS patients (n = 16)
Serum pepsinogen I <20 μg/liter	6	5	11 (69%)
Serum gastrin >100 pmoles/liter	4	2	6 (38%)
Serum pepsinogen I <20 μg/liter + serum gastrin >100 pmoles/liter	4	2	6 (38%)
Parietal cell antibodies	1	1	2 (13%)
Intrinsic factor antibodies	0	0	0

In this study the degree of hypopepsinogenemia appeared to correlate with some serologic parameters, such as erythrocyte sedimentation rate, IgA level, and, in patients with primary SS, high SS-B antibody titer. This does not mean that the chronic gastritis in SS is solely due to the SS, however. In fact, it is very probable that other factors, e.g., age, contribute to the gastric pathology seen in this disease.

The frequency of atrophic gastritis is age-dependent. In a population study (31), atrophic gastritis was found in 41% of the subjects aged 41–65 years, which roughly corresponds to the age distribution of the SS patients in the present study. In our age-matched rheumatic disease controls, atrophic gastritis was found in 35%, which corresponds to the age-expected figure. This is, however, significantly less than that found among the SS patients (81%), suggesting that the age factor can only be a contributory one.

In patients with secondary SS, the associated connective tissue/autoimmune disease may contribute to the gastric changes. However, there were no obvious differences in the gastric mucosal findings between our primary and secondary SS patients. Moreover, the control rheumatic disease patients without SS had no more atrophic gastritis than expected on the basis of age. These findings are in keeping with those of our previous study (8) which showed that serum pepsinogen I levels, reflecting gastric secretory capacity and degree of chronic gastritis (21,26,28,30), were similar in rheumatoid arthritis patients without SS and in healthy controls, whereas matched rheumatoid arthritis patients with SS had significantly depressed pepsinogen levels.

The role of antirheumatic medication in the pathogenesis of the gastric changes in SS is unclear. The present results suggest that medication is of minor importance, however, since the control rheumatic disease patients, who were receiving antirheumatic medication, had no increased frequency of atrophic gastritis. In addition, no obvious relationship was observed between the type, dosage, and duration of medication and the histologic findings in SS. Finally, 4 of the patients with primary SS were not regularly receiving any medication, but had endoscopically and histologically verified atrophic gastritis.

Previous studies have demonstrated achlorhydria (6,7), chronic inflammatory cell infiltration of

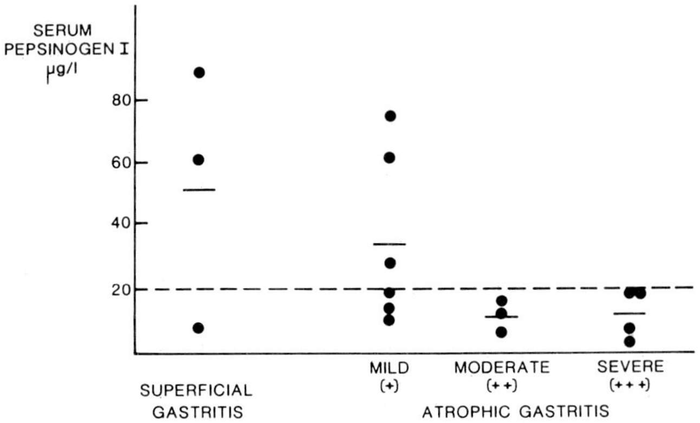

Figure 4. Relationship between serum level of pepsinogen I and type of gastritis in Sjögren's syndrome.

Table 6. Laboratory findings in Sjögren's syndrome (SS) patients

Condition	Primary SS (n = 8)	Secondary SS (n = 8)	All SS patients (n = 16)
Erythrocyte sedimentation rate >30 mm/hour	5	7	12 (75%)
C-reactive protein >5 mg/liter	3	4	7 (44%)
Rheumatoid factor, Rose-Waaler titer >80	5	4	9 (56%)
IgG >16.3 gm/liter*	6	4	10 (63%)
IgM >2.9 gm/liter*	2	3	5 (31%)
IgA >5.8 gm/liter*	2	1	3 (19%)
Antinuclear antibodies, titer ≥100	2	1	3 (19%)
Complement C4 <0.20 gm/liter	5	4	9 (56%)
SS-B antibodies >0.35 absorbance units (ref. 37)	3	2	5 (31%)
SS-A antibodies + (ref. 24)	1	2	3 (19%)
β_2-microglobulin >2.5 mg/liter*	3	5	8 (50%)

* Reference value is the mean + 2 SD of that found in healthy controls (refs. 38,39).

gastric mucosa (7,10,11), and parietal cell antibodies (7,9) in patients with SS, whereas pernicious anemia is a rare finding (32,33). None of the SS patients in the present series had overt pernicious anemia, but interestingly, there was a significant positive correlation between serum pepsinogen I and vitamin B_{12} levels.

High frequencies of parietal cell antibodies have been reported in patients with SS (7,9). Among our SS patients we found only 2 (13%) with parietal cell antibodies; of the 13 SS patients with atrophic gastritis, only 1 (8%) had these antibodies. This frequency is considerably lower than that reported earlier (37–67%) in individuals with chronic atrophic gastritis not selected for family history of pernicious anemia (34–36). Although the frequency of parietal cell antibodies will, obviously, depend on the severity of atrophic gastritis, the low frequency of autoantibodies we found in gastritis associated with SS suggests that the pathogenesis of atrophic gastritis in this disease could differ from that of "seropositive" gastritis. Further studies on this question are needed.

ACKNOWLEDGMENTS

We thank Drs. P. Sipponen and I. Kääriäinen for their advice.

REFERENCES

1. Bloch KJ, Buchanan WW, Wohl MJ, Bunim JJ: Sjögren's syndrome: a clinical, pathological, and serological study of sixty-two cases. Medicine (Baltimore) 44:187–231, 1965
2. Pavlidis NA, Karsh J, Moutsopoulos HM: The clinical picture of primary Sjögren's syndrome: a retrospective study. J Rheumatol 9:685–690, 1982
3. Alexander EL, Provost TT, Stevens MB, Alexander GE: Neurologic complications of primary Sjögren's syndrome. Medicine (Baltimore) 61:247–257, 1982
4. Moutsopoulos HM, Webber BL, Vlagopoulos TP, Chused TM, Decker JL: Differences in the clinical manifestations of sicca syndrome in the presence and absence of rheumatoid arthritis. Am J Med 66:733–736, 1979
5. Gumpel JM: Sjögren's syndrome. Br Med J 285:1598, 1982
6. Morgan AD, Raven RW: Sjögren's syndrome: a general disease. Br J Surg 40:154–162, 1952
7. Buchanan WW, Cox AG, Harden RM, Glen AIM, Anderson JR, Grey KG: Gastric studies in Sjögren's syndrome. Gut 7:351–354, 1966
8. Maury CPJ, Räsänen V, Teppo A-M, Helve T, Wegelius O: Serum pepsinogen I in rheumatic diseases: reduced levels in Sjögren's syndrome. Arthritis Rheum 25:1059–1063, 1982
9. Adams JF, Glen AIM, Kennedy EH, MacKenzie IL, Morrow JH, Anderson JR, Grey KG, Middleton DG: The histological and secretory changes in the stomach in patients with autoimmunity to gastric parietal cells. Lancet I:401–402, 1964
10. Von Jebavy M, Hradsky M, Herout B: Gastric biopsy in patients with Sjögren's syndrome. Z Med Lab Diagn 16:930–935, 1961
11. Kilpi A, Bergroth V, Konttinen YT, Maury CPJ, Reitamo S, Wegelius O: Lymphocyte infiltrations of the gastric mucosa in Sjögren's syndrome: an immunoperoxidase study using monoclonal antibodies in the avidin-biotin-peroxidase method. Arthritis Rheum 26:1196–1200, 1983
12. Alspaugh MA, Talal N, Tan EM: Differentiation and characterization of autoantibodies and their antigens in Sjögren's syndrome. Arthritis Rheum 19:216–222, 1976
13. Akizuki M, Boehm-Truitt MJ, Kassan SS, Steinberg AD, Chused TM: Purification of an acidic nuclear protein antigen and demonstration of its antibodies in subsets of patients with sicca syndrome. J Immunol 119:932–938, 1977
14. Moutsopoulos HM, Mann DL, Johnson AM, Chused TM: Genetic difference between primary and secondary sicca syndrome. N Engl J Med 301:761–763, 1979
15. Whitehead R: Mucosal biopsy of the gastrointestinal tract, Major Problems in Pathology. Second edition. Vol. 3. Edited by JL Bennington. Philadelphia, WB Saunders, 1979, p 11
16. Morson BC, Dawson IMP: Gastrointestinal Pathology. Second edition. Oxford, Blackwell, 1979, p 91
17. Clamp JR: Analysis of glycoproteins. Biochem Soc Symp 40:3–16, 1974
18. Bhatti T, Chambers RE, Clamp JR: The gas chromatographic properties of biologically important N-acetylglucosamine derivatives, monosaccharides, disaccharides, trisaccharides, tetrasaccharides and pentasaccharides. Biochim Biophys Acta 222:339–347, 1970
19. Maury CPJ: Carbohydrate patterns of endoscopic mucosal biopsies in cancer of the stomach and chronic gastritis. Clin Chim Acta 126:155–159, 1982
20. Hartree EF: Determination of protein: a modification of the Lowry method that gives a linear photometric response. Anal Biochem 48:422–427, 1972
21. Samloff IM, Liebman WM: Radioimmunoassay of group I pepsinogens in serum. Gastroenterology 66:494–502, 1974
22. Räsänen V: A radioimmunoassay for group I pepsinogens in human serum. J Clin Chem Clin Biochem 18:700, 1980
23. Evrin PE, Wibell L: The serum levels and urinary excretion of β_2-microglobulin in apparently healthy subjects. Scand J Clin Lab Invest 29:69–74, 1972
24. Kurata N, Tan EM: Identification of antibodies to nuclear acidic antigens by counterimmunoelectrophoresis. Arthritis Rheum 19:574–580, 1976
25. Teppo A-M: Enzyme immunoassay of antibodies to

Sjögren's syndrome B antigen. Clin Chem 27:1341–1345, 1981

26. Varis K, Samloff IM, Ihamäki T, Siurala M: An appraisal of tests for severe atrophic gastritis in relatives of patients with pernicious anemia. Dig Dis Sci 24:187–191, 1979
27. Michalski JP, Daniels TE, Talal N, Grey HM: $Beta_2$ microglobulin and lymphocytic infiltration in Sjögren's syndrome. N Engl J Med 293:1228–1231, 1975
28. Stemmerman GN, Samloff IM, Nomura A, Walsh JH: Serum pepsinogen I and gastrin in relation to extent and location of intestinal metaplasia in the surgically resected stomach. Dig Dis Sci 25:680–687, 1980
29. Nomura AMY, Stemmerman GN, Samloff IM: Serum pepsinogen I as a predictor of stomach cancer. Ann Intern Med 93:537–540, 1980
30. Samloff IM, Varis K, Ihamäki T, Siurala M, Rotter J: Relationships among serum pepsinogen I, serum pepsinogen II and gastric mucosal histology: a study in relatives of patients with pernicious anemia. Gastroenterology 83:204–209, 1982
31. Siurala M, Isokoski M, Varis K, Kekki M: Prevalence of gastritis in a rural population: bioptic study of subjects selected at random. Scand J Gastroenterol 3:211–223, 1968
32. Williamson J, Paterson RW, McGavin DD, Whaley K: Sjögren's syndrome in relation to pernicious anemia and idiopathic Addison's disease. Br J Ophthalmol 54:31–36, 1950
33. Wegelius O, Fyhrquist F, Adner P-L: Sjögren's syndrome associated with vitamin B_{12} deficiency. Acta Rheum Scand 16:184–190, 1970
34. Coghill NF, Doniach D, Roitt IM: Autoantibodies in simple atrophic gastritis. Gut 6:48–53, 1965
35. Fisher JM, Taylor KB: A comparison of autoimmune phenomena in pernicious anemia and chronic atrophic gastritis. N Engl J Med 272:499–503, 1965
36. Varis K, Krohn K, Isokoski M, Siurala M: Circulating antibodies in gastritis. Acta Med Scand 185:369–372, 1969
37. Manthorpe R, Teppo A-M, Bendixen G, Wegelius O: Antibodies to SS–B in chronic inflammatory connective tissue diseases: relationship with HLA–Dw2 and HLA–Dw3 antigens in primary Sjögren's syndrome. Arthritis Rheum 25:662–667, 1982
38. Teppo A-M, Maury CPJ: Serum prealbumin, transferrin and immunoglobulins in fatty liver, alcoholic cirrhosis and primary biliary cirrhosis. Clin Chim Acta 129:279–286, 1983
39. Maury CPJ, Helve T, Sjöblom C: Serum β_2-microglobulin, sialic acid, and C-reactive protein in systemic lupus erythematosus. Rheumatol Int 2:145–149, 1982

PHAGOCYTOSIS AND INTRACELLULAR KILLING BY POLYMORPHONUCLEAR CELLS FROM PATIENTS WITH RHEUMATOID ARTHRITIS AND FELTY'S SYNDROME

FERDINAND C. BREEDVELD, MARIA T. VAN DEN BARSELAAR, PETER C. J. LEIJH, ARNOLD CATS, and RALPH VAN FURTH

The present in vitro study concerned the phagocytosis and intracellular killing by polymorphonuclear cells (PMN) of 5 patients with rheumatoid arthritis (RA) and 12 patients with Felty's syndrome (FS). PMN phagocytosis was assessed by microbiologic and morphologic methods, and intracellular killing was measured independently of continuous phagocytosis of viable bacteria (*Staphylococcus aureus*). PMN from patients with RA or FS ingested *S aureus* opsonized with immunoglobulins and complement as effectively as did PMN from healthy donors. However, the capacity of patient PMN to ingest *S aureus* opsonized with sera lacking complement activity, e.g., heat-inactivated donor serum and the sera of 2 patients with FS, was lower than that of healthy donor PMN. This decreased ingestion is associated with diminished expression of Fc receptors on the membrane of PMN from patients who have RA or FS. As with sera lacking complement activity, decreased capacity to ingest *S aureus* was observed after preloading donor PMN with immune aggregates, which also decreased the expression of Fc receptors. PMN from patients with RA or FS were found to be as active in killing *S aureus* as cells from healthy donors.

Patients with rheumatoid arthritis (RA) or Felty's syndrome (FS) have frequent bacterial infections (1–3). It has been shown that this susceptibility to infections cannot be related solely to the degree of leukopenia (4,5). Although susceptibility to infections has been reported to be due to polymorphonuclear cell (PMN) dysfunction, the published results are not consistent, and both a normal and a decreased rate of phagocytosis by PMN from RA and FS patients have been described (6–16). The bactericidal activity of RA and FS PMN has also been found to be normal in some studies (12,17,18) and decreased in others (9,13). This decreased phagocytosis and bactericidal activity has been attributed to previous phagocytosis of immune complexes.

The conflicting results concerning the phagocytic and bactericidal activities of PMN from RA and FS patients might be due to the assay methods used and to the simultaneous measurement of phagocytosis and intracellular killing, which will mask any defect in either of the phases of the phagocytic process. Phagocytosis of particles opsonized with immunoglobulins and complement is initiated by binding of the coated particles to C3 and Fc receptors in the membrane of the phagocyte. Recently, decreased expression of Fc receptors on PMN from patients with RA or FS has been ascribed to previous ingestion of immune complexes (19).

In the present study, the phagocytosis and

From the Departments of Rheumatology and Infectious Diseases, University Hospital, Leiden; the Department of Rheumatology and the Department of Internal Medicine and Infectious Diseases, University of Leiden, The Netherlands.

Ferdinand C. Breedveld, MD: Department of Rheumatology, University Hospital, Leiden; Maria T. van den Barselaar: Technologist, Department of Infectious Diseases, University Hospital, Leiden; Peter C. J. Leijh, PhD: Department of Infectious Diseases, University Hospital, Leiden; Arnold Cats, MD: Professor of Medicine and Chairman, Department of Rheumatology, University of Leiden; Ralph van Furth, MD: Professor of Medicine and Chairman, Department of Internal Medicine and Infectious Diseases, University of Leiden, The Netherlands.

Address reprint requests to F. C. Breedveld, MD, Department of Rheumatology, University Hospital, PO Box 9600, 2300 RC, Leiden, The Netherlands.

Submitted for publication June 11, 1984; accepted in revised form October 19, 1984.

intracellular killing of *Staphylococcus aureus* by PMN from patients with RA or FS were investigated using various in vitro methods. Since the ingestion of immune aggregates by PMN from these patients might affect cell functions, the effect of immune aggregates on the functional activities of donor PMN was also studied. In addition, the involvement of complement in the ingestion of *S aureus* by PMN and the effect of immune aggregates on this involvement were investigated.

PATIENTS AND METHODS

Patients. Five patients with definite RA, according to the American Rheumatism Association criteria (20), and 12 patients with FS (definite RA with spontaneous, sustained leukopenia of $<2.0 \times 10^9$ PMN/liter and splenomegaly) were investigated. At the time of investigation, none of the patients was receiving corticosteroids or cytostatic drugs, and none had an infection. None of the patients had taken antibiotics for at least 3 weeks prior to the beginning of the study.

Isolation of PMN. Eighty milliliters of heparinized blood was added to a 5% solution of dextran in buffered saline (molecular weight 2,000,000; 3 ml of solution to 10 ml of blood) and incubated for 30 minutes at 37°C. Leukocytes were collected from the leukocyte-rich plasma by centrifugation for 10 minutes at 110*g*, washed twice with phosphate buffered saline (PBS) containing 0.5 units of heparin/ml, and suspended in Hanks' balanced salt solution (HBSS) containing 0.1% gelatin (gelatin-HBSS) at a concentration of 1×10^7 PMN/ml. The cell preparations contained at least 90% PMN. The viability of the PMN, determined by trypan blue exclusion, was always >98%.

Preparation of sera. In all experiments, we used sera prepared from the blood of patients or healthy AB donors. The blood was clotted for 1 hour at room temperature, centrifuged for 20 minutes at 1,100*g*, and stored in 2-ml aliquots at −20°C until use (no longer than 2 months). Heat-inactivated serum was prepared by heating the serum for 30 minutes at 56°C. Human IgG was isolated from heat-inactivated donor serum by ammonium sulfate precipitation and anion exchange chromatography on DEAE cellulose. Aggregated human IgG (AIgG) was prepared by heating a solution of 17.4 mg/ml of purified human IgG at 63°C for 30 minutes.

Serologic studies. Rheumatoid factor was determined by latex fixation, according to established methods (21), and antinuclear antibodies were determined by indirect immunofluorescence (22). The serum concentrations of IgM, IgG, and IgA were measured by agarose gel electrophoresis and immunoelectrophoresis (23). Immune complexes were measured by the C1q binding assay (C1q-BA) (24); the amount of immune complexes was expressed as microgram equivalents of a standard of aggregated IgG (25). Complement activity was expressed as the total hemolytic complement activity (CH50), determined by the method of Mayer (26); C1q, C1 inhibitor, C3, and C4 levels were measured by radial immunodiffusion using monospecific antisera (27). C3–C9 levels were determined hemolytically (28). Functional activities of C1 inhibitor (29) and C2 (30) were assessed using appropriate hemolytic assays.

Demonstration of intracytoplasmic immunoglobulins on fixed PMN. Intracytoplasmic immunoglobulins were studied in cytocentrifuge preparations of PMN suspensions, which were dried at room temperature, fixed in 96% alcohol containing 5% acetic acid at −20°C for 15 minutes, and washed in PBS for 1 hour at 4°C. The PMN preparations were incubated with fluorescein isothiocyanate–labeled antisera against human IgG (Nordic, Tilburg, The Netherlands), IgA, or IgM (Dakopats, Copenhagen, Denmark) for 30 minutes at room temperature in a moist chamber. After a 10-minute wash in PBS, the preparations were immersed in a drop of 90% glycerol, and the fluorescence was scored semiquantitatively as grade 0 = no fluorescence, grade 1 = small inclusions, grade 2 = more and clear inclusions, grade 3 = many large inclusions. At least 300 cells in each preparation were scored. The percentage of cells assigned to each grade was multiplied by that grade number, and the fluorescence score for each experimental condition was expressed as the sum of these products.

Fc receptors. The presence of Fc receptors on PMN was demonstrated by means of a rosetting technique using ox erythrocytes coated with rabbit IgG anti-ox erythrocytes, as previously described (19).

Microorganisms. *S aureus* (type 42D) were stored on agar slants at 4°C, cultured overnight in Nutrient Broth No. 2 (Oxoid, Ltd., London, England), harvested by centrifugation for 10 minutes at 1,500*g*, washed twice with PBS, and suspended at a concentration of 10^7 microorganisms/ml in gelatin-HBSS. Preopsonization of microorganisms was performed by incubating 5×10^6 bacteria/ml with 10% serum for 30 minutes at 37°C, under rotation at 4 revolutions per minute. Excess serum was removed by centrifugation, at 1,500*g* for 10 minutes, and 2 washes with ice-cold gelatin-HBSS. Finally, the bacteria were resuspended at a concentration of 10^7 microorganisms/ml in gelatin-HBSS.

Phagocytosis. *Microbiologic assay*. Phagocytosis was determined by measuring the decrease in the number of viable extracellular bacteria during incubation of 5×10^6 PMN/ml with 5×10^6 bacteria/ml and 10% serum, for 60 minutes at 37°C, and rotation at 4 rpm (31). At various times, samples were subjected to differential centrifugation for 4 minutes at 110*g* to separate PMN and bacteria; the number of viable bacteria in the supernatant was then determined microbiologically. Phagocytosis at a given time was expressed as the percentage decrease from the initial number of viable extracellular bacteria.

Morphologic assay. Phagocytosis was also measured morphologically. For these studies, 5×10^6 PMN/ml and 5×10^6 *S aureus*/ml were incubated in the presence of 10% serum for 60 minutes at 37°C, and at 4 rpm. The suspension was then cooled to 4°C and subjected to differential centrifugation for 4 minutes at 110*g*. The PMN were incubated with 1 unit of lysostaphin/ml (Sigma, St. Louis, MO) for 5 minutes at 37°C to lyse all extracellular *S aureus* (32), and washed once with HBSS before cytopreparations were made. After fixation and Giemsa staining, phagocytosis, expressed as the number of intracellular bacteria per 100 PMN, was determined microscopically.

Intracellular killing. Intracellular killing of *S aureus*

Table 1. Clinical, hematologic, and serologic data on 12 patients with Felty's syndrome (FS) and 5 patients with rheumatoid arthritis (RA)*

Patient no., age/sex	Years duration of RA and of FS	PMN, $\times 10^6$/liter	ESR, mm/hour	Infections	Spleen size	ANA titer	RF titer	Treatment, daily dose
Felty's syndrome								
1, 66/F	31, 5	1,020	128	Pneumonia, cystitis, ulcerations, skin abscesses, died of septicemia	+	$1:10^{-2}$	$1:2^{-17}$	Ibuprofen 500 mg
2, 68/F	13, ½	1,020	133	Osteomyelitis, ulcerations, skin abscesses, died of septicemia	+	$1:10^{-2}$	$1:2^{-16}$	Naproxen 750 mg, D-penicillamine 500 mg
3, 53/F	7, 2	1,700	83	Cystitis	+	$1:10^{-3}$	$1:2^{-15}$	None
4, 75/M	33, 22	360	60	None	+	$1:10^{-2}$	$1:2^{-10}$	Paracetamol 1,500 mg
5, 59/F	13, 4	1,250	59	Cystitis, sinusitis	+	1:1	$1:2^{-10}$	Ibuprofen 800 mg
6, 61/F	13, 2	1,800	60	Cystitis	+	$1:10^{-2}$	$1:2^{-14}$	Naproxen 750 mg
7, 77/F	37, 4	1,160	97	Cystitis	+	$1:10^{-2}$	$1:2^{-16}$	Paracetamol 2,000 mg
8, 79/F	4, 2	500	32	Bronchitis, diverticulitis	+	1:1	$1:2^{-14}$	Indomethacin 50 mg, chloroquine 100 mg
9, 77/F	29, 10	1,500	23	Cystitis, bronchitis	+	1:10	$1:2^{-10}$	Azapropazone 600 mg, chloroquine 200 mg
10, 36/F	13, 3	1,980	82	Ulcerations, skin abscesses	+	$1:10^{-3}$		Indomethacin 100 mg, chloroquine 100 mg
11, 51/M	30, 15	100	60	Ecthyma gangrenosum, septic arthritis	+	$1:10^{-3}$	$1:2^{-12}$	Ibuprofen 600 mg
12, 68/M	25, 9	600	68	None	+	1:10	$1:2^{-10}$	Naproxen 500 mg
Rheumatoid arthritis								
1, 73/M	3, NA	3,220	128	None	–	–	$1:2^{-12}$	Indomethacin 150 mg, sodium aurothiomalate 50 mg
2, 82/F	21, NA	5,680	63	Cystitis	–	–	$1:2^{-11}$	Ibuprofen 800 mg, chloroquine 100 mg
3, 80/M	16, NA	4,250	140	Bronchitis	–	1:10	$1:2^{-12}$	Naproxen 1,000 mg
4, 62/F	13, NA	3,440	30	None	–	–	$1:2^{-7}$	Ibuprofen 700 mg, sodium aurothiomalate 50 mg
5, 78/M	20, NA	4,280	72	None	–	$1:10^{-2}$	$1:2^{-12}$	Paracetamol 1,500 mg, D-penicillamine 250 mg

* PMN = polymorphonuclear cells; ESR = erythrocyte sedimentation rate. Spleen measured by isotope scanning, + = enlarged; – = normal. Antinuclear antibody (ANA) titer is the highest dilution giving a positive reaction. Rheumatoid factor (RF) titer, by latex fixation, is the highest dilution giving a positive reaction. NA = not applicable.

can be determined by measuring the decrease in the number of viable intracellular bacteria during incubation of PMN containing *S aureus* (33). For this purpose, 5×10^6 PMN/ml was incubated with 5×10^6 preopsonized bacteria/ml for 3 minutes at 37°C, and at 4 rpm; phagocytosis was stopped by shaking the tube in crushed ice. The noningested bacteria were removed by differential centrifugation (4 minutes at 110*g*) and 2 washes with ice-cold HBSS. The cells containing ingested bacteria were reincubated at 37°C and 4 rpm in HBSS containing 10% serum. At 0, 60, and 120 minutes, a 0.5-ml sample was taken. Intracellular killing was stopped by adding 0.5 ml of ice-cold HBSS, and the suspension was centrifuged for 4 minutes at 110*g*. After removal of the supernatant, distilled water containing 0.01% bovine albumin was added to disrupt the PMN, and the number of viable intracellular bacteria was determined by a microbiologic plate method. Intracellular killing is expressed as the percentage decrease from the initial number of viable intracellular bacteria.

Statistical analysis. For statistical analysis of the occurrence of cytoplasmic immunoglobulins and circulating immune complexes, multiple regression analysis was used; the results are expressed as the correlation coefficient (r) and the *P* value for regression.

RESULTS

Clinical, hematologic, and serologic data obtained on our patients are listed in Table 1. Felty's

Table 2. Additional serologic data on 12 patients with Felty's syndrome and 5 patients with rheumatoid arthritis*

Patient no.	CIg (normal <10)	C1q-BA (normal <10 μg eq/ml)	CH50 (normal 256–580 units/ml)	C4 (normal 16.3–30.1 mg %)	C3 (normal 54.7–73.3 mg %)
Felty's syndrome					
1	ND	583	1	2	56
2	639	1,117	1	12	86
3	671	687	51	12	68
4	0	20	331	13	59
5	89	83	576	32	104
6	583	104	407	32	106
7	597	798	148	10	74
8	166	165	395	39	114
9	60	0	317	10	71
10	700	800	110	17	68
11	ND	478	282	24	100
12	0	0	890	23	103
Rheumatoid arthritis					
1	650	630	79	22	83
2	76	63	548	39	108
3	61	189	471	24	101
4	4	0	396	34	194
5	75	4	879	22	88

* Cytoplasmic immunoglobulins (CIg) were scored semiquantitatively; the value represents the sum of the scores for IgG, IgA, and IgM. C1q-BA = C1q binding assay. See Patients and Methods for details. ND = not done.

syndrome patients 1, 2, 8, and 11 were admitted to the hospital because of severe infections; patients 1 and 2 eventually died of septicemia from large skin ulcers infected with *S aureus*. The other patients did not develop major infections. Felty's syndrome patients 1 and 2 were the only patients considered to have active rheumatoid disease, i.e., weight loss, severe arthralgias, joint swelling, high erythrocyte sedimentation rate, anemia, and dermal vasculitis.

Additional serologic data on all patients are shown in Table 2. Ten patients with FS and 3 patients with RA had circulating immune complexes, as measured by the C1q-BA. All patients had normal or elevated serum levels of IgG, IgM, and IgA (data not shown).

Determination of the complement activity revealed an extremely low total hemolytic complement activity (CH50) in FS patients 1 and 2. Normal or elevated C3 concentrations were found in all sera; 6 patients with FS had decreased C4 activity in their sera. Detailed investigation of the sera of FS patients 1 and 2 revealed not only low C4 concentrations (Table 2), but also decreased C2 activity, 730 units/ml and 728 units/ml, respectively (normal 1,830–2,330), and normal levels of C1q, C1 inhibitor, and the C3–9 complex. A pattern of decreased C4 and C2 concentration with normal amounts of the other complement components implies complement activation via the classical pathway (34).

Cytoplasmic immunoglobulins in PMN. Cytoplasmic immunoglobulins were detected in PMN from 12 of the 15 patients investigated (Table 2). IgG, IgA, and IgM were always present simultaneously. There was a linear relationship between the sum of the score for phagocytosed cytoplasmic IgG, IgM, and IgA and the levels of circulating immune complexes in each serum (C1q-BA: $r = 0.86$, $P < 0.001$) (Table 2). The immunofluorescence score for PMN of healthy controls was always <10.

Phagocytosis of *S aureus* by PMN. Phagocytosis of *S aureus* by RA and FS PMN, measured microbiologically at a bacteria:cell ratio of 1:1 in the presence of donor or autologous serum, was normal for all patients (data not shown). Incubation of 5×10^6 donor PMN/ml and 5×10^6 bacteria/ml in the presence of 10% of each patient serum showed no difference in phagocytosis whether in the presence of patient serum or donor serum. In control experiments to investigate a possible bactericidal activity of patient serum, a suspension of 5×10^6 *S aureus*/ml in gelatin-HBSS was incubated with 10% patient serum. The number of viable bacteria increased in all cases, except with the

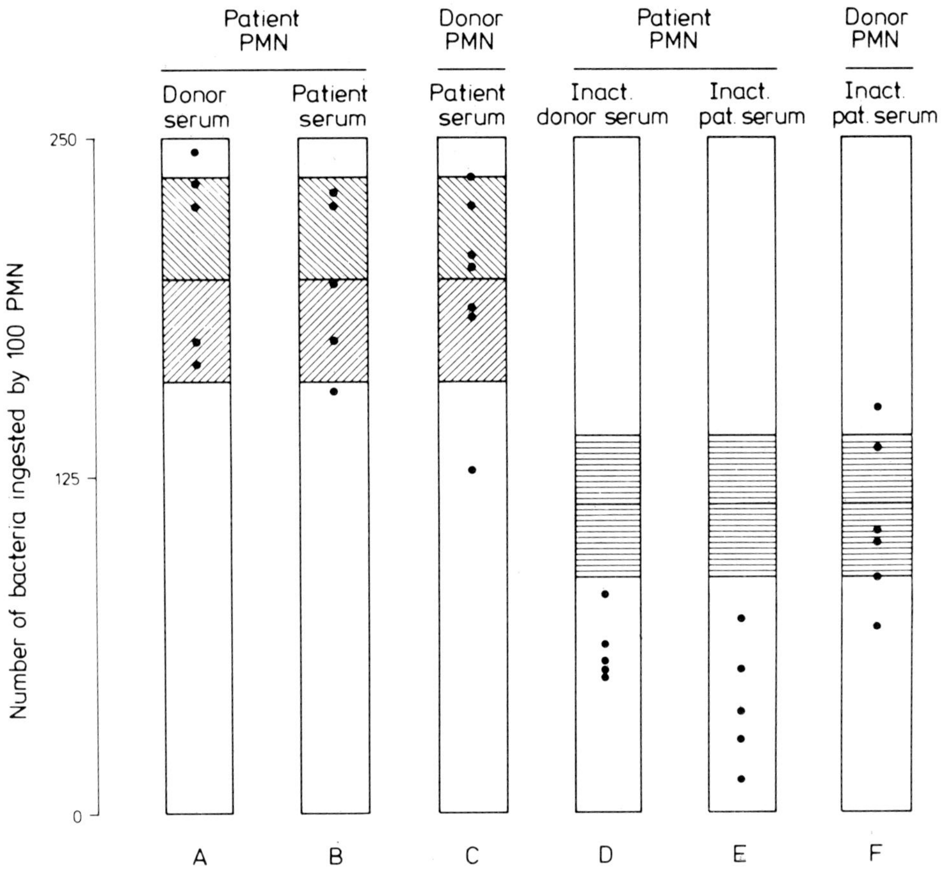

Figure 1. Morphologic assessment of phagocytosis of *Staphylococcus aureus* by polymorphonuclear cells (PMN). (See Patients and Methods for details.) Hatched areas represent ingestion of *S aureus* by PMN of healthy donors in the presence of either 10% fresh donor serum (**A**, **B**, and **C**) or 10% heat-inactivated donor serum (**D**, **E**, and **F**), mean ± 1 SD. Phagocytosis by PMN of **A**, Felty's syndrome (FS) patients in the presence of 10% fresh donor serum; **B**, FS patients in the presence of 10% fresh autologous patient serum; **C**, healthy donors in the presence of 10% serum from FS patients; **D**, FS patients in the presence of 10% heat-inactivated donor serum; **E**, FS patients in the presence of 10% heat-inactivated autologous patient serum; and **F**, healthy donors in the presence of 10% heat-inactivated patient serum.

sera of FS patients 1, 2, and 10, for which the number of viable bacteria decreased in the absence of PMN. This decrease was found to be due to agglutination of bacteria and subsequent sedimentation during centrifugation, as observed microscopically.

Because of this effect on the number of bacteria in the supernatant seen with the 3 FS patients' sera, no conclusions can be drawn concerning phagocytosis by PMN in the presence of these particular sera. To overcome this problem, which obscures any findings about phagocytosis based on the microbiologic assay, phagocytosis was also measured morphologically. The results showed that in the presence of donor and autologous patient serum, PMN from FS patients ingest *S aureus* to the same degree as normal donor PMN (Figures 1A and B). Because FS patients 1 and 2 died during the period of this study, it was impossible to perform these experiments with PMN from these patients. Donor PMN ingested *S aureus* in the presence of patient serum (including serum from FS patient 2) as effectively as in the presence of donor serum, except in the case of the serum from FS patient 1, which showed a slight decrease of ingestion (Figure 1C).

To investigate phagocytosis by patient PMN in the absence of complement, 5×10^6 PMN and 5×10^6

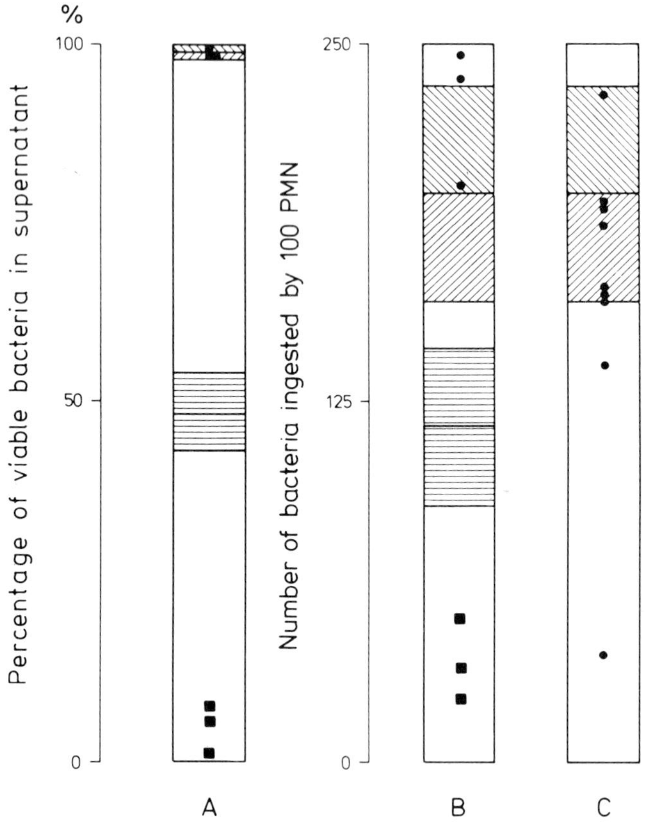

Figure 2. Phagocytosis of *Staphylococcus aureus*, in the presence of fresh and heat-inactivated donor serum, by healthy donor polymorphonuclear cells (PMN) loaded with immune aggregates, as assessed microbiologically (**A**) and morphologically (**B** and **C**). (See Patients and Methods for details.) Hatched areas represent ingestion of *S aureus* by PMN of healthy donors in the presence of either 10% fresh donor serum (oblique hatching) or 10% heat-inactivated serum (horizontal hatching), mean ± 1 SD of 10 experiments. **A**, Microbiologic assessment: the decrease in the number of viable extracellular bacteria during incubation of aggregate-loaded PMN in the presence of 10% fresh donor serum (●) or 10% heat-inactivated donor serum (■). **B**, Morphologic assessment: the number of bacteria ingested by aggregate-loaded PMN in the presence of 10% fresh donor serum (●) or 10% heat-inactivated donor serum (■). **C**, Morphologic assessment: the number of bacteria ingested by aggregate-loaded PMN in the presence of 10% fresh Felty's syndrome (FS) patient serum (●); phagocytosis was decreased in the presence of sera from FS patients 1 and 2.

S aureus were incubated in the presence of heat-inactivated donor serum or autologous patient serum. These incubations all resulted in a significant decrease in phagocytosis of *S aureus* by patient PMN, compared with that by donor PMN under similar conditions ($P < 0.002$) (Figures 1D–F). The sera of FS patients 1 and 2 were not used in these experiments. In a limited number of experiments, phagocytosis was also determined after incubation of PMN with bacteria for 120 minutes. The results of these experiments showed no differences compared with those obtained at 60 minutes (data not shown).

Effect of various bacteria:cell ratios on the ingestion of *S aureus* by PMN from FS patients. To find out whether the capacity of the patient PMN to ingest *S aureus* was lower than that of PMN from healthy donors, PMN from FS patients 3, 10, and 11 were allowed to ingest bacteria in the presence of donor or autologous serum at bacteria:PMN ratios of 10:1 and 100:1, and phagocytosis was measured microbiologically. The results indicated that ingestion of *S aureus* by PMN from these patients and healthy donors was the same (data not shown).

Effect of intracellular AIgG on the ingestion of *S aureus*. Since PMN from RA and FS patients contain cytoplasmic immunoglobulins, a series of experiments was performed to find out whether ingested immune aggregates affect the subsequent ingestion of microorganisms. For this purpose, 5×10^6 donor PMN/ml were incubated with 1.7 mg/ml AIgG at 37°C for 30 minutes, and then washed twice to remove free aggregates. After this procedure, the cells showed strong immunofluorescence for cytoplasmic IgG, and the percentage of PMNs forming rosettes by means of their Fc receptors decreased from 79.2% (SD 7.2) to 22.6% (SD 8.8), means of 4 experiments. In control experiments, donor PMN were incubated with PBS under the same conditions; the percentage of PMNs forming rosettes did not change. Incubation of 5×10^6 aggregate-loaded PMN/ml and 5×10^6 *S aureus*/ml in the presence of 10% fresh donor serum, followed by measurement of phagocytosis with both the microbiologic and the morphologic assay, showed that ingestion of bacteria was comparable with that of donor PMN without immune aggregates (Figures 2A and B). Incubation in the presence of 10% heat-inactivated serum instead of fresh serum resulted in total inhibition of the phagocytosis of *S aureus* (Figures 2A and B).

In similar experiments performed with 10% FS sera, the ingestion of *S aureus* was comparable with that by donor sera, except in the case of sera from FS patients 1 and 2, which showed ingestion comparable with that observed using 10% heat-inactivated donor serum (Figure 2C). These results indicate that PMN containing immune aggregates are as active as cells without aggregates in terms of phagocytosis in the presence of an intact complement system, whereas

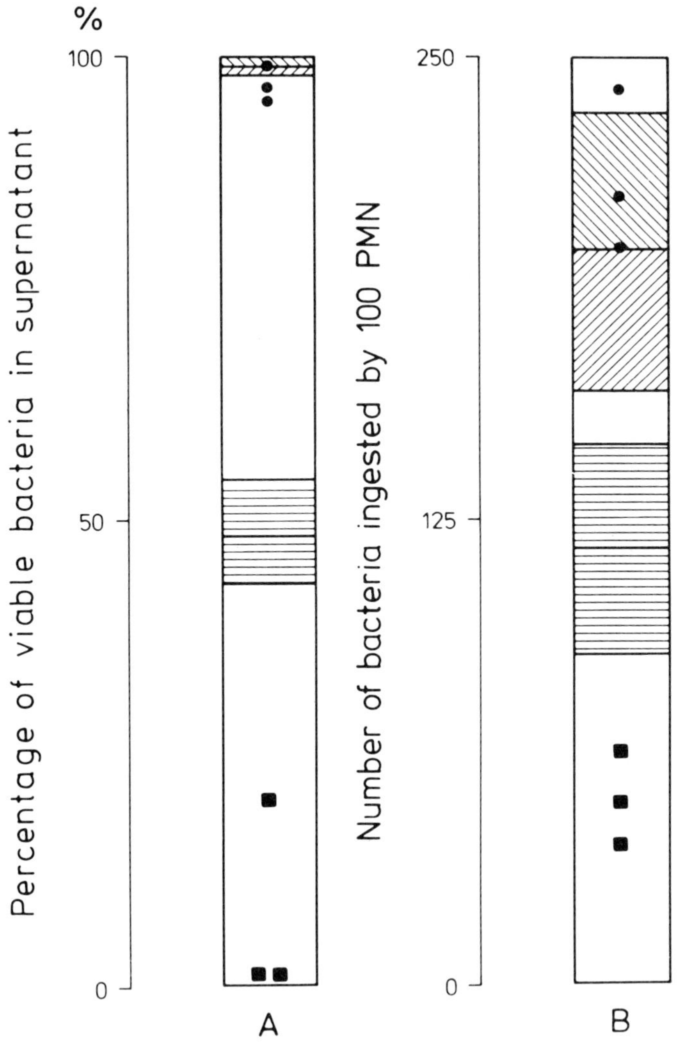

Figure 3. Phagocytosis of *Staphylococcus aureus* by polymorphonuclear cells (PMN) of healthy donors in the simultaneous presence of bacteria, serum, and aggregated human IgG (AIgG), as measured microbiologically (**A**) and morphologically (**B**). (See Patients and Methods for details.) Hatched areas represent the ingestion of *S aureus* by PMN of healthy donors in the presence of either 10% fresh donor serum (oblique hatching) or 10% heat-inactivated serum (horizontal hatching), mean ± 1 SD of 10 experiments. **A,** Microbiologic assessment: the decrease in number of viable extracellular bacteria during incubation of PMN with AIgG and 10% fresh donor serum (●) or 10% heat-inactivated serum (■). **B,** Morphologic assessment: the number of bacteria ingested by PMN in the presence of AIgG and 10% fresh donor serum (●) or 10% heat-inactivated donor serum (■).

ingestion in the presence of sera lacking complement activity is impaired.

Effects of extracellular AIgG on the ingestion of *S aureus*. To investigate the effect of extracellular immune aggregates on the phagocytosis of *S aureus*, 5×10^6 donor PMN/ml were incubated with 5×10^6 bacteria/ml, 1.7 mg/ml AIgG, and 10% fresh or heat-inactivated donor serum, for 60 minutes at 37°C, and at 4 rpm. The microbiologic and morphologic assays performed after coincubation of cells, bacteria, and aggregates in the presence of fresh serum showed that AIgG does not affect ingestion under these conditions (Figures 3A and B). However, phagocytosis was strongly affected when heat-inactivated serum and AIgG were present simultaneously (Figures 3A and B).

Intracellular killing. Incubation of RA and FS PMN containing bacteria, i.e., after phagocytosis by PMN of bacteria opsonized with donor serum for 3 minutes at 37°C, resulted in intracellular killing of *S aureus* similar to that by donor PMN; PMN from FS patients 1, 2, and 8 displayed a slightly decreased intracellular killing activity (Figure 4A; RA patients not shown). When the killing assay was performed after phagocytosis of bacteria opsonized with autologous patient serum, no killing by the PMN from FS patients 1 and 2 was seen (Figure 4B). A similar absence of killing was found for donor PMN when the killing assay was performed after phagocytosis of bacteria opsonized with serum from FS patient 1 or FS patient 2 (data not shown).

To investigate the decreased intracellular killing of bacteria opsonized with sera from FS patients 1 and 2 in more detail, control experiments were performed to determine the number of bacteria ingested at the start of the assay. Microscopic analysis of the PMN after 3 minutes of ingestion of bacteria showed intracellular bacteria at the start of the killing assay except when PMN were allowed to ingest bacteria preopsonized with sera from either FS patient 1 or FS patient 2, in which case large clumps of PMN and extra- and intracellular bacteria as well as areas of PMN without bacteria were observed. On the basis of these data, we concluded that the results of the intracellular killing assay performed after phagocytosis of bacteria opsonized with serum from FS patients 1 and 2 must be unreliable because of the presence of extracellular bacteria in the killing assay.

Effect of AIgG on the intracellular killing of *S aureus* by PMN. To investigate the effect of ingested immune aggregates on the intracellular killing of bacteria by PMN, 5×10^6 donor PMN/ml were incubated with 1.7 mg AIgG/ml at 37°C for 30 minutes and washed to remove free aggregates. Aggregate-loaded PMN were allowed to ingest bacteria opsonized with

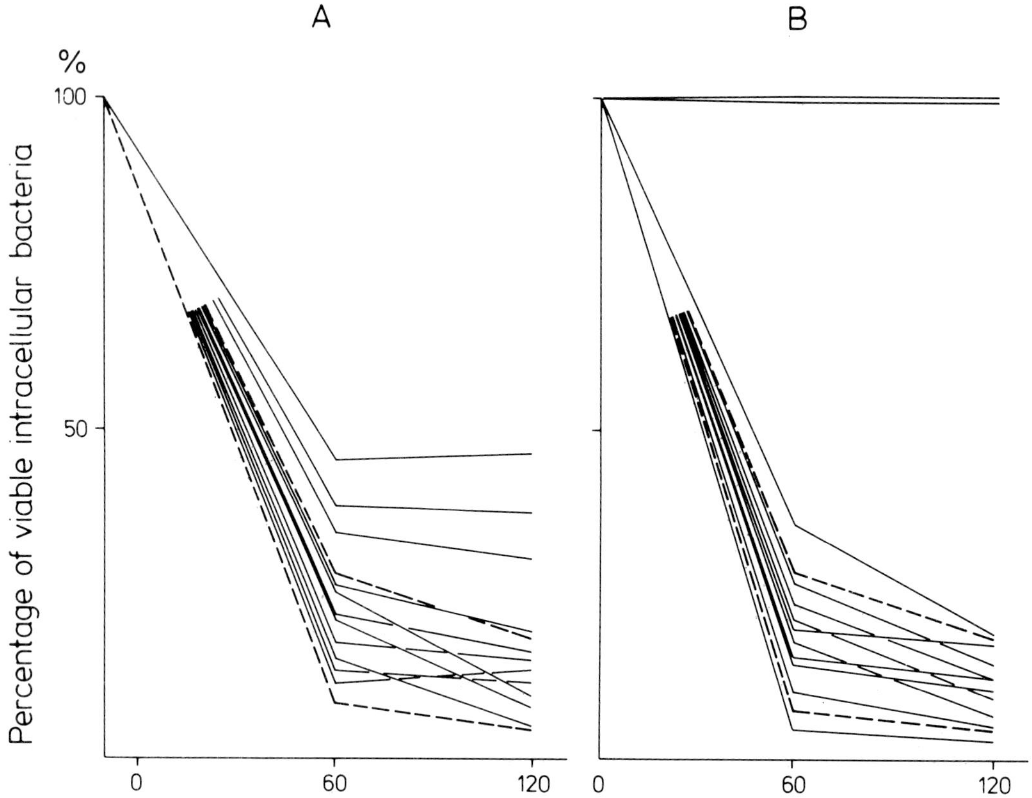

Figure 4. Intracellular killing of *Staphylococcus aureus* by polymorphonuclear cells (PMN) of Felty's syndrome patients. (See Patients and Methods for details.) The area between the dashed lines represents the decrease in the number of viable intracellular bacteria during incubation of donor PMN containing bacteria. **A,** Bacteria preopsonized with donor serum; **B,** Bacteria preopsonized with autologous patient serum. Numbers on the ordinate are the sampling times in minutes.

fresh donor serum for 3 minutes at 37°C before the killing assay was performed. Preincubation of the PMN with immune aggregates had almost no effect on the capacity of these cells to kill ingested *S aureus* (data not shown).

DISCUSSION

When PMN from RA and FS patients ingest immune complexes in vivo, the expression of Fc receptors on the cell membrane is decreased (19). Our findings indicate that the decreased expression of Fc receptors leads to impaired phagocytosis by patient PMN in the absence of complement, i.e., Fc receptor–mediated phagocytosis, compared with that of PMN of healthy donors. However, patient PMN have the same capacity as those of healthy donors to phagocytose microorganisms in the presence of an opsonizing serum containing immunoglobulins and complement.

A decrease in the expression of Fc receptors associated with impaired Fc receptor–mediated ingestion of bacteria was also observed for donor PMN after the ingestion of immune aggregates. Moreover, ingestion of bacteria was reduced in the presence of extracellular immune aggregates, due to competitive binding of aggregated IgG and IgG-coated bacteria to Fc receptors; these results are in agreement with previous reports (35,36). Serum from 2 patients (FS patients 1 and 2) agglutinated *S aureus*, thus disturbing the conditions for microbiologic assessment of phagocytosis and intracellular killing. This agglutination may be ascribed to interaction between antibacterial antibodies (expected to be present in high concentration in these patients with *S aureus*–infected skin ulcers) and rheumatoid factor. The ability of rheumatoid factor to enhance bacteria agglutination by antibacterial antibodies has been reported previously (37). Other factors present in the serum of FS patients 1 and 2, which may cause abnormal processing of bacteria by PMN, cannot be excluded, but the agglutination of *S aureus* by the sera makes it impossible to form any conclusion regarding such factors.

Furthermore, the present study showed not only that PMN from FS and RA patients have the same capacity to kill intracellular bacteria as PMN from healthy donors, but also that ingested immune complexes do not affect this functional activity. This observation differs from the findings of others (9,13), whose results must be questioned since, in the microbiologic assay they used, phagocytosis and intracellular killing were measured simultaneously.

Clinically, the 12 FS patients we investigated form a representative group for this syndrome. As has been reported in other series, our patients also had high titers of rheumatoid factor (4), antinuclear antibodies (38), circulating immune complexes, and cytoplasmic immune complexes in the PMN (39). Joint destruction was severe in most FS patients. Major infections were seen in FS patients 1, 2, 8, and 11, two of whom (patients 1 and 2) died of *S aureus* septicemia arising from skin ulcers. The sera of these 2 patients differed from those of the other patients; these sera induced agglutination of *S aureus* and were almost unable to activate complement via the classical pathway. The hypocomplementemia of these sera prevented C3 receptor–mediated phagocytosis, which, in turn, has a strong inhibitory effect on the phagocytic activity of patient PMN because of their decreased capacity to ingest bacteria via Fc receptors. Therefore, the lethal infections of FS patients 1 and 2 appear to be due to a decreased phagocytosis of bacteria by PMN. FS patients 8 and 11 developed infections together with extreme leukopenia.

The occurrence of infections in patients with FS compared with patients with RA, and the factors related to this, are presently being investigated in a larger group of FS and RA patients. Preliminary results indicate that FS patients' increased susceptibility to infections, compared with that of RA patients, is paralleled by the use of corticosteroids and immunosuppressive agents, the disabling joint destruction and sedentary lives of most FS patients, leukopenia of $<500 \times 10^6$/liter, and hypocomplementemia. In the clinical condition represented by FS patients 1 and 2, i.e., recurrent infections in patients with high levels of circulating immune complexes and with hypocomplementemia, therapy must be directed toward the restoration of C3 receptor–mediated phagocytosis. If the circulating immune complexes could be removed from the circulation and fresh serum supplied, serum complement activity might become normal, after which phagocytosis would improve and infections could be treated more efficiently.

ACKNOWLEDGMENTS

We are indebted to Dr. Mohammed R. Daha for the detection of serum complement activity, to Geertruida J. M. Lafeber for the detection of cytoplasmic immunoglobulins and the quantification of cells bearing Fc receptors, and to Gerda J. C. van den Hout for technical assistance.

REFERENCES

1. Baum J: Infection in rheumatoid arthritis. Arthritis Rheum 14:135–137, 1971
2. Barnes CG, Turnbull AL, Vernon-Roberts B: Felty's syndrome. Ann Rheum Dis 30:359–374, 1971
3. Moore RA, Brunner CM, Sandusky WR, Leavell BS: Felty's syndrome: long-term follow-up after splenectomy. Ann Intern Med 75:381–385, 1971
4. Ruderman M, Miller LM, Pinals RS: Clinical and serologic observations on 27 patients with Felty's syndrome. Arthritis Rheum 11:377–384, 1968
5. Thorne C, Urowitz MB: Long-term outcome in Felty's syndrome. Ann Rheum Dis 41:486–489, 1982
6. Bodel PT, Hollingsworth JW: Comparative morphology, respiration and phagocytic function of leucocytes from blood and joint fluid in rheumatoid arthritis. J Clin Invest 45:580–589, 1966
7. Brandt L, Hedberg H: Impaired phagocytosis by peripheral blood granulocytes in systemic lupus erythematosus. Scand J Haematol 6:348–353, 1969
8. Turner RA, Schumacher HR, Myers AR: Phagocytic function of polymorphonuclear leukocytes in rheumatic diseases. J Clin Invest 52:1632–1635, 1973
9. Gupta RC, Laforce FM, Mills DM: Polymorphonuclear leukocyte inclusions and impaired bacterial killing in patients with Felty's syndrome. J Lab Clin Med 88:183–193, 1976
10. Corberand J, Amiques J, De Larrard B, Pradere J: Neutrophil function in rheumatoid arthritis. Scand J Rheumatol 6:49–52, 1977
11. Hällgren R, Håkansson L, Venge P: Kinetic studies of phagocytosis. I. The serum independent particle uptake by PMN from patients with rheumatoid arthritis and systemic lupus erythematosus. Arthritis Rheum 21:107–113, 1978
12. Wilton JMA, Gibson T, Chuck CM: Defective phagocytosis by synovial fluid and blood polymorphonuclear leukocytes in patients with rheumatoid arthritis. I. The nature of the defect. Rheumatol Rehabil Suppl:25–35, 1978
13. Bültmann B, Geitner R, Seibold H, Kratsch G, Haferkamp O: Interaction of circulating immune complexes with granulocyte function in patients with rheumatoid arthritis. Klin Wochenschr 58:727–732, 1980

14. Wynne KM, Dieppe PA, Scott J, Huskisson EC: Cellular phagocytic studies in rheumatoid arthritis patients treated with levamisol. Ann Rheum Dis 40:382–387, 1981
15. Attia WM, Shams AH, Ali MKH: Studies of phagocytic cell function in rheumatoid arthritis. I. Phagocytic and metabolic activities of neutrophils. Allergy Appl Immunol 48:279–282, 1982
16. Spisani S, Divigo L, Corazza G, Carletti R, Traniello S: The effect of rifamycin SV on neutrophil functions in patients with rheumatoid arthritis. Scand J Rheumatol 11:65–69, 1982
17. El-Ghobarey AF, Mavrikakis ME, MacLeod M: Clinical and laboratory studies of levamisol in patients with rheumatoid arthritis. Q J Med 187:385–400, 1978
18. Uden A, Trang L, Venizelos N, Plamblad J: Neutrophil functions and clinical performance after total fasting in patients with rheumatoid arthritis. Ann Rheum Dis 42:45–51, 1983
19. Breedveld FC, Lafeber GJM, De Vries E, Leijh PCJ, Daha MR, Cats A: Fc receptors on granulocytes from patients with rheumatoid arthritis and Felty's syndrome. J Clin Exp Immunol 55:677–683, 1984
20. Ropes MW, Bennett GA, Cobb S, Jacox R, Jessar RA: 1958 revision of diagnostic criteria for rheumatoid arthritis. Bull Rheum Dis 9:175–176, 1958
21. Valkenburg HA: The Epidemiology of Chronic Rheumatism. Vol. I. Edited by MR Jeffrey, J Ball, under direction of JH Kellgren. Oxford, Blackwell Scientific, 1963, p 377
22. Heymans W, Schuit HRE, Mandema E, Nienhuis RLF, Feltkamp TEW, Holborow EJ, Johnson GD: Comparative study for the detection of antinuclear factors with the fluorescent antibody technique. Ann Rheum Dis 23:73–77, 1964
23. Briët E, Van Nieuwkoop JA, Jol-van den Zijde CM, Den Ottolander GJ, Radl J: Chronic lymphocytic leukemia and IgG heavy chain disease. Scand J Haematol 25:244–250, 1980
24. Zubler RH, Lange G, Lambert PH, Miescher PA: Detection of immune complexes in unheated sera by a modified ^{125}I-C1q binding test: effect of heating on the binding of C1q by immune complexes and application of the test to systemic lupus erythematosus. J Immunol 116:232–235, 1976
25. Kauffmann RH, Van Es LA, Daha MR: Aggregated human immunoglobulin G stabilized by albumin: a standard for immune complex detection. J Immunol Methods 31:11–22, 1979
26. Mayer MM: Complement and complement function, Experimental Immunochemistry. Edited by EA Kabat, MM Mayer. Springfield, Illinois, Charles C. Thomas, 1961
27. Mancini G, Carbonara AO, Heremans JF: Immunochemical quantitation of antigens by single radial immunodiffusion. Immunochemistry 2:235–254, 1965
28. Daha MR, Van Es LA: Relative resistance of the F-$\overline{42}$-stabilized classical pathway C3 convertase to inactivation by C4-binding protein. J Immunol 125:2051–2054, 1980
29. Gigli I, Ruddy S, Austin KF: The stoichiometric measurement of the serum inhibitor of the first component of complement by inhibition of immune hemolysis. J Immunol 100:1154–1164, 1968
30. Polley MJ, Müller-Eberhard HJ: Enhancement of the hemolytic activity of the second component of human complement by oxidation. J Exp Med 126:1013–1025, 1967
31. Leijh PCJ, Van den Barselaar MTh, Van Zweth TL, Dubbeldeman-Rempt I, Van Furth R: Kinetics of phagocytosis of Staphylococcus aureus and Escherichia coli by human granulocytes. Immunology 37:453–465, 1977
32. Van Furth R, Diesselhof-den Dulk MMC: Method to prove ingestion of particles by macrophages with light microscope. Scand J Immunol 12:265–269, 1980
33. Leijh PCJ, Van den Barselaar MTh, Dubbeldeman-Rempt I, Van Furth R: Kinetics of intracellular killing of Staphylococcus aureus and Escherichia coli by human granulocytes. Eur J Immunol 10:750–757, 1980
34. Sandberg AL, Osler AG: Dual pathways of complement interaction with guinea pig immunoglobulins. J Immunol 107:1268–1273, 1971
35. Griffin FM: Effects of soluble immune complexes on Fc receptor- and C3b receptor-mediated phagocytosis by macrophages. J Exp Med 152:905–919, 1980
36. Starkebaum G, Jimenez RAH, Arend WP: Effect of immune complexes on human neutrophil phagocytic function. J Immunol 128:141–147, 1982
37. Messner RP, Laxdal T, Quie PG, Williams RC: Serum opsonin, bacteria and polymorphonuclear leukocyte interactions in subacute bacterial endocarditis: anti-γ-globulin factors and interactions with specific opsonins. J Clin Invest 47:1109–1119, 1968
38. Wiik A, Munthe E: Complement-fixing granulocyte-specific antinuclear factors in neutropenic cases of rheumatoid arthritis. Immunology 26:1127–1134, 1974
39. Hurd ER, Andreis M, Ziff M: Phagocytosis of immune complexes by polymorphonuclear leucocytes in patients with Felty's syndrome. Clin Exp Immunol 28:413–425, 1977

HUMAN RHEUMATOID ARTHRITIC CARTILAGE AND ITS NEUTRAL PROTEOGLYCAN–DEGRADING PROTEASES

The Effects of Antirheumatic Drugs

JOHANNE MARTEL-PELLETIER, JEAN-MARIE CLOUTIER, DAVID S. HOWELL, and JEAN-PIERRE PELLETIER

Measurements were made of the neutral proteoglycan–digesting protease activity in the cartilage matrix breakdown observed in the rheumatoid arthritic process. Normal knee (tibial plateau) cartilage specimens were obtained from 7 fresh cadavers and 29 cartilage specimens were obtained from 23 patients diagnosed as having rheumatoid arthritis (RA). The total neutral metalloproteoglycan–degrading enzyme (NMPE) activity in RA cartilages exhibited roughly an eightfold elevation over that of control subjects. The active form of the NMPE for diseased cartilage was higher than that observed for normal cartilage, but was not statistically different. A very low level of activity was detected for serine proteases and no variation was observed between normal and diseased cartilages. Data obtained from RA cartilages were also analyzed with respect to the relationship between enzyme activities and the patients' medications. Four groups of patients were then selected according to their drug treatments: S + G patients received steroid and gold therapy; S patients received steroids only; NS + NG patients did not receive steroid or gold therapy; G patients received gold therapy alone. The total NMPE activity for each of these groups remained at a very high level. The active enzyme activity measured in S + G and S patients was decreased to a level not different from that of normal controls. Specimens from NS + NG patients presented a significantly higher level of the active form of the enzyme ($P < 0.05$) when compared with either normal controls, S + G, or S patients. No significant difference was noted in the level of serine protease activity between the RA cartilage and normal cartilage. These data strongly support the role of NMPE in the destruction of RA cartilage. Steroids, whether alone or associated with gold compounds, are able to suppress the activity of the active form of the NMPE.

Presented in part at the 30th Annual Scientific Meeting of the Orthopedic Research Society, Atlanta, GA, February 1984.

From the Department of Medicine and Surgery, University of Montreal, Notre Dame and St. Luc Hospitals, Montreal, Canada and the Department of Medicine, University of Miami, School of Medicine, Miami, Florida.

Supported by a grant from the Medical Research Council of Canada.

Johanne Martel-Pelletier, PhD: Assistant Professor of Medicine, Notre Dame Hospital, University of Montreal, School of Medicine; Jean-Marie Cloutier, MD: Professor of Surgery, St. Luc Hospital, University of Montreal, School of Medicine; David S. Howell, MD: Professor of Medicine, University of Miami, School of Medicine; Jean-Pierre Pelletier, MD: Assistant Professor of Medicine, Notre Dame Hospital, University of Montreal, School of Medicine.

Address reprint requests to J. Martel-Pelletier, PhD, Unité des Maladies Rhumatismales, Hôpital Notre-Dame, 1560 est, rue Sherbrooke, Montreal, Quebec, Canada H2L 4K8.

Submitted for publication May 21, 1984; accepted in revised form October 11, 1984.

Cartilage destruction is a major characteristic of rheumatoid arthritis (RA). The mechanism involved seems to be a degradation of the cartilage matrix components by a number of proteolytic enzymes that are found in one or more cellular elements of the diseased joint (1). Although some of the enzymes have been partially characterized, their cellular origins and individual roles in the pathogenic sequence of cartilage degradation have not yet been established.

Chondrocytes have the capacity to degrade their own matrix probably via the synthesis of proteolytic enzymes (2–5). Some of these enzymes hydrolyse peptides which are bound in the core protein of the proteoglycan (PG) subunits. A mechanism, independent of the direct diffusion of degrading enzyme into the cartilage matrix, and one which includes the participation of chondrocytes, has been found (6–8). It was demonstrated that cartilage matrix degradation, mediated by chondrocytes, can be enhanced by a soluble factor. This factor is released from the inflamed synovial membrane of rheumatoid joints. Moreover, this increased degradation can be inhibited by hydrocortisone-related compounds (9).

Neutral proteoglycanases have been found in cartilage tissue. For instance, neutral metalloproteases, capable of degrading proteoglycans, have been described and identified in human articular cartilage (10,11). We have recently demonstrated that human osteoarthritic cartilage contains neutral metalloproteoglycan–degrading enzymes (NMPE) (5). The activity of these enzymes was directly correlated with many parameters of the disease severity. This study focused attention on the quantitative net neutral protease activity in the cartilage matrix during the rheumatoid arthritic process in humans. The relationship between neutral enzyme activity and the medication taken by these patients was also investigated.

There was an observable increase in the level of NMPE activity, especially when RA cartilages were compared with normal human articular cartilages. RA patients treated with steroids were found to have a significantly lower level of the active form of the metalloenzymes. The possible significance of this finding and its helpfulness in understanding the matrix destruction that occurs in rheumatoid cartilage is outlined.

PATIENTS AND METHODS

Chemicals. The chemicals used were either American Chemical Society certified or were the best grade commercially available. Phenylmethylsulfonyl fluoride (PMS-F) was purchased from Sigma Chemical Co., St. Louis, MO; p-aminophenylmercuric acetate (APMA), cetylpyridinium chloride (CPC), and carbazole from Eastman Kodak, Rochester, NY.

Patients and tissue preparation. The subjects studied were patients from both St. Luc and Notre Dame Hospitals, Montreal, Quebec, Canada. All were classified as having either definite or classic rheumatoid arthritis determined by the established criteria of the American Rheumatism Association (12). Although the indications for surgical intervention were not uniform from a clinical and biochemical evaluation, at the time of surgery, all patients had active synovitis in the joint under study.

Twenty-nine tibial plateaus from 23 patients (18 female, 5 male, mean age 62, range 44–80), were obtained at the time of surgery for total knee replacement. Previous medications were documented. Therapy consisted of 1 or more of the basic treatments for rheumatoid arthritis, i.e., 1) therapeutic doses (ranging from moderate to high) of nonsteroidal antiinflammatory drugs (NSAIDs), 2) steroids (prednisone) in a daily dosage of 5 to 10 mg taken orally, and/or 3) gold salts (sodium aurothiomalate) as a standard course, i.e., weekly injections of 50 mg intramuscularly for 20 weeks, followed by 50 mg every 2–4 weeks for an indefinite period. None of the patients had received any other type of treatment (chloroquine, D-penicillamine, immunosuppressive agents, levamisole) for RA in the preceding 6 months. Patients had, in the past, used 1 or more antirheumatic drugs, but only those drugs in use at the time of hospitalization and those used for at least 6 months previously are listed.

We grouped the RA patients according to their previous medication. Because all 23 patients were taking nonsteroidal antiinflammatory compounds, these drugs were not used as a variable. Cartilage specimens from RA patients were then divided into 4 broad groups—S + G: patients who were receiving steroid and gold therapies, 8 specimens from 7 female patients; S: patients who underwent steroid therapy solely, 10 specimens from 7 patients (5 female, 2 male); NS + NG: patients who received neither steroid nor gold compounds, i.e., they were receiving a support therapy of nonsteroidal antiinflammatory drugs only, 8 specimens from 6 patients (5 female, 1 male); G: patients who received only gold salts, 3 specimens from 3 patients (1 female, 2 male). Caution should be used in interpreting the statistical accuracy of the results from group G: because gold compounds are seldom used alone in the treatment of RA patients, this group had only 3 such specimens. The accuracy of the statistical data on 3 specimens may or may not be relevant. Therefore, these results are mentioned only in the text.

Immediately after the resection of the knee the specimens were kept on ice, washed with cold physiologic saline solution, scraped with a policeman, and dissected. The cartilage tissue from the tibial surfaces was shaved from the bone with a scalpel. Care was taken to remove the cartilage sections in areas away from the invading pannus tissue. Histologic experiments showed no evidence of invading pannus nor of any surface adhering inflammatory cells. The diced cartilage was weighed, frozen, and stored at −80°C until further use.

Normal control cartilages from 7 age-matched patients were obtained from the knee joint at autopsy, within 12 hours of death. Cartilage that appeared macroscopically normal and was without any evidence of fibrillation was chosen. Samples were taken from the same site previously described for RA specimens.

Enzyme assay. The neutral proteoglycan–degrading protease assay was described in detail in an earlier study (5). In summary, the cartilage tissue was homogenized in 7 volumes of Tris buffer (Tris-HCl 50 m*M*, $CaCl_2$ 10 m*M*, NaCl 150 m*M*, NaN_3 0.02% weight/volume and gentamycin 40 μg [Schering Corp.]) at pH 7.4 and incubated at 37°C for 42 hours. Aliquots subjected to incubation were first submitted to either: (a) APMA (1 m*M*); (b) APMA (1 m*M*) plus o-phenanthroline (5 m*M*); (c) no addition; (d) o-phenanthroline (5 m*M*); or (e) APMA (1 m*M*), o-phenanthroline (5 m*M*) plus PMS-F (1 m*M*).

To determine any possible interference of the serine proteases with the level of the active metalloenzymes by an in vitro activation, we conducted the following test. We repeated the experiment, already knowing that the NMPE (active form) activity was high, but this time we added PMS-F (1mM) under conditions c and d stated above. No change in the level of the active form was noted.

After the incubation period, proteolytic activity was quantitated via the degradative products released from the endogenous PG. The quantification method uses the precipitation of PG with CPC at a final concentration of 1.7%. This was followed by the release of the PG-digested products with trichloroacetic acid, in solution, at a final concentration of 9%. The degradation of these PG was quantitated by their uronic acid content (13) analyzed in the last supernatant. A unit of PG-degrading enzyme activity was defined as the release of 1 μg of uronic acid per hour. All homogenates subjected to the above-described conditions were assayed in this manner. The activity was expressed in units/gm (wet weight) of cartilage.

PG-degrading enzyme activity was calculated for the following: 1) total NMPE—the digestion found in group a minus that found in group b, 2) active NMPE—group c minus group d, 3) latent NMPE—the difference between total and active forms, and 4) serine proteases—group b minus group c. All activities were corrected for non-enzymatic release of the proteoglycans. This was done under a 42-hour test period at 4°C.

Analytic study of the whole cartilage and the PG-digested products of NMPE. DNA determination was made on each cartilage sample using the method of Bonting and Jones (14). The DNA unit used was μg/mg wet weight of cartilage. Uronic acid measurement was carried out on a whole cartilage sample (10 mg wet weight) and was used as an index of PG content. Too little tissue was left for further quantification using any other parameter.

Statistical analysis. Mean values and standard errors of the resulting data were calculated for both patient and control samples. To test the equality of means, an analysis of variance was performed. When significant P values, <0.05, were obtained in any combination of the groups studied, a Scheffe's multiple comparison (15) was done to assess which group(s) was (were) responsible for the significant difference.

RESULTS

Biochemical data. Table 1 shows the PG content (expressed as uronic acid) in the diseased cartilage compared with that of normal controls. These results were consistent with the findings published by other authors (16). The uronic acid content of the cartilage of the diseased joints was significantly lower ($P < 0.001$) than that of the controls. This reduction was greater in groups where the patients received NSAIDs alone, compared with the 2 groups of patients (S + G and S) treated with steroids. The uronic acid value for patients receiving gold compound alone (G) was lower (1.14 ± 0.08) than that of the control values. Rheumatoid cartilage samples showed a lower DNA content (0.47 ± 0.02 μg/mg wet weight; mean ± SEM) than the normal controls (0.54 ± 0.04), but no statistical difference could be noted between these 2 sets of data. The treatment applied did not seem to affect the DNA content, with values roughly in the same range, i.e., S + G, 0.46 ± 0.05; S, 0.45 ± 0.03; NS + NG, 0.48 ± 0.04; G, 0.53 ± 0.12.

Neutral protease activity. Table 2 illustrates the trend of the neutral enzyme activity in normal and rheumatoid arthritic cartilages. The major neutral enzyme activity appeared in the category of metalloproteases, i.e., activated by APMA (1 mM) and inhibited by o-phenanthroline (5 mM). A very low level of serine

Table 2. Neutral metalloproteoglycan-degrading protease (NMPE) activity

	Normal subjects	Rheumatoid arthritis patients	P*
No. of specimens	7	29	
Total NMPE†	1.16 ± 0.37‡	9.95 ± 1.34	<0.003
Active NMPE	0.10 ± 0.10	1.68 ± 0.40	NS
Serine protease	0.36 ± 0.18	0.48 ± 0.17	NS

* Probability values were calculated by the analysis of variance followed by Scheffe's procedure comparing the values for the rheumatoid arthritis specimens with those from normal tissues. NS = not significant.
† Enzyme activity was measured as described in Patients and Methods after 42 hours incubation at 37°C, and expressed as units/gm of cartilage (wet weight).
‡ Values expressed as mean ± SEM.

Table 1. Uronic acid content

	Normal subjects	RA	RA subgroups* S + G	S	NS + NG
No. of specimens	7	29	8	10	8
Uronic acid, μg/mg wet weight	3.82 ± 0.23†	1.80 ± 0.15	1.80 ± 0.24	2.34 ± 0.31	1.31 ± 0.15
P‡	–	<0.001	<0.001	<0.001	<0.001

* RA = rheumatoid arthritis; S + G = patients receiving steroid and gold therapies; S = patients receiving steroid therapy; NS + NG = patients who received neither steroid nor gold compounds.
† Values expressed as mean ± SEM.
‡ Probability values were calculated by analysis of variance followed by Scheffe's procedure comparing the values for the RA specimens with those from normal tissues. When RA specimens from subgroups were compared with one another, no significant difference was noted.

protease activity was recorded in our cartilage specimens.

The patients with diseased cartilage exhibited a very high level of total NMPE activity. The mean value of all patients with arthritic disease was significantly increased over the mean value of the control group ($P < 0.003$). One should particularly note the level of the active form of the NMPE. Thus, the RA cartilage samples showed a higher mean value (1.68 ± 0.40) than that noted for normal cartilage (0.10 ± 0.10), but the analysis of variance showed no significant difference ($P < 0.07$). Serine proteases showed an insignificant difference in activity between normal subjects and diseased specimens. Similar serine levels were noted for both RA specimens and normal controls.

For comparison purposes, the data obtained in this study were divided into 4 groups, each specifying an individual drug therapy. Figure 1 presents the distribution of the total NMPE activity of RA cartilages (divided into 3 broad groups) and that of normal control cartilages. Total NMPE activity was high in every RA group and did not seem influenced by different therapies. All RA groups presented similar amounts of enzyme. The multiple comparison procedure showed the 4 RA groups as a subset, which was significantly different from the normal control group. The total NMPE activity of group G also presented a higher level (7.56 ± 4.09) than the one found for the control group.

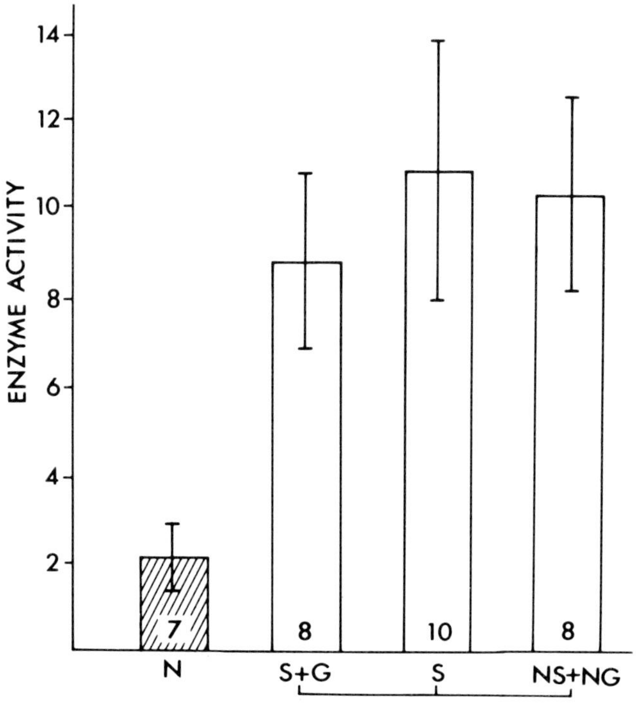

Figure 1. Total neutral metalloproteoglycan–degrading enzyme activity in human articular cartilage specimens. N = normal controls (crossline column); S + G = patients receiving steroid and gold therapies; S = patients receiving steroid therapy; NS + NG = patients receiving nonsteroidal antiinflammatory compounds. The assay is described in Patients and Methods. Enzyme activity is expressed as units/gm of cartilage (wet weight). Results are given as the mean ± SEM. The number of tissue specimens is indicated in the lower part of each column. Using analysis of variance and subsequent Scheffe's multiple comparison, there are two subsets: N and (S + G, S, NS + NG), statistically different at $P < 0.05$.

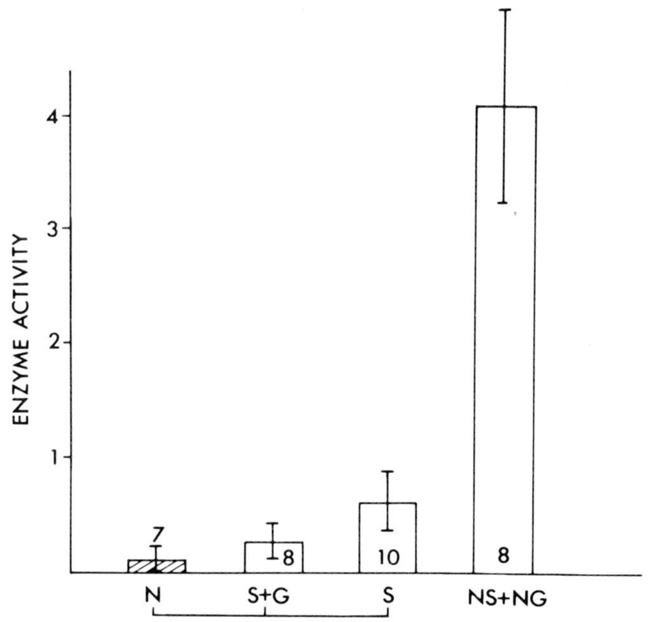

Figure 2. Neutral metalloproteoglycan–degrading enzyme activity in human articular cartilage specimens. Results are given as the mean ± SEM. The number of tissue specimens is indicated in the lower part of each column (except N column; number shown above column). Using analysis of variance and subsequent Scheffe's multiple comparison, there are two subsets: (N, S+G, S) and NS + NG, statistically different at $P < 0.05$. See Figure 1 for definitions.

Figure 2 illustrates the level of the active form of the NMPE for the 4 groups. In contrast to the total NMPE activity, the level of the active form showed a wide variation with respect to the different medications. Our results revealed that patients receiving steroids along with gold (S + G; 0.27 ± 0.15) or those receiving steroids alone (S; 0.60 ± 0.29) formed a subset. This subset had a significantly lower level of activity observed than that noted from group NS + NG, which was comparatively high (4.0 ± 0.85) (Figure 2). The values of group G (2.36 ± 1.41) were in the same range as those of group NS + NG. Cartilage from patients taking steroids showed about the same level of NMPE activity as that found in normal cartilage. No significant difference was recorded among groups S + G, S, and normal subjects. However,

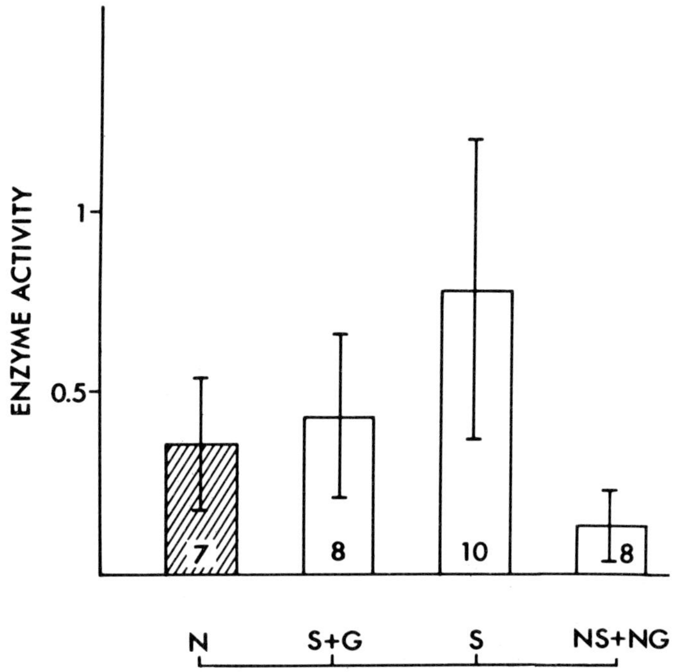

Figure 3. Serine protease activity in human articular cartilage specimens. Results are given as the mean ± SEM. The number of tissue specimens is indicated in the lower part of each column. Using analysis of variance and subsequent Scheffe's multiple comparison, there was no statistical difference between any of the groups listed. See Figure 1 for definitions.

group NS + NG showed a significant increase in active enzyme activity, especially when the group was compared with the normal controls.

Serine proteases had a low level of activity. This was observed not only in normal controls (0.36 ± 0.18) but also in RA cartilages, regardless of the treatment (Figure 3). Although an increase in activity was seen in group S, statistically it was not different from any of the other 3 groups studied. The mean value for group G was 0.23 ± 0.23.

DISCUSSION

The operative mechanism in the process of irreversible cartilage damage in inflammatory arthritis is largely unknown. Generalized damage of the rheumatoid cartilage includes a "thinning" of the cartilage, a dramatic decrease of metachromatic proteoglycans, and a degradation of surface collagen. PG loss appears in the early stages of the disease and even precedes collagenolysis (1). Several enzymatic mechanisms, such as those dependent on synovial fluid proteases of diverse origin and the enzymes which come from the inflammatory synovium, pannus cells, or chondrocytes, have been considered to play a role in cartilage degradation.

In chronic inflammatory arthritis, an obvious source of proteolytic enzymes is their release from the inflammatory cells present in the synovial fluid. Therefore, the enzyme diffusion into the cartilage might be responsible for the matrix degradation. Some of these enzymes, such as leukocyte elastase, have been found in the synovial fluid in rabbit models of arthritis (17). The presence of enzyme inhibitors (α_1-antitrypsin and α_2-macroglobulins) in the synovial fluid is responsible for the inactivation of these neutral enzymes. Neutral proteases capable of degrading PG have been isolated from mononuclear cells (18). Again, most of this activity is inactivated by the same enzyme inhibitors.

Both the breakdown of matrix components and the progressive cartilage erosion brought about by rheumatoid pannus have been reported by many authors (19,20). However, cartilage degradation due solely to an enzymatic invasion from the pannus area is unlikely. Erosion has also been seen on the free surface of the cartilage, which is some distance from the synovium (6,19). It has been proposed that chondrocytes participate in these erosions by destroying their own matrix (6). The histologic observation of the early collagen degradation and of the loss of matrix proteoglycans around the chondrocytes (21), analyzed in RA cartilage, adds some credence to the hypothesis that matrix degradation may be mediated by these cells.

The primary stimulus that activates chondrocytes in the diseased cartilage is not known. It seems that self-propagating cartilage damage must be attributed to endogenous enzyme activation. It has been demonstrated that synovial factors and the factors derived from mononuclear cells and from macrophages stimulated the chondrocytes to either degrade their own matrices or to secrete proteases (22–24).

It is likely that PG breakdown occurs by a proteolytic action on the core protein. This protein is readily destroyed by many proteases. There are only a few enzymes, isolated from articular cartilage or chondrocytes in culture, to which one can attribute the PG degradation. Muirden et al (25) found an increased amount of cathepsin D in the cartilage of patients with rheumatoid arthritis. However, it is unlikely that those acid proteases had an important role in extracellular rather than intracellular digestion, since the pH of the cartilage matrix lies in the neutral range. Hembry et al (26) have performed experiments in which they demonstrated that the proteolytic action of cathepsin D was limited to the intrachondrocytic degradation of proteoglycans in lysosomes. Therefore neutral proteases seem the most likely candidates responsible for the loss of matrix proteoglycans in the injured joint.

Our results have clearly demonstrated that human RA cartilage contains a substantial amount of neutral proteases, which are capable of degrading PG. The total NMPE in rheumatoid cartilage was enhanced 8-9 times over that of normal controls (Table 2). Our findings are in accordance with previous reports that suggested the major fraction of neutral protease activity found in articular cartilage does respond to metalloprotease inhibitors (27). The total NMPE activity present in these RA cartilages was not affected by the patients' medication (steroid and/or gold salts). Although there was a slight decrease in total NMPE when steroids and gold agents were used in combination, one could not correlate the combination with a further suppression of this enzyme activity. If, as previously reported, the cartilage breakdown and possibly the synthesis of proteolytic enzymes by chondrocytes are under the control of stimulating factors in RA tissue (22–24), there are at least 2 possible explanations for the apparent lack of suppression of total NMPE in patients receiving either steroids or steroids in conjunction with gold.

One explanation may be that even though the cartilage specimens used came from 23 different patients, the patients themselves had at least 2 features in common. They all had long-standing rheumatoid arthritis and all, technically speaking, had had unsuccessful results with medical therapy. That is, the patients needed surgery because of either their lack of therapeutic response to or an inadequate dosage in their medication.

The second explanation can be related to the fact that steroids inhibit the synthesis and/or the release of chondrocytic-activating factor(s) (9). It has also been postulated that there is a direct chondrocytic inhibition of the synovial factor(s) action (28). As yet, little is known about this mechanism in vivo. The above observations were based on in vitro experiments and the response was visible at very high drug concentrations. It is therefore possible that the therapeutic level was not enough to suppress the release and/or action of the activating factor(s) in our study. These two explanations may be operative; however, they may play only a small role in regard to the entire degenerative process of this disease.

The NMPE detected in tissues or in cell cultures occurred mostly as latent enzymes, which could be activated by trypsin or mercurial compounds. We have previously reported the presence in human OA cartilage of NMPE in both latent and active forms (5). In addition to the prominent increase in total NMPE activity, rheumatoid cartilage exhibited an increase in the active enzyme level—especially so in the specimens taken from patients receiving NSAIDs only (NS + NG, Figure 2). This quantitatively high increase in the enzyme activity level can be relevant in the degradative process.

It has not yet been established how the latent enzyme is activated in vivo. The latency could be explained by the presence of a pro-enzyme (zymogen), which in turn causes a proteolytic cleavage to yield the active form (29). Activation of neutral metalloproteases, from a latent to an active form, may be affected by a number of proteinases of which the serine type seems the most likely candidate. Despite the fact that serine proteases show a clear capacity to activate synovial collagenase (30), there is no evidence that they activate the NMPE in the RA matrix cartilage. So far, in our assay, we have been unable to demonstrate an in vitro, serine enzyme activation of the NMPE.

In this study, only trace amounts of serine proteases were found in normal and RA cartilages (Table 2). The various medications received had no significant effect on the serine level (Figure 3). Even if the chondrocytic production of plasminogen activator has been shown to be stimulated by a substance that is isolated from cultured synovium (31), there is little evidence to prove that chondrocytes actually initiate in vivo protease activity. Recently, Vater et al (32) have reported that latent collagenase can be activated by a protein called procollagenase activator. Even if purely speculative at this stage, it is possible that a similar mechanism might be responsible for activating the NMPE in RA cartilage.

The present study emphasized the steroid-induced suppression of the active NMPE activity. Our data demonstrated that active NMPE activity was altered to a normal level in groups S + G and S (Figure 2). This was, moreover, paralleled by a less severe depletion of the uronic acid content in these specimens (Table 1). However, with this observation, we are not excluding the possibility that the combination of steroid, gold, and NSAIDs affects NMPE activity. It is possible that the predominant effect of these steroids operates on the activation step. It has been shown that activators, such as the plasminogen activator, are inhibited by steroid agents (33). On the other hand, McGuire et al (34) have suggested that the steroid-induced reduction of matrix degradation is due to an increased concentration of free endogenous inhibitors. Our data do not allow us to determine which hypothesis is correct, nor whether activators or inhibitors are likely to play a significant role in the progressive tissue damage of RA. However, the suppressive effect of steroid compounds on the active enzyme activity confirms the reported protective effect that low steroid doses seem to have on RA cartilage breakdown (35). This may also explain the beneficial effect that low prednisone doses have on hand/wrist erosions in RA patients (36).

Nevertheless, the fact that total NMPE is enhanced in RA cartilage and that the active form is significantly increased in the degradative RA (NSAID group), may be relevant in explaining the disease process. The effect of steroids on the active form of the NMPE gives us an additional insight in determining the possible mechanism of action of these drugs.

ACKNOWLEDGMENTS

The authors thank Dr. R. Vauclair, Head of the Department of Pathology, Notre Dame Hospital, for supplying the postmortem specimens. The technical assistance of W. Nedwetsky and F. Mineau and the assistance of D. Fournier in preparing the manuscript are greatly appreciated.

REFERENCES

1. Barret AJ: The enzymatic degradation of cartilage matrix, Dynamics of Connective Tissue Macromolecules. Edited by PMC Burleigh, AR Poole. Amsterdam, North Holland, 1975, pp 189–215
2. Malemud CJ, Norby DP, Sapolsky AI, Matsuta K, Howell DS, Moskowitz RW: Neutral proteinases from articular chondrocytes in culture. I. A latent collagenase that degrades human cartilage type II collagen. Biochim Biophys Acta 657:517–529, 1981
3. Sapolsky AI, Malemud CJ, Norby DP, Moskowitz RW, Matsuta K, Howell DS: Neutral proteinases from articular chondrocytes in culture. II. Metal-dependent latent neutral proteoglycanase and inhibitory activity. Biochim Biophys Acta 658:138–147, 1981
4. Pelletier J-P, Martel-Pelletier J, Howell DS, Ghandur-Mnaymneh L, Enis JE, Woessner JF Jr: Collagenase and collagenolytic activity in human osteoarthritic cartilage. Arthritis Rheum 26:63–68, 1983
5. Martel-Pelletier J, Pelletier J-P, Cloutier JM, Howell DS, Ghandur-Mnaymneh L, Woessner JF Jr: Neutral proteases capable of proteoglycan digesting activity in osteoarthritic and normal human articular cartilage. Arthritis Rheum 27:305–312, 1984
6. Fell HB, Jubb RW: The effect of synovial tissue on the breakdown of articular cartilage in organ culture. Arthritis Rheum 20:1359–1371, 1977
7. Dingle JT, Saklatvala J, Hembry R, Tyler J, Fell HB, Jubb R: A cartilage catabolic factor from synovium. Biochem J 184:177–180, 1979
8. Steinberg J, Sledge CB, Noble J, Stirrat CR: A tissue culture model of cartilage breakdown in rheumatoid arthritis. I. Quantitative aspects of proteoglycan release. Biochem J 180:403–412, 1979
9. Steinberg JJ, Kincaid SB, Sledge CB: Inhibition of cartilage breakdown by hydrocortisone in a tissue culture model of rheumatoid arthritis. Ann Rheum Dis 42:323–330, 1983
10. Sapolsky AI, Keiser H, Howell DS, Woessner JF Jr: Metalloproteases of human articular cartilage that digest cartilage proteoglycan at neutral and acid pH. J Clin Invest 58:1030–1041, 1976
11. Sapolsky AI, Howell DS: Further characterization of a neutral metalloprotease isolated from human articular cartilage. Arthritis Rheum 25:981–988, 1982
12. Ropes MW, Bennett GA, Cobb S, Jacox R, Jessar RA: 1958 revision of diagnostic criteria for rheumatoid arthritis. Arthritis Rheum 2:16–20, 1959
13. Bitter T, Muir M: A modified uronic acid carbazole reaction. Anal Biochem 4:330–334, 1962
14. Bonting SL, Jones M: Determination of microgram quantities of deoxyribonucleic acid and protein in tissues grown in vitro. Arch Biochem Biophys 66:340–353, 1957
15. Scheffe HA: The Analysis of Variance. New York, Wiley, 1959
16. Jacoby RK, Jayson MIV: Synthesis of glycoaminoglycan in adult human articular cartilage in organ culture from patients with rheumatoid arthritis. Ann Rheum Dis 35:32–36, 1976
17. Sandy JD, Sriramata A, Brown HLG, Lowther DA: Evidence of polymorphonuclear-leucocyte-derived proteinases in arthritic cartilage. Biochem J 193:193–202, 1981
18. Mohr W, Westerhellweg J, Wessinghage D: Polymorphonuclear granulocytes in rheumatic tissue destruction. III. An electron microscopic study of PMNs at the pannus-cartilage junction in rheumatoid arthritis. Ann Rheum Dis 40:396–399, 1981
19. Kobayashi I, Ziff M: Electron microscopic studies of the cartilage-pannus junction in rheumatoid arthritis. Arthritis Rheum 18:475–483, 1975
20. Harris ED Jr, Glauert AM, Murley AHG: Intracellular collagen fibers at the pannus-cartilage junction in rheumatoid arthritis. Arthritis Rheum 20:657–665, 1977
21. Mitchell NS, Shepard N: Changes in proteoglycan and collagen in cartilage in rheumatoid arthritis. J Bone Joint Surg 60A:349–354, 1978
22. Deshmukh-Phadke K, Nanda S, Lee K: Macrophage factor that induces neutral protease secretion by normal rabbit chondrocytes: studies of some properties and effects on metabolism of chondrocytes. Eur J Biochem 104:175–180, 1980
23. Ridge SC, Oronsky AL, Kerwar SS: Induction of the

synthesis of latent collagenase and latent neutral protease in chondrocytes by a factor synthesized by activated macrophages. Arthritis Rheum 23:448–454, 1980
24. Saklatvala J, Dingle JT: Identification of catabolin, a protein from synovium which induces degradation of cartilage in organ culture. Biochem Biophys Res Commun 96:1225–1231, 1980
25. Muirden KD, Deutschmann PH, Phillips M: Articular cartilage in rheumatoid arthritis: ultrastructure and enzymology. J Rheumatol 1:1–33, 1974
26. Hembry RM, Knight CG, Dingle JT, Barret AJ: Evidence that extracellular cathepsin D is not responsible for the resorption of cartilage matrix in culture. Biochim Biophys Acta 714:307–312, 1982
27. Woessner JF Jr, Sellers A: Metalloproteases are responsible for the degradation of connective tissue matrix proteins. Fed Proc 39:1020, 1980
28. Sheppard H, Pibworth LMC, Hazleman B, Dingle JT: The effects of anti-rheumatoid drugs on the production and action of porcine catabolin. Ann Rheum Dis 4:463–468, 1982
29. Nagase H, Jackson RC, Brinckerhoff CE, Vater CE, Harris ED Jr: A precursor form of latent collagenase produced in a cell-free system with mRNA from rabbit synovial cells. J Biol Chem 256:11951–11954, 1981
30. Werb Z, Mainardi CL, Vater CA, Harris ED Jr: Endogenous activation of latent collagenase by rheumatoid synovial cells: evidence for a role of plasminogen activator. N Engl J Med 296:1017–1023, 1977
31. Meats JE, McGuire MB, Russell RGG: Human synovium releases a factor which stimulates chondrocyte production of PGE and plasminogen activator. Nature 286:891–892, 1980
32. Vater CA, Nagase H, Harris ED Jr: Purification of an endogenous activator of procollagenase from rabbit synovial fibroblast culture medium. J Biol Chem 258:9374–9382, 1983
33. Hamilton JA, Bootes A, Philips PE, Slywka J: Human synovial fibroblast plasminogen activator: modulation of enzyme activity by antiinflammatory steroids. Arthritis Rheum 24:1296–1303, 1981
34. McGuire MB, Murphy G, Reynolds JJ, Russell RGG: Production of collagenase and inhibitor (TIMP) by normal rheumatoid and osteoarthritic synovium in vitro: effects of hydrocortisone and indomethacin. Clin Sci 61:703–710, 1981
35. Masi AT: Low dose glucocorticoid therapy in rheumatoid arthritis (RA): transitional or selected add-on therapy? J Rheumatol 10:675–678, 1983
36. Harris ED Jr, Emkey RD, Nichols JE, Newberg A: Low dose prednisone therapy in rheumatoid arthritis: a double blind study. J Rheumatol 10:713–721, 1983

CARTILAGE NUCLEOSIDE TRIPHOSPHATE PYROPHOSPHOHYDROLASE

II. Role in Extracellular Pyrophosphate Generation and Nucleotide Metabolism

LAWRENCE M. RYAN, ROBERT L. WORTMANN, BARBARA KARAS, and DANIEL J. McCARTY, Jr.

Extracellular generation of inorganic pyrophosphate (PPi) in cartilage organ culture is markedly augmented by ATP. ATP, not an ATP metabolite (ADP, AMP, adenosine), is necessary for this augmentation. Excess PPi production is effectively blocked by known inhibitors of nucleoside triphosphate (NTP) pyrophosphohydrolase (EDTA, EGTA, dithiothreitol). Excess ^{32}P-PPi is generated directly from γ^{32}P-ATP by cartilage, as substrate and product have similar specific activities. These findings strongly favor ecto-NTP pyrophosphohydrolase as the source of extracellular PPi generation in the presence of NTP. Additionally, active nucleotide and nucleoside catabolism is demonstrated in these cartilage organ cultures.

Calcium pyrophosphate dihydrate (CPPD) crystal deposition disease is defined by the presence of CPPD crystals in articular fluid or tissues. These crystals often cause an inflammatory arthritis (pseudogout) and even more frequently, are associated with a chronic degenerative arthritis in a distribution of affected joints different from that of primary osteoarthritis. The inorganic pyrophosphate (PPi) which participates in crystal formation appears to originate from articular cartilage itself, although the mechanism of its generation is unclear (1,2).

Tenenbaum et al (3) have reported increased activity of nucleoside triphosphate pyrophosphohydrolase (NTPPPHase) in Triton X-100 extracts of degenerated articular cartilage from patients with CPPD deposition in comparison with extracts from osteoarthritic or normal cartilage. This enzyme generates PPi from the nucleoside triphosphates in the reaction:

$$\text{nucleoside triphosphate (NTP)} \rightleftharpoons \text{nucleoside monophosphate (NMP)} + \text{PPi}$$

Tenenbaum et al also noted increased 5′nucleotidase (5′NT) and decreased inorganic pyrophosphatase (PPiase) in CPPD cartilage.

Abnormalities of these 3 enzymes theoretically could lead to increased PPi accumulation in tissue by the following mechanisms: 1) increased NTP pyrophosphohydrolase activity could generate increased amounts of PPi; 2) removal of the NMP coproduct by 5′NT could favor NTP degradation; and 3) low PPiase activity could decrease PPi removal. We have characterized NTPPPHase as an ecto-enzyme in canine cartilage organ culture (4). Therefore, in the presence of suitable substrate, the nature and concentration of which are still obscure, PPi could be generated by this enzyme extracellularly in cartilage.

The PPi which appears in the presence of NTP may result from 2 processes other than ecto-

From the Section of Rheumatology, Department of Medicine, The Medical College of Wisconsin, Milwaukee, Wisconsin, and Wood Veterans Administration Medical Center, Wood, Wisconsin.

Supported by USPHS grants AM-18074-11 and AM-31395; a Merit Review grant from the Veterans Administration; and a grant from the Wisconsin Chapter of The Arthritis Foundation.

Lawrence M. Ryan, MD, FACP: Associate Professor of Medicine, Section of Rheumatology, and recipient of New Investigator Award, NIADDK; Robert L. Wortmann, MD, FACP: Assistant Professor of Medicine, Section of Rheumatology; Barbara Karas, MA: Research Associate, Section of Rheumatology; Daniel J. McCarty, Jr., MD, FACP: Will and Cava Ross Professor and Chairman, Department of Medicine, Medical College of Wisconsin.

Address reprint requests to Lawrence M. Ryan, MD, Section of Rheumatology, Medical College of Wisconsin, 8700 W. Wisconsin Avenue, Milwaukee, WI 53226.

Submitted for publication July 9, 1984; accepted in revised form October 16, 1984.

NTPPPHase. First, since spontaneous "background" extracellular PPi elaboration occurs in the absence of exogenous NTP (1,2), it is possible that part or all of the PPi liberated in the presence of NTP results from augmented endogenous secretion by chondrocytes stimulated by the NTP or by an NTP metabolite. Second, extracellular ATP has been demonstrated to increase the permeability of some cell types (5,6) and cause degranulation of others (7), thus providing another route by which extracellular PPi could appear following exposure of cells to NTP.

We sought to determine the role of NTPPPHase in NTP-stimulated extracellular PPi generation. All excess PPi generated by cartilage in the presence of exogenous ATP was derived directly from ATP via NTPPPHase since 1) ATP metabolites did not stimulate significant PPi elaboration; 2) elaboration of excess PPi in the presence of ATP is substantially depressed by the addition of known NTPPPHase inhibitors; and 3) ^{32}P-PPi elaborated by chondrocytes in the presence of γ^{32}P-ATP has a specific activity similar to that of the initial ^{32}P-ATP. Additionally, extracellular nucleotide catabolism occurred in cartilage, as has been demonstrated in other tissues.

MATERIALS AND METHODS

Reagents. $Na_4P_2O_7 \cdot 10\ H_2O$, ATP, ADP, AMP, adenosine, dithiothreitol, theophylline, adenosine diphosphonate (AMPCP), dipyridamole, cysteine, and tetramisole were purchased from Sigma Chemical Co. (St. Louis, MO). Erythro-9-[3-(2-hydroxy-nonyl)] adenine (EHNA) was purchased from Burroughs Wellcome (Research Triangle Park, NC); γ^{32}P-ATP was obtained from New England Nuclear (Boston, MA). All reagents were prepared in doubly deionized, glass-distilled, charcoal-filtered water.

Assays for PPi and ATP metabolites. PPi was determined by a modification of the method of Cheung and Suhadolnik (8). Briefly, ^{14}C-UDPG was quantitatively converted enzymatically to ^{14}C-glucose-1-PO_4 and UTP in the presence of PPi. Differential charcoal adsorption of ^{14}C before and after reaction in the assay was directly related to PPi concentration. Appropriate standard PPi determinations at concentrations from 0.5–20 μM were made with each assay. Standard stock PPi solutions (16 mm) were assayed for inorganic phosphate content by the method of Fiske and SubbaRow (9) before and after hydrolysis by yeast inorganic pyrophosphatase or by acid hydrolysis as described previously (10). This is necessary since stock $Na_4P_2O_7 \cdot 10\ H_2O$ powder readily gains or loses waters of hydration (10), which makes calculations of molarity by weight inaccurate.

Concentrations of ATP and its metabolites were determined by high performance liquid chromatography (HPLC) (Varian 5300, Sunnyvale, CA). Samples were prepared for analysis using 6% trichloroacetic acid and 0.5*M* tri-N-octyl amine in freon as described by Chen et al (11). Samples were analyzed immediately or stored at −20°C. ATP, ADP, AMP, and IMP were chromatographed with a Micropak AX-10 anion exchange column and a gradient of 0.01*M* KH_2PO_4, pH 2.85 (buffer A) and 0.75*M* KH_2PO_4, pH 4.4 (buffer B) at a flow rate of 2.0 ml/minute. A linear gradient was developed over 37.5 minutes at 5% B to 100% B followed by elution with 100% B for 12.5 minutes (12). Nucleosides and bases were quantified with a MCH-10 reverse phase column isocratically using 0.05*M* KH_2PO_4, pH 6.0 (buffer C) for 11 minutes and then buffer C in 25% methanol (volume/volume) for 15 minutes at a flow rate of 2.0 ml/minute (13).

Cartilage organ cultures. Hyaline articular cartilage was obtained from the femoral condyles and fibrocartilage from the menisci of freshly killed adult mongrel dogs and transported in Dulbecco's modified Eagle's medium (DMEM) supplemented with 10% fetal calf serum (FCS). Cartilage was minced with a scalpel using sterile techniques into ≈5-mg fragments and washed 3 times with DMEM over 1 hour prior to study in order to remove debris and FCS, which contains NTP pyrophosphohydrolase activity. Control cartilage specimens were incubated in a sevenfold (volume/wet weight) volume of DMEM containing 50 m*M* Tris, pH 7.2 at 37°C in a 10% CO_2 atmosphere for 30–240 minutes, as previously described (2). Experimental plates contained cartilage from the same animal incubated with identical media to which 1 m*M* ATP, ATP metabolites, and/or inhibitors of NTP pyrophosphohydrolase had been added in various combinations.

At the conclusion of incubations, media was immediately removed and centrifuged. A portion of the supernatant was frozen at –20°C for PPi analysis. The remainder was extracted for HPLC. PPi production was expressed as nmoles/hour/mg wet weight of cartilage.

Effect of ATP metabolites on PPi production. To determine whether a metabolite of ATP is indirectly stimulating PPi extrusion from cartilage, canine cartilage was incubated in the presence of 1.0 m*M* adenosine, AMP, or ADP in single experiments. With each metabolite a companion plate containing cartilage from the same animal was incubated in 1 m*M* ATP. Results were expressed as:

$$\% = \frac{PPi_{M}\ (\text{nmoles/hour/100 mg cartilage})}{PPi_{ATP}\ (\text{nmoles/hour/100 mg cartilage})} \times 100$$

Inhibitors of nucleoside production. Nucleosides are produced during incubation of cartilage with ATP (see Results). To determine its effect upon PPi elaboration, nucleoside production was inhibited by 0.5 m*M* AMPCP (inhibits 5′NT), by 0.5 m*M* AMPCP plus 1 m*M* AMP (further inhibits 5′NT), by 10 μM dipyridamole (inhibits transport of adenosine into cells where it is further catabolized), or by EHNA (inhibits intracellular adenosine deaminase). Portions of cartilage from the same dog were incubated in DMEM containing ATP or ATP plus inhibitor in single experiments. Results were expressed as:

$$\%\ \text{PPi generation} = \frac{PPi_{I}\ (\text{nmoles/hour/100 mg cartilage})}{PPi_{ATP}\ (\text{nmoles/hour/100 mg cartilage})} \times 100$$

where PPi_I = PPi produced on the plate with inhibitor plus 1 m*M* ATP, and PPi_{ATP} = PPi produced on the plate with ATP alone.

Inhibitors of NTP pyrophosphohydrolase. The following were studied to assess their effect upon PPi generation by ATP: (a) known inhibitors of NTPPPHase (14) (10 m*M* EGTA, 10 m*M* dithiothreitol, 5 m*M* EDTA and 1 m*M* cysteine); (b) an inhibitor of alkaline phosphatase which does not affect NTPPPHase (14) (2 m*M* tetramisole); and (c) an inhibitor of Na^+, K^+ ATPase (15) (0.1 m*M* ouabain). PPi production in the presence of ATP and ATP plus inhibitor was measured on 2 aliquots of cartilage from the same dog. Results were expressed as:

$$\% \text{ PPi production} = \frac{\text{PPi produced per hour with inhibitor} + 1 \text{ m}M \text{ ATP}}{\text{PPi produced per hour with 1 m}M\text{ ATP}} \times 100$$

Specific activity of ^{32}P-PPi produced in the presence of ^{32}P-ATP. If the PPi generated by cartilage in the presence of ATP is derived entirely from ATP via NTP pyrophosphohydrolase, then the specific activity of the ^{32}P-PPi produced from γ^{32}P-ATP substrate should be identical to that of the starting ^{32}P-ATP. Production of endogenous unlabeled PPi would dilute ^{32}P-PPi produced via NTP pyrophosphohydrolase, thereby lowering the specific activity of the total ^{32}P-PPi produced. Organ cultures of articular cartilage were incubated with 1 m*M* γ^{32}P-ATP in DMEM. The specific activity of the starting ^{32}P-ATP was determined as follows: ATP was measured by the method of Bucher (16) as modified by Adams (17). ^{32}P-ATP counts were determined in 100 μl of media after precipitation of contaminating ^{32}P inorganic phosphate (Pi) (18) by measuring Cerenkov radiation in 0.5 *N* HCl in a Packard Tri-Carb scintillation counter with a 50–1,000 window at 50% gain. The specific activity of the media PPi at the conclusion of the organ culture incubations was determined as follows: PPi concentration was measured as previously described. ^{32}P-PPi counts were determined by differential counting of ^{32}P-Pi precipitated by the method of Sugino and Miyoshi (18) before and after incubation with Type III yeast inorganic PPiase (Sigma) in a mixture containing 50 μl media, 50 μl of 100μ/ml PPiase, and 100 μl of 13 m*M* $MgCl_2$, 15 m*M* Tris Cl, 5 m*M* EDTA, pH 7.2, for 1 hour at room temperature.

Table 1. Appearance of PPi and ATP catabolites in media of cartilage specimens incubated with ATP*

Substrate	Hours of incubation 0	2	4
ATP	882 ± 257	586 ± 394	435 ± 303
ADP	53 ± 20	85 ± 17	102 ± 44
AMP	12 ± 9	19 ± 3	20 ± 9
Adenosine	11 ± 7	83 ± 25	120 ± 39
Inosine	<2	74 ± 49	181 ± 137
Hypoxanthine	<2	54 ± 23	136 ± 74
PPi	1.8 ± 1.5	182 ± 75	275 ± 71

* Values represent media concentration (μM), mean ± SD (n = 5). PPi = inorganic pyrophosphate. For comparison, plates containing cartilage but no ATP routinely increased media PPi concentration by 2 μM after 4 hours. ATP incubated in media alone exhibited no spontaneous breakdown to PPi during a 4-hour incubation.

Table 2. NTP pyrophosphohydrolase activity of articular hyaline and fibrocartilage*

	Dog 1	Dog 2	Dog 3
Inner ⅔ meniscus	105	68	192
Outer ⅓ meniscus	105	115	241
Femoral condyle cartilage	84	111	–

* Inorganic pyrophosphate produced/hour/100 mg wet weight of cartilage incubated in DMEM plus ATP, in nmoles.

RESULTS

When hyaline articular cartilage was incubated in the presence of 1 m*M* ATP, PPi was liberated linearly over the next 4-hour period, or until nearly 300 μM PPi had accumulated in the media (Table 1). Both articular hyaline and fibrocartilages generated PPi (Table 2). Concurrently, nucleoside and nucleotide coproducts appeared in the media (Table 1). Mean measurements for 5 consecutive incubations of cartilage specimens from different dogs are summarized in Table 1. PPi generation from ATP varied widely and raised media PPi concentrations between 75 and 250 μM after 2 hours of incubation (28–90 nmoles PPi generated/hour/100 mg wet weight cartilage). In each incubate, ATP degradation exceeded PPi accumulation, implying avenues of degradation other than the pyrophosphohydrolase reaction. The generation of significant levels of ADP reinforces this inference. The difference between ATP degradation and PPi production cannot be explained by hydrolysis of a portion of the newly-formed PPi since ^{32}P-PPi added to the media was not substantially hydrolyzed, precipitated, or adsorbed during the incubation period (data not shown).

Addition of ATP metabolites did not cause the same increase in PPi elaboration into the cartilage culture media (Table 3) as did ATP. However, minor increases in PPi generation were observed with cAMP, adenosine, and especially ADP. Addition of compounds known to interfere with nucleoside and nucleotide metabolism did not prevent the enhanced PPi liberation seen in the presence of ATP (Table 4). The inhibitors effectively slowed primary nucleotide catabolism at the concentrations noted: AMPCP increased AMP accumulation 146% by inhibiting 5′NT; dipyridamole increased extracellular adenosine accumulation 117% by preventing adenosine ingress into cells; and

Table 3. Effect of ATP metabolites upon pyrophosphate (PPi) generation by canine hyaline articular cartilage

Additive	% PPi generated*	No.
ADP	4.8	2
AMP	0.3	4
Adenosine	0.8	1
cAMP	1.8	1
None	0.3	2

* $\% = \frac{PPi_M}{PPi_{ATP}}$; PPi_M = PPi produced by plate containing 1 m*M* metabolite; PPi_{ATP} = PPi produced by companion plate containing 1 m*M* ATP.

Table 5. Inhibition of cartilage NTP pyrophosphohydrolase

Inhibitor	% PPi production*
Dithiothreitol (10 m*M*)	13
Ouabain (0.1 m*M*)	63
EDTA (10 m*M*)	1
EGTA (5 m*M*)	5
Tetramisole (2 m*M*)	81
Cysteine (1 m*M*)	80

* % pyrophosphate (PPi) production = $\frac{\text{PPi production in presence of inhibitor + 1 m}M\text{ ATP}}{\text{PPi production in presence of 1 m}M\text{ ATP}} \times 100.$

EHNA decreased inosine accumulation 94% by inhibiting adenosine deaminase.

We studied the effect produced by addition of NTPPPH inhibitors, upon ATP-induced PPi generation. EDTA (10 m*M*) and EGTA (5 m*M*) inhibited PPi production by 99 and 95%, respectively (Table 5). Incubation of cartilage with these chelators for one-half hour prior to adding ATP maximized inhibition. Dithiothreitol inhibited 90% of NTPPPHase activity in cartilage extracts (14) and inhibited PPi production by 87% in our study. Other substances tested, including ouabain, tetramisole, and cysteine, were weak PPi production inhibitors.

If PPi is generated entirely by cleavage of the α-β pyrophosphate bond of ATP, then the specific activity of γ^{32}P-ATP added to cartilage media and ^{32}P-PPi generated from it should be identical. Results of studies of 5 femoral condylar cartilage specimens from different dogs are summarized in Table 6. Ninety-seven ± 20% (mean ± SD) of the PPi produced was radiolabeled, indicating a direct origin from ATP via NTP pyrophosphohydrolase.

DISCUSSION

Howell et al first reported spontaneous extracellular release of PPi by human osteoarthritic cartilage in culture (1), and we have previously demonstrated that normal articular hyaline and fibrocartilage from several species spontaneously elaborates PPi (2). When any one of a number of nucleoside triphosphates is added to the incubation media, PPi generation is markedly augmented (4). This augmentation presumably results from the action of ecto–NTP pyrophosphohydrolase, which cleaves nucleoside triphosphates into nucleoside monophosphates and PPi (3,4,14).

We have further studied the interaction of ATP and cartilage to determine whether PPi is derived entirely or partially via NTPPPHase or whether PPi production is an independent process resulting from chondrocyte stimulation by ATP or an ATP metabolite.

During in vitro incubation of cartilage with exogenous ATP, PPi was generated linearly, which confirmed our prior results (4). ATP is concomitantly catabolized to nucleotides, nucleosides, and purine bases. Since ATP degradation always exceeded PPi accumulation, and since ADP appeared in the media, it is clear that extracellular ATP is also catabolized by an ATPase, nonspecific phosphatase, or a protein kinase. Similar amounts of PPi generation were not observed when nucleoside or nucleotide catabolites of ATP were substituted for ATP. Moreover, inhibition of various steps in ATP degradation with AMPCP, dipy-

Table 4. Pyrophosphate (PPi) generation from cartilage in the presence of inhibitors of nucleotide and nucleoside catabolism

Additive	% PPi generated*
1 m*M* ATP	100
125 μM AMPCP + 1 m*M* ATP	119
500 μM AMPCP + 1 m*M* ATP	97
500 μM AMPCP + 1 m*M* AMP + 1 m*M* ATP	85
5 μM EHNA + 1 m*M* ATP	92
10 μM dipyridamole + 1 m*M* ATP	115

* $\% = \frac{PPi_I}{PPi_{ATP}}$; PPi_I = PPi produced by plate with inhibitor + 1 m*M* ATP; PPi_{ATP} = PPi produced on plate with 1 m*M* ATP alone. AMPCP = adenosine diphosphonate.

Table 6. Specific activity of ^{32}P-PPi generated in the presence of γ^{32}P-ATP

Dog	PPi (μM)	Hours incubated	Specific activity PPi / Specific activity ATP*
1	40	2	0.66
2	50	2	1.16
3	64	2	1.16
4	137	2	1.04
5	40	1	0.83

* ^{32}P-PPi counts per nmole pyrophosphate (PPi) divided by ^{32}P counts per nmole ATP. See Table 1 for definitions.

ridamole, or EHNA did not interfere with PPi production. These two latter lines of evidence indicate that ATP and not an ATP derivative is essential for augmented PPi production.

Muniz et al (14) reported that divalent cation chelators and dithiothreitol are excellent inhibitors of NTPPPHase in human cartilage extracts. EDTA, EGTA, and dithiothreitol all blocked excess PPi generation in our organ cultures, further supporting the role of NTPPPHase in PPi generation. However, the effects of these inhibitors are highly nonspecific in living cells and results must be interpreted cautiously. Tetramisole and ouabain, which inhibit other phosphatases, only moderately affected PPi generation from ATP. Cysteine was not an effective inhibitor in canine cartilage organ culture, in contrast to findings in detergent extracts of human cartilage (14). These variances may be a result of species difference or represent the enhanced inhibition by cysteine in detergent extracts in comparison with native preparations, as described for cartilage extracellular fluid alkaline phosphatase (19).

Studies of the specific activity of ^{32}P-PPi generated in the presence of γ ^{32}P-ATP showed that excess extracellular PPi is not derived from unlabeled intracellular or extracellular pool. The similar specific activities of ^{32}P-PPi product and the ^{32}P-ATP substrate indicate that the majority of PPi is formed from the γ, and probably β, phosphate of ATP.

The function of this enzyme is unclear. It has been identified in multiple nonarticular tissues (19, 20), as well as in cartilage (3,4,14,21) and matrix vesicles (22–24). Flodgaard and Torp-Pedersen hypothesized that it represents a membrane-associated, ATP-dependent, calcium pump (25). Its ecto-position makes this function less likely. It may represent a means of salvaging purines which escape from damaged cells, as suggested by Tran-Thi et al (26). Our data support this possibility by clearly demonstrating that in cartilage, nucleoside triphosphates can be converted sequentially to nucleoside monophosphates, then to nucleosides which gain access to cells, and finally to purine bases which may be re-utilized (Table 1).

The significance of NTP pyrophosphohydrolase in the pathogenesis of CPPD crystal deposition disease is uncertain, since a naturally occurring extracellular substrate has not been identified. It seems likely that exogenous ATP leads directly to PPi production via NTP pyrophosphohydrolase. A concerted effort to identify possible natural substrates seems justified. Perhaps chondrocytes may become "leaky" under certain physiologic or pathologic conditions, much as endothelial cells or platelets release ATP in response to trauma or enzymatic insult (27). Leaked substrate could be converted to PPi which might accumulate in areas relatively deficient in pyrophosphatase, as discussed by Howell et al (24).

Tenenbaum et al (3) reported and Muniz et al (14) confirmed an excess of 5′NT in extracts of cartilage from patients with CPPD deposition. They hypothesized that 5′NT might accelerate AMP removal, thereby favoring further PPi production (3). Our studies indicate that in the presence of supraphysiologic concentrations of AMP and a specific inhibitor of 5′NT, PPi generation from ATP is not appreciably altered (Table 4). Assuming that human and canine cartilage behave similarly, this finding may diminish the potential import of 5′NT in influencing PPi production. However, 5′NT may be an important modulator at lower concentrations of NTP.

NTP pyrophosphohydrolase activity in normal canine cartilage is adequate to hydrolyze large amounts of substrate at physiologic pH. The excess NTP pyrophosphohydrolase noted in extracts of cartilage from patients with CPPD deposition disease may, therefore, be less important than postulated. Perhaps an excess of substrate is more crucial in the generation of extracellular PPi in CPPD deposition disease.

ACKNOWLEDGMENTS

We wish to acknowledge the helpful suggestions of Dr. Herman Cheung, the donation of canine cartilage by Dr. Garrett Gross, and the manuscript preparation by Dorothy Shrode.

REFERENCES

1. Howell DS, Muniz O, Pita JC, Enis JE: Extrusion of pyrophosphate into extracellular media by osteoarthritic cartilage incubates. J Clin Invest 56:1473–1480, 1975
2. Ryan LM, Cheung HS, McCarty DJ: Release of pyrophosphate by normal mammalian articular hyaline and fibrocartilage in organ culture. Arthritis Rheum 24:1522–1527, 1981
3. Tenenbaum J, Muniz O, Schumacher HR, Good AE, Howell DS: Comparison of pyrophosphohydrolase activities from articular cartilage in calcium pyrophosphate deposition disease and primary osteoarthritis. Arthritis Rheum 24:492–500, 1981
4. Ryan LM, Wortmann RL, Karas B, McCarty DJ Jr: Cartilage nucleoside triphosphate (NTP) pyrophosphohydrolase. I. Identification as an ecto-enzyme. Arthritis Rheum 27:404–409, 1984
5. Stewart C, Gosic G, Hempling H: Effect of exogenous ATP on the volume of TA_3 ascites cells. J Cell Physiol 73:125–132, 1969

6. Makan N: Induction of permeability change and restoration of membrane permeability barrier in transformed cell cultures. Exp Cell Res 114:417–427, 1978
7. Dahlquist R, Diamant B, Kruger P: Increased permeability of the rat mast cell membrane to sodium and potassium caused by extracellular ATP and its relationship to histamine release. Int Arch Allergy Appl Immunol 46:655–675, 1974
8. Cheung CP, Suhadolnik RJ: Analysis of inorganic pyrophosphate at the picomole level. Anal Biochem 83:61–63, 1977
9. Fiske CH, SubbaRow Y: The colorimetric determination of phosphorus. J Biol Chem 66:375–400, 1925
10. Ryan LM, Kozin F, McCarty DJ: Quantification of human plasma inorganic pyrophosphate. I. Normal values in osteoarthritis and calcium pyrophosphate dihydrate crystal deposition disease. Arthritis Rheum 22:886–891, 1979
11. Chen SC, Brown PR, Rosie DM: Extraction procedures for use prior to HPLC nucleotide analysis using microparticle chemically bonded packings. J Chromatogr Sci 15:218–221, 1977
12. Edelson EH, Lawless JG, Wehr CT, Abbott SR: Ion-exchange separation of nucleic acid constituents by high-performance liquid chromatography. J Chromatogr 174:409–419, 1979
13. Hartwick RA, Brown PR: Evaluation of microparticle chemically bonded reversed-phase packings in high-pressure liquid chromatography analysis of nucleosides and their bases. J Chromatogr 126:679–691, 1976
14. Muniz O, Pelletier J-P, Martel-Pelletier J, Morales S, Howell DS: NTP pyrophosphohydrolase in human chondrocalcinotic and osteoarthritic cartilage. I. Some biochemical characteristics. Arthritis Rheum 27:186–192, 1984
15. Manery JF, Dryden EE: Ecto-enzymes concerned with nucleotide metabolism, Physiological and Regulatory Functions of Adenosine and Adenine Nucleotides. Edited by HP Baer, GI Drummond. New York, Raven Press, 1981, pp 323–339
16. Bucher T: Uber ein phosphatubertragendes garungsfermeut. Biochim Biophys Acta 1:292, 1947
17. Adams H: Adenosine 5′-triphosphate determination with phosphoglycerate kinase, Methods of Enzymatic Analysis. Edited by HU Bergmeyer. New York, Academic Press, 1963, pp 539–543
18. Sugino Y, Miyoshi Y: The specific precipitation of orthophosphate and some biochemical applications. J Biol Chem 239:2360–2364, 1964
19. Howell DS, Blanco L, Pita JC, Muniz O: Further characterization of a nucleational agent in hypertrophic cell extracellular cartilage fluid. Metab Bone Dis Relat Res 1:155–159, 1978
20. Torp-Pedersen C, Flodgaard H, Saermark T: Studies on a Ca^{2+}-dependent nucleoside triphosphate pyrophosphohydrolase in rat liver plasma membranes. Biochim Biophys Acta 571:94–104, 1979
21. Cartier P, Picard J: La mineralization du cartilage ossifiable. III. La mecanisme de la reaction ATP asique du cartilage. Bull Soc Chem Biol 37:1159–1176, 1955
22. Hsu H: Purification and partial characterization of ATP pyrophosphohydrolase from fetal bovine epiphyseal cartilage. J Biol Chem 258:3463–3468, 1983
23. Siegel S, Hummel C, Carty P: The role of nucleoside triphosphate pyrophosphohydrolase in in vitro nucleoside triphosphate-dependent matrix vesicle calcification. J Biol Chem 258:8601–8607, 1983
24. Howell DS, Martel-Pelletier J, Pelletier J-P, Morales S, Muniz O: NTP pyrophosphohydrolase in human chondrocalcinotic and osteoarthritic cartilage. II. Further studies on histologic and subcellular distribution. Arthritis Rheum 27:193–199, 1984
25. Flodgaard H, Torp-Pedersen C: A calcium-dependent adenosine triphosphate pyrophosphohydrolase in plasma membrane from rat liver. Biochem J 171:817–820, 1978
26. Tran-Thi T, Phillips J, Schulze-Specking A, Rosenack J, Decker K: Properties and biosynthetic connection of the nucleotide pyrophosphatases of rat liver plasma membrane and endoplasmic reticulum. Hoppe-Selyers Z Physiol Chem 362:305–316, 1981
27. Pearson JD, Gordon JL: Vascular endothelial and smooth muscle cells in culture selectively release adenine nucleotides. Nature 281:384–386, 1979

CARTILAGE RESPONSE TO MECHANICAL FORCE IN HIGH-DENSITY CHONDROCYTE CULTURES

G. P. J. VAN KAMPEN, J. P. VELDHUIJZEN, R. KUIJER, R. J. VAN DE STADT, and C. A. SCHIPPER

High-density cultures of chick embryonic chondrocytes were exposed to intermittent compressive force (ICF) of physiologic magnitude for 24 hours. Proteoglycan synthesis was significantly increased in chondrocyte cultures exposed to ICF as compared with control cultures. Similar effects were found in explants of epiphyseal cartilage. Proteoglycans extracted with guanidine-HCl from cultures exposed to ICF aggregated better with hyaluronic acid than did control cultures, as shown by Sepharose 2B gel chromatography. In addition, the amount of non-extractable proteoglycans was increased in ICF cultures. We conclude that ICF not only increases the synthesis of proteoglycans but also improves the aggregating capacity of proteoglycans and the coherence of proteoglycans with other matrix components. High-density cultures of epiphyseal chondrocytes provide a suitable model to study the processes involved in the perception of and the subsequent cellular response to compressive force by cartilage.

The ability of cartilage to function as a weight-bearing tissue is related to its chemical composition and the macromolecular organization of its constituents (1). The extracellular matrix of cartilage is primarily composed of collagen and proteoglycan, which account for 50–60% and 10–40% of the dry weight, respectively (2). Collagen confers tensile strength (3) and proteoglycans provide the elasticity and the ability to resist compression (4,5). Proteoglycan monomers which have an average molecular weight of $1–2 \times 10^6$ daltons (6) possess a high fixed negative charge density, which renders them highly hydrophilic (7).

In cartilage the proteoglycans form predominantly very large aggregates, in which many individual monomers are noncovalently associated with hyaluronic acid (8,9). A proteoglycan monomer consists of a protein core which contains 3 regions: the hyaluronic acid binding region with a few short keratan sulfate chains, an intermediate keratan sulfate–rich fragment, and a chondroitin sulfate–rich fragment of variable size (10,11). The proteoglycan–hyaluronic acid interaction is stabilized by 2 glycoproteins (9,12–16).

The initial in vivo response of articular cartilage to repetitive trauma is enhanced matrix production without cell proliferation (17), whereas a decrease in loading provokes degenerative changes in the articular cartilage (18,19). This study reports the in vitro response of high-density chondrocyte cultures to intermittent compression. We reported earlier that under in vitro conditions, intermittent compressive force (ICF) decreased cell proliferation of chondrocytes cultured in a monolayer (20). Matrix production, however, should be studied using high-density chondrocyte cultures (21–25). We developed a suitable model (24) and reported that high-density chondrocyte cultures exposed to intermittent compressive force showed a decrease in cell proliferation and an increase in matrix

From the Vrije Universiteit, Amsterdam, The Netherlands and the Jan van Breemen Institute, Amsterdam, The Netherlands.

G. P. J. van Kampen, PhD: Department of Oral Cell Biology, School of Dentistry, Vrije Universiteit; J. P. Veldhuijzen, PhD: Department of Oral Cell Biology, School of Dentistry, Vrije Universiteit; R. Kuijer: Center for Rheumatology and Rehabilitation, Jan van Breemen Institute; R. J. van de Stadt, PhD: Center for Rheumatology and Rehabilitation, Jan van Breemen Institute; C. A. Schipper: Department of Oral Cell Biology, School of Dentistry, Vrije Universiteit.

Address reprint requests to J. P. Veldhuijzen, PhD, Department of Oral Cell Biology, School of Dentistry, Vrije Universiteit, PO Box 7161, 1007 MC, Amsterdam, The Netherlands.

Submitted for publication April 12, 1984; accepted in revised form September 25, 1984.

production (26). The present in vitro investigation describes the changes in the nature of the proteoglycans synthesized by high-density chondrocyte cultures when exposed to intermittent compressive force.

MATERIALS AND METHODS

From the epiphyses of 15-day-old chick embryos the segments farthest from the diaphysis, containing the flattened chondrocytes (27) (also referred to as proliferative cells), were dissected. These epiphyseal segments were digested with collagenase (300 units/ml; CLS II, Worthington Biochemicals, Freehold, NJ) to isolate the chondrocytes. The isolated single cells were suspended in culture medium M199 (Gibco, Grand Island, NY) supplemented with 250 μg L-glutamine/ml, (Merck, Darmstadt, FRG) and 50 μg L–ascorbic acid/ml (Merck). Preincubation of 2×10^5 cells in a 5-μl drop of M199 for 18 hours resulted in identical, high-density cultures of cohering chondrocytes which can be handled individually (24). The zone of flattened cells excised from the epiphyses was cultured as an explant, after a 30-minute collagenase treatment to remove damaged and noncartilage cells.

Individual high-density chondrocyte cultures and explants were cultured for 24 hours in polystyrene tubes with 2 ml of culture medium M199 containing 10% fetal calf serum (Gibco). Control cultures and explants were cultured in a humidified (98%) incubator (5% CO_2 in air) at 37°C. Experimental cultures were exposed to ICF during the 24-hour culture period and compared with control cultures.

ICF was applied to cultures and explants in the test tubes by compressing the gas phase (75% N_2, 20% O_2, and 5% CO_2) above the culture medium. Tubes exposed to ICF were closed with a rubber cap. A hypodermic needle (18G 1½) was inserted through the rubber cap and connected to an air chamber via a hose (ϕ 6 mm). Two electromagnetic valves in the air chamber controlled the flow of the gas mixture. One valve controlling the inflow was connected via a reducer to the gas mixture under compression, while the other valve controlled the outlet to air. Both valves were opened alternately by an electric circuit with a frequency of 0.3 Hz, thus providing an intermittent compressive force. The pressure changes were monitored by a manometer connected to the system, and the pressure differential at its peak measured 130 mb. As was reported by Rodan and coworkers (28), this pressure was calculated to be equivalent to the weight-bearing force of the chicken epiphyseal plate, taking into account the weight of a chicken and the cross-section of the plate.

For determination of cellular activity, 6 control and 6 ICF cultures were labeled during the entire culture period or pulse labeled for the last 90 minutes of the culture period with 5 μCi ^{35}S-sulfate/ml (66 mCi/mmole) and 5 μCi ^{3}H-glucosamine/ml (34.6 Ci/mmole) or 1 μCi ^{3}H-thymidine/ml (5 Ci/mmole). The radiochemicals were purchased from The Radiochemical Centre, Amersham, UK. Cell proliferation was measured by determining the amount of ^{3}H-thymidine incorporated into DNA. Matrix deposition was determined after papain digestion of the cultures and measurement of the incorporation of ^{35}S-sulfate and ^{3}H-glucosamine into cetylpyridinium chloride precipitable glycosaminoglycans (24). The results were analyzed statistically by the Wilcoxon rank sum test.

The aggregating capacity of proteoglycans with hyaluronic acid was studied in 60 control and 60 ICF cultures that had been labeled with ^{35}S-sulfate during a 24-hour experiment. The proteoglycans synthesized during this period were extracted (at 4°C) with guanidine-HCl. Guanidine-HCl solutions (0.15*M* potassium acetate, 0.01*M* EDTA, pH 6.8; special Aristar grade, BDH Chemicals Poole, UK) were filtered through charcoal to remove ultraviolet absorbing material, after which 5 m*M* iodoacetic acid, 0.1*M* caproic acid, 5 m*M* benzamidine-HCl, and 50 mg trypsin inhibitor per liter were added.

Control and ICF cultures were extracted under associative conditions in 4 ml of 0.5*M* guanidine-HCl with magnetic stirring for 24 hours. After centrifugation at 56,000*g* for 60 minutes, the supernatants were stored at −20°C (associative extracts). The remaining pellets were extracted under dissociative conditions in 4 ml of 4.0*M* guanidine-HCl with 0.15*M* potassium acetate and 0.01*M* EDTA (pH 6.8) supplemented with the same inhibitor cocktail as described above, with magnetic stirring for 72 hours, and subsequently centrifuged. The supernatants were then dialyzed against 15 volumes of 0.15*M* potassium acetate to associative conditions for 18 hours (reassociated-dissociative extracts). The associative extracts and reassociated-dissociative extracts were extensively dialyzed against distilled water and freeze-dried.

The freeze-dried extracts were dissolved in 1 ml of the elution buffer containing 0.15*M* potassium acetate and 1 m*M* NaN_3. The total amount of incorporated ^{35}S-sulfate was determined by liquid scintillation counting. Aliquots were centrifuged in a Janetski centrifuge and 250-μl aliquots from the supernatants were subjected to downward column chromatography on Sepharose 2B (149×0.7 cm, Pharmacia Fine Chemicals, Piscataway, NJ) with 0.15*M* potassium acetate (pH 6.8) supplemented with 1 m*M* NaN_3 as an eluant. The flow rate was 2 ml per hour, and 700-μl fractions were collected. From each fraction the amount of ^{35}S-sulfate was determined using Picofluor 15 in an A300 CD Tricarb liquid scintillation counter (Packard, Downers Grove, IL).

Twenty microliters of hyaluronic acid (1 mg/ml) was added to 400-μl aliquots of the reassociated-dissociative extracts from control and ICF cultures and mixed for 24 hours. These samples were chromatographed as described above.

RESULTS

The data for cell proliferation and proteoglycan synthesis in control and ICF cultures are presented in Figure 1. Incorporation of ^{3}H-thymidine into DNA, a parameter for cell proliferation, was decreased by 20% with ICF ($P < 0.01$), whereas incorporation of ^{35}S-sulfate into glycosaminoglycans, a parameter for proteoglycan synthesis, was increased by 40% ($P < 0.01$). The ratios of ^{35}S-sulfate incorporation into glycosam-

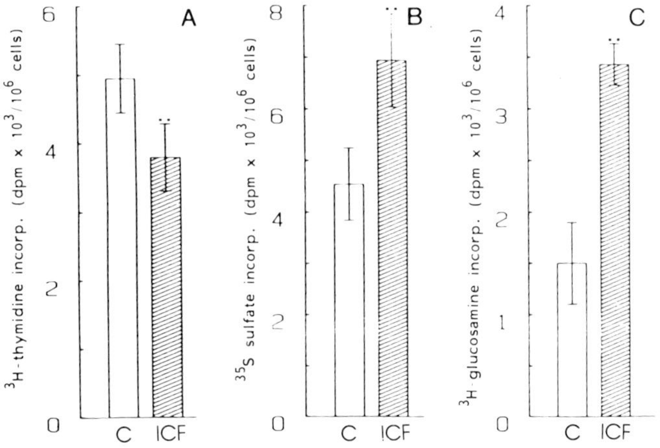

Figure 1. Cell proliferation and proteoglycan synthesis of control (C) and experimental (intermittent compressive force, ICF) chondrocyte cultures, pulse labeled for 90 minutes, after a 24-hour culture period. **A**, ^{3}H-thymidine incorporation into DNA. **B**, ^{35}S-sulfate incorporation into glycosaminoglycans. **C**, ^{3}H-glucosamine incorporation into glycosaminoglycans. Values shown are mean ± SD of 6 cultures. ** = $P < 0.01$.

inoglycans and ^{3}H-glucosamine incorporation into glycosaminoglycans did not differ significantly in either control or ICF cultures.

The effect of ICF on proteoglycan synthesis and cell proliferation in explants, derived from the zone of flattened chondrocytes from the epiphyses, was also examined. Figure 2 shows that ICF stimulated ^{35}S-sulfate incorporation (120% increase, $P < 0.01$), whereas ^{3}H-thymidine incorporation was not significantly changed.

The effect of ICF on the aggregating capacity and the extractability of proteoglycans from the matrix was studied by Gu-HCl extraction. In a typical experiment, the amount of ^{35}S-sulfate incorporated into the extractable pools of proteoglycans (0.5*M* and 4.0*M* Gu-HCl) yielded an average of 477,200 disintegrations per minute for control aggregates. For cultures subjected to ICF, this figure was 411,700 dpm. It should be noted that ICF did significantly stimulate the incorporation of ^{35}S-sulfate into the total pool of extractable and non-extractable proteoglycans after papain digestion (Figure 1B).

The ratio between the amount of label present in the associative (0.5*M* Gu-HCl) and the reassociated-dissociative (4.0*M* Gu-HCl) extracted proteoglycans was comparable in control and ICF cultures: 71%:29% and 74%:26%, respectively (Table 1).

The amount of proteoglycan aggregates and monomers in the guanidine-HCl extracts was determined by Sepharose 2B column chromatography. The profiles for the associative extracts are shown in Figure 3A. In Figure 3B the profiles of the reassociated-dissociative extracts are presented. From Figure 3A it can be seen that although the profiles followed the same pattern, the amount of label present in all fractions of the ICF cultures was lower than in the corresponding fractions of the control cultures. The

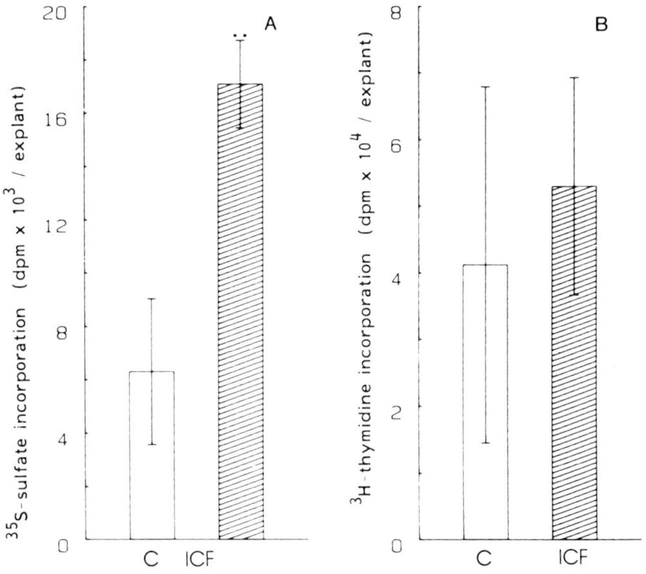

Figure 2. Proteoglycan synthesis and cell proliferation of control (C) and experimental (intermittent compressive force, ICF) explants of epiphyseal cartilage during a 24-hour culture period. **A**, ^{35}S-sulfate incorporation into glycosaminoglycans. **B**, ^{3}H-thymidine incorporation into DNA. Values shown are mean ± SD of 6 cultures. ** = $P < 0.01$.

Table 1. Percent distribution of ^{35}S-sulfate incorporation into proteoglycans of control and experimental (intermittent compressive force, ICF) cultures, measured after guanidine-HCl extraction, and percent distribution of label in proteoglycans in aggregate form and as monomers after Sepharose 2B column chromatography of the various guanidine-HCl extracts

	Gu-HCl extraction	% extractable proteoglycans	Column chromatography: Aggregates	Column chromatography: Monomers
Control	0.5*M*	71	35	65
	4.0*M*	29	23	77
Total in aggregate form (control)			31	
ICF	0.5*M*	74	45	55
	4.0*M*	26	55	45
Total in aggregate form (ICF)			48	

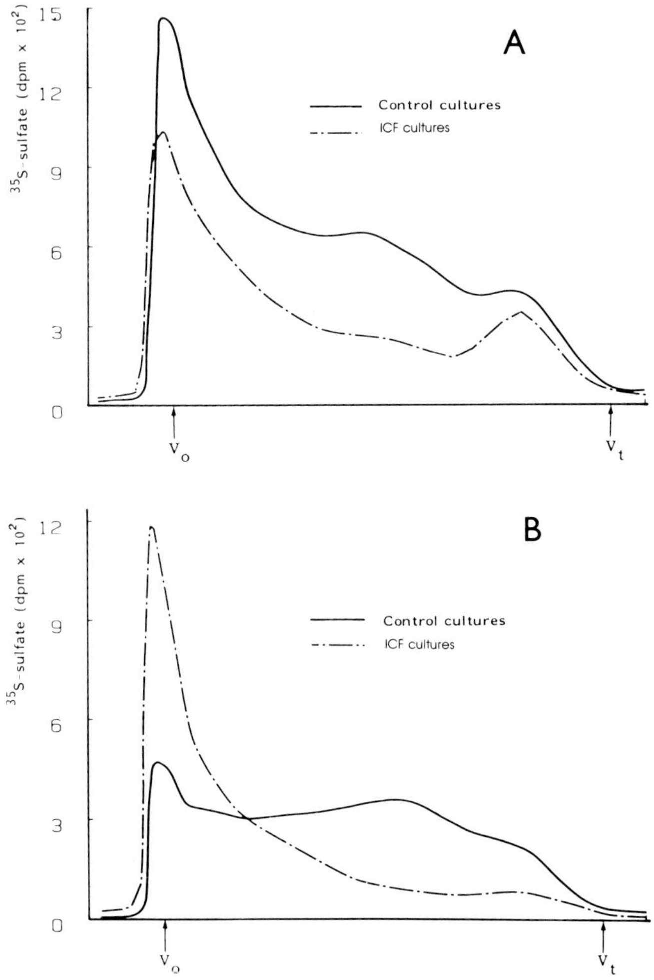

Figure 3. Elution profiles of guanidine-HCl–extracted fractions from control and experimental (intermittent compressive force, ICF) chondrocyte cultures. **A**, Associative fractions (extracted with 0.5*M* Gu-HCl). **B**, Reassociated-dissociative fractions (extracted with 4.0*M* Gu-HCl). Aggregates of proteoglycan and hyaluronic acid elute in the void volume (V_0).

peak in the void volume (V_o) corresponded with the large aggregates of proteoglycans and hyaluronic acid, whereas the proteoglycan monomers eluted between V_t and V_o.

The percentage distribution of the proteoglycan aggregates and monomers found after column chromatography is shown in Table 1. From the associative extracts (0.5*M* Gu-HCl) of control cultures, 35% of the label was found in the proteoglycan aggregates and 65% in the monomers. In ICF cultures the distribution was 45% and 55% in aggregates and monomers, respectively.

The proteoglycans in the reassociated-dissociated extracts (4.0*M* Gu-HCl) showed an increased aggregating capacity after ICF exposure, as indicated by the larger peak in the void volume after column chromatography (Figure 3B). Table 1 shows that 23% of the label was measured in the peak in the void volume (large aggregates) of control cultures, whereas this value was 55% in ICF cultures. When these data are compiled, it can be calculated that in control cultures, 31% of the total extractable proteoglycans were present in the aggregate form, whereas in ICF cultures this percentage increased to 48% (Table 1).

To determine whether the aggregating capacity of the proteoglycan monomers was influenced by the amount of hyaluronic acid present in the reassociated-dissociative extracts, reassociation in the presence of 1% hyaluronic acid was performed. These extracts were also chromatographed and the profiles were compared with those shown in Figure 3B. No significant differences were found.

DISCUSSION

We have found that there is an increase in the incorporation of ^{35}S-sulfate into glycosaminoglycans synthesized and deposited in the matrix by high-density cultures of epiphyseal chondrocytes in vitro, when the cells are exposed to intermittent compression of physiologic magnitude for 24 hours. The same phenomenon was observed in explants, indicating that neither the presence of preexisting matrix nor the isolation procedure influenced the cellular response to ICF.

It has been suggested that intermittent compression may improve exchange of nutrients and catabolites. Joint motion has been considered to be important for the pumping of nutrient molecules from the synovial space into cartilage and for movement of catabolites from the cartilage into synovial space (29), since nutrition of normal adult articular cartilage is derived chiefly from the synovial fluid (30). However, on the basis of the relatively high diffusion coefficients of small ionic and non-ionic solutes, Maroudas (31) stated that compressive force will not appreciably increase the rate of transport of nutrients in articular cartilage above that which can be achieved by diffusion alone. Since high-density chondrocyte cultures and explants of whole cartilage responded to ICF in a similar manner, whereas the former contained much less matrix than the latter, we conclude that the exchange of metabolites provides no or only a minor contribution to the ICF effect.

The ratio of ^{35}S-sulfate incorporation to ^{3}H-glucosamine incorporation was not significantly changed as a result of the stimulus. This means that the sulfation rate of the glycosaminoglycans did not change. Therefore, it is concluded that the amount of sulfated glycosaminoglycans synthesized is increased after ICF. The increase in negatively charged groups provides a higher water-binding capacity, which will improve the resilience to compression (4,5,7).

Our results are corroborated by in vivo experiments. Changes in knee cartilage of normal dogs after a few weeks of immobilization were accompanied by a decrease of uronic acid in the tissue and suppression of net synthesis of proteoglycans (18). Joint motion in the absence of normal loading did not maintain normal articular cartilage, which was reversed during normal loaded motion of the joint (19). Repetitive impulsive loading of the knee joints of rabbits did not change the amount of collagen in the cartilage, but the synthesis of sulfated glycosaminoglycans was increased (32).

From Figure 1B it can be concluded that as a result of ICF, the amount of label incorporated into glycosaminoglycans of the total proteoglycan population (measured after papain digestion) had increased significantly. However, ICF did not increase the amount of label incorporated into the guanidine-HCl extractable proteoglycans. From the data presented in Figure 3A, it is also clear that it is more difficult to extract proteoglycans with 0.5*M* guanidine-HCl from the matrix of ICF cultures than from control cultures. We conclude, therefore, that exposure to ICF leads to an increase in non-extractable proteoglycans which are firmly anchored in the matrix, probably via improved binding to collagen.

ICF also changes the aggregating characteristics of the guanidine-extractable proteoglycans. Column chromatography showed that the relative amount of label present in large proteoglycan aggregates after associative extraction (0.5*M* Gu-HCl) was enhanced after ICF (45% versus 35%; Table 1), indicating that the binding of proteoglycans to hyaluronic acid is also improved after ICF. This conclusion is corroborated by the data from the reassociated-dissociative extracts (4.0*M* Gu-HCl). After reassociation of the dissociative extracts, the percentage distribution of the label showed that more proteoglycan–hyaluronic acid aggregates were formed in the reassociated extracts of ICF cultures than of control cultures (55 versus 23%; Figure 3B and Table 1).

This difference in proteoglycan and hyaluronic acid aggregation is not caused by a low amount of hyaluronic acid. Addition of hyaluronic acid during the reassociation of the dissociative extracts did not change the data, as presented in Figure 3B and Table 1. Thus, the improved aggregating capacity after ICF is probably caused by alterations in the hyaluronic acid binding region of the proteoglycan protein core. This conclusion is corroborated by the in vivo experiments of Palmoski et al (18,19), who reported a defective macromolecular organization, i.e., an impaired proteoglycan aggregation, in knee cartilage of normal dogs after a few weeks of immobilization.

We conclude that under our experimental conditions, the in vivo effects of intermittent compressive force can be mimicked and studied in detail in vitro. Chondrocytes in our high-density tissue culture model respond to a mechanical stimulus of physiologic magnitude in a manner comparable with the in vivo response. The chondrocytes respond to intermittent compressive force by an increased synthesis of glycosaminoglycans in matrix proteoglycans. In addition, ICF improved both the aggregating capacity of proteoglycans with hyaluronic acid and the coherence of proteoglycans with other matrix components. This in vitro model opens the possibility for further study of chondrocyte perception of mechanical stimuli and the subsequent cellular response.

REFERENCES

1. Freeman MAR, Kempson G: Load carriage, Adult Articular Cartilage. Edited by MAR Freeman. London, Pitman Medical, 1973, pp 228–246
2. Strider W, Pal S, Rosenberg L: Comparison of proteoglycans from bovine articular cartilage. Biochim Biophys Acta 379:271–281, 1975
3. Kempson GE, Muir H, Polland C, Tuke M: The tensile properties of the human femoral condyles related to the content of collagen and glycosaminoglycans. Biochim Biophys Acta 297:456–472, 1973
4. Kempson GE, Muir H, Swanson SV, Freeman MAR: Correlations between the compressive stiffness and chemical constituents of human articular cartilage. Biochim Biophys Acta 215:70–77, 1970
5. Kempson GE, Tuke MA, Barrett AJ, Horsfield PM: Effects of proteolytic enzymes on the mechanical properties of adult human articular cartilage. Biochim Biophys Acta 428:741–760, 1976
6. Rosenberg L, Hellman W, Kleinschmidt AK: Macromolecular models of protein polysaccharides from bovine nasal cartilage based on electron microscopic studies. J Biol Chem 245:4123–4130, 1970
7. Maroudas A: Physicochemical properties of articular cartilage, Adult Articular Cartilage. Edited by MAR Freeman. London, Pitman Medical, 1973, pp 131–170

8. Hardingham TE, Muir H: The specific interaction of hyaluronic acid with cartilage proteoglycan. Biochim Biophys Acta 279:401–405, 1972
9. Hascall VC, Heinegard D: Aggregation of cartilage proteoglycans. I. The role of hyaluronic acid. J Biol Chem 249:4232–4241, 1974
10. Hardingham TE, Ewins RJF, Muir H: Cartilage proteoglycans: structure and heterogeneity of the protein core and the effects of specific protein modifications on the binding to hyaluronate. Biochem J 457:127–143, 1976
11. Heinegard D, Axelson I: Distribution of keratan sulfate in cartilage proteoglycans. J Biol Chem 252:1971–1979, 1977
12. Hascall VC, Sajdera SW: Protein-polysaccharide complex from bovine nasal cartilage: the function of glycoprotein in the formation of aggregates. J Biol Chem 244:2384–2396, 1969
13. Heinegard D, Hascall VC: Aggregation of cartilage proteoglycans. III. Characteristics of proteins isolated from trypsin digests of aggregates. J Biol Chem 249: 4250–4256, 1974
14. Hardingham TE, Muir H: Structure and stability of proteoglycan aggregation. Ann Rheum Dis (suppl) 34: 26–28, 1975
15. Baker JR, Caterson B: The isolation and characterization of the link proteins from proteoglycan aggregates of bovine nasal cartilage. J Biol Chem 254:2387–2393, 1979
16. Tang LH, Rosenberg L, Reiner A, Poole AR: Proteoglycans from bovine nasal cartilage: properties of a soluble form of link protein. J Biol Chem 254:10523–10531, 1979
17. Muir H: Molecular approach to the understanding of osteoarthrosis. Ann Rheum Dis 36:199–208, 1979
18. Palmoski M, Perricone E, Brandt KD: Development and reversal of a proteoglycan aggregation defect in normal canine knee cartilage after immobilization. Arthritis Rheum 22:508–517, 1979
19. Palmoski MJ, Colyer RA, Brandt KD: Joint motion in the absence of normal loading does not maintain normal articular cartilage. Arthritis Rheum 23:325–334, 1980
20. Veldhuijzen JP, Bourret LA, Rodan GA: In vitro studies of the effect of intermittent compressive forces on cartilage cell proliferation. J Cell Physiol 98:299–306, 1979
21. Oakes BW, Handley CJ, Lisner F, Lowther DA: An ultrastructural and biochemical study of high density primary cultures of embryonic chick chondrocytes. J Embryol Exp Morphol 38:239–263, 1977
22. Kuettner KE, Pauli BU, Gall G, Memoli VA, Schenk RK: Synthesis of cartilage matrix by mammalian chondrocytes in vitro. I. Isolation culture characteristics and morphology. J Cell Biol 93:743–750, 1982
23. Kuettner KE, Memoli VA, Pauli BU, Wrobel NC, Thonar EJMA, Daniel JC: Synthesis of cartilage matrix by mammalian chondrocytes in vitro. II. Maintenance of collagen and proteoglycan phenotype. J Cell Biol 93:751–757, 1982
24. Van Kampen GPJ, Veldhuijzen JP: Aggregated chondrocytes as a model system to study cartilage metabolism. Exp Cell Res 140:440–443, 1982
25. Amadio PC, Ehrlich MG, Mankin HJ: Matrix synthesis in high density cultures of bovine epiphyseal chondrocytes. Connect Tissue Res 11:11–19, 1983
26. Van Kampen GPJ, Veldhuijzen JP: An in vitro model to study factors affecting the matrix production and cell proliferation of chondrocytes, Current Advances in Skeletogenesis. Edited by M Silbermann, HC Slavkin. Amsterdam, Excerpta Medica, 1982, pp 356–361
27. Holtrop ME: The ultrastructure of the epiphyseal plate. I. The flattened chondrocyte. Calcif Tissue Res 9:131–139, 1972
28. Rodan GA, Mensi T, Harvey A: A quantitative method for the application of compressive forces to bone in tissue culture. Calcif Tissue Res 18:125–131, 1975
29. Ekholm R: Nutrition of articular cartilage: an autoradiographic study. Acta Anat (Basel) 24:329–338, 1955
30. Hodge JA, McKibbin B: The nutrition of mature and immature cartilage in rabbits. J Bone Joint Surg 51B:140–147, 1969
31. Maroudas A: Transport through articular cartilage and some physiological implications, Normal and Osteoarthrotic Articular Cartilage. Edited by SY Ali, MW Elves, DM Leaback. London, Institute of Orthopedics, 1974, pp 33–47
32. Radin EL, Ehrlich MG, Chernack R, Abernethy P, Paul IL, Rose RM: Effect of repetitive impulsive loading on the knee joints of rabbits. Clin Orthop 131:288–293, 1978

A LONGITUDINAL STUDY OF HIGH AND LOW AVIDITY ANTIBODIES TO DOUBLE-STRANDED DNA IN SYSTEMIC LUPUS ERYTHEMATOSUS

HUGH McGRATH, Jr. and JOSEPH J. BIUNDO, Jr.

The role of avidity in the pathogenicity of double-stranded DNA/anti–double-stranded DNA immune complexes in systemic lupus erythematosus (SLE) has been controversial. We used polyethylene glycol to identify low avidity antibodies and the standard Farr assay to detect high avidity antibodies against double-stranded DNA in a longitudinal study of sera from 19 patients with SLE. We found that high and low avidity antibodies to double-stranded DNA did not move independently, but instead, rose and fell in a parallel and relatively fixed manner in these patients. The mechanisms responsible for the changes in titer of anti–double-stranded DNA antibody appeared nondiscriminatory in regard to avidity. In addition, the humoral immune response in SLE depicted by these antibody measurements appeared atypical, lacking maturational features.

It is well known that circulating antibodies to double-stranded DNA (dsDNA) are present in patients with systemic lupus erythematous (SLE) (1,2). They may be associated with certain disease manifestations (3,4) and their levels may fluctuate with disease activity (5,6). Qualitative properties of these antibodies are believed to influence their pathogenicity (7,8). Avidity, which refers to the composite forces that bind antigen to antibody, is a qualitative property that has been closely studied in recent years. Although a number of investigators have stressed the importance of avidity, its role in disease mechanisms in SLE has been highly debated. In conflicting studies, both high avidity (9–11) and low avidity (12–14) anti-dsDNA antibodies have been shown to correlate independently with nephritis or disease activity. A major obstacle to resolution of this problem has been the lack of a simple assay that will differentiate high and low avidity antibodies in this complex multivalent system (15,16).

We recently developed a method that detects low avidity antibodies to dsDNA (17). We used polyethylene glycol to precipitate both high and low avidity ^{3}H-dsDNA/anti-dsDNA immune complexes from sera, but the contribution of high avidity antibodies to binding values in this test is small. The polyethylene glycol (PEG) assay measures large lattices which may be favored by the presence of high numbers of cross-reacting low avidity antibodies. The standard Farr assay measures only high avidity antibodies to dsDNA because the ammonium sulfate salt used in the Farr assay dissociates low avidity bonds (18–20). We have shown that both excess dsDNA and salt will dissociate the low avidity dsDNA antibodies measured by the PEG assay but not detected by the Farr assay. This finding has been confirmed by others (21). Low avidity bonds are preserved by polyethylene glycol.

The Farr and PEG assays have been used together in this study to observe the changes that occur in the high and low avidity anti-dsDNA antibody populations, during periods of up to 3½ years, in patients with SLE.

From the Department of Medicine, Section of Rheumatology, Louisiana State University, New Orleans.

Supported by a grant from the Baton Rouge Chapter of the Louisiana Lupus Foundation, and by the National Institutes of Health research support grant BRSG SO-RR-5376, with funds provided by the Division of Research Resources.

Hugh McGrath, Jr., MD: Assistant Professor of Medicine, Louisiana State University Medical School; Joseph J. Biundo, Jr., MD: Professor of Medicine and Chief, Section of Rheumatology, Department of Medicine, Louisiana State University Medical School.

Address reprint requests to Hugh McGrath, Jr., MD, Department of Medicine, Louisiana State University Medical Center, 1542 Tulane Avenue, New Orleans, LA 70112.

Submitted for publication January 30, 1984; accepted in revised form October 3, 1984.

PATIENTS AND METHODS

Patients and sera. We measured binding levels of high and low avidity antibody using the Farr and PEG assays, respectively, for up to a 3½-year period of disease in patients with SLE. One hundred seventy-six serum specimens from 19 SLE patients, and 25 serum specimens from 25 normal human subjects were studied. All SLE patients (ages 16–67) fulfilled the American Rheumatism Association's revised criteria for SLE (22). All but 1 were women. Four patients were white and 15 were black. All had at least intermittently active disease assessed by clinical and serologic variables, including antibody to DNA using the *Crithidia luciliae* (CL) assay (23). The sera were stored at −20°C and, before use, were inactivated at 56°C for one-half hour and then briefly spun on a table-top centrifuge to remove aggregates.

DNA. Tritium-labeled *Escherichia coli* dsDNA (^{3}H–*E coli* dsDNA) was obtained in several lots (New England Nuclear, Boston, MA) and purified by passage through an 8 × ½-cm column of nitrocellulose in two times standard saline citrate, pH 6.7, for removal of single-stranded DNA (ssDNA) (24). The purified dsDNA was tested in the Farr assay against 5 serum specimens that contained only anti-ssDNA antibodies. These sera bound up to 30% of ssDNA but did not bind purified dsDNA.

The Farr assay (25). Twenty-five microliters of sera, diluted 1:10 with borate buffered saline (BBS) (0.03*M* borate, 0.15*M* NaCl, pH 7.8), were added to 15 ng of ^{3}H-dsDNA in 75 μl of BBS. The mixture was incubated in a 0.4-ml stoppered polyethylene tube for 1 hour at 37°C. One hundred microliters of 100% cold-saturated ammonium sulfate (SAS) was added, and the mixture was vortexed and then incubated for 24 hours at 4°C. After centrifugation at 8,000*g* for 15 minutes at 4°C, the supernatant was discarded and the precipitate washed twice with 50% SAS, followed each time with centrifugation. The washed precipitate was solubilized in 300 μl of distilled water for 1 hour at 37°C. The dissolved material was added to 1 ml of water and 10 ml of Beckman EP Liquid Scintillation Cocktail, mixed, and counts per minute were then determined in a Beckman LS-250 liquid scintillation system. Background binding of normal human serum (NHS) in the Farr assay was 8 ± 3%. In both the Farr and PEG assays, the binding by SLE sera was corrected for the background binding of NHS. Thus, % ^{3}H-DNA bound =

$$\frac{\text{Counts in SLE precipitate} - \text{counts in NHS precipitate}}{\text{Total counts} - \text{counts in NHS precipitate}} \times 100$$

The PEG assay. This procedure was basically the same as in the Farr assay, with the following differences: Serum dilution was 1:5 and 7% PEG was used instead of SAS. To eliminate nonspecific binding of dsDNA to lipoproteins, dextran sulfate was used in a final concentration of 50 μg/ml (26). The precipitate was washed with 3.5% polyethylene glycol and solubilized by adding 300 μl of 0.1*M* NaOH and then incubating at 56°C for 1 hour. Background binding of normal human sera in the PEG assay was 3 ± 2%.

The CL, C3, and C4 assays. The CL assay and the C3 and C4 level determinations were done with commercially available, standard kits (Meloy Laboratories, Springfield, VA) by means of the manufacturer's recommended protocol. Normal values for C3 ranged from 86–202 mg/dl and for C4, 15–53 mg/dl.

Dissociation studies. The Farr and PEG assays were done both with and without the addition of either unlabeled dsDNA or NaCl to determine the ease with which the dsDNA/anti-dsDNA complexes could be dissociated by these substances under these assay conditions. For dissociation with unlabeled DNA, 15 ng of ^{3}H-dsDNA in 75 ml of BBS was added to 25 μl of an SLE serum dilution, and the mixture was vortexed and then incubated for 1 hour at 37°C. Three micrograms of unlabeled calf thymus dsDNA (type I; Sigma, St. Louis, MO) was added in 25 μl of BBS to bring the thymus dsDNA to a final concentration that was 200× that of the ^{3}H-dsDNA. Twenty-five microliters of BBS alone was added to controls. These mixtures were vortexed, incubated at room temperature for 2 hours, and then incubated overnight at 4°C. Precipitates were washed, collected, and counted.

For the salt dissociation study, the same procedure was followed except that instead of calf thymus dsDNA, 25 μl of 2.4*M* NaCl was added to bring the final molarity of the NaCl in the mixture to 0.6. Incubation was for 2 hours at room temperature.

Statistical analysis. Correlation coefficients (r values) were obtained for the combined Farr and PEG assay paired samples in each individual. A pooled correlation coefficient was then obtained for the combined correlation coefficients of the 19 patients.

RESULTS

Sensitivity of Farr and PEG assays. Sensitivity was greatest for the Farr assay, with 90% of the 176 sera exhibiting above normal binding, while 74% did so in the PEG assay. In 24 sera, there was significant binding at some point in the Farr assay, but not in the PEG assay (Figures 1A, B, and F).

The correlation of Farr assay to PEG assay. High and low avidity antibody binding levels measured by the Farr and PEG assays rose and fell in parallel. Figures 1A–F show high and low avidity binding levels plotted against disease course. The pooled correlation coefficient between the Farr assay and the PEG assay was 0.74 ($P < 0.001$), with 6 patients having individual r values >0.95.

The pattern of the Farr to PEG binding remained consistent in each patient throughout the course of his/her disease (Figures 1A–F). Thus, when Farr binding was greater than PEG binding in 1 sample, it tended to remain so throughout the serial study. The converse was also true. In 3 patients in whom the Farr and PEG binding were essentially equal, this pattern persisted throughout the course of disease also (Figure 1E). These easily identifiable avidity patterns were compared with disease manifestations (Table 1). There was no apparent correlation between avidity pattern and disease manifestation.

Dissociation studies. Table 2 gives the results of dissociation studies that show the effect of either salt or excess DNA on dissociation of anti-dsDNA as measured by the Farr and PEG assays. There was

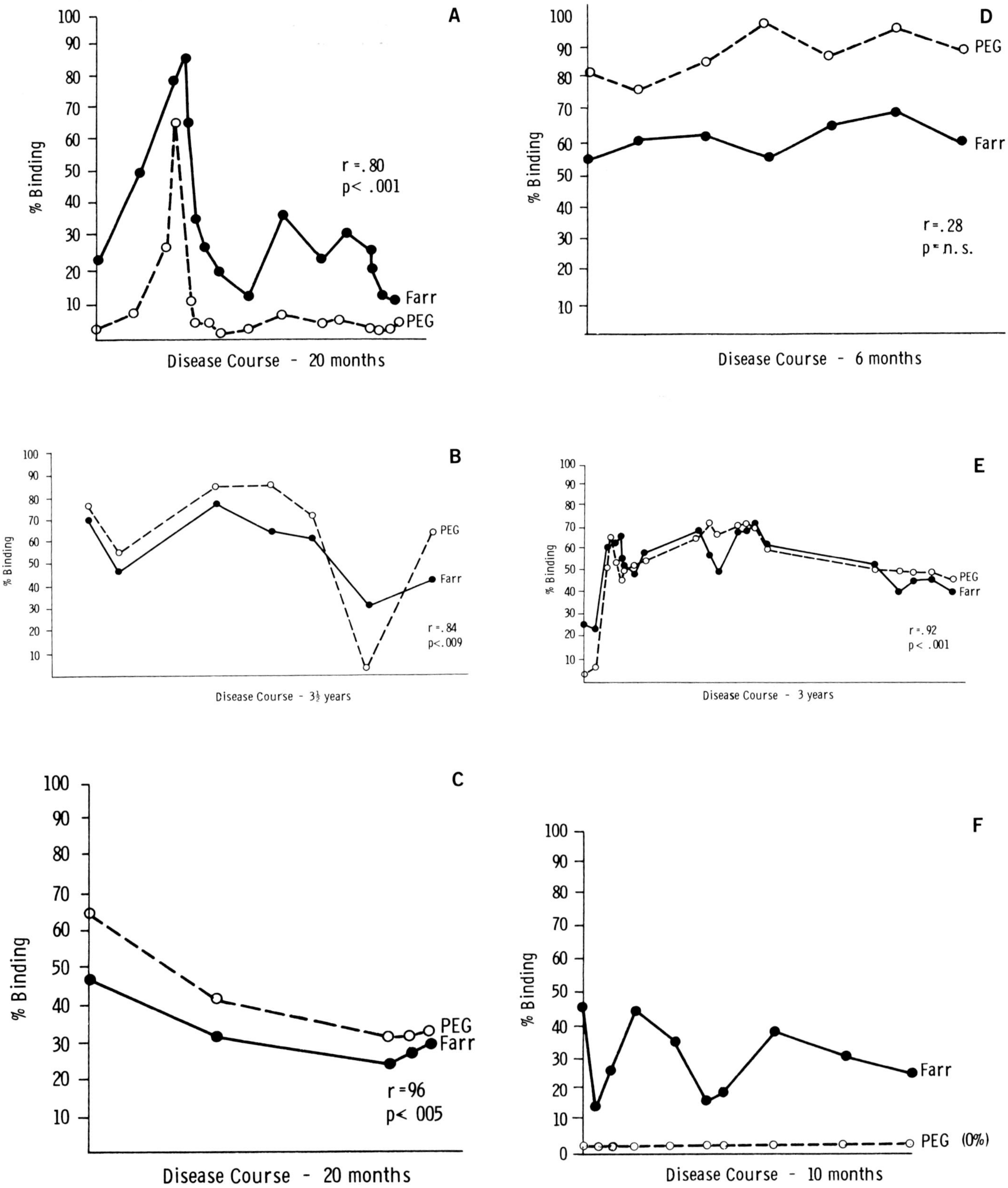

Figure 1 **A–F**, Binding percentages of high and low avidity antibodies, determined by the Farr and polyethylene glycol (PEG) assays during the course of disease in 6 patients with systemic lupus erythematosus. Patient represented in **D** had the lowest and only nonsignificant correlation coefficient of the 19 patients studied. Patient represented in **F** showed no binding of double-stranded DNA by the PEG assay. NS = not significant.

rapid dissociation from ^{3}H–*E coli* dsDNA of those antibodies measured by the PEG assay, but slow dissociation of those measured by the Farr assay.

Additional controls. The effect of pH was evaluated in the PEG assay. Recent studies suggested that changes in pH may occur during incubation of sera at 37°C and that these changes may affect binding in the PEG assay (27). We found that the change in DNA binding as the pH increased from 7–8 was less than 10%; moreover, incubation of serum for 1 hour at 37°C increased the pH by only 0.1 unit, from pH 7.8 to pH 7.9.

DISCUSSION

The parallel rise and fall of high and low avidity antibodies was unexpected. Although studies correlating high avidity and those correlating low avidity of circulating anti-dsDNA antibody with severity of disease have been nearly equally divided, all have implied an independent role for each of these 2 antibody populations (9–14,28). In the present study, neither high nor low avidity antibody could be independently correlated during the course of disease because both moved synchronistically throughout this time. The mechanisms responsible for the rise and fall of anti-dsDNA antibody levels in SLE appeared nondiscriminatory in regard to avidity.

The discordance of results among earlier studies and with our study on the role of avidity may, in part, be explained by the complicated techniques—Sips transformation (11,12), Scatchard analysis (10), and dilutional assays (9)—previously used in this complex multivalent system. But the discordance may also be due to the use of the Farr assay in several of these studies for assessment of both high and low avidity antibody binding because low avidity antibodies go undetected by the Farr assay (17,19).

Table 1. Comparison of Farr assay and polyethylene glycol (PEG) assay binding avidity patterns and disease manifestations in systemic lupus erythematosus

	Avidity pattern		
Disease manifestations	Farr > PEG (10 patients)	PEG > Farr (6 patients)	Farr = PEG (3 patients)
CNS involvement*	5	4	1
Nephritis†	7	4	1
Pulmonary disease‡	6	4	1
Decreased complement	8	5	2

* CNS = central nervous system. Seven patients had seizures, 1 had aseptic meningitis, 1 had hemiparesis, and 1 had headaches and abnormal electroencephalogram results.
† All patients had >5 gm protein/24-hour urine specimen, 4 had nephrotic syndrome, and 2 patients had biopsy-proven lupus glomerulonephritis.
‡ Eight patients had pleuritis and 2 patients had diffuse interstitial pneumonitis.

Table 2. Kinetics of complexes of ^{3}H-dsDNA/anti-dsDNA; comparison of the polyethylene glycol (PEG) and Farr assays before and after dissociation

	% DNA dissociated*		% salt dissociated†	
Patient	PEG	Farr	PEG	Farr
1	87	16	ND	ND
2	88	47	ND	ND
3	80	11	ND	ND
4	54	8	ND	ND
5	94	43	88	8
6	81	42	80	5
7	93	23	96	27
Average	81	27	88	13

* % ^{3}H-dsDNA dissociated after addition of excess DNA and incubation for one-half hour at 37°C.
† % ^{3}H-dsDNA dissociated after addition of 0.6*M* NaCl and incubation for 2 hours at room temperature. ND = not done.

The parallel rise and fall of these 2 antibody populations resulting in a fixed pattern of Farr assay to PEG assay binding for each patient has other implications. Normal immune responses are characterized by increases of antibody affinity with time. Avidity is dependent in part on affinity, and yet the SLE patients in the present study showed no changes in antibody avidity with time. DeHeer and Edgington have reported a failure of anti-dsDNA antibody affinity to increase with time in the New Zealand black/New Zealand white (NZB/NZW) mouse (29). It actually decreased with time. They attributed this to an inability of the B cell to produce high affinity antibody. A similar abnormality of the B cell might help to explain our findings in the present study, but our study differed in that we measured avidity, not affinity, and we found neither an increase nor a decrease of avidity with time.

An alternative explanation derives from studies by Aarden (30), who showed that low avidity antibody to dsDNA can sometimes react as high avidity antibody to ssDNA. If ssDNA were the primary antigen to which high avidity antibodies were directed, dsDNA could be a secondary antigen toward which low avidity interactions might be expected. In this case the immune response would be mature as regards avidity because antibody against the primary antigen would be of high avidity. This principle could, of course, apply to any other unknown primary antigen.

Polyclonal B cell activators might also have played a role in this phenomenon. They have been implicated recently in numerous studies involving NZB/NZW mice (31,32) as well as in studies of SLE patients (33,34). Because they trigger activation of B cells, which is immunologically nonspecific (35), qualitative changes in avidity toward any one antigen might never occur. Low avidity antibody could persist and the avidity pattern remain relatively stable, as observed here.

The observations in this study were based on the combined use of the PEG and Farr assays, a now recognized means of differentiating high and low avidity antibodies to dsDNA in SLE sera (17–20). Each of these assays has repeatedly been shown to measure separate antibody populations that differ in their ability to resist dissociation by salt or excess DNA (17–20). Salt lability is used as a measure of avidity in this system (21) because the interaction of dsDNA with antibody to dsDNA consists purely of Coulombic (electrostatic) forces (36). Dissociation with excess dsDNA is used similiarly and has been stated by Griffiths et al to be the most appropriate method for measuring the avidity of anti-dsDNA antibody (15).

Studies with the CL assay have further corroborated the distinctiveness of these two antibody populations (21); antibodies detected by the CL and PEG assays, but not by the Farr assay, are easily eluted from the dsDNA on the CL substrate by salt solutions or excess DNA. Antibodies detected by both the Farr and the CL assays cannot be so eluted. In other words, the antibodies detected by the Farr assay have been shown to bind with relatively greater avidity to the dsDNA within the CL substrate than do those antibodies measured by the PEG assay. In the same study, antibodies detected by the PEG assay and missed by the Farr assay were characterized by Celada plots and found to be of low avidity (37). More recently, a monoclonal antibody that binds to double-stranded DNA in both the CL and PEG assays but not in the Farr assay was developed (21).

We repeated dissociation studies in the present investigation and again showed rapid salt dissociation of those antibodies measured by the PEG assay and almost no dissociation of those detected by the Farr assay. Excess dsDNA also dissociated complexes measured by the PEG assay more effectively than those measured by Farr, although this difference was less dramatic than with salt.

We found the Farr to be the more sensitive of the 2 assays. Since a single high avidity antibody can bring down an entire molecule of dsDNA in the Farr assay, this finding was not unexpected (30). Many antibodies are required to form the large lattices needed for precipitation in polyethylene glycol (26). If antibodies are of low avidity because of an inability to bind with both arms to one DNA molecule (38), this would also confer an increased capacity for the cross-linking necessary to build lattices.

In summary, high and low avidity antibodies to dsDNA measured by the Farr and PEG assays, respectively, rose and fell in parallel rather than independently during the SLE disease course. The mechanism responsible for changes in the levels of anti-dsDNA antibody appeared nondiscriminatory with regard to avidity. In addition, the humoral immune response depicted by these antibody measurements appeared atypical, lacking maturational features.

ACKNOWLEDGMENTS

We are indebted to David Zelman, MD for his earlier participation in this study, to Elizabeth Bak for her excellent technical assistance, and to Dr. Robert Elston for his expert statistical advice. We also thank Roxanne Roig-Smith and Frank DeVay for their most helpful assistance.

REFERENCES

1. Koffler D, Schur PH, Kunkel HG: Immunological studies concerning the nephritis of systemic lupus erythematosus. J Exp Med 26:607–624, 1967
2. Stollar DB: Nucleic acid antigens, The Antigens. Vol. I. Edited by M Sela. New York, Academic Press, 1973, p 1
3. Tan EM, Schur PH, Carr RI, Kunkel HG: Deoxyribonucleic acid (DNA) and antibodies to DNA in the serum of patients with systemic lupus erythematosus. J Clin Invest 45:1732–1740, 1966
4. Miniter MF, Stollar BD, Agnello V: Reassessment of the clinical significance of native DNA antibodies in systemic lupus erythematosus. Arthritis Rheum 9:959–968, 1979
5. Pearson L, Lightfoot RW Jr: Correlation of DNA-anti-DNA association rates with clinical activity in systemic lupus erythematosus (SLE). J Immunol 126:16–19, 1981
6. Swaak AJG, Aarden LA, Statius van Eps LW, Feltkamp TEW: Anti-dsDNA and complement profiles as prognostic guides in systemic lupus erythematosus. Arthritis Rheum 22:226–235, 1979
7. Sontheimer RD, Gilliam JN: DNA antibody class, subclass, and complement fixation in systemic lupus erythematosus with and without nephritis. Clin Immunol Immunopathol 10:459–467, 1978
8. Rothfield NF, Stollar BD: The relation of immunoglobulin class, patterns of antinuclear activity, and complement-fixing, antibodies to DNA in sera from patients with systemic lupus erythematosus. J Clin Invest 46:1785–1794, 1967
9. Gershwin ME, Steinberg AD: Qualitative characteristics of anti-DNA antibodies in lupus nephritis. Arthritis Rheum 17:947–954, 1974
10. Leon SA, Green A, Ehrlich GE, Poland M, Shapiro B: Avidity of antibodies in SLE: relation to severity of renal involvement. Arthritis Rheum 20:23–29, 1977
11. Winfield JB, Faiferman I, Koffler D: Avidity of anti-

DNA antibodies in serum and glomerular eluates from patients with systemic lupus erythematosus: association of high avidity antinative DNA antibody with glomerulonephritis. J Clin Invest 59:90–96, 1977
12. Soothill JF, Steward MW: The immunopathological significance of the heterogeneity of antibody affinity. Clin Exp Immunol 9:193–199, 1971
13. Steward MW, Glass DN, Maini RN, Scott JT: Role of low avidity antibody to native DNA in human and murine lupus syndrome (abstract). J Rheumatol 1:75, 1974
14. Johnson GD, Edmonds JP, Holborow EJ: Precipitating antibody to DNA detected by two-stage electroimmunodiffusion. Lancet ii:883–885, 1973
15. Griffiths ID, Holian J, Maini RN, Glass DN, Scott JT: Anti-DNA antibodies: qualitative aspects of measurement using ^{125}I-labeled DNA. Ann Rheum Dis (suppl) 36:122–128, 1977
16. Aarden LA, Lakmaker F, DeGroot ER, Feltkamp TEW: Avidity of antibodies to DNA in relation to SLE. Behring Inst Mitt 64:36–44, 1979
17. Riley RL, McGrath H Jr, Taylor RP: Detection of low-avidity anti-DNA antibodies in systemic lupus erythematosus. Arthritis Rheum 22:219–225, 1979
18. Tron F, Bach JF: Relationships between antibodies to native DNA and glomerulonephritis in systemic lupus erythematosus. Clin Exp Immunol 28:426–432, 1977
19. Aarden LA, Lakmaker F, DeGroot ER, DeSwaak AJG, Feltkamp TEW: Detection of antibodies to DNA by radioimmunoassay and immunofluorescence. Scand J Rheumatol [Suppl] 11:12–19, 1975
20. Riley RL, Addis DJ, Taylor RP: Stability of DNA/anti-DNA complexes. II. Salt lability and avidity. J Immunol 124:1–7, 1980
21. Smeenk R, Van der Lilij G, Aarden L: Avidity of antibodies to dsDNA: comparison of IFT on Crithidia luciliae, Farr assay and PEG assay. J Immunol 128:73–78, 1982
22. Tan EM, Cohen AS, Fries JM, Masi AT, McShane DJ, Rothfield NF, Schaller JG, Talal N, Winchester RJ: The 1982 revised criteria for the classification of systemic lupus erythematosus. Arthritis Rheum 25:1271–1277, 1982
23. Aarden LA, DeGroot ER, Feltkamp TEW: Immunology of DNA. III. Crithidia luciliae, a simple substrate for the determination of anti-dsDNA with the immunofluorescence technique. Ann NY Acad Sci 254:505–510, 1975
24. Klamerth O: Biochemistry: separation of high-molecular deoxyribonucleic acid and ribonucleic acid. Nature 208:1318–1319, 1965
25. Wold RT, Young FE, Tan EM, Farr RS: Deoxyribonucleic acid antibody, a method to detect its primary interaction with deoxyribonucleic acid. Science 161:806–807, 1968
26. Smeenk R, Aarden L: The use of polyethylene glycol precipitation to detect low-avidity anti-DNA antibodies in systemic lupus erythematosus. J Immunol 39:165–180, 1980
27. Smeenk R, Van der Lilij G, Aarden L: Measurement of low avidity anti-dsDNA by the Crithidia luciliae test and the PEG assay. Clin Exp Immunol 50:603–610, 1982
28. Devens B, Chia D, Barnett EV: Anti-DNA antibody: avidity and valence measurements, studies using sera from immunized rabbits and from two systemic lupus erythematosus patients. J Immunol 19:187–203, 1978
29. DeHeer DH, Edgington TS: Aberrant maturation of the immune response to the thymus-independent antigen DNP-Lys-Ficoll by New Zealand black mice. Clin Immunol Immunopathol 15:472–480, 1980
30. Aarden LA: Measurement of anti-DNA antibodies. Ann Rheum Dis (suppl) 36:91–96, 1977
31. Cohen L, Ziff M: Abnormal polyclonal B cell activation in NZB/NZW F mice. J Immunol 119:1534–1537, 1977
32. Hang L, Slack JH, Amundson C, Izui S, Theofilopoulos AN, Dixon FJ: Induction of murine autoimmune disease by chronic polyclonal B cell activation. J Exp Med 157:874–883, 1983
33. Fauci AS, Steinberg AD, Haynes BF, Whalen G: Immunoregulatory aberrations in systemic lupus erythematosus. J Immunol 121:1473–1479, 1978
34. Levinson AI, Dziarski A, Pincus T, DeHoratius RJ, Zweiman B: Heterogeneity of polyclonal B cell activity in systemic lupus erythematosus. J Clin Lab Immunol 5:17–22, 1981
35. Coutinho A, Moller G: Immune activation of B cells: evidence for "one non-specific triggering signal" not delivered by Ig receptors. Scand J Immunol 3:133–151, 1974
36. DeGroot ER, Lamers MC, Aarden LA, Smeenk RJT, Van Oss CJ: Dissociation of DNA/anti DNA complexes at high pH. Immunol Commun 9:515–528, 1980
37. Celada FD, Strom R: Determination of avidity of anti-albumin antibodies in the mouse. Immunology 17:189–198, 1969
38. Hornick CL, Karush F: Antibody affinity. III. The role of multivalence. Immunochemistry 9:325–330, 1972

SPONTANEOUS IN VITRO PRODUCTION OF ANTI-DNA AND ANTI-RNA BY SYSTEMIC LUPUS ERYTHEMATOSUS AND NORMAL PERIPHERAL BLOOD MONONUCLEAR CELLS

MICHAEL R. LIEBLING, CURTICE WONG, and JEAN RADOSEVICH

The spontaneous in vitro production of anti-DNA and anti-RNA by peripheral blood mononuclear cells (PBMC) from patients with systemic lupus erythematosus (SLE) and from normal subjects was evaluated employing sensitive solid-phase assays that are specific for these antibodies. PBMC from SLE patients produced more IgG anti-DNA and anti-RNA than did normal PBMC ($P < 0.01$). In vitro production of IgG anti-DNA appeared to correlate with serum DNA bindings ($r = 0.72$, $P < 0.005$). Similar amounts of IgM anti-DNA and anti-RNA were produced by both SLE and normal PBMC. However, IgM anti-DNA antibodies always appeared to be directed against determinants on denatured DNA. Only PBMC from SLE patients produced IgG antibodies to native DNA.

Systemic lupus erythematosus (SLE) is characterized by the serologic finding of antibodies to nucleic acids and to proteins associated with nucleic acids. Explanations of these findings have focused, in part, on abnormalities of immunoregulation noted in vitro (1–10). Interpretation of these immunoregulatory abnormalities has been clouded by at least 3 factors. First, many of the studies have employed lectin-induced activation or suppression of the cultured cells. The relevance of these findings to the basal, unstimulated state of these cells (and by inference, their in vivo status) has not always been clear. Second, other studies have examined either total immunoglobulin responses or antibody responses to antigens that do not appear to play a significant role in the pathogenesis of SLE (11).

Finally, when in vitro antibody production to nucleic acid antigens has been examined, either the methodology has been difficult to reproduce in other laboratories or insufficient data have been presented to allow evaluation of the specificity of the response toward a given nucleic acid as opposed to other closely related antigens (9,10,12,13). The latter point is important if meaningful studies aimed at the specific suppression of pathologic antibody responses are to proceed in this disease.

In an attempt to rectify some of these difficulties and to further investigate immune regulation of pathogenic antibody production in SLE, we have developed extremely sensitive, specific, and reproducible solid-phase radioimmunoassays for antibodies to DNA and RNA. These assays have enabled us to examine the spontaneous production of these 2 presumably pathologic antibodies by human peripheral blood mononuclear cells (PBMC) obtained from SLE patients and from normal individuals.

From the Department of Medicine, Division of Rheumatology, UCLA School of Medicine, Los Angeles, California.

Michael R. Liebling, MD; Curtice Wong, BS; Jean Radosevich, MS.

Address reprint requests to Michael R. Liebling, MD, Associate Chief, Division of Rheumatology, Department of Medicine, Harbor–UCLA Medical Center, 1000 West Carson Street, Torrance, CA 90509.

Submitted for publication March 16, 1984; accepted in revised form October 11, 1984.

PATIENTS AND METHODS

Patients. All but 1 patient had a history of manifesting 4 or more of the American Rheumatism Association revised criteria for SLE (14). The patient who did not fulfill 4 criteria, did, however, manifest the following 3: a positive antinuclear antibody test (1:320) with a homogeneous pattern on rat liver substrate, thrombocytopenia, and pericarditis. Activity of disease was estimated by the method of Urowitz et al (15). Patients and controls were not age- and sex-matched prior to the study. However, the mean ages of the 2 groups proved to be similar, 35.2 ± 3.1 (mean ± SE) for the patients and 30.0 ± 1.2 for the controls. There were 1 man and 24 women in the patient group, while the control group contained 3 men and 14 women.

Serum DNA binding. A modified Farr assay was employed (16), using heat-denatured calf thymus DNA (Worthington Biochemicals, Freehold, NJ). The DNA solution, 1 mg/ml in 0.01*M* phosphate buffered saline (PBS), pH 7.4, was boiled for 10 minutes, rapidly cooled in an ice bath, sonicated for 10 minutes by a sonifier cell disrupter (Model 140D; Heat Systems-Ultrasonics, Inc., Plainview, NY), and radiolabeled with ^{125}I using the method of Commerford (17).

Solid-phase radioimmunoassays for total IgG and IgM production. A modification of the method of Stevens was employed (18). Briefly, 96-well, V-bottom microtiter plates (Dynatech, Alexandria, VA) were coated with rabbit anti-human IgG, γ-chain–specific, or rabbit anti-human IgM, μ-chain–specific (Miles-Yeda, Rehovot, Israel) which had been purified by $(NH_4)_2SO_4$ precipitation followed by diethylaminoethyl (DEAE) chromatography (19). The protein concentration of the solution used to coat the wells was 1 mg/ml. Five percent bovine serum albumin (BSA) diluted in PBS was employed to fill any unoccupied binding sites on the plastic.

The coated wells were then filled with 300 μl of a 1:100 dilution of culture supernatants or a range of known concentrations of human IgG or IgM, purified by standard techniques (19). These were allowed to incubate overnight at room temperature in a moist chamber. The wells were then washed 3 times with 1% BSA and exposed to 300 μl of radiolabeled rabbit anti-human IgG or IgM, γ- or μ-chain–specific, for 5 hours at room temperature. These antibodies had been purified as noted above and radiolabeled with ^{125}I by the lactoperoxidase method of Marchalones (20). The specific activity ranged between 1,700–3,000 counts per minute/ng of protein. The plate was then washed 3 times with BSA, followed by 8 washings with tap water, after which individual wells were counted in a gamma counter.

All supernatant determinations were performed in triplicate while determinations on known concentrations of human IgG or IgM were performed in duplicate. From the samples containing the known concentrations of Ig, a standard curve was generated by plotting cpm versus ng/ml of IgG or IgM. The cpm obtained with individual culture supernatants was then used to enter the standard curve so that the immunoglobulin concentration in the given supernatant could be determined.

Solid-phase radioimmunoassays for antibodies to DNA and RNA. Ninety-six–well, V-bottom microtiter plates were exposed to solutions of calf thymus DNA or yeast RNA (Worthington) 1 mg/ml in PBS, 300 μl per well, in a moist chamber overnight at room temperature. The remaining solution was then aspirated and the wells filled with 25% glutaraldehyde (Fisher, Fairlawn, NJ). After 1½–2 hours of incubation at room temperature in a hood, the glutaraldehyde was aspirated and the wells filled with 0.2*M* glycine-HCl buffer, pH 2.8. Fifteen to twenty minutes later, the glycine buffer was aspirated until dry. The wells were then washed 3 times with 1% BSA. The resultant plate coatings were termed glutaraldehyde-linked DNA (GL-DNA) or glutaraldehyde-linked RNA (GL-RNA). The glutaraldehyde linking step was employed in these assays because it significantly enhanced reproducibility. Utilizing this method with ^{125}I-labeled DNA, it was found that an average of 3.5 ± 0.07 μg of DNA was bound to each well.

The wells were then coated with 5% BSA to fill any remaining binding sites, washed 3 times with 1% BSA, and aspirated to dryness. A solution of 1% BSA–2% rabbit gamma globulin (Sigma, St. Louis, MO) in PBS was then used to coat the wells in an attempt to take up any nonspecific binding sites on the relatively "sticky" DNA or RNA. This step decreased background counts and also improved reproducibility. Three hundred microliters of supernatant or, where appropriate, diluted sera was added to the wells and incubated at room temperature in a moist chamber overnight. The wells were then aspirated and washed 3 times in 1% BSA.

Rabbit anti-human IgG, γ-chain–specific, or rabbit anti-human IgM, μ-chain–specific antibody (Miles-Yeda), was purified and labeled as above. Three hundred microliters of the labeled rabbit antibody was added to wells of microtiter plates and incubated at room temperature for 5 hours in a moist chamber. The antibody solution was aspirated, and the wells were washed 3 times with 1% BSA and 8 times with tap water. The individual wells were then counted in a gamma counter. All determinations were performed in triplicate.

Assessment of antibodies to native DNA (nDNA) and denatured DNA (ssDNA). Calf thymus DNA was denatured by the methods discussed below. A solution containing 1 mg/ml of this ssDNA was then used to coat a microtiter plate as described above. All subsequent procedures in the radioimmunoassay were the same.

Individual supernatants were simultaneously tested for anti-DNA antibody content both on plates coated with nDNA and on ssDNA-coated plates. Supernatants with binding to the nDNA-coated plates which statistically significantly exceeded the binding to ssDNA-coated plates were thought to contain antibodies specific for nDNA. The quantity of nDNA was calculated as follows:

$$\text{cpm nDNA} = \text{cpm bound to nDNA-coated plate} - \text{cpm bound to ssDNA-coated plate}$$

The quantity of nDNA in terms of ng/culture was then determined by the methods outlined below.

Quantitation of antibodies to DNA and RNA. We initially attempted to estimate the quantity of specific antibody produced by the cultures by using a standard curve generated in the same manner as that used in determinations of total IgG and IgM. This method assumes that since the same radiolabeled rabbit anti-human IgG or IgM is used in both the anti-DNA and the total Ig assays, these labeled rabbit antibodies "see" the same number of determinants on the Ig molecules in each assay. The counts in the 2 assays are then equated and the quantity of specific anti-DNA antibody can be read directly off the standard curve for IgG or IgM. Unfortunately, this assumption is incorrect primarily because the plate coatings in each assay (e.g., DNA and rabbit anti-human IgG) are different and probably allow a different degree of access to the bound antibody molecules.

We have demonstrated this phenomenon and attempted to correct for it by employing affinity column–purified IgG anti-DNA antibody kindly donated by Drs. Eugene Barnett and Osamu Taniguchi of UCLA (21). An aliquot of this antibody preparation was labeled with ^{125}I by the iodogen technique (22). The percentage of purified antibody active in our radioimmunoassay was determined by assessing the number of counts bound to GL-DNA or to anti-IgG–coated plates and calculating:

$$\frac{^{125}\text{I anti-DNA bound to GL-DNA} - \text{background cpm}}{^{125}\text{I anti-DNA bound by anti-human IgG} - \text{background cpm}} \times 100$$

This percentage was 3.83 ± 0.21 (mean ± SD). It remained the same irrespective of the IgG concentration of the anti-DNA preparation over a range of 1–50 ng/ml.

The unlabeled, purified, anti-DNA preparation was then used in our radioimmunoassays for anti-DNA and IgG. Since it was known from the previous experiment what proportion of the counts detected in the IgG assay were specifically attributable to functioning anti-DNA antibody, we could compare that number of counts with the number of counts obtained in the anti-DNA assay and come up with a second ratio:

$$\frac{\text{cpm IgG} - \text{cpm background}}{\text{cpm DNA} - \text{cpm background}}$$

This ratio always hovered around 1.5 (1.51 ± 0.02, mean ± SD). Once again, this occurred irrespective of the IgG concentration of the anti-DNA preparation. Therefore, to determine the true quantity of anti-DNA bound in our radioimmunoassay we multiplied the cpm found in the anti-DNA assay by a factor of 1.5 and then used the resultant cpm to enter the standard IgG curve and obtain an accurate figure for ng/ml of IgG anti-DNA.

Although this calibration method was mildly cumbersome, it was only necessary to use it when a new batch of rabbit anti-human IgG plate coating was prepared, i.e., approximately once every 3 months.

We recognize, of course, that IgM anti-DNA cannot be quantitated by the above method (nor, for that matter, can either IgG or IgM anti-RNA). Therefore, the quantity of these antibodies produced by a given culture was estimated by employing the original standard curve method described above. However, even when the levels of IgG anti-DNA were estimated by this latter method, there was no difference in the number of patients or normal subjects producing this antibody, nor was there any change in the significance of the statistical comparison between the 2 groups.

The lower levels of sensitivity for these assays of anti-DNA and anti-RNA production were between 100–200 pg per culture.

Culture conditions. After Ficoll-Hypaque separation (23), washing, and counting, 2.0 × 10^6 viable PBMC were placed in 12 × 75-mm sterile culture tubes (Falcon Labware, Oxnard, CA). Enough RPMI 1640 supplemented with 10% fetal calf serum, 25 mM HEPES buffer, and penicillin-streptomycin (Gibco, Grand Island, NY) was added to the cells to bring the final volume to 2.0 ml/tube. The cultures were incubated in air at 37°C for 1 hour, washed once, and then reincubated under the same conditions. After 8 days, the supernatants were harvested for analysis. Cell viability after 8 days of culture, determined by trypan blue exclusion, averaged 95.5% and 96.5% on 2 separate occasions.

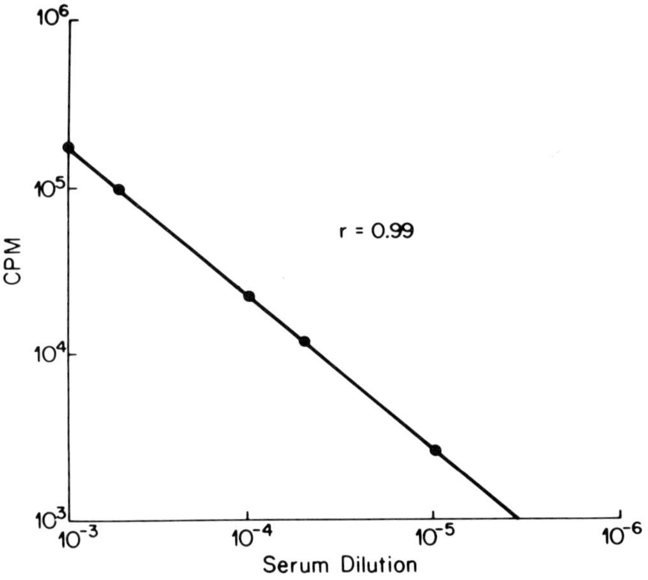

Figure 1. Linearity of solid-phase IgG anti-DNA radioimmunoassay. CPM = counts per minute above background. Each point is the mean of triplicate determinations; the SE of each was less than ±2.3%. The line was drawn using linear regression analysis.

Nucleic acids. Calf thymus DNA, yeast RNA, and poly(dG · dC) (Boehringer, Indianapolis, IN) were used. Denatured DNA was prepared by heating the calf thymus DNA solution (1 mg/ml in PBS) to 100°C for 10 minutes, followed by rapid cooling in ice. No sonication step was performed for preparations not destined for Farr assay.

For inhibition experiments, both ssDNA and DNA digested with bovine pancreatic DNase I (dDNA) were employed to examine the specificity of antibody binding. Limit digests of calf thymus DNA were obtained in the following manner: 0.2 ml of crystalline DNase I (Worthington) diluted to 250 μg/ml in 0.1M Tris-HCl, pH 7.4, was added to 0.8 ml of calf thymus DNA, 1 mg/ml in 0.1M Tris-HCl, pH 7.4. $MgCl_2$ was then added to a final concentration of 0.01M. The digestion was allowed to proceed for 1 hour at 37°C. An additional 50 μg of DNase I was then added, and

Table 1. Reproducibility of anti-DNA/anti-RNA assays

	IgG		IgM	
	Anti-DNA	Anti-RNA	Anti-DNA	Anti-RNA
Intra-assay coefficient of variation, %*	2.7	3.3	3.7	3.9
Inter-assay coefficient of variation, %†	6.5	8.3	9.0	8.2

* Average coefficient of variation derived from pentuplicate determinations performed on supernatants from 4 individuals on the same day.
† Average coefficient of variation derived from assays performed on supernatants from 7 individuals on 3 separate occasions.

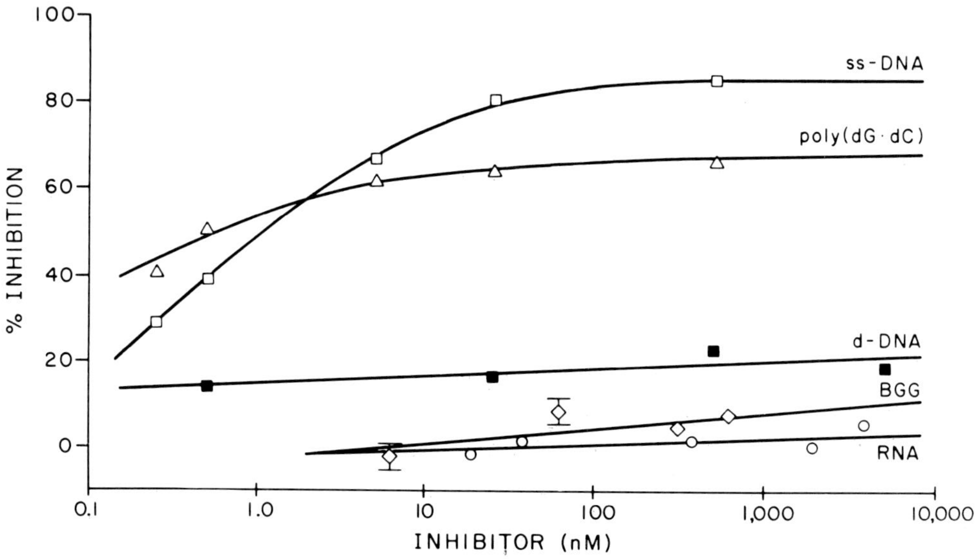

Figure 2. Specificity of assay, showing inhibition of binding of patient serum to native glutaraldehyde-linked DNA–coated microtiter plate by single-stranded DNA (ssDNA), native DNA [poly(dG · dC)], digested DNA (dDNA), bovine gamma globulin (BGG), and yeast RNA. All points represent the mean of triplicate determinations; the SE of each was less than or equal to ±2% inhibition except where bars denote larger variations. For dDNA, RNA, and BGG, straight lines were drawn using linear regression analysis.

the mixture was allowed to digest for 1 more hour at 37°C. DNase activity and undigested polynucleotides were eliminated by precipitation with 10% trichloroacetic acid followed by centrifugation and subsequent dilution of the supernatant. The final dilution was made in 5% BSA/PBS. The pH of the highest concentration of dDNA used in inhibition experiments was always ≥7.38. For inhibition experiments, all other nucleic acids were solubilized in 5% BSA diluted in PBS. With the exception of dDNA, the molecular weights of individual nucleic acid preparations used in inhibition experiments were determined in the following manner. After filtration on a Sepharose 4B column (2.5 × 100 cm; eluted with 0.01*M* PBS, pH 7.4), the nucleic acid peaks were collected in 5-ml fractions. Aliquots of selected fractions were then evaluated by agarose gel electrophoresis on 0.7% gels using λ-phage DNA and Hae III digestion fragments of ϕ X 175 phage DNA as molecular weight markers (24). The molecular weight of dDNA was estimated from the fact that limit digests of DNA are known to predominantly contain tetranucleotides (25).

Statistical analysis. For comparisons between the means of separate groups, the Wilcoxon rank sum test was used (26). Correlation coefficients and their statistical significance were determined by linear regression analysis (26). Variation about the mean found in tables, figures, and text is always expressed as mean ± SE unless otherwise noted.

RESULTS

Preliminary studies. The radioimmunoassays for anti-DNA and anti-RNA were linear over more than 2 orders of magnitude (Figure 1). They were also quite reproducible (Table 1). Moreover, inhibition studies with several different polynucleotides demonstrated that the assays were highly specific and could distinguish antibodies directed against DNA from those directed against RNA (Figures 2 and 3). Five sera other than the one shown in Figures 2 and 3 were tested in a similar manner. In all instances, the amount of inhibition was significantly higher when the appropriate inhibitor (DNA for GL-DNA–coated plates and RNA for GL-RNA–coated plates) was employed. Similar specificity was demonstrated in supernatant studies (Table 2).

Moreover, inhibition by native DNA [poly (dG · dC)] was always greater than that produced by pure single-stranded DNA (dDNA) when tested on GL-DNA plates. Indeed, as shown in Figure 2, summing the inhibition produced by the native and pure single-stranded DNAs at each concentration gave levels of inhibition that were greater than or equal to that produced by ssDNA at the same concentration. This would suggest that the ssDNA preparation was inhibiting binding by antibodies directed against both single-stranded and double-stranded determinants.

Finally, we attempted to examine the nature of the GL-DNA plate coating with respect to native configuration. Using previously described methods (27), predigestion of GL-nDNA–coated wells with S1 nuclease (1,000 units/ml) failed to reduce the binding produced by a serum containing antibodies to both ss-

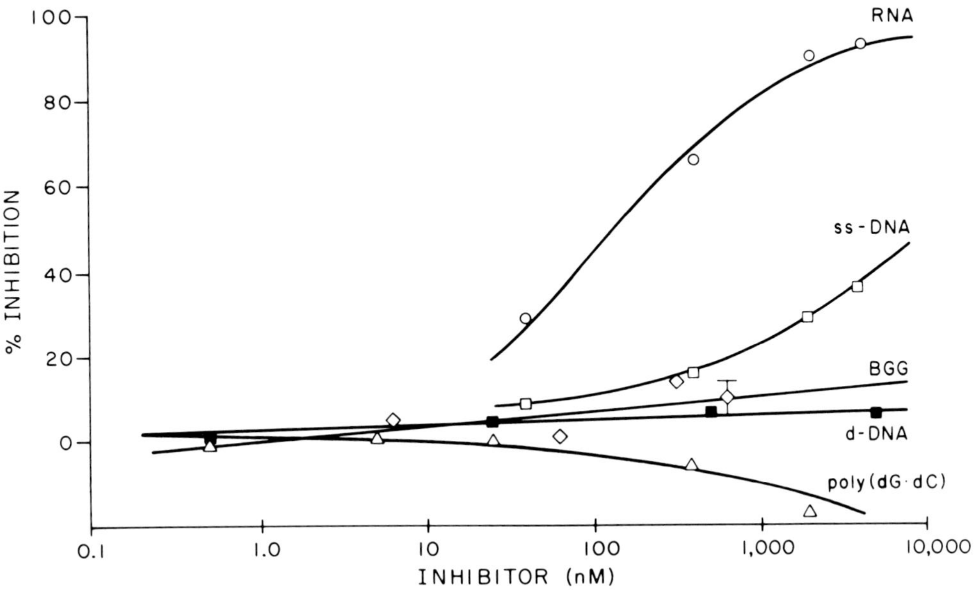

Figure 3. Specificity of assay, showing inhibition of binding of patient serum to glutaraldehyde-linked RNA–coated microtiter plate by yeast RNA, single-stranded DNA (ssDNA), bovine gamma globulin (BGG), digested DNA (dDNA), and native DNA [poly(dG · dC)]. All points represent the mean of triplicate determinations; the SE of each was less than or equal to ±3% except where bars denote larger variations. For dDNA and BGG, straight lines were drawn using linear regression analysis.

and nDNA. In a control experiment, exposure of GL-ssDNA–coated wells to the same experimental conditions resulted in a decrease of 92% in the binding of the above-mentioned serum (data not shown).

Antibody production by SLE and normal PBMC. Using these assays, we were able to examine spontaneous anti-DNA, anti-RNA, total IgG, and total IgM production by PBMC from 17–25 SLE patients and 16–17 normal individuals. As might be expected, the PBMC from the SLE patients produced significantly greater ($P < 0.01$) amounts of both IgG anti-DNA and anti-RNA than did the normal PBMC (Figures 4a and b). Interestingly, the 2 groups did not differ significant-

Table 2. Inhibition of binding of patient's culture supernatant to native glutaraldehyde-linked DNA–coated microtiter plates by various polynucleotides*

Polynucleotide	Concentration (n*M*)	% inhibition (mean ± SE)
Poly(dG · dC)	500	46.2 ± 1.4
	25	16.2 ± 0.2
dDNA	500	25.1 ± 0.3
	25	11.2 ± 0.1
ssDNA	500	60.4 ± 0.7
	25	21.4 ± 0.4
RNA	500	21.4 ± 0.2
	25	7.9 ± 0.3

* Poly(dG · dC) = native DNA; dDNA = digested DNA; ssDNA = denatured or single-stranded DNA.

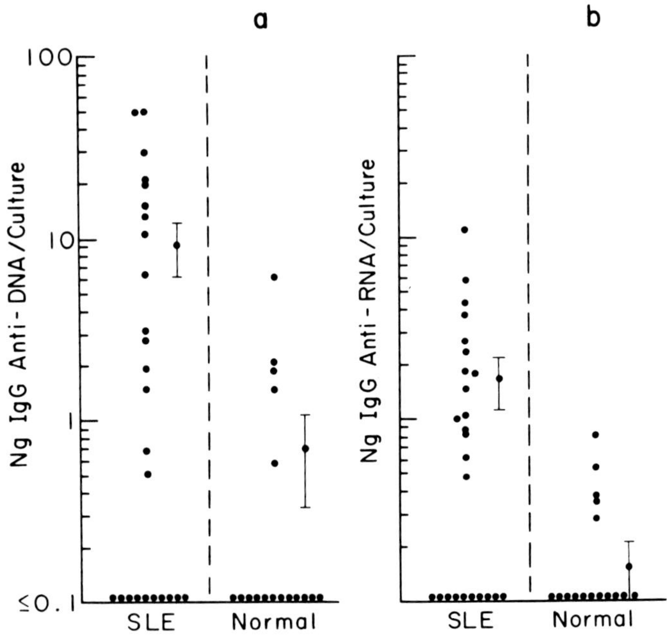

Figure 4. a, IgG anti-DNA production by systemic lupus erythematosus (SLE) and normal peripheral blood mononuclear cells (PBMC). **b,** IgG anti-RNA production by SLE and normal PBMC. Represents the quantity of antibody found in 2 ml of supernatants from 8-day cultures of 2 × 10⁶ cells. The anti-DNA assays were performed on microtiter plates coated with native calf glutaraldehyde-linked DNA.

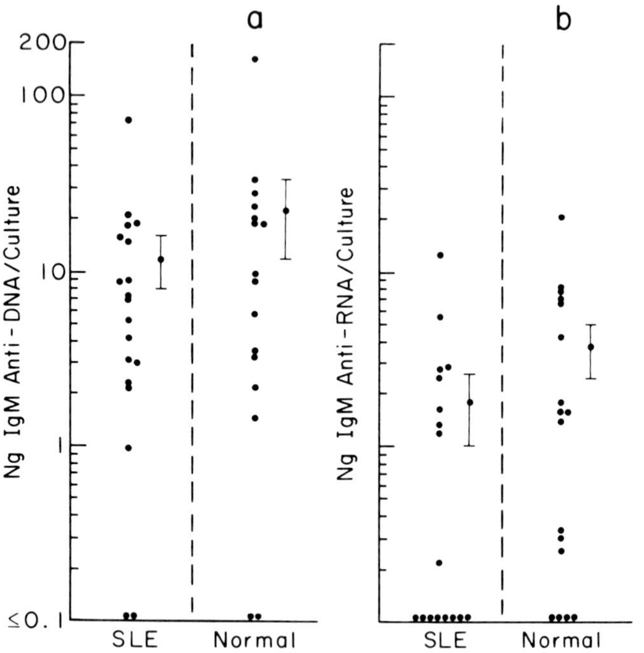

Figure 5. a, IgM anti-DNA production by systemic lupus erythematosus (SLE) and normal peripheral blood mononuclear cells (PBMC). **b,** IgM anti-RNA production by SLE and normal PBMC. Represents the quantity of antibody found in 2 ml of supernatants from 8-day cultures of 2×10^6 cells. The anti-DNA assays were performed on microtiter plates coated with native calf thymus glutaraldehyde-linked DNA.

ly in the ability of their PBMC to produce IgM anti-DNA or anti-RNA (Figures 5a and b). Moreover, the 2 groups did not differ significantly in total production of IgG or IgM (Table 3).

Several important differences between the SLE and normal groups were noted, however. First, total autoantibody production (anti-DNA + anti-RNA) by SLE PBMC represented a significantly greater proportion of total IgG production than did autoantibody production by normal PBMC (Table 3). Perhaps more importantly, 53% of the SLE PBMC that produced antibodies to DNA made antibodies directed against determinants found only on the nDNA-coated plates. None of the normal PBMC produced these antibodies (Table 3). Moreover, none of the IgM anti-DNA antibodies produced by either SLE or normal PBMC appeared to be directed against these native determinants (Table 3). Finally, the quantity of these antibodies directed against determinants found only on nDNA-coated plates ranged between 13% and 100% (mean 64.3 ± 17.4%) of the total anti-DNA produced.

In a further attempt to determine whether our system was detecting true antibody production as opposed to release of preformed or adherent antibody, we lysed PBMC from 4 SLE patients after 20 hours or after 8 days of incubation and tested the supernatants for anti-DNA antibody and total IgG. Lysis was accomplished by freezing and thawing the cultures. The results (Table 4) clearly demonstrate that <23% of the total amount of IgG or IgG anti-DNA found at 8 days of incubation can be detected after 20 hours of incubation. Thus, release of preformed or cell receptor–bound antibody cannot account for the vast majority of the antibody detected at 8 days. Therefore, in vitro production must be responsible for at least 77% of the IgG antibody detected in our system.

Assessment of interference by rheumatoid factor. In these assays, IgG or IgM rheumatoid factor produced by PBMC in vitro could conceivably interfere with the accurate determination of anti-DNA or anti-

Table 3. Total immunoglobulin and autoantibody production by systemic lupus erythematosus (SLE) and normal peripheral blood mononuclear cells (PBMC)

	SLE (mean ± SE)		Normal (mean ± SE)	
	IgG	IgM	IgG	IgM
Total Ig produced (ng/culture)	1,013 ± 139	975 ± 415	930 ± 230	1,393 ± 216
Total autoantibody (ng/culture)*	14.8 ± 3.7†	15.5 ± 5.5	1.0 ± 0.4	25.4 ± 11.2
Anti-DNA antibody‡	9.0 ± 2.9†	12.6 ± 4.4	0.8 ± 0.4	21.8 ± 10.0
Anti-nDNA§	3.2 ± 0.4	–	–	–
Number producing anti-nDNA¶	8/24 (8/15)	0/24	0/17	0/17

* Sum of anti-DNA and anti-RNA produced by PBMC cultures.
† Significantly different compared with normal, $P < 0.01$.
‡ Quantity of antibody bound to microtiter plates coated with native calf thymus glutaraldehyde-linked DNA (GL-DNA).
§ Quantity of anti-native DNA (anti-nDNA) antibody bound to microtiter plates coated with native calf thymus GL-DNA over and above that bound to plates coated with denatured calf thymus GL-DNA. Difference between the 2 bindings had to be significant at $P = 0.05$ in order to be counted.
¶ Number of individuals who produced antibodies directed at determinants found only on native calf thymus GL-DNA–coated plates, but not on denatured calf thymus GL-DNA–coated plates. The fraction in parentheses represents the number of individuals who produced antibody to nDNA over the number who produced detectable antibody to either nDNA or ssDNA.

Table 4. Antibody detected in supernatants after lysis of cultures following incubation*

Incubation time	IgG anti-DNA (ng/culture)	Total IgG (ng/culture)
20 hours	0.7 ± 0.1	122 ± 6
8 days	4.3 ± 0.8	540 ± 80

* Mean ± SE of duplicate determinations on supernatants from 4 patients with systemic lupus erythematosus.

RNA. The following experiment was performed to determine whether such interference was occurring. Human IgG was isolated by ammonium sulfate precipitation and DEAE chromotography (18). The isolated human IgG was then aggregated by incubation of a 1 mg/ml solution at 60°C for 10 minutes. This solution of aggregated IgG was used to coat microtiter plates overnight. The plates were then exposed to 5% BSA for 1 hour to fill any empty binding sites on the surface of the wells. Control plates were coated with 5% BSA. Supernatants from 11 SLE patients and 6 normal subjects were exposed to the aggregate and the BSA-coated wells overnight in an attempt to absorb any rheumatoid factor in the supernatants. Absorbed and unabsorbed supernatants were then tested for IgG and IgM anti-DNA antibody content by the methods described above.

These supernatants had been tested previously, and each group was approximately equally divided between those which contained significant amounts of anti-DNA and those which contained little, if any, anti-DNA. The results (Table 5) demonstrate that neither IgG nor IgM rheumatoid factor appeared to contribute significantly to the amount of anti-DNA detected in the culture supernatants of these individuals. The aggregate-absorbed supernatants from each subject were compared with both the unabsorbed and

Table 5. Quantity of anti-DNA antibody in culture supernatants after absorption with aggregated IgG (AIgG) or bovine serum albumin (BSA)*

	Unabsorbed supernatants†	Supernatants absorbed with	
		AIgG	BSA
IgG anti-DNA (ng/culture)	4.86 ± 2.03	4.77 ± 1.77	4.48 ± 1.75
IgM anti-DNA (ng/culture)	14.51 ± 5.54	14.83 ± 6.24	11.42 ± 4.35

* Mean ± SE of duplicate determinations on 11 systemic lupus erythematosus patients and 6 normal subjects.
† Quantity of anti-DNA found in unabsorbed supernatants is not significantly different from that found in supernatants absorbed with AIgG or BSA.

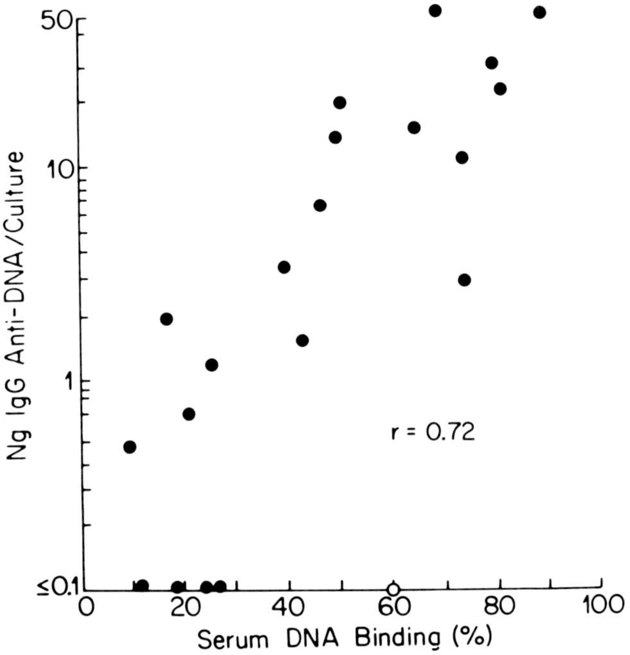

Figure 6. Correlation of the IgG anti-DNA content of systemic lupus erythematosus culture supernatants with simultaneous serum DNA binding by Farr assay; r = 0.72, $P < 0.001$.

BSA-absorbed supernatants from the same individual by paired *t*-test (26). The aggregate-absorbed supernatants still demonstrated no significant differences from the 2 controls in the amount of anti-DNA antibody detected by the radioimmunoassay.

Correlation of in vitro findings with serologic and clinical findings. DNA bindings were performed on serum samples obtained at the same time or within 1 week of collection of PBMC for culture. In vitro IgG anti-DNA production showed a significant correlation with serum DNA bindings ($r = 0.72$, $P < 0.001$) (Figure 6). Despite the statistical correlation, an individual was identified who demonstrated no detectable in vitro production of IgG anti-DNA, but whose serum DNA binding was considerably elevated at 60% (Figure 6, open circle). This finding was demonstrated in the same individual on 2 subsequent occasions. Moreover, this patient produced no IgM anti-DNA in vitro to account for elevated serum DNA binding. Production of IgG and IgM by this patient's PBMC was not deficient. In addition, a $1:10^5$ dilution of his serum still produced significant binding in our IgG anti-DNA solid-phase assay. Therefore, it was unlikely that interfering substances such as C1q or lipoprotein were fallaciously elevating the Farr assay result. Finally, Farr binding assays and solid-phase assays were performed on the sera of 25 SLE patients in an attempt to eliminate the possibility that the 2 assays were detecting totally distinct populations of anti-DNA antibodies. The results obtained from the 2 assays were found to correlate significantly ($r = 0.75$, $P < 0.001$).

In vitro production of IgM anti-DNA by SLE PBMC showed no correlation with serum DNA binding. It should be noted that none of the normal subjects had serum DNA binding outside the normal range, i.e., <20%, and there was no correlation of serum DNA binding with in vitro production of either IgG or IgM anti-DNA by normal PBMC. Finally, with respect to clinical parameters, neither prednisone dosage nor disease activity was found to correlate with in vitro production of IgG or IgM anti-DNA by SLE PBMC.

DISCUSSION

Utilizing our present assay systems, we found that both normal and SLE PBMC were capable of spontaneously producing antibodies to DNA and RNA. The major differences between the 2 groups were the significantly greater quantities of IgG autoantibodies produced by the SLE PBMC and the reactivity of some of these SLE antibodies with determinants found only on nDNA-coated plates.

The first finding is reminiscent of the early "switch" to IgG antibody production found in the New Zealand black/New Zealand white mouse model of SLE (28). It is also compatible with the findings of others that suggest chronic polyclonal activation of SLE B cells, since an IgG response is generally considered a chronologically more mature response than is an IgM response to the same antigen. In this respect, it is of interest that 10 patients and 12 normal subjects failed to produce detectable quantities of IgG anti-DNA (Figure 4). Of the 10 SLE patients, 5 produced inadequate amounts of both total IgG and total IgM (<200 ng/culture of each) and another patient produced inadequate quantities of total IgG alone. None of these patients were hypogammaglobulinemic (28).

From these data it appears that culture artifact is a possible explanation for the lack of production of IgG anti-DNA by the cells of these 5 or 6 patients. Conversely, none of the 12 normal individuals demonstrated inadequate production of total IgG or total IgM. Moreover, cells from 11 of these normal subjects produced readily detectable quantities of IgM anti-DNA (Figure 5). This would suggest that lack of production of IgG anti-DNA by normal PBMC was due to a lack of switching from IgM to IgG rather than to a lack of autoantibody repertoire or culture artifact.

Only PBMC from SLE patients produced antibodies to determinants found solely on nDNA-coated microtiter wells. This result was consistent with the findings of others that anti-nDNA antibody is found almost exclusively in the sera of patients with SLE. The antigen with which these antibodies reacted in our assay was thought to be nDNA. We were able to demonstrate that there was no loss of binding when this antigen was exposed to quantities of S1 nuclease adequate to digest 92% of similarly bound ssDNA. This enzyme is specific for ssDNA and will not affect truly nDNA. However, Steinman et al (29) stated that nDNA derived from natural sources always contains regions of ssDNA digestible with S1 nuclease. If this is indeed the case, the ss regions in the GL-nDNA are apparently not accessible to the enzyme after undergoing binding to a solid phase. Similar results have been found by other investigators under a variety of solid-phase assay conditions (27,30,31).

One further comment is appropriate with respect to the specificity of the nDNA-coated plates as indicated by the competitive inhibition studies. Both digested DNA and single-stranded DNA were chosen as inhibitors in order to examine the reactivity of the GL-DNA plates with antibodies to denatured DNA.

Antibodies to denatured DNA are generally divided into 2 classes (32). The first reacts exclusively with denatured DNA, combining primarily with bases and oligonucleotides. The combining site for these antibodies appears to be no larger in size than 4–6 nucleotides (32). DNA digests contain nucleotides of this size in abundance, and for this reason, dDNA was used in the inhibition experiments to examine this specificity (25). The second class of antibodies to denatured DNA recognizes sites on both native and denatured DNA but usually reacts most effectively with denatured DNA (32,33). Single-stranded DNA was chosen as an inhibitor to examine the reactivity of nDNA-coated plates with these antibodies. The results of the inhibition experiments with these antigens (Figure 2) indicate that antibodies binding to nDNA-coated plates were preferentially inhibited by native DNA when compared with pure denatured DNA. Also, any binding to nDNA-coated plates that was inhibited by ssDNA appeared to be predominantly attributable to antibodies which cross-reacted with sites on native DNA.

Nevertheless, binding to nDNA-coated plates was inhibited to a minor degree (≤22%, Figure 2) by dDNA. Thus, while ssDNA regions on calf thymus nDNA may not be accessible to S1 nuclease when bound to a solid phase, a few ssDNA determinants may still be accessible to anti-DNA antibodies. Moreover, as previously noted, a significant proportion of antibodies reactive with nDNA have equal or greater reactivity with ssDNA. It is for these reasons that we used both nDNA- and ssDNA-coated plates and defined the quantity of anti-nDNA in a specimen as the amount of antibody bound to an nDNA-coated plate over and above that which bound to an ssDNA-coated plate.

If, as some investigators suggest, antibody binding to ssDNA is actually due to aggregated molecules or hairpin segments of ssDNA producing native determinants rather than to true ssDNA per se, then our methods may well have underestimated both the quantity and number of individuals producing anti-nDNA (34,35). Recognizing this possibility, we chose to err in the conservative, rather than in the speculative direction.

We are not aware of other published studies that quantitatively examine the correlation between spontaneous in vitro production of antibody by human PBMC and the serum level of that antibody. Nies et al (36) touched on this point with respect to the anti-tetanus response, but only in a qualitative way and without a definitive conclusion. That a correlation exists between the levels of anti-DNA binding in the sera of SLE patients and the quantity of IgG anti-DNA produced by their PBMC is intriguing in its own right. Indeed, in the mouse, in vitro antibody production by spleen cells either after booster immunization or during spontaneous autoantibody production often does not reflect serum levels of the same antibody (37–39). Information on synthesis of antibody by mouse PBMC in these situations is unavailable.

Recent studies in humans would suggest that spontaneous in vitro production of anti–keyhole limpet hemocyanin and anti-tetanus antibodies by SLE or normal PBMC also correlate poorly with simultaneous serum levels of these antibodies, even after booster immunization (Louie J: personal communication). Thus, our results and those of others suggest that in SLE there is a selective release from sequestered sites of primed, autoantibody-producing cells. This may prove to be yet another defect of immune regulation in SLE. Its significance remains speculative at this time.

Finally, it may be important to discuss our rationale for examining anti-RNA antibody production. Anti-RNA has not been demonstrated to be a particularly pathologic antibody system. It is, however, found in the sera of as many as 75% of SLE patients (40). Moreover, it is another polynucleotide. Because of these 2 qualities, i.e., its wide distribution and polynucleotide nature, it was thought that anti-RNA would provide an excellent method of confirming data on anti-DNA antibody production by SLE and normal PBMC. More importantly, perhaps, the ability to measure the spontaneous, in vitro production of these 2 antibodies will permit in vitro investigation of specific suppression of anti-DNA antibody production (41).

REFERENCES

1. Budman DR, Merchant EB, Steinberg AD, Doft B, Gershwin ME, Lizzio E, Reeves JP: Increased spontaneous activity of antibody-forming cells in the peripheral blood of patients with active SLE. Arthritis Rheum 20:829–834, 1977
2. Waldman TA, Broder S: Suppressor cells in the regulation of immune response. Prog Clin Immunol 3:155–163, 1978
3. Sakane T, Steinberg AD, Green I: Studies of immune functions of patients with systemic lupus erythematosus. I. Dysfunction of suppressor T-cell activity related to impaired generation of, rather than response to, suppressor cells. Arthritis Rheum 21:657–664, 1978
4. Abdou NI, Sagawa A, Pascual E, Herbert J, Sadegher S: Suppressor T-cell abnormality in idiopathic systemic lupus erythematosus. Clin Immunol Immunopathol 6: 192–197, 1976
5. Bresnihan B, Jasin HE: Suppressor function of peripheral blood mononuclear cells in normal individuals and in patients with systemic lupus erythematosus. J Clin Invest 59:106–111, 1977
6. Tardieu M, Dupuy JM: Suppressor activity of lymphocytes from patients with systemic lupus erythematosus. Clin Immunol Immunopathol 11:125–131, 1978
7. Newman B, Blank S, Lomnitzer R, Disler P, Rabson AR: Lack of suppressor cell activity in systemic lupus erythematosus. Clin Immunol Immunopathol 13:187–193, 1979
8. Krakauer RS, Clough JD, Alexander T, Sundeen J, Sauder DN: Suppressor cell defect in SLE: relationship to native DNA binding. Clin Exp Immunol 40:72–76, 1980
9. Clough JD, Frank SA, Calabrese LH: Deficiency of T cell mediated regulation of anti-DNA production in systemic lupus erythematosus. Arthritis Rheum 23:24–29, 1980
10. Sagawa A, Abdou NI: Suppressor-cell dysfunction in systemic lupus erythematosus: cells involved and in vitro correction. J Clin Invest 62:789–796, 1978
11. Gladman D, Keystone E, Urowitz M, Cane D, Poplonski L: Impaired antigen specific suppressor cell activity in patients with systemic lupus erythematosus. Clin Exp Immunol 40:77–86, 1980
12. Bell DA, Clark C, Blomgren SE, Vaughan JH: Anti-

DNA antibody production by lymphoid cells of NZB/W mice and human systemic lupus erythematosus. Clin Immunol Immunopathol 1:293–298, 1973
13. Takeuchi T, Abe T, Koide J, Hosono D, Morimoto C, Homma M: Cellular mechanisms of DNA-specific antibody synthesis by lymphocytes from systemic lupus erythematosus patients. Arthritis Rheum 27:766–773, 1984
14. Tan EM, Cohen AS, Fries JF, Masi AT, McShane DJ, Rothfield NF, Schaller JG, Talal N, Winchester RJ: The 1982 revised criteria for the classification of systemic lupus erythematosus. Arthritis Rheum 25:1271–1277, 1982
15. Urowitz MB, Gladman DD, Goldsmith C, Tozman ES: Lupus activity criteria count (abstract). Arthritis Rheum (suppl) 25:S78, 1982
16. Wold RT, Young FE, Tan EM, Farr RS: Deoxyribonucleic acid antibody: a method to detect its primary interaction with deoxyribonucleic acid. Science 161:806–807, 1968
17. Commerford SD: Iodination of nucleic acids in vitro. Biochemistry 10:1993–2000, 1971
18. Stevens RH: Quantitative radioimmunoassays for the antibodies and immunoglobulin produced in vitro, Manual of Clinical Immunology. Second edition. Edited by NR Rose, H Freidman. Washington, DC, American Society for Microbiology, 1980, pp 157–162
19. Garvey SJ, Cremer NE, Susdorf DH: Methods in Immunology. Reading, WA Benjamin, Inc., 1977, pp 218–219, 223–230
20. Marchalones JJ: An enzymatic method for the trace iodination of immunoglobulins and other proteins. Biochem J 113:299–305, 1969
21. Taniguchi O, Chia D, Barnett EV: Auto-anti-anti-DNA antibodies from SLE patients and normals (abstract). Arthritis Rheum (suppl) 25:S30, 1982
22. Fraker P, Speck JC Jr: Protein and cell membrane iodinations with a sparingly soluble chloramide, 1,3,4,6-tetrachloro-3a,6a-diphenylglycouril. Biochem Biophys Res Commun 80:849–857, 1978
23. Territo MC, Cline M: Macrophage activation and function, Manual of Clinical Immunology. Second edition. Edited by NR Rose, H Freidman. Washington, DC, American Society for Microbiology, 1980, p 304
24. Maniatis T: Molecular Cloning, A Laboratory Manual. Cold Spring Harbor, NY, Cold Spring Harbor Laboratory Publications, 1982, pp 150–172
25. Matsuda M, Ogoshi H: Specificity of DNase I: estimation of nucleosides present at the 5′-phosphate terminus of limit digests of DNA by DNase I. J Biochem (Tokyo) 59:230–235, 1966
26. Brown BW Jr, Hollander W: Statistics, A Biomedical Introduction. New York, John Wiley & Sons, 1977, pp 85–108, 109–118, 261–291
27. Eaton RB, Schneider G, Schur PH: Enzyme immunoassay for antibodies to native DNA: specificity and quality of antibodies. Arthritis Rheum 26:52–62, 1983
28. Talal N: Autoimmunity. Prog Clin Immunol 2:101–162, 1975
29. Steinman CR, Deesomchok U, Spiera H: Detection of anti-DNA antibody using synthetic antigens: characterization and clinical significance of binding of poly(deoxyadenylate-deoxythymidylate) by serum. J. Clin Invest 57:1330–1341, 1976
30. Klotz JL, Minami RM, Teplitz RL: An enzyme-linked immunoabsorbent assay for antibodies to native and denatured DNA. J Immunol Methods 29:155–165, 1979
31. Swenk R: Low Avidity Antibodies to ds DNA. Amsterdam, Rodopi, 1982, p 149
32. Stollar BD: The Antigens. Edited by M Sella. New York, Academic Press, 1973, pp 44–46
33. Koffler D, Carr RI, Agnello V, Thoburn R, Kunkel HG: Antibodies to polynucleotides in human sera: antigenic specificity and relation to disease. J Exp Med 134:294–310, 1971
34. Aarden LA, Lakaker F, Feltkamp TEW: Immunology of DNA. II. The effect of size and structure of the antigen on Farr assay. J Immunol Methods 10:39–48, 1976
35. Stollar BD, Papalian M: Secondary structure in denatured DNA is responsible for its reaction with anti-native DNA antibodies of systemic lupus erythematosus sera. J Clin Invest 66:210–219, 1980
36. Nies K, Boyer R, Stevens R, Louie J: Anti-tetanus toxoid antibody synthesis after booster immunization in systemic lupus erythematosus: comparison of in vitro and in vivo responses. Arthritis Rheum 23:1343–1350, 1980
37. Henry C, Lucas A: The relation of idiotypic expression to isotype and allotype in the anti-p-azobenzenearsonate response. Eur J Immunol 12:175–183, 1982
38. Sigal NH: Regulation of azophenylarsonate-specific repertoire expression. I. Frequency of cross-reactive idiotype-positive B cells in A/J and Balb/c mice. J Exp Med 156:1352–1365, 1982
39. Datta SK, Stollar D, Schwartz RS: Normal mice express idiotypes related to auto-antibody idiotypes of lupus mice. Proc Natl Acad Sci USA 80:2723–2727, 1983
40. Pillarisetty RJ, Talal N: Clinical studies of antibodies binding polyriboadenylic acid in systemic lupus erythematosus. Arthritis Rheum 19:705–710, 1976
41. Liebling MR, Wong C: Specific suppression of anti-DNA in vitro (abstract). Clin Res 31:45A, 1983

INTRAARTICULAR VOLUME AND CLEARANCE IN HUMAN SYNOVIAL EFFUSIONS

WAYNE J. WALLIS, PETER A. SIMKIN, WIL B. NELP, and DAVID M. FOSTER

Intraarticular volumes were measured by radiolabeled albumin (RISA) distribution in chronic knee effusions from 11 rheumatoid arthritis patients and 9 osteoarthritis patients. Volumes of synovial fluid obtained at joint aspiration were substantially less than those found by RISA dilution. Up to 24 hours was needed for full distribution of RISA throughout the intraarticular compartment. Measured ^{123}I and RISA radioactivity over the knee described monoexponential rate constants, λ (minute^{-1}). The clearance of ^{123}I and RISA from synovial effusions was derived by the formulation volume (ml) × λ (minute^{-1}) = clearance (ml/minute). RISA clearance in rheumatoid effusions was significantly greater than that found in osteoarthritis effusions. Intraarticular volume and isotope clearance were easily quantified and provide measures for further evaluating the microvascular physiology of synovial effusions.

Radiolabeled compounds exit synovial effusions at rates which can be used to quantify the microvascular physiology of synovitis. Studies conducted with small solutes (^{23}Na, ^{131}I, and ^{133}Xe) and radiolabeled proteins (albumin and immunoglobulins) have all revealed the monoexponential decline in radioactivity characteristic of first-order kinetics (1–6). These constant rates mean that the departure of each solute from the joint cavity can be expressed as a single half-life (minutes) or, alternatively, a removal rate constant (minutes^{-1}) (7).

One cannot fully interpret such rate constants, however, without knowing the distribution volume of the isotope. For example, a value of 0.05 minutes^{-1} would correspond to an articular clearance rate of 0.5 ml/minute from a small intraarticular volume of 10 ml, but would reflect the much higher clearance of 5 ml/minute from a swollen volume of 100 ml. Such compartmental clearances are calculated easily from the product of compartmental volume, V (ml), and the rate constant of solute removal, λ (minute^{-1}), as follows:

$$V \text{ (ml)} \times \lambda \text{ (minute}^{-1}\text{)} = \text{clearance (ml/minute)}$$

Identical synovial clearances could result from a large effusion with a slow removal rate or from a small effusion with a rapid removal rate. These simple examples emphasize the importance of volume considerations in evaluating isotope clearance from synovial effusions.

In this report we describe a method of determining intraarticular volume and synovial clearances. We hypothesized that articular solute clearances would reflect the microvascular physiology of synovitis more accurately than rate constants of isotope removal. We determined the removal rate constants of ^{131}I-labeled albumin (RISA) and free ^{123}I from the synovial effusions of individuals with rheumatoid arthritis (RA) and osteoarthritis (OA). In the same effusions we also derived, by isotope dilution, the

From the Departments of Medicine, Radiology, and Bioengineering, University of Washington, Seattle.

Supported in part by NIH grants AM-22186, AM-32811, T32-AM-07108, and RR-37, and by a grant from the Western Washington Chapter of the Arthritis Foundation.

Wayne J. Wallis, MD: Acting Instructor in Medicine; Peter A. Simkin, MD: Professor of Medicine; Wil B. Nelp, MD: Professor of Medicine and Rheumatology and Director, Division of Nuclear Medicine; David M. Foster, PhD: Research Associate Professor of Bioengineering.

Address reprint requests to Peter A. Simkin, MD, School of Medicine, Department of Medicine, Division of Rheumatology, RG-28, University of Washington, Seattle, WA 98195.

Submitted for publication May 21, 1984; accepted in revised form October 23, 1984.

apparent distribution volume of RISA within the articular cavity and synovial tissues. These values have enabled us to calculate the albumin and iodine clearances from synovial effusions.

PATIENTS AND METHODS

Patient selection. Individuals with clinically evident knee effusions and rheumatoid arthritis or osteoarthritis were referred by physicians at the rheumatology clinics of the Affiliated Hospitals of the University of Washington. Fully informed consent was granted by all study participants through a protocol approved by the University Human Subjects Committee. Patients were admitted to the Clinical Research Center of University Hospital, where a history was taken and physical examination performed prior to each study.

Rheumatoid arthritis patients. Eleven individuals with classic or definite rheumatoid arthritis (8) and chronic stable knee effusions were included in this investigation. The age, sex, duration of disease, and patient's estimate of both the duration of the effusion and duration of recent morning stiffness are reported in Table 1. Six of 8 patients who had undergone previous joint aspiration for knee effusion had also received intraarticular corticosteroids an average of 7.5 months prior to study. Each patient's medication regimen was continued during the period of study in order to sustain the steady-state effect of outpatient therapy. Eight patients were receiving gold or penicillamine, 4 took oral prednisone ≤15 mg per day, and all were receiving aspirin and/or other nonsteroidal antiinflammatory drugs.

Physical examination findings, including height, weight, girth of the knee at mid-patella, range of motion, and the presence of laxity and crepitation, are shown in Table 1. Synovial (Baker's) cysts were detected by physical examina-

Table 1. Clinical features of rheumatoid arthritis (RA) and osteoarthritis (OA) patients with synovial effusions

Patient	Age/sex	Disease duration, years	Duration of effusion, months	Morning stiffness, minutes	Previous joint aspiration/injection (months before study)	Medications*	Height, cm	Weight, kg	Knee girth, cm	Range of motion, degrees	Laxity/crepitance	Cyst
RA												
1	64/F	5	15	90	+/+ (2)	NSAID, gold, ASA	160	46.8	38	120	−/+	−
2	62/M	18	12	240	+/+ (3)	DP, ASA, Pred (10 mg/day)	178	91.8	43	75	−/−	−
3	67/F	11	24	0	−/−	ASA	168	55.9	41	135	+/+	+
4	66/F	45	156	120	+/+ (4)	NSAID, Pred (3 mg/day)	163	56.8	39	125	+/+	+
5	41/M	5	6	120	−/−	NSAID	168	58.6	38	90	−/−	−
6	64/F	15	36	30	+/+ (6)	NSAID, DP, ASA	155	46.4	36	120	+/+	+
7	60/M	18	60	120	+/+ (6)	Gold, ASA	170	60.0	35	100	−/−	+
8	39/F	19	72	15	+/−	Gold, ASA	170	53.2	37	110	−/−	+
9	21/M	1.4	18	360	+/−	Gold, ASA, Pred (15 mg/day)	193	85.9	45	135	−/−	−
10	60/F	10	72	0	−/−	DP, ASA	152	76.8	39	135	+/+	−
11	60/M	20	42	0	+/+ (24)	NSAID, gold, Pred (5 mg/day)	188	95.5	44	135	−/−	+
Mean ± SE	55 ± 4	15 ± 4	47 ± 13	100 ± 34†			170 ± 4	67 ± 5	40 ± 1	116 ± 6		
OA												
1	41/F	0.4	2	10	−/−	None	183	110.9	51	135	−/−	−
2	75/M	3	36	15	−/−	NSAID, Pred (12.5 mg/day)	160	67.3	37	135	−/+	−
3	74/F	5	36	20	−/−	NSAID	163	63.2	39	135	−/+	−
4	54/M	3	36	20	−/−	NSAID	173	104.5	46	135	−/+	−
5	45/M	8	6	20	+/−	ASA	183	100.0	44	135	−/−	−
6	57/M	20	19	0	+/+ (2)	NSAID	180	74.5	39	135	+/−	+
7	86/F	3	72	0	−/−	NSAID	150	69.1	41	100	+/+	−
8	60/M	16	120	0	−/−	None	173	84.1	41	130	+/−	+
9	27/F	6	1	10	−/−	NSAID	168	65.9	39	95	+/+	−
Mean ± SE	58 ± 6	7 ± 2	37 ± 13	11 ± 3†			170 ± 4	82 ± 6	42 ± 1	126 ± 5		

* NSAID = nonsteroidal antiinflammatory drug; ASA = aspirin; DP = D-penicillamine; Pred = prednisone.
† $P < 0.05$, RA patients versus OA patients. Differences between RA and OA groups were not significant for any other parameters.

tion (RA patients 3, 4, 7, 8, and 11), scintigraphic imaging (RA patients 3 and 7), or previous arthrography (RA patients 6 and 7). Serum rheumatoid factor by latex agglutination was positive at a titer $\geq$1:640 within the year prior to study in all but 1 individual (RA patient 9). The mean serum hemoglobin level was 13 gm/dl.

Osteoarthritis patients. Nine individuals with chronic osteoarthritis and stable knee effusions are also characterized in Table 1. Many of these patients had suffered significant trauma to the knee. Although the values were not statistically different than those of RA patients, the OA group had joint disease of shorter duration (P = 0.08), weighed more (P = 0.07), and had knees of greater girth (P = 0.21) and wider range of motion (P = 0.25). OA patient 2 was receiving prednisone therapy for idiopathic thrombocytopenic purpura during the study. OA patient 6 was undergoing regular outpatient peritoneal dialysis for end-stage renal disease and had a massive effusion and synovial cyst. OA patient 7 had mild incidental hypothyroidism detected during the study of her effusion, when synovial fluid (SF) was found to string more than 3 feet from the aspirating syringe (9). The diagnosis of hypothyroidism was confirmed by thyroid function tests. OA patient 8 had a synovial (Baker's) cyst detected by physical examination.

Radionuclide preparation. The sodium salt of iodine-123 dissolved in water (^{123}I; half-life 13.3 hours) (Mediphysics, Emeryville, CA) was sterilized by passage through a 0.22-μm filter and tested by the limulus assay for absence of endotoxin. ^{131}I-labeled human serum albumin (^{131}I; half-life 193.9 hours; RISA concentration 10 mg/ml in H_2O, pH 7.6, with 9 mg/ml benzyl alcohol as preservative) was purchased from E. R. Squibb Co., New Brunswick, NJ. The nuclide solutions (30 μCi of each) were combined, and the total volume brought to 3 ml by the addition of isotonic saline. One milliliter was stored as a quantitative standard and the remaining 2 ml, containing 20 μCi of ^{123}I and 20 μCi of RISA, was used for intraarticular injection. The specific activity of injectate (μCi ^{131}I/mg albumin) varied with the age of the RISA preparation in different studies.

Study protocol. Investigations were all initiated in the morning, with patients fasting prior to study to assure a stable blood glucose level. Patients drank 0.3 ml of Lugol's solution 1 hour prior to study and each day during the ensuing 2 weeks, in order to block thyroidal uptake of radioiodine. Samples of venous blood were obtained through an antecubital in-dwelling heparin-flushed cannula, with the patient reclining on an examining table.

The knee was positioned at 30° of flexion and the medial suprapatellar aspect superficially anesthetized with 2% lidocaine. An 18-gauge intravenous catheter was then passed into the joint space until synovial fluid returned freely, and a 5-ml aliquot was withdrawn for study. The 2-ml double radionuclide solution was then injected into the knee, followed by barbitage to promote intraarticular mixing and then injection of 3 ml saline. The latter was employed to flush all injectate from the dead space of the catheter and to sustain the steady-state volume and hydrostatic pressure of the initial synovial effusion. The catheter was promptly withdrawn and intraarticular mixing and distribution of the injectate was again promoted by massage as well as passive flexion and extension of the knee for 5 minutes.

Radioactivity in the joint space and its rate of disappearance were measured with a sodium iodide crystal (thyroid probe) 28 cm over the patella. At this distance the collimator subtended a flat field response 18 cm in diameter at the surface of the patella, and the relative counting efficiency of 16% varied 0.8% per vertical cm. Thus, small differences with repositioning of the knee created little change in relative count rate. The counting of the 2 isotopes was done using gamma spectrometry and dual channel analysis. The photo peak was centered at 364 keV, with a window equal to the full width at half maximum of the photo peak. The ^{123}I activity was similarly counted, with the photo peak centered at 150 keV. The compton scatter of the ^{131}I into the ^{123}I photo peak was subtracted. This scatter fraction averaged 19% and was determined by counting a fixed ^{131}I source in 1 ml of water 28 cm from the crystal surface.

Counts were obtained at 5-minute intervals over the first 3 hours and then every 2–4 hours until midnight. Further counting resumed the following morning for total periods ranging from 24–96 hours. In selected individuals, serial joint imaging was accomplished with a Picker 4/11 gamma camera (Picker Corp., New Haven, CT) and a computer (MDS Simul; Media Data Systems, Ann Arbor, MI) calibrated for both isotopes. Between counting intervals, study patients were encouraged to ambulate at their normal level of activity.

Aliquots of synovial fluid (0.2 ml) were obtained at 1 and 24 hours by repeat arthrocentesis with a 22-gauge needle and tuberculin syringe. From 1 consenting individual with seronegative rheumatoid arthritis (RA patient 9), additional aliquots of synovial fluid (0.2 ml) were obtained every 24 hours over 3 days from bilateral, clinically identical knee effusions. From 4 OA patients and 4 RA patients, additional synovial fluid samples were taken at 24, 48, and 72 hours after injection. At the end of each study, the entire synovial fluid volume (V_A) of the effusion was aspirated as thoroughly as possible. ^{123}I and ^{131}I radioactivities of the synovial fluid samples (0.1 ml) and the quantitative standard (0.1 ml) were measured in a Packard well-type scintillation detector using dual channel analysis. For external surface counting and well counting, counting statistics had a relative error of $\leq$5%.

Characterization of synovial fluid RISA activity. Studies were conducted to determine if intraarticular RISA became aggregated or deiodinated within the joint space. ^{131}I activity in 1 synovial fluid sample obtained from RA patient 6, 24 hours after RISA injection was analyzed by sucrose density gradient ultracentrifugation. Hyaluronidase (0.1 mg, type I-S; Sigma, St. Louis, MO) was added to 2 ml of synovial fluid and incubated at 37°C for 60 minutes. Hyaluronidase-treated synovial fluid (0.4 ml) diluted 1:1 (volume/volume) with phosphate buffered saline (PBS) and 0.4 ml RISA reagent diluted 1:9 (v/v) in PBS were characterized on 5–30% sucrose gradients in borate buffered saline, and run at 37,000 revolutions per minute at 4°C for 16 hours in a SW41Ti rotor and Beckman L2-6513 ultracentrifuge (Beckman Instruments, Spinco Division, Palo Alto, CA).

Serial samples were collected and analyzed for radioactivity on an automatic gamma counter (Searle Radiographics, Des Plaines, IL). RISA activity in the injection solution and in synovial fluid (24-hour aspirate) remained monomeric without significant aggregation. In addition, ^{131}I activities in the RISA reagent and in 2 synovial fluid samples

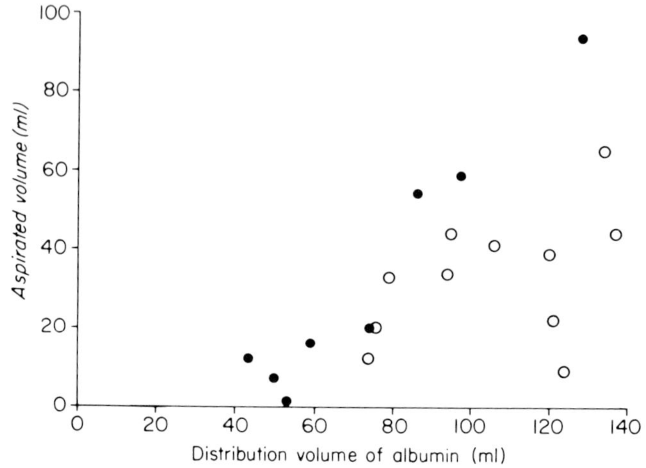

Figure 1. Intraarticular volumes. Volume of synovial fluid obtained at the termination of each study (V_A) markedly underestimated the apparent intraarticular distribution volume of ^{131}I-labeled human serum albumin (V_{R24}). V_A closely correlated with V_{R24} in effusions from osteoarthritis patients (●) (r = 0.98). Aspirated volumes in effusions from rheumatoid arthritis patients (○) were less predictive of distribution volumes. One patient with a massive effusion and a synovial cyst (osteoarthritis patient 6) is not included in this figure.

taken 24 hours after injection were studied by trichloroacetic acid (TCA) precipitation. In all 3 samples, the TCA-precipitable ^{131}I activity was >99%.

Clearance kinetics. External radioactivities over the knee for ^{123}I and ^{131}I were graphed and the removal rate constants for each isotope (corrected for physical decay) were obtained by regression analysis on a VAXII/780 computer using the SAAM 27 computer program (10). The R^2 of the "best fit" regressions of declining RISA radioactivity was 0.94 ± 0.03 (mean ± SE) in RA and 0.98 ± 0.01 in OA. Similarly, the R^2 of the ^{123}I regressions was 0.93 ± 0.02 in RA and 0.92 ± 0.03 in OA. In all cases, ^{123}I and ^{131}I radioactivities declined monoexponentially. Disappearance half-lives were calculated from the removal rate constants using the expression, half-life ($t_{1/2}$) = 0.693/λ.

Apparent distribution volumes for intraarticular RISA (V_{R24}) were calculated from the equation

$$V_{R24} = A_0 \times V_0/A_{24}$$

where A_0 and V_0 represent the activity (counts per minute/ml) and volume (ml) of the injectate, and A_{24} represents the activity of the SF aspirate obtained at 24 hours, corrected for isotope cleared from the joint (aspirated activity extrapolated back to time zero). A_{24} was obtained by multiplying the 24-hour aliquot (cpm/ml) by the externally monitored radioactivity at time zero (cpm) (N_0) and dividing by RISA N_{24} (both N taken from the computer-derived regression line of external RISA activity). Clearance of RISA from synovial effusions (ml/minute) was derived from the product of V_{R24} (ml) and RISA (minutes^{-1}). Iodine clearance was calculated from the product of V_{R24} and λ^{123}I.

Statistical analysis included linear regression and Student's 1-tailed *t*-test, using the SPSS (11) and BMDP (12) programs on a CDC-3000 computer.

RESULTS

Intraarticular volume in OA and RA synovial effusions. Preliminary studies revealed that RISA distribution volumes obtained by sampling synovial fluid 1 hour after injection were significantly smaller than those obtained at 24 hours. After 1 hour, the RISA distribution volume in all 9 OA effusions was 74 ± 33 ml (mean ± SEM), and after 24 hours, it was 109 ± 35 ml. In the 11 RA effusions the 1-hour RISA distribution volume,

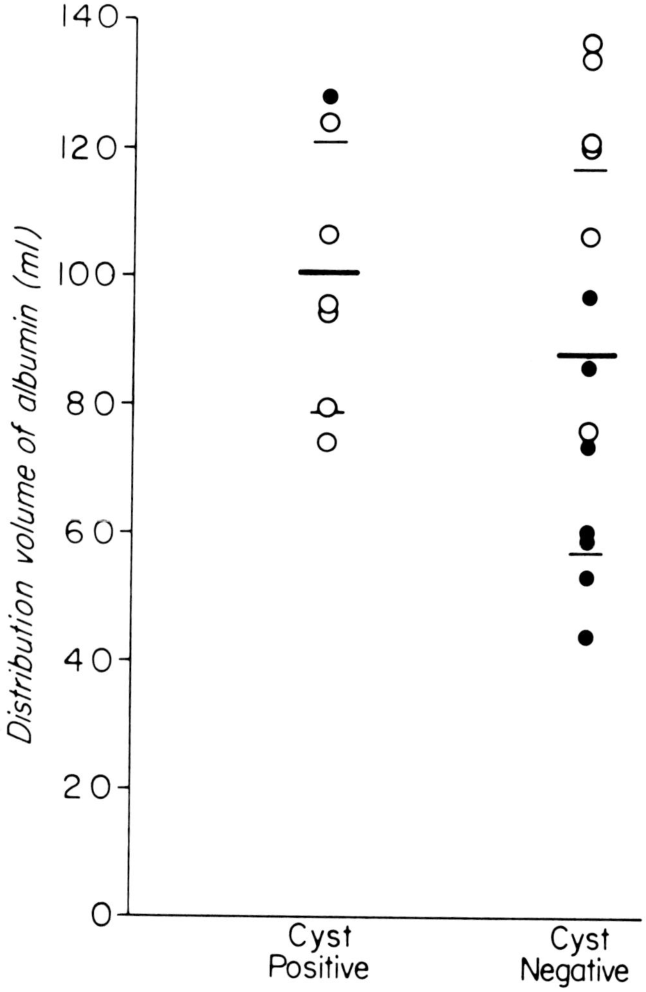

Figure 2. Popliteal cysts and intraarticular volumes. The presence of a popliteal cyst (detected by physical examination, previous arthrography, or scintigraphic imaging) did not significantly change the apparent distribution volume of intraarticular ^{131}I-labeled human serum albumin. Most cysts were found in individuals with rheumatoid arthritis (○). Osteoarthritis patient 6 is not included in the osteoarthritis data (●).

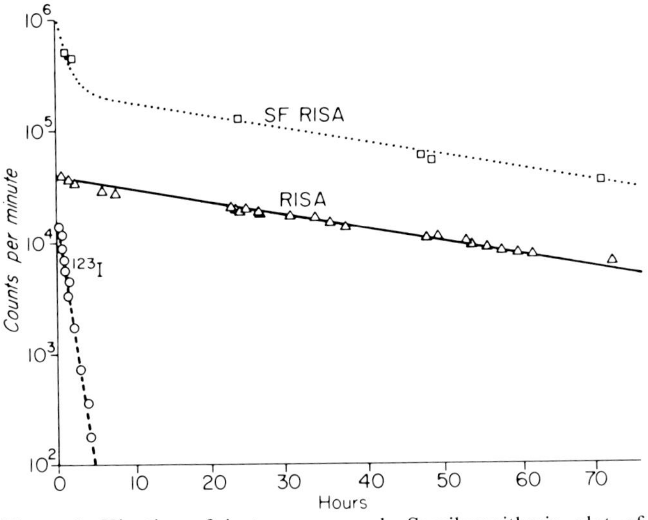

Figure 3. Kinetics of isotope removal. Semilogarithmic plot of activity over time for ^{123}I and ^{131}I-labeled human serum albumin (RISA) after injection into the stable knee effusion of an individual with osteoarthritis (OA patient 4). Externally monitored radioactivity of RISA (△) and ^{123}I (○) describes monoexponential plots with RISA intraarticular half-life approximately 36 times that of ^{123}I. Synovial fluid (SF) RISA activity (□) (counts per minute/ml) declined rapidly (distribution phase) and subsequently paralleled externally monitored RISA at 24 hours. Plots are corrected for Compton scatter and isotope physical decay.

45 ± 10 ml, was significantly less than the V_{R24}, 105 ± 7 ml. RISA distribution volumes were also derived from synovial fluid samples taken at 48, 72, and 96 hours in 4 patients with OA and 4 with RA. The derived distribution volumes at these later times did not significantly differ from those obtained at 24 hours.

The volume of synovial fluid aspirated from OA effusions was consistently less than that determined by RISA distribution, but a close correlation was observed between aspirated volume and V_{R24} ($P = 0.001$, $r = 0.98$) (Figure 1). Osteoarthritis V_A averaged 28 + 60, or −19% (geometric mean + 1 SD) of V_{R24}. Aspirated volume from RA effusions correlated less consistently with RISA distribution volume ($P = 0.091$, $r = 0.43$), primarily because V_A markedly underestimated V_{R24} in 2 individuals (RA patients 7 and 8). The geometric mean V_A in rheumatoid arthritis was 27 + 22 or −12% of V_{R24}. The presence of a synovial cyst (as defined in Patients and Methods) did not significantly affect V_{R24} (Figure 2).

Kinetics and clearance of radionuclide removal from synovial effusions. In accordance with previous findings (7), radioactivity over the knee from each isotope (free ^{123}I and albumin-bound ^{131}I) declined

Table 2. Intraarticular volumes and isotope clearance determinations in rheumatoid arthritis (RA) and osteoarthritis (OA) patients with synovial effusions*

Patient	V_A (ml)	V_{R24} (ml)	RISA $t_{1/2}$ (minutes)	RISA (R^2)	Iodine $t_{1/2}$ (minutes)	^{123}I (R^2)	C_{RISA} (ml/minutes)	C_I (ml/minutes)
RA								
1	44	137	1,540	0.98	69	0.91	0.062	1.37
2	39	120	877	0.99	35	0.94	0.095	2.40
3	34	94	1,050	0.95	53	0.98	0.062	1.22
4	33	79	877	0.91	69	0.88	0.062	0.79
5	20	76	1,260	0.92	41	0.92	0.042	1.29
6	44	95	1,506	0.66	69	0.92	0.044	0.95
7	12	74	976	0.99	53	0.81	0.053	0.96
8	9	124	613	0.99	29	0.97	0.140	2.98
9	65	134	1,174	0.99	29	0.99	0.079	3.22
10	22	121	1,358	0.98	29	0.98	0.062	2.90
11	41	106	900	0.99	24	0.90	0.082	3.07
Mean ± SE	33 ± 5	105 ± 7	1,102 ± 83†	0.94 ± 0.03	45 ± 5	0.93 ± 0.02	0.071 ± 0.028‡	1.92 ± 0.30
OA								
1	59	97	2,772	0.96	41	0.92	0.024	1.65
2	20	74	1,733	0.99	41	0.98	0.030	1.26
3	1	53	2,235	0.98	33	0.90	0.016	1.59
4	12	43	1,414	0.91	58	0.99	0.021	0.52
5	54	86	1,690	0.99	23	0.99	0.035	2.58
6	267	379	2,310	0.99	46	0.73	0.114	5.69
7	16	59	1,611	0.98	46	0.98	0.025	0.89
8	94	128	1,650	0.99	41	0.85	0.054	2.18
9	7	60	1,414	0.99	12	0.97	0.029	3.36
Mean ± SE	59 ± 28	109 ± 35	1,870 ± 155†	0.98 ± 0.01	38 ± 5	0.92 ± 0.03	0.039 ± 0.030‡	2.19 ± 0.52

* V_A = volume of synovial fluid by joint aspiration (at end of study); V_{R24} = apparent intraarticular distribution volume of ^{131}I-labeled human serum albumin (RISA) 24 hours after injection; $t_{1/2}$ = half-life of isotope marker in the knee as measured by external gamma emission counting; C_{RISA} = clearance of albumin; C_I = clearance of iodine. See text for clearance calculation methods.
† $P < 0.005$, RA patients versus OA patients.
‡ $P < 0.05$, RA patients versus OA patients.

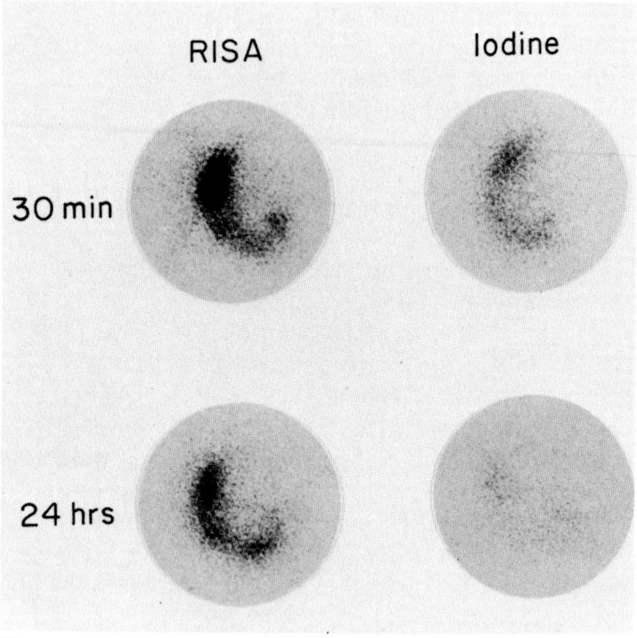

Figure 4. Articular scans. Lateral knee scintigraphic imaging of the intraarticular ^{123}I and ^{131}I-labeled human serum albumin (RISA) indicates that RISA activity declines more slowly with time than ^{123}I. These images (from osteoarthritis patient 8) suggest that both isotopes are largely confined to the intracapsular compartment. ^{123}I activity imaged at 24 hours represents Compton scatter from RISA into the ^{123}I energy window.

over time in monoexponential fashion (see example in Figure 3). The average elimination half-life for RISA was 1,102 ± 83 (mean ± SE) minutes in RA effusions and 1,870 ± 155 minutes in OA effusions. The corresponding mean half-life for ^{123}I was 45 ± 5 minutes in RA effusions and 38 ± 5 minutes in OA effusions. Table 2 illustrates the marked differences in rate constants of isotope removal, both between individuals and between diagnostic groups. In addition, the distribution image of both radionuclides did not expand beyond the immediate articular region with serial joint scans (Figure 4). As in any study utilizing radiolabeled proteins in vivo, we necessarily assumed that the administered radioalbumin was not deiodinated within the joint.

Intraarticular volume, defined by apparent distribution volume of injected RISA, was multiplied by the removal rate constants obtained for RISA and ^{123}I to derive the synovial clearances in ml/minute. The product of V_{R24} (ml) and $\lambda^{123}I$ (minutes^{-1}) is the synovial iodine clearance (ml/minute). The product of V_{R24} (ml) and RISA yields RISA clearance (ml/minute). The mean iodine clearance in RA effusions (1.92 ± 0.30 ml/minute) was comparable with that found in OA effusions (2.19 ± 0.52 ml/minute) (Table 2). Figure

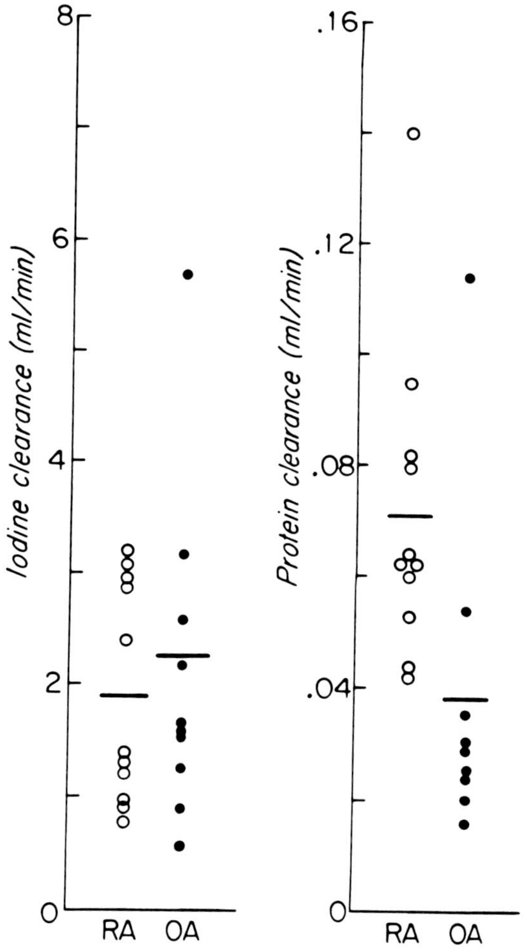

Figure 5. Synovial clearances of iodine and radioalbumin. Scattergrams of calculated ^{123}I clearance and ^{131}I-labeled human serum albumin clearance from the synovial effusions of individuals with osteoarthritis (OA) and rheumatoid arthritis (RA). Synovial ^{123}I clearances were comparable from RA and OA knee joints (P = 0.663), while synovial protein clearance was significantly higher in RA than in OA joints (P = 0.024).

5 emphasizes the wide distribution of synovial iodine clearance values found in our sample of rheumatoid synovial effusions. The mean RISA clearance in RA patients (0.071 ± 0.028 ml/minute) was significantly greater than that found in OA patients (0.039 ± 0.030 ml/minute). Protein clearance was greater in every RA effusion than in every OA effusion except that from OA patient 6, who had a massive effusion and a RISA distribution volume of 379 ml.

Recirculation of RISA from plasma to synovial fluid. In order to assess the possible contribution of recirculated RISA, we measured radioactivity in serial samples of synovial fluid from both the injected knee

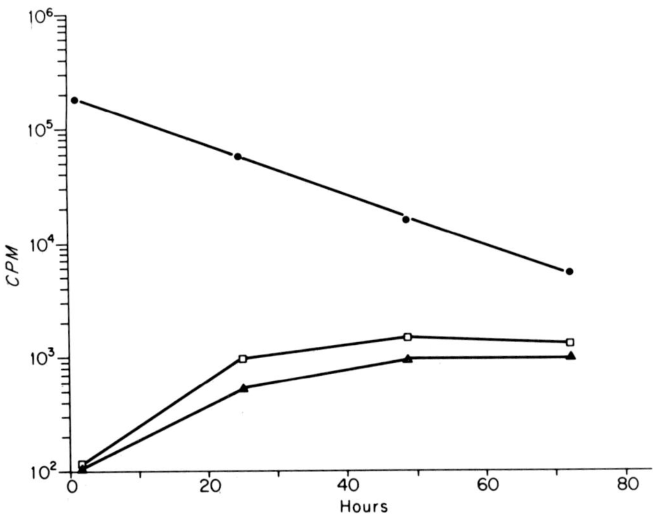

Figure 6. Radioalbumin recirculation. Semilogarithmic plot of ^{131}I-labeled human serum albumin (RISA) activity (counts per minute/ml) in serial samples obtained from synovial fluid of the injected knee (●), and serum (□) and synovial fluid (▲) from a clinically similar contralateral knee effusion from an individual with seronegative rheumatoid arthritis. Assuming that the effusion volumes and exchange rates were identical at both knees, then recirculation of RISA accounts for approximately 1%, 6%, and 18% of synovial fluid activity in the injected knee at 24, 48, and 72 hours, respectively.

effusion and a similar contralateral knee effusion in 1 consenting individual with seronegative rheumatoid arthritis (RA patient 9). Serial plasma samples were also studied. The history and physical findings of both effusions were essentially identical, and the synovial fluid leukocyte counts differed by <10% (28,130 and 30,400). Synovial fluid RISA in the contralateral, uninjected knee was 15, 55, 62, and 74% of plasma activity 1, 24, 48, and 72 hours, respectively, after injection. Assuming that the RISA transsynovial exchange kinetics and synovial fluid RISA distribution volumes were approximately equal in both knees, then recirculation of RISA from peripheral blood constituted <1% of synovial fluid RISA activity 24 hours after injection. At 48 and 72 hours, this figure increased to 6% and 18%, respectively (see Figure 6). RISA recirculation was thus an insignificant factor in determining synovial fluid RISA activity during the 24-hour observation period used for the present study.

DISCUSSION

A simple and accurate measure of intraarticular volume provides a useful tool for studying the local physiology of joint disease. In this report we have introduced an isotopic method for quantifying intraarticular volume in the knees of patients with rheumatoid arthritis or osteoarthritis. Volumes derived by RISA distribution have been contrasted with volumes obtained at aspiration, and distribution volumes have enabled us to quantify the clearance of albumin and iodine from human synovial effusions.

Previous work in our laboratory on the kinetics of transsynnovial solute exchange included volume considerations (13,14). Isotonic saline was injected into normal and diseased knees while solute entry and exit were evaluated by serial sampling. Those early studies with artificial effusions revealed that variations in injected volume significantly affected the exchange rates of solutes crossing the synovial tissue barrier. The experiments described in this report extend and refine those early observations by considering the volumes and exchange rates of natural synovial effusions unchanged by saline injection or by serial aspiration.

These studies were designed to minimize distortion of the baseline pathophysiologic condition. All effusions were clinically stable prior to study, and synovial fluid volume and hydrostatic pressure were maintained by saline replacement of the initial synovial fluid aspirate. All patients remained ambulatory, and medication regimens were unchanged throughout the period of observation. We assume, therefore, that the synovial effusions remained in a steady state, clinically and physiologically, throughout the period of study.

Measurement of volume by isotope dilution requires a marker which is physiologically inert at the studied site. Because albumin is the most abundant protein in both plasma and synovial fluid and is critical in the regulation of transvascular fluid balance, we chose radiolabeled albumin for measurements of intraarticular volume. We have assumed that exogenous RISA is handled like endogenous albumin within the joint space, i.e., without substantial local aggregation, degradation, nonspecific binding, or consumption by joint tissues. These assumptions are supported by sucrose density gradient analysis, which indicates that synovial fluid RISA does not become aggregated within the joint, and by protein precipitation studies, which suggest that synovial fluid ^{131}I radioactivity remains bound to albumin within the knee. In addition, studies with scintigraphic imaging indicate that RISA does not diffuse into periarticular tissues. These results suggest that the injected RISA behaves like monomeric endogenous albumin and constitutes a stable and appropriate marker for defining intraarticular volume.

Solute distribution and clearance from joints reflects organ-level physiology. We presume that the articular tissue, although histologically diverse, may be approached as a single functional unit isolated from adjacent tissues by a relatively impermeable joint capsule. Images obtained by scintigraphic scanning support our view that the joint constitutes a discrete anatomic and functional unit (Figure 4). The isotope markers used for these studies, ^{123}I and RISA, are highly water-soluble and easily distribute throughout the articular compartment. Unlike xenon (15), neither is preferentially sequestered in periarticular fatty stores.

Recirculation of injected radionuclide from plasma to synovial fluid, after initial clearance from synovial fluid, has been considered to be a significant obstacle in studies of articular clearance kinetics (16). Through study of one individual's bilateral knee effusions we determined that, at the doses of isotope used in these studies, recirculation constitutes $<1\%$ of detectable radioactivity over the knee, up to 24 hours after injection.

Serial determinations of apparent RISA distribution volume were made in preliminary studies and revealed that volumes expanded for up to 24 hours and were stable thereafter. Scintigraphic imaging of intraarticular RISA did not reveal changes in the geometry of RISA distribution after 24 hours. On the basis of these findings, the calculated distribution volume V_{R24} was chosen as the most physiologically appropriate volume for characterizing synovial effusions. We believe V_{R24} reflects the total volume of synovial fluid continuous with the interstitial fluid in adjacent synovial tissues. Since tight junctions are not observed between the synovial lining cells, synovial fluid may be considered a fluid-phase extension of the extracellular matrix in synovial tissues (17). Volumes obtained by isotope distribution will therefore vary with the extent to which the isotope marker has equilibrated within intracapsular tissues. Our findings indicate that radiolabeled albumin completes this process by 24 hours and that distribution volumes remain constant thereafter.

Average aspirated synovial fluid volume, V_A, substantially underestimates the intraarticular volume defined by RISA distribution. The aspirated volume of synovial fluid in OA effusions was generally less than half the volume obtained by RISA distribution. The aspirated synovial fluid volume from rheumatoid effusions was an even smaller and more variable fraction of V_{R24} (Figure 1). Aspirated volume underestimates intraarticular distribution volume because it necessarily neglects the volume of synovial tissue interstitial fluid. The interstitial portion of the intraarticular volume is of considerable physiologic interest since it represents the site where nutrient exchange between plasma and synovial fluid occurs. Spuriously low aspirated volume readings in some effusions may have resulted from obstructing rice bodies (18), synovial plicae (19), or popliteal cysts sequestered by one-way valves (20). Factors such as posterior recesses and the complexity of knee joint geometry clearly render additional portions of the intraarticular space inaccessible for sampling.

Intraarticular volume determination by dilution of injected marker has been described previously. Rekonen et al (21) found average intraarticular apparent distribution volumes of 49 ml in the knee effusions of 17 individuals with rheumatoid arthritis, using a small solute (^{113}indium) that was allowed to distribute within the knee for 2 minutes before resampling. Wigginton et al (22) evaluated methotrexate distribution within 4 rheumatoid effusions by serial arthrocentesis, and described a mean intraarticular apparent distribution volume of 69 ml. These figures are lower than volumes obtained by RISA dilution in our investigations. We suspect that this difference chiefly reflects selection of an inadequate time for full distribution throughout the intracapsular space, although differences in the study populations may also be important.

In this report we have introduced a method of quantifying intraarticular volume. Determinations of intraarticular volumes and isotope removal rate constants have enabled us to derive the iodine clearance and albumin clearance from relatively unperturbed synovial effusions in vivo. Aspirated volumes of synovial fluid were considerably less than intraarticular volume defined by isotope distribution. Mean iodine clearance in rheumatoid effusions was comparable with that found in osteoarthritis effusions, while mean albumin clearance was significantly greater.

ACKNOWLEDGMENTS

We thank the patients who generously consented to participate in these studies, many kind physicians for patient referrals, Chris Pickerell for able technical assistance, and Nisa Rachie for skillful word processing.

REFERENCES

1. Harris R, Millard JB: Clearance of radioactive sodium from the knee joint. Clin Sci Mol Med 15:9–15, 1956
2. Scholer JF, Lee PR, Polley HF: The absorption of heavy water and radioactive sodium from the knee joint of normal persons and patients with rheumatoid arthritis. Arthritis Rheum 2:426–432, 1959
3. Kremer D, Deodhar SD, Dick WC: A function of synovial membrane of normal and diseased humans in relation to the movement of small-molecular weight ions. Clin Sci Mol Med 44:611–615, 1973
4. Ahlstrom S, Gedda PO, Hedberg H: Disappearance of radioactive serum albumin from joints in rheumatoid arthritis. Acta Rheum Scand 2:129–136, 1956
5. Rodnan GP, Maclachlan MJ: The absorption of serum albumin and gamma globulin from the knee joint of man and rabbit. Arthritis Rheum 3:152–157, 1960
6. Brown DL, Cooper AG, Bluestone R: Exchange of IgM and albumin between plasma and synovial fluid in rheumatoid arthritis. Ann Rheum Dis 20:644–651, 1969
7. Simkin PA, Nilson KL: Trans-synovial exchange of large and small molecules, The Biology of the Joint. Edited by P Hasselbacher. Clin Rheum Dis 7:99–130, 1981
8. Blumberg BS, Bunim JJ, Calkins E, Pirani CL, Zvaifler NJ: ARA nomenclature and classification of arthritis and rheumatism (tentative). Arthritis Rheum 7:93–97, 1964
9. Dorwart BB, Schumacher HR: Joint effusions, chondrocalcinosis and other rheumatic manifestations in hypothyroidism. Am J Med 59:780–790, 1975
10. Berman M, Weiss MF: SAAM Manual. DHEW Publication No. (NIH) 78-180. Government Printing Office
11. Nie NH, Hull CH: SPSS Update 7-9: New Procedures and Facilities for Releases. St. Louis, McGraw-Hill, 1981
12. Department of Biomathematics, University of California, Los Angeles: BMDP Statistical Software. Berkeley, University of California Press, 1981
13. Simkin PA, Pizzorno JE: Transynovial exchange of small molecules in normal human subjects. J Appl Physiol 36:581–587, 1974
14. Simkin PA: Synovial permeability in rheumatoid arthritis. Arthritis Rheum 22:689–696, 1979
15. Phelps P, Steele AD, McCarty DJ: Significance of xenon-133 clearance rate from canine and human joints. Arthritis Rheum 15:360–370, 1972
16. Llew M, Dick MC: Anatomy and physiology of blood flow, The Biology of the Joint. Edited by P Hasselbacher. Clin Rheum Dis 7:131–148, 1981
17. Hadler NM: The biology of the extracellular space, The Biology of the Joint. Edited by P Hasselbacher. Clin Rheum Dis 7:71–97, 1981
18. Popert HA, Scott DL, Wainright AC, Walton KW, Williamson N, Chapman JH: Frequency of occurrence, mode of development and significance of rice bodies. Ann Rheum Dis 41:109–117, 1982
19. Fujikawa K, Mikura Y: Synovial pleat syndrome, Topical Reviews in Rheumatic Disorders. Vol. 2. Edited by V Wright. Bristol, England, John Wright and Sons, 1982, pp 167–187
20. Jayson MIV, Dixon ASJ: Valvular mechanisms in juxta-articular cysts. Ann Rheum Dis 29:415–420, 1970
21. Rekonen A, Oka M, Kuikka J: Measurement of synovial fluid volume by a radioisotope method. Scand J Rheumatol 2:33–35, 1973
22. Wigginton SM, Chu BCF, Weisman MH, Howell SB: Methotrexate pharmacokinetics after intraarticular injection in patients with rheumatoid arthritis. Arthritis Rheum 23:119–122, 1980

GOVERNMENT AFFAIRS

FDA ARTHRITIS ADVISORY COMMITTEE MEETING

HAROLD E. PAULUS

The Food and Drug Administration Arthritis Advisory Committee met October 25 and 26, 1984 to consider the following issues.

Phenylbutazone and oxyphenbutazone. On December 28, 1983, based on his interpretation and extrapolation of spontaneously reported postmarketing data on deaths due to phenylbutazone/oxyphenbutazone–associated bone marrow suppression, Sidney M. Wolfe, MD, Director of the Health Research Group, petitioned the FDA to immediately remove these drugs from the market as imminent hazards, prior to the due-process procedures normally involved in the withdrawal of FDA approval of a drug. Following a public hearing in January 1984 and after FDA analysis of available data, the Secretary of Health and Human Services denied the petition, but recommended a revision of the labeling of these drugs to include additional information about risks and appropriate uses in order to discourage their prescription for minor or self-limiting conditions.

The Arthritis Advisory Committee reviewed the revised labeling information. (It should be noted that the "label" is a legal document that specifically limits the claims that the manufacturer can make about a drug and, to some extent, limits the manufacturer's liability.) The FDA estimates that there are about 16 deaths due to marrow suppression per million patients receiving these drugs, but that this risk is approximately sixfold greater in women over the age of 60. The Committee agreed that the revised label should include a statement such as, "Because of the increased risk of agranulocytosis, thrombocytopenia, and aplastic anemia, Butazolidin is not generally recommended as initial therapy for any of its indications." Warning statements about these risks are being strengthened and prominently displayed in the label. Regular monitoring of complete blood counts and white blood cell differential and platelet counts is recommended, but the frequency of monitoring is left to the physician's discretion.

An informative package insert for the patient is to be prepared and distributed to all patients by the pharmacist dispensing the medication. Educational workshops for physicians are to be conducted under the auspices of the American Medical Association. It is hoped that these actions will decrease the inappropriate use of phenylbutazone and oxyphenbutazone but permit appropriate use for patients who truly need these drugs.

Step-use of nonsteroidal antiinflammatory drugs (NSAIDs). The Committee considered whether to attempt to develop differential labeling based on differences in the profiles of adverse reactions (obtained from voluntary reporting Adverse Drug Reaction [ADR] Registries) to the various NSAIDs in order to establish a stepwise preferred sequence for the use of these drugs in individual patients, which would be similar to the "step-use" recommendations for antihypertensive drugs. After reviewing available data, the Committee decided that there was not enough evidence to justify the ranking decisions for most of the NSAIDs.

The "not for initial use" stipulation was discussed, and there was a consensus that it should be used sparingly and be modified to indicate that a drug

Harold E. Paulus, MD: American Rheumatism Association Representative to the FDA Arthritis Advisory Committee, UCLA School of Medicine, Center for the Health Sciences, Los Angeles, CA 90024.

is *generally* not for initial use, in order to avoid excessive intrusion into the practice of medicine.

A suggestion was introduced that all new drugs be labeled "not for initial use" during the dangerous interval following approval, and that the stipulation be removed when sufficient experience has accumulated that would document their safety in general clinical practice.

General warning regarding effect of NSAIDs on renal function. The following general warning was approved in principle and will be added to the labeling of all NSAIDs.

> In patients with prerenal conditions leading to a reduction in renal blood flow or blood volume, the renal prostaglandins have a supportive role in the maintenance of renal perfusion. In these patients, administration of an NSAID may cause a dose-dependent reduction in prostaglandin formation and may precipitate overt renal decompensation. Patients at greatest risk of this reaction are those with heart failure, decreased renal function, hypertension, liver dysfunction; those taking diuretics; and the elderly. Discontinuation of NSAID therapy is typically followed by recovery to the pretreatment state.

Additional risk factors include the use of maximum doses of NSAID, oliguria, sepsis with volume depletion, and the postoperative state when associated with third space fluid sequestration. Monitoring of serum creatinine is not included in the general warning but was considered to be prudent in patients with predisposing conditions or circumstances.

Auranofin. The manufacturer reviewed currently available information about the efficacy and safety of auranofin in the treatment of rheumatoid arthritis, emphasizing controlled clinical comparisons with gold sodium thiomalate (GST) therapy. Prospective controlled comparisons of these 2 gold-containing drugs have involved 893 patients worldwide. Depending on the study, the efficacy of auranofin was either equal to or modestly less than that of GST, but the proportion of patients discontinuing treatment because of toxicity was significantly less among those taking auranofin. All of the toxic reactions commonly associated with GST were seen with auranofin, but their prevalence was generally lower. For example, in patients taking auranofin versus those taking GST, respectively, proteinuria occurred in 0.9% versus 5.4%, rash in 26% versus 39%, white blood count of $<3,000/mm^3$ in 1.3% versus 2.2%, platelet count of $<100,000/mm^3$ in 0.9% versus 2.2%. No drug-related deaths occurred with either therapy in these controlled prospective trials. However, auranofin is now being marketed in a number of countries, and 2 deaths attributed to auranofin-associated thrombocytopenia have recently been reported, under the conditions of general marketed use, among an estimated total of about 30,000 patients who have received auranofin.

Because of incomplete absorption, the body burden of gold from 6-mg daily doses of oral auranofin is about 10–15% of that from 50-mg weekly intramuscular injections of GST; steady-state serum gold levels confirm this relationship. The above data have led the FDA and the Committee to postulate that auranofin therapy is not unique, but is a more convenient method of administering low-dose gold therapy with, perhaps, slightly less efficacy and substantially less dose-related toxicity than standard doses of GST. It remains to be determined whether the frequency of the rare, lethal, gold-associated bone marrow aplasias is also dose-related, or is truly idiosyncratic and independent of dose.

Based on this reasoning, pending experience in a large number of patients, it seems prudent to apply the same caution to the use of auranofin as is applied to the use of GST. The FDA and the sponsor are negotiating the specific language of the label, particularly regarding the indications, warnings, and suggested intervals for laboratory monitoring; preparation of an information sheet to be made available for physicians to give to their patients, if they wish to do so; and constraints regarding promotion of the drug. (Resolution of these issues is likely to be followed by release of the drug.)

BRIEF REPORT

MYOCARDITIS IN ADULT STILL'S DISEASE

ILAN BANK, CHARLES C. MARBOE, RITA F. REDBERG, and JERRY JACOBS

Cardiopulmonary manifestations in adult Still's disease include pleuritis, pneumonitis, and pericarditis (1–3). In children with Still's disease, myocarditis may lead to congestive heart failure and arrhythmias (4,5), but these manifestations have not been reported in adult patients. We describe a patient with adult Still's disease and biopsy-proven, clinically significant myocarditis that responded favorably to steroid treatment.

Case report. A 21-year-old man noted the onset of fever, myalgias, arthralgias, pleuritic chest pain, and a fleeting rash on his upper extremities. Oral ampicillin and erythromycin treatment had no effect and he was admitted to another hospital. He was febrile (102.4°F), and a mild exudative pharyngitis and bibasilar chest dullness were noted. A chest radiograph revealed cardiomegaly and bibasilar interstitial infiltrates with small pleural effusions. An electrocardiogram showed sinus tachycardia and elevated ST segments in V_2 through V_4.

The white blood cell count was 62,000/ml with a shift to the left; other laboratory values included: hematocrit 41.6%, erythrocyte sedimentation rate 40–110 mm/hour, hemoglobin 12.1 gm/dl, aspartate transaminase 64 units/dl (normal 20–50), alkaline phosphatase 267 units/dl (normal 25–100), lactate dehydrogenase 580 units/dl (normal 40–200), and bilirubin 0.7 mg/dl.

Negative results were obtained on the following: blood cultures, viral stool cultures, throat cultures, purified protein derivative, latex fixation test, monospot, lupus erythematosus preparation, antinuclear antibody, the Farr test, total hemolytic complement, VDRL, tests for *Salmonella* agglutinins, the Weil-Felix reaction test, tests for *Toxoplasma*, and herpes virus cultures. He was immune to rubella. A bone marrow biopsy revealed myeloid hyperplasia. Transbronchial aspirate and biopsy revealed bronchial inflammation and interstitial pneumonitis; stains were negative for *Pneumocystis carinii* and *Legionella pneumophila*. A therapeutic trial with broad spectrum intravenous antibiotics for 1 week failed to lower his temperature or improve his toxic-appearing condition.

He was transferred to Columbia Presbyterian Medical Center for further evaluation. In addition to the previously described findings, shotty lymphadenopathy, hepatomegaly, and a diffuse maculopapular rash were noted. His cardiac examination revealed sinus tachycardia. No murmur, rub, or gallop was noted on admission, but an S_4 gallop rhythm developed during the hospital stay. Antibiotics were discontinued, and the spiking fever persisted. He developed small effusions in the knee and a pericardial friction rub; echocardiography revealed a moderate to large pericardial effusion. Skin biopsy findings showed a perivascular mononuclear infiltrate. A diagnosis of adult Still's disease was made and salicylate treatment at therapeutic blood levels resulted in some symptomatic improvement; the fever, however, abated only upon addition of indomethacin.

By the sixth week of hospitalization, the rash, arthralgias, and pericarditis had resolved. A repeat

From the Columbia Presbyterian Medical Center, Columbia University, College of Physicians and Surgeons, New York, New York.

Ilan Bank, MD: Fellow in Rheumatology; Charles C. Marboe, MD: Assistant Professor of Pathology; Rita F. Redberg, MD: Resident in Medicine; Jerry Jacobs, MD: Professor of Clinical Pediatrics.

Address reprint requests to Charles C. Marboe, MD, Columbia University, College of Physicians and Surgeons, Black Building 813, 630 West 168th Street, New York, NY 10032.

Submitted for publication July 9, 1984; accepted in revised form October 11, 1984.

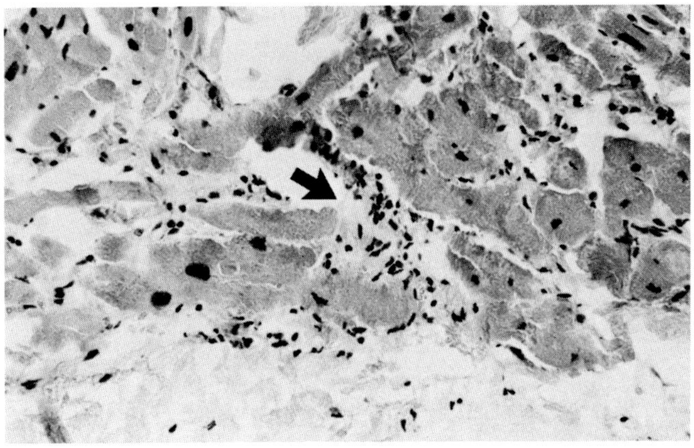

Figure 1. Microscopic sections of the endomyocardial biopsy specimen, showing a diffuse interstitial mononuclear cell infiltrate associated in some areas with proliferating fibroblasts and immature connective tissue (**arrow**). Biopsy was taken after 4 weeks of indomethacin and salicylate therapy, and this histologic appearance is consistent with partial healing in an acute immune-associated myocarditis (hematoxylin-phloxine-saffron stained, original magnification × 250).

echocardiogram showed resolution of the pericardial fluid. His exercise tolerance, however, remained reduced; extreme fatigue, dyspnea, and tachycardia were present after minimal exertion. By radiographic criteria, the heart was moderately enlarged, and radionuclide angiography revealed a decreased ejection fraction (39%) and anterolateral hypokinesis. The electrocardiogram showed diffuse inversion of the T-waves.

Percutaneous transvenous endomyocardial biopsy revealed mild edema and a diffuse mononuclear cellular infiltrate associated in some areas with proliferating fibroblasts, immature connective tissue, and capillaries (Figure 1). Patches of virtually acellular, dense connective tissue and moderate hypertrophy of some myocardial fibers were also present. Prednisone, 60 mg daily, was begun and the patient was followed at the clinic. Marked improvement was noted on a slowly tapering regimen of daily steroids. After 7 months of treatment, his exercise tolerance level was normal and the ejection fraction was 53%. Ten months after his disease onset, while receiving 10 mg of prednisone daily, he developed arthritis of the wrists and knees with morning stiffness, limitation of motion, and inflammatory effusions (white blood cell count from a knee effusion: 18,000 with 60% segments and 40% mononuclear cells). The aggressive nature of his arthritis has necessitated high doses of indocin, intraarticular steroids, and recently, chrysotherapy. So far there has been no evidence of a flare of his myocarditis, and the electrocardiogram result has reverted to normal.

Discussion. Adult Still's disease was delineated as a distinct entity by Bywaters (1). The clinical syndrome is characterized by high fever, a blotchy transient rash, and arthritis. The etiology is unknown, although findings suggestive of immune complex involvement (6) and a viral etiology (7) have been reported.

Several studies have emphasized the systemic nature of the disease (2,3). Myocarditis has not been reported, but is a recognized complication of the systemic form of juvenile rheumatoid arthritis, Still's disease (4). The histologic features found in this patient are similar to those features described in Still's disease and rheumatoid heart disease (4,8).

While most of the manifestations of this patient's disease (pneumonitis, rash, pericarditis) responded to salicylates and indomethacin, his cardiac symptoms did not, which prompted an endomyocardial biopsy. This modality has been used as a diagnostic tool and a guide for treatment in both acute inflammatory myocarditis (9) and in chronic myocarditis (10). The findings in the biopsy corresponded to an acute exacerbation of a "chronic" myocarditis on the basis of the presence of both an inflammatory infiltrate and areas of dense connective tissue. According to a recent study (10), patients with this clinicopathologic picture have been those most likely to benefit from steroid therapy. In addition, children with myocarditis as part of Still's disease have benefited from treatment with steroids (4). These considerations and the good response of this patient to prednisone suggest that steroid treatment may be indicated in adult Still's disease with clinically significant myocarditis.

REFERENCES

1. Bywaters EGL: Still's disease in the adult. Ann Rheum Dis 30:121–133, 1971
2. Esdaile JM, Tannenbaum H, Hawkins D: Adult Still's disease. Am J Med 68:825–830, 1980
3. Bajak JS, Aptekar RG, Decker JL, Wolff SM: Juvenile rheumatoid arthritis presenting in the adult as fever of unknown origin. Medicine (Baltimore) 52:431–444, 1973
4. Miller JJ, French JW: Myocarditis in juvenile rheumatoid arthritis. Am J Dis Child 131:205–209, 1977
5. Bernstein B, Takahaihi M, Hanson V: Cardiac involvement in juvenile rheumatoid arthritis. J Pediatr 85:313–317, 1974
6. Elkon KB, Hughes GRV, Bywaters EGL, Ryan PFJ, Inman RD, Bowley NB, James MP, Eady RAJ: Adult-onset Still's disease. Arthritis Rheum 25:647–654, 1982

7. Harth M, Thompson JM, Ralph ED: Adult-onset Still's disease. Can Med Assoc J 120:1507–1510, 1979
8. Lebowitz WB: The heart in rheumatoid arthritis: a clinical and pathological study of sixty-two cases. Ann Intern Med 58:102–123, 1963
9. Mason JW, Billingham ME, Ricci DR: Treatment of acute inflammatory myocarditis assisted by endomyocardial biopsy. Am J Cardiol 45:1037–1044, 1980
10. Fenoglio JJ Jr, Ursell PC, Kellogg CF, Drusin RE, Weiss MB: Diagnosis and classification of myocarditis by endomyocardial biopsy. N Engl J Med 308:12–18, 1983

BRIEF REPORT

A PERSISTENT ADENOVIRUS TYPE 1 INFECTION IN SYNOVIAL TISSUE FROM AN IMMUNODEFICIENT PATIENT WITH CHRONIC, RHEUMATOID-LIKE POLYARTHRITIS

KEVIN J. FRASER, BARRY J. CLARRIS, KENNETH D. MUIRDEN, J. ROBERT E. FRASER, and IAN JACK

Microbiologic studies of patients with rheumatoid arthritis (RA) have failed to establish a causal link with any specific infective agent, though most of the evidence points to viruses rather than prokaryotes. On several occasions, virus-like particles have been detected in rheumatoid synovial tissue, using electron microscopy (1–3). However, the only successful isolations of live viruses reported so far have involved unrelated species, namely, cytomegalovirus (4) and parvovirus (5). These findings could reflect opportunistic colonization, but it is possible that more than one agent could initiate the pathogenesis of RA, in which case either or both of these viruses could qualify as potential causative agents.

In this report, we describe the isolation of another virus from arthritic synovial tissue—a human adenovirus that, hitherto, has been associated only with respiratory tract infections. The patient presented an unusual combination of chronic, erosive, rheumatoid-like polyarthritis and an immunodeficiency condition classified as "acquired" hypogammaglobulinemia. Strong evidence is presented indicating that the adenovirus persisted in the patient's synovium, since cultured synovial cells obtained from 2 surgical procedures, 16 months apart, yielded viruses of the same serotype.

Case report. Our patient, born in 1940, had suffered from recurrent respiratory infections since the age of 12; he later developed bronchiectasis. This had been effectively controlled by antibiotics and physiotherapy, and the patient showed no symptoms of active respiratory disease during the time of our study. At the age of 29, he first noted pain, stiffness, and swelling in the right wrist and knee. A synovial biopsy that was performed early in the course of the disease showed synovial hyperplasia, villus proliferation, and infiltration of the synovium with lymphocytes, but only a few plasma cells.

Radiographs obtained in 1977 showed small erosions of the lateral femoral condyle and the right medial tibial plateau, but none in the hands or feet. There was no evidence of sacroiliitis, and the chest was reported as "clear." By 1981, radiographs revealed involvement of the finger joints, wrists, elbows, shoulders, and knees, and there were prominent erosive changes in the left wrist, right shoulder, and both knees. The rheumatoid factor test had given consistently negative results, and the erythrocyte sedimentation rate was only mildly elevated. A synovectomy of the right knee was performed in May 1981. Until this time, treatment had included nonsteroidal antiinflammatory drugs (aspirin and indomethacin) and prednisolone (5 mg/day). Penicillamine (375 mg/day) was begun shortly before the operation.

From the Department of Medicine, University of Melbourne and the Virus Laboratory, Royal Children's Hospital, Victoria, Australia.

Supported in part by the National Health and Medical Research Council of Australia.

Kevin J. Fraser, MB, FRACP: Rheumatologist, Austin Hospital, Heidelberg, Victoria, Australia; Barry J. Clarris, PhD: Senior Research Fellow in Rheumatology, Royal Melbourne Hospital, Victoria, Australia; Kenneth D. Muirden, MD: Head, Rheumatology Unit, Royal Melbourne Hospital, Victoria, Australia; J. Robert E. Fraser, MD: Deputy Director, Department of Medicine, University of Melbourne, Victoria, Australia; Ian Jack, MSc: Deputy Director, Microbiology (Virology), Royal Children's Hospital, Parkville, Victoria, Australia.

Address reprint requests to Barry J. Clarris, PhD, University of Melbourne, Department of Medicine, Royal Melbourne Hospital, Victoria, 3050, Australia.

Submitted for publication July 12, 1984; accepted in revised form October 23, 1984.

Laboratory investigations preceding the synovectomy revealed a low total serum globulin (20 gm/liter), which had also been noted in 1979. Immunoglobulin levels, determined by radial immunodiffusion, were markedly reduced: IgA was <0.25 gm/liter, IgG <2.50 gm/liter, and IgM was <0.25 gm/liter. T lymphocytes (E-rosette–forming cells) and B lymphocytes (Ig-positive) were quantitated at 56% and 14%, respectively, of the total lymphocytes. The patient's blood group was A+, but no anti-B isoagglutinins could be detected in the serum.

These findings, together with the patient's history of recurrent respiratory tract infections, were consistent with the diagnosis of "acquired" hypogammaglobulinemia (6). A total replacement of the same (right) knee joint became necessary 16 months after the synovectomy.

Samples of the synovial tissues excised during each operation were dissected into explants of approximately 1 mm^3. These were cultured at 37°C in 5% CO_2 in Eagle's basal medium supplemented with 20% fetal bovine serum and neomycin sulfate (100 μg/ml). A number of synovial cell lines from nonrheumatoid donors were cultured concurrently. The medium was replenished at 2–4-day intervals. All culturing was performed by 1 person, and no other work with viruses was performed in the culture laboratory during this period of time. The progress of the cultures was monitored using phase-contrast microscopy. After the second operation, lymphocytes were prepared on a Ficoll-Hypaque gradient, cultured alone for several days, and then co-cultured with human fetal fibroblasts.

When changes consistent with virus-induced cytopathology appeared in the synovial explant cultures, supernatants were passaged onto monolayer cultures of nonrheumatoid synovial fibroblasts, human fetal fibroblasts, or Vero cells (transformed African green monkey kidney). The supernatants were also cultured for aerobic and anaerobic bacteria, *Mycoplasma* spp., and *Ureaplasma*. Samples of the supernatants were subjected to standard virologic procedures, culminating in type-specific neutralization of the cytopathic effects, in cell cultures using a panel of antisera to the adenovirus types 1–10 (the serotypes most commonly encountered in Melbourne, Austra-

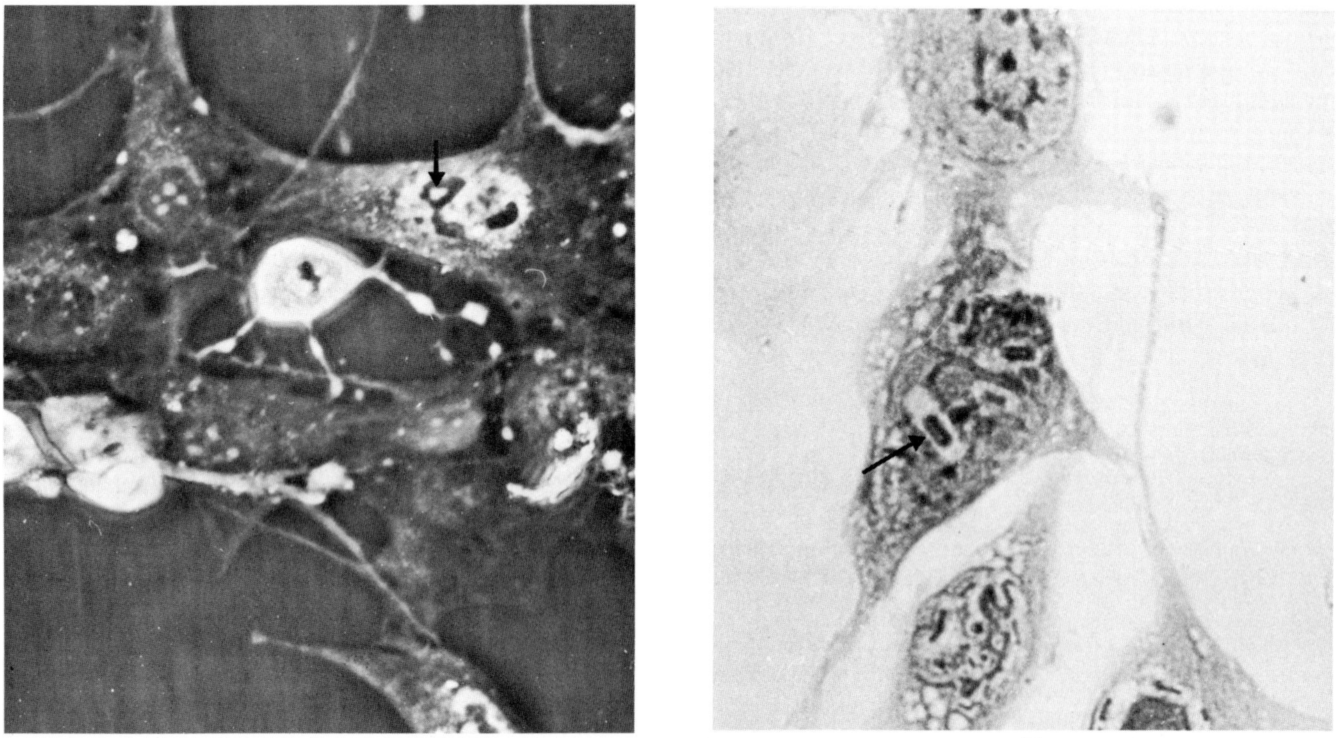

A B

Figure 1. Cytopathic effects in synovial fibroblasts, occurring 3 days after inoculation with infected supernatants, shown using negative phase-contrast microscopy (**A**), and hematoxylin and eosin stain (**B**). Note the clustering and rounding of cells (**A**) and the intranuclear inclusions, some of which are in clear capsules (**arrows**) (original magnification × 530).

lia). Transmission electron microscopy was performed on cultured cells which had developed nuclear changes.

Results. The histologic appearance of stained synovial sections from the 2 operations was similar to that of the biopsy sample taken early in the course of the patient's disease. Subsequent electron microscopy of these specimens failed to show viral particles in either sample.

Some of the explants from the excised synovial tissue failed to produce outgrowth. The others generated cell sheets, but migration from most was rather slow, compared with our usual experience with cultures of both RA and non-RA synovial tissue. Identical media supported normal growth of concurrent synovial cultures, and appropriate microbiologic cultures excluded other infections. Cytopathic changes appeared about 3 weeks after plating. Coveıage of the culture surfaces was then still <20%, and the cell population consisted mainly of fibroblast-like cells, most of the macrophage-like cells seen early in culture having lysed or detached. Fibroblasts first retracted, then clustered together, and finally detached. In a further 3 weeks, cell destruction was total. The changes seen in explant cultures from the second surgical specimen were virtually the same as those seen in the first.

There was no evidence of viral infection in cultures of peripheral blood lymphocytes. Two serum samples were collected 1 month apart, after the second operation. Using neutralization techniques, we found no evidence of circulating antibodies to adenovirus 1 when serum dilutions of 1:8 were reacted with $30 TCID_{50}$ of the patient's virus isolate.

Transfer of culture medium successfully and repeatedly produced similar cytopathic effects in nonrheumatoid synovial fibroblasts, human fetal fibroblasts, and in Vero cells. In each of these cell types, intranuclear inclusions of various shapes developed approximately 24 hours before the more gross cytopathic effects (Figure 1A). Some of these inclusions were enclosed in clear capsules. Stained preparations showed intranuclear pleomorphic inclusions with a basophilic/eosinophilic pattern (Figure 1B).

Electron microscopy of synovial fibroblasts from transmission experiments (after both operations) showed intranuclear, icosahedron-like particles, 70–80 nm in diameter, and crystalline inclusions (Figure 2) that strongly resembled those in cultured cells infected with adenovirus type 5, as noted by Betz and Maurin (7). However, the agent in both isolates was specifically neutralized by antiserum to adenovirus type 1, a strain not previously associated with this kind of crystalline inclusion.

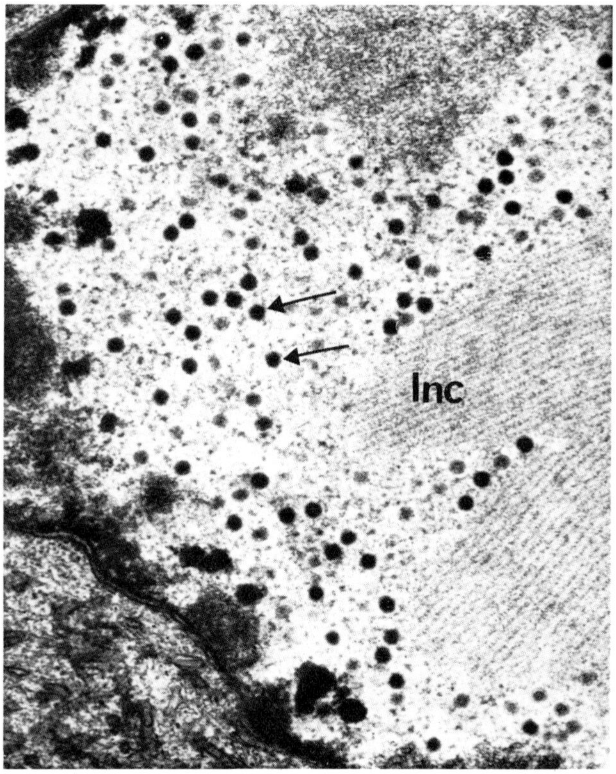

Figure 2. Electron micrograph showing intranuclear particles with adenovirus-like structure (**arrows**) and crystalline inclusions (**Inc**), occurring 3 days after inoculation of synovial fibroblasts with supernatants from those cell cultures which showed nuclear changes suggestive of virus infection (magnification × 50,000).

Discussion. Grahame et al (8) reported the repeated isolation of rubella virus from the joint fluids of 6 polyarthritic patients who had no evidence of natural rubella infection or of vaccination at disease onset, and had no apparent immune defects. Thus, it is clear that at least 1 recognized arthritogenic virus can persist in joints for long periods of time, though there are no grounds for supposing that rubella will invariably be found in such patients. Adenovirus type 7 has been strongly associated with several cases of acute arthritis, but these were all of a self-limiting type, with no erosive lesions (9). It is widely recognized that some adenovirus serotypes, including type 1, may cause chronic, persistent infections of tonsils and other lymphoid tissues, though there is no evidence that these infections spread to other body tissues.

In a previous study (3), we detected intranuclear particles with adenovirus morphology in electron micrographs of long-term synovial cell cultures from a patient with seropositive RA. However, this finding could not be confirmed by isolation of virus, nor could it be reproduced in a second primary synovial culture from the same patient, or in a study of 5 other RA patients (unpublished observations).

In the present study, a human adenovirus of a specific serotype not previously associated with either transient or chronic arthritis was found in synovial tissue from a patient with polyarthritis. Moreover, it seems that the infection was not transient, in that it persisted for at least 16 months. Apart from the interest inherent with this first report of an adenovirus present at the site of a lesion, the finding is of particular interest in relation to the recent isolation of a parvovirus from rheumatoid synovial cells (5); adenovirus infections often occur in association with a defective adeno-associated virus, which has been identified as a parvovirus. Using electron microscopy, we have examined the available material for parvovirus, but none could be detected; however, this will receive further study.

The relationship between the arthritis and the immunodeficiency in this patient is not clear. Speculation has persisted for some time, however, that an RA-like disease occurring with congenital and "acquired" forms of agammaglobulinemia may be related to an infectious agent and that the association might provide a clue to the pathogenesis of RA in general (10,11). In these earlier cases, the arthritis had many features of rheumatoid disease, but the erosions seen in our patient are most unusual (6,11). The humoral defect in our patient might have allowed for a freer dissemination of the virus which, in other cases, might remain restricted to the upper respiratory tract. Even though it was localized in the synovium, the role of the virus in synovitis is not clear, but it is possible that the virus contributed to the uncommon degree of erosive change.

Further investigation of this patient was, unfortunately, not possible, largely because of his reluctance to participate. Should further surgery become necessary, additional serologic assessment, which in retrospect, might have provided data of further interest, will be pursued. If possible, future evaluation will also include examination for virus in his sputum, nasopharynx, urine, and feces. Opportunities to repeat the present work with similar patients are likely to be rare. However, a selective IgA deficiency is relatively common in patients with RA and systemic lupus erythematosus (12), and in continuing this line of investigation, such patients might be helpful. If further evidence of adenovirus infection is found in rheumatoid joint tissues, more sophisticated study using complementary DNA probes for the group-specific portion of the 32 known adenovirus serotypes might well be warranted.

Acknowledgments. The authors are grateful to Dr. D. Birch for the *Mycoplasma* and *Ureaplasma* cultures, Dr. R. Pavillard for bacteriology, and K. Rogers for electron microscopy.

REFERENCES

1. Györkey F, Sinkovics JG, Min KW, Györkey P: A morphologic study on the occurrence and distribution of structures resembling viral nucleocapsids in collagen diseases. Am J Med 53:148–158, 1972
2. Schumacher HR: Synovial membrane and fluid morphologic alterations in early rheumatoid arthritis: microvascular injury and virus-like particles. Ann NY Acad Sci 256:39–64, 1975
3. Clarris BJ, Fraser JRE, Moran CJ, Muirden KD: Rheumatoid synovial cells from intact joints: morphology, growth and polykaryocytosis. Ann Rheum Dis 36:293–301, 1977
4. Hamerman D, Gresser I, Smith C: Isolation of cytomegalovirus from synovial cells of a patient with rheumatoid arthritis. J Rheumatol 9:658–664, 1982
5. Simpson RW, McGinty L, Simon L, Smith CA, Godzeski CW, Boyd RJ: Association of parvoviruses with rheumatoid arthritis of humans. Science 223:1425–1428, 1984
6. Hermans DE, Diaz-Buxo JA, Stobo JD: Idiopathic late-onset immunoglobulin deficiency: clinical observations in 50 patients. Am J Med 61:221–237, 1976
7. Betz A, Maurin J: Les inclusions intranucleaires eosinophiles d'aspect cristallin produites par les adenovirus de types 5 et 6. Ann Inst Pasteur 101:120–124, 1961
8. Grahame R, Armstrong R, Simmons N, Wilton JMA, Dyson M, Laurent R, Millis R, Mims CA: Chronic arthritis associated with the presence of intrasynovial rubella virus. Ann Rheum Dis 42:2–13, 1983
9. Panush RS: Adenovirus arthritis. Arthritis Rheum 17:534–536, 1974
10. Good RA, Rotstein J: Rheumatoid arthritis and agammaglobulinemia. Bull Rheum Dis 10:203–206, 1960
11. Williams RC: Rheumatoid arthritis as a systemic disease. Philadelphia, WB Saunders, 1974, pp 140–142
12. Fraser KJ: IgA immunoglobulins and autoimmunity. Lancet 2:804–805, 1969

BRIEF REPORT

RAYNAUD'S PHENOMENON OF A SINGLE DIGIT FOLLOWING LOCAL INTRADERMAL BLEOMYCIN SULFATE INJECTION

EDWIN A. SMITH, FRANK E. HARPER, and E. CARWILE LeROY

Bleomycin sulfate, administered parenterally alone and in combination with vinblastine sulfate for treatment of various neoplastic diseases, has been associated with the development of Raynaud's phenomenon (1–5). Additionally, bleomycin therapy has been associated with a number of varied skin reactions, including hyperpigmentation, sclerosis, gangrene, indurated plaques, and hyperpigmented nodules (6).

Several recent reports have described the use of intralesional injections of bleomycin sulfate for treatment of cutaneous warts, and have noted no complications (7–10). We describe a patient who received this treatment and subsequently developed Raynaud's phenomenon, which was limited to the injected digit.

Case report. A 23-year-old, healthy woman sought medical treatment for a wart located over the palmar aspect of the proximal interphalangeal joint (PIP) of the right index finger. An initial, unsuccessful, attempt at electrocautery was followed by multiple local liquid nitrogen treatments over the ensuing 5 months; each treatment was unsuccessful. Four months later, after regrowth of the wart, the patient received a single injection of bleomycin sulfate (1 mg) into the wart. Approximately 2 months thereafter, she began to notice cold-induced, intermittent blanching followed by cyanosis and rubor, which was limited to the injected finger. Additionally, fissures developed in the skin of the involved finger, and ultimately, desquamation of the distal pad without frank ischemic ulceration occurred.

The patient noted that none of her other fingers or her toes showed cold sensitivity. There was no history of occupational exposure to hazardous chemicals, toxins, dusts, or vibrating machinery. The patient denied previous frostbite or traumatic injury. There was no history of blood dyscrasia, hypercoagulability, illicit or medicinal use of drugs, including conjugated estrogens, or tobacco use. She denied pain or paresthesias in her shoulders or arms, or symptoms of connective tissue disease, including arthritis, rash, pleuritic chest pain, weight loss, fever, and dysphagia. There was no family history of connective tissue disease or cold sensitivity.

On physical examination she appeared to be well. Her vital signs were: blood pressure 112/66, pulse rate 72, temperature 98.6°F, and respirations 16. Examination of her skin revealed a cool, cyanotic index finger on the right hand with desquamation of the distal pad and slight thickening of skin distal to the PIP joint. There were no digital tip ulcers or trophic scars (Figure 1). There was no evidence of sclerodactyly, proximal skin thickening, or telangiectasias. All other fingers and all toes appeared normal. Brachial, ulnar, and radial pulses of both arms were 2+ and equal. Allen's test revealed no occlusion of the radial or ulnar artery. Hyperabduction, military, and Adson's maneuvers for thoracic outlet syndromes were negative. There were no vascular bruits. Heart exami-

From the Department of Medicine, Division of Rheumatology and Immunology, Medical University of South Carolina, Charleston, South Carolina.

Edwin A. Smith, MD: Fellow in Rheumatology; Frank E. Harper, MD: Assistant Professor of Medicine; E. Carwile LeRoy, MD: Professor of Medicine.

Address reprint requests to Edwin A. Smith, MD, Medical University of South Carolina, Division of Rheumatology and Immunology, 171 Ashley Avenue, Charleston, SC 29425.

Submitted for publication July 31, 1984; accepted in revised form October 19, 1984.

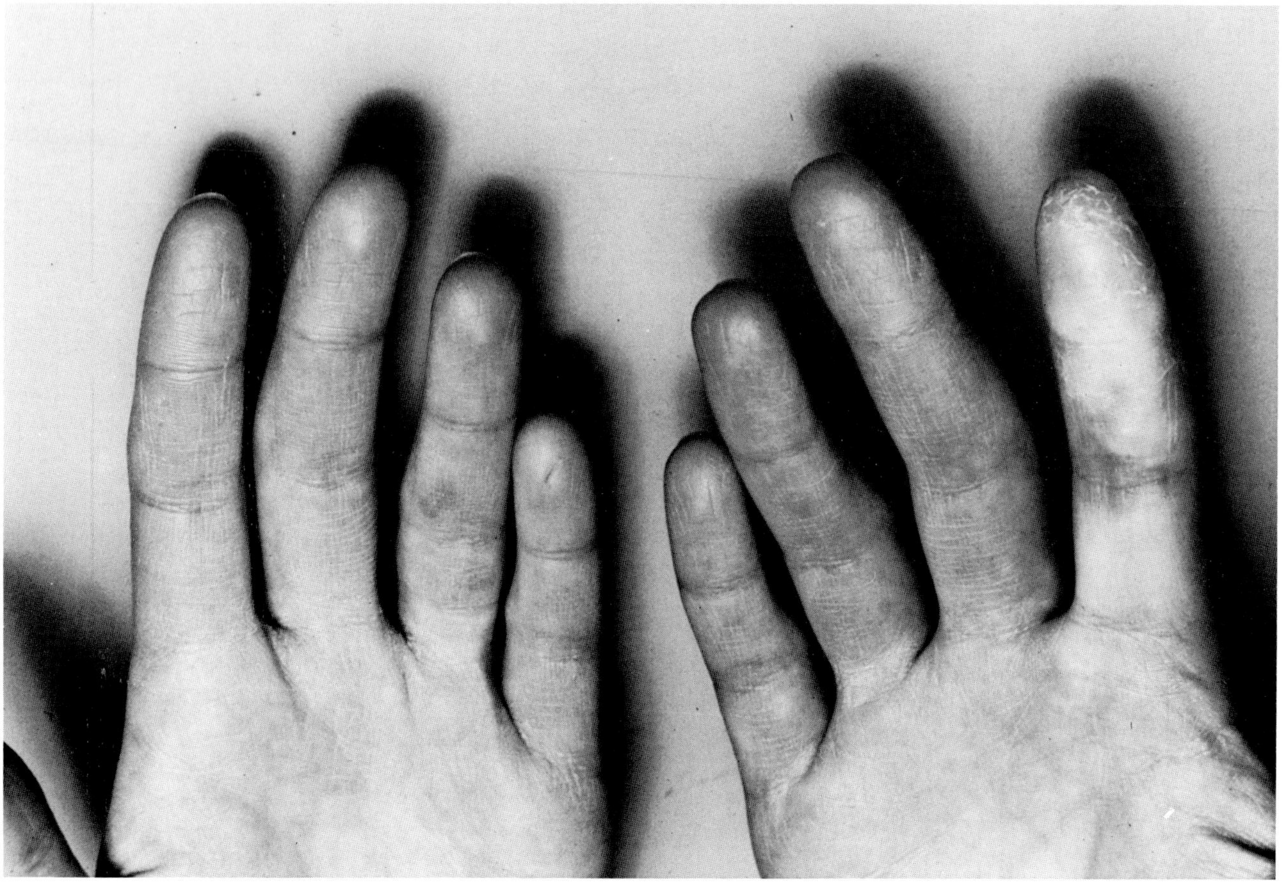

Figure 1. Hands of a 23-year-old woman approximately 2 months after receiving a single injection of bleomycin sulfate into a wart located over the palmar aspect of the proximal interphalangeal joint of her right index finger. There is pallor and skin thickening of the right index finger; the other fingers are unaffected.

nation revealed no murmurs. Results of the remainder of the physical examination were entirely normal.

Laboratory tests were negative for antinuclear antibodies, rheumatoid factor (by latex fixation), cryoglobulins, and cold agglutinins. Results of the complete blood count, urinalysis, and serum protein electrophoresis were normal. The Westergren erythrocyte sedimentation rate was normal. A chest radiograph showed normal results and revealed no cervical rib. Results of M-mode and 2-dimensional echocardiography were normal. In vivo nailfold capillary microscopy revealed a normal capillary pattern.

Discussion. Combination systemic chemotherapy for testicular cancer, using bleomycin and vinblastine, has been associated with a substantial incidence of Raynaud's phenomenon (22 of 60 patients); arteriography in these patients showed restricted blood flow to the digits (1). Various types of skin lesions have been associated with bleomycin administration, including development of infiltrated plaques, nodules, and bands occurring on the hands (6). Histologically, these lesions may resemble sclerodermatous skin with dense collagen and areas of homogenization, particularly around vessels and adnexal structures, and evidence of thickened vascular walls.

In our patient, although a cause and effect relationship cannot be clearly established, the temporal relation of bleomycin injection with the appearance of Raynaud's phenomenon suggests that the drug had a toxic effect on the blood vessels of the involved finger. Cold injury to the finger, resulting from the previous liquid nitrogen cryosurgery, is a consideration, though we believe this is less likely because of the time relationships involved. Moreover, Raynaud's phenomenon has not been reported as a complication of cryosurgery for cutaneous warts.

Although cutaneous reactions to bleomycin rarely occur at systemic doses of less than 150 mg, soft tissue injections of small doses in direct proximity to digital vessels may be sufficient to cause vascular injury. In light of the benign, self-limited nature of cutaneous warts, we believe that injection of bleomycin into warts on the digits should be avoided.

Acknowledgments. We would like to thank Judy Anderson and Carol Cook for their secretarial assistance.

REFERENCES

1. Vogelzang NJ, Bosl GJ, Johnson K, Kennedy BJ: Raynaud's phenomenon: a common toxicity after combination chemotherapy for testicular cancer. Ann Intern Med 95:288–292, 1981
2. Teutsch C, Lipton A, Harvey HA: Raynaud's phenomenon as a side effect of chemotherapy with vinblastine and bleomycin for testicular carcinoma. Cancer Treat Rep 61:925–926, 1977
3. Rothberg H: Raynaud's phenomenon after vinblastine-bleomycin chemotherapy (letter). Cancer Treat Rep 62:569–570, 1978
4. Soble AR: Chronic bleomycin-associated Raynaud's phenomenon (letter). Cancer Treat Rep 62:570, 1978
5. Chernicoff DP, Burkowski RM, Young JR: Raynaud's phenomenon after bleomycin treatment (letter). Cancer Treat Rep 62:570–571, 1978
6. Cohen IS, Mosher MB, O'Keefe EJ, Klaus SN, DeConti RC: Cutaneous toxicity of bleomycin therapy. Arch Dermatol 107:553–555, 1973
7. Bremner RM: Warts: treatment with intralesional bleomycin. Cutis 18:264–266, 1976
8. Abbott LG: Treatment of warts with bleomycin. Aust J Dermatol 19:69–71, 1978
9. Shumack PH, Haddock MJ: Bleomycin: an effective treatment for warts. Aust J Dermatol 20:41–42, 1979
10. Cordero AA: The common wart: intralesional treatment with bleomycin sulfate. Cutis 26:319–324, 1980

BRIEF REPORT

CONCURRENT SYSTEMIC LUPUS ERYTHEMATOSUS AND COMMON VARIABLE HYPOGAMMAGLOBULINEMIA

ANTHONY STEIN, ALAN WINKELSTEIN, and AMRIT AGARWAL

Both systemic lupus erythematosus (SLE) and common variable hypogammaglobulinemia (CVH) are classified as disorders resulting from malfunctions of B lymphocytes. The former is typified by excessive activity of this host defense system, which results in polyclonal hypergammaglobulinemia and the formation of antibodies against endogenous antigens. In contrast, CVH patients show reduced levels of immunoglobulins, are unable to mount appropriate antibody responses to exogenous antigens, and may incur repeated pyogenic infections.

Although it is distinctly uncommon for SLE to evolve into CVH, we recently had the opportunity to study this process. A patient presented with clinical findings typical of SLE. Over a 17-year period, she gradually developed severe panhypogammaglobulinemia with recurrent pyogenic infections. Concomitant with the onset of the immune deficiency, symptoms referable to her SLE abated.

Case report. A 36-year-old white woman was diagnosed as having systemic lupus erythematosus in October 1967. At that time, she presented with symmetric arthritis primarily involving the knees, ankles, and the proximal interphalangeal joints. Her articular manifestations were associated with weight loss, a generalized erythematous rash, and a history of Raynaud's phenomenon. Laboratory tests revealed a hemoglobin value of 10 gm/dl, a white blood cell count of 3,950, positive antinuclear antibody (ANA) and lupus erythematosus cell preparations, and a false-positive serologic test for syphilis. Results of renal function tests, including creatinine clearance and 24-hour urinary protein determinations, were normal. Gamma globulin determination by electrophoresis was 3.19 gm/dl.

In May 1968, she had a lupus flare and prednisone was prescribed; steroid therapy in varying doses (5–40 mg/day) has been maintained throughout her illness. During the early period of her disease, she experienced several recurrences of SLE manifestations, an episode of acute parotitis, and ischemic leg ulcers. However, at no time during the course of her disease did she manifest significant renal disease. For the repeated flares of SLE, azathioprine was prescribed in June 1969 and was continued until 1979. Several gamma globulin determinations were made during her illness (Figure 1).

In March 1971, the patient was treated for an episode of pneumococcal pneumonia. The following October, she developed an episode of cryptococcal meningitis which responded to therapy with amphotericin B and 5-fluorocytosine. Coincidentally with the cryptococcal infection, she had an episode of herpes zoster, primarily involving the vulva. Unfortunately, no immunologic studies were performed at this time. Between 1976 and 1982, she developed avascular necrosis involving both femoral heads, the left knee, and the left humeral head. Both femoral heads were surgically replaced. Her lupus remained relatively

From the Department of Medicine, Montefiore Hospital, University of Pittsburgh School of Medicine, Pittsburgh, Pennsylvania.

Supported in part by NIH grant CA-2449.

Anthony Stein, MD: Resident in Medicine; Alan Winkelstein, MD: Professor of Medicine, Head, Clinical Immunology Unit; Amrit Agarwal, MD: Clinical Assistant Professor of Medicine.

Address reprint requests to Alan Winkelstein, MD, Department of Medicine, Montefiore Hospital, University of Pittsburgh School of Medicine, Pittsburgh, PA 15243.

Submitted for publication August 8, 1984; accepted in revised form October 11, 1984.

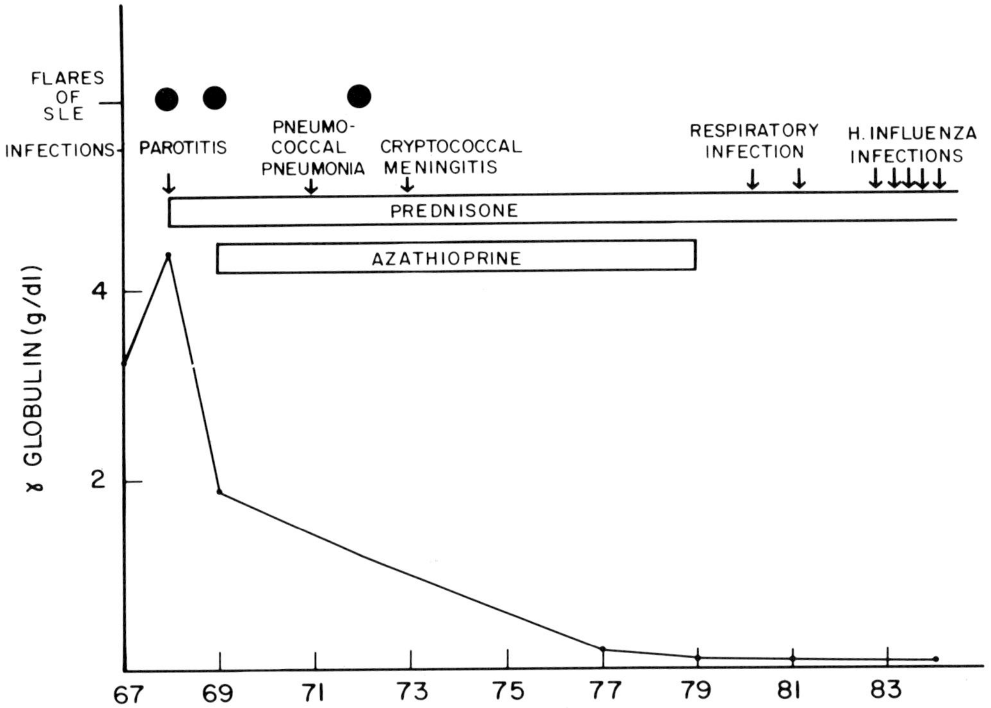

Figure 1. Serial gamma globulin measurements, 1967–1983, determined by protein electrophoresis. Exacerbation of systemic lupus erythematosus (SLE), the courses of therapy for this connective tissue disease, and episodes of severe infections are depicted at the top of the figure.

quiescent during this interval, and she did not experience any other serious infections until 1979.

Hypogammaglobulinemia was first diagnosed in 1977 when her gamma globulin level was found to be 0.4 gm/dl by protein electrophoresis. No further evaluations were performed at that time. Between 1980 and 1981, she had 2 episodes of respiratory infection which required hospitalization. Specific bacterial diagnosis was not made during either of these episodes, but she showed a prompt response to systemic antibiotics.

Between January and November 1983, she experienced 5 separate episodes of infection with *Hemophilus influenzae*. This included 3 occurrences of pneumonia, 1 of septic arthritis, and 1 of cellulitis of the hand. Two of these infections were further complicated by *H influenzae* septicemia. Blood counts obtained during each of these episodes of infection showed either a normal or elevated neutrophil count, indicating no quantitative abnormalities in this defense system.

Laboratory evaluation in November 1983 showed a hemoglobin level of 15 gm/dl; hematocrit 44.6%; white blood cells 15,300 with 70% neutrophils, 11% bands, and 16% lymphocytes. The test for ANA was positive at a titer of 1:80 with a speckled pattern. Complement components C3 and C4 were within the normal range. Gamma globulin quantitation by protein electrophoresis was 0.14 gm/dl.

Immunoglobulins were analyzed by serum protein electrophoresis, immunoelectrophoresis, and quantitative radial immunodiffusion. T and B cell analysis was performed using monoclonal antibodies OKT3, OKT4, OKT8, OKT11 (Ortho Diagnostics, Raritan, NJ), and Leu-12 (Becton Dickinson, Monoclonal Center, Mountainville, CA). All cells were analyzed on an Ortho Spectrum III analyzer. Quantitative immunoglobulins showed an IgG of <200 mg/dl; both IgA and IgM were undetectable. Immunoelectrophoresis failed to demonstrate a monoclonal protein. Lymphocyte subset analysis showed a markedly reduced number of B cells (1.6%).

Total T cells (OKT3) were slightly above the normal range (84.7%) and there was an excess of T suppressor (OKT8) cells (61.7%) and an inverted T helper/T suppressor ratio (0.42). When these values were correlated with her lymphocyte count, the total T cell count was 2,073/mm^3 with 641 T helper cells (normal 400–1,500) and 1,510 T suppressor cells (normal 250–750). B cells were quantitated at 39/mm^3 (normal >150).

In view of the patient's severe hypogammaglobulinemia, intravenous gamma globulin replacement therapy was begun, and she is currently receiving 100 mg/kg of gamma globulin intravenously every 3 weeks. She is also receiving antibiotics for a cough productive of purulent sputum. Her steroid dose has been reduced gradually; she is currently receiving 2.5 mg of prednisone daily. At present, her lupus appears to be inactive. While receiving the replacement gamma globulin therapy, she has not incurred any severe infections over the past 9 months.

Discussion. The transition of the hyperreactivity of B cells seen in SLE into the hyporeactive state characteristic of CVH is distinctly uncommon. Only 3 other cases have been reported (1,2) and in only 1 was there a profound reduction in all 3 immunoglobulin classes (2). The salient features of the previously reported cases, along with those of the present patient, are summarized in Table 1.

There are features common to all of these patients. As noted, each of the patients presented with SLE symptoms, and only after several years did immune deficiency develop. The interval between the diagnosis of lupus and the onset of CVH ranged from 7–11 years. All patients were treated with corticosteroids and a cytotoxic immunosuppressant. Finally, there were distinct abnormalities involving B lymphocytes and T suppressor cells. It is interesting that in our patient and in 2 of the other patients, the ANA remained positive despite the low levels of IgG.

Although all 4 patients were treated with immunosuppressants, it is unlikely that either steroids, azathioprine, or chlorambucil produced a sufficiently severe and sustained decrease in immunoglobulin production to account for the immune deficiency disorder. In general, the effects of these medications are reversed shortly after they are discontinued (3,4). In our patient, azathioprine was stopped approximately 2 years before she manifested symptoms related to her hypogammaglobulinemia. Although she has taken steroids throughout the duration of her illness, only small quantities were administered during the several years preceding the onset of her hypogammaglobulinemia. It is unlikely that this had a significant effect on immunoglobulin production (2).

Phenotypic studies of this patient showed a marked decrease in the numbers and percentage of B lymphocytes and a similar increase in the total number of T suppressor cells. Functional assays in 2 previously described patients detected excessive T suppressor cell activities coupled with hyporesponsiveness of B cells (1). In the other patient, phenotypic analysis failed to show any abnormalities, but subnormal B cell proliferative responses to *Staphylococcus aureus* were noted (2).

The significance of these lymphocyte abnormalities in any of these patients is not clearly defined. There is considerable debate on whether either or both of these diseases are the result of a primary defect of B lymphocytes or are a secondary abnormality resulting from deranged T suppressor cell functions. In a proportion of patients with CVH, there is excessive T suppressor cell activity which appears to depress the ability of both autologous and allogenic B cells to synthesize immunoglobulins (5). It has also been postulated that depressed T suppressor cell responses may be a prime factor in the B cell hyperreactivity present in lupus (6–8). However, other investigators have concluded that primary B cell abnormalities are responsible for the abnormal immunoglobulin produc-

Table 1. Hypogammaglobulinemia in patients with systemic lupus erythematosus (SLE)

Patient	Age/sex	Onset of SLE	Treatment of SLE	Onset of hypogamma-globulinemia	Disappearance of SLE symptoms	Immunologic abnormalities	Ref. no.
1	16/F	1966	Prednisone, chlorambucil	1971*	1968	↓ B cell response, ↑ T suppression, ↓ T helper activity	1
2	32/F	1969	Prednisone	1976†	Still present	↓ B cell response, ↑ T suppression, ↓ T helper activity	1
3	34/M	1973	Prednisone, azathioprine	1980	1975	↓ B cell response to *S aureus*	2
4	36/F	1967	Prednisone, azathioprine	1977	1979	↓ B cell number, ↑ T suppressor cells	This report

* IgA initially noted to be low in 1971. In 1976, she was found to have dysgammaglobulinemia with ↑ IgM.
† IgG levels flucuated about lower levels of normal.

tion which is characteristic of both diseases (9–11). These conflicting data do not allow conclusions to be made regarding the primary abnormalities in these 4 patients. Nevertheless, the findings of an apparent association between these 2 disorders in this small group of patients should alert physicians to a new long-term sequela of lupus. Furthermore, as more data are accumulated, this association may provide information about the pathogenesis of both immune-related disorders.

Acknowledgment. The excellent secretarial assistance of Mary T. Almade is greatly appreciated.

REFERENCES

1. Ashman RF, White RH, Wiesenhutter C, Cantor Y, Lasarow E, Liebling M, Talal N: Panhypogammaglobulinemia in systemic lupus erythematosus: in vitro demonstration of multiple cellular defects. J Allergy Clin Immunol 70:465–473, 1982
2. Sussman GL, Rivera VJ, Kohler PF: Transition from systemic lupus erythematosus to common variable hypogammaglobulinemia. Ann Intern Med 99:32–55, 1983
3. Haynes BF, Katz P, Fauci AS: Mechanisms of corticosteroid action on lymphocyte subpopulations. Cell Immunol 44:169–178, 1979
4. Levy J, Barnett EV, MacDonald NS, Klinenberg JR, Pearson CM: The effects of azathioprine on gammaglobulin synthesis in man. J Clin Invest 51:2233–2238, 1972
5. Waldmann TA, Broder S, Krakauer R, MacDermott RP, Durm M, Goldman C, Meade B: The role of suppressor cells in the pathogenesis of common variable hypogammaglobulinemia and in the immunodeficiency associated with myeloma. Fed Proc 35:2067–2072, 1976
6. Sagawa A, Abdou NI: Suppressor-cell dysfunction in systemic lupus erythematosus: cells involved and in vitro correction. J Clin Invest 62:789–796, 1978
7. Fauci AS, Steinberg AD, Haynes BF, Whalen G: Immunoregulatory aberrations in systemic lupus erythematosus. J Immunol 121:1473–1479, 1978
8. Gottlieb AB, Lahita RG, Chiorazzi N, Kunkel HG: Immune function in systemic lupus erythematosus. J Clin Invest 63:885–892, 1979
9. Siegal FP, Siegal M, Good RA: Role of helper, suppressor and B cell defects in the pathogenesis of hypogammaglobulinemias. N Engl J Med 299:172–178, 1978
10. Nies KM, Stevens RH, Louie JS: Impaired immunoglobulin M synthesis by peripheral blood lymphocytes in systemic lupus erythematosus: a primary B-cell defect. Clin Immunol Immunopathol 19:118–130, 1981
11. Bell DA: Cell-mediated immunity in rheumatoid arthritis and systemic lupus erythematosus: too little or too much. J Rheumatol 6:484–488, 1979

BRIEF REPORT

BOWEL INVOLVEMENT IN SYSTEMIC LUPUS ERYTHEMATOSUS: CROHN'S DISEASE OR LUPUS VASCULITIS?

DAFNA D. GLADMAN, THEODORE ROSS, BEVERLEY RICHARDSON, and SAVITA KULKARNI

Gastrointestinal involvement in systemic lupus erythematosus (SLE) has long been recognized, and the gastrointestinal features of this disease have been recently reviewed (1). All parts of the bowel may be involved; the most common presentation is with abdominal pain (1,2). There have been at least 2 reports of patients with presumed coexistence of SLE and Crohn's disease, although pathologic information was not available (3,4). We have recently encountered an SLE patient whose presentation and radiologic features suggested Crohn's disease, but in whom the pathologic findings disclosed vasculitis of the large bowel.

Case report. A 36-year-old woman was well until May 1983, when she first presented with fever and polyarthritis. Investigations revealed a hemoglobin level of 10.2 gm/dl, white blood cell (WBC) count 2.8×10^9/liter, erythrocyte sedimentation rate (ESR) elevated at 52 mm/hour, positive lupus erythematosus (LE) cell preparation, positive antinuclear antibodies (ANA), and depressed serum complement levels. Abnormal findings on liver function tests were attributed to salicylate-induced hepatotoxicity, and she was thought to have SLE. She refused further investigations at the time, but improved with indomethacin therapy.

In July 1983, she presented to another hospital with weakness and occasional blood in the stool. She denied having abdominal pain, nausea, or vomiting, but had had a 9-kg weight loss in the preceding 4 weeks. She had no further joint pains. Laboratory investigations revealed a hemoglobin level of 8.0 gm/dl, WBC count of 3.9×10^9/liter, and ESR of 100 mm/hour. A positive Coombs' test result and LE cell preparation were detected. ANA were positive at a titer of 1:1,280, and anti-DNA antibody by the *Crithidia* method was positive at 1:40. Radiologic examination of the chest and the large bowel revealed no abnormality.

A diagnosis of SLE was made, and therapy with prednisone, 40 mg/day, was begun. There was improvement in the anemia, but she presented to Women's College Hospital in September 1983, with generalized malaise, weakness, diarrhea, abdominal pain, and a further weight loss of 3 kg. There were no joint complaints. She denied presence of a skin rash, Raynaud's phenomenon, or serositis, but had had buccal mucosal ulcerations.

Physical examination showed that she was emaciated. Her blood pressure was 110/80, pulse 120 and regular. There was nasal septal erythema. Cardiovascular examination results were unremarkable. There was no abdominal organomegaly, no tenderness or rebound tenderness, and bowel sounds were normal. There was no lymphadenopathy. Neurologic examination revealed hyperreflexia, marked muscle wasting, and generalized weakness. The grip strength was reduced, but there were no actively inflamed joints.

Investigations in the hospital revealed a hemoglobin level of 9.5 gm/dl, WBC count 6.5×10^9/liter

From the Departments of Medicine, Surgery, and Pathology, Women's College Hospital, and the University of Toronto, Toronto, Ontario, Canada.

Dafna D. Gladman, MD, FRCP(C), FACP: Associate Professor of Medicine, University of Toronto and Associate, Canadian Arthritis Society; Theodore Ross, MD, FRCS(C): Lecturer, Department of Surgery, University of Toronto; Beverley Richardson, MD, FRCP(C): Assistant Professor of Medicine, University of Toronto; Savita Kulkarni, MD, FRCP(C): Associate Pathologist, Women's College Hospital.

Address reprint requests to Dr. D. Gladman, Women's College Hospital, Burton Hall, Suite 226, 60 Grosvenor St., Toronto, Ontario, M5S 1B6, Canada.

Submitted for publication May 29, 1984; accepted in revised form November 20, 1984.

(normal differential), and normal results on liver and kidney function tests. The ANA was positive, as was the LE cell preparation, but antibody to extractable nuclear antigen was not detected. Serum complement was reduced. DNA binding was normal. Bone marrow examination revealed slightly hypercellular marrow. Flexible sigmoidoscopy to 40 cm revealed scattered telangiectatic vessels, aphthous ulcers, and pseudopolyps with "mucosal bridging." A biopsy specimen taken from the sigmoid showed evidence of chronic inflammation in the lamina propria and the muscularis layers.

The findings were considered to be compatible with Crohn's colitis, but vasculitis could not be excluded as the etiology. Barium enema revealed narrowing, cobblestoning, and mucosal irregularity compatible with severe granulomatous colitis. The prednisone dosage was increased first to 60 mg/day, then to intravenous methylprednisolone, 20 mg every 6 hours. There was improvement in the abdominal pain and the diarrhea, followed by a weight gain of 5 kg.

However, 2 weeks later, the patient was awakened by severe abdominal pain. Examination revealed guarding, diffuse tenderness, and loss of bowel sounds. Three views of the abdomen revealed free air under the diaphragm, suggesting an acute perforation. At laparotomy a purulent peritonitis was seen and a perforation of the transverse colon was detected. The whole large bowel, from the cecum to the distal sigmoid colon, was found to be involved in a severe pathologic process, with the area distal to the mid-transverse colon being most severely affected. A subtotal colectomy and ileostomy were performed, and the operative picture was consistent with Crohn's disease. Subsequent assessment of the rectal stump, which measured 20 cm, revealed normal rectal mucosa with pseudopolyps in the proximal 3 cm.

Macroscopic examination of the descending and transverse colon showed diffuse ulceration, some cobblestoning, and many pseudopolyps (Figure 1). The colon was narrowed in the central area, where a perforation measuring 1 cm in diameter was seen. The ascending colon revealed normal mucosa with focal ulceration.

Microscopic examination of the colon revealed areas of mucosal ulcerations. Mucosal goblet cell population was well preserved, and neither transmural inflammation nor granulomata were seen. Instead, there were markedly dilated vessels and a dense infiltrate of lymphocytes and plasma cells. In the non-ulcerated areas, folded and hyperplastic mucosa was noted. The underlying submucosa was markedly edematous and contained dilated blood vessels and

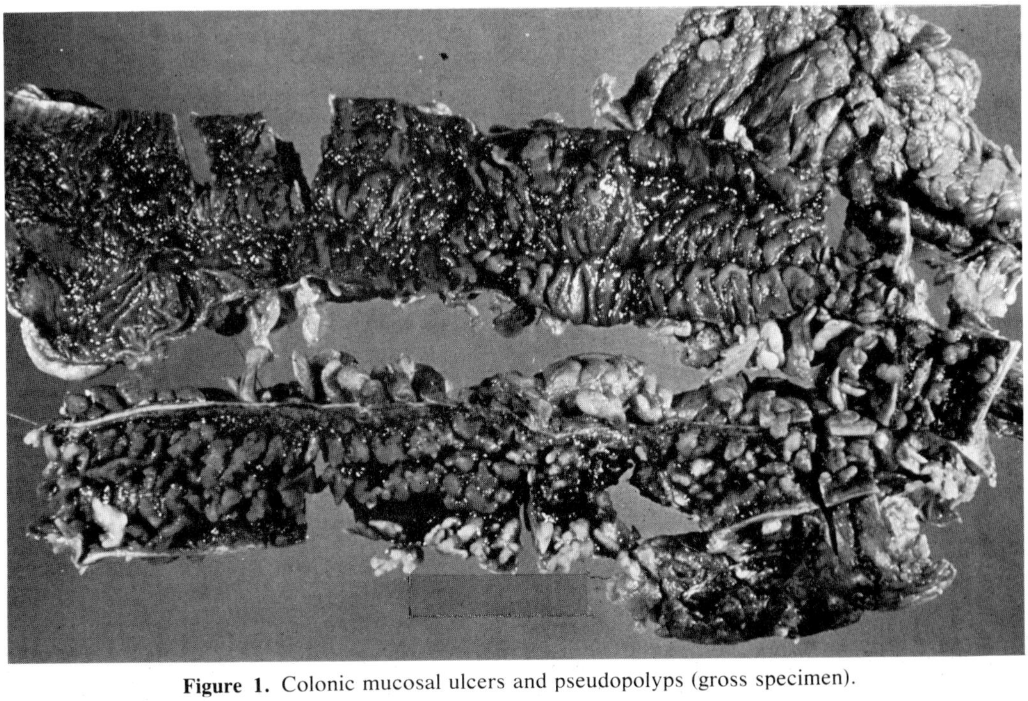

Figure 1. Colonic mucosal ulcers and pseudopolyps (gross specimen).

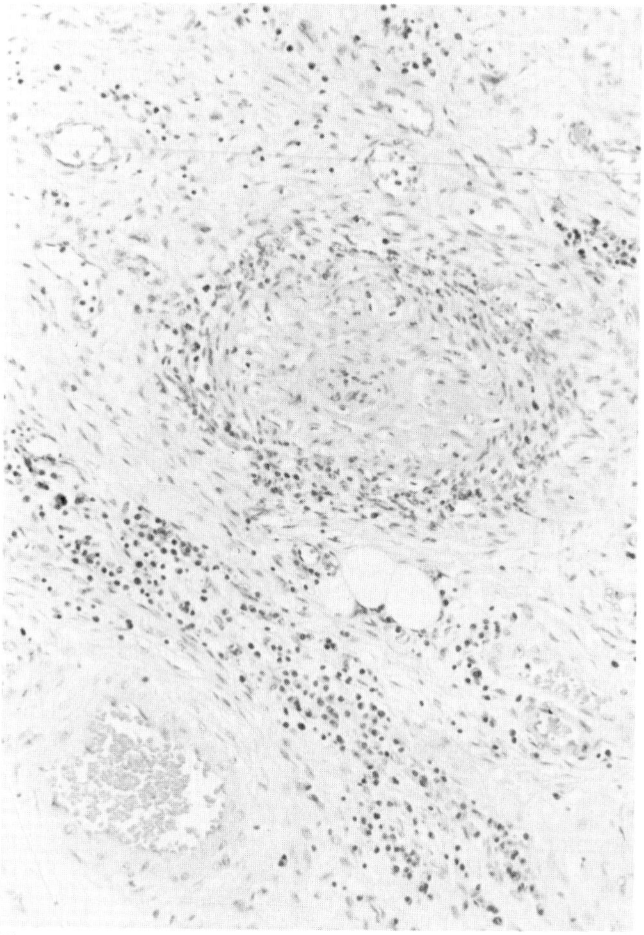

Figure 2. A submucosal artery infiltrated by inflammatory cells (hematoxylin and eosin stained, low power).

lymphatic vessels. The arterioles revealed intimal proliferation and breaking of the elastic lamina. Focally the vessels were infiltrated with a few polymorphonuclear cells and macrophages (Figure 2).

Definite fibrinoid necrosis was not seen, but occasional arterioles and venules revealed recent organizing thrombus due to inflammation of the wall. Similar changes were seen in some vessels in the serosa. Occasional mesenteric vessels revealed intimal proliferation. Ultrastructural examination revealed deposition of fibrin and accumulation of polymorphonuclear cells in the walls of small arterioles and capillaries. In the small capillaries there were electron-dense nodular deposits between the endothelium and the basement membrane (Figure 3). Immunofluorescence studies demonstrated deposits of IgG in vessel walls. No C3 was detected.

Postoperatively the patient had improved hemoglobin and WBC, and a decrease in ESR. Both LE cell preparation and ANA became negative, and the complement levels returned to normal. Five months postoperatively, a laparotomy with an ileorectal anastomosis was performed. At that time chronic sterile periileostomy abscesses were found. Despite these, her ileorectal anastomosis healed without complications. All tests for evidence of SLE produced negative results. The patient has continued steroid therapy with a reducing dose, with the SLE remaining under good control.

Discussion. Our patient fulfilled 4 of the American Rheumatism Association criteria for the classification of SLE (5), namely, arthritis, Coombs' positive hemolytic anemia, positive ANA, and positive LE cell preparation. We therefore consider her to have definite SLE. She was initially thought to have lesions compatible with Crohn's disease based on the findings on sigmoidoscopy and barium enema, and was treated accordingly. However, the pathologic findings did not confirm Crohn's disease but, rather, were typical of vasculitis, with inflammatory cell infiltrates in vessel walls, and with both immunofluorescence and electron microscopic confirmation of immune deposits. Similar lesions in venules of the submucosa and muscularis externa in a patient with lupus and a protein-losing enteropathy have been reported by Weiser et al (6).

Lupus enteritis is a term used by Hoffman and Katz to denote the gastrointestinal tract lesions reported in SLE (1). In their review of the clinical syndromes reported in SLE, they note that the majority of patients with gastrointestinal involvement had perforation or infarction. The reported pathologic findings have been those of vasculitis. It has been suggested that lupus enteritis may resemble regional ileitis, as in our patient.

There have been 2 reported cases in which suspected Crohn's disease and SLE may have coexisted. The first (3) was a report of a 20-year-old man who presented with acute abdominal pain, anemia, leukopenia, and an abnormal urinary sediment. A localized area of nonspecific ileitis was found at laparotomy. He also demonstrated a biologic false-positive test for syphilis, circulating anticoagulant, abnormal serum proteins, and cryoglobulins. No definite diagnosis of either Crohn's disease or SLE could be made.

The second report (4) describes a 35-year-old man with an established diagnosis of SLE (pleurisy, arthralgia, hematuria and proteinuria, and positive LE cell preparation), who developed abdominal pain and was found to have 2 areas of edema and red-purple discoloration in the distal ileum associated with nar-

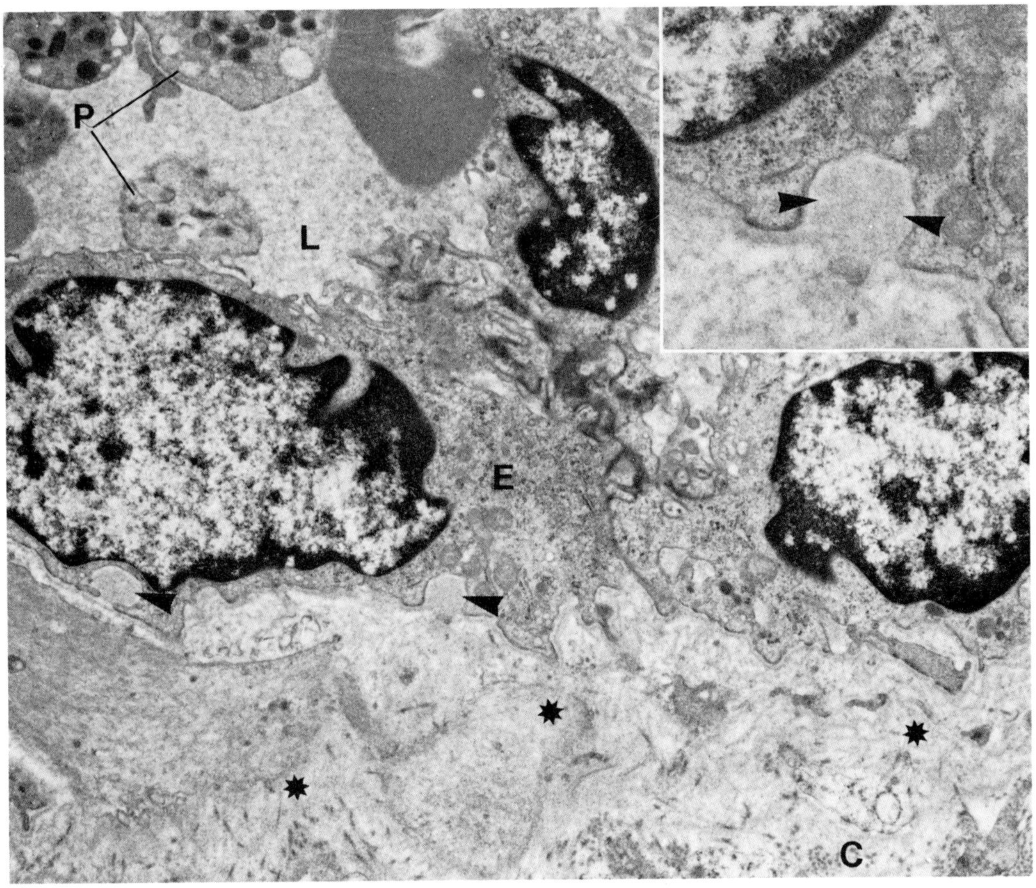

Figure 3. Electron-dense deposits (**arrowheads**) are seen in the capillary wall between the endothelial cells (**E**) and the laminated basement membrane (*). The lumen of the vessel (**L**) contains platelets (**P**). Perivascular collagen (**C**) is seen as well (original magnification × 11,000). **Inset** shows the dense deposits at a higher magnification (original magnification × 33,000).

rowing of the lumen. Regional ileitis was diagnosed on clinical grounds. Despite increasing doses of prednisone, the patient become azotemic and died of pulmonary edema. At autopsy, there were superficial erosions and submucosal scarring seen in the terminal ileum, with a "skip lesion" 15 cm proximally. Although no specific lesions of regional ileitis were seen, the authors attributed the lesions to that diagnosis and suggested that the lesions had improved with steroid therapy. However, it is just as likely that any vasculitic lesions might have responded to that therapy. Thus, the lack of definite changes of Crohn's disease in these cases suggests that the association between SLE and Crohn's disease is still unproven.

Zizic et al (2) have suggested that patients with SLE and gastrointestinal vasculitis often have evidence of vasculitis elsewhere. This was not the case in our patient. She presented with gastrointestinal complaints at a time when her initial manifestations of SLE were under control, without evidence of cutaneous vasculitis. In this patient vasculitis of the colon appeared to be the major manifestation. Indeed, the perforation occurred concurrently with a generalized improvement: the abdominal pain had decreased, the diarrhea had lessened, and she had gained weight.

There have been reports suggesting that steroid therapy may predispose to perforation (7). However, in our patient, the extent of disease in the removed bowel and the presence of acute inflammation do not support this possibility. In fact, we believe the bowel perforation occurred as a result of her underlying disease, which we were attempting to control with steroid therapy.

It is of interest that after the removal of the diseased bowel, the patient's laboratory indicators of active disease improved. Thus, the LE cell preparation and antinuclear antibody, as well as the anti-DNA antibody, disappeared, and the complement levels returned to normal.

This case illustrates the fact that although lupus enteritis may resemble Crohn's disease, it results from a vasculitic process. It further demonstrates that unlike Crohn's disease and ulcerative colitis, where a perforation is less likely to occur in conjunction with clinical improvement, lupus enteritis may be complicated by perforation even when the disease appears to be well controlled.

REFERENCES

1. Hoffman BI, Katz WA: The gastrointestinal manifestations of systemic lupus erythematosus: a review of the literature. Semin Arthritis Rheum 9:237–247, 1980
2. Zizic TM, Classen JN, Stevens MB: Acute abdominal complications of systemic lupus erythematosus and polyarteritis nodosa. Am J Med 73:525–531, 1982
3. Shafer RB, Gregory DH: Systemic lupus erythematosus presenting as regional ileitis. Minn Med 53:789–792, 1970
4. Dubrow MH, McPherson JR, Bowie JW: Lupus erythematosus presenting as an acute abdomen. Minn Med 49:577–579, 1966
5. Tan EM, Cohen AS, Fries JF, Masi AT, McShane DJ, Rothfield NF, Schaller JG, Talal N, Winchester RJ: The 1982 revised criteria for the classification of systemic lupus erythematosus. Arthritis Rheum 25:1271–1277, 1982
6. Weiser MM, Andres GA, Brentjens JR, Evans JT, Reichlin M: Systemic lupus erythematosus and intestinal venulitis. Gastroenterology 81:570–579, 1981
7. Cushman P Jr: Glucocorticosteroids and the gastrointestinal tract: current status. Gut 11:534–539, 1970

SPECIAL ARTICLE

RHEUMATOLOGY TRAINING AT INTERNAL MEDICINE AND FAMILY PRACTICE RESIDENCY PROGRAMS

DON L. GOLDENBERG, RAPHAEL J. DEHORATIUS, STEPHEN R. KAPLAN, JOHN MASON, ROBERT MEENAN, SUSAN G. PERLMAN, and JOHN B. WINFIELD

The Medical Research Education Subcommittee of the American Rheumatism Association surveyed a random selection of large and small programs in internal medicine and family practice residency programs in order to evaluate their rheumatology training. Formal rheumatology training is offered in 90% of these residency programs, but many available positions are not being filled. A full-time staff rheumatologist was present at 69% of large internal medicine programs, 32% of small internal medicine programs, and 11% of family practice programs. The methods of rheumatology training are similar in most programs, although small internal medicine programs and family practice programs more often utilize physicians' offices or outside medical centers for the rheumatology elective training. A majority of the directors of these residency programs thought that many basic skills and techniques were not taught adequately and that the training of their rheumatology residents was not equal to that of residents in cardiology or gastroenterology.

Don L. Goldenberg, MD: Chairman, American Rheumatism Association Medical Research Education Subcommittee, Associate Professor of Medicine, Clinical Program Director, Arthritis Center, Boston University School of Medicine, Boston, Massachusetts; Raphael J. DeHoratius, MD: Professor of Medicine, Director, Division of Clinical Immunology/Rheumatology, Hahnemann University, Philadelphia, Pennsylvania; Stephen R. Kaplan, MD: Professor of Medicine, Brown University Program in Medicine, Providence, Rhode Island; John Mason, MA: Medical Sociologist, Research Associate, Arthritis Center, Boston University School of Medicine; Robert Meenan, MD: Associate Professor of Medicine, Associate Director, Multipurpose Arthritis Center, Boston University School of Medicine; Susan G. Perlman, MD: Assistant Professor of Clinical Medicine, Section of Arthritis and Connective Tissue Diseases, Department of Medicine, Northwestern University, Chicago, Illinois; John B. Winfield, MD: Chairman, American Rheumatism Association Education Committee, Professor of Medicine, Director, Multipurpose Arthritis Center, University of North Carolina School of Medicine, Chapel Hill.

Address reprint requests to Don L. Goldenberg, MD, Boston University School of Medicine, Arthritis Center, K5, 71 East Concord Street, Boston, MA 02118.

Submitted for publication June 21, 1984; accepted in revised form October 23, 1984.

Rheumatic diseases affect about 10% of the population (1). Five to ten percent of office visits to general physicians are related to musculoskeletal problems (2), and a small minority of these patients will be referred to physicians with specialized training in these disorders (3). The National Arthritis Plan suggested that every primary and family physician be trained in the diagnosis and treatment of the common musculoskeletal conditions (4). Rheumatology training of generalists occurs to a limited extent in medical school (5), but it is likely that the most intensive training in rheumatology occurs during residencies in internal medicine and family practice. Little is known, however, about the content or process of training in rheumatic diseases at this critical stage of medical education (6–8). Thus, the Medical Education Research Subcommittee of the American Rheumatism Association (ARA) designed and conducted a survey to evaluate the current status of rheumatology education in internal medicine and family practice programs in the United States. The results of this survey provide an overview of house staff training in rheumatology and support conclusions about the general physician's education in rheumatology in the United States.

METHODS

Seven committee members designed the questionnaire to determine basic information regarding rheumatology education. "Rheumatology" was not defined in any descriptive fashion, although aspects of rheumatology training that the committee believed to be important were indirectly conveyed to the respondents. These were specified in a question about the level of training in the following areas of rheumatology: musculoskeletal examination, differential diagnosis of acute arthritis, differential diagnosis of rheumatoid arthritis, management of rheumatoid arthritis, laboratory tests in the rheumatic diseases, synovial fluid analysis, joint aspiration technique, diagnosis and management of tendinitis, general principles of occupational and physical therapy, and psychosocial aspects of chronic disease. The respondents were asked to rate the level of training (good, fair, poor) in each of these areas, and were asked to compare the training of their residents in rheumatology with the training of residents in other medical subspecialty areas such as cardiology or gastroenterology.

Program variables were surveyed by questions that could be answered by yes, no, or a numeric value. These questions included: the total number of residents in the program, the total number of residents in a rheumatology elective each year, the percentage of available rheumatology elective slots filled each year, the duration of rheumatology training, specific assignments during the rheumatology training, including inpatient and outpatient consultations and longitudinal care, private office experiences, rheumatology attending rounds, teaching conferences, and orthopedic training. Furthermore, the availability of other electives in orthopedics, physical and rehabilitation medicine, gerontology, cardiology, pulmonary medicine, gastroenterology, nephrology, oncology, hematology, endocrinology, and infectious diseases was surveyed. A description of the training program, including medical school affiliation and faculty rheumatologists, was provided. The specific weekly activities of rheumatology faculty in the following areas were also determined: house officer teaching conferences, inpatient consultations, hospital-based clinic, hospital-based clinical and basic research, and general medical attending responsibilities.

The 1,125 internal medicine and family practice programs listed in the 1982–1983 Directory of Residency Programs (9) were initially grouped by the following variables: (a) internal medicine or family practice; (b) large or small (small was defined as fewer than 30 residents; large was defined as equal to or greater than 30 residents total in each residency program); (c) general geographic location. Since there were not many large family practice programs, we later grouped all family practice programs into 1 category and compared them with large internal medicine and small internal medicine programs. Two hundred twenty-four programs were randomly selected to receive the questionnaire.

Completed questionnaires were received from 177 programs, a 79% response rate. The questionnaires were answered by the internal medicine or family practice director at 80% of the programs, and the other questionnaires were completed by the rheumatology program director or by an associate director of the residency training program. The number of respondents from the 3 general categories included: 61 large internal medicine programs (35%), 44 small internal medicine programs (25%), and 72 family practice programs (40%).

The survey data were analyzed by applying chi-square tests for nominal data or counts and analysis of variance for continuous variables, to look for overall differences across the 3 program types. If a significant difference was found, initial analysis was followed by explicit paired comparisons using chi-square for counts and *t*-tests for continuous data. All differences reported as significant displayed P values ≤ 0.01. This conservative significance level was chosen rather than the more traditional 0.05 level, in order to adjust for multiple comparisons.

RESULTS

General characteristics and faculty of the residency programs. The mean number of house officers in all of the programs surveyed was 36, with a range of 3–225. The mean number of internal medicine house officers was 37, whereas the mean number of family practice house officers was 18. Seventy-three percent of the respondents reported that their program was a major affiliate of a medical school, and another 23% reported that their residency program had some affiliation with a medical school.

Eighty-three percent of the large internal medicine programs, 70% of the small internal medicine programs, but only 13% of the family practice programs had a rheumatology department affiliated with their residency program (Table 1). A full-time staff rheumatologist was present at 69% of the large internal medicine programs, 32% of the small internal medicine programs, and 11% of the family practice programs. Each family practice program with a full-time rheumatologist was directly affiliated with a major medical center and an internal medicine training program. Large internal medicine programs were more likely to be affiliated with a rheumatology fellowship program and have more than 2 full-time staff rheumatologists. Overall, 65 residency programs (37% of those surveyed) did not have a full-time staff rheumatologist and 20 (14%) did not have a full-time or a part-time staff rheumatologist.

Table 1. Rheumatology faculty manpower

	% of programs		
	Large internal medicine (n = 61)	Small internal medicine (n = 44)	Family practice (n = 72)
Rheumatology department	83	70	13*
Full-time staff rheumatologist	69*	32	11
>2 full-time staff rheumatologists	38*	9	6

* Significant difference compared with other 2 programs ($P < 0.01$).

The family practice and small internal medicine programs without a full-time staff rheumatologist provided formal rheumatology education by employing a part-time rheumatologist or by sending their residents to training sites outside their own medical center. Eighteen of the 20 programs that did not have a full-time or part-time faculty rheumatologist were contacted by telephone in order to determine who provided rheumatology education to their residents. Ten of these programs sent their residents to an affiliated medical center that did have a staff rheumatologist and an existing rheumatology training program. Five of the 18 programs sent their residents to the private practice of a rheumatologist or an internist. Three of the 18 programs reported that they provided no formal staff-supervised rheumatology training.

The weekly teaching activities of the staff rheumatologists at large internal medicine programs more often included inpatient consultations, didactic teaching conferences, and arthritis clinics, when compared with the teaching activities of rheumatologists at small internal medicine and at family practice programs (Table 2). Less than 20% of the rheumatologists affiliated with family practice and small internal medicine programs participated in weekly clinical or basic research, whereas approximately 70% of rheumatologists at large internal medicine programs were involved in these investigative activities (Table 2).

Content of rheumatology residency education. Formal training in rheumatology was available at 92% of all programs surveyed, including 93% of the internal medicine programs and 90% of the family practice programs. Three-fourths of the trainees received their formal rheumatology education during a 1- or 2-month elective. Most respondents reported that their programs provided a balance of inpatient and ambulatory patient training experience, although the family practice programs were more likely to provide only ambulatory training.

During any single academic year, approximately one-quarter of residents at large internal medicine, small internal medicine, and family practice programs received some formal rheumatology education. In contrast, the mean percentage of house officers who received an orthopedic elective each year was 45% of residents at family practice programs, 9% at small internal medicine programs, and 4% at large internal medicine programs. Whereas more than 75% of available rheumatology elective positions were filled by residents at more than three-quarters of the large internal medicine programs, only about one-third of the small internal medicine and one-quarter of the family practice programs had filled more than 75% of their available elective positions (Table 3). In contrast, fewer than one-quarter of available elective positions were filled at 8% of large internal medicine programs, and at 42% of family practice programs.

The specific content of formal rheumatology training at most programs included teaching conferences, inpatient consultations, and attending rounds and ambulatory clinics (Table 4). Compared with the large internal medicine programs, family practice residency programs and small internal medicine programs more often provided some training in a private practice office setting. Family practice programs more often provided specific orthopedic training within their rheumatology elective in comparison with the internal medicine programs, while large internal medicine programs more commonly presented weekly teaching conferences.

Perceived training quality. Quality of training in 10 specific educational variables was assessed by the program directors (Table 5). Approximately two-thirds of program directors at all residency programs surveyed considered the training of their residents in the

Table 2. Weekly activities of staff rheumatologists*

	Large internal medicine programs (n = 61)	Small internal medicine programs (n = 44)	Family practice programs (n = 72)
Teaching conferences	78†	49	52
Inpatient consultations	95	88	68†
Arthritis clinic (hospital-based)	89†	58	38
Clinical research	76†	20	16
Basic research	66†	17	16
Attending rounds	84	63	49†

* % who participate in each of these activities weekly.
† Significant difference compared with other 2 programs ($P < 0.01$).

Table 3. Percentage of available rheumatology elective positions filled

	% of programs		
	Large internal medicine (n = 61)	Small internal medicine (n = 44)	Family practice (n = 72)
<25%	8	18	42
25–50%	2	24	22
50–75%	11	20	9
>75%	79*	38	27

* Significant difference compared with other 2 programs ($P < 0.01$).

Table 4. Rheumatology elective curriculum

Training variable	% of programs offering training variable		
	Large internal medicine (n = 61)	Small internal medicine (n = 44)	Family practice (n = 72)
Teaching conferences	98*	81	83
Inpatient consultations	97	97	89
Attending rounds	93	86	80
Outpatient clinics	95	86	90
Emergency room	48	50	35
Private office	42*	67	78
Orthopedics	42	19	54

* Significant difference compared with other 2 programs ($P < 0.01$).

general principles of occupational and physical therapy and the psychosocial aspects of chronic disease to be inadequate. However, there were significant differences in the inadequacies perceived by the program directors relative to the type and size of the program. For example, a significantly greater number of directors at family practice and small internal medicine programs, in comparison with those at large internal medicine programs, considered their residents' training inadequate in the interpretation of laboratory tests, performance and interpretation of synovial fluid analysis, and the technique of joint aspiration (Table 5). In contrast, the family practice program directors, in comparison with the directors of the large and small internal medicine programs, more often believed that their residents' training in the diagnosis and management of tendinitis and the psychosocial aspects of chronic disease was adequate. In general, however, there were significant inadequacies perceived with regard to each important training variable assessed. This perception of inadequacy was especially striking with regard to the basic techniques of a musculoskeletal examination and joint aspiration.

The program directors also were asked to assess the perceived adequacy of their rheumatology training programs relative to that of cardiology and gastroenterology. Only 10% of respondents reported that the training received in rheumatology was slightly or much better than that received in cardiology and gastroenterology, whereas 39% of the respondents believed the rheumatology training was slightly or much worse than cardiology and gastroenterology training. When program directors were asked what they considered to be the single most important change in current rheumatology training that would help to improve the rheumatology skills of their residents, 40% of the respondents stated that exposure to more patients with arthritis was most important, 25% believed more general interest in rheumatology throughout the residency program was most important, 19% thought that more emphasis on ambulatory rheumatology was most important, and only 15% stated that a larger rheumatology faculty was most important.

Table 5. Perceived "inadequacies" of rheumatology house officer training*

Specific training variable	% of respondents who rated skill inadequate		
	Large internal medicine programs (n = 61)	Small internal medicine programs (n = 44)	Family practice programs (n = 72)
Musculoskeletal examination	33	50	39
Differential diagnosis of acute arthritis	12	23	31
Differential diagnosis of rheumatoid arthritis	12	23	31
Management of rheumatoid arthritis	25	30	43
Laboratory tests in the rheumatic diseases	15†	34	46
Synovial fluid analysis	25†	55	70
Joint aspiration technique	33†	52	61
Diagnosis and management of tendinitis	53	57	33†
General priniciples of occupational and physical therapy	76	82	68
Psychosocial aspects of chronic disease	61	73	41†

* For each training variable listed, the program directors rated their residents' education as good, fair, or poor. "Inadequate" represents the sum of fair and poor responses for each variable.
† Significant difference compared with other 2 programs ($P < 0.01$).

DISCUSSION

After evaluating rheumatology education in U.S. medical schools, the Undergraduate Education Subcommittee of the Education Committee of the ARA reported that 10% of medical schools provided no formal rheumatology education and that 13% did not have a rheumatologist on their full-time faculty (5). Furthermore, 22% of the schools did not have a rheumatology fellowship program and 38% had 2 or fewer full-time rheumatologists. Only 62% of the schools provided specific training in musculoskeletal examination. An intense 1- or 2-month rheumatology elective was available to students at most medical schools, but fewer than 20% of the medical students participated in such electives. Three-fourths of the rheumatology program directors at the medical schools believed the educational impact of rheumatology on students was inadequate, primarily because of a lack of significant exposure to rheumatology patients.

The current study, the first to evaluate the rheumatology training of residents in internal medicine and family practice programs throughout the United States, found similar educational deficiencies. While some formal rheumatology education is offered in 90% of these residency programs, the availability, utilization, and content of this education varies significantly with specific program characteristics. Those family practice and small internal medicine programs without a full-time staff rheumatologist (Table 1) utilized part-time rheumatologists or sent their residents to other programs for formal rheumatology education. Since formal training in rheumatology is not required, only about one-quarter of residents each year participate, a situation analogous to that in medical student rheumatology education (5). Whereas there are far too few elective positions available in rheumatology at U.S. medical schools (5), there is an underutilization of available electives in rheumatology at the level of residency training, especially in family practice and small internal medicine programs (Table 3).

Furthermore, residents were often considered by program directors to be inadequately trained in the techniques of musculoskeletal examination, synovial fluid analysis, and joint aspiration. Ambulatory-oriented skills, such as the diagnosis and management of tendinitis and the psychosocial aspects of chronic disease, were more often judged to be inadequately taught in the internal medicine programs, whereas the interpretation of laboratory tests and synovial fluid analysis were more often judged to be inadequately taught in the family practice programs. In general, the program directors believed their residents were not as well trained in rheumatology as they were in cardiology or gastroenterology.

These perceived inadequacies may correlate with the inefficient utilization of available elective training positions in rheumatology. Recent studies have concluded that a formal educational program in rheumatology is important if basic skills are to be acquired during residency training (6–8). In contrast, significant education may be acquired by "osmosis" in medical subspecialties such as cardiology and gastroenterology, which are emphasized during general inpatient medical training. Rheumatology training skills, including a familiarity with many common musculoskeletal conditions such as soft tissue rheumatism and osteoarthritis, can best be provided in ambulatory sites over a long time frame. Therefore, residency programs should focus greater emphasis on ambulatory rheumatology training. The Internal Medicine Residency Review Committee recommends that "most rotations on subspecialties should be at least six weeks duration (9)." However, a 6-week rotation may not be optimal or practical in the provision of basic rheumatology training to most internal medicine residents.

The Family Practice Residency Review Committee recommends that the curriculum in internal medicine should include both inpatient and outpatient experiences in medical subspecialties and that the faculty should include both general internists and subspecialists (9). In contrast, 160–200 hours of orthopedic training is required. Thus, formal training in orthopedics is provided for all family practice residents, and in a much greater degree than comparable rheumatology training. The family practice residents may receive substantial education in certain rheumatic conditions during their orthopedic training, although the content of this training is not known.

The validity of the information gathered by this survey is subject to the accuracy of the program directors' responses. Formal validity testing is not possible in such a survey. However, certain features of the questionnaire design and analysis should have served to increase validity. For example, most questions offered clear-cut dichotomous choices. The fact that our analyses focused on comparisons of program types, e.g., family practice versus internal medicine, tends to balance inaccuracies and reduce threats to validity. Furthermore, we are now in the process of followup site visits to a sample of the responding programs. These site visits will validate the reliability of the program directors' responses and, more importantly, will provide an instrument to evaluate the impact of these rheumatology training variables on residents' performance.

In conclusion, our survey of residency training at family practice and internal medicine programs found that formal training in rheumatology is offered at the great majority of programs throughout the United States, although currently the available educational positions are not fully utilized. Program directors thought that the rheumatology education of their trainees was not adequate in regard to a number of specific variables, and that they would benefit from greater exposure to rheumatology and a greater mastery of basic rheumatology skills.

REFERENCES

1. Bennett PH, Wood PHN: Population Studies of the Rheumatic Diseases. Amsterdam, Excerpta Medica, 1968
2. DeLozier JE, Gagnon RO: National Ambulatory Medical Care Survey. DHEW Publication No. 761772. Rockville, Maryland, US Department of Health, Education and Welfare, 1975
3. Ogryzlo MA: Editorial: specialty of rheumatology—manpower requirements. J Rheumatol 2:1–4, 1975
4. Engleman EP: The National Arthritis Plan: an overview. Arthritis Rheum 20:1–6, 1977
5. Goldenberg DL, Mason JH, DeHoratius R, Goldberg V, Kaplan SR, Keiser H, Lockshin MD, Rynes R, Sandson JI, Schumacher HR, Skosey J: Rheumatology education in United States medical schools. Arthritis Rheum 24:1561–1566, 1981
6. Goldenberg DL, Meenan RF, Allaire S, Cohen AS: The educational impact of a rheumatology elective. Arthritis Rheum 26:658–663, 1983
7. Eyanson S, Brandt KD: Some effects on houseofficers of an elective rheumatology rotation. J Rheumatol 7:251–257, 1980
8. Strosberg MA, Strosberg JM: Do family practice residents in the United States learn clinical rheumatology? An important question. J Rheumatol 7:923–926, 1980
9. 1982–1983 Directory of Residency Training Programs. Chicago, American Medical Association, 1982

LETTERS

Comment on article by Faure et al

To the Editor:

We would like to comment on the report of Faure et al (1) regarding lymphocyte typing after an intravenous pulse of methylprednisolone in a patient with Still's disease. They found that an initially reversed helper/inducer:suppressor/cytotoxic cell ratio (OKT4:OKT8 or Leu 3a:Leu 2a) became normal during a prolonged period of lymphopenia which occurred after an intravenous pulse of methylprednisolone.

We have studied 9 children with various rheumatic diseases, including systemic onset juvenile rheumatoid arthritis, for the effects of steroid pulses on T cells. We consistently found a transient lymphopenia and decreased Leu 3a:Leu 2a ratio at 5 hours after a pulse, and a return to pre-pulse values by 48 hours (2). This is consistent with previous reports on normal volunteers (3–5) and on patients with rheumatoid arthritis observed for 21 days after a pulse (6). This phenomenon has also been reported in patients receiving alternate-day prednisone (7). Thus, the persisting lymphopenia found by Faure et al (1) is unusual and not consistent with general experience.

Second, the initial OKT4:OKT8 ratio of their patient was 0.7, while in our experience, patients with juvenile rheumatoid arthritis have variable but usually normal ratios which change with disease activity (unpublished data).

Third, their patient's increase in Leu 7–positive cells from 1–27% over 13 days is intriguing in light of the findings of Katz et al (8), who reported a transient "relative" increase in a natural killer (NK) cells 4 hours after a pulse of steroids, and a return to pre-pulse values by 24 hours. As in other studies (8,9), the absolute NK cell number as well as cytotoxic activity per cell was unchanged throughout. The continued increase in Leu 7–positive cells noted by Faure et al (1) may reflect general clinical improvement, and not be specifically related to steroid therapy.

We suggest that changes in OKT4:OKT8 or Leu 3a:Leu 2a ratios may reflect improvement in the disease independently of the drug administered. The question of whether these determinations add any information to the clinical evaluation and standard laboratory tests needs further investigation.

Barry Lee Myones, MD
University of North Carolina
Chapel Hill, NC
Earl D. Silverman, MD
Stanford University
Stanford, CA
John J. Miller, III, MD, PhD
Children's Hospital at Stanford
Palo Alto, CA

1. Faure G, Bene MC, Bordigoni P: Peripheral T cell subset modifications induced by steroid pulse in a case of Still's disease (letter). Arthritis Rheum 27:718–719, 1984
2. Silverman ED, Myones BL, Miller JJ III: Lymphocyte subpopulation alterations induced by intravenous megadose pulse methylprednisolone. J Rheumatol 11:287–290, 1984
3. Fauci AS, Dale DC: The effect of in vivo hydrocortisone on subpopulations of human lymphocytes. J Clin Invest 53:240–246, 1974
4. Webel ML, Ritts RE Jr, Taswell HF, Donadio JV Jr, Wood JE: Cellular immunity after intravenous administration of methylprednisolone. J Lab Clin Med 83:383–392, 1974
5. Zweiman B, Atkins PC, Bedard PM, Flaschen SL, Lisak RP: Corticosteroid effects on circulating lymphocyte subset levels in normal humans. J Clin Immunol 4:151–155, 1984
6. Fan PT, Yu DTY, Clements PJ, Fowlston S, Eisman J, Bluestone R: Effects of corticosteroids on the human immune response: comparison of one and three daily 1 gram intravenous pulses of methylprednisolone. J Lab Clin Med 91:625–634, 1978
7. Fauci AS, Dale DC: Alternate day prednisone therapy and human lymphocyte subpopulations. J Clin Invest 55:22–32, 1975
8. Katz P, Zaytoun AM, Lee JH Jr: The effects of in vivo hydrocortisone on lymphocyte-mediated cytotoxicity. Arthritis Rheum 27:72–78, 1984
9. Onsrud M, Thorsby E: Influence of in vivo hydrocortisone on some human blood lymphocyte subpopulations. I. Effect on natural killer cell activity. Scand J Immunol 13:573–579, 1981

Popliteal cyst presenting as an anterior tibial mass

To the Editor:

O'Dell et al recently reported the case of a young girl with juvenile rheumatoid arthritis, who developed a popliteal cyst presenting as an anterior lower leg mass (1). We wish to report a similar case.

A 58-year-old man with seropositive rheumatoid arthritis of 5 years duration, treated with naproxen and salazosulfapyridine, was admitted to our hospital with an acute synovitis of extensor tendons of the left fingers, and pain and swelling of the right leg. Three months prior to admission, he had been treated by osmic acid synoviorthesis for a right popliteal cyst, and 1 month prior to admission, a right olecranon bursitis was treated surgically, with incomplete healing and intermittent purulent flow.

Physical examination revealed the presence of a tender mass over the right anterior tibia, about 15 cm below the patella, and a synovitis of the extensor tendons, with warmth. There was still an olecranon bursitis, without any tenderness.

Initial laboratory data included an erythrocyte sedimentation rate of 132 mm/hour, hemoglobin level of 9.2 gm/100 ml, and white blood cell count of 4,200/ml with 75% polymorphonuclear cells. Radiographs of the legs showed chronic arthritis of both knees, with no abnormalities of the bone.

Aspiration of the leg mass yielded a purulent fluid, and culture demonstrated *Staphylococcus aureus*; cystography revealed that the shin mass was an anterior dissection of the popliteal cyst (Figure 1).

Antibiotic therapy (fusidic acid and cephalexin) was started, and a surgical drainage procedure with wide debridement was performed, along with a synovectomy of the left extensor tendons.

The anterior dissection of a popliteal cyst is unusual (2); O'Dell found only 1 other case in the English literature (3). Possibly, additional cases of this complication have occurred but have not been published.

The diagnosis was not difficult in our patient because we were aware of the presence of a popliteal cyst. The infection may have caused rapid enlargement of the anterior dissection (4). A septic hematogenous spread from a chronic infection of the olecranon bursitis must be suspected. We don't think the previous synoviorthesis of the cyst could have caused the infection, since it was performed much earlier, and we are not aware of osmic acid synoviorthesis ever having led to septic complication (5).

If clinical examination leads to an unconfirmed suspicion of popliteal cyst as the cause of a shin mass, puncture and cystogram can easily be performed to verify the diagnosis.

A. Thevenon, MD
P. Hardouin, MD
B. Duquesnoy, MD
Hôpital de la Charité
Lille, France

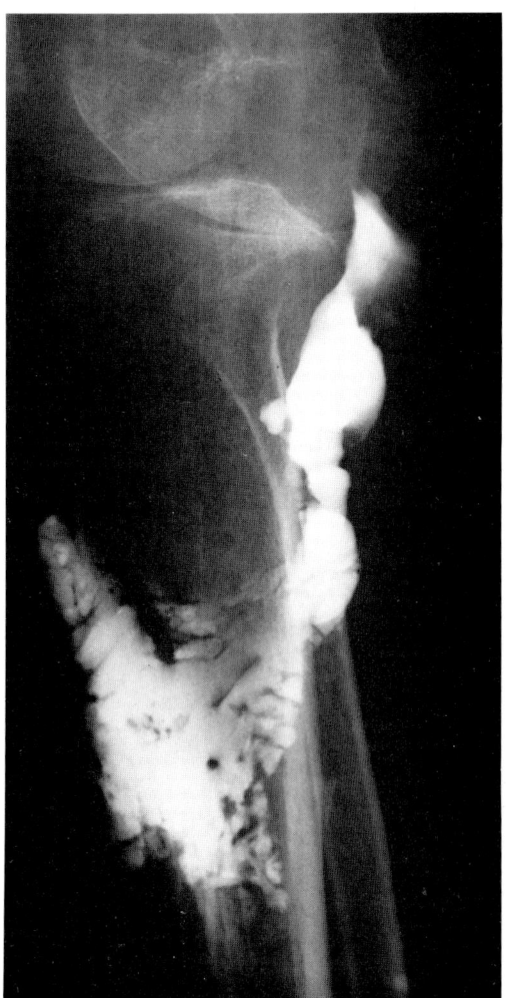

Figure 1. Cystogram showing the anterior dissection of the popliteal cyst.

1. O'Dell JR, Andersen PA, Hollister JR, West SG: Anterior tibial mass: an unusual complication of popliteal cysts. Arthritis Rheum 27:113–115, 1984
2. Hench PK, Smith JL: Atypical syndromes associated with synovial cysts of the knee (abstract). Arthritis Rheum 12:302–303, 1969
3. Jayson MIV, Dixon AS: Valvular mechanisms in juxta-articular cysts. Ann Rheum Dis 29:415–420, 1970
4. Stewart IM, Swinson DR, Hardinge K: Pyogenic arthritis presenting as a ruptured popliteal cyst. Ann Rheum Dis 38:181–182, 1979
5. Delcambre B, DeFrance D, Douchy P, Robert d'Eshougues J: Les synoviorthèses à l'acide osmique dans le traitement de la maladie rhumatoïde: remarques et bilan de 5 années d'utilisation. Lille Méd 21:813–820, 1976

Comment on article by Brenner et al

To the Editor:

Brenner et al recently reported that T-enriched peripheral blood mononuclear cells (PBMC) from patients with Reiter's syndrome responded better to formalin-treated *Yersinia enterocolitica* serotype 3 (Ye3) than did similarly enriched cells from HLA–B27 positive controls (Brenner MB, Kobayashi S, Weisenhutter CW, Huberman AK, Bales P, Yu DTY: In vitro T lymphocyte proliferative response to Yersinia enterocolitica in Reiter's syndrome: lack of response in other HLA–B27 positive individuals. Arthritis Rheum 27:250–257, 1984). This difference was not seen if non-enriched PBMC were used, nor was it seen if heat-killed Ye3 were used. They suggested that this represented a disease-specific response to a Ye3 antigen present on formalin-killed but not heat-killed organisms, and that the response was detectable only by the T-enriched populations.

An examination of the data reveals an alternative interpretation. Lymphocyte response was assessed in the conventional way by the incorporation of tritiated thymidine into proliferating lymphocytes. The results were expressed as average counts per minute of stimulated cells, minus background. Although stated to be consistently less than 4,000 cpm, this latter figure is not provided for individual groups.

Even without knowledge of the actual background levels, it can be seen from Table 1 that all subjects responded

Table 1. Response of peripheral blood mononuclear cells (PBMC) to heat- and formalin-killed *Yersinia enterocolitica* serotype 3 (Ye3)

		Counts per minute of cultured cells from:	
Antigen	Cells used	Reiter's patients	B27+ controls
Ye3 formalin	PBMC	28,531	29,943
Ye3 formalin	T-enriched PBMC	27,409	5,414
Ye3 heat	T-enriched PBMC	21,888	15,383

to both heat- and formalin-killed Ye3 antigens, with a significant elevation of cpm.

However, when lymphocytes depleted of non–T cells were studied, Reiter's patients maintained their response to formalin-killed *Yersinia*, while the response of the controls was reduced by the procedure. This emphasis is different from that of Brenner et al.

The change in response in the B27 positive control subjects remains an interesting finding, but may have more to do with qualities of antigen-presenting cells in the 2 groups. We agree that the response is likely to reflect exposure to a cross-reacting antigen on a locally prevalent organism, but we remain unconvinced that the evidence clearly demonstrates a difference in sensitivity between the 2 groups of subjects to a specific *Yersinia* antigen.

Stephen Aaron, FRCP(C)
University of Alberta
Edmonton, Alberta
Canada

Tender point count

To the Editor:

Since Smythe first proposed it as a diagnostic sign in 1972 (1), the "tender point count" has been an essential criterion for fibrositis diagnosis in studies published on the disorder (2–6). Although Smythe originally required 12 of 14 possible tender areas for diagnosis, other investigators have required less; as few as 4 tender points have been accepted as meeting the tender point criterion (2,3).

Although the presence of tender points is uncommon in a healthy, young population (2), there are no published data concerning the frequency of tender points in patients with rheumatic disease in whom joint disease could be associated with musculoskeletal tenderness.

To investigate the frequency of tender points in a rheumatic disease population, 980 consecutive patients attending a private practice rheumatic disease clinic were examined by the same physician for tenderness in the 14 areas suggested by Smythe, using his methodology (7). Sixty-eight percent (669 of 980) had no tender points. This group included 165 of 248 patients with definite or classic rheumatoid arthritis (66.6%) and 128 of 185 patients with

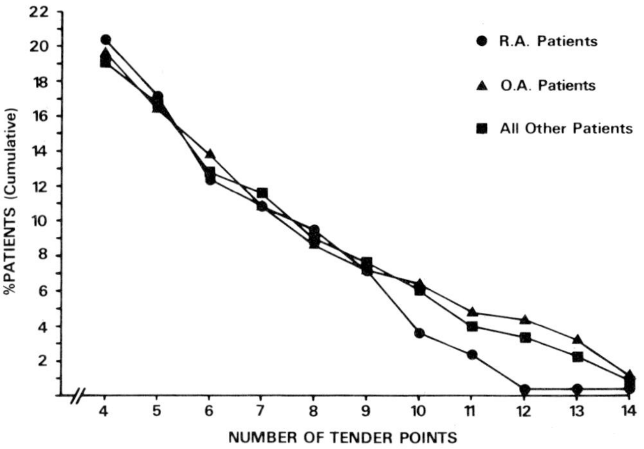

Figure 1. The tender point count in 980 consecutive rheumatic disease patients. RA = rheumatoid arthritis; OA = osteoarthritis.

peripheral joint osteoarthritis (69.2%). Four or more tender points were found in 19–21% of patients, and only 11–12% had 7 or more tender points. A tender point count of 12 or greater was unusual (Figure 1). There was no statistically significant difference in the proportion or distribution of tender points among the disease groups, as shown in Figure 1. These data suggest that, except in fibrositis patients, a high number of tender points is uncommon. Thus, the identification of multiple tender points in patients with musculoskeletal pain suggests the possibility of the diagnosis of fibrositis.

Frederick Wolfe, MD
University of Kansas School of Medicine
Wichita, KS

1. Smythe HA: Nonarticular rheumatism and fibrositis, Arthritis and Allied Conditions. Edited by DJ McCarty. Philadelphia, Lea & Febiger, 1972, pp 874–884
2. Yunus M, Masi AT, Calabro JJ, Miller KA, Feigenbaum SL: Primary fibromyalgia (fibrositis): clinical study of 50 patients with matched normal controls. Semin Arthritis Rheum 11:151–171, 1981
3. Payne TC, Leavitt F, Garron DC, Katz RS, Golden HE, Glickman PB, Vanderplate C: Fibrositis and psychogenic disturbance. Arthritis Rheum 25:213–217, 1982
4. Campbell SM, Clark S, Tindall EA, Forehand ME, Bennett RM: Clinical characteristics of fibrositis. Arthritis Rheum 26:817–824, 1983
5. Wolfe F, Cathey M: Prevalence of primary and secondary fibrositis. J Rheumatol 10:965–968, 1983
6. Wolfe F, Cathey M, Kleinheksel S, Amos S, Hoffman R, Young D, Hawley D: Psychological status in primary fibrositis and fibrositis associated with rheumatoid arthritis. J Rheumatol 11:500–505, 1984
7. Smythe HA: Fibrositis and other diffuse musculoskeletal syndromes, Textbook of Rheumatology. Edited by WN Kelley, ED Harris Jr, S Ruddy, CB Sledge. Philadelphia, WB Saunders, 1980, 485–493

Angiotensin converting enzyme inhibitors and rheumatoid arthritis

To the Editor:

Dr. Israeli Jaffe reported the results of an open-label study of the non-sulfhydryl angiotensin converting enzyme (ACE) inhibitor MK 421 (Enalapril) in 3 patients whose rheumatoid arthritis was persistent and unresponsive to standard therapies (Jaffe I: Angiotensin converting inhibitors in rheumatoid arthritis [letter]. Arthritis Rheum 27:840, 1984). In that trial, MK 421 showed no beneficial effect upon disease activity as measured by standard clinical and biochemical criteria. Jaffe concluded that this "open study strongly suggest[s] that the anti-rheumatoid activity of captopril is due to the presence of the active sulfhydryl group, and not to its property of ACE inhibition."

The study may not justify such a strong conclusion: the enrollment of patients who were eventual nonresponders to, or experienced adverse side effects with, D-penicillamine treatment constitutes a selection bias, the 16-week treatment period (including the first 2 weeks at a lower dose) was too short to ascertain D-penicillamine–like efficacy, and the study was an open-label trial with very few subjects.

The role of an active sulfhydryl group in the activity of anti-rheumatoid drugs is, of course, unknown. Both clozic (Dixon JS, Sitton NG, Surrall KE, Martin MFR, Pickup ME, Bird HA: The effect of drugs on serum histidine levels in rheumatoid arthritis. Rheumatol Int 3:145–149, 1983) and hydroxychloroquine are long-acting agents (or disease-modifying anti-rheumatic drugs), but neither contains a sulfhydryl group. It is therefore premature to reject the possibility that ACE inhibitors possess inherent anti-rheumatoid activity.

Allen Traficante, MD
Michael A. Catalano, MD
George E. Ehrlich, MD
Ciba-Geigy Pharmaceuticals Corporation
Summit, NJ

BOOK REVIEW

Differential Diagnosis in Rheumatology: An Atlas for the Physician. *Andrei Calin. Philadelphia, JB Lippincott, 1984. 220 pages. Illustrated. $35.00.*

The purpose of this book, as stated by the author, is to review common rheumatic complaints and arrive at correct diagnoses, emphasizing the history and physical examination. The intended readership is non-rheumatologist, either medical students or postgraduate generalists. Are the aims accomplished for this audience?

Chapters 1–4 display an overview approach to a rheumatologic differential diagnosis from the perspective of a very capable and seasoned clinician. The book's two major strengths in these sections are the general points on history-taking and the chapter on how to conduct the joint examination. The author very appropriately sounds the theme of all rheumatology teachers—when in doubt, "just you wait" for the diagnosis. If the organization were tightened and some of the jargon were eliminated—"enthesopathic diseases," for example—these chapters would be improved. The chapter focusing on the diagnostic discrimination among rheumatoid arthritis, polymyalgia rheumatica, localized nonarticular problems, and fibrositis emphasizes the history more than the physical examination—a debatable point. Two errors should be pointed out: fibrositis is not the same as psychogenic rheumatism, and adhesive capsulitis is not more common than bicipital tendinitis.

The real meat of this volume, chapters 5–11, is an attempt to focus on regions from which a primary complaint arises, then present a typical example (short history with physical findings), and subsequently arrive at a specific diagnosis. The illustrations are the major strengths here. They are carefully chosen, well presented, and valid; they do illustrate the author's points. The weaknesses are primarily a lack of consistency in approach and the absence of a context in which the student or generalist will grasp the expert author's essential points. Too many suggestions are couched in the terms "is typically seen" or "is characteristically involved." Certainly, this section would have been improved if the author stressed, in a consistent manner, the importance and timing of further diagnostic tests, such as biopsies, angiograms, or laboratory studies.

This reviewer, therefore, has some doubts about whether the author's goal can be accomplished in this volume. With the style and format used, a great deal of knowledge about rheumatic diseases is already taken for granted. The author is obviously skilled and experienced, yet the approach in these chapters appears too short-circuited or truncated to allow that information to be placed meaningfully within the context of the "uninitiated." How to take the expert's approach and make it function within the framework of a novice is a difficult problem; this author has that goal in mind, but more structure and consistency are required to accomplish the task.

Michael H. Weisman, MD
University of California
San Diego, CA

arthritis
and
rheumatism

Official Journal of the American Rheumatism Association Section of the Arthritis Foundation

ANTIBODIES TO HUMAN T CELL LEUKEMIA VIRUS ARE ABSENT IN PATIENTS WITH SYSTEMIC LUPUS ERYTHEMATOSUS

TAKAO KOIKE, MASARU KAGAMI, KATSUHIKO TAKABAYASHI, NAOKI MARUYAMA, HISAO TOMIOKA, and SHO YOSHIDA

It has been anticipated that type C oncornaviruses, which participate in the pathogenesis of murine systemic lupus erythematosus (SLE), would be found to have a role in the development of SLE in humans. In studies of tissues from SLE patients, type C–related proteins have been identified. Using information obtained on the recent isolation of the human T cell leukemia virus (HTLV), together with that from studies of murine SLE, we attempted to clarify the role of antibodies to HTLV in the pathogenesis of human SLE. Using a solid-phase enzyme-linked immunosorbent assay and sodium dodecyl sulfate–polyacrylamide gel electrophoretic techniques, we were unable to find evidence of the participation of antibodies to HTLV proteins in the development of human SLE.

The participation of type C oncornaviruses in the pathogenesis of human systemic lupus erythematosus (SLE) has been investigated (1–5), principally because of their role in the murine model of SLE (6–8).

From the Second Department of Internal Medicine, School of Medicine, Chiba University and Department of Pathology, Chiba Rosai Hospital, Chiba, Japan.

Supported by grants from the Ministry of Health and Welfare, Science and Culture, Japan, and from the Japan Medical Research Foundation.

Takao Koike, MD: Instructor of Internal Medicine; Masaru Kagami, MD: Research Fellow in Clinical Immunology; Katsuhiko Takabayashi, MD: Fellow in Clinical Immunology; Naoki Maruyama, MD: Director of Pathology, Chiba Rosai Hospital; Hisao Tomioka, MD: Assistant Professor of Internal Medicine; Sho Yoshida, MD: Professor of Medicine.

Address reprint requests to Takao Koike, MD, Second Department of Internal Medicine, School of Medicine, Chiba University, 1-8-1 Inohana, Chiba 280, Japan.

Submitted for publication August 15, 1984; accepted in revised form October 26, 1984.

Recently, a novel human type C retrovirus, the human T cell leukemia virus (HTLV), was isolated from patients with leukemia and lymphoma (9). The role of this virus in the development of certain types of human T cell leukemia/lymphoma has been well characterized (10,11).

We searched for antibodies to HTLV proteins in sera from patients with SLE in an attempt to elucidate the participation of type C virus and antibodies in human SLE. We found no evidence of the presence of anti-HTLV antibodies in the sera of SLE patients.

PATIENTS AND METHODS

Sera were obtained from patients with SLE, classified according to the American Rheumatism Association criteria (12), and from patients with adult T cell leukemia (ATL) and their family members.

The HTLV-producer, human cell line MT-2, was kindly provided by Professor I. Miyoshi, Kochi Medical School, Nangoku, Japan.

Viral antigens were purified according to the method of Saxinger and Gallo (13). Briefly, the viral particles were obtained by zonal ultracentrifugation (20–55%) of the medium from a 72-hour culture of MT-2 cells. The virus peak was centrifuged at 30,000 revolutions per minute for 1.5 hours, and the pellet was disrupted by the addition of Triton X-100 and KCl.

Antibodies to HTLV antigens were measured by a solid-phase enzyme-linked immunosorbent assay (ELISA) described by Saxinger and Gallo (13), with modifications. Each well of the polyvinyl chloride plates (Flow Laboratories, McLean, VA) was first coated with 50 μl of HTLV antigen solution, 5 μg/ml in 0.01*M* phosphate buffered saline (PBS), pH 7.4, by incubation for 1 hour at room temperature. After discarding the antigen solution, 200 μl of 10% fetal calf serum (FCS) was added to each well, and the preparations were incubated for 1 hour at room temperature to block nonspecific binding of immunoglobulins to the well surface. After 5 washes in PBS, 50 μl of test serum (diluted with PBS containing 10% FCS) was added to each well, and the preparations were incubated for 1 hour at room temperature. The preparations were washed 5 times in PBS, and 50 μl of mouse monoclonal anti-human IgG (Wako Chemical Co., Tokyo, Japan) labeled with alkaline phosphatase (Sigma, St. Louis, MO) was added to each well. After the plate was incubated for 1 hour, 100 μl of p-nitrophenyl phosphate in 1*M* diethanolamine buffer, pH 9.0, was added to each well, and the plate was incubated an additional 1 hour.

Optical absorbance was measured at 405 nm by a Micro-ELISA Auto Reader, MR580 (Dynatech, Alexandria, VA). The values of anti-HTLV antibodies were expressed as a unit of the standard serum containing 100 units/ml of antibody, which corresponds to 200 ng/ml of IgG measured by a solid-phase ELISA.

RESULTS

Figure 1 illustrates the representative HTLV antigen binding of serum from an adult T cell leukemia patient, using ELISA techniques. This ATL serum had antibodies reactive with HTLV proteins. Sodium dodecyl sulfate–polyacrylamide gel electrophoretic

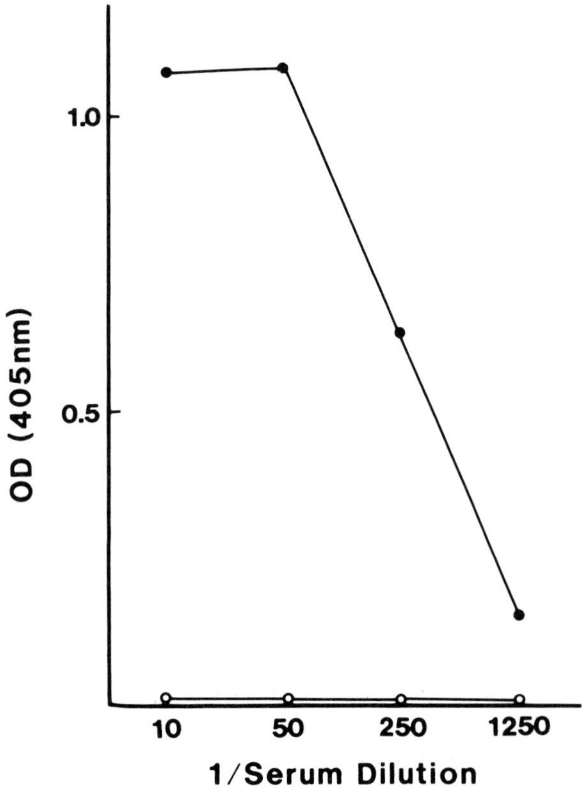

Figure 1. Binding of the human T cell leukemia virus antigen by antibodies in sera of a representative patient with adult T cell leukemia (●) and a healthy individual (○).

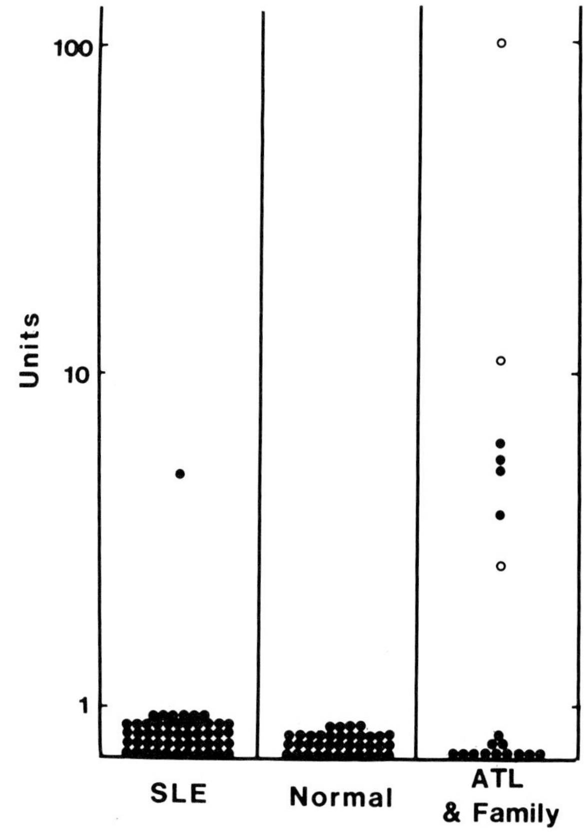

Figure 2. Levels of anti–human T cell leukemia virus antibodies in sera from 51 systemic lupus erythematosus (SLE) patients, 37 healthy individuals, and 3 adult T cell leukemia (ATL) patients (○) and 16 of their family members (●).

(SDS-PAGE) analysis of the HTLV antigens used in this study identified the major viral structure proteins p15, p19, p23, and gp65. The proteins p15, p19, and p23 seem to be identical with the *gag* gene product, and gp65 seems to be identical with the *env* gene product of the HTLV, which have been reported by Seiki et al (14) and Hattori et al (15), respectively. SDS-PAGE was also used to analyze the ATL patient serum used as a standard in this study, and we confirmed that the standard had antibodies to these structure proteins of the HTLV genome (data not shown).

To determine whether SLE serum contained antibodies to the HTLV antigens, we performed the same ELISA studies on sera from 51 patients with active SLE who had no history of leukemia/lymphoma or blood transfusion, 3 patients with ATL and 16 of their family members, and sera from 37 healthy individuals. As shown in Figure 2, all 3 ATL patient sera tested and 4 (25%) of the 16 sera from ATL patient family members were positive for antibodies to the HTLV antigens. Of the 51 SLE patient sera tested, only 1 (1.96%) was positive for antibodies to HTLV structure proteins, and none of the 37 sera from healthy individuals was positive for these antibodies. No evidence of leukemia or lymphoma was observed in the antibody-positive SLE patient.

DISCUSSION

It can be said that an endogenous type C virus is involved in the murine model of SLE, since 1) type C virus–like particles and high concentrations of murine viral antigens are present in the tissues of New Zealand black mice (6); 2) a spontaneously expressed xenotropic virus can be isolated from virtually all tissues of New Zealand black mice affected with SLE (7); and 3) the pathogenesis of immune complex glomerulonephritis is significantly related to the deposition of viral envelope glycoprotein gp70 in the glomeruli of mice with SLE (8).

Much effort has been directed toward study of the participation of the virus (especially the type C oncornavirus) in the pathogenesis of human SLE, principally because of its role in murine SLE. Strand and August (1), using competitive radioimmunoassay techniques, found that tissues from SLE patients contained type C–related proteins. Mellors and Mellors (2) reported that an antigen recognized by antisera produced against the p30 (core proteins) of some mammalian (murine and feline) type C viruses was located in some renal glomeruli of humans with SLE; the antigen existed in the form of immune complexes. Furthermore, Panem et al (3) found a putative human type C virus isolated in glomeruli of all of their 11 SLE patients studied.

The human T cell leukemia virus is an exogenously acquired human type C RNA tumor virus that affects T cells, and it is isolated from patients with leukemia and lymphoma (9). Epidemiologic studies on the distribution of antibodies to HTLV in humans revealed clusters of positive sera in groups of patients with adult T cell leukemia, a unique leukemia of T cell origin that has been recognized in Japan, and in some family members of ATL patients in certain parts of Japan where the disease is endemic (16). Recently, Seiki et al (14) isolated molecular clones containing provirus genomes of HTLV and determined the complete nucleotide sequence of HTLV. Analyses of this sequence revealed 3 large open-reading frames, which, from their sequence characteristics and location in the viral genome, were concluded to be *gag*, *pol*, and *env* genes (11,14,15).

It has also been shown that sera from patients with ATL contained antibodies which were reactive with the gene products of *gag* and *env* (13,15). Very recently, Miyoshi et al (including author TK of the present study) (17) reported evidence for the deposition of HTLV antigens, apparently as immune complexes, in the glomeruli of an ATL patient.

Based on observations of the participation of endogenous type C virus or the virus gene products and their corresponding antibodies in the development of murine SLE, together with data from the recently isolated human type C retrovirus (the HTLV), we attempted to clarify the role of HTLV and its antibodies in the pathogenesis of human SLE. We designed a solid-phase ELISA technique for the detection of antibodies to HTLV. Using this assay and SDS-PAGE, we confirmed the presence of antibodies in the sera of ATL patients and their family members, and we found the antibodies to be reactive with HTLV gene products p15, p19, p23, and gp65. Our assay revealed no anti-HTLV antibodies in the sera of our normal healthy population, and of 51 patients with active SLE, only 1 patient showed positive results.

According to the results of our studies, there is no evidence to indicate that the type C virus or its antibodies participate in the development of human SLE. However, the HTLV nucleic acid sequence has not been found in normal human DNA, and researchers have concluded that HTLV is not an endogenous human type C virus (10,11). Therefore, whether the true endogenous type C virus of human origin participates in human SLE is still to be determined.

ACKNOWLEDGMENTS

We are grateful for the support and advice of Professor M. Taniguchi, Department of Immunology, School of Medicine, Chiba University and Dr. Takashi Yoshiki, Department of Pathology, Sapporo City General Hospital. We also thank M. Ohara, Kyushu University, for reading the manuscript.

REFERENCES

1. Strand M, August JT: Type-C RNA virus gene expression in human tissue. J Virol 14:1584–1596, 1974
2. Mellors RC, Mellors JW: Antigen related to mammalian

type-C RNA viral p30 proteins is located in renal glomeruli in human systemic lupus erythematosus. Proc Natl Acad Sci USA 73:233–237, 1976
3. Panem S, Ordonez NG, Kirstein WH, Katz AI, Spargo BH: C-type virus expression in systemic lupus erythematosus. N Engl J Med 295:470–475, 1976
4. Imamura M, Phillips PE, Mellors RC: The occurrence and frequency of type C virus-like particle in placentas from patients with SLE and from normal subjects. Am J Pathol 83:383–394, 1976
5. Phillips PE: Type C oncornavirus studies in systemic lupus erythematosus. Arthritis Rheum (suppl) 21:S76–S88, 1978
6. Mellors RC, Huang CY: Immunopathology of NZB/BL mice. V. Virus like (filterable) agent separable from lymphoma cells and identifiable by electron microscopy. J Exp Med 124:1031–1038, 1966
7. Levy JA, Pincus T: Demonstration of biological activity of a murine leukemia virus of New Zealand black mice. Science 170:326–327, 1970
8. Yoshiki T, Mellors RC, Strand M, August JT: The viral envelope glycoprotein of murine leukemia virus and the pathogenesis of immune complex glomerulonephritis of New Zealand mice. J Exp Med 140:1011–1027, 1974
9. Poiesz BJ, Ruscetti FW, Gazdar AF, Bunn PA, Minna JD, Gallo RC: Detection and isolation of type C retrovirus particles from fresh and cultured lymphocytes of a patient with cutaneous T-cell lymphoma. Proc Natl Acad Sci USA 77:7415–7419, 1980
10. Reitz MS Jr, Poiesz BJ, Ruscetti FW, Gallo RC: Characterization and distribution of nucleic acid sequences of a novel type C retrovirus isolated from neoplastic human T lymphocytes. Proc Natl Acad Sci USA 78:1887–1891, 1981
11. Yoshida M: Human leukemia virus associated with adult T-cell leukemia. Gann 74:777–789, 1983
12. Tan EM, Cohen AS, Fries JF, Masi AT, McShane DJ, Rothfield NF, Schaller JG, Talal N, Winfield RJ: The 1982 revised criteria for the classification of systemic lupus erythematosus. Arthritis Rheum 25:1271–1277, 1982
13. Saxinger C, Gallo RC: Methods in laboratory investigation: application of the indirect enzyme-linked immunosorbent assay microtest to the detection and surveillance of human T cell leukemia-lymphoma virus. Lab Invest 49:371–377, 1983
14. Seiki M, Hattori S, Hirayama Y, Yoshida M: Human adult T cell leukemia virus: complete nucleotide sequence of the provirus genome integrated in leukemia cell DNA. Proc Natl Acad Sci USA 80:3618–3622, 1983
15. Hattori S, Imagawa K, Shimizu F, Hashimoto E, Seiki M, Yoshida M: Identification of envelope glycoprotein encoded by env gene of human T-cell leukemia virus. Gann 74:790–793, 1983
16. Hinuma Y, Nagata K, Hanaoka M, Nakai M, Matsumoto T, Kinoshita I, Shirakawa S, Miyoshi I: Adult T-cell leukemia: antigen in an ATL cell line and detection of antibodies to the antigen in human sera. Proc Natl Acad Sci USA 78:6476–6480, 1981
17. Miyoshi I, Yoshimoto S, Ohtsuki Y, Fujishita M, Akagi T, Yoshiki T, Koike T: Adult T-cell leukemia antigen in renal glomeruli. Lancet I:769–770, 1983

WHEN DOES RHEUMATOID DISEASE START?

K. AHO, T. PALOSUO, V. RAUNIO, P. PUSKA, A. AROMAA, and J. T. SALONEN

Stored serum specimens collected in connection with a community-oriented epidemiologic study were available from 30 subjects who later developed seropositive rheumatoid arthritis. In 9 of these pre-rheumatoid specimens, the Rose-Waaler test result was positive, and in 16, the latex fixation test was positive. Two-thirds of the samples were positive when the interval between taking the blood specimen and onset of the disease was <4 years, and one-third were positive when the interval was ≥4 years. The occurrence of rheumatoid factor preceded the onset of clinical disease more often in males than in females.

Recent discussion on the pathogenesis of rheumatoid arthritis (RA) has focused on the relationships between host genetic factors, immunologically-mediated tissue injury, and an inciting agent (1).

The main humoral feature seen in RA is rheumatoid factor (RF) with autologous IgG (2,3). The resulting complexes can activate complement in rheumatoid joints and extraarticularly, with all the inflammatory consequences. In fact, IgG autosensitization may be the main driving force in the perpetuation of the chronic immune reaction in rheumatoid synovium (4). Several other antibodies are also found with significantly higher frequency in RA patients than in other subjects (5). They may be only secondary manifestations of the inflammatory process, but they can provide additional clues to pathogenetic mechanisms. A basic problem in understanding the immunologic evolution of rheumatoid lesions is knowing what extraneous agent(s) constitutes the original stimulus that generates the above responses, or whether they arise de novo.

Autoantibodies have been detected several years before actual diagnosis in subjects with hypothyroidism; it has been suggested that the prolonged autoimmune process results in disease (6,7). The same may be true for certain other organ-specific autoimmune diseases (8). It is difficult to draw parallels between the slowly evolving endocrinopathies and RA, in which the onset can be fixed with an accuracy of weeks or at least of a few months. However, it would be important to know at what phase the immunologic markers of RA appear. No hard facts about this are available.

In this study we investigated the occurrence of RF prior to the onset of clinical RA.

PATIENTS AND METHODS

Two independent, cross-sectional surveys of random population samples were carried out in 1972 and 1977 in 2 provinces in eastern Finland in connection with the North Karelia project, a community-based preventive study on

From the National Public Health Institute, Helsinki; the Social Insurance Institution of Finland, Helsinki; and the Department of Community Health, University of Kuopio, Kuopio, Finland.

Supported by a grant from the Medical Research Council, the Academy of Finland.

K. Aho, MD: Professor and Head, Department of Immunobiology, National Public Health Institute; T. Palosuo, MD: Head of Laboratory, Department of Immunobiology, National Public Health Institute; V. Raunio, MD: Professor and Deputy Director, National Public Health Institute; P. Puska, MD: Professor and Head, Department of Epidemiology, National Public Health Institute; A. Aromaa, MD: Director, Medical Research Group, Social Insurance Institution of Finland; J. T. Salonen, MD, MPH: Professor of Epidemiology, Department of Community Health, University of Kuopio.

Address reprint requests to Dr. K. Aho, National Public Health Institute, SF-00280, Helsinki 28, Finland.

Submitted for publication May 21, 1984; accepted in revised form November 7, 1984.

cardiovascular diseases (9). A total of 11,873 persons aged 25–59 (born 1913–1947) participated in the baseline survey performed in 1972. A different sample of 10,199 persons aged 30–64 (born 1913–1947) participated in the 5-year follow-up survey carried out in 1977.

Participants in these surveys who either had established RA during the survey or who later developed RA were identified by linking the data from these surveys with those of the Finnish Sickness Insurance Register (up to the end of year 1982), using the unique identification number assigned to each Finnish citizen. Since 1966, under the Sickness Insurance Act, no charges are made for drugs prescribed for certain chronic diseases, including RA. The sickness insurance covers the entire population of Finland, and virtually all patients fulfilling the criteria take advantage of the program. Eligibility requires a comprehensive document written by the attending physician and approved by an expert adviser on behalf of the sickness insurance system.

These written documents were used to select the study subjects, using the following criteria: 1) the patient had been granted the right to free medication because of RA (all patients had polyarthritis, and in most of them it was symmetric); 2) tests for RF were known to be positive at some phase of the disease; and 3) the onset of the disease (including transient joint swellings occasionally preceding the persistent arthritis) was unequivocally known to have occurred during the period after sampling of the blood.

Sera from about 1,500 subjects chosen from the baseline survey (in 1972) had been tested for RF in connection with studies reported in part elsewhere (10). Eight of them had developed RA which met the above criteria after the initial survey. Serum from the remaining subjects in the baseline survey was no longer available. In the 1977 survey population there were 24 subjects who later developed RA; serum was available from 22 of them.

The documents recommending free medication for these 30 subjects originated from the Rheumatism Foundation Hospital (5 subjects), Kuopio University Central Hospital (6 subjects), a specialist rheumatologist working in a general hospital (7 subjects) and at an outpatient clinic for rheumatic diseases (4 subjects), a specialist in internal medicine working in a general hospital (4 subjects), a general practitioner working at an outpatient clinic for rheumatic diseases (2 subjects) and at a communal health center (1 subject), and a specialist in internal medicine in private practice (1 subject).

Stored serum specimens from an additional 21 subjects who had participated in the 1977 survey, who already had established RA based on the same criteria when the blood specimen was taken, and who were known to be RF-positive at some phase were used as controls.

The Rose-Waaler test for RF was performed on microtiter plates with U-shaped wells. Sheep red blood cells were sensitized with one-third of the minimum agglutinating dose. The plates were stored overnight at 4°C in a refrigerator, after which the readings were made on the basis of sedimentation patterns. Titers ≥64 were regarded as positive; such titers are seen in about 2% of nonrheumatoid subjects.

The latex fixation test was performed on heat-inactivated 1:20 diluted serum with equipment devised for the VDRL test for syphilis. The baseline specimens were tested using Hyland (Costa Mesa, CA) reagents, and the followup specimens were tested using reagents from Behringwerke (Marburg, West Germany). About 5% of control sera from the baseline survey reacted with the Hyland reagents (10), while the test using the Behringwerke reagents yielded a slightly lower frequency of positive reactions.

RESULTS

Testing for RF was performed on sera from the 30 subjects who developed seropositive RA a few months to 9 years after the survey (Table 1). Fifteen of the subjects were men and 15 were women. The mean age of the men at the onset of RA was 51; that of the women was 49.

The Rose-Waaler test was positive in 9 instances, and the latex fixation test was positive in 16 (Table 2). All samples that were positive by the Rose-Waaler test were also positive by the latex fixation test. The Rose-Waaler titers in the positive

Table 1. Occurrence of rheumatoid factor in individual subjects, in relation to the interval to onset of clinical disease

Sample year	Sex	Age at onset	Rose-Waaler titer	Latex fixation test	Interval to onset (years)
1972	M	41	0	+	5
	F	58	0	−	9
	M	57	0	−	6½
	M	47	0	−	½
	F	51	0	−	¼
	F	40	0	−	3
	M	41	64	+	2
	M	58	0	−	9
1977	M	68	32	+	4
	F	48	0	+	1¼
	F	44	0	−	5
	M	41	0	+	½
	F	60	256	+	5
	F	46	0	−	2
	M	32	64	+	½
	F	33	128	+	3
	M	62	0	+	½
	M	44	256	+	5
	F	54	0	−	4
	M	43	32	+	4
	F	57	0	−	4
	F	54	0	−	4
	M	61	128	+	3½
	F	56	0	−	4
	F	38	0	−	4
	M	41	256	+	⅓
	M	57	32	+	1
	F	40	128	+	4
	M	65	256	+	1½
	F	62	0	−	4

Table 2. Occurrence of rheumatoid factor in pre–rheumatoid arthritis (RA) sera

	No. of samples	Positive samples: Rose-Waaler	Positive samples: Latex fixation
Time to onset of RA			
<4 years	14	6	10
≥4 years	16	3	6
Sex			
Male	15	6	12
Female	15	3	4
Age at onset of RA			
<50	15	6	10
≥50	15	3	6

samples ranged from 64–256; the mean log titer of the positive samples was 150.

Two-thirds of the sera were RF-positive when the interval between blood sampling and the onset of clinically manifest arthritis was <4 years, and one-third were positive when the interval was 4 years or longer (Table 2). In 6 cases the interval was <1 year; 4 of these patients were RF-positive. Positive RF reactions preceded the clinical disease more often in males than in females and more often in subjects under 50 years of age than in subjects 50 years or older at the onset of RA (Table 2).

The interval between blood sampling and the onset of RA was, on the average, shorter in males than in females (<4 years in 9 males and 5 females). When the interval was controlled for by stratification into 5 periods (<2 years, 2–2½, 3–3½, 4–4½, and ≥5 years), the proportion of men with positive tests was 8.6 times greater than that of women (Mantel-Haenszel chi-square 5.48; $P < 0.05$).

Stored serum specimens from the 21 control patients with established RA who were known to be RF-positive at some phase since the time of the survey were analyzed using the same tests. The Rose-Waaler test was positive in 9 instances, and the latex fixation test was positive in 15. The Rose-Waaler titers in the positive specimens ranged from 64–1,024. The mean log titer of the positive samples was 220, only slightly higher than in the pre-rheumatoid sera.

DISCUSSION

Many early studies dealing with clinical correlations of rheumatoid factor showed a lower frequency of positive reactions in patients with recently diagnosed arthritis than in those with disease of longer duration (11). However, many of the seronegative cases with short duration were most likely transient, infection-associated arthropathies rather than RA. With increasing knowledge of the clinical, immunologic, and immunogenetic characteristics of the inflammatory arthritis syndromes, the concept of RA has emerged more clearly (12). In cohort studies, the RF test has been positive when first performed in the majority of cases, although a minority of patients have developed seropositivity only later in the disease (13–15).

Followup of subjects with false-positive RF reactions encountered in population surveys has demonstrated the subsequent development of RA in a few cases (16,17). Thus, the appearance of RF can, at least occasionally, herald other manifestations of the disease. In a few other patients, however, the serologic conversion has been observed to occur simultaneously with or after the development of clinical arthritis (18).

Recently, there has been renewed interest in the relative times of appearance of immunologic parameters such as antiglobulins, antibodies against Epstein-Barr virus–induced nuclear antigen, and circulating immune complexes in early RA (19–22). In the present work we extended these studies beyond the onset of clinical disease. Only patients in whom the disease onset could be fixed unequivocally to the period after blood sampling were included as study subjects.

Our findings indicate that the appearance of RF positivity frequently precedes the onset of clinical RA by years. Similar conclusions were reached in a smaller population series, in which serial blood samples from all the study subjects had been tested (23). It would be interesting to learn whether there are eventual changes in titer due to possible tissue deposition in conjunction with the onset of arthritis, but the data do not allow conclusions concerning this.

The occurrence of RF preceded the clinical disease more often in men than in women. In this regard it should be recalled that certain systemic manifestations of RA, such as pleuropulmonary manifestations, are more frequent in men, and they occasionally precede the joint disease (24). It is possible that the recognized syndromes represent only the tip of the iceberg, and that low-grade involvement of the lower respiratory tract occurs very frequently.

Taking into account the incidence of seropositive RA and the frequency of positive RF reactions in the population, it can be estimated on the basis of the present data that only a small minority, roughly 5%, of the subjects with false-positive RF reactions will develop RA. In subjects with strong positive reactions this figure is probably higher (23). The very fact that followup studies comprising only a few thousand person-years have revealed such cases strongly supports our contention that RF reactivity frequently precedes clinical RA by long periods.

A key question is whether the RF differs between those subjects who will develop RA and the rest of the population, either in its genesis and/or in some molecular characteristic. Certain inferences can be drawn by comparing RF from patients with established RA with that from subjects with false-positive reactions (of whom the great majority will not develop RA). IgG rheumatoid factor (IgG-RF) represents one obvious potential answer. However, subjects with RA and those with false-positive RF reactions do not seem to differ with respect to the occurrence of IgG-RF (25,26).

The association of RA with certain HLA–D locus antigens clearly indicates that there is a genetic component operating in this disease. However, RF in healthy subjects is determined predominantly by environmental factors (27,28). How can the pieces of the puzzle be arranged to give a meaningful picture of the whole?

One tentative model postulates the existence of a distinct form of abortive RA (benign polyarthritis), which will evolve into chronic RA under appropriate conditions (29). In this model, pre-morbid factors, such as preexisting autoantibodies, will direct the subsequent development of the disease. The right type of autoantibody being present at the right time in the right place (e.g., inflammatory joint exudate) will complete a vicious circle.

Experimental evidence has identified 3 types of environmental stimuli that can induce RF production: immunization with aggregated or altered IgG in the form of antigen–antibody complexes, polyclonal B cell activation, and unexplained cross-reaction between IgG and exogenous antigens (3). However, the problem of the very frequent occurrence of RF in patients with RA remains. Several possible explanations, not mutually exclusive, have been proposed to account for this (30): (a) a genetic predisposition of RA patients to produce autoreactive antiglobulins; (b) a hitherto unknown, very efficient antigenic stimulus, possibly of viral origin, that maintains a hyperimmune state with a continuing in vivo formation of antigen–antibody complexes; and (c) specific conditions in the diseased joints and other organs that lead to enzymatic degradation or denaturation of IgG. A further possibility along different lines is that an abortive RA selects its pathogenetic autoantibody, RF, which renders the disease chronic.

Whatever the mechanisms considered in the induction of RF, it is clear that the crux of the immunologic reactivity in RA is not to be found in the early phases of joint disease, but frequently far earlier. This imposes investigative constraints, but also opens new prospects concerning hypotheses on the pathogenesis of RA. Practical implications with respect to patients presenting with recent joint afflictions are clear: if the test for RF is negative, it is unlikely that it will become positive later.

REFERENCES

1. Bennett JC: The etiology of rheumatoid arthritis, Textbook of Rheumatology. Edited by WN Kelley, ED Harris Jr, S Ruddy, CB Sledge. Philadelphia, WB Saunders, 1981, pp 887–895
2. Natvig JB, Mellbye OJ: Immunology in the pathogenesis of rheumatoid arthritis. Triangle 18:39–44, 1979
3. Carson DA: Rheumatoid factor, Textbook of Rheumatology. Edited by WN Kelley, ED Harris Jr, S Ruddy, CB Sledge. Philadelphia, WB Saunders, 1981, pp 677–690
4. Roitt IM, Hay FC, Nineham LJ, Male DK: Rheumatoid arthritis, Clinical Aspects of Immunology. Fourth edition. Edited by PJ Lachmann, DK Peters. Oxford, Blackwell Scientific Publications, 1982, pp 1161–1195
5. Holborow EJ: Autoantibodies in rheumatoid arthritis. Clin Immunol Allergy 1:127–138, 1981
6. Doniach D, Bottazzo GF, Russell RCG: Goitrous autoimmune thyroiditis (Hashimoto's disease). Clin Endocrinol Metab 8:63–80, 1979
7. Lamberg B-A: Aetiology of hypothyroidism. Clin Endocrinol Metab 8:3–19, 1979
8. Smith CID, Hammarström L: When does an autoimmune disease start? Immunology Today 4:273–274, 1983
9. Puska P, Salonen JT, Nissinen A, Tuomilehto J, Vartiainen E, Korhonen H, Tanskanen A, Rönnqvist P, Koskela K, Huttunen J: Changes in risk factors for coronary heart disease during 10 years of a community intervention programme (North Karelia project). Br Med J 287:1840–1844, 1983
10. Aho K, Salonen JT, Puska P: Autoantibodies predicting death due to cardiovascular disease. Cardiology 69:125–129, 1982
11. Sievers K: The rheumatoid factor in definite rheumatoid arthritis. Acta Rheumatol Scand (suppl 9):1–121, 1965
12. Masi AT, Feigenbaum SL: Seronegative rheumatoid arthritis: fact or fiction? Arch Intern Med 143:2167–2172, 1983

13. Otten HA, Boerma FW: Significance of the Waaler-Rose test, streptococcal agglutination, and antistreptolysin titre in the prognosis of rheumatoid arthritis. Ann Rheum Dis 18:24–28, 1959
14. Jacoby RK, Jayson MIV, Cosh JA: Onset, early stages, and prognosis of rheumatoid arthritis: a clinical study of 100 patients with 11-year follow-up. Br Med J 2:96–100, 1973
15. Masi AT, Maldonado-Cocco JA, Kaplan SB, Feigenbaum SL, Chandler RW: Prospective study of the early course of rheumatoid arthritis in young adults: comparison of patients with and without rheumatoid factor positivity at entry and identification of variables correlating with outcome. Semin Arthritis Rheum 5:299–326, 1976
16. Kellgren JH: Epidemiology of rheumatoid arthritis. Arthritis Rheum 9:658–674, 1966
17. Thorsteinsson J, Björnsson OJ, Kolbeinsson A, Allander E, Sigfusson N, Olofsson O: A population study of rheumatoid factor in Iceland. Ann Clin Res 7:183–194, 1975
18. Hall AP: Observations on subjects developing a positive test for rheumatoid factor in a prospective study (abstract). Arthritis Rheum 12:301, 1969
19. Male D, Young A, Pilkington C, Sutherland S, Roitt IM: Antibodies to EB virus- and cytomegalovirus-induced antigens in early rheumatoid disease. Clin Exp Immunol 50:341–346, 1982
20. Hay FC, Young A, Jones MG, Nineham LJ, Male DK, Roitt IM: Anti-globulins and circulating complexes in early rheumatoid arthritis. Clin Exp Immunol 54:723–730, 1983
21. Jones VE, Jacoby RK, Wallington T, Holt P: Immune complexes in early arthritis. I. Detection of immune complexes before rheumatoid arthritis is definite. Clin Exp Immunol 44:512–521, 1981
22. Jones VE, Jacoby RK, Cowley PJ, Warren C: Immune complexes in early arthritis. II. Immune complex constituents are synthesized in the synovium before rheumatoid factors. Clin Exp Immunol 49:31–40, 1982
23. Aho K, Palosuo T, Niemelä J, Takala J: Rheumatoid factor seroconversions in relation to clinical rheumatoid arthritis. Ann Clin Res (in press)
24. Turner-Warwick M, Evans RC: Pulmonary manifestations of rheumatoid disease. Clin Rheum Dis 3:549–564, 1977
25. Palosuo T, Aho K, Punsar S: IgG-rheumatoid factor in a population of elderly males: relationship to IgM-rheumatoid factor and rheumatoid arthritis. Clin Exp Rheumatol 1:311–315, 1983
26. Palosuo T, Aho K, Raunio V, Kaarela K: IgG-rheumatoid factor in seronegative rheumatoid arthritis (abstract). Scand J Rheumatol (suppl 52):79, 1984
27. O'Brien WM, Bennett PH, Burch TA, Bunim JJ: A genetic study of rheumatoid arthritis and rheumatoid factor in Blackfeet and Pima Indians. Arthritis Rheum 10:163–179, 1967
28. Aho K, Sistonen P, Takala J, Sievers K: Genetics of autoantibodies in relation to disease. Acta Med Scand 211:213–218, 1982
29. Aho K, Raunio V: EB-virus and rheumatoid arthritis: new insights into their interrelation. Med Biol 60:49–52, 1982
30. Aho K, Somer T, Salo OP: Rheumatoid factor and immuno-conglutinin responses following various vaccinations. Proc Soc Exp Biol Med 124:229–233, 1967

NIFEDIPINE AND ESOPHAGEAL DYSFUNCTION IN PROGRESSIVE SYSTEMIC SCLEROSIS

A Controlled Manometric Study

ANDRÉ KAHAN, BRUNO BOUR, DANIEL COUTURIER, BERNARD AMOR, and CHARLES J. MENKES

We evaluated the effect of the calcium channel blocking agent, nifedipine, on esophageal dysfunction in 15 patients with progressive systemic sclerosis, using a double-blind, randomized, crossover, placebo-controlled manometric study. Nifedipine significantly decreased lower esophageal sphincter pressure in these patients; this reduced lower esophageal sphincter pressure may cause gastroesophageal reflux. Thus, nifedipine may have detrimental effects on progressive systemic sclerosis patients.

The pathogenesis of esophageal dysfunction in progressive systemic sclerosis (scleroderma; PSS) has not been well elucidated (1,2). PSS is characterized by vascular and microvascular abnormalities (1–4), excessive fibroblastic activity (5,6), and collagen deposition in numerous organs (1,2,7). The possibility that the lesions in target organs are a reflection of a primary fibrous tissue overgrowth leading to secondary vascular compromise has not been ruled out. Nevertheless, a growing body of evidence based on studies of several organs involved in PSS suggests that the vascular system per se may be the primary target organ and that the lesions are a manifestation of focal ischemic injury resulting from functional, with or without accompanying structural, vascular disease (1–4,8–14).

Nifedipine, a calcium channel blocking agent, is effective in the treatment of coronary vasospasm (15–18). We (19–21) and others (22–25) have shown that nifedipine is effective in the treatment of idiopathic Raynaud's phenomenon and Raynaud's phenomenon occurring with progressive systemic sclerosis. Thus, if a microvascular abnormality is a contributor to the pathogenesis of scleroderma, nifedipine may be useful in the treatment of patients with early disease.

However, nifedipine may have detrimental effects caused by its direct action on the lower esophageal sphincter. The actions of nifedipine on smooth muscle cells are well documented (15–18). Several studies have shown that the drug decreases the lower esophageal sphincter pressure (LESP) in patients with achalasia (26,27). If nifedipine also decreases the LESP in patients with progressive systemic sclerosis, this could lead to gastroesophageal reflux.

In the present investigation, we used a controlled, double-blind, randomized, crossover manometric study to evaluate the effect of nifedipine on 15 patients with progressive systemic sclerosis and esophageal dysfunction. Our trial demonstrates that nifedipine significantly decreases the lower esophageal sphincter pressure in patients with PSS.

PATIENTS AND METHODS

Patients. Fifteen patients with progressive systemic sclerosis and diffuse scleroderma were studied. All patients satisfied the American Rheumatism Association preliminary criteria for classification of definite systemic sclerosis (28). None of the patients had the CREST syndrome variant (calcinosis, Raynaud's phenomenon, esophageal dysmo-

Presented in part at the 48th Annual Meeting of the American Rheumatism Association, Minneapolis, MN, June 1984.

From the Departments of Rheumatology and Gastroenterology, René Descartes University, School of Medicine, Hôpital Cochin, Paris, France.

André Kahan, MD: Department of Rheumatology; Bruno Bour, MD: Department of Gastroenterology; Daniel Couturier, MD: Department of Gastroenterology; Bernard Amor, MD: Department of Rheumatology; Charles J. Menkes, MD: Department of Rheumatology.

Address reprint requests to André Kahan, MD, Department of Rheumatology, Hôpital Cochin, 27 Rue du Fg Saint-Jacques, 75674 Paris Cedex 14, France.

Submitted for publication June 11, 1984; accepted in revised form December 20, 1984.

tility, sclerodactyly, telangiectasias) of PSS (29). The presence of the esophageal symptoms of heartburn and dysphagia was determined by direct questioning. All patients had abnormal results on basal esophageal manometric studies. Informed consent was obtained from all participants.

Thirteen of the 15 patients were women. The mean age (±SD) was 47.4 ± 12.1 years (range 18–67). The duration of disease ranged from 2–24 years (mean ± SD, 11.5 ± 7.6 years). All 15 patients had Raynaud's phenomenon, and 8 had a history of digital ulcers. All patients had normal serum creatinine concentrations (76 ± 13 μmoles/liter, mean ± SD). Three patients had associated Sjögren's syndrome. Four patients had pulmonary involvement (abnormal forced vital capacity, lung diffusion capacity, or chest roentgenogram results); none of the patients had evidence (auscultation, electrocardiographic, roentgenographic, or echocardiographic) of significant pulmonary hypertension (1,2). Six of the 15 PSS patients reported a history of dysphagia with solid foods, 5 of them also had heartburn, i.e., a retrosternal burning pain radiating into the neck, with sour and bitter regurgitation.

Evaluation of esophageal dysfunction. The methods we used have been described in detail previously (30–32). In summary, patients were evaluated in the fasting state and in a supine position, using a triple-lumen assembly (inside diameter of each lumen, 1.1 mm) with radially oriented side ports (diameter, 1 mm) spaced 5 cm apart. Radial side-hole recording orifices were used to minimize the effects of LESP asymmetry as a source of recording error between pull-throughs. The polyvinyl catheters were perfused with distilled water (22°C) at 0.6 ml/minute, using a low-compliance pneumohydraulic capillary system (32). Occlusion of any orifice caused a rise in the recording pressure to >800 cm H_2O/second. Polyvinyl catheters were connected in series with Statham transducers (model P 23ID) and pressure tracings were recorded on a Beckman polygraph (model R 511A). The manometric system was calibrated in cm H_2O, with end-expiratory gastric pressure set at 0 as a reference point.

For manometry, the catheter assembly was passed via the mouth. The LESP was recorded by the conventional station pull-through technique and by a rapid pull-through technique (31). The station pull-through technique consisted of withdrawal of the radial recording tips through the LES in 0.5-cm increments, with a pause of 20 seconds or longer at each station; we assessed resting LESP by measuring peak LESP at the pressure inversion point. The rapid pull-through technique featured continuous manual withdrawal of the recording sensors through the LES at an approximate rate of 0.5–1.0 cm/second during a 10–15-second interval of suspended respiration. In our study and in those of others (30,31), LESP values measured by the rapid pull-through technique were similar to those determined by the station pull-through technique.

We averaged the pressure values obtained from the 3 radial recording sites to obtain a representative LESP value. At least 3 pull-throughs were performed. Using this method, reproducible LESP were obtained in normal subjects. LESP between 10–30 cm H_2O were considered normal. We also assessed LES relaxation following deglutition (several dry swallows were obtained in each patient).

To record esophageal peristalsis, the recording sensors were stationed in the distal esophagus, _
respectively, above the LES. Waves wer(
each lumen in response to 3 dry swallows (sp
apart). Waves were analyzed for amplitude
averaging, respectively, the height from the mean esophageal baseline to the peak and the width from the extrapolated onset of the rapid upstroke to the return to baseline. In the distal esophagus, peristaltic waves of 40–80 cm H_2O lasting 2–4 seconds were considered normal. Speed of contraction propagation was calculated in cm/second by dividing the 5-cm distance between 2 pressure orifices by the time required for the pressure front of the contractile wave to travel this distance.

Finally, the amplitude and duration of waves were recorded in the upper esophagus (5 cm below the upper esophageal sphincter).

The tracing was read by 2 of the authors, who were unaware of the patient's symptoms.

Protocol. Our protocol for manometry required that the patient take no medication (including alcohol, coffee, or cigarettes) for 48 hours before the study. After a baseline manometric recording, each patient received a single oral dose of 20 mg nifedipine or placebo; the manometric study was done 90 minutes after each drug or placebo administration. Nifedipine and placebo were assigned on a random, double-blind basis and were administered at the same time at 3-day intervals.

Statistical methods. The Student's *t*-test for paired data was used to evaluate the significance of the differences between the values at baseline and those obtained after placebo or nifedipine administration. P values <0.05 were considered significant.

RESULTS

Esophageal manometric findings. Results of the manometric studies are shown in Table 1. Baseline esophageal dysfunction was demonstrated by decreased or absent distal peristalsis in all 15 PSS patients. Eight patients had distal aperistalsis; 7 patients had a decrease in esophageal contraction amplitude, 5 of whom also had an increase in the duration of waves. Ten patients had normal baseline LESP (group I), and 5 had low basal LESP (group II). Four of the 10 patients with normal baseline LESP and 4 of the 5 patients with low baseline LESP had distal aperistalsis. Two patients with low baseline LESP and distal aperistalsis had heartburn and a history of dysphagia. Two patients with normal baseline LESP and distal aperistalsis had dysphagia, 1 of whom also had heartburn. Two patients with normal baseline LESP and low-amplitude distal esophageal contractions had heartburn and dysphagia.

Twelve patients had normal baseline upper esophageal peristalsis; 3 patients had a decrease in amplitude of peristaltic contractions in the upper esophagus (5 cm below the upper esophageal sphincter).

Table 1. Manometric characteristics of 15 patients with progressive systemic sclerosis and diffuse scleroderma, at baseline and after placebo and nifedipine administration*

	n	Baseline	Placebo	Nifedipine
LESP				
All patients	15	13.9 ± 7.7	13.8 ± 8.3	10.2 ± 5.7†
Group I	10	18.0 ± 5.8	18.2 ± 6.3	12.9 ± 5.1‡
Group II	5	5.6 ± 2.0	5.0 ± 2.2	4.9 ± 2.2
Waves				
Amplitude, 1 cm above LES	15	7.7 ± 8.7	7.5 ± 8.4	7.0 ± 7.9
Amplitude, 6 cm above LES	15	7.7 ± 8.8	7.6 ± 8.7	6.6 ± 7.6
Amplitude, 11 cm above LES	15	8.1 ± 9.1	8.1 ± 9.0	8.5 ± 9.7
Duration, 1 cm above LES	7	5.1 ± 1.8	4.5 ± 1.2	5.4 ± 1.0
Duration, 6 cm above LES	7	4.8 ± 1.1	4.6 ± 1.1	4.8 ± 0.9
Duration, 11 cm above LES	7	4.4 ± 1.4	4.5 ± 1.4	4.2 ± 1.0
Amplitude, 5 cm below UES	15	48.1 ± 26.1	47.1 ± 25.8	49.4 ± 25.9
Duration, 5 cm below UES	14	2.5 ± 0.7	2.5 ± 0.6	2.6 ± 0.8

* Amplitude in cm H_2O; duration in seconds. Eight patients had distal esophageal aperistalsis; the amplitude of distal esophageal contractions in these 8 patients was considered to be 0, and was taken into account in calculating the mean amplitude of distal esophageal waves in all 15 patients. The mean duration of distal esophageal contractions was calculated using the values obtained in the other 7 patients. One patient had upper esophageal aperistalsis; the amplitude of upper esophageal contractions in this patient was considered to be 0, and was taken into account in calculating the mean amplitude of upper esophageal waves (5 cm below the upper esophageal sphincter [UES]) in all 15 patients. The mean duration of upper esophageal waves was calculated using the values obtained in the other 14 patients. Group I = 10 patients with normal baseline lower esophageal sphincter pressure (LESP), in cm H_2O; Group II = 5 patients with low baseline LESP. Values are mean ± SD.
† $P < 0.005$ versus placebo; $P < 0.0025$ versus baseline.
‡ $P < 0.0025$ versus placebo; $P < 0.0025$ versus baseline.

The mean (±SD) baseline LESP of the total group was 13.9 ± 7.7 cm H_2O; it was 13.8 ± 8.3 cm H_2O in the placebo-treated patients and 10.2 ± 5.7 cm H_2O in the nifedipine-treated patients (Figure 1 and Table 1). Nifedipine treatment significantly decreased LESP when compared with values at baseline ($P < 0.0025$) and after placebo treatment ($P < 0.005$). The mean LESP values at baseline and after placebo treatment did not differ significantly.

Nifedipine induced a 25–50% decrease in LESP in 6 of the 10 patients with normal baseline LESP (group I) and in 1 of the 5 patients with low baseline LESP (group II). In group I, nifedipine significantly decreased LESP (12.9 ± 5.1 cm H_2O, mean ± SD) when compared with placebo (18.2 ± 6.3 cm H_2O; $P < 0.0025$) and with baseline values (18.0 ± 5.8 cm H_2O; $P < 0.0025$) (Table 1).

Other manometric characteristics were not significantly changed in the treated patients (Table 1). Nifedipine did not significantly modify the amplitude, duration, or speed of waves in the distal esophagus, or the LES relaxation. The amplitude and duration of waves in the upper esophagus (5 cm below the upper esophageal sphincter) were similar at baseline and after placebo and nifedipine administration.

DISCUSSION

Esophageal involvement occurs in up to 90% of patients with progressive systemic sclerosis (1,2,7,33–44). Esophageal manometric studies often demonstrate abnormalities in the portion of the esophagus containing smooth muscle (the distal one-half to two-thirds), with diminished amplitude or absence of peristaltic waves. A decrease or absence of pressure in the lower esophageal sphincter is frequently noted (1,2,35–39,41–44). These abnormalities may lead to dysphagia, heartburn, and reflux esophagitis. Patients may have dysphagia secondary to either an esophageal stricture or to disturbed esophageal peristalsis. The incomplete functioning of the lower esophageal sphincter allows gastroesophageal reflux; weakened peristaltic contractions in the lower esophagus fail to clear this refluxed gastric acid, and acid remains in contact with the esophageal mucosa for a longer period of time, causing esophagitis (1,2,42–44).

Several reports have emphasized the possible vascular and microvascular pathogenesis of progressive systemic sclerosis (1–4). On histopathologic examination, the digital arteries of patients with scleroderma reveal striking intimal hyperplasia, leading in the majority of cases to severe attenuation of the arterial lumen (45). Similar histopathologic changes are evident in the small arteries of the gastrointestinal tract, lungs, and kidneys (4,7). Transient nonperfusion or Raynaud's phenomenon of the digits (1,2), kidneys (10,11), lungs (12,13), and heart (8,9) probably accounts for many of the morphologic changes observed in these organs (1,2).

Recent findings of an ultrastructural study of

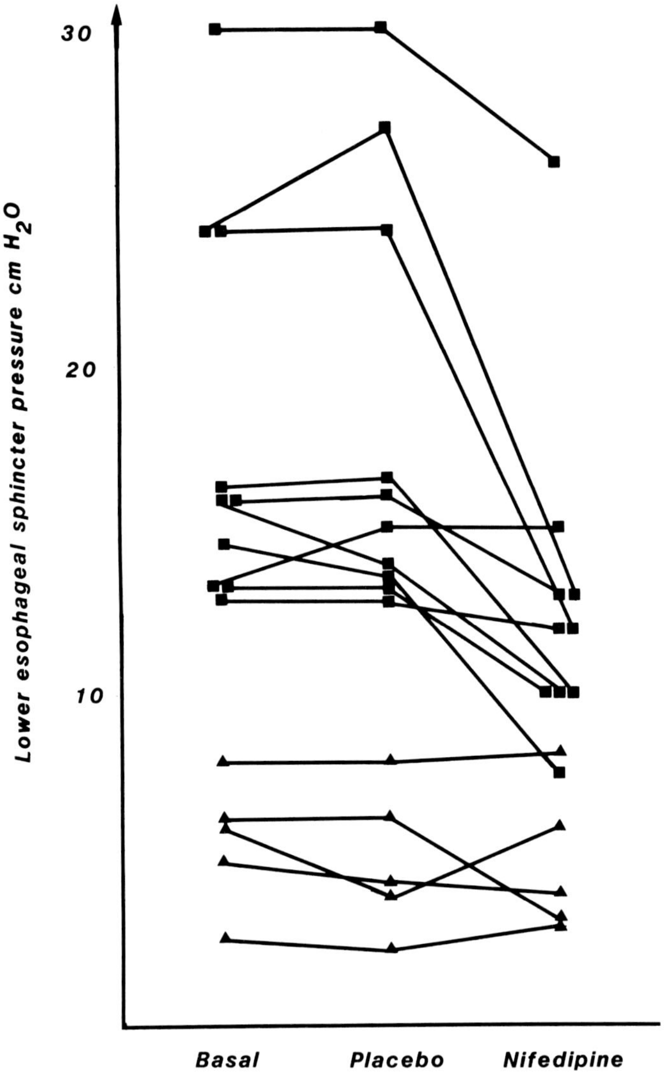

Figure 1. Effect of nifedipine on lower esophageal sphincter pressure (LESP) in 15 patients with progressive systemic sclerosis and diffuse scleroderma. Lower esophageal sphincter pressure in each individual patient is shown for the baseline state and after placebo and nifedipine administration. ■ = group I: 10 patients with normal baseline LESP; ▲ = group II: 5 patients with low baseline LESP.

the esophagus (46) also supported a primary vascular cause, rather than a neurogenic (47) or myopathic process, of esophageal dysfunction in progressive systemic sclerosis. Thus, a functional, with or without accompanying structural, vascular disease may be an important contributor to the pathogenesis of PSS. The calcium channel blocking agent, nifedipine, which causes vasodilation (15–25), may be effective in early stages of the disease in preventing some vasospastic events that could lead to the long-term damage often found in scleroderma; thus, we would recommend the use of nifedipine in the treatment of early PSS.

However, our manometric findings should be taken into account when nifedipine is being considered as a treatment for patients with scleroderma. The major observation in this study was that nifedipine significantly decreased the lower esophageal sphincter pressure in these patients. It should be emphasized that nifedipine-induced reduction in LESP was striking in patients with normal baseline LESP. This effect is probably due to the block of calcium transmembrane influx, which determines the LES tone, both under baseline conditions and after administration of some agonists (48,49).

Thus, nifedipine, which decreases the LESP, may have a detrimental effect on patients with progressive systemic sclerosis. An incompletely functioning lower esophageal sphincter fails to provide a barrier to reflux of gastric acid into the esophagus, which may cause esophagitis. Moreover, gastroesophageal reflux may be responsible for chronic aspiration; thus, nifedipine may also enhance chronic aspiration and pulmonary disease in PSS patients (50).

The effectiveness of cimetidine in the treatment of gastroesophageal reflux has been demonstrated in progressive systemic sclerosis patients (51). Thus, the use of an H-2 receptor antagonist may prevent some of the deleterious effects of nifedipine: in early scleroderma, when nifedipine can be an effective treatment for vascular features of the disease, an H-2 receptor antagonist may be used to minimize esophageal damage and the potential gastroesophageal reflux that may accompany ongoing pulmonary aspiration, pulmonary hypertension, and/or pulmonary fibrosis.

Recent studies (52) have shown that various mechanisms, such as transient complete LES relaxation, transient increase in intraabdominal pressure, or spontaneous free reflux associated with a low resting LESP, may cause gastroesophageal reflux in patients with symptomatic reflux esophagitis (without progressive systemic sclerosis). Further studies with continuous monitoring of LESP and esophageal pH (52) are needed to determine whether nifedipine can modify transient LES relaxation unrelated to swallowing in patients with early PSS.

In summary, when nifedipine is used in treating scleroderma patients, the physician should consider both the generalized potential effects on the disease and the local effects on the esophagus. On the one hand, since a vascular abnormality may be a contributor to the pathogenesis of progressive systemic sclerosis, nifedipine, which causes relief of artery spasm, may be beneficial in the treatment of early scleroderma. However, our controlled manometric study does document that nifedipine has a deleterious effect on lower esophageal sphincter pressure, which could contribute to gastroesophageal reflux leading to esophagitis and chronic aspiration and pulmonary disease. Thus, it appears that the use of nifedipine for generalized scleroderma may be helpful if protective mechanisms, i.e., H-2 receptor antagonists, liquid antacids, and the use of postural esophageal drainage, are added. A long-term controlled study of nifedipine in patients with early PSS and esophageal dysfunction is warranted.

ACKNOWLEDGMENTS

We thank Drs. F. Delrieu and L. Saporta for encouraging their patients to participate in these studies and for helpful discussions and Magali Vallet-Amor for expert secretarial assistance.

REFERENCES

1. LeRoy EC: Scleroderma (systemic sclerosis), Textbook of Rheumatology. Edited by WN Kelley, ED Harris Jr, S Ruddy, CB Sledge. Philadelphia, WB Saunders, 1981, pp 1211–1230
2. Rodnan GP: Progressive systemic sclerosis (scleroderma), Arthritis and Allied Conditions. Ninth edition. Edited by DJ McCarty. Philadelphia, Lea & Febiger, 1979, pp 762–809
3. Campbell PM, LeRoy EC: Pathogenesis of systemic sclerosis: a vascular hypothesis. Semin Arthritis Rheum 4:351–368, 1975
4. Norton WL, Nardo JM: Vascular disease in progressive systemic sclerosis (scleroderma). Ann Intern Med 73:317–324, 1970
5. LeRoy EC: Connective tissue synthesis by scleroderma skin fibroblasts in cell culture. J Exp Med 135:1351–1362, 1972
6. Buckingham RB, Prince RK, Rodnan GP, Taylor F: Increased collagen accumulation in dermal fibroblast cultures from patients with progressive systemic sclerosis (scleroderma). J Lab Clin Med 92:5–21, 1978
7. D'Angelo WA, Fries JF, Masi AT, Shulman LE: Pathologic observations in systemic sclerosis (scleroderma): a study of fifty-eight autopsy cases and fifty-eight matched controls. Am J Med 46:428–440, 1969
8. Bulkley BH, Ridolfi RL, Salyer WR, Hutchins GM: Myocardial lesions of progressive systemic sclerosis: a cause of cardiac dysfunction. Circulation 53:483–490, 1976
9. Alexander EL, Firestein GS, Leitl G, Wagner HN, Hochberg MC, Heuser RR, Stevens MB, Weiss J, Becker L: Scleroderma heart disease: evidence for cold-induced abnormalities of myocardial function and perfusion (abstract). Arthritis Rheum (suppl) 24:S58, 1981
10. Kovalchik MT, Guggenheim SJ, Silverman MH, Robertson JS, Steigerwald JC: The kidney in progressive systemic sclerosis: a prospective study. Ann Intern Med 89:881–887, 1978
11. Cannon PJ, Hassar M, Case DB, Casarella WJ, Sommers SC, LeRoy EC: The relationship of hypertension and renal failure in scleroderma (progressive systemic sclerosis) to structural and functional abnormalities of the renal cortical circulation. Medicine (Baltimore) 53:1–46, 1974
12. Furst DE, Davis JA, Clements PJ, Chopra SK, Theofilopoulos AN, Chia D: Abnormalities of pulmonary vascular dynamics and inflammation in early progressive systemic sclerosis. Arthritis Rheum 24:1403–1408, 1981
13. Wise RA, Wigley F, Newball HH, Stevens MB: The effect of cold exposure on diffusing capacity in patients with Raynaud's phenomenon. Chest 81:695–698, 1982
14. Kahaleh MB, Sherer GK, LeRoy EC: Endothelial injury in scleroderma. J Exp Med 149:1326–1335, 1979
15. Antman EM, Stone PH, Muller JE, Braunwald E: Calcium channel blocking agents in the treatment of cardiovascular disorders. I. Basic and clinical electrophysiologic effects. Ann Intern Med 93:875–885, 1980
16. Stone PH, Antman EM, Muller JE, Braunwald E: Calcium channel blocking agents in the treatment of cardiovascular disorders. II. Hemodynamic effects and clinical applications. Ann Intern Med 93:886–904, 1980
17. Henry PD: Comparative pharmacology of calcium antagonists: nifedipine, verapamil and diltiazem. Am J Cardiol 46:1047–1058, 1980
18. Braunwald E: Mechanism of action of calcium-channel-blocking agents. N Engl J Med 307:1618–1627, 1982
19. Kahan A, Weber S, Amor B, Saporta L, Hodara M, Degeorges M: Etude contrôlée de la nifédipine dans le traitement du phénomène de Raynaud. Rev Rhum Mal Osteoartic 49:337–343, 1982
20. Kahan A, Weber S, Amor B, Menkes CJ, Saporta L, Hodara M, Degeorges M: Nifedipine for Raynaud's phenomenon (letter). Lancet 1:131, 1983
21. Kahan A, Amor B, Menkes CJ: Nifedipine treatment for Raynaud's phenomenon (letter). Arthritis Rheum 27:959–960, 1984
22. Smith CD, McKendry RJR: Controlled trial of nifedipine in the treatment of Raynaud's phenomenon. Lancet 2:1299–1301, 1982
23. Rodeheffer RJ, Rommer JA, Wigley F, Smith CR: Controlled double-blind trial of nifedipine in the treatment of Raynaud's phenomenon. N Engl J Med 308:880–883, 1983
24. Winston EL, Pariser KM, Miller KB, Salem DN, Creager MA: Nifedipine as a therapeutic modality for

Raynaud's phenomenon. Arthritis Rheum 26:1177–1180, 1983
25. Sauza J, Kraus A, González-Amaro R, Alarcón-Segovia D: Effect of the calcium channel blocker nifedipine on Raynaud's phenomenon: a controlled double blind trial. J Rheumatol 11:362–364, 1984
26. Bortolotti M, Labo G: Clinical and manometric effects of nifedipine in patients with esophageal achalasia. Gastroenterology 80:39–44, 1981
27. Gelfond M, Rozen P, Gilat T: Isosorbide dinitrate and nifedipine treatment of achalasia: clinical, manometric and radionuclide evaluation. Gastroenterology 83:963–969, 1982
28. Subcommittee for Scleroderma Criteria of the American Rheumatism Association Diagnostic and Therapeutic Criteria Committee: Preliminary criteria for the classification of systemic sclerosis (scleroderma). Arthritis Rheum 23:581–590, 1980
29. Rodnan GP, Jablonska S, Medsger TA Jr: Classification and nomenclature of progressive systemic sclerosis (scleroderma). Clin Rheum Dis 5:5–13, 1979
30. Dodds WJ: Instrumentation and methods for intraluminal esophageal manometry. Arch Intern Med 136:515–523, 1976
31. Dodds WJ, Hogan WJ, Stef JJ, Miller WN, Lydon SB, Arndorfer RC: A rapid pull-through technique for measuring lower esophageal sphincter pressure. Gastroenterology 68:437–443, 1975
32. Arndorfer RC, Stef JJ, Dodds WJ, Linehan JH, Hogan WJ: Improved infusion system for intraluminal esophageal manometry. Gastroenterology 73:23–27, 1977
33. Stevens MB, Hookman P, Siegel C, Esterly JR, Schulman LE, Hendrix TR: Aperistalsis of the esophagus in patients with connective tissue disorders and Raynaud's phenomenon. N Engl J Med 270:1218–1222, 1964
34. Poirier TJ, Rankin GB: Gastrointestinal manifestations of progressive systemic scleroderma based on a review of 364 cases. Am J Gastroenterol 58:30–44, 1972
35. Treacy WL, Baggenstoss AH, Slocumb CH, Code CF: Scleroderma of the esophagus: a correlation of histologic and physiologic findings. Ann Intern Med 59:351–356, 1963
36. Atkinson M, Summerling MD: Oesophageal changes in systemic sclerosis. Gut 7:402–408, 1966
37. Saladin TA, French AB, Zarafonetis CJD, Pollard HJ: Esophageal motor abnormalities in scleroderma and related diseases. Dig Dis Sci 11:522–535, 1966
38. Garrett JM, Winkelmann RK, Schlegel JF, Code CF: Esophageal deterioration in scleroderma. Mayo Clin Proc 46:92–96, 1971
39. Turner R, Lipshutz W, Miller W, Rittenberg G, Schumacher HR, Cohen S: Esophageal dysfunction in collagen disease. Am J Med Sci 265:191–199, 1973
40. Orringer MB, Dabich L, Zarafonetis CJD, Sloan H: Gastroesophageal reflux in esophageal scleroderma: diagnosis and implications. Ann Thorac Surg 295:120–130, 1976
41. Clements PJ, Kadell B, Ippoliti A, Ross M: Esophageal motility in progressive systemic sclerosis (PSS): comparison of cineradiographic and manometric evaluation. Dig Dis Sci 24:639–644, 1979
42. Atkinson M: Oesophageal motor changes in systemic disease. Clin Gastroenterol 5:119–133, 1976
43. Mukhopadhyay AK, Graham DY: Esophageal motor dysfunction in systemic diseases. Arch Intern Med 136:583–588, 1976
44. Myers AR: Progressive systemic sclerosis: gastrointestinal involvement. Clin Rheum Dis 5:115–129, 1979
45. Rodnan GP, Myerowitz RL, Justh GO: Morphologic changes in the digital arteries of patients with progressive systemic sclerosis (scleroderma) and Raynaud's phenomenon. Medicine (Baltimore) 59:393–408, 1980
46. Russell ML, Friesen D, Henderson RD, Hanna WM: Ultrastructure of the esophagus in scleroderma. Arthritis Rheum 25:1117–1123, 1982
47. Cohen S, Fisher R, Lipshutz W, Turner R, Myers A, Schumacher R: The pathogenesis of esophageal dysfunction in scleroderma and Raynaud's disease. J Clin Invest 51:2663–2668, 1972
48. Fox JE, Daniel EE: The role of Ca^{++} in the genesis of lower esophageal sphincter tone and contraction (abstract). Gastroenterology 74:1035, 1978
49. Rattan S, Goyal RK: Influence of verapamil on the stimulated lower esophageal sphincter pressure (abstract). Gastroenterology 74:1082, 1978
50. Denis P, Ducrotte P, Pasquis P, Lefrançois R: Esophageal motility and pulmonary function in progressive systemic sclerosis. Respiration 42:21–24, 1981
51. Petrokubi RJ, Jeffries GH: Cimetidine versus antacid in scleroderma with reflux esophagitis: a randomized double-blind controlled study. Gastroenterology 77:691–695, 1979
52. Dodds WJ, Dent J, Hogan WJ, Helm JF, Hauser R, Patel GK, Egide MS: Mechanisms of gastroesophageal reflux in patients with reflux esophagitis. N Engl J Med 307:1547–1552, 1982

RELATIONSHIP BETWEEN NAILFOLD CAPILLARY ABNORMALITIES AND ORGAN INVOLVEMENT IN SYSTEMIC SCLEROSIS

MICHAEL LOVY, DARYL MacCARTER, and JAMES C. STEIGERWALD

Nailfold capillary abnormalities in 42 consecutive patients with systemic sclerosis were studied by wide-field capillary microscopy, and capillary abnormalities were correlated with organ involvement. Twenty-eight patients had diffuse skin disease, and 14 had the CREST variant of systemic sclerosis (calcinosis, Raynaud's phenomenon, esophageal dysmotility, sclerodactyly, telangiectasias) with anticentromere antibodies. Nailfold capillary enlargement and loss were graded from photographs. There was no correlation between the severity of either nailfold capillary loss or enlargement and duration of disease, number of organ systems involved, or acroosteolysis. The presence of telangiectasias correlated with extreme capillary enlargement ($P < 0.025$). Based on these findings it can be concluded that nailfold capillary changes in individual patients with systemic sclerosis are not useful in predicting organ involvement.

Distinctive changes in the appearance of nailfold capillaries have been noted in patients with a variety of connective tissue diseases including scleroderma or systemic sclerosis, adult and childhood dermatomyositis, Raynaud's disease, systemic lupus erythematosus, and mixed connective tissue disease (1–6). The combination of capillary enlargement in association with areas of capillary loss has been seen in over 80% of patients with systemic sclerosis (1–5). These nailfold capillary abnormalities may be useful in the early recognition of connective tissue diseases and especially in identifying patients at risk of developing systemic sclerosis (3,7). Previous studies have also suggested that the severity of nailfold capillary abnormalities correlated with the extent of systemic involvement in systemic sclerosis (2) and in childhood dermatomyositis (6). The purpose of this study was to reexamine the relationship between nailfold capillary abnormalities and organ involvement in a group of patients with systemic sclerosis.

From the University of Colorado Health Sciences Center, Denver.

Michael Lovy, MD: Fellow in Rheumatology; Daryl MacCarter, MD: Clinical Assistant Professor of Medicine; James C. Steigerwald, MD: Associate Professor of Medicine, Rheumatology Division.

Address reprint requests to Dr. James C. Steigerwald, Box B115, University of Colorado Health Sciences Center, 4200 East Ninth Avenue, Denver, CO 80262.

Submitted for publication May 21, 1984; accepted in revised form October 23, 1984.

PATIENTS AND METHODS

Patients. Forty-two consecutive patients seen in the Scleroderma Clinic or admitted to the Clinical Research Center at the University of Colorado Health Sciences Center during a recent 8-month period were studied. All patients satisfied the preliminary criteria for the classification of definite systemic sclerosis (8). Twenty-eight of the 42 patients had diffuse disease with skin involvement of the proximal extremities or trunk. The remaining 14 patients fulfilled at least 3 of 5 criteria for the CREST variant of systemic sclerosis (calcinosis, Raynaud's phenomenon, esophageal dysmotility, sclerodactyly, telangiectasias). The sera of these 14 patients also contained anticentromere antibodies. One patient each also had fascioscapulohumeral dystrophy, ulcerative colitis, and polymyalgia rheumatica. Thirty-three of the patients were women. The median age of the patients was 52 years (range 27–75), and the duration of disease from the onset of symptoms varied from 1–35 years (mean 8.9).

Clinical and laboratory evaluation. All 42 patients had been evaluated during the previous year in the Clinical Research Center, with a complete history, physical examination, and the following studies performed: complete blood count, urinalysis, creatinine phosphokinase, aldolase, 24-hour urine collection for creatinine clearance rate, antinucle-

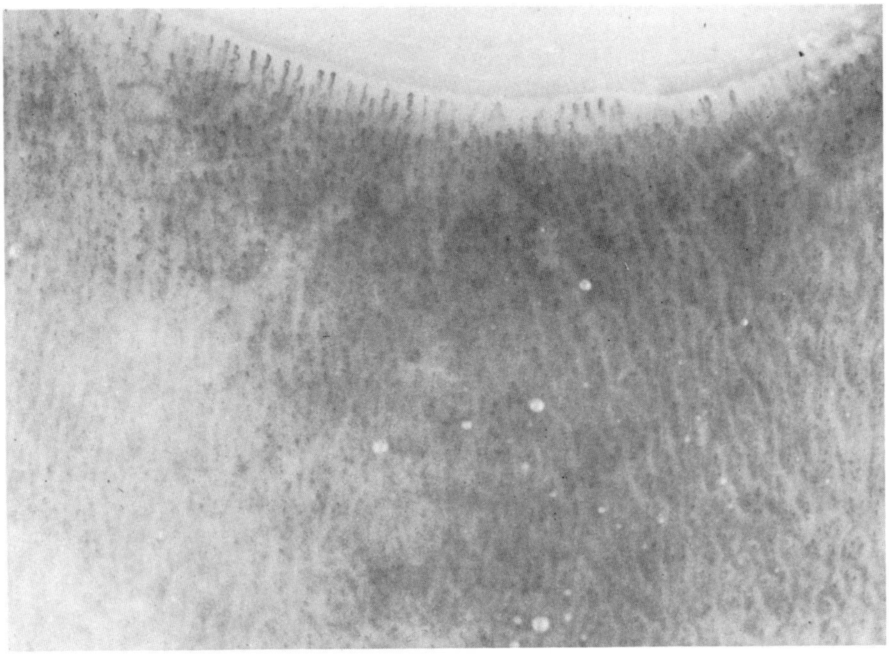

Figure 1. Nailfold capillary pattern of a normal subject (class I).

ar antibody titer using both mouse kidney and HEp-2 cells as substrates, immunodiffusion test for antibodies to SS-A SS-B, Scl–70, Sm, and RNP, and DNA binding by a millipore filter technique. Roentgenograms of the chest and hands and cineesophagogram with upper gastrointestinal tract series and small bowel follow-through were also performed, as were pulmonary function tests including oxygen desaturation with exercise, measured by ear oximetry. All patients also had an electrocardiogram.

Clinical organ involvement was totaled for each patient, based on results of the above tests, to include: 1) diffuse skin involvement: proximal extremity or trunk; 2)

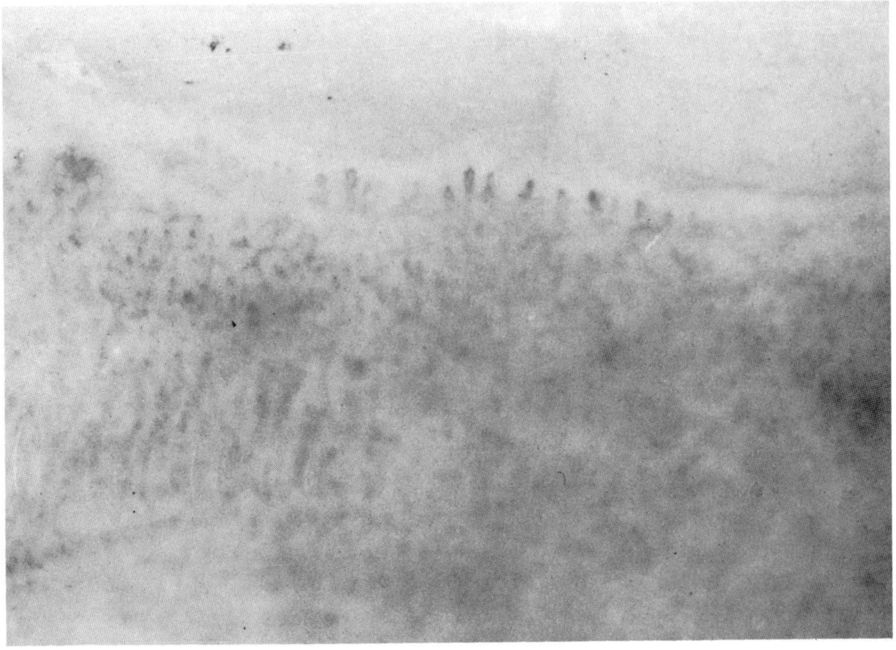

Figure 2. Definitely enlarged capillaries along the edge of the nailfold (class II).

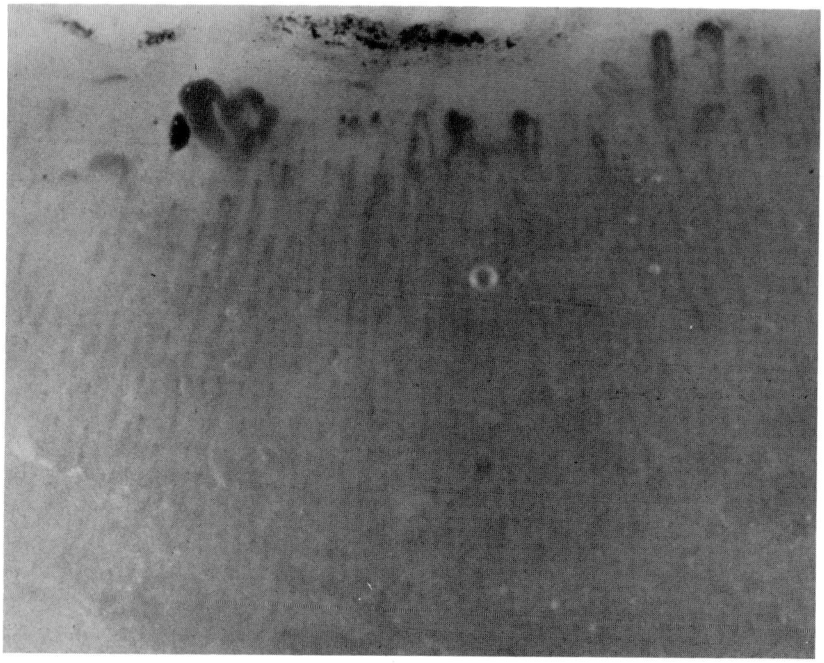

Figure 3. Extreme enlargement of capillaries (class III).

gastrointestinal: decreased motility of the lower two-thirds of the esophagus, widened duodenum, or pseudosacculation of the colon; 3) pulmonary: bibasilar interstitial fibrosis on chest roentgenogram, diffusion capacity or total lung capacity <70% of predicted, or >10% oxygen desaturation with exercise; 4) cardiac: pericarditis, congestive heart failure, or conduction defects without other cause; 5) muscle: creatinine phosphokinase more than 2 times normal, myositis on muscle biopsy, or weakness with either electromyographic or biopsy abnormalities consistent with myositis; 6) joint: swelling in a joint without evidence of infections, crystalline arthritis, or avascular necrosis; 7) renal: >25% deterioration in creatinine clearance and diastolic blood pressure elevation above 90 mm mercury occurring in a 6-month period. Since

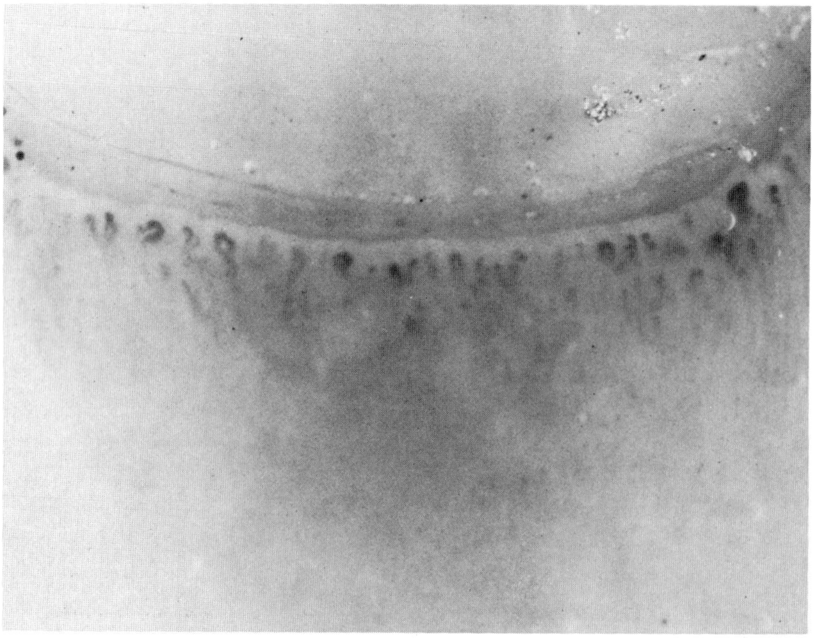

Figure 4. Moderate loss of capillaries in addition to definite enlargement.

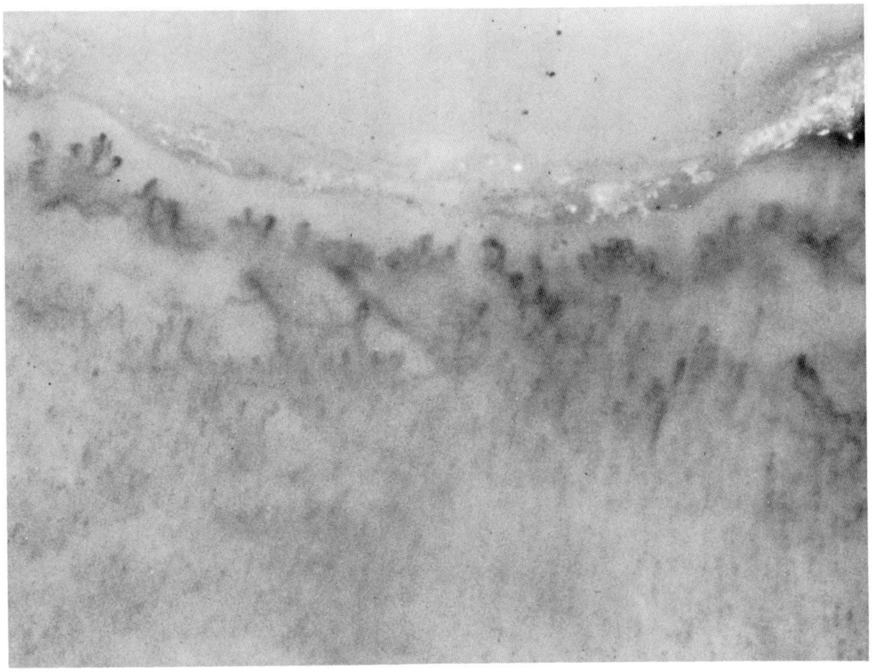

Figure 5. Extreme loss of capillaries.

patients had Raynaud's phenomenon, it was not included in the totals for organ involvement.

Nailfold microscopy technique. Widefield nailfold capillary microscopy was performed using a 35-mm single lens reflex camera with bellows and a 58-mm macrolens (Topcon, Tokyo Optical) and Bowens macrolight (Bowen, London, UK). All 10 digits were inspected after placing a drop of type B immersion oil on the nailfold area. Digits with the most severe capillary changes as well as the fourth digit of each hand were photographed using Ektachrome 200 film. The nailfold capillary abnormalities were graded from photographs, simultaneously by all 3 authors, without knowledge of the clinical details. The severity of changes was graded according to the capillary classification of Maricq (9) as follows: capillary enlargement: none (class I), definite enlargement (class II), extreme enlargement (class III); capillary loss: none, moderate loss, and extensive loss. Examples of each with more detailed descriptions are shown in Figures 1–5.

Table 1. Correlation between nailfold capillary microscopy results and organ system involvement in 42 systemic sclerosis patients

	Capillary enlargement		
No. of systems involved	None	Definite	Extreme
All patients			
0–2*	5	16	6
3–4*	4	6	5
Patients with diffuse skin disease (n = 28)			
0–2†	4	10	1
3–4†	4	5	4
Patients with CREST syndrome (n = 14)			
0–2‡	1	6	5
3–4‡	0	1	1

* $\chi^2 = 1.44$; $P > 0.30$.
† $\chi^2 = 3.34$; $P > 0.20$.
‡ $\chi^2 = 0.19$; $P > 0.80$. CREST = calcinosis, Raynaud's phenomenon, esophageal dysmotility, sclerodactyly, telangiectasias.

RESULTS

Thirty-six of the 42 patients (86%) exhibited either nailfold capillary enlargement or avascular areas or capillary loss. Thirty-two of the 36 exhibited both capillary enlargement and loss, 3 had moderate capillary loss without enlargement, and 1 patient had enlarged capillaries but no evidence of capillary loss. There was a statistically significant difference (Mann-Whitney test) in the duration of disease between the group of patients without capillary loss and those with extreme loss. Those with extreme capillary loss had had their disease for a mean of 10 years, while those with no loss had a mean disease duration of only 5

Table 2. Correlation between telangiectasias and nailfold capillary enlargement in 42 systemic sclerosis patients

	Nailfold capillary enlargement		
	None	Definite	Extreme
Telangiectasias*	2	11	11
No telangiectasias*	7	11	0

* $\chi^2 = 13.19$; $P < 0.025$.

years ($P < 0.04$). There was no difference in disease duration among groups of patients with varying degrees of capillary enlargements.

Chi-square analysis was used to compare the number of organ systems involved among patients within each category of capillary enlargement (Table 1). No significant correlation was found between either the presence or severity of capillary enlargement and the extent of organ involvement. Similar analyses were performed separately for the 28 patients with diffuse skin disease and the 14 patients with the CREST variant of systemic sclerosis (Table 1). These also failed to demonstrate a statistically significant difference between number of organ systems involved and severity of capillary enlargement. Correlation of the severity of capillary enlargement and the number of organ systems involved, excluding skin and gastrointestinal tract, was also examined in a similar fashion and failed to show any statistically significant relationships.

Similar chi-square analysis was performed to examine the relationship between nailfold capillary loss and organ involvement for the entire group of 42 patients, the 28 patients with diffuse skin disease, and the 14 patients with CREST. Again, no statistically significant correlations could be made.

The presence of telangiectasias did correlate with the presence and severity of nailfold capillary enlargement (Table 2). All patients with extremely enlarged (class III) capillary loops had telangiectasias, whereas the definitely enlarged capillaries (class II) were evenly distributed between patients with and those without telangiectasias. Although acroosteolysis was seen frequently in patients with severe capillary loss, statistical analysis did not show any significant correlation.

DISCUSSION

The pattern and frequency of nailfold capillary abnormalities in our study of 42 patients were similar to those previously described (2,3). One of those previous studies (2) found no relationship between the degree of capillary involvement and the duration of a patient's illness. Similarly, we found no correlation between disease duration and the varying degrees of capillary enlargement. In our study, however, patients with severe capillary loss did have a longer disease duration than patients without any nailfold capillary loss.

We also found a correlation between presence of telangiectasias and nailfold capillary enlargement, suggesting that the nailfold changes may reflect a more generalized vascular abnormality in the skin and mucus membranes. This correlation also emphasizes the value of a careful search for telangiectasias in patients presenting with Raynaud's phenomenon and other symptoms possibly related to systemic sclerosis.

In contrast to the results of a previous study (2), we were unable to demonstrate any association between nailfold capillary abnormalities and organ involvement in our group of 42 systemic sclerosis patients. The previous study included 13 patients with Raynaud's syndrome, 3 patients with dermatomyositis, 25 patients with diffuse scleroderma, and 3 patients with the CREST variant of systemic sclerosis. Because our group of 42 patients included a larger number of patients with the CREST variant (14 of 42), we performed a separate analysis comparing patients who had diffuse scleroderma with those who had the CREST variant. Again, we were unable to show any statistically significant correlations between nailfold capillary changes and organ involvement. Thus, the higher proportion of CREST patients in our study group does not explain the differing results. The criteria for organ involvement, the grouping of patients according to nailfold capillary dilatation used for chi-square analysis, and the mean duration of disease in our study were also similar to those in the previous study. Thus, we are unable to offer an obvious explanation for the differing results in the 2 studies.

In view of our results, however, it seems apparent that nailfold capillary changes in the individual patient with a diagnosis of systemic sclerosis are frequently not useful in predicting organ involvement.

REFERENCES

1. Maricq HR, LeRoy EC: Patterns of finger capillary abnormalities in connective tissue disease by "wide-field" microscopy. Arthritis Rheum 16:619–628, 1973
2. Maricq HR, Spencer-Green G, LeRoy EC: Skin capillary abnormalities as indicators of organ involvement in scleroderma (systemic sclerosis): Raynaud's syndrome and dermatomyositis. Am J Med 61:862–870, 1976
3. Maricq HR, LeRoy EC, D'Angelo WA, Medsger TA Jr, Rodnan GP, Sharp GC, Wolfe JF: Diagnostic potential of in vivo capillary microscopy in scleroderma and related disorders. Arthritis Rheum 23:183–189, 1980
4. Kenik JG, Maricq HR, Boles GG: Blind evaluation of the

diagnostic specificity of nailfold capillary microscopy in the connective tissue diseases. Arthritis Rheum 24:885–891, 1981

5. Vayssairat M, Fiessinger JN, Priollet P, Goldberg J, Housset E: Interet de la capillaroscopie pour le diagnostic de la sclerodermie generalisee. Rev Med Interne 3:333–340, 1981
6. Spencer-Green G, Crowe WE, Levinson JE: Nailfold capillary abnormalities and clinical outcome in childhood dermatomyositis. Arthritis Rheum 25:954–958, 1982
7. Maricq HR, Weinberger AB, LeRoy EC: Early detection of scleroderma spectrum disorders by in vivo capillary microscopy: a prospective study of patients with Raynaud's phenomenon. J Rheumatol 9:289–291, 1982
8. Subcommittee for Scleroderma Criteria of the American Rheumatism Association Diagnostic and Therapeutic Criteria Committee: Preliminary criteria for the classification of systemic sclerosis (scleroderma). Arthritis Rheum 23:581–590, 1980
9. Maricq HR: Widefield capillary microscopy: technique and rating scale for abnormalities seen in scleroderma and related disorders. Arthritis Rheum 24:1159–1165, 1981

SELECTIVE INHIBITION OF EXCESSIVE SCLERODERMA FIBROBLAST COLLAGEN PRODUCTION BY LYMPHOKINES FROM NORMAL HUMAN MONONUCLEAR CELLS

SERGIO A. JIMENEZ, WILLIAM M. McARTHUR, REZA I. BASHEY, and JOEL ROSENBLOOM

We studied the effects of lymphokines from mitogen-stimulated normal human mononuclear cells on collagen production by confluent monolayer cultures of scleroderma dermal fibroblasts. We examined 10 cell lines obtained from patients with early onset, rapidly progressive disease. All cell lines exhibited increased collagen production, compared with cell lines from age- and sex-matched normal individuals. We found that supernatants from phytohemagglutinin-stimulated mononuclear cells caused >45% inhibition of collagen production by the cultured scleroderma fibroblasts; the degree of inhibition was concentration-dependent. Partially purified lymphokine preparations produced 84–94% inhibition of collagen production by scleroderma cells. The lymphokine effects were shown to be selective for collagen, since the synthesis of noncollagenous proteins was not significantly affected. The results suggest that lymphokines from normal mononuclear cells can modulate the excessive collagen biosynthesis that is characteristic of scleroderma fibroblasts, and these lymphokines may have a place as possible therapeutic agents for this incurable disease.

From the Collagen Research Laboratories, Rheumatology Section, Department of Medicine, School of Medicine, and the Center for Oral Health Research, School of Dentistry, University of Pennsylvania, Philadelphia.

Supported by NIH grants AM-19106 and AM-19616.

Sergio A. Jimenez, MD: Associate Professor and Director, Collagen Research Laboratories, School of Medicine; William M. McArthur, PhD: Associate Professor, School of Dentistry; Reza I. Bashey, PhD: Research Associate Professor, School of Dentistry; Joel Rosenbloom, MD, PhD: Professor and Director, Center for Oral Health Research.

Address reprint requests to Sergio A. Jimenez, MD, Room 570, Maloney Bldg., Hospital of the University of Pennsylvania, 3600 Spruce Street, Philadelphia, PA 19104.

Submitted for publication July 19, 1984; accepted in revised form November 19, 1984.

Scleroderma, or progressive systemic sclerosis (PSS), is a connective tissue disease of unknown etiology, characterized by the deposition of excessive amounts of collagen and other connective tissue macromolecules in the skin and various internal organs (1). Although the pathogenesis and mechanisms responsible for the excessive connective tissue accumulation in PSS are not known, it is apparent that many of the clinical manifestations of the disease result from tissue damage caused by progressive fibrosis of the affected organs. The mechanisms responsible for the excessive collagen accumulation in sclerodermatous tissues are not entirely known, but several studies have suggested that increased collagen production by scleroderma fibroblasts may be one important factor (2–5). Since the first description of scleroderma in 1753 (6), multiple forms of therapy have been advocated. At present, however, there is no effective treatment for the disease, and frequently, the relentless progression of the fibrotic process causes severe functional and structural alterations in multiple organs and eventually results in death.

We have recently discovered that supernatants from mitogen-stimulated normal human mononuclear cells cause, in a dose-dependent manner, potent and selective inhibition of collagen production by normal human dermal fibroblasts. Addition of samples containing active supernatants to confluent cultures of normal human dermal fibroblasts resulted in >50% inhibition of collagen production by these cultures, with minimal effects on cell viability and total protein synthesis (7). Our findings have been confirmed recently by Hart et al (8,9).

Further studies showed that the active factor, which we termed "collagen synthesis inhibitory factor'' (CSIF), was produced predominantly by T lymphocytes, and that various mitogens enhanced its production by these cells. In addition, we demonstrated that CSIF was a protein, since its activity was abolished by trypsin digestion and its production was inhibited by the protein synthesis inhibitors puromycin and cycloheximide (10). Purification and characterization of CSIF by ammonium sulfate fractionation, gel filtration chromatography, and isoelectric focusing showed that the protein had a molecular weight of approximately 55,000 and a pI of 6.2 (11).

The purpose of the present study was to determine if CSIF could also modulate the excessive collagen biosynthesis that is characteristic of PSS fibroblasts. The results reported here demonstrate that CSIF is a potent and selective inhibitor of collagen production by scleroderma dermal fibroblasts. These findings suggest the possibility of a novel therapeutic approach for PSS—using lymphocyte products capable of modulating fibroblast biosynthesis to inhibit the excessive collagen accumulation characteristic of the disease.

PATIENTS AND METHODS

Selection of patients. All dermal fibroblast cell lines were obtained from patients who fulfilled the recently described American Rheumatism Association criteria for the diagnosis of PSS (12). We studied only patients who had active and rapidly progressive disease and who had not received any treatment known to influence connective tissue metabolism. In all cases, the disease duration from the onset of symptoms to the time of study was less than 1 year. After informed consent was obtained, full-thickness skin biopsy specimens were obtained from the leading edge of affected skin from untreated patients. Monolayer cultures of dermal fibroblasts were established from these specimens, as described in a previous publication (13). All aspects of the research were carried out according to the guidelines of the Declaration of Helsinki.

Isolation of mononuclear cells and generation of lymphokines. Normal human mononuclear cell suspensions were obtained from heparinized (10 IU/ml) peripheral blood obtained by venipuncture from healthy volunteers. Mononuclear cells were separated from the granulocytes and erythrocytes by centrifugation (400*g*) of the whole blood over a lymphocyte separation medium (LSM solution, a Ficoll preparation; Litton Bionetics, Kensington, MD) for 30 minutes at 22°C. Mononuclear lymphocytes and monocytes were recovered at the LSM–plasma interface and washed twice within Hanks' balanced salt solution (HBSS), by centrifugation. Viablility of mononuclear cells was >98%, measured by trypan blue exclusion.

Cells were suspended to a final concentration of 1×10^6 cells/ml in RPMI 1640 medium supplemented with glutamine (2 m*M*), penicillin (100 units/ml), and streptomycin (100 μg/ml) and incubated at 37°C for 72 hours in 5% CO_2, 95% air. Phytohemagglutinin-P (PHA; Difco, Detroit, MI), 1 μg/ml, was added to half of the mononuclear cell cultures; the other half served as nonstimulated controls. At the end of the incubation, cells and media were separated by centrifugation, and the media were exhaustively dialyzed against HBSS.

To test the mitogenic response of the mononuclear cells, samples from triplicate cultures of both PHA-stimulated and nonstimulated controls received ^{3}H-thymidine (New England Nuclear, Boston, MA), 0.5 μCi/ml, 16 hours before termination of the incubation period. The degree of ^{3}H-thymidine incorporation into the cultures was assessed by collecting the cells on 24-mm glass-fiber filters, rinsing them repeatedly with physiologic saline, and counting the dried filters in a liquid scintillation counter. The stimulation index was defined as the ratio of ^{3}H-thymidine incorporation in PHA-containing cultures compared with control cultures. Only cultures having a simulation index of at least 10 were used as a source of stimulated supernatants.

Partial purification of lymphokines. Partial purification of lymphokines from control and PHA-stimulated mononuclear cell supernatants was accomplished as described in detail elsewhere (11). Briefly, supernatants were obtained from nonstimulated and PHA-stimulated mononuclear cells cultured for 48 hours in the presence of 1% bovine serum albumin (BSA), instead of serum, to facilitate purification and were fractionally precipitated with increasing concentrations of ammonium sulfate. The fraction precipitating between 30% and 75% ammonium sulfate, which contained most of the collagen synthesis inhibitory activity, was utilized for these experiments.

Fibroblast cultures and labeling conditions. Fibroblasts were obtained from skin biopsy specimens from normal individuals and patients with PSS, as described previously (13), and were grown in Eagle's minimal essential medium (EMEM) supplemented with 10% fetal calf serum (FCS), in 5% CO_2. The cells were used between passage 6 and passage 14. Routinely, the cells were plated at a density of 19,000/cm^2 in 30-mm plastic culture dishes, were cultured for 5 days to allow them to reach confluency, and then the experiments with the mononuclear preparations were begun. Previous experiments demonstrated that under these conditions, the cultures were contact-inhibited, since they did not display detectable cell division as measured by serial cell counts, DNA assays, or ^{3}H-thymidine incorporation. To avoid any influence of the supernatants on fibroblast proliferation, which may have obscured their effects on collagen synthesis, only confluent cultures were used in these studies.

The media were removed, and 1.5 ml of fresh media containing various dilutions of the mononuclear supernatants, 5% FCS, and 50 μg/ml ascorbate in EMEM were added. In certain experiments, 10% FCS was used, but because the results were essentially identical, the lower serum concentration was used for all subsequent experiments.

After 2 days of culture, the media were again replaced with the same media, which, in addition, contained 2–4 μCi/ml ^{14}C-proline and 100 μg/ml β-aminopropionitrile, and the incubation was continued for 24 hours. Control experiments showed that PHA alone, at concentrations

Table 1. Clinical data of progressive systemic sclerosis patients studied*

Culture code	Sex/age	Disease duration (months)	Biopsy site	Progressive scleroderma	Raynaud's phenomenon	Pigmentary changes	Arthritis	Visceral involvement			
								GI	Lung	Heart	Kidney
S1 (KA)	M/43	8	Forearm	+	–	+	–	+	–	+	–
S2 (JL)	F/52	3	Forearm	+	+	+	+	+	+	–	–
S3 (PH)	M/28	3	Forearm	+	+	+	+	+	+	–	–
S4 (GP)	M/56	11	Forearm	+	+	+	–	+	+	–	–
S5 (OG)	F/36	9	Forearm	+	+	+	+	+	–	–	–
S6 (DT)	F/53	10	Forearm	+	+	+	+	+	–	–	–
S7 (AW)	F/52	4	Forearm	+	+	–	+	+	+	+	–
S8 (MY)	F/57	5	Forearm	+	+	+	+	+	+	–	–
S9 (SO)	F/28	5	Forearm	+	+	+	+	+	+	–	–
S10 (MM)	F/66	3	Forearm	+	–	+	–	+	–	–	–

* Disease onset was considered to have occurred when development of proximal scleroderma was first documented by a physician. In some cases, Raynaud's phenomenon or dysphagia preceded the development of proximal dermal sclerosis. GI = gastrointestinal tract.

present in the stimulated mononuclear cell supernatants, did not have a discernible effect on collagen production by normal or PSS fibroblasts.

To examine the effects of the supernatants on biosynthesis of noncollagenous proteins, cultures were processed exactly as described above except that the labeling was performed with 5 μCi/ml of either ^{3}H-tyrosine or ^{3}H-fucose. After labeling for 24 hours, the media were removed, and the cell layers were detached with a rubber policeman. To avoid proteolytic cleavage of the labeled noncollagenous proteins, trypsin was not used. Samples of media and suspended cell layers were extensively dialyzed against distilled H_2O, and aliquots were counted in a scintillation counter. Because most of the radioactivity incorporated into nondialyzable

Table 2. ^{14}C-hydroxyproline production by cultured dermal fibroblasts from age- and sex-matched normal controls and progressive systemic sclerosis (PSS) patients*

Normal fibroblasts			PSS fibroblasts		
Cell line	Age/sex	^{14}C-hydroxyproline	Cell line	Age/sex	^{14}C-hydroxyproline
N1	46/M	9.23	S1 (KA)	43/M	12.65
		7.96			12.97
					11.51
N2	32/M	9.24	S3 (PH)	28/M	11.23
		8.42			10.38
					9.80
N3	56/M	5.99	S4 (GP)	56/M	7.76
		6.10			7.21
N4	32/F	8.40	S5 (OG)	36/F	14.81
		6.81			15.75
N5	56/F	6.23	S2 (JL)	52/F	8.45
		6.33			8.38
					9.55
			S6 (DT)	53/F	8.74
			S7 (AW)	52/F	14.77
			S8 (MY)	57/F	10.19
					9.04
N6	28/F	9.41	S9 (SO)	28/F	27.75
		8.15			14.25
					18.68
N7	62/F	9.75	S10 (MM)	66/F	12.47
					12.50
Mean ± SD		7.84 ± 1.39	Mean ± SD		12.22 ± 4.54†

* ^{14}C-hydroxyproline expressed as disintegrations per minute × 10^3/dish. Each value represents the average of results of experiments performed either in duplicate or in triplicate. See Patients and Methods for details.
† Significant compared with normal, $P < 0.005$ using Student's t-test.

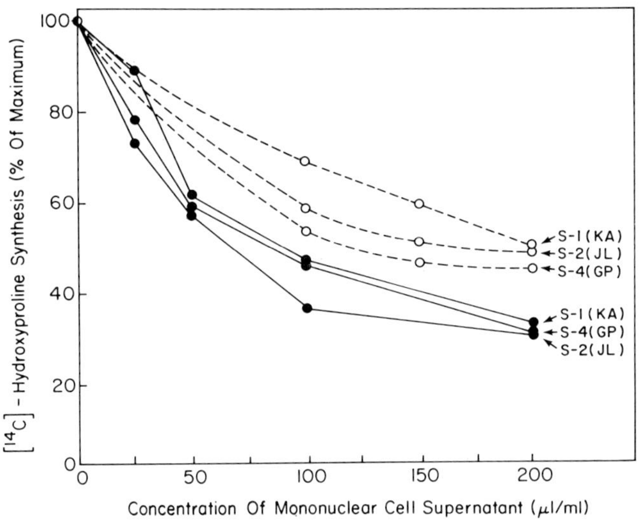

Figure 1. Dose-dependent inhibition of progressive systemic sclerosis (PSS) fibroblast collagen production by supernatants from phytohemagglutinin (PHA)–stimulated normal human mononuclear cells. Confluent cultures of 3 PSS cell lines were incubated with 2 preparations of supernatants from PHA-stimulated normal human mononuclear cells as described in Patients and Methods. Collagen production was assessed after incubation with various concentrations of the supernatants and labeling with ^{14}C-proline, by assaying aliquots of the culture media for their ^{14}C-hydroxyproline content. Each value shown is an average of 2 separate cultures. ○– – –○ = preparation 1; ●——● = preparation 2.

macromolecules appeared in the culture media, only these results are shown.

To examine the effects of the supernatants on fibroblast proliferation and viability, separate plates were cultured exactly as described above except that the isotopes were omitted. At the end of the experiment, the media were aspirated, and the cell layers were detached by trypsinzation. The fibroblasts were resuspended in fresh media and their viability determined by trypan blue exclusion. Subsequently, the numbers of cells in each plate were counted with a hemacytometer.

Gel electrophoresis. Electrophoresis of labeled proteins from the media of PSS fibroblast cultures incubated under control conditions or in the presence of 200 µl/ml of partially purified PHA-stimulated supernatants was performed on 5% polyacrylamide slab gels in sodium dodecyl sulfate (SDS). After electrophoresis, the gels were processed for fluorography and scanned at 585 nm on a linear drive densitometer. The relative proportions of radioactivity in each band were calculated from densitometric tracings, using a planimeter.

Assays. The amount of ^{14}C-hydroxyproline, representing the collagen produced by the cultured fibroblasts at the end of the 24-hour incubation with ^{14}C-proline, was measured by a specific chemical assay (14). Only the culture media were assayed since, as shown previously, >85% of the total collagen produced by the control or experimental cultures was released into the media under the conditions used (7).

RESULTS

Clinical characteristics of patients studied. Table 1 shows the clinical characteristics of the patients whose dermal fibroblasts were studied. In all these patients with active, rapidly progressive disease, the onset of PSS symptoms was considered to have occurred when skin sclerosis extending proximally to the wrists or ankles was documented by a physician. Many patients showed clinical evidence of internal organ involvement at the time the biopsy was obtained (Table 1). All scleroderma cell lines used in these studies displayed increased collagen production, compared with cell lines obtained from age- and sex-matched controls (Table 2). The average collagen production by the 10 PSS cell lines tested was >160% of the average collagen production by the 7 normal cell lines; some PSS cell lines (S5, S7, and S9) produced 2–3-fold more collagen than did their matched normal counterparts.

Table 3. Effects of supernatants from nonstimulated or phytohemagglutinin (PHA)–stimulated mononuclear cells on ^{14}C-hydroxyproline production by progressive systemic sclerosis fibroblasts*

	^{14}C-hydroxyproline (dpm × 10^{-3})		
Cell line	Media alone	Media + PHA-stimulated supernatants	% change
S1 (KA)			
Expt. 1	11.51	5.39	−53.2
Expt. 2	3.77	1.71	−54.6
Expt. 3	3.18	1.66	−47.8
S2 (JL)			
Expt. 1	8.45	3.83	−54.6
Expt. 2	4.01	1.30	−67.6
Expt. 3	3.45	1.71	−50.4
S3 (PH)			
Expt. 1	10.66	4.27	−59.9
Expt. 2	4.86	2.08	−57.2
Expt. 3	4.54	2.39	−47.4
S4 (GP)			
Expt. 1	6.28	1.98	−68.5
Expt. 2	3.93	1.79	−54.4
Expt. 3	2.50	0.74	−70.4
S5 (OG)			
Expt. 1	8.06	3.85	−52.2
Expt. 2	3.29	1.33	−59.5
S6 (DT)			
Expt. 1	8.73	3.92	−55.1
Expt. 2	4.71	2.40	−49.0

* Confluent monolayer cultures of dermal fibroblasts were incubated and labeled as described in Patients and Methods. All experiments performed in duplicate. Values shown are the average of 2 determinations, which differed from each other by <15%. The higher incorporation obtained in experiment 1 reflects the use of a higher isotope concentration during labeling.

Table 4. Effects of partially purified supernatants from nonstimulated and phytohemagglutinin (PHA)–stimulated normal human mononuclear cells on ^{14}C-hydroxyproline production by progressive systemic sclerosis (PSS) fibroblasts*

	^{14}C-hydroxyproline (dpm $\times 10^{-3}$)				
Cell line	Media alone	Media + nonstimulated supernatants	% change	Media + PHA-stimulated supernatants	% change
S1 (KA)	9.34	4.36	−53.3	0.67	−92.8
	8.22	3.47	−57.5	0.53	−93.6
S7 (AW)	7.69	6.15	−20.0	1.32	−83.8
	7.32	6.04	−17.5	1.20	−83.6
S8 (MY)	9.30	4.31	−53.6	0.92	−90.1
	8.87	4.36	−50.3	0.89	−89.9
S9 (SO)	14.53	5.43	−62.6	1.10	−92.4
	13.97	5.03	−64.0	0.95	−93.2
S10 (MM)	11.95	4.69	−60.8	0.99	−91.2
	11.03	5.38	−51.2	1.16	−89.5

* Supernatants were obtained and partially purified by fractional ammonium sulfate precipitation. Aliquots of the fractions precipitating between 30% and 75% ammonium sulfate were added to confluent cultures of PSS fibroblasts, and their effects on collagen synthesis by these cells were measured. See Patients and Methods for details.

Effects of mononuclear cell supernatants on PSS fibroblast collagen synthesis and dose-response. Dose-response experiments were carried out using 2 different preparations of supernatants from PHA-stimulated mononuclear cells. We examined the effects of various concentrations of the supernatants, ranging from 0–200 μl/ml, on ^{14}C-hydroxyproline production by 3 PSS cell lines. The results shown in Figure 1 demonstrate that both preparations caused a dose-dependent inhibition of ^{14}C-hydroxyproline production by the PSS fibroblasts. Although 1 of the preparations appeared to exert a more potent inhibitory effect, near maximal inhibition was obtained with both supernatants at a concentration of 200 μl/ml. Therefore, all subsequent studies were performed using this concentration.

Table 3 shows the effects of active supernatants obtained from PHA-stimulated normal human mononuclear cells on collagen production by confluent cultures of 6 scleroderma cell lines. At a concentration of 200 μl/ml, these supernatants caused a 47.4–70.4% inhibition of ^{14}C-hydroxyproline production by the PSS fibroblasts. All 6 cell lines were tested on at least 2 separate occasions, and they showed similar results. Supernatants from nonstimulated mononuclear cells did not cause a significant decrease in collagen production by the scleroderma cells.

Effects of mononuclear cell supernatants on fibroblast viability and proliferation. Mononuclear cell supernatants, whether obtained from nonstimulated or PHA-stimulated cells, did not have a significant effect on cell viability or fibroblast proliferation when added to confluent cultures of normal or PSS fibroblasts. The number of viable fibroblasts present in the cell layers of parallel cultures incubated with control medium or with media containing supernatants from nonstimulated or from PHA-stimulated mononuclear cells were counted as described in Patients and Methods.

In 15 separate experiments involving 4 normal fibroblastic cell lines, the mean number of viable cells/culture after incubation with media alone, with supernatants from nonstimulated mononuclear cells, and with PHA-stimulated mononuclear cells was $380 \pm 105 \times 10^3$, $386 \pm 116 \times 10^3$, and $391 \pm 101 \times 10^3$, respectively. There were no statistically significant differences between these values when evaluated by Student's *t*-test ($P = 0.89$ for control versus nonstimulated supernatants and $P = 0.78$ for control versus stimulated supernatants). When 3 PSS cell lines were similarly examined in 6 separate experiments, the values obtained were $221 \pm 145 \times 10^3$, $242 \pm 159 \times 10^3$, and $219 \pm 128 \times 10^3$ for cultures incubated with media alone, with supernatants from nonstimulated mononuclear cells, and with PHA-stimulated mononuclear cells, respectively. These values were not statistically different from each other ($P = 0.85$ for control versus nonstimulated supernatants and $P = 0.98$ for control versus stimulated supernatants).

Effects of partially purified mononuclear cell supernatants on PSS fibroblast collagen production. In the experiments shown in Table 4, we examined the effects of partially purified supernatants from nonstim-

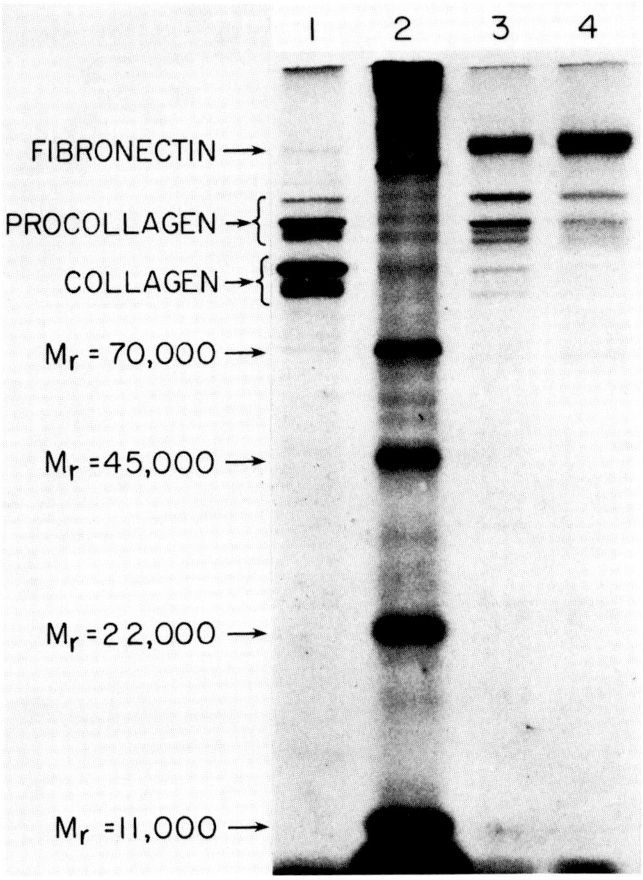

Figure 2. Fluorograph of sodium dodecyl sulfate–polyacrylamide slab gel electrophoresis of media proteins from confluent cultures of fibroblasts incubated in media alone or in media with 200 μl/ml of partially purified phytohemagglutinin (PHA)–stimulated supernatant, labeled with 4 μCi/ml ^{14}C-proline as described in Patients and Methods. Lane 1, standard chick tendon type I procollagen and collagen; Lane 2, molecular weight standard; Lane 3, medium from control cultures; Lane 4, medium from cultures incubated in the presence of PHA-stimulated supernatant.

ulated and from PHA-stimulated mononuclear cells on collagen production by 5 scleroderma cell lines. The supernatants obtained from mononuclear cells cultured with 1% BSA instead of serum were fractionally precipitated with increasing concentrations of ammonium sulfate, and the fractions precipitating between 30% and 75% ammonium sulfate, which contained most of the CSIF activity, were tested. These preparations showed greater inhibitory effects on collagen production by PSS fibroblasts than did the unpurified samples. Purified preparations of nonstimulated mononuclear cell supernatants caused 17.5–64.0% inhibition of collagen production, whereas those from PHA-stimulated cells caused 83.6–93.6% inhibition. In 4 of the 5 cell lines tested, the inhibition was 90% or greater.

Gel electrophoresis and autoradiography of labeled proteins from PSS fibroblast cultures. To further characterize the effects of mononuclear cell supernatants on collagen biosynthesis by PSS fibroblasts, the newly synthesized molecules from the media of fibroblast cultures incubated with partially purified mononuclear cell supernatants were examined by electrophoresis on SDS-slab gels, with subsequent fluorography. As shown in Figure 2, the partially purified PHA-stimulated supernatant caused a selective decrease in the proportion of radioactivity migrating in the procollagen region without a discernible reduction in radioactivity migrating in the region of fibronectin. In addition, no detectable increase in radioactivity corresponding to collagen-cleaved products was observed. When the relative proportions of fibronectin and procollagen were calculated from the densitometric tracings of the fluorographs, we found that the ratio of fibronectin to procollagen was 0.64 in control cultures. In contrast, this ratio increased fourfold to 2.57 in the cultures incubated with the partially purified PHA-stimulated supernatant. These results indicate that the active supernatants caused selective inhibition of PSS fibroblast collagen production relative to noncollagenous proteins. The results also showed that the observed decrease in collagen production was not due to increased extracellular degradation of the newly synthesized molecules.

Effects of mononuclear cell supernatants on synthesis of noncollagenous proteins by normal and PSS fibroblasts. To exclude the possibility that the inhibition of collagen production was due to a general toxic effect on fibroblast protein biosynthesis, the effects of PHA-stimulated mononuclear cell supernatants on production of noncollagenous proteins by normal and PSS cells were examined. For this purpose, normal and PSS fibroblast cultures were labeled with either ^{3}H-tyrosine, an amino acid which is incorporated preferentially into noncollagenous proteins, or with ^{3}H-fucose, a monosaccharide incorporated exclusively into noncollagenous glycoproteins. The results shown in Table 5 demonstrate that supernatants containing CSIF did not significantly inhibit the incorporation of these 2 precursors into macromolecules biosynthesized by the PSS fibroblasts. The incorporation of ^{3}H-tyrosine was only minimally decreased (<15%), whereas the incorporation of ^{3}H-fucose was moderately increased (up to 42.9%).

Table 5. Effects of supernatants from phytohemagglutinin (PHA)–stimulated normal human mononuclear cells on the incorporation of ^{3}H-tyrosine and ^{3}H-fucose into media macromolecules by 2 cell lines of normal and progressive systemic sclerosis (PSS) dermal fibroblasts*

	^{3}H-tyrosine (cpm $\times 10^{-3}$)			^{3}H-fucose (cpm $\times 10^{-3}$)		
Cell line	Media alone	Media + PHA-stimulated supernatant	% change	Media alone	Media + PHA-stimulated supernatant	% change
Normal						
N3	149.20	140.96	−5.5	80.12	86.79	+8.3
	145.01	134.31	−7.4	70.83	82.26	+16.1
N4	153.84	150.27	−2.3	69.13	98.80	+42.9
	152.78	130.62	−14.5	68.27	83.55	+22.4
PSS						
S1 (KA)	171.40	148.61	−13.3	67.80	85.85	+26.6
	148.39	135.29	−8.8	65.28	81.97	+25.6
S9 (SO)	183.17	162.26	−11.4	92.88	96.25	+3.6
	175.18	151.75	−13.4	79.49	84.45	+6.2

* Supernatants were added to confluent cultures of fibroblasts and labeled with 5 μCi/ml of isotope to study biosynthesis of noncollagenous proteins. See Patients and Methods for details. Values represent total radioactivity incorporated into nondialyzable media macromolecules.

DISCUSSION

The results presented here demonstrate that lymphokines obtained from normal human mononuclear cells are capable of influencing the biosynthetic behavior of sclerodermatous fibroblasts in a manner similar to that of normal fibroblasts, which was previously described by us and by others (7–11). Addition of supernatants from PHA-stimulated cells to monolayer cultures of PSS dermal fibroblasts consistently resulted in >45% inhibition of collagen production by the scleroderma cells. These effects were concentration-dependent, as shown in Figure 1. When partially purified supernatants from PHA-stimulated mononuclear cells were used, the effects were more dramatic. In 4 of 5 cell lines studied, the inhibition of collagen production was >90%. These results are more remarkable since all the cell lines studied were obtained from patients with rapidly progressive disease and, in most cases, with characteristic PSS internal organ involvement. Furthermore, all PSS dermal fibroblasts tested exhibited increased collagen production in culture, compared with normal fibroblasts (Table 2). Although unpurified supernatants from nonstimulated mononuclear cells did not cause significant inhibition of collagen production by PSS cells, the partially purified preparations of the same materials were inhibitory. These findings are probably due to the concentration of small amounts of CSIF produced by the nonstimulated mononuclear cells during the ammonium sulfate fractionation. However, the possibility that the purification procedure removed other factors which may either stimulate fibroblast collagen production or render the inhibitory factor inactive cannot be excluded and is under investigation.

Although we cannot completely exclude the possibility that other products from mitogen-stimulated mononuclear cells, such as interleukin-2 or γ-interferon, may be able to influence the biosynthetic behavior of PSS fibroblasts, the biochemical characteristics of CSIF suggest that it is a separate factor capable of modulating PSS fibroblast biosynthetic activity. The molecular weight (55,000 daltons) and pI (6.2) determined for purified CSIF preparations (11) indicate that it probably represents a separate mononuclear cell product distinct from interleukin-2 (MW = 15,000; pI = 6.8) and γ-interferon (MW = 40,000–45,000; pI = 8.6). However, conclusive elucidation of this problem will be obtained only by using monoclonal antibodies against interleukin-2 and γ-interferon and studying the effects of recombinant preparations of these substances on fibroblasts. This work is now in progress.

One important finding in the studies reported here was the demonstration that the effects of CSIF were selective for collagen, since the incorporation of ^{3}H-tyrosine, an amino acid nonprevalent in collagen, and that of ^{3}H-fucose, a monosaccharide not known to be incorporated into collagen, were not significantly inhibited by the partially purified supernatants. In fact, the incorporation of ^{3}H-fucose appeared to be consistently increased in cultures exposed to CSIF. Further confirmation of the selective effect of CSIF was obtained from the densitometric analysis of the fluorographs (shown in Figure 2), which demonstrated a fourfold increase in the fibronectin:collagen ratio in the cultures incubated with the partially purified PHA-stimulated supernatant.

Although other investigators have described the stimulation of fibroblast collagen production by mononuclear cell supernatants (15,16) or by direct contact with mononuclear cells (17), the possibility that the effects were due to stimulation of fibroblast proliferation rather than to a net increase in collagen production/cell was not rigorously excluded. In those studies, the fibroblast cultures examined were not confluent, and it is likely that a substantial increase in the fibroblast population may have occurred under those conditions. In fact, in the study by Wahl et al (16), there was a marked increase in production of noncollagenous proteins, and the proportion of collagen from the total protein synthesized in the presence of active mononuclear cell supernatants actually decreased compared with control conditions.

An alternative explanation for these discrepancies may be related to the production by mononuclear cells of separate factors that may either stimulate or inhibit fibroblast proliferation and/or collagen production. This possibility is supported by the previous demonstration by Neilson et al (18) that mononuclear cells are able to produce distinct factors that bidirectionally modulate fibroblast proliferation. Careful analysis of the results described by Hibbs et al (17) indicates that similar heterogeneity may exist for factors affecting collagen production. Although those authors emphasized the presence of collagen stimulatory activity in their co-culture studies, when higher concentrations of the active samples were examined (1:5 dilution), a profound inhibition of collagen production (>70%) was demonstrated. Subsequent studies by the same group of investigators have indeed demonstrated the existence of both stimulatory and inhibitory factors in antigen- and mitogen-activated mononuclear cell supernatants (19).

Despite the discrepancies discussed above, the findings described in this paper clearly show that mononuclear cell supernatants contain factors capable of potent and selective inhibition of collagen production by PSS fibroblasts. An attractive hypothesis that can be formulated to explain the excessive collagen accumulation characteristic of PSS is that mononuclear cells from PSS patients may have a defect in production of CSIF. When we performed studies to test this hypothesis, however, we failed to show significant differences in the amount of CSIF produced by either PSS or normal mononuclear cells that were stimulated by PHA (unpublished observations). These results, however, do not completely exclude the possibility that the in vivo response of PSS mononuclear cells may be different from that elicited in vitro under maximal nonphysiologic stimulation with PHA. This aspect may have relevance to the pathogenesis of PSS and clearly needs further study.

The potent and selective inhibition of PSS fibroblast collagen production by lymphokines obtained from normal human mononuclear cells demonstrated here suggests the feasibility of a novel therapeutic approach for PSS—using these substances to modulate the excessive collagen production characteristic of scleroderma fibroblasts. These findings are encouraging since, at the present time, there is no therapeutic modality which can effectively prevent the frequently progressive fibrosis that is characteristic of the disease.

ACKNOWLEDGMENTS

We appreciate the technical assistance of Ruth Herold, Mary Dixon, and Ronald Yankowski, and the expert assistance of Esther Lobb in the preparation of the manuscript.

REFERENCES

1. LeRoy EC: Scleroderma (systemic sclerosis), Textbook of Rheumatology. Edited by WN Kelley, ED Harris Jr, S Ruddy, CB Sledge. Philadelphia, WB Saunders, 1981, pp 1211–1230
2. LeRoy EC: Increased collagen synthesis by scleroderma skin fibroblasts in vitro: a possible defect in the regulation or activation of the scleroderma fibroblast. J Clin Invest 54:880–889, 1974
3. Jimenez SA, Bashey RI: Collagen synthesis by scleroderma fibroblasts in culture (letter). Arthritis Rheum 20:902–903, 1977
4. Buckingham RB, Prince RK, Rodnan GP, Taylor F: Increased collagen accumulation in dermal fibroblast cultures from patients with progressive systemic sclerosis (scleroderma). J Lab Clin Med 92:5–21, 1978
5. Uitto J, Bauer EA, Eisen AZ: Scleroderma: increased synthesis of triple helical type I and type III procollagens associated with unaltered expression of collagenase by skin fibroblasts in culture. J Clin Invest 64:921–930, 1979
6. Rodnan GP, Benedeck TG: An historical account of the study of progressive systemic sclerosis (diffuse scleroderma). Ann Intern Med 57:305–319, 1962

7. Jimenez SA, McArthur W, Rosenbloom J: Inhibition of collagen synthesis by mononuclear cell supernatants. J Exp Med 150:1421–1431, 1979
8. Hart PH, Powell LW, Cooksley WGE, Halliday JW: Mononuclear cell factors that inhibit fibroblast collagen synthesis. I. In vitro conditions determining their production and expression. Scand J Immunol 18:41–49, 1983
9. Hart PH, Powell LW, Cooksley WGE, Halliday JW: Mononuclear cell factors that inhibit fibroblast collagen synthesis. II. Properties of the factors. Scand J Immunol 18:51–58, 1983
10. McArthur W, Derr K, Dixon M, Jimenez SA, Rosenbloom J: Immune modulation of connective tissue functions: studies on the production of collagen synthesis inhibitory factor by populations of human peripheral blood mononuclear cells. Cell Immunol 74:126–139, 1982
11. Rosenbloom JR, McArthur W, Malamud D, Jimenez SA: Characterization of a lymphokine produced by human T cells which inhibits collagen synthesis. Cell Immunol 81:192–198, 1983
12. Subcommittee for Scleroderma Criteria of the American Rheumatism Association Diagnostic and Therapeutic Criteria Committee: Preliminary criteria for the classification of systemic sclerosis (scleroderma). Arthritis Rheum 23:581–590, 1980
13. Bashey RI, Jimenez SA: Increased sensitivity of scleroderma fibroblasts to stimulation of protein and collagen synthesis by serum. Biochem Biophys Res Commun 76:1214–1222, 1977
14. Juva K, Prockop DJ: Modified procedure for the assay of [^{3}H]- or [^{14}C]-labeled hydroxyproline. Anal Biochem 15:77–80, 1966
15. Johnson RL, Ziff M: Lymphokine stimulation of collagen accumulation. J Clin Invest 58:240–246, 1976
16. Wahl SM, Wahl LM, McCarthy JB: Lymphocyte-mediated activation of fibroblast proliferation and collagen production. J Immunol 121:942–946, 1978
17. Hibbs MS, Postlethwaite AE, Mainardi CL, Seyer JM, Kang AH: Alterations in collagen production in mixed mononuclear leukocyte-fibroblast cultures. J Exp Med 157:47–59, 1983
18. Neilson EG, Phillips SM, Jimenez SA: Lymphokine modulation of fibroblast proliferation. J Immunol 128:1484–1486, 1982
19. Postlethwaite AE, Smith GN, Mainardi CL, Seyer JM, Kang AH: Lymphocyte modulation of fibroblast function in vitro: stimulation and inhibition of collagen production by different molecules. J Immunol 132:2470–2477, 1984

SYNOVIAL FLUID CRYSTALS IN OSTEOARTHRITIS

PAUL A. GIBILISCO, H. RALPH SCHUMACHER, JR., JOSEPH L. HOLLANDER, and KEITH A. SOPER

Apatite crystals, calcium pyrophosphate dihydrate crystals, or both were observed in knee joint effusions from 60% of 100 consecutive osteoarthritis (OA) patients. Crystals were more common in patients with more severe OA and in joints that had received previous intraarticular steroid injections. Whether the latter was predominantly related to an effect of the steroid or to the fact that steroids were used in more severe cases was not clear. Crystals existed in many effusions without elevated synovial fluid leukocyte counts. A subgroup of 7 patients had both types of crystals, more crystal phagocytosis, and more severe OA.

Apatite and calcium pyrophosphate dihydrate (CPPD) crystals have been described in osteoarthritic synovial fluids in several reports (1–4). Although their frequency and significance are not known, such crystals have been proposed as possible factors in the production or exacerbation of osteoarthritis. We have studied 100 consecutive osteoarthritis patients with knee joint effusions, to determine how often crystals are present and to begin to evaluate their possible significance.

From the Arthritis Section, Department of Medicine, Veterans Administration Medical Center and Hospital of the University of Pennsylvania, Philadelphia.

Supported in part by NIH grant 1-R21-AG-02815-01.

Paul A. Gibilisco, MD: former Rheumatology Fellow, Veterans Administration Medical Center and Hospital of the University of Pennsylvania (current address: 185 Albert Street, Torrington, CT 06790); H. Ralph Schumacher, Jr., MD: Professor of Medicine, University of Pennsylvania School of Medicine, and Director, Arthritis–Immunology Center, Veterans Administration Medical Center; Joseph L. Hollander, MD: Emeritus Professor of Medicine, University of Pennsylvania School of Medicine; Keith A. Soper, MA: Biostatistician, Clinical Epidemiology Unit, University of Pennsylvania.

Address reprint requests to H. Ralph Schumacher, Jr., MD, Director, Arthritis–Immunology Center, VA Medical Center, University and Woodland Avenues, Philadelphia, PA 19104.

Submitted for publication June 26, 1984; accepted in revised form November 7, 1984.

MATERIALS AND METHODS

One hundred consecutive osteoarthritis (OA) patients with knee joint effusions were studied over a period of 2 years at the Philadelphia VA Medical Center and at the adjacent Hospital of the University of Pennsylvania. Current radiographs of the affected joints were available in 72 patients and were graded for severity of osteoarthritis on a scale of 1–4 (5). Each patient's age, disease duration, and information on previous intraarticular steroid injections were recorded. Pain severity on weight-bearing was graded on a scale of 0–3 (0 = no pain; 1 = mild pain; 2 = moderate pain; 3 = intolerable pain). Morning stiffness was also graded on a 0–3 scale (1 = <15 minutes; 2 = 15–30 minutes; 3 = >30 minutes). Crepitus was graded as 0–3 (1 = palpable with weight-bearing but not at rest; 2 = palpable with weight-bearing and at rest; 3 = audible on range of motion test without palpation).

Joints were thoroughly aspirated; synovial fluid volume and leukocyte count (white blood cells/mm^3) were recorded promptly after aspiration in all 100 patients. The absolute leukocyte count for each synovial fluid effusion was calculated (absolute white blood cell count = leukocytes/mm^3 × aspirated volume in mm^3).

In 52 of the patients, an aliquot of each effusion was centrifuged at 1,800 revolutions per minute for 10 minutes, and the supernatant was analyzed for lactic acid dehydrogenase, acid phosphatase, alkaline phosphatase, and total protein. To another 1–5-cc aliquot of synovial fluid, 0.03 cc of hyaluronidase (Wyeth, Philadelphia, PA) was added, followed by centrifugation at 1,000 rpm for 10 minutes. The sediment was examined for birefringent crystals by compensated polarized light microscopy, and for calcium-containing compounds, including clumps of apatite crystals, with von Kossa's and alizarin red stains (6,7). Percentages of crystals phagocytosed by leukocytes were estimated when possible by counting 100 CPPD crystals or apatite-like clumps and classifying each as intra- or extracellular.

In 80 patients with sufficient synovial fluid sediments, these sediments were studied by transmission electron microscopy (TEM) (7–9). Apatite was tentatively identified by +2 and +3 clumps on calcium stains (7) and ultimately confirmed by TEM in all cases. CPPD was identified by compensated polarized light microscopy, calcium stains, and in some cases by TEM.

The presence of osteoarthritis was established by typical history and physical findings. All 100 patients had chronic knee pain that was increased on activity. Many had OA at other sites, and none had evidence of any other cause for arthritis. Past or current radiographs had shown at least grade 1 OA in the knees. OA was confirmed radiographically in the 72 patients who had recently had radiographs taken. All 100 patients had synovial fluid leukocyte counts of $<2,000/mm^3$. OA patients who had leukocyte counts $>2,000/mm^3$ were previously eliminated from this study because of the possibility of coexisting diseases. Patients with chondrocalcinosis detectable on roentgenograms were also excluded.

Continuous variables which followed an approximately normal distribution were analyzed using the *t*-test when there were 2 groups and by 1-way analysis of variance when there were more than 2 groups (10). Continuous variables which have a highly nonsymmetric distribution, such as white blood cell counts, were analyzed using nonparametric methods: the Wilcoxon test when there were 2 groups and the Kruskal-Wallis test when there were more than 2 groups (11).

Categorical variables were analyzed using Fisher's exact test (11) and chi-square statistics. The association between previous steroid injections and presence of crystals, after adjustment for other predictors of crystal presence (OA grade, sex, duration, and crepitus), was analyzed using the multivariate technique of logistic regression (12). All *P* values were 2-sided.

RESULTS

As shown in Table 1, 60% of the patients studied had crystals identified in their synovial fluid. Twenty-two percent of the patients with crystals had CPPD crystals alone, 30% had apatite crystals alone, and 48% had both types of crystals.

Table 2 gives a comparison of patients with no crystals and those with crystals, on several variables.

Table 1. Presence and type of crystals found in synovial effusions from 100 osteoarthritis patients

	No. patients (%)
No crystals	40 (40)
Crystals	60 (60)
Apatite alone	18 (30)
CPPD alone*	13 (22)
Apatite + CPPD	29 (48)

* CPPD = calcium pyrophosphate dihydrate.

Table 2. Characteristics of 100 osteoarthritis (OA) patients by presence or absence of crystals in synovial fluid

Variable*	No crystals	Crystals	*P*
n	40	60	–
OA grade (0–4)	1.86 ± 0.85	2.61 ± 0.97	0.001†
% male	45	35	0.426
Age	61 ± 15	68 ± 17.5	0.019†
Disease duration (years)	4.0 ± 5.0	5.5 ± 7.0	0.108
Crepitus grade (0–3)	1.85 ± 0.80	2.25 ± 0.70	0.010†
SF absolute WBC (millions)	1.2 ± 5.0	1.0 ± 1.9	0.342
SF WBC ($\times 10^3$/ml)	200 ± 228	150 ± 188	–
SF volume (ml)	6.0 ± 6.0	5.0 ± 9.5	–
Previous intraarticular steroids	6/40 (15%)	29/60 (48%)	0.001†

* OA grade and crepitus variables are not skewed; values shown are mean ± SD. Age, OA duration, SF absolute WBC (synovial fluid absolute white blood cell count), SF WBC, and SF volume variables are skewed; values shown are median ± interquartile range.
† Statistically significant difference.

Patients with crystals had radiographic evidence of significantly more severe osteoarthritis, were older, had more crepitus, and were more likely to have had previous intraarticular steroid injections than patients without crystals. There were no statistically significant differences between the 2 groups in their levels of synovial fluid protein, alkaline phosphatase, acid phosphatase, or lactic dehydrogenase.

Table 3 shows the mean and median absolute synovial fluid leukocyte counts in patients with apatite alone, those with CPPD alone, and those with both apatite and CPPD. Absolute synovial fluid leukocyte counts were a skewed variable in this study; therefore, they were better summarized with the median rather than the mean. There was no significant difference in the absolute synovial fluid leukocyte counts of patients with and those without crystals. Also, there was no significant difference among patients with apatite alone, those with CPPD alone, and those with both crystals.

Table 3. Synovial fluid absolute white blood cell count (SF absolute WBC) of 100 osteoarthritis patients, by presence and type of crystals in effusions*

		SF absolute WBC (millions)	
	No. patients	Mean ± SD	Median ± interquartile range
No crystals	40	3.19 ± 4.99	1.20 ± 5.0
Crystals			
Apatite alone	18	2.18 ± 3.41	0.78 ± 2.0
CPPD alone	13	1.85 ± 2.75	1.00 ± 2.5
Apatite + CPPD	29	4.73 ± 11.40	1.00 ± 2.2

* Based on medians, $P = 0.344$, crystals versus no crystals; $P = 0.532$, comparison between crystal types. CPPD = calcium pyrophosphate dihydrate.

Table 4. Correlation between radiographic grade of osteoarthritis (OA) and presence of apatite or calcium pyrophosphate dihydrate crystals*

OA grade	No. of patients	No. (%) with crystals
1	14	4 (29)
2	28	17 (61)
3	21	14 (67)
4	9	9 (100)
Total	72	44 (61)

* Significant positive association ($P < 0.001$) between higher grade of OA and presence of crystals.

Table 4 gives the correlations between radiographic grades of osteoarthritis and the presence of apatite and/or CPPD crystals. Higher radiographic grades of OA were associated with increased frequency of crystals in the synovial fluid. Twenty-nine percent of the patients with grade 1 OA had crystals, while 100% of those with grade 4 disease had crystals ($P < 0.001$).

Figure 1 shows the percentage of crystals phagocytosed in patients with apatite alone, those with CPPD alone, and those with both apatite and CPPD crystals, by radiographic grade of osteoarthritis. Patients with higher radiographic grades of OA were more likely to have predominantly (>50%) intracellular crystals. Predominantly intracellular crystals were found in 7 patients, all of whom had radiographic grade 3 or 4 disease. In addition, these 7 patients all had apatite and CPPD crystals occurring together and had significantly higher absolute synovial fluid leukocyte counts than patients with more extracellular crystals.

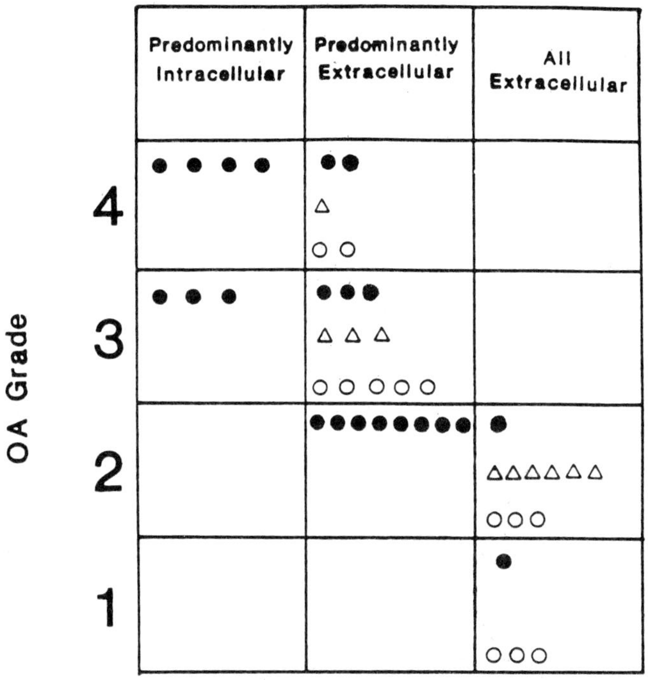

Figure 1. Osteoarthritis (OA) grade, by type and location of apatite and calcium pyrophosphate dihydrate (CPPD) crystals. ○ = apatite alone; △ = CPPD alone; ● = apatite + CPPD.

Since patients with crystals were more likely to have had previous intraarticular steroid injections than were patients without crystals ($P < 0.001$), we also compared several other variables in patients with and without previous intraarticular steroid injections (Table 5). Patients with previous injections had radiographic evidence of significantly more severe osteoar-

Table 5. Characteristics of osteoarthritis (OA) patients with versus those without previous intraarticular (IA) steroid injections

Variable*	No IA steroids	IA steroids	P
n	65	35	–
OA grade (0–4)	2.0 ± 0.91	2.77 ± 0.94	0.001†
% male	43	31	0.355
Age	61 ± 15.0	69 ± 13.0	0.002†
Disease duration (years)	4 ± 4.5	7 ± 5.0	0.004†
Crepitus grade (0–3)	1.91 ± 0.79	2.43 ± 0.61	0.001†
Morning stiffness grade (0–3)	1.52 ± 0.81	2.06 ± 0.73	0.002†
Pain on weight-bearing grade (0–3)	2.11 ± 0.75	2.46 ± 0.61	0.020†
LDH (IU/liter)	142 ± 72.0	186 ± 99.5	0.004†
SF absolute WBC (millions)	1.0 ± 1.72	1.2 ± 3.90	0.044†

* OA grade, crepitus, morning stiffness, and pain on weight-bearing variables are not skewed; values shown are mean ± SD. Age, disease duration, lactic dehydrogenase (LDH), and synovial fluid absolute white blood cell count (SF absolute WBC) variables are skewed; values shown are median ± interquartile range.
† Statistically significant difference.

Table 6. Osteoarthritis (OA) patients with versus those without previous intraarticular (IA) steroids, compared by presence or absence of synovial fluid crystals, with stratification by OA grade

	Grade 1–2 OA, no. (%)*			Grade 3–4 OA, no. (%)†		
	No crystals	Crystals	Total	No crystals	Crystals	Total
No IA steroids	19 (90)	10 (48)	29 (69)	3 (43)	10 (43)	13 (43)
IA steroids	2 (10)	11 (52)	13 (31)	4 (57)	13 (57)	17 (57)

* $P = 0.006$, Fisher's 2-sided exact test.
† $P = 1.000$, Fisher's 2-sided exact test.

thritis, were older, had longer disease duration, more symptoms, and higher synovial fluid lactic dehydrogenase and absolute leukocyte counts.

In addition, we examined whether apatite crystals alone, CPPD crystals alone, or apatite and CPPD crystals together were more common in patients with previous intraarticular steroid injections. There were no significant differences in presence of the different crystals.

We next considered whether the observed association between previous intraarticular steroid injections and the presence of crystals might have arisen solely because both are associated with OA grade or some other measure of disease severity. After adjustment for radiographic grade of OA using logistic regression, intraarticular steroids had a borderline significant ($P = 0.064$) association with the presence of crystals. By the same logistic regression model, no other variable (age, disease duration, sex, crepitus, etc.) showed any significant association with crystal presence.

The group of patients who had previous intraarticular steroids was compared with those who did not, according to presence or absence of crystals. The results are shown in Table 6, for patients with grade 1–2 OA and those with grade 3–4 disease. The grades were pooled because of relatively small sample sizes. There was a highly statistically significant association between previous injections and presence of synovial fluid crystals in affected joints of patients with grade 1–2 disease ($P = 0.006$). However, this was not found in patients with grade 3–4 disease ($P = 1.0$).

DISCUSSION

A striking finding in this study was the presence of either apatite, CPPD, or both types of crystals in 60% of the 100 osteoarthritic knees studied, even though only 1 effusion from each patient was examined. Dieppe and coworkers in England (3,4) identified CPPD or apatite crystals in 14 of 34 (41%) osteoarthritic synovial fluids. They used polarized light and both scanning and transmission EM, but did not perform initial screening with a calcium stain, as we did with alizarin red and von Kossa's stains. Halverson and McCarty, using a semiquantitative radionuclide binding technique, reported binding, presumably due to hydroxyapatite, in 29% of a variety of noninflammatory joint fluids and in none of the inflammatory fluids (13). Presence of the presumed apatite and/or CPPD correlated with higher radiologic grades of osteoarthritis. Further studies quantifying numbers of crystals would be of interest.

It should be noted that our patients were selected by the presence of knee effusions, so crystals may not be equally prominent in all osteoarthritic joints. The correlation between presence of crystals and higher radiologic grade of osteoarthritis would be consistent with the thesis that the crystals contribute to the severity, or that crystal presence results from more severe disease. Prospective studies that include examinations of more mildly involved joints should be helpful. It is of interest that in an autopsy study (14,15) we found that joint calcification, as manifested by roentgenograms, alizarin red and von Kossa staining of tissues, and limited electron microscopy of cartilage correlated strongly with severity of osteoarthritis.

The correlation between crystal presence and previous steroid injections is also of interest. This relationship could be due in part to more severe OA, requiring more injections, but it is also possible that the local steroids contributed to the crystal precipitation or release into the joint space. Correlation between crystal presence and previous steroid injections was only of borderline significance after correction for radiographic grade of OA, when the entire group was considered. The correlation between crystal presence and intraarticular steroid use was stronger in patients with grade 1–2 OA than in those with grade 3–4 disease, suggesting that, at least in these patients, the injections may in fact have been an important factor. McCarty (16) and Hardin et al (17) have described radiographic evidence of the appearance of calcification around joints after injection with depot corticosteroids. Whether this would be associated with demonstrable apatite crystals in joint fluid is not known.

Unfortunately, we did not record the frequency with which joints had been injected. The only way to definitely establish whether there is a cause/effect relationship between injections and crystal presence is to conduct a prospective clinical trial in which 1 group of patients does not receive intraarticular steroids and another group receives them as needed. The findings in patients with grade 1–2 OA would be of particular interest.

We could not demonstrate any higher median synovial fluid absolute leukocyte counts in patients with crystals versus those without. A contribution of crystals to inflammation in some osteoarthritis patients must still be considered, however. It should be noted that patients with synovial leukocyte counts $>2{,}000/mm^3$ were excluded from this study. Crystal phagocytosis by synovial cells has been described (2), and it could also contribute to joint disease (18), even without being reflected by synovial fluid leukocytosis.

This study again confirms that, as with monosodium urate crystals in gout (19), CPPD and apatite crystals can exist in synovial effusions with little readily detectable inflammatory cell response. Crystals were seen to be phagocytosed by some cells in many fluid samples with varying leukocyte counts. One surprising and incompletely explained finding was that crystals were predominantly extracellular in all patients with grade 1–2 OA in whom phagocytosis was studied. Patients with more severe OA had higher percentages of crystals in cells. The group with predominantly intracellular crystals all had grade 3–4 radiographic OA, all had both CPPD and apatite crystals, and this subgroup of 7 patients did have significantly higher leukocyte counts. We do not have data as to what cell types contained the crystals. Whether increased phagocytosis is a result of increased numbers of or different properties of crystals, or is related to an increase in leukocytes due to some other cause, is not yet clear.

REFERENCES

1. Schumacher HR: Osteoarthritis: the role of articular crystals. Ariz Med 25:22–25, 1978
2. Schumacher HR: Pathogenesis of crystal-induced arthritis. Clin Rheum Dis 3:105–131, 1977
3. Dieppe PA, Crocker PR, Corke CF, Doyle DV, Huskisson EC, Willoughby DA: Synovial fluid crystals. Q J Med 48:533–553, 1979
4. Huskisson EC, Dieppe PA, Tucker AK, Cannell LB: Another look at osteoarthritis. Ann Rheum Dis 38:423–428, 1979
5. Kellgren JH, Lawrence JS: Radiological assessment of osteoarthritis. Ann Rheum Dis 16:494–502, 1957
6. Mallory FB: Pathological Technique. Philadelphia, WB Saunders, 1942, p 144
7. Paul H, Reginato AJ, Schumacher HR: Alizarin red S staining as a screening test to detect calcium compounds in synovial fluid. Arthritis Rheum 26:191–200, 1983
8. Schumacher HR, Smolyo AP, Tse RL, Maurer K: Arthritis associated with apatite crystals. Ann Intern Med 87:411–416, 1977
9. Schumacher HR, Miller JL, Ludivico C, Jessar RA: Erosive arthritis associated with apatite crystal deposition. Arthritis Rheum 24:31–37, 1981
10. Winer BJ: Statistical Principles in Experimental Design. Second edition. New York, McGraw-Hill, 1971, pp 160–166
11. Siegal S: Non-Parametric Statistics. New York, McGraw-Hill, 1956, pp 116–127
12. Schlesselman J: Case-Control Studies—Design, Conduct, and Analysis. Oxford, Oxford University Press, 1982
13. Halverson PB, McCarty DJ: Identification of hydroxyapatite crystals in synovial fluid. Arthritis Rheum 22: 389–395, 1979
14. Gordon GV, Villanueva T, Schumacher HR, Gohel V: Autopsy study correlating degree of osteoarthritis, synovitis and evidence of articular calcification. J Rheumatol 11:681–686, 1984
15. Schumacher HR, Gibilisco P, Reginato A, Cherian V, Gordon G: Implications of crystal deposition in osteoarthritis. J Rheumatol (suppl) 10:40–41, 1983
16. McCarty DJ: Treatment of rheumatoid joint inflammation with triamcinolone hexacetonide. Arthritis Rheum 15:157–173, 1972
17. Hardin JG Jr, Grelier JM, Andriopoulos N: Controlled study of long-term effects of "total hand" injection: a preliminary report (abstract). Arthritis Rheum 19:800–801, 1976
18. Wigley FM, Fine IT, Newcombe DS: The role of the human synovial fibroblast in monosodium urate crystal-induced synovitis. J Rheumatol 10:602–611, 1983
19. Agudelo CA, Weinberger A, Schumacher HR, Turner R, Molina J: Definitive diagnosis of gout by identification of urate crystals in asymptomatic metatarsophalangeal joints. Arthritis Rheum 22:559–560, 1979

BLASTOMYCOSIS PRESENTING AS MONARTICULAR ARTHRITIS

The Role of Synovial Fluid Cytology

ALFRED L. GEORGE, JR., J. TAYLOR HAYS, and BARNEY S. GRAHAM

Joint complaints are common among patients with blastomycosis; however, true arthritis is infrequently documented by synovial fluid analysis. Of 72 individuals with blastomycosis who were patients at the Vanderbilt School of Medicine affiliated hospitals during the period 1957–1983, 6 (8%) had arthritis at presentation. In 5 patients (7%), monarticular arthritis was the chief complaint leading to hospitalization. Cytologic examination of synovial fluid was performed in 4 patients and demonstrated characteristic organisms each time. Three patients had negative 10% potassium hydroxide smears, and 2 had negative synovial fluid cultures. Blastomycosis should be considered in the differential diagnosis of acute arthritis. In patients with blastomycotic arthritis, cytologic examination of synovial fluid can add to the diagnostic yield of synovial fluid fungal cultures and potassium hydroxide preparations.

Blastomycosis is a fungal infection caused by *Blastomyces dermatitidis* (1). The illness can affect multiple organs including lung, skin, bone, and genitourinary tract. Joint involvement has been infrequently reported and has only rarely been noted as a presenting manifestation of disseminated disease. We discuss 5 patients with systemic blastomycosis in whom monarticular arthritis was the initial complaint, and we review the diagnostic implications suggested by these cases.

From the Departments of Medicine, Metropolitan Nashville General Hospital and Vanderbilt University Hospital, Vanderbilt University School of Medicine, Nashville, Tennessee.

Alfred L. George, Jr., MD: Resident in Medicine, Vanderbilt University Hospital; J. Taylor Hays, MD: Instructor of Medicine (former Chief Medical Resident), Metropolitan Nashville General Hospital; Barney S. Graham, MD: Fellow in Infectious Diseases (former Chief Medical Resident), Vanderbilt University Hospital.

Address reprint requests to Barney S. Graham, MD, Department of Medicine, Vanderbilt University Hospital, Nashville, TN 37232.

Submitted for publication July 2, 1984; accepted in revised form November 14, 1984.

METHODS

Data were compiled from 4 Nashville hospitals: Vanderbilt University Hospital (VUH), Nashville Veterans Administration Hospital (NVAH), Metropolitan Nashville General Hospital (MNGH), and St. Thomas Hospital. The records of all patients with a discharge diagnosis of blastomycosis or with a culture positive for *Blastomyces dermatitidis* between 1957 and February 1984 were reviewed. The records of patients who exhibited symptoms suggestive of bone or joint involvement were evaluated to determine the specific clinical syndrome on presentation, the methods used to determine joint infection, and the outcome of the illness.

The diagnosis of blastomycotic joint infection required culture-positive synovial fluid or microscopic evidence of the yeast in synovial fluid and culture-positive tissue from another site. Arthritis was defined as pain in a joint with limited mobility and a synovial effusion.

Cytologic preparations were made by staining air-dried synovial fluid smears with methenamine silver, periodic acid–Schiff (PAS) reagent, or Wright's stain.

RESULTS

Seventy-two patients with blastomycosis, ranging in age from 2–75 years, were discovered. There were 54 men. Eight patients (11%) had joint pain on admission to the hospital. In 2 instances, this pain was from periarticular soft tissue involvement, so true arthritis with synovial effusion was present at the time of admission in only 6 patients (8%). Five patients (7%) had proven blastomycotic arthritis. One patient with arthritis had only bacterial cultures performed on her synovial fluid and is not included in our analysis. Other sites were involved with the following frequencies: lung in 51 patients (71%), skin in 27 patients (38%), bone in 12 patients (17%), oropharynx in 6 patients (8%), genitourinary tract in 4 patients (6%), deep soft tissue in 4 patients (6%), and other visceral organs in 4 patients (6%). Of the 5 patients with blastomycotic arthritis at the time of admission, 4 had pulmonary involvement (patients 1, 2, 3, and 5), 4 had osteomyelitis (patients 1, 2, 4, and 5), 3 had skin lesions (patients 2, 3, and 4), and 1 had lymph node and epididymal involvement (patient 4). All 5 patients with blastomycotic arthritis were treated with amphotericin B, and they recovered fully.

The results of synovial fluid analyses are illustrated in Table 1. Synovial fluid cytology was the only method that yielded no false-negative results. In 2 patients, synovial fluid fungal cultures were negative, with concomitant positive cultures from another site and positive synovial fluid cytology (patients 2 and 5).

Information on patient 5 has been previously reported (2). A review of the specific findings on patients 1–4 follows.

Patient 1. Patient 1, a 57-year-old white man, presented to MNGH after 1 week of progressive pain and swelling of his left ankle. He had no other complaints initially, but later in the hospitalization he reported a 2-week history of night sweats, exertional dyspnea, and an increasingly productive cough.

He was thin and had a swollen, tender left ankle. Blood pressure was 140/80 mm Hg, pulse rate 92/minute, and oral temperature 36.1°C. Examination results were otherwise unremarkable. Peripheral white blood cell (WBC) count was 8,900 cells/mm^3 with a normal differential. Roentgenograms demonstrated a 1.5-cm lytic lesion of the distal left fibula and regional soft tissue swelling. A bone scan showed this lesion to be "cold."

He was admitted for bone biopsy and was treated with intravenous oxacillin. Routine chest roentgenogram revealed bilateral interstitial infiltrates. An arthrocentesis was performed and yielded grossly purulent fluid. Microscopic examination revealed 52,900 WBC/mm^3 (79% neutrophils) and 400 red blood cells (RBC)/mm^3. A Gram stain of synovial fluid was negative, but examination of a 10% potassium hydroxide (KOH) preparation demonstrated budding yeasts. Similar organisms were seen in sputum KOH preparations. Amphotericin B therapy was begun, and gradual improvement in the ankle swelling was observed. *Blastomyces dermatitidis* was isolated from cultures of sputum and synovial fluid. Complete resolution of the patient's arthritis, lytic bone lesion, and pulmonary infiltrates was achieved after treatment with amphotericin B.

Comment. This man sought medical care because of arthritis. He had septic arthritis, osteomyelitis, and pneumonitis caused by *B dermatitidis*. Diagnosis was made by microscopic examination of a 10% KOH preparation of synovial fluid.

Patient 2. This 69-year-old black man was admitted for evaluation of left knee pain and swelling. Medical history was remarkable only for mild degenerative arthritis. Six weeks prior to entering the hospital he had noted the onset of pain, warmth, redness, and swelling in the left knee. After an unsuccessful trial of cephalexin, he came to NVAH. At the time of presentation, he also reported a 6-week history of fever, chills, anorexia, and 15-lb. weight loss, but he denied night sweats, cough, hemoptysis, or chest pain.

He was thin and had an oral temperature of 38.2°C. The left knee was swollen, with a synovial effusion. There was exquisite tenderness of the proximal left tibia and warm erythema over the upper calf. A 1.5-cm crusted plaque was noted above the left eyebrow. Peripheral WBC count was 9,300 cells/mm^3 with a normal differential; the hematocrit was 31.4%. A chest roentgenogram revealed diffuse, fine nodular interstitial infiltrates. Roentgenograms of the left knee demonstrated mottling of the proximal tibia. Arthrocentesis yielded cloudy yellow fluid with 6,425 WBC/mm^3 (99% neutrophils) and 65,000 RBC/mm^3. No crystals were seen by polarized light microscopy, and results of a Gram stain examination were negative.

The patient was initially treated with intravenous oxacillin. A bone scan showed increased radio-

Table 1. Results of synovial fluid examinations in patients with arthritis and blastomycosis

Patient	Potassium hydroxide preparation	Culture	Cytology
1	+	+	Not done
2	–	–	+
3	–	+	+
4	+	+	+
5	–	–	+

isotope labeling of the proximal left tibia, consistent with osteomyelitis. Although 10% KOH preparations of synovial fluid produced negative findings, cytologic staining with PAS and methenamine silver revealed numerous yeast forms. Subsequent histologic examination and culture of a biopsy specimen from the patient's skin lesion demonstrated *Blastomyces dermatitidis*. Synovial fluid fungal cultures were negative. Treatment with amphotericin B resulted in resolution of his skin lesion, pulmonary infiltrates, osteomyelitis, and arthritis.

Comment. Patient 2 sought medical attention because of arthritis. His illness also included asymptomatic pneumonitis, a culture-positive skin lesion, and osteomyelitis. Examination of special stains of synovial fluid smears revealed yeast forms, even though synovial fluid 10% KOH preparations and cultures were negative.

Patient 3. A 60-year-old black woman was admitted to MNGH for evaluation of an acutely painful and swollen right ankle. Her health had been generally good except for mild, non–insulin-dependent diabetes mellitus. Three months prior to admission, she developed an area of induration over her left hip, which drained purulent material upon incision. Bacterial culture of the exudate was negative. She was treated with cloxacillin, but after 1 week, she still had a low-grade fever. A chest roentgenogram showed a diffuse increase in interstitial markings. An intermediate-strength tuberculin skin test produced negative results. Kinyoun stains and 10% KOH preparations of the sputum were examined and were negative. Three weeks after her initial visit, she was lost to followup. Two months later, she returned with a 1-week history of increasing pain, accompanied by warmth and swelling, in her right ankle.

She was obese and ill-appearing, with an oral temperature of 37°C. An open wound without drainage was present over the left greater trochanter; there were no other skin lesions. The right ankle was swollen, hot, and painful on passive motion. A peripheral WBC count was 15,100 cells/mm^3; the hematocrit was 35.6%. Serum chemistry findings were normal except for a glucose level of 348 mg/dl. A chest roentgenogram showed increased interstitial markings without significant interval change. A roentgenogram of the right ankle showed no bony abnormalities. Joint aspiration yielded <1 cc of purulent synovial fluid. Examination of a Gram stain, Kinyoun stain, and 10% KOH preparation of synovial fluid revealed no organisms. Examination with polarized light microscopy showed no crystals.

She was treated with indomethacin, oxacillin, and gentamicin. Dyspnea and marked hypoxemia developed over the next week, at which time an open lung biopsy was performed. Microscopic examination

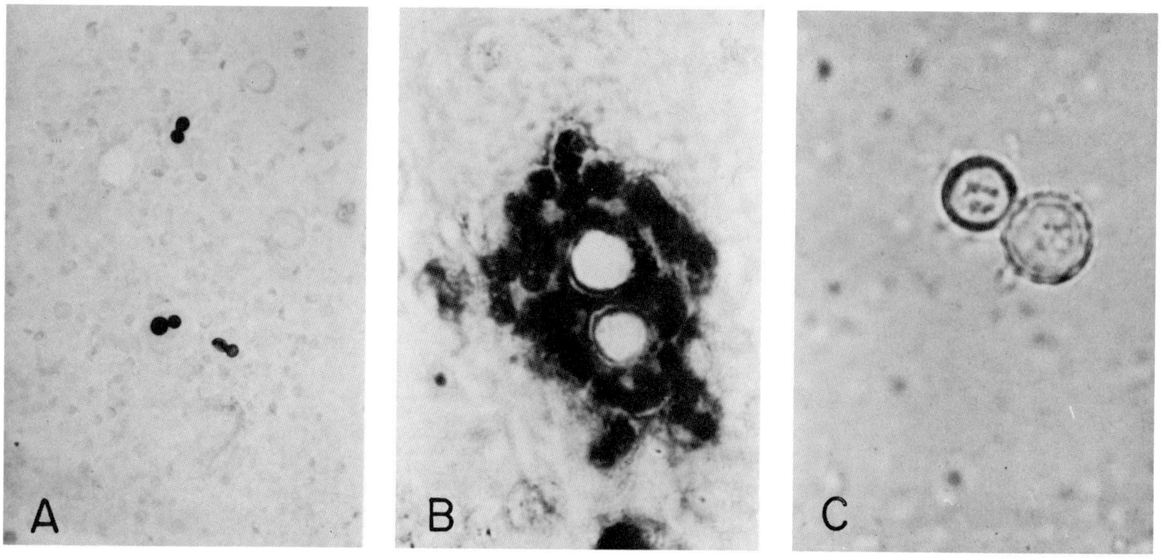

Figure 1. Appearance of *Blastomyces dermatitidis* in synovial fluid smears. Note the doubly refractile wall, multiple nuclei, and broad-based buds. **A**, Patient 3 (methenamine silver stain, original magnification × 400). **B**, Patient 4 (Wright's stain, original magnification × 1,000). **C**, Patient 4 (10% potassium hydroxide stain, original magnification × 1,000).

of special stains of this specimen revealed budding yeast resembling *Blastomyces dermatitidis*. Synovial fluid fungal cultures later yielded *B dermatitidis*. A smear of synovial fluid from the initial arthrocentesis was then stained with methenamine silver, and microscopic examination revealed the characteristic broad-based budding yeast (Figure 1A). Treatment with amphotericin B resulted in complete resolution of her illness.

Comment. Retrospective cytologic examination in this patient demonstrated *B dermatitidis*, after 10% KOH preparations had been negative for the organism. Cytologic examination of synovial fluid smears on admission would have obviated the need for an open lung biopsy, and earlier treatment may have avoided the life-threatening respiratory decompensation that occurred during hospitalization.

Patient 4. Patient 4, a 64-year-old white man, was admitted to VUH because of pain of 5 weeks duration in the left elbow, both hands, and right knee. During this time he also noted the development of multiple skin lesions with purulent drainage over his extremities. One week prior to admission, he developed dysuria. He had been wheelchair-bound for 2 years and had become demented. He had mild glucose intolerance.

The temperature was 37.6°C orally. There were several small, nontender, violaceous nodules over the extremities. The left testicle was enlarged, tender, and firm, and there was scrotal erythema. The only synovial effusion was in the right second metacarpophalangeal joint, which also had limited mobility. Chest roentgenogram results were normal; WBC count was 10,500 cells/mm^3 with a normal differential. Roentgenograms of the right hand and ankle were diagnostic of osteomyelitis.

Aspiration of the right second metacarpophalangeal joint yielded 10 cc of pus. Examination of KOH and Wright's stained preparations revealed the characteristic forms of *B dermatitidis* (Figures 1B and C). Synovial fluid culture also yielded the organism. Involvement of skin, lymph nodes, and epididymis was proven histologically from biopsy specimens. He received 2,500 mg of amphotericin B and was cured.

Comment. This patient was brought for medical care because of arthritis. Several joints were painful, but only 1 had an effusion. He had skin, genitourinary tract, bone, and joint infection with *Blastomyces dermatitidis*. The nature of his illness was first revealed by examination of synovial fluid.

Table 2. Frequency of joint pain and synovial fluid analysis in patients with blastomycosis

Reference	Frequency of joint complaints	No. of synovial fluid examinations	No. of cases diagnosed from synovial fluid examination
Kunkel et al, 1954 (7)	2/90	NA	NA
Cherniss and Waisbren, 1955 (6)	6/40	NA	NA
VA Cooperative Study, 1964 (5)	6/198	0	0
Sanders, 1967 (10)	9/74	6	4
Witorsch and Utz, 1968 (3)	6/40	2	1
Duttera and Osterhout, 1969 (9)	6/63	NA	NA
Vanek et al, 1970 (11)	2/10	2	2
Fountain, 1973 (12)	3/25	2	2
Cush et al, 1976 (8)	7/44	NA	NA
Present report	8/72	5	5
Total	55/656 (8.4%)	17	14/17 (82%)

* NA = information not available.

DISCUSSION

Blastomycosis is a primary pulmonary infection that commonly disseminates to skin, bone, and multiple other organs (3). The syndrome can range from an asymptomatic, self-limited pneumonia to a rapidly progressive, fatal, systemic illness (1). Because it is an uncommon infection with protean manifestations, there is often delay in diagnosis (4).

Joint pain has been reported in 3–15% of patients who have blastomycosis (3,5–9). The frequency of blastomycotic arthritis, however, is not known since synovial fluid has rarely been examined (Table 2). Only 14 cases of documented joint involvement by *Blastomyces dermatitidis* could be found in the English literature since 1950 (2,3,10–17). Our series of patients demonstrated a frequency of joint pain (11%) similar to that found in the previously reported patients. More importantly, in each of the 5 patients in our group who underwent synovial fluid examination, *B dermatitidis* was identified.

Two processes contribute to the pathogenesis of joint involvement in blastomycosis. Direct extension from juxtaarticular osteomyelitis is well recognized (ref. 10 and our patients 1, 2, and 4), and hematogenous seeding is also thought to occur (refs. 7, 10, and 12 and our patient 3). The arthritis is usually monarticular, most commonly affecting the knee, ankle, or elbow (18). The small joints of the hands and feet are involved in rare instances (ref. 16 and our patient 4). The joint pain is generally severe and relatively acute in onset (18). Four of our 5 patients sought medical attention within 1 week of the beginning of their arthritis; the only one who did not was a man with documented dementia. Nearly all patients (90%) have signs of extraarticular blastomycotic infection at the time of their joint complaint (ref. 18 and our patients 1–5).

The diagnosis of blastomycotic arthritis requires synovial fluid analysis. The diagnostic yield is high (82%) when synovial fluid from a symptomatic joint is examined in the setting of blastomycosis (Table 2). The synovial fluid is typically purulent with a high polymorphonuclear leukocyte count. Examination of synovial fluid smears prepared with 10% KOH might reveal the broad-based budding yeast with its doubly refractile wall and multiple nuclei (ref. 18 and our patients 1 and 4) (Figure 1C). Cytologic analysis of synovial fluid can also be diagnostically useful (patients 2–5 (Figures 1A and B), as it is for sputum (19,20), bronchial washings (21), and pleural fluid (22) from patients with blastomycosis. Cytologic examination can reveal the organism even when 10% KOH preparations (patients 2 and 3) or cultures (patients 2 and 5) are negative. An additional advantage of cytologic preparations over KOH preparations is their permanence, which allows the use of multiple stains and examination by several individuals, resulting in more accurate and reproducible information.

Papanicolau, Giemsa-Wright, methenamine silver, and PAS are the agents commonly used to stain fungi. Methenamine silver offers the greatest contrast between stained organisms and background material, and thereby is the most sensitive (ref. 23 and Figure 1A). Synovial fluid fungal cultures should be performed to confirm the diagnosis of blastomycosis. *Blastomyces dermatitidis* will form colonies on the appropriate media within 4–7 days (3).

Blastomycosis should be considered in any patient with a monarthritis-pneumonitis syndrome; it is the diagnosis of exclusion if a suggestive skin lesion or osteomyelitis is also present. Eleven percent (8 of 72) of our patients with blastomycosis complained of joint pain; 8% (6 of 72) had frank arthritis; and 7% (5 of 72) had documented blastomycotic arthritis. Arthritis may be the presenting manifestation of the illness and is usually monarticular, involving the knee, ankle, elbow, or, less frequently, the small joints of the hands. Pulmonary involvement is usually present, and concomitant infection of skin and bone is common.

Analysis of synovial fluid has resulted in a diagnosis in 82% of patients with blastomycosis and arthritis (Table 2). The method is rapid, accurate, and safe. Its use will allow for early initiation of specific therapy and will obviate the need for more invasive diagnostic tests. Cytologic examination of synovial fluid can increase the diagnostic yield when added to the routine performance of KOH preparations and fungal cultures.

ACKNOWLEDGMENTS

We are grateful to Dr. William Schaffner for editorial comments and to Dr. Ann Melly for assistance in preparation of illustrations. We thank Stacy Dunaway and Sherry Bachus for typing the manuscript.

REFERENCES

1. Sarosi GA, Davies SF: Blastomycosis. Am Rev Respir Dis 120:911–938, 1979
2. Tustin AW, Kaiser AB, Bradsher RW, Herrington JL: Unusual fungal infections following jejunoileal bypass surgery. Arch Intern Med 140:643–645, 1980
3. Witorsch P, Utz JP: North American blastomycosis: a study of 40 patients. Medicine (Baltimore) 47:169–200, 1968
4. Cope JR: Blastomycosis: diagnostic difficulties. South Med J 74:284–287, 1980
5. Blastomycosis Cooperative Study of the Veterans Administration: Blastomycosis: a review of 198 collected cases in Veterans Administration hospitals. Am Rev Respir Dis 89:659–672, 1964
6. Cherniss EI, Waisbren BA: North American blastomycosis: a clinical study of 40 cases. Ann Intern Med 44:105–123, 1955
7. Kunkel WM, Weed LA, McDonald JR, Clagett OT: North American blastomycosis—Gilchrist's disease: a clinicopathologic study of ninety cases. Int Abstr Surg 99:1–26, 1954
8. Cush R, Light RW, George RB: Clinical and roentgenographic manifestations of acute and chronic blastomycosis. Chest 69:345–349, 1976
9. Duttera MJ, Osterhout S: North American blastomycosis: a survey of 63 cases. South Med J 62:295–301, 1969
10. Sanders LL: Blastomycosis arthritis. Arthritis Rheum 10:91–98, 1967
11. Vanek J, Schwarz J, Hakin S: North American blastomycosis: a study of ten cases. Am J Clin Pathol 54:384–400, 1970
12. Fountain FF: Acute blastomycotic arthritis. Arch Intern Med 132:684–688, 1973
13. Marx FJ, Berenbaum AA: Systemic blastomycosis: cause of an obscure infection in a nonendemic area. N Engl J Med 251:56–60, 1954

14. Liggett AS, Silberman Z: Blastomycosis of the knee joint. J Bone Joint Surg 52A:1445–1449, 1970
15. Maioriello RP, Merwin CF: North American blastomycosis presenting as an acute panniculitis and arthritis. Arch Dermatol 102:92–96, 1970
16. Claflin K, Milbauer J, Sullivan B: Ketoconazole and blastomycotic osteomyelitis (letter). Ann Intern Med 98:260–261, 1983
17. Stelling CB, Woodring JH, Rehm SR, Hopper DW, Noble RC: Miliary pulmonary blastomycosis. Radiology 150:7–13, 1984
18. Bayer AS, Scott VJ, Guze LB: Fungal arthritis. IV. Blastomycotic arthritis. Semin Arthritis Rheum 9:145–151, 1979
19. Johnston WW, Amatulli J: The role of cytology in the primary diagnosis of North American blastomycosis. Acta Cytol (Baltimore) 14:200–204, 1970
20. Sutliff WD, Cruthirds TP: Blastomyces dermatitidis in cytologic preparations. Am Rev Respir Dis 108:149–151, 1973
21. Sanders JS, Sarosi GA, Nollett DJ, Thompson JI: Exfoliative cytology in the rapid diagnosis of pulmonary blastomycosis. Chest 72:193–196, 1977
22. Covell JL, Lowry EH, Feldman PS: Cytologic diagnosis of blastomycosis in pleural fluid. Acta Cytol (Baltimore) 26:833–836, 1982
23. Schwarz J: The diagnosis of deep mycoses by morphologic methods. Hum Pathol 13:519–533, 1982

Erratum

Figures 12A and 12C were inadvertently transposed in the article by Dr. Neil D. Broom which appeared in the September 1984 issue of *Arthritis and Rheumatism* (Broom ND: The altered biomechanical state of human femoral head osteoarthritic articular cartilage. Arthritis Rheum 27:1028–1039, 1984). The corrected figure is shown below.

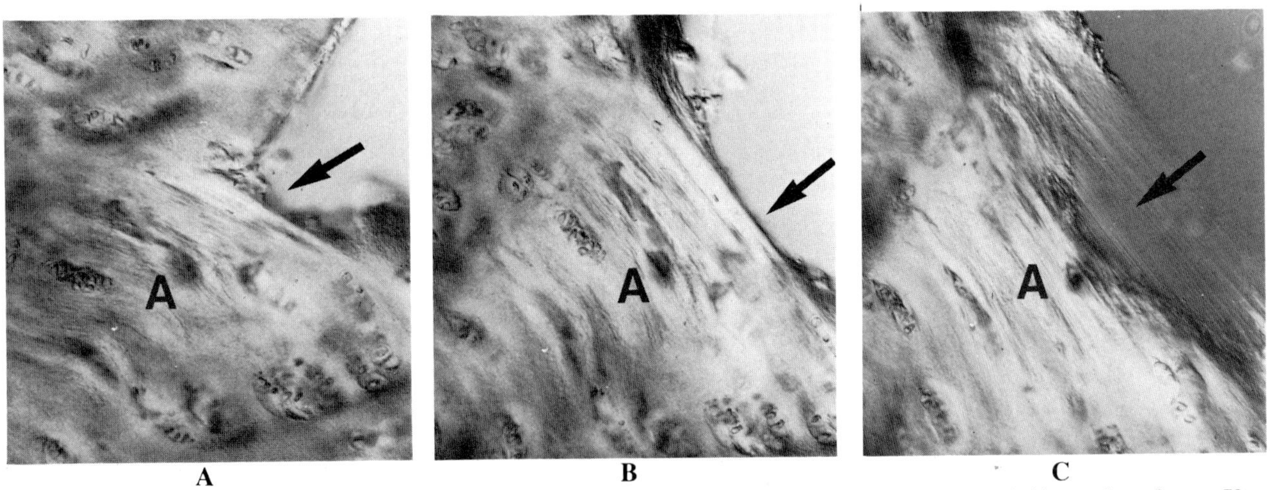

Figure 12. Sequence showing propagation of transverse notch through middle zone radial array (**A**) in osteoarthritic cartilage from a 72-year-old woman. **Arrows** indicate transverse direction and notch root. **A**, Unloaded tissue; **B**, Initial loading to first onset of rupture; **C**, Propagation of notch though radial array in transverse direction (differential interference contrast, original magnification × 120).

INDUCTION OF CHRONIC POLYARTHRITIS IN RABBITS BY HYPERIMMUNIZATION WITH *ESCHERICHIA COLI*

I. Pathologic and Serologic Features in Two Breeds of Rabbits

SHIGEHISA AOKI, KOJI IKUTA, TSUNEMASA NONOGAKI, and YOSHITAKE ITO

Hyperimmunization of 147 rabbits (outbred Japanese white rabbits and New Zealand white [NZW] rabbits bred in a closed colony) with heat-killed *Escherichia coli* 0:14 in Freund's incomplete adjuvant resulted in the animals developing a chronic polyarthritis resembling rheumatoid arthritis (RA). While both Japanese white and NZW rabbits showed a high incidence of the induced arthritis, a higher proportion of NZW rabbits developed the disease, suggesting that genetic influence is important in the development of RA-like illness. This experimental model may be useful for the study of RA.

Attempts to produce a pathologic condition resembling rheumatoid arthritis (RA) in laboratory animals have been both numerous and varied (1). It has been difficult, however, to find animal models that have both the morphologic and serologic characteristics associated with human RA (2).

We discovered, while investigating pyelonephritis caused by enterobacteriaceae (3,4), that arthritis developed in 1 of the rabbits immunized with heat-killed *Escherichia coli* 0:14. Based on this observation, we immunized additional rabbits over prolonged periods of time with the same bacterial antigen, which resulted in the development of a chronic polyarthritis having a morphologic and serologic resemblance to RA (5). This study was carried out to further characterize rabbit arthritis induced by hyperimmunization with heat-killed *E coli* 0:14, and to examine breed differences in the animals' susceptibility to the development of joint lesions.

From the Department of Pathology, Aichi Medical University, Nagakute-cho, Aichi-ken, Japan.

Supported in part by the Research Grant for the Intractable Diseases from the Ministry of Health and Welfare, and the Research Grant from the Ministry of Education, Science, and Culture, Japan.

Shigehisa Aoki, MD; Koji Ikuta, MD; Tsunemasa Nonogaki, PhD; Yoshitake Ito, PhD.

Address reprint requests to Shigehisa Aoki, MD, Department of Pathology, Aichi Medical University, Nagakute-cho, Aichi-ken 480-11, Japan.

Submitted for publication July 2, 1984; accepted in revised form November 14, 1984.

MATERIALS AND METHODS

Animals. One hundred fifty outbred Japanese white rabbits and 50 New Zealand white (NZW) rabbits bred in a closed colony at the Livestock Division, Department of Agriculture and Forestry, Tokyo were used. Rabbits of both sexes, each weighing about 2,000 gm at the beginning of the experiment, were caged individually and fed a commercial pellet diet, with water ad libitum.

Antigen. A strain of *E coli* 0:14 obtained through the courtesy of the Research Institute of Microbial Diseases, Osaka University, Japan was inoculated into tryptic soy broth (Difco, Detroit, MI). After overnight growth, bacteria were incubated at 37°C for 24 hours on trypticase soy agar (Baltimore Biological Laboratories, Baltimore, MD). Cultures were harvested in saline (10 ml per plate) and heated at 100°C for 2 hours. Large quantities of bacteria were stored in a cold room after freeze-drying to render them stable for prolonged periods of time. Heat-killed *E coli* 0:14 antigens containing both O antigen and common enterobacterial antigen (CA) (6,7) were adjusted to a concentration of 960 μg/ml, and this saline suspension showed a median lethal dose for mice of 180 μg. A single preparation of bacteria as described above was used for immunization of both strains of rabbits.

Immunization. One hundred seventeen Japanese white rabbits were injected intramuscularly, into multiple sites on the back, at monthly intervals with 2 ml of heat-killed *E coli* 0:14 (960 μg) suspended in Freund's incomplete adjuvant. The adjuvant was mixed with an equal volume of the antigen solution. Immunization was continued in each animal until the time of killing. Twenty-three additional

Japanese white rabbits of both sexes, injected with Freund's incomplete adjuvant alone, and 10 untreated rabbits of both sexes were used as controls.

After completion of the experiments with Japanese white rabbits, 30 NZW rabbits were similarly sensitized, and additional experiments were carried out with 10 NZW rabbits of both sexes, injected with adjuvant alone, and 10 normal NZW rabbits of both sexes, as controls. Blood was obtained at approximately 1-month intervals from each animal, via ear artery puncture. Sera were frozen and stored at −20°C.

Serologic methods. The antibody to the O antigen was titrated by bacterial agglutination. Titration of the CA antibody was done by the hemagglutination method using tanned sheep erythrocytes coated with the antigen from heat-killed heterologous enteric bacteria (7). The serologic method for quantitating a rheumatoid factor–like substance (RFLS) (8,9) analogous to human rheumatoid factor consisted of the hemagglutination of tanned sheep erythrocytes coated with aggregated (heated at 70°C for 10 minutes) rabbit gamma globulin (rabbit Cohn fraction II; Miles, Elkhart, IN), carried out primarily according to the method of Heller et al (10).

Histologic examination. Different animals were killed at various intervals, weekly until 1 month after initial immunization or monthly thereafter, in order to detect the development of various stages of arthritis. After dissection, the larger joints, including both shoulders, elbows, knees, and hips, were fixed in formol saline, decalcified, and sections were prepared. Sections were stained with hematoxylin and eosin, Masson's trichrome, and phosphotungstic acid hematoxylin (PTAH). In all experiments, arthritis was evaluated histologically.

RESULTS

Arthritis and serologic features in Japanese white rabbits. In the affected animals, marked ankylosis in both knee joints, resulting in stretched hind limbs, was seen 9 months after initial immunization (Figure 1). Autopsy of the affected animals revealed large amounts of fibrous connective tissue, which filled the knee joint space and adhered to the surface of the articular cartilage (Figure 2). In the shoulder joints of the same animals, articular cartilage was replaced by fibrous pannus, which extended across the joint surface and occasionally destroyed the bony endplate.

Grossly apparent lesions of small joints such as the wrists, ankles, forepaws, and hind paws were not generally noted. Therefore, the larger joints, i.e., the

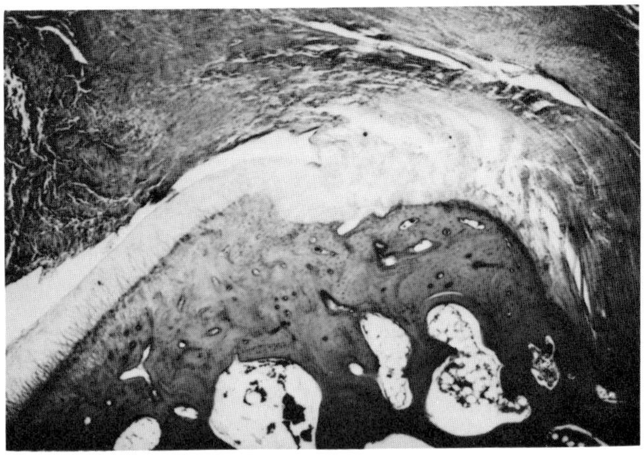

Figure 2. Histologic specimen from the right knee joint of the animal shown in Figure 1. A large amount of connective tissue pannus has occurred within the joint space, and articular cartilage is partially replaced by scar tissue (hematoxylin and eosin stained, magnification × 25).

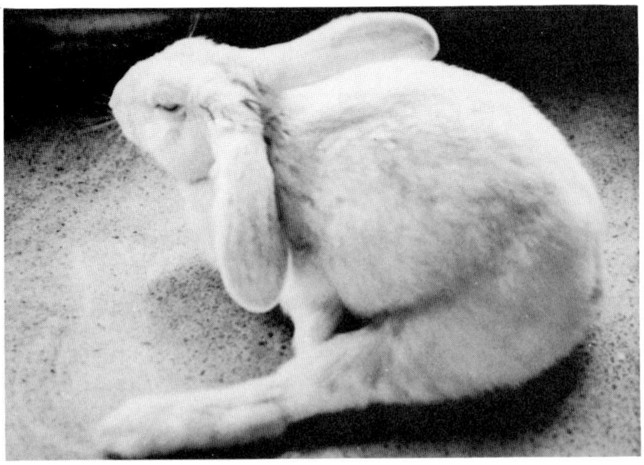

Figure 1. Typical affected Japanese white rabbit with chronic polyarthritis after 9 months of immunization with *Escherichia coli*. Because of severe ankylosis of the knee joints, both hind limbs remain stretched.

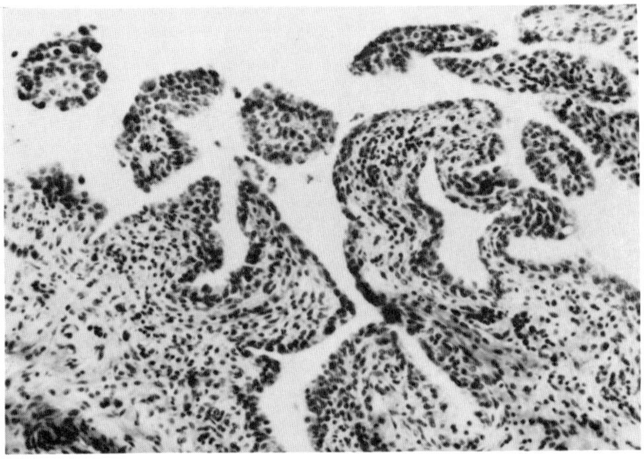

Figure 3. Histologic specimen showing chronic arthritis in the right shoulder joint of a Japanese white rabbit after 4 months of immunization with *Escherichia coli*. Hyperplastic villi are seen, with infiltration by lymphocytes and plasma cells (hematoxylin and eosin stained, magnification × 100).

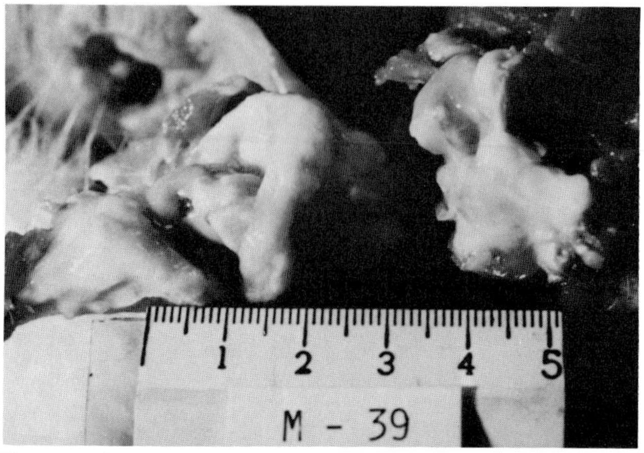

Figure 4. Specimens from both shoulder joints of the same animal shown in Figure 3, showing thickened synovial tissue and pannus formation.

shoulders, elbows, knees, and hips, were studied histologically in the rabbits killed at various intervals since initial immunization, in order to elucidate the developmental process of the arthritis.

Nonpurulent synovitis with proliferation of synovial lining cells and inflammatory cell infiltration, including aggregation of lymphocytes, occurred within 2 months of immunization. Fibrinous synovitis, confirmed by PTAH stain, was also seen after 2 months. Thereafter, hyperplastic synovial villi covered with proliferating lining cells were seen, and granulation tissue, accompanied by lymphocyte and plasma cell infiltration, increased in subsynovial tissue (Figure 3).

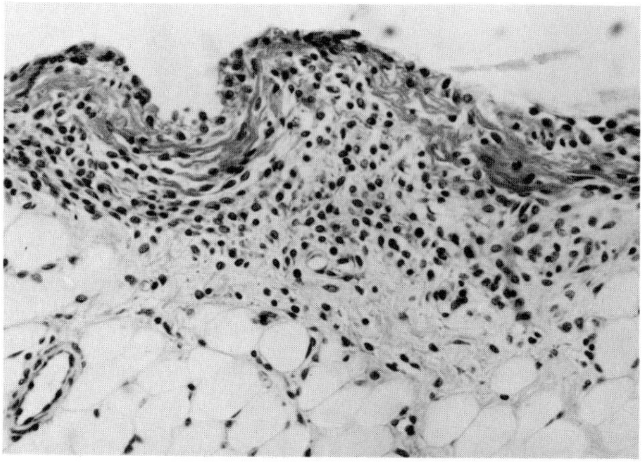

Figure 5. Histologic specimen from the right knee joint of a Japanese white rabbit after 7 months of immunization with *Escherichia coli*, showing chronic arthritis with longstanding fibrin deposition in the superficial layer of the synovium (hematoxylin and eosin stained, magnification × 200).

Table 1. Frequency of development of arthritis and pannus formation in Japanese white and New Zealand white (NZW) rabbits, after 1–7 months of immunization with *Escherichia coli*

	Japanese white rabbits		NZW rabbits	
	Frequency of arthritis (%)	Frequency of pannus formation (%)	Frequency of arthritis (%)	Frequency of pannus formation (%)
Males	47.7	10.5	71.4	21.4
Females	61.5	25.6	85.7	42.9
Total	56.9	20.7	78.6	32.1

Granulation tissue extending from the margins of the synovial membrane was found growing over the surfaces of articular cartilage after 4 months of immunization (Figure 4). In those places where the pannus came in contact with the cartilage, the latter was destroyed, producing small, localized areas of erosion.

After 7 months of immunization, affected synovial membranes became thickened and fibrous, and articular cartilage, partially replaced by fibrous pannus, was seen. Both old and new lesions were frequently present in a single affected joint. In areas with relatively new lesions, chronic synovitis was observed, with fibrin deposition in the superficial layer of the synovial membranes and subsynovial granulation tissue infiltrated by lymphocytes and plasma cells (Figure 5).

Of the Japanese white rabbits autopsied after periods of immunization ranging from a few weeks to 27 months, nonpurulent arthritis was observed in 64.1% (75 of 117) of the animals, while pannus formation occurred in 23% (27 of 117). However, of the 58 Japanese white rabbits killed after periods of immunization ranging from 1–7 months, nonpurulent arthritis was observed in 56.9% (33 of 58) of the animals, while the incidence of pannus formation was 20.7% (12 of 58) (Table 1).

Table 2. Bacterial agglutination titer (after 3 months of immunization with *Escherichia coli*) and frequency of arthritis in 78 outbred Japanese white rabbits*

Bacterial agglutination titer	No. of immunized rabbits	Frequency of arthritis (%)
>5,000	30	86.7
1,000–5,000	33	75.8
<1,000	15	46.7
Total	78	74.4

* Rabbits were immunized for 3–27 months before being killed; all sera were titrated after 3 months of immunization.

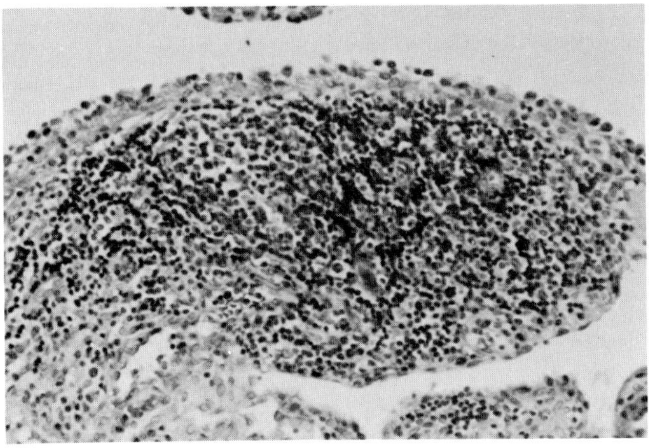

Figure 6. Histologic specimen from the right elbow joint of a New Zealand white rabbit after 6 months of immunization with *Escherichia coli*, showing chronic arthritis with lymphoid cell aggregation appearing as a follicle within the synovial villus (hematoxylin and eosin stained, magnification × 100).

The nonpurulent synovitis was first seen approximately 2 months after the initial immunization, with a peak incidence of 80% (12 of 15) being recorded at 8–9 months after the start of the experiment. Females were more frequently affected than males (Table 1). The nonpurulent arthritis was entirely absent in the control animals immunized over a 24-month period with Freund's incomplete adjuvant alone and in the untreated controls.

Serologically, the titers of the O antibody, measured by bacterial agglutination after 3 months of immunization, ranged from 1:80 to 1:20,480. The CA antibody titers, also after 3 months of immunization, correlated with those of the O antibody, though the CA titers were slightly lower. Untreated control animals generally exhibited O and CA antibody titers <1:40.

To study the relationship between the O antibody titers and the occurrence of arthritis, all rabbits immunized for 3–27 months were divided into 3 groups according to the antibody titer values, as follows: >1:5,000, 1:1,000 to 1:5,000, and <1:1,000. Of 30 rabbits showing antibody titers >1:5,000, 86.7% developed arthritis; of 33 rabbits with titers ranging from 1:1,000 to 1:5,000, 75.8% developed arthritis; and of the 15 animals with values <1:1,000, the incidence was 46.7% (Table 2).

RFLS was positive in the sera from 82 (70.1%) of the 117 Japanese white rabbits. In the same group, RFLS was positive in 80% of the 75 arthritic rabbits and in 28.6% of the 42 non-arthritic animals. In general, the RFLS in the sera of immunized animals was first detected 2 months after initial immunization, and the titer increased as immunization progressed.

Arthritis and serologic features in NZW rabbits. Nonpurulent synovitis with superficial fibrin deposition was observed 1 month after initial immunization in NZW rabbits. After 3 months of immunization, 1 rabbit showed arthritis of both hind limbs, with the left side remaining stretched. In both hips and knee joints of this affected animal, pannus formation was seen and granulation tissue extending to the articular cartilage from the area of synovitis was observed histologically. Marked lymphoid cell aggregation, appearing as follicles in the synovial villus, was found after 6 months of immunization (Figure 6). At this stage, multiple erosions and irregular destruction of the articular cartilage

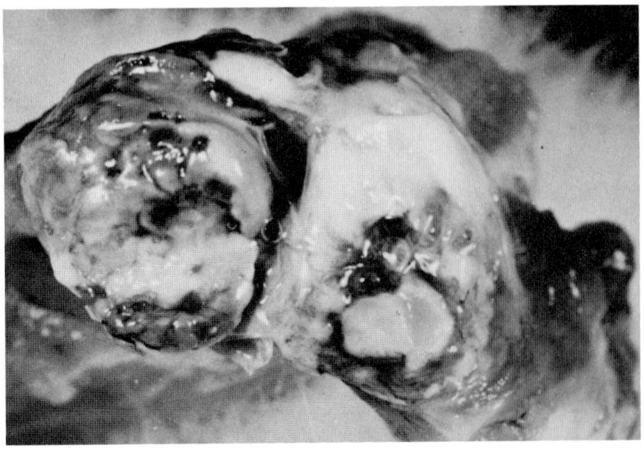

A

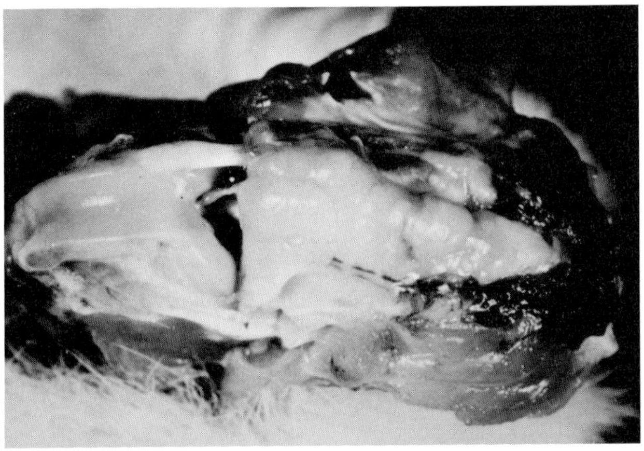

B

Figure 7. **A**, Specimen demonstrating severe arthritis in the left knee joint of a New Zealand white (NZW) rabbit after 6 months of immunization with *Escherichia coli*, showing multiple erosions and irregular destruction of the articular cartilage, accompanied by partial fibrous pannus. **B**, Left knee joint of a normal NZW rabbit, with the cartilage appearing markedly different from that shown in **A**.

occurred, accompanied by partial fibrous pannus (Figure 7A). This finding was shown more clearly when the destroyed knee joint was compared with the knee joint of a normal NZW rabbit (Figure 7B).

Histologically, the articular cartilage in grossly destroyed joints was replaced by fibrous pannus, and fibrous connective tissue came in contact with the bone. This finding was observed more easily when Masson's trichrome stain was used. Nonpurulent arthritis was absent in the control animals immunized over an 8-month period with Freund's incomplete adjuvant alone and in untreated control animals.

In the 30 NZW rabbits autopsied after an 8-month period of immunization, nonpurulent arthritis was observed in 76.7% (23 of 30) of the animals, and the incidence of pannus formation was 30% (9 of 30). Of the 28 NZW rabbits killed after periods of immunization ranging from 1–7 months, nonpurulent arthritis was observed in 78.6% (22 of 28) of the animals, and the incidence of pannus formation was 32.1% (9 of 28) (Table 1). As in the Japanese white rabbits, females were more frequently affected than males.

Serologically, the O antibody titer after 3 months of immunization was >1:1,280 for most of the immunized NZW rabbits. The CA antibody titers, also after 3 months of immunization, correlated with those of the O antibody, as was seen in the Japanese white rabbits. Most normal control NZW rabbits showed O and CA antibody titers <1:40. RFLS was positive in 82.8% of the sera from the 30 immunized rabbits. As with the Japanese white rabbits, the RFLS in NZW rabbits was positive after 2 months of immunization. Of the group of 30 NZW rabbits, the RFLS in the 23 arthritic animals was positive in 87%, and among the 7 non-arthritic rabbits, the incidence of positivity was 57%.

DISCUSSION

Although a number of bacteria and bacterial components have been studied in relation to their ability to induce a chronic synovitis similar to RA in experimental animals (1), it has not previously been documented, except in earlier studies in our laboratory (5), that hyperimmunization with heat-killed *E coli* is capable of inducing a chronic polyarthritis resembling RA. In the present experiment, we demonstrated that rabbits immunized with whole heat-killed *E coli* 0:14 suspended in Freund's incomplete adjuvant developed a chronic polyarthritis which appeared within 1–2 months after initial immunization. The synovitis was characterized by hyperplasia of the synovial cells, superficial fibrin deposition, and inflammatory cell infiltration including lymphoid cell aggregation. Inflammation in the larger joints advanced to pannus formation after an additional 2 months, finally resulting in articular cartilage destruction and fibrous ankylosis.

The heat-killed *E coli* 0:14 used as the antigen for immunization in our study is rich not only in heat-stable O antigen, but also in antigens common to the enterobacteriaceae (6,7), both of which are known to produce endotoxic reactions. It has been reported that bacterial endotoxins can induce proliferation of synovial cells (11) and synovitis (12). It is also considered possible that direct action against the synovium by the heat-killed *E coli* 0:14 containing endotoxic substances may participate in the formation of arthritis.

Gram-negative bacilli (13) and their cell wall lipopolysaccharides (14), as well as representative acid-fast bacteria (13), demonstrate adjuvant ability which stimulates the immune response of animals to such antigens. Therefore, it is conceivable from the present experiments that a cell wall component of *E coli* 0:14 itself was the adjuvant of significance in the induction of an immunologic synovitis and the continued formation of immune complexes stimulating the production of RFLS.

Intensive investigations have been focused on the production of lesions similar to RA in experimental animals, mainly by means of infection due to microorganisms, injection of noninfectious antigens, and immunologic reactions such as *Erysipelothrix* arthritis (15), *Mycoplasma* arthritis (16), streptococcal cell wall–induced arthritis (17), adjuvant arthritis (18), collagen arthritis (19), and antigen-induced arthritis (20). Although the pathoanatomic features of arthritis experimentally produced in animals by the methods described above resemble, in some respects, those of human RA, RFLS is usually absent from or inconsistently demonstrated in sera in these animal models. Abruzzo and Christian (8) succeeded in producing RFLS which resembled human RF, by long-term immunization of rabbits with formalin-killed *E coli*, but failed to produce arthritis in the animals.

In our experiments, the chronic polyarthritis that developed in rabbits immunized over prolonged periods of time with heat-killed *E coli* resembled RA not only pathomorphologically, but also serologically.

However, the distribution of arthritis in our study was different from the pattern of small joint involvement in human RA. In this investigation, histologic study of small joints was not performed since no grossly apparent lesions were observed on these joints; the possibility of histologic involvement will be examined in future studies. In addition, the significance of RFLS in the pathogenetic mechanism of this model will be assessed by immunohistologic study.

In outbred Japanese white rabbits, animals showing a high incidence of induced arthritis also had high levels of antibodies against the *E coli* antigen. However, when these results were compared with those obtained using NZW rabbits bred in a closed colony, the frequency of arthritis in the NZW rabbits was higher than that found in the Japanese white rabbits.

Blackham et al (21) reported that Old English rabbits were more susceptible to antigen-induced arthritis than either NZW or Dutch rabbits and that NZW rabbits were more sensitive than Dutch rabbits. Oldham and Coombs (22) also found that Old English rabbits were more susceptible to serum sickness arthritis than a number of other breeds tested, including NZW rabbits. However, they noted that the greatest incidence of joint lesions in Old English rabbits was similar to that found in the relatively closed breeding colony of NZW rabbits. These data indicate that immunologically-mediated arthritis is at least partially under genetic control.

The possibility that rheumatoid inflammation might be the result of many different etiologic agents and hence related to the presence of persistent bacterial debris, including peptidoglycan, in the joints of genetically susceptible individuals has often been proposed (23–25). The gastrointestinal tract is a possible continuing source of bacterial antigen. For example, postdysenteric Reiter's syndrome (26,27), arthritis after intestinal bypass surgery for morbid obesity (28), and juvenile rheumatoid arthritis with IgA deficiency (29) are all diseases which indicate that the gastrointestinal tract is a source of bacterial components capable of initiating arthritis. Lehman et al (30) reported the development of polyarthritis in rats following systemic injection of cell wall fragments from *Lactobacillus casei* commonly found in the gastrointestinal flora.

Perlmann et al (31) observed, in patients with ulcerative colitis, an increase in antibody titers against not only the polysaccharides of the mucous membrane of the colon, but also against those of *E coli* 0:14. The arthritis associated with ulcerative colitis, in which the intestinal barrier to enteric bacterial flora is impaired, may be related to continuing antigenic stimuli due to bacterial components, including endotoxins released from the dead organisms. Our results also suggest that an ordinary bacterium in the intestine may play a role in the pathogenetic mechanism of arthritic disease associated with RA.

Because of the similarities between the arthritic conditions we were able to induce in rabbits experimentally and those in human RA, it is anticipated that further study of the effects of hyperimmunization with *E coli* in animal models will contribute to the understanding of human rheumatoid disease.

ACKNOWLEDGMENTS

We wish to thank Atsuo Mori and Hiroshi Tanaka for their expert technical assistance.

REFERENCES

1. Gardner DL: The experimental production of arthritis: a review. Ann Rheum Dis 19:297–317, 1960
2. Imrei RC: Animal models of arthritis. Lab Anim Sci 26:345–351, 1967
3. Aoki S, Merkel M, Aoki M, McCabe WR: Immunofluorescent localization of bacterial antigen in pyelonephritis. I. The use of antisera against the common enterobacterial antigen in experimental renal lesions. J Lab Clin Med 70:204–212, 1967
4. Aoki S, Imamura S, Aoki M, McCabe WR: "Abacterial" and bacterial pyelonephritis: immunofluorescent localization of bacterial antigen. N Engl J Med 281:1375–1382, 1969
5. Aoki S, Ikuta K, Aoyama G: Induction of chronic polyarthritis in rabbits. Nature 237:168–169, 1972
6. Kunin CM, Beard MV, Halmagyi NE: Evidence for a common hapten associated endotoxin in fractions of E. coli and other enterobacteriaceae. Proc Soc Exp Biol Med 111:160–166, 1962
7. Aoki S, Merkel M, McCabe WR: Immunofluorescent demonstration of the common enterobacterial antigen. Proc Soc Exp Biol Med 121:230–234, 1966
8. Abruzzo JL, Christian CL: The induction of a rheumatoid factor-like substance in rabbits. J Exp Med 114:791–806, 1961
9. Christian CL: Rheumatoid factor properties of hyperimmune rabbit sera. J Exp Med 118:827–844, 1963
10. Heller G, Jacobson SA, Kolodny HM, Kammerer WH: The hemagglutination test for rheumatoid arthritis. II. The influence of human plasma fraction II (gamma globulin) on the reaction. J Immunol 72:66–78, 1954
11. Lewis DC, Jasin HE, Ziff M: Cellular responses in the

synovial membrane: arthritis produced by endotoxin and by phytohemagglutinin (abstract). Arthritis Rheum 9:863–864, 1966
12. Hollingsworth JW, Atkins E: Synovial inflammatory response to bacterial endotoxin. Yale J Biol Med 38: 241–256, 1965
13. Munoz J: Effect of bacteria and bacterial products on antibody response. Adv Immunol 4:397–440, 1964
14. Johnson AG: Adjuvant action of bacterial endotoxins on the primary antibody response, Bacterial Endotoxins. Edited by M Landy, W Braun. Rahway, NJ, Quinn & Boden Co., 1964, pp 252–262
15. Collins DH, Goldie W: Observations on polyarthritis and on experimental erysipelothrix infection of swine. J Pathol Bacteriol 50:323–353, 1940
16. Decker JL, Barden JA: Mycoplasma arthritis in the pig, Infection and Immunology in the Rheumatic Diseases. Edited by DC Dumonde. Oxford, Blackwell Scientific Publications, 1976, pp 191–193
17. Cromartie WJ, Craddock JG, Schwab JH, Anderle SK, Yang CH: Arthritis in rats after systemic injection of streptococcal cells or cell walls. J Exp Med 146.1585–1602, 1977
18. Pearson CM: Development of arthritis, periarthritis and periostitis in rats given adjuvants. Proc Soc Exp Biol Med 91:95–101, 1956
19. Trentham DE, Townes AS, Kang AH: Autoimmunity to type II collagen: an experimental model of arthritis. J Exp Med 146:857–868, 1977
20. Dumonde DC, Glynn LE: The production of arthritis in rabbits by an immunological reaction to fibrin. Br J Exp Pathol 43:373–383, 1962
21. Blackham A, Farmer JB, Radziwonik H, Westwick J: The role of prostaglandins in rabbit mono-articular arthritis. Br J Pharmacol 51:35–44, 1974
22. Oldham G, Coombs RRA: Early rheumatoid-like joint lesions in rabbits injected with foreign serum or milk proteins. III. Influence of concomitant IgE-like antibodies and of the breed of rabbit. Int Arch Allergy Appl Immunol 61:81–90, 1980
23. Hadler NM: A pathogenetic model for erosive synovitis: lessons from animal arthritides. Arthritis Rheum 19:256–266, 1976
24. Bennett JC: The infectious etiology of rheumatoid arthritis: new considerations. Arthritis Rheum 21:531–538, 1978
25. Bennett JC: The etiology of rheumatoid arthritis, Textbook of Rheumatology. Edited by WN Kelley, ED Harris Jr, S Ruddy, CB Sledge. Philadelphia, WB Saunders, 1981, pp 887–895
26. Catterall RD: The role of microbial infection in Reiter's syndrome, Infection and Immunology in the Rheumatic Diseases. Edited by DC Dumonde. Oxford, Blackwell Scientific Publications, 1976, pp 147–150
27. Good AE: Enteropathic arthritis, Textbook of Rheumatology. Edited by WN Kelley, ED Harris Jr, S Ruddy, CB Sledge. Philadelphia, WB Saunders, 1981, pp 1063–1075
28. Shagrin JW, Frame B, Duncan H: Polyarthritis in obese patients with intestinal bypass. Ann Intern Med 75:377–380, 1971
29. Cassidy JT, Petty RE, Sullivan DB: Occurrence of selective IgA deficiency in children with juvenile rheumatoid arthritis. Arthritis Rheum 20:181–183, 1977
30. Lehman TJA, Allen JB, Plotz PH, Wilder RL: Polyarthritis in rats following the systemic injection of Lactobacillus casei cell walls in aqueous suspension. Arthritis Rheum 26:1259–1265, 1983
31. Perlmann P, Hammarström S, Lagercrantz R, Gustafsson BE: Antigen from colon of germfree rats and antibodies in human ulcerative colitis. Ann NY Acad Sci 124:377–394, 1965

ETIOPATHOGENESIS OF THE RHEUMATOID ARTHRITIS–LIKE DISEASE IN MRL/l MICE

I. The Histomorphologic Basis of Joint Destruction

FRANK X. O'SULLIVAN, HANS-GEORG FASSBENDER, STEFFEN GAY, and WILLIAM J. KOOPMAN

MRL/l mice spontaneously develop a hindlimb arthropathy, as well as a number of immunologic abnormalities, including circulating rheumatoid factors. Although previous studies have suggested that this arthropathy is primarily an inflammatory process, we performed a comprehensive histomorphologic study which indicated that inflammation is a late manifestation of MRL/l arthritis. The pathologic changes that occur in the joints of these mice can be divided into 3 stages. The first stage develops between the ages of 7 and 13 weeks and consists of synovial cell proliferation in the joint recesses. The second stage is characterized by continued proliferation of synovial cells which take on an appearance similar to that of transformed mesenchymal cells. The earliest destructive changes occur in the second stage and include marginal erosions, followed soon after by progressive destruction of articular and meniscal cartilage. The final stage is characterized by a diminution of synovial cell proliferation, extensive cartilage destruction, formation of scar tissue and fibrocartilage, and a very moderate infiltration of the synovial stroma by mononuclear and polymorphonuclear inflammatory cells. Throughout the disease progression there is a striking dissociation between inflammatory cell infiltration or exudation and tissue destruction. The histomorphologic similarities between human rheumatoid synovitis and the arthritis of MRL/l mice, as well as the presence of rheumatoid factors, make this mouse strain an excellent model for studying human rheumatoid arthritis.

Historically, the joint destruction which occurs in rheumatoid arthritis (RA) has been attributed to complex cellular interactions among acute and chronic inflammatory cells, proliferating synovial lining cells, chondrocytes, macrophages and other monocytic modulatory cells, and to the production of a variety of humoral factors such as proteolytic enzymes and soluble mediators (1–3). However, the elucidation of the precise mechanisms of destruction has been hampered by the lack of an appropriate spontaneous animal model. Until recently, the only available animal models have been based on the induction of inflammatory synovitis by a variety of exogenous agents (4–7). However, the development of the MRL/l mouse strain by Murphy and Roths (8) has addressed this problem. These mice, already useful as a model for SLE (9), spontaneously develop inflammatory arthritis of the hindlimbs, possess serum IgG and IgM rheumatoid factors (10,11), and develop antibodies to types I and II collagen (12), thus exhibiting the combined morphologic and immunologic similarities to the human disease that experimentally-induced arthritides lack

From the Division of Clinical Immunology and Rheumatology, Department of Medicine, University of Alabama at Birmingham, and the World Health Organization Center for Classification and Diagnostic Criteria of Rheumatoid Arthritis and Allied Diseases, Mainz, West Germany.

Supported in part by NIDR grant DE-02670 and NIH grant R01 AM-32073.

Frank X. O'Sullivan, MD: Fellow; Hans-Georg Fassbender, MD: Professor of Pathology, World Health Organization Center for Classification and Diagnostic Criteria of Rheumatoid Arthritis and Allied Diseases; Steffen Gay, MD: Professor of Medicine; William J. Koopman, MD: Professor of Medicine and Director, Division of Clinical Immunology and Rheumatology, Department of Medicine, University of Alabama at Birmingham.

Address reprint requests to Frank X. O'Sullivan, MD, University of Alabama at Birmingham, Division of Clinical Immunology and Rheumatology, Department of Medicine, 601 MEB, University Station, Birmingham, AL 35294.

Submitted for publication August 6, 1984; accepted in revised form November 9, 1984.

We have developed an interest in the biochemical and immunologic abnormalities seen in the MRL/l mouse strain. We therefore carried out a detailed histomorphologic examination of the arthritic process in these mice to precisely describe the pathologic changes which occur in their joints. We found destruction of articular bone and cartilage associated with proliferating synovial cells which resemble transformed mesenchymal cells, in a manner very similar to that described in RA in humans (1). Moreover, the joint destruction in these mice occurs without the direct participation of inflammatory cells. The findings of this study provide further support for the use of the MRL/l mouse strain as a model for human rheumatoid arthritis.

MATERIALS AND METHODS

Mice. MRL/Mp-lpr/lpr (MRL/l) mice were originally obtained from the pedigreed stock of the Jackson Laboratories, Bar Harbor, ME, and were bred and maintained in our rodent colony. They were allowed standard laboratory rodent chow and water ad libitum.

Histologic studies. Twenty male and female MRL/l mice, ages 7 through 25 weeks, were examined. The age and sex of mice examined in this study are listed in Table 1. After the mice were killed, the hindlimbs were removed, excess tissue and bone was trimmed proximal and distal to the knees, and whole knee joints were fixed for 24 hours in neutral buffered formalin.

After decalcification in dilute formic acid, the knees were routinely processed for paraffin embedding, and serial 5 μm–thick sections were taken sagittally through the entire knee. Representative sections were stained with hematoxylin and eosin, and examined for the presence or absence of the following features: synovial cell proliferation, destruction of articular and meniscal cartilage and subchondral bone, infiltration of synovial stroma by acute and/or chronic inflammatory cells, and periarticular inflammation (vasculitis, myositis, tendinitis, or perineuritis).

RESULTS

Four animals were examined at 7 weeks of age, and no detectable abnormalities were found. Inflammatory infiltrates were not present, and the synovial membranes were without evidence of synovial cell proliferation. No articular cartilage destruction had occurred, and there was no evidence of periarticular inflammation (Figure 1).

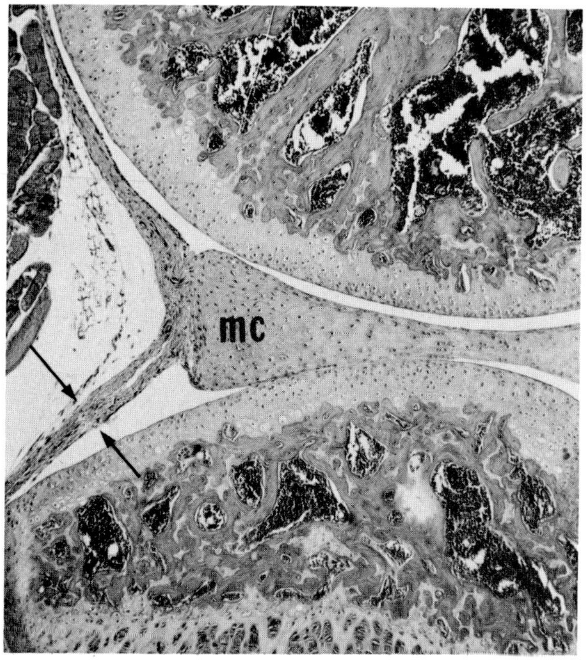

Figure 1. Histologic specimen of a normal knee joint from an MRL/l mouse aged 7 weeks. The joint capsule has a normal synovial lining membrane **(arrows)**. mc = meniscal cartilage (hematoxylin and eosin stained, magnification × 160).

Of the 7 animals examined at 13–14 weeks of age, 5 displayed early synovial pathology. Synovial cell proliferation was easily recognizable and most prominent in the joint recesses. Early subchondral bone destruction was noted in these areas, producing marginal erosions (Figure 2A). Small synovial villi were occasionally seen projecting into the joint cavity (Figure 2B), and proliferating synovial lining cells could be seen adhering to meniscal cartilage and patellar tendon (Figures 2B and C). The articular cartilage was, for the most part, intact. The synovial stroma was devoid of inflammatory cells, and there was no evidence of periarticular vasculitis, perineuritis, or focal myositis. The remaining 2 animals displayed more advanced changes which will be described later.

Although there were only minimal destructive changes at this stage of the disease process, it is important to note the intriguing appearance of the proliferating synovial lining cells. In areas of apparent ongoing proliferation and early destruction, these cells were found to have plentiful cytoplasm and large, pale

Table 1. Age and sex of MRL/l mice

Age (weeks)	Sex	No. animals
7	F	2
7	M	2
13–14	F	7
16	F	2
19	F	3
21–25	F	4

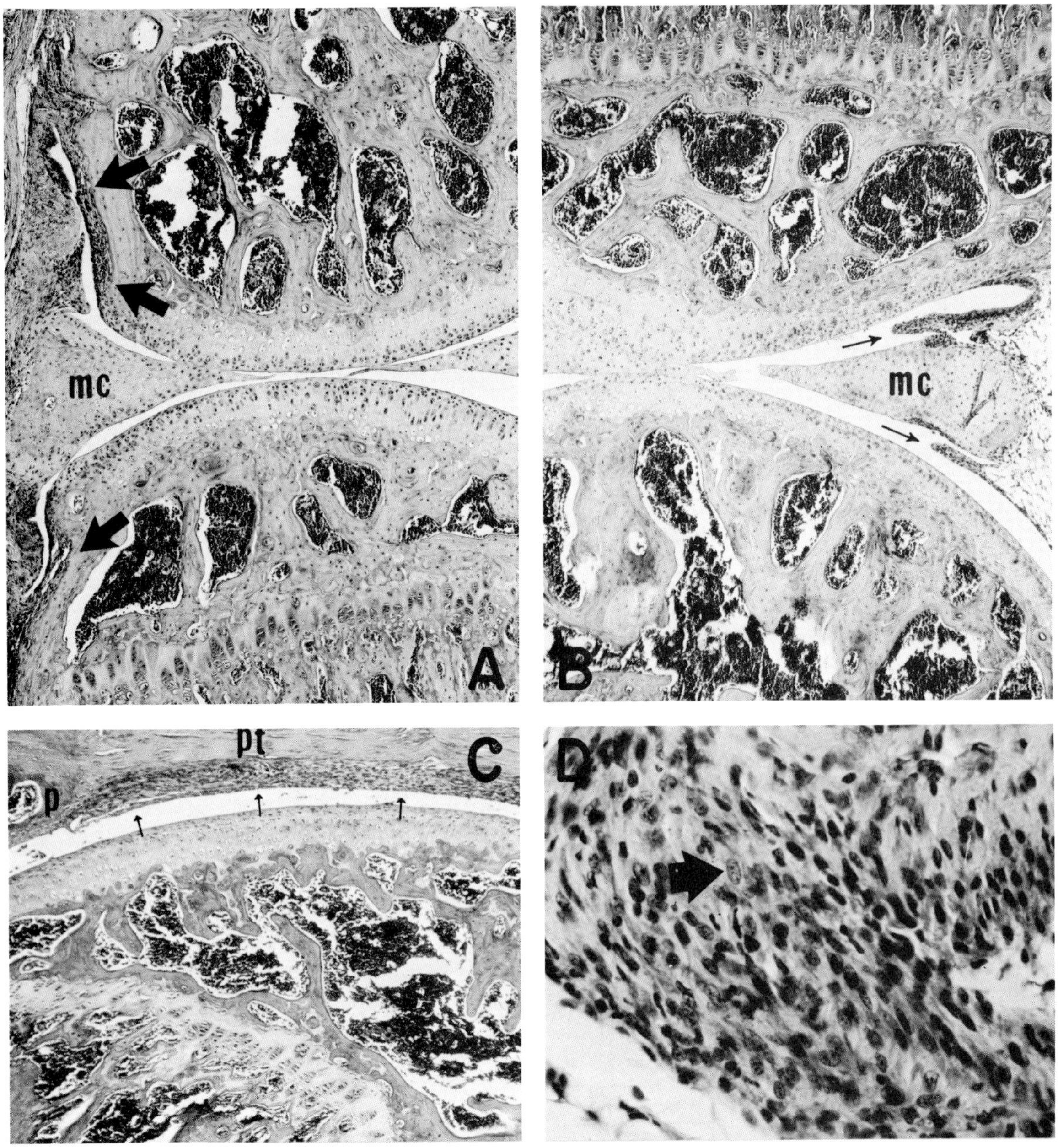

Figure 2. Rheumatoid arthritis–like disease, stage 1: histologic specimens. **A**, Thirteen-week-old MRL/l mouse with synovial cell proliferation in joint recesses, with associated marginal erosions (**arrows**). mc = meniscal cartilage (hematoxylin and eosin stained, magnification × 150). **B**, Fourteen-week-old mouse with small villi of proliferating synovial cells (**arrows**) extending into the joint space (hematoxylin and eosin stained, magnification × 150). **C**, Thirteen-week-old mouse with proliferating synovial cells densely adherent to patellar tendon (**pt**) (**arrows**). p = patella (hematoxylin and eosin stained, magnification × 150). **D**, Thirteen-week-old mouse, high-power view of proliferating synovial cells. **Arrow** demonstrates a typical proliferating synovial cell with large nucleus and prominent nucleoli (hematoxylin and eosin stained, magnification × 600).

nuclei with multiple prominent nucleoli, and appeared to be densely adherent to underlying tissue (Figure 2D).

In the remaining 2 animals age 13–14 weeks, as well as in all the animals ages 16 and 19 weeks, an aggressive destructive process was present. Proliferating synovial lining cells continued to be associated with cartilage and subchondral bone destruction (Figures 3A, B, and C) and could even be seen eroding into the marrow space (Figure 3B). In addition, they began

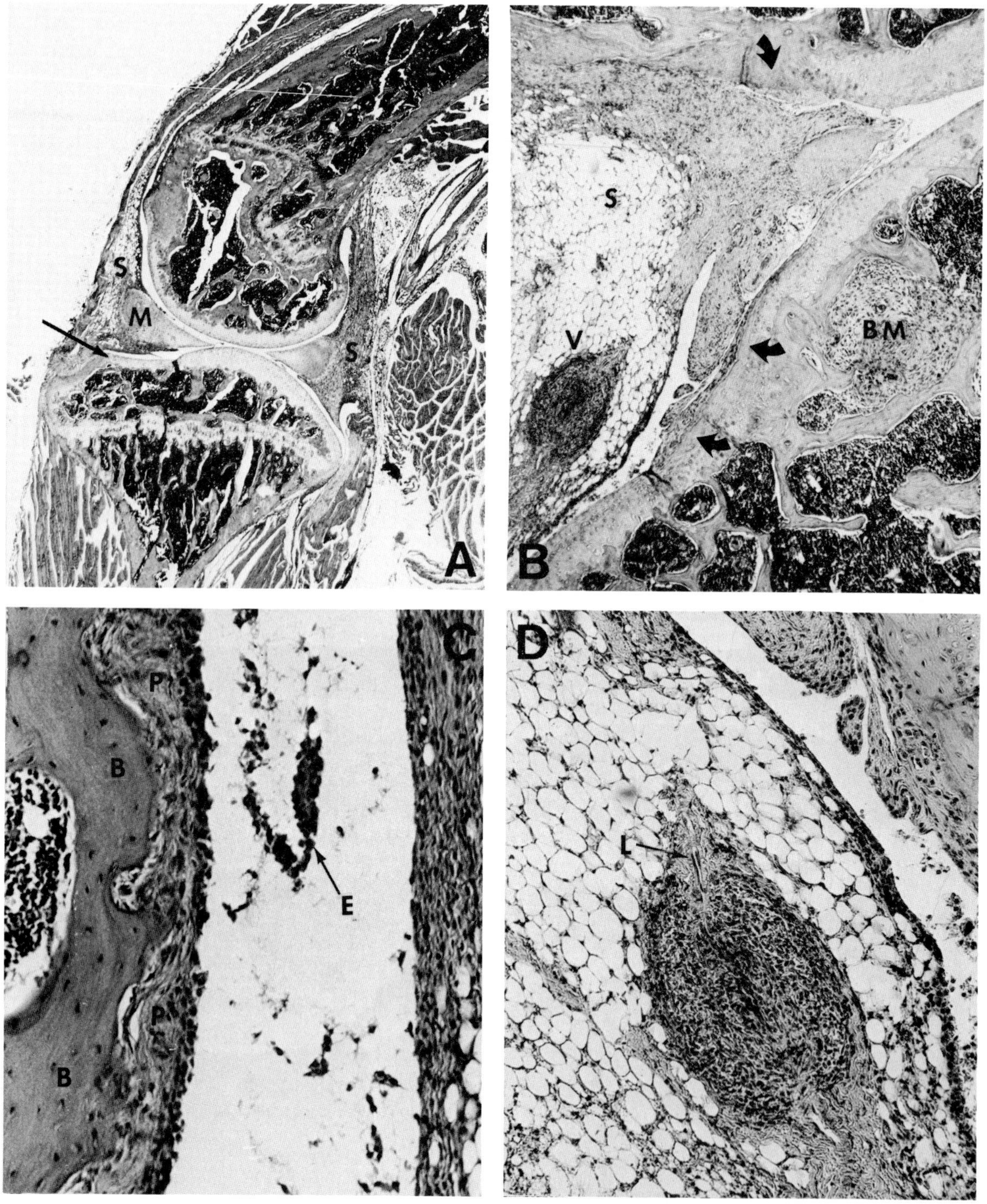

Figure 3. Rheumatoid arthritis–like disease, stage 2: histologic specimens. **A**, Sixteen-week-old MRL/l mouse with proliferating synovial cells filling synovial stroma **(S)** and adhering to meniscal cartilage **(M)**. **Arrow** indicates articular cartilage destruction (hematoxylin and eosin stained, magnification × 25). **B**, Nineteen-week-old mouse with more extensive articular cartilage loss **(arrows)**, invasion of bone marrow **(BM)** by proliferating synovial cells and fibrous tissue, and vasculitis **(V)** involving a stromal vessel (hematoxylin and eosin stained, magnification × 150). **C**, Nineteen-week-old mouse. Articular cartilage has been replaced by pannus **(P)** which appears to be associated with destruction of bone matrix **(B)**. E = exudate (hematoxylin and eosin stained, magnification × 500). **D**, High-power view of stromal vasculitis seen in Figure 3B. L = vessel lumen (hematoxylin and eosin stained, magnification × 400).

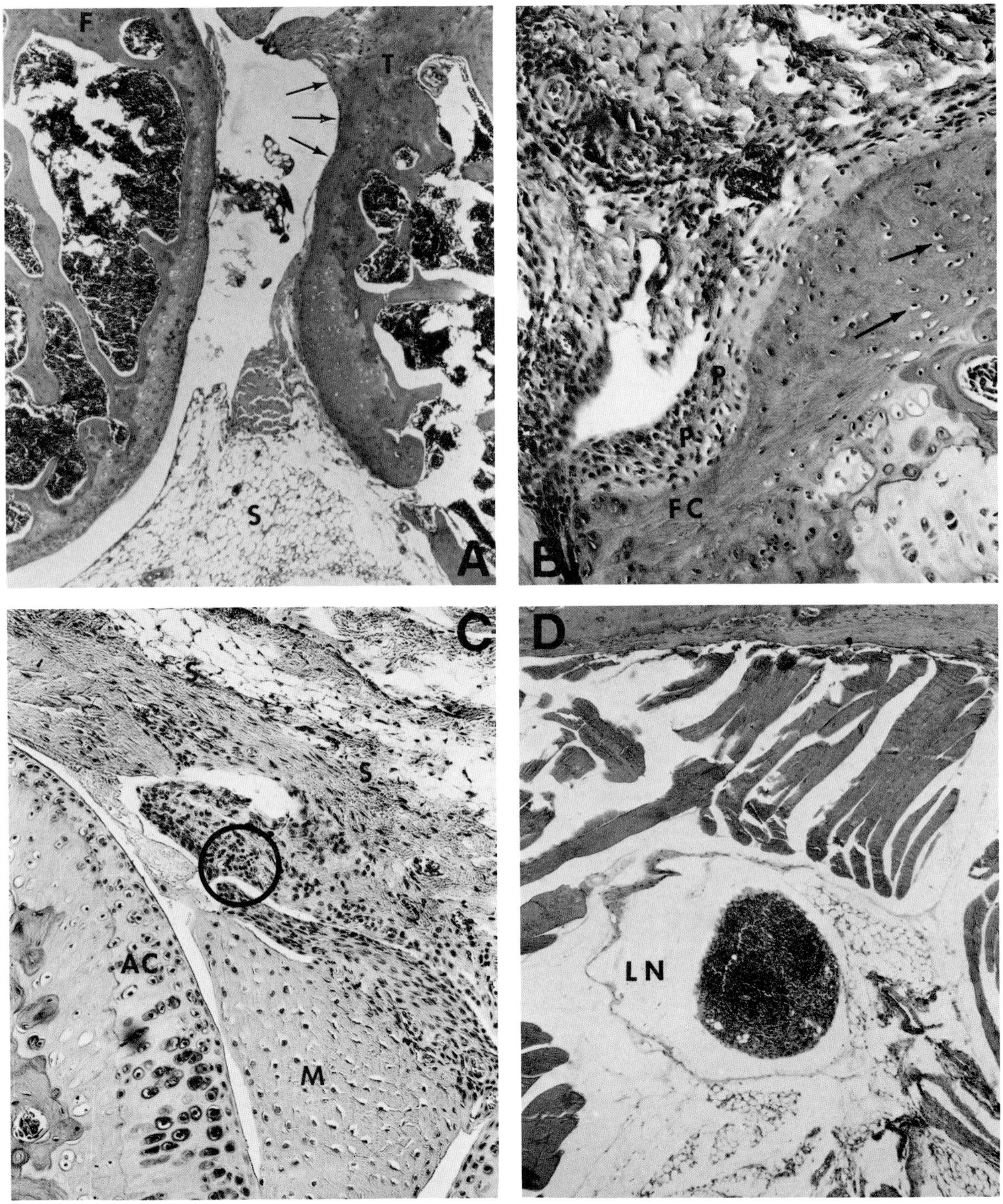

Figure 4. Rheumatoid arthritis–like disease: histologic specimens. **A**, Stage 3. Articular cartilage of the femur (**F**) of a 19-week-old MRL/l mouse is attenuated and has an irregular surface. The articular surface of the tibia (**T**) has been destroyed and remodeled with fibrocartilage (**arrows**). Few inflammatory or proliferating synovial cells are present. S = synovial stroma (hematoxylin and eosin stained, magnification × 165). **B**, Stage 3. Twenty-five-week-old mouse with late stage of cartilage destruction with formation of fibrocartilage (**FC**) and chondrocyte degeneration (**arrows**) remote from areas of proliferating synovial cells. P = pannus (hematoxylin and eosin stained, magnification × 500). **C**, Stage 3. Nineteen-week-old mouse demonstrating synovial stroma containing actively proliferating synovial cells which form villi and, in this case, containing a focus of inflammatory cells (**circle**). M = meniscal cartilage; AC = articular cartilage (hematoxylin and eosin stained, magnification × 400). **D**, Stage 2. Popliteal lymph node (**LN**) from a 16-week-old mouse (hematoxylin and eosin stained, magnification × 200).

to fill the joint space in the form of villi and as sheets of cells tightly attached to articular cartilage (Figure 3C). Articular cartilage destruction was limited to the area immediately adjacent to adherent proliferating synovial cells, and abundant degenerating chondrocytes were noted. No definite inflammatory cells were seen intermingled with proliferating synovial lining cells, although the synovial stroma contained a few lymphocytes and plasma cells. Occasional instances of vasculitis were noted in the synovial stroma, usually in the form of focal arteriolitis, appearing as endothelial cell proliferation surrounded by a few mononuclear cells and nuclear dust (Figure 3D).

In all 4 mice age 21–25 weeks (and also in 1 19-week-old mouse), synovial lining cell proliferation was less prominent, but extensive destructive changes were seen (Figure 4A). In addition to articular cartilage destruction adjacent to adherent synovial lining cells, balloon-like degeneration of chondrocytes still surrounded by normal-appearing cartilage was seen in areas somewhat remote from the sites of direct cartilage destruction by proliferating synovial cells (Figure 4B). The synovial stroma contained more numerous lymphocytes, plasma cells, and a few polymorphonuclear leukocytes but few, if any, were located in areas of proliferating synovial lining cells (Figure 4C). There was extensive joint derangement with evidence of new bone formation, as well as development of periarticular fibrous scar tissue and fibrocartilage (Figures 4A and B).

Throughout the entire series of animals, neither classic perineuritis nor focal myositis was noted. On several sections, popliteal lymph nodes appeared as areas of diffuse lymphoid hyperplasia adjacent to synovial stromal tissue (Figure 4D).

DISCUSSION

Initial interest in the MRL/l mouse strain focused on the lupus-like diathesis and massive lymphoproliferation which occur in these mice. However, detection of the spontaneous development of hindlimb arthritis and high levels of circulating rheumatoid factors have led Andrews and colleagues (10) and Hang et al (11) to suggest that the MRL/l mouse may serve as a reasonable animal model for human rheumatoid arthritis. Consequently, we performed a comprehensive study of the arthritic process in the MRL/l mouse, in order to more firmly establish the validity of this mouse as an animal model for human RA.

In the initial description of the arthritic disease of the MRL/l mouse strain the majority of old, sick, MRL/l mice were found to have a hindlimb arthropathy resembling human RA, and a high incidence of circulating IgG and IgM rheumatoid factors was noted (10). A subsequent, more detailed study of the rheumatoid arthritis–like features of MRL/l mice included a specific histologic description of hindlimb arthritis and emphasized the presence of subsynovial and periarticular inflammatory infiltrates as criteria for arthritis (11). In that study, 75% of 12–16-week-old mice were found to have subsynovial or periarticular inflammation, and 45% had synovial cell proliferation and articular erosions. By the age of 20–24 weeks, 82% had subsynovial or periarticular inflammation, and 54% had synovial proliferation and erosions. Subsynovial infiltrates containing lymphocytes, plasma cells, larger mononuclear cells, and occasional polymorphonuclear leukocytes were described but were not related to age or degree of joint destruction. Rheumatoid factor levels were measured, and a strong correlation was noted between the presence of arthritis and IgM rheumatoid factor.

In contrast, our study reveals that joint destruction is more closely related to the presence of transformed-appearing proliferating synovial cells than to the presence of subsynovial or periarticular inflammation. Moreover, there is no apparent involvement of inflammatory cells at the immediate site of destruction. The moderate inflammatory infiltrates that finally do appear are remote from areas of cartilage and bone destruction, and actually appear to be sequelae of the primary destructive process.

The earliest pathologic change appearing in MRL/l mouse joints, and the first stage in the destructive process, is synovial cell proliferation in the joint recesses, with associated subchondral bone destruction producing marginal erosions. Initially, the articular cartilage is spared. The second, and most destructive, phase occasionally develops by 13 weeks of age and is firmly established by 16 weeks. Sheets of proliferating synovial cells can be seen adhering to and associated with destruction of subjacent cartilage, both on the articular surfaces and on the meniscal structures. These changes may persist up to 19 weeks of age.

At this stage of the disease, the appearance of the synovial cells is noteworthy. The abundant cytoplasm and large, pale nuclei with multiple prominent nucleoli are reminiscent of the appearance of transformed mesenchymal cells. In some studies of human rheumatoid synovium, a fleeting phase of synovial cell proliferation has been observed in which similar synovial cells appear, followed by the formation of pannus.

During the active, proliferative phase, ultrastructual studies of the proliferating human synovial cells reveal the presence of lysosomes and phagolysosomes (1).

In the final stage of destruction, extensive structural damage has occurred, and actively proliferating synovial cells are less prominent. Attempted healing occurs as evidenced by the presence of scar tissue and fibrocartilage in areas of serious articular cartilage destruction. There is also evidence of chondrocyte obsolescence in areas of intact cartilage that are remote from proliferating synovial cells or pannus, suggesting that humoral factors are being elaborated that are capable of reaching distant chondrocytes and, in some way, causing their degeneration.

Perhaps the most striking feature of arthritis in the MRL/l mouse is the clear-cut dissociation between destruction and overt inflammation. In the second stage of disease, there is a dearth of inflammatory cells in the synovial stroma in spite of florid synovial cell proliferation and cartilage destruction. Even in the final stage of disease, no obvious inflammatory cells are noted in proximity to bony or cartilaginous erosions, though variable numbers of mononuclear or polymorphonuclear inflammatory cells are seen infiltrating the synovial stroma. These findings are in contrast to those in type II collagen–induced arthritis, in which bone and cartilage destruction are associated with the presence of intense synovial inflammatory infiltrates (4,13).

Several older animals were noted to have focal vasculitis in periarticular tissue; however, older MRL/1 females are known to have systemic vasculitis (10), so it is not clear whether the vascular lesions seen in this study are associated with the arthritis, or are simply a manifestation of systemic vasculitis.

The dissociation between the destructive process and inflammation in joints of MRL/l mice differs somewhat from earlier observations in RA, in which cartilage destruction and synovial cell proliferation were described as being generally associated with infiltration of the synovial stroma by mononuclear inflammatory cells and by proliferation of small stromal vessels which are also surrounded by mononuclear inflammatory cells (3,14). Moreover, in human rheumatoid synovium, macrophage-like HLA–DR+ cells interdigitating with OKT4+ lymphocytes have been detected (15). Whether similar interactions may be occurring in the synovial stroma of MRL/l mice in numbers too low to be detectable by light microscopy remains to be seen.

The main similarities between the arthritis in MRL/l mice and that of human RA revealed by this study include the following: 1) the histologic appearance of actively proliferating synovial lining cells which resemble transformed mesenchymal cells, 2) the proclivity for proliferating synovial cells to adhere to and to be associated with destruction of adjacent articular cartilage and subchondral bone, and 3) the formation of fibrous scar tissue and fibrocartilage in areas of extensive destruction.

The observations in MRL/l mice of articular cartilage destruction adjacent to proliferating synovial cells and of degenerating chondrocytes in cartilage remote from sites of active destruction suggest that types of cellular interactions similar to those thought to be responsible for joint destruction in human RA may be operative in MRL/l mice. For example, purified catabolin, which may be identical to interleukin-1 (16), is capable of stimulating human chondrocytes to degrade matrix proteoglycans in organ explants, followed some days later by collagen breakdown (17).

It is tempting to postulate that similar mechanisms are operative in the MRL/l mouse, with local production of interleukin-1–like humoral factors contributing to tissue injury. Proof that these events occur in the arthritis of MRL/l mice will require further investigation. Nevertheless, the findings of this study strongly suggest that the MRL/l mouse strain is the best available animal model for human RA.

ACKNOWLEDGMENTS

The authors wish to thank Brenda Gilmore and Melody Edwards for their expert assistance in the preparation of the manuscript, and Francis R. Denys for his expert technical assistance.

REFERENCES

1. Fassbender H-G: Histomorphologic basis of articular cartilage destruction in rheumatoid arthritis. Coll Relat Res 3:141–155, 1983
2. Harris ED Jr: Pathogenesis of rheumatoid arthritis. Clin Orthop 182:14–23, 1984
3. Zvaifler NJ: The immunopathology of joint inflammation in rheumatoid arthritis. Adv Immunol 13:265–336, 1973
4. Trentham DE, Townes AS, Kang AH: Autoimmunity to type II collagen: an experimental model of arthritis. J Exp Med 146:857–868, 1977
5. Chang Y, Pearson CM, Abe C: Adjuvant polyarthritis. IV. Induction by a synthetic adjuvant: immunologic, histopathologic, and other studies. Arthritis Rheum 23:62–71, 1980
6. Taylor G, Taylor-Robison D, Keystone ED: Effects of lymecycline on Mycoplasma pulmonis-induced arthritis in mice. Br J Exp Pathol 59:204–212, 1978

7. Cooke TD, Hurd ER, Ziff M, Jasin HE: The pathogenesis of chronic inflammation in antigen-induced arthritis. II. Preferential localization of antigen-antibody complexes to collagenous tissues. J Exp Med 135:323–338, 1972
8. Murphy ED, Roths JB: Autoimmunity and lymphoproliferation: induction by mutant gene lpr, and acceleration by a male-associated factor in strain BXSB mice, Genetic Control of Autoimmune Disease. Edited by NR Rose, RE Bigazzi, NL Warner. New York, Elsevier/North-Holland, 1978, pp 207–219
9. Theofilopoulous AN, Dixon FJ: Etiopathogenesis of murine SLE. Immunol Rev 55:179–216, 1981
10. Andrews BS, Eisenberg RA, Theofilopoulous AN, Izui S, Wilson CB, McConahey PJ, Murphy ED, Roths JB, Dixon FJ: Spontaneous immune lupus-like syndromes: clinical and immunopathological manifestations in several strains. J Exp Med 148:1198–1215, 1978
11. Hang L, Theofilopoulous AN, Dixon FJ: A spontaneous rheumatoid arthritis-like disease in MRL/l mice. J Exp Med 155:1690–1701, 1982
12. Phadke K, Fouts R, Parrish J, Baker RS: Autoreactivity to collagen in a murine lupus model. Arthritis Rheum 27:313–319, 1984
13. Caulfield JP, Hein A, Dynesius-Trentham R, Trentham DE: Morphologic demonstration of two stages in the development of type II collagen-induced arthritis. Lab Invest 46:321–343, 1982
14. Van Boxel JA, Paget SA: Predominantly T cell infiltrate in rheumatoid synovial membranes. N Engl J Med 293:517–520, 1975
15. Janossy G, Duke O, Poulter L, Panayi G, Bafill M, Goldstein G: Rheumatoid arthritis: a disease of T lymphocyte/macrophage immunoregulation. Lancet 2:839–842, 1981
16. Mizel SB, Dayer JM, Krane SM, Mergenhagen SE: Stimulation of rheumatoid synovial cell collagenase and prostaglandin production by partially purified lymphocyte-activating factor (IL-l). Proc Natl Acad Sci USA 78:2474–2477, 1981
17. Dingle JT: Catabolin—a cartilage catabolic factor from synovium. Clin Orthop 156:219–231, 1981

THE AUTOLOGOUS MIXED LYMPHOCYTE REACTION IS DECREASED IN FREUND'S ADJUVANT–INJECTED RATS OF ARTHRITIS-SUSCEPTIBLE AND -INSUSCEPTIBLE STRAINS

WILLIAM E. CROWE, JACK R. BATTISTO, and R. N. SMITH

We examined the T–non-T cell autologous mixed lymphocyte reaction (AMLR) of spleen cells from rats with arthritis induced by Freund's complete adjuvant in an effort to establish an animal model for the study of the relationship between the AMLR and autoimmune disease. We found that the splenic T–non-T AMLR was markedly decreased in rats with adjuvant-induced arthritis and that this decrease was mediated by suppressor cells within the nylon-wool–adherent stimulator cell population. However, we also found a similar decrease in the AMLR of arthritis-resistant Fisher 344 rats that received Freund's complete adjuvant but did not develop arthritis. Control animals with local inflammation induced by turpentine, a nonarthritogenic inflammatory substance, had normal AMLR, whereas other controls given Freund's incomplete adjuvant, also a nonarthritogenic substance, had a modest responder cell–mediated decrease in AMLR. These studies help to clarify the relationship between the decreased AMLR and the pathogenesis of adjuvant-induced arthritis by demonstrating that: 1) the acute-phase inflammatory response does not reduce the AMLR; and 2) the decreased AMLR can occur in the absence of overt autoimmune disease. This latter observation calls into question the proposed pathogenetic relationship between the AMLR and autoimmune disease states.

The autologous mixed lymphocyte reaction (AMLR) is the in vitro phenomenon of T cell proliferation in response to autologous Class II (Ia/DR) antigen–bearing cells (B cells, macrophages, dendritic cells, or activated T cells). The AMLR was originally detected in mice (1) and, subsequently, was detected in humans (2). The cells that proliferate in the AMLR have been shown to be capable of immunomodulation. The type of cell generated (helper or suppressor) appears to be dependent upon the cell type used to stimulate the reaction. The T–non-T AMLR (in which the non-T stimulator cell population is primarily B cells) is thought to generate helper cells (3,4), whereas the T–T AMLR, in which the stimulator cells are mitogen-activated T cells, causes a population of suppressor cells to proliferate (5). Thus, the different types of AMLR may be involved in the initiation and cessation of immunologic reactions. However, since the AMLR has not yet been shown to occur under physiologic conditions, its role in vivo is not clear.

The relevance of the AMLR to immunoregulation is supported by the observation that the T–non-T AMLR is decreased in a number of autoimmune diseases (6–10). This association of decreased AMLR with autoimmune disease suggests that the impaired immunoregulation caused by the abnormal AMLR may be related to the pathogenesis of these disorders. However, this central question of the relationship between the AMLR and autoimmune disease has not been rigorously tested because previously available animal models have not provided an approach for doing so.

From the Research Division, Cleveland Clinic Foundation and the Departments of Medicine and Reproductive Biology, Case Western Reserve University, Cleveland, Ohio.

William E. Crowe, MD: Department of Medicine, Case Western Reserve University; Jack R. Battisto, PhD: Research Division, Cleveland Clinic Foundation; R. N. Smith, PhD: Department of Reproductive Biology, Case Western Reserve University.

Address reprint requests to William E. Crowe, MD, Cleveland Metropolitan General/Highland View Hospital, Hamann Building, Room 540, 3395 Scranton Road, Cleveland, OH 44109.

Submitted for publication June 19, 1984; accepted in revised form November 7, 1984.

The rat model of adjuvant-induced arthritis (AIA) is ideal for such studies. AIA, a well-established experimental model of arthritis, is induced by a single injection of Freund's complete adjuvant (FCA) (11,12). The arthritis begins approximately 10 days after the injection, is maximal at 20 days postinjection, involves all peripheral joints, lasts 6–8 weeks, and then usually remits. The histopathology resembles that of rheumatoid arthritis, and hypersensitivity to type II collagen has been demonstrated and is thought to play a central pathogenetic role (13–15). Inbred strains of AIA-susceptible and -resistant rats, as well as a variety of arthritogenic and nonarthritogenic stimuli, are available.

We investigated the T–non-T AMLR in rats with AIA in order to develop a model for the study of the relationship between the AMLR and autoimmune disease. In the present study, we determined the tritiated thymidine (^{3}HTdR) uptake occurring in the T–non-T AMLR of spleen cells from: 1) both normal and arthritic arthritis-susceptible DA rats; 2) both normal and FCA-injected arthritis-resistant Fisher 344 (F344) rats; and 3) DA rats that had been injected with turpentine or Freund's incomplete adjuvant (FIA), 2 nonarthritogenic stimuli of inflammation.

We found the AMLR to be decreased both in arthritic DA rats and in FCA-treated nonarthritic F344 rats, but not in turpentine-injected DA rats showing an equal amount of local inflammation. In addition, we produced syngeneic MLRs by mixing arthritic responder cells with normal stimulators and vice versa. These studies determined that the decreased AMLR seen in both the arthritic DA rats and the FCA-treated F344 rats was due to the nylon-wool–adherent stimulator cell population. Furthermore, we observed that the addition of arthritic nylon-wool–adherent cells to a normal T–non-T AMLR dramatically decreased thymidine uptake, suggesting the presence of a suppressor cell population. We also found that the AMLR was decreased in cells derived from DA rats injected with FIA, but that this decrease was mediated by the responder cell population.

MATERIALS AND METHODS

Animals. For this study we used inbred 12–24-week-old rats of the DA and F344 strains. They were kept in conventional housing and fed pelleted chow. In previous studies (16), we determined that the DA rats are 100% susceptible to AIA and that the F344 rats are 100% resistant.

Adjuvants. FCA consisted of Freund's adjuvant (Difco, Detroit, MI) to which was added 10 mg/ml heat-killed *Mycobacterium butyricum* (Difco). The mixture was stirred overnight at room temperature before use. Freund's incomplete adjuvant (Difco) consisted of mineral oil and emulsifier without mycobacteria.

Induction of arthritis. On day 0, we injected 0.25 ml of FCA intradermally into the right hind footpad. By day 14, all susceptible rats had active arthritis of all extremities.

T–non-T AMLR. Normal or adjuvant-injected rats were anesthetized with ether and then killed by cardiac puncture. Whole spleen cell suspensions were prepared by pressing through stainless steel mesh, and after washing, the cells were cultured in RPMI 1640 supplemented with 0.19% sodium bicarbonate, 15 m*M* HEPES buffer, 1% penicillin/streptomycin, and 10% fetal bovine serum. T cell–enriched and –depleted fractions were prepared using nylon-wool columns, as has been described (17). The whole spleen cell suspensions were incubated for 45 minutes on nylon-wool columns (2 gm scrubbed nylon-wool [Fenwal Laboratories, Deerfield, IL] in a 50-ml plastic syringe) at 37°C in 5% CO_2.

The nonadherent, T-enriched responder population was recovered by slow rinse with media (2 ml/minute), the rate of which was controlled by placing a 22-gauge needle on the syringe.

The adherent, non-T stimulator population was then prepared by agitation of the column with a sterile pipette and forceful expression of medium using the syringe piston. The stimulator cells were then irradiated with 2,000R using a Mark I cesium irradiator (2,970R/minute; JL Shepard and Associates, Glendale, CA).

Responder cells (2×10^5) were cultured in 200 μl of medium with an equal number of stimulators in standard 96-well microtiter plates (Nunc/Gibco, Grand Island, NY). On day 5, 10 μl of medium containing 1 μCi of ^{3}HTdR (Schwartz-Mann, Spring Valley, NY) was added to each well. After 24 hours, samples were harvested by standard methods onto glass-fiber filters, using a semiautomated harvester. ^{3}HTdR uptake was then determined by liquid scintillation counting, and the results were expressed as counts per minute. Statistical analysis of results was performed using the Mann-Whitney U test.

RESULTS

Initially, we performed dose- and time-response studies of normal rat splenic T–non-T AMLR, and we determined that the maximum ^{3}HTdR uptake occurred on day 6, at a responder:stimulator ratio of 1:1 (data not shown). All further studies were performed under these conditions unless stated otherwise.

We then compared the AMLR of normal DA rats with that of arthritic DA rats. The arthritic rats had been injected with FCA 14 days earlier. This interval of time was chosen because, by day 14, all FCA-injected DA rats would have developed severe arthritis of all extremities. We found the AMLR of the arthritic animals to be markedly depressed (75%) when compared with that of the normal animals (Table 1).

To determine whether the decrease in the AMLR was due to a change in the kinetics of the

Table 1. The splenic T–non-T autologous mixed lymphocyte reaction is decreased (due to the stimulator cell population) in DA rats with adjuvant-induced arthritis

Spleen cells in culture		^{3}H-thymidine uptake‡	% reduction from normal
Responder*	Stimulator†		
Normal	Normal	102.1 ± 25.9	–
Arthritic	Arthritic	25.4 ± 21.5§	75
Arthritic	Normal	86.6 ± 31.7	15
Normal	Arthritic	35.6 ± 9.8§	65

* The uptake of normal responder cells cultured alone was 12.4 ± 3.3 SD. For arthritis induction, Freund's complete adjuvant was administered 14 days prior to study; the uptake of arthritic responder cells cultured alone was 6.2 ± 2.7 SD.
† The uptake of irradiated normal and arthritic (Freund's complete adjuvant–induced) stimulator cells cultured alone was ≤0.4.
‡ Values are counts per minute × 10^{-3}, mean ± SD of 5 experiments.
§ Statistically significant compared with normal, $P < 0.01$.

reaction, we studied the AMLR time-response curves of splenic cells from arthritic animals and found that this reaction had the same temporal profile as that of normal animals (i.e., optimal proliferation on day 6) (data not shown).

The chronologic relationship between the decrease in the AMLR and the degree of arthritis was also studied. A decreased AMLR was observed on day 7 (prior to overt arthritis), and on days 14 and 21 (when arthritis was in its early active phase), but not at 9 weeks (when the arthritis was quiescent) (data not shown). To provide uniform comparisons, all data presented are from rats that were killed 14 days after adjuvant injection.

We then attempted to determine whether the decreased AMLR was due to one or both of the interacting cell populations. In these studies, responder cells from normal animals were co-cultured with stimulator cells from arthritic animals and vice versa (Table 1). These studies showed that the decreased AMLR was mediated primarily by the stimulator cell population since: 1) the AMLR of normal responders cultured with arthritic stimulators was decreased in an amount comparable with that obtained from co-culture of arthritic responders with arthritic stimulators, and 2) when arthritic responders and normal stimulators were co-cultured, a normal AMLR resulted.

We next added nylon-wool–adherent cells derived from arthritic rats to a normal T–non-T AMLR to determine whether this fraction contained suppressor cells. Indeed, the addition of these cells dramatically decreased a normal AMLR (Table 2), demonstrating the presence of suppressor cells.

Having established that the AMLR is decreased in rats with AIA and that this is due to cell-associated suppression, we investigated the relationship between the change in AMLR and the presence of arthritis by studying the AMLRs of arthritis-resistant F344 rats in both the normal state and at 14 days after FCA injection. We found that the AMLR was decreased by 50% in the FCA-injected animals and that this decrease was also mediated by the stimulator cell population (Table 3).

Further experiments were conducted to determine whether the decreased AMLR is a nonspecific response to inflammation or a more specific response to some component of FCA. In our first studies, we injected DA rats with turpentine to stimulate inflammation. Turpentine is a stimulus commonly used in studies of the acute-phase response in rats; it is nonarthritogenic and is chemically unrelated to FCA. We compared the AMLRs of normal DA rats with those of DA rats that had been injected with turpentine

Table 2. Nylon-wool–adherent cells from arthritic rats suppress normal T–non-T autologous mixed lymphocyte reaction

Splenic cells in culture		^{3}H-thymidine uptake (cpm × 10^{-3})	
Responder	Stimulator		
Nonadherent cells from normal rats (2 × 10^5)	Irradiated nylon-wool–adherent cells, (n) × 10^5	Expt. 1	Expt. 2
Present	None	6.1	4.8
Absent	Normal (2.0)	0.2	0.4
Absent	Arthritic (2.0)	0.3	0.3
Present	Normal (2.0)	32.3	34.6
Present	Normal (4.0)	32.0	36.4
Present	Normal (2.0) + arthritic (2.0)	13.4	10.1

Table 3. Decreased splenic T–non-T autologous mixed lymphocyte reaction in arthritis-resistant, Freund's complete adjuvant–injected Fisher 344 rats (attributable to changes in the stimulator cell population)

Spleen cells in culture		^{3}H-thymidine uptake‡	% reduction from normal
Responder*	Stimulator†		
Normal	Normal	30.7 ± 1.6	–
FCA-treated	FCA-treated	15.1 ± 7.4§	49
FCA-treated	Normal	31.0 ± 13.7	0
Normal	FCA-treated	15.3 ± 10.7§	50

* The uptake of normal responder cells cultured alone was 7.2 ± 1.9 SD. Freund's complete adjuvant (FCA) was administered 14 days prior to study; the uptake of FCA-treated responder cells cultured alone was 10.1 ± 4.2 SD.
† The uptake of irradiated normal and FCA-treated stimulator cells cultured alone was ≤0.7.
‡ Values are counts per minute × 10^{-3}, mean ± SD of 3 experiments.
§ Statistically significant compared with normal, $P < 0.01$.

Table 4. Normal splenic T–non-T autologous mixed lymphocyte reaction in DA rats with turpentine-induced inflammation

	^{3}H-thymidine uptake*		
Spleen cells in culture	Normal	Turpentine, day 2	Turpentine, day 14
Responder T cells alone	10.6 ± 4.0	15.2 ± 4.7	15.5 ± 1.9
Stimulator non-T cells alone	0.5	0.2	0.4
Responder + stimulator	66.8 ± 19.6	52.8 ± 20.7†	64.9 ± 7.8†

* Values are counts per minute × 10^{-3}, mean ± SD of 7 experiments on normal rats, of 4 experiments at 2 days postinjection, and of 3 experiments at 14 days postinjection.
† Not significantly different from normal values.

either 2 days or 14 days previously. The 2-day interval was chosen because it is representative of the maximal acute-phase response, and the 14-day interval was chosen to allow comparison of these data with those obtained from the 14-day studies using FCA injections.

We found the AMLR to be normal in turpentine-injected animals whether studied at 2 days or 14 days after injection (Table 4), suggesting that the decreased AMLR seen in FCA-injected animals is not attributable solely to local inflammation.

To determine which component of FCA (mineral oil, emulsifier, or *Mycobacterium*) was responsible for the decreased AMLR, we studied the AMLR of DA rats injected 14 days previously with FIA, which consists only of mineral oil and emulsifier. Although these animals showed a decreased AMLR (Table 5), it was a modest decrease (35%) and was due to changes in the responder population. Thus, *Mycobacterium* appears to be the component of FCA that is essential for the stimulator cell–mediated decrease in AMLR seen in FCA-injected animals.

DISCUSSION

In this study, we have shown that the splenic T–non-T AMLR is markedly decreased in DA rats with AIA and that this decrease is mediated by the stimulator cell population. Additionally, we have shown that the AMLR is similarly decreased in arthritis-resistant F344 rats injected with FCA, and that this effect is also mediated by the stimulator cell population. Furthermore, we have shown that nylon-wool–adherent cells derived from arthritic DA rats are capable of suppressing a normal T–non-T AMLR, suggesting that the decreased AMLR of arthritic rats is due to the action of nylon-wool–adherent suppressor cells.

Table 5. The splenic T–non-T autologous mixed lymphocyte reaction is decreased (due to changes in the responder cell population) in DA rats injected with Freund's incomplete adjuvant

Spleen cells in culture			
Responder*	Stimulator†	^{3}H-thymidine uptake‡	% reduction from normal
Normal	Normal	59.8 ± 4.8	–
FIA-treated	FIA-treated	37.5 ± 13.9§	37
FIA-treated	Normal	40.5 ± 13.1§	32
Normal	FIA-treated	53.8 ± 13.0	10

* The uptake of normal responder cells cultured alone was 10.4 ± 4.9 SD. Freund's incomplete adjuvant (FIA) was administered 14 days prior to study; the uptake of FIA-treated responder cells cultured alone was 13.8 ± 2.3 SD.
† The uptake of irradiated normal and FIA-treated stimulator cells cultured alone was always <1.5.
‡ Values are counts per minute × 10^{-3}, mean ± SD of 5 experiments.
§ Statistically significant compared with normal, $P < 0.01$.

The cell type(s) which mediates the suppression is not known. Negative and positive selection studies to determine whether the suppressor is a macrophage, an activated T cell, or a B cell (the major constituents of nylon-wool–adherent cell fractions) are in progress in our laboratory.

The mechanism of action of the suppressor cells is unknown as well. Our further studies are aimed at determining whether: (a) this effect is mediated by soluble factors or by cell contact; (b) the stimulator population actually contains the suppressor cells or if it activates suppressor cells present in the responder cell population; (c) this effect occurs due to neutralization of helper factors, such as interleukin-2.

A critical question concerning the pathogenesis of autoimmunity is whether the decrease in AMLR is related to autoimmune disease (Figure 1). The decreased AMLR may be: (a) an essential step in the pathogenesis of autoimmunity; (b) an event that modifies the severity of autoimmune processes but is not

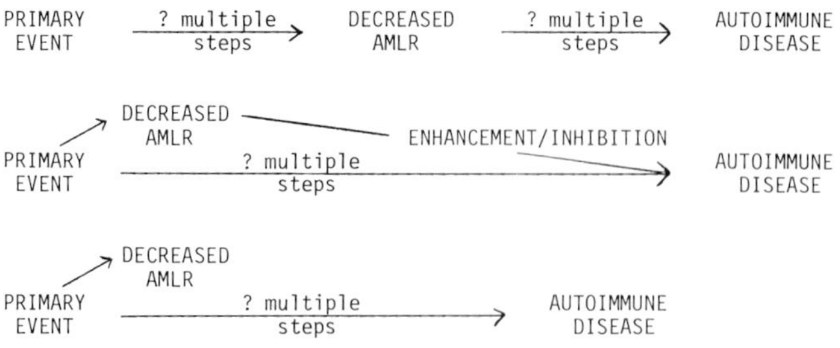

Figure 1. Schematic representation of the possible relationships between the autologous mixed lymphocyte reaction (AMLR) and autoimmune disease. The decreased AMLR may be: an essential pathogenetic step (top); a modulatory event (middle); or an unrelated response to the primary event (bottom).

required for their occurrence; (c) caused by the event initiating the autoimmune disease, but otherwise unrelated to the occurrence or severity of disease.

Our studies of arthritis-resistant rats demonstrate that the decreased AMLR can occur without overt arthritis. This would appear to make the first hypothesis untenable, but in reality it does not, because the event responsible for the arthritis resistance of F344 rats is not known.

In our studies utilizing nonarthritogenic stimuli of inflammation, we sought to determine whether the decreased AMLR was due to systemic effects of the local inflammatory response at the injection site. To investigate this, we induced clinically comparable local inflammation with 2 different nonarthritogenic substances (FIA and turpentine). We found that injection of turpentine had no effect on the AMLR either on day 2 (the acute phase) or on day 14. However, FIA caused a modest decrease in AMLR, but in this case, the effect was mediated by the responder cell population; thus, the mechanism is different from that by which FCA decreases the AMLR. Overall, these data demonstrate that the stimulator cell–mediated decrease in AMLR seen in FCA-treated animals is not due to the effects of either acute or chronic local inflammation. Further investigation aimed at determining the identity of the suppressor cell, as well as its site and mode of action, may help to clarify the cause of the reduced AMLR and its ultimate relationship to autoimmune conditions.

ACKNOWLEDGMENT

The authors wish to thank Mary Lou Adams for her excellent secretarial assistance in the preparation of this manuscript.

REFERENCES

1. Howe ML, Goldstein AL, Battisto JR: Detection of self recognition cells by in vitro isogeneic lymphocyte interaction, Proceedings of the Fifth Leucocyte Culture Conference, Ottawa, June 25–27, 1970. New York, Academic Press, 1970, p 515
2. Opelz G, Kiuchi M, Takasugi M, Terasaki PI: Autologous stimulation of human lymphocyte subpopulation. J Exp Med 142:1327–1333, 1975
3. Damle NK, Hansen JA, Good RA, Gupta S: Monoclonal antibody analysis of human T lymphocyte subpopulations exhibiting autologous mixed lymphocyte reaction. Proc Natl Acad Sci USA 78:5096–5098, 1981
4. Yu DTY, Chiorazzi N, Kunkel HG: Helper factors derived from autologous mixed lymphocyte cultures. Cell Immunol 50:305–313, 1980
5. Damle NK, Gupta S: Autologous mixed lymphocyte reaction in man. V. Functionally and phenotypically distinct human T-cell subpopulations respond to non-T and activated T cells in AMLR. Scand J Immunol 16:59–68, 1982
6. Sakane T, Steinberg AD, Green I: Failure of autologous mixed lymphocyte reactions between T and non-T cells in patients with systemic lupus erythematosus. Proc Natl Acad Sci USA 75:3464–3468, 1978
7. Smith JB, Pasternak RC: Syngeneic mixed lymphocyte reaction in mice: strain distribution, kinetics, participating cells, and absence in NZB mice. J Immunol 121: 1889–1892, 1978
8. Miyasaka N, Sauvezie B, Pierce DA, Daniels TE, Talal N: Decreased autologous mixed lymphocyte reaction in Sjögren's syndrome. J Clin Invest 66:928–933, 1980
9. James SP, Elson CO, Waggoner JG, Jones EA, Strober W: Deficiency of autologous mixed lymphocyte reaction in patients with primary biliary cirrhosis. J Clin Invest 66:1305–1310, 1980
10. Beck P, Burmester GR, Ledwoch A, Urban C, Kalden JR: Autologous and allogeneic reactivity in patients with rheumatoid arthritis. J Lab Clin Immunol 6:27–34, 1981
11. Pearson CM: Development of arthritis, periarthritis and periostitis in rats given adjuvant. Proc Soc Exp Biol Med 91:95–101, 1956
12. Pearson CM: Arthritis in animals, Arthritis and Allied Conditions. Ninth edition. Edited by DJ McCarty. Philadelphia, Lea & Febiger, 1979, pp 308–319
13. Trentham DE, McCune WJ, Susman P, David JR: Autoimmunity to collagen in adjuvant arthritis of rats. J Clin Invest 66:1109–1117, 1980
14. Welles WL, Battisto JR: Immunological protocols can diminish or abrogate the expression of adjuvant arthritis, Immunoregulation and Autoimmunity. Edited by RS Krakauer, MK Cathcart. New York, Elsevier/North-Holland, 1980, pp 139–147
15. Welles WL, Battisto JR: Suppression of adjuvant arthritis by antibodies specific for collagen type II. Immunol Commun 10:673–685, 1981
16. Battisto JR, Smith RN, Beckman K, Sternlicht M, Welles WL: Susceptibility to adjuvant arthritis in DA and F_{344} rats: a dominant trait controlled by an autosomal gene locus linked to the major histocompatibility complex. Arthritis Rheum 25:1194–1200, 1982
17. Handwerger BS, Schwartz RH: Separation of murine lymphoid cells using nylon wool columns: recovery of the B cell-enriched population. Transplantation 18:544–547, 1974

COMPARATIVE MEASUREMENT EFFICIENCY AND SENSITIVITY OF FIVE HEALTH STATUS INSTRUMENTS FOR ARTHRITIS RESEARCH

MATTHEW H. LIANG, MARTIN G. LARSON, KAREN E. CULLEN, and JULIE A. SCHWARTZ

Five health status instruments were administered in random order to 50 arthritis patients before and after total joint arthroplasty. Relative efficiency and sensitivity in measurement of change in pain, mobility and physical function, social role and social activity, and global health were assessed. The instruments had highly correlated scores, but had differences in certain dimensions. Inter-instrument differentials were larger for social and global outcomes than for pain or mobility. No single instrument consistently outperformed the others. A method for determining relative efficiency is described.

Over the last 10 years, the measurement of outcome in chronic disease has been pursued actively. For the rheumatic diseases, specific instruments measuring quality of life or health status have recently been developed, building on a strong tradition of concern with the accurate measurement of musculoskeletal function. Evaluating the results of health care in its multiple dimensions and from the patient's perceptions represents an important shift in health care assessment which has posed new questions. Among these are whether the new instruments have sufficient sensitivity to measure clinically important changes (1,2) and which instruments are most efficient for detecting these changes.

We present the results of a study of the relative measurement sensitivity of 5 widely-used health status indicators as applied to patients with end-stage joint disease who were undergoing primary total joint replacement. This population was chosen because total joint replacement is a unique pulse intervention in arthritis management, resulting in nearly certain improvement in pain and function (3). Patients predictably attain much of their expected improvement by 3 months after discharge. Thus, the population provided a high likelihood of change on which the instruments could be tested.

These results should assist the investigator who is planning a study in which improved functional performance is likely and who must choose among the many available instruments. Our premise is that, all other things being equal, the statistically most powerful instrument, with highest probability of demonstrating significant change, would be the most desirable.

PATIENTS AND METHODS

Five health status instruments which fulfill the minimum requirement of measurement reliability and validity were studied: the Functional Status Index (FSI) (4), the Health Assessment Questionnaire (HAQ) (5), the Arthritis Impact Measurement Scales (AIMS) (6,7), the Index of Well-Being (IWB; also referred to as the Quality of Well-Being Instrument) (8), and the Sickness Impact Profile (SIP) (9). The first 3 instruments were developed for patients with rheumatoid arthritis and have been used extensively. The

From the Departments of Medicine, Rheumatology/Immunology, and Orthopedic Surgery and the Robert B. Brigham Multipurpose Arthritis Center, Brigham and Women's Hospital, Harvard Medical School, and the Department of Biostatistics, Harvard School of Public Health, Boston, Massachusetts.

Supported by NIH Multipurpose Arthritis Center grant AM-20580 and Biomedical Research Support grant RR-05669.

Matthew H. Liang, MD, MPH; Martin G. Larson, ScD; Karen E. Cullen, MEd; Julie A. Schwartz, BS.

Address reprint requests to Matthew H. Liang, MD, Robert B. Brigham Multipurpose Arthritis Center, Brigham and Women's Hospital, 75 Francis Street, Boston, MA 02115.

Submitted for publication March 27, 1984; accepted in revised form October 23, 1984.

last 2 scales, though not arthritis-specific, have had even wider usage, including among patients with arthritis and orthopedic disorders.

Patient selection criteria. Consecutive patients scheduled for primary total joint replacement of the hip or knee were screened for the study. Eligibility criteria were: age 50–80, primary diagnosis of rheumatoid arthritis (RA) or osteoarthritis (OA), either primary or secondary, and identification early enough to be interviewed 2 weeks before surgery. Subjects with cognitive impairments, language barriers, or visual or hearing deficits were excluded because their responses to questionnaires might not be reliable. Patients with previous joint surgery were excluded so as not to confound expected functional results. All patients were seen in our 96-bed referral unit devoted to the management of arthritis and related disorders. Information about comorbid conditions was abstracted from medical records. Informed consent was obtained.

Description of instruments. The Functional Status Index measures dependence, pain, and difficulty experienced in the performance of 18 activities of daily living. Each activity is rated between 0 and 4 on each dimension. Studies on patients with rheumatoid arthritis show validity and a high degree of inter-observer reliability. In self-assessed format, it takes 10–20 minutes to complete. The 18 activities were grouped into 5 subscales, and the average of dependence and difficulty scores was used for each subscale. Pain scores were averaged across all activities.

The Health Assessment Questionnaire is an arthritis-specific scale that measures performance in activities of daily living, emphasizing difficulty and the need for equipment and physical assistance to complete tasks. Scores on 8 subscales are averaged to create a disability index. The possible scores range from 0 to 3 on each scale. A visual analog subscale measures pain intensity. The HAQ is self-administered and requires 8–10 minutes to complete.

The Arthritis Impact Measurement Scale has 48 multiple-choice questions with 9 subscales measuring physical, social, and mental health status. The possible range of scores on each subscale is 0–10; subscale results are averaged to obtain a total score. The AIMS is self-administered and takes 15–20 minutes to complete.

The Index of Well-Being defines function by 3 scales with ordinal categories: physical activity, mobility, and social activity. Accompanying these is a list of symptom/problem complexes used to generate a weighted score. It is administered by trained interviewers in 10–20 minutes.

The Sickness Impact Profile assesses function in terms of yes/no responses on 136 health-related behaviors divided into 12 major categories of activities of daily living. A total score is computed by summing category scores. Scores are then standardized to a percentage (0–100) of the maximum possible score. Questions in 3 of the categories (sleep and rest, emotional, and alertness behaviors) were not used in this study. The instrument can be completed in 15–30 minutes.

All 5 instruments were administered in random order to each patient approximately 2 weeks before and 3 months after discharge from hospitalization for joint surgery. The IWB was administered in person or by phone by a trained research assistant and randomized to before or after completion of the other 4 instruments, which are self-administered. The mode and order of administration were the same preoperatively and postoperatively.

Dimensions of function. Since the number of subscales and their substance differed for each instrument, the first task was to create new measures with comparable content across instruments. Three dimensions of function or "health status" were chosen: Mobility, including ambulatory and physical activity such as bed and chair transfers; Social, including social activities, social role, and home management functions; and Pain. Table 1 shows the groupings of subscales for each instrument (IWB and SIP do not have a Pain dimension). Each dimension score was formed as the average of the relevant subscale scores. In addition, Global Status scores were computed according to published specifications for each instrument.

Scores on all dimensions were linearly transformed to a common range of possible values, 0–100. A score of 0 indicates no dysfunction or no pain, whereas 100 indicates maximum dysfunction or pain. The latter term is specific to each instrument, so the "internal" scaling may produce differences between instruments in terms of mean values and standard deviations. We chose to retain these differences, rather than submerge them by scaling all values to a common mean and standard deviation. Either approach could be used without affecting the main comparisons between instruments (see below). This transformation has no effect on the tests of hypothesis, the computation of correlations, or the relative efficiency measures to be defined.

Statistical methods. Data analysis was performed on an IBM 4341 computer using the SAS package of statistical programs (10). Means and standard deviations were computed for preoperative scores and for changes in scores on each patient; changes were computed as preoperative minus postdischarge, such that positive change indicates improvement. Paired t-statistics, based on within-patient changes (11), are presented for evaluating the average change in functional status. Pearson product-moment correlations were calculated to assess whether scores on different instruments reflected measurement of similar aspects of function.

This report compares each instrument with the FSI in terms of Relative Efficiency (RE) to detect change in Mobility, in Pain, in Social Function, and in Global Status. The choice of "standard" was arbitrary and does not imply any preference for the FSI. Relative Efficiency was computed by squaring the ratio of appropriate t-statistics, e.g., RE(AIMS versus FSI) = $(t_{AIMS}/t_{FSI})^2$. These equations would exactly equal ratios of coefficients of variation (11) if all patients completed all parts of every instrument at both assessments. Because some responses were missing or invalid, we based the RE computations on t-statistics, which include a sample-size factor, thereby reducing the efficiency of instruments with "bad data." The largest adjustment made in this study was about 30%, in favor of the AIMS versus FSI on the change in Pain scores.

An RE >1 (or RE <1) means that the instrument was a more (or less) efficient tool for measuring change than the FSI. Relative Efficiencies may be computed for any pair of instruments using the data from this study. Stated simply,

Table 1. Functional dimensions: component subscales*

	Instrument				
Dimension	AIMS	FSI	HAQ	IWB	SIP
Mobility	Mobility, physical activity	Mobility	Arising, walking	Mobility, physical activity	Mobility, ambulation
Social	Social role, social activity	Chores, social activity	Reaching/bending, social activity	Social activity	Work, recreation, home management, social interaction
Global	Above + dexterity, depression, pain (excludes social activity)	Above + dexterity, personal care	Above + eating, dressing, grip, hygiene	Above + symptom complex weighted	Above + body care, communication, eating
Pain	Specific subscale	Pain dimension	Visual analog	–	–

* AIMS = Arthritis Impact Measurement Scales; FSI = Functional Status Index; HAQ = Health Assessment Questionnaire; IWB = Index of Well-Being; SIP = Sickness Impact Profile.

the instrument with highest relative efficiency should give the best trade-off between sample size and statistical power (11) to detect change between assessments. The instrument with highest RE has the highest power for a fixed sample size, or requires fewer patients to achieve a fixed level of statistical power.

RESULTS

Of 201 consecutive surgical candidates screened for this study, 113 failed to meet entry criteria because of prior joint replacement (56 patients), age (39 patients), diagnoses other than RA or OA (12 patients), cognitive problems (2 patients), and miscellaneous reasons (4 patients). Of 88 who met the eligibility criteria, 12 refused to participate, 3 could not be contacted in time before surgery, and 7 did not undergo total hip or knee surgery. Sixty-six patients agreed to participate, but 16 were dropped because surgery was cancelled or questionnaires were not returned. This resulted in a final sample of 50 subjects. The mean age of the subjects was 66.3 years (SD = 6.8); 31 subjects were female, and 40 had a diagnosis of osteoarthritis. Similar characteristics were found among the 31 eligible patients who had total joint replacement but were excluded from the final sample.

Fifty percent of the subjects had hip replacements, and 50% had knee replacements. The mean number of involved (tender/swollen) joints was 6.2 (SD = 2.0) for RA patients and 1.8 (SD = 0.9) for OA patients. The most prevalent concomitant diagnoses were pulmonary disease (12%) and cardiac disease (12%). Table 2 presents additional patient characteristics.

Preoperative functional assessment. Univariate statistics for preoperative scores on the dimensions of Mobility, Pain, Social Function, and Global Health are presented in Table 3. Substantial Mobility impairment was registered by the AIMS (mean = 55.1) and HAQ (mean = 45.7), both arthritis-specific instruments. The 2 general health instruments registered intermediate levels of impairment, with means of 33.3 on the IWB and 22.3 on the SIP. In contrast, the FSI registered the lowest average level of impairment (mean = 19.1). Correlations between scores on different instruments are shown in Table 4. Inter-instrument correlations were quite high, ranging from r = 0.49 (HAQ, SIP) to r = 0.84 (AIMS, SIP), the average correlation being r = 0.65 over 10 unique pairs.

Table 2. Characteristics of subjects (n = 50)

Age (mean)	66.3
Female/male (%)	62/38
Education completed (%)	
Less than high school	22
High school	52
College	10
Graduate school	16
Marital status (%)	
Married	68
Widowed	18
Never married	8
Separated	4
Divorced	2
Current employment status (%)	
Full-time	24
Part-time	8
Housewife	16
Not employed	50
Other	2
Reason for non-employed status (n = 26) (%)	
Arthritis	10
Other health reasons	2
Retired naturally	36
Not related to health	4
Osteoarthritis/rheumatoid arthritis (%)	80/20
Concurrent diagnosis (%)	
Pulmonary disease	12
Cardiac disease	12
Neurologic disease	4
Trauma	6
Miscellaneous diagnoses	12

Table 3. Subjects' preoperative function, as measured by 5 assessment instruments*

	Instrument				
Dimension	AIMS	FSI	HAQ	IWB	SIP
Mobility					
n	50	48	50	49	50
Mean	55.1	19.1	45.7	33.3	22.3
SD	25.3	13.1	25.4	21.5	14.1
Pain					
n	49	45	48	–	–
Mean	57.6	24.4	46.4	–	–
SD	20.7	16.0	24.0	–	–
Social					
n	50	48	50	49	50
Mean	24.1	22.5	47.0	45.4	21.4
SD	12.4	21.1	30.1	23.8	13.4
Global					
n	50	48	50	49	50
Mean	36.8	16.2	37.3	61.3	15.2
SD	17.3	12.5	23.4	8.2	9.3

* n values represent the number of valid scores; see Table 1 for abbreviations.

Pain scores before surgery were also high, mean values being 57.6 on the AIMS and 46.4 on the HAQ, but the FSI had a lower average (24.4). Correlations of Pain scores were strong and nearly equal: r = 0.52 (AIMS, HAQ), r = 0.53 (FSI, HAQ), and r = 0.65 (AIMS, FSI). Two instruments registered substantial impairment of Social Function, the IWB (mean = 45.4) and the HAQ (mean = 47.0), but the mean values for other instruments were in the low 20s. The average inter-instrument correlation of Social scores was r = 0.44; specific correlations ranged from r = 0.21 (AIMS, FSI) to r = 0.69 (HAQ, SIP).

Only the IWB had a high mean value (61.3) for Global impairment. Two arthritis-specific instruments had mean values in the mid 30s (36.8 for the AIMS, 37.3 for the HAQ), whereas the FSI and SIP averages were much lower, 16.2 and 15.2, respectively. Correlations of Global dysfunction scores were high, from r = 0.50 (FSI, IWB) to r = 0.87 (AIMS, SIP). The IWB stood apart in this aspect: its average correlation with the other 4 instruments was just 0.58, while the average correlation was 0.80 among the AIMS, FSI, HAQ, and SIP.

These results demonstrate 3 features of the preoperative assessments. First, there were moderate to high levels of impairment and pain intensity. Second, the 5 instruments registered different average levels of impairment, and the relative ordering of instruments by level of impairment registered varied across functional dimensions. Finally, the instruments generally had highly correlated scores; their measures of dysfunction were mutually consistent on each dimension.

Measuring change. Each instrument detected statistically significant improvement in Mobility (Table 5). Approximately equal Relative Efficiencies were found for the AIMS (RE = 0.85), FSI (RE = 1.00 by definition), and SIP (RE = 1.11), but the HAQ (RE = 0.48) and IWB (RE = 0.45) were less efficient. Percentage change (100 × mean change/preoperative mean) varied from 35.2% (AIMS) to 71.2% (FSI). Correlations of Mobility change scores (Table 6) were lower than those for preoperative scores (Table 4), and changes registered on the HAQ and IWB were poorly correlated with changes measured by the other instruments. Differences in relative efficiency for the Mobility data were associated with different gradations of the measurement scales. The HAQ and IWB had much cruder scales, mapping 6 or 7 preoperative values into only 8 or 9 distinct change scores, whereas the other instruments all had 20 or more distinct values for the changes in Mobility.

The 3 instruments having Pain scales all registered statistically significant reduction in Pain scores (Table 5). Percentage changes were on the order of 50% from preoperative levels: 43.4% for AIMS, 45.9% for HAQ, and 59.8% for FSI. The FSI had the highest efficiency, the AIMS (RE = 0.79) performed almost as well, but the HAQ (RE = 0.57) was less efficient. Correlations of change in Pain scores, shown in Table 6, were r = 0.31 (AIMS, FSI), r = 0.43 (AIMS, HAQ),

Table 4. Inter-instrument correlations of functional scores at preoperative assessment*

	Instrument			
Dimension	AIMS	FSI	HAQ	IWB
Mobility (n)				
FSI	0.74 (48)			
HAQ	0.61 (50)	0.58 (48)		
IWB	0.76 (49)	0.50 (47)	0.51 (49)	
SIP	0.84 (50)	0.60 (48)	0.49 (50)	0.82 (49)
Pain (n)				
FSI	0.65 (45)			
HAQ	0.52 (47)	0.53 (43)		
Social (n)				
FSI	0.21 (48)			
HAQ	0.53 (50)	0.54 (48)		
IWB	0.30 (49)	0.42 (47)	0.46 (49)	
SIP	0.49 (50)	0.41 (48)	0.69 (50)	0.39 (49)
Global (n)				
FSI	0.84 (48)			
HAQ	0.84 (50)	0.75 (48)		
IWB	0.62 (49)	0.50 (47)	0.60 (49)	
SIP	0.87 (50)	0.73 (48)	0.78 (50)	0.59 (49)

* n values represent the number of valid scores; see Table 1 for abbreviations.

Table 5. Functional change and Relative Efficiencies for its detection, by assessment instrument*

Dimension	Instrument				
	AIMS	FSI	HAQ	IWB	SIP
Mobility					
n	50	46	50	49	50
Mean change	19.4	13.6	19.3	13.4	11.9
SD	20.5	12.7	27.0	19.3	11.0
t-statistic	6.69	7.26	5.05	4.86	7.65
Relative Efficiency	0.85	1.00	0.48	0.45	1.11
Pain					
n	49	37	44	–	–
Mean change	25.0	14.6	21.3	–	–
SD	23.3	10.5	22.1	–	–
t-statistic	7.51	8.46	6.39	–	–
Relative Efficiency	0.79	1.00	0.57	–	–
Social					
n	50	46	50	49	50
Mean change	2.6	10.7	12.3	15.3	6.4
SD	10.6	17.7	26.9	35.7	12.8
t-statistic	1.73	4.10	3.23	3.00	3.54
Relative Efficiency	0.18	1.00	0.62	0.54	0.74
Global					
n	50	47	50	49	50
Mean change	11.5	5.4	7.8	16.4	6.0
SD	13.1	12.1	16.8	13.7	7.4
t-statistic	6.21	3.06	3.28	8.38	5.73
Relative Efficiency	4.12	1.00	1.15	7.50	3.51

* n values represent the number of valid scores; see text for calculation of Relative Efficiency. See Table 1 for abbreviations.

and r = 0.03 (FSI, HAQ). Differential relative efficiency was not associated with the gradation of pain scales: the HAQ had the largest number of distinct values but the lowest efficiency.

Postoperative improvement in Social scores was found, with all instruments except the AIMS detecting significant change (Table 5). Percentage changes from mean preoperative levels were between 10.8% (AIMS) and 47.6% (FSI). The most efficient instrument for detecting change in Social Function was the FSI (RE = 1.00), followed by the SIP (RE = 0.74), HAQ (RE = 0.62), and IWB (RE = 0.54), while the AIMS (RE = 0.18) was considerably less efficient. Reduced efficiency of the HAQ and IWB may be due to crude measurement scales which mapped changes into just 6 or 7 distinct values, but this does not explain the poor RE of the AIMS which, along with the FSI and SIP, registered 30 or more distinct values for Social Function change. Correlations across instruments (Table 6) were low, ranging from r = −0.18 (FSI, IWB) to r = 0.39 (AIMS, HAQ), and may reflect different content of the subscales for each instrument.

There were also significant improvements in Global dysfunction scores with each instrument (Table 5). Percentage change from preoperative level ranged from 20.9% (HAQ) to 39.5% (SIP). Relative Efficiency to measure Global change was diverse: the FSI (RE = 1.00) and HAQ (RE = 1.15) were much less efficient than the SIP (RE = 3.51), AIMS (RE = 4.12), or IWB (RE = 7.50). Correlations of changes in Global scores (Table 6) were lower than the cross-sectional correlations based on preoperative data (Table 4); they ranged from r = −0.16 (FSI, IWB) to r = 0.50 (AIMS, HAQ). All instruments had finely-graded measurement scales for Global scores, so differential RE was not due to crude scaling of values. The low RE of FSI and HAQ may result from the fact that their Global scores did not incorporate pain.

DISCUSSION

There is an abundance of instruments to measure "quality of life" or "health status." Scores on different instruments often correlate highly, providing evidence of convergent validity and suggesting that instruments (or subscales) are interchangeable to some degree. When selecting an instrument for use in medical research, one should examine closely its appropriateness for the target population and the type of intervention, and its measurement efficiency for detecting differences of the size expected to occur between groups. If repeated measures of function are sought, one needs to consider each instrument's efficiency for detecting changes over time (12). To date, there have been little or no data on the latter point.

This paper reports the relative efficiency of 5 instruments for measuring changes in pain and function among patients undergoing total joint replacement. Self-reported levels of pain and impairment

Table 6. Inter-instrument correlations of functional change*

Dimension	AIMS	FSI	HAQ	IWB
Mobility (n)				
FSI	0.42 (46)			
HAQ	0.34 (50)	0.18 (46)		
IWB	0.30 (49)	−0.12 (45)	0.04 (49)	
SIP	0.55 (50)	0.42 (46)	0.28 (50)	0.32 (49)
Pain (n)				
FSI	0.31 (37)			
HAQ	0.43 (44)	0.03 (35)		
Social (n)				
FSI	−0.03 (46)			
HAQ	0.39 (50)	0.26 (46)		
IWB	0.15 (49)	−0.18 (45)	0.12 (49)	
SIP	0.33 (50)	0.12 (46)	0.31 (50)	0.29 (49)
Global (n)				
FSI	0.32 (47)			
HAQ	0.50 (50)	0.44 (47)		
IWB	0.25 (49)	−0.16 (46)	0.31 (49)	
SIP	0.54 (50)	0.02 (47)	0.31 (50)	0.33 (49)

* n values represent the number of valid scores; see Table 1 for abbreviations.

were quite high preoperatively, generally with strong correlations among scores derived from different instruments. Yet the instruments clearly had distinct metric properties as judged by measures of central location (median, mean) and spread (range, standard deviation).

Marked improvements in pain level and functional performance were found 3 months after discharge. The AIMS, FSI, and SIP were about equally efficient in detecting changes in Mobility scores, but the HAQ and IWB were only about half as efficient as the other 3 instruments. Thus, the HAQ and IWB are judged to be poor candidates for use when mobility change is a major functional outcome. Three instruments were compared for Pain assessment. Relative to the FSI, the AIMS was 79% efficient, whereas the HAQ was only 57% efficient. The HAQ has a single visual analog scale to measure pain intensity, and may fail to cover all aspects of arthritis pain.

The AIMS was inefficient (RE = 0.18) compared with the FSI for measuring change in Social Function, while efficiency of the other instruments was between 0.54 (IWB) and 0.74 (SIP). These differences are difficult to interpret since Social Function has many facets. Selection of subscales of Social Function for a specific research project must be guided by a clear definition of which aspects of this broad area are most important to assess.

Our final comparison involved the Global indices of functional impairments. The FSI and HAQ performed equally, but were less than one-third as efficient as the SIP, AIMS, or IWB. These results were surprising because the FSI had high relative efficiency on other dimensions of function. We believe the explanation is that Global indices for the FSI and HAQ did not include Pain subscales, but did include subscales measuring upper body function, which was not changed much by lower extremity joint replacement. In contrast, the more efficient instruments for detecting change in Global dysfunction either included Pain (as a subscale in AIMS, as a symptom/problem in IWB), or weighted the Global score heavily toward mobility and physical activities (SIP).

In this study, reduction of pain and improved physical function in patients who had joint replacement surgery were measured by 5 health status instruments. However, the tools differed in their relative efficiencies to detect change on specific dimensions of function. This study provides a method for determining efficiency quantitatively and highlights the need to carefully review instruments for research applications, to ensure that key aspects of function are represented by specific subscales. The issue is critical in situations where the expected changes are smaller than those seen in joint replacement, settings that include medical and rehabilitative management of arthritis.

REFERENCES

1. Liang MH, Jette AM: Measuring functional ability in chronic arthritis: a critical review. Arthritis Rheum 24:80–86, 1981
2. Liang MH, Cullen KE, Larson MG: In search of a more perfect mousetrap (health status or quality of life instrument). J Rheumatol 9:775–779, 1982
3. Liang MH, Cullen KE, Poss R: Primary total joint replacement: evaluation of patients. Ann Intern Med 97:735–739, 1982
4. Jette AM: Functional status instrument: reliability of a chronic disease evaluation instrument. Arch Phys Med Rehabil 61:395–401, 1980
5. Fries JF, Spitz P, Kraines RG, Holman HR: Measurement of patient outcome in arthritis. Arthritis Rheum 23:137–145, 1980
6. Meenan RF, Gertman PM, Mason JM: Measuring health status in arthritis: the arthritis impact measurement scales. Arthritis Rheum 23:146–152, 1980
7. Meenan RF, Gertman PM, Mason JH, Dunaif R: The arthritis impact measurement scales: further investigations of a health status measure. Arthritis Rheum 25: 1048–1053, 1982
8. Kaplan RM, Bush JW, Berry CC: Health status: types of validity for an index of well-being. Health Serv Res 11:478–507, 1976
9. Bergner M, Bobbitt RA, Pollard WE, Martin DP, Gilson BS: The sickness impact profile: validation of a health status measure. Med Care 14:57–67, 1976
10. Statistical Analysis System: SAS User's Guide. Cary, North Carolina, SAS Institute, 1982
11. Snedecor GW, Cochran WG: Statistical Methods. Ames, Iowa State University Press, 1967
12. Liang MH, Cullen KE, Larson MG: Measuring function and health status in rheumatic disease clinical trials. Clin Rheum Dis 9:531–539, 1983

PROTEOGLYCAN DEPLETION, RATHER THAN FIBRILLATION, DETERMINES THE EFFECTS OF SALICYLATE AND INDOMETHACIN ON OSTEOARTHRITIC CARTILAGE

MARSHALL J. PALMOSKI and KENNETH D. BRANDT

The effects of salicylate and indomethacin on glycosaminoglycan (GAG) synthesis by atrophic and osteoarthritic (OA) canine cartilage were examined in vitro by transecting distal femora at the metaphysis and incubating the knuckle, with its overlying cap of articular cartilage, in medium containing sodium salicylate or indomethacin, and $^{35}SO_4$. Atrophic cartilage had an intact articular surface, but its uronic acid content averaged 65% of the control level, and GAG synthesis was decreased to 50% of control values. Both salicylate and indomethacin decreased net GAG synthesis in the atrophic cartilage by an additional 10%. OA cartilage showed surface disruption, a uronic acid content 49% of the control value, and a 49% increase in net GAG synthesis. Salicylate and indomethacin profoundly decreased GAG synthesis in the OA cartilage. However, GAG synthesis and uronic acid content of cartilage which had been lacerated in vitro immediately prior to culture (to stimulate fibrillation) were normal and not affected by either drug. The data emphasize the importance of matrix proteoglycan content in protecting the chondrocyte from the suppressive effects of salicylate and indomethacin on GAG metabolism, and suggest that the lower proteoglycan content of OA cartilage may be more important than fibrillation in rendering it vulnerable to the metabolic effects of these drugs.

From the Rheumatology Division, Indiana University School of Medicine, Indianapolis.

Supported in part by grants from the National Institute of Arthritis, Metabolism and Digestive Diseases (AM-20582 and AM-7448) and awards from the Arthritis Foundation and the Grace M. Showalter Trust.

Marshall J. Palmoski, PhD: Associate Professor of Medicine and Anatomy (current address: Department of Pharmacology, Bristol-Myers Co., PO Box 4755, Syracuse, NY 13221); Kenneth D. Brandt, MD: Professor of Medicine and Head, Rheumatology Division, Indiana University School of Medicine.

Address reprint requests to Kenneth D. Brandt, MD, Rheumatology Division, Indiana University School of Medicine, 541 Clinical Drive, Indianapolis, IN 46223.

Submitted for publication August 13, 1984; accepted in revised form November 9, 1984.

We have previously reported that aspirin, when fed to dogs in quantities sufficient to achieve a serum salicylate concentration of 20–25 mg%, aggravated the degeneration of articular cartilage in osteoarthritic (OA) joints, although it had no effect on normal cartilage from the contralateral knees (1). In vitro studies have shown that the marked augmentation of glycosaminoglycan (GAG) synthesis in slices of cartilage from osteoarthritic joints was suppressed by salicylate to a much greater extent than GAG synthesis in normal cartilage, and that this difference was associated with greater uptake of the drug by fibrillated cartilage than by normal cartilage (2). Other data are consistent with the concept that the suppressive effects of salicylate and also of indomethacin on GAG synthesis in normal cartilage are inversely related to the proteoglycan content of the extracellular matrix, and indicate that the proteoglycan content of cartilage may affect its permeability to these drugs (3,4).

To determine whether the augmented effect of salicylate on osteoarthritic cartilage was due to decreased proteoglycan content and/or to disruption of surface integrity, providing increased access of the drug to the chondrocytes, we examined the effects of salicylate on GAG synthesis in normal cartilage which had been lacerated in vitro to simulate fibrillation, as well as on osteoarthritic cartilage and atrophic cartilage, which had an intact surface but a reduced proteoglycan content.

MATERIALS AND METHODS

Experimental groups and procedures. Fourteen adult mongrel dogs, whose weights ranged from 23–30 kg, were used. Four animals (the Cru-X group) underwent transection of the right anterior cruciate ligament, as previously described (1). All Cru-X animals bore weight on the operated limb by the third day after surgery and were maintained in pens (8 × 10′) for 16 weeks, at which time they were killed with an overdose of sodium pentothal.

The right hind legs of 4 additional dogs (the IK group) were immobilized in a cast with approximately 90° of hip and knee flexion, to induce articular cartilage atrophy (5). These animals were killed after 6 weeks of confinement in pens, as described above.

A third group of 4 dogs (the Lac group) was killed with an overdose of sodium pentothal within 5 days after procurement. At the time of death, both knees of each animal were opened aseptically and the distal femurs were removed at the metaphysis with a bone saw. After the femurs were cleaned of adhering soft tissue, the articular cartilage of the central weight-bearing regions of the medial and lateral condyles of the right knee of each dog in the Lac group was lacerated with a scalpel at approximately 1-mm intervals, with care taken not to penetrate the subchondral bone.

Culture technique. The medial and lateral condyles of both knees of each dog in the above 3 experimental groups were separated through the intercondylar groove with a bone saw, and were placed separately in breakers containing 15 ml of Ham's F-12 nutrient mixture, pH 7.4, supplemented with 10% newborn calf serum, streptomycin (50 μg/ml), penicillin (50 units/ml) (all obtained from Gibco, Grand Island, NY), and ascorbic acid (50 μg/ml). In half of the experiments, the medial condyles were incubated with gentle rocking for 24 hours at 37°C in 5% CO_2, 95% air in medium containing sodium salicylate ($10^{-3}M$) or indomethacin ($4 \times 10^{-6}M$), with Na_2-$^{35}SO_4$ (10 μCi/ml) added for the final 8 hours of incubation, while the lateral condyles were cultured in an identical fashion, but without the drug added. In the remaining experiments, the conditions were reversed, i.e., the lateral condyles were incubated in medium which contained drug, while the medial condyles were cultured in the absence of drug.

Characterization of medial and lateral condyles. The remaining 2 dogs were killed, and cartilage from both knees was obtained and was used to provide comparisons between medial and lateral femoral condyles with respect to uronic acid content and GAG biosynthesis in the absence of drug.

Determination of net glycosaminoglycan synthesis. Following incubation of the tissues as described above, the medium was decanted and the condyles were rinsed with 0.9% saline. The spent medium and rinse were combined and dialyzed against 200 volumes of 0.05*M* sodium acetate, pH 6.8, for 48 hours at 4°C in Spectrapor No. 3 dialysis tubing (approximate molecular weight cutoff = 3,500 daltons; Spectrum Medical Industries, Los Angeles, CA).

The articular cartilage was then shaved with a scalpel from the central, habitually-loaded surface of each condyle. Cartilage from each condyle was pooled separately. Portions (approximately 15 mg) of the shaved cartilage were weighed and used for determination of uronic acid content. Representative full-thickness samples of the cartilage from the central weight-bearing regions of each condyle were obtained with a Craig biopsy needle and were placed in 10% buffered formalin for histologic study, while the remainder was divided into 3 approximately equal portions (20–30 mg wet weight each) which were used to assay net GAG synthesis.

The triplicate samples were suspended in 3 ml of 0.1*M* borate buffer, pH 8.0, containing 0.02*M* calcium chloride, and were digested under toluene for 24 hours at 55°C with pronase (200 μg/10 mg cartilage wet weight; Calbiochem-Behring, San Diego, CA). The digests were placed in Spectrapor No. 3 membrane tubing and dialyzed overnight at 4°C against running tap water, following which aliquots (0.1 ml) were added to 10 ml of Ready-Solv HP 60 (Beckman Instruments, Irvine, CA) and counted in a Beckman liquid scintillation spectrometer. Results (nondialyzable counts per minute) were adjusted for differences in wet weight of the cartilage.

Determination of uronic acid content. Portions (approximately 15 mg) of cartilage were placed in 2 changes of acetone for 24 hours, dried to constant weight in vacuo at 80°C, and digested with pronase as above. The GAGs were isolated from the pronase digests by precipitation with 9-aminoacridine hydrochloride, and were converted to their sodium salts with Bio-Rad AG-50 (Na′) (6). After the resin was removed by filtration, the uronic acid content of the filtrate was determined (7).

Histologic examination. Histologic sections (6μ) of full-thickness samples of the articular cartilage were examined microscopically after staining with Safranin O–fast green.

RESULTS

Gross observations. None of the knee joints contained an effusion. At the time of death, articular cartilage from the control knees of the Cru-X and IK dogs, and from both knees of the Lac dogs, was grossly normal. In all 4 Cru-X dogs, marginal osteophytes were present on medial and lateral femoral condyles of the unstable knees and the cartilage surface was dull and rough. In contrast, the unstable knees of IK dogs had no osteophytes and the cartilage was smooth, although it appeared thinner than in the control knees.

Histology and histochemistry. In all control samples, the cartilage surface and tidemark were intact, and Safranin O staining was normal. All samples of cartilage from the unstable knees of dogs from the Cru-X group showed a reduction in Safranin O staining in comparison with the contralateral control cartilage. Horizontal flaking of the cartilage surface was noted in all samples, but no vertical fibrillation was seen. The cartilage thickness was comparable with that of the

Table 1. Comparison of articular cartilage from medial and lateral femoral condyles of knees of normal dogs

Dog	Source of cartilage*	Uronic acid content, % of tissue dry weight	Net glycosaminoglycan synthesis†
1	RMC	4.1	12,432 ± 1,021
	RLC	4.0	12,805 ± 858
	LMC	4.2	13,301 ± 1,231
	LLC	4.1	13,110 ± 1,410
2	RMC	3.9	18,567 ± 823
	RLC	3.8	17,492 ± 1,210
	LMC	4.0	17,890 ± 1,390
	LLC	3.8	18,420 ± 1,521

* RMC = right medial condyle; RLC = right lateral condyle; LMC = left medial condyle; LLC = left lateral condyle.
† Nondialyzable ^{35}S cpm/10 mg wet weight of cartilage. Values represent mean ± SEM of triplicate samples.

contralateral control knees, and the tidemark was intact in all cases. No brood capsules were observed.

Cartilage from the scored condyles of dogs from the Lac group showed cuts extending to varying depths below the surface. None penetrated the tidemark. Safranin O staining adjacent to the cuts and throughout the matrix was normal. In dogs from the IK group, the thickness of cartilage from the immobilized leg was decreased to about 70% of that of cartilage from the contralateral knee, and Safranin O staining was reduced. The articular surface, however, was intact in all samples of atrophic cartilage.

Comparison of cartilage from medial and lateral femoral condyles of normal dogs. Studies utilizing 2 normal dogs indicated that there was no difference between the medial and lateral femoral condyles with respect to uronic acid content or net glycosaminoglycan synthesis (Table 1). In all cases, the uronic acid content was about 4% of the tissue dry weight, while net glycosaminoglycan synthesis in the medial condyles averaged 103 ± 2% of that in the lateral condyles. Cartilage from the contralateral (control) knees of dogs in all 3 experimental groups exhibited normal uronic acid content (4.1 ± 0.1% of the tissue dry weight) (Table 2).

Table 2. Uronic acid content of osteoarthritic, lacerated, and atrophic articular cartilage

Group (no. of dogs)*	Source of cartilage	Uronic acid content: % of tissue dry weight ± SEM	Uronic acid content: % of control
Cru-X (4)	Control knee	4.1 ± 0.2	–
	Experimental knee	2.0 ± 0.5	49
Lac (4)	Control knee	4.3 ± 0.1	–
	Experimental knee	4.5 ± 0.2	96
IK (4)	Control knee	4.0 ± 0.1	–
	Experimental knee	2.6 ± 0.2	65

* Cru-X = anterior cruciate ligament transection (osteoarthritic); Lac = cartilage lacerated in vitro; IK = immobilized knee (atrophic); control = cartilage from contralateral knee.

Uronic acid content and GAG synthesis in the experimental groups, and drug effects. *Cartilage from dogs in the Cru-X group.* The uronic acid content of osteoarthritic cartilage from the knees of dogs in the Cru-X group averaged 49% of that of cartilage from the contralateral knees of the same animals, while glycosaminoglycan synthesis was increased. In the 4 dogs in this group, net GAG synthesis in the osteoarthritic cartilage was 49 ± 5% greater than that in the corresponding control knee ($P < 0.01$). Both salicylate and indomethacin strikingly decreased glycosaminoglycan synthesis in OA cartilage (to 9% and 22%, respectively, of that in osteoarthritic samples cultured in the absence of the drugs) (Tables 3 and 4).

Cartilage from dogs in the Lac group. Uronic acid content and net GAG synthesis in experimental knees of the dogs with lacerated cartilage were similar to that of control knees (Table 2). GAG synthesis was not affected by either salicylate or indomethacin (Tables 3 and 4).

Cartilage from dogs in the IK group. The uronic acid content of the atrophic cartilage in immobilized knees was reduced to 65% of that in the contralateral knees of dogs in the IK group (Table 2). In contrast to the osteoarthritic samples, in which GAG synthesis was increased, in the IK cartilage GAG synthesis was only 50 ± 4% of control values ($P < 0.01$) (Tables 3 and 4). Both salicylate and indomethacin caused a further decrease in GAG synthesis in the atrophic cartilage, but this decrease was less than that seen when the osteoarthritic cartilage was incubated with the drugs ($P < 0.01$). Thus, in the absence of salicylate, GAG synthesis in IK cartilage averaged 48% of that in control cartilage, while in the presence of salicylate it averaged 37% of that in control cartilage (Table 3). Indomethacin, too, further reduced GAG synthesis in the atrophic cartilage by an additional 10% over the reduction seen without the drug (Table 4).

Neither salicylate nor indomethacin affected net GAG synthesis in control cartilage of the contralateral knees of dogs from any of the experimental groups.

DISCUSSION

The results of this study confirm our previous finding that the proteoglycan content of the matrix

Table 3. Effect of salicylate on glycosaminoglycan synthesis by osteoarthritic, lacerated, and atrophic articular cartilage

Dog	Source of cartilage*	Uronic acid content, % of tissue dry weight	Net glycosaminoglycan synthesis† — No salicylate added: ^{35}S cpm/10 mg wet weight of cartilage	% of control	Salicylate, $10^{-3}M$: ^{35}S cpm/10 mg wet weight of cartilage	% of control	$\frac{\text{Salicylate}}{\text{No salicylate}} \times 100$
3	Control knee	4.1	17,414 ± 1,542	–	16,989 ± 1,342	–	98
	Cru-X knee	1.5	26,295 ± 2,742	151	2,209 ± 275	13	8
4	Control knee	3.9	12,630 ± 1,421	–	11,560 ± 748	–	92
	Cru-X knee	1.8	17,452 ± 982	138	1,695 ± 350	16	10
5	Control knee	4.2	22,560 ± 2,404	–	23,576 ± 1,032	–	105
	Lac knee	4.4	23,070 ± 962	102	22,149 ± 760	94	96
6	Control knee	4.5	17,983 ± 842	–	16,783 ± 1,213	–	93
	Lac knee	4.7	16,366 ± 1,732	91	16,191 ± 683	96	99
7	Control knee	4.1	28,345 ± 2,978	–	30,047 ± 3,083	–	106
	IK knee	2.8	15,196 ± 1,543	54	12,420 ± 1,501	41	82
8	Control knee	4.0	31,224 ± 3,211	–	29,685 ± 2,450	–	95
	IK knee	2.5	13,114 ± 942	42	9,836 ± 1,021	33	75

* Cru-X = anterior cruciate ligament transection (osteoarthritic); Lac = cartilage lacerated in vitro; IK = immobilized knee (atrophic); control = cartilage from contralateral knee.
† Values represent mean ± SEM of triplicate samples.

affects the susceptibility of articular cartilage to the effects of nonsteroidal antiinflammatory drugs on GAG biosynthesis (3,4). In addition, our present findings suggest strongly that disruption of the cartilage surface (fibrillation) in osteoarthritis is less important than loss of proteoglycans in determining the effects of salicylate and indomethacin on cartilage GAG metabolism. Thus, GAG synthesis in cartilage which had been lacerated in vitro to simulate fibrillation, but whose uronic acid content was normal, was not affected by either salicylate or indomethacin. In contrast, GAG synthesis in atrophic cartilage, whose uronic acid content was diminished even though the articular surface was intact, was decreased by both drugs.

We recognize that laceration of normal cartilage with a scalpel only crudely simulates osteoarthritic fibrillation. However, both conditions cause an increase in the surface area:volume ratio of the carti-

Table 4. Effect of indomethacin on glycosaminoglycan synthesis by osteoarthritic, lacerated, and atrophic articular cartilage

Dog	Source of cartilage*	Uronic acid content, % of tissue dry weight	Net glycosaminoglycan synthesis† — No indomethacin added: ^{35}S cpm/10 mg wet weight of cartilage	% of control	Indomethacin, $4 \times 10^{-6}M$: ^{35}S cpm/10 mg wet weight of cartilage	% of control	$\frac{\text{Indomethacin}}{\text{No indomethacin}} \times 100$
9	Control knee	4.3	8,064 ± 951	–	8,231 ± 1,021	–	102
	Cru-X knee	2.6	11,802 ± 1,432	146	2,351 ± 121	29	20
10	Control knee	4.2	17,458 ± 1,234	–	16,253 ± 2,340	–	93
	Cru-X knee	2.0	28,457 ± 3,213	162	6,401 ± 324	39	23
11	Control knee	4.1	8,609 ± 897	–	8,519 ± 449	–	99
	Lac knee	4.3	9,162 ± 749	106	8,494 ± 782	100	93
12	Control knee	4.3	20,285 ± 1,317	–	20,622 ± 1,604	–	102
	Lac knee	4.5	21,348 ± 1,027	105	20,289 ± 1,747	98	95
13	Control knee	3.8	27,672 ± 1,725	–	28,788 ± 505	–	104
	IK knee	2.1	12,452 ± 1,432	45	10,086 ± 1,492	35	81
14	Control knee	4.2	34,525 ± 3,021	–	33,230 ± 3,141	–	96
	IK knee	2.8	20,066 ± 1,901	58	15,490 ± 1,238	47	77

* Cru-X = anterior cruciate ligament transection (osteoarthritic); Lac = cartilage lacerated in vitro; IK = immobilized knee (atrophic); control = cartilage from contralateral knee.
† Values represent mean ± SEM of triplicate samples.

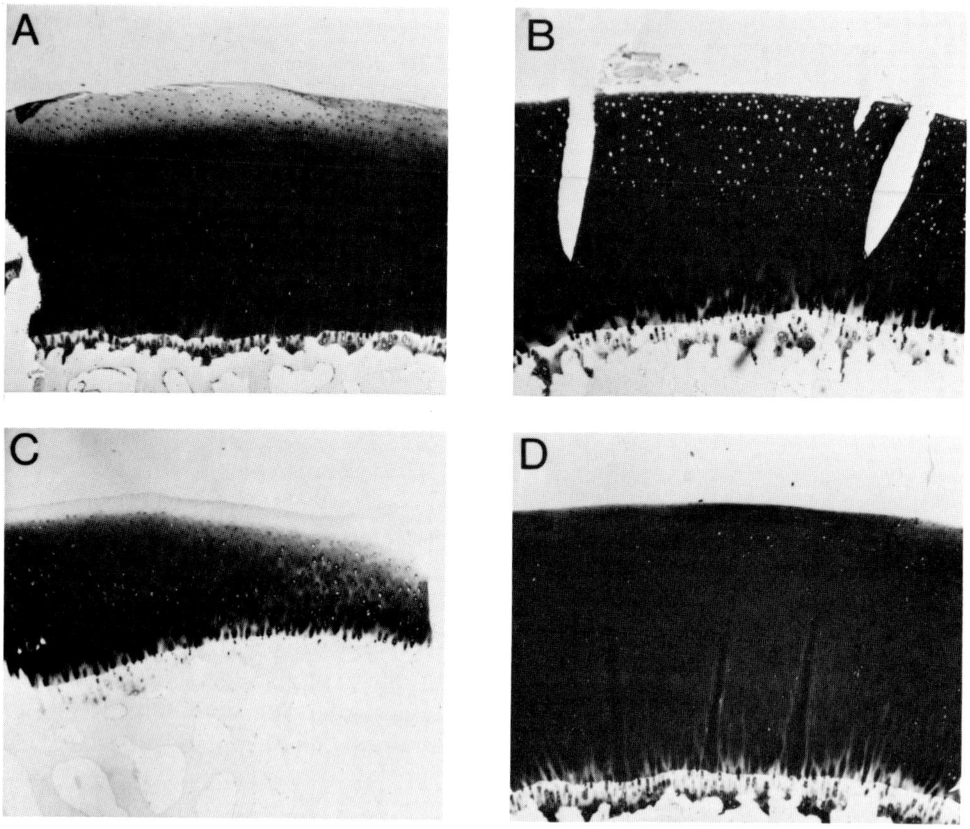

Figure 1. Canine knee cartilage, stained with Safranin O–fast green. **A**, 16 weeks after anterior cruciate ligament transection. **B**, Articular surface lacerated at time of killing. **C**, Ipsilateral leg immmobilized for 6 weeks. **D**, Representative control knee.

lage, which may affect uptake of drug from the culture medium. It is particularly notable, therefore, that the above differences in GAG synthesis occurred despite the fact that this ratio was increased to a much greater extent by laceration than by cruciate ligament transection, which produced only mild surface disruption (Figure 1).

The data in this study are consistent with our previous findings that aspirin, when fed to dogs in quantities sufficient to achieve a serum salicylate concentration of approximately $10^{-3}M$, aggravated the degeneration of articular cartilage from habitually loaded areas of immobilized (8) or unstable joints (1), although it had no effect on normal articular cartilage from analogous sites in the contralateral knees of the same animal. It should be pointed out that the culture system employed herein, using *whole* femoral condyles, more closely resembles the in vivo conditions than do tissue slices in organ culture, since salicylate has been reported to *suppress* GAG synthesis in vitro in slices of cartilage from the weight-bearing surfaces of normal canine joints (9).

The in vitro laceration technique used here is similar to that described by Meachim (10), in which multiple superficial slices are made across the articular surface at close intervals. Notably, the laceration procedure itself had no effect on the uronic acid content of the cartilage or on GAG synthesis (Tables 2–4). Mankin and Boyle (11) reported an enhanced rate of GAG synthesis 1 day after scarification of rabbit femoral cartilage, with a return to control levels of synthesis within another 24 hours. Their study, however, utilized immature rabbits, and GAG synthesis was measured in tissue slices, which may account for the difference between their results and ours.

In this study, salicylate and indomethacin caused significantly more marked suppression of GAG synthesis in OA cartilage than in atrophic cartilage (Tables 3 and 4). It seems unlikely that this was due only to the small difference in the uronic acid content of the tissues (2.0 and 2.6% of the tissue dry weight, for osteoarthritic and atrophic cartilage, respectively). The marked effect of these drugs on osteoarthritic cartilage thus suggests that the OA chondrocyte itself may be more vulnerable to the effects of these agents than the normal chondrocyte.

ACKNOWLEDGMENTS

We are grateful to James Bean for technical support and to Roberta Fehrman for secretarial assistance.

REFERENCES

1. Palmoski MJ, Brandt KD: In vivo effect of aspirin on canine osteoarthritic cartilage. Arthritis Rheum 26:994–1001, 1983
2. Palmoski MJ, Colyer RA, Brandt KD: Marked suppression by salicylate of the augmented proteoglycan synthesis in osteoarthritic cartilage. Arthritis Rheum 23:83–91, 1980
3. Palmoski MJ, Brandt KD: Relationship between matrix proteoglycan content and the effects of salicylate and indomethacin on articular cartilage. Arthritis Rheum 26:528–531, 1983
4. Palmoski MJ, Brandt KD: Effects of salicylate and indomethacin on glycosaminoglycan and prostaglandin E_2 synthesis in intact canine knee cartilage ex vivo. Arthritis Rheum 27:398–403, 1984
5. Palmoski MJ, Perricone E, Brandt KD: Development and reversal of a proteoglycan aggregation defect in normal canine knee cartilage after immobilization. Arthritis Rheum 22:508–517, 1979
6. Tsiganos CP, Muir H: Studies on protein-polysaccharides from pig laryngeal cartilage: extraction and purification. Biochem J 113:879–884, 1969
7. Bitter T, Muir H: A modified uronic acid carbazole reaction. Anal Biochem 4:330–334, 1962
8. Palmoski MJ, Brandt KD: Aspirin aggravates the degeneration of canine joint cartilage caused by immobilization. Arthritis Rheum 25:1333–1342, 1982
9. Palmoski MJ, Brandt KD: Effects of salicylate on proteoglycan metabolism in normal canine articular cartilage in vitro. Arthritis Rheum 22:746–754, 1979
10. Meachim G: Effect of scarification on articular cartilage in the rabbit. J Bone Joint Surg 45B:150–161, 1963
11. Mankin HJ, Boyle CJ: The acute effects of lacerative injury on DNA and protein synthesis in articular cartilage, Cartilage, Degradation and Repair. Edited by CAC Bassett. National Research Council, National Academy of Sciences, 1967, pp 185–199

ROLE OF SYNOVIAL MEMBRANE INFLAMMATION IN CARTILAGE MATRIX BREAKDOWN IN THE POND-NUKI DOG MODEL OF OSTEOARTHRITIS

JEAN-PIERRE PELLETIER, JOHANNE MARTEL-PELLETIER, LATIFA GHANDUR-MNAYMNEH, DAVID S. HOWELL, and J. FREDERICK WOESSNER, JR.

Using the Pond-Nuki procedure, osteoarthritis was induced in 26 crossbred dogs. Their right knees were subjected to anterior cruciate ligament sectioning, and their left knees received a sham operation. The unoperated knees of 7 additional dogs served as controls. Cartilage and synovial membranes were excised 2, 4, and 8 weeks after surgery. Collagenolytic activity, determined by direct tissue assay, was higher at all times tested in osteoarthritic cartilage and synovia than in sham operated and control specimens. The increased collagenolytic activity of the cartilage did not correlate with the collagenolytic activity of the synovium, but it did correlate (r = 0.57) with the degree of synovial inflammation, which was graded histologically. Treatment for 4 weeks with prednisone (0.20–0.25 mg/kg/day) blocked the increased collagenolytic activity of the cartilage. Our results indicate that stimulating factors may, but collagenolytic enzymes probably do not, diffuse from the synovium to the cartilage and modulate tissue breakdown. Prednisone may also suppress cartilage breakdown by either acting at the level of the synthesis or by acting on the release/action of the stimulating factors.

From the Department of Medicine, University of Montreal, Notre-Dame Hospital, Montreal, Canada, and the Departments of Biochemistry, Medicine, and Pathology, University of Miami, School of Medicine, Miami, Florida.

Supported by research grants from the Canadian Arthritis Society and the NIH (AM-16940 and AM-08662).

Jean-Pierre Pelletier, MD: Assistant Professor of Medicine, Notre-Dame Hospital, University of Montreal, School of Medicine; Johanne Martel-Pelletier, PhD: Assistant Professor of Medicine, Notre-Dame Hospital, University of Montreal, School of Medicine; Latifa Ghandur-Mnaymneh, MD: Associate Professor of Pathology, University of Miami, School of Medicine; David S. Howell, MD: Professor of Medicine, University of Miami, School of Medicine; J. Frederick Woessner, Jr., PhD: Professor of Biochemistry and Medicine, University of Miami, School of Medicine.

Address reprint requests to J-P. Pelletier, MD, Unité des Maladies Rhumatismales, Hôpital Notre-Dame, 1560 Est, Rue Sherbrooke, Montreal, Quebec, Canada H2L 4K8.

Submitted for publication February 27, 1984; accepted in revised form September 13, 1984.

Of the diseases of the human joint, osteoarthritis is the most frequently seen. It is a slow, progressive disease that is associated with pain, stiffness, and limited capacity to move the joint. The principal pathologic change is a progressive degradation of the articular cartilage. The exact mechanisms by which these changes take place are still unknown.

Proteolytic enzymes, which are active at neutral pH, are thought to be responsible for the breakdown of the cartilage matrix. Collagenase, collagenolytic enzymes, and neutral proteoglycanase activity have been found to be increased in human osteoarthritic cartilage (1–4). The levels of these enzymes have been directly correlated with the severity of the disease (1,2). Using the Pond-Nuki dog model of osteoarthritis (5), we have recently shown a correlation between the collagenolytic enzyme activity and the early breakdown of the cartilage collagen network (6). The increased enzyme activity was also correlated with the appearance of cartilage lesions. Therefore, one may propose that collagen degradation is accomplished by proteolytic enzymes that infiltrate the cartilage either from internal sources (chondrocytes) or from external sources (synovial fluid, synovium, infiltrating mononuclear cells).

There is an increasing body of literature which shows that neutral proteases that are capable of degrading the cartilage matrix can be synthesized by articular chondrocytes (7–9). The chondrocytic synthesis of proteases as well as the degradation of the cartilage matrix can be stimulated by factors released from the inflamed synovium or by macrophages (10–17). Chronic inflammation of the synovial membrane is frequently observed in human osteoarthritis (18,19) and has also been reported in the Pond-Nuki model (6,20). It is therefore possible that these factors may also play an important role in cartilage breakdown in osteoarthritis.

In the present study, we have used the Pond-Nuki dog model to examine possible correlations between the collagenolytic activity in the cartilage and the enzyme activity in the synovial membrane, as well as correlations between the collagenolytic activity in the cartilage and the degree of inflammation in the synovial membrane.

MATERIALS AND METHODS

Animals. Thirty-three adult crossbred dogs, weighing 20–25 kg, were used. The absence of joint disease was established by clinical examination. Seven of the 33 dogs were used as controls. The Pond-Nuki operation (5) was performed on the right knee of the other 26 animals. After the dogs were anesthetized with intravenous Nembutal (25 mg/kg), the anterior cruciate ligament was sectioned by a stab incision. A sham operation was performed on the left knee, leaving the anterior cruciate ligament intact. After surgery, the dogs were housed in a kennel and allowed to exercise freely. Starting 1 day after the operation, 6 dogs were treated with oral prednisone (0.20–0.25 mg/kg/day; Upjohn, Montreal, Canada). These animals were killed at the end of the fourth week postsurgery.

Preparation of specimens. The animals were killed by an intravenous overdose of Nembutal. Six were killed 2 weeks after surgery, 13 (including the 6 prednisone-treated dogs) were killed 4 weeks after surgery, and 7 were killed 8 weeks after surgery. The knee joints were immediately opened aseptically, and the proximal end of the tibia and the distal end of the femur were both removed. The samples were rinsed with cold physiologic saline and placed on ice for dissection.

Articular cartilage was microdissected from the central weight-bearing surface of the medial femoral condyles of the right and left knees. The specimens were rinsed with cold physiologic saline, immediately frozen at −80°C, and stored until assayed for collagenolytic activity.

The synovial membrane specimens were carefully dissected from the underlying tissues, under a microscope (Stereozoom; Bausch and Lomb, Rochester, NY). Samples were taken from the suprapatellar notch as well as from the medial tibiofemoral compartments and rinsed in cold saline. Portions were taken for histologic study, and the remainder were frozen at −80°C for enzyme assay.

Histology. The central weight-bearing surface of each lateral femoral condyle was used for histologic study of osteoarthritic lesions. The condyles under study were taken from the operated knees. Two sagittal sections (including the underlying bone), which appeared to be the most representative of specimens, were selected from each joint. The sections were fixed in 10% formaldehyde, embedded in paraffin, cut at a thickness of 6μ, and double-stained with Safranin O and hematoxylin and eosin.

Synovial membrane specimens were fixed, embedded, cut, and stained as described above. Each specimen was analyzed for its degree of histologic change. The grading system was modified from that described by Goldenberg and Cohen (21). In assessing the overall grade, 2 specimens from each knee were considered as a unit. The severity of synovitis was graded from 0–10 by adding the scores of 3 histologic criteria: 1) synovial lining cell hyperplasia was graded 0–2+, where 0 = 1–2 layers of cells, 1+ = 3–5 layers, 2+ = ≥ 6 layers. The layers were counted from the surface of the membrane to the subsynovial tissue. 2) Villous hyperplasia was graded 0–3+, where 0 = not present, 1+ = few, scattered, and short, 2+ = marked (finger-like), 3+ = marked and diffuse. 3) Cellular infiltration, the degree of infiltration by perivascular lymphocytes and mononuclear and polymorphonuclear leukocytes, was graded from 0–5+, where 0 = normal and 5+ = marked cellular infiltration mixed with lymphoid follicles.

Enzyme assays. Collagenolytic activity was assessed by measuring the amount of digestion of endogenous collagen when tissue homogenates were incubated under physiologic conditions as previously described (1). Briefly, cartilage specimens (50 mg wet weight) were homogenized in 10 volumes of 0.01*M* $CaCl_2$ containing Triton X-100 (0.25%). After centrifugation, the pellet was resuspended in Tris-HCl buffer (0.05*M* Tris-HCl, 0.15*M* NaCl, 0.01*M* $CaCl_2$, 0.02% [weight/volume] NaN_3, pH 7.5) and 20 μg of gentamycin (40 mg/ml; Schering, Montreal, Canada). Aliquots (50 μl) were placed in test tubes, grouped in pairs, and run in duplicate. Group 1 was treated with aminophenylmercuric acetate (APMA) at a final concentration of 0.001*M*, to activate the latent enzyme. Group 2 received APMA (0.001*M*) and EDTA (final concentration 0.025*M*) to provide a blank. After incubation for 18 hours at 37°C, the test tubes were centrifuged. The supernatants and pellets were hydrolyzed in 6*N* HCl and assayed for hydroxyproline content. The enzyme activity was expressed as the percent of total hydroxyproline solubilized. The level of collagenolytic activity was obtained from subtracting the value of group 2 from that of group 1.

We measured the collagenolytic activity in synovial membranes using the same procedure, with 2 changes: 100 mg wet weight tissue was used instead of 50 mg, and 5 volumes of Tris buffer was used to homogenize the synovial membranes, compared with the 10 volumes used for cartilage.

DNA content was determined on 50-μl aliquots of tissue homogenates using the method of Bonting and Jones (22), with calf thymus DNA as a standard.

Statistical analysis. Student's *t*-test was used for statistical analysis; *P* values <0.05 were considered significant. Regression lines were fitted to the equation $y = mx + b$, using the method of least squares and assuming errors in both x and y. The *P* value for the correlation coefficient was calculated using the "r test" (23).

RESULTS

Histologic changes. Histologic modifications observed in osteoarthritic cartilage from the operated knees were similar to those previously described (6), and presented changes that were analogous to those seen in human osteoarthritic cartilage. Cartilage specimens taken from control knees appeared normal.

Synovial membranes obtained from control knees appeared normal and were graded 0. Microscopic examination of the synovial membranes from the sham operated joints revealed only a very mild synovitis, mainly related to a small mononuclear cell infiltration (Figure 1). In contrast, a significant degree of inflammation was shown in most of the specimens from operated knees. This was characterized by synovial lining cell hyperplasia and inflammatory cell infiltration (Figure 2). The infiltrates consisted mainly of mononuclear and plasmocytic cells. Marked membrane thickening was also observed in samples taken at 4 and 8 weeks postsurgery. This was due to an increase in the subsynovial connective tissue.

The mean histologic scores (±SEM) for membranes from operated knees at 2, 4, and 8 weeks were 4.8 ± 0.8, 5.4 ± 1.0, and 4.7 ± 0.9, respectively. In each case, these values were higher than those for the sham operated knees (1.8 ± 0.6, 1.3 ± 0.5, and 0.5 ± 0.3, mean ±SEM, at 2, 4, and 8 weeks, respectively). Specimens obtained from the prednisone-treated animals (killed at 4 weeks) had a mean score (±SEM) of 5.0 ± 0.7; this corresponded to the degree of inflammation observed at 4 weeks in operated animals (Figure 3).

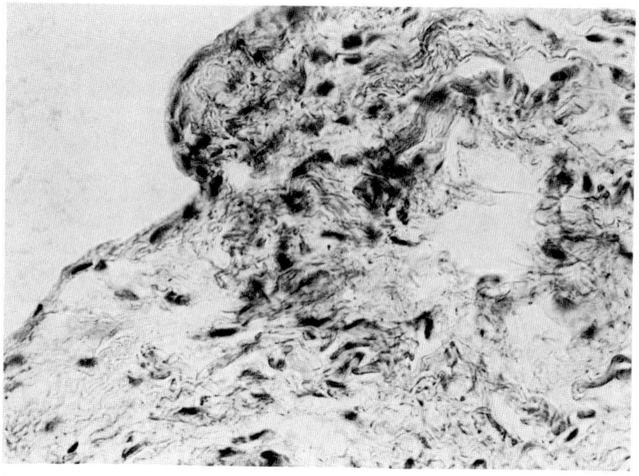

Figure 1. Synovial membrane specimen from a sham operated knee, obtained 4 weeks after surgery. There is no synovial lining cell hyperplasia, and only a very light cellular infiltration is observed in the underlying tissue. By histologic criteria, this illustrates a low grade synovitis (hematoxylin and eosin stained, original magnification × 120).

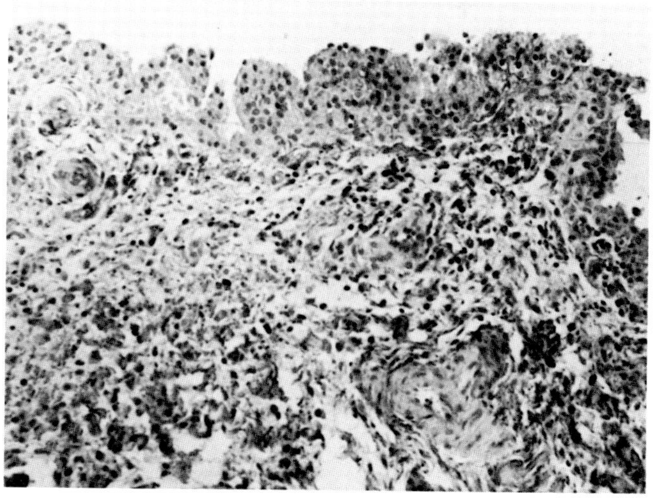

Figure 2. Synovial membrane specimen from an operated knee, obtained 4 weeks after ligament sectioning. There is synovial lining cell proliferation with palisading and a marked, mixed cellular infiltration consisting mainly of lymphocytes and plasmocytes in the underlying tissue (hematoxylin and eosin stained, original magnification × 160).

DNA analysis. Table 1 shows the DNA content of articular cartilage and synovial membranes. The cartilage DNA content both of the operated and the sham operated knees was not different from that of the control knees. Prednisone treatment had no effect on cartilage DNA content. There was no significant dif-

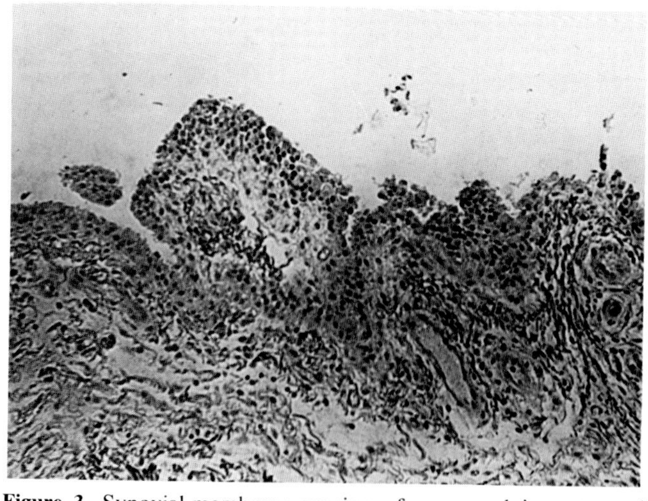

Figure 3. Synovial membrane specimen from a prednisone-treated dog, obtained 4 weeks after ligament sectioning. There is synovial lining cell proliferation and a mixed cellular infiltration of mononuclear cells in the underlying tissue (hematoxylin and eosin stained, original magnification × 165).

Table 1. DNA content of articular cartilage and synovial membrane of 33 adult crossbred dogs*

		Articular cartilage					Synovial membrane				
Week	No. of dogs	Controls	Sham	Operated	P†	P‡	Controls	Sham	Operated	P†	P‡
–	7	0.61 ± 0.11	–	–	–	–	0.83 ± 0.06	–	–	–	–
2	6	–	0.65 ± 0.08	0.61 ± 0.11	NS	NS	–	0.83 ± 0.06	1.51 ± 0.18	<0.005	<0.02
4	7	–	0.62 ± 0.01	0.60 ± 0.06	NS	NS	–	0.99 ± 0.06	1.51 ± 0.10§	<0.001	<0.005
8	7	–	0.60 ± 0.10	0.57 ± 0.05	NS	NS	–	0.84 ± 0.09	1.35 ± 0.22	<0.05	<0.05
Steroid-treated dogs											
4	6	–	0.66 ± 0.03	0.62 ± 0.03	NS	NS	–	0.89 ± 0.09	1.09 ± 0.09§	<0.05	NS

* Values are mean μg of DNA/mg wet weight of tissue (±SEM). P values for both the articular cartilage and synovial membranes of control knees compared with sham operated knees were not significant (NS).
† Operated knees compared with control knees.
‡ Operated knees compared with sham operated knees.
§ $P < 0.02$, operated (treated) knees compared with operated (untreated) knees.

ference in synovial DNA content between controls and sham operated knees. However, when membranes of operated knees were compared with those of sham operated and control knees, a significant increase was noted at 2, 4, and 8 weeks after surgery. The maximum was observed at 2 and 4 weeks, but the DNA content did not return completely to normal levels, indicating that some residual inflammation was still present. Prednisone treatment significantly ($P < 0.02$) reduced the DNA content of the synovial membranes of operated knees by 4 weeks.

Collagenolytic activity. Table 2 illustrates the collagenolytic activity in cartilage and in synovium. The cartilage collagenolytic activity of sham operated knees was low at all times and was not significantly different from that of the controls. At 2, 4, and 8 weeks after surgery, a significantly higher level of activity was recorded in cartilage specimens of the operated knees compared with the sham operated knees or with the control knees. The enzyme activity was significantly elevated in all stages of the disease. However, no significant difference was noted during the progression of the disease, i.e., when the enzyme activity levels at 2, 4, and 8 weeks were compared with each other.

Collagenolytic activity of the synovial specimens (Table 2) showed a pattern similar to that of the cartilage specimens: 1) no significant difference was found between control and sham operated knees; 2) a significantly higher level of activity was found in membranes of operated knees at all stages; and 3) no changes were found in the progression of the disease from 2 to 8 weeks.

Specimens taken from prednisone-treated animals were also assayed for collagenolytic activity (Table 2). The cartilage collagenolytic activity was not significantly increased in operated knees compared with sham operated (treated) knees or with control knees, i.e., prednisone suppressed the increase that was normally found in operated knees. Activity in the synovium remained significantly elevated in operated knees despite the prednisone treatment. Thus, prednisone can decrease the enzyme level in cartilage but has no effect on the enzyme level in the synovial membrane.

Correlation studies of cartilage and synovium. For each operated knee, the histologic grading of the synovial membrane inflammation was compared with the collagenolytic activity (Figure 4). No significant correlation was found (r = −0.23; n = 20). Moreover,

Table 2. Collagenolytic activity (aminophenylmercuric acetate–activated) of articular cartilage and synovial membrane of 33 crossbred dogs*

		Articular cartilage					Synovial membrane				
Week	No. of dogs	Controls	Sham	Operated	P†	P‡	Controls	Sham	Operated	P†	P‡
–	7	0.95 ± 0.23	–	–	–	–	1.18 ± 0.18	–	–	–	–
2	6	–	0.87 ± 0.21	3.43 ± 0.60	<0.001	<0.005	–	1.63 ± 0.37	3.12 ± 0.47	<0.005	<0.05
4	7	–	0.77 ± 0.17	2.76 ± 0.67	<0.02	<0.05	–	1.85 ± 0.27	3.51 ± 0.49	<0.001	<0.02
8	7	–	0.81 ± 0.26	2.95 ± 0.69	<0.01	<0.02	–	1.75 ± 0.30	3.44 ± 0.30	<0.001	<0.005
Steroid-treated dogs											
4	6	–	0.80 ± 0.22	1.37 ± 0.29	NS	NS	–	1.83 ± 0.35	3.22 ± 0.32	<0.005	<0.02

* Activity is expressed as % of collagen digested (mean ± SEM). P values for both the articular cartilage and synovial membranes of control knees compared with those of sham operated knees were not significant (NS).
† Operated knees compared with control knees.
‡ Operated knees compared with sham operated knees.

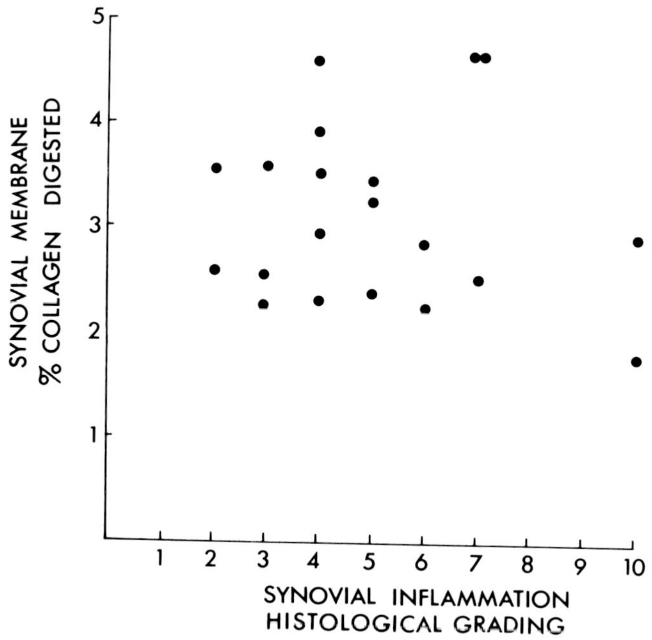

Figure 4. Relationship between the synovial inflammation, graded histologically (see Materials and Methods), and the collagenolytic activity of the synovial membrane. No significant correlation was found (r = −0.23; n = 20).

no significant correlation was found when the separate scores for synovial cell plus villous hyperplasia (r = 0.19; n = 20), or those for cellular infiltration (r = 0.03; n = 20), were compared with collagenolytic activity. Figure 5 shows that, for the operated knees, a negative

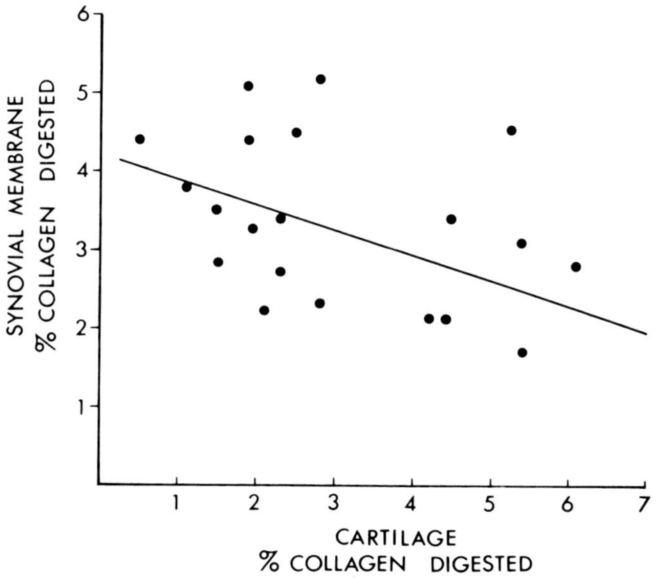

Figure 5. Relationship between the levels of collagenolytic activity of cartilage and of synovial membrane. There was a negative trend of the linear regression curve, but no significant correlation was noted (r = −0.36; n = 20).

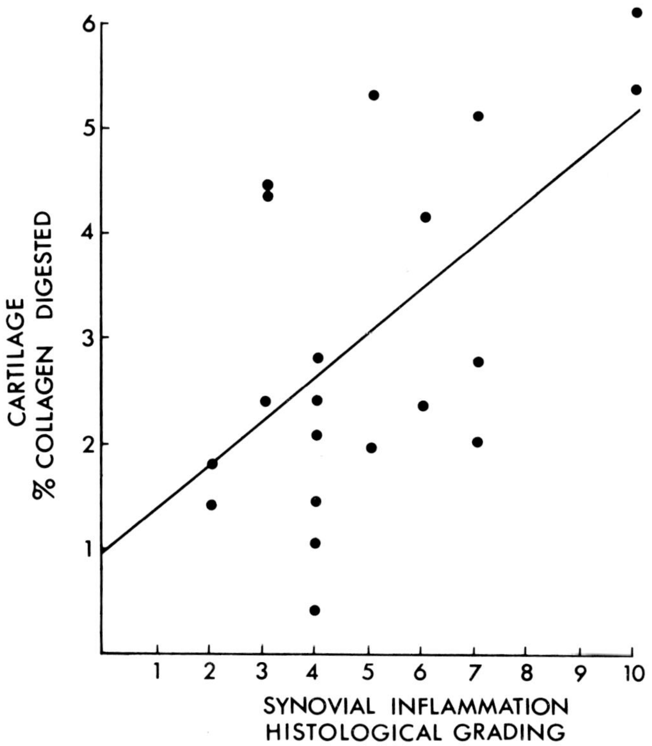

Figure 6. Relationship between the degree of synovial inflammation, graded histologically (see Materials and Methods), and the collagenolytic activity of the cartilage. A positive, direct correlation was found (r = 0.57, $P < 0.01$; n = 20).

slope occurred (r = −0.36; n = 20) when the cartilage collagenolytic activity was plotted against the synovial membrane collagenolytic activity, but the correlation was not significant.

When we compared the histologic grade of synovial inflammation and the cartilage collagenolytic activity of the operated knees (Figure 6), a direct linear relationship was found, with a statistical significance of $P < 0.01$ (r = 0.57; n = 20). When synovial cell hyperplasia and cellular infiltration were analyzed separately, it was not possible to relate the collagenolytic activity with either.

DISCUSSION

Osteoarthritis is characterized by a progressive degradation of articular cartilage. Concomitant changes of the joint include subchondral bone sclerosis, osteophyte formation, and, often (13 of 15 cases, ref. 18), a mild to moderate degree of synovitis. Ultrastructural studies have revealed that early changes in osteoarthritic cartilage are characterized by increased chondrocytic metabolism and breakdown of the collagen meshwork, which is first noted at pericellular/perilacunar areas in the middle zone (6,24,25). These changes eventually spread to the entire matrix. There is no significant change in the collagen content of osteoarthritic cartilage compared with normal cartilage (26). The collagen is mainly type II, as is found in normal cartilage. However, immunofluorescence methods of analysis detect a few areas of type I collagen surrounding the clones or brood capsules (27).

Ehrlich et al (3) have demonstrated that osteoarthritic cartilage, in tissue cultures, produces increased amounts of collagenase. Using a direct tissue assay, we have demonstrated a positive correlation between the histologic severity of human osteoarthritic lesions and their levels of metalloproteases acting on collagen and on proteoglycan (1,2). In the dog model, we have shown that collagenolytic activity in cartilage is elevated at the time when early osteoarthritic changes are detected (6).

Since the chondrocytes are capable of secreting collagenase and since the early collagen damage is seen immediately around the chondrocytes, it is reasonable to propose that activated chondrocytes are responsible for matrix degradation in osteoarthritis. However, since synovial inflammation has been shown both in experimentally induced osteoarthritis (6,20) and in primary human osteoarthritis (18,19), a diffusion of enzymes from the synovium to the cartilage cannot be ruled out. Moreover, it is known that inflamed synovia can produce factors that stimulate chondrocytes to degrade their matrix (10,13,15). Therefore, we have considered 2 possibilities: 1) that enzymes diffuse from the synovium to the cartilage matrix, and 2) that soluble factors, released by the inflamed synovium, stimulate the chondrocytes to synthesize more enzymes.

Our present measurements of collagenolytic activity confirm our previous findings: there is an increase in the collagenolytic activity in the cartilage of the operated knees at 2, 4, and 8 weeks after surgery (6). We have previously shown that approximately 25% of the collagenolytic activity is in an active form and the remainder is in a latent, proenzyme form (6). Further, we have found that human articular cartilage contains the inhibitor TIMP (tissue inhibitor of metalloproteinases) that stoichiometrically inactivates collagenolytic activity (28). TIMP can be slowly inactivated by aminophenylmercuric acetate, but the TIMP–enzyme complex is essentially irreversible (29). Therefore, when the tissue homogenates are activated, TIMP is destroyed and the latent enzyme becomes activated. Enzyme that was already active is probably lost, at least in part, by binding to TIMP before it is destroyed. Our measurement of enzyme activity is thus the measurement of a composite of latent activity plus part of the active enzyme. By analogy to the processes in the involuting rat uterus (30), we assume that in vivo, about 30–40% of the collagenolytic activity would be in an active state due to the action of activating proteases present in the tissue.

The present study shows that cartilage DNA content is not significantly altered in osteoarthritis (Table 1). This agrees with previous reports that there are no significant changes in the DNA concentration of human osteoarthritic cartilage (31), except in severe lesions (2). These results indicate that the increased enzyme activity found in the dog cartilage is not related to increased cellularity but to an activation of the existing chondrocytes to secrete more enzymes.

The histologic study of synovial specimens shows that the operated knees have a significant inflammatory reaction. The histologic grading does not show any change in inflammatory intensity from 2, 4, or 8 weeks. However, the intensity is much more pronounced in the operated than in the sham operated knees. Therefore, the inflammation was not solely related to the surgical procedure. The wear and tear of the synovial membrane caused by the instability of the joint, consequent to sectioning the anterior cruciate ligament, may play a role in the observed changes. The release of cartilage breakdown products or of mechanical wear particles into the synovial fluid at a time when the lesions appear (usually 2–4 weeks) could also play a role.

The collagenolytic activity of the synovial membrane is significantly elevated in operated knees compared with sham operated or control knees (Table 2). The increase in this enzyme activity was concomitant with, but was not proportional to, the increase in synovial membrane DNA (Table 1). This finding indicates that the increased activity is related partly to the increased tissue cellularity and partly to an increased enzyme synthesis. It is not possible to establish a clear correlation between the enzyme activity of the synovial membrane and the histologic grade of inflammation (Figure 4).

To evaluate a possible role of the synovial membrane in the increased collagenolytic activity of the cartilage, we have studied 2 correlations: 1) the enzyme level in cartilage versus the enzyme level in the synovial membrane (Figure 5), and 2) the histologic grade of synovial inflammation versus the collagenolytic activity of the cartilage (Figure 6). There was no correlation between the 2 enzyme activities in their respective tissues. This would serve as an argument against there being a simple diffusion of the enzyme from the synovium to the cartilage. Even if the enzymes were released into the synovial fluid, they would likely be inactivated by α_2-macroglobulins. However, there was a direct correlation between membrane inflammation and cartilage enzyme content. Possibly, the membrane releases soluble factors which stimulate the chondrocytes to synthesize enzymes. Hydrocortisone is known to inhibit this process (10,32).

A second part of our study was an investigation of the effect of prednisone on collagenolytic activity. No significant changes in the DNA content of the cartilage were produced by prednisone treatment of the dogs. The degree of inflammation, graded histologically, in synovial specimens from operated knees of prednisone-treated animals at 4 weeks was not significantly reduced (5.0 versus 5.4 for untreated operated knees). However, the membrane DNA increase was reduced in prednisone-treated animals. This indicates that the steroid was effective to a certain extent in reducing the total cell content of the inflamed synovium. Even though the histologic scores of the treated animals were unaltered, the DNA content did change. It is probable that the DNA measurement is more precise and quantitative than the histologic evaluation in determining the total cell content of the synovial membrane. This is partly because the whole tissue is analyzed in measurements of DNA, whereas only a focal aspect is used for histologic evaluations. Prednisone treatment did not lower the collagenolytic activity of the synovial membrane, but it was effective in reducing the collagenolytic activity of the cartilage to a level similar to that in controls (Table 2). This decrease in cartilage enzyme while the membrane enzyme remains elevated is a further argument against the synovium being the source of the cartilage enzyme.

In this experimental model of osteoarthritis, if one assumes that chondrocytes are responsible for an increased synthesis of cartilage collagenolytic enzymes, there are 2 possible explanations for the action of prednisone. The first is that prednisone directly inhibits chondrocytic enzyme synthesis by either acting at the level of cellular receptors or doing so intracellularly (33). The second is that it inhibits synthesis and/or release of chondrocyte-activating factor(s) from the inflamed synovium.

We have demonstrated that the collagenolytic activity of cartilage is correlated with synovial inflammation but not with synovial enzyme content. We have also demonstrated that prednisone can effectively decrease the level of cartilage collagenolytic activity, although it does not suppress the level of the synovial enzyme activity. These results are consistent with the hypothesis that in osteoarthritis, synovial inflammation may play an important role in breaking down the cartilage matrix. This inflammation may be a phenomenon that is secondary to the actual release of matrix breakdown products into the synovial fluid. Once the inflammation starts, it may trigger a vicious circle whereby the synovium, via its released factors, stimulates the chondrocytes to secrete proteolytic enzymes, which in turn, break down the extracellular matrix of the cartilage.

ACKNOWLEDGMENTS

The authors thank François Mineau and Johanne Harnois for their technical assistance, Mrs. M. P. Faure for the microscopy preparations, Diane Fournier for her secretarial assistance, and Valentina Nedwetsky for reviewing the manuscript.

REFERENCES

1. Pelletier J-P, Martel-Pelletier J, Howell DS, Ghandur-Mnaymneh L, Enis JE, Woessner JF Jr: Collagenase and collagenolytic activity in human osteoarthritic cartilage. Arthritis Rheum 26:63–68, 1983
2. Martel-Pelletier J, Pelletier J-P, Cloutier J-M, Howell DS, Ghandur-Mnaymneh L, Woessner JF Jr: Neutral proteases capable of proteoglycan digesting activity in osteoarthritic and normal human articular cartilage. Arthritis Rheum 27:305–312, 1984
3. Ehrlich MG, Houle PA, Vigliani G, Mankin HJ: Correlation between articular cartilage collagenase activity and osteoarthritis. Arthritis Rheum 21:761–766, 1978
4. Ehrlich MG, Mankin HJ, Jones H, Wright R, Crispen C, Vigliani G: Collagenase and collagenase inhibitors in osteoarthritic and normal human cartilage. J Clin Invest 59:226–233, 1977
5. Pond MJ, Nuki G: Experimentally induced osteoarthritis in the dog. Ann Rheum Dis 32:387–388, 1973
6. Pelletier J-P, Martel-Pelletier J, Altman RD, Ghandur-Mnaymneh L, Howell DS, Woessner JF Jr: Collagenolytic activity and collagen matrix breakdown of the articular cartilage in the Pond-Nuki dog model of osteoarthritis. Arthritis Rheum 26:866–874, 1983
7. Malemud CJ, Norby DP, Sapolsky AI, Matsuta K,

Howell DS, Moskowitz RW: Neutral proteinases from articular chondrocytes in culture. I. A latent collagenase that degrades human cartilage type II collagen. Biochim Biophys Acta 657:517–529, 1981
8. Sapolsky AI, Malemud CJ, Norby DP, Moskowitz RW, Matsuta K, Howell DS: Neutral proteinases from articular chondrocytes in culture. II. Metal-dependent latent neutral proteoglycanase, and inhibitory activity. Biochim Biophys Acta 658:138–147, 1981
9. Morales TI, Kuettner KE: The properties of the neutral proteinase released by primary chondrocyte culture and its action on proteoglycan aggregates. Biochim Biophys Acta 705:92–101, 1982
10. Steinberg JJ, Sledge CB: Synovial factors and chondrocyte mediated breakdown of cartilage: inhibition by hydrocortisone. J Orthop Res 1:13–21, 1983
11. Saklatvala J, Sarsfield SJ: Lymphocytes induce resorption of cartilage by producing catabolin. Biochem J 202:275–278, 1982
12. Jasin HE, Dingle JT: Human mononuclear cell factors mediate cartilage matrix degradation through chondrocyte activation. J Clin Invest 68:571–581, 1981
13. Saklatvala J: Characterization of catabolin, the major product of pig synovial tissue that induces resorption of cartilage proteoglycan in vitro. Biochem J 199:705–714, 1981
14. Ridge SC, Oronsky AL, Kerwar SS: Induction of the synthesis of latent collagenase and latent neutral protease in chondrocytes by a factor synthesized by activated macrophages. Arthritis Rheum 23:448–454, 1980
15. Dingle JT, Saklatvala J, Hembry R, Tyler J, Fell HB, Jubb R: A cartilage catabolic factor from synovium. Biochem J 184:177–180, 1979
16. Deshmukh-Phadke K, Lawrence M, Nanda S: Synthesis of collagenase and neutral proteases by articular chondrocytes: stimulation by a macrophage-derived factor. Biochem Biophys Res Commun 85:490–496, 1978
17. Fell HB, Jubb RW: The effect of synovial tissue on the breakdown of articular cartilage in organ culture. Arthritis Rheum 20:1359–1371, 1977
18. Goldenberg DL, Egan MS, Cohen AS: Inflammatory synovitis in degenerative joint disease. J Rheumatol 9:204–209, 1982
19. Howell DS, Sapolsky AI, Pita JC, Woessner JF Jr: The pathogenesis of osteoarthritis. Semin Arthritis Rheum 5:365–383, 1976
20. McDevitt C, Muir H: An experimental model of osteoarthritis: early morphological and biochemical changes. J Bone Joint Surg 59B:24–35, 1977
21. Goldenberg DL, Cohen AS: Synovial membrane histopathology in the differential diagnosis of rheumatoid arthritis, gout, pseudo-gout, systemic lupus erythematosus, infectious arthritis and degenerative joint disease. Medicine (Baltimore) 57:239–252, 1978
22. Bonting SL, Jones M: Determination of microgram quantities of deoxyribonucleic acid and protein in tissue grown in vitro. Arch Biochem Biophys 66:340–353, 1957
23. Colton T: Statistics in Medicine. Boston, Little, Brown & Co., 1974, pp 188–217
24. Weiss C: Ultrastructural characteristics of osteoarthritis. Fed Proc 32:1459–1466, 1973
25. Weiss C, Mirow S: An ultrastructural study of osteoarthritic changes in the articular cartilage of human knees. J Bone Joint Surg 54A:954–970, 1972
26. Mankin HJ, Lippiello L: Biochemical and metabolic abnormalities in articular cartilage from osteoarthritic human hips. J Bone Joint Surg 52A:424–434, 1970
27. Gay S, Muller PK, Lemmen C, Remberger K, Matzen K, Kuhn K: Immuno-histological study on collagen in cartilage-bone metamorphosis and degenerative osteoarthritis. Klin Wochenschr 54:969–976, 1976
28. Dean DD, Woessner JF Jr: Extracts of human articular cartilage contain an inhibitor of tissue metalloproteinases. Biochem J 218:277–280, 1984
29. Cawston TE, Murphy G, Mercer E, Galloway NA, Hazleman BL, Reynolds JJ: The interaction of purified rabbit bone collagenase with purified rabbit bone metalloproteinase inhibitor. Biochem J 211:313–318, 1983
30. Woessner JF Jr: Total, latent and active collagenase during the course of post-partum involution of rat uterus. Biochem J 180:95–102, 1979
31. Mankin HJ, Dorfman H, Lippiello L, Zarins A: Biochemical and metabolic abnormalities in articular cartilage from osteoarthritic human hips. II. Correlation of morphology with biochemical and metabolic data. J Bone Joint Surg 53A:523–537, 1971
32. Steinberg JJ, Kincaid SB, Sledge CB: Inhibition of cartilage breakdown by hydrocortisone in a tissue culture model of rheumatoid arthritis. Ann Rheum Dis 42:323–330, 1983
33. Phadke K, Nanda S, Lee K: Release of proteases from cartilage cells as a result of activation by a macrophage factor—effects of some anti-inflammatory drugs. Biochem Pharmacol 28:3671–3673, 1979

THE SPECIFICITY OF ANTIBODIES TO THE $F(ab')_2$ FRAGMENT OF HUMAN IgG

RALPH HEIMER, LAWRENCE D. WOLFE, and JOHN L. ABRUZZO

The specificity of IgG anti-$F(ab')_2$ antibodies was examined in unfractionated sera of patients with rheumatoid arthritis and also with affinity-purified antibody preparations. Examination of the sera by an enzyme-linked immunosorbent assay, using pooled human $F(ab')_2$ fragments absorbed to microtiter plates, revealed that IgG anti-$F(ab')_2$ antibodies cross-react with human and rabbit IgG and rabbit $F(ab')_2$. IgG anti-$F(ab')_2$ antibodies were purified by affinity chromatography and, when tested by a fluid-phase inhibition enzyme-linked immunosorbent assay, were found to be of 2 types. One fraction, similar to pepsin agglutinator, reacted with human $F(ab')_2$ fragment alone. The other fraction was cross-reactive with human IgG and yet failed to react with idiotopes on Fab or epitopes on Fc fragments. The IgG anti-$F(ab')_2$ antibodies we purified had no reactivity toward a human immune complex prepared from tetanus toxoid and antitoxoid.

Antibodies to $F(ab')_2$ fragments of pooled human IgG are elevated in patients with rheumatoid arthritis (RA) (1–7), patients with subacute bacterial endocarditis (2,7), the elderly (8), and patients with infertility linked to anti-sperm antibody production (9). Some of these antibodies appear to be cytotoxic to B lymphocytes (10). Cross-reactivity with $F(ab')_2$ fragments of IgG of other species has been reported recently (11–14). Previous studies have stressed circumstantial evidence that some of these antibodies recognize idiotopes present in $F(ab')_2$ fragments prepared from pooled human IgG (3,6). Other antibodies of this family react only with $F(ab')_2$ but not with intact IgG or Fab fragments, indicating recognition of epitopes accessible only after some structural modification of IgG (1,2,15). Previous studies of specificity of anti-$F(ab')_2$ antibodies, however, are difficult to interpret, because of use of assay procedures which are susceptible to interference by rheumatoid factors (RF) (1–3,7,16). The assay difficulties are compounded by the problems of separating RF from purified anti-$F(ab')_2$ antibodies (3). We directed our research to preparing purified anti-$F(ab')_2$ antibodies free of RF, foregoing, however, attempts to fully recover a subset "hidden" within complexes (6) and possibly associated with antiidiotypic activity. This report describes a purification protocol and details specificity studies of purified antibodies with a panel of inhibitors using isotype-specific enzyme-linked immunosorbent assays (ELISA).

From the Department of Biochemistry and the Department of Medicine, Jefferson Medical College of Thomas Jefferson University, Philadelphia, Pennsylvania.

Supported by NIH grant AM-26409 and by a grant from the Eastern Pennsylvania Chapter of the Arthritis Foundation.

Ralph Heimer, PhD; Lawrence D. Wolfe, PhD; John L. Abruzzo, MD.

Address reprint requests to Ralph Heimer, PhD, Department of Biochemistry, Jefferson Medical College of Thomas Jefferson University, 1020 Locust Street, Philadelphia, PA 19107.

Submitted for publication May 21, 1984; accepted in revised form November 7, 1984.

MATERIALS AND METHODS

Sera. Sera in this study were obtained from 7 patients with classic RA who were seropositive for RF and from 2 seronegative, apparently healthy volunteers. The sera were kept at −20°C until use.

Antisera. Affinity-purified goat anti-human IgM and anti-human IgG antibodies (Tago, Inc., Burlingame, CA) were absorbed with pooled $F(ab')_2$ fragments of human IgG to make them specific for the Fc fragments of the above isotypes. Rabbit anti-human IgG (Fd fragment–specific) was obtained from Calbiochem-Behring, La Jolla, CA. Rabbit anti-goat IgG and goat anti-human IgG (Fc fragment–specific) were obtained from Cappel Laboratories, West Chester, PA. The specificity of these antibodies was confirmed by immunoelectrophoresis. Affinity-purified antibodies were conjugated to alkakine phosphatase (Sigma, St. Louis, MO) with glutaraldehyde according to the recommendations of the manufacturer, to obtain an approximate enzyme activity of 500 units/mg.

Assays. ELISA for anti-$F(ab')_2$ antibodies and RF were carried out in rigid flat-bottom polystyrene microtiter plates (Immulon; Dynatech Laboratories, Inc., Alexandria, VA). $F(ab')_2$ for anti-$F(ab')_2$ antibody assays and Fc for RF assays, each at 500 ng/well, were adsorbed for 12 hours. After washing with Buffer A (0.05*M* Tris [hydroxymethyl] aminomethane, 0.15*M* NaCl, 1% sodium azide, pH 7.4) containing 0.05% Tween 20 (Buffer A–Tween), sera or purified antibodies (diluted in 0.1% egg albumin) were allowed to bind for 2 hours.

For an assay of RF, 0.01 units of goat anti-human IgM or rabbit anti-human Fd fragment linked to alkaline phosphatase was added for 2 hours, washed with Buffer A–Tween 20, and further incubated with 0.1 mg/well p-nitrophenyl phosphate (Sigma).

For IgM and IgG anti-$F(ab')_2$ antibody assays, we adapted the radioimmunoassay described previously (5) to conditions for ELISA. In this method, an excess unlabeled goat anti-Fc fragment antibody was interposed between binding of anti-$F(ab')_2$ antibodies and the addition of the enzyme-conjugated antibody. This step minimizes interference by RF. After a 2-hour incubation with goat anti-Fc antibody, the presence of the anti-$F(ab')_2$ antibodies was determined with alkaline phosphatase–linked rabbit anti-goat IgG and/or goat anti-human IgM. In inhibition experiments, highly purified IgG anti-$F(ab')_2$ antibody was measured directly with enzyme-linked goat anti-human Fc. All ELISA were quantitated by measuring absorbance at 405 nm with a Titertek Multiscan Monitor (Flow Laboratories, McLean, VA).

Isotype-specific radioimmunoassays (RIA) for IgG anti-$F(ab')_2$ were carried out as described previously (5).

Antigens and inhibitors. Human IgG was purified from pooled Cohn fraction II (United States Biochemical Corp., Cleveland, OH) or individual serum by passage through a DEAE-AffiBlue ion exchange column (Bio-Rad Laboratories, Richmond, CA), pH 8.0, in 0.02*M* K_2HPO_4 buffer. All preparations were absorbed with pooled IgG-Sepharose to remove RF and other antibodies reacting with intact IgG. Rabbit IgG was purified from serum by adsorption to protein A–Sepharose.

$F(ab')_2$ fragments were prepared from purified IgG of pooled Cohn fraction II which had been digested with pepsin and gel-filtered through Sephadex G-200 (Pharmacia Fine Chemicals, Piscataway, NJ) as described previously (5). The $F(ab')_2$ preparations were examined by sodium dodecyl sulfate–polyacrylamide gel electrophoresis (SDS-PAGE) under nonreducing conditions and found to give a single broad band. Preparations were also tested on microtiter plates with anti-Fc antibodies conjugated with alkaline phosphatase, without finding detectable amounts of undigested IgG and Fc' fragments. The $F(ab')_2$ preparations were absorbed with IgG-Sepharose and $F(ab')_2$-Sepharose prior to use as antigen or inhibitor to remove RF and anti-$F(ab')_2$ antibodies.

Fab fragments of human IgG were obtained from Rockland, Inc. (Gilbertsville, PA). The material was tested by SDS-PAGE under reducing and nonreducing conditions and found to be free of intact IgG or Fc fragments. The material reacted with rabbit anti-human IgG (Fd fragment–specific), but not with goat anti-human IgG (Fc fragment–specific).

Fc fragments, prepared by plasmin cleavage of pooled human IgG, were obtained from Alpha Therapeutics Corp. (Los Angeles, CA). On SDS-PAGE, in the absence of reducing agents, the antigen appeared to be a single material with an estimated molecular weight of 5×10^4. The material did not react with anti-human $F(ab')_2$ antibodies by ELISA.

Light chains were prepared from pooled human IgG by a modification of the method of Fleischman et al (17). Reduction was carried out for 1 hour at room temperature with 10 m*M* dithiothreitol in 0.5*M* Tris-HCl, pH 8.0. Twenty millimoles of iodoacetamide was added and the solution was incubated for 30 minutes at 4°C, dialyzed against 1*M* acetic acid, and then fractionated on Sephadex G-200. Light chains were dialyzed against Buffer A and shown by SDS-PAGE to be free of intact IgG and free gamma chains.

Immune complexes were prepared from tetanus toxoid obtained from the Massachusetts Department of Public Health, Boston. The material was radiolabeled with ^{125}Na by the method of Fraker and Speck (18) and moved on SDS-PAGE in the presence of 2-mercaptoethanol as a major component at approximately 180,000 daltons. Antibody to tetanus toxoid was purified from human tetanus immune globulin (Wyeth Laboratories, Inc., Marietta, PA) on a column of tetanus toxoid conjugated to CNBr-activated Sepharose. Soluble immune complexes were formed by mixing 50 μg of tetanus toxoid with 350 μg of affinity-purified antitoxoid. This ratio (Ab6:Ag1) appears to correspond to the equivalence point when studied by precipitin reactions in the presence of 3% polyethylene glycol (PEG). The complexes remained soluble in the absence of PEG.

Purification of anti-$F(ab')_2$ antibodies. The purification procedure is outlined in Figure 1. Briefly, 2 ml of serum from patients with RA or 6 ml of serum from healthy volunteers was diluted fivefold in Buffer A–Tween and incubated for 2 hours at room temperature with 10 mg of Fc fragments of IgG covalently linked to 1 gm CNBr-activated Sepharose. After washing with Buffer A–Tween, bound anti-Fc antibodies were eluted with glycine-HCl buffer (0.1*M*, pH 2.0), and neutralized immediately with 3*M* Tris. The fraction that had not bound to Fc-Sepharose was incubated for 2 hours at room temperature with 10 mg $F(ab')_2$ covalently linked to CNBr-activated Sepharose.

After washing with Buffer A–Tween, bound material was eluted sequentially with acetate buffer (0.1*M*, pH 5.0), followed by glycine-HCl buffer. One milligram of egg albumin was added to each milliliter of eluate. Fractions eluted from immunoadsorbents were concentrated in a Savant Speed Vac Concentrator and 200-μl aliquots of these fractions were layered on a 10–40% sucrose gradient in Buffer A. The samples were ultracentrifuged in a Beckman SW 50L rotor at 30,000 revolutions per minute for 18 hours at 4°C. Fractions were collected by puncturing the bottom of the

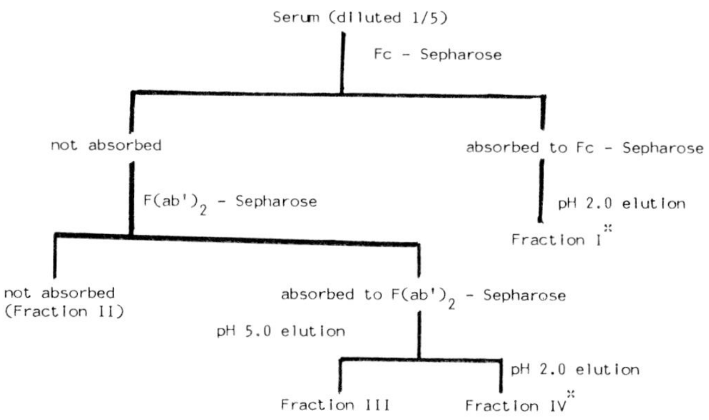

Figure 1. Purification of anti-F(ab′)$_2$ antibodies. Fractions I and IV were further purified by sucrose density gradient ultracentrifugation prior to testing specificity with various inhibitors.

tube and were screened by ELISA for IgM and IgG antibodies to F(ab′)$_2$ or Fc fragments. The IgG concentration of some of the fractions was determined by ELISA, using microtiter wells containing adsorbed protein A, and adsorbed IgG was detected with alkaline phosphatase–conjugated F(ab′)$_2$ fragments of goat anti-human IgG.

RESULTS

Specificity of IgG anti-F(ab′)$_2$ antibodies in serum. To test for the specificity of these antibodies with IgG isotype–specific RIA, RA patient sera, diluted 1:5, were absorbed with various antigens (1 mg each) covalently linked to Sepharose CL–4B. Following incubation at 4°C for 18 hours, the absorbed sera were tested for residual anti-F(ab′)$_2$ antibody activity by comparing antibody levels with those of controls prepared from similarly diluted sera which had been exposed to egg albumin–Sepharose.

The loss of reactivity due to exposure to F(ab′)$_2$-Sepharose was set at 100% inhibition. The results (Table 1) indicate that more anti-F(ab′)$_2$ antibody was consistently absorbed by human F(ab′)$_2$-Sepharose than by human IgG, rabbit IgG, or rabbit F(ab′)$_2$-Sepharose. Since the 5 sera tested contained considerable amounts of RF, it remained uncertain whether reactivity with human and rabbit IgG was due to RF itself, or whether a considerable portion of anti-F(ab′)$_2$ antibodies was directed against epitopes shared by human and rabbit IgG and their F(ab′)$_2$ fragments.

Purification of IgG anti-F(ab′)$_2$ antibodies. When F(ab′)$_2$-Sepharose was used for the purification of anti-F(ab′)$_2$ antibodies from diluted sera which contained large amounts of RF, preparations obtained were heavily contaminated with RF. A more successful purification protocol was eventually devised (Figure 1) in which sera, diluted 1:5, were exposed initially to Fc-Sepharose to remove substantial amounts of RF.

The sera were then exposed to F(ab′)$_2$-Sepharose from which anti-F(ab′)$_2$ antibodies and further quantities of RF were removed by a 2-step elution. The progress of the purification was followed by isotype-specific ELISA, in wells coated with Fc fragments for estimating RF and in wells coated with F(ab′)$_2$ fragments for estimating anti-F(ab′)$_2$ antibodies. The results of the fractionation of 2 ml of serum from patient SL, who had RA and high levels of RF, are detailed in Table 2. A substantial portion of the initial IgG anti-F(ab′)$_2$ antibody activity (titer 1:320) was recovered from F(ab′)$_2$-Sepharose after elution at pH 2.0 (fraction IV, titer 1:80). This fraction was free of IgG-RF. Considerable IgG anti-F(ab′)$_2$ antibody activity was recovered also in the initial absorption step with Fc-Sepharose by elution at pH 2.0 (fraction I, titer 1:40).

Using our fractionation protocol (Figure 1 and Table 2), IgG anti-F(ab′)$_2$ antibodies were prepared from the sera of 2 RA patients (including SL) and from

Table 1. Percent inhibition of serum IgG anti-F(ab′)$_2$ antibody activity by absorption with human IgG-Sepharose, rabbit IgG-Sepharose, and rabbit F(ab′)$_2$-Sepharose*

Patient	Human IgG-Sepharose	Rabbit IgG-Sepharose	Rabbit F(ab′)$_2$-Sepharose
LH	46	26	14
LB	79	39	59
JC	32	18	18
FB	17	3	7
DH	19	13	8

* The activity of serum IgG anti-F(ab′)$_2$ antibody following absorption with the above listed antigens was compared with that of human F(ab′)$_2$-Sepharose–exposed serum (100% inhibition).

Table 2. The fractionation of serum from rheumatoid arthritis patient SL, using Fc-Sepharose followed by F(ab′)$_2$-Sepharose*

	Titer			
	RF		Anti-F(ab′)$_2$ antibodies	
	IgM	IgG	IgM	IgG
Initial serum	40,960	640	640	320
Fraction I	640	40	20	40
Fraction II	10,240	320	40	<5
Fraction III	1,280	40	20	<5
Fraction IV	40	<5	20	80

* Fractionation was done by the same method as in Figure 1. Enzyme-linked immunosorbent assay performed on fractions adjusted to initial serum volume. The titers were determined by the amount of dilution of sample required for an absorbance of 0.500 at 405 nm. RF = rheumatoid factor.

Table 3. Purification of IgG anti-F(ab')$_2$ antibodies*

Serum source	Titer		
	Initial	Fraction I	Fraction IV
SL (RA)	320	40	80
DW (RA)	640	80	320
RH (normal)	40	<5	<5
SP (normal)	320	160	20

* The titers were determined by the amount of dilution of sample required for an absorbance of 0.500 at 405 nm in enzyme-linked immunosorbent assay for IgG anti-F(ab')$_2$ antibody; fractions refer to material eluted at pH 2.0 from Fc-Sepharose (fraction I) and F(ab')$_2$-Sepharose (fraction IV) (see Figure 1). Volumes of all fractions were adjusted to correspond to that of initial serum. RA = rheumatoid arthritis.

2 normal sera (Table 3). It can be seen that IgG anti-F(ab')$_2$ antibody activity was recovered to a substantial extent in fraction IV in the 2 RA patients' sera. In contrast, anti-F(ab')$_2$ antibody recovery was best in fraction I in the 2 normal sera.

Specificity of IgG anti-F(ab')$_2$ antibodies recovered in fraction IV. IgG anti-F(ab')$_2$ antibodies purified as indicated in Figure 1, and representing material recovered as fraction IV, were purified further by sucrose density gradient ultracentrifugation. Fractions devoid of IgM anti-F(ab')$_2$ or IgM anti-Fc antibody were tested with a panel of potential inhibitors. The concentration of each antibody preparation chosen (1.6 pmoles) was on the linear portion of a dose-response curve obtained by ELISA. The concentration of all inhibitors was fixed at 560, 280, 140, and 70-fold molar excess relative to antibody. The assays were carried out at room temperature for 2 hours in the presence of 1 mg/ml of egg albumin in Buffer A–Tween.

The amount of IgG anti-F(ab')$_2$ bound to microtiter wells coated with F(ab')$_2$ fragments was measured with enzyme-conjugated goat anti-human Fc fragment. Absorbance at 405 nm, obtained when inhibitors were used in the absence of anti-F(ab')$_2$ antibodies, were subtracted from test results. Figure 2 gives the results of 1 set of experiments and is representative of 3 separate experiments with the same 2 RA sera (SL and DW). Only human F(ab')$_2$ fragment was an effective inhibitor. Pooled human IgG and rabbit F(ab')$_2$ fragments were relatively poor inhibitors and light chains, Fab and Fc fragments, and rabbit IgG did not inhibit at all. An immune complex prepared from tetanus toxoid–antitoxoid had no greater inhibitory activity than the affinity-purified anti–tetanus toxoid IgG itself.

The same 2 preparations (patients SL and DW) were also tested in the presence of autologous IgG which had been pre-absorbed with pooled F(ab')$_2$-Sepharose and pooled Fc-Sepharose. No inhibition was found. When the 2 antibody preparations were added separately to a normal serum which had been diluted 1:10 and absorbed to remove endogenous anti-F(ab')$_2$ antibodies, levels of antibody activity also remained unchanged.

The 2 purified IgG anti-F(ab')$_2$ antibody preparations (fraction IV) obtained from the sera of normal individuals (RH and SP) and tested in concentrations equal to those in Figure 2 reacted similarly to the 2 preparations obtained from patients with RA, with respect to lack of inhibition by light chains, Fab and Fc

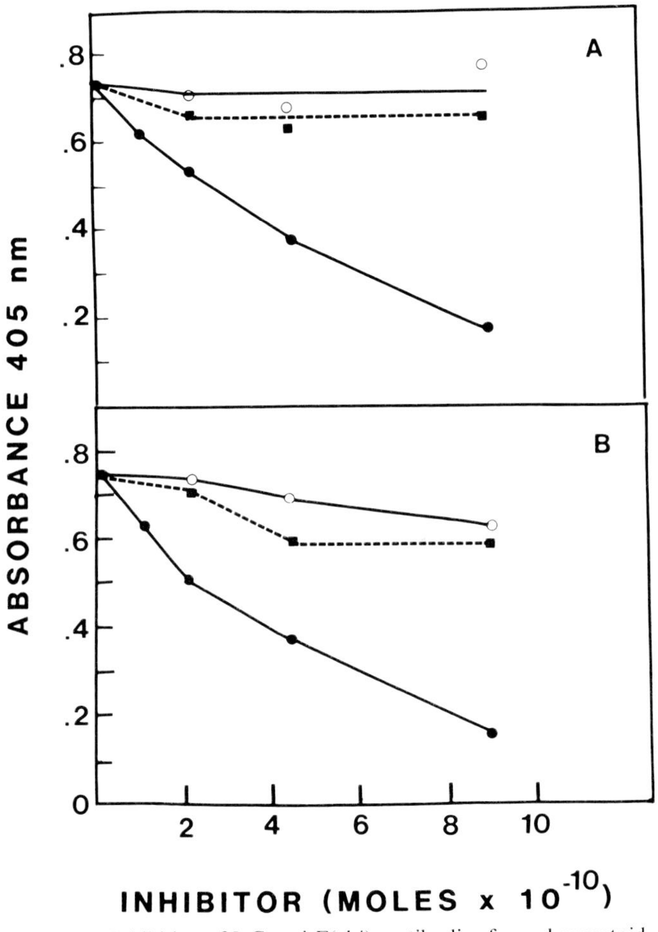

Figure 2. Inhibition of IgG anti-F(ab')$_2$ antibodies from rheumatoid arthritis patients DW (**A**) and SL (**B**) by pooled human F(ab')$_2$ fragments (●——●), rabbit F(ab')$_2$ fragments (○——○), and human IgG (■---■). IgG anti-F(ab')$_2$ antibody in fraction IV (further purified by sucrose density gradient ultracentrifugation) was examined by enzyme-linked immunosorbent assay in the presence of 113–900 pmoles inhibitor (70–560-fold excess with respect to antibody present).

fragments, and rabbit IgG. Relative to the inhibition obtained with $F(ab')_2$ fragments (100%), 1 preparation (from SP) was 40% inhibited by a 560-fold molar excess of rabbit $F(ab')_2$ fragment and preparations from SP and RH were inhibited 50–60% by a 560-fold molar excess of pooled human IgG.

Specificity of IgG anti-$F(ab')_2$ antibodies recovered in fraction I. Fraction I was also subjected to sucrose density gradient ultracentrifugation to remove IgM antibodies. Each of these preparations, however, retained small amounts of IgG-RF (titers ≤ 1:40). IgG anti-$F(ab')_2$ antibody reactivity was not inhibited in the presence of 560-fold and 140-fold molar excess of pooled human Fab and Fc fragments or rabbit IgG and rabbit $F(ab')_2$ fragments. Unlike the fraction IV preparation, similar amounts of pooled human IgG and anti–tetanus toxoid antibody inhibited the IgG anti-$F(ab')_2$ antibody activity between 29 and 80%, relative to $F(ab')_2$, whose inhibitory action was set at 100% (Table 4). The immune complex prepared from tetanus toxoid–antitoxoid was no more inhibitory than the antibody itself.

DISCUSSION

Serum IgG anti-$F(ab')_2$ antibody activity appears to be directed against epitopes present on the surface, as well as in the interior of the $F(ab')_2$ portion of IgG. This heterogeneity is seen when sera are analyzed for this antibody after absorption with immobilized human or rabbit IgG and $F(ab')_2$ fragments thereof. There appears to be considerable variation among human sera in response to these absorptions, as some serum antibodies are extensively cross-reactive with rabbit IgG and rabbit $F(ab')_2$ fragments (Table 1). Cross-reactivity with $F(ab')_2$ fragments of IgG of other species has been reported recently (11–14).

The effectiveness of absorbing sera that contain soluble IgG with immobilized IgG may, however, be compromised. Additionally, endogenous RF may also affect the absorptions. To better define the specificities of IgG anti-$F(ab')_2$ antibodies, attempts were made to purify these, preferably free of RF, and then to test specificity in the presence of known quantities of soluble inhibitors.

Table 4. Percent inhibition of IgG anti-$F(ab')_2$ antibody activity in fraction I*

Serum source	Pooled human IgG	Anti–tetanus toxoid antibody
SL (RA)	29	34
DW (RA)	78	39
SP (normal)	42	80

* The numbers represent the percent inhibitory activity tested at 400-fold molar excess relative to input antibody in fraction I, and also relative to inhibition by human $F(ab')_2$ fragment (100%). RA = rheumatoid arthritis.

Initially we encountered difficulties, as did other investigators (3), in obtaining purified anti-$F(ab')_2$ antibodies without concomitant RF impurities. Eventually we developed a purification protocol in which we made use of the fact that RF are usually low affinity antibodies, which can be removed from solid-phase IgG at pH 5.0. This selective elution facilitated the purification of anti-$F(ab')_2$ antibodies free of IgG-RF activity (Table 2). The activity of the highly purified IgG anti-$F(ab')_2$ antibody preparations was virtually unaffected by the presence of a 560-fold molar excess of pooled human IgG (Figure 2), human Fab and Fc fragments, light chains, as well as a soluble complex of tetanus toxoid and human anti–tetanus toxoid at equivalence. The anti-$F(ab')_2$ antibody activity was also unaffected when added to 1:5 diluted serum, depleted of RF and anti-$F(ab')_2$ antibody by appropriate absorptions. Moreover, rabbit IgG and their $F(ab')_2$ fragments were also ineffective inhibitors.

It would appear that nearly all IgG anti-$F(ab')_2$ antibodies from the 2 patients with RA present in fraction IV, and accounting for substantial antibody activity when compared with whole serum (Table 3), are directed against epitopes uncovered by pepsin digestion at pH 4.0. These epitopes are inaccessible to antibody in the intact IgG molecule. To that extent, fraction IV from these 2 sera behaved as if it contained mainly the previously described pepsin agglutinator (PA), but the activity varied from the original description (2) and a later study (7) of these antibodies by remaining unreactive with immune complexes. In previous work, the specificity of PA was tested in whole serum using only insoluble immune complexes. Thus, other anti-$F(ab')_2$ antibodies and RF may have influenced the analysis. On the basis of our findings, a revised definition of PA would have these antibodies react with $F(ab')_2$ fragments exclusively.

The IgG anti-$F(ab')_2$ antibodies of fraction IV of the 2 normal individuals appeared to be heterogeneous, since they exhibited PA activity and considerable cross-reactivity with IgG. In view of the lack of reactivity with Fab fragments, it is unlikely that the cross-reacting antibodies are antiidiotypic antibodies. Because of lack of reactivity with Fc fragments, the location of the reactive epitope for the subset of anti-$F(ab')_2$ antibody reacting with intact IgG may be in the hinge region.

Fraction I, obtained in our purification procedure by absorption to Fc-Sepharose, also contained considerable quantities of IgG anti-$F(ab')_2$ antibodies (Table 3). The latter may co-purify with IgM-RF which can bind immune complexes, including those which may contain anti-$F(ab')_2$ antibodies (6). When fraction I was further purified by sucrose density gradient ultracentrifugation, all of the IgM-RF activity was removed, leaving IgG-RF and IgG anti-$F(ab')_2$ antibodies which were demonstrable by separate ELISA, using either Fc or $F(ab')_2$ fragments absorbed to microtiter wells. In ELISA, anti-$F(ab')_2$ antibody activity was unaffected by the addition of 560-fold excess Fab and Fc fragments, as well as the tetanus toxoid immune complex preparation. Despite such lack of reactivity, varying degrees of inhibition were observed when the preparations were tested in the presence of pooled IgG or an affinity-purified antitoxoid IgG preparation (Table 4). Fraction I, therefore, was quite similar to fraction IV, except that there was less PA present and, more importantly, there were antibodies cross-reacting with intact IgG. Because of lack of reactivity with Fab fragments, fraction I, like fraction IV, contains no measurable antiidiotypic antibodies.

In a recent report (6), it was suggested that antibody activity to reduced and alkylated pooled human $F(ab')_2$ fragments was detectable both in the free form and also in complexes as "hidden antibody" and that free antibody predominated over hidden antibody in RA sera but not in normal sera. It was suggested that the hidden antibodies might be the result of interaction between idiotypes and antiidiotypes. Our failure to encounter a significant contribution to anti-$F(ab')_2$ activity by antiidiotypic antibodies among the affinity-purified fractions may be attributed to our purification procedure, since we made no attempts to dissociate by acid hidden anti-$F(ab')_2$ antibodies.

The emphasis in this report has been on IgG anti-$F(ab')_2$ antibodies. This is not to say that IgM anti-$F(ab')_2$ antibodies are less important, but rather that IgM anti-$F(ab')_2$ antibodies were not readily purified by our procedures. A report on the specificity of these antibodies in whole serum has been published elsewhere (13).

In summary, on the basis of our results, albeit with a limited sample, we suggest that IgG anti-$F(ab')_2$ antibodies make up a heterogeneous population. A substantial portion of the IgG anti-$F(ab')_2$ antibody activity is due to PA. Moreover, PA is redefined here as antibodies reacting with epitopes which become accessible on pepsin digestion but remain inaccessible when on intact IgG or IgG immune complexes. A subset of IgG anti-$F(ab')_2$ antibodies, especially those found in fraction I, appears to be cross-reactive with human IgG, but because of lack of reactivity with Fab fragments cannot be considered to be antiidiotypic. Sera also contain other IgG anti-$F(ab')_2$ antibodies with cross-reactivity for rabbit IgG and rabbit $F(ab')_2$ fragments, but these could not be purified effectively by affinity chromatography using Fc-Sepharose followed by $F(ab')_2$-Sepharose. In contrast to the work of others (3,6,16), we found no evidence suggestive of reactivity with idiotypes. This may be explained in part by our use of pooled and absorbed $F(ab')_2$ fragments as immunoabsorbents and test antigens.

REFERENCES

1. Osterland CK, Harboe M, Kunkel HG: Anti-gamma-globulin factors in human sera revealed by enzymatic splitting of anti-Rh antibodies. Vox Sang 8:113–152, 1963
2. Harboe M, Rau B, Aho K: Properties of various anti-gammaglobulin factors in human sera. J Exp Med 121:503–519, 1965
3. Nasu H, Chia DS, Knutson DW, Barnett EV: Naturally occurring human antibodies to the $F(ab')_2$ portion of IgG. Clin Exp Immunol 42:378–386, 1980
4. Natvig JB: Heterogeneity of anti-gammaglobulin factors detected by pepsin digested human gamma-G-globulin. Acta Pathol Microbiol Scand 66:369–381, 1966
5. Heimer R, Wolfe LD, Abruzzo JL: IgM and IgG anti-$F(ab')_2$ antibodies in rheumatoid arthritis and systemic lupus erythematosus. Arthritis Rheum 25:1298–1306, 1982
6. Birdsall HH, Lidsky MD, Rossen RD: Anti-Fab′ antibodies in rheumatoid arthritis: measurement of the relative quantities incorporated in soluble immune complexes in sera and supernatants from cultured peripheral blood lymphocytes. Arthritis Rheum 26:1481–1492, 1983
7. Davey MP, Korngold L: Association of anti-$F(ab')_2$ antibodies (pepsin agglutinators) with immune complexes as determined by enzyme linked immunosorbent assays. Int Arch Allergy Appl Immunol 67:278–283, 1982
8. Lawrence TG Jr, Williams RC Jr: Studies of human anti-gamma globulin factors reacting with pepsin-digested gamma globulins. J Exp Med 125:233–248, 1967
9. Mathur S, Khansari N, Genco PV, Williamson HO,

Perry LC, Cracker AJ, Rust PF, Fudenberg HH: Association of antibodies to Fab with sperm antibodies and HLA (abstract). Fed Proc 42:1209, 1983
10. Nasu H, Chia D, Iwaki Y, Barnett EV, Terasaki PL: Cytotoxicity of anti-Fab antibodies against B lymphocytes in rheumatoid arthritis. Arthritis Rheum 24:1278–1282, 1981
11. Olds LC, Miller JJ: Anti-$F(ab')_2$ antibodies that interfere with interpretation of the anti-C3 assay for immune complexes in children with rheumatic diseases. Arthritis Rheum 27:330–336, 1984
12. Wolfe LD, Abruzzo JL, Heimer R: Specificity of anti-$F(ab')_2$ antibodies (abstract). Fed Proc 42:931, 1983
13. Wolfe LD, Abruzzo JL, Heimer R: Specificities of IgM anti-$F(ab')_2$ antibodies. Immunol Commun 13:15–27, 1984
14. Ling NR, Drysdale P: Antibodies in human sera to $F(ab')_2$ fragments of monoclonal and polyclonal IgG. Int Arch Allergy Appl Immunol 66:459–463, 1981
15. Waller M, Blaylock K: Further studies on the anti-globulin factors in human serum to the pepsin digested fragment of the Ri anti-Rh antibody. J Immunol 97:438–443, 1966
16. Nasu H, Chia DS, Taniguchi O, Barnett EV: Characterization of anti-$F(ab')_2$ antibodies in SLE patients: evidence for crossreacting auto-anti-idiotypic antibodies. Clin Immunol Immunopathol 25:80–90, 1982
17. Fleischman JB, Pain R, Porter RR: Reduction of gamma globulins. Arch Biochem Biophys (suppl) 1:174–187, 1961
18. Fraker PH, Speck JC Jr: Protein and cell membrane iodinations with sparingly soluble chloroamide, 1,3,4,6 tetrachloro-3a, 6a-diphenylglycoluril. Biochem Biophys Res Comm 80:849–857, 1978

SPECIAL ARTICLE

WINNERS OF THE 1984 SLIDE COMPETITION

SIDNEY BLOCK and the AUDIOVISUAL AIDS SUBCOMMITTEE OF THE ARA EDUCATION COMMITTEE

The American Rheumatism Association Audiovisual Aids Subcommittee regularly seeks slides to consider for additions to the 1981 Revised Clinical Slide Collection on the Rheumatic Diseases. To stimulate slide submission, the Subcommittee holds an annual slide competition. The first competition was held in 1983 (Block S, Audiovisual Aids Subcommittee of the ARA Education Committee: Winners of the 1983 Slide Competition. Arthritis Rheum 27:456–458, 1984). We are pleased to present here the results of the second annual competition.

During 1983 and early 1984, the Audiovisual Aids Subcommittee received over 200 slides, most of them from members of the ARA. In May 1984, 7 slides from this group were chosen as being deserving of special recognition. These slides were displayed with the slide collection exhibit and were presented at a plenary session at the 1984 American Rheumatism Association Annual Meeting in Minneapolis, Minnesota. They are reproduced in Figures 1–7.

By the time of the 1985 Annual Meeting of the ARA, the winning slides of the 1983 and 1984 competitions, as well as other selected slides, will be assembled for sale as the first supplement to the 1981 Collection. Some slides will represent improvements over those on the same subject currently in the Collection, but most will cover additional topics. This supplement, and future supplements, will include revised syllabus pages for easy insertion into the Collection's looseleaf binder.

The Subcommittee also plans to have available by the 1985 meeting a cassette tape rendition of the

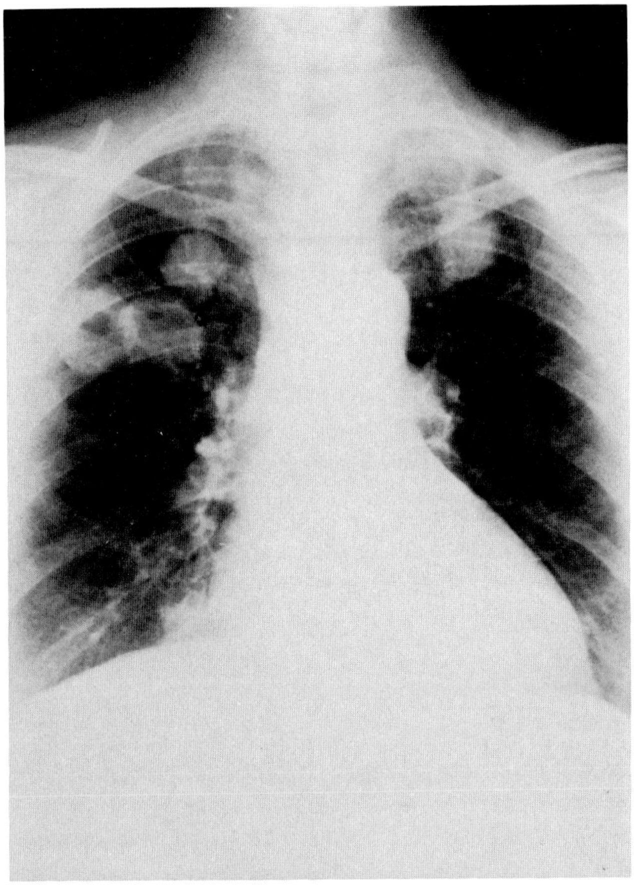

Figure 1. Radiograph of a patient with Wegener's granulomatosis. Submitted by William Beetham, MD, Burlington, MA.

Members of the Audiovisual Aids Subcommittee of the American Rheumatism Association Education Committee: William Beetham, MD; Sidney Block, MD: Chair; Joseph Croft, MD; William Ginsburg, MD; Timothy Harrington, MD; Bernhard Singsen, MD.

Submitted for publication September 21, 1984; accepted December 20, 1984.

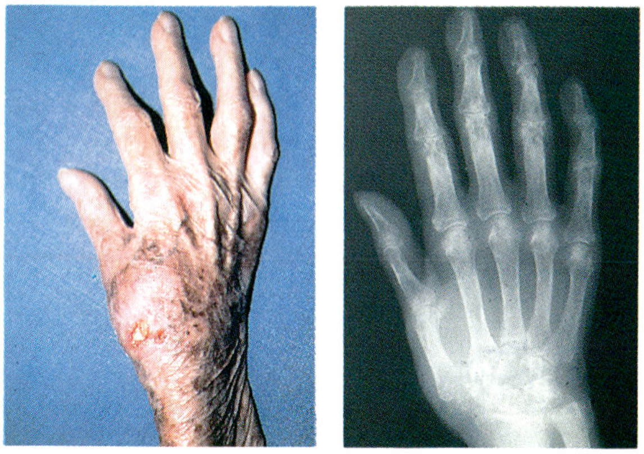

Figure 2. Tuberculosis wrist. **Left:** gross view. **Right:** radiograph. Submitted by Joseph Croft, MD, Washington, DC.

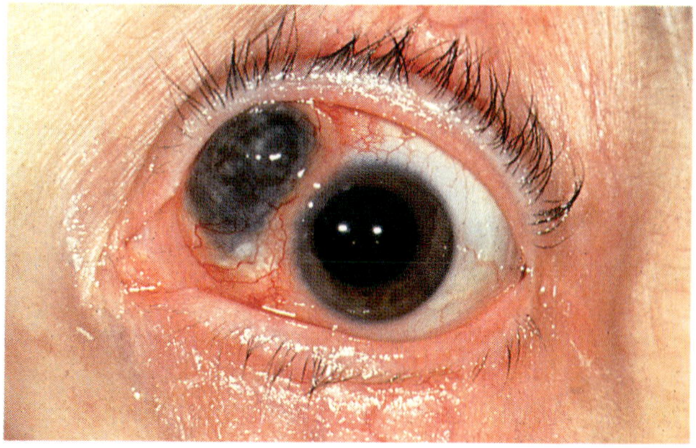

Figure 3. Scleromalacia perforans. Submitted by Gene Hunder, MD, Rochester, MN.

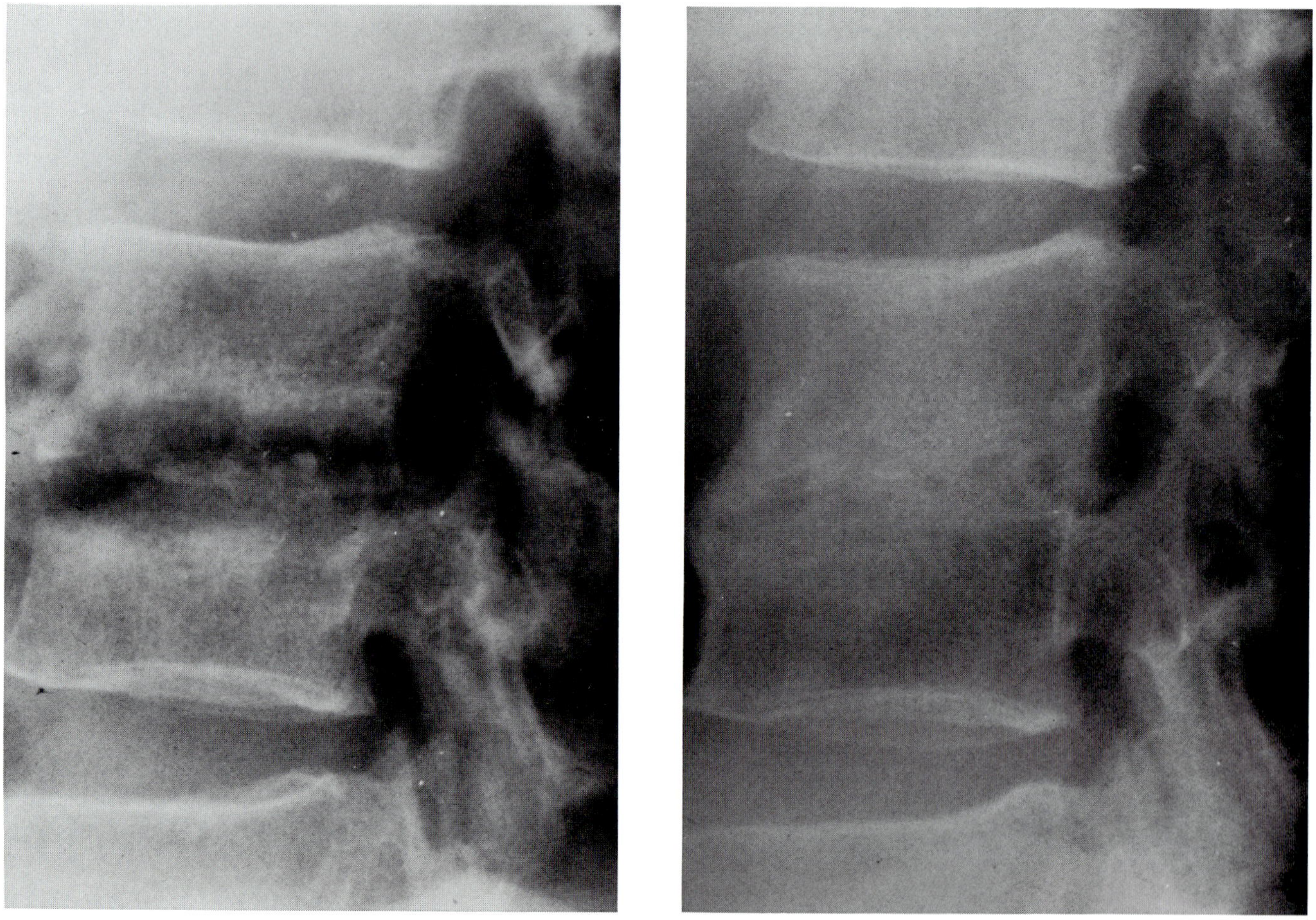

Figure 4. Radiographs of a patient with septic disc. **Left:** early. **Right:** late. Submitted by Richard McLeod, MD, Rochester, MN.

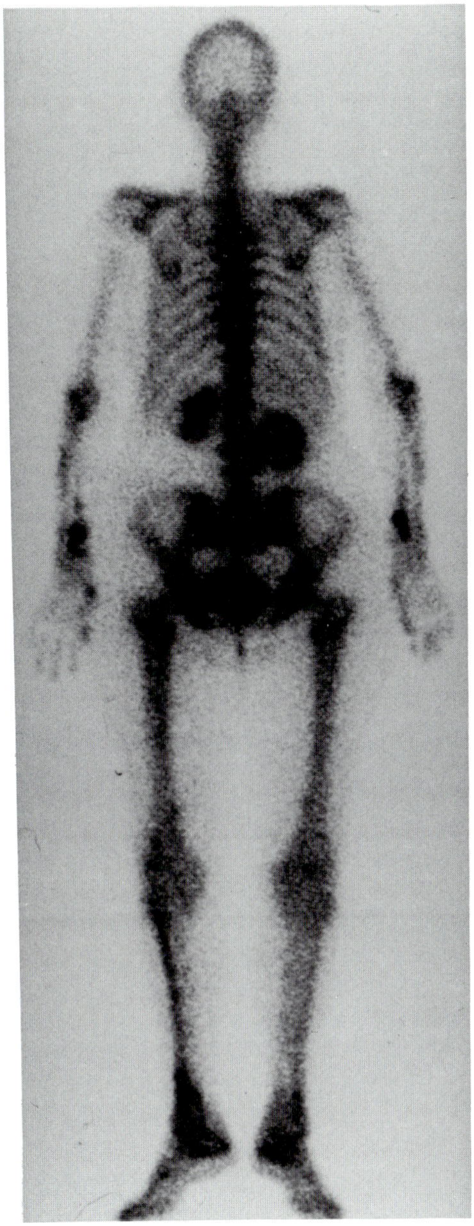

Figure 5. Bone scan of a patient with hypertrophic pulmonary osteoarthropathy. Submitted by Allen Segal, DO, Cleveland, OH.

syllabus to allow the student easier review of the Collection in a dark room. The tape will operate with automatic carousel and self-contained projection units (e.g., caramate) designed to accept tone-keyed slide advancement signals.

The Audiovisual Aids Subcommittee will continue upgrading the 1981 Revised Collection by replacing current slides with better ones ("hit list," Table 1) and by adding new topics that should be covered. Examples of desired slides that would expand the Collection are listed in the "wish list" (Table 2). The lists are by no means complete, but the Subcommittee hopes they will serve to stimulate readers to submit slides for consideration.

The Audiovisual Aids Subcommittee appreciates the contributions made by the ARA membership. The Subcommittee urges you to take and submit slides or original radiographs. (Submit entries to Dr. Sidney R. Block, Chair, American Rheumatism Association Audiovisual Aids Subcommittee, Arthritis Foundation, 1314 Spring St. NW, Atlanta, GA 30309.) Also, when you see good slides or radiographs made by others, urge them to submit them. The Subcommittee will return all original material not added to the Collection. Original materials deemed worthy of inclusion will be retained for future best-quality reproduction, but the donors will receive as many first-production duplicates as they need.

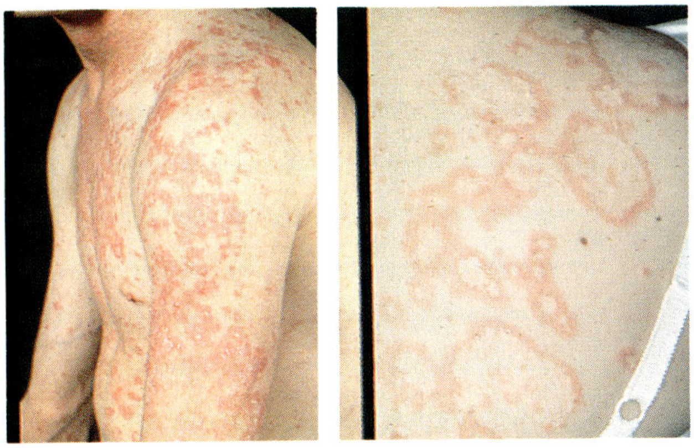

Figure 6. Subacute cutaneous lupus erythematosus. Submitted by Richard Sontheimer, MD, Dallas, TX.

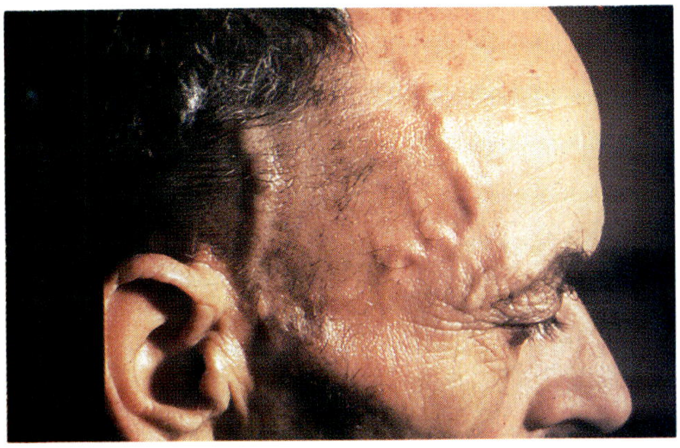

Figure 7. Temporal arteritis. Submitted by Kenneth Wilske, MD, Seattle, WA.

Table 1. Hit list

Section 2: Rheumatoid arthritis	
2-1*	Hand, fusiform swelling
2-3	Hand, inflammation (scan)
2-5	Hand, swan-neck deformity
2-6	Hand, boutonnière deformity
2-28	Subcutaneous nodule (microscopic)
2-42	Foot deformities
2-49	Hip, early erosions (x-ray)
2-57	Cervical spine, atlantoaxial subluxation (x-ray)
2-61	Mucin clot test
Section 3: Juvenile rheumatoid arthritis	
3-3	Micrognathia
Section 4: Spondylarthropathies	
4-2	Ankylosing spondylitis: lumbar spine ankylosis, with patient flexing
Section 5: Systemic lupus erythematosus	
5-1	Butterfly rash, discoid type
Section 6: Dermatomyositis/polymyositis	
6-2	Hand, edema and rash
Section 7: Scleroderma	
7-2	Raynaud's phenomenon: hands, cyanosis
7-10	Acrosclerosis
7-11	Sclerodactyly and terminal digit resorption
Section 9: Vasculitis	
9-3	Henoch-Schönlein syndrome: legs, purpura (prefer child's legs)
9-73	Kawasaki disease: skin and mucous membrane
9-74	Kawasaki disease: strawberry tongue
Section 11: Crystal-associated arthropathies	
11-4	Gout: tophi, ear
Section 13: Degenerative diseases	
13-14	Spondylosis: cervical vertebrae, foraminal encroachment (x-ray)
13-15	Apophyseal disease: cervical vertebrae (x-ray)
13-51	Diffuse idiopathic skeletal hyperostosis: lumbar spine (x-ray)
13-53	Diffuse idiopathic skeletal hyperostosis: cervical spine (x-ray)
13-84	Knee, meniscus tear (arthrogram)
Section 14: Metabolic and primary bone diseases	
14-1	Avascular necrosis: systemic lupus erythematosus, hips (x-ray)
14-19	Bone: osteomalacia (microscopic)
Section 16: Infiltrative and systemic disease	
16-53	Shoulder-hand syndrome: hand, edema
16-54	Shoulder-hand syndrome: wrist, osteopenia (x-ray)
Section 17: Tumor-associated rheumatic syndromes	
17-1	Hypertrophic pulmonary osteoarthropathy: fingers, clubbing
17-22	Leukemia: forearm, periostitis and osteopenia (x-ray)

* Numbers of current slides.

Table 2. Wish list

Section 1: Normal
Arthrogram: knee
X-ray: hip, foot, hand, lumbosacral spine, pelvis
Section 2: Rheumatoid arthritis
Temporomandibular joint disease (x-ray)
"Bullseye" lesion of Plaquenil eye toxicity
Surgical exposure of median nerve compression
Section 3: Juvenile rheumatoid arthritis
Slit lamp view of iritis
Section 4: Spondylarthropathies
Psoriasis (bone scan)
Ankylosing spondylitis (bone scan)
Section 5: Systemic lupus erythematosus
Neonatal lupus erythematosus, skin lesions
Section 9: Vasculitis
Giant cell arteritis, scalp gangrene
Giant cell arteritis, tongue blanching
Weber-Christian disease (gross)
Lymphomatoid granulomatosis, skin lesions and pathology
Section 11: Crystal-associated arthropathies
Gout: arthroscopy
Section 12: Infectious arthritis
Psoas abscess (computed tomography scan)
Gonococcal arthritis (Gram stain joint fluid)
Joint fluid: normal/inflammatory/septic: comparison
Section 13: Degenerative diseases
Herniated disc (computed tomography scan)
Spinal stenosis (computed tomography scan)
Traumatic bursitis
Section 14: Metabolic and primary bone diseases
Paget's disease: skull, long bone, pelvis (x-ray)
Paget's disease (bone scan)
Osgood-Schlatter disease (x-ray and clinical)
Section 15: Heritable disorders of connective tissue
Marfan's syndrome
Section 17: Tumor-associated rheumatic syndromes
Osteoid osteoma (x-ray/tomogram/scan)
Metastatic cancer (scan)

BRIEF REPORT

SYSTEMIC LUPUS ERYTHEMATOSUS IN A PREMATURE INFANT

NANCY P. CUMMINGS, JEFFREY HANSEN, and J. ROGER HOLLISTER

Systemic lupus erythematosus (SLE) in young children is a rare occurrence (1–3). In 101 patients evaluated at the Mayo Clinic between 1945 and 1970, only 9 children were under 9 years of age at the time of diagnosis (3). To date, the youngest patient described with a definite diagnosis of SLE presented at 11 months of age (4). We report a case of a premature infant who at age 3 months developed signs and symptoms consistent with a diagnosis of SLE.

Case report. The infant, a male weighing 920 gm, was born to a 24-year-old healthy mother in January 1982. The pregnancy was uneventful until 2 months prior to delivery when the mother fell and experienced spontaneous onset of labor. A cesarean section for a double footling breech presentation was performed. Apgar scores were 0 at 5 and 10 minutes and 5 at 20 minutes. Estimated gestational age was 28 weeks. The neonatal course was complicated by hyperbilirubinemia which was treated with phototherapy, respiratory distress syndrome requiring intubation and ventilation, and pneumothorax requiring thoracostomy tube insertion, a patent ductus arteriosus which required surgical ligation, and intraventricular hemorrhage with resultant mild hydrocephalus.

During the first 2 months of the infant's life, grade III retrolental fibroplasia was noted, and it progressed to total retinal detachment in the left eye and partial retinal detachment in the right eye. Bronchopulmonary dysplasia developed. Between the ages of 2 and 3 months, the infant improved and showed steady weight gain.

At 3 months, the infant became irritable. His platelet count had decreased from 180,000/mm^3 to 90,000/mm^3; urinalysis revealed proteinuria and hematuria. Urine collection demonstrated 1.43 gm of protein/m^2/24 hours; total serum protein was 3.2 gm/dl. A blood culture grew *Escherichia coli*. The infant was treated with intravenous ampicillin and gentamicin.

Further laboratory investigations conducted several days later revealed that the platelet count had fallen to a low of 46,000/mm^3. Serum electrolytes, blood urea nitrogen, creatinine, and liver function test results were within normal limits; negative results were also obtained on tests for VDRL, purified protein derivative, and a urine culture for cytomegalovirus. Immunologic evaluation revealed LE cells, antinuclear antibodies (ANA) at >1:256 dilution, antibodies to double-stranded DNA (dsDNA; 33% bound at a 1:40 dilution, normal <10%), C3 level of 32 mg/dl (infant normal range 33–109), and C4 level of 9 mg/dl (infant normal range 5–33). Other nuclear antigen antibodies (SS-B, SS-A, Sm, and RNP) were not present. A renal biopsy specimen appeared normal by light microscopy, but electron microscopy revealed small subendothelial deposits in the glomerular basement membrane and microtubular inclusions, which were consistent with early focal proliferative nephritis.

At age 4 months, the platelet count had fallen to 17,000/mm^3. Bone marrow aspirate revealed increased numbers of megakaryocytes. Anti-platelet antibodies

From the Department of Pediatrics, National Jewish Hospital and Research Center/National Asthma Center, and The University of Colorado Medical School, and the Department of Perinatology, The Children's Hospital, Denver, Colorado.

Nancy P. Cummings, MD; Jeffrey Hansen, MD; J. Roger Hollister, MD.

Address reprint requests to J. Roger Hollister, MD, Department of Pediatrics, National Jewish Hospital and Research Center/National Asthma Center, 3800 East Colfax Avenue, Denver, CO 80206.

Submitted for publication March 19, 1984; accepted in revised form December 12, 1984.

were present. Prednisone, 2 mg/kg/day, was instituted. By 4½ months, the thrombocytopenia resolved and the proteinuria improved. At 5½ months, the infant was discharged from the hospital receiving a tapering dosage of prednisone, which was discontinued at 7 months.

Two weeks after the discontinuation of prednisone, the platelet count dropped to 45,000/mm^3. The urinalysis results remained normal, but ANA were present at a 1:1,280 dilution with a homogeneous pattern, dsDNA were 66% bound at a 1:40 dilution, and anti-platelet antibodies were present. Prednisone was restarted and continued until the age of 12 months.

At 14 months, limitation of movement in the left hip was noted and arthroscopy revealed aseptic necrosis. Marked generalized lymphadenopathy and hepatosplenomegaly were noted, which decreased following the prednisone treatment. From age 14 months to 24 months, 4 surgical procedures were required for retrolental fibroplasia. The prednisone dosage was increased during the surgical periods. The child experienced recurrent episodes of erythema multiforme and transient joint swellings involving the elbows, wrists, and ankles. He was maintained on a regimen of prednisone ranging from 0.5–1 mg/kg every other day.

At age 24 months, the child was below the third percentile for both height and weight. Developmental evaluation was thought to be normal for his age and for the degree of blindness. Results of urinalysis and tests for total hemolytic complement were normal, but ANA were still present at >1:256 dilution, and dsDNA were bound 57.5% at a 1:10 dilution. Chromosomal analysis with banding revealed no abnormalities.

Both parents were in good health and denied any family history of collagen vascular disease. On repeated laboratory evaluations, the mother's serum was negative for ANA including antibodies to SS-A and SS-B.

Discussion. This infant demonstrated 5 of the criteria for the diagnosis of SLE (5): nonerosive arthritis, nephritis, thrombocytopenia, immunologic disorder (positive LE cell preparation and dsDNA in abnormal titers), and the presence of ANA. In addition, serum complement levels were low, anti-platelet antibodies were present, and a renal biopsy specimen showed changes consistent with a diagnosis of early-stage focal proliferative lupus nephritis (6).

In children, SLE is predominantly a disease of adolescent females, with the peak age of onset being 12 years. The female preponderance of 9:1 in teenagers and adults is less evident during the first decade of life, when females with SLE exceed males by only 3:1. Sixty to 80 percent of patients will have clinical findings of renal involvement (as was present in this child) at the time of diagnosis (1–4).

SLE in children under 2 years of age is rare and has been reported in only 2 patients. One was an 11-month-old girl who presented with oral ulcerations, alopecia, thrombocytopenia, and positive ANA. She died of sepsis at age 15 months (4). The second patient was a full-term infant presenting with proteinuria at 3 months of age, who had some similarities to our patient (7). Laboratory investigation revealed hemolytic anemia, leukopenia, thrombocytopenia, hypocomplementemia, and the presence of ANA and dsDNA. A renal biopsy specimen demonstrated membranous glomerulopathy. However, that child also had chromosomal abnormalities, and his mother had immunologic abnormalities including positive ANA and rheumatoid factor. The boy was not monitored long enough to assure that the antibodies were not passively acquired.

Whereas neonatal lupus resulting from passive antibody transmission from the mother to the fetus, associated with discoid rash, cytopenias, and complete heart block has been described (8–10), our patient had a clinical spectrum typical of idiopathic SLE. Antibodies to SS-A, both in the neonate and in the mother, have been shown to have a strong association with the transient neonatal lupus syndrome (9,10). The diagnosis of SLE should not be made on the basis of serologic abnormalities until sufficient time has elapsed for the disappearance of proteins transmitted through the placenta. However, in the case reported here, neither the patient nor his mother had evidence of SS-A antibodies, nor did the child have the discoid skin lesions or heart block associated with neonatal lupus, thus making the more common passively acquired syndrome unlikely.

Our patient's subsequent clinical disease demonstrated the idiopathic nature of his illness with the characteristics present in older children and adults with SLE, particularly arthritis, nephritis, and thrombocytopenia. In addition, he demonstrated lymphadenopathy and hepatosplenomegaly, which may be more characteristic of childhood SLE. Avascular necrosis, a complication of both steroid administration and SLE, was also present in this child, and may be more frequent in pediatric patients with SLE (11,12).

The susceptibility to SLE is affected by a multitude of genetic factors including age, race, sex, and family history, none of which appear to be pertinent in this child's case. However, a large number of environmental and infectious factors have been implicated as precipitating factors in the disease. It is tempting to speculate that this child's difficult neonatal course, which included prematurity, ventilation, surgery, and *E coli* sepsis, may have played a role in the expression of SLE.

This case emphasizes that idiopathic SLE as well as neonatal lupus can develop in very young infants. In infants with unexplained multisystem disease, an investigation with immunologic evaluation for the possibility of SLE should be considered.

Acknowledgment. The authors wish to thank Gale Waldstein for assistance in the interpretation of the renal biopsy.

REFERENCES

1. King KK, Kornreich HK, Bernstein BH, Singsen BH, Hanson V: The clinical spectrum of systemic lupus erythematosus in childhood. Arthritis Rheum 20:287–294, 1977
2. Norris DG, Colon AR, Stickler GB: Systemic lupus erythematosus in children: the complex problems of diagnosis and treatment encountered in 101 such patients at the Mayo Clinic. Clin Pediatr (Phila) 9:774–778, 1977
3. Abeles M, Urman JD, Weinstein A, Lowenstein M, Rothfield NF: Systemic lupus erythematosus in the younger patient: survival studies. J Rheumatol 7:515–522, 1980
4. Grossman J, Schwartz RH, Callerame ML, Condemi JJ: Systemic lupus erythematosus in a 1-year-old child. Am J Dis Child 129:123–125, 1975
5. Tan EM, Cohen AS, Fries JF, Masi AT, McShane DJ, Rothfield NF, Schaller JG, Talal N, Winchester RJ: The 1982 revised criteria for the classification of systemic lupus erythematosus. Arthritis Rheum 25:1271–1277, 1982
6. Baldwin DS, Gluck MC, Lowenstein J, Gallo GR: Lupus nephritis: clinical course as related to morphologic forms and their transitions. Am J Med 62:12–30, 1977
7. Ty A, Fine B: Membranous nephritis in infantile systemic lupus erythematosus associated with chromosomal abnormalities. Clin Nephrol 12:137–141, 1979
8. Bremers HH, Golitz LE, Weston WL, Hays WG: Neonatal lupus erythematosus. Cutis 24:287–290, 1979
9. Kephart DC, Hood AF, Provost TT: Neonatal lupus erythematosus: new serologic findings. J Invest Dermatol 77:331–333, 1981
10. Reed BR, Lee LA, Harmon C, Wolfe R, Wiggins J, Peebles C, Weston WL: Autoantibodies to SS-A/Ro in infants with congenital heart block. J Pediatr 103:889–891, 1983
11. Hurley RM, Steinberg RH, Patriquin H, Drummond KN: Avascular necrosis of the femoral head in childhood systemic lupus erythematosus. Can Med Assoc J 111:781–784, 1974
12. Klipper AR, Stevens MB, Zizic TM, Hungerford DS: Avascular necrosis of the bone in systemic lupus erythematosus. Medicine (Baltimore) 55:251–257, 1976

BRIEF REPORT

MENINGOCOCCEMIA PRESENTING AS SEPTIC ARTHRITIS, PERICARDITIS, AND TENOSYNOVITIS

MICHAEL S. ROSEN, ALLEN R. MYERS, and BURTON DICKEY

There have been infrequent reports of meningococcemia mimicking gonococcemia (1–8). In this paper we extend such observations by reporting a case of tenosynovitis and septic arthritis in a young woman with meningococcemia.

Case report. The patient, a 32-year-old black woman, was well until 1 day prior to admission, when she awoke with a temperature of 103°F, chills, myalgias, and pain in her left wrist, right ankle, and both knees. That evening she developed nausea and watery diarrhea. On the following day she presented to Germantown Hospital and Medical Center emergency room, with persistent arthralgias and myalgias and onset of severe anterior pleuritic chest pain. She denied having abdominal pain, vaginal discharge, rash, sore throat, dysuria, shortness of breath, cough, stiff neck, headache, or photophobia. She was sexually active, and her last known menstrual period was 1 month prior to admission. She denied contact with persons with meningococcal disease. Her medical history was significant for bilateral ectopic pregnancies, bilateral oophorectomy, and an appendectomy. She took no medications and had no allergies.

Physical examination revealed a well-developed woman who appeared moderately ill. Her blood pressure was 80/50, pulse rate 132, temperature 100°F orally, and her respiratory rate was 24 and shallow. The skin was dry and there was no rash. Her pharynx was clear. There was no adenopathy and her neck was supple. The chest was clear to auscultation and percussion, and there were no rubs. Her chest wall was diffusely tender. The cardiac examination revealed a regular rate and rhythm with no murmurs, gallops, or rubs. Abdominal examination revealed tenderness in both lower quadrants, with guarding but no rebound. A pelvic examination showed a white vaginal discharge, tenderness on cervical motion, and bilateral lower quadrant tenderness. There were no palpable masses. Results of the rectal examination were negative. The joint examination revealed a tender left knee without obvious effusion, a tender right ankle, and warmth and tenderness along the dorsal aspect of her left hand following the course of the extensor tendon of her left wrist. The neurologic examination findings were within normal limits.

Admission laboratory data revealed a white blood cell (WBC) count of 14,800/mm^3 with 62% neutrophils, 30% bands, 6% lymphocytes, 4% monocytes; hemoglobin 11.2 gm/dl; hematocrit 33.2%; platelets 157,000/mm^3; prothrombin time 10.9 seconds; partial thromboplastin time 31 seconds; sodium 140 mEq/liter; potassium 3.9 mEq/liter; HCO_2 25 mEq/liter; chloride 105 mEq/liter; blood urea nitrogen 15 mg/dl; serum glucose 146 mg/dl. Results of a chest radiograph were within normal limits. Electrocardiogram (EKG) showed sinus tachycardia but otherwise normal findings. Urinalysis revealed trace ketones, 2+ protein, and no cells. Erythrocyte sedimentation rate was 87 mm/hour.

At admission a pelvic ultrasound was per-

From the Departments of Medicine, Germantown Hospital Medical Center and Temple University Hospital, Philadelphia, Pennsylvania.

Michael S. Rosen, MD: Chief Medical Resident, Temple University Hospital; Allen R. Myers, MD: Professor and Acting Chairman, Department of Medicine, Temple University School of Medicine; Burton Dickey, MD: Resident in Internal Medicine, Temple University Hospital.

Address reprint requests to Allen R. Myers, MD, Professor and Acting Chairman, Department of Medicine, Temple University Hospital, 3400 N. Broad Street, Philadelphia, PA 19140.

Submitted for publication August 15, 1984; accepted in revised form November 26, 1984.

formed, revealing no abnormality. Cultures were obtained from blood, urine, cervix, rectum, and throat, and she was started on a regimen of penicillin, 2 million units every 6 hours, for a presumed diagnosis of disseminated gonococcal infection. By the following day, she was afebrile and normotensive and felt much improved, with a decrease in her arthralgias and myalgias. However, she complained of persistent chest pain and increased pain and swelling of her right ankle. A right ankle effusion was noted on physical examination. Arthrocentesis of that ankle revealed purulent fluid with 117,000 WBC/mm^3 with 98% neutrophils. Gram stain revealed many intracellular gram-negative diplococci.

The next day her chest pain increased and a repeat EKG was performed, demonstrating diffuse S-T segment elevation. Subsequently, an echocardiogram showed a moderate-sized posterior pericardial effusion. Later that day, all of the initial 4 blood culture bottles were reported as showing positive results for *Neisseria meningitidis*, type C. All other cultures demonstrated no growth. A lumbar puncture was performed, revealing 22,000 WBC/mm^3 with 85% neutrophils and 15% lymphocytes. Cerebrospinal fluid glucose was 26 mg% and protein was 71 mg%. Gram stain and cultures were negative. Over the ensuing days, her chest pain gradually improved with indomethacin therapy, and her ankle effusion slowly resolved with successive daily arthrocenteses. CH50 was 41 units/ml (normal 20–40). Immune complexes by Raji cell assay were negative. She received a 10-day course of antibiotics and was discharged in excellent condition.

Discussion. Meningococcal arthritis is considered to be a reasonably common complication of meningococcal disease, occurring in 11% of adult patients (1). Only rarely, however, has it been clinically confused with disseminated gonococcemia (1–8). This presentation occurs predominantly in young patients without meningitis who develop a monarticular or oligoarticular arthritis involving mainly large joints, usually knees, but occasionally ankles, wrists, or elbows. It is frequently (79% of cases) associated with a rash. Our patient's course was also initially misdiagnosed as gonococcemia, based on the findings of a vaginal discharge and pelvic pain, along with an oligoarticular polyarthritis. In addition, her condition was unique in its similarity to gonococcal arthritis in that she had an acute tenosynovitis of the left wrist. To the best of our knowledge, this has not been previously reported in meningococcal disease.

The pathogenesis of this syndrome is unclear, although there may be similarities to disseminated gonococcemia. Direct invasion by bacteria may play a role in some patients, although in an extensive review of the literature, Schaad (1) noted that when evaluated, only 21.2% of patients had a positive joint fluid Gram stain or culture. Immune mechanisms have also been suspected in the etiology of the arthritis. Bryerson et al (9) investigated 4 patients with arthritis developing late in the course of meningococcal meningitis. Meningococcal antigen was detected in blood initially in all patients and was cleared from the circulation rapidly. One week later antibody was detected, along with a fall in C3. At that time meningococcal antigen, antibody, and C3 were detected in synovial cells. Histologic examination of skin lesions also revealed meningococcal antigen, antibody, and C3. Furthermore, circulating immune complexes were detected by Davis et al (10) by C1q binding and polyethylene glycol methods in a patient with late-onset monarticular arthritis.

It has been noted that the presumed allergic complications of meningococcal disease—arthritis, pericarditis, and cutaneous vasculitis—are seen more frequently with group C disease (9,11–13). It is suspected that a bacterial cell wall polysaccharide antigen in group C meningococcus is responsible for the eventual formation of immune complexes. There has been a similar debate regarding the pathogenesis of gonococcal arthritis (14). Like gonococcal arthritis, meningococcal arthritis has an excellent prognosis with regard to joint function, with residua noted in only 0.7% of the patients (1).

One feature helpful in distinguishing meningococcemia from gonococcemia is the presence of pericarditis, as seen in our patient. This is seen in 4–19% of cases of meningococcal disease (12,15–18). In contrast, although EKG changes are common in gonococcemia, documented pericarditis is rare (19).

Although our patient had no skin lesions, they can be helpful in distinguishing between gonococcemia and meningococcemia. Skin lesions in gonococcemia, seen in 50% of patients (20), generally occur in the distal extremities (21) and consist of early petechial lesions which develop into papules or pustules on an erythematous or hemorrhagic base. Occasionally, bullae can be seen (19). Meningococcal skin lesions, seen in 79% of patients, are usually more generalized in distribution and consist of petechiae or maculopapular lesions. Eleven percent of patients develop more distal purpura or ecchymotic lesions, and this portends a more ominous prognosis (22).

Another symptom which simulated gonococcal

disease in our patient was abdominal pain. Although the etiology in her case was never proved, it might have been due to peritonitis from meningococcus, as described in 2 prior reports (23,24).

In retrospect, meningococcal disease might have been suspected in our patient on the basis of hypotension (80/50) and tachycardia (136 beats/minute). These imply a picture of early septic shock, and are thus more consistent with meningococcus than with gonococcemia.

In conclusion, although there have been other reports of meningococcemia resembling gonococcemia, this is the first case of meningococcemia presenting with tenosynovitis. In a patient with fever, polyarthritis, and tenosynovitis, meningococcemia may rarely be the cause of the syndrome, especially in the presence of clinical pericarditis.

Acknowledgment. We appreciate the assistance of E. Lobb in preparation of the manuscript.

REFERENCES

1. Schaad V: Arthritis in disease due to Neisseria meningitidis. Rev Infect Dis 2:880–887, 1980
2. Feldman H: Meningococcus and gonococcus: never the twain. . .well hardly ever. N Engl J Med 285:518–519, 1971
3. Young E, Morton G: Meningococcal arthritis simulating gonococcemia. South Med J 68:636–638, 1975
4. Eichner HL, Deller JJ Jr: Meningococcal arthritis: report of two cases. Arthritis Rheum 13:272–275, 1970
5. Byeff P, Suskiewicz L: Meningococcal arthritis. JAMA 235:2752, 1976
6. Pinals R: Meningococcemia presenting as acute polyarthritis. J Rheumatol 4:420–424, 1977
7. Fernando N, Gupta Y, Kothari N, Weinstein M: Purulent meningococcal arthritis in an adult. J Med Soc NJ 77:590–591, 1980
8. Fam A, Tenenbaum J, Stern J: Clinical forms of meningococcal arthritis: a study of five cases. J Rheumatol 6:567–573, 1979
9. Bryerson A, Whittle A, Greenwood B: Allergic complications of meningococcal disease. II. Immunological investigations. Br Med J 2:737–740, 1973
10. Davis J, Peters N, Mohammed I, Major G, Holborow E: Circulating immune complexes in a patient with meningococcal disease. Br Med J 1:1445–1446, 1976
11. Evans-Jones L, Whittle H, Onyewotu I, Egler L, Greenwood B: Comparative study of group A and group C meningococcal infection. Arch Dis Child 52:320–323, 1977
12. Morse J, Oretsky N, Hudson J: Pericarditis as a complication of meningococcal meningitis. Ann Intern Med 74:212–217, 1971
13. Edwards E: Immunological investigations of meningococcal disease. II. Some characteristics of group C antigen of Neisseria meningitidis in the sera of patients with fulminant meningococcemia. J Infect Dis 129:538–544, 1974
14. O'Brien J, Goldenberg D, Rice P: Disseminated gonococcal infection: a prospective analysis of 49 patients and a review of pathophysiology and immune mechanisms. Medicine (Baltimore) 62:395–406, 1983
15. Pierce I, Cooper E: Meningococcal pericarditis. Arch Intern Med 129:918–922, 1972
16. Rao V, Rajashekaroiah K, Rice T, Riaz M, Towne W, Kallick C: Primary meningococcal pericarditis. South Med J 73:1276–1278, 1980
17. Miller G, Witham C: Delayed febrile pleuropericarditis after sepsis. Ann Intern Med 79:194–197, 1973
18. Varriale P, Kumar R, Kwa R: Primary meningococcal pericarditis with tamponade. NY State J Med 81:79–81, 1981
19. Holmes K, Counts G, Beaty H: Disseminated gonococcal infection. Ann Intern Med 74:979–993, 1971
20. Brogadir S, Schimmer B, Myers A: Spectrum of gonococcal arthritis-dermatitis syndrome. Semin Arthritis Rheum 8:177–183, 1979
21. Myers AR: Septic arthritis, Textbook of Rheumatology. Vol. 2. Edited by WN Kelley, ED Harris Jr, S Ruddy, CB Sledge. Philadelphia, WB Saunders, 1981, pp 1551–1572
22. Toews W, Bass J: Skin manifestations of meningococcal infections: an immediate indicator of prognosis. Am J Dis Child 127:173–176, 1974
23. Bar-Meir S, Chojkier M, Groszmann R, Atterbury C, Conn A: Spontaneous meningococcal peritonitis: a report of two cases. Digestive Diseases 23:119–122, 1978
24. Bannatyne R, Lakdawalla N, Ein S: Primary meningococcal peritonitis (letter). Can Med Assoc J 117:436, 1977

BRIEF REPORT

RELATIONSHIP OF AUTOANTIBODY EXPRESSION AND HLA PHENOTYPE IN JAPANESE PATIENTS WITH CONNECTIVE TISSUE DISEASES

MASAHIKO NISHIKAI and SUSUMU SEKIGUCHI

Genetic factors have long been considered to play a role in the pathogenesis of connective tissue diseases (1). Recent studies have shown that genetic influences coded by the major histocompatibility complex (MHC) appear to have a profound relationship to the development of these diseases (2). At the same time, autoantibodies which possess a high degree of disease specificity have been reported in connective tissue diseases (3,4). Several alleles in the HLA–D region may exert major influence on the expression of those antibodies.

This report describes the relationship between such autoantibodies and HLA antigens, including DQ locus (second D locus) B cell alloantigens, in Japanese patients with connective tissue diseases. The differences between these findings and findings in white patients are discussed.

MATERIALS AND METHODS

Autoantibodies. Estimation of autoantibodies to the low molecular weight ribonucleoproteins, Sm, nuclear RNP (nRNP), Ro (SS-A), and La (SS-B), was carried out as reported previously (4). Briefly, the Ouchterlony double immunodiffusion technique was used to monitor antigen identity. Agarose (0.6%; Bio-Rad, Richmond, CA) in 0.01*M* phosphate buffered saline, pH 7.4, containing 0.1% sodium azide was utilized. Native calf thymus tissue extract (200 μl; 60 mg protein/ml) (4) was added to wells as an antigen source. To each well was added 200 μl of patient serum.

Patients. Study patients were individuals who attended our rheumatic disease clinic. They included 5 patients with anti-Sm, 30 with anti-nRNP, 5 with anti-La, and 50 with anti-Ro. Sixty-two normal, race-matched individuals served as controls. All patients with anti-Sm also had anti-nRNP. Anti-Ro was also present in 4 of the 5 patients who had anti-La.

Four of the patients with anti-Sm had systemic lupus erythematosus (SLE), and 1 had SLE-scleroderma overlap. Anti-nRNP–positive patients included 16 with SLE, 8 with mixed connective tissue disease (MCTD), and 6 with other connective tissue diseases. Of the anti-La–positive patients, 3 had SLE, 1 had Sjögren's syndrome, and 1 had SLE–Sjögren's syndrome overlap. Anti-Ro–positive patients included 14 with primary Sjögren's syndrome, 22 with Sjögren's syndrome–rheumatoid arthritis (RA) overlap, and 14 with Sjögren's syndrome–SLE overlap.

Diagnoses of SLE and RA were made using the American Rheumatism Association criteria (5,6). All of the RA patients with Sjögren's syndrome had typical erosive changes shown in their joint radiographs. Diagnosis of MCTD was made on the basis of the presence of components of 3 connective tissue diseases, SLE, scleroderma, and polymyositis, and the presence of anti-nRNP and the absence of anti-Sm. Sjögren's syndrome was diagnosed using the criteria of the Research Committee for Sjögren's Syndrome in

Masahiko Nishikai, MD: Chief, Rheumatology Section, Department of Internal Medicine, The Second Tokyo National Hospital, Tokyo, Japan; Susumu Sekiguchi, MD: Professor of Laboratory Medicine, National Defense Medical College, Saitama, Japan.

Address reprint requests to Masahiko Nishikai, MD, Rheumatology Section, Department of Internal Medicine, The Second Tokyo National Hospital, 2-5-1 Higashigaoka, Meguro-ku Tokyo, 152 Japan.

Submitted for publication July 9, 1984; accepted in revised form December 14, 1984.

Japan (7), which are a modification of the criteria of Shearn (8).

HLA typing. Heparinized blood was used to separate lymphocytes and T and B cells by standard techniques from the NIH and Eighth International Histocompatibility Workshop. Typing was done using the microdroplet lymphocytotoxicity test (9). The 568 anti-HLA (TE-10 and TB-25) sera used were those submitted to the Second Asia and Oceania Histocompatibility Workshop and those kindly supplied by Dr. P. I. Terasaki of the University of California, Los Angeles. HLA specificities of the control subjects had been determined previously, in accordance with the standards of the Seventh and Eighth International Histocompatibility and Japanese Workshops.

Statistical analysis. Groups were compared using the chi-square test.

RESULTS

Prevalence of HLA antigens in the patient groups and healthy controls is shown in Table 1. The presence of autoantibodies to Sm, nRNP, La, and Ro correlated with HLA–B61(40) ($P < 0.00005$; relative risk = 20.8), DQw3(MT4) ($P < 0.0005$; relative risk = 6.9), DRw8 ($P < 0.005$; relative risk = 11.8), and B7 ($P < 0.05$; relative risk = 2.9), respectively, in these Japanese subjects. However, results related to anti-Sm and anti-La are tentative because of the small number of patients tested.

DISCUSSION

There are some differences in the frequency of occurrence of HLA antigens among the Japanese population compared with whites. For example, HLA–B8 and DR3 are frequently found in white patients with various autoimmune diseases, but are found very rarely in Japanese patients (Table 1).

Reports on the relationship between autoantibody expression and HLA antigens in white patients are small in number and controversial. With regard to anti-Sm, Ahearn et al (10) could find no correlated HLA antigen. In contrast, Schur et al (11) described a strong correlation with DR7. HLA–B61(40) was found to be correlated with anti-Sm in our Japanese series.

Correlations between HLA antigens and anti-nRNP have not been found in whites (10,12); however, anti-nRNP was correlated with the DQ locus B cell antigen, DQw3 in our Japanese series.

HLA–Dw2 and Dw3 (13) and HLA–DR3 (14) have been reported to be related antigens in white patients with positive anti-La. In our Japanese patients, the strongest MHC determinant for anti-La was HLA–DRw8.

HLA–DR3 and DR2 have been reported to correlate with anti-Ro in white patients (12,14). In our Japanese patients with anti-Ro, a relatively weak correlation with B7 was found. The lack of correlation with HLA–DR3 in our series is not surprising, since

Table 1. Frequencies of and correlations between autoantibodies and HLA antigens in Japanese patients with connective tissue diseases

HLA antigen	Anti-Sm (n = 5)	P*	Anti–nuclear RNP (n = 30)	P*	Anti-La (n = 5)	P*	Anti-Ro (n = 50)	P*	Local controls (n = 62)
B7	0	NS	4 (13%)	NS	0	NS	16 (32%)	<0.05	9 (14%)
B8	1 (20%)	NS	1 (3%)	NS	0	NS	1 (2%)	NS	1 (2%)
B39(16)	0	NS	5 (17%)	NS	2 (40%)	<0.05	3 (6%)	NS	3 (5%)
B61(40)	4 (80%)	<0.00005	8 (27%)	NS	0	NS	12 (24%)	NS	10 (16%)
DR1	0	NS	2 (7%)	NS	0	NS	13 (24%)	NS	8 (13%)
DR2	1 (20%)	NS	13 (43%)	NS	1 (20%)	NS	21 (42%)	NS	22 (35%)
DR3	1 (20%)	NS	2 (7%)	NS	0	NS	0	NS	0
DR4	4 (80%)	NS	20 (67%)	NS	1 (20%)	NS	24 (48%)	NS	30 (48%)
DR5	0	NS	2 (7%)	NS	0	NS	6 (12%)	NS	4 (6%)
DRw6	0	NS	5 (17%)	NS	2 (40%)	<0.05	1 (2%)	NS	5 (8%)
DR7	0	NS	0	NS	1 (20%)	NS	0	NS	0
DRw8	0	NS	6 (20%)	NS	3 (60%)	<0.005	12 (24%)	NS	7 (11%)
DRw9	1 (20%)	NS	4 (13%)	NS	0	NS	8 (16%)	NS	13 (21%)
DRw10	0	NS	0	NS	0	NS	1 (2%)	NS	1 (2%)
DRw13	2 (40%)	NS	5 (17%)	NS	1 (20%)	NS	1 (2%)	NS	15 (24%)
DRw52	1 (20%)	NS	15 (50%)	NS	4 (80%)	NS	22 (44%)	NS	31 (50%)
DRw53	5 (100%)	NS	25 (83%)	NS	3 (60%)	NS	31 (62%)	NS	41 (66%)
DQw1	2 (50%)	NS	20 (67%)	NS	3 (60%)	NS	39 (78%)	NS	48 (77%)
DQw3	5 (100%)	<0.05	28 (93%)	<0.0005	4 (80%)	NS	23 (46%)	NS	30 (48%)

* P values are versus normal Japanese controls. NS = not significant ($\chi^2 < 3.84$, $P > 0.05$).

this antigen is found only very rarely in the Japanese population.

Our study has shown that autoantibody expressions are related to the different genetic influences coded by HLA antigens (10–15). The prevalence of autoantibodies to Sm, nRNP, Ro, and La in our Japanese subjects is not very different from that in series of white subjects (data not shown). Nonetheless, our findings show that even among different races, autoantibody expression is partially controlled immunogenetically, although by different HLA antigens. This is compatible with the fact that differences also exist among races in the prevalence of the various symptoms and laboratory findings in the same diseases. In addition, we have shown that discrete antibody expression in a Japanese population is at least partially controlled by the distinct immunogenetic background of that population.

Further study on the relationship between autoantibodies and immunogenetic background may enable us to classify the connective tissue diseases into subsets, which could lead to a better understanding and better management of the patients in each subset.

REFERENCES

1. Arnett FC, Shulman LE: Studies in familial systemic lupus erythematosus. Medicine (Baltimore) 55:313–322, 1976
2. Stastny P: HLA-D in the rheumatic diseases. J Reticuloendothel Soc 26:601–607, 1979
3. Tan EM, Kunkel HG: Characterizations of a soluble nuclear antigen precipitating with sera of patients with systemic lupus erythematosus. J Immunol 96:464–471, 1966
4. Nishikai M, Reichlin M: Heterogeneity of precipitating antibodies in polymyositis and dermatomyositis: characterization of the Jo-1 antibody system. Arthritis Rheum 23:881–888, 1980
5. Tan EM, Cohen AS, Fries JF, Masi AT, McShane DJ, Rothfield NF, Schaller JG, Talal N, Winchester RJ: The 1982 revised criteria for the classification of systemic lupus erythematosus. Arthritis Rheum 25:1271–1277, 1982
6. Ropes MW, Benett GA, Cobb S, Jacox R, Jessar RA: 1958 revision of diagnostic criteria for rheumatoid arthritis. Bull Rheum Dis 9:175–176, 1958
7. Research Committee for Sjögren's Syndrome: Diagnostic criteria for Sjögren's syndrome, Annual Report of the Ministry of Health and Welfare of Japan, 1978, p 6
8. Shearn MA: Sjögren's Syndrome. Philadelphia, WB Saunders, 1971, p 11
9. Terasaki PI, Bernoco D, Park MS, Ozturk G, Iwaki Y: Microdroplet testing for HLA A-B-C-D antigens. Am J Clin Pathol 69:103–120, 1978
10. Ahearn JM, Provost TT, Dorsch CA, Stevens MB, Bias WB, Arnett FC: Interrelationships of HLA–DR, MB, and MT phenotypes, autoantibody expression, and clinical features in systemic lupus erythematosus. Arthritis Rheum 25:1031–1040, 1982
11. Schur PH, Myer I, Garonoy M, Carpenter CB: Associations between systemic lupus erythematosus and major histocompatibility complex: clinical and immunological considerations. Clin Immunol Immunopathol 24:263–275, 1982
12. Bell DA, Maddison PJ: Serologic subsets in systemic lupus erythematosus: an examination of autoantibodies in relationship to clinical features of disease and HLA antigens. Arthritis Rheum 23:1268–1273, 1980
13. Manthorpe R, Teppo A-M, Bendixen G, Wegelius O: Antibodies to SS–B in chronic inflammatory connective tissue diseases: relationship with HLA–Dw2 and HLA–Dw3 antigens in primary Sjögren's syndrome. Arthritis Rheum 25:662–667, 1982
14. Wilson RW, Provost TT, Bias WB, Alexander EL, Edlow DW, Hochberg MC, Stevens MB, Arnett FC: Sjögren's syndrome: influence of multiple HLA–D region alloantigens on clinical and serologic expression. Arthritis Rheum 27:1245–1253, 1984
15. Arnett FC, Hirsch TJ, Bias WB, Nishikai M, Reichlin M: The Jo-1 antibody system in myositis: relationships to clinical features and HLA. J Rheumatol 8:925–930, 1981

BRIEF REPORT

AORTIC REGURGITATION IN GIANT CELL ARTERITIS

ALICE V. KLINKHOFF, GRAHAM D. REID, and MICHAEL MOSCOVICH

Giant cell arteritis (GCA) is a generalized large vessel vasculitis occurring in elderly persons. Temporal artery involvement, with headaches and blindness resulting from involvement of the posterior ciliary and ophthalmic arteries, is a frequent finding (1–7). A feature of GCA that is not widely recognized is that it affects the large arteries diffusely and may be the cause of claudication, aneurysmal dilatation, and aortic aneurysm dissection and rupture (2,8–14). We describe a patient with known GCA who developed progressive aortic dilatation and, eventually, aortic regurgitation while being treated with low-dose prednisone. Aortic regurgitation as a manifestation of GCA has been described previously in only 6 patients.

Case report. In 1977 a 65-year-old white woman developed severe temporal headaches with scalp tenderness. Temporal artery biopsy showed a granulomatous inflammation of the media and adjacent internal elastic lamina, with focal destruction of the latter. A heavy lymphohistiocytic infiltrate with occasional multinucleated giant cells was present. The histologic features were those of GCA. She took prednisone, 20 mg daily, for 3 months, and over the next 7 years the dosage was gradually reduced to 2.5 mg daily. The erythrocyte sedimentation rate (ESR), which was initially 104 mm/hour, never fell below 35 mm/hour. In June 1982 she developed exertional dyspnea without chest pain, ankle swelling, orthopnea, or syncopal episodes. There was no history of hypertension or rheumatic fever, and a heart murmur had not previously been heard. In January 1983 she was referred for evaluation of increasing exertional dyspnea and aortic regurgitation.

During the month prior to hospitalization she had noted shoulder-girdle morning stiffness lasting 1 hour, myalgia, and a 5-lb weight loss. She denied having fever, headaches, visual symptoms, or jaw claudication.

On examination she was afebrile. The right temporal artery was palpable but not tender or enlarged, and no bruit was heard. The left temporal artery had previously been biopsied. Ocular examination findings were unremarkable. Examination of the joints and muscles showed no abnormalities. Blood pressure was 180/80 in both arms. Peripheral pulses were bounding in quality, and symmetric. The cardiac apex was visible in the sixth intercostal space in the midclavicular line. There was a grade 3/6 diastolic decrescendo murmur maximal at the second right intercostal space and a grade 3/6 systolic murmur in the same location radiating to the carotid arteries. The abdominal aorta was palpably enlarged with a bruit, but no other bruits were heard.

Relevant laboratory data included: ESR 38 mm/hour (Westergren), hemoglobin 13.4 gm/dl, white blood cell count 9,200/mm^3, normal platelet count, normal alkaline phosphatase, and a negative serologic test for syphilis. Electrocardiogram demonstrated Q waves consistent with an old anterior infarction. Cardiac ultrasound confirmed aortic regurgitation and demonstrated no valvular vegetations. Chest radiographs from 1972 and 1977 were available for compari-

From the Divisions of Rheumatology and Cardiology, Department of Medicine, Vancouver General Hospital, University of British Columbia, Vancouver, British Columbia, Canada.

Alice V. Klinkhoff, MD: Fellow of the Canadian Arthritis Society; Graham D. Reid, MB; Michael Moscovich, MD.

Address reprint requests to Dr. Graham Reid, The Arthritis Centre, 895 West 10th Avenue, Vancouver, British Columbia, V5Z 1L7, Canada.

Submitted for publication June 19, 1984; accepted in revised form November 20, 1984.

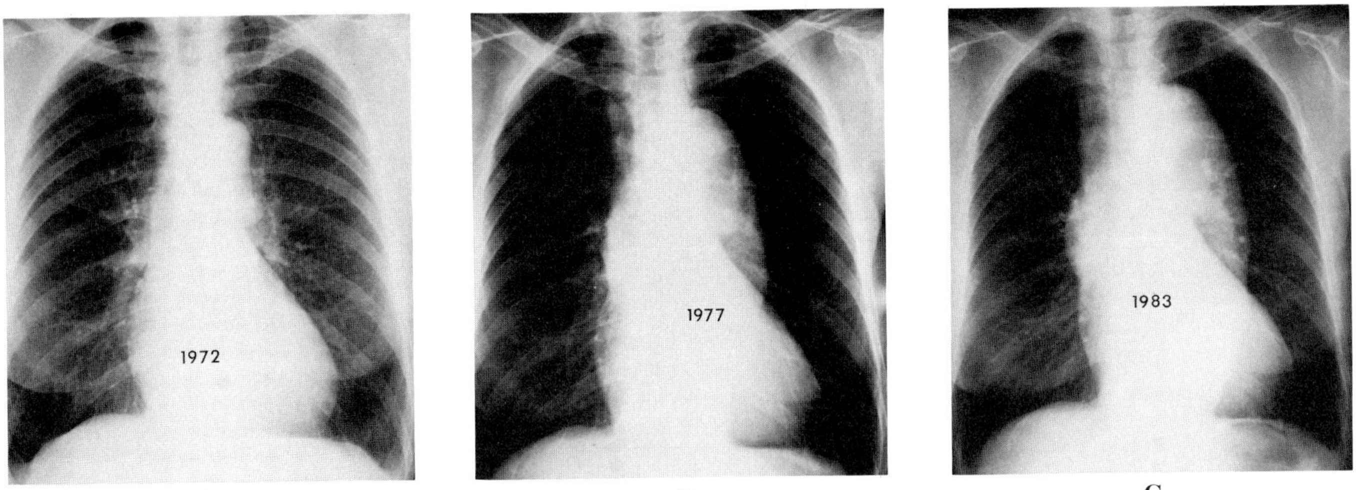

A B C

Figure 1. Chest radiographs taken in 1972 (**A**), 1977 (**B**), and 1983 (**C**), revealing progressive widening of the mediastinum with aneurysmal dilatation of the aorta and cardiomegaly.

son with recent radiographs. These revealed progressive widening of the mediastinum with aneurysmal dilatation of the aorta since 1977, and cardiomegaly (Figure 1). Arteriography of the coronary vessels, ascending, and descending aorta showed a large aneurysm of the ascending aorta with dilatation of the aortic ring and gross regurgitation of contrast material into the left ventricle (Figure 2). The aorta and its branch vessels were dilated. Additional findings included coronary artery disease with obstruction of the anterior descending and circumflex arteries.

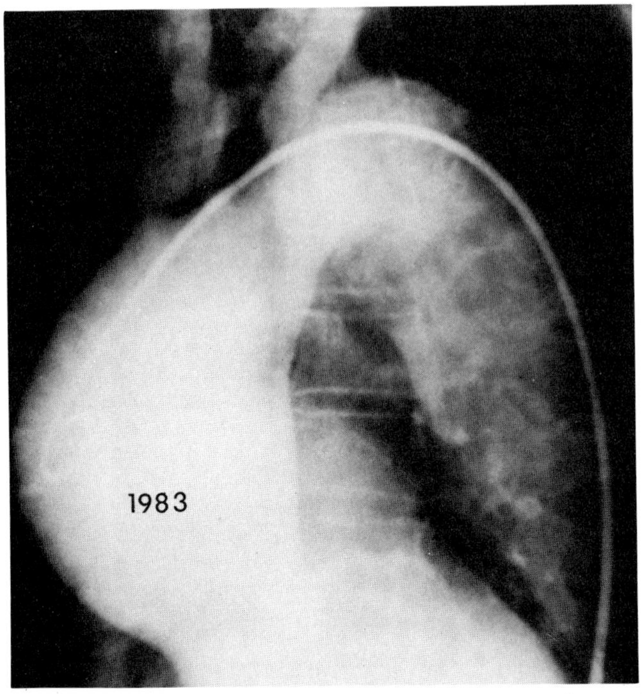

Figure 2. Arteriography of the coronary vessels, ascending, and descending aorta, showing a large aneurysm of the ascending aorta with dilatation of the aortic ring and gross regurgitation of contrast material into the left ventricle.

She was treated with prednisone, 60 mg daily. At followup 6 months later she was taking prednisone, 20 mg daily. Polymyalgic symptoms had resolved and the cardiac status remained unchanged. The ESR was 15 mm/hour. Repeat chest radiographs showed no further increase in aortic dilatation.

Discussion. Our patient had proven GCA and, over a 7-year period, had taken less than the recommended dosage of prednisone. While under observation she developed symptomatic aortic regurgitation and polymyalgic symptoms. The dramatic aortic dilatation is clearly demonstrated in serial radiographs taken over a 5-year period. While we could not confirm a diagnosis by biopsy, the sequence of events and radiologic findings are most compatible with a diagnosis of polymyalgia rheumatica and aortic regurgitation developing secondary to GCA of the ascending aorta.

Involvement of major arteries in GCA is well documented (8,15–17). Of 248 GCA patients in 1 study, 34 were judged clinically to have involvement of the aorta or its major branches (17). In 10 patients this was confirmed by angiography, which showed typical arterial occlusions or aneurysmal dilatation. Three patients in that series died; each of them had giant cell arteritis at autopsy. These 3 deaths were caused by acute dissection of an aortic aneurysm which occurred while patients were taking low doses of prednisone. A Swedish autopsy study described large vessel involvement in 16 patients who died with

Table 1. Review of reported cases of aortic regurgitation attributed to giant cell arteritis*

Patient no., reference	Age	Temporal artery biopsy	ESR	Disease duration (years)	Radiologic findings	Treatment	Course
1, Paulley and Hughes (9)	72	+	33	6	Aneurysmal dilatation of aortic arch	Prednisone, 80 mg/day	Several months followup: doing well taking prednisone, 20 mg/day
2, How and Strachan (19)	65	+	Normal	2.5	Dilatation of aorta	Prednisolone, 9 mg/day	1.5 years followup: no deterioration of aortic regurgitation
3, Castleman and McNeely (20)	66	ND	57	7	Aneurysmal dilatation of ascending and descending aorta; angiography: aortic regurgitation, ascending and descending aneurysm	Aortic valve replacement, aneurysmectomy of ascending and descending aorta	Died 19 days postsurgery; post mortem: giant cell aortitis
4, Fauchald et al (10)	NA	+	NA	NA	NA	Prednisone, 40–60 mg/day, decreased over 4 weeks to 5–12.5 mg/day	NA
5, Fauchald et al (10)	NA	+	NA	NA	NA	Prednisone, 40–60 mg/day, decreased over 4 weeks to 5–12.5 mg/day	Died; post mortem: dissecting aortic arch aneurysm
6, Fauchald et al (10)	NA	+	NA	NA	NA	Prednisone, 40–60 mg/day, decreased over 4 weeks to 5–12.5 mg/day	NA
7, Present report	72	+	38	7	Aneurysmal dilatation of aortic arch; angiography: aortic regurgitation, ascending aortic aneurysm	Prednisone, 60 mg/day, decreased over 6 months to 20 mg/day	6 months followup: stable aortic regurgitation

* ESR = erythrocyte sedimentation rate; ND = not done; NA = information not available.

known GCA; in 12 of these there was aortic involvement (18). Other researchers have reported asymmetric pulse volumes, vascular bruits, claudication, and aortic aneurysmal dilatation and dissection (8–11,13).

Aortic regurgitation secondary to GCA has been described previously in 6 patients (9,10,19,20). These cases are summarized in Table 1. Of the 7 patients (including our own), none was known to have a heart murmur prior to the onset of symptoms of GCA. In 6 of 7, biopsy of temporal arteries had confirmed the diagnosis of GCA. In patient 3, who had a compatible clinical history and giant cell aortitis at autopsy, a temporal artery biopsy was not performed during life, and at autopsy the temporal arteries were normal. Additional information is available on patients 1, 2, 3, and 7 (our patient). All were women. Two of them (patients 1 and 3) were hypertensive. The duration of symptoms of GCA prior to institution of appropriate therapy was prolonged in patients 1, 2, and 3 (range 2.5–7 years). No patient suffered ophthalmologic or neurologic complications during the period prior to treatment.

In 3 patients (patients 2, 3, and 7) symptoms were related primarily to the aortic regurgitation itself, and only careful history-taking revealed the possibility of GCA. In patient 2, aortic regurgitation was an incidental finding when she presented with myalgia and headaches. All 7 patients had the typical diastolic aortic regurgitation murmur and in 4 (patients 1, 2, 3, and 7) there was radiologically evident dilatation of the ascending aorta.

Six of the 7 patients received steroid treatment for GCA. Although patient 3 had a suggestive clinical history, a markedly elevated ESR, and progressive aortic regurgitation, GCA was not diagnosed, and she did not receive prednisone. Our patient took only 20 mg of prednisone daily after the initial diagnosis of GCA, and this dose was gradually reduced to 2.5 mg daily when aortic regurgitation was first detected. Similarly, patients 4, 5, and 6 developed aortic regurgitation while being followed for known GCA. Treatment in these patients had included prednisone at an initial dose of 40–60 mg daily, which was reduced to 5–12.5 mg daily over a period of 1–4 weeks.

Two patients (patients 3 and 5) died from complications of giant cell aortitis. Patient 3 died 19 days after aortic valve replacement and aortic aneurysm resection, from rupture of the aortotomy suture line. Patient 5 died from a dissecting aortic arch aneurysm.

Three patients (patients 1, 2, and 7) had stable aortic regurgitation when followed up 3 months to 2 years after diagnosis and treatment. At followup, 2 patients (patients 1 and 7) were taking prednisone, 20 mg daily; the dosage taken by patient 2 was not specified.

Although the ESR is generally a sensitive indicator of disease activity in GCA, in 3 patients (patients 1, 2, and 7) symptoms of GCA and aortic regurgitation developed in spite of a normal or only moderately increased ESR. In patient 1, the ESR was never known to be higher than 33 mm/hour. In patient 2, an illness characterized by anorexia, weight loss, and elevated ESR had previously been investigated without diagnosis. When the patient was first seen with aortic regurgitation, the ESR was "normal," despite a diagnostic temporal artery biopsy.

GCA should be considered in the evaluation of aortic regurgitation in elderly patients. When following patients with GCA, careful attention should be given to the cardiovascular findings since major vessel involvement is associated with significant morbidity and mortality. It is important to be aware that large vessel arteritis can progress with low-dose prednisone therapy and that the ESR is not a reliable indicator of disease activity.

The long-term prognosis of aortic regurgitation in this group of patients is not known, but surgery probably should not be contemplated until the patient has had the benefit of an adequate course of steroid therapy.

Addendum. Since this report was prepared, an abstract, describing 16 patients with aortic insufficiency seen over a 30-year period at the Mayo Clinic, has been presented (21).

REFERENCES

1. Hamilton CR, Shelley WM, Tumulty PA: Giant cell arteritis: including temporal arteritis and polymyalgia rheumatica. Medicine (Baltimore) 50:1–27, 1971
2. Cooke WT, Cloake PCP, Govan ADT, Colbeck JC: Temporal arteritis: a generalized vascular disease. Q J Med 15:47–75, 1946
3. Huston KA, Hunder GG, Lie JT, Kennedy BA, Elveback CR: Temporal arteritis: a 25 year epidemiologic, clinical, and pathological study. Ann Intern Med 88:162–167, 1978
4. Hollenhorst RW, Brown JR, Wagener HP, Schick RM: Neurologic aspects of temporal arteritis. Neurology 10:490–498, 1960
5. Whitfield AGW, Bateman M, Cooke WT: Temporal arteritis. Br J Ophthalmol 47:555–556, 1963
6. Parsons-Smith G: Sudden blindness in cranial arteritis. Br J Ophthalmol 43:204–216, 1959
7. Meadows SP: Temporal or giant cell arteritis. Proc R Soc Med 329–333, 1966
8. Mowat AG, Hazleman BL: Polymyalgia rheumatica: a clinical study with particular reference to arterial disease. J Rheumatol 2:190–202, 1974
9. Paulley JW, Hughes JP: Giant-cell arteritis, or arteritis of the aged. Br Med J 2:1562–1567, 1960
10. Fauchald P, Rygvold O, Oystese B: Temporal arteritis and polymyalgia rheumatica: clinical and biopsy findings. Ann Intern Med 77:845–852, 1972
11. Harris M: Dissecting aneurysm of the aorta due to giant cell arteritis. Br Heart J 30:840–844, 1968
12. Reid JV: Dilatation of the aorta due to granulomatous (giant cell) aortitis. Br Heart J 19:206–210, 1957
13. Hunder GG, Ward LE, Burbank MK: Giant cell arteritis producing an aortic arch syndrome. Ann Intern Med 66:578–582, 1967
14. Garret R: Chronic diffuse giant cell mesaortitis with dissecting aneurysm and rupture. Am J Clin Pathol 38:406–414, 1962
15. Hamrin B, Jonsson N, Landberg T: Involvement of large vessels in polymyalgia arteritica. Lancet 1:1193–1196, 1965
16. Harrison RJ, Harrison CV, Kopelman H: Giant cell arteritis with aneurysms: effects of hormone therapy. Br Med J 2:1593–1595, 1955
17. Klein RG, Hunder GG, Stanson AW, Sheps SG: Large artery involvement in giant cell (temporal) arteritis. Ann Intern Med 83:806–812, 1975
18. Oestberg G: Arterial lesions in polymyalgia arteritica. Pathol Microbiol 43:182–186, 1975
19. How J, Strachan RW: Aortic regurgitation as a manifestation of giant cell arteritis. Br Heart J 40:1052–1054, 1978
20. Castleman B, McNeely B: Case records of the Massachusetts General Hospital. N Engl J Med 284:1201–1210, 1971
21. Bowles C, Hunder GG: Aortic valve involvement in temporal arteritis (abstract). Arthritis Rheum (suppl) 27:S86, 1984

BRIEF REPORT

WRIST DROP IN PROGRESSIVE SYSTEMIC SCLEROSIS (SCLERODERMA): COMPLETE RUPTURE OF THE EXTENSOR TENDON MECHANISM

LEWIS H. ROSENBAUM, WILLIAM M. SWARTZ, GERALD P. RODNAN, and THOMAS A. MEDSGER, Jr.

Although rupture of individual tendons at the wrist is a well-recognized occurrence in patients with rheumatoid arthritis (RA) (1), and has also been noted rarely in systemic lupus erythematosus (SLE), a complete extensor tendon rupture leading to wrist drop has not been reported previously. We describe here a young woman with arthritis and tenosynovitis due to progressive systemic sclerosis (PSS or scleroderma), who developed a spontaneous wrist drop following complete rupture of the extensor tendon mechanism of her wrist.

Case report. In April 1977, CC, a 24-year-old secretary, developed Raynaud's phenomenon, involving her fingers and toes, and digital pitting scars. Thereafter, she noted morning stiffness, arthralgias, myalgias, and intermittent swelling of her fingers and hands. Treatment with prednisone, 40 mg/day, diminished the rheumatic symptoms.

In February 1978, she first experienced dysphagia. Examination at that time revealed sclerodactyly and flexion contractures of her fingers and elbows. The metacarpophalangeal and proximal interphalangeal joints of her hands and the wrist joints were tender, but were not swollen. Roentgenograms of the hands and wrists showed no articular abnormalities, but loss of the distal digital tufts was noted. Distal esophageal mobility was markedly reduced on manometric study. The dosage of prednisone was gradually reduced.

We first evaluated this woman in July 1978, when she had fever (102°F), malaise, recurrent polyarthralgia, and weight loss (10 pounds). She complained of dry mouth and "scratchy" eyes. At this time, scleroderma involved the fingers, hands, forearms, and face. There was no salivary gland enlargement or glossitis. There were partially reducible flexion contractures of the proximal interphalangeal joints, and a 30° loss of wrist motion in both flexion and extension. There was no synovial thickening of the wrists or other joints or tendon sheaths, but prominent tendon friction rubs were palpated over the wrist extensors, distal forearms, and anterior tibialis tendons, bilaterally.

Serum antinuclear antibody was present at a titer of 1:300 and in a speckled pattern, the rheumatoid factor titer was 1:40, and tests for anti–extractable nuclear antigen and anti-DNA antibodies were negative. Serum C3 and C4 levels were slightly reduced at 78 mg/dl and 14 mg/dl, respectively. Roentgenograms of the hands and wrists showed diffuse osteoporosis without joint space narrowing or erosions. A lip biopsy disclosed lymphocytic infiltration of minor salivary glands consistent with Sjögren's syndrome.

Treatment with 40 mg of prednisone per day was reinstituted, but subsequent reduction below 15 mg/day resulted in the recurrence of fever, malaise,

From the Division of Rheumatology & Clinical Immunology, Department of Medicine, and the Department of Plastic and Reconstructive Surgery, University of Pittsburgh School of Medicine, Pittsburgh, Pennsylvania.

Supported by grants from the RGK Foundation, Austin, Texas, and the Arthritis Foundation, Western Pennsylvania Chapter.

Lewis H. Rosenbaum, MD: Fellow, Division of Rheumatology & Clinical Immunology; William M. Swartz, MD: Assistant Professor of Plastic Surgery; Thomas A. Medsger, Jr., MD: Associate Professor of Medicine, Division of Rheumatology & Clinical Immunology.

Dr. Rodnan is deceased.

Address reprint requests to Dr. Lewis H. Rosenbaum, Suite 260, 4400 Town Center Professional Building, Southfield, MI 48075.

Submitted for publication November 7, 1983; accepted in revised form November 26, 1984.

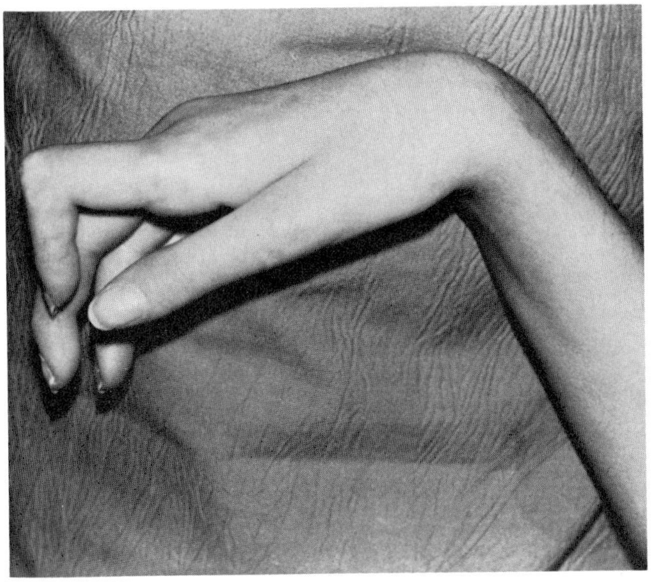

Figure 1. Right wrist drop in a 24-year-old woman with progressive systemic sclerosis. Note the absence of gross swelling of the wrist joint, which was normal on examination.

and polyarthralgia. Attempts to institute D-penicillamine therapy in August 1978, and again in October 1979, resulted in the prompt development of oral ulceration. A 3-month trial of azathioprine, 2 mg/kg daily, was completed without beneficial effect. In May 1980, D-pencillamine was reintroduced at a dosage of 125 mg daily, and this dosage was tolerated without recurrence of oral ulcerations. Slowly, over the next 10 months, an increase in dosage to 500 mg/day was achieved. Thereafter, gradual softening of the skin of the hands and forearms was noted, and after 1 year of treatment, only sclerodactyly and facial skin thickening remained. The total skin score, an estimate of the degree and extent of skin thickening on physical examination, declined from 31 to 8 during this period (2). Prednisone was reduced to a dosage of 12.5 mg/day without incident.

In June 1981, 13 months after the initiation of D-penicillamine, the patient noted the abrupt onset of a painless inability to extend the right wrist (Figure 1). She had received no corticosteroid injection, and she denied local trauma or signs of infection. A radial nerve palsy was suspected, and a wrist splint was applied for several weeks. Although the right forearm extensor muscles appeared to contract appropriately,

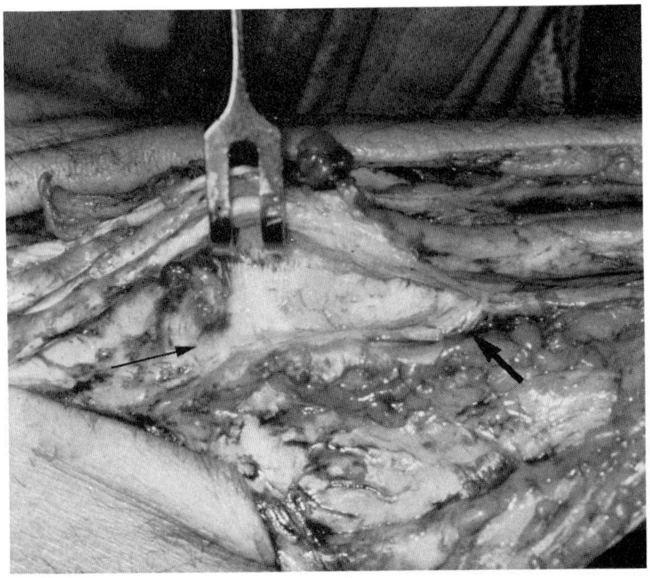

Figure 2. Deep dissection of the right forearm during surgery. The attenuated end of ruptured tendon (**thick arrow**) overlies a synovial mass (**thin arrow**).

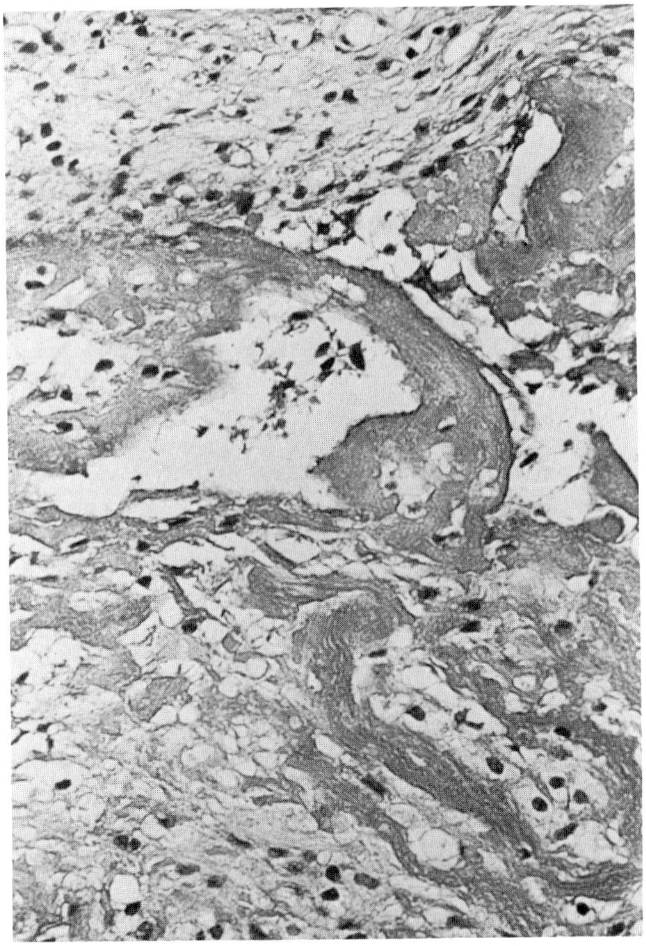

Figure 3. Photomicrograph of wrist synovium, illustrating absence of synovial lining cell hypertrophy and marked surface fibrin deposition (hematoxylin and eosin stained, original magnification × 25).

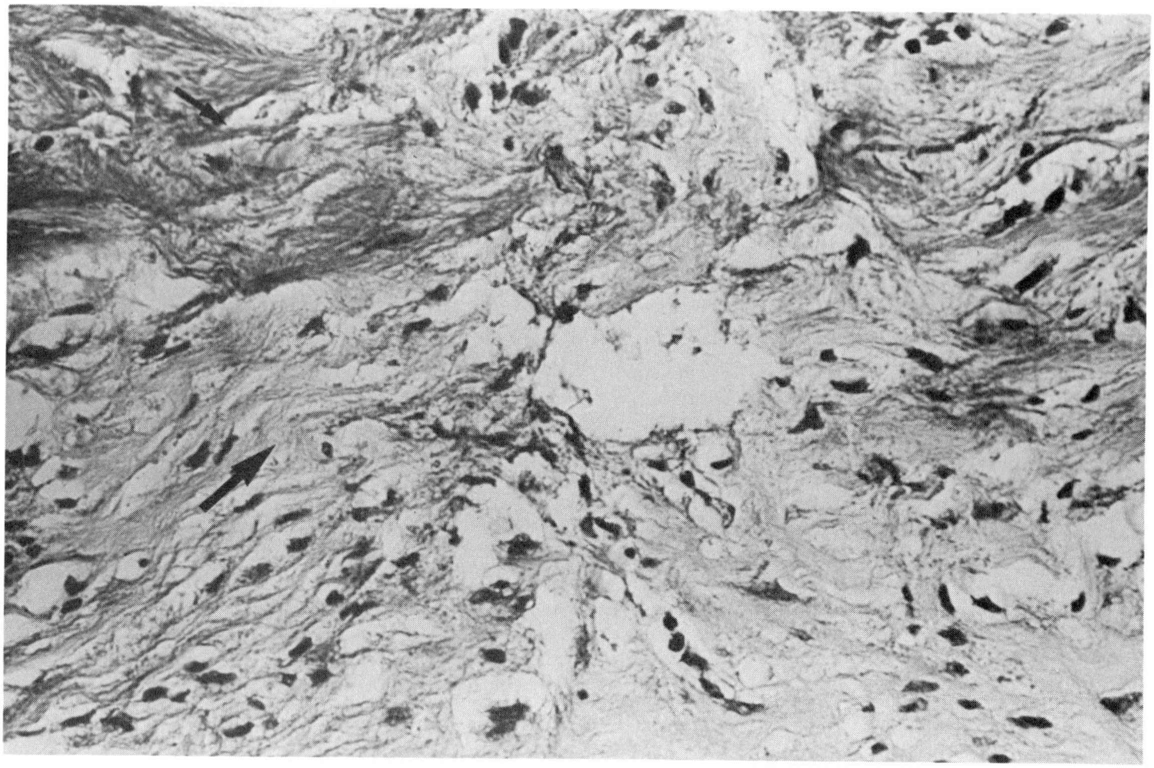

Figure 4. Photomicrograph of wrist extensor tendon. Note prominent infiltration of the tendon (**smaller arrow**) by prominent granulation-like fibroblastic tissue (**larger arrow**) (hematoxylin and eosin stained, original magnification × 25).

no wrist extension was possible. Electromyographic and nerve conduction studies confirmed normal radial nerve function.

A complete rupture of the wrist extensor tendon mechanism was suspected, and the area was surgically explored. A grey, gelatinous mass of synovium, originating in the wrist joint, was seen to be bulging beneath the dorsal retinaculum (Figure 2). The extensor digitorum communis, extensor carpi radialis longus and brevis, extensor indicis proprius, and extensor pollicis longus tendons were all ruptured, with their proximal ends attenuated and intimately adherent to the synovial mass. No reconstruction could be attempted because of the extensive destruction of the tendons, and power of the flexor muscles was not deemed satisfactory to allow a successful tendon transfer.

Histopathologic examination of the synovium and tenosynovium about the wrist joint revealed mild, chronic synovitis with minimal lining cell proliferation. Fibrin deposits were present on the surface of the synovium (Figure 3). No subsynovial collections of lymphocytes or plasma cells were seen. There was nonspecific degeneration of tendons with increased fibrous tissue and infiltration of granulation-like fibroblastic tissue (Figure 4).

Discussion. Rheumatic complaints are often an early manifestation of progressive systemic sclerosis. Since, occasionally, there is objective evidence of polyarthritis, a number of these patients are first thought to have rheumatoid arthritis (2). Despite certain early similarities, the sequelae of arthritis and tenosynovitis are quite different in PSS than in RA. In the former, fibrosis of paraarticular structures and, to a lesser extent, synovial inflammation are associated with the development of contractures, rather than erosion, joint laxity, or subluxation that occurs in RA patients. Fibrinous deposits on the synovial surfaces of joints and tendon sheaths are responsible for palpable, and at times audible, joint and tendon friction rubs in patients with PSS, especially those with widespread, diffuse scleroderma (3).

Our patient had the typical histologic features of PSS involving the synovium, with bland inflammation, surface fibrin deposition, and minimal synovial lining hyperplasia. Although it could be argued that this patient had both PSS and RA, the histologic features and absence of juxtaarticular erosions suggest that PSS is the best unifying diagnosis. Mixed connective tissue disease was not considered further because of the absence of the anti-RNP antibody and other lupus-like manifestations. Rupture of a digital extensor tendon was recently reported in a patient who had PSS complicated by amyloidosis (4). In our patient, the excised tissue failed to reveal amyloid on staining with Congo red and thioflavin T.

Attenuation or rupture of tendons in PSS alone has not been reported previously, which is in contrast with the relatively frequent rupture of the extensor tendons of the thumb and fingers in RA (1) and the occasional occurrence of such tendon ruptures in SLE (5). Individual tendon rupture, rather than rupture of the entire tendon mechanism, is the rule in RA. It is possible that our patient's therapy may have played a role in the development of this complication. It has been suggested that corticosteroids contribute to tendon rupture in RA and SLE (5,6). These compounds are presumed to impair tendon healing through their catabolic effects and the induction of a negative nitrogen balance.

D-penicillamine has been shown to interfere with collagen cross-linking (7) and to increase the proportion of soluble tissue collagen, leading to thinning and friability of the skin (8). Several studies have indicated a beneficial effect of D-penicillamine in the treatment of PSS (9–11), and our patient had a striking reduction in skin thickness while receiving this drug. D-penicillamine–treated rats have been reported to have significantly less peritendinous scarring than controls, following a surgically-induced tendon injury (12). It is thus possible that in our patient, D-penicillamine may have impeded the scarring of tendons injured by tenosynovial inflammation and granulation tissue.

Multiple tendon ruptures of the extensor mechanism of the wrist are indeed an unusual event. We hypothesize that rupture occurred in our patient because of invasion of the tendon by granulation tissue, thus undermining its structure. The contributions of D-penicillamine and corticosteroids in this case are unknown. One might expect that RA patients would also have rupture of the entire tendon mechanism, since they often take these medications. Instead, individual tendon rupture is the rule in RA. Physicians should be aware that wrist drop may be related to an extensor tendon rupture and that prompt evaluation is necessary if surgical repair is to be attempted.

REFERENCES

1. Clayton ML, Ferlic DC: The wrist in rheumatoid arthritis. Clin Orthop 106:192–197, 1975
2. Steen VD, Medsger TA Jr, Rodnan GP: D-penicillamine therapy in progressive systemic sclerosis (scleroderma). Ann Intern Med 97:652–659, 1982
3. Rodnan GP, Medsger TA Jr: The rheumatic manifestations of progressive systemic sclerosis (scleroderma). Clin Orthop 57:81–91, 1968
4. Rodnan GP: The nature of joint involvement in progressive systemic sclerosis (diffuse scleroderma): clinical study and pathologic examination of synovium in twenty-nine patients. Ann Intern Med 56:422–439, 1962
5. Horwitz HM, DiBeneditto JD Jr, Allegra SR, Baumann HM: Scleroderma, amyloidosis, and extensor tendon rupture. Arthritis Rheum 25:1141–1143, 1982
6. Kahn MA, Ballou SP: Tendon rupture in systemic lupus erythematosus. J Rheumatol 8:308–310, 1981
7. Halpern AA, Horowitz BG, Nagel DA: Tendon ruptures associated with corticosteroid therapy. West J Med 127:378–382, 1977
8. Nimni ME: A defect in the intramolecular and intermolecular cross-linking of collagen caused by penicillamine. I. Metabolic and functional abnormalities in soft tissues. J Biol Chem 243:1457–1466, 1968
9. Uitto UJ, Helin P, Rasmussen O, Lorenzen I: Skin collagen in patients with scleroderma: biosynthesis and maturation in vitro, and the effect of D-penicillamine. Ann Clin Res 2:228–234, 1970
10. Asboe-Hansen G: Treatment of generalized scleroderma with inhibitors of connective tissue formation. Acta Derm Venereol (Stockh) 55:461–465, 1975
11. Bora FW Jr, Lane JM, Prockop DJ: Inhibitors of collagen biosynthesis as a means of controlling scar formation in tendon injury. J Bone Joint Surg 54:1501–1508, 1972
12. Jayson MIV: The effects of D-penicillamine on collagen in systemic sclerosis and rheumatoid arthritis, Symposium on Penicillamine Research in Rheumatoid Disease. Spatind, Norway, March 7–10, 1976

BRIEF REPORT

COMBINATION IMMUNOSUPPRESSIVE TREATMENT OF STEROID-RESISTANT DERMATOMYOSITIS/POLYMYOSITIS

DANIEL J. WALLACE, ALLAN L. METZGER, and KATHY K. WHITE

Dermatomyositis (DM) and polymyositis (PM) are inflammatory autoimmune muscle disorders in which the majority of patients respond to high-dose corticosteroids (1). Those infrequent patients who do not respond to steroids or whose dosage requirements are unsafe, generally improve with the addition of immunosuppressive agents such as chlorambucil, cyclophosphamide, azathioprine, or methotrexate (2–5). Perhaps up to 5% of all DM/PM patients will not adequately respond to the above regimen, do not have an underlying malignancy, and will require further aggressive treatment. We report the successful management of 2 patients with refractory inflammatory myositis, using steroids in combination with 2 simultaneously administered immunosuppressive agents, chlorambucil and methotrexate.

Case reports. Patient 1, a 42-year-old white woman, was in excellent health until September 1980, when she developed polyarthritis and fever. In November 1980, she was hospitalized for bilateral interstitial pulmonary infiltrates, fever, and hypoxemia with a PO_2 value of 58 mm Hg while breathing room air. The test result for antinuclear antibody (ANA) was positive with a titer of 1:1,280 (speckled pattern); results of the anti-DNA (Farr), anti–extractable nuclear antigen, and complement studies were within normal limits. The creatine phosphokinase (CPK) level was 3,678 units/liter (normal <180). Bronchoscopy and a biopsy specimen revealed evidence of fibrosing alveolitis and prednisone, 60 mg/day, was started. Since her sputum cultures were positive for *Mycobacterium tuberculosis*, isoniazid and rifampin were prescribed. With therapy, the CPK level dropped to 767 units/liter in 1 month and her pulmonary disease completely resolved.

In February 1981, she developed fever, edematous fingers, a heliotrope rash around her eyes, and Gottron's lesions on the metacarpal and the interphalangeal joints. She received 3 intravenous pulses of 1 gm of methylprednisolone, and her CPK decreased from 2,000 to 525. However, her muscle weakness persisted and the prednisone dosage could not be tapered below 40 mg/day.

Over the next 2 months, methotrexate, 15 mg/week, was given intravenously; however, after 120 mg of methotrexate over 8 weeks and 40 mg of prednisone/day, the CPK value rose to 16,070, and by March 1981 the patient was barely able to walk.

Again, 1 gm of intravenous methylprednisolone was given daily for 3 days, without improvement, and subsequently, from June 1981 to August 1981 she underwent fifteen 40 ml/kg plasmaphereses with albumin replacement. Her CPK dropped from 13,900 to 2,500 with 15 mg of methotrexate weekly and 25 mg of prednisone daily. Over the next 6 months she remained on the above regimen; her CPK level stabilized between 2,000 and 3,000 units/liter, and her muscle strength was 3+/5. In February 1982, she underwent an additional 6 plasmaphereses which were of no benefit; her CPK level was up to 17,770, and 60 mg of prednisone daily was started along with 150 mg of oral azathioprine daily.

By November 1982, her CPK value was in the

From the Division of Rheumatology, Department of Medicine, Cedars-Sinai Medical Center, UCLA School of Medicine, Los Angeles, California.

Daniel J. Wallace, MD, FACP: Assistant Clinical Professor of Medicine; Allan L. Metzger, MD: Associate Clinical Professor of Medicine; Kathy K. White, BS, RDH.

Address reprint requests to Daniel J. Wallace, MD, Cedars-Sinai Medical Center, 8737 Beverly Boulevard, Suite 203, Los Angeles, CA 90048.

Submitted for publication September 9, 1984; accepted in revised form November 26, 1984.

1,000–2,000 range while she received prednisone, 20 mg/day, and azathioprine, 250 mg/day. A third course of pulse steroids was given in November 1982 without effect on either muscle strength or CPK level.

In December 1982, an electromyogram of the right upper and lower extremities was performed. Increased irritability and increased polyphasic potentials were noted. No positive sharp waves or fasciculations were seen. In March 1983, her CPK level was 15,000; a biopsy specimen from the right quadriceps muscle revealed multifocal inflammation with segmental fibrinoid necrosis, and regeneration was found along with variable fiber atrophy and rounding.

After 1 year, the azathioprine was stopped and oral cyclophosphamide was begun at a dosage of 100 mg daily; later it was administered at doses of 350–500 mg intravenously every 2 to 3 weeks. Her weakness persisted and the CPK level never fell below 4,000 while she was taking 20–60 mg of prednisone in addition to cyclophosphamide.

In November 1983, the patient's heliotrope rash and Gottron's rash were quite active, proximal muscle strength was grade 4/5, and her CPK level was 3,600 units/liter. She was started on a regimen of prednisone, 60 mg/day, 15 mg of oral methotrexate weekly, and 6 mg of chlorambucil daily.

Within 1 month, the CPK level was less than 1,000, and it became normal by 5 months. After 1 year of this combined therapy, the patient's rashes have disappeared, and her most recent CPK test value was normal for the first time in 4 years. She is currently receiving 15 mg of prednisone daily, chlorambucil, 4 mg daily, and methotrexate, 12.5 mg/week orally. She has no muscle pain or stiffness, is able to function fully as a homemaker and dental hygienist, and has no systemic or drug-related complaints. We anticipate gradually lowering her steroid dosage and administering methotrexate less frequently.

Patient 2, a 29-year-old black woman, was in excellent health until October 1981, when she developed knee effusions, fatigue, and weakness. In January 1982, her proximal muscle strength was grade 4/5, and bilateral pleural effusions, mild anemia, and 3+ proteinuria were noted. Her CPK level was 14,000 units/liter, Westergren erythrocyte sedimentation rate 120 mm/hour, and a biopsy specimen from the left quadriceps muscle revealed extensive degeneration along with focal necrosis, basophilic changes, sarcolemmal proliferation, and an inflammatory infiltrate. Results of ANA, rheumatoid factor, C3, T4, complement determinations, and hepatitis serologies were negative.

She started receiving 80 mg of prednisone/day, and the CPK value became normal 4 months later. The prednisone dose was decreased to 50 mg, she became weak, and her CPK level rose to 2,300 by July 1982. Methotrexate was started intramuscularly at 25–50 mg weekly, and the CPK level decreased to 150 units/liter 5 months later (December 1982). However, she subsequently experienced a disease flare on this regimen, and the serum CPK value increased to 20,000. She was hospitalized in February 1983 with bilateral pleural effusions, myocarditis, fever, and weakness. Results of all cultures and immunologic studies were negative. She received 3 daily intravenous 1-gm methylprednisolone pulses, and the CPK level dropped to 1,947 within 2 months.

Azathioprine was begun at a daily dose of 150 mg in addition to 40 mg of prednisone; over the next 2 months her CPK value remained stable, but she became weaker. In June 1983, chlorambucil, 6 mg/day, was substituted for azathioprine. In August 1983, her CPK level was 2,935 and methotrexate (15 mg/week orally) was added to the chlorambucil and 35 mg/day of prednisone. Within 2 months, her CPK level was 160 and it has remained normal since. After more than 1 year of treatment, she is totally asymptomatic taking prednisone, 15 mg/day, methotrexate, 15 mg/week orally, and 4 mg of chlorambucil/day. Her most recent CPK value was 57, and she is working full-time as a secretary, without muscular or systemic complaints. No drug toxicity has occurred.

Discussion. Dermatomyositis/polymyositis (DM/PM) is generally considered an immunologic autoreactive disorder in which muscle inflammation results from cytotoxic lymphocytes specifically sensitized to striated muscle antigens (6). Both of our patients fulfilled the criteria of Bohan and Peter for the diagnosis of inflammatory myositis (7), and had extramuscular manifestations of autoimmune disease, although the dominant pathologic finding in both patients was myositis. Our patients failed to respond to 6-week courses of high-dose corticosteroids, in addition to pulse methylprednisolone, apheresis, cyclophosphamide, azathioprine, or methotrexate used alone. Only when the combination of prednisone, chlorambucil, and methotrexate was instituted, did these patients' diseases enter remission.

Since DM/PM is rare (prevalence 1:12,000 [8]), only a few therapeutic studies have documented the efficacy of high-dose prednisone (1–2 mg/kg/day) in managing the acute stage of this disorder (4,5). Up to 15–25% of idiopathic adult DM/PM patients are unresponsive to corticosteroid therapy alone or develop unacceptable steroid toxicity; in these patients, the additive efficacy of cyclophosphamide (4), chlorambucil (4), azathioprine (3), total body irradiation (9), thymectomy (10), pulse methylprednisolone (11), hydroxychloroquine (12), antilymphocyte globulin (13), and cyclosporin A (14) have been reported. One of us (DJW) has critically reviewed the role of plasmapheresis in DM/PM and is skeptical about its usefulness (15). Another of us (ALM) has conducted a large study on the use of methotrexate in corticosteroid-resistant DM/PM and reported that the majority of patients had an excellent response to a combination of prednisone and parenteral methotrexate (2).

Recently, McCarty and Carrera (16) suggested that refractory rheumatoid arthritis will respond to the simultaneous use of several remittive agents, including low-dose prednisone, cyclophosphamide, azathioprine, and hydroxychloroquine. In an effort to mimic this "additive, if not synergistic anti-rheumatic effect," our 2 DM/PM patients were treated with a modification of the McCarty regimen.

The remarkable response observed by combining an alkylating agent and an anti-metabolite with corticosteroid therapy in steroid-resistant inflammatory myositis has now been documented.

The 5-year survival rate of DM/PM patients ranges from 40–86% (4,8,17). However, the quality of life in these patients is often poor, and the side effects and complications of repeated courses of high-dose corticosteroids are often quite debilitating. Thus, since up to 5,000 of the estimated 20,000 Americans with DM/PM will either be unresponsive to steroids or develop toxic reactions to these agents, alternative therapy is essential to the overall management of this immunologic muscle disease. The long-term potential serious toxicity of corticosteroids should be minimized due to the "steroid-sparing" effect of both chlorambucil and methotrexate (2,4). The individual toxicity of these agents may include sterilization, bone marrow suppression, oncogenesis, and cirrhosis. The combined use of an alkylating agent with an anti-metabolite, particularly in low doses, does not seem to augment or potentiate their respective individual or additive toxicities. Moreover, it is our purpose to minimize the side effects and remote risks of oncongenesis of these agents by gradually decreasing their individual dosages and frequencies.

We are keenly aware of the overtly aggressive therapeutic approach we have proposed. Nevertheless, in rare instances of DM/PM, this regimen seems indicated in the following situations: steroid-resistant disease that has not responded to the long-term addition of a single immunosuppressive agent (with or without pulse steroid and/or plasmapheresis), the development of profound steroid and/or immunosuppressive toxicity or allergy, or the failure of any conventional program to adequately improve the quality of life of the DM/PM patient. We suggest that more experience with similar aggressive regimens be recorded and that critical controlled studies be conducted.

Acknowledgments. We wish to thank Dr. James R. Klinenberg for his help in reviewing the manuscript and Dr. Daniel J. McCarty for suggesting the patients' treatment regimen to us.

REFERENCES

1. Hudgson P: Polymyositis and dermatomyositis in adults. Clin Rheum Dis 10:85–93, 1984
2. Metzger AL, Bohan A, Goldberg LS, Bluestone R, Pearson CM: Polymyositis and dermatomyositis: combined methotrexate and corticosteroid therapy. Ann Intern Med 81:182–189, 1974
3. Bunch TW: Prednisone and azathioprine for polymyositis: long-term followup. Arthritis Rheum 24:45–48, 1981
4. Bohan A, Peter JB, Bowman RL, Pearson CM: A computer assisted analysis of 153 patients with polymyositis and dermatomyositis. Medicine (Baltimore) 56:255–286, 1977
5. Ansell BM: Management of polymyositis and dermatomyositis. Clin Rheum Dis 10:205–213, 1984
6. Dawkins RL, Mastalgia FL: Cell mediated cytotoxicity in polymyositis. N Engl J Med 288:434–438, 1973
7. Bohan A, Peter J: Polymyositis and dermatomyositis. N Engl J Med 292:344–347, 403–407, 1975
8. De Vere R, Bradley WG: Polymyositis: its presentation, morbidity and mortality. Brain 98:637–666, 1975
9. Hubbard WN, Walport MJ, Halnan KE, Beaney RP, Hughes GRV: Remission from polymyositis after total body irradiation. Br Med J 284:1915–1916, 1982
10. Behan PD, Currie S: Clinical Neuro-Immunology. London, Saunders, 1978
11. Yanagisawa T, Sueishi M, Nawata Y, Akimoto T, Nozaki T, Koike T, Tomioka H, Kumagai A: Methylprednisolone pulse therapy in dermatomyositis. Dermatologica 167:47–51, 1983
12. Woo TY, Callen JP, Voorhees JJ, Bickers DR, Hawkins C: Cutaneous lesions of dermatomyositis are improved by hydroxychloroquine. J Am Acad Dermatol 10:592–600, 1984
13. Gumpel JM, Martin J, Smith DS, Denman AM: Intensive immunosuppression versus prednisolone in the treatment of connective tissue diseases. Ann Rheum Dis 41:557–562, 1982
14. Zabel P, Leimenstoll G, Gross WL: Cyclosporin for acute dermatomyositis (letter). Lancet 1:343, 1984
15. Wallace DJ, Klinenberg JR: Apheresis. DM 30:1–45, 1984
16. McCarty DJ, Carrera GF: Intractable rheumatoid arthritis: treatment with combined cyclophosphamide, azathioprine and hydroxychloroquine. JAMA 248:1718–1723, 1982
17. Riddoch D, Morgan-Hughes JA: Prognosis in adult polymyositis. J Neurol Sci 36:71–80, 1975

LETTERS

Diagnosis of Sjögren's syndrome

To the Editor:

We are writing in response to Dr. Eversmeyer's letter (1), which we did not have an opportunity to see before publication. He comments on an earlier published paper (2) dealing with labial salivary gland (LSG) biopsy in the diagnosis of Sjögren's syndrome (SS). We agree with his basic premise that "for a diagnostic test to be clinically applicable, it must not only increase our objectivity, but also influence our decision-making in our approach to the patient." Dr. Eversmeyer does not question the objectivity of the LSG biopsy, but he asserts that results from this test do not influence therapeutic decision-making and that there is no specific treatment available for SS. These statements are in sharp contrast with 13 years' experience in our multidisciplinary Sjögren's syndrome clinic; moreover, his remarks appear to relate only to secondary SS and do not consider primary SS.

Primary SS (oral and ocular components without connective tissue disease) occurs at least as frequently as secondary SS (a connective tissue disease along with either or both of the other 2 components), and the oral and ocular features of primary SS are generally more severe than those of secondary SS (3–5). To determine whether the usual diagnostic criteria—the objective presence of 2 of 3 components of the triad making up the disease (2,3)—are fulfilled, an LSG biopsy is necessary for diagnosing all cases of primary SS and, in addition, those cases of secondary SS in which a clearly-defined connective tissue disease is present in the absence of keratoconjunctivitis sicca.

As well as providing clear evidence of the most disease-specific diagnostic criterion for the salivary component of primary or secondary SS, results from an LSG biopsy influence clinical decision-making. For example, patients who do not have a clear diagnosis of connective tissue disease but complain of dry mouth and/or dry eyes may be diagnosed as having primary SS based only on these symptoms and a brief clinical examination. Such a decision (an unfortunately frequent event) could overlook the most common causes of these symptoms (side effects from single or combined drug therapy, meibomitis, or allergic conjunctivitis), thus denying the patient treatment for a reversible condition and burdening him or her with the diagnosis of a "benign" but incurable chronic disease.

An alternative decision might be to disregard the patient's symptoms because definitive signs are not observed and the symptoms may seem to be of neurotic origin. In such a case, a patient with primary SS would continue to have these chronic, troubling symptoms without appropriate treatment, and would suffer the frustration of not knowing their cause. The problem would continue and likely progress until irreversible damage occurs to the patient's teeth and/or conjunctivae (a common event). Indeed, establishing the diagnosis of primary SS affects clinical decision-making.

Dr. Eversmeyer correctly points out that only 5 diseases other than SS were diagnosed in our series of 362 LSG biopsies, but fails to note the 169 LSG biopsies which indicated various degrees of nonspecific chronic sialadenitis and atrophy, thus ruling out the salivary component of SS. Some of these biopsies came from patients who had previously been given the diagnosis of primary SS based on symptoms as described above. Labial salivary gland biopsy is, therefore, a cost-effective diagnostic technique because it can provide clinically useful information to either establish or rule out the salivary component of SS.

While SS is not curable, it is certainly treatable to the extent of both significantly reducing patients' symptoms and preventing irreversible damage to their teeth and eyes. In our experience, there are 3 major oral effects of SS: dryness, chronic or recurrent oral mucosal candidiasis, and dental caries in cervical and incisal locations. The first can be reduced by stimulating residual gland function, the second can be treated with appropriate antifungal drugs, and the third prevented with fluorides and dental care.

We have found that common causes of eye symptoms mimicking the ocular component of SS are meibomitis and conjunctival inflammation arising from acquired hypersensitivity to preservatives in artificial tears (often self-prescribed). There are also a number of less frequently occurring ocular diseases which may produce dry eye symptoms, and all of these require specific diagnosis and treatment. Appropriate treatment of primary SS, and of conditions that mimic SS, requires a clear and objective diagnosis.

A diagnosis of Sjögren's syndrome is difficult for any particular clinical practitioner to make because its diagnostic criteria cross specialty boundaries. The LSG biopsy, if properly performed and interpreted, has an essential role in the diagnosis of primary SS and a frequently helpful role in diagnosing secondary SS. Once accurate diagnosis is secured, significant preventive and symptom-reducing treatment can be provided.

Troy E. Daniels, DDS
John P. Whitcher, MD
University of California
Sjögren's Syndrome Clinic
San Francisco, CA

1. Eversmeyer WH: Comment on Daniels article (letter). Arthritis Rheum 27:1320, 1984
2. Daniels TE: Labial salivary gland biopsy in Sjögren's syndrome: assessment as a diagnostic criterion in 362 suspected cases. Arthritis Rheum 27:147–156, 1984
3. Bloch KJ, Buchanan WW, Wohl MJ, Bunin JJ: Sjögren's syndrome: a clinical, pathological, and serological study of sixty-two cases. Medicine (Baltimore) 44:187–231, 1965
4. Daniels TE, Silverman S Jr, Michalski JP, Greenspan JS, Sylves-

ter RA, Talal N: The oral component of Sjögren's syndrome. Oral Surg 39:875–885, 1975
5. Moutsopoulos HM, Weber BL, Vlagopoulos TP, Chused TM, Decker JL: Differences in the clinical manifestations of sicca syndrome in the presence and absence of rheumatoid arthritis. Am J Med 66:733–736, 1979

Aortic arch syndrome associated with anticardiolipin antibodies and the lupus anticoagulant: comment on Ferrante paper

To the Editor:

The case reported by Ferrante, Myerson, and Goldman in 1982 (1) was that of a 19-year-old woman with systemic lupus erythematosus, who developed an aortic arch syndrome with obstruction of the left subclavian artery by thrombus. The left brachial, radial, and ulnar pulses were absent, and the patient complained of numbness of her left hand.

We recently encountered a similar patient with a lupus-like illness, with occluded left axillary and subclavian arteries, also giving rise to an aortic arch syndrome. In addition to involvement of a major vessel arising from the aortic arch, she experienced recurrent cerebrovascular accidents (computerized tomography results were positive), had a false-positive result on VDRL testing, and had antibodies to cardiolipin and demonstrated the presence of the lupus anticoagulant in serum studies.

The patient, a 50-year-old white woman, initially presented in 1976, at age 42, with polyarthralgias, weakness, and lethargy. Three years later, in 1979, she developed a right-sided hemiparesis accompanied by hemianesthesia and a right homonymous hemianopia. Several months later, she complained of headaches and diplopia. Laboratory investigations showed a moderately elevated erythrocyte sedimentation rate (39 mm/hour), positive antinuclear factor (ANF), and a reduced C3 of 480 mg% (normal >700 mg/liter).

Over the next 2 years, she developed Raynaud's phenomenon, dry gritty eyes, lapses of memory, and incoordination. Migrainous headaches became more frequent, and polyarthralgias and myalgias were prominent. Systemic steroid therapy (prednisone, 10 mg daily) was begun in mid-1982. By then, she had become hypertensive (200/110 mm Hg), with mitral incompetence, and she was treated with diuretic therapy (furosemide, 40 mg daily).

Livedo reticularis and an erythematous rash (not involving the face) were noted. When admitted to the Hammersmith Hospital in 1983, she had absent left brachial and radial pulses, and an arch aortogram showed complete occlusion of the left axillary artery extending from the subclavian artery which showed severe stenosis. There was no evidence of atheromatous disease in any vessels. Computerized tomography showed multiple widespread cerebral infarcts.

Laboratory studies showed the following results: negative DNA binding of 8–12% (normal <30%), negative antibodies to extractable nuclear antigens, and negative rheumatoid factor (latex agglutination). The ANF was still weakly positive (1:40), with a positive Coombs' test, and at this stage, it was noted that the antibodies to cardiolipin were strongly positive. The test for lupus anticoagulant was positive, partial thromboplastin time was 49 seconds (control 15), and she also had a false-positive result on VDRL. The serum cholesterol value averaged 5.9 mmoles/liter over a 9-month period.

She was treated with steroids (prednisone, 10 mg daily), regular pulses of cyclophosphamide (500 mg), and plasma exchanges.

Although our patient was 52 years of age, her symptoms had begun when she was 42. There was no clinical or radiologic evidence of atherosclerosis in any other major vessels of the arch or abdominal aorta. Serum cholesterol values, taken over a 9-month period, were within the normal range. Her clinical symptoms were those of a lupus-like disease.

The other case of active systemic lupus erythematosus (SLE) with involvement of the major arch vessels was reported by Lessof and Glynn (2). Their patient also had a false-positive Wasserman reaction, a common finding in patients who demonstrate the lupus anticoagulant and antibodies to cardiolipin. Although Ferrante and his colleagues mention the importance of this in their case report, it did not appear in the investigations performed on their patient.

We have recently documented a close relationship between antibodies to cardiolipin and the lupus anticoagulant (3). There appears to be a strong association between the presence of these antibodies and thromboses, commonly venous thromboses, in SLE and other autoimmune conditions (4,5). We have, however, also noted their association with arterial occlusions, particularly cerebral (as in our patient) (6), as well as mesenteric, with large bowel infarctions (7), and with occlusions of other peripheral arteries, not infrequently resulting in gangrene of the extremities (8). This has also been documented by Jindal et al (9). Involvement of major vessels in SLE and lupus-like conditions may be associated with high titers of these antibodies (10).

We are presently evaluating differing forms of therapy in order to determine the most effective way of reducing high antibody levels or of eliminating their effects.

Out thanks to Dr. K. T. Rajan for referring this patient to us.

Ronald A. Asherson, MB, ChB, FCP(SA)
E. Nigel Harris, MPhil, DM, MD
Azzudin E. Gharavi, MD
Helen E. Englert, MB, BS
Graham R. V. Hughes, MD, FRCP
The Royal Postgraduate School of Medicine
Hammersmith Hospital
London, UK

1. Ferrante FM, Myerson GE, Goldman JA: Subclavian artery thrombosis mimicking the aortic arch syndrome in systemic lupus erythematosus. Arthritis Rheum 25:1501–1504, 1982
2. Lessof MH, Glynn LE: The pulseless syndrome. Lancet i:799–801, 1959
3. Harris EN, Loizou S, Englert H, Derue G, Chan JK, Gharavi AE, Hughes GRV: Anticardiolipin antibodies and lupus anticoagulant (letter). Lancet ii:1099, 1984
4. Harris EN, Gharavi AE, Boey ML, Patel BM, Mackworth-Young CG, Loizou S, Hughes GRV: Anticardiolipin antibodies: detection by radioimmunoassay and association with thrombosis in systemic lupus erythematosus. Lancet ii:1211–1214, 1983
5. Boey ML, Colaco CB, Gharavi AE, Elkon KB, Loizou S, Hughes GRV: Thrombosis in systemic lupus erythematosus: striking association with the presence of circulating lupus anticoagulant. Br Med J 287:1021–1023, 1984
6. Harris EN, Gharavi AE, Asherson RA, Boey ML, Hughes GRV: Cerebral infarction in systemic lupus: association with anticardiolipin antibodies. Clin Exp Rheumatol 2:47–51, 1984
7. Asherson RA, Mackworth-Young CG, Harris EN, Gharavi AE, Boey ML, Hughes GRV: Multiple venous and arterial thromboses associated with the lupus anticoagulant and antibodies to cardiolipin in the absence of SLE. Rheumatol Int 5:91–93, 1985
8. Hughes GRV, Asherson RA: Atypical lupus with special reference to ANA negative lupus and lupus subsets, Advances in Nephrology. Edited by JP Grunfeld, MH Maxwell. Chicago, Year Book Medical Publishers, 1985, pp 333–346
9. Jindal MK, Martin MFR, Gayner A: Gangrene developing after minor surgery in a patient with undiagnosed systemic lupus erythematosus and lupus anticoagulant. Ann Rheum Dis 42:347–349, 1983
10. Asherson RA, Harris EN, Gharavi AE, Hughes GRV: Clinical manifestations associated with the lupus anticoagulant and elevations of antibodies to cardiolipins in SLE and other conditions, Progress in Rheumatology. Vol. II. Edited by I Machtey, Israel, Hasharon Hospital, 1984, pp 323–329

Nephrotic syndrome induced by tiopronin: association with the HLA–DR3 antigen

To the Editor:

The role of tiopronin as a useful disease-remittive drug in rheumatoid arthritis (RA) has been established in clinical trials (1–3). Pasero et al (4), in a multicenter trial comparing tiopronin treatment with D-penicillamine treatment, have demonstrated comparable efficacy. In Pasero's study, proteinuria ranging from 2–3 gm/day (but not associated with nephrotic syndrome) occurred in 4 patients in the tiopronin-treated group. We describe a patient who developed nephrotic syndrome during treatment with tiopronin, and was also found to have the HLA–DR3 antigen.

In October 1983, a 60-year-old woman was diagnosed as having definite RA, according to American Rheumatism Association criteria (5). Treatment with tiopronin was started, with gradually increasing doses, until she was taking 1 gm/day. After 3 months of treatment, the patient was clinically improved, but in February 1984, she developed a generalized edema and was hospitalized.

At that time, laboratory investigations revealed the following: serum creatinine of 2 mg/100 ml, creatinine clearance of 46 ml/minute, proteinuria at 4.5 gm/24 hours (moderately selective according to Cameron's index), hypoalbuminemia at 1.9 gm/100 ml, hypercholesterolemia at 550 mg/100 ml. Immunologic studies revealed normal levels of C3, C4, and CH50, and tests for fluorescent antinuclear antibodies, anti–double-stranded DNA, cryoglobulins, and circulating immune complexes (C1q and conglutinin binding tests) showed negative results. HLA identification showed that she had A29,B17,B37,Cw4,DR3,DR5,MT1,MT2.

A renal biopsy was performed, and under light microscopy, the sample showed normal glomeruli. Immunofluorescence analysis of the specimen gave negative results using antisera against IgG, IgM, IgA, C1q, C3, C4, and fibrinogen. Using electron microscopy, the only abnormality noted was a complete loss of the foot processes of the epithelial cells (foot process disease) (Figure 1). Withdrawal of the tiopronin (total cumulative dose 70 gm) and institution of prednisone treatment (1 mg/kg/day) completely resolved the nephrotic syndrome within 1 month.

There are many similarities in the nephrotic syndrome induced by tiopronin and that induced by D-penicillamine, both drugs having a chemical structural affinity (6–11). First, the highest incidence of disease occurs during the first year of treatment, showing no correlation between mean daily dose and toxicity. Second, the glomerular injury is mediated by an immunologic mechanism,,and it appears to be self-limiting upon withdrawal of the offending drug.

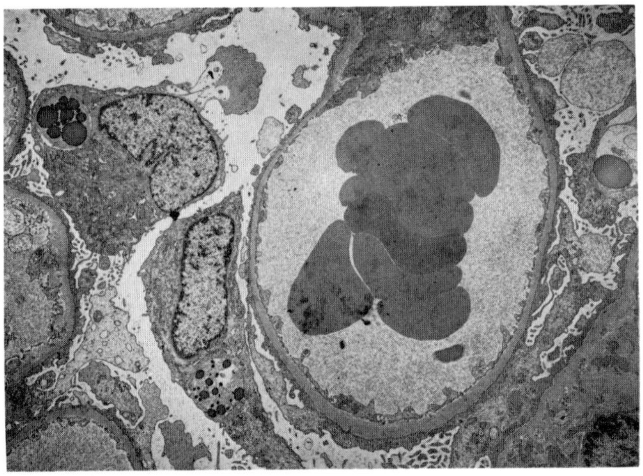

Figure 1. Electron micrograph of renal biopsy specimen from a 60-year-old woman with tiopronin-induced nephrotic syndrome, showing complete loss of the foot processes of epithelial cells (original magnification × 5,000).

Third, the morphologic basis of glomerulopathy consists of both membranous and minimal change glomerular lesions.

The pathogenesis of tiopronin-induced nephropathy is still unclear. The renal injury may be an immune complex–mediated membranous nephropathy similar to the D-penicillamine–induced lesions. The antigenic role of tiopronin has been demonstrated by Stratta et al (9), who have shown a positive result on immune complex elution testing after incubation of kidney sections with tiopronin. According to Lupo et al (8), in tiopronin-induced minimal change nephropathy, a sensitization mechanism similar to that described in minimal change nephropathy associated with exposure to allergens may occur. In patients with HLA–DR3, Speerstra et al (12) showed that there is an increased risk of nephrotic syndrome during treatment with D-penicillamine. Our observation suggests a similar immunogenetic susceptibility for the renal damage induced by tiopronin; however, further studies will be necessary to prove whether this association is statistically significant.

Carlo Salvarani, MD
PierLuigi Macchioni, MD
Fulvia Rossi, MD
Ido Iori, MD
Giordano Filippi, MD
Hospital of Reggio Emilia
Reggio Emilia, Italy

1. Pasero G, Ciompi ML: Thiopronine therapy in rheumatoid arthritis (letter). Arthritis Rheum 22:803–804, 1979
2. Pasero G, Pellegrini P, Ciompi ML, Colamussi V, Barbieri P, Mazzoni MR: La tiopronine, nouveau traitement de fond de la polyarthrite rhumatoïde: étude ouverte de 158 cas. Rev Rhum Mal Osteoartic 47:163–168, 1980
3. Amor B, Mery C, de Gery A: La tiopronine: nouvel antirhumatismal à action lente dans la polyarthrite rhumatoïde. Rev Rhum Mal Osteoartic 47:157–162, 1980
4. Pasero G, Pellegrini P, Ambanelli U, Ciompi ML, Colamussi V, Ferraccioli G, Barbieri P, Mazzoni MR, Menegale G, Trippi D: Controlled multicenter trial of tiopronin and D-penicillamine for rheumatoid arthritis. Arthritis Rheum 25:923–929, 1982
5. Ropes MW, Bennett GA, Cobb S, Jacox R, Jessar RA: 1958 revision of diagnostic criteria for rheumatoid arthritis. Bull Rheum Dis 9:175–176, 1958
6. Bacon PA, Tribe CR, Mackenzie JC, Verrier-Jones J, Cumming RH, Amer B: Penicillamine nephropathy in rheumatoid arthritis. Q J Med 45:661–684, 1976
7. Falck HM, Tornroth T, Koch B, Wegelius O: Fatal renal vasculitis and minimal change glomerulonephritis complicating treatment with penicillamine. Acta Med Scand 205:133–138, 1979
8. Lupo A, Faraggiana T, Loschiavo C, Parolini C, Maschio G: Nephrotic syndrome during 2-mercapto-propionyl-glycine (thiola) therapy. Nephron 28:96–99, 1981
9. Stratta P, Coratelli P, Camussi G, Passavanti G, Segoloni GP, Coppo R, Amerio A, Vercellone A: Sindrome nefrosica durante trattamento con 2-mercaptopropionilglicina. Minerva Nefrol 25:87–92, 1978
10. Fruttero B, Dall'Aglio PP, Bruno M, Rossi E, Pozzo L, Ferrari C, Linari F, Migone L: Sindrome nefrosica indotta dalla 2-mercapto-propionil-glicina. Symposium on Metabolic, Physiochemical and Therapeutical Aspects of Urolithiasis. Edited by F Linari, M Brund, B Fruttero, M Marancella. Milan, Italy, Wichtig, 1983, pp 131–135
11. Rizzoni G, Pavanello L, Dussini N, Chiandetti L, Zacchello G: Nephrotic syndrome during treatment with alpha-mercaptopropionylglycine. J Urol 122:381–382, 1979
12. Speerstra F, Reekers P, Van de Putte LBA, Vandenbroucke JP, Rasker JJ, de Rooij DJRAM: HLA-DR antigens and proteinuria induced by aurothioglucose and D-penicillamine in patients with rheumatoid arthritis. J Rheumatol 10:948–953, 1983

Idiopathic thrombocytopenic purpura with high-titer, speckled pattern antinuclear antibodies: possible marker for systemic lupus erythematosus

To the Editor:

Idiopathic thrombocytopenic purpura (ITP) has been associated, in a small number of patients, with the subsequent development of systemic lupus erythematosus (SLE) (1,2). Several histologic features resembling those described in SLE have been found in the spleens of some ITP patients (3), supporting the concept that an ITP-like syndrome can be the initial manifestation of SLE. Since SLE is a chronic and potentially fatal disease, it is of prognostic importance to identify ITP patients who are at risk of developing SLE. In this report we provide evidence suggesting that ITP patients presenting with high-titer, speckled pattern, antinuclear antibodies (ANA) appear to be at risk of developing SLE.

Between 1976 and 1983, we studied 18 patients in whom the diagnosis of ITP was made. All patients presented with easy bruising, petechiae and/or bleeding, and platelet counts ranging from 5,000–15,000/mm^3. None of the patients had ingested drugs known to induce thrombocytopenia, nor did they have evidence of any other underlying disease. All patients were female, with a mean age of 29 years (range 16–38). Patients were followed for a mean of 3.4 years (range 10 months–7 years). At the time of diagnosis of ITP, all patients had serum drawn for rheumatoid factor (latex fixation), complement levels (C3 and C4), antibodies to double-stranded DNA, and ANA determinations. In those sera exhibiting speckled pattern ANA, the presence or absence of antibodies directed against the nuclear antigens RNP and/or Sm was determined (4). The diagnosis of SLE was established using the American Rheumatism Association preliminary criteria (5). Presence of 4 or more criteria was required before the diagnosis of SLE was made.

Table 1. Serologic characteristics of idiopathic thrombocytopenic purpura patients at the time of diagnosis

Rheumatoid factor*	<1:20
C3/C4 levels (mg/dl), mean ± SD†	112 ± 30/26 ± 10
Anti-DNA antibodies‡	<20%
Positive antinuclear antibodies	
Diffuse	2/18 (titer 1:80)
Speckled	4/18 (titers 1:160–1:640)

* Latex fixation test.
† Radial immunodiffusion technique. Normal levels: C3, 70–140 mg/dl; C4, 16–30 mg/dl.
‡ Farr technique. Normal level: 15–20% binding.

The serologic characteristics of this group of patients are presented in Table 1. None of the patients had circulating rheumatoid factor (IgM) in their serum. Serum levels of C3 and C4 were within normal limits, and circulating antibodies to double-stranded DNA were undetectable.

Six of the 18 patients had positive ANA determinations. Two had the diffuse pattern of immunofluorescence (with titers of 1:80), and 4 had speckled pattern ANA with titers ranging between 1:160–1:640. Of the 4 patients with speckled pattern ANA, 1 had high-titer antibody to Sm, while another had high-titer antibody to RNP. The remaining 2 patients had negative Sm and RNP determinations. Only 1 patient had a serologic marker (Sm antibody) that might be considered characteristic of SLE (6).

Thus, 6 of 18 patients (33%) with the diagnosis of ITP had positive ANA determinations. It should be emphasized, however, that none of these patients had signs or symptoms of SLE at the time of initial consultation.

Four patients later developed SLE. The mean time from the initial diagnosis of ITP to the development of SLE was 2.3 years (range 8 months–4 years). All of the patients who developed SLE had presented initially with high-titer, speckled pattern ANA. The 2 patients presenting with diffuse pattern ANA had not developed any signs or symptoms of SLE at the followup examination 3 years later.

Thus, this pilot prospective study suggests that ITP patients who have high-titer, speckled pattern ANA at the time of initial diagnosis may be at risk of developing SLE. Recently, a similar (but larger) study that supports our findings was reported in abstract form. Peebles et al (7) reported on the significance of ANA in patients with immune thrombocytopenia. Twenty-four of 117 patients with ITP (20%) were found to have positive ANA, a frequency similar to ours. Five of the 24 patients with positive ANA had the speckled pattern, with antibodies directed against various nuclear antigens. Four of these 5 patients developed SLE. Furthermore, SLE did not develop in the remaining 19 patients with positive ANA. These findings are almost identical to those reported here.

Given the association between these 2 diseases (1,2), the presence of a serologic marker that would allow the identification of the subset of ITP patients who are at risk of developing SLE may be of prognostic significance. Large, controlled studies are needed in order to determine the precise incidence of ANA positivity in ITP patients, and the percent of those patients who will develop SLE.

H. Daniel Perez, MD
Ernest Katler, MD
Stephen Embury, MD
University of California, San Francisco
San Francisco General Hospital
San Francisco, CA

1. Rabinowitz Y, Dameshek W: Systemic lupus erythematosus after "idiopathic" thrombocytopenic purpura: a review. Ann Intern Med 52:1–28, 1960
2. Budman DR, Steinberg AD: Hematologic aspects of systemic lupus erythematosus: current concepts. Ann Intern Med 80:220–229, 1977
3. Breckenridge RT, Moore RD, Ratnoff OD: A study of thrombocytopenia: new histologic criteria for the differentiation of idiopathic thrombocytopenia and thrombocytopenia associated with disseminated lupus erythematosus. Blood 30:39–53, 1967
4. Sharp GC, Irvin WS, Tan EM, Gould RG, Holman HR: Mixed connective tissue disease: an apparent distinct rheumatic disease syndrome associated with a specific antibody to an extractable nuclear antigen (ENA). Am J Med 52:148–159, 1972
5. Cohen AS, Reynolds WE, Franklin EC, Kulka JP, Ropes MW, Shulman LE, Wallace SL: Preliminary criteria for the classification of systemic lupus erythematosus. Bull Rheum Dis 21:643–648, 1971
6. Notman DD, Kurata N, Tan EM: Profiles of antinuclear antibodies in systemic rheumatic diseases. Ann Intern Med 83:464–469, 1975
7. Peebles CL, Anderson MJ, Tan EM, McMillan R, Curd JC: Significance of fluorescent antinuclear antibodies in patients with immune thrombocytopenia (abstract). Arthritis Rheum (suppl) 27:S42, 1984

Autoantibodies during captopril treatment

To the Editor:

In a recent brief report, Reidenberg et al described the development of antinuclear antibody (ANA) in patients treated with high doses of captopril (1). They concluded that this was not a result of any linkage between the gene for susceptibility to ANA development and the gene for slow acetylation.

In a prospective study conducted at this institution (2), we described the development of ANA in 13 of 89 patients treated with captopril. The ANA were mainly of the IgM class, did not fix complement, and were transiently present. In addition, low avidity anti–double-stranded DNA antibodies, exclusively of the IgM class and not complement-fixing, developed in 3 patients. In 5 patients, perinuclear factors developed during captopril treatment (3).

Based on these data, we hypothesize that captopril induces dose-related alterations in immunoregulation, resulting in autoimmune phenomena, as has been shown for methyldopa (4). Indeed, alterations in lymphocyte reactivity during captopril treatment have been demonstrated (5,6). In agreement with the data of Reidenberg et al, we did not find an association between captopril-induced side effects and ANA development (2). In a report on cutaneous side effects, captopril-induced in vitro lymphocyte transformation and positive findings of intracutaneous skin test were described in patients with skin rashes due to captopril (7), indicating drug-specific allergic reactions.

In conclusion, treatment with high doses of captopril seems to result in immunoregulatory disturbances such as the development of multiple autoantibodies, and some of the side effects of captopril are associated with a drug-specific immune response.

Cees G. M. Kallenberg, MD
University Hospital
Groningen, The Netherlands

1. Reidenberg MM, Case DB, Drayer DE, Reis S, Lorenzo B: Development of antinuclear antibody in patients treated with high doses of captopril. Arthritis Rheum 27:579–581, 1984
2. Kallenberg CGM, Hoorntje SJ, Smit AJ, Weening JJ, Donker AJM, Hoedemaeker PhH, The TH: Antinuclear and antinative DNA antibodies during captopril treatment. Acta Med Scand 211:297–300, 1982
3. Hoorntje SJ: Merits and demerits of the converting-enzyme inhibitor captopril in antihypertensive treatment. Thesis, Groningen, The Netherlands, 1981, pp 32–33
4. Kirtland HH, Mohler DN, Horwitz DA: Methyldopa inhibition of suppressor-lymphocyte function. N Engl J Med 302:825–829, 1980
5. Kallenberg CGM, van der Laan S, de Zeeuw D: Captopril and the immune system. Lancet II:92, 1981
6. Delfraissy JF, Galanaud P, Balavoine JF, Wallon C, Dermont J: Captopril and immune regulation. Kidney Int 25:925–929, 1984
7. Smit AJ, van der Laan S, de Monchy J, Kallenberg CGM, Donker AJM: Cutaneous reactions to captopril: predictive value of skin tests. Clin Allergy 14:413–419, 1984

Systemic lupus erythematosus and Down's syndrome

To the Editor:

The recent report by Yancey et al (1) describes an inflammatory arthropathy associated with Down's syndrome. Their estimated prevalence of arthritis in Down's syndrome appeared to be much higher than the prevalence of juvenile rheumatoid arthritis (JRA) in the general population. It remains uncertain whether this arthropathy represents JRA occurring in a genetically predisposed population, or a separate illness occurring as a result of the known genetic and immunologic abnormalities in Down's syndrome (2). Previously described abnormalities in Down's syndrome include chronic active hepatitis and multiple serologic abnormalities (3), psoriatic arthritis (4), gouty arthritis (5), an increased incidence of thyroid antibodies (6), and an increased incidence of alopecia areata (7). We recently treated a patient with Down's syndrome who developed an inflammatory polyarthritis with additional clinical and serologic features of SLE.

The patient is a 20-year-old white woman with Down's syndrome, congenital heart disease, and suspected Eisenmenger's syndrome with pulmonary hypertension. In August 1981, she was hospitalized with congestive heart failure. Daily temperatures elevated to 39°C were noted. Multiple blood cultures revealed no abnormalities. Daily fevers persisted, and in November 1981, she developed a gradual onset of pain and swelling in multiple joints. Evaluation revealed moderate swelling of the proximal interphalangeal, metacarpophalangeal, wrist, elbow, ankle, and subtalar joints bilaterally. Mild ulnar drift was noted. There were flexion contractures of both elbows and limited mobility of the shoulders. Effusions were present in both knees and there was metatarsophalangeal tenderness. Persistent malar erythema and patchy alopecia were present without mucous membrane lesions. There was mild axillary adenopathy. The lungs were clear. P_2 was increased, and there was a grade 3/6 systolic mumur at the left sternal border. There was no abdominal organomegaly.

Laboratory studies revealed the following values: a hemoglobin of 10.8 gm/dl, hematocrit 32.7%, white blood cells (WBC) 7,400/mm^3 with 7% bands, 84% segmented neutrophils, and 9% lymphocytes. Persistent leukopenia was subsequently noted with the WBC count ranging from 2,800–4,200 cells/mm^3. Erythrocyte sedimentation rate was increased at 67 mm/hour. A test for antinuclear antibodies was positive at a titer of 1:160 with a homogenous pattern. Anti-DNA antibody (*Crithidia luciliae* method) was positive at a titer of 1:10 initially and subsequently increased to 1:80. Lupus erythematosus cell preparation was positive. Complement C3 and C4 levels were normal. Rheumatoid factor was negative. Direct Coombs' test result was negative. Liver enzyme values and renal function were normal. Radiographs of the hands and wrists revealed fusiform swelling of the proximal interphalangeal joints and periarticular demineralization without erosive changes or periostitis.

She was treated with salicylates with marked symptomatic improvement evidenced by diminished articular swelling and resolution of the daily fevers. Her course was complicated by gastrointestinal bleeding necessitating the cessation of aspirin. She has subsequently been treated with choline magnesium trisalicylate and hydroxychloroquine and has continued to do well.

The patient fulfilled 5 of the 11 American Rheumatism Association revised criteria for SLE (8). One hundred sixty-one patients with Down's syndrome were evaluated at the

Geisinger Medical Center between 1973 and 1982, but no other instances of SLE were detected. Although no previous association between Down's syndrome and SLE has been suggested, the patient described by McCulloch et al (3) had chronic active hepatitis with hyperglobulinemia, antinuclear antibodies, anti-DNA antibodies, antithyroid antibodies, hypocomplementemia, and circulating immune complexes.

The occurrence of an arthropathy which may be immunologically mediated, SLE, and other autoimmune phenomena in Down's syndrome is of considerable interest. Further investigation of this unique group of patients may improve our understanding of the relationships between the immune response, heredity, and the pathogenesis of rheumatic disease.

C. Michael Franklin, MD
Dennis Torretti, MD
Geisinger Medical Center
Danville, PA

1. Yancey CL, Zmijewski C, Athreya BH, Doughty RA: Arthropathy of Down's syndrome. Arthritis Rheum 27:929–934, 1984
2. Spina CA, Smith D, Korn E, Fahey JL, Brossman HJ: Altered cellular immune functions in patients with Down's syndrome. Am J Dis Child 135:251–255, 1981
3. McCulloch AJ, Ince PG, Kendall-Taylor P: Autoimmune chronic active hepatitis in Down's symdrome. J Med Genet 19:232–234, 1982
4. Angevine CD, Pless IB, Baum J, Jacox RF: Psoriatic arthritis in a child. Arthritis Rheum 16:278–283, 1973
5. Nishida Y, Akaoka I, Nishizawa T, Maruki M, Aikawa T, Mitamura T, Yokohari R, Horiuchi Y: A case of gouty arthritis associated with Down's syndrome. J Ment Defic Res 20:277–283, 1976
6. Vanhaelst L, Hayez F, Bonnyns M, Bastenie PA: Thyroid autoimmune disease and thyroid function in families of subjects with Down's syndrome. J Clin Endocrinol Metab 30:792–797, 1970
7. DuViviev A, Munro DD: Alopecia areata, autoimmunity, and Down's syndrome. Br Med J [Clin Res] 1:191–192, 1975
8. Tan EM, Cohen AS, Fries JF, Masi AT, McShane DJ, Rothfield NF, Schaller JG, Talal N, Winchester RJ: The 1982 revised criteria for the classification of systemic lupus erythematosus. Arthritis Rheum 25:1271–1277, 1982

Low plasma renin activity in lupus-prone mice: a metabolic abnormality in MRL/Mp-lpr/lpr mice?

To the Editor:

Numerous immunopathologic studies have shown that murine systemic lupus erythematosus is an excellent model for investigation of the pathogenesis and modes of treatment of the human disease. Female (New Zealand black × New Zealand white)F_1 ([NZB × NZW]F_1) hybrid and MRL/MpJ-lpr/lpr (MRL-lpr) and male BXSB/Mp mice develop immune complex nephritis early in life (1,2). Additional abnormalities include production of various autoantibodies (3), immune complex deposition in the dermal–epidermal junction (4), vascular lesions (5), and lymphoproliferative disease (2).

In a recent study of hypertension in lupus-prone mice (6), we observed that MRL-lpr mice had low or virtually undetectable plasma renin activity (PRA), as measured by the low pH activation of plasma renin and by radioimmunoassay of angiotensin I generated (ng/ml of plasma) during 1 hour of incubation at 37°C (kit from New England Nuclear, Boston, MA). The MRL/lpr mice had extremely low PRA, regardless of the degree of renal or lymphoproliferative disease. By contrast, MRL/MpJ-+/+ congenic partners, which lack the lpr gene, had normal PRA (6).

We have now examined other non–lupus-prone strains of mice which bear the autosomal mutant gene lpr (lymphoproliferation): AKR/J-lpr/lpr (AKR-lpr), C57BL/6J-lpr/lpr (C57BL/6-lpr), and C3H/HeJ-lpr/lpr (C3H-lpr); control C3H/HeJ-+/+ (C3H-+) mice and C3H/HeJ-gld/gld (C3H-gld) mice bearing the non-allelic mutation, generalized lymphoproliferative disease (7,8), were also evaluated (Table 1).

Both male and female MRL-lpr mice had low or undetectable PRA, whereas normal PRA was found in the other strains of homozygous lpr mice. (The range of normal adult mouse PRA values in our laboratory is 6–16 ng/ml.) PRA in other lupus-prone strains declined during the development of severe renal disease (6).

The reasons for the low PRA in MRL-lpr mice are unknown. Renin secretion could be reduced by defects in the synthetic process in the juxtaglomerular apparatus or by an inherent problem in the secretory release mechanism. Secretion of renin could also be limited by reduced adrenergic activity, by abnormalities in prostaglandin metabolism, or by salt and water retention. Inhibitors or substrate limitation might also play a role.

Table 1. Plasma renin activity (measured by angiotensin I generated during incubation) in MRL-lpr mice and other strains with lymphoproliferation

Strain	Age (months)/sex	n	Angiotensin I (ng/ml in 1 hour), mean ± SD
MRL-lpr	4–5/F	11	1 ± 1
MRL-lpr	4–5/F	3	2 ± 2
MRL-lpr	7/F	7	2 ± 3
MRL-lpr	5/M	5	2 ± 1
C3H-lpr	6/F	4	10 ± 3
AKR-lpr	6/F	4	6 ± 3
C57BL/6-lpr	7/F	5	6 ± 3
C3H-gld*	6/M	4	5 ± 2
MRL-+	6/M	8	16 ± 7
C3H-+	5/M	4	9 ± 5

* See reference 8.

It will be of interest to determine if the low PRA in MRL-lpr mice reflects a disturbance in renal hemodynamics or a more generalized biosynthetic metabolic disorder, e.g., in the arachidonic acid pathway, and how such abnormalities contribute to immune complex renal disease and autoimmune disease.

Ulrich H. Rudofsky, BS
Robert L. Dilwith, BS
Albert M. Magro, PhD
Wadsworth Center for Laboratories and Research
New York State Department of Health
Albany, NY
John B. Roths, BA
Jackson Laboratory
Bar Harbor, ME

1. Howie JB, Heyler BJ: The immunology and pathology of NZB mice. Adv Immunol 9:216–266, 1968
2. Murphy ED, Roths JB: Autoimmunity and lymphoproliferation: induction by mutant gene lpr, and acceleration by a male-associated factor in BXSB mice, Genetic Control of Autoimmune Diseases. Edited by N Rose, P Bigazzi, N Warner. New York, Elsevier/North Holland, 1978, pp 206–221
3. Theofilopoulos AN, Dixon FJ: Autoimmune diseases: immunopathology and etiopathogenesis. Am J Pathol 108:321–365, 1982
4. Sommer VM, Rudofsky UH, Gabrielsen AE: Immune complexes in skin of NZB/NZW mice. Clin Exp Immunol 22:461–467, 1975
5. Dixon FJ: Murine SLE models and autoimmune disease. Hosp Pract 17:63–73, 1982
6. Rudofsky UH, Dilwith RL, Roths JB, Lawrence DA, Kelley VE, Magro AM: Differences in the occurrence of hypertension among (NZB × NZW)F_1, MRL-lpr, and BXSB mice with lupus nephritis. Am J Pathol 116:107–114, 1984
7. Izui S, Kelley VE, Masuda K, Yoshida H, Roths JB, Murphy ED: Induction of various autoantibodies by mutant gene lpr in several strains of mice. J Immunol 133:227–233, 1984
8. Roths JB, Murphy ED, Eicher EM: A new mutation, gld, that produces lymphoproliferation and autoimmunity in C3H/HeJ. J Exp Med 159:1–20, 1984

Botticelli and arthritis

To the Editor:

When my colleagues and I reviewed Botticelli's paintings for evidence of arthritis for our paper on the probable depiction of juvenile arthritis in his work (1), we discarded "The Birth of Venus" both because the convex contour is present in only one side of the fingers, indicating flexion rather than actual swelling of the fingers, and because the model for this painting is known to have been Simonetta Vespucci, who died suddenly at age 23 and did not have arthritis (2). Therefore, I disagree with Dequeker's notion that "The Birth of Venus" represents arthritis (3).

In my own personal analysis, none of the other paintings by Botticelli that were referred to by Leden (4) represent arthritis, again, because of the presence of the convex contour in only one side of the fingers. In my opinion, the painting he does present as an example of arthritis in Botticelli's work clearly shows flexion of the fingers, as indicated both by its position as well as by the shadowing of the 2 distal phalanxes.

None of the classic works mentioned by Dr. Leden as suggesting a chronic deforming joint disease is so striking to me as the account of the arthritis of Byzantine Emperor Constantine IX Monomachus (c. 980–1055) by his advisor, and perhaps physician, Michael Psellus (5).

I do agree with Dr. Leden, however, that bone remains may be the best source of information about the presence of arthritis in ancient times. Indeed, a recent investigation in a Roman cemetery in England disclosed evidence of rheumatoid arthritis in 2 of 416 skeletons from adult Brythonic Celts studied (6). The skeletons, which were particularly well-preserved in the British museum, gave the unusual opportunity to make this finding despite the brittleness of rheumatoid arthritis–affected bones.

It seems, therefore, that the question of the existence of rheumatoid arthritis in ancient times has been answered positively by various means. The questions now are: how far back does the disease go, and how was it dealt with in ancient days? We know with certainty, for instance, that Indians from Mesoamerica performed therapeutic arthrocentesis probably long before the arrival of Cortés (7).

The quest for arthritis and other rheumatic conditions as depicted in art has shown us how artists, keen observers of nature, were able to "describe," or at least record, these conditions long before physicians did. It has been a lesson in humility, but on the other hand, it is a quest that has, I am sure, given Dequeker, myself, and many others, much pleasure.

Donato Alarcón-Segovia, MD
Instituto Nacional de la Nutrición "Salvador Zubirán"
Mexico City, Mexico

1. Alarcón-Segovia D, Laffón A, Alcocer-Varela J: Probable depiction of juvenile arthritis by Sandro Botticelli. Arthritis Rheum 26:1266–1268, 1983
2. Arciniegas G: Biografía del Caribe. Bogota, Colombia, Plaza & James Editores, 1984, pp 21–22
3. Dequeker J: Arthritis in the paintings of Sandro Botticelli (letter). Arthritis Rheum 27:1196–1197, 1984
4. Leden I: Doubts about Sandro Botticelli's depiction of juvenile rheumatoid arthritis (letter). Arthritis Rheum 27:1197–1198, 1984
5. Caughey DE: The arthritis of Constantine IX. Ann Rheum Dis 33:77–80, 1974
6. Thould AK, Thould BT: Arthritis in Roman Britain. Br Med J 287:24–31, 1983
7. Alarcón-Segovia D: Descriptions of therapeutic arthrocentesis and of synovial fluid in a Nahuatl text from prehispanic Mexico. Ann Rheum Dis 39:291–293, 1980

arthritis
and
rheumatism
Official Journal of the American Rheumatism Association Section of the Arthritis Foundation

THE IMMUNOREACTIVITY, LIGAND, AND CELL BINDING CHARACTERISTICS OF RHEUMATOID SYNOVIAL FLUID FIBRONECTIN

STEVEN CARSONS, BEVERLY B. LAVIETES, HERBERT S. DIAMOND, and SANDRA G. KINNEY

Fibronectin promotes macrophage adherence and expression of Fc receptors, is chemotactic for fibroblasts, and is an opsonin for fibrin and denatured collagen. These properties suggest a role for fibronectin in the modulation of joint inflammation. Since structural modification of the fibronectin molecule has been shown to result in loss or de novo acquisition of opsonic and chemotactic activity, we determined the functional and immunochemical properties of fibronectin isolated from the inflamed joint. Eighty-six percent of synovial fluids obtained from patients with active rheumatoid arthritis (RA) contained fibronectin fragments, and 39% of the fluids no longer displayed the dimeric form. Compared with native fibronectin, RA peptides were as active in promoting synoviocyte chemotaxis and in glycosaminoglycan binding, but displayed lower affinity for fibrin and gelatin. Although comparable with intact protein in augmenting monocyte attachment to gelatin, the RA synovial fluid peptides did not augment monocyte attachment to fibrin. Analysis of whole synovial fluid and isolated fibronectins by enzyme immunoassay showed that the increased fibronectin immunoreactivity, previously reported in RA synovial fluid, measures intact and nearly intact protein and does not measure extensively degraded fragments.

Presented in part at the VIII Pan-American Congress of Rheumatology, Washington, DC, June 1982.

From the Division of Clinical Immunology, Department of Medicine, Long Island Jewish–Hillside Medical Center, New Hyde Park, New York, and the State University of New York, Stony Brook, New York.

Supported by Multipurpose Arthritis Center grant P60-AM-20625 and grants from the Kroc Foundation and the Arthritis Foundation, New York Chapter.

Steven Carsons, MD: Physician-in-Charge, Division of Clinical Immunology, Long Island Jewish–Hillside Medical Center, and Professor of Medicine, SUNY, Stony Brook; Beverly B. Lavietes, PhD: Research Scientist, Long Island Jewish–Hillside Medical Center, and Assistant Professor of Medicine, SUNY, Stony Brook; Herbert S. Diamond, MD: Chairman, Department of Medicine, Long Island Jewish–Hillside Medical Center, and Professor of Medicine, SUNY, Stony Brook; Sandra G. Kinney, MS: Research Technician, Long Island Jewish–Hillside Medical Center.

Address reprint requests to Steven Carsons, MD, Division of Clinical Immunology, Long Island Jewish–Hillside Medical Center, New Hyde Park, NY 11042.

Submitted for publication August 22, 1984; accepted in revised form December 14, 1984.

Arthritis and Rheumatism, Vol. 28, No. 6 (June 1985)

Known effects of fibronectin on the promotion of fibroblast and monocyte adherence and migration (1–4) suggest that the high levels of fibronectin in rheumatoid arthritis (RA) synovial fluid (5–9) may influence the function of cells that compose the proliferated synovial lining. In addition, the opsonic activity of fibronectin that is displayed for denatured collagen and fibrin (10–12) may facilitate the clearance of these proteins from the inflamed joint.

Fibronectin binding to macromolecules and cells is mediated by protease-resistant domains interconnected by flexible protease-sensitive polypeptide regions (13). Since fibronectin is readily cleaved by proteases in vitro, it has been suggested that fibronectin is fragmented at inflammatory sites in vivo (14,15). Such fragments could lose certain biologic functions or could acquire new biologic activities (15). For instance, the amino-terminal end of each monomer is composed of a 30-kd domain, which mediates binding to fibrin, and a 40-kd domain, which binds to collagen. These domains can be specifically cleaved by plasmin and chymotrypsin, respectively. The remaining carboxy-terminal ends of the molecule lose the ability to bind cells to these ligands (16), whereas the dissociated gelatin-binding fragment acquires cell transformation–enhancing activity (17).

Elevated levels of immunoreactive fibronectin have been found in human rheumatoid synovial fluid (5–9), but whether this fibronectin is altered in structure or function in this inflammatory environment remains to be demonstrated.

We report here on the immunoreactivity, polypeptide structure, and ligand-binding affinities of synovial fluid fibronectin isolated from patients with rheumatoid arthritis. We also report the results of our investigations on its role in synoviocyte chemotaxis and monocyte/macrophage attachment.

PATIENTS AND METHODS

Human plasma. Outdated normal human plasma was obtained from the New York Blood Center and was stored at −20°C until use.

Human synovial fluid. After obtaining informed consent, synovial fluid was taken from patients with active rheumatoid arthritis or noninflammatory osteoarthritis, who were undergoing diagnostic and/or therapeutic arthrocentesis. Fluid was drawn into plastic syringes and placed directly into tubes containing the protease inhibitors EDTA, phenylmethylsulfonyl fluoride (PMSF), and Trasylol (final concentrations 5.7 m*M*, 1 m*M*, and 500 units/ml, respectively; Sigma, St. Louis, MO). The fluids were centrifuged at 500*g* to remove cellular elements, and the supernatants were frozen at −20°C. Whole fluids undergoing electrophoresis were pretreated with hyaluronidase (3 mg/ml, bovine testicular; Millipore, Inc., Bedford, MA) and diluted in Laemmli sample buffer (see below).

Isolation of plasma and synovial fluid fibronectin by gelatin-Sepharose chromatography. Gelatin (type I; Sigma) was coupled to CNBr-Sepharose 4B (Pharmacia Fine Chemicals, Piscataway, NJ), according to the manufacturer's instructions, and poured into a 0.9 × 15-cm column. One milliliter of normal plasma or synovial fluid per milliliter of beads was applied to the column. Protein was sequentially eluted with 0.05*M* Tris-HCl, 1 m*M* PMSF, pH 7.2 (buffer A), and then 1*M* NaCl and either 8*M* urea or 1.0*M* arginine-HCl in buffer A. Some samples were prechromatographed on Sepharose 4B. Pooled fractions were dialyzed against buffer A and concentrated, when necessary, by immersible membrane ultrafiltration (CX; Millipore). Lower molecular weight peptides of 50–100 kd were separated by gel filtration on a 1.6 × 70-cm Sephacryl S-200 column (Pharmacia), using a 0.1*M* Tris–0.15*M* NaCl buffer, pH 7.3.

Affinity chromatography on heparin–Sepharose 6BCl. Synovial fluid, plasma, or fibronectin that had been isolated from the above fluids was applied to a 0.9 × 15-cm heparin-Sepharose column (Pharmacia). Unbound protein was eluted in 0.01*M* phosphate, 1 m*M* PMSF, pH 7.3 (buffer B). Elution of bound protein was achieved by a stepwise increase in ionic strength by adding NaCl in buffer B to final molarities of 0.15*M*, 0.5*M*, 1.0*M*, and 1.5*M*, or by using a linear NaCl gradient. Protein in the eluates was monitored by absorbance at 280 nm. Fractions were pooled, dialyzed against phosphate buffered saline (PBS), and concentrated. Fibronectin was quantitated by electroimmunoassay (5) or enzyme-linked immunosorbent assay (ELISA). The fibronectin concentration of purified solutions was determined assuming $A^{1\%}_{cm}$ at 280 nm = 12.8 (18).

Rabbit anti-human fibronectin. Rabbit anti-human fibronectin was prepared by multiple-site injections of a total of 1 mg of purified plasma fibronectin in Freund's complete adjuvant into 6-week-old male New Zealand white rabbits. At 4 and 6 weeks postinjection, booster injections of 500 μg of fibronectin in incomplete adjuvant were administered. Rabbit serum was made monospecific by absorption ×2 with fibronectin-depleted human plasma (a byproduct of the plasma fibronectin isolation procedure). Immunoelectrophoresis against whole human plasma yielded 1 arc, and immunoprecipitation of ^{35}S-methionine-labeled fibroblast-conditioned medium yielded 1 band at 230 kd after sodium dodecyl sulfate–polyacrylamide gel electrophoresis (SDS-PAGE) and fluorography.

Goat anti-rabbit IgG. Commercially prepared goat anti-rabbit immunoglobulin fraction (Pel-Freez, Rogers, AR) was obtained and further purified by affinity chromatography on protein A–Sepharose 4B (Pharmacia) and by gel filtration on Sephacryl S-300 (Pharmacia). Purified IgG was labeled with ^{125}I (New England Nuclear, Boston, MA), by the iodine monochloride method (19), to a specific activity of 28.9 μCi/μg, or was linked to alkaline phosphatase with glutaraldehyde (20).

Measurement of fibronectin immunoactivity and ligand binding by ELISA (21). Microtiter plate wells (Dynatech, Alexandria, VA) were coated with purified plasma fibronectin (200 ng/well) by overnight incubation at 4°C. The plates were washed 3 times with 0.05% Triton-X100 in PBS (PBS-Triton), dried at room temperature, and stored at 4°C. A 1:20,000 dilution of rabbit anti-human fibronectin antiserum was incubated with increasing concentrations of purified fibronectin standard, unknown synovial fluid, purified protein samples, or buffer for 90 minutes at 20°C in 12 × 75-mm polypropylene tubes. Antigen–antibody mixtures were then transferred to the fibronectin-coated microtiter plate wells and incubated for 30 minutes at 37°C. Plates were then washed with PBS-Triton, and goat anti-rabbit IgG conjugated to alkaline phosphatase (as above, or purchased from Sigma) was added to each well and incubated 90 minutes at 37°C. After washing, paranitrophenyl phosphate (Sigma) was added (1 mg/ml 0.05*M* sodium bicarbonate, 1 m*M* $MgCl_2$, pH 9.8), and incubation was continued for 15 minutes at 37°C. The reactions were terminated by adding 50 μl of 4*N* NaOH, and the absorbance was read at 405 nm.

To estimate fibronectin binding to fibrin and gelatin, wells were coated with 500 μg of fibrin or 1 mg of gelatin (1). A series of fibrin- and gelatin-coated wells were incubated with increasing concentrations of purified normal plasma fibronectin and isolated synovial fluid fibronectin having identical immunoreactivity (as determined in the competitive binding ELISA described above). After washing with PBS-Triton, bound fibronectin was detected by sequential incubation with rabbit anti-human fibronectin, goat anti-rabbit IgG conjugated to alkaline phosphatase, and substrate (see above).

SDS-PAGE. Using cylindrical gels, SDS-PAGE was performed according to the method of Weber and Osborne (22), with an acrylamide concentration of 5%. Slab gel electrophoresis was performed using a discontinuous Laemmli buffer system (23). Samples were reduced with dithiothreitol. Gels were stained with Coomassie brilliant blue or silver (Bio-Rad, Richmond, CA). Molecular weight standards were purchased from Bio-Rad.

Localization of fibronectin antigen according to molecular size was accomplished by SDS-PAGE followed by labeling with antifibronectin, according to the method of Olden and Yamada (24), or by immunoblotting, as described by Towbin et al (25). Peaks from radiodensitometric plots were excised and weighed to obtain a relative proportion of each polypeptide present. Apparent molecular weights were calculated from molecular weight standards on replicate lanes.

Proteolysis of fibronectin. Paired aliquots (100 μg of protein) of purified plasma fibronectin and synovial fluid fibronectin were incubated with porcine plasmin (Sigma), 4.2 units/mg (10:1 weight:weight), for 10, 30, 60, and 180 minutes. Proteolysis was stopped by the addition of 2 m*M* PMSF and Trasylol (500 units/ml). Samples were analyzed by SDS-PAGE.

Effect of fibronectin on synoviocyte migration. Human synoviocytes derived from explants of rheumatoid synovium, obtained at the time of surgery, were maintained in culture as described (26). Early (the first through the third) passage cultures were used. Flasks (75 mm) were rinsed with Dulbecco's modified Eagle's medium (DMEM; Gibco, Grand Island, NY) and then incubated with 4 ml of trypsin-EDTA (Gibco) for 3 minutes at 37°C. Synoviocytes were washed with an equal volume of DMEM, resuspended, and incubated in DMEM–10% fetal bovine serum (FBS; Gibco) for 20 minutes. The cells were washed and resuspended in DMEM without FBS to a concentration of 2×10^5/ml.

After filling the lower portions of blind chemotaxis chambers (Nucleopore, Inc., Cabin John, MD) with 0.2 ml of chemoattractant and placement of an 8-μm polycarbonate membrane (polyvinyl pyrrolidone–free; Nucleopore), cell suspensions (0.5 ml) were placed in the upper portion. Chambers were incubated for 2.5 hours in 10% CO_2 at 37°C. Filters were stained with hematoxylin, mounted on slides, and the mean number of cells in 20 high power fields (×400) was counted. Each experiment was performed in triplicate chambers.

Monocyte attachment to gelatin and fibrin. Tissue culture plate wells (16 mm; Becton-Dickinson, Oxnard, CA) were gelatin-coated by incubation with 0.5 ml of gelatin (30 mg/ml) in distilled water for 2 hours at 37°C, followed by 2 hours incubation at 40°C.

Plates were coated with fibrin using human fibrinogen purchased from Calbiochem (San Diego, CA), which was further purified and rendered fibronectin-free by DEAE-Sephacel and gelatin-Sepharose chromatography. Fibrinogen was converted to fibrin by treatment with thrombin (1 unit/ml) for 60 minutes at 37°C. The wells were washed with PBS containing 1 unit of Hirudin (Calbiochem) and then dried.

Gelatin- and fibrin-coated wells were incubated with buffer or fibronectin preparations for 1 hour at 22°C, aspirated, and washed with DMEM. To evaluate the effect of fibronectin fragments on monocyte adherence mediated by intact fibronectin, wells were pretreated with buffer (control) or with the relevant fragment before incubation with intact fibronectin.

Peripheral blood mononuclear cells were obtained by density gradient centrifugation (27). Viability, assessed by trypan blue exclusion, was 96–99%.

One milliliter of cell suspension (4×10^5 cells) was added per well and incubated for 1 hour at 37°C in 10% CO_2. Nonadherent cells were aspirated, the wells were washed with DMEM, and adherent cells were fixed with glutaraldehyde (1.25%). Data are expressed as adherent cells per 5 high power fields (×400). Each point represents data from duplicate or triplicate wells.

RESULTS

Polypeptide composition of synovial fluid fibronectin. Fibronectin was isolated from synovial fluid by gelatin-Sepharose affinity chromatography.

SDS-PAGE analysis of bound material that eluted with 8*M* urea revealed fibronectin fragments in 16 of 18 reduced samples (86%) from patients with active RA (Figures 1 and 2). Polypeptides of 210–215 kd and 190–205 kd were predominant (Figure 1, lanes b, e, h, and j; Figure 2, lanes B and C), although faint bands of 145–180 kd and 50–100 kd were also noted. In 61% (8 of 13) of the samples examined both with and without reduction, dimeric fibronectin was present in the nonreduced state (Figure 1, lane i) in addition to the lower molecular weight bands. In 5 preparations, only bands of 215 kd and 200 kd were present both with (Figure 2, lanes B and C) and without (Figure 2, lanes E and F) reduction.

Electrophoresis of whole synovial fluid followed by reaction of fixed gels with antifibronectin allowed molecular size estimation of the major antigenic forms. The predominant bands seen on Coomassie blue–stained gels were immunoreactive. When RA synovial fluid and whole normal plasma were electrophoresed in parallel gel lanes and the relative areas of the major immunoreactive bands were compared, the RA fluid sample contained a doublet at 210–220 kd and an increase in material of 170–190 kd.

Unbound immunoreactive fibronectin fragments recovered in 1*M* NaCl gelatin-Sepharose eluates were present in 5–10-fold higher concentration in eluates from RA fluid, compared with normal plasma. Gel filtration of these eluates (Figure 3) showed fibronectin immunoreactivity in multiple column fractions corresponding to 50–100 kd. Immunoblotting procedures localized the major immunoreactive species to 66 kd (Figure 4).

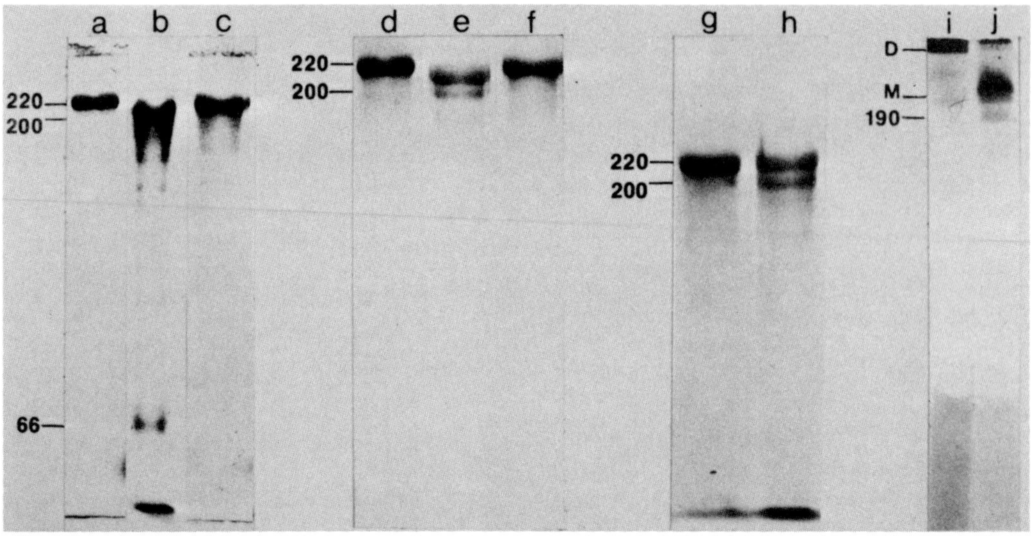

Figure 1. Polypeptide composition of synovial fluid fibronectin: 8*M* urea eluates from gelatin-Sepharose columns electrophoresed on polyacrylamide gels and stained with Coomassie brilliant blue. Molecular weight markers are shown to the left. Lane a, plasma fibronectin; lane b, rheumatoid arthritis (RA) synovial fluid fibronectin (Table 1, sample 4); lane c, osteoarthritis (OA) synovial fluid fibronectin (Table 1, sample 8); all on 3% stacking gel, 9% separating slab gel. Lane d, plasma fibronectin; lane e, RA synovial fluid fibronectin (Table 1, sample 1); lane f, OA synovial fluid fibronectin; all on 3% stacking gel, 7% separating slab gel. Lane g, plasma fibronectin; lane h, RA synovial fluid fibronectin (Table 1, sample 3), showing a polypeptide pattern identical to that observed without reducing agent; both on 3% stacking gel, 6% separating slab gel. Lane i, nonreduced RA synovial fluid fibronectin; lane j, reduced RA synovial fluid fibronectin. Note a large amount of material corresponding to the fibronectin dimer (D) at the top of lane i; both on 5% cylindrical gel. M = monomer.

Plasmin digestion of synovial fluid and plasma fibronectin. Plasmin treatment of native plasma fibronectin for 30 minutes generated high molecular weight polypeptides with migration patterns nearly identical to the major fibronectin species isolated from RA synovial fluid. Plasmin digestion of plasma fibronectin generated a 34-kd polypeptide which was not seen in plasmin-treated RA synovial fluid fibronectin even after prolonged digestion. In addition, other minor differences between the polypeptide patterns of plasma and synovial fluid fibronectin were noted.

Immunoreactivity of synovial fluid fibronectin. Consistent with previously published results (5–9), we found that RA synovial fluid contained higher amounts of fibronectin antigen than did normal plasma, when measured by ELISA. The shapes of the dilution-binding curves for RA synovial fluid and normal plasma, however, were similar (Figure 5, panels B and C). Fibronectin immunoreactivity in noninflammatory osteoarthritic synovial fluid was equal to that of normal plasma (Figure 5, panel A).

Isolated rheumatoid fibronectin polypeptides displayed immunoreactivity similar to that of purified plasma fibronectin peptides; however, the immunoreactivity of unbound fibronectin peptides was consider-

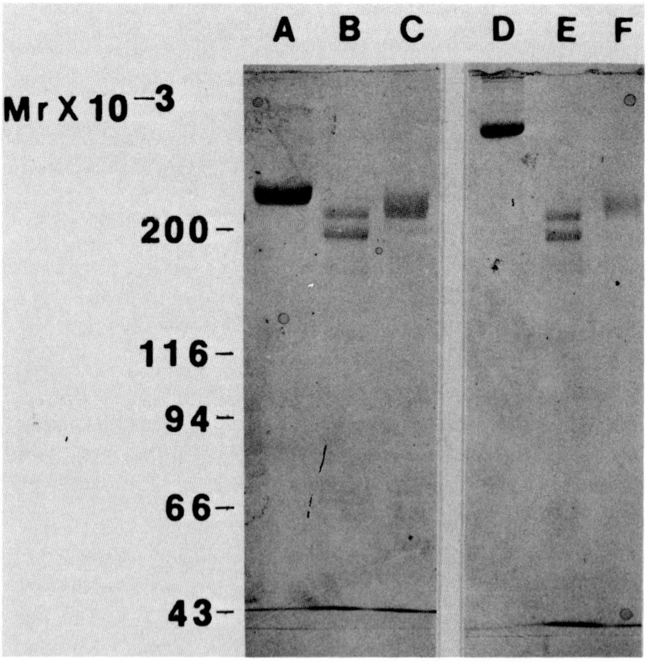

Figure 2. Polypeptide composition of synovial fluid fibronectin (see Figure 1 for details). Lane A, reduced purified plasma fibronectin; lanes B and C, reduced isolated rheumatoid arthritis (RA) synovial fluid fibronectins; lane D, nonreduced purified plasma fibronectin; lanes E and F, isolated nonreduced RA synovial fluid fibronectins; all on 6% separating gel.

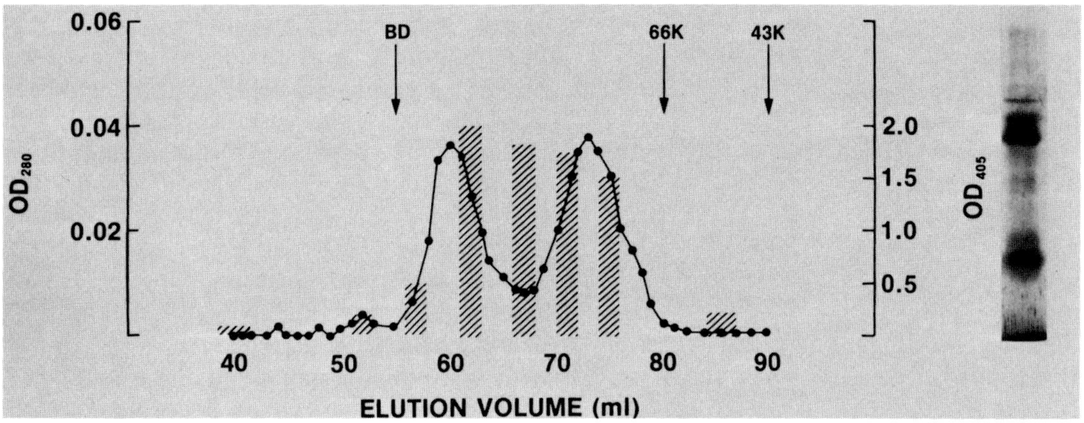

Figure 3. Sephacryl S-200 chromatography of the 1*M* NaCl fraction obtained during the isolation of rheumatoid arthritis (RA) synovial fluid fibronectin (Table 1, sample 7). Protein eluted in 0.1*M* Tris–0.15*M* NaCl, pH 7.4, is indicated by the solid line profile (at OD 280). Hatched bars represent immunoreactive fibronectin in pooled, concentrated fractions, determined by enzyme-linked immunosorbent assay (at OD 405). There is approximately a 5–10-fold enrichment of immunoreactive fibronectin in the RA synovial fluid 1*M* NaCl eluate, compared with the plasma 1*M* NaCl eluate, after normalization to the total fibronectin applied to the column. BD = blue dextran.

ably reduced (Figures 6A and B). Collection of synovial fluid into heparin tubes or treatment of synovial fluid with hyaluronidase before ELISA did not alter immunoreactivity (Figure 5, panel C).

Binding of synovial fluid fibronectin to gelatin, heparin, and fibrin. Recovery of bound fibronectin (defined as material that eluted with 8*M* urea) during isolation from synovial fluid was compared with the recovery of fibronectin from normal plasma as an estimate of relative gelatin binding (Table 1). Recovery of bound fibronectin from normal human plasma ranged from 68–95%, with a mean ± SD of 78 ± 12%. Fibronectin recovery from noninflammatory osteoarthritic fluid was 88%. Recovery of bound fibronectin from 7 RA fluids was highly variable, ranging from 45–125%.

Measurement of fibronectin by ELISA in the 0.05*M* Tris flow-through material and in the 1*M* NaCl eluates (Table 1) revealed that in normal human plasma (samples 9 and 10) and in 3 RA fluids (samples 1, 2, and 4), for which the mean recovery of bound fibronectin was 93%, unbound fibronectin antigen measured <1% (mean). In 4 RA fluids (samples 3, 5, 6, and 7), for which the mean recovery of bound fibronectin was 58%, a mean of 12% (range 3–37) of immunoreactive fibronectin was unbound. Inclusion of the unbound fraction increased recovery to 70%.

When gelatin-binding fibronectin polypeptides were chromatographed on heparin-Sepharose, recovery of protein isolated from 3 RA synovial fluids (Figure 7A) was 56 ± 6% (mean ± SD), which was

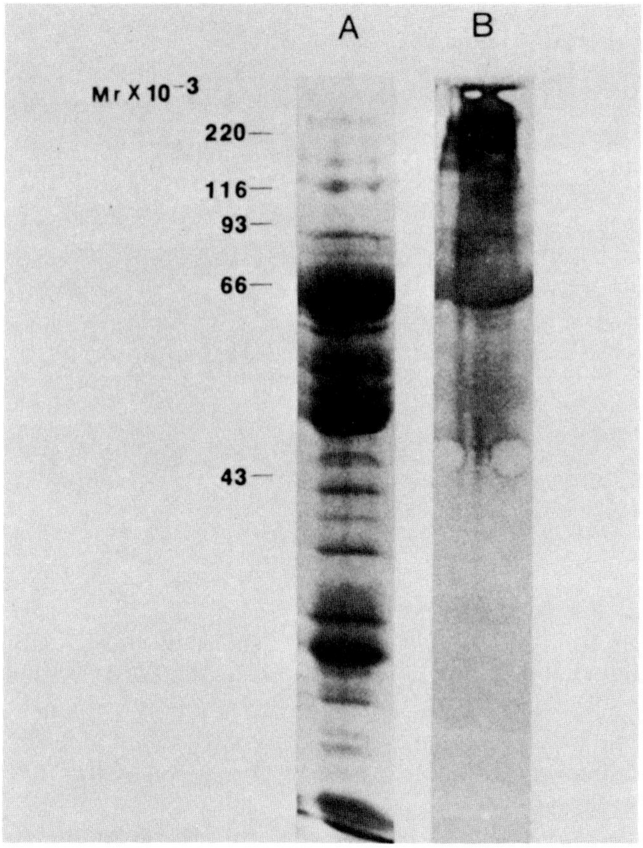

Figure 4. Sodium dodecyl sulfate–polyacrylamide gel electrophoresis of gelatin-Sepharose 1*M* NaCl eluate (10% gel). Lane A, total protein, by Coomassie brilliant blue staining; lane B, immunoblot of lane A transferred to nitrocellulose and stained with antifibronectin. The predominant immunoreactive band is observed at approximately 66 kd.

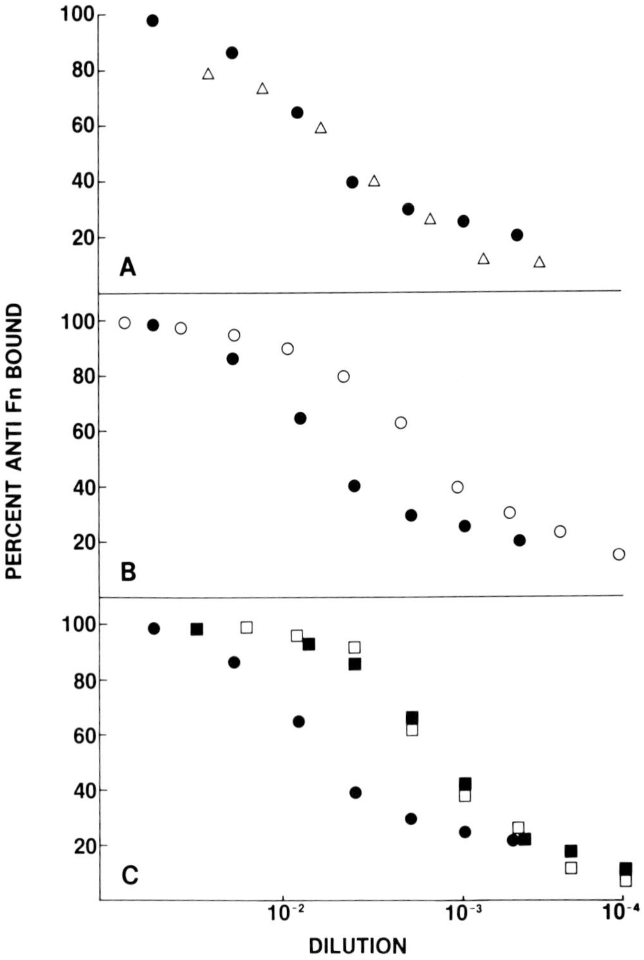

Figure 5. Dilution-binding curves of whole normal human plasma (●) and synovial fluid in a competitive binding fibronectin enzyme-linked immunosorbent assay, showing the percent of antifibronectin (anti Fn) antibody bound by soluble antigen (see Patients and Methods). Panel A, osteoarthritis synovial fluid (△) (Table 1, sample 8); panel B, rheumatoid arthritis (RA) synovial fluid (○) (Table 1, sample 7); panel C, RA synovial fluid with (□) and without (■) hyaluronidase (Table 1, sample 4).

similar to that from plasma fibronectin, 63 ± 25% (mean ± SD); however, synovial fluid fibronectin eluted at a slightly lower ionic strength (0.46*M* versus 0.50*M* NaCl). Chromatography of whole RA synovial fluid on heparin-Sepharose (Figure 7B) resulted in the elution of all immunoreactive fibronectin with 0.5*M* NaCl.

A modified ELISA was used to quantitate fibronectin binding to solid-phase gelatin and fibrin (Figure 8). Dilution-binding curves revealed that isolated rheumatoid synovial fluid fibronectin had a threefold lower affinity for gelatin than did purified normal plasma fibronectin of equivalent protein concentration and immunoreactivity. For the same sample, fibrin binding was decreased sixfold.

Cell-binding activity. The chemotactic property of fibronectin was used to assess the activity of the cell-binding domain of synovial fluid fibronectin (Figure 9, panels A–D) (4). Plasma fibronectin was chemotactic for early passage human rheumatoid synoviocytes, and the activity was comparable with that of zymosan-activated serum (panel A). Heat treatment of plasma fibronectin at 56°C for 30 minutes did not alter the chemotactic activity (panel B).

Whole rheumatoid synovial fluid (1:100 dilution) was chemotactic for synoviocytes (panel C). Heating whole synovial fluid for 30 minutes at 56°C to destroy residual complement activity reduced chemo-

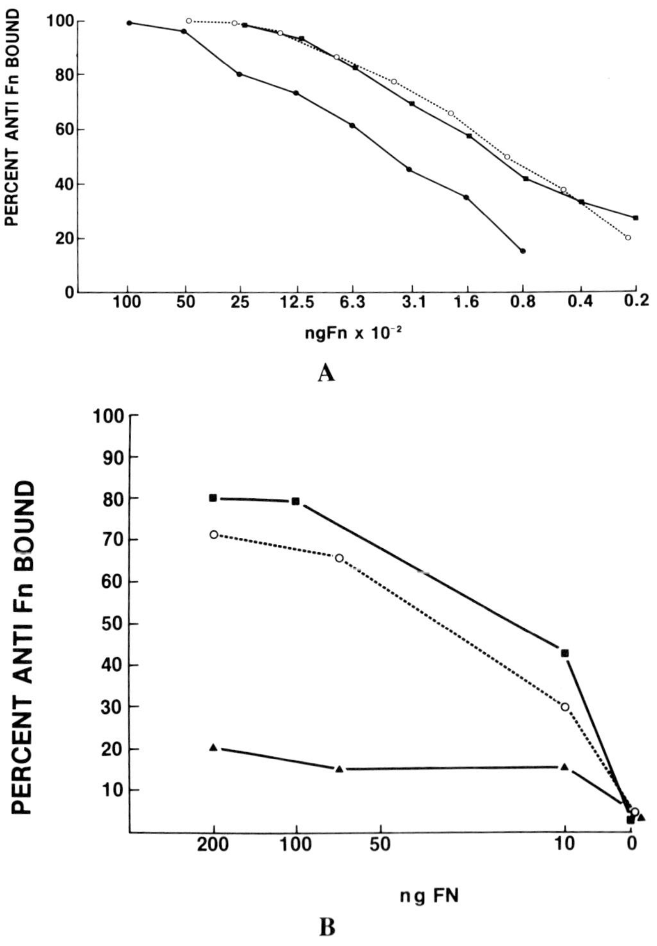

Figure 6. Dilution-binding curves of purified fibronectins (Fn). **A**, ○ = purified plasma fibronectin; ■ = purified rheumatoid arthritis (RA) synovial fluid fibronectin (Table 1, sample 4; *cf* Figure 1, lane b). ● = unbound fibronectin species from RA sample 7, Table 1 (*cf* Figure 5, panel B). **B**, ○ = purified plasma fibronectin; ■ = purified RA synovial fluid fibronectin; ▲ = gelatin-Sepharose unbound synovial fluid fibronectin peptides, purified by chromatography on antifibronectin-Sepharose.

Table 1. Recovery of fibronectin from synovial fluid and plasma*

Sample, diagnosis	Vol. (ml)	Protein (mg/ml)	Fn (μg/ml)	Total Fn (μg)	Unbound Fn (μg)	Bound Fn (μg)†	% recovery Total	% recovery Unbound	% recovery Bound
1, RA	7	54	1,000	7,000	110	8,500	126	1.0	125
2, RA	13	39	1,000	13,000	100	15,000	115	<1	115
3, RA	12	23	790	9,500	300	8,200	94	3.5	90
4, RA	11	81	300	3,300	0	3,000	81	0	81
5, RA	7	45	650	34,000	1,360	2,300	88	37	51
6, RA	8	84	700	5,600	70	2,600	49	3	46
7, RA	10	35	900	9,000	230	4,000	51	6	45
Total 1–7‡		52 ± 23	760 ± 245				86 ± 29	7 ± 13	78 ± 32
8, OA	3	33	300	900	<1	800	88	0	88
9, NHP	100	ND	340	34,000	14	25,300	74	<1	74
10, NHP	100	ND	320	32,000	340	21,800	70	1.6	68
11, NHP	200	ND	350	70,000	ND	67,000	95	ND	95
12, NHP	100	ND	350	35,000	ND	26,800	76	ND	76
Total 9–12‡			340 ± 14				79 ± 11	1	78 ± 12

* Vol. = total volume; Fn = fibronectin; RA = rheumatoid arthritis synovial fluid; OA = osteoarthritis synovial fluid; NHP = normal human plasma; ND = not done.
† Bound fibronectin eluted from the column with 8*M* urea.
‡ Data expressed as mean, or mean ± SD.

tactic activity by 24%. Subsequent gelatin-Sepharose treatment removed 98.5% of immunoreactive fibronectin and abolished the remainder of the synovial fluid chemotactic activity.

The chemotactic activity of isolated RA fibronectin fragments of 190–205 kd was nearly equivalent to that of plasma fibronectin (Figure 9, panel D, lanes 1 and 2). The weakly bound gelatin-Sepharose fraction

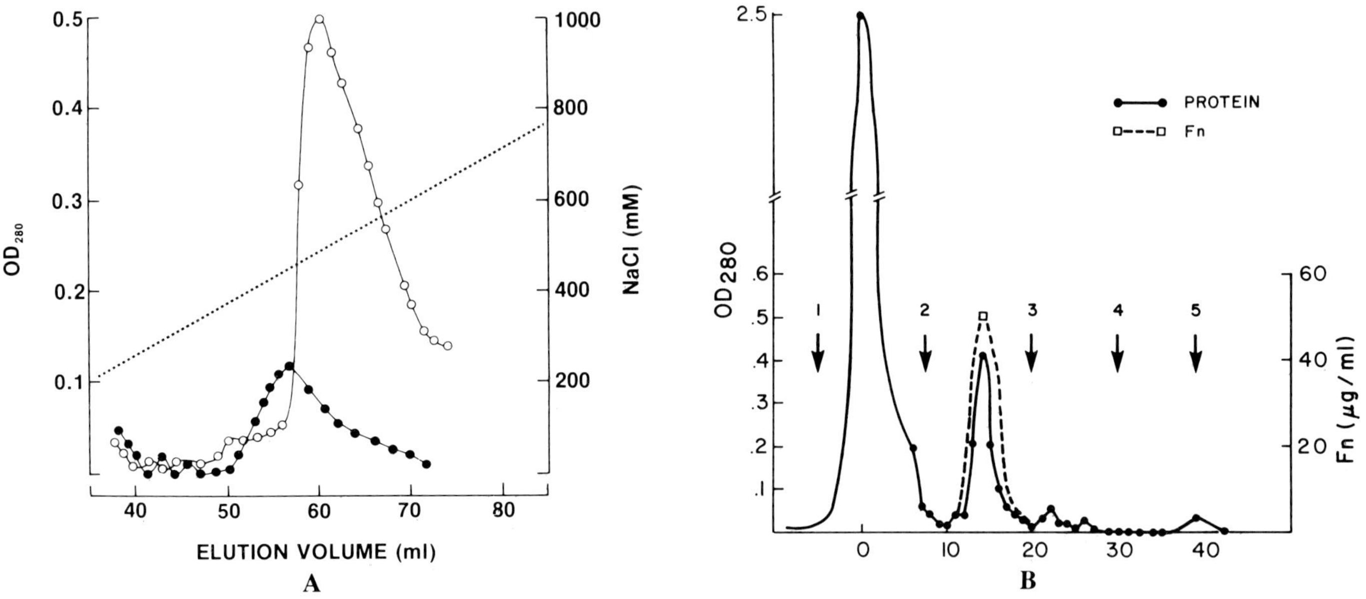

Figure 7. A, Chromatography of purified rheumatoid arthritis (RA) synovial fluid fibronectin, 3.6 mg (●——●) (*cf* Figure 1, lane h) and purified normal human plasma fibronectin, 6.6 mg (○——○) on a 1.5 × 9.0-cm column of heparin-Sepharose 6BCl. Protein was eluted in a linear gradient (0.1–1.0*M* NaCl) in 0.01*M* phosphate, pH 7.3. Synovial fluid fibronectin elutes with 0.46*M* NaCl; plasma fibronectin elutes with 0.50*M* NaCl. **B**, Chromatography of whole RA synovial fluid on heparin-Sepharose. Buffers 1–5 (arrows) in 0.01*M* phosphate buffer are: 0.15*M*, 0.5*M*, 1.0*M*, 1.5*M* NaCl, and 4*M* urea, respectively. All immunoreactive fibronectin (Fn) eluted with 0.5*M* NaCl. Protein was detected by absorbance at 280 nm. Numbers across the x-axis represent the elution volume.

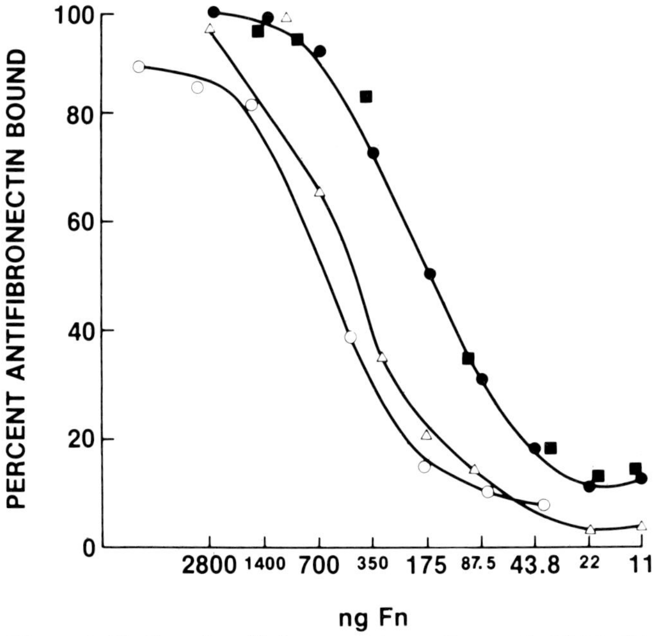

Figure 8. Binding of purified normal plasma fibronectin (Fn) (solid symbols) and purified rheumatoid arthritis (RA) synovial fluid fibronectin (Table 1, sample 4) (open symbols) to gelatin (triangles and squares) and fibrin (circles) surfaces (plasma Fn curves superimposed to allow comparisons). Incremental amounts of purified fibronectins were added to either gelatin- or fibrin-coated microtiter wells. Fibronectin binding to gelatin or fibrin was determined as the proportion of antifibronectin bound to the well. RA synovial fluid fibronectin binding to gelatin was one-third, and binding to fibrin one-sixth, that of plasma fibronectin. Purified RA and plasma fibronectins had nearly identical immunoreactivity (see Figure 6A).

(50–100 kd) was chemotactic at a tenfold higher molar concentration than fibronectin monomer (panel D, lane 3).

Role of synovial fluid fibronectin in monocyte attachment. Preincubation of gelatin-coated surfaces with RA synovial fluid enhanced the attachment of monocytes in a dose-dependent manner (Table 2, experiment 1). Monocyte attachment to gelatin surfaces incubated with RA synovial fluid at dilutions of 1:2, 1:4, and 1:8 increased by 247%, 187%, and 120%, respectively ($P < 0.002$, $P < 0.01$, $P > 0.05$, respectively). Prior depletion of fibronectin by affinity chromatography on gelatin-Sepharose abrogated the enhanced monocyte attachment to gelatin surfaces.

Equivalent dilutions of normal human plasma (Table 2, experiment 2) were less active ($P < 0.002$) in promoting monocyte attachment to gelatin. Fibronectins isolated from plasma and those from RA fluid, however, were equivalent in their ability to promote monocyte attachment.

Monocytes, which have a fibrin receptor on their surfaces (28), bound to fibrin-coated surfaces in medium alone (Table 2, experiment 3). Treatment of fibrin-coated surfaces with intact plasma fibronectin produced a significant enhancement of monocyte attachment to fibrin (mean for experiments 3 and 4 = 138%). Neither the 200-kd fragments isolated from RA synovial fluid (experiment 3) nor the 200-kd fragments produced by in vitro plasmin digestion of plasma fibronectin (experiment 4) were capable of enhancing monocyte binding to fibrin.

Since fibronectin fragments coexist with intact fibronectin in synovial fluid, we investigated whether fragments could block functions of the intact molecule. We examined the effect of preincubation of fibrin-coated wells with 30-kd fibrin-binding fragments before incubation with intact fibronectin, and we compared the attachment of monocytes to these wells with attachment to those treated with native fibronectin alone. The 30-kd amino-terminal fragments used were

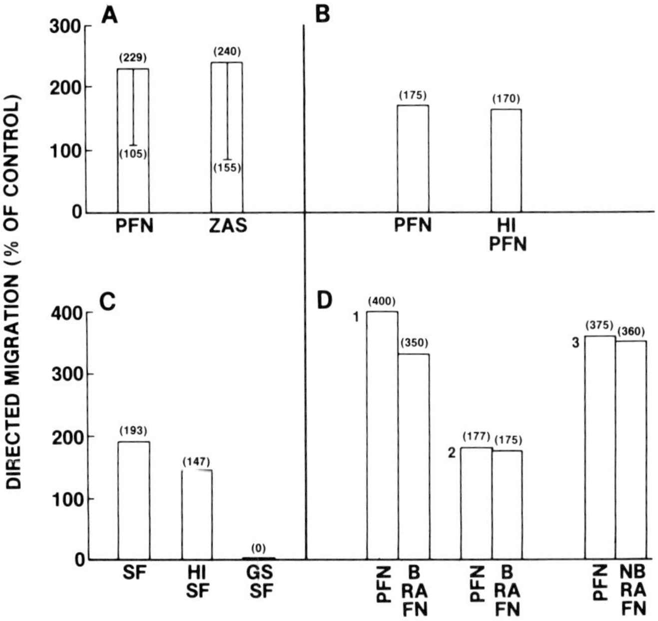

Figure 9. Effect of fibronectin peptides on chemotaxis of early passage human synoviocytes. Panel A, purified plasma fibronectin (PFN) (2 μg) had chemotactic activity similar to that of zymosan-activated serum (ZAS); panel B, heat inactivation of purified fibronectin (HI PFN) did not significantly alter chemotactic activity; panel C, whole rheumatoid arthritis (RA) synovial fluid (SF) diluted 1:100 was chemotactic for synoviocytes. Heat inactivation of synovial fluid (HI SF) reduced chemotactic activity by 24%, whereas subsequent fibronectin depletion by gelatin-Sepharose (GS SF) abrogated chemotactic activity; panel D, chemotactic activity of fibronectins isolated from synovial fluid. High molecular weight gelatin-Sepharose–bound fragments (B RA FN) (Table 1, samples 1 and 4) at 4×10^{-8} moles (lanes 1 and 2) and low molecular weight unbound (NB) fragments at 4×10^{-7} moles (lane 3) possessed chemotactic activity similar to that of purified plasma fibronectin (2-μg samples).

Table 2. Fibronectin-mediated monocyte attachment to gelatin and fibrin*

Source	Dil./μg	Cells/5 hpf	% DMEM	*P*
Gelatin-coated surface				
Experiment 1				
DMEM	0	15 ± 4	–	–
RA SF	1:2	37 ± 12	247	<0.002
RA SF	1:4	28 ± 7	187	<0.01
RA SF	1:8	18 ± 7	120	>0.05
Fn Dep	1:2	15 ± 5	100	>0.05
Experiment 2				
DMEM	0	7 ± 3	–	–
NHP	1:4	18 ± 5	257	<0.01
RA SF	1:4	28 ± 7	400	<0.002
P Fn	50	22 ± 11	314	<0.004
RA Fn	50	22 ± 13	314	<0.004
Fibrin-coated surface				
Experiment 3				
DMEM	0	29 ± 6	–	–
P Fn	100	37 ± 7	128	<0.03
RA Fn	100	29 ± 7	100	>0.05
Experiment 4				
DMEM	0	15 ± 3	–	–
P Fn	50	22 ± 5	147	<0.02
200 kd†	50	16 ± 5	107	>0.05
Experiment 5				
DMEM	0	8 ± 3	–	–
Tris/P Fn‡	50	21 ± 7	263	–
30 kd/P Fn§	50	14 ± 4	175	0.02¶

* Dil./μg = dilution of plasma or synovial fluid or amount of protein (in μg); hpf = high power field (data expressed as mean ± SD); DMEM = Dulbecco's modified Eagle's medium; *P* = significance versus DMEM value for experiment; RA = rheumatoid arthritis; SF = synovial fluid; Fn Dep = fibronectin depleted; NHP = normal human plasma; P Fn = purified fibronectin; RA Fn = rheumatoid arthritis fibronectin.
† 200-kd fibronectin fragments produced by in vitro plasmin digestion.
‡ Fibrin wells sequentially incubated with Tris buffer and intact fibronectin (50 μg).
§ Fibrin wells sequentially incubated with 30-kd fragment (13 μg) and intact fibronectin (50 μg).
¶ Versus Tris buffer control.

formed in vitro by 15-minute plasmin digestion of plasma fibronectin followed by separation on Sephadex G-100. Monocyte attachment to fibrin surfaces pretreated with 30-kd fragments was inhibited by 54% ($P = 0.02$) (Table 2, experiment 5).

DISCUSSION

Elevated levels of immunoreactive fibronectin in rheumatoid synovial fluid have been well documented (5–9). The purpose of this study was to investigate the structural and functional properties of fibronectin isolated from inflammatory synovial fluid.

We found that fibronectin isolated from inflammatory RA fluid contained polypeptides of smaller apparent molecular weight than the native plasma fibronectin monomer. Since fibronectin that is newly synthesized by metabolically labeled RA tissue explants is intact (230–240 kd) (26), these smaller peptides probably arise from proteolytic cleavage.

Sixty-one percent of RA samples examined before disulfide bond reduction contained molecules that co-migrated with fibronectin dimer, indicating an intact interchain disulfide bond at the carboxy-terminal (29). This area of the molecule contains the major heparin- and cell-binding sites (30). The presence of 190–210-kd peptides as the highest molecular weight species in 39% of nonreduced samples indicates proteolytic cleavage interior to the interchain disulfide bond.

Plasmin or trypsin treatment of plasma fibronectin in vitro (13,31) produces fragments of strikingly similar molecular size, as demonstrated by co-migration of rheumatoid synovial fluid fibronectin peptides with 30-minute plasmin digests of native fibronectin. A 30-kd peptide similar to that formed by digestion of plasma fibronectin has not been recovered from synovial fluid, indicating that it may have undergone either transglutaminase-mediated cross-linking (32) to collagen or fibrin in synovium, or further degradation. A monoclonal antibody specific for the fibronectin N-terminal domain would be useful in the detection of such a fragment.

Clemmensen and Andersen (8) have also demonstrated increased fibronectin polypeptide heterogeneity in RA synovial fluid, whereas Vartio et al (7) found no significant differences when they compared isolated synovial fluid fibronectin with plasma fibronectin. We have found intact synovial fluid fibronectin in patients with a diagnosis of RA, but without synovial inflammation, undergoing reconstructive surgery for end-stage disease (Carsons SE, Lavietes B: unpublished observations). Differences in fibronectin heterogeneity reported in the above-referenced studies may be secondary to variations in disease activity and to the degree of inflammation present in vivo.

Mosher and Johnson (33) have hypothesized that lower molecular weight fibronectin species in plasma may be derived from tissue undergoing active proteolysis. Therefore, it was somewhat surprising that the fibronectin we recovered from inflammatory synovial fluid was not more extensively degraded, especially in view of fibronectin's protease sensitivity and the extensive antigenic heterogeneity of synovial fluid fibrinogen (34). Susceptibility of fibronectin to proteases at sites of inflammation in vivo may be modulated by local concentrations of protease inhibitors (35) or differences in fibronectin glycosylation (36).

Gelatin-Sepharose binding of the 190–220-kd peptides indicates that these fibronectin fragments possess collagen-binding domains. Although other proteins of similar molecular weight, such as procollagens I and III (190 and 170 kd, respectively) (37), chondronectin (180 kd) (38), or thrombospondin (160 kd) (39), could theoretically be co-isolated by gelatin-Sepharose chromatography, antibody labeling of gels demonstrates that the 190–220-kd peptides possess fibronectin antigenic determinants.

Immunoreactivity of the major fibronectin species isolated from rheumatoid synovial fluid was similar to that of purified plasma fibronectin. This is consistent with the findings of Vuento et al (40), who showed that the immunoreactivity of 180–200-kd fragments generated by plasmin in vitro was nearly identical to that of intact protein. The elevated levels of immunoreactive fibronectin measured in RA synovial fluid accurately reflect increased concentrations of intact or nearly intact protein. Unbound peptides recovered from RA fluids demonstrated reduced immunoreactivity in the ELISA assay. Thus, extensive proteolytic cleavage results in reduced apparent levels of synovial fluid fibronectin.

The relative affinity of isolated synovial fluid fibronectin species for gelatin, fibrin, and heparin was compared with that of plasma fibronectin, using solid-phase enzyme-linked binding assays and affinity chromatography. Although synovial fluid fibronectin peptides were isolated by affinity chromatography on gelatin, they demonstrated reduced affinity for gelatin when compared with native plasma fibronectin in a solid-phase binding assay. This may be due, in part, to loss of the dimeric form, which has been shown to be necessary for maximal gelatin binding (41).

Synovial fluid fibronectin peptides demonstrated an even greater reduction in fibrin binding. This is consistent with loss of the amino-terminal, which contains the high-affinity fibrin-binding site (42). In contrast, binding of synovial fluid fibronectin to heparin did not markedly differ from that of plasma fibronectin despite loss of the low-affinity heparin-binding site in the amino-terminal fragment (43). The presence of the high-affinity carboxy-terminal heparin-binding domain probably accounts for nearly maximal heparin binding.

The chemotactic activity of rheumatoid synovial fluid fibronectin provides evidence for the presence of an intact cell-binding site (4). Passaged human synoviocytes exhibit fibroblastic morphology in culture (26), and fibroblast chemotactic activity of purified fibronectin (Figure 9, panel A) has been shown to be dependent on the cell-binding domain present on a 140-kd carboxy-terminal fragment (4). Rheumatoid synovial fluid fibronectin (190–220 kd) displayed chemotactic activity similar to that of intact plasma fibronectin, both mediating 200–400% of control migration at concentrations equivalent to 4.5×10^{-8} moles of monomer (Figure 9, panel D, lanes 1 and 2). Although a higher concentration (10^{-7} moles) was required, unbound fragments of lower molecular weight (50–100 kd) also mediated enhanced synoviocyte migration, suggesting that a portion of these fragments had intact cell-binding domains (Figure 9, panel D, lane 3).

Fibronectin was shown to be responsible for part of the chemotactic activity of whole RA synovial fluid since fibronectin depletion of heat-inactivated synovial fluid abrogated its chemotactic activity (Figure 9, panel C). Fibronectin distribution is heterogeneous in rheumatoid synovium, and differences in local fibronectin concentration may modulate synoviocyte migration in the diseased tissue. The increased deposition that is seen in the proliferated lining and surrounding inflamed blood vessels (26,44) may mediate the recruitment of additional connective tissue cells and macrophages (14) to these areas.

Fibronectin is also the major synovial fluid protein that mediates the attachment of human blood monocytes to denatured collagen. In fact, because of the elevated fibronectin concentration, RA synovial fluid has greater monocyte attachment–promoting activity than is found in equal dilutions of normal plasma. Isolated synovial fluid fibronectin peptides, including those composed entirely of 190–220-kd fragments, are equivalent to purified plasma fibronectin in the promotion of monocyte attachment (based on weight).

Rourke et al (45) showed that 170–210-kd fibronectin fragments produced by in vitro plasmin digestion were able to mediate the uptake of gelatinized erythrocytes by rat peritoneal macrophages. Molnar et al (46) measured the uptake of latex particles by liver slices and defined a 190–200-kd fragment as the minimal unit required for gelatin-coated particles to retain their opsonic activity. Synovial fluid fibronectin, however, does not augment monocyte attachment to fibrin. Since synovial fluid fibronectin possesses a functionally active cell-binding domain, the defect may lie in an inability of this form of the protein to bind fibrin, thus preventing it from forming an effective molecular link between substrate-bound fibrin and the monocyte.

Our data and data from the studies cited above suggest that synovial fluid fibronectin has the potential to mediate the binding and opsonization of denatured collagen in the diseased joint. The inability of synovial fluid fibronectin to enhance monocyte binding to fibrin may result in the persistence of fibrin in inflamed joints. The inhibition of fibronectin-mediated monocyte attachment by small fibronectin fragments containing the fibrin-binding site may be an additional mechanism that interferes with fibrin opsonization. Although Ehrlich et al (47) did not directly address fibrin binding in their studies, their results showed depression of sheep red blood cell uptake by the rat reticuloendothelial system after treatment with fibronectin fragments produced by plasmin treatment.

In summary, rheumatoid synovial fluid contains fibronectin fragments which display alterations in biologic activity in vitro. The studies reported here suggest that these molecular forms may play a significant role in the modulation of synovial inflammation and repair in vivo.

ACKNOWLEDGMENTS

We thank Ann Scozzari and Lesley Carsons for typing the manuscript and Barbara Diamond for photographic assistance.

REFERENCES

1. Bevilacqua MP, Amrani D, Mosesson MW, Bianco C: Receptors for cold-insoluble globulin (plasma fibronectin) on human monocytes. J Exp Med 153:42–60, 1981
2. Yamada KM: Immunological characterization of a major transformation-sensitive fibroblast cell surface glycoprotein: localization, redistribution, and role in cell shape. J Cell Biol 78:520–541, 1978
3. Klebe RJ: Isolation of a collagen-dependent cell attachment factor. Nature 250:248–251, 1974
4. Postlethwaite AE, Keski-Oja J, Balian G, Kang AH: Induction of fibroblast chemotaxis by fibronectin: localization of the chemotactic region to a 140,000-molecular weight non gelatin-binding fragment. J Exp Med 153:494–499, 1981
5. Carsons S, Mosesson MW, Diamond HS: Detection and quantitation of fibronectin in synovial fluid from patients with rheumatic disease. Arthritis Rheum 24:1261–1267, 1981
6. Lu-Steffes M, Iammartino AJ, Schmid FR, Castor CW, Davis L, Entwhistle R, Anderson B: Fibronectin in rheumatoid and non-rheumatoid arthritic synovial fluids and in synovial fluid cryoproteins. Ann Clin Lab Sci 12:178–185, 1982
7. Vartio T, Vaheri A, Von Essen R, Isomaki H, Stenman S: Fibronectin in synovial fluid and tissue in rheumatoid arthritis. Eur J Clin Invest 11:207–212, 1981
8. Clemmensen I, Andersen RB: Different molecular forms of fibronectin in rheumatoid synovial fluid. Arthritis Rheum 25:25–31, 1982
9. Scott DL, Farr M, Crockson AP, Walton KW: Synovial fluid and plasma fibronectin levels in rheumatoid arthritis. Clin Sci 62:71–76, 1982
10. Hormann H, Jelinic V: Fibronectin. VII. Binding of cold-insoluble globulin and of denatured collagen by macrophages. Hoppe Seyler's Z Physiol Chem 361:379–387, 1980
11. Saba TM, Gregory TJ, Blumenstock FA: Human host defense mechanisms as they relate to surgery and trauma. Surg Annu 12:1–80, 1980
12. Czop JK, Kadish JL, Austen KF: Augmentation of human monocyte independent phagocytosis by fragments of human plasma fibronectin. Proc Natl Acad Sci USA 78:3649–3653, 1981
13. Sekiguchi K, Hakomori S: Domain structure of human plasma fibronectin: differences and similarities between

human and hamster fibronectins. J Biol Chem 258:3967–3973, 1983
14. Norris DA, Clark RA, Swigart LM, Huff JC, Weston WL, Howell SE: Fibronectin fragment(s) are chemotactic for human peripheral blood monocytes. J Immunol 129:1612–1618, 1982
15. Vartio T, Vaheri A, De Petro G, Barlati S: Fibronectin and its proteolytic fragments: potential as cancer markers. Invasion Metastasis 3:125–138, 1983
16. Yamada K: Cell surface interactions with extracellular materials. Annu Rev Biochem 52:761–799, 1983
17. De Petro G, Barlati S, Vartio T, Vaheri A: Transformation enhancing activity in plasma of tumor patients: relationship with fibronectin fragments. Int J Cancer 31:157–162, 1983
18. Chen AB, Amrani DL, Mosesson MW: Heterogeneity of the cold-insoluble globulin of human plasma (CIg), a circulating cell surface protein. Biochim Biophys Acta 493:310–322, 1977
19. Bale WF, Helmkarp RW, David TP, Izzo MJ, Contreras MA, Spar IC: High specific activity labeling of protein by the iodine monochloride method. Proc Soc Exp Biol Med 122:407–413, 1966
20. Engvall E: Enzyme Immunoassay: ELISA and EMIT. Methods Enzymol 70:419–439, 1980
21. Rennard SI, Berg R, Martin GR, Foidart JM, Robey PG: Enzyme-linked immunoassay (ELISA) for connective tissue components. Anal Biochem 104:205–214, 1980
22. Weber K, Osborne M: Proteins and sodium dodecyl sulfate: molecular weight determinations on polyacrylamide gels and related procedures, The Proteins. Vol. 1. Edited by H Neurath, RH Hill. New York, Academic Press, 1975, p 197
23. Laemmli UK: Cleavage of structural proteins during the assembly of the head of bacteriophage T4. Nature 227:680–685, 1970
24. Olden K, Yamada K: Direct detection of antigens in sodium dodecyl sulfate–polyacrylamide gels. Anal Biochem 78:483–490, 1977
25. Towbin H, Staehelin T, Gordon T: Electrophoretic transfer of proteins from polyacrylamide gels to nitrocellulose sheets: procedure and some applications. Proc Natl Acad Sci USA 76:4350–4354, 1979
26. Lavietes B, Carsons SE, Diamond H, Laskin R: Synthesis, secretion, and deposition of fibronectin in cultured human synovium. Arthritis Rheum (in press)
27. Boyum A: Isolation of mononuclear cells and granulocytes from human peripheral blood. Scand J Clin Lab Invest [Suppl] 97:77, 1968
28. Sherman LA: Binding of soluble fibrin to macrophages. Ann NY Acad Sci 408:610–620, 1983
29. Mosesson MW, Amrani DL: The structure and biologic activities of plasma fibronectin. Blood 56:145–158, 1980
30. Ruoslahti E, Hayman EG, Engvall E, Cothran WC, Butler WT: Alignment of biologically active domains in the fibronectin molecule. J Biol Chem 256:7277–7281, 1981
31. Jilek F, Hormann H: Cold-insoluble globulin: plasminolysis of cold-insoluble globulin. Hoppe Seyler's Z Physiol Chem 358:133–136, 1977
32. Mosher DF, Schad PE, Vann JM: Cross-linking of collagen and fibronectin by factor XIIIa: localization of participating glutaminyl residues to a tryptic fragment of fibronectin. J Biol Chem 255:1181–1188, 1979
33. Mosher D, Johnson R: In vitro formation of disulfide-bonded fibronectin multimers. J Biol Chem 258:6595–6601, 1983
34. Gormsen J, Andersen RB, Feddersen C: Fibrinogen-fibrin breakdown products in pathologic synovial fluids: an immunologic study. Arthritis Rheum 14:503–512, 1971
35. Ohlsson K: α_1-antitrypsin and α_2-macroglobulin: interactions with human neutrophil collagenase and elastase. Ann NY Acad Sci 256:409–419, 1975
36. Bernard BA, Yamada KM, Olden K: Carbohydrates selectively protect a specific domain of fibronectin against proteases. J Biol Chem 257:8549–8554, 1982
37. Carter WB, Hakomori SI: A new cell surface, detergent-insoluble glycoprotein matrix of human and hamster fibroblasts: the role of disulfide bonds in stabilization of the matrix. J Biol Chem 256:6953–6960, 1981
38. Hewitt AT, Varner HH, Silver MH, Dissace W, Wilkes CM, Martin GR: The isolation and partial characterization of chondronectin, an attachment factor for chondrocytes. J Biol Chem 257:2330–2339, 1982
39. Hayashi M, Yamada K: Domain structure of the carboxyl-terminal half of human plasma fibronectin. J Biol Chem 258:3332–3340, 1983
40. Vuento M, Salonen E, Salminen K, Pasanen M, Stenman UK: Immunochemical characterization of human plasma fibronectin. Biochem J 191:719–727, 1980
41. Amrani D, Homandberg G, Tooney M, Wolfenstein-Todel C, Mosesson M: Separation and analysis of the major forms of plasma fibronectin. Biochim Biophys Acta 748:308 320, 1983
42. Seidl M, Hormann H: Affinity chromatography of immobilized fibrin monomer. IV. Two fibrin-binding peptides of a chymotryptic digest of human plasma fibronectin. Hoppe Seyler's Z Physiol Chem 364:83–92, 1983
43. Richter H, Seidl M, Hormann H: Location of heparin-binding sites of fibronectin: detection of hitherto unrecognized transamidase sensitive site. Hoppe Seyler's Z Physiol Chem 362:399–408, 1981
44. Scott DL, Delamere JP, Walton KW: The distribution of fibronectin in the pannus in rheumatoid arthritis. Br J Exp Pathol 62:362–368, 1981
45. Rourke FJ, Blumenstock FA, Kaplan JE: Effect of fibronectin fragments on macrophage phagocytosis of gelatinized particles. J Immunol 132:1931–1937, 1984
46. Molnar J, Lai MZ, Siefring GE, Lorand L: Enzymatic modifications of human plasma fibronectin in relation to opsonizing activity. Biochemistry 22:5704–5709, 1983
47. Ehrlich MI, Krushell JS, Blumenstock FA, Kaplan JE: Depression of phagocytosis by plasmin degradation products of plasma fibronectin. J Lab Clin Med 98:263–270, 1981

REDUCED JOINT COUNT INDICES IN THE EVALUATION OF RHEUMATOID ARTHRITIS

M. J. EGGER, D. A. HUTH, J. R. WARD, J. C. READING, and H. J. WILLIAMS

Two types of summary measures of joint disease were evaluated in 2 controlled clinical trials in rheumatoid arthritis patients. One measure was based solely on the clinical/biologic judgment approach; the other combined this methodology with statistical approaches using reliability and factor analyses. "Signal joint" indices, summarizing disease activity in 2–5 key joints, were found to be insensitive to deterioriation of nonsignal joints. Therefore, they are not recommended as replacements for the complete articular survey in rheumatoid arthritis. A reduced version of the complete articular survey was found to be desirable based on its validity, reliability, accuracy, precision, and sensitivity to active drugs. Its sensitivity can be slightly higher or lower than that of the full joint survey.

The assessment of joint involvement in rheumatoid arthritis has been the single most important variable by which an individual patient's disease is evaluated. The patient is seeking relief of pain and functional loss and the physician is attempting to achieve the same objectives in addition to controlling inflammation. However, there is no single, uniform measure used in day-to-day management of rheumatoid arthritis or in therapeutic studies for evaluation of particular treatments. Indices of arthritis activity which involve counting or scoring every joint for involvement by pain, tenderness, and/or swelling have been developed by the Cooperating Clinics Committee of the American Rheumatism Association (ARA) (1), by Lansbury and Haut (2), by Ritchie et al (3), and by the Cooperative Systematic Studies of the Rheumatic Diseases group (CSSRD) (4–7). These complete joint assessments are time-consuming to perform and suffer from limited reliability in joints that are difficult to examine for swelling, such as the glenohumeral and metatarsophalangeal (MTP) joints.

An alternative approach would involve a more concise and limited description of joint inflammation. Ward et al (4) have explored the use of a small number of representative "signal" joints (SJ) which are chosen by the clinician to characterize an individual patient's disease. SJ indices and other summary measures have been a recent source of substantial discussion (8–11).

In order to examine the utility and reliability of various joint count indices, we examined joint counts and summative scores, based on SJ counts and on the "reduced joint survey" (RJS), a 36-joint subset of the full joint survey, by a secondary analysis of 2 controlled clinical trials. These abbreviated measures were compared with traditional complete joint surveys, and recommendations for the uses and limitations of reduced joint counts were developed.

METHODS

Data sources. Scores on the proposed indices, traditional CSSRD joint counts and scores, and a modified Ritchie index (4) were calculated from data gathered during 2 controlled clinical trials of rheumatoid arthritis treatments:

From the University of Utah School of Medicine, Salt Lake City.

Supported by NIH contract N01AM1-2204 from the National Institute of Arthritis, Diabetes and Digestive and Kidney Diseases.

M. J. Egger, PhD: Department of Family and Community Medicine, Division of Biostatistics; D. A. Huth, BS: Department of Family and Community Medicine, Division of Biostatistics; J. R. Ward, MD: Department of Medicine; J. C. Reading, PhD: Department of Family and Community Medicine, Division of Biostatistics; H. J. Williams, MD: Department of Medicine.

Address reprint requests to M. J. Egger, PhD, Family and Community Medicine, Division of Biostatistics, University of Utah Medical Center, Salt Lake City, UT 84132.

Submitted for publication January 30, 1984; accepted in revised form December 14, 1984.

azathioprine (AZA) versus D-penicillamine (DP) (7) and auranofin versus parenteral gold sodium thiomalate (GST) versus placebo (6). Both studies were prospective, randomized, double-blind trials by the multi-institutional Cooperative Systematic Studies of the Rheumatic Diseases group. In the AZA–DP study, 206 patients who had been treated unsuccessfully with gold received either 1.25–1.5 mg/kg/day AZA or 10–12 mg/kg/day DP with appropriate placebo for 24 weeks. In the 21-week study of gold therapy, 208 patients received either auranofin (3 mg orally, twice daily) plus placebo injections, weekly intramuscular injections of GST (10 mg on the first injection, 25 mg on the second injection, and 50 mg on each of 19 subsequent injections) plus placebo tablets, or both placebo tablets and placebo injections.

Active disease at entry into each study was defined as a minimum of 6 swollen joints capable of response to an active drug and at least 2 of the following: (a) ≥9 joints tender on pressure, (b) at least 45 minutes of morning stiffness, (c) Westergren erythrocyte sedimentation rate of ≥28 mm/hour. To minimize the effects of interobserver variability (12), patients' joint counts were performed by the same clinician at the first and last visits. Traditional CSSRD joint counts and scores (5) were calculated for those patients who continued in the AZA–DP study for at least 24 weeks or in the gold study for at least 20 weeks. All 4 active drugs have been shown to cause significantly greater improvement than placebo in randomized, controlled clinical trials (5–7,13).

Conceptual taxonomy. A taxonomy of summary measures of articular response is presented in Figure 1. Condensation of the information from joint surveys has been achieved in the past by 3 methods: (a) clinical/biologic judgment (10), as in the Ritchie index (3), (b) statistical analyses, such as discriminant analysis, as was done in the indomethacin study conducted by the Cooperating Clinics of the ARA (14), and (c) simple summation of the number of active, responsive joints or their pain/tenderness or swelling scores, as was done in the original 7-day variability study by the Cooperating Clinics of the ARA (1) and extended by the CSSRD (5).

Simple summation effectively gives each joint equal weight in quantifying a patient's joint activity. The clinical/biologic judgment approach chooses joints and assigns them weights based on a subjective judgment of each individual joint's biologic importance (10). The statistical approach chooses and weights joints to maximize a statistical criterion.

Used alone, the statistical approach produces measures of articular responses which tend to lack face validity or intuitive reasonableness (see refs. 8,10,15). For example, the coefficients and subsets of joints produced by a reliability or factor analysis may well be statistically optimal but clinically nonsensical, e.g., 10 × first proximal interphalangeal joint scores + 0.5 × third metacarpophalangeal joint scores + 25.7 × wrist scores. The use of weights from discriminant analysis is further flawed by poor criterion validity (16). Because of the absence of a standard criterion for joint improvement, these weights maximize the ability to identify which patients were in which *treatment* group, and thus will differ depending on which treatments are under study.

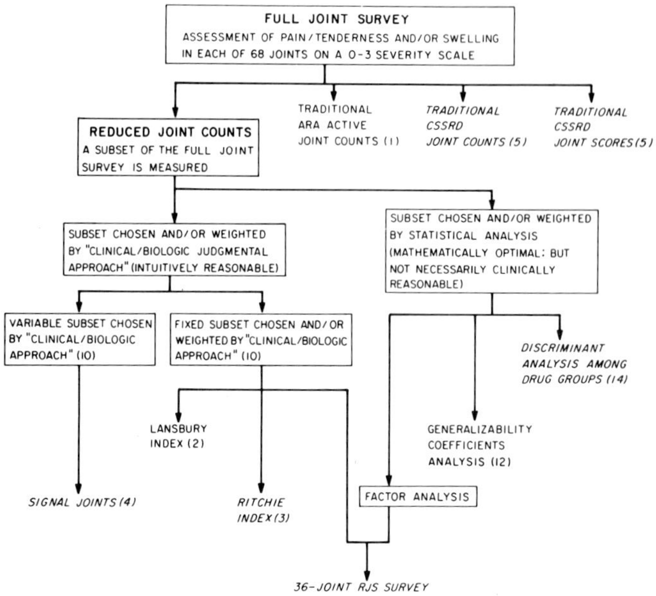

Figure 1. Measures of articular response. Measures shown in italics are discussed in this report. Numbers in parentheses are reference numbers. ARA = American Rheumatism Association; CSSRD = Cooperative Systematic Studies of the Rheumatic Diseases; RJS = reduced joint survey.

A discriminant analytic summary measure was considered for this study, but was dropped because of the above considerations and the results of a pilot study which produced large variances. However, the RJS measure discussed in the next section combines the statistical and clinical/biologic judgment approaches.

Index definitions. The present report compares traditional CSSRD indices and a modified Ritchie index with the proposed SJ and RJS indices. Traditional CSSRD joint counts and scores (5) assess pain/tenderness and swelling separately, as opposed to the original ARA joint count (1) which combined these and other indications of joint activity. Traditional CSSRD joint counts are the total number of active, responsive joints (excluding joints with mechanical problems prohibiting complete response to active drugs). Traditional CSSRD joint scores summate the total severity of the above joints, with individual joints scored from 0 (uninvolved) to 3 (most severe) (5). CSSRD defines "active" joints as those currently showing disease activity, as opposed to "involved" joints which have been affected, but are not necessarily active at the present time. "Responsive" joints are involved, active joints which are considered to be capable of responding to an active drug.

The Ritchie index (3) measures tenderness, not swelling, and pools groups of joints such as all metacarpophalangeal (MCP) joints in a single score, so that it summates 26 tenderness scores. Our modified Ritchie index omits evaluation of joints of the cervical spine and includes separate calculations of pain/tenderness and swelling.

In contrast to the Ritchie index, in which a fixed subset of joints is evaluated, the SJ method described by Ward et al (4) entails the use of 2–5 actively involved and potentially responsive joints, representing no more than 30% of a patient's disease, chosen by the individual physician to characterize a particular patient's response to drug therapy (4). Clinicians chose SJs at the first and last visits in the AZA–DP and gold studies. Pain/tenderness and swelling were evaluated by separate indices.

RJS indices were defined by a combination of the statistical and clinical/biologic judgment approaches: multiple factor and reliability analyses (8) led to identification of 5 chief groupings of joints which seemed to improve or deteriorate together, as well as a list of joints which did not contribute to the reliability of the summary joint scores. The 5 joint groupings were the MCP joints of the hand, interphalangeal (IP) joints of the hand, MTP joints of the feet, IP joints of the feet, and large joints such as wrists, elbows, ankles, and knees. Joints judged to provide little statistical and clinical information about improvement were eliminated from the survey. The 36 joints which remained were: the distal IP joint of the thumb, individual proximal IP and MCP joints of the hand, individual MTP joints of the feet, and the wrists, elbows, ankles, and knees. These joints were weighted equally in separate RJS indices for pain/tenderness and swelling. SJ and RJS counts and scores were defined analogously to the traditional CSSRD joint counts and scores, as the count of affected joints and the sum of joint severity ratings, respectively.

Standardization of indices. To standardize the range of values across indices, each index was divided by the total number of joints utilized by that index. For example, consider a patient with 10 involved joints out of 68, of which all 10 are tender, 7 of the 10 are swollen, and 1 of the swollen joints is nonresponsive. Suppose the joint swelling scores of the 9 tender, responsive joints are 3, 2, 3, 1, 2, 2, 0, 0, and 0, and the first and fourth joints had been chosen as signal joints. The traditional CSSRD joint swelling count and cumulative joint swelling score would be calculated as 6 and 13, respectively, with analogous signal joint count and score of 2 and 4. The standardized indices used for this study would be 6/68 = 0.09 and 13/68 = 0.19 for the traditional measures and 2/2 = 1.0 and 4/2 = 2.0 for the signal joint measures. Note that standardized joint *counts* will never be larger than 1.0, and standardized joint *scores* will never be larger than 3.0.

Table 1. Response indices by treatment at beginning and end of auranofin versus gold sodium thiomalate (GST) trial in rheumatoid arthritis patients*

Variable	Placebo (n = 23) First visit	Placebo (n = 23) Δ (adjusted)	Auranofin (n = 37) First visit	Auranofin (n = 37) Δ (adjusted)	GST (n = 38) First visit	GST (n = 38) Δ (adjusted)	P, ANCOVA (K-W)†
Pain/tenderness							
RJS count	0.60 ± 0.05	−0.02 ± 0.05	0.61 ± 0.04	−0.15 ± 0.04	0.59 ± 0.04	−0.23 ± 0.04	0.003 (0.027)
SJ count	1.00 ± 0.00	−0.13 ± 0.07	0.99 ± 0.01	−0.29 ± 0.06	0.96 ± 0.02	−0.32 ± 0.06	0.094 (0.096)
Traditional count	0.49 ± 0.05	0.01 ± 0.04	0.48 ± 0.04	−0.12 ± 0.03	0.45 ± 0.04	−0.18 ± 0.03	<0.001 (0.007)
RJS score	0.95 ± 0.09	−0.08 ± 0.08	0.93 ± 0.08	−0.29 ± 0.06	0.87 ± 0.08	−0.41 ± 0.06	0.005 (0.075)‡
SJ score	2.08 ± 0.11	−0.47 ± 0.14	1.95 ± 0.10	−0.85 ± 0.11	1.93 ± 0.11	−1.00 ± 0.11	0.017 (0.032)
Traditional score	0.75 ± 0.08	−0.03 ± 0.06	0.73 ± 0.08	−0.22 ± 0.05	0.66 ± 0.07	−0.31 ± 0.05	0.002 (0.037)
Modified Ritchie score	1.03 ± 0.08	0.01 ± 0.07	1.04 ± 0.09	−0.28 ± 0.05	0.96 ± 0.07	−0.44 ± 0.05	<0.0001 (0.003)
Swelling							
RJS count	0.50 ± 0.04	−0.10 ± 0.04	0.59 ± 0.04	−0.10 ± 0.04	0.53 ± 0.04	−0.20 ± 0.03	0.083 (0.177)
SJ count	0.91 ± 0.04	−0.11 ± 0.06	1.00 ± 0.004	−0.18 ± 0.04	0.96 ± 0.03	−0.25 ± 0.04	0.137 (0.150)
Traditional count	0.32 ± 0.03	−0.07 ± 0.03	0.40 ± 0.03	−0.07 ± 0.03	0.36 ± 0.03	−0.13 ± 0.03	1.73 (0.227)
RJS score	0.74 ± 0.08	−0.10 ± 0.06	0.82 ± 0.06	−0.19 ± 0.04	0.75 ± 0.07	−0.30 ± 0.04	0.119 (0.120)
SJ score	1.56 ± 0.14	−0.22 ± 0.11	1.86 ± 0.07	−0.60 ± 0.08	1.72 ± 0.08	−0.76 ± 0.08	<0.001 (<0.001)
Traditional score	0.47 ± 0.05	−0.12 ± 0.04	0.54 ± 0.04	−0.12 ± 0.03	0.50 ± 0.06	−0.20 ± 0.03	0.159 (0.148)
Modified Ritchie score	0.72 ± 0.07	−0.11 ± 0.05	0.86 ± 0.05	−0.19 ± 0.04	0.77 ± 0.05	−0.32 ± 0.04	0.005 (0.007)

* Joint counts and scores were divided by the total number of joints in the survey, yielding "per joint" counts and scores. "Per joint" indices were then averaged for all patients and adjusted for first visit by analysis of covariance (ANCOVA). Figures are group means ± SE. At entry, all groups showed statistical equivalence for each response index. RJS = reduced joint survey; SJ = signal joint.

† *P* values are for the test of differences among groups by ANCOVA, with *P* values for Kruskal-Wallis (K-W) nonparametric tests in parentheses.

‡ *P* values for ANCOVA and Kruskal-Wallis test are on opposite sides of 0.05.

Standardized SJ counts for swelling will be less than 1.0 when not all signal joints exhibit swelling or when a previously swollen signal joint has ceased swelling. Standardized indices identify the average contribution *per joint* to a patient's joint count or score, as if all joints were equally diseased. Analogous counts and scores were constructed for the pain/tenderness dimension of joint inflammation.

Statistical methods. The initial sample of 414 (206 + 208) patients entered into the 2 controlled clinical trials of treatments of rheumatoid arthritis was reduced (by dropout, changes in observers, and other protocol violations), to 134 subjects in the AZA–DP study and 161 in the gold study. In 55 and 63 patients in the respective studies, signal joints were not identified at the first visit, because of late institution of the signal joint procedure relative to the rest of the protocol. This left 23 patients in the placebo group, 37 receiving auranofin, 38 receiving GST, 38 receiving AZA, and 41 receiving DP, for a total of 177 patients in the 2 studies.

In an attempt to utilize the patients lost due to the above-described administrative error, signal joints were chosen once at patient entry and independently at patient exit. The difference in a priori versus post hoc choice of signal joints was analyzed to assess the effect of including those patients who had signal joints chosen at trial end but not at entry. Signal joints identified post hoc were found to be qualitatively different from those identified at entry. Therefore, the following analysis includes only those 177 patients who had signal joints chosen at entry and in whom there was no violation of protocol.

The frequency at which a joint was chosen as the signal joint in the AZA–DP and gold studies was tabulated. Unusually over- or under-favored joints were tested against the proportion expected from random choice based on the distribution of active, responsive joints, the assumption that signal joints represent 30% of a patient's diseased joints, and a binomial formula.

Evaluation of the proposed indices was performed using standard reliability/validity criteria, specifically, the definitions of Tugwell and Bombardier (15). Reliability analyses used to develop the RJS measure included alpha coefficients, point biserial correlations for individual joints versus the full survey, and factor analysis; these are detailed elsewhere (8). Convergent construct validity (15), or agreement with other accepted measures, was examined using Pearson correlations of proposed and traditional indices. Discriminant validity, or issues of precision and power to detect an active drug, was compared for the proposed and

Table 2. Response indices by treatment at beginning and end of azothioprine versus D-penicillamine trial in rheumatoid arthritis patients*

Variable	Azathioprine (n = 38) First visit	Azathioprine (n = 38) Δ (adjusted)	D-penicillamine (n = 41) First visit	D-penicillamine (n = 41) Δ (adjusted)	*P*, ANCOVA (K-W)†
Pain/tenderness					
RJS count	0.64 ± 0.04	−0.23 ± 0.05	0.66 ± 0.04	−0.20 ± 0.04	0.666 (0.776)
SJ count	0.98 ± 0.02	−0.35 ± 0.06	0.93 ± 0.03	−0.30 ± 0.06	0.560 (0.384)
Traditional count	0.54 ± 0.04	−0.19 ± 0.04	0.56 ± 0.04	−0.17 ± 0.04	0.742 (0.802)
RJS score	0.98 ± 0.07	−0.40 ± 0.08	1.07 ± 0.09	−0.39 ± 0.07	0.914 (0.810)
SJ score	2.01 ± 0.12	−0.88 ± 0.12	1.93 ± 0.11	−0.87 ± 0.11	0.951 (0.779)
Traditional score	0.82 ± 0.07	−0.33 ± 0.07	0.89 ± 0.08	−0.32 ± 0.07	0.886 (0.922)
Modified Ritchie score	1.12 ± 0.08	−0.41 ± 0.07	1.09 ± 0.08	−0.42 ± 0.07	0.935 (0.731)
Swelling					
RJS count	0.53 ± 0.03	−0.20 ± 0.03	0.55 ± 0.04	−0.19 ± 0.03	0.965 (0.848)
SJ count	0.99 ± 0.01	−0.31 ± 0.05	0.95 ± 0.03	−0.23 ± 0.05	0.296 (0.202)
Traditional count	0.40 ± 0.03	−0.15 ± 0.02	0.41 ± 0.03	−0.16 ± 0.02	0.930 (0.709)
RJS score	0.84 ± 0.08	−0.38 ± 0.05	0.84 ± 0.07	−0.38 ± 0.05	0.954 (0.810)
SJ score	2.00 ± 0.10	−0.91 ± 0.10	1.79 ± 0.11	−0.80 ± 0.10	0.433 (0.278)
Traditional score	0.61 ± 0.06	−0.28 ± 0.03	0.60 ± 0.05	−0.28 ± 0.03	0.978 (0.871)
Modified Ritchie score	0.91 ± 0.07	−0.34 ± 0.05	0.81 ± 0.06	−0.37 ± 0.05	0.667 (0.735)

* Joint counts and scores were divided by the total number of joints in the survey, yielding "per joint" counts and scores. "Per joint" indices were then averaged for all patients and adjusted for first visit by analysis of covariance (ANCOVA). Figures are group means ± SE. At entry, all groups showed statistical equivalence for each response index. RJS = reduced joint survey; SJ = signal joint.

† *P* values are for the test of differences among groups by ANCOVA, with *P* values for Kruskal-Wallis (K-W) nonparametric tests in parentheses.

traditional joint indices by analysis of covariance (ANCOVA), with verification by the Kruskal-Wallis test to control for violations of assumptions. Precision was further described by tabulating coefficients of variation (17) for differences between drug groups and ratios of F-statistics from ANCOVA. To permit comparison of the proposed measures with the measures actually used in the drug studies, descriptive statistics and differences between first and last visit adjusted by ANCOVA are given in Tables 1 and 2, showing only those patients for whom both traditional and proposed indices could be computed.

The problem of multiple inference, i.e., performance of so many statistical tests at significance level alpha that some of the results are significant by chance alone, arose in 3 separate areas: the evaluation of clinician preferences for signal joints, the correlations which establish convergent construct validity, and the drug efficacy comparisons. A blanket significance level of $\alpha = 0.05$ or $\alpha = 0.01$ was not sufficient to control for the probability of spurious significance in this study. Therefore, the significance level is controlled within each table so that <1 spuriously significant result is expected for each research question. For clinician preference of signal joints, alpha is dropped to 0.005; for correlations, it is dropped to 0.001. Exact P values are reported for drug efficacy comparisons in Tables 1 and 2, since these are what would appear in a clinical report.

RESULTS

Reliability and validity. Assessment of discriminant validity, or precision, and sensitivity of these reduced indices to an active drug is shown in Table 3. The relative precision of traditional versus proposed indices is calculated as the ratio of squared coefficients of variation of differences between groups, with improvement at last visit corrected for severity at first visit by ANCOVA. This ratio is approximately the sample size inflation factor necessary to achieve the same significance level and power if traditional indices were replaced by either SJ or RJS indices. Table 3 shows that both SJ and RJS indices had precision comparable with traditional measures. Our modified Ritchie index also performed quite favorably. Both proposed indices exhibited instances of substantial savings in sample size, and there were cases in which traditional measures reported a difference between groups which was severely underestimated by the SJ or RJS index.

Convergent construct validity (17) of SJ and RJS indices was fair to excellent compared with the complete traditional joint count and score and a modified Ritchie index, as measured by Pearson correlations. RJS indices were more highly correlated with SJ and with the full joint survey indices than the latter 2 measures were correlated with each other. All correlations were statistically significant, except at study entry, where SJ counts had low correlation with other indices as an artifact of uniform involvement of signal joints.

Table 3. Sample size inflation factors for reduced joint count surveys versus traditional indices, in controlled trials of treatments for rheumatoid arthritis*

	Gold treatment trial				Azathioprine–D-penicillamine trial
	Placebo–auranofin	Placebo–GST	Auranofin–GST	Summary	
Pain/tenderness					
SJ count/traditional count	2.02	3.34	16.32†	3.09	0.31
SJ score/traditional score	1.44	1.56	1.93	1.56	5.38
SJ score/Ritchie index	2.53	3.20	5.15	3.16	1.74
RJS count/traditional count	1.44	1.21	0.94	1.23	0.58
RJS score/traditional score	1.30	1.17	0.98	1.18	1.77
RJS score/Ritchie index	2.28	2.40	2.62	2.40	1.77
Swelling					
SJ count/traditional count	0.002‡	0.55	2.02	0.88	0.006‡
SJ score/traditional score	0.001‡	0.15	1.61	0.23	0.0009‡
SJ score/Ritchie index	0.21	0.66	2.76	0.71	0.30
RJS count/traditional count	12.11‡	0.67	0.72	0.70	4.04‡
RJS score/traditional score	0.12‡	0.77	0.94	0.86	0.22‡
RJS score/Ritchie index	27.35†	3.31	1.61	2.61	54.61‡

* Values are ratios of squared coefficients of variation ($CV^2 = SE^2/\Delta^2$), where Δ is the estimated index difference between treatment groups as calculated by analysis of covariance (ANCOVA). For example, the number of patients needed to compare pain/tenderness in the placebo and auranofin groups at $\alpha = 0.05$ with 90% power using the signal joint count is 2.02 times the number of patients required if the traditional joint count were used. The summary column is the ratio of F-statistics from ANCOVA in the gold study. GST = gold sodium thiomalate; SJ = signal joint; RJS = reduced joint survey.

† The estimated index difference (Δ) is less than its standard error.

‡ Estimated Δs are close to 0.

We judged that the index based on signal joints would comprehensively summarize the intuitive clinical concept of "disease activity" if the clinicians' choices of SJs met the following criteria: 1) Choice of SJs must include diseased joints which are easily observed and which constitute good signals of a patient's disease progression or response to treatment. 2) Clinicians' choices of SJs must be sufficiently predictable to assure reproducibility of summary scores by trained physicians on similar patients in similar experiments. Therefore, we tabulated the frequency of choice of each joint as a signal joint and tested to see which joints were significantly preferred (see Methods). Wrists, knees, ankles, elbows, and the first through third MCP joints were favored, controlling for the frequency with which joints were involved and responsive. Thus, the numbers represent clinician preference, not simply the disease process. Only the wrists achieved statistically significant clinician preference ($\alpha = 0.005$), with a statistically significant lack of preference for IP joints of the hands and feet.

The overall ratio of signal joints to responsive joints was 0.11 in both studies, indicating that the "30%-of-disease" instructions for choice of SJs could not always be followed. This will tend to inappropriately reduce the statistical significance for joints which were preferred 20–40% of the time. As a consequence, the large joints and first through third MCP joints were probably more preferred than the statistical model showed. Joints on the right side tended to be slightly more favored than joints on the left side, perhaps reflecting the fact that more patients were right-handed. In the 2 studies, clinicians chose a mean and median of 4 joints as SJs. The frequent choice of large joints suggests that without other instructions, clinicians will choose SJs that represent the worst of a patient's disease. In fact, SJs did tend to be more severely afflicted than the "average" responsive joint at the first visit (see Tables 1 and 2).

DISCUSSION

This study investigated 2 "streamlined" indices of joint disease that combine statistical and clinical/biologic judgment approaches to data condensation in 2 controlled clinical trials of treatments for rheumatoid arthritis. With signal joints chosen by the clinician, SJ counts and scores primarily summarize the patient's disease in large joints and are moderately sensitive to the effects of active drugs. They are less precise than indices from the full joint survey for pain/tenderness, but more precise for swelling. RJS counts and scores, based on a 36-joint survey, eliminate joints which provide little information on the overall disease process. Their precision is more nearly representative of the full joint survey. Since this study incorporated multiclinic variability, the indices should be even more precise when utilized at single institutions.

One advantage of SJ and RJS indices in clinical trials is cost-effectiveness. They would reduce clinician time required for completion of case report forms, as well as costs of data storage and analysis. They eliminate the necessity to estimate scores for joints that are difficult to evaluate, such as the IP joints of the foot, the hips, acromioclavicular joints, and temporomandibular joints. This benefit carries over to clinical practice.

While the signal joint method is flexible in allowing the clinician to tailor a measure of significant improvement for each patient at any stage of the disease, it is limited in its capacity to describe deterioration, particularly when non-signal joints deteriorate. The SJ approach allows clinicians to choose the studied joints, causing the results of the study to be dependent on the characteristics of the clinicians involved and their method of clinical practice. Although clinicians in these studies were fairly consistent in choosing as signal joints the large joints representing the worst of a patient's disease, the use of SJs could conceivably reduce the reproducibility of a clinical trial. A more serious concern is that although in this investigation and previous work (4) clinicians favored SJs characterizing large joint disease, factor and reliability analyses indicate that it may be equally important to follow the progress of disease in the hands and feet. Thus, SJs, as presently defined, cannot be recommended as a substitute for the full joint survey.

In contrast, RJS indices reflect the range of joint disease progression. Their validity has been well established. They share the inter- and intra-observer reliability of the full joint survey, since for both measures, observers score joints individually. Their precision has been assessed in 2 controlled clinical trials of active drugs and is comparable with, though occasionally reduced from, that of the full joint survey. Index precision in the AZA–DP trial should not be equated with statistical significance of the drug comparisons since both drugs were active. Thus, RJS indices can be utilized reasonably by both the clinician and researcher in quantifying the status of joint disease in rheumatoid arthritis.

REFERENCES

1. The Cooperating Clinics Committee of the American Rheumatism Association: A seven-day variability study of 499 patients with peripheral rheumatoid arthritis. Arthritis Rheum 8:302–335, 1965
2. Lansbury J, Haut DD: Quantitation of the manifestations of rheumatoid arthritis. 4. Area of joint surfaces as an index to total joint inflammation and deformity. Am J Med Sci 232:150–155, 1956
3. Ritchie DM, Boyle JA, McInnes JM, Jasani MK, Dalakos TG, Grieveson P, Buchanan WW: Clinical studies with the articular index for the assessment of joint tenderness in patients with rheumatoid arthritis. Q J Med 37:393–406, 1968
4. Ward JR, Niethammer TA, Egger MJ: Can we just measure signal joints? Should ring size and walking time be analyzed only in selected patients? Controversies in the Clinical Evaluation of Analgesic–Anti-Inflammatory–Antirheumatic Drugs. Edited by HE Paulus, GE Ehrlich, E Lindenlaub. New York, FK Schattauer Verlag, 1980
5. Williams HJ, Ward JR, Reading JC, Egger MJ, Grandone JT, Samuelson CO, Furst DE, Sullivan JM, Watson MA, Guttadauria M, Cathcart ES, Kaplan SB, Halla JT, Weinstein A, Plotz PH: Low-dose D-penicillamine therapy in rheumatoid arthritis: a controlled, double-blind clinical trial. Arthritis Rheum 26:581–592, 1983
6. Ward JR, Williams HJ, Egger MJ, Reading JC, Boyce E, Altz-Smith M, Samuelson CO Jr, Willkens RF, Solsky MA, Hayes SP, Blocka KL, Weinstein A, Meenan RF, Guttadauria M, Kaplan SB, Klippel J: Comparison of auranofin, gold sodium thiomalate, and placebo in the treatment of rheumatoid arthritis: a controlled clinical trial. Arthritis Rheum 26:1303–1315, 1983
7. Paulus HE, Williams HJ, Ward JR, Reading JC, Egger MJ, Coleman ML, Samuelson CO Jr, Willkens RF, Guttadauria M, Alarcon GS, Kaplan SB, MacLaughlin EJ, Weinstein A, Wilder RL, Solsky MA, Meenan RF: Azathioprine versus D-penicillamine in rheumatoid arthritis patients who have been treated unsuccessfully with gold. Arthritis Rheum 27:721–727, 1984
8. Egger MJ, Ward JR, Reading JC, Williams HJ, Coleman ML: Evaluation of summary indices of response in controlled clinical trials (abstract). Controlled Clin Trials 3:154, 1982
9. Buchanan WW: Assessment of joint tenderness, grip strength, digital joint circumference and morning stiffness in rheumatoid arthritis. J Rheumatol 9:763–765, 1982
10. Buchanan WW, Tugwell P: Traditional assessments of articular diseases. Clin Rheum Dis 9:515–529, 1983
11. Tugwell P, Bombardier C: Practical issues in clinical trials as applied to current state of the art in rheumatology trials. Br J Rheumatol (suppl) 22:9–13, 1983
12. Eberl DR, Fasching V, Rahlfs V, Schleyer I, Wolf R: Repeatability and objectivity of various measurements in rheumatoid arthritis: a comparative study. Arthritis Rheum 19:1278–1286, 1976
13. Urowitz MB, Hunter T, Bookman AAM, Gordon DA, Smythe HA, Ogryzlo MA: Azathioprine in rheumatoid arthritis: a double blind study comparing full dose to half dose. J Rheumatol 1:274–281, 1974
14. Cooperating Clinics of the ARA Committee: A three-month trial of indomethacin in rheumatoid arthritis, with special reference to analysis and inference. Clin Pharmacol Ther 8:11–37, 1967
15. Tugwell P, Bombardier C: A methodologic framework for developing and selecting endpoints in clinical trials. J Rheumatol 9:758–762, 1982
16. Bombardier C, Tugwell P: A methodological framework to develop and select indices for clinical trials: statistical and judgmental approaches. J Rheumatol 9:753–757, 1982
17. Snedecor GW, Cochran WG: Statistical Methods. Seventh edition. Ames, The Iowa State University Press, 1980, p 37

A COMPARISON OF THE SPECIFICITY OF THE 1971 AND 1982 AMERICAN RHEUMATISM ASSOCIATION CRITERIA FOR THE CLASSIFICATION OF SYSTEMIC LUPUS ERYTHEMATOSUS

CONSTANCE M. PASSAS, ROBERT L. WONG, MARGARET PETERSON, MARCIA A. TESTA, and NAOMI F. ROTHFIELD

The specificity of the preliminary and the revised American Rheumatism Association criteria for the classification of systemic lupus erythematosus (SLE) was tested in 207 of our patients with other rheumatic diseases which were considered to be important in the differential diagnosis of SLE. Using the preliminary criteria, the data revealed that 5 patients were falsely classified as having SLE (2 with scleroderma, 2 with Raynaud's disease, and 1 with systemic necrotizing vasculitis), whereas using the revised criteria, only 2 patients (1 with scleroderma and 1 with systemic necrotizing vasculitis) were falsely classified. The calculated specificity was 99% for the revised criteria and 98% for the preliminary criteria. Thus, the data revealed that the specificity of the revised criteria is high and comparable with that of the preliminary criteria when applied to a group of patients with related rheumatic diseases.

From the Division of Rheumatic Diseases, Department of Medicine, and the Department of Research in Health Education, University of Connecticut School of Medicine, Farmington.

Supported in part by NIH Multipurpose Arthritis Center grant AM-20621, an Arthritis Research Center grant from the Arthritis Foundation, and grants from the Connecticut Chapter of the Arthritis Foundation and the Connecticut Chapter of the Lupus Foundation of America.

Constance M. Passas, MD: Fellow, Division of Rheumatic Diseases, Department of Medicine; Robert L. Wong, MD: Fellow, Division of Rheumatic Diseases, Department of Medicine; Margaret Peterson, PhD: Assistant Professor, Department of Research in Health Education; Marcia A. Testa, PhD: Assistant Professor, Department of Research in Health Education and Director of Statistical Core, NIH Multipurpose Arthritis Center; Naomi F. Rothfield, MD: Professor and Chief of the Division of Rheumatic Diseases, Department of Medicine.

Address reprint requests to Dr. Naomi Rothfield, Division of Rheumatic Diseases, University of Connecticut School of Medicine, Farmington, CT 06032.

Submitted for publication May 21, 1984; accepted in revised form October 23, 1984.

The American Rheumatism Association (ARA) revised criteria for the classification of systemic lupus erythematosus (SLE) have recently been published (1). The ARA preliminary criteria for the classification of systemic lupus erythematosus have been in use since publication of the criteria in 1971, and the revision was believed to be necessary in order to include newer tests such as anti-DNA, anti-Sm, and antinuclear antibodies (ANA). In addition, it was believed that laboratory tests and clinical manifestations should be regrouped in order to increase the specificity and the sensitivity of the preliminary criteria (2). We have used our own patients to test the sensitivity of the revised criteria and the preliminary criteria and have shown that the revised criteria are marginally more sensitive (3). This increased sensitivity was due to the addition of ANA as a criterion in the revised criteria.

We have now tested the specificity of the revised and preliminary criteria on a group of non-SLE patients who were followed during the same period of time by the same faculty and fellows as the SLE patients who were studied previously for sensitivity of the criteria. The data suggest that compared with the preliminary criteria, the revised criteria are marginally more sensitive and of comparable specificity.

PATIENTS AND METHODS

Patients. All outpatients or hospitalized patients at the University of Connecticut Health Center followed by faculty members of the Division of Rheumatic Diseases during the period of January 1, 1981 through December 30, 1983 were considered for study. These patients were selected at random from a computerized printout of all patients followed during that period. Diagnosis was provided by the faculty member following the patient. The sample size for each disease group was chosen to obtain a minimum of 30 patients when possible. When more than 30 patients were available, the number chosen was inversely relative to the sample size to maximize statistical power and for practical convenience. Charts were reviewed in alphabetical order. In addition, an attempt was made to enter a larger sample in the more common diseases which might be confused with SLE. Five major groups of diseases were included: 1) definite or classic rheumatoid arthritis, defined by criteria (4), 2) scleroderma, defined by ARA criteria (5), 3) Raynaud's disease, defined by uniform database for rheumatic diseases (6), 4) patients with CREST (calcinosis, Raynaud's phenomenon, esophageal dysmotility, sclerodactyly, and telangiectasias) and undifferentiated connective tissue disease or overlap diseases which did not satisfy criteria for any single diagnostic group, and 5) patients with systemic necrotizing vasculitis (Tables 1 and 2).

Data entry and analysis. The charts of the 207 patients were reviewed and information was entered into a database booklet by a fellow or faculty member. The database booklet listed the 36 elements of the 2 sets of SLE criteria exactly as defined in the literature (1,2). For each element, the reviewer entered one of the following: "yes," "no," "unclear," or "unknown." Unclear entries were defined as results which were neither yes, no, or unknown. Unknown was defined as information which was not available. For arthritis as defined by the revised criteria (nonerosive arthritis involving 2 or more peripheral joints, characterized by tenderness, swelling, or effusion), an additional entry was allowed i.e., "unclear because no x-ray done."

Prior to keypunching, all data entries were reviewed for omissions, errors, and discrepancies. After transfer to punch cards, the data entries were reviewed again and the cards were corrected. The SPSS software package (7) was used for tabulation of elements and subsequent classification using the 2 sets of criteria.

Serologic tests. Anti-DNA antibodies were considered present when the result of our tests indicated >33% binding (8). Anti-Sm was considered present when a titer of ≥1:2 was obtained in our laboratory using counterimmunoelectrophoresis (9). A positive ANA was defined as a titer of >1:16 in our laboratory by indirect immunofluorescence and using mouse liver as substrate. A false-positive test for syphilis was considered present only if it occurred twice during a ≥6-month interval as defined in both criteria. If the test was only ordered once and was positive, the result was entered as unclear. Specificity was determined using the following standard format:

$$\text{Specificity} = \frac{\text{True-negatives}}{\text{True-negatives} + \text{false-positives}}$$

Table 1. Patients

Diagnosis	Number
Rheumatoid arthritis	99
Raynaud's syndrome	43
Scleroderma	36
Overlap syndromes	14
Sjögren's + Raynaud's	1
Dermatomyositis/scleroderma	1
Polymyositis/scleroderma	1
CREST*	11
Systemic necrotizing vasculitis	15
Wegener's	4
Takayasu's	1
Polyarteritis nodosa	2
Medium and small vessel vasculitis	8
Total	207

* CREST = calcinosis, Raynaud's phenomenon, esophageal dysmotility, sclerodactyly, telangiectasias. Five patients had CREST; 2 patients had REST; 1 patient had CREST + Sjögren's; 2 patients had CREST + scleroderma; 1 patient had CREST + Sjögren's + myositis.

Table 2. Characteristics of the study population (n = 207)

	Number	%
Female/male	160/47	77.3/22.7
Age <16 years at diagnosis	2	1.0
White	192	92.8
Black	10	4.8
Hispanic	4	1.9
Oriental	1	0.5
Years disease duration, mean ± SD (range)	5.0 ± 6.5 (<1–38)	
Followup by clinic physician, mean ± SD (range)	2.7 ± 2.8 (<1–15)	
Age at diagnosis, mean ± SD (range)	45.2 ± 14.6 (5–79)	

RESULTS

False-positives are shown in Table 3. Patients with established non-SLE diseases who met 4 or more ARA criteria for the classification of SLE were considered false-positives. Using the preliminary criteria, there were 5 false-positives: 2 patients with scleroderma, 2 with Raynaud's disease, and 1 patient with systemic medium and small vessel necrotizing vasculitis. Using the revised criteria, there were 2 false-positives: 1 patient (patient 1) with scleroderma and the above patient (patient 5) with vasculitis who also met the preliminary criteria.

Patient 1 had classic scleroderma with multisystem involvement (pulmonary, cardiac, renal, and skin) and malignant hypertension with renal failure which required dialysis and angiotensin converting enzyme-blocking agents. With the presence of a positive ANA (titer 1:124), patient 1 fulfilled the revised criteria. With the presence of Raynaud's phenomenon, the patient met the preliminary criteria. The duration of observation of this patient was 2 years. The patient with systemic vasculitis was followed for 6 years.

The 2 patients with Raynaud's disease and the second patient with scleroderma satisfied the preliminary but not the revised criteria because of alopecia

Table 3. False-positives

	Patient no.	Diagnosis	Criteria
Preliminary criteria	1	Scleroderma	Arthritis, Raynaud's phenomenon, renal disease, serositis (pleuritis + pericarditis)
	2	Scleroderma	Arthritis, Raynaud's phenomenon, alopecia, serositis (pleuritis)
	3	Raynaud's phenomenon	Arthritis, Raynaud's phenomenon, alopecia, photosensitivity
	4	Raynaud's phenomenon	Arthritis, Raynaud's phenomenon, alopecia, photosensitivity, butterfly rash
	5	Medium and small vessel vasculitis	Blush, oral ulcer, psychosis, hematologic disorder (thrombocytopenia), immunologic disorder (false-positive serologic test for syphilis)
Revised criteria	1	Scleroderma	Arthritis, serositis (pleuritis + pericarditis), renal disease (proteinuria + casts), antinuclear antibody
	5	Medium and small vessel vasculitis	Blush, oral ulcer, psychosis, hematologic disorder (thrombocytopenia), immunologic disorder (false-positive serologic test for syphilis)

and Raynaud's phenomenon, which are not in the revised criteria. One patient with Raynaud's and 1 patient with scleroderma were followed for 1 year; a second patient with Raynaud's has been followed for 10 years. The mean duration of followup for the entire group of 207 patients was 2.7 years.

Serologic tests were not performed on all patients (Table 4). The ANA was the test most frequently ordered (35/36 scleroderma patients, 40/43 Raynaud's phenomenon patients, 83/99 rheumatoid arthritis patients, 14/14 patients with overlap diseases, 13/15 vasculitis patients).

The specificity of the revised criteria at diagnosis was 99.5% and at latest observation was 99%. The specificity of the preliminary criteria at diagnosis was 99.5% and at latest observation was 97.6%.

DISCUSSION

The magnitude of the specificity of a test is dependent upon the magnitude of the sensitivity. Comparisons between different tests should take into account this relationship by using techniques such as those described by Galen and Gambino (10), if comparisons at fixed levels of either sensitivity or specificity are not possible.

In our previous study (3), we showed that the sensitivity of the preliminary and revised criteria was 87% and 91%, respectively, a difference that is not statistically significant. For the present analysis, this difference was considered minimal and essentially provided us with the opportunity to compare specificity values between revised and preliminary criteria using a fixed value for sensitivity.

Therefore, if the sensitivities are considered to be comparable, the preliminary and revised criteria appear to provide nearly identical specificity for the diagnosis of SLE. It is possible that there would have been more false-positive results if all patients had all 4 of the tests included in the immunologic disorder criterion (LE cell preparation), anti-Sm, anti-DNA, and false-positive test for syphilis). In addition, the

Table 4. Immunologic disorder criteria by diagnostic group

		Number positive/number tested*				
	Number	LE preparation	STS	Anti-DNA	Anti-Sm	ANA
Scleroderma	36	0/11	0/11	1/18	1/23	29/35
Raynaud's phenomenon	43	1/17	0/6	0/26	0/25	21/40
Rheumatoid arthritis	99	2/16	0/15	0/27	0/10	55/83
Overlap syndromes	14	0/7	1/4	0/10	0/10	13/14
Systemic vasculitis	15	0/10	1/10	0/10	0/7	5/13

* LE = lupus erythematosus; STS = serologic test for syphilis; ANA = antinuclear antibody.

observation period was of relatively short duration (2.7 years) and more false-positives could appear with a longer period of observation.

The criteria were established to develop a uniform standard for the definition and classification of SLE. They were revised to include more specific and sensitive serologic tests (ANA, anti-DNA, anti-Sm) which have become routine in the evaluation of SLE patients and to exclude alopecia and Raynaud's phenomenon due to their lack of specificity.

Our data suggest that the deletion of alopecia and Raynaud's phenomenon did lead to slightly increased specificity in that 3 of 5 patients who met the preliminary criteria did not meet the revised criteria because of this deletion.

We used 207 patients to study specificity compared with the control group of 162 patients used in the SLE criteria study by Tan et al (1). A major difference between the 2 control groups was the difference in number of Raynaud's patients. Only 2 Raynaud's patients were used in the SLE criteria, whereas we had 43 Raynaud's patients in our specificity testing. We believed this was an important group to include because Raynaud's phenomenon may be the first manifestation of either SLE or scleroderma and because Raynaud's occurred in 31% of our SLE patients studied for criteria sensitivity testing (3) and in 29% of the SLE patients used in the development of the revised criteria (1).

We have previously shown that the addition of the ANA test as a criterion marginally increased the sensitivity of the revised criteria over the preliminary criteria (3). In this study we show that the specificity of the revised criteria (99.5%) was essentially the same as that of the preliminary criteria (97.6%). Moreover, our patient with scleroderma was classified as having SLE using the revised criteria because of positive ANA, a test known to have low specificity. It appears that the specificity of each element can affect the specificity of the criteria. It may be advisable to include specificity of each element as a weighting factor when classifying patients according to criteria.

ACKNOWLEDGMENT

We wish to thank Susan Christensen for secretarial help with the manuscript.

REFERENCES

1. Tan EM, Cohen AS, Fries JF, Masi AT, McShane DJ, Rothfield NF, Schaller JG, Talal N, Winchester RJ: The 1982 revised criteria for the classification of systemic lupus erythematosus. Arthritis Rheum 25:1271–1277, 1982
2. Cohen AS, Reynolds WE, Franklin EC, Kulka JP, Ropes MW, Shulman LE, Wallace SL: Preliminary criteria for the classification of systemic lupus erythematosus. Bull Rheum Dis 21:643–648, 1971
3. Levin RE, Weinstein A, Peterson M, Testa MA, Rothfield NF: A comparison of the sensitivity of the 1971 and 1982 ARA criteria for the classification of systemic lupus erythematosus. Arthritis Rheum 27:530–538, 1984
4. Ropes MW, Bennett GA, Cobb S, Jacox R, Jessar RA: 1958 revision of diagnostic criteria for rheumatoid arthritis. Bull Rheum Dis 9:175–176, 1958
5. Masi AT, Rodnan GP, Medsger TA Jr, Altman RD, D'Angelo WA, Fries JF, LeRoy EC, Kirsner AB, MacKenzie AH, McShane DJ, Myers AR, Sharp GC: Preliminary criteria for the classification of systemic sclerosis (scleroderma). Bull Rheum Dis 31:1–6, 1981
6. ARA Glossary Committee: Signs and Symptoms. Vol. 1. Dictionary of the Rheumatic Diseases. New York, Contact Associates, 1982
7. Nie NH, Hull CH, Jenkins JG, Steinbrenner K, Bent DH: SPSS Statistical Package for the Social Sciences. Second edition. New York, McGraw-Hill, 1975
8. Weinstein A, Bordwell B, Stone B, Tibbetts C, Rothfield NF: Antibodies to native DNA and serum complement (C3) levels: application to diagnosis and classification of systemic lupus erythematosus. Am J Med 74:206–216, 1983
9. Weinstein A, Sullivan M: Antibodies to the Sm antigen in systemic lupus erythematosus: clinical significance (abstract). Arthritis Rheum 22:672, 1979
10. Galen RS, Gambino SR: Beyond Normality: The Predictive Value and Efficiency of Medical Diagnoses. New York, Wiley, 1975

RELATIONSHIP BETWEEN CIRCULATING INTERFERON AND ANTI-INTERFERON ANTIBODIES AND IMPAIRED NATURAL KILLER CELL ACTIVITY IN SYSTEMIC LUPUS ERYTHEMATOSUS

WILMER L. SIBBITT, Jr., DWAYNE L. GIBBS, CAROL KENNY, ARTHUR D. BANKHURST, ROBERT P. SEARLES, and KENNETH D. LEY

Interferon (IFN) production and response are impaired in a high percentage of systemic lupus erythematosus (SLE) patients. In addition, elevated serum levels of α-IFN or anti–α-IFN antibodies are present in some SLE patients. This study examined the relationship of circulating IFN and anti-IFN antibodies to the impairment of natural killer (NK) cell function in SLE. All 15 SLE patients studied had measurable circulating α-IFN, while the normal controls had minimal serum IFN. Neither patient nor control sera contained any detectable anti–α-IFN activity. However, most of the SLE patients demonstrated defects in NK cell function. Because these defects in NK cell function appeared to be associated with circulating IFN, but not anti-IFN, antibodies, the effect of prolonged in vitro IFN exposure on NK cell function of peripheral blood mononuclear cells was determined. It was found that prolonged exposure to IFN induced both an apparent defect in IFN response and a definite impairment of baseline NK cell function. These results suggest that prolonged elevation of circulating α-IFN levels could be responsible, in part, for the defects in natural cytotoxicity present in SLE.

Systemic lupus erythematosus (SLE) is a chronic inflammatory disease characterized by multiple abnormalities of the immune system including decreased suppressor cell function (1), B cell activation (2,3), and impairment of natural killer (NK) cell activity (4,5). The NK cell has many important functions including elimination of virus-infected cells (6), rejection of neoplastic cells (7), and prevention of tumor metastasis (8). Recently, the NK cell has been shown to be an important regulator of B cell function (9,10). It is possible that the abnormalities in NK cell function in SLE could contribute to the relatively uncontrolled B cell activity present in this autoimmune disease.

The cause of the abnormality in NK cell activity is unclear, but it has been shown to be related in some instances to the presence of circulating anti–NK cell antibodies (11,12) or immune aggregates (13). However, these factors alone do not seem to be entirely responsible for the dysfunction of the NK cell in SLE (14). Indeed, other abnormalities in the NK cell subpopulation, which appear to be independent of these circulating factors, are present (14).

The NK cell is modulated by numerous soluble factors including interleukin-2 (IL-2) (15) and interferon (IFN) (16). Both factors greatly accentuate NK cell activity and may be necessary for normal NK cell function (15). Significantly, production of these factors is often impaired in SLE (17,18). However, impaired production of these lymphokines in SLE does not appear to be directly related to dysfunction of the NK cell (19–21). This suggests that other circulating serum factors may be involved.

Although IFN production is decreased in SLE (21), serum IFN levels are often elevated (22). In addition, sera of some SLE patients contain anti-interferon antibodies (23). Since NK cells respond to

From the Department of Medicine, University of New Mexico, Albuquerque and Lovelace Medical Foundation, Research Division, Albuquerque, New Mexico.

Supported by NIH grant R01-CA-24873-07 and a grant from the Arthritis Foundation. Dr. Sibbitt is a Postdoctoral Fellow of the Arthritis Foundation.

Address reprint requests to Wilmer L. Sibbitt, Jr., MD, Department of Medicine, Division of Clinical Immunology, and Rheumatic Diseases, University of New Mexico, Albuquerque NM 87131.

Submitted for publication March 30, 1984; accepted in revised form January 3, 1985.

IFN and may actually produce IFN themselves (24), the presence of circulating anti-interferon antibodies could contribute to impaired NK cell function. This study was designed to determine the importance of circulating anti-interferon antibodies and serum interferon in the impairment of NK cell function in SLE.

PATIENTS AND METHODS

Study population. Fifteen SLE patients and 15 normal controls were studied. All patients included in this study fulfilled the criteria for SLE defined by the American Rheumatism Association (25). Clinical activity was scored according to the method of Barada et al (3), where 0 = complete remission, 1 = mild activity, 2 = moderate activity, and 3 = severe systemic disease. No patients were being treated with cytotoxic agents and only 3 patients were receiving corticosteroids at the time of the study. Patients receiving corticosteroids were asked to refrain from taking the morning dose until a blood sample was obtained. Blood samples were collected by phlebotomy and sera were immediately frozen and stored at −70°C until use.

Peripheral blood mononuclear cells (PBMC). PBMC were isolated from heparinized whole blood by centrifugation on Ficoll-Hypaque gradients (26). Cells from the interface were washed 3 times with phosphate buffered saline and resuspended in RPMI 1640 (Gibco, Grand Island, NY) which contained penicillin (100 IU/ml), streptomycin (100 μg/ml), and 10% heat-inactivated human AB serum. Cell viability was >99% as determined by trypan blue exclusion and contained 2–20% monocytes as shown by peroxidase staining (27). Glass-wool adherent cells were removed as previously described (28). Final suspensions contained 0–1% monocytes. Subsequently, in certain experiments, the nonadherent PBMC were cultured for 1–6 days in the presence of IL-2 (10 units/ml; American Biological Associates, Buffalo, NY) as has been described before in detail (29). Peak activation of NK cell activity occurred at day 3 of culture, as previously described (29).

Assay for human α-IFN. Alpha-IFN titers in serum were determined in 96-well microtiter plates by a cytopathic effect (CPE) inhibition assay (30). The samples were serially diluted and placed into the appropriate microtiter wells. Each plate also contained as a control a reference preparation of α-IFN (E04, α-IFN, British 69/19, NIH, Bethesda, MD). Each well was seeded with WISH cells (American Type Culture, CCL25). The wells were challenged with vesicular stomatitis virus and the percent CPE was noted. The titer in units per milliliter was calculated for each sample by comparison of the dilution with the standard control sample. The identity of the serum α-IFN was confirmed by neutralization of IFN activity by specific sheep anti-human α-IFN and antibody (catalog numbers 6-026-502-568 and 6-027-501-568, NIH).

Assay for antibody to human α-IFN. Sera from patients were diluted in microtiter plates and 10 units of purified α-IFN (Interferon Sciences, New Brunswick, NJ) was added to each well. Each plate contained cell and virus control wells, an IFN standard, and 2 sheep sera: 1 a sheep antiserum to human α-IFN and 1 a control sheep antiserum to mock human α-IFN (NIH standard, NIH). The latter was raised to those components of crude human α-IFN preparations which did not bind to anti-IFN globulin bound to Sepharose 4B. The plate was challenged with WISH cells and stained as described for the IFN assay. Antibody titer was defined as the highest dilution of serum which neutralized 10 units of IFN by restoring the viral cytopathic effect, corrected to 1 unit of IFN and 1 ml volume.

^{51}Cr release assay. The ^{51}Cr release assay used for the determination of NK activity was performed as previously described (12). K562 was used as the target cell (31). Target cells were radiolabeled by incubation of 10×10^6 cells with 0.1 ml $Na_2{}^{51}CrO_4$ (specific activity 1.0 mCi/ml; New England Nuclear, Boston, MA) in 0.2 ml fetal calf serum for 45 minutes at 37°C, followed by 3 washings with media. Target cells, 1×10^4, were mixed with various effector cell preparations to achieve effector:target ratios of 100:1, 50:1, 25:1, and 12.5:1 in sterile round-bottom microtiter plates (Linbro, Flow Laboratories, Hamden, CT). A final volume of 0.2 ml per well was obtained. The plates were incubated for 4 hours at 37°C in humidified air/5% CO_2. After incubation, the plates were centrifuged at 400g for 10 minutes and 0.1 ml of supernatant was carefully removed. The supernatants were counted in an automatic gamma scintillation counter. All samples were run in sextuplet. The percent NK activity was calculated as: % NK activity =

$$\frac{\text{Experimental }^{51}\text{Cr release} - \text{spontaneous }^{51}\text{Cr release}}{\text{Maximum }^{51}\text{Cr release} - \text{spontaneous }^{51}\text{Cr release}} \times 100$$

A lytic unit (LU) was defined as the number of effector cells necessary to result in 30% lysis of 1.0×10^4 target cells. These values were determined by linear regression analysis from individual effector:target titration curves. Relative NK activity was expressed in LU/10^7 cells. In some instances, α-IFN (100 units/ml; Interferon Sciences) was used to pretreat effector cells for 8 hours prior to determination of NK activity in order to quantitate IFN response, as has been previously described (19). Percent IFN enhancement of NK activity was calculated as: % NK enhancement =

$$\frac{\text{LU IFN}/10^7\text{ cells} - \text{LU baseline}/10^7\text{ cells}}{\text{LU baseline}/10^7\text{ cells}} \times 100$$

Statistical analysis. P values between the means of paired groups of data were calculated using the Student's paired t-test. Linear regression analysis was used to compute r and P values for linear correlation comparisons.

RESULTS

NK activity in SLE. The NK activity of PBMC was significantly decreased in SLE patients compared with that in normal controls (Table 1). In this group of SLE patients, NK activity bore no clear relationship to clinical disease activity ($P > 0.05$). Of the 15 SLE patients studied, 8 had impaired NK cell activity (<15 LU/10^7 cells), while all 15 normal controls demon-

Table 1. Natural killer (NK) cell activity in systemic lupus erythematosus (SLE) patients*

	Baseline NK activity (LU/10^7 cells)	IFN-NK activity (LU/10^7 cells)	Disease activity†
SLE patient			
1	38.4	38.7	2
2	10.0	12.5	2
3	12.5	12.5	2
4	41.6	41.6	1
5	50.0	83.3	2
6	18.8	16.6	2
7	40.0	24.4	2
8	41.6	55.5	1
9	10.0	83.3	1
10	4.7	3.3	2
11	13.3	16.6	3
12	83.0	166.0	2
13	11.2	16.6	2
14	6.6	33.3	3
15	4.0	5.0	2
Mean ± SD	24.9 ± 23.0‡	40.6 ± 42.9‡	1.9 ± 0.59‡
Normal controls, mean ± SD (n = 15)	58.4 ± 36.8	188.4 ± 194.0	0.0 ± 0.0

* LU = lytic units; IFN = interferon.
† Defined in Patients and Methods.
‡ $P < 0.05$ versus normal controls.

strated NK activity >15 LU/10^7 cells. Nine SLE patients had impaired NK cell response to IFN (<30% enhancement) (Table 2), while all 15 normal controls had an IFN response >50% enhancement. Twelve of 15 SLE patients demonstrated a defect in NK cell function defined as either a decrease in NK cell activity or an impaired response to IFN (Tables 1 and 2). Thus, over 80% of the SLE patients had some defect in NK cell function.

IFN and anti-IFN antibody levels in SLE. All of the SLE patients studied demonstrated some serum IFN activity (Table 2). The average IFN activity present in SLE sera was 52.3 ± 23.6 units/ml (mean ± SD). In normal control sera, in contrast, the activity was <16.0 units/ml in all cases ($P < 0.05$). The identity of this IFN was confirmed by the addition of specific anti–α-IFN antibody, which neutralized the serum IFN activity. None of the SLE or normal control sera contained any intrinsic anti–α-IFN antibody activity. Thus, all 12 patients with impaired NK cell function demonstrated circulating α-IFN. These results suggested that circulating IFN may be important in the pathogenesis of impaired NK cell function in SLE. Serum anti–α-IFN antibodies were not present in any of the SLE patients tested, suggesting that specific anti-IFN antibodies were not important in the induction of NK cell abnormalities in SLE.

Effect of α-IFN on NK cell activity. Because abnormalities in NK cell function in SLE seemed to be related to the presence of serum IFN, the effect of α-IFN on the NK cell activity of normal control PBMC was determined. Since NK cell activity rapidly deteriorates with prolonged culture (32), optimum NK cell activity was maintained by the addition of IL-2 (10 units/ml) at the beginning of the culture period. As can be seen in Table 3, preincubation with α-IFN consistently resulted in a definite enhancement of NK activity. However, the relative enhancement of NK cell activity by IFN was dramatically decreased at all IFN preincubation periods.

Interestingly, during 6 days of preincubation with IFN, there was a gradual decrease in baseline and IFN-stimulated NK cell activity. No significant cell death as detected by trypan blue exclusion was present during this period, suggesting that impairment of NK cell function was not secondary to simple depletion of effector cells occurring through cell death. These results suggest that prolonged in vitro exposure to IFN could result in both an apparent insensitivity to IFN and an actual decrease in NK cell function.

DISCUSSION

The present study demonstrates that NK cell activity and IFN response are often impaired in SLE. In many of our patients these abnormalities appeared to be associated with the presence of circulating α-IFN, which attained levels as high as 96 units/ml in some patients. Anti–α-IFN antibodies did not appear to be related to the presence of impaired NK cell function in any of the SLE patients studied. These results suggest that IFN, but not anti-IFN, antibodies are associated with an impairment of NK cell activity in SLE.

Preincubation of normal control PBMC with IFN resulted in an immediate increase in NK cell activity. However, prolonged preincubation with IFN induced both an apparent insensitivity to IFN and an actual decrease in baseline unstimulated NK cell activity of PBMC maintained in prolonged culture with IL-2. These results suggest that continuous exposure of PBMC to circulating endogenous α-IFN in SLE could result in defective NK cell activity and an insensitivity to IFN.

The defects in cellular immune response induced by IFN could occur via several mechanisms.

Table 2. Relationship of serum α-IFN and anti–α-IFN antibodies to impaired natural killer (NK) cell function in systemic lupus erythematosus (SLE) patients*

	NK cell activity (LU/10^7)	IFN response (% enhancement)	Serum IFN (IU/ml)	Anti-IFN antibodies (present/absent)
SLE patient				
1	38.4	7.8	96	Absent
2	10.0	25.0	96	Absent
3	12.5	0.0	96	Absent
4	41.6	0.0	64	Absent
5	50.0	66.0	64	Absent
6	18.8	−11.7	48	Absent
7	40.0	−39.0	48	Absent
8	41.6	33.4	48	Absent
9	10.0	730.0	48	Absent
10	4.6	−29.7	32	Absent
11	13.3	24.8	32	Absent
12	83.0	100.0	24	Absent
13	11.2	48.2	24	Absent
14	6.6	500.0	16	Absent
15	4.0	20.0	16	Absent
Mean ± SD	24.9 ± 23.0†	93.3 ± 21.7†	52.3 ± 23.6†	Absent
Normal controls, mean ± SD (n = 15)	188.4 ± 194.0	218.0 ± 132.0	All <16	Absent

* LU = lytic units; IFN = interferon.
† $P < 0.05$ versus normal controls.

The insensitivity to IFN present in SLE may be only an apparent defect resulting from prior IFN priming from endogenously elevated levels of circulating IFN. The present study has demonstrated that both chronic and acute IFN exposure can induce this apparent defect. If the NK cell were already primed by prior exposure to IFN, then very little further IFN enhancement could be expected. Indeed, recent studies have demonstrated that PBMC from SLE patients with elevated levels of circulating IFN had already been primed by IFN and contained increased intracellular levels of 2′-5′ adenylate synthetase, which is a rather specific indicator of prior IFN priming (33).

Another possibility is that prolonged incubation with IFN decreased the number of IFN surface receptors, which then resulted in an apparent decrease in the IFN response. A reduction of IFN surface receptors by previous exposure to IFN has recently been reported (34) and may explain the defect in IFN response apparent in many SLE patients (35).

IFN can also induce the release of natural killer cytotoxic factor from NK cells (36,37). It is possible that prolonged IFN exposure could deplete the NK cell of intracellular natural killer cytotoxic factor or could interfere with other intracellular processes (38). However, since no significant cell death was noted by trypan blue exclusion, it is unlikely that prolonged exposure to IFN resulted in accelerated death of the NK effector cells.

Another possibility is that exposure to IFN

Table 3. Effect of interferon (IFN) exposure on baseline and IFN-augmented natural killer (NK) cell activity in 3 normal controls

	NK cell activity (lytic units/10^7 cells), mean ± SD*									
	In vitro incubation without IFN					In vitro incubation with IFN				
	Time 0	16 hours	36 hours	72 hours	144 hours	Time 0	16 hours	36 hours	72 hours	144 hours
Baseline	50.0 ± 15.2	52.4 ± 7.1	61.9 ± 2.3	47.2 ± 6.4	42.7 ± 8.9	68.4 ± 10.1	71.4 ± 8.2	51.4 ± 5.2	32.4 ± 6.2	24.1 ± 6.1
IFN augmentation	71.4 ± 10.2	73.8 ± 8.1	75.6 ± 9.5	72.0 ± 5.6	69.8 ± 9.2	71.4 ± 8.9	75.6 ± 11.6	55.6 ± 7.1	35.1 ± 10.1	29.2 ± 7.1
% enhancement	42.1	40.2	25.6	53.7	55.8	4.3	5.8	8.1	9.3	20.7

* All cultures contained 10 units/ml of interleukin-2 as described in Patients and Methods.

could have activated suppressor cells, which then suppressed NK cell function. Indeed, prolonged exposure of murine spleen cells to IFN has been shown to inhibit NK cell activity, and this inhibition appeared to be mediated by T lymphocytes (39). The fact that both in vivo (40,41) and in vitro exposure of NK effectors to IFN over prolonged periods resulted in similar suppression of NK cell activity suggests that this same effect may be present in human systems. These mechanisms may be particularly important in the autoimmune diseases, in which chronically elevated levels of circulating α-IFN are present.

In conclusion, the present study has demonstrated that elevated levels of circulating α-IFN were present in many patients with SLE and that the elevated levels were often associated with defects in NK cell function. Although anti-IFN antibodies have been reported to be present in some SLE patients (23), no such antibodies were detected in this series of patients; thus, there was no association between these antibodies and any defects in NK cell function. However, prolonged in vitro exposure of PBMC to IFN resulted in a relative impairment of both NK cell activity and IFN response. These results suggest that the elevated levels of IFN in the sera of many SLE patients may be related to the impairment of NK cell function.

REFERENCES

1. Ruíz-Arguelles A, Alarcón-Segovia D, Llorente L, Del Giudice-Knipping JA: Heterogeneity of the spontaneously expanded and mitogen-induced generation of suppressor cell function of T cells on B cells in systemic lupus erythematosus. Arthritis Rheum 23:1004–1009, 1980
2. Takeuchi T, Abe T, Kiyotuki M, Toguchi T, Koide J, Morimoto C, Homma M: In vitro immune response of SLE lymphocytes: the mechanism involved in B-cell activation. Scand J Immunol 16:369–377, 1982
3. Barada FA Jr, Andrews BS, Davis JS IV, Taylor RP: Antibodies of Sm in patients with systemic lupus erythematosus: correlation of Sm antibody titers with disease activity and other laboratory parameters. Arthritis Rheum 24:1236–1244, 1981
4. Hoffman T: Natural killer function in systemic lupus erythematosus. Arthritis Rheum 23:30–35, 1980
5. Neighbour PA, Grayzel AJ, Miller AE: Endogenous and interferon-augmented natural killer cell activity of human peripheral blood mononuclear cells in vitro: studies of patients with multiple sclerosis, systemic lupus erythematosus or rheumatoid arthritis. Clin Exp Immunol 49:11–21, 1982
6. Fujimiya LA, Babiuk LA, Rouse BT: Direct lymphocytotoxicity against herpes simplex virus infected cells. Can J Microbiol 24:1076–1081, 1978
7. Marx J: Natural killer cells help defend the body. Science 7:624–626, 1980
8. Hanna N, Burton RC: Definite evidence that natural killer (NK) cells inhibit experimental tumor metastasis in vivo. J Immunol 127:1754–1759, 1981
9. Tilden AB, Abo T, Balch CM: Suppressor cell function of human granular lymphocytes identified by the HNK-1 (Leu-7) monoclonal antibody. J Immunol 130:1171–1175, 1983
10. Si L, Whiteside TL: Tissue distribution of human NK cells studied with anti-leu-7 monoclonal antibody. J Immunol 130:2149–2155, 1983
11. Goto M, Tanimoto K, Horiuchi Y: Natural cell mediated cytotoxicity in systemic lupus erythematosus: suppression by antilymphocyte antibody. Arthritis Rheum 23: 1274–1281, 1980
12. Sibbitt WL Jr, Froelich CJ, Bankhurst AD: Natural cytotoxicity in systemic lupus erythematosus: mechanisms of suppression by inhibitory serum factors. Clin Exp Immunol 53:363–370, 1983
13. Karsh J, Dorval G, Osterland CK: Natural cytotoxicity in rheumatoid arthritis and systemic lupus erythematosus. Clin Immunol Immunopathol 19:437–441, 1981
14. Sibbitt WL Jr, Froelich CJ, Bankhurst AD: Abnormal interferon modulation of natural cytotoxicity in systemic lupus erythematosus: relation to suppressive serum factors. Arthritis Rheum 26:1452–1459, 1983
15. Kuribayashi K, Gillis S, Kern DE, Henney CS: Murine NK cell cultures: effects of interleukin-2 and interferon on cell growth and cytotoxic reactivity. J Immunol 126:2321–2327, 1981
16. Targan S, Stebbing N: In vitro interactions of purified cloned human interferons on NK cells: enhanced activation. J Immunol 129:934–935, 1982
17. Alcocer-Varela J, Alarcón-Segovia D: Decreased production of response to interleukin-2 by cultured lymphocytes from patients with systemic lupus erythematosus. J Clin Invest 69:1388–1392, 1982
18. Neighbour PA, Grayzel AI: Interferon production in vitro by leucocytes from patients with systemic lupus erythematosus and rheumatoid arthritis. Clin Exp Immunol 25:576–582, 1981
19. Sibbitt WL Jr, Likar L, Spellman CW, Bankhurst AD: Impaired natural killer cell activity in systemic lupus erythematosus: relationship to interleukin-2 production. Arthritis Rheum 26:1316–1320, 1983
20. Strannegard O, Hermodsson S, Westberg G: Interferon and natural killer cells in systemic lupus erythematosus. Clin Exp Immunol 50:246–252, 1982
21. Tsokos GC, Rook AH, Djeu JY, Balow JB: Natural killer cells and interferon responses in patients with systemic lupus erythematosus. Clin Exp Immunol 50: 234–245, 1982
22. Preble OT, Black RJ, Friedman RM, Klippel JH, Vilcek

J: Systemic lupus erythematosus: presence in human serum of an unusual acid-labile leukocyte interferon. Science 216:429–431, 1982
23. Panem S, Check IJ, Henriksen D, Vilcek J: Antibodies to alpha-interferon in a patient with systemic lupus erythematosus. J Immunol 129:1–3, 1982
24. Herberman RB, Holden HT: Natural killer cells as antitumor effector cells. JNCI 62:441–444, 1979
25. Tan EM, Cohen AS, Fries JF, Masi AT, McShane DJ, Rothfield NM, Schaller JG, Talal N, Winchester RJ: The 1982 revised criteria for the classification of systemic lupus erythematosus. Arthritis Rheum 25:1271–1277, 1982
26. Boyum AJ: Isolation of mononuclear cells and granulocytes from human blood. Scand J Clin Lab Invest [Suppl] 21:77–89, 1968
27. Yam LT, Li CY, Crosby WH: Cytochemical identification of monocytes and granulocytes. Am J Pathol 55: 283–290, 1971
28. Sibbitt WL Jr, Bankhurst AD, Williams RC Jr: Studies of cell subpopulations mediating mitogen hyporesponsiveness in Hodgkin's disease. J Clin Invest 61:55–63, 1978
29. Miyasaka N, Darnell B, Baron S, Talal N: Interleukin 2 enhances natural killing of normal lymphocytes. Cell Immunol 84:154–162, 1984
30. Rubenstein S, Famillett PC, Pestha S: A convenient assay for interferon. J Virol 37:766–768, 1981
31. Klein E, Ben-Bassat H, Newmann H: Properties of the K562 cell line derived from a patient with chronic myeloid leukemia. Int J Cancer 18:421–431, 1976
32. Suzuki T, Handa K, Itoh K, Kumagi K: Natural killer (NK) cells as a responder to interleukin 2 (IL-2). J Immunol 130:981–897, 1983
33. Preble OT, Rothko K, Klippel JH, Friedman RM, Johnston MI: Interferon-induced 2′-5′ adenylate synthetase in vivo and interferon production in vitro by lymphocytes from systemic lupus erythematosus patients with and without circulating interferon. J Exp Med 157:2140–2146, 1983
34. Branca AA, Baglioni C: Down-regulation of the interferon receptor. J Biol Chem 257:13197–13200, 1982
35. Sibbitt WL Jr, Mathews PM, Bankhurst AD: The natural killer cell in systemic lupus erythematosus: defects in effector lytic activity and response to interferon and interferon inducers. J Clin Invest 71:1230–1239, 1983
36. Sibbitt WL Jr, Mathews PM, Bankhurst AD: Impaired release of a soluble natural killer cytotoxic factor in systemic lupus erythematosus. Arthritis Rheum 27: 1095–1100, 1984
37. Mathews PM, Sibbitt WL Jr, Froelich CJ, Bankhurst AD: Interferon enhances the production of NK cytotoxic factor by NK cells (abstract). Clin Res 31:90A, 1983
38. Cooper HL, Faghani R, London J, Trepel J, Lester E: Effect of interferon on protein synthesis in human lymphocytes: enhanced synthesis of eight specific peptides in T cells and activation dependent inhibition of overall protein synthesis. J Immunol 128:828–833, 1982
39. Riccardi C, Vose BM, Herberman RB: Modulation of IL 2-dependent growth of mouse NK cells by interferon and T lymphocytes. J Immunol 130:228–232, 1983
40. Maluish AE, Ortaldo JR, Conlon JE, Sherwin SA, Leavitt R, Strong DM, Weirnik P, Oldhun RK, Herberman RB: Depression of natural killer cytotoxicity after in vivo administration of recombinant leukocyte interferon. J Immunol 131:503–507, 1983
41. Melder RJ, Ho M: Modulation of natural killer cell activity in mice after interferon induction: depression of activity and depression of in vitro enhancement by interferon. Infect Immun 36:990–995, 1982

CRICOPHARYNGEAL OBSTRUCTION IN INFLAMMATORY MYOPATHY (POLYMYOSITIS/DERMATOMYOSITIS)

Report of Three Cases and Review of the Literature

LAWRENCE J. KAGEN, RAYMOND B. HOCHMAN, and ELLIOT W. STRONG

Three adults, 2 of whom had polymyositis and 1 with dermatomyositis, developed dysphagia during the course of their illness. Results of esophageal manometry supplemented with esophageal radiography indicated the presence of cricopharyngeal achalasia. Because of the severity of this disorder, which is associated with aspiration of esophageal contents into the airways, surgery to divide the cricopharyngeal musculature was performed in 2 patients, giving complete relief of their symptoms. Prednisone dosage was not increased to treat this condition since it arose not from weakness but from obstruction. A biopsy specimen taken from 1 patient demonstrated inflammatory changes in the obstructing muscle. A review of these 3 patients and 3 previously reported cases indicates that cricopharyngeal obstruction can be a dominant cause of dysphagia in patients with myositis. The recognition of this entity is important in the management of patients with myositis because: 1) it has serious and potentially life-threatening implications; and 2) in certain cases, it can be effectively treated with surgery.

Dysphagia may arise from several causes in patients with myositis. A decrease in the strength of the pharyngeal musculature, disordered motility of the esophagus, vallecular pooling, and tongue weakness may all interfere with normal swallowing (1). Recently, emphasis has been placed on the high frequency of distal esophageal dysfunction in patients with this type of disease (2,3). Dysphagia also has been shown to be indicative of a poor prognosis in patients with inflammatory myopathy (4).

We have observed cricopharyngeal achalasia as a mechanism of obstruction in 3 patients with inflammatory myopathy. In this report, we describe these occurrences and show that, in certain cases, surgery may relieve this condition.

CASE REPORTS

Patient 1. This 77-year-old white woman had polymyositis which had begun insidiously, with myalgia and weakness, 4–5 years earlier. At that time, she complained of tiredness, trouble lifting dishes from a closet, and a slight difficulty in walking. Initially, her physicians detected no other signs of myopathy, although elevation of her creatine phosphokinase (CPK) level to 172 mU/ml (normal 80) was noted. Because of a history of epigastric distress, a series of radiographs of the gastrointestinal (GI) tract was performed. A small hiatus hernia was shown, but the swallowing mechanism was otherwise normal.

Over the next 2 years, her feelings of muscle weakness and fatigue increased, and 2 years from the time of symptom onset, a biopsy of the left deltoid muscle was performed. The biopsy specimen showed myositis with mononuclear cell infiltrates in interstitial foci and around blood vessels, along with degeneration and myofiber necrosis. At that time, her serum CPK level had increased to 600 mU/ml. Prednisone therapy

From the Departments of Medicine and Surgery, The Hospital for Special Surgery, The New York Hospital–Cornell Medical Center, and the Memorial Sloan-Kettering Cancer Center, New York, New York.

Lawrence J. Kagen, MD; Raymond B. Hochman, MD; Elliot W. Strong, MD.

Address reprint requests to Dr. Lawrence J. Kagen, The Hospital for Special Surgery, 535 East 70th Street, New York, NY 10021.

Submitted for publication October 5, 1984; accepted in revised form December 20, 1984.

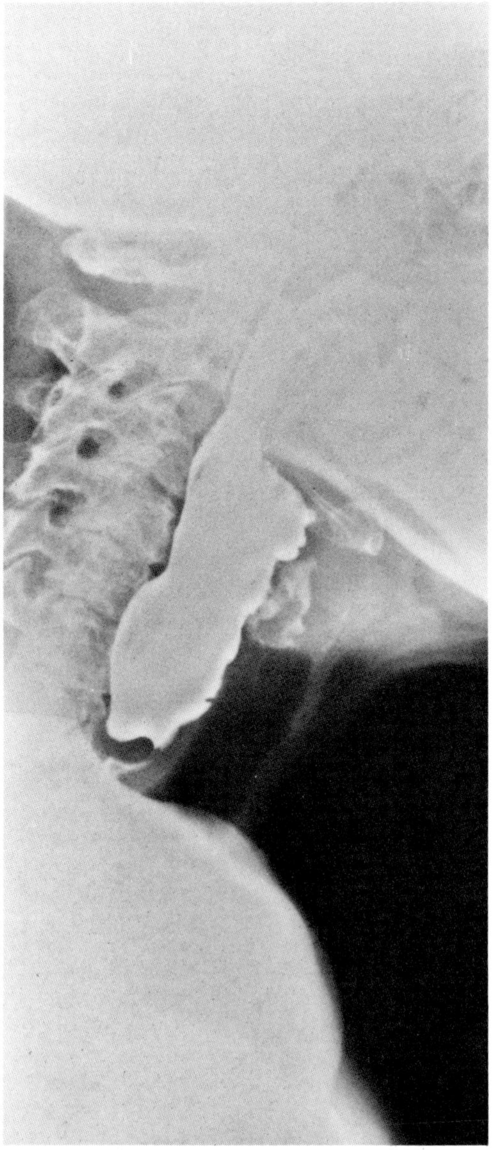

Figure 1. Barium esophagram, lateral view, of patient 1, demonstrating marked cricopharyngeus muscle impression, and patulous dilatation of the proximal hypopharynx.

was begun at a dosage of 30 mg, taken on alternate days, and she showed improvement in muscle strength. The dosage was subsequently tapered to a maintenance level of 15 mg on alternate days. At the time of diagnosis of polymyositis, isotope scans and radiographs of her abdominal organs, as well as a chest radiograph, appeared normal. She had no skin lesions.

For 2–3 years prior to evaluation by us, her general condition improved somewhat, but she had developed difficulty in swallowing liquids as well as solids. Occasionally, liquids and chewed food were expelled through the nose after an attempt to swallow. She felt as though she were choking on her own oral secretions. During the previous year, she lost 18 pounds.

At the time of initial examination by us, she showed moderately reduced muscle strength in all muscle groups tested; her gait was normal. She was able to walk on toes and heels and arise from both the supine and seated positions without using her hands, but she was unable to rise from a deep squat. Laboratory evaluation showed the following results: normal complete blood count, a Westergren erythrocyte sedi-

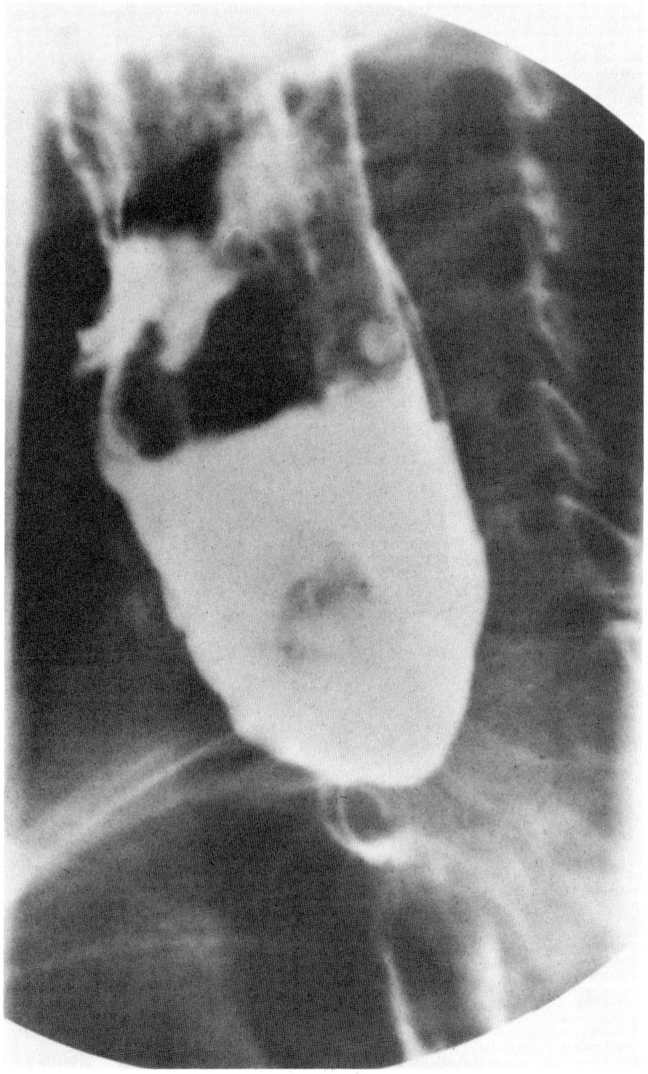

Figure 2. Barium esophagram, oblique view, of patient 1, demonstrating patulous proximal hypopharynx and normal distal esophagus with prominent cricopharyngeus.

mentation rate (ESR) of 32 mm, normal urinalysis findings; blood chemistries were normal except for a slightly elevated lactic dehydrogenase (LDH) level at 227 mU/ml. CPK was normal at 195 mU/ml, and serum glutamic oxaloacetic transaminase (SGOT) was normal at 27 mU/ml.

Radiographic studies of her esophagus (Figures 1 and 2) showed marked hypertrophy of the distal pharyngeal muscular ring, consistent with a diagnosis of cricopharyngeal sphincter hypertrophy. There was also significant proximal pharyngeal patulous dilatation. During the act of swallowing, there was aspiration of barium into the laryngotracheal airway and regurgitation into the nasopharynx.

Esophageal manometry showed normal peristalsis at 20 mm Hg, except in the upper third, where motility was simultaneous and spontaneous, reflecting a myopathy. At 16 cm from the incisor teeth, pressure was elevated (25 mm Hg), and the muscle failed to relax. Achalasia occurred in 14 of 15 swallows evoking premature contractions and no relaxation.

The patient underwent esophagoscopy and cricopharyngeal myotomy. The muscle specimen that was removed (Figures 3 and 4) demonstrated areas of necrosis, inflammatory cell infiltration, and an increase in connective tissue. Her postoperative course was uneventful, and she was discharged 4 days postsurgery, on a soft diet regimen. Her ability to swallow has subsequently improved. Repeat esophagram 9 weeks postoperatively demonstrated a normal swallowing mechanism with slight nasopharyngeal reflux and a minimal cricopharyngeus indentation without radiographic evidence of obstruction.

Six months postoperatively, her clinical status is stable. She takes 10 mg of prednisone on alternate days, and her swallowing function appears normal.

Patient 2. This 47-year-old white woman with dermatomyositis had been in good health until 2 years prior to admission. At that time, she developed a noticeable pruritic rash, characterized by erythema and swelling periorbitally, erythema of the neck and chest, and redness and swelling over the knuckles of

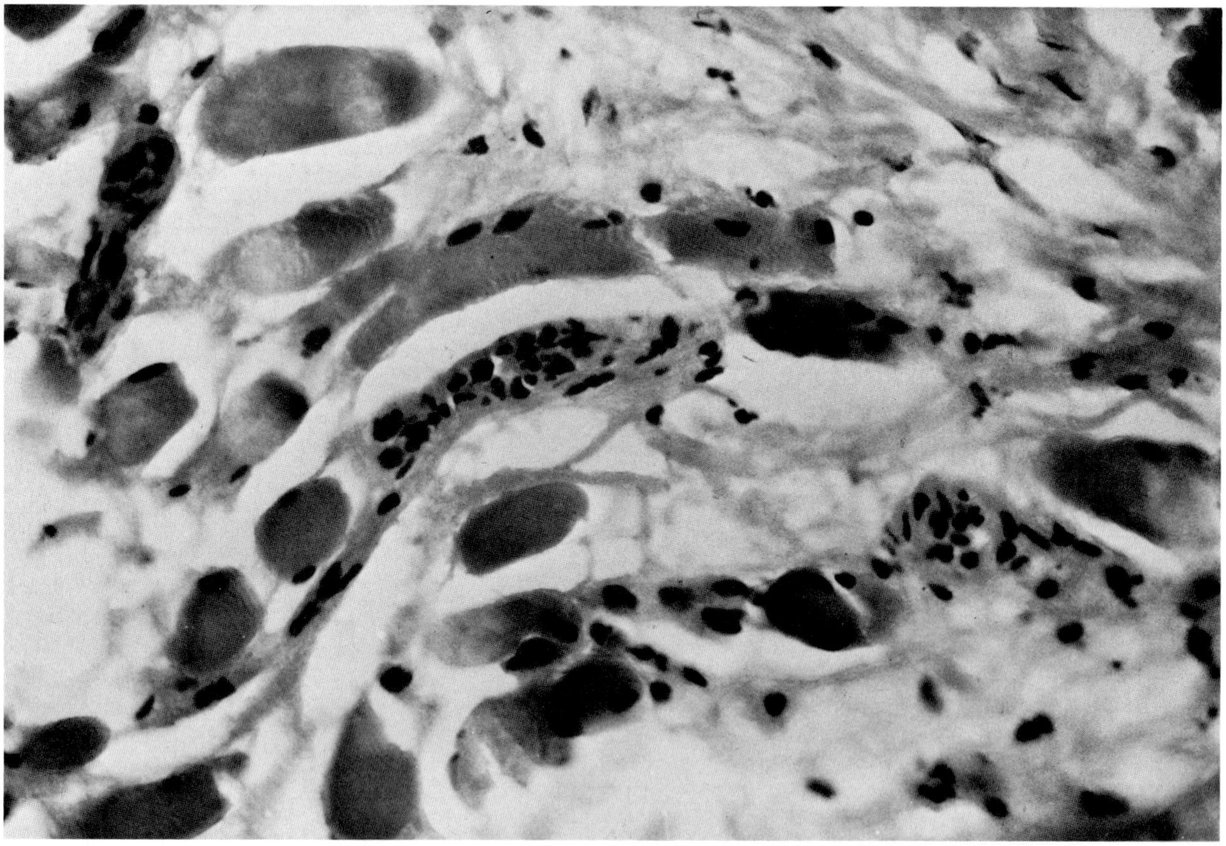

Figure 3. High power magnification of histologic section of cricopharyngeus muscle taken from patient 1, revealing fiber necrosis, mononuclear cell infiltrate, and prominent connective tissue (hematoxylin and eosin stained).

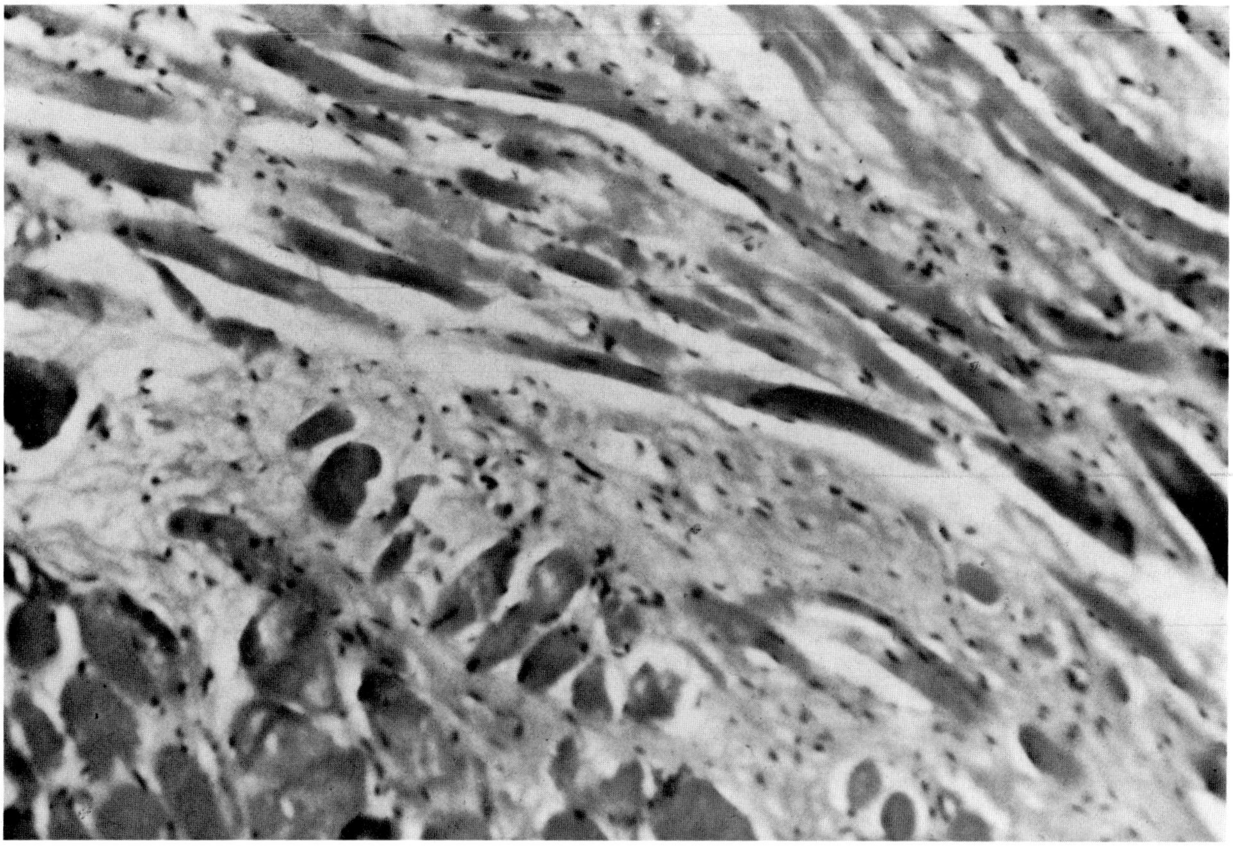

Figure 4. Low power magnification of histologic section of cricopharyngeus muscle taken from patient 1, revealing prominent connective tissue, fiber degeneration, and mononuclear cell infiltrate (hematoxylin and eosin stained).

the hands. Within 2 weeks, myalgia of the proximal musculature of the upper and lower extremities became prominent. She showed moderate weakness of the proximal musculature of her arms and legs. CPK was 3,000 mU/ml, LDH was 1,160 mU/ml, and SGOT was 194 mU/ml.

At that time, a biopsy of the quadriceps femoris muscle demonstrated myofiber necrosis and mononuclear cell infiltrates. A series of radiographs of the GI tract obtained at that time demonstrated moderately decreased esophageal motility without obstruction. She was begun on prednisone therapy, 60 mg/day. Muscle strength improved and the rash faded, but within the next 2 years she had 2 further episodes of disease exacerbation, each of which was responsive to an increased prednisone dose.

Toward the conclusion of this second cycle of illness, while receiving 50 mg of prednisone per day, she developed, over a period of several days, an acute difficulty in swallowing. She felt an obstruction behind her sternum when she attempted to swallow, with a feeling that there was "something swelling" in that region. In addition, attempts to swallow led to aching substernal pain. She stopped eating solids, and restricted herself to fluids, which, after some attempts at swallowing, flowed out of her nose.

At this time, however, her peripheral strength was improving: she was able to lift both arms over her head and elevate both legs above the bed to a heel height of 20 inches, neither of which was she able to do the previous month. Barium swallow radiography demonstrated sharp obstruction of flow at the cricopharyngeus area and aspiration of radiopaque material into both lungs. Complete blood count and urinalysis performed at this time gave normal results, as did evaluation of her serum chemistries.

Esophageal manometry demonstrated achalasia at the level of the cricopharyngeus, with failure of relaxation and with premature contraction. The patient underwent cricopharyngeal myotomy, after which she had complete relief of symptoms. Her ability to swallow returned to normal, and she again returned to a full diet. Over the course of the followup period, she initially exhibited several minor exacerbations and remissions of myositis, which after 3 years, entered a period of sustained remission. Swallowing remained normal throughout this time. At present, 10 years later, she takes no medication and maintains full activity. Followup roentgenographic studies of the upper GI tract have shown no abnormality.

Patient 3. This 41-year-old white male plumber had a 4-month history of muscle weakness and diffuse myalgia of the proximal and distal musculature of his arms and legs. Coincident with this, he had trouble lifting his tools and pipes at work, and he also had difficulty in ascending stairs. Within 1–2 months, he developed difficulty in swallowing solid foods, but no difficulty in swallowing liquids. Laboratory evaluation performed elsewhere revealed an elevated serum CPK level. A biopsy sample taken from the deltoid muscle showed interstitial mononuclear cell infiltrates and myofiber necrosis. He was begun on prednisone, 50 mg/day, which he independently reduced and then discontinued because he felt that it was not helping. After stopping prednisone, his myalgia increased, and within 2 weeks, prednisone, 30 mg/day, was reinstituted and maintained. A series of radiographs of the GI tract, performed 3 months previously, showed no esophageal abnormality.

At the time of his initial evaluation by us, his weight was 151 pounds (approximately his normal), and he had weakness of the proximal extremity musculature with difficulty going up 1 step and difficulty arising from a squat. His complete blood count and ESR were normal, as were his serum chemistries (CPK 60 mU/ml, LDH 125 mU/ml, and SGOT 16 mU/ml).

An electromyogram gave results suggestive of inflammatory myopathy, with increased insertional activity, small, narrow, fragmented motor unit potentials, and early recruitment pattern.

Endoscopy of the upper GI tract revealed no abnormality. Esophageal manometry demonstrated cricopharyngeal achalasia, with a lack of expected relaxation of the cricopharyngeal area during swallowing, and with increased pressure to 35 mm Hg. During approximately 50% of his attempts to swallow, partial or inadequate relaxation did occur. In addition, low-amplitude, broad-based, discoordinate pharyngeal waves were noted.

Because his symptoms were not severe and there was no evidence of aspiration, a surgical procedure was not performed. He was maintained under close followup observation.

DISCUSSION

Disorders of the swallowing mechanism are known to occur as the result of abnormalities in the nasopharynx as well as in the upper and lower esophagus. Weakness or dysfunction of the nasopharyngeal and upper esophageal mechanisms as well as of lower smooth muscle portions of the esophagus may play a role in the development of dysphagia. In addition, other abnormalities, such as dilatation, stricture, or hiatus hernia, may be present as complicating factors.

The precise incidence of dysphagia among patients with myositis is not known, but reports based upon a retrospective review of symptoms indicate that it is rather uncommon. It was found in 12% of the patients in a large series reported by Bohan and coworkers (4), whereas series based upon physiologic studies of esophageal function and prospective questioning suggest a greater frequency of the disorder.

In one prospective study of 12 patients with polymyositis (2), 8 patients had manometrically observed abnormalities of the esophageal smooth muscle, with impaired peristalsis, and 8 patients had abnormalities of the striated muscle segment of the esophagus. Of these patients, 5 were thought to have esophageal dysphagia. Using techniques of cineradiography, de Merieux et al (3) found abnormalities of the distal esophagus in 14 of 16 patients with polymyositis or dermatomyositis. Proximal esophageal dysfunction was present in 70% of these patients.

The cricopharyngeal muscle is considered to be the upper esophageal sphincter, although there are difficulties in its anatomic definition (5,6). In a large series of patients without myopathy who had gastrointestinal evaluations reviewed by videorecording techniques, 77 of 618 were found to have a visible cricopharyngeal muscle (6). It was seen as an obstruction to the pharyngeal bolus or as an indentation in the pharyngeal swallow. It was most often found at the C5–C6 level. Of these patients, only 15% reported dysphagia (6). Abnormalities in the function of the cricopharyngeus increase with age (7), and have been observed in relation to neurologic diseases (8–10), reflux (11), and surgery, as well as other causes.

As far as we can determine, the first report of the syndrome of cricopharyngeal achalasia in myositis was that of a 44-year-old woman with acute polymyositis and dysphagia in whom carcinoma of the esophagus was initially suspected (12). Although manometric studies were not reported, her physicians theorized that inflammation and edema of the cricopharyngeus may have caused the pseudostricture appearance suggestive of a neoplasm (12).

In 1973, Porubsky and colleagues (13) described a 54-year-old man with dermatomyositis who developed rapid and total esophageal obstruction while receiving, and improving with, initial prednisone therapy. Cricopharyngeal myotomy was performed, and the excised muscle demonstrated an inflammatory cell infiltrate. His dysphagia was relieved by this procedure, and he continued to do well in this regard for the next 6 months of followup.

In 1980, an 82-year-old woman with cricopharyngeal achalasia and polymyositis was described (14). At the time of her evaluation, it was thought that she did not have active muscle disease. Cricopharyngeal myotomy was performed, and the muscle specimen that was removed demonstrated fibrosis and minimal evidence of round cell infiltration. The patient was thought to have obstruction secondary to fibrosis of the inlet muscle mechanism.

Our observations presented here represent the first grouping of patients with cricopharyngeal obstruction in relation to inflammatory muscle disease. In 1 case, histologic evidence of myositis was observed in the affected muscle. In 2 cases, spillover of oropharyngeal contents into the airways was concomitantly present, posing the hazard of aspiration pneumonitis. Pulmonary infection has been previously observed in this setting (15).

Our 3 patients were adults: 2 were women, 1 was a man, and all were white (Table 1). At the time they developed symptoms of dysphagia, they had had myopathy for 4 months, 2 years, and 5 years. In 2 patients, dysphagia was acute and associated with pain on swallowing. All 3 patients were receiving prednisone at the time of onset of dysphagia symptoms, and all 3 were thought to be improving from their recently active myopathy. Surgery was performed on 2 patients, with excellent results; patient 1 was followed for 6 months postsurgery and patient 2 was followed for 10 years. These patients did not, for any other reasons, require an increase in prednisone dosage. In all 3 patients, radiographic series of the GI tract with esophageal study was obtained at the onset of illness, 3, 24, and 60 months prior to the development of swallowing difficulty, and failed to show evidence of achalasia at that time. This further suggests a relationship between the development of cricopharyngeus muscle dysfunction and the occurrence of myositis.

Our case reports, together with previous reports, suggest that cricopharyngeal obstruction due to inflammation and/or fibrosis of the cricopharyngeus apparatus may occur during the course of polymyositis and dermatomyositis in adults. Two such patients were over age 70, and 4 were younger (age range 41–54). It is of interest that in 5 of the 6 patients, symptomatic obstruction was noted during a period of remission or inactivity of their peripheral muscle disease.

The syndrome of cricopharyngeal achalasia in myositis is important for several reasons. First, aspiration of esophageal contents into the airways may occur

Table 1. Summary of clinical characteristics of cricopharyngeal obstruction in myositis

Patient (ref.)	Age/sex	Diagnosis	Duration of myopathy at onset of dysphagia	Therapy	Esophageal radiography result	Esophageal manometry result	Surgical result
1 (this report)	77/F	Polymyositis	5 years*	Prednisone 15 mg on alternate days	Diagnostic	Diagnostic	Excellent
2 (this report)	47/F	Dermatomyositis	2 years*	Prednisone 50 mg/day	Suggestive of obstruction	Diagnostic	Excellent
3 (this report)	41/M	Polymyositis	4 months*	Prednisone 30 mg/day	Negative	Diagnostic	Surgery not done
4 (12)	44/F	Polymyositis	1 week	None	Obstructive†	Not reported	Surgery not done
5 (13)	54/M	Dermatomyositis	8 months*	Prednisone 60 mg/day	Diagnostic	Not reported	Excellent
6 (14)	82/F	Polymyositis	2 years*	Not stated	Diagnostic	Not reported	Improvement

* Myopathy believed to be in remission, improving, or inactive at the time of onset of dysphagia.
† Diagnosis of cricopharyngeus obstruction suggested by the authors but not demonstrated with certainty.

with this syndrome, and may result in pulmonary infection and damage. Second, this syndrome, if severe, may best be treated with surgical management, which offers the chance of complete amelioration of symptoms without the need for an increase in prednisone dosage, if not otherwise required. The surgical procedure has been well tolerated by these chronically ill patients with little morbidity. The diagnosis of cricopharyngeus muscle dysfunction, if suspected, can be confirmed by roentgenographic study of swallowing, along with esophageal manometry. At present, we do not know how frequently this mechanism is responsible for dysphagia in patients with inflammatory muscle disease.

REFERENCES

1. Kagen LJ: Polymyositis and dermatomyositis, Arthritis and Allied Conditions. Tenth edition. Edited by DJ McCarty. Philadelphia, Lea & Febiger, 1984, pp 971–993
2. Jacob H, Berkowitz D, McDonald E, Bernstein LH, Beneventano T: The esophageal motility disorder of polymyositis. Arch Intern Med 143:2262–2264, 1984
3. De Merieux P, Verity MA, Clements PJ, Paulus HE: Esophageal abnormalities and dysphagia in polymyositis and dermatomyositis: clinical, radiographic, and pathologic features. Arthritis Rheum 26:961–968, 1983
4. Bohan A, Peter JB, Bowman RL, Pearson CM: A computer-assisted analysis of 153 patients with polymyositis and dermatomyositis. Medicine (Baltimore) 56:255–286, 1977
5. Ellis FH Jr: Upper esophageal sphincter in health and disease. Surg Clin North Am 51:553–565, 1971
6. Curtis DJ, Cruess DF, Berg T: The cricopharyngeal muscle. AJR 142:497–500, 1984
7. Pitcher JL: Dysphagia in the elderly: causes and diagnosis. Geriatrics 28:64–69, 1973
8. O'Connor AF, Adrian GM: Cinefluorography in the diagnosis of pharyngeal palsies. J Laryngol Otol 90:1015–1019, 1976
9. Donner MW, Silbiger ML: Cinefluorographic analysis of pharyngeal swallowing in neuromuscular disorders. Am J Med Sci 251:600–616, 1966
10. Schleider MA, Nagurney JT: Progressive supranuclear ophthalmoplegia. JAMA 237:994–995, 1977
11. Henderson RD, Woolf C, Marryatt G: Pharyngoesophageal dysphagia and gastroesophageal reflux. Laryngoscope 86:1531–1539, 1976
12. Thomas FB, LeBauer S, Greenberger NJ: Polymyositis masquerading as carcinoma of the cervical esophagus. Arch Intern Med 129:984–986, 1972
13. Porubsky ES, Murray JP, Pratt LL: Cricopharyngeal achalasia in dermatomyositis. Arch Otolaryngol 98:428–429, 1973
14. Dietz F, Logeman JA, Sahgal V, Schmid FR: Cricopharyngeal muscle dysfunction in the differential diagnosis of dysphagia in polymyositis. Arthritis Rheum 23:491–495, 1980
15. Dickey BF, Myers AR: Pulmonary disease in polymyositis/dermatomyositis. Semin Arthritis Rheum 14:60–76, 1984

DECREASED CORONARY RESERVE IN PRIMARY SCLERODERMA MYOCARDIAL DISEASE

ANDRÉ KAHAN, ALAIN NITENBERG, JEAN-M. FOULT, BERNARD AMOR, CHARLES-J. MENKES, JEAN-Y. DEVAUX, FRANÇOISE BLANCHET, JEANNINE PERENNEC, GENEVIÈVE LUTFALLA, and JEAN-C. ROUCAYROL

We assessed coronary reserve, by measuring the increase in coronary sinus blood flow (CSBF) after intravenous administration of dipyridamole (0.14 mg/kg/minute for 4 minutes), in 7 patients with primary scleroderma myocardial disease (PSMD) and in 7 control subjects. Coronary reserve was greatly impaired in PSMD: before administration of dipyridamole, CSBF was similar in patients with PSMD (89 ± 32 ml/minute/100 gm, mean ± SD) and in controls (100 ± 15 ml/minute/100 gm); after dipyridamole infusion, CSBF was significantly lower in patients with PSMD (191 ± 45 ml/minute/100 gm) than in controls (399 ± 58 ml/minute/100 gm) ($P < 0.01$). Six of the 7 patients with PSMD had angiographically normal epicardial coronary arteries and normal left ventricular function. Decreased coronary reserve may be an important contributor to the pathogenesis of primary scleroderma myocardial disease.

Primary cardiac involvement is common in progressive systemic sclerosis (PSS), being present in up to 50% of autopsied subjects (1–3). When clinically evident, cardiac involvement has been shown to indicate a poor prognosis for survival (4,5). Symptoms of primary scleroderma myocardial disease (PSMD) include chest pain, dyspnea, palpitations, congestive heart failure, syncope, and sudden death (1–3,6,7). Angina pectoris and myocardial infarctions have been seen in PSS patients with normal coronary arteries (1,7,8).

The standard noninvasive clinical tests for primary scleroderma myocardial disease (physical examination, chest radiograph, electrocardiogram [EKG]) are less sensitive than myocardial perfusion scintigraphy, radionuclide ventriculography, echocardiography, and Holter monitoring (2,3,9–14). Coronary angiography usually demonstrates normal extramural coronary arteries (2,3); occasionally, slow run-off of dye has been noted (15), a finding which might reflect increased vascular resistance of a functional as well as a structural type (16).

The pathogenesis of primary scleroderma myocardial disease remains uncertain. Several reports, however, have emphasized a vascular and microvascular dysfunction in progressive systemic sclerosis. On histopathologic examination, PSS is characterized by microvascular abnormalities (2,3,17,18), by excessive fibroblastic activity (19,20), and by collagen depo-

Presented in part at the 48th Annual Meeting of the American Rheumatism Association, Minneapolis, MN, June 1984.

From the Departments of Rheumatology, Cardiology, and Nuclear Medicine, René Descartes University School of Medicine, Hôpital Cochin, Paris, and INSERM U 251, Xavier Bichat University and INSERM U 2, Paris 12 University, Paris, France.

André Kahan, MD: Department of Rheumatology, Hôpital Cochin; Alain Nitenberg, MD: INSERM U 251, Xavier Bichat University; Jean-M. Foult, MD: INSERM U 251, Xavier Bichat University; Bernard Amor, MD: Professor of Rheumatology, Department of Rheumatology, Hôpital Cochin; Charles-J. Menkes, MD: Professor of Rheumatology, Department of Rheumatology, Hôpital Cochin; Jean-Y. Devaux, MD: Department of Nuclear Medicine, Hôpital Cochin; Françoise Blanchet, MD: INSERM U 251, Xavier Bichat University; Jeannine Perennec, MD: INSERM U 2, Paris 12 University; Geneviève Lutfalla, MD: Department of Cardiology, Hôpital Cochin; Jean-C. Roucayrol, MD: Professor of Biophysics, Department of Nuclear Medicine, Hôpital Cochin.

Address reprint requests to André Kahan, MD, Department of Rheumatology, Hôpital Cochin, 27 rue du faubourg Saint Jacques, 75674 Paris Cedex 14, France.

Submitted for publication September 4, 1984; accepted in revised form December 20, 1984.

sition in numerous organs (2,5). The characteristic manifestation of myocardial involvement in PSS is myocardial fibrosis unrelated to evident disease or narrowing in the large coronary arteries (1–3,6,8,16,21–24). Myocardial fibrosis tends to be patchy and to involve the epicardium as frequently as the endocardium, and the right ventricle as well as the left.

Extramural coronary arteries are usually normal in PSS (1,8,15,21,23,24). Reports of intramural coronary artery involvement vary among several series of patients. Concentric intimal hypertrophy, narrowing, fibrosis, and fibrinoid necrosis of intramural coronary arteries and arterioles have been noted (21,25). On the other hand, Bulkley et al (1) have emphasized the paucity of small vessel abnormalities in 52 PSS patients. When present, myocardial necrosis has a specific appearance displaying myofibrillar degeneration with contraction band formation, a histologic lesion seen in the setting of ischemic injury followed by reperfusion (1). Bulkley et al (1) noted pathologic findings consistent with progression from contraction band necrosis through replacement fibrosis in the hearts of PSS patients.

Thus, despite the usual finding of normal extramural coronary arteries, much of the clinical and pathologic presentation of primary scleroderma myocardial disease mimics ischemic heart disease, a finding which may be accounted for by a Raynaud's-like phenomenon of the coronary vasculature (3), with or without accompanying structural vascular disease. To further investigate the possible coronary vascular and microvascular dysfunction in primary scleroderma myocardial disease, we assessed coronary reserve, by measuring the increase in coronary sinus blood flow after intravenous administration of dipyridamole, in 7 patients with progressive systemic sclerosis and diffuse scleroderma and in 7 control subjects. All patients with progressive systemic sclerosis had evidence of primary scleroderma myocardial disease, documented using noninvasive procedures.

Our study demonstrates that coronary reserve is greatly impaired in progressive systemic sclerosis patients who have normal findings on coronary angiogram and normal left ventricular function. This decreased coronary reserve may be an important contributor to the pathogenesis of primary scleroderma myocardial disease.

PATIENTS AND METHODS

Progressive systemic sclerosis patients. Seven female patients with PSS and diffuse scleroderma were studied. All patients satisfied the American Rheumatism Association preliminary criteria for classification of systemic sclerosis (26). None of the patients had the CREST syndrome variant (calcinosis, Raynaud's phenomenon, esophageal dysmotility, sclerodactyly, telangiectasias) of progressive systemic sclerosis (27). The mean age was 50 years (range 41–53). The duration of disease ranged from 3–24 years (mean ± SD 12.9 ± 8.1 years). At the time of the study, none of the patients was taking medication for cardiac disease. Selection of PSS patients for cardiac catheterization was primarily based on evidence of primary scleroderma myocardial disease, documented using noninvasive procedures. All patients gave informed consent for all procedures.

Control subjects. During the same period, 7 control subjects (6 female, 1 male; mean age 46 years, range 31–54) with normal left ventricular function and normal results on coronary arteriography underwent the same catheterization procedure. Four control subjects had mild mitral stenosis (pulmonary wedge pressure inferior to 15 mm Hg) with normal cardiac output, 1 had mild pulmonary stenosis (right ventricular systolic pressure = 45 mm Hg), 1 had Roger's disease (small ventricular septal defect without left to right shunt, shown by oximetry), and 1 had patent foramen ovale.

Noninvasive tests. All patients with PSS had the following performed: physical examination, pulmonary function testing (routine spirometry with forced vital capacity [FVC], forced volume in 1 second, and single-breath diffusing capacity for carbon monoxide [DLco] [28]), electrocardiograms, standard anteroposterior and lateral chest roentgenograms, 2-dimensional echocardiograms, resting thallium-201 myocardial single photon emission computed tomographic scintigrams, and ^{99m}technetium multiple-gated equilibrium blood pool imaging.

Thallium-201 myocardial single photon emission computed tomography (29,30) was performed with the subject at rest, using a gamma camera equipped with a rotating gantry (CGR Gammatome T 9000). A 75-MBq (2.0 mCi) activity of thallium-201 was injected intravenously. Acquisition began within 15 minutes following the tracer administration. Thallium images were acquired for 20 minutes. Thirty-two images were recorded on a 180° rotation basis, each of them digitized in a 64 × 64 matrix. Approximately two million counts were accumulated in 1 study. About 20 transverse slices (6 mm thick) were reconstructed on a minicomputer (CGR IMAC) and then 2 sets of oblique views (left anterior and right anterior) were displayed and used for interpretation. The left myocardium was divided into 9 segments. Tracer activity was visually graded in 5 steps (2.0 = normal perfusion, 0 = no tracer activity) by 3 independent observers. Scores for each segment were averaged. Thallium defects were defined as mean scores of <1.5.

Each patient subsequently underwent supine resting radionuclide ventriculography with a gamma camera (CGR Acticamera), using in vitro labeling of red blood cells with 555 MBq (15 mCi) of ^{99m}technetium. Resting gated blood pool images were acquired for 300,000 counts in each of the 16 frames. The best left anterior oblique view with a 10° caudal tilt was used in order to separate the ventricles from the atrial images. Left ventricular ejection fraction was determined by a 2–region-of-interest method with an automatic thresholding technique for background subtraction.

Normal resting left ventricular function was defined as an ejection fraction of ≥55%.

All noninvasive studies were analyzed by independent observers who had no knowledge of the other test results.

All 7 PSS patients included in the final catheterization study had evidence of primary scleroderma myocardial disease (chest pain, dyspnea, palpitations, and 1 or more abnormalities on EKG, chest radiograph, echocardiogram, thallium-201 myocardial single photon emission computed tomographic scintigram, or ^{99m}technetium multiple-gated equilibrium blood pool imaging); none of them had evidence of significant pulmonary or renal involvement.

Catheterization procedure. Using 1% lidocaine as local anesthesia, a 7F high fidelity double-tipped micromanometer catheter (PC-770, Millar Instruments, Houston, TX) was placed in the left ventricle through a femoral artery and positioned to simultaneously record left ventricular and aortic pressures. A 7F sheath was placed in the other femoral artery for left ventriculography and coronary arteriography catheters. A 7F Swan-Ganz thermodilution catheter (Edwards Laboratory) was placed into the pulmonary artery via a femoral vein for cardiac output determinations (Cardiac Output Computer 9520 A; Edwards Laboratory, Saint-Ouen l'Aumone, France). A 7F coronary sinus thermodilution catheter (Wilton Webster Laboratories, Altadena, CA) was inserted in the left subclavian vein and positioned into the coronary sinus for coronary sinus blood flow (CSBF) measurements; the position of the catheter was periodically controlled by fluoroscopy in order to place the proximal thermistor in front of the posterior interventricular vein arrival site into the coronary sinus.

Protocol. After left ventricular angiography (1 ml/kg body weight ioxaglate) and coronary arteriography were performed, resting left ventricular and aortic pressures, cardiac output, and coronary sinus blood flow were measured. This was done after a delay of 30 minutes, in order to eliminate the effects of contrast material (31). Arterial, pulmonary, and coronary sinus blood samples were collected. The whole procedure was repeated after a right atrial infusion of dipyridamole, 0.14 mg/kg/minute for 4 minutes. The coronary sinus blood flow was also recorded during a contrast medium injection into the left coronary artery after dipyridamole infusion.

Data analysis. Cardiac output was determined by the thermodilution method. Coronary sinus blood flow was measured by the continuous thermodilution method (32). Heart rate, left ventricular end diastolic pressure (LVEDP), left ventricular systolic pressure, mean aortic pressure (MAP), systemic vascular resistance, and maximum velocity of shortening (33) were calculated by a catheterization data analysis computer system (Hewlett Packard 5600 M), which performed on-line analysis on 9 beats, for averaging of variations in respiration.

Left ventricular end diastolic volume and left ventricular end systolic volumes (LVESV) and ejection fraction were calculated from the monoplane angiogram in a 30° right anterior oblique projection using the area length method (34). Left ventricular mass was calculated according to the equation of Trenouth et al (35), which was used to quantitate the equatorial end systolic wall thickness. Average left ventricular end systolic equatorial stress (σES) was calculated according to the equation of Falsetti et al (36), using the left ventricular end systolic pressure corresponding to the left ventricular end systolic volume (the left ventricular pressure and a frame marker were recorded during the left ventricular angiography), and allowed the calculation of the end systolic wall stress:end systolic volume ratio (σES:LVESV) (37). Left ventricular compliance was assessed by the volume elastic constant α (38), and myocardial stiffness was evaluated by the elastic stiffness constant k (39).

Coronary sinus blood flow was assumed to be representative of the total left ventricular myocardial blood flow, and values were expressed for 100 gm left ventricular mass (40,41). Coronary resistance was calculated as:

$$\frac{\text{MAP} - \text{LVEDP (mm Hg)}}{\text{CSBF (ml/minute/100 gm)}}$$

Oxygen content of arterial and coronary venous blood samples was determined by a galvanic cell method (Lex O_2 Con K; Waltham Instruments, Waltham, MA). Myocardial oxygen consumption was calculated as arterial–coronary sinus oxygen content difference (a–cs O_2 D, ml/100 ml) multiplied by coronary sinus blood flow (ml/minute/100 gm). Arterial plasma lactate concentration (lact a) and coronary sinus lactate concentration (lact cs) were measured by an enzymatic method (Boehringer Mannheim Laboratories, Mannheim, FRG). Lactate extraction was calculated as:

$$\frac{\text{lact a} - \text{lact cs}}{\text{lact a}}$$

Transarterial left ventricular endomyocardial biopsy. Left ventricular endomyocardial biopsy was performed on PSS patients at the end of the study, using a King's College bioptome (42) introduced through a sheath positioned into the left ventricle via a femoral artery. Two to 3 specimens were obtained from each patient and immediately dropped into 10 ml of the patient's procainized blood; the specimens were then fixed with a sodium cacodylate–3% glutaraldehyde solution at 4°C. The myocardium was studied by light and electron microscopy. The amount of interstitial fibrous tissue was determined morphometrically by the point-counting method (43).

Table 1. Selected clinical characteristics of 7 patients with diffuse scleroderma

Disorder	No.
Raynaud's phenomenon	7
Dyspnea	7
Chest pain	6
Palpitations	2
Systemic hypertension	0
Electrocardiographic abnormalities	4
Echocardiographic pericardial disease	2
Tomographic thallium-201 myocardial perfusion scintigram abnormalities	7
Decreased left ventricular ejection fraction (radionuclide ventriculography)	1

Table 2. Left ventricular function, control subjects and progressive systemic sclerosis (PSS) patients*

	Control subjects (n = 7)	PSS patients (n = 7)	*P*†
LVEDV	76 ± 16	74 ± 17	NS
LVESV	31 ± 9	31 ± 14	NS
EF	61 ± 5	60 ± 8	NS
LVM	61 ± 9	63 ± 20	NS
σES	210 ± 46	202 ± 51	NS
σES:LVESV	4.80 ± 0.90	4.48 ± 0.56	NS
α	0.024 ± 0.007	0.024 ± 0.003	NS
k	14.3 ± 1.6	14.1 ± 2.2	NS

* Values are mean ± SD. LVEDV = left ventricular end diastolic volume, ml/m^2; LVESV = left ventricular end systolic volume, ml/m^2; EF = ejection fraction, %; LVM = left ventricular mass, gm/m^2; σES = average left ventricular end systolic equatorial stress, gm/cm^2; α = volume elastic constant/1 ml; k = elastic stiffness constant.
†NS = not significant.

Statistical analysis. Mean values and standard deviations were calculated for each parameter. Statistical comparisons were made with Student's *t*-test and the Wilcoxon rank sum test. *P* values <0.05 were considered significant.

RESULTS

Clinical findings of noninvasive procedures. Selected clinical characteristics of the PSS population at the time of study are shown in Table 1. None of the PSS patients had either a history of systemic hypertension or a blood pressure above 140/90 mm Hg during the evaluation. All 7 patients met previously published clinical criteria for cardiac involvement in progressive systemic sclerosis (2,3,14,44,45). None of the patients had congestive heart failure. Six patients had chest pain consistent with angina pectoris. Four patients had abnormal findings on EKG, including 1 with a pseudo-infarction pattern, 2 with ST segment depression, and 1 with left bundle branch block. None of the patients had cardiac enlargement documented by standard chest roentgenograms. Echocardiograms showed minimal posterior pericardial disease in 2 patients.

All 7 patients had abnormalities on resting thallium scan: all had diffuse defects (39 defects were found in a total of 63 segments). Resting left ventricular ejection fraction, assessed by radionuclide ventriculography, was normal in 6 PSS patients (61 ± 10%, mean ± SD). Five patients had hypokinetic regional left ventricular wall motion when at rest; these abnormalities were associated with defects shown on thallium scan in the same territories. These results are in agreement with those of other investigators, who have demonstrated a high prevalence of abnormalities of myocardial perfusion that can be detected by means of radionuclide techniques in patients with PSS (14).

Chest radiographs showed normal findings in 5 patients, and showed mildly abnormal interstitial markings in 2.

Pulmonary function findings were normal in 5 patients. One patient had mild restrictive lung disease (FVC 75% of predicted normal); 1 had an isolated decrease in DLco (70% of predicted normal). None of the patients had either physical findings of severe pulmonary hypertension or electrocardiographic evidence of right ventricular hypertrophy.

All 7 patients had normal serum creatinine concentrations (65 ± 17 μmoles/liter, mean ± SD).

Table 3. Hemodynamic data at baseline and after dipyridamole infusion, in control subjects versus progressive systemic sclerosis (PSS) patients*

	Baseline			After dipyridamole		
	Control subjects (n = 7)	PSS patients (n = 7)	*P*†	Control subjects (n = 7)	PSS patients (n = 7)	*P*
CI	3.57 ± 0.37	3.31 ± 0.82	NS	4.80 ± 0.76	4.39 ± 1.00	NS
HR	86 ± 14	92 ± 11	NS	109 ± 20	107 ± 17	NS
LVSP	126 ± 15	123 ± 15	NS	118 ± 13	116 ± 17	NS
LVEDP	7 ± 2	8 ± 5	NS	6 ± 4	6 ± 4	NS
MAP	99 ± 8	96 ± 9	NS	89 ± 7	88 ± 11	NS
SVR	17.4 ± 1.8	19.9 ± 6.4	NS	11.6 ± 1.5	13.4 ± 4.1	NS
V_{max}	1.84 ± 0.33	1.70 ± 0.22	NS	2.26 ± 0.54	2.08 ± 0.73	NS

* Values are mean ± SD. CI = cardiac index, l/minute/m^2; HR = heart rate, beats/minute; LVSP = left ventricular systolic pressure, mm Hg; LVEDP = left ventricular end diastolic pressure, mm Hg; MAP = mean aortic pressure, mm Hg; SVR = systemic vascular resistance, mm Hg/liter/minute; V_{max} = maximum velocity of shortening/1 second.
† NS = not significant.

Coronary arteriography and left ventricular function. The coronary arteriogram results were normal in all but 1 PSS patient, who had 80% stenosis of a small lateral artery. This stenosis did not correlate with a thallium perfusion defect nor a wall motion abnormality.

Results of left ventricular angiography are summarized in Table 2. Volume, ejection fraction, and left ventricular mass were within the normal range in all but 1 PSS patient, whose left ventricular end diastolic volume and left ventricular mass were increased to 109 ml/m^2 and 107 gm/m^2, respectively, and ejection fraction decreased to 46%. End systolic stress and σES: LVESV ratio did not differ significantly between PSS patients and control subjects. The diastolic properties of the left ventricle, i.e., α and k values, were similar in PSS patients and control subjects, except in the PSS patient with increased left ventricular end diastolic volume, and decreased ejection fraction, who showed a mild increase of α and k.

Hemodynamic data. Hemodynamic data did not differ significantly between PSS patients and control subjects, either under baseline conditions or after dipyridamole infusion (Table 3).

Coronary sinus blood flow and coronary resistance. Under resting conditions, coronary sinus blood flow was similar in PSS patients (89 ± 32 ml/minute/100 gm, mean ± SD) and control subjects (100 ± 15 ml/minute/100 gm) (Table 4 and Figure 1). After administration of dipyridamole, however, coronary sinus blood flow in PSS patients was significantly lower than in controls (191 ± 45 versus 399 ± 58 ml/minute/100 gm), $P < 0.01$ (Table 4 and Figure 1). Under baseline

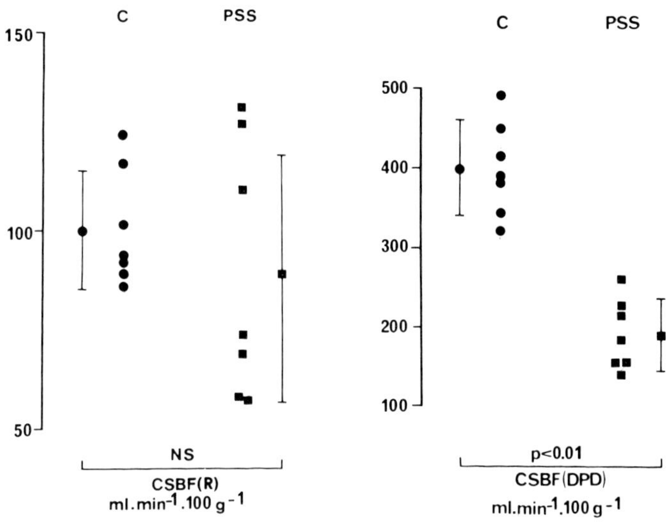

Figure 1. Alterations in coronary sinus blood flow (CSBF) induced by dipyridamole (DPD) in control subjects (C) and progressive systemic sclerosis (PSS) patients. CSBF at rest (R) was similar in control subjects and PSS patients (*P* not significant [NS]). In contrast, CSBF after dipyridamole infusion was significantly lower in PSS patients than in controls ($P < 0.01$).

conditions, coronary resistance was similar in PSS patients (1.19 ± 0.40 mm Hg/ml/minute/100 gm, mean ± SD) and control subjects (0.92 ± 0.10 mm Hg/ml/minute/100 gm) (Table 4 and Figure 2). After administration of dipyridamole, coronary resistance in PSS patients (0.44 ± 0.11) was significantly higher than in control subjects (0.21 ± 0.03), $P < 0.01$ (Table 4 and Figure 2). After dipyridamole infusion, a contrast medium injection into the left coronary artery (46) failed to increase coronary sinus blood flow in all

Table 4. Coronary circulation and myocardial metabolism, at baseline and after dipyridamole infusion, in control subjects versus progressive systemic sclerosis (PSS) patients*

	Baseline			After dipyridamole		
	Control subjects (n = 7)	PSS patients (n = 7)	*P*†	Control subjects (n = 7)	PSS patients (n = 7)	*P*
CSBF	100 ± 15	89 ± 32	NS	399 ± 58	191 ± 45	<0.01
CR	0.92 ± 0.10	1.19 ± 0.40	NS	0.21 ± 0.03	0.44 ± 0.11	<0.01
a O_2	17.48 ± 0.95	15.04 ± 1.75	0.02	16.54 ± 0.83	14.26 ± 1.66	<0.02
cs O_2	4.69 ± 0.34	4.50 ± 0.35	NS	12.71 ± 0.37	10.19 ± 1.98	<0.05
a–cs O_2 D	12.56 ± 0.84	10.54 ± 1.46	<0.02	3.51 ± 0.39	4.12 ± 0.64	NS
$M\dot{V}O_2$	12.88 ± 2.10	9.06 ± 2.42	<0.01	13.87 ± 1.38	7.86 ± 2.10	<0.01
Lactate extraction	0.62 ± 0.14	0.47 ± 0.22	NS	0.56 ± 0.22	0.54 ± 0.37	NS

* Values are mean ± SD. CSBF = coronary sinus blood flow, ml/minute/100 gm; CR = coronary resistance, mm Hg/ml/minute/100 gm; a O_2 = arterial O_2 content, ml/100 ml; cs O_2 = coronary sinus oxygen content, ml/100 ml; a–cs O_2 D = arterial–coronary sinus oxygen content difference, ml/100 ml; $M\dot{V}O_2$ = myocardial oxygen consumption, ml/minute/100 gm.
† NS = not significant.

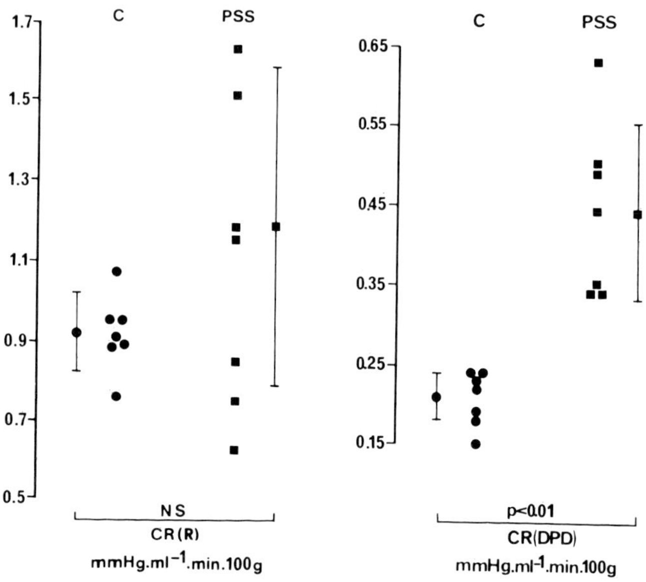

Figure 2. Alterations in coronary resistance (CR) induced by dipyridamole in control subjects and PSS patients. CR at rest was similar in control subjects and PSS patients. In contrast, CR after dipyridamole infusion was significantly higher in PSS patients than in controls ($P < 0.01$). See Figure 1 for definitions.

patients and controls, suggesting that maximal coronary vasodilation had been reached with dipyridamole.

Myocardial metabolism. Under resting conditions, arterial–coronary sinus oxygen content difference was significantly lower in PSS patients than in controls (Table 4); at baseline, arterial oxygen content was significantly lower in PSS patients than in control subjects, whereas coronary sinus oxygen content was similar in PSS patients and in controls (Table 4). Since almost all of the PSS patients had normal pulmonary function, the decreased arterial oxygen content was probably caused by anemia (hemoglobin 12.3 ± 1.1 gm/dl [mean ± SD] in PSS patients and 14.2 ± 0.7 gm/dl in control subjects).

After dipyridamole infusion, arterial–coronary sinus oxygen content difference decreased in all patients and controls; a–cs O_2 D was higher in PSS patients than in control subjects, but the difference was not statistically significant. It should be emphasized that, during coronary vasodilation by dipyridamole, coronary sinus oxygen content was significantly lower in PSS patients than in control subjects (10.19 ± 1.98 ml/100 ml versus 12.71 ± 0.38 ml/100 ml, mean ± SD), $P < 0.05$ (Table 4). The individual coronary sinus oxygen content values after dipyridamole administration were strikingly lower in 5 PSS patients, compared with controls (Figure 3).

Myocardial oxygen consumption was significantly lower in PSS patients than in control subjects, under resting conditions as well as during dipyridamole-induced coronary vasodilation, $P < 0.01$ (Table 4).

Lactate extraction was similar in PSS patients and in control subjects, both at rest and after dipyridamole administration (Table 4). However, lactate extraction decreased from 0.44 to 0.07 after dipyridamole infusion in 1 PSS patient, and she developed chest pain without any modification seen on EKG. Another PSS patient also experienced isolated chest pain without EKG alteration. These 2 patients had normal coronary angiogram results.

Endomyocardial biopsy. Examination by light microscopy showed increased fibrotic tissue in 4 PSS patients, compared with controls. In 1 endomyocardial specimen, a typical vascular lesion of PSS (with concentric intimal hypertrophy) was found (Figure 4).

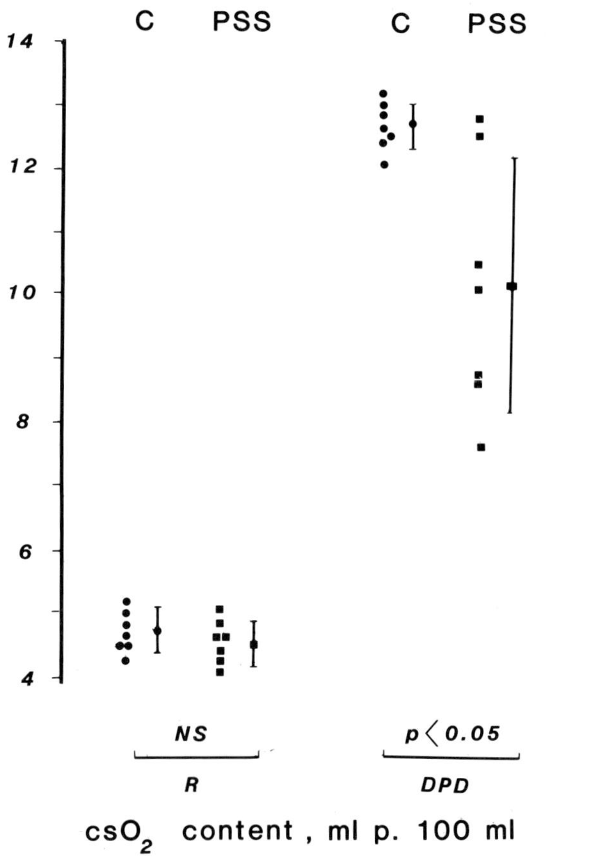

Figure 3. Increase in coronary sinus oxygen content (csO_2) induced by dipyridamole in control subjects and PSS patients. At rest, csO_2 was similar in control subjects and PSS patients. After dipyridamole infusion, csO_2 was significantly lower in PSS patients than in controls ($P < 0.05$). See Figure 1 for definitions.

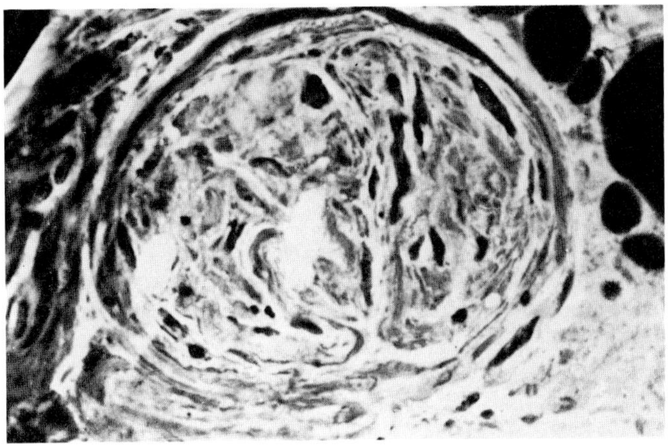

Figure 4. Light microscopy of a coronary arteriole from a patient with primary scleroderma myocardial disease, showing marked intimal proliferation (toluidine blue stained, original m[illegible] 800).

Electron microscopy of myocardial cells showed mitochondrial alterations in 3 patients, myofibrillar damage in 4 patients, and cell clearing in 4. Endomyocardial biopsy findings were considered normal in 1 patient.

DISCUSSION

The pathogenesis of primary scleroderma myocardial disease has not been well elucidated. The cause of the myocardial necrosis and fibrosis that occurs in the setting of normal extramural coronary arteries is not fully understood, and the possibility that these lesions are a reflection of a primary fibrous tissue overgrowth leading to secondary vascular compromise is still reasonable. Nevertheless, a growing body of evidence from studies of the heart and other organs involved in progressive systemic sclerosis suggests that the vascular system, per se, may be the primary target organ in PSS and that the myocardial lesion is a manifestation of focal ischemic injury resulting from functional, with or without accompanying structural, vascular disease (1–3,15,17,18,25,47).

Transient nonperfusion or Raynaud's phenomenon of the digits and kidneys and possibly the lungs is a recognized feature of PSS and probably accounts for many of the morphologic changes observed in these organs (1,3,5,48). Bulkley et al (1) reported a high prevalence of myocardial contraction band necrosis—a histologic lesion seen in the setting of ischemic injury followed by reperfusion (1,3,49)—and speculated that myocardial fibrosis results from intermittent spasm of the small coronary arteries, a form of "myocardial Raynaud's phenomenon" (1). Additional support for this hypothesis has been provided by other investigators (50) who demonstrated cold-induced abnormalities on thallium perfusion in patients with progressive systemic sclerosis.

The major observation in this study was that coronary reserve, assessed by dipyridamole-induced coronary vasodilation, was greatly impaired in patients with primary scleroderma myocardial disease. Under baseline conditions, coronary sinus blood flow was similar in PSS patients and in control subjects; after dipyridamole infusion, coronary sinus blood flow was significantly lower in PSS patients than in controls ($P < 0.01$).

Such a reduction of coronary reserve has been previously described in patients with coronary artery disease, in patients with normal coronary arteries and left ventricular hypertrophy secondary to aortic valve disease or arterial hypertension, and in patients with cardiomyopathies involving hypertrophism and dilation (41,51–57).

The extent of the dipyridamole-induced vasodilation in control subjects was similar to that found in other studies, which report comparable values of myocardial blood flow (300–400 ml/minute/100 gm) and coronary resistance (55,58). We could assert that maximal coronary vasodilation was reached with the dose of dipyridamole used, since a superinduced vasodilator stimulus, i.e., a contrast medium injection into the left coronary artery (46), failed to increase the coronary sinus blood flow either in control subjects or in PSS patients. Thus, the decreased coronary reserve in PSS patients could not result from a resistance to the dipyridamole vasodilator effect.

Coronary reserve is reduced in the presence of proximal flow limiting coronary stenosis (51,59,60); such a mechanism could not account for the decreased coronary reserve in PSS patients, however, since 6 of the 7 patients had normal findings on coronary angiogram.

When large coronary arteries are free of lesions, decreased coronary reserve may be attributed to a low aortic pressure or to an increase in coronary resistance due to augmentation of myocardial tissue pressure. These mechanisms could be excluded in our PSS patients, however, since all parameters of left ventricular function and hemodynamic data (particularly mean aortic pressure, heart rate, left ventricular mass, and left ventricular end diastolic pressure) did not significantly differ between PSS patients and control subjects (Tables 2 and 3). It should be noted that although light microscopy evidenced increased fibrotic tissue in 4 PSS patients, elastic properties of the left ventricle were unaffected in all but 1 patient. This probably results from the rather rough diastolic indices used, which are unable to detect minor alterations.

Since obstructive coronary lesions were not present in 6 of the 7 PSS patients, the reduced coronary reserve may be attributed to abnormalities of small intra-myocardial vessels not visualized by coronary arteriography (61), i.e., small vessel disease.

A possible cause of the decreased coronary reserve in PSS patients could be the increased fibrotic tissue, which could reduce the number of functional vessels or impair the arteriolar vasodilation. This augmentation of the fibrotic tissue could also be the explanation for the decreased myocardial oxygen consumption in PSS patients. However, indirect measurements of myocardial function were similar in PSS patients and in control subjects. This would imply that in PSS patients, the heart uses oxygen more efficiently; such a hypothesis has been suggested for myocardial adaptation in cardiac hypertrophy (62).

Alternatively, the decreased coronary reserve in PSS patients could be due to abnormalities of small coronary vessels in the functional myocardium. This hypothesis is supported by the lower decrease in the arterial–coronary sinus oxygen content difference after dipyridamole infusion in PSS patients compared with control subjects, which suggests a limitation of vasodilation in territories where the oxygen demand is normal, thus excluding the fibrotic zones. Moreover, 1 PSS patient, with normal coronary arteriography results, who experienced chest pain without EKG alteration after dipyridamole infusion, evidenced a strikingly decreased lactate extraction. Finally, in 1 left ventricular endomyocardial biopsy specimen, a typical vascular lesion of PSS was found.

These results suggest that the decreased coronary reserve in PSS patients is due to primary abnormalities of small coronary vessels in the functional myocardium. Whether this is a vasospastic or structural process impeding maximal flow in the small arteries cannot be established from this study. It remains to be determined whether additional factors such as immune-mediated injury (45) have a role in the pathogenesis of decreased coronary reserve in primary scleroderma myocardial disease.

There are some limitations to our studies, which should be addressed. First, the present study is based on the assumption that the coronary sinus blood flow represents the myocardial flow of the left ventricle. This assertion is sustained by anatomic (40) and clinical (41) studies, provided that the proximal thermistor of the thermodilution catheter takes into account the flow issuing from the posterior interventricular vein. Furthermore, values of resting coronary sinus blood flow in control subjects in our study were similar to the findings of other investigators (32).

Second, we assumed that our control subjects had normal coronary reserve, even though none was free of heart disease. The cardiac abnormalities in these control subjects did not involve the coronary arteries or the left ventricle; moreover, coronary blood flow and coronary resistance in our control subjects, at baseline and after dipyridamole infusion, were similar to those observed in other studies (55,58).

Third, PSS patients in this study had evidence of primary scleroderma myocardial disease documented by noninvasive procedures. Consequently, it would be difficult to extrapolate our results to an unselected population of progressive systemic sclerosis patients.

In summary, the results of the present study demonstrate that coronary reserve is strikingly reduced in PSS patients with normal left ventricular function and normal findings on coronary angiogram. This markedly impaired coronary reserve could explain the observations of chest pain, alterations on thallium scans, and progressive myocardial damage resulting from episodes of imbalance between myocardial oxygen supply and demand. Thus, this decreased coronary reserve may be an important contributor to the pathogenesis of primary scleroderma myocardial disease.

ACKNOWLEDGMENTS

We thank Drs. F. Delrieu and L. Saporta for encouraging their patients to participate in these studies and for helpful discussions. The expert secretarial assistance of Magali Vallet-Amor is gratefully acknowledged.

REFERENCES

1. Bulkley BH, Ridolfi RL, Salyer WR, Hutchins GM: Myocardial lesions of progressive systemic sclerosis: a cause of cardiac dysfunction. Circulation 53:483–490, 1976
2. Botstein GR, LeRoy EC: Primary heart disease in systemic sclerosis (scleroderma): advances in clinical and pathologic features, pathogenesis, and new therapeutic approaches. Am Heart J 102:913–919, 1981
3. Bulkley BH: Progressive systemic sclerosis: cardiac involvement. Clin Rheum Dis 5:131–149, 1979
4. Medsger TA Jr, Masi AT, Rodnan GP, Benedek TG,

Robinson H: Survival with systemic sclerosis (scleroderma): a life-table analysis of clinical and demographic factors in 309 patients. Ann Intern Med 75:369–376, 1971
5. Rodnan GP: Progressive systemic sclerosis, Arthritis and Allied Conditions. Ninth edition. Edited by DJ McCarty. Philadelphia, Lea & Febiger, 1979, pp 762–809
6. Sackner MA, Heinz ER, Steinberg AJ: The heart in scleroderma. Am J Cardiol 17:542–559, 1966
7. Oram S, Stokes W: The heart in scleroderma. Br Heart J 23:243–259, 1961
8. Bulkley BH, Klacsmann PG, Hutchins GM: Angina pectoris, myocardial infarction and sudden cardiac death with normal coronary arteries: a clinicopathologic study of 9 patients with progressive systemic sclerosis. Am Heart J 95:563–569, 1978
9. Clements PJ, Furst DE, Cabeen W, Tashkin D, Paulus HE, Roberts N: The relationship of arrhythmias and conduction disturbances to other manifestations of cardiopulmonary disease in progressive systemic sclerosis (PSS). Am J Med 71:38–46, 1981
10. Eggebrecht RF, Kleiger RE: Echocardiographic patterns in scleroderma. Chest 71:47–51, 1977
11. Gottdiener JS, Moutsopoulos HM, Decker JL: Echocardiographic identification of cardiac abnormality in scleroderma and related disorders. Am J Med 66:391–398, 1979
12. Smith JW, Clements PJ, Levisman J, Furst D, Ross M: Echocardiographic features of progressive systemic sclerosis (PSS): correlation with hemodynamic and postmortem studies. Am J Med 66:28–33, 1979
13. Bletry O, Scheuble C, Lévèque D, Guillevin L, Cérèze P, Godeau P: Cardiomyopathie sclérodermique: étude prospective utilisant des explorations non traumatisantes (phonocardiographie, échocardiographie): intérêt des paramètres diastoliques de fonction ventriculaire. Ann Med Interne (Paris) 133:84–91, 1982
14. Follansbee WP, Curtiss EI, Medsger TA Jr, Steen VD, Uretsky BF, Owens GR, Rodnan GP: Physiologic abnormalities of cardiac function in progressive systemic sclerosis with diffuse scleroderma. N Engl J Med 310:142–148, 1984
15. Gupta MP, Zoneraich S, Zeitlin W, Zoneraich O, D'Angelo W: Scleroderma heart disease with slow flow velocity in coronary arteries. Chest 67:116–119, 1975
16. Tambe AA, Demany MA, Zimmerman HA, Mascarenhas E: Angina pectoris and slow flow velocity of dye in coronary arteries: a new angiographic finding. Am Heart J 84:66–71, 1972
17. Campbell PM, LeRoy EC: Pathogenesis of systemic sclerosis: a vascular hypothesis. Semin Arthritis Rheum 4:351–368, 1975
18. Norton WL, Nardo JM: Vascular disease in progressive systemic sclerosis (scleroderma). Ann Intern Med 73:317–324, 1970
19. LeRoy EC: Connective tissue synthesis by scleroderma skin fibroblasts in cell culture. J Exp Med 135:1351–1362, 1972
20. Buckingham RB, Prince RK, Rodnan GP, Taylor F: Increased collagen accumulation in dermal fibroblast cultures from patients with progressive systemic sclerosis (scleroderma). J Lab Clin Med 92:5–21, 1978
21. D'Angelo WA, Fries JF, Masi AT, Shulman LE: Pathologic observations in systemic sclerosis (scleroderma): a study of fifty-eight autopsy cases and fifty-eight matched controls. Am J Med 46:428–440, 1969
22. Sackner MA, Akgun N, Kimbel P, Lewis DH: The pathophysiology of scleroderma involving the heart and respiratory system. Ann Intern Med 60:611–630, 1964
23. Nasser WK, Mishkin ME, Rosenbaum D, Genovese PD: Pericardial and myocardial disease in progressive systemic sclerosis. Am J Cardiol 22:538–542, 1968
24. Weiss S, Stead EA, Warren JV, Bailey OT: Scleroderma heart disease with a consideration of certain other visceral manifestations of scleroderma. Arch Intern Med 71:749–776, 1943
25. James TN: De subitaneis mortibus. VIII. Coronary arteries and conduction system in scleroderma heart disease. Circulation 50:844–856, 1974
26. Subcommittee for Scleroderma Criteria of the American Rheumatism Association Diagnostic and Therapeutic Criteria Committee: Preliminary criteria for the classification of systemic sclerosis (scleroderma). Arthritis Rheum 23:581–590, 1980
27. Rodnan GP, Jablonska S, Medsger TA Jr: Classification and nomenclature of progressive systemic sclerosis (scleroderma). Clin Rheum Dis 5:5–13, 1979
28. Weinberger SE, Johnson TS, Weiss ST: Use and interpretation of the single-breath diffusing capacity. Chest 78:483–488, 1980
29. Holman BL, Hill TC, Wynne J, Lovett RD, Zimmerman RE, Smith EM: Single-photon transaxial emission computed tomography of the heart in normal subjects and in patients with infarction. J Nucl Med 20:736–740, 1979
30. Maublant J, Cassagnes J, LeJeune JJ, Mestras D, Veyre A, Jallut H, Meyniel G: A comparison between conventional scintigraphy and emission tomography with thallium-201 in the detection of myocardial infarction. J Nucl Med 23:204–208, 1982
31. Karliner JS, Bouchard RJ, Gault JH: Haemodynamic effects of angiographic contrast material in man: a beat-by-beat analysis. Br Heart J 34:347–355, 1972
32. Ganz W, Tamura K, Marcus HS, Donoso R, Yoshida S, Swan HJC: Measurement of coronary sinus blood flow by continuous thermodilution in man. Circulation 44:181–195, 1971
33. Pollack GH: Maximum velocity as an index of contractility in cardiac muscle. Circ Res 26:111–127, 1970
34. Dodge HT, Sandler H, Baxley WA, Hawley RR: Usefulness and limitations of radiographic methods for determining left ventricular volume. Am J Cardiol 18:10–24, 1966
35. Trenouth RS, Phelps NC, Neill WA: Determinants of

left ventricular hypertrophy and oxygen supply in chronic aortic valve disease. Circulation 53:644–650, 1976
36. Falsetti HL, Mates RE, Grant C, Greene DG, Bunnell IL: Left ventricular wall stress calculated from one-plane cineangiography: an approach to force velocity analysis in man. Circ Res 26:71–83, 1970
37. Carabello BA, Nolan SP, McGuire LB: Assessment of preoperative left ventricular function in patients with mitral regurgitation: value of the end-systolic wall stress-end-systolic volume ratio. Circulation 64:1212–1217, 1981
38. Gaasch WH, Battle WE, Oboler AA, Banas JS Jr, Levine HJ: Left ventricular stress and compliance in man: with special reference to normalized ventricular function curves. Circulation 45:746–762, 1972
39. Mirsky I, Cohn PF, Levine JA, Gorlin R, Herman MV, Kreulen TH, Sonnenblick EH: Assessment of left ventricular stiffness in primary myocardial disease and coronary artery disease. Circulation 50:128–136, 1974
40. Hood WB Jr: Regional venous drainage of the human heart. Br Heart J 30:105–109, 1968
41. Pasternac A, Noble J, Streulens Y, Elie R, Henschke C, Bourassa MG: Pathophysiology of chest pain in patients with cardiomyopathies and normal coronary arteries. Circulation 65:778–789, 1982
42. Olsen EG: Diagnostic value of the endomyocardial bioptome. Lancet 1:658–660, 1974
43. Weibel ER, Kistler GS, Scherle WF: Practical stereological methods for morphometric cytology. J Cell Biol 30:23–38, 1966
44. Medsger TA Jr, Masi AT: Epidemiology of systemic sclerosis (scleroderma). Ann Intern Med 74:714–721, 1971
45. LeRoy EC: The heart in systemic sclerosis. N Engl J Med 310:188–190, 1984
46. Mishima M, Inoue M, Hori M, Tsujioka K, Kuruya T, Kodama K, Nanto S, Abe H: Validity of contrast hyperemia for clinical assessment of coronary flow reserve: the optimal dose of contrast medium and reproducibility of the technique. Cathet Cardiovasc Diagn 9:553–568, 1983
47. Kahaleh MB, Sherer GK, LeRoy EC: Endothelial injury in scleroderma. J Exp Med 149:1326–1335, 1979
48. Cannon PJ, Hassar M, Case DB, Casarella WJ, Sommers SC, LeRoy EC: The relationship of hypertension and renal failure in scleroderma (progressive systemic sclerosis) to structural and functional abnormalities of the renal cortical circulation. Medicine (Baltimore) 53:1–46, 1974
49. Jennings RB, Sommers HM, Herdson PB, Kattenbach JP: Ischemic injury of myocardium. Ann NY Acad Sci 156:61–78, 1969
50. Alexander EL, Firestein GS, Leitl G, Wagner HN, Hochberg MC, Heuser RR, Stevens MB, Weiss J, Becker L: Scleroderma heart disease: evidence for cold-induced abnormalities of myocardial function and perfusion (abstract). Arthritis Rheum (suppl) 24:S58, 1981
51. White CW, Wright CB, Doty DB, Hiratza LF, Eastham CL, Harrison DG, Marcus ML: Does visual interpretation of the coronary arteriogram predict the physiologic importance of a coronary stenosis? N Engl J Med 310:819–824, 1984
52. Neill WA, Fluri-Lundeen JH: Myocardial oxygen supply in left ventricular hypertrophy and coronary heart disease. Am J Cardiol 44:746–753, 1979
53. Marcus ML, Doty DB, Hiratza LF, Wright CB, Eastham CL: Decreased coronary reserve: a mechanism for angina pectoris in patients with aortic stenosis and normal coronary arteries. N Engl J Med 307:1362–1366, 1982
54. Pichard AD, Gorlin R, Smith H, Ambrose J, Meller J: Coronary flow studies in patients with left ventricular hypertrophy of the hypertensive type: evidence for an impaired coronary vascular reserve. Am J Cardiol 47:547–554, 1981
55. Opherk D, Mall G, Zebe H, Schwarz F, Weihe E, Manthey J, Kübler W: Reduction of coronary reserve: a mechanism for angina pectoris in patients with arterial hypertension and normal coronary arteries. Circulation 69:1–7, 1984
56. Pichard AD, Smith H, Holt J, Meller J, Gorlin R: Coronary vascular reserve in left ventricular hypertrophy secondary to chronic aortic regurgitation. Am J Cardiol 51:315–320, 1983
57. Foult JM, Nitenberg A, Huyghebaert MF: Coronary reserve in patients with nonobstructive cardiomyopathy (abstract). J Am Coll Cardiol 3:595, 1984
58. Domenech RJ, Goich J: Effect of heart rate on regional coronary blood flow. Cardiovasc Res 10:224–231, 1976
59. Gould KL, Lipscomb K: Effects of coronary stenoses on coronary flow reserve and resistance. Am J Cardiol 34:48–55, 1974
60. Gould KL, Lipscomb K, Hamilton GW: Physiologic basis for assessing critical coronary stenosis: instantaneous flow response and regional distribution during coronary hyperemia as measures of coronary flow reserve. Am J Cardiol 33:87–94, 1974
61. James TN: Small arteries of the heart. Circulation 56:2–14, 1977
62. Swynghedauw B, Schwartz K, Apstein CS: Decreased contractility after myocardial hypertrophy: cardiac failure or successful adaptation? Am J Cardiol 54:437–440, 1984

COLLAGEN SYNTHESIS REGULATION BY THE AMINOPROPEPTIDE OF PROCOLLAGEN I IN NORMAL AND SCLERODERMA FIBROBLASTS

JEROME S. PERLISH, RUPERT TIMPL, and RAUL FLEISCHMAJER

The effect of the aminopropeptide of type I procollagen, Col 1(I), on collagen synthesis by normal and scleroderma fibroblasts was investigated. Collagen synthesis was inhibited by about 42% when normal fibroblasts were labeled with ^{3}H-proline in the presence of 4 μM Col 1(I). In contrast, collagen synthesis by scleroderma fibroblasts was inhibited to a lesser degree, about 19%. Furthermore, scleroderma fibroblasts with elevated rates of collagen synthesis (2.5–5 times normal) were inhibited by only about 10%. The data suggest that the increased accumulation of collagen in the skin of scleroderma patients may be related to a defect in the regulation of collagen synthesis by the aminopropeptide.

Scleroderma is a disorder characterized by excessive deposition of collagen in various organs of the body. It is well established that fibroblasts isolated from the skin of scleroderma patients synthesize more collagen than do fibroblasts from the skin of normal controls (1–4). The increased dermal activity in scleroderma appears to be more prominent in the lower levels of the skin (2,3,5). It has recently been suggested that in scleroderma, the high production of collagen by fibroblasts is the result of a selection process (6).

From the Department of Dermatology, Mount Sinai School of Medicine, New York, New York and the Max Planck Institut fur Biochemie, Munich, West Germany.

Supported by NIH grant AM-27608, a grant from the Scleroderma Society of Greater New York, Inc., and the Deutsche Forschungsgemeinschaft.

Jerome S. Perlish, PhD; Rupert Timpl, PhD; Raul Fleischmajer, MD.

Address reprint requests to Jerome S. Perlish, PhD, Mount Sinai School of Medicine, Department of Dermatology, One Gustave L. Levy Place, New York, NY 10029.

Submitted for publication July 31, 1984; accepted in revised form December 6, 1984.

Human dermal fibroblasts synthesize collagen in a precursor form known as procollagen. Procollagen is characterized by propeptide extensions at both the amino and carboxyl ends of the molecule. These propeptide extensions are cleaved by specific proteases during the conversion of procollagen into collagen (7).

It has been suggested that the aminopropeptides may play a role in regulating collagen synthesis (8–10). Using cultured fibroblasts from normal skin, it has been demonstrated that the free aminopropeptides of type I and type III procollagens reduce collagen synthesis, presumably by a feedback mechanism (8,9). In this regard, increased collagen accumulation was observed with dermatosparactic sheep fibroblasts, due to a decrease in the release of the aminopropeptide (10). The regulation mechanism of collagen synthesis in scleroderma remains unknown, although normalization of collagen synthesis was noted in vitro in the presence of the aminopropeptide of type I procollagen for a single line of scleroderma fibroblasts (11).

The present study was undertaken to determine whether the aminopropeptide of type I procollagen plays a role in the regulation of collagen synthesis in scleroderma skin fibroblasts.

MATERIALS AND METHODS

Cell culture. Skin biopsy specimens were taken from involved areas of the forearms of female scleroderma patients ranging in age from 22–79 years. Normal specimens were taken from matched volunteers. Primary cultures were established in 60 × 15-mm culture dishes in Ham's F-10 medium containing glutamine (Flow Laboratories, Rockville, MD) and supplemented with 10% fetal calf serum, 100 units/ml penicillin, and 50 μg/ml streptomycin. All explants were kept at 37°C under an atmosphere of 95% O_2–5% CO_2 and fed twice a week until confluent. Stock cultures were established from these primary cultures.

We have previously demonstrated that fibroblasts from different levels of the dermis differ in their degrees of collagen synthesis in culture (2). Scleroderma fibroblasts from the reticular dermis accumulated more collagen in culture than those from the papillary dermis. For this reason, fibroblasts isolated from the reticular dermis were chosen for the present study.

Preparation of aminopropeptide. The N-terminal noncollagenous fragment of the aminopropeptide of procollagen type I, Col 1(I), was prepared by collagenase digestion from the insoluble residue of dermatosparactic sheep skin. It was purified by chromatography on DEAE cellulose and by molecular sieve chromatography (12).

Labeling studies. Fibroblasts from previously established stock cultures (normal + scleroderma) were grown to confluency in 96-well Falcon plastic culture plates. Cells were preincubated for 24 hours in Dulbecco's modified Eagle's medium (Flow Laboratories) supplemented with 10% fetal calf serum, 400 units/ml penicillin, 50 μl/ml ascorbate, and 50 μg/ml β-aminopropionitrile. The preincubation was followed by 24-hour incubation in fresh medium containing 10 μCi/ml L-^{3}H-proline with and without 4 μ*M* Col 1(I). Following labeling, cells were scraped and the contents of the wells transferred to tubes containing cold 0.1*M* EDTA, phenylmethanesulfonyl fluoride (3 mg/liter), p-chloromercuribenzoate (3 mg/liter), and iodoacetamide ($5 \times 10^{-4}M$). All samples were dialyzed exhaustively at 4°C against tap water followed by distilled water, in order to remove all unincorporated label. Aliquots were assayed for total ^{3}H-proline content with a Beckman LS100 liquid scintillation counter. Cells were counted using a Fuchs Rosenthal Ultra Plane hemacytometer.

Microassay for collagen determination. Collagen synthesis was determined using an assay described by Webster and Harvey (13). Following labeling with ^{3}H-proline as described above, the collagen was extracted from each microwell by the addition of 100 μl of cold acetic acid (1*M*) containing pepsin (1 mg/ml). The samples were shaken for 16 hours at 4°C. The contents of each well were placed in polypropylene tubes, to which 800 μl of acetic acid (0.5*M*) containing neutral salt–soluble rat skin collagen (200 μg/ml) was added as carrier. The tubes were centrifuged and the supernatants placed in fresh tubes. Collagen was precipitated from the supernatants by the addition of 250 μl NaCl in 0.5*M* acetic acid (25% weight/volume). The tubes were allowed to stand for 2 hours, followed by centrifugation at 4,000*g* for 30 minutes, and the precipitates were dissolved in 0.15*M* NaCl, 0.05*M* Tris-HCl, pH 7.5. Collagen was precipitated by the addition of 4.5*M* NaCl in the Tris buffer. The samples were allowed to stand for 2 hours and were then centrifuged at 4,000*g* for 30 minutes. The collagen precipitate was washed with 20% ethanol and centrifuged at 4,000*g* for 30 minutes. Following washing, the precipitates were dissolved in acetic acid (0.5*M*), transferred to scintillation vials containing Liquiscint (National Diagnostics, Somerville, NJ), and measured in a Beckman LS100 liquid scintillation counter.

RESULTS

Effect of Col 1(I) on collagen synthesis by normal and scleroderma fibroblasts. Five normal and 6 scleroderma lines of dermal fibroblasts derived from the reticular dermis were used. All cell lines were in the second–fourth passage. Confluent cultures were grown in the presence and absence of the aminopropeptide Col 1(I). Incorporation of ^{3}H-proline into collagen and isolation of ^{3}H-collagen were used to measure newly synthesized collagen. The data in Table 1 show an average of 42% inhibition of collagen synthesis by normal fibroblasts when grown in the presence of 4 μ*M* Col 1(I). Similarly-treated scleroderma fibroblasts were inhibited by 4–19%, except that 1 line, scleroderma line 6, was inhibited by 53% (Table 2). It should be noted that this particular scleroderma fibroblast line synthesized collagen at a rate lower than all other lines studied. Several of the scleroderma lines studied were found to be high collagen-producers (Table 2). When high collagen-producing cells were grown in the presence of 4 μ*M* Col 1(I), collagen synthesis was affected minimally. The inhibitory effect was greater in scleroderma lines with normal collagen production, but except in scleroderma line 6, it was still not as great as the effect observed with the normal controls.

Col 1(I) inhibition of collagen synthesis versus protein synthesis. Two normal and 1 scleroderma fibroblast lines were studied with respect to both protein and collagen synthesis in the presence and absence of

Table 1. Effect of Col 1(I) peptide (4 μ*M*) on collagen synthesis by normal dermal fibroblasts in culture

Subject	Addition	Collagen synthesis, cpm/10^3 cells (n)*	% change	P†
1	−	340 ± 37 (6)	−14	NS
	+	294 ± 28 (6)		
2	−	478 ± 50 (6)	−44	<0.05
	+	267 ± 57 (3)		
3	−	237 ± 6.6 (6)	−5	NS
	+	226 ± 7.3 (4)		
4	−	669 ± 37 (5)	−57	<0.005
	+	291 ± 8.7 (3)		
5	−	366 ± 17 (4)	−67	<0.001
	+	119 ± 40 (4)		
Mean	−	412 ± 32 (27)	−42	<0.001
	+	241 ± 20 (20)		

* Values are mean ± SEM for the number of determinations shown in parentheses.
† Level of significance: NS = not significant.

Table 2. Effect of Col 1(I) peptide (4 μM) on collagen synthesis by scleroderma fibroblasts in culture

Subject	Addition	Collagen synthesis, cpm/10^3 cells (n)*	% change	Mean % change	P†
High producers‡					
1	–	2,097 ± 82 (6)	–4		NS
	+	2,011 ± 115 (5)			
2	–	994 ± 66 (4)	–8	–10	NS
	+	912 ± 117 (5)			
3	–	635 ± 26 (7)	–17		<0.01
	+	525 ± 17 (3)			
Normal producers					
4	–	363 ± 51 (6)	–12		NS
	+	318 ± 35 (6)			
5	–	344 ± 13 (6)	–19	–28	<0.01
	+	279 ± 13 (6)			
6	–	145 ± 11 (6)	–53		<0.005
	+	69 ± 6 (5)			
Normal controls (n = 5)	–	412 ± 32 (27)	–42	–42	<0.001
	+	241 ± 20 (20)			

* Values are mean ± SEM for the number of determinations shown in parentheses.
† Level of significance: NS = not significant.
‡ Collagen accumulation in excess of 500 cpm/10^3 cells.

Col 1(I). This was done in order to determine the specificity of the inhibition reaction. Fibroblasts were incubated for 24 hours in medium containing ^{3}H-proline. Nondialyzable ^{3}H-proline was then taken as a measure of total protein synthesis. ^{3}H-collagen was also determined for these cultures. The data presented in Table 3 show that collagen accounted for 5–6.8% of the total protein synthesized by normal fibroblasts, but it accounted for 8.4% of the protein synthesis of scleroderma fibroblasts. In the presence of 4 μM Col 1(I), protein synthesis did not appear to be affected, while collagen synthesis was significantly depressed in the normal cells (by 57% and 67%, respectively).

DISCUSSION

The aminopropeptide is released from procollagen by a specific neutral protease (7,14). The segment that has been cleaved consists of 2 noncollagenous and 1 collagenous sequence (8,12,15,16). The N-terminal end is noncollagenous and has been termed Col 1(I). This noncollagenous segment is followed by a collagenous segment which, in turn, is followed by another short, noncollagenous segment before being joined to the telopeptide region of the collagen α1(I) chain. The molecular weight of Col 1(I) has been determined to be 10,000 (14).

It has been suggested that the aminopropeptide may have a regulatory function in the synthesis of type I collagen (8–11,17). In in vitro experiments with normal fibroblasts, Col 1(I) was shown to significantly inhibit collagen synthesis. Wiestner et al (10) demonstrated a correlation between a slow rate of release of the aminopropeptide and an increased rate of synthesis of type I collagen in dermatosparactic sheep fibro-

Table 3. Inhibitory effect of Col 1(I) on collagen and total protein synthesis

Fibroblasts	Col 1(I) (4 μM)	^{3}H-collagen, cpm/10^3 cells (n)*	P†	^{3}H-proline, cpm/10^3 cells	P†	Collagen % of total protein
Normal	–	669 ± 37 (5)	<0.005	13,237 ± 792	NS	5.05
	+	291 ± 8.7 (3)		14,595 ± 116		1.99
Normal	–	366 ± 17 (4)	<0.001	5,373 ± 334	NS	6.81
	+	119 ± 40 (4)		5,031 ± 50		2.37
Scleroderma	–	2,097 ± 82 (6)	NS	25,068 ± 3,518	NS	8.36
	+	2,011 ± 115 (5)		26,491 ± 2,182		7.59

* Values are mean ± SEM for the number of determinations shown in parentheses.
† Level of significance: NS = not significant.

blasts. These studies suggest that a certain amount of the aminopropeptide is required for the proper control of type I collagen synthesis. It is therefore possible that during the normal conversion of procollagen into collagen, the aminopropeptide which is released by the action of procollagen N-proteinase controls the production of procollagen by feedback inhibition. A defect in this mechanism, as seen in dermatosparaxis, could then account for increased collagen synthesis by the fibroblasts.

Scleroderma is characterized by an increased accumulation of collagen in various organs of the body. We therefore decided to determine the effect of Col 1(I) on collagen synthesis in scleroderma fibroblasts. An earlier report involving a single scleroderma patient (11) suggested that scleroderma fibroblasts respond normally to the inhibitory effect of Col 1(I). Comparing 6 scleroderma cell lines and 5 normal cell lines, we have been able to demonstrate that Col 1(I) does inhibit collagen synthesis in scleroderma fibroblasts, but not as strongly as in normal controls.

Several investigators have suggested that fibroblasts derived from the scleroderma dermis are metabolically heterogeneous (2,3,6,18,19). Different rates of growth have been noted in fibroblasts isolated from the papillary and reticular dermis (18,19). Variable rates of collagen synthesis have been noted in both normal and scleroderma fibroblasts isolated from different levels of the dermis (2,3,6); however, this was not confirmed in another study on normal fibroblasts from the papillary and reticular dermis, which demonstrated similar rates of collagen synthesis at confluent densities (19). It has been suggested that scleroderma skin contains low and high collagen-producing fibroblasts (2,6). Peptide Col 1(I) was found to depress collagen synthesis in the normal lines, while the scleroderma lines, particularly the high producing lines, were affected to a lesser degree (Table 3). It is possible that in scleroderma, certain populations of fibroblasts are characterized by excessively elevated rates of collagen synthesis, and these particular populations may have a defect in the regulatory mechanism of collagen synthesis by aminopropeptide.

Paglia et al (20,21) have demonstrated that the aminopropeptide inhibits translation of collagen messenger RNA (mRNA) isolated from the calvaria of embryonic chickens. Several investigators have reported increased procollagen mRNA levels in scleroderma skin fibroblasts (22,23). The increased rates of collagen synthesis in scleroderma may be explained by these elevated levels of mRNA. The lack of inhibition we have observed with Col 1(I) in scleroderma fibroblasts could then indicate a defect in the regulatory mechanism of collagen synthesis at this level.

REFERENCES

1. LeRoy EC: Increased collagen synthesis by scleroderma skin fibroblasts in vitro: a possible defect in the regulation or activation of the scleroderma fibroblast. J Clin Invest 54:880–889, 1979
2. Fleischmajer R, Perlish JS, Krieg T, Timpl R: Variability in collagen and fibronectin synthesis by scleroderma fibroblasts in primary culture. J Invest Dermatol 76: 400–403, 1981
3. Buckingham RB, Prince RK, Rodnan GP, Taylor F: Increased collagen accumulation in dermal fibroblast cultures from patients with progressive systemic sclerosis (scleroderma). J Lab Clin Med 92:5–21, 1978
4. Uitto J, Bauer EA, Eisen AZ: Scleroderma: increase in biosynthesis of triple helical type I and type III procollagen associated with unaltered expression of collagenase by skin fibroblasts in culture. J Clin Invest 64:921–930, 1979
5. Perlish JS, Bashey RI, Stephens RE, Fleischmajer R: Connective tissue synthesis by cultured scleroderma fibroblasts. I. In vitro collagen synthesis by normal and scleroderma dermal fibroblasts. Arthritis Rheum 19: 891–901, 1976
6. Botstein GR, Sherer GK, LeRoy EC: Fibroblast selection in scleroderma: an alternative model of fibrosis. Arthritis Rheum 25:189–195, 1982
7. Lapiere CM, Lenaers A, Kohn LD: Procollagen peptides: an enzyme excising the coordination peptides of procollagen. Proc Natl Acad Sci USA 68:3054–3058, 1971
8. Wiestner M, Krieg T, Hörlein D, Glanville RW, Fietzek P, Müller PK: Inhibitory effect of procollagen peptides on collagen biosynthesis in fibroblast cultures. J Biol Chem 254:7016–7023, 1979
9. Kühn K, Wiestner M, Krieg T, Müller PK: Structure and function of the amino terminal propeptide of type I and III collagen. Connect Tissue Res 10:43–50, 1982
10. Wiestner M, Rohde H, Helle O, Krieg T, Timpl R, Müller PK: Low rate of procollagen conversion in dermatosparactic sheep fibroblasts is paralleled by increased synthesis of type I and type III collagens. EMBO J 1:513–516, 1982
11. Krieg T, Hörlein D, Wiestner M, Müller PK: Aminoterminal extension peptides from type I procollagen normalize excessive collagen synthesis of scleroderma fibroblasts. Arch Dermatol Res 263:171–180, 1978

12. Becker U, Timpl R, Helle O, Prockop DJ: NH_2-terminal extensions on skin collagen from sheep with a genetic defect in conversion of procollagen into collagen. Biochemistry 15:2853–2862, 1976
13. Webster DF, Harvey W: A quantitative assay for collagen synthesis in microwell fibroblast cultures. Anal Biochem 96:220–224, 1979
14. Timpl R, Glanville RW: The aminopropeptide of collagen. Clin Orthop 158:224–242, 1981
15. Fessler LI, Morris NP, Fessler JH: Procollagen: biological scission of amino and carboxyl extension peptides. Proc Natl Acad Sci USA 72:4905–4909, 1975
16. Pesciotta DM, Silkowitz MH, Fietzek PP, Graves PN, Berg RA, Olsen BR: Purification and characterization of the amino-terminal propeptide of pro α1(I) chains from embryonic chick tendon procollagen. Biochemistry 19: 2447–2454, 1980
17. Perlish JS, Fleischmajer R, Timpl R, Carter V: Effect of Col 1(I) peptide on the synthesis of collagen by scleroderma skin fibroblasts in culture (abstract). Arthritis Rheum (suppl) 26:S30, 1983
18. Harper RA, Grove G: Human skin fibroblasts derived from papillary and reticular dermis: differences in growth potential in vitro. Science 204:526–527, 1979
19. Tajima S, Pinnell SR: Collagen synthesis by human skin fibroblasts in culture: studies of fibroblasts explanted from papillary and reticular dermis. J Invest Dermatol 77:410–412, 1981
20. Paglia LM, Wilczek J, Diaz de Leon L, Martin GR, Hörlein D, Müller PK: Inhibition of procollagen cell-free synthesis by amino-terminal extension peptides. Biochemistry 18:5030–5034, 1979
21. Paglia L, Wiestner M, Duchene M, Ouellette L, Hörlein D, Martin GR, Müller PK: Effects of procollagen peptides on the translation of type II collagen messenger ribonucleic acid and on collagen biosynthesis in chondrocytes. Biochemistry 20:3523–3527, 1981
22. Graves PN, Weiss IK, Perlish JS, Fleischmajer R: Increased procollagen mRNA levels in scleroderma skin fibroblasts. J Invest Dermatol 80:130–132, 1983
23. Kähäri VM, Vuorio T, Näntö-Salonen K, Vuorio E: Increased type I collagen mRNA levels in cultured scleroderma fibroblasts. Biochim Biophys Acta 78:183–186, 1984

CORONARY ARTERITIS IN MICE FOLLOWING THE SYSTEMIC INJECTION OF GROUP B *LACTOBACILLUS CASEI* CELL WALLS IN AQUEOUS SUSPENSION

THOMAS J. A. LEHMAN, SHARYN M. WALKER, VLADIMIR MAHNOVSKI, and DEBORAH McCURDY

We describe the induction of an asymmetric, focal, inflammatory coronary arteritis by a single intraperitoneal injection of group B *Lactobacillus casei* cell wall fragments in various inbred mouse strains. This coronary arteritis resembles the arteritis which is responsible for the 1–2% fatality rate among children with mucocutaneous lymph node syndrome. Coronary arteritis developed in 18 of 26 C57BL/6, 14 of 26 A/J, 7 of 15 Balb/c, and 8 of 15 C3Heb/FeJ mice injected. It also developed in 2 of 4 "nude" A/J background mice and 3 of 4 "nude" C57BL/6 mice, but in 0 of 15 C3H/HeJ mice. Lesions were evident as early as 3 days following injection. The development of arteritis was accompanied by disruption of the arterial intima and media with true aneurysm formation. Measurement of serial IgG and IgM titers indicated no relationship between the development of coronary arteritis and immunoglobulin response to *L casei* cell walls or the development of antibodies cross-reactive with normal myocardium. The absence of disease in only the C3H/HeJ mice, which are known to have defective macrophages, suggests that macrophages may play an essential role in the pathogenesis of coronary arteritis.

Coronary arteritis is a life-threatening potential complication of many rheumatic diseases. It most frequently occurs as a complication of mucocutaneous lymph node syndrome (MLNS) (1,2) or polyarteritis nodosa (3). However, it may complicate systemic lupus erythematosus (4,5), Takayasu's arteritis (6), rheumatoid arthritis (7), and other rheumatic diseases (8,9). Aneurysmal dilatation resulting from coronary arteritis occurs in at least 15% of children with MLNS (2), and 1–2% of MLNS cases are fatal. Most of the fatalities in children with MLNS are caused by myocardial infarctions which result from thrombosis of the inflamed coronary arteries (10,11). In this paper we describe an asymmetric, focal, inflammatory coronary arteritis and myocarditis occurring in mice following the intraperitoneal injection of group B *Lactobacillus casei* cell wall fragments in aqueous suspension.

Group B *L casei* is a common component of the normal enteric flora of both humans and rodents (12). However, it shares with group A *Streptococcus pyogenes* both a high cell wall rhamnose content and resistance to degradation by lysozyme (13). Both

From the Divisions of Rheumatology and Research Immunology, Department of Pediatrics, and the Department of Laboratories, Childrens Hospital of Los Angeles, and the University of Southern California School of Medicine, Los Angeles.

Thomas J. A. Lehman, MD: Assistant Professor of Pediatrics, Childrens Hospital of Los Angeles and the University of Southern California School of Medicine; Sharyn M. Walker, PhD: Associate Professor of Microbiology and Associate Member of the Division of Research Immunology, Department of Pediatrics, the University of Southern California School of Medicine; Vladimir Mahnovski, MD: Associate Clinical Professor of Pathology, Childrens Hospital of Los Angeles and the University of Southern California School of Medicine; Deborah McCurdy, MD: Research Fellow, Division of Rheumatology, Department of Pediatrics, Childrens Hospital of Los Angeles.

Address reprint requests to Thomas J. A. Lehman, MD, Division of Rheumatology, Childrens Hospital of Los Angeles, 4650 Sunset Blvd., Los Angeles, CA 90027.

Submitted for publication October 12, 1984; accepted in revised form December 6, 1984.

group B *L casei* and group A *S pyogenes* have been shown to induce chronic polyarthritis in rats (14,15). In addition, group A *S pyogenes* has been shown to induce a rheumatic fever–like illness in mice, with the development of "Aschoff-like" lesions, myocarditis and, in some mice, coronary arteritis (16).

The induction of coronary arteritis by a single intraperitoneal injection of group B *L casei* cell wall materials is important because it provides an opportunity to examine both the evolution and natural history of coronary arteritis and the effect of therapeutic regimens on its healing, without placing human subjects at risk. The knowledge gained may make possible the development of therapeutic regimens to prevent the occurrence of coronary artery lesions or to promote their healing in an optimal manner. In addition, since injection of identical material leads to arthritis in rats but to arteritis in mice, careful study of how the immune and reticuloendothelial systems of rats and mice differ in their response to injection of these cell wall materials may yield important information regarding the pathogenesis of both arteritis and arthritis.

MATERIALS AND METHODS

Inbred mouse strains. Male and female 6–8-week-old C57BL/6, Balb/c, A/J, C3H/HeJ, and C3Heb/FeJ mice were obtained from Jackson Laboratories (Bar Harbor, ME). T cell–deficient, "nude" C57BL/6 background (nC57BL/6) and "nude" A/J background (nA/J) mice were obtained from Dr. Elliot Parks of the Scripps Clinic and Research Foundation, La Jolla, CA.

Preparation of bacteria and bacterial cell wall fragments. Group B *L casei* (ATCC 11578) cells and cell wall–associated material were obtained and prepared as previously described (14). In brief, following growth in *Lactobacillus* MRS broth (Difco, Detroit, MI), the cells were harvested and the cytoplasmic membrane disrupted by detergent lysis with 4% sodium dodecyl sulfate (SDS) overnight at room temperature. Identification and purity of the cultures were confirmed by the Childrens Hospital of Los Angeles microbiology laboratories. The cell wall–associated material was washed extensively to remove the SDS, then incubated sequentially with DNase, RNase, and trypsin to remove cytoplasmic materials. This cell wall–associated material was sonicated for 2 hours using a W-375 sonicator (Heat Systems Ultrasonic, Syracuse, NY) with cooling by a dry ice–ethanol bath.

After the sonicated material was centrifuged for 1 hour at 20,000*g*, the material remaining in the supernatant was utilized for the induction of coronary arteritis. Although this material may contain small amounts of cellular materials closely bound to the cell wall, the successive treatment with SDS, DNase, RNase, and trypsin would remove all lipids, nucleic acids, and proteins, leaving the cell wall backbone and any associated polysaccharides. The amount of cell wall material injected was quantitated by determining the total amount of carbohydrate in the cell wall preparation by the phenol–sulfuric acid extraction colorimetric method (17).

Injection of *L casei* cell wall fragments. All mice received 500 μg of group B *L casei* cell wall–associated material suspended in 1 ml of sterile phosphate buffered saline (PBS), prepared as described above, as a single intraperitoneal injection on day 0.

Histologic evaluation. Representative animals were killed on days 5, 10, 14, 28, and 56 after injection. In addition, 3 C57BL/6 mice were killed on each of days 1–5 after injection in order to determine the time at which inflammation became apparent. At the time of killing, sections of heart, lung, liver, spleen, kidney, the hind limb, and in some cases, brain and testis were obtained. Tissue specimens were fixed in 10% phosphate buffered formalin, stained with hematoxylin and eosin, trichrome, or a modified Gomori aldehyde–fuchsin stain by routine histologic techniques (18), and examined by light microscopy.

Antibody production. Mice from each inbred strain were bled on days 5 and 14 following injection. In addition, mice of the inbred A/J, C57BL/6, and Balb/c strains were bled on days 28 and 56. Antibodies directed against group B *L casei* cell wall materials were quantitated by solid-phase enzyme-linked immunosorbent assay (ELISA). In brief, a 1 mg/ml solution of *L casei* cell wall–associated material in carbonate buffer was incubated for 2 hours at room temperature in 96-well Dynatech Immulon I plates (Dynatech, Mclean, VA). The wells were washed 3 times with "wash-block" buffer containing 0.5% Tween 20 and 1% bovine serum albumin (BSA), then incubated for 30 minutes with this same buffer. Following this, the wells were again washed, then incubated for 1 hour with the primary mouse sera diluted 1:50 in 1% BSA. The plates were washed and 100 μl of the appropriate second antibody diluted 1:1,000 (peroxidase-labeled goat anti-mouse IgG, heavy and light chain specific, or anti-mouse IgM, mu chain specific; Kirkegard and Perry, Gaithersburg, MD) was added to each well and incubated at room temperature for 1 hour. A uniform amount of orthophenylenediamine was then added to each well and the optical density at 405 nm determined after 30 minutes with a Dynatech MR 600 automated spectrophotometer. The background value of sera from a group of control, uninjected mice of the same strain was subtracted from the reported values.

Preparation of crude myocardial antigen. A preparation of crude myocardial antigen was utilized for the detection of antibodies cross-reactive with normal myocardium by ELISA, as described below. This crude myocardial antigen was obtained as follows: mice of the appropriate strain were killed by cervical dislocation and their hearts removed using an aseptic technique. The hearts were dissected free from adherent adipose and connective tissue, freed of blood by cutting them into large fragments, and then rinsed with 0.067*M* PBS. The hearts were then minced and the fragments rinsed and then collected by centrifugation at 500 revolutions per minute for 5 minutes. This rinsing procedure was repeated 3 times.

The resultant small fragments were subjected to sonication at full power using a ¾″ probe with the W-375 sonicator for 15 minutes, with cooling of the sonication vessel in an ice water–ethanol bath. The sonicated suspen-

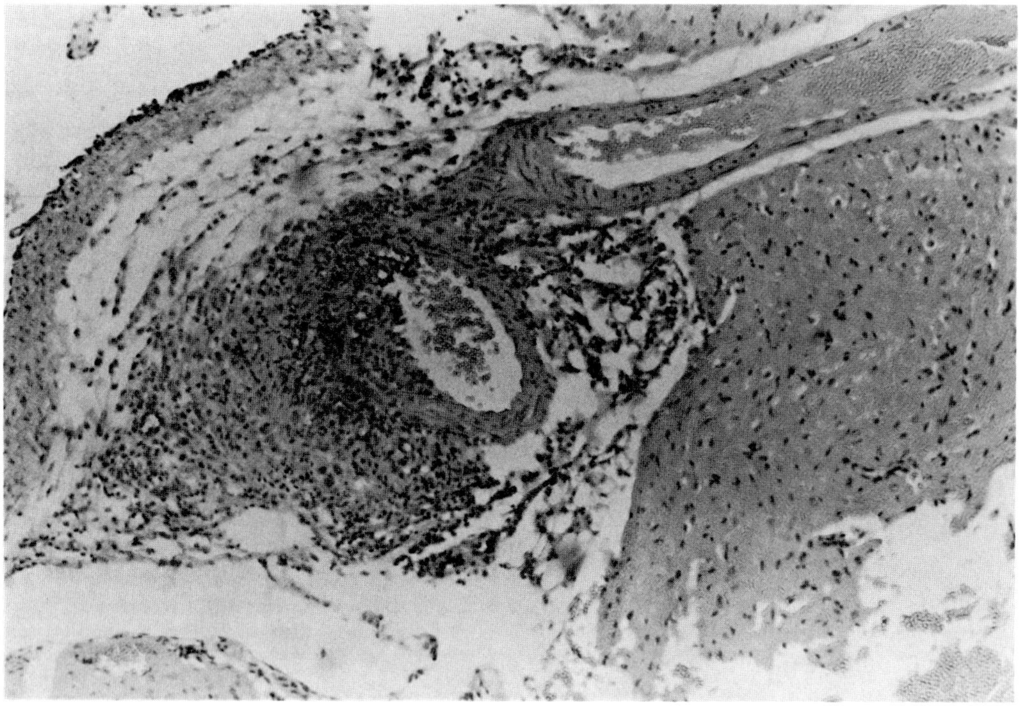

Figure 1. Coronary artery of a C57BL/6 mouse 14 days after intraperitoneal injection of group B *Lactobacillus casei,* illustrating asymmetric invasion of the vessel wall (hematoxylin and eosin stained, original magnification × 100).

sion was then centrifuged for 30 minutes at 2,000 rpm to remove all large tissue fragments. The protein concentration of the supernatant containing sonicated myocardial fragments was determined using the spectrophotometric Bio-Rad protein assay with a bovine serum albumin standard curve (19).

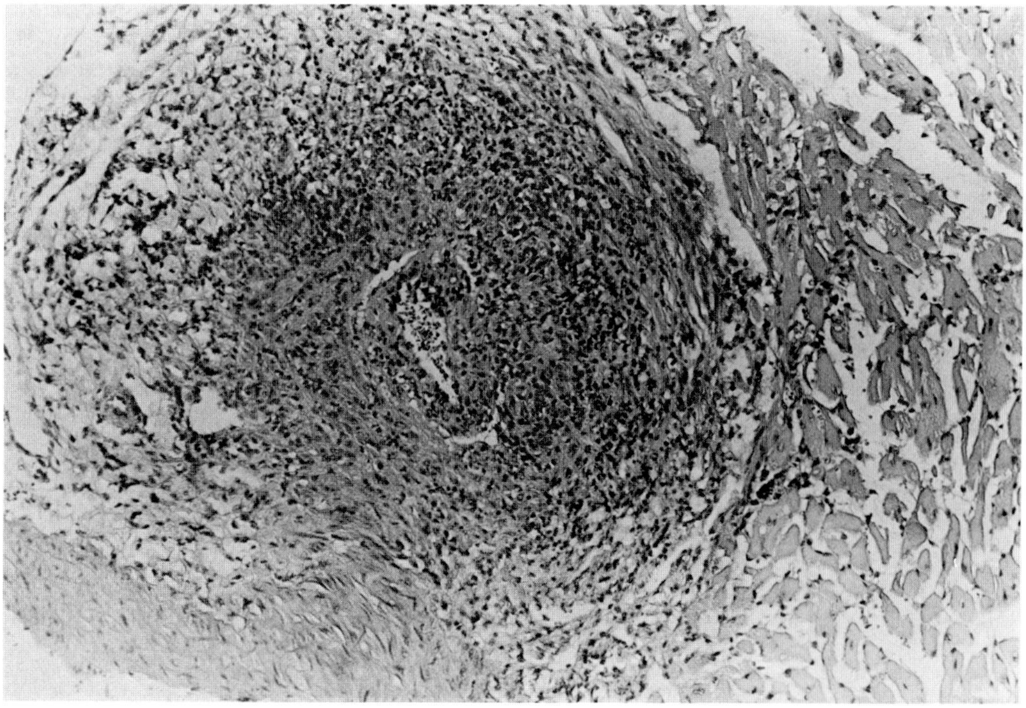

Figure 2. Coronary artery of a C57BL/6 mouse 28 days after intraperitoneal injection of group B *Lactobacillus casei,* illustrating circumferential invasion and narrowing of the vessel (hematoxylin and eosin stained, original magnification × 200).

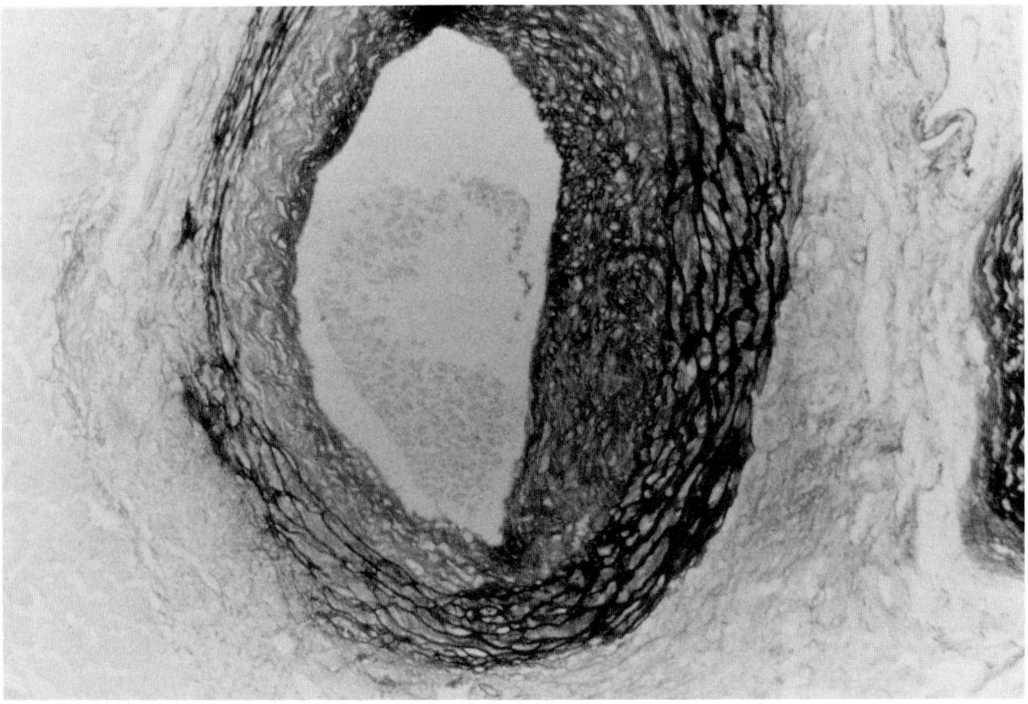

Figure 3. Coronary artery of a C57BL/6 mouse 56 days after intraperitoneal injection of group B *Lactobacillus casei*, illustrating disruption of the lamina interna and externa with marked intimal proliferation (modified aldehyde-fuchsin stain, original magnification × 250).

Measurement of antibodies cross-reactive with normal myocardium. Antibodies directed against the crude myocardial antigen preparation were quantitated by ELISA as described above for the detection of antibodies to *L casei*, with the exception that a 1 mg/ml solution of crude mouse heart extract from a mouse of the appropriate strain was prepared in carbonate buffer and utilized as the antigen bound to the plates.

Immunofluorescent dectection of antibodies cross-reactive with normal myocardium. To confirm the absence of antibodies cross-reactive with normal myocardium, small sections of normal mouse heart from mice of the appropriate strains were snap-frozen at −70°C in OCT compound (Lab-Tek Products, Naperville, IL) using liquified nitrogen. Thin sections were then cut from these hearts with a cryostat and incubated for 1 hour at room temperature with a 1:10 dilution of sera from either syngeneic normal mice or syngeneic mice which had been injected with group B *L casei* cell walls and had developed coronary arteritis. These sections were then rinsed thoroughly with PBS and incubated for 1 hour with a 1:20 dilution of fluorescein-labeled goat anti-mouse IgG, heavy and light chain specific, or anti-mouse IgM, mu chain specific (Kirkegard and Perry).

RESULTS

Development of coronary arteritis. Invasion of the vessel wall by an inflammatory mononuclear cell infiltrate was evident in the coronary arteries of 18 of 26 C57BL/6 inbred mice killed on or after the fourteenth day following injection of group B *L casei* cell wall fragments. The inflammatory lesion consisted of a focal, often circumferential, asymmetric invasion of all layers of the vessel wall by a predominantly mononuclear cell infiltrate (Figures 1 and 2). The accompanying intimal proliferation often produced narrowing of the vascular lumen (Figure 3). Aldehyde-fuchsin staining revealed disruption of the arterial intima and media with true aneurysm formation (Figure 4). In addition, most mice exhibited a mild myocarditis; in some mice, myocardial changes suggestive of recent infarction were present. Control C57BL/6 mice injected with PBS only (n = 15) or with an equivalent dose of another strain of *Lactobacillus*, ATCC 25302 (which was not arthritogenic in rats [13]) (n = 15) did not develop coronary arteritis.

Accumulation of inflammatory mononuclear cells in the adventitia of the coronary arteries was apparent in C57BL/6 mice killed on day 3 after intraperitoneal injection of *L casei* cell wall–associated material, but not in those killed earlier. No polymorphonuclear cells were present at day 3, and only rare polymorphonuclear cells were seen during the subsequent evolution of the lesion. The lesions progressed from focal, asymmetric invasion of the arterial wall on day 14 (Figure 1) to circumferential lesions associated with marked proliferation of the intima and media accompanied by narrowing or even complete obstruc-

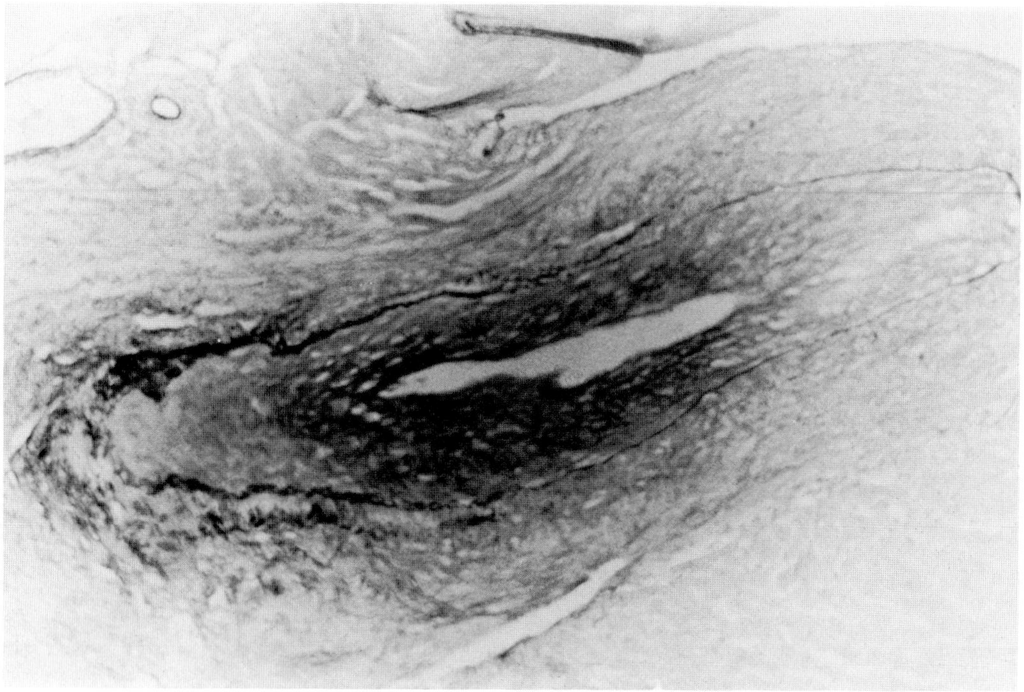

Figure 4. Coronary artery of a C57BL/6 mouse 28 days after intraperitoneal injection of group B *Lactobacillus casei*, illustrating disruption of the lamina interna and externa with intimal proliferation and true aneurysm formation (modified aldehyde-fuchsin stain, original magnification × 250).

tion of the vascular lumen by day 28 (Figure 2). These lesions were accompanied by a marked proliferation of the adventitial fibrous tissue surrounding the coronary arteries. By day 56 the fibrous tissue surrounding the coronary arteries had become quite dense. Within the inflamed arteries, narrow, irregular channels were present, representing either marked narrowing of the vessel by intimal proliferation or recanalization subsequent to thrombosis.

Coronary artery lesions identical to those described above were found in similar percentages of the A/J, Balb/c, and C3Heb/FeJ inbred mice following the intraperitoneal injection of group B *L casei* cell wall fragments (Table 1). In addition, "Aschoff-like" lesions were found in the left ventricular outflow tract of 2 of 26 A/J mice (Figure 5), but not in other inbred mouse strains. The nA/J and nC57BL/6 inbred mouse strains also developed coronary arteritis following the injection of group B *L casei* cell walls. However, these lesions were less intense than those seen in mice of the background strains receiving similar amounts of *L casei* cell walls. In contrast, none of 15 C3H/HeJ mice developed coronary arteritis after injection of group B *L casei* cell wall–associated materials. No sex predilection was found in the development of coronary arteritis.

The hind limb sections revealed no evidence of synovial inflammation at any time. In addition the

Table 1. The induction of coronary arteritis and antibody responses in selected strains of inbred mice following the injection of *Lactobacillus casei* cell walls

Strain	Incidence of arteritis (%)	IgG response* Day 5	IgG response* Day 14	IgM response* Day 5	IgM response* Day 14
A/J	14/26 (54%)	0.129 ± 0.057 (12)	0.691 ± 0.030 (8)	0.543 ± 0.124 (12)	0.196 ± 0.131 (8)
C57BL6	18/26 (69%)	0.179 ± 0.064 (18)	0.818 ± 0.123 (7)	0.191 ± 0.027 (18)	0.088 ± 0.040 (7)
Balb/c	7/15 (47%)	0.148 ± 0.098 (8)	0.273 ± 0.139 (8)	0.446 ± 0.177 (8)	0.203 ± 0.095 (8)
C3Heb/FeJ	8/15 (53%)	0.421 ± 0.035 (6)	1.086 ± 0.045 (6)	0.438 ± 0.174 (6)	0.298 ± 0.187 (6)
C3H/HeJ	0/15 (0%)	0.480 ± 0.228 (6)	1.106 ± 0.100 (6)	0.632 ± 0.134 (6)	0.253 ± 0.077 (6)
"Nude" A/J	2/4 (50%)	0.260 ± 0.087 (4)	0.350 ± 0.117 (4)	0.270 ± 0.165 (4)	0.270 ± 0.269 (4)
"Nude" C57BL/6	3/4 (75%)	0.012 ± 0.060 (4)	0.014 ± 0.051 (4)	0.019 ± 0.037 (4)	0.007 ± 0.154 (4)

* Expressed in optical density units ± 1 SD; numbers in parentheses are n values.

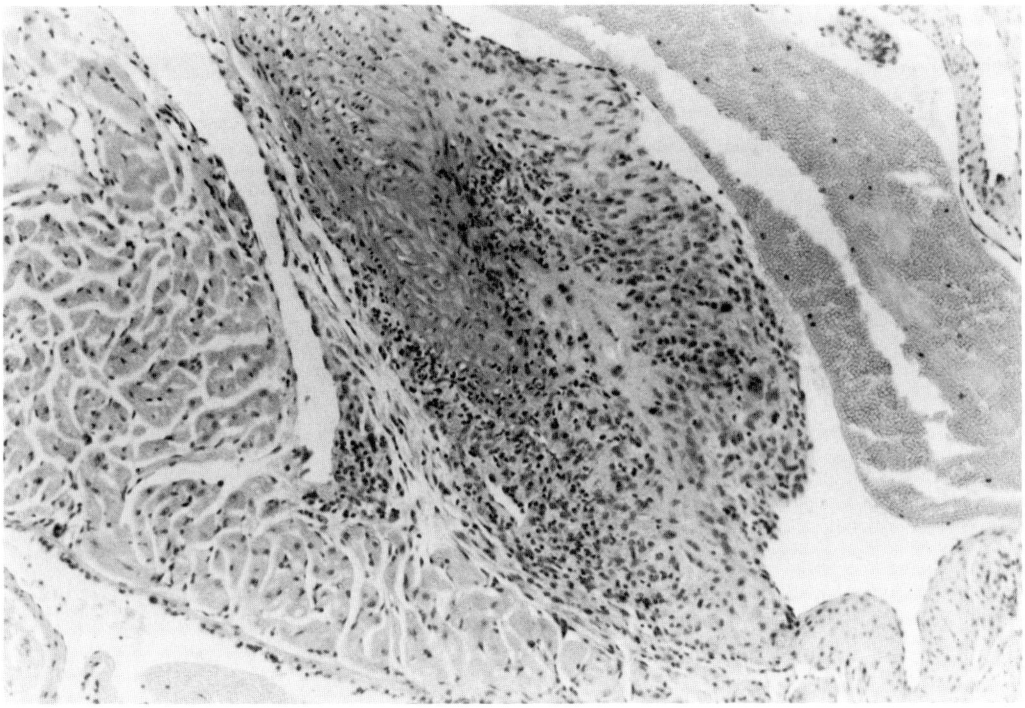

Figure 5. An "Aschoff-like" lesion in the left ventricular outflow tract of an A/J mouse 14 days after intraperitoneal injection of group B *Lactobacillus casei* (hematoxylin and eosin stained, original magnification × 100).

kidney, brain, lung, and testis sections were without abnormality. Sections of liver occasionally revealed small areas of perivascular inflammation. These liver lesions were a consistent finding in A/J mice, but not in the other strains.

Immunoglobulin response. All of the C57BL/6, A/J, C3H/HeJ, and C3Heb/FeJ mice tested had a brisk IgG antibody response directed against group B *L casei* cell wall materials, which peaked 14–28 days after injection (Table 1). The antibody response of the Balb/c strain was modest compared with that of the other strains. Nonetheless, mice of this inbred strain had coronary artery lesions which did not differ from those seen in the other strains. On day 14, the mean IgG antibody titer of the C3H/HeJ mice, which did not have evident coronary arteritis, was not significantly different from the mean titer of the C3Heb/FeJ inbred mice, which did have the disease ($P > 0.05$). IgM antibody responses to group B *L casei* cell wall materials peaked at about the fifth day following injection and declined thereafter in all strains that had intact T cell–mediated immunity (Table 1). In contrast, the nC57BL/6 and nA/J inbred mouse strains did not manifest a significant IgG or IgM antibody response following injection of group B *L casei* cell wall fragments ($P > 0.05$).

Antibodies directed against syngeneic normal mouse heart were not found by either ELISA or immunofluorescence in the sera of mice who had developed coronary arteritis. Although a small amount of nonspecific sticking of IgG to snap-frozen myocardium (by immunofluorescence) and the crude myocardial extract (by ELISA) was found, this did not differ in amount between control and *L casei*–injected mice (data not shown).

DISCUSSION

In recent publications it has been demonstrated that group B *L casei* cell wall fragments share with group A *S pyogenes* cell wall fragments the ability to induce polyarthritis in rats (14,20). In this paper we have demonstrated that group B *L casei* cell wall fragments also share with group A *S pyogenes* cell wall fragments the ability to induce coronary arteritis in mice. However, the coronary arteritis reported by others, after injection of group A *S pyogenes* cell walls in outbred mice (16), differs from that found in this study. Following the injection of group B *L casei* cell wall fragments, coronary arteritis was a pronounced feature of the lesions, while severe myocarditis and the development of "Aschoff-like" lesions, prominent findings in the mice injected with group A *S pyogenes* (16), were rare. The explanation for the ability of cell wall materials from these 2 distinct gram-positive bacteria to produce similar-appearing chronic inflammatory lesions in mice may lie in the resistance of their cell wall materials to degradation by macrophages and their high cell wall polysaccharide rhamnose content (13). Why intraperitoneal injection of the identical material will produce coronary arteritis without evidence of synovial inflammation in mice, but chronic polyarthritis without evidence of coronary arteritis in rats, is unknown.

The development of an acute and chronic coronary arteritis accompanied by aneurysmal dilatation and/or thrombosis in A/J, Balb/c, C57BL/6, C3Heb/FeJ, nA/J, and nC57BL/6 inbred mice following the intraperitoneal injection of group B *L casei* cell wall materials provided the opportunity to evaluate the occurrence of disease in inbred mouse strains lacking normal complement systems (A/J), macrophages (C3H/HeJ), and T cell–mediated immunity (nA/J, nC57BL/6). In addition, we were able to compare the humoral immune responses of these strains. The A/J, Balb/c, C57BL/6, and C3Heb/FeJ inbred mouse strains manifested a vigorous IgG and IgM antibody response directed against group B *L casei* cell wall–associated materials. However, the nA/J and nC57BL/6 inbred mouse strains, which did not develop a significant humoral response, also developed coronary arteritis. Further, C3H/HeJ mice mounted an antibody response to group B *L casei* cell wall materials equivalent to that seen in C3Heb/FeJ mice but, unlike the C3Heb/FeJ mice, did not develop coronary arteritis.

The presence of disease in the "nude" nA/J and nC57BL/6 inbred mouse strains suggests that intact T cell–mediated immunity may not be required for the development of coronary arteritis. However, intraperitoneal injection of bacterial products into "nude" mice may induce T cell maturation (21); therefore, it cannot be concluded that the development of coronary arteritis is "T-independent." It has been suggested that the myocarditis which accompanies rheumatic fever may be the result of the induction of antibodies cross-reactive with myocardium (22). However, no such antibodies were found in affected mice of the C57BL/6, A/J, or Balb/c inbred strains by ELISA or immunofluorescence methods in this study.

Among the inbred mouse strains tested, only the C3H/HeJ strain consistently failed to develop coronary arteritis or myocarditis. The macrophages of C3H/HeJ mice are defective in their ability to process lipopolysaccharide antigens, have diminished cytotoxic activity, and have fewer Fc receptors than normal macrophages (23). The failure to develop disease in only this inbred mouse strain, of all those tested, may indicate that macrophages and/or macrophage antigen processing are important in the pathogenesis of coronary arteritis.

In previous descriptions of a rheumatic fever–like myocarditis accompanied by coronary arteritis in outbred mice following the intraperitoneal injection of group A *S pyogenes* cell wall fragments, it was noted that group A *S pyogenes* cell wall fragments were resistant to macrophage degradation (24,25) and persisted in the mediastinal lymph nodes and adjacent tissues for up to 10 weeks after injection (26). It was proposed that the myocardial lesions were probably due to a direct toxic effect of the cell wall materials associated with the prolonged release by macrophages of large amounts of inflammatory enzymes. The failure of C3H/HeJ mice to develop coronary arteritis after the injection of group B *L casei* cell wall fragments in the present study provides additional evidence that macrophages may play an essential role in the pathogenesis of coronary arteritis following the injection of gram-positive bacterial cell wall fragments.

Coronary arteritis in mice following the subcutaneous injection of cortisone acetate (27), or the intraperitoneal injection of an extract of *Candida albicans* (28), has previously been described. The arteritis which occurred after the injection of cortisone acetate did not histologically resemble that which accompanies MLNS. The arteritis which developed after the injection of *C albicans* did resemble MLNS, but it has not been subsequently reported, and its significance is uncertain.

This experimental model in which coronary arteritis is induced in inbred mice by the intraperitoneal injection of group B *L casei* cell wall–associated materials is important because it provides an opportunity to study the natural history, pathogenesis, and response to therapy of coronary artery inflammation in an animal model. Careful study of this animal model may provide fundamental information which will increase our understanding of the pathogenesis, natural history, and appropriate therapy of coronary arteritis in humans, issues about which very little is currently known. Additionally, since the lesions which occur in this model and in MLNS are histologically similar, the model provides a useful opportunity to evaluate the effects of various therapeutic regimens on the healing of coronary arteritis, without placing human subjects at risk.

ACKNOWLEDGMENT

The authors wish to thank Heidi Wietting for her excellent technical assistance.

REFERENCES

1. Kato H, Koike S, Yamamoto M, Ito Y, Yano E: Coronary aneurysms in infants and young children with mucocutaneous lymph node syndrome. J Pediatr 86: 892–898, 1975
2. Kato H, Ichinose E, Yoshioka F, Takechi T, Matsunaga S, Suzuki K, Rikitake N: Fate of coronary aneurysms in Kawasaki disease: serial coronary angiography and long term followup study. Am J Cardiol 49:1758–1766, 1982
3. Holsinger DR, Osmundson PJ, Edwards JE: The heart in periarteritis nodosa. Circulation 25:610–618, 1962
4. Bonfiglio TA, Botti RE, Hagstrom JWC: Coronary arteritis, occlusion, and myocardial infarction due to lupus erythematosus. Am Heart J 83:153–158, 1972
5. Homcy CJ, Liberthson RR, Fallon JT, Gross S, Miller LM: Ischemic heart disease in systemic lupus erythematosus in the young patient: report of six cases. Am J Cardiol 49:478–484, 1982
6. Rosen N, Gaton E: Takayasu's arteritis of coronary arteries. Arch Pathol 94:225–229, 1972
7. Karten I: Arteritis, myocardial infarction and rheumatoid arthritis. JAMA 210:1717–1720, 1979
8. Cohle SD, Titus JL, Espinola A, Jachimczyk JA: Sudden unexpected death due to coronary giant cell arteritis. Arch Pathol Lab Med 106:171–172, 1982
9. Ahronheim JH: Isolated coronary periarteritis: report of a case of unexpected death in a young pregnant woman. Am J Cardiol 40:287–290, 1977
10. Kawasaki T, Kosaki F, Okawa S, Shigematsu I, Yanagawa H: A new infantile acute febrile mucocutaneous lymph node syndrome (MLNS) prevailing in Japan. Pediatrics 54:271–276, 1974
11. Tanaka N, Sekimoto K, Naoe S: Kawasaki disease. Arch Pathol Lab Med 100:81–86, 1976
12. London JC: The ecology and taxonomic status of the lactobacilli. Annu Rev Microbiol 30:279–301, 1976
13. Lehman TJA, Allen JB, Plotz PH, Wilder RL: Bacterial cell wall composition, lysozyme resistance, and the induction of chronic arthritis in rats. Rheumatol Int (in press)
14. Lehman TJA, Allen JB, Plotz PH, Wilder RL: Polyarthritis in rats following the systemic injection of Lactobacillus casei cell walls in aqueous suspension. Arthritis Rheum 26:1259–1265, 1983
15. Cromartie WJ, Craddock JG, Schwab JH, Anderle S, Yang CH: Arthritis in rats after systemic injection of streptococcal cells or cell walls. J Exp Med 146:1585–1602, 1977
16. Cromartie WJ, Craddock JG: Rheumatic like cardiac lesion in mice. Science 154:283–284, 1966
17. Dubois M, Giles KA, Hamilton JK, Rebers PA, Smith F: Colorimetric method for determination of sugars and related substances. Anal Chem 28:350–356, 1956
18. Luna LG, editor: Manual of Histological and Special Staining Techniques, Armed Forces Institute of Pathology. New York, Mc-Graw Hill, 1968
19. Bradford M: A rapid and sensitive method for the quantitation of microgram quantities of protein utilizing the principle of protein-dye binding. Anal Biochem 72:248–254, 1976
20. Lehman TJA, Allen JB, Plotz PH, Wilder RL: Lactobacillus casei cell wall–induced arthritis in rats: cell wall fragment distribution and persistence in chronic arthritis–susceptible LEW/N and –resistant F344/N rats. Arthritis Rheum 27:939–942, 1984
21. Ishikawa H, Saito K: Congenitally athymic nude (nu/nu) mice have Thy-l-bearing immunocompetent helper T cells in their peritoneal cavity. J Exp Med 151:965–968, 1980
22. Rijn I, Zabriskie JB, McCarty M: Group A streptococcal antigens cross-reactive with myocardium. J Exp Med 146:579–599, 1977
23. Oppenheim JJ, Potter M: Immunity and inflammation, Cellular Functions in Immunity and Inflammation. Edited by JJ Oppenheim, DL Rosentreich, M Potter. New York, Elsevier/North-Holland, 1981, pp 1–26
24. Schwab JH, Ohanian SH: Degradation of streptococcal cell wall antigens in vivo. J Bacteriol 94:1346–1352, 1967
25. Smialowicz RJ, Schwab JH: Processing of streptococcal cell walls by rat macrophages and human monocytes in vitro. Infect Immun 17:591–598, 1977
26. Ohanian SH, Schwab JH, Cromartie WJ: Relation of rheumatic-like cardiac lesions of the mouse to localization of group A streptococcal cell walls. J Exp Med 129:37–48, 1969
27. Ashburn AD, Williams WL, Smith-Vaniz GT: Arteritis of coronary arteries in mice receiving a single dose of cortisone. Anat Rec 160:1–11, 1968
28. Murata H: Experimental Candida-induced arteritis in mice: relation to arteritis in the mucocutaneous lymph node syndrome. Microbiol Immunol 23:825–831, 1979

CARTILAGE SURFACE CHARGE

A Possible Determinant in Aging and Osteoarthritic Processes

ZAHAVA LAVER-RUDICH and MICHAEL SILBERMANN

Polycationic labels such as cationized ferritin and colloidal iron were used to evaluate the surface negative charges over the mandibular condyles of ICR mice. The effects of neuraminidase, hyaluronidase, pronase, and collagenase on the binding of cationized ferritin and colloidal iron particles to the condylar articular surface were also studied. The results of this study clearly indicate that the surface area of the cartilaginous condyle is negatively charged and that its composition consists mainly of a collagenous material embedded within a proteinaceous matrix. With age, a substantial decrease in the density of negative charges took place along the surface area and, in particular, in the context of sialic acid residues. It is, therefore, possible that the reduction in cartilage surface charge might be associated with the onset of osteoarthritic changes commonly seen in aging humans and experimental animals.

The articular portion of condylar cartilage differs in its structure and function from the rest of the organ and plays a special role in joint biomechanics and cartilage nutrition (1–6). Alterations in the chemical composition of the latter constitute one of the earliest changes noticed in age-related osteoarthritis (7–11). Age-related degenerative changes in articular cartilages (2,9,12–16) which precede osteoarthritis (17–19) resemble, to a great extent, those changes observed in the joints of animals submitted to glucocorticoid treatment (20).

Previous studies have indicated a close correlation between age-related changes in cartilage and the alterations in the glycosaminoglycan content of this tissue (2,4,21,22). Polycationic labels such as the cationized ferritin (CF), which labels all anionic groups at physiologic pH (23), and colloidal iron (CI) hydroxide particles, which normally label only the carboxylic group of sialic acids at pH 1.8 (24), have been used to study changes in the chemical nature of articular cartilages (6,25).

In the present study, we applied the cationized ferritin and colloidal iron labeling techniques and used a variety of enzymes, such as neuroaminidase, hyaluronidase, pronase, and collagenase, to evaluate the age-related changes in the charge properties of the articular cartilage.

From the Laboratory for Musculoskeletal Research, the Rappaport Family Institute for Research in the Medical Sciences, and the Faculty of Medicine, Technion-Israel Institute of Technology, Haifa, Israel.

Supported in part by a research grant from the David Ben-Gurion Research Fund of the Histadrut (General Federation of Labor), Israel.

Zahava Laver-Rudich, PhD: Research Associate (present address: Department of Virology, Weizmann Institute of Science, PO Box 26, Rehovot 76100, Israel); Michael Silbermann, DMD, PhD: Associate Professor and Head, Division of Morphological Sciences.

Address reprint requests to Dr. Michael Silbermann, Division of Morphological Sciences, Faculty of Medicine, Technion-Israel Institute of Technology, PO Box 9649, Haifa 31096, Israel.

Submitted for publication April 9, 1984; accepted in revised form November 14, 1984.

MATERIALS AND METHODS

Mice. Pregnant ICR mice were obtained from the Animal Breeding Center of the Weizmann Institute of Science (Rehovot, Israel), and the offspring (male and female) were maintained in our laboratory up to the age of 12 months. One hundred fifteen animals were used; the offspring were divided into 3 experimental groups: 50 neonatal mice (5–7 days old), 40 young-adult animals (2–3 months old), and 25 older mice (12 months old).

Mandibular condyles (2 from each animal) were obtained while the animals were anesthetized with ether. All the specimens were immediately placed in petri dishes containing cacodylate buffer (0.1*M*, pH 7.3). After an additional brief rinsing with cacodylate buffer, the tissues were treated by 1 of the following procedures.

Longer washing procedure using cacodylate buffer. In order to eliminate the possibility of nonspecific absorption, specimens were washed at 37°C with 0.1*M* cacodylate buffer (agitated gently in a water bath) for periods ranging from 30–120 minutes. The tissues were then treated with Karnovsky's fixative (26) for 90 minutes at room temperature and were washed 3 times with 0.1*M* cacodylate buffer, pH 7.3. To date, it has not been determined to what extent aldehyde fixation blocks a significant portion of the positive-charge groups of protein constituents, yet aldehyde is still an essential component of whatever fixative is used. The specimens were then labeled with cationized ferritin and processed for electron microscopy. An additional group of specimens underwent a similar washing procedure using distilled water instead of cacodylate buffer.

Surface-charged labeling of articular cartilage. *Labeling with cationized ferritin.* Fixed or unfixed condyles were incubated with 0.5 mg/ml CF (Miles-Yeda, Rehovot, Israel) in 0.1*M* cacodylate buffer, pH 7.3, for 20 minutes at room temperature. They were then washed 3 times with 0.1*M* cacodylate buffer, postfixed in 1% OsO_4 in 0.1*M* cacodylate for 2 hours at 4°C, dehydrated through graded alcohols, during which time the condyles were stained en bloc with saturated uranyl acetate in 70% methanol for 1 hour, and embedded in Epon.

Labeling with colloidal iron hydroxide. Positively-charged CI was prepared according to the procedure of Gasic et al (24) and used undialyzed at pH 1.8. Aldehyde-fixed tissue specimens were washed twice with distilled water, incubated with CI for 5–10 minutes at room temperature, washed with 12% acetic acid, and washed again with distilled water. The labeled specimens were then processed for electron microscopy as described above.

Effects of various enzymes on the binding of cationized ferritin and colloidal iron. Unfixed tissue specimens were used for this series of experiments.

Vibrio cholerae neuraminidase, free of proteases, aldolase, and lecithinase C (Behringwerke, Marburg-Lahn, West Germany), was applied for 60 minutes at 37°C in 10-ml Erlenmeyer flasks containing 2 ml of the enzyme at a concentration of 50 units/ml in 0.1*M* cacodylate buffer, pH 7.3. For control purposes, heat-inactivated enzymes (boiled for 10 minutes prior to use) in cacodylate buffer were used. The specimens were incubated in a water bath with continuous agitation, thereafter were washed 3 times with 0.1*M* cacodylate buffer, fixed for 90 minutes in Karnovsky's solution at room temperature, washed with cacodylate buffer, and then labeled with either CF or CI. The labeled specimens were then processed for electron microscopy.

Hyaluronidase (552 USP units/mg; Worthington Biochemicals Corp., Freehold, NJ) was applied for 30, 60, and 120 minutes at 37°C at a concentration of 1 mg/ml in 0.1*M* cacodylate buffer. Subsequently, the tissues were labeled with CF and processed as described above. Controls consisted of heat-inactivated hyaluronidase and cacodylate buffer.

Chromatographically pure collagenase (425 units/mg; Worthington) was applied for 15, 30, and 60 minutes at 37°C at a concentration of 0. 2 mg/ml. Controls consisted of heat-inactivated collagenase and cacodylate buffer. Tissues were then labeled with CF and processed for electron microscopy.

Pronase (120 PUK/mg; Calbiochem, San Diego, CA) was applied for 15, 30, and 60 minutes at 37°C in a water bath with continuous shaking. Subsequently, the tissues were labeled with CF. Controls consisted of heat-inactivated pronase and cacodylate buffer. All specimens were processed for electron microscopy as described above.

When the various enzymes were evaluated on fixed specimens, it became apparent that they had no apparent effect on the tissues' charge properties.

Decalcification with EDTA. Specimens obtained from older animals were also decalcified with 10% EDTA in phosphate buffered saline, pH 7.4, for 3–5 days at 4°C. The EDTA was removed by extensive washings with 0.1*M* cacodylate. The specimens were labeled with CF and processed for electron microscopy. Parallel experiments with undecalcified specimens showed that the decalcification procedure had no effect on the binding of CF.

Processing for electron microscopy. Cross-sections of the articular cartilage, 1 μm thick, were obtained for orientation purposes and were stained with 1% toluidine blue.

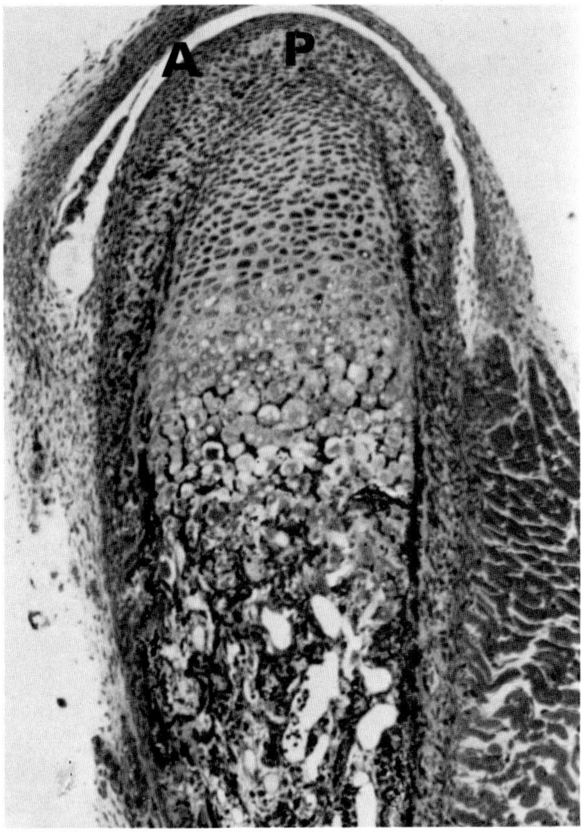

Figure 1. Frontal section through the mandibular condyle of a 1-week-old normal mouse. Note the well-organized perichondrium (**P**) surrounding the core of a well-developed cartilage. A = articular surface (1% toluidine blue stained, magnification × 96).

Sections 600Å thick (gray interference color) were cut with an LKB Ultratome III and mounted on uncoated 300-mesh copper grids. Sections were stained with uranyl acetate and lead citrate (27) and were examined with a Jeol 100B electron microscope at 80 kV.

RESULTS

Surface charge of mandibular condylar cartilage cationized ferritin labeling. The superficial zone of the mandibular condyles of neonatal mice consisted of a perichondrium formed by 3–4 rows of fibroblast-like cells which were very close to the surface (Figure 1). Most of the surface was covered by a layer of amorphous material with a high-affinity binding capacity for CF particles (Figure 2). Further away from the articular surface, the matrix revealed granular structures with abundant collagen fibers perpendicular or parallel to the articular surface. Most of the CF particles were confined to the superficial layer of the cartilage: the fibroblast cells and the collagen fibers underneath them (Figure 3). Fixed specimens revealed a pronounced difference in labeling pattern in comparison with their unfixed homologs. In the former specimens, the ferritin particles were evenly distributed along the cell membranes, but to a lesser extent in the intercellular matrix (Figure 4). In unfixed specimens, the ferritin particles appeared in the form of large, irregular patches (Figure 5). No ferritin particles were noted beyond the perichondrial zone in either the fixed or the unfixed specimens. These findings were not affected by pre-washing the specimens with either cacodylate buffer or distilled water for as long as 90 minutes.

In young-adult mice, the most superficial layer of the articular zone appeared acellular and consisted of an amorphous material where electron-dense particles were intermingled with fine fibrillar material (Figure 6). In contrast to the observations made in neonatal mice, in young-adult animals the CF labeling pattern in fixed and unfixed condyles appeared very similar (Figure 7). Of particular interest was the fact that the CF labeling was no longer associated with the cells, but was confined solely to the acellular matrix. Also, the surface area showed small irregularities in the form of tufts, blisters, and small, shallow clefts, all of which were labeled with ferritin particles. There,

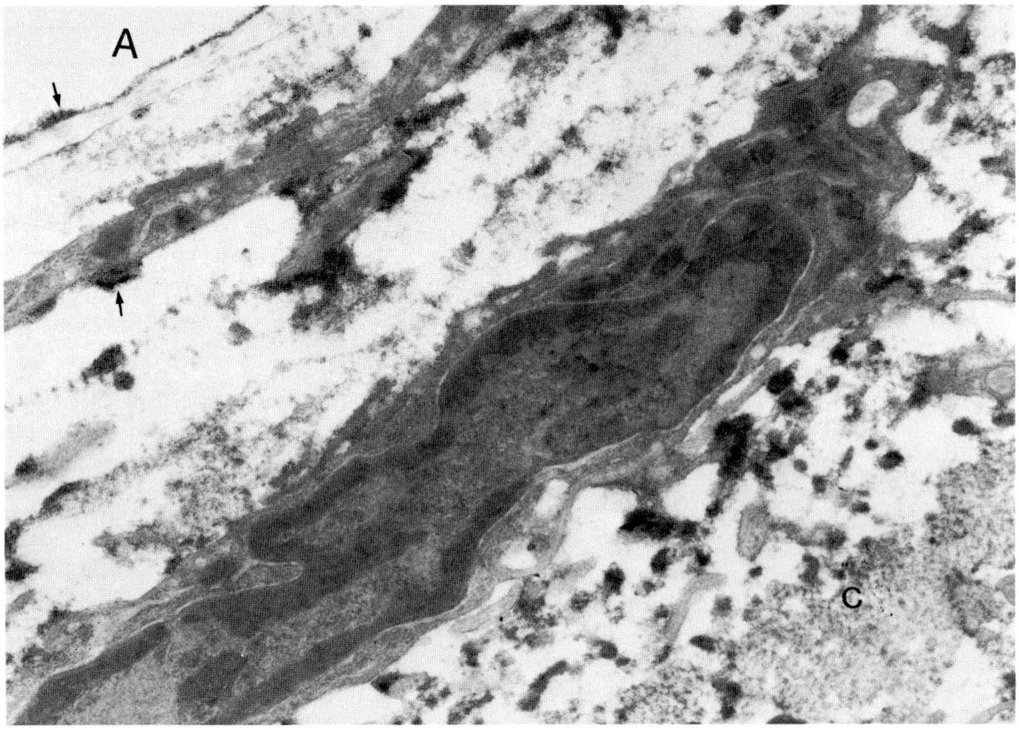

Figure 2. Electron micrograph of a part of the articular area (**A**) of the mandibular head of a 5-day-old mouse. Area was first labeled with cationized ferritin (CF), washed briefly, and subsequently fixed with Karnovsky's fixative. The CF particles are seen on the membrane surfaces of cells (**arrows**), in the matrix of the deeper layers, and on collagen fibers (**C**) (uranyl acetate and lead citrate stained, original magnification × 16,000).

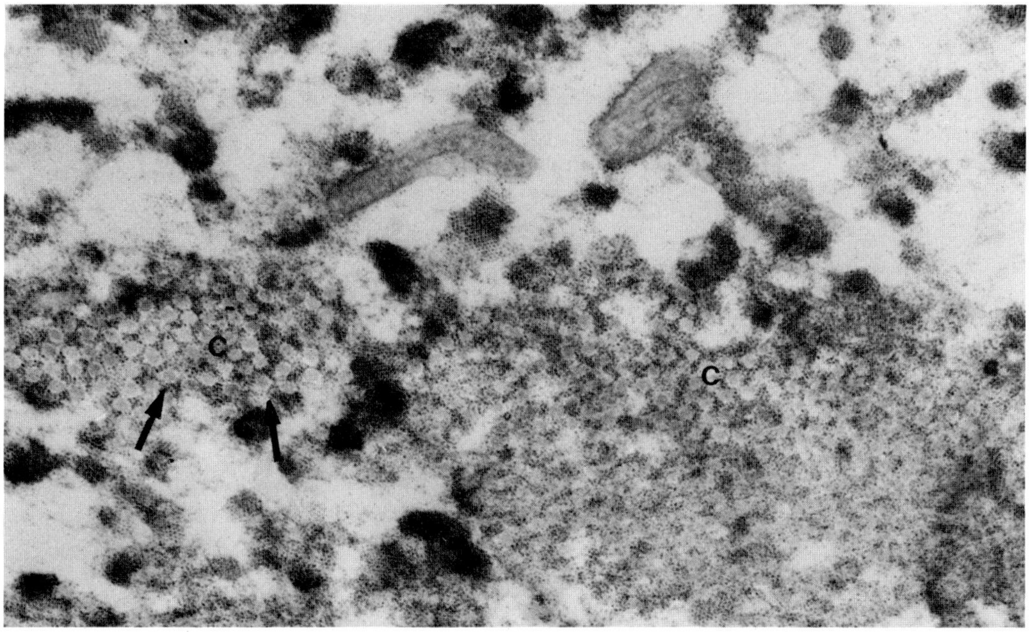

Figure 3. Electron micrograph of a part of the perichondrial zone of the mandibular head of a 5-day-old mouse. Area was labeled with cationized ferritin, washed briefly, and fixed in Karnovsky's fixative. The ferritin particles align with the collagen fibers (**C**) (**arrows**) (uranyl acetate and lead citrate stained, magnification × 60,000).

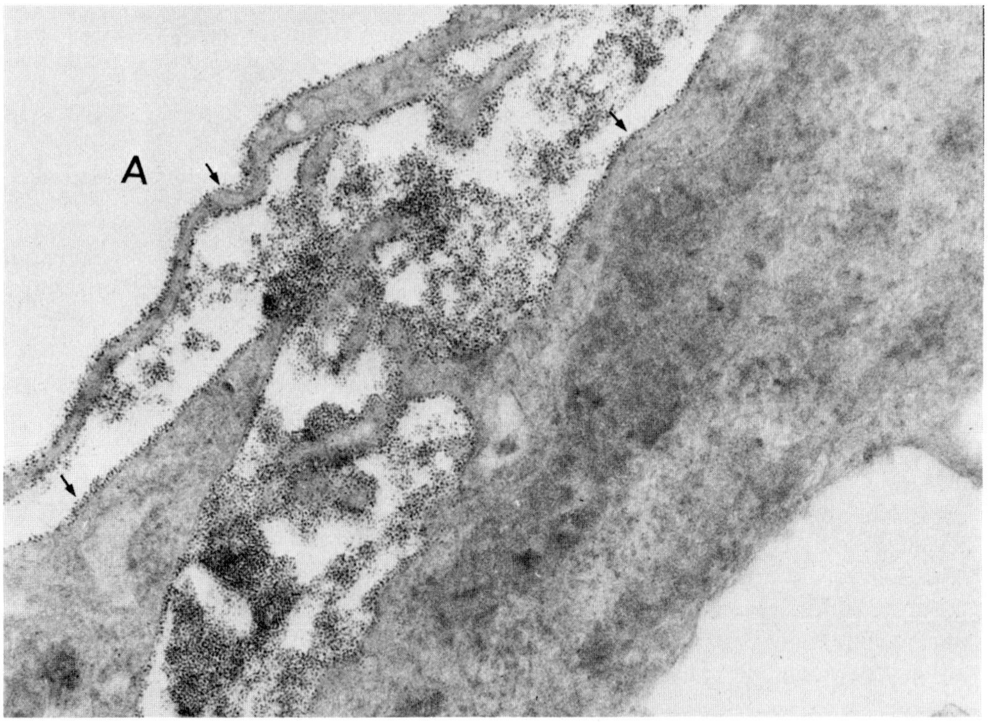

Figure 4. Electron micrograph of a part of the condylar cartilage of a 5-day-old mouse. The tissue was first fixed in Karnovsky's fixative, washed briefly, and only then labeled with cationized ferritin (CF). The ferritin particles are evenly distributed along the membrane surface of the cells (**arrows**). There is no penetration of CF particles into the deeper layers. A = articular surface (uranyl acetate and lead citrate stained, magnification × 45,000).

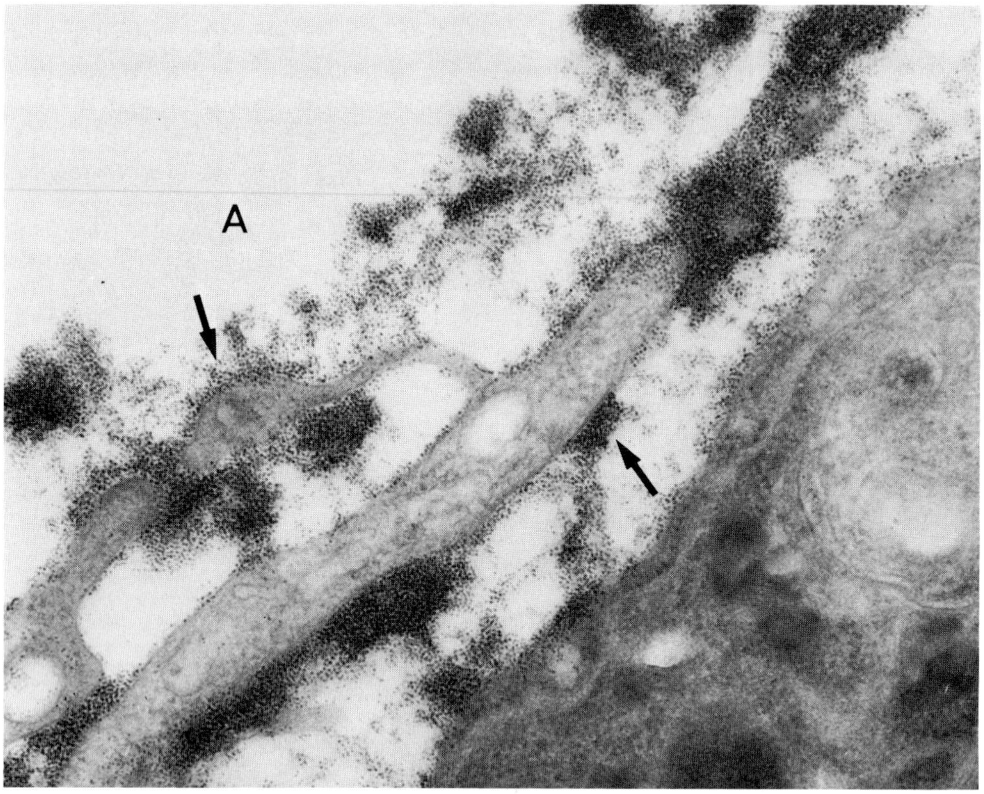

Figure 5. Electron micrograph of a part of the mandibular head cartilage of a 5-day-old mouse. Area was first labeled with cationized ferritin, washed briefly, and then fixed with Karnovsky's fixative. Note the distribution of the ferritin particles, forming clusters on the membrane surfaces of the cells (**arrows**). A = articular surface (uranyl acetate and lead citrate stained, magnification × 50,000).

again, the CF labeling was not affected by previous washings with either cacodylate buffer or distilled water.

During maturation and with the onset of aging, the superficial zone increased in size and comprised electron-dense material (Figure 8). By the end of the first year, the articular surface revealed signs of fibrillation. A consistent feature in this age group was a marked decrease in the width of the ferritin layer (Figure 9) in comparison with that noted in young-adults (Figure 7). In the mature mice, no ferritin particles could be detected beyond the superficial layer. In those cases where the articular surface was disrupted, the ferritin particles were confined only to the undamaged surface areas, whereas no particles could be detected in the adjacent clefts or cracks (Figure 10).

Colloidal iron labeling. Since the labeling procedure with CI was performed at pH 1.8, all tissues had to undergo fixation. At such an acidic pH, the CI particles were positively charged, while the sulfonic and sialic acids were negatively charged. Throughout our study, the CI particles were confined to the surface area, yet there was a substantial difference in the degree of labeling in specimens from neonatal mice versus those obtained from older mice. In neonatal condyles, the iron particles formed a rather dense and continuous layer, with occasional clusters (Figure 11), while in specimens from aged animals, the binding capacity for CI decreased markedly (Figure 12).

Effects of various enzymes on the binding of CF and CI onto the mandibular condylar surface. Treatment with neuraminidase and hyaluronidase for 30 and 60 minutes did not affect the binding capacity for CF in either neonatal or old mice. The CI binding, on the other hand, was completely abolished by the neuraminidase treatment. In contrast, pronase treatment (60 minutes) led to a remarkable change in the CF labeling in all age groups. Following pronase treatment, the articular surfaces in young-adult and older mice underwent dramatic structural changes and showed only a narrow layer of ferritin particles, con-

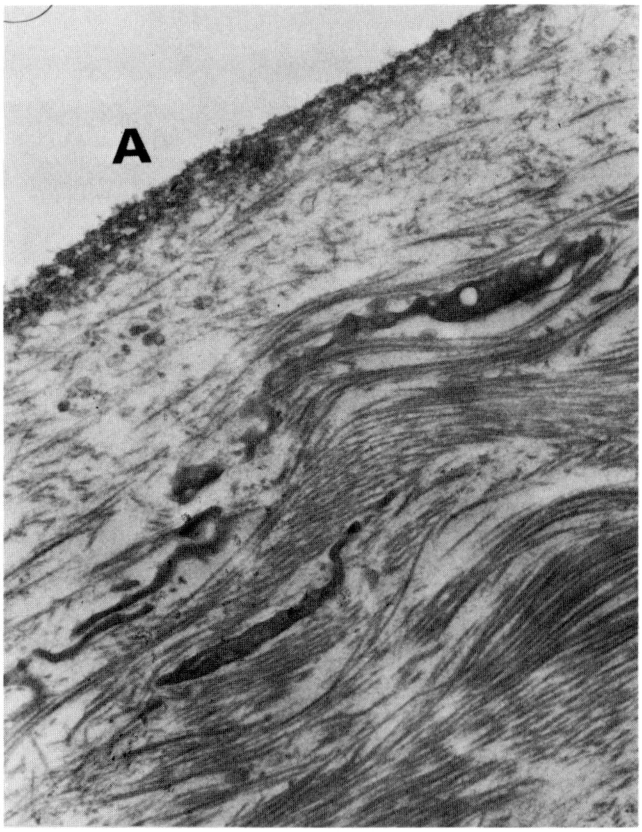

Figure 6. Electron micrograph of a part of the cartilage of the mandibular condyle (in Karnovsky's fixative) of a 2-month-old mouse. Note the well-defined layer of amorphous material at the surface. In the deeper layers, note the densely packed collagen fibers running parallel and tangentially to the surface. A = articular surface (uranyl acetate and lead citrate stained, magnification × 12,000).

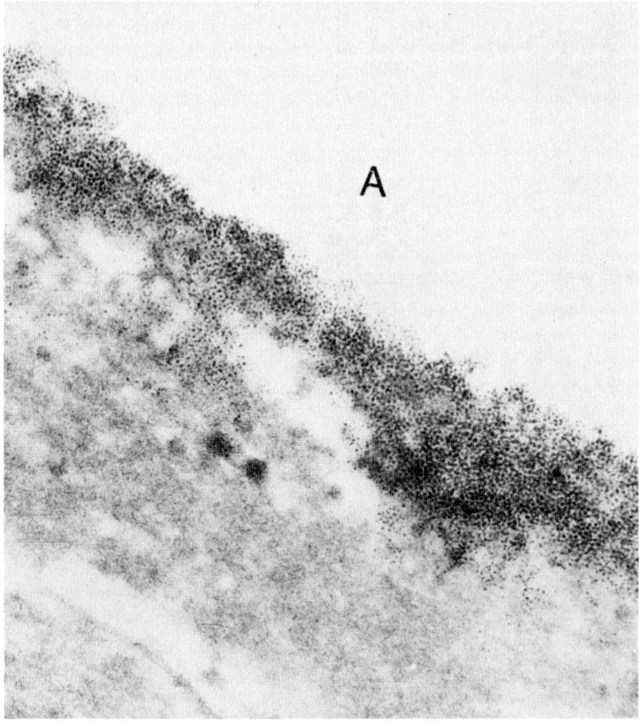

Figure 7. Electron micrograph of a part of the mandibular head of a 2-month-old mouse (in Karnovsky's fixative and labeled with cationized ferritin). A thick layer of ferritin particles is seen along the articular surface (**A**); no particles are seen underneath the surface area (uranyl acetate and lead citrate stained, magnification × 60,000).

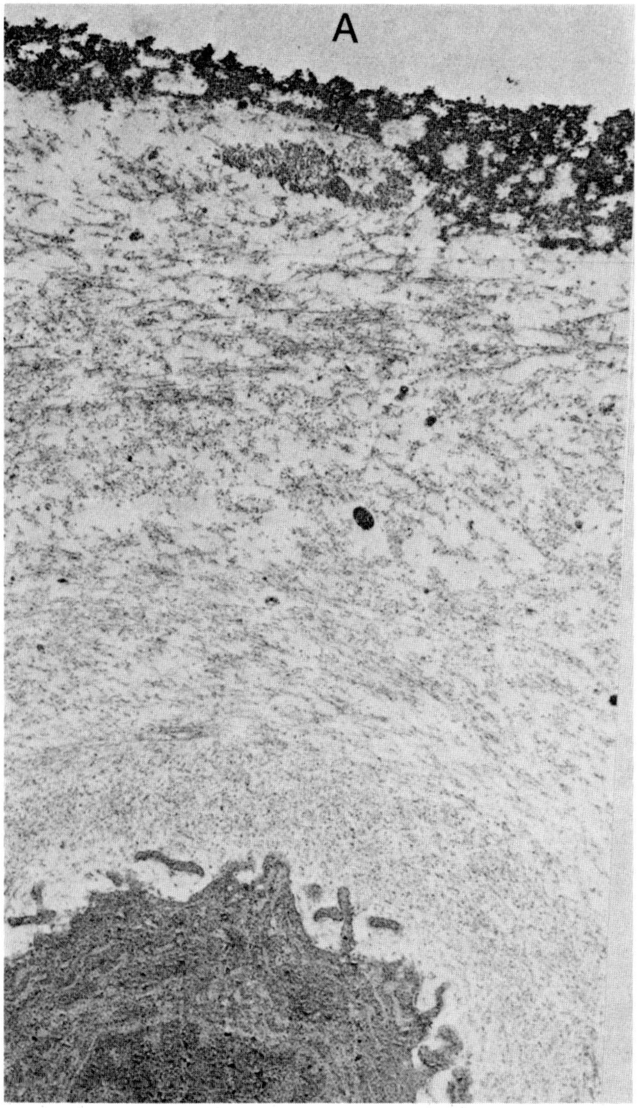

Figure 8. Electron micrograph of a part of the mandibular condyle of a 12-month-old mouse. Note the increased thickness of the most superficial layer compared with layer from 2-month-old mice seen in Figure 6. A = articular surface (uranyl acetate and lead citrate stained, magnification × 8,000).

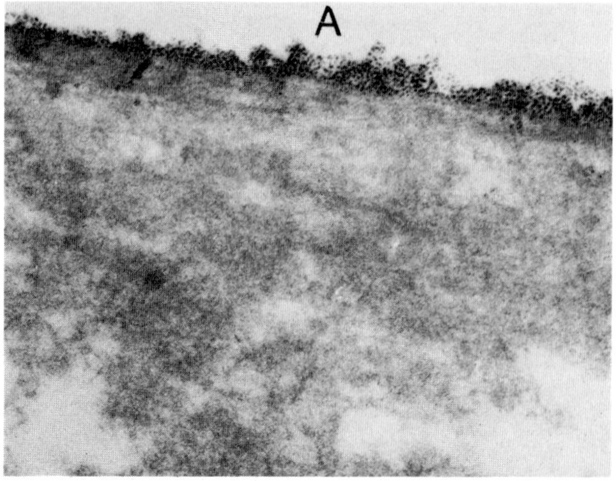

Figure 9. Electron micrograph of a part of the mandibular head of a 12-month-old mouse. Area was first fixed and then stained with cationized ferritin (CF). The binding capacity was diminished for CF compared with that of the 2-month-old mice (Figure 6). No CF particles could be seen beyond the surface. A = articular surface (uranyl acetate and lead citrate stained, magnification × 60,000).

It was consistently evident that the specimens from the neonatal mice were very sensitive to collagenase treatment, although pronase also caused marked derangements. Both enzymes provoked severe damage concomitant with many surface discontinuities and the presence of CF particles within the deeper layers of the tissue (Figure 13). Likewise, collagenase treatment also brought about marked changes in the labeling of CF. Following 60 minutes of collagenase treatment, most of the filamentous material and fibers beneath the articular surface were digested. The clusters of ferritin particles that were seen underneath the articular area were largest closest to the surface area and smaller at deeper levels within the tissue (Figure 14).

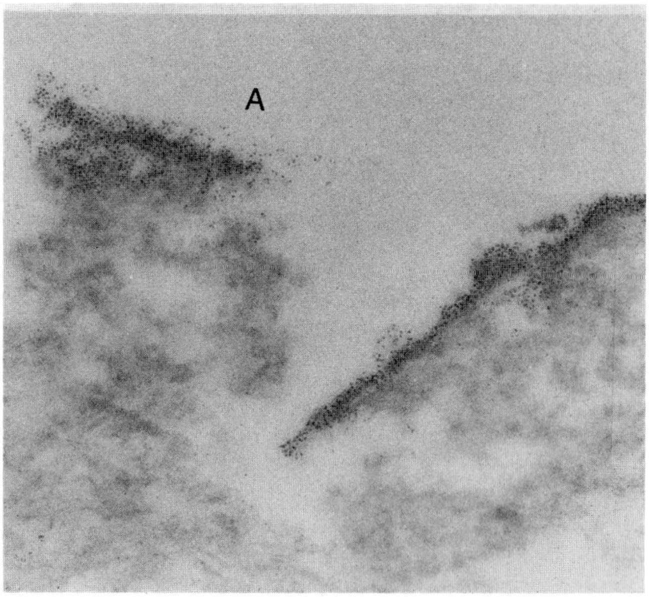

Figure 10. Electron micrograph of a part of the superficial layer of the mandibular condyle of a 12-month-old mouse. Area was fixed and stained with cationized ferritin (CF). The CF particles were confined to the surface, with no penetration into existing cracks along the articular surface (**A**) (uranyl acetate and lead citrate stained, original magnification × 60,000).

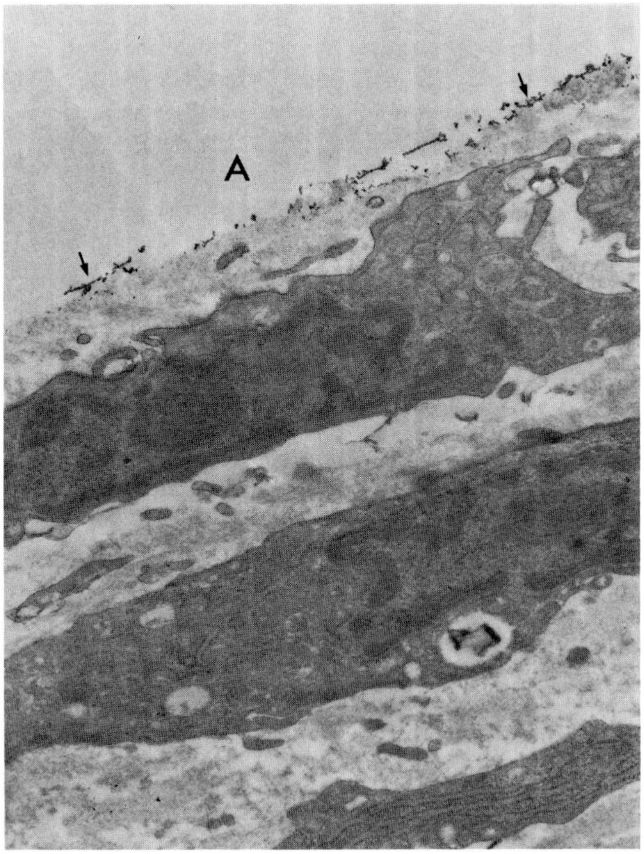

Figure 11. Electron micrograph of a part of the mandibular head cartilage of a 5-day-old mouse that was fixed and labeled with colloidal iron (CI). The CI particles appear in small clusters (**arrows**) that are randomly distributed over the articular surface (**A**). The CI particles were confined to the surface and could not be seen beyond the superficial layer (uranyl acetate and lead citrate stained, magnification × 12,000).

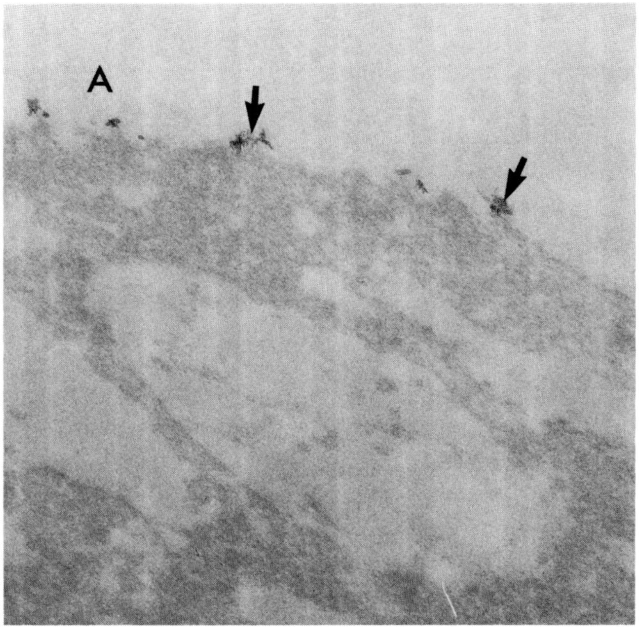

Figure 12. Electron micrograph of a part of the articular cartilage of the mandibular condyle of a 12-month-old mouse. Area was fixed and stained with colloidal iron (CI). Note the diminished binding capacity for CI (**arrows**) compared with younger mice (Figure 11). A = articular surface (uranyl acetate and lead citrate stained, magnification × 60,000).

age to the entire perichondrium, to the cells, and their intercellular matrix, thus enabling the ferritin particles to penetrate into the deeper layers of the cartilage. Similar enzyme treatment of fixed specimens did not affect the CF labeling pattern in any age group. In the present study, we did not perform any biochemical studies to assess which and how much of the various charge constituents were removed by the various enzymatic treatments.

DISCUSSION

The present ultrastructural study investigated the chemical nature of the articular surface of mandibular condyles by cytochemical methods using cationized ferritin and colloidal iron. Our results reiterate that the condylar articular surface is negatively charged and that prolonged washings of unfixed specimens with either buffer solution or distilled water do not adversely affect the binding capacity of either CF or CI. Hence, it seems reasonable to assume that the anionic sites along the condylar surface refer to actual structural elements, rather than to an absorbed film of synovial fluid (28).

Of interest was the finding that fixed specimens from neonatal mice revealed a different pattern of CF labeling when compared with unfixed tissues, suggesting that the labeling pattern in the unfixed specimens could be the result of a rearrangement of mobile sites, as has been suggested in regard to anionic sites on the surface of malignant cells (29) or vascular endothelium (30).

Furthermore, remarkable differences in both structure and labeling patterns were noted in cartilage from mature and old mice. In condyles of neonatal mice, one could not identify any distinct structure confining the joint surface, whereas in condyles of mature animals, the cartilages were covered by a distinct layer which was composed mostly of an electron-dense, amorphous material containing fine fila-

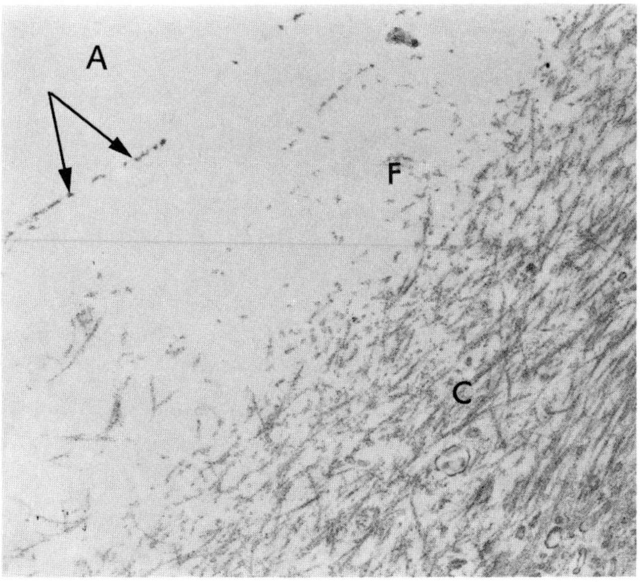

Figure 13. Electron micrograph of a pronase-treated articular cartilage of a 12-month-old mouse. Area was labeled with cationized ferritin (CF). Only a very narrow layer of ferritin particles (**arrows**) can be seen along the articular surface (**A**). Fine filaments (**F**) are seen underneath the surface area. With increasing depth, the collagen fibers (**C**) are densely packed. All constituents were labeled with CF (uranyl acetate and lead citrate stained, original magnification × 15,000).

ments. This kind of a developmental process appeared to further intensify with the aging of the animals.

However, the overall thickness of the ferritin particles layer, as well as its rate of penetration into the cartilaginous tissue, decreased with age. Hence, in neonatal mice the ferritin particles were noted both along the surface as well as within the deeper layers of the tissue, yet in older animals the ferritin and CI particles were confined solely to the superficial layer of the mandibular condyle.

It should be noted, however, that based on Danon's exclusion theory (30), positive CI particles may not enter the matrix and, therefore, may be localized on the surface at localized negative sites. Taking into consideration the above possibility, the present findings tend to suggest that with increasing age, the amount of negative charges over the articular surface is reduced, a feature that has been similarly reported in human specimens (31).

Ficat and Maroudas (21) have indicated that fibrillation of the articular cartilage is usually accompanied by a local reduction of fixed charge density and of glycosaminoglycans and, consequently, by a reduction in labeling when stained with CF and/or CI. A similar feature has been reported in cases of experimentally induced arthritis (32). It therefore seems logical to assume that the decrease in the concentration of negative charges of articular cartilages could be one of the first local biochemical changes that precede the onset of degenerative joint disease. It should be noted, however, that the latter studies referred to bulk density rather than to surface tissue charge density.

Condyles of old mice also experienced a decrease in the number of sialyl groups. It has been documented that old red blood cells (33) and endothelial cells in old animals (34) undergo similar changes with regard to their surface charge and sialic acid content. Thus, the sialic acid residues seem to play an important role in maintaining the cells' viability and functional capacity, and any factor affecting their number and/or distribution might enhance the development of cellular and tissue degeneration (35–37). Neuraminidase digestion, while removing almost all the CI particles, did not significantly affect the CF labeling, which could indicate that the tissue contains different carriers for anionic groups, such as aspartic or glutamic acids, that are insensitive to sialidase.

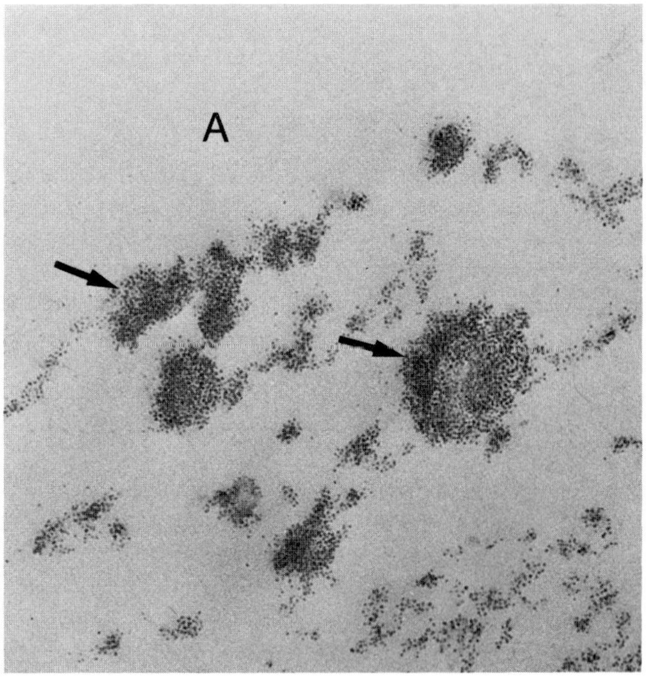

Figure 14. Electron micrograph of a collagenase-treated part of the mandibular condyle of a 12-month-old mouse. Area was labeled with cationized ferritin. Clusters of ferritin particles are seen, forming a discontinuous layer with numerous gaps at the articular surface. The clusters of ferritin (**arrows**) appear to relate to their size, so that the largest remain superficial and the smallest occur deeply. A = articular surface (uranyl acetate and lead citrate strained, magnification × 60,000).

Hyaluronidase, like neuraminidase, did not affect the CF labeling in any of the groups tested. These findings appear inconsistent with those of Appleton (6), who indicated that the mandibular joint contains a hyaluronate-protein layer that is bound to the articular surface, from which it can be removed by hyaluronidase treatment. Dearden et al (38) have reported that with aging, costal cartilages experience an increase in the amount of hyaluronidase-resistant material. It might, therefore, be possible that in the mandibular condyles of mice, hyaluronate contributes to the negative charges of the articular surface, but that the latter component is hyaluronidase-resistant. Pronase and collagenase induced substantial changes in both the morphology and the labeling pattern of the articular cartilage.

Despite the fact that both enzymes led to the disruption of the surface area, and thereby to the penetration of ferritin particles into deep layers within the cartilage, their effects appeared additive. Following collagenase treatment, ferritin clusters within the tissue showed a size-related gradient, whereby the largest aggregates remained superficial, while the smaller ones penetrated deeper into the tissue.

By and large, the present findings are in agreement with those of Ohno et al (10), who related intrinsic collagenase activity to cartilage pathology, and the distribution of degradable materials to their size. Moreover, collagenase digestion potentiates the penetration of high molecular weight substances into the tissue (39).

It is generally agreed that protease and collagenase are actively involved in the pathogenesis of joint diseases and, in particular, osteoarthritis. However, the origin of these enzymes and the degree of susceptibility to these enzymes are not as yet fully understood. Stephens et al (40) have hypothesized that the pathogenesis of osteoarthritis might, at least in part, be involved in the inability of chondrocytes to manufacture protease inhibitors that are normally found in cartilage. In considering the origin of collagenase in articular cartilage, one cannot exclude the synovial membrane, yet it seems reasonable to assume that in cases of osteoarthritis, collagenase might originate from an endogenous source (41). The fact that chondrocytes are capable of collagenase synthesis has been shown in an in vitro system (42).

Since the articular surface of the mandibular condyles of mice appears to be highly sensitive to both protease and collagenase, while being resistant to hyaluronidase and neuraminidase, it therefore seems likely that the most superficial layer of this articular cartilage comprises a proteinaceous-collagenous complex. The present study also gives clear indication of a marked difference in the permeability properties of aging cartilages, as well as changes in their labeling patterns using CF and CI. Alterations in the surface charge properties due to aging or mechanical or chemical factors may lead to changes in the structural and permeability properties of the articular cartilage and subsequently, to a series of destructive processes that are encountered more frequently in older humans.

ACKNOWLEDGMENTS

The authors wish to thank Matilda Brenman for technical assistance, Eli Engel for photographic work, and Ruth Singer for her excellent assistance in the preparation of this manuscript.

REFERENCES

1. Stockwell RA: Biology of Cartilage Cells. London, Cambridge University Press, 1979
2. Balazs EA, Bloom GD, Swann DA: Fine structure and glycosaminoglycan content of the surface layer of articular cartilage. Fed Proc 25:1813–1816, 1966
3. Weiss C, Rosenberg L, Helfet AJ: An ultrastructural study of normal young adult human articular cartilage. J Bone Joint Surg 50A:663–674, 1968
4. Venn M, Maroudas A: Chemical composition and swelling of normal and osteoarthritic femoral head cartilage. Ann Rheum Dis 36:555–563, 1977
5. Moskowitz RW: Cartilage and osteoarthritis: current concepts (editorial). J Rheumatol 4:329–331, 1977
6. Appleton J: The fine structure of a surface layer over the fibrous articular tissue of the rat mandibular condyle. Arch Oral Biol 23:719–723, 1978
7. Kimura H, Tateishi H, Ziff M: Surface ultrastructure of rheumatoid articular cartilage. Arthritis Rheum 20:1085–1098, 1977
8. Stockwell RA: Changes in the acid glycosaminoglycan content of the matrix of aging human articular cartilage. Ann Rheum Dis 29:509–515, 1970
9. Weiss C: Ultrastructural characteristics of osteoarthritis. Fed Proc 32:1459–1466, 1973
10. Ohno O, Tateishi H, Cooke D: Pathogenesis of chronic inflammation in experimental ferritin-induced arthritis. Arthritis Rheum 21:81–91, 1978
11. Moskowitz RW: Clinical and laboratory findings in osteoarthritis, Arthritis and Allied Conditions. Ninth edition. Edited by DJ McCarty. Philadelphia, Lea & Febiger, 1979, pp 1161–1180
12. Bonner WM, Jonsson H, Malanos C, Bryant M: Changes in the lipids of human articular cartilage with age. Arthritis Rheum 18:461–473, 1975

13. Shitama K: Calcification of aging articular cartilage in man. Acta Orthop Scand 50:613–619, 1979
14. Roughley PJ, White RJ: Age-related changes in the structure of the proteoglycan subunits from human articular cartilage. J Biol Chem 255:217–224, 1980
15. Moffet BC, McCabe JB: Histologic age changes in adult human temporomandibular joints (abstract). Anat Rec 142:259, 1962
16. Silbermann M, Livne E: Age-related degenerative changes in the mouse mandibular joint. J Anat 129:507–520, 1979
17. Silberberg R, Silberberg M, Volgel A, Wettstein W: Ultrastructure of articular cartilage of mice of various ages. Am J Anat 109:251–275, 1961
18. Silberberg M, Silberberg R: Age changes of bones and joints in various strains of mice. Am J Anat 68:69–95, 1941
19. Sokoloff L: Nature of degenerative joint disease in small laboratory animals. I. Pathological anatomy of degenerative joint disease in mice. Arch Pathol Lab Med 62:118–128, 1956
20. Silbermann M: Experimentally induced osteoarthritis in the temporomandibular joint of the mouse. Acta Anat (Basel) 96:9–24, 1976
21. Ficat C, Maroudas A: Cartilage of the patella: topographical variations of glycosaminoglycan content in normal and fibrillated tissue. Ann Rheum Dis 34:515–519, 1975
22. Thompson RC, Oegema TR: Metabolic activity of articular cartilage in osteoarthritis: in vitro study. J Bone Joint Surg 61A:407–416, 1979
23. Danon D, Goldstein L, Marikovsky Y, Skutelsky E: Use of cationized ferritin as a label of negative charges on cell surface. J Ultrastruct Res 38:500–510, 1972
24. Gasic GJ, Berwick L, Sorrentino M: Positive and negative collidal iron and a cell-surface electron stain. Lab Invest 18:63–71, 1968
25. Stanescu R, Leibovich SJ: The negative charge of articular cartilage surfaces. J Bone Joint Surg 64A:388–398, 1982
26. Karnovsky MJ: A formaldehyde-glutaraldehyde fixative of high osmolarity for use in electron microscopy (abstract). J Cell Biol 27:137a, 1965
27. Reynolds ES: The use of lead citrate at high pH as an electron-opaque stain in electron microscopy. J Cell Biol 17:208–212, 1963
28. Swann DA: Macromolecules of synovial fluid, Joints and Synovial Fluid. Edited by L Sokoloff. New York, Academic Press, 1978, pp 407–435
29. Marikovsky Y, Inbar M, Danon D, Sachs L: Distribution of surface charge and concanavalin A-binding sites on normal and malignant transformed cells. Exp Cell Res 89:359–367, 1974
30. Danon D, Laver-Rudich Z, Skutelsky E: Surface charge properties of endothelium of the aorta in young and old animals. Rheinisch-Westfälische Akademie der Wissenschaften Westdeutscher-Verlag 63:541–552, 1978
31. Stockwell RA, Scott JC: Observations on the acid glycosaminoglycan (mucopolysaccharide) content of the matrix of aging cartilage. Ann Rheum Dis 24:341–350, 1965
32. McDevitt CA, Muir H: Biochemical changes in the cartilage of the knee in experimental and natural osteoarthritis in the dog. J Bone Joint Surg 58B:94–101, 1976
33. Yaari A: Mobility of human red blood cells of different age groups in electric field. Blood 33:159–165, 1969
34. Laver-Rudich Z, Skutelsky E, Danon D: Age-related changes in aortic intima of rats. J Gerontol 33:337–346, 1978
35. Durocher JR, Rayne RC, Conrad ME: Role of sialic acid in erythrocyte survival. Blood 45:11–21, 1975
36. Gattegno L, Bladier D, Cornillot T: The role of sialic acid in the determination of survival of rabbit erythrocytes in the circulation. Carbohydr Res 34:361–369, 1974
37. Jancik J, Schauer R: Sialic acid: a determination of the lifetime of rabbit erythrocytes. Hoppe Seylers Z Physiol Chem 355:385–400, 1974
38. Dearden LC, Bonucci E, Cuicchio M: An investigation of aging in human costal cartilage. Cell Tissue Res 152:305–337, 1974
39. Lotke PA, Granda JL: Alterations in the permeability of articular cartilage by proteolytic enzymes. Arthritis Rheum 15:302–308, 1972
40. Stephens RW, Ghoch P, Taylor TKF: The pathogenesis of osteoarthritis. Med Hypotheses 5:809–816, 1979
41. Harris ED Jr, Cohen GL, Krane SM: Synovial collagenase: its presence in culture from joint disease of diverse etiology. Arthritis Rheum 12:92–102, 1969
42. Ehrlich MG, Mankin HJ, Jones H, Wright R, Crispen C, Vigliana G: Collagenase and collagenase inhibitors in osteoarthritic and hormonal human cartilage. J Clin Invest 59:226–233, 1977

EFFECTIVENESS OF CYCLOSPORIN THERAPY FOR BEHÇET'S DISEASE

ROBERT B. NUSSENBLATT, ALAN G. PALESTINE, CHI-CHAO CHAN, MANABU MOCHIZUKI, and KIM YANCEY

Behçet's disease is a clinical entity with mouth and genital ulcers, skin lesions, and both anterior and posterior uveitis as its major criteria. It has been theorized that Behçet's disease is immune complex mediated, and is characterized by multiple attacks which often lead to severe visual handicap. Behçet's disease patients with severe ocular involvement and cytotoxic and/or systemic corticosteroid agent failures were treated with cyclosporin (CsA). CsA therapy effectively abrogated the acute phase of the ocular attack and either totally prevented, or markedly reduced, the recurrences of these attacks. Generally, patients tolerated the medication well; occasionally however, renal toxicity secondary to cyclosporin therapy prevented prescription of a maximally effective therapeutic dose of the drug. CsA levels in plasma were dose-dependent for each patient, but the dosage per kg of CsA needed to obtain a specific plasma level varied greatly from patient to patient. Circulating immune complex levels were not universally elevated during the acute ocular attack. However, increases in circulating immune complex concentrations were noted after treatment with CsA was begun and the disease became clinically inactive. These data, as well as the effectiveness of CsA, an agent with predominantly anti–T cell effects, raise a question as to whether circulating immune complexes are centrally relevant to the pathogenesis of this disorder, and if T cell mediation of this disease must be contemplated.

From the National Eye Institute, Clinical Ophthalmic Immunology and Experimental Immunology Sections and the National Cancer Institute, Dermatology Branch, Bethesda, Maryland.

Robert B. Nussenblatt, MD; Alan G. Palestine, MD; Chi-Chao Chan, MD; Manabu Mochizuki, MD; Kim Yancey, MD.

Address reprint requests to Robert B. Nussenblatt, MD, National Institutes of Health, National Eye Institute, Bldg. 10, Rm. 10N202, Bethesda, MD 20205.

Submitted for publication June 11, 1984; accepted in revised form December 12, 1984.

Behçet's disease is a disorder involving many organ systems. Though these symptoms were known in ancient times, a Turkish dermatologist, Hulusi Behçet, was the first to recognize recurrent intraocular inflammatory disease associated with mouth and genital ulcers as a distinct entity (1). The customarily followed criteria for the diagnosis of Behçet's disease are those outlined by the Behçet Syndrome Research Committee of Japan (2), which include skin manifestations as a major criteria.

Though relatively uncommon in the United States, Behçet's disease is the most common form of endogenous uveitis seen in many Japanese ophthalmology clinics and is a serious problem in countries bordering the Mediterranean Sea (3). Severe visual impairment is secondary to multiple ocular attacks involving the posterior segment of the eye, whereas attacks of the anterior segment alone generally do not result in visual loss (4). Posterior pole involvement is more common in men. The proposed therapies for this sight-threatening disorder have been varied, reflecting, perhaps, the frequently unsatisfactory therapeutic responses. Mamo and Azzam (5), as well as others (6), have suggested that cytotoxic agents, particularly chlorambucil, were effective in the treatment of this disorder. O'Duffy and colleagues (7) reported an improvement in visual acuity in 5 of 7 eyes in patients treated with chlorambucil. However, a recent report by Tabbara (8) would suggest that this is not the case. Presently, the standard therapy in Japan has been colchicine, which has been noted to decrease the number of ocular attacks (9).

The underlying mechanisms of action in this multi-organ disease still remain conjectural. The hypotheses have included environmental, as well as endogenous, causes (4). It has been suggested that the ocular component of this disease is immune complex mediated (10). We have demonstrated that circulating lymphocytes from patients with this disease have positive in vitro cell-mediated immune responses to retinal antigens (11), including the uveitogenic retinal S antigen. Our finding that experimental autoimmune uveitis, induced by the retinal S antigen, was totally abrograted by cyclosporin (11) suggested that this agent might be beneficial in certain uveitic entities. We report here our experience with cyclosporin, an agent that appears to affect the T cell predominantly (12), in the treatment of this entity.

PATIENTS AND METHODS

Patients. Seven patients with Behçet's disease are described. All patients entered a National Institutes of Health program, IND #16451, for the therapy of endogenous uveitis and gave written consent before therapy commenced. The criteria utilized for the diagnosis of the disease were those outlined in reference 2. Three of the patients had the complete type of the disease; 4 patients with 3 of the major symptoms (including intra-ocular inflammatory disease) had the incomplete type of the entity. All patients had posterior pole manifestations of their disease and all previously had received either cytotoxic or systemic oral corticosteroid (40–60 mg/day) therapy, or both and were considered therapeutic failures either because of poor control of their ocular disease or because of side effects. Additionally, all patients were admitted into the study only during active intra-ocular inflammatory disease.

Standard laboratory tests to evaluate renal, hematopoietic, and hepatic function were performed. All patients received a standard ocular evaluation, which included a slit lamp examination, and an examination while the pupils were dilated, which included evaluation of the posterior pole with either a Hruby lens, contact lens, or indirect ophthalmoscopy. Ocular inflammatory activity for the anterior and posterior segment was judged on the basis of previously reported criteria (13,14). Patients entering the study received 10 mg/kg/day of cyclosporin, orally. Patients previously taking cytotoxic agents had at least 2 weeks of a "washout" period before beginning cyclosporin. In patients who were taking systemic corticosteroids at study entry, these drugs were tapered as rapidly as was medically indicated. All patients were initially treated only with cyclosporin.

Immune complex determination. Both the Raji cell assay and C1q assay were utilized in the determination of circulating immune complexes. Sera were drawn from patients before and after initiation of cyclosporin therapy. The pre-cyclosporin sera were always drawn during an acute attack. Raji cell radioimmunoassays for the detection of IgG and IgA containing circulating immune complexes (CIC) were performed using previously described techniques (15–17). All serum samples were tested in duplicate. Statistical analysis of immune complex data was performed using a modification of the method of Woodroffe et al (18). Briefly, a daily 95% upper confidence limit (U_i—in counts per minute) is developed with a panel of normal controls. The mean of duplicate values of each test serum (T_i—in cpm) is divided by U_i. If this ratio ($T_i:U_i$) is greater than 1.0, the value of the test sample exceeds the 95% upper confidence limit and is considered abnormal.

The ^{125}I-C1q binding assay for the detection of IgG or IgM containing circulating immune complexes was performed using previously described techniques (1). The 95% upper confidence limit of C1q binding activity in normal human sera in this assay is 10%.

In vitro proliferation responses to the retinal S antigen. In vitro responses to the retinal S antigen were determined by methodology reported elsewhere (11). Briefly, 2×10^5 cells in 0.2 cc of medium per microtiter well (Falcon, Oxnard, CA) were incubated for 5 days in the presence of S antigen (5 mg/ml), with tritiated thymidine added 14 hours before the termination of culture. The proliferative responses are presented as stimulation indices. A stimulation index >2 has been calculated to fall beyond twice the standard deviation obtained from cultures of lymphocytes from controls. These results are therefore beyond the 95% confidence limits established, and were considered to be significant responses.

Plasma cyclosporin concentration. Plasma cyclosporin levels were measured in heparinized blood samples obtained at the trough period, i.e., 24 hours after the last ingestion of the medication. These specimens were equilibrated at room temperature for 1 hour and centrifuged at 2,000 rpm at 25°C. The plasma was removed and immediately frozen at −25°C. The determination of the cyclosporin present was performed using Sandimmune radioimmunoassay kits. Samples were diluted 1:10 and 100 μl was added to 100 μl of anti-CsA antibody and 0.7 ml of Tris buffer, pH 8.4. One hundred microliters of tritiated CsA tracer was added and the assay was incubated for 2 hours at room temperature.

The specimens were then placed in a 40°C water bath for 15 minutes. A mixture of 0.5 cc of 1% charcoal and 0.5% human serum was added, the specimens were incubated for 12 minutes, and centrifuged at 2,500 rpm. One milliliter of the supernatant was removed and counted in a gamma counter. A standard curve was prepared with each assay and a logit best fit line was determined. Patient plasma levels were then determined by interpolation with the standard curves. Plasma levels of 50–200 ng/ml are considered to be within therapeutic range, as recently reported (19).

RESULTS

Seven patients meeting the criteria for either the complete or incomplete form of Behçet's disease were enrolled in the study. A synopsis of the pertinent clinical and therapeutic findings is seen in Tables 1 and 2. Although none of the patients was oriental, patient 1 was of Greek ancestry, an ethnic group considered to have a higher prevalence of this disease. Of the

Table 1. National Eye Institute patients with Behçet's disease treated with cyclosporin (CsA)

Patient (age/sex)	Pre-CsA visual acuity	Duration and frequency of ocular attacks	In vitro S antigen response	Previous drug therapy
1 (35/M)	20/70 20/400	10 years, every 3 weeks	Positive	Prednisone, chlorambucil
2 (36/M)	20/30 20/70	2 years, every 2 months	Positive	Prednisone, chlorambucil
3 (32/F)	20/70 20/40	5 years, every 2–3 months	Positive	Prednisone, chlorambucil
4 (41/M)	Light perception 20/200	10 years, smoldering with exacerbations	Positive	Prednisone, chlorambucil
5 (25/M)	20/60 20/400	2 years, every 6 months	Negative	Prednisone, panretinol photocoagulation (left eye), chlorambucil
6 (32/F)	20/70 CF2'*	3 years, every 2 weeks	Negative	Prednisone
7 (22/F)	20/40 20/40	2 years, smoldering with exacerbations	Negative	Prednisone, chlorambucil

* Counting fingers at 2 feet.

remaining 6 patients, 5 were of northern European extraction, and 1 was Hispanic. All of the patients had been having ocular attacks on frequent, recurrent bases. The use of cyclosporin as the sole systemic agent for their uveitis led to a rapid decrease in their ocular inflammatory responses. Additionally, patients noted a rapid increase in their visual acuity, sometimes quite dramatic, as in patient 6 whose visual acuity went from counting fingers at 2 feet to 20/25 within 1 week's time. Patient 1, who presented with a hypopyon uveitis, as well as posterior pole involvement, was noted to have resolution of his hypopyon in 2 days, while the usual course of his previous anterior segment attacks took well over a week to resolve with alternative therapy.

The number of ocular attacks in these patients has diminished markedly over the average interval of 13 months that the patients have been receiving cyclosporin. Four patients have had no attacks while receiving cyclosporin, while 3 others have had ocular attacks, including 1 patient with a mild vitreal response. This was in marked distinction to the multiple attacks that these patients suffered with previous medications. Attempts to discontinue cyclosporin in 3 patients resulted in a recurrence of an ocular attack within 2–14 days.

Those patients with the non-ocular complications of Behçet's disease at the initiation of cyclosporin therapy noted an improvement in these conditions as well. Mouth ulcers were noted to decrease in number and severity. Patients have noted having occasional mouth ulcers while being free of any ocular inflammatory activity. Patient 1 noted complete improvement of severe arthritic complaints which had been associated with his uveitis. Patient 3 had resolution of vaginal ulcers which had previously been refractory to therapy.

Fluorescein angiography. Though all patients noted an improvement in visual acuity, the fluorescein angiographic findings after the initiation of cyclosporin varied considerably. Some patients were noted to have a marked improvement in retinal vascular leakage associated with their increase in visual acuity. However, others were noted to have an increase in visual acuity with continued leakage detected by fluorescein angiographic examinations.

In vitro responses to the S antigen. Four of the 7 patients had positive in vitro cell-mediated responses to the S antigen. Their clinical courses have not appeared to be different from the courses of patients who did not have positive responses initially.

Determination of circulating immune complexes. Circulating immune complexes were looked for in the sera of patients during an acute ocular attack before cyclosporin therapy, and when their ocular conditions became quiescent while they were receiving cyclosporin. The results can be seen in Table 3.

The patients with acute ocular attacks did not have elevated levels of circulating immune complexes. Only patient 3 had elevated immune complexes determined by the C1q binding assay; patient 2's level was borderline. Changes in the level of circulating immune

Table 2. Effects of cyclosporin (CsA) therapy on patients with Behçet's disease

Patient	Best vision post-CsA therapy	Duration of CsA therapy (months)	Side effects attributable to CsA therapy	Ocular attacks with CsA	Average CsA dose	Serum creatinine levels with CsA
1	20/50–70 20/200	21	Gingivitis, anemia, hirsutism	None, 1 attack while not taking CsA	7 mg/kg	1.4
2	20/25 20/30	17	Hirsutism	Mild vitritis while decreasing dose with no change in visual acuity	4–5 mg/kg	1.3
3	20/20 20/20	15	Hirsutism, hidradenitis, epigastric discomfort	0	6.5 mg/kg	1.4
4	Light perception 20/40 (4/83) 20/60 (9/83)	13	Increased serum creatinine	1 while not taking CsA, smoldering at lower dose	3 mg/kg, 20 mg prednisone	2.5
5	20/15 20/100	8	Transient hypertension, fatigue, decreased appetite, scrotal abscess(?)	0	9 mg/kg	1.2
6	20/15 20/25	9	Tingling of extremities	1	10 mg/kg	1.3
7	20/16 20/25	6	None	0	10 mg/kg	1.1

complexes were noted, however, after cyclosporin therapy was initiated. Patient 1 was noted to have an increase in circulating immune complexes by all of the assays utilized, thereby suggesting that immune complexes bearing IgA, IgG, and IgM were possibly present. Patient 4 was found to have an almost fourfold increase in the level of circulating immune complexes using the C1q binding assay. Patient 3, who was found to have elevated circulating immune complexes on the basis of the C1q binding assay, was noted to have a similar level after the initiation of cyclosporin therapy.

Plasma cyclosporin levels. Plasma cyclosporin levels were determined 24 hours after the last ingestion of cyclosporin. These trough levels are shown on Table 4. The level of cyclosporin in plasma appeared to be dose-dependent for each patient. However, the amount of cyclosporin present for each cyclosporin dose per kg varied to some degree from patient to patient. Levels for all patients fell within the generally accepted guidelines for the proper therapeutic concentration of cyclosporin.

Secondary effects of cyclosporin. To date, none of the patients has required discontinuation of cyclosporin because of secondary effects of the drug. Gingivitis and hypertrichosis were the most common secondary effects seen in this group of patients. Additionally, a transient fatigue and tingling of extremities were also noted, these being previously reported in other uveitis patients treated with cyclosporin (20). An increase in the serum creatinine level was noted in patient 4, who has a horseshoe kidney. This patient's renal function appeared to be exquisitely sensitive to cyclosporin. He required frequent changes of dosage and ultimately was administered a dosage of cyclosporin far below that of the therapeutic optimum, accompanied by the addition of prednisone (see case report). The other patients, however, continued to receive only cyclosporin.

Case report: patient 7. This 22-year-old woman began to note difficulties with her left eye in February 1983. At that time, a nongranulomatous iritis was

Table 3. Circulating immune complex determinations in Behçet's disease patients

Patient	Raji cell assay (IgA)*		Raji cell assay (IgG)		C1q binding assay (%)†	
	Pre-CsA	Post-CsA	Pre-CsA	Post-CsA	Pre-CsA	Post-CsA
1	0.72	1.08	0.69	1.12	7.0	23.9
2	0.73	0.89	0.44	0.46	10.3	4.0
3	0.58	0.65	0.62	0.66	19.4	15.5
4	0.62	0.66	0.49	0.43	8.7	34.1
5	0.59	0.62	0.53	0.61	3.0	3.7
6	0.56	0.79	0.44	0.63	5.8	8.1
7	ND	ND	ND	ND	ND	ND

* Values >1.0 considered elevated. CsA = cyclosporin; ND = not done.
† Values >10% binding considered elevated.

Table 4. Plasma cyclosporin (CsA) levels of Behçet's disease patients

Patient	Date	CsA level (ng/ml)	CsA dose (mg/kg)	Date CsA therapy begun
1	6/83	150	14	3/82
	8/83	90	15	
	12/83	52	15	
2	7/83	167	10	8/82
	12/83	91	4.5	
3	2/83	89	4.5	10/82
	12/83	17	4.5	
4	1/83	233	10	1/83
	3/83	130	9	
	3/83	200	5	
	4/83	93	2.5	
	4/83	54	3	
	8/83	66	3.5	
	1/84	91	3	
5	6/83	243	10	5/83
	9/83	104	8.5	
	1/84	119	8.5	
6	9/83	70	10	8/83
	11/83	92	8.5	
	2/84	137	10	
			15	
7	5/84	88	10	3/84
	6/84	89	10	
	9/84	49	10	

noted in that eye. She was initially treated with topical corticosteroid and mydriatic therapy. In spite of this therapy, when she was seen again 5 days later, she had developed a bilateral anterior and posterior uveitis with retinal vasculitis in both eyes and neovascularization of the right optic disc. At the same time oral and vaginal ulcers were present and a diagnosis of Behçet's disease was made.

In mid-February 1983, she received an injection of 1 cc of Kenalog subconjunctivally in the left eye because of the severe vitreal and posterior pole involvement, including cystoid macula edema. Because of her poor response to topical and local therapy, oral corticosteroids were prescribed in late February and she did well until April of 1983, when examination of the eyes revealed numerous white retinal lesions in her right eye.

The patient was evaluated for cytomegalovirus but titers were not supportive of this diagnosis. She continued to receive 40 mg of prednisone every other day, as well as topical mydriatics and corticosteroids. In May 1983, oral chlorambucil (6 mg daily) was prescribed and her oral corticosteroids were reduced to 30 mg every other day.

By the middle of May she had developed a vitreous hemorrhage in the right eye, which originated from her disc neovascularization. This ultimately cleared by early June and the patient underwent panretinal photocoagulation treatment in the right eye. No further vitreal hemorrhages were noted. However, her inflammatory disease waxed and waned in spite of continued systemic therapy, as well as repeated subconjunctival injections of corticosteroids. Cystoid macula edema was a chronic problem in both eyes and was not controlled by therapy. Chlorambucil was discontinued in early March 1984 because of inefficacy. This was accompanied by a gradual reduction of her prednisone dosage as well. She was again noted to have episodes of numerous vaginal ulcers and multiple ocular flares, leading to secondary glaucoma. The intra-ocular pressure was poorly controlled with medication for glaucoma, and surgery could not be considered because of the active ocular inflammatory state. Her vision was 20/40 in both eyes and she had bilateral cystoid macula edema with a vitreal reaction.

The patient began taking 650 mg of cyclosporin daily (10 mg/kg/day) on March 23, 1984, and her vision improved to 20/20 in the right eye and 20/25 in the left after 10 days of therapy. Additionally, active skin ulcers with pustules disappeared. The patient was averaging approximately 1 ocular attack every 2 weeks prior to therapy and has not had an attack since she started taking cyclosporin, with a 6-month followup. Additionally, after she had taken the medication for approximately 1 month, her macula edema began to disappear. She was also able to undergo filtering surgery in both eyes for her glaucoma. Since that time her intra-ocular pressure has been normal without any medication. By September 1984, the visual acuity in her right eye had improved to 20/16 −1 with a near vision of J1+. The anterior segment had no inflammatory disease while the vitreous had a very occasional cell with no haze. The fundus showed no evidence of cystoid macula edema. The patient is receiving a maintenance dosage of 650 mg/day of cyclosporin.

Case report: patient 4. This 41-year-old Hispanic man first developed painful mouth ulcers which required morphine in 1970. Approximately 3 months after this episode, he developed a severe retinitis in the right eye and vitritis in the left. He was treated with systemic corticosteroids and his ocular condition improved. Over the ensuing 4 years he suffered multiple ocular inflammatory attacks which led to a progressive decrease in visual acuity in both eyes.

In 1974, because of the increasing number of ocular attacks, a thorough evaluation was made which excluded toxoplasmosis, histoplasmosis, syphilis, tuberculosis, sarcoidosis, and diabetes as possible causes of his ocular disease, but did reveal a horseshoe kidney and intermittent hypertension (155/110).

From 1975–1976, because of the continuing ocular attacks, he had therapeutic trials of cyclophosphamide and chlorambucil, with a minimal effect. Subsequently, the patient underwent cataract surgery (January 1977, right eye; April 1977, left eye). The ocular flares continued monthly, including hypopyon uveitis, as well as multiple bouts of mouth ulcers and arthritic complaints which were treated with systemic corticosteroids and antibiotics. The multiple attacks in the right eye ultimately resulted in optic atrophy in that eye with a best visual acuity of 20/400.

The patient was first seen at the National Eye Institute in January 1983, because of an exacerbation of ocular inflammatory disease in his left eye. His visual acuity in the left eye at that time was 20/200 (near vision J8) and he was taking 100 mg of prednisone daily. The vitreous cavity had 3+ cells and debris, while there was 3+ disc pallor in the right eye and a normal disc on the left. There was a markedly atrophic-appearing retina in the right eye while the left eye appeared to have cotton wool spots and hemorrhages surrounding the disc, as well as arterial sheathing.

Cyclosporin (10 mg/kg/day) was begun while his prednisone was tapered. His serum creatinine level was 1.3 mg/dl. Ten days after cyclosporin therapy was started, the visual acuity in the right eye remained at light perception and vision in his left eye had improved to 20/80. There were trace to 1+ cells and haze in the left vitreal cavity. No cystoid macula edema nor any hemorrhages or exudates were apparent. In March 1983, the patient was noted to have a visual acuity of 20/50 +1 in the left eye with a near vision of J3. The serum creatinine level was elevated to 2.2 mg/dl. The patient's cyclosporin dosage was decreased sequentially from 7 mg/kg/day to 2.5 mg/kg/day because of serum creatinine levels of 2.0 and a creatinine clearance of <50 ml/minute. His visual acuity stabilized at 20/40 and there were no ocular attacks. Cyclosporin therapy was discontinued in April 1983 when the patient's serum creatinine level was 2.5 mg/dl.

Two days after discontinuation of the drug, the patient noted a marked drop in visual acuity in his left eye (20/200) and a severe inflammatory response was noted. Cyclosporin was restarted at 3 mg/kg/day, and the patient noted some increase in his visual acuity, but 1 week after the medication was restarted his creatinine level climbed from 1.9 to 2.3 mg/dl. Therefore, the cyclosporin dosage was decreased to 2 mg/kg/day. His visual acuity still improved to 20/100 with a near vision of J6 on this regimen. By late April 1983, however, his serum creatinine level stabilized at 1.8 mg/dl at this dosage and his vision continued to improve to 20/60 by May 1983. But by June 1983, his visual acuity decreased and a regimen of alternating doses of cyclosporin between 2 mg/kg/day and 3 mg/kg day was established. Visual acuity improved to 20/50, and the creatinine level stayed below 1.8. In August 1983, he noted eye pain and a drop in visual acuity (20/400). Multiple retinal lesions and an active ocular inflammatory response were noted. Cyclosporin was increased to 3.5 mg/kg/day. Because of the recurrent ocular attacks and the impression that cyclosporin could not be given without the occurrence of renal complications, a regimen of 20 mg of prednisone daily was added to the 3 mg/kg/day of cyclosporin. His visual acuity remained at 20/200 on this regimen. Flares of ocular disease occurred in October and December of 1983, his prednisone dosage was increased, and there was a slight increase in visual acuity to 20/100.

DISCUSSION

The ocular complications of Behçet's disease can lead to severe visual handicap, even when appropriate systemic antiinflammatory or immunosuppressive therapy is instituted. It has been calculated that this handicap will occur in 5 years in those patients with posterior segment involvement (21). The recurrent nature of the posterior ocular attack is of major concern, since the anterior segment inflammatory attacks are not statistically associated with permanent visual loss. Cyclosporin appeared effective in not only altering the acute episodes of attacks involving the posterior pole, but also in decreasing markedly, or abrogating totally, the recurrence rate of these attacks. It should be emphasized that this was observed in patients who had already received conventional therapy for their disorder.

Additionally, we have noted an improvement in the non-ocular signs and symptoms of Behçet's disease in our patients treated with cyclosporin. Patient 1 noted that the arthritic complaints associated with the disease activity have disappeared while he is taking cyclosporin. Mucosal ulcerations, both oral and genital, have also improved. Similar positive results appear to be noted in a parallel pilot study in the treatment of ocular Behçet's disease in Japan (Masuda K, Tokyo University: personal communication).

The etiology of this disease remains unknown.

The disease has been associated with HLA–B51 (22). It would seem likely that the disease initiation is a combination of a genetic propensity and an exogenous stimulus. Recently it has been noted that *Streptococcus anhemolyticus* fragments have been found in the blood of a high percentage of patients with Behçet's disease, suggesting a possible bacterial role in at least the initiation of this disease process (23). Additionally, the multiple approaches to therapy of this condition reflect the difficulty in managing its ocular complications, and as well, the various immune alterations observed in Behçet's disease. Matsumura and Mizushima (24), as well as others (25), have noted the increased chemotactic activity of polymorphonuclear leukocytes from Behçet's disease patients compared with those of controls. It was subsequently reported by Mizushima and colleagues (9) that colchicine, a strong inhibitor of chemotaxis, had a beneficial effect on the course of this disease. Mamo and Azzam (5) and other investigators (6) have suggested that cytotoxic agents, particularly the alkylating agents, were particularly beneficial in this disorder. Indeed, in 1981, the International Uveitis Study Group suggested that the diagnosis of this ocular disease was one of the few indications where such agents might be considered before a trial of systemic steroids (O'Connor GR: personal communication). However, others have not found these agents to be effective (7,26).

Though systemic corticosteroid administration may be utilized, particularly during the acute attacks of this disorder, others have not found it to be of long-term benefit (4). Other regimens have included plasmapheresis (27), transfer factor, and fresh plasma or whole blood. More recently Bredinin, a new agent similar to azathioprine, is undergoing a clinical trial in the treatment of this disease (Kogure M, Women's Medical College of Tokyo: personal communication). The efficacy of various treatment modes is difficult to assess since to date, well-controlled clinical trials have not been carried out.

Perhaps the most widely held hypothesis concerning the mechanism of tissue damage in Behçet's disease has been that this is an immune complex mediated disease (type III hypersensitivity reaction). Immune complexes, as well as damaged membrane fragments, have been reported in the blood of patients with Behçet's disease (28). Gamble and coworkers (29) observed the deposition of IgG, the third and fourth components of complement, and fibrin in the kidney and lung biopsy specimens taken from one patient with Behçet's disease, who had uni-ocular uveitis with scarring of the peripheral retina, alterations not totally typical of the ocular presentation of this disease. The assumption has been that the ocular manifestations of this disease are immune complex mediated as well. More recently, however, T cell aberrations have been noted in patients with this condition. Sakane and colleagues (30) have reported abnormalities of suppressor cell activity and in the autologous mixed lymphocyte reaction in the pre-active stage of Behçet's disease. Ohno (31) reported that T cells from patients with Behçet's disease spontaneously produce gamma interferon, a finding suggesting a derangement in the normally exquisite T cell regulatory process.

The evidence presented in this report that cyclosporin was exceptionally effective in modulating the disease process would suggest strongly that T cell alterations play a central role in the expression of the ocular component of this disease, and perhaps in its non-ocular aspects as well. Furthermore, using 3 sensitive radioimmunoassays, CIC were found in the sera of a minority of our patients, and when present, these immunoreactants were in rather modest levels. In fact, only one patient in this series had evidence of CIC during the active phase of the disease (patient 3; ^{125}I-C1q binding assay determination = 19.4%). Interestingly, 3 of 6 patients had evidence of CIC in at least one radioimmunoassay when serum samples were obtained while their disease was controlled with cyclosporin. Dumonde and colleagues (32) recently described a positive correlation between good visual outcome and CIC in retinal vasculitis patients. Our findings would suggest a similar mechanism, though the number of patients in this study is too small to definitely answer this question. It is interesting to note that circulating immune complexes may not be as readily demonstrated in those Behçet's disease patients with ocular disease compared with those without ocular manifestations, suggesting differences in immune mechanisms (Mizushima Y, Marianna University, Kawasaki, Japan: personal communication).

The treatment of the ocular complications of Behçet's disease requires a long-term commitment to a regimen. The potential side effects of any medication, therefore, become most important. Several patients included in this study developed many of the complications associated with both systemic corticosteroid and cytotoxic agent therapy. Except in 1 patient, the secondary effects of cyclosporin have not been problematic to date. However, the potential alterations in renal function associated with cyclosporin therapy require regular monitoring. As outlined in the case report of patient 4, this complication did not permit a therapeutically effective dose of cyclosporin to be maintained. Cyclosporin levels in the plasma of this patient vary, in general, with the dosage taken, but the plasma levels for the same amount of cyclosporin per kilogram varies considerably from patient to patient. How effective plasma levels will be in determining the therapeutic zone within which there will be minimal secondary complications still remains to be seen, since similar cyclosporin plasma levels may produce a marked reduction in kidney function in one patient, while in others no obvious alterations are noted.

Cyclosporin would appear to be an effective alternative medication for the potentially devastating ocular complications of Behçet's disease. However, to date, we do not seem to have induced a tolerant immune state in these patients, and all patients have required continued therapy. Just how effective this therapy will be compared with the more classic therapies for this disease must be evaluated in a controlled, randomized trial. Such studies are currently underway in Japan (Nakajima A, Urayama A, Tokyo: personal communication) and in England (von Graffenried B, Basel: personal communication).

REFERENCES

1. Behçet H: Uber Rezidivierende, Aphthose Durch ein Virus verursachte Geschwure am Mund, am Auge und an den Genitalien. Dermatol Wochenschr 105:1152–1157, 1937
2. Editorial: Behçet's disease. Jpn J Ophthalmol 18:291–294, 1974
3. James DG, Spitere MA: Behçet's disease. Ophthalmology 89:1279–1284, 1982
4. Mishima S, Masuda K, Izawa Y, Mochizuki M, Nanba K: Behçet's disease in Japan: ophthalmologic aspects. Trans Am Ophthalmol Soc 77:225–279, 1979
5. Mamo JG, Azzam SA: Treatment of Behçet's disease with chlorambucil. Arch Ophthal 84:446–450, 1970
6. Tricoulis D: Treatment of Behçet's disease with chlorambucil. Br J Ophthalmol 60:55–57, 1976
7. O'Duffy JD, Robertson DM, Goldstein NP: Chlorambucil in the treatment of uveitis and meningoencephalitis of Behçet's disease. Am J Med 76:75–84, 1984
8. Tabbara KF: Chlorambucil in Behçet's disease, a reappraisal. Ophthalmology 90:906–908, 1983
9. Mizushima T, Matsumura N, Mori M, Shimizu T, Fukushima B: Colchicine in Behçet's disease (letter). Lancet ii:1037, 1977
10. O'Connor GR: Epidemiology and pathogenesis of the ocular and cerebral forms of Behçet's disease, Behçet's Disease. Edited by G Inaba. Tokyo, University of Tokyo Press, 1982, pp 115–126
11. Nussenblatt RB, Rodrigues MM, Wacker WB, Cevario SJ, Salinas-Carmona MC: Cyclosporin A: inhibition of experimental autoimmune uveitis in Lewis rats. J Clin Invest 67:1228–1231, 1981
12. Borel JF, Lafferty KJ: Cyclosporin: speculation about its mechanism of action. Transplant Proc 15:1881–1885, 1983
13. Hogan MJ, Kimura SJ, Thygeson P: Signs and symptoms of uveitis I. Anterior uveitis. Am J Ophthalmol (suppl) 47:155–170, 1959
14. Kimura SJ, Thygeson P, Hogan MJ: Signs and symptoms of uveitis. II. Classification of the posterior manifestations of uveitis. Am J Ophthalmol (suppl) 47:171–176, 1959
15. Lawley TJ, Moutsopoulos HM, Katz SI, Theofilopoulos AN, Chused TM, Frank MM: Demonstration of circulating immune complexes in Sjögren's syndrome. J Immunol 123:1382–1387, 1979
16. Hall RP, Lawley TJ, Heck JA, Katz SI: IgA containing circulating immune complexes in dermatitis herpetiformis, Henoch-Schönlein purpura, systemic lupus erythematosus, and other diseases. Clin Exp Immunol 40:431–437, 1980
17. Yancey KB, Cason JC, Hall RP, Lawley TJ: Dietary gluten challenge does not influence the levels of circulating immune complexes in patients with dermatitis herpetiformis. J Invest Dermatol 80:468–471, 1983
18. Woodroffe AJ, Border WA, Theofilopoulos AN, Gotze O, Glasscock RJ, Dixon FH, Wilson CB: Detection of circulating immune complexes in patients with glomerulonephritis. Kidney Int 12:268–278, 1977
19. Kahan BD, Van Buren CT, Wideman CA, Cooley DA, Frazier OH: Nephrotoxicity of cyclosporine (letter). N Engl J Med 312:48, 1985
20. Nussenblatt RB, Palestine AG, Rook AH, Scher I, Wacker WB, Gery I: Treatment of intraocular inflammatory disease with cyclosporin A. Lancet ii:235–238, 1983
21. Shimizu T, Ehrlich GE, Inaba G, Hayashi K: Behçet's disease. Semin Arthritis Rheum 8:223–260, 1979
22. Ohno S, Sugiura S, Ohguchi M, Aoki K: Close association of HLA-5 with Behçet's disease, Immunology and Immunopathology of the Eye. Edited by AM Silverstein, GR O'Connor. New York, Masson Publishing, 1979, pp 15–17
23. Namba K, Ueno T, Matsumi F, Okita M, Yumita A, Hayashi K: Behçet's disease and streptococcus infection. Jpn J Ophthalmol 87:124–132, 1984
24. Matsumura N, Mizushima Y: Leucocyte movement and colchicine treatment in Behçet's disease. Lancet ii:813, 1975
25. Sobel JD, Haim S, Obedeanu N, Meshulam T, Merzbach D: Polymorphonuclear leucocyte function in Behçet's disease. J Clin Pathol 30:250–253, 1977
26. Wong VG: Immunosuppressive therapy of ocular inflammatory diseases. Arch Ophthalmol 81:628–637, 1969
27. Saraux H, LeHoang P, Audebert A-A, Canuel C, Cava-

lier J: Interet de la plasmapherese dans le traitement du syndrome de Behçet. Bull Soc Ophtalmol Fr 82:41–44, 1982

28. Lehner T, Almeida JD, Levinsky J: Damaged membrane fragments and immune complexes in the blood of patients with Behçet's syndrome. Clin Exp Immunol 34: 206–212, 1978
29. Gamble CN, Wiesner KB, Shapiro RF, Boyer WJ: The immune complex pathogenesis of glomerulonephritis and pulmonary vasculitis in Behçet's disease. Am J Med 66:1031–1039, 1979
30. Sakane T, Kotani H, Takada S, Tsunematsu T: Functional aberration of T cell subsets in patients with Behçet's disease. Arthritis Rheum 25:1343–1351, 1982
31. Ohno S: Immunological aspects of Behçet's, Vogt-Koyanagi, and Harada's diseases. Trans Ophthalmol Soc UK 101:335–341, 1981
32. Dumonde DC, Kasp-Grochowska E, Graham E, Sanders MD, Faure JP, De Kozak Y, Van Tuyen V: Anti-retinal autoimmunity and circulating immune complexes in patients with retinal vasculitis. Lancet ii:787–792, 1982

OUTCOMES OF SELF-HELP EDUCATION FOR PATIENTS WITH ARTHRITIS

KATE LORIG, DEBORAH LUBECK, R. GUY KRAINES, MITCHELL SELEZNICK, and HALSTED R. HOLMAN

Behavioral and health status outcomes of an unreinforced, self-help education program for arthritis patients taught by lay persons were examined in 2 ways: a 4-month randomized experiment and a 20-month longitudinal study. At 4 months, experimental subjects significantly exceeded control subjects in knowledge, recommended behaviors, and in lessened pain. These changes remained significant at 20 months. The course was inexpensive and well-accepted by patients, physicians, and other health professionals.

As the prevalence of chronic disease increases, so does the potential usefulness of health education. An informed patient can, in theory, play an important role in reducing predisposing factors and in managing established illness.

While there is evidence that patient education can change behaviors and health status in some settings (1,2), this is not clear in the case of arthritis education. Arthritis education increases knowledge (3,16) and sometimes influences health behaviors, such as compliance with treatment regimens, the practice of joint protection, or exercise (6,9,12,15,17,18, and Harlowe D, Yu P: unpublished observations). Some investigators have reported improvements in psychosocial factors, such as coping, family communication, or depression (6,7,9,11,15,17). Finally, a few studies demonstrated improvements in health status measures, such as mobility and pain (14,16,19). However, others suggested that no change in health behaviors occurred (13–19), and 1 study reported increased pain among the participants (20). Together, these studies indicate that arthritis patient education may be effective in changing certain behaviors and possibly physical or psychological health status.

With the emergence of arthritis as the largest cause of disability in the United States, the potential role of arthritis patient education assumes increased importance. If benefits can be shown from an inexpensive, replicable program, then patient education might be a useful part of a therapeutic program. Our study explored this possibility. It differed from previous studies in that it utilized both a randomized design and a longitudinal 20-month followup, and measured outcomes in terms of knowledge, behaviors, and health status. While former studies had 1 or more of these features, none had all 5. The experience with the first 286 patients over a 20-month period is reported.

METHODS

The Arthritis Self-Management Program (ASMP) is a community-based patient education course developed by the Stanford Arthritis Center (SAC). Two general assumptions underlie the ASMP: 1) patients can learn the general principles of managing arthritis, including aspects of the use of drugs, and 2) knowledgable patients practicing self-care will experience improved physical function, less pain, and reduced health care costs. Other assumptions which generated the program were that 1) health education should be widely available and low in cost in order to avoid dependence on the expensive and limited time of health professionals, 2) trained lay persons could effectively deliver structured health education programs, and 3) such lay instructors would be accept-

From the Department of Medicine, Stanford University, Stanford, California.

Supported by NIH Multipurpose Arthritis Center grant 20610-05 and an Arthritis Health Professionals grant from the Arthritis Foundation.

Kate Lorig, RN, DrPH; Deborah Lubeck, PhD; R. Guy Kraines, MS; Mitchell Seleznick, MD; Halsted R. Holman, MD.

Submitted for publication January 27, 1984; accepted in revised form January 3, 1985.

able both to the patients and the professional community. There is research evidence that role models (in this case leaders with similar backgrounds and disease problems) have powerful effects in bringing about behavior change (21–24).

The ASMP was based on a needs assessment conducted on 100 patients with arthritis and 50 practicing rheumatologists (25). This assessment revealed that pain was the main concern of patients, followed, in turn, by disability, fear, depression, and deformity. Physicians generally agreed that these were primary concerns. The course emphasized the nature of arthritis, the appropriate use of medication, range of motion and isometric exercises, Benson (26) and Paul (27) relaxation techniques, joint protection, nutrition, interaction of patients with physicians, and evaluation of nontraditional treatments. The content of the program has been published as *The Arthritis Helpbook* (28) which is widely available.

As conducted by the SAC, each course had 15–20 participants plus family members if they wished. All diagnoses were confirmed by the participant's physician, who also consented to the patient's participation. Each course was taught by a pair of trained lay leaders, ranging in age from 21–84 years, who had received 20 hours of training and a teaching manual (29). Approximately one-half of the 21 leaders had arthritis, and one-fourth were active or retired health professionals; few had previous experience in health education.

The course was given in 6 sessions spread over 4 months, usually in a community setting, without subsequent reinforcement. The ASMP teaching methods were based on a standardized educational protocol (29) emphasizing group discussion, practice, the use of contracts and diaries to improve compliance, and weekly feedback. Methods were taken from a number of sources, including the models of social learning theory (30), learned helplessness (31), and personal constructs (32). Program costs were approximately $15–20 per participant.

The project was approved by the Stanford Committee for the Protection of Human Subjects in Research. All participants gave written informed consent.

Subjects were recruited by public service announcements in the mass media, from a community clinic, and from senior citizen centers. All applicants were promised that they would receive the course immediately or after 4 months service as controls.

Table 1. Study design and number of subjects completing questionnaires at 4, 8, and 20 months*

	0 months		4 months		8 months	20 months
Intervention with pre-test	O	X	O		O	O
n	134		129		124	115
Intervention, no pre-test		X	O			
n	49		48			
Control subjects with pre-test	O		O	X		
n	65		61			
Control subjects, no pre-test			O	X		
n	38		32			

* O = time of data collection; X = time of intervention.

Table 2. Demographic profile of Arthritis Self-Management Program participants

Sex, F/M (%)	83/17
Age	
Mean ± SD	67.4 ± 11.84
Median	68.0
Range	23–94
Race, white/nonwhite (%)	97/3
Years of schooling	
Mean ± SD	14.6 ± 3.13
Median	15.0
Range	0–22
Diagnosis, OA/RA/UA (%)*	77.3/10.7/12.0

* OA = osteoarthritis; RA = rheumatoid arthritis; UA = arthritis, not otherwise specified.

The measured outcome variables included: 1) knowledge of arthritis, 2) practice of exercise and relaxation, 3) walking, 4) pain, 5) disability, 6) locus of control, 7) the number of visits to a physician for treatment of arthritis, and 8) the participant's satisfaction with the physician.

Most variables were assessed by instruments which had been tested in other studies for reliability and, where appropriate, for validity. The knowledge instrument developed by Stanford contained 10 multiple choice questions primarily concerned with arthritis self-help knowledge. The original Wallston Health Locus of Control scale (33) was used, as was the short version of the Rand Health Insurance Study Patient Satisfaction instrument developed by John Ware and colleagues (Ware J, Snyder MK, Wright RW: unpublished observations). Because pain is subjective, it was measured by 2 scales: a double-anchored visual analog scale which had been used in previous arthritis studies (34–36) and an ordinal scale which asked patients to rank their pain as mild, moderate, or severe. This technique of cross-validation on subjective measures is suggested by Cook and Campbell (37). The Stanford Health Assessment Questionnaire, a physical disability scale, assessed performance of common functions of daily living such as eating, bathing, reach, grip, and walking, thereby acting as a measure of disease severity (38). The behavior scales reported the monthly frequency of various self-management antivities. A chart check to validate the self-report of visits to physicians on an independent sample of 29 arthritis patients yielded a correlation r = 0.79.

Two types of studies were conducted, in part, simultaneously. The first was a 4-month prospective comparison of control and treatment groups. The second was a longitudinal comparison of baseline attributes of participants from the treatment group with their attributes at 4, 8, and 20 months from baseline. Table 1 depicts the 2 study designs.

A Solomon 4-group design was used for the first 4 months of the study (39,40). Participants were randomized to 1 of 4 groups: a pre-test and post-test intervention group, a pre-test and post-test control group, a post-test only intervention group, and a post-test only control group. The 4-group design has the advantage of traditional randomized trials, as well as allowing study of the effects of pre-tests on outcome. Such effects were not found in this study. The disadvantage of the design is the loss of statistical power due to the lack of pre-test data on all the participants.

In the first study, 2 types of analysis were performed: 1) a Wilcoxon rank sum test, a non-parametric test based on differences of medians which corrects for outliers, and 2) an analysis of covariance. Only the former has been applied to data from the longitudinal portion of the study.

Of the first 286 subjects, 94% completed the 4-month portion of the study. Of the 134 subjects in the pre-tested intervention group, 96% completed 4 months of the study, 93% completed 8 months, and 84% completed 20 months. There were no baseline differences in knowledge, behaviors, or health status between those completing and those not completing 20 months in the study. Demographic information is reported in Table 2.

RESULTS

The 4-month randomized study. Table 3 presents the baseline data from the randomized study, comparing mean scores of participants who completed the ASMP (n = 129) with controls who received no intervention (n = 61). It should be noted that despite randomization, significant baseline differences were found for the assessment of pain when measured by the visual analog scale.

Table 4 compares the mean change scores (4-month scores minus baseline scores) of those who received the ASMP with those who did not. The treatment group increased both their knowledge and practice of self-management behaviors, whereas the control group did not. When measured by visual analog scale, pain decreased in the treatment group by more than twice the amount of the control group; when measured by ordinal scale, pain remained unchanged in the control group, but decreased significantly in the treatment group. Significant changes were not seen in disability or number of visits to a physician.

Table 3. Four-month randomized study baseline data (mean ± standard deviation) for control and treatment groups

	Control group (n = 61)	Treatment group (n = 129)	*P**
Behavior variables			
Knowledge (0–10 scale)	4.11 ± 1.92	4.69 ± 1.81	0.06
Arthritis exercise (times/month)	13.80 ± 18.78	12.18 ± 15.13	0.55
Relaxation (times/month)	10.37 ± 17.84	6.62 ± 11.98	0.13
Health variables			
Pain (visual analog scale, 0–10)	3.58 ± 2.39	4.43 ± 2.17	0.03
Pain (ordinal scale, 0–3)	1.96 ± 0.85	2.18 ± 0.66	0.10
Disability (0–3 scale)	0.53 ± 0.53	0.62 ± 0.55	0.23
Number of visits to physician during previous 4 months	2.02 ± 3.06	1.33 ± 1.82	0.29

* Value using Wilcoxon rank sum test.

Because of the differences between control and treatment groups in baseline reports of pain, a covariance analysis was carried out using multiple linear regression analysis relating each of the 2 measures of pain at 4 months to their baseline values and to the presence or absence of the course. In these analyses, pain improvement by the visual analog scale was not statistically significant ($P = 0.40$), whereas improvement by the ordinal scale remained significant ($P = 0.01$). Similar analyses using baseline values as independent variables did not change disability outcomes but brought the decline in visits to physicians by the treatment group to a significance level of $P = 0.06$.

For the treatment group, the mean decrease in pain was 23% when measured by the visual analog scale and 20% by the ordinal scale. For those people whose pain decreased (n = 89), no changes were found in use of medications, nor were visits to physicians more frequent than for patients whose pain did not decrease. Thus, the pain decrease was not likely to have resulted from an intensification of medical treatment.

The 20-month longitudinal study. Table 5 presents change score comparisons between baseline and 4, 8, and 20 months for all participants who initially received the intervention and who completed 20 months of the study (n = 115). Comparisons were made by the *t*-test for paired differences.

Knowledge of self-management behaviors declined over time but remained significantly above the initial levels at 20 months ($P < 0.01$). Though the frequency of exercise declined at 20 months, it remained significant. The percentage of people exercising also exceeded baseline at both 8 months ($P < 0.001$) and 20 months ($P < 0.05$). A similar pattern was seen for the practice of relaxation. Locus of control did not change, indicating that the general sense of self-responsibility was not affected.

Utilizing both scales, a significant decline in pain was sustained at 20 months. Physical disability declined only at 4 months; however, the percentage of persons who reported disability decreased from 86% at baseline to 76% at 20 months. At 4 and 8 months, extrapolated annual visits to physicians for treatment of arthritis declined by 1.05 and 0.84 visits, respectively. However, at 20 months, visit rates were similar to baseline.

Table 4. Four-month randomized study of mean score changes (mean ± standard deviation) for control and treatment groups

	Control group (n = 61)	Treatment group (n = 129)	P*
Behavior variables			
Knowledge (0–10 scale)	0.10 ± 1.48	1.39 ± 2.00	<0.0001
Arthritis exercise (times/month)	−4.23 ± 18.82†	12.85 ± 25.36	<0.0001
Relaxation (times/month)	−5.21 ± 15.96	4.63 ± 15.10	<0.0001
Health variables			
Pain (visual analog scale, 0–10)	−0.43 ± 1.68	−1.04 ± 2.11	0.04
Pain (ordinal scale, 0–3)	−0.02 ± 0.80	−0.45 ± 0.77	0.002
Disability (0–3 scale)	−0.02 ± 0.24	−0.06 ± 0.34	0.45
Number of visits to physician during previous 4 months	−0.26 ± 3.07	−0.46 ± 1.98	0.61

* Value using Wilcoxon rank sum test.
† Minus signs represent score decrease.

Other relevant results from this study were: 1) When comparing pre-tested and non–pre-tested groups of both control and treatment subjects, no effects of pre-tests on outcome were found. 2) As a check on acquiescent response, data were collected on the use of self-massage, which was not taught in the course; no change was seen. 3) In terms of changes in the 13 outcome variables, there were no significant differences among the 24 courses taught by a total of 20 persons. 4) To test for other explanatory effects, a multiple regression analysis was done on the 4-month data for the 8 key behavior and health status variables. The effects of the course remained significant after controlling for age, diagnosis, and level of education. Other findings of this analysis were that younger patients learned slightly better than older patients ($P < 0.02$), that older patients tended to be more satisfied with their physicians ($P < 0.05$), and that patients with higher levels of education reported less pain ($P < 0.01$). 5) While we found no differences in outcomes between osteoarthritis patients and rheumatoid arthritis patients, the number of rheumatoid arthritis patients was too small to draw conclusions from this study.

DISCUSSION

This study was the initial part of an evaluation of health education for persons with arthritis. The format had the attributes of medium-sized classes, lay teachers, and heterogeneity of participants in terms of

Table 5. Longitudinal study of mean score changes (mean ± standard deviation) between baseline and 4-, 8-, and 20-month assessments

	Baseline scores	Mean change in scores*		
	0 months (n = 115)	4 months (n = 115)	8 months (n = 115)	20 months (n = 115)
Behavior variables				
Knowledge (0–10 scale)	4.94 ± 1.66	1.25 ± 1.92†	1.40 ± 2.14†	1.08 ± 2.04†
Arthritis exercise (times/month)	12.08 ± 15.32	14.33 ± 26.25†	10.88 ± 26.10†	4.09 ± 20.05‡
Relaxation (times/month)	7.12 ± 12.52	4.64 ± 15.52†	2.78 ± 14.34	3.24 ± 15.59‡
Health variables				
Pain (visual analog scale, 0–10)	4.48 ± 2.13	−1.03 ± 2.07†	−1.01 ± 2.24†	−1.09 ± 2.65†
Pain (ordinal scale, 0–3)	2.15 ± 0.67	−0.39 ± 0.72†	−0.42 ± 0.85†	−0.34 ± 0.88†
Disability (0–3 scale)	0.63 ± 0.55	−0.07 ± 0.33‡	−0.05 ± 0.38	−0.03 ± 0.39
Number of visits to physician during previous 4 months	1.25 ± 1.88	−0.39 ± 2.04	−0.17 ± 2.10	0.06 ± 2.36

* Minus values represent decrease in score.
† $P < 0.01$ using t-tests for paired differences.
‡ $P < 0.05$ using t-tests for paired differences.

type and severity of arthritis. This approach was chosen because it approximates attributes assumed to be desirable in health education for persons with chronic illness: voluntary participation, group learning, teaching by trained lay persons, and applicability to a broad range of patients. Should such an approach succeed, it would be a useful example of relatively inexpensive health education which might be incorporated in health services.

The results are encouraging, though certainly not definitive. They showed growth in knowledge and adoption of taught behaviors to be statistically significantly greater in the treatment group during the randomized portion of the study, with persistence of all effects for the 20 months of the longitudinal study. Health status effects were less dramatic. When corrected for baseline values, pain in the treatment group was significantly reduced when measured by the ordinal scale, but was not reduced when measured by the visual analog scale. However, pain was diminished for 20 months, as measured by both scales in the longitudinal study. All of these results occurred without formal reinforcement.

Unfortunately, baseline differences in visual analog pain scores occurred despite randomization. Therefore, it is unclear whether reduction of pain in the experimental group was directly attributable to the intervention. However, pain reduction measured by the ordinal scale was significant both in comparison with controls and over time. Since they are subjective, pain scales elude validation except possibly by concordance of reports using different instruments. Visual analog and ordinal scales are the common forms of measurement. In our study, concordance between the 2 scales was only partial.

Aside from a formal test of knowledge, our data were obtained by self-reports. We chose this method because evaluation of health education programs is essential and self-report is probably the only economic and logistically feasible method. Validity of the self-reports is, therefore, a major issue. In our case, the Stanford Health Assessment Questionnaire has been validated by trained professional observers in the clinic and in the home. The self-reports of visits to physicians were validated by chart checks. Experience elsewhere indicates that patients tend to underreport physician visits initially but become more accurate in subsequent reports (41,42); that bias would work against finding a significant reduction in visits in this study. Questions concerning frequency of exercise, relaxation, and medications were not formally validated. Data on self-massage suggest the absence of an acquiescent response.

A final possible limiting factor is the relative homogeneity of the study sample; most of the subjects were white, well-educated, and middle class. Generalization of the ASMP to other populations and geographic sites is currently under study.

Two matters of particular concern to us were patients' attitudes toward physicians at the end of the study and physicians' attitudes toward their patients' participation. In neither instance did a problem arise. When measured by the 7 subscales of the Rand Satisfaction Instrument (humaneness, quality of care, conduct, access, convenience, facilities, and insurance coverage), there was no difference between the treatment and control groups at the end of 4 months. Conversely, more than 200 physicians have had patients participate in the ASMP, and 3 Kaiser Hospitals and 3 community hospitals have adopted the program to be regularly offered to their patients. Only 1 complaint about adverse effects of the course on a patient has been registered with us by a physician.

No conclusions can be drawn concerning clinical significance of the results. Increased knowledge and new, presumably healthy, behaviors are not formal clinical outcomes; pain is, but conclusions about its alteration remain tentative. The number of visits to physicians was reduced and disability declined without reaching statistical significance. These findings provide a basis for further efforts to understand the cause of the changes and to enhance them through reinforcement. Such efforts are underway.

REFERENCES

1. Mazzuca SA: Does patient education in chronic disease have therapeutic value? J Chronic Dis 35:521–529, 1982
2. Green LW, Squyres WD, D'Altroy LH, Herber B: What do recent evaluations of patient education tell us? Patient Education. Edited by WD Squyres. New York, Spring Publishing Co., 1980, pp 11–44
3. Holstein DJ, Morri AD, Moeschberger M: Effects of an organized educational program on patient understanding of rheumatoid arthritis and compliance with medical treatment, 12th Scientific Meeting of the Allied Health Professions Section of the Arthritis Foundation, Miami, 1976
4. Vignos P, Parker W, Thompson H: Evaluation of a clinic education program for patients with rheumatoid arthritis. J Rheumatol 3:155–156, 1976
5. Stross J, Middelson WM: Educating patients with osteoarthritis. J Rheumatol 4:313–316, 1977

6. Kaye R, Hammond A: Rheumatoid arthritis. JAMA 239:2966–2967, 1978
7. Udelman H, Udelman D: Group therapy with rheumatoid arthritis patients. Am J Psychother 32:288–299, 1978
8. Schmitt A, McBrair W: Assessing the quality of education provided to rheumatoid arthritis patients in a suburban rural setting, 14th Scientific Meeting of the Allied Health Professions Section of the Arthritis Foundation, Denver, 1979
9. Gross M, Brandt KD: Educational support groups for patients with ankylosing spondylitis: a preliminary report. Patient Counsel Health Ed 3:6–12, 1981
10. Gunter-Hunt G, Ferguson K: The impact of an educational program for patients receiving oral corticosteroid therapy, 16th Scientific Meeting of the Arthritis Health Professions Association, Boston, 1981
11. Kaplan S, Kozin F: A controlled study of group counseling in rheumatoid arthritis. J Rheumatol 8:91–99, 1981
12. Knudson KG, Spiegel TM, Furst DE: Outpatient education program for rheumatoid arthritis patients. Patient Counsel Health Ed 3:77–82, 1981
13. Monternach CA, Mitz BG, Lightfoot RW Jr: A controlled study of outpatient education for women with rheumatoid arthritis, 16th Scientific Meeting of the Arthritis Health Professions Association, Boston, 1981
14. Bielicki B, Belch P, Schumacher HR: Patient education in gout: what does it accomplish? (abstract). Arthritis Rheum (suppl) 25:S87, 1982
15. Wetstone SL, Sheehan J, Votaw R, Peterson M: Computer-based education in rheumatoid arthritis (abstract). Arthritis Rheum (suppl) 25:S26, 1982
16. Potts M, Brandt K: Analysis of education support groups for patients with rheumatoid arthritis. Patient Counsel Health Ed 4:161–166, 1983
17. Schwartz L, Marcus R, Condon R: Multidisciplinary group therapy for rheumatoid arthritis. Psychosomatics 19:289–293, 1978
18. Ferguson K, Bole GG: Family support, health beliefs, therapeutic compliance, in patients with rheumatoid arthritis. Patient Counsel Health Ed 1:101–105, 1979
19. Doyle TH, Granada JL: Influence of two management approaches of the health status of women with osteoarthritis (abstract). Arthritis Rheum (suppl) 25:S56, 1982
20. Parker J, Singsen B, Hewett J, Moeschberger M, Walker S, Hazelwood S, Hall P: Patient education for rheumatoid arthritis: short term positive adverse consequences (abstract). Arthritis Rheum (suppl) 25:S38, 1982
21. Bandura A, Jeffrey RW, Wright CL: Efficacy of participant modeling as a function of response induction aids. J Abnorm Psychol 83:56–64, 1974
22. Cox CA: A pilot study: using the elderly as community health educators. Int J Health Educ 12:49–52, 1979
23. Lorig K, Garcia WE: Cuidaremos: the HECO approach to breast self-examination. Int Q Commun Health Educ 1:125–134, 1980–81
24. Zapka J, Mazur R: Peer sex education training and evaluation. Am J Public Health 67:450–454, 1977
25. Lorig K, Cox T, Cuevas Y, Kraines RG, Britton MC: Converging and diverging beliefs about arthritis: caucasian patients, Spanish-speaking patients, and physicians. J Rheumatol 11:76–79, 1984
26. Benson H: The Relaxation Response. New York, Avon Books, 1976
27. Paul G: Insight vs. Desensitization: An Experiment in Anxiety Reduction. Stanford, Stanford University Press, 1966
28. Lorig K, Fries JF: The Arthritis Helpbook. Reading, MA, Addison-Wesley, 1980
29. Lorig K: Arthritis Self-Help Course Leader's Manual. Atlanta, Arthritis Foundation, 1981
30. Rotter JB: Social Learning and Clinical Psychology. Englewod Cliffs, NJ, Prentice-Hall, 1954
31. Seligman M: Helplessness. San Francisco, WH Freeman, 1975
32. Kelly G: The Psychology of Personal Constructs. New York, WW Norton & Co., 1955
33. Wallston BS, Wallston KA, Karland GD, Maides SA: Development and validation of the health locus of control (HLC) scale. J Consult Clin Psychol 44:580–585, 1976
34. Downie WW, Leatham PA, Rhind VM, Wright V, Branco JA, Anderson JA: Studies with pain rating scales. Ann Rheum Dis 37:378–381, 1978
35. Downie WW, Leatham PA, Rhind VM, Pickup ME, Wright V: The visual analogue scale in the assessment of grip strength. Ann Rheum Dis 37:382–384, 1978
36. Dixon JS, Bird HA: Reproducibility along a 10 cm vertical analogue scale. Ann Rheum Dis 40:87–89, 1981
37. Cook TD, Campbell DT: Quasi-experimentation. Chicago, Rand McNally, 1979
38. Fries JF, Spitz P, Kraines RG, Holman HR: Measurement of patient outcome in arthritis. Arthritis Rheum 23:137–145, 1980
39. Solomon RL: An extension of control groups design. Psychol Bull 46:137–150, 1949
40. Campbell DT, Stanley JC: Experimental and Quasi-Experimental Design for Research. Chicago, Rand McNally, 1963
41. Marquis KH, Cannell CF, Laurent A: Health Events in Household Interviews. National Center for Health Statistics, USDHEW Publication no. (HSM) 72-1028. Vital and Health Statistics, series 2, no. 45. Rockville, Maryland, 1974
42. Cannell CF: A Summary of Studies of Interviewing Methodology. National Center for Health Statistics, USDHEW Publication no. (HRA) 77-1343. Vital and Health Statistics, series 2, no. 69. Rockville, Maryland, 1977

UTILIZATION OF NONSTEROIDAL ANTIINFLAMMATORY DRUGS

CARLENE BAUM, DIANNE L. KENNEDY, and MARY B. FORBES

Information derived from pharmaceutical marketing databases on the use of 12 nonsteroidal antiinflammatory drugs in 1983 is presented. Estimates of population exposure, regularity of treatment, average daily dose, age and sex distributions of users, concomitant use of other drugs, associated diagnoses, and trends in use are provided. Utilization patterns were similar for 8 of the nonsteroidal antiinflammatory drugs, with differing patterns seen for mefenamic acid, oxyphenbutazone, phenylbutazone, and zomepirac.

Nonsteroidal antiinflammatory drugs (NSAIDs) are among the most frequently used drugs in the United States. Five of the 50 drug products most often dispensed during 1983 were NSAIDs: Motrin (#9), Naprosyn (#20), Feldene (#27), Indocin (#28), and Clinoril (#41). Approximately 66.5 million prescriptions for nonsalicylate NSAIDs were dispensed by retail pharmacies in 1983, representing over 4% of the total prescription market. Consumers spent over one billion dollars for these prescriptions.

The opinions expressed in this paper are those of the authors and not necessarily those of the Food and Drug Administration. The authors assume responsibility for the accurate transcription of all data and the mathematical calculations performed by the Drug Use Analysis Branch.

From the Drug Use Analysis Branch and the Adverse Reactions and Poisoning Surveillance Branch, Division of Drug and Biological Product Experience, Center for Drugs and Biologics, Food and Drug Administration, Rockville, Maryland.

Carlene Baum, PhD: Technical Information Specialist, Drug Use Analysis Branch; Dianne L. Kennedy, RPh, MPH: Chief, Drug Use Analysis Branch; Mary B. Forbes, RPh: Pharmacist, Adverse Reactions and Poisoning Surveillance Branch.

Address reprint requests to Carlene Baum, PhD, Drug Use Analysis Branch, HFN-737, FDA, 5600 Fishers Lane, Rockville, MD 20857.

Submitted for publication May 25, 1984; accepted in revised form December 14, 1984.

This article provides an overview of the utilization of nonsteroidal antiinflammatory drugs, including a review of trends in the total number of NSAID prescriptions from 1973 to 1983 and more detailed prescription data for 1983. Information on how the drugs are being used, as well as how much they are used is also provided. Only nonsalicylate prescription drugs are discussed (e.g., aspirin is not included), and with the exception of population exposure estimates, data reflect only outpatient use. Benoxaprofen is not covered in this review since it was withdrawn from the market shortly after its introduction in 1982. Zomepirac was withdrawn the following year, but is included since it was on the market for 3 years and represented a major drug exposure during that time.

METHODS

Data were drawn from 3 subscription databases purchased by the Food and Drug Administration from IMS America, Ltd. (1–3). The *National Prescription Audit* (*NPA*) (1) provides information on prescriptions dispensed by chain and independent pharmacies in the continental United States; other outlets such as discount stores and supermarkets with pharmacies are not included. Since 1981, IMS has received monthly data tapes on approximately 4.3 million prescriptions dispensed by a panel of 1,200 computerized pharmacies. Because data collection is dependent upon computerized pharmacies, the panel does not represent a true random sample; however, IMS does ensure that the panel is representative of US pharmacies in terms of geographic region, type of ownership, and pharmacy size. Prior to 1981, data were obtained from a representative sample of 800 pharmacies, each of which was audited for 2 days per month. Therefore, changes from 1980–1981 in the number of prescriptions reported by the *NPA* may reflect methodologic revisions, as well as actual changes in drug use. The *NPA* provided data for the current study on the number of prescriptions, the percentage that were new prescriptions, average prescription size, and average daily dose prescribed by physicians.

The *US Pharmaceutical Market—Drugstore and Hospital Purchases* (2) provides national estimates of pharmaceutical purchases based on invoices from a drugstore panel of 840 retail outlets and 439 warehouses and a hospital panel of 350 hospitals and 362 wholesalers. It covers a broader range of drugstore outlets than the *National Prescription Audit* and represents hospital use as well, but contains more limited summary figures. Dollar costs are summarized for products and classes, but information on drug quantity is presented only for the individual strengths and package sizes of each manufacturer (e.g., 565,000 bottles containing 500 tablets of Upjohn's 600-mg ibuprofen). Data on individual drug quantity were used to calculate the total kilograms of each NSAID purchased by drugstores and hospitals in 1983. The kilogram data were then used to estimate population exposure through a method based on the concept of the defined daily dose (DDD) developed and routinely used by European drug researchers (4). A DDD for a particular drug represents the average maintenance dose for the main indication based upon an analysis of the medical literature. DDDs are presented not as a recommended dose but only as a measurement tool. Drug exposure is generally expressed as DDDs/1,000 population/day. An estimate for a given drug would be calculated as follows:

1) Total kilograms of drug available during the year ÷ DDD for drug = total DDDs/year;
2) Total DDDs/year ÷ 365 = DDDs/day;
3) DDDs/day ÷ population size = DDDs/person/day; and
4) DDDs/person/day × 1,000 = DDDs/1,000 population/day.

DDDs established by European researchers (5) were used where possible; however, DDDs have not been published for meclofenamate, piroxicam, and zomepirac, so the official labeling for these drugs was used.

Figures were also calculated from *National Prescription Audit* data on the average prescribed daily doses (PDDs) in the US as specified by the prescribing physicians. Since the daily doses actually prescribed for American patients are higher than the defined daily doses for most NSAIDs, estimates of PDDs/1,000 population/day were also calculated. More detailed information on the use and limitations of pharmaceutical purchase data for assessing population exposure is presented elsewhere (6).

The 2 preceding databases provide information on the extent of drug utilization, but not on more qualitative aspects of drug use, such as who is using the drug or what the drug is being used for. The *National Disease and Therapeutic Index* (*NDTI*) (3) does give this type of information. The *NDTI* is based on case history information from over 2,000 office-based physicians who report on each private patient seen or contacted in any way. Since between 4–36% of NSAIDs recorded during a physician–patient contact are issued by means other than a formal prescription (e.g., hospital order, sample), drug reports do not equate to written prescriptions. In addition, refill prescriptions not involving a physician–patient contact are not included in *NDTI* data. By convention, the *NDTI* employs the term "mentions" for such reports; mentions reflect usage, but should not be interpreted as directly equivalent to prescriptions or patients. We used data from the *National Disease and Therapeutic Index* to characterize the age and sex distributions of NSAID users, associated diagnoses (as coded in the *International Classification of Diseases–Seventh Revision* [7]), drug therapy for arthritis, and concomitant use of other drugs.

All 3 databases group individual drug products according to the Uniform System of Classification (developed by IMS America, Ltd. in conjunction with the Pharmaceutical Marketing Research Group, Ambler, PA). Within this system, the category for systemic antiarthritics includes some products that are not NSAIDs (i.e., gold therapies). In addition, some NSAIDs are categorized as synthetic non-narcotic analgesics rather than systemic antiarthritics (mefenamic acid and zomepirac), while some NSAIDs appear in both categories. For example, naproxen is categorized and promoted as an antiarthritic under the trade name Naprosyn and as an analgesic under the trade name Anaprox. All estimates presented in this paper are based on analgesic and antiarthritic data combined, with the exception of those data for concomitant use of other drugs.

Table 1. Prescriptions for nonsteroidal antiinflammatory drugs in 1983*

Generic and trade names	Total no. prescriptions (in millions)	% new prescriptions	Mean no. of tablets in prescription
Fenoprofen Nalfon Nalfon-200	3.3	47	56.1
Ibuprofen Motrin Rufen	19.8	52	56.8
Indomethacin Indocin Indocin SR	9.1	50	51.3
Meclofenamate Meclomen	1.8	48	58.6
Mefenamic acid Ponstel	0.7	59	29.5
Naproxen Naprosyn Anaprox	11.5	51	45.6
Oxyphenbutazone Tandearil	0.6	73	35.8
Phenylbutazone Azolid Azolid-A Butagen Butazolidin Butazolidin alka	2.6	76	34.0
Piroxicam Feldene	7.6	41	28.3
Sulindac Clinoril	5.8	41	53.7
Tolmetin Tolectin Tolectin DS	2.4	45	61.1
Zomepirac Zomax	1.4	67	35.4

* Based on data from reference no. 1.

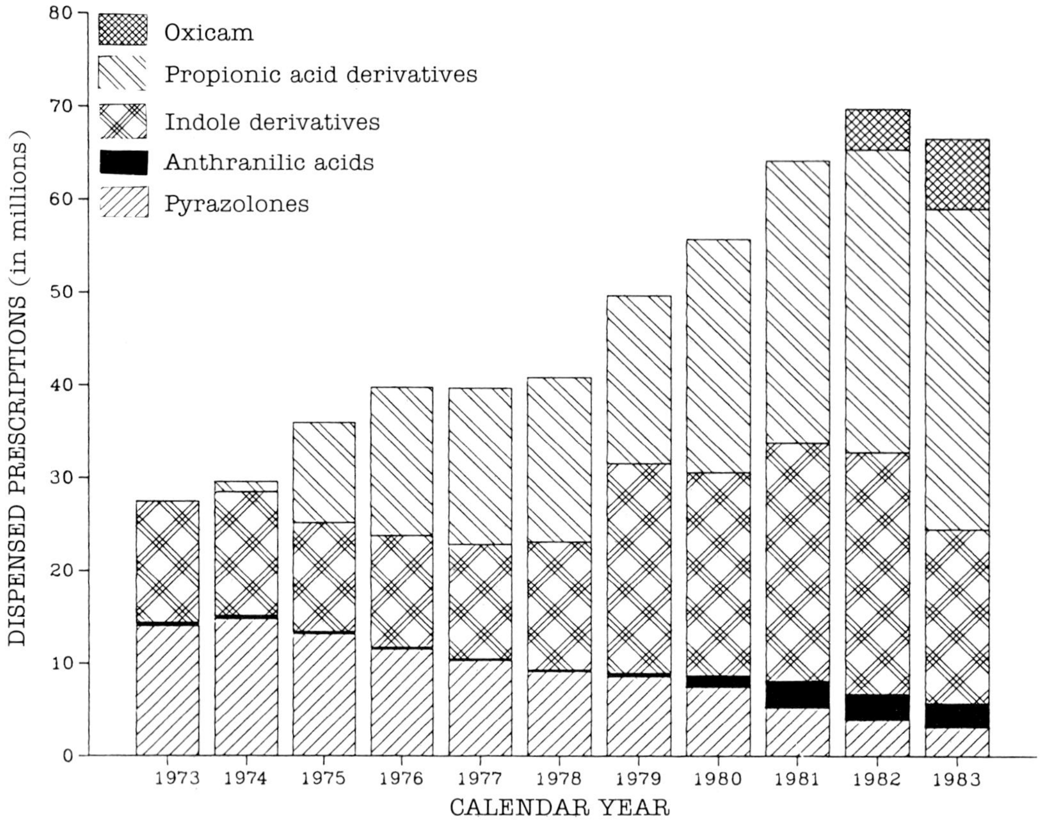

Figure 1. Prescriptions for nonsteroidal antiinflammatory drugs (by chemical class) dispensed by retail pharmacies from 1973–1983.

RESULTS

Table 1 provides a breakdown of total NSAID prescriptions in 1983 by individual generic name and also indicates the percentage of each that were new prescriptions (rather than refills). The latter data provide an indication of whether a drug is for long-term use or for acute conditions, but should be used for comparative purposes (rather than taken as an estimate of the percentage of use that is actually new therapy) because some portion of new prescriptions are written for continued therapy. The percentage of new NSAID prescriptions was around 50%, with 4 exceptions: mefenamic acid, oxyphenbutazone, phenylbutazone, and zomepirac had a higher percentage of new prescriptions.

Differences in the mean number of tablets or capsules in a prescription paralleled differences in the " % new Rxs," with fewer units included in prescriptions for mefenamic acid, oxyphenbutazone, phenylbutazone, and zomepirac. Prescription size was also relatively low for piroxicam, but was comparable with the other NSAIDs considering its once-a-day dosage.

Trends in NSAID use. Figure 1 displays data from the *NPA* on trends in the total number of prescriptions. For simplification of graphic display, data were grouped into 5 chemical classes: pyrazolones, anthranilic acids, indole derivatives, propionic acid derivatives, and oxicam.

In 1983, there were 12 nonsalicylate NSAIDs on the market (zomepirac was withdrawn during the latter part of the year). In 1973, there were only 4. The bottom bar on the graph represents the 2 pyrazolones: phenylbutazone (approved by the FDA in 1952) and oxyphenbutazone (approved in 1960). No new pyrazolones have since been introduced, and there has been a steady decline in the number of prescriptions for these drugs over the 11-year period. One anthranilic acid, mefenamic acid, which was approved in 1965, was available in 1973. Mefenamic acid is a very small proportion of the class, and as will be discussed later, is not used in the same way as the other NSAIDs. In

Table 2. Population exposure to nonsteroidal antiinflammatory drugs

Drug	kg*	DDD (mg)†	DDDs/ 1,000 population/day	US PDD (mg)‡	PDDs/ 1,000/population/day
Fenoprofen	98,600	1,200	0.97	1,563	0.74
Ibuprofen	473,600	800	6.98	1,715	3.26
Indomethacin	15,500	100	1.83	106	1.72
Meclofenamate	6,800	200§	0.40	245	0.33
Mefenamic acid	5,000	1,000	0.06	1,025	0.06
Naproxen	149,700	500	3.53	825	2.14
Oxyphenbutazone	2,100	300	0.08	352	0.07
Phenylbutazone	7,600	300	0.30	371	0.24
Piroxicam	3,800	20§	2.24	22	2.04
Sulindac	52,400	200	3.09	388	1.59
Tolmetin	51,800	700	0.87	1,165	0.52
Zomepirac	6,400	400§	0.19	430	0.18
Total			20.54		12.89

* Total kilograms of drug purchased by retail pharmacies and hospitals during 1983 (2).
† DDD = defined daily dose.
‡ Based on data from reference no. 1. PDD = prescribed daily dose.
§ No published DDD; developed in-house based on official labeling.

mid-1980 the second anthranilic acid, meclofenamate, was approved.

Indomethacin was the only other NSAID on the market in 1973. Although there has been a decline in prescriptions for indomethacin over the past 10 years, it still ranks third among the 12 NSAIDs. Three additional indole derivatives have been approved by the FDA since 1973: tolmetin in March 1976, sulindac in November 1978, and zomepirac in October 1980.

The first propionic acid derivative, ibuprofen, was approved in September 1974. Two additional members of this class, naproxen and fenoprofen, were introduced in 1976. In April 1982, piroxicam was approved and represented a new chemical class. Benoxaprofen, a propionic acid derivative, was also approved in April 1982, but was withdrawn later that year and, as noted previously, is not included in the current data.

Table 3. Drugs used concomitantly with antiarthritic nonsteroidal antiinflammatory drugs (NSAIDs)*

	% of mentions
Used alone	68
Used with other drugs	32
Corticoids	6
Codeine and combination analgesics (oral)	4
Muscle relaxants without analgesics	3
Other NSAI antiarthritics	3
Propoxyphenes	2
Aspirin, APC, etc.	1

* NSAIDs categorized in the Uniform System of Classification (7) as synthetic non-narcotic analgesics rather than systemic antiarthritics are not included. Based on data from reference no. 3. APC = acetylsalicylic acid, phenacetin, and caffeine.

The number of prescriptions for NSAIDs as a group increased steadily from 1973 to 1982, but decreased in 1983. This decrease is entirely attributable to the withdrawal of zomepirac from the market in 1983. If zomepirac use is not considered in the estimates, prescriptions for the remaining NSAIDs increased 2.2% from 1982 to 1983.

As noted previously, the *NPA* methodology was revised in 1981, so 1980–1981 changes should be interpreted with caution; however, the 1981 data shown in Figure 1 appear to be fairly congruent with overall trends for NSAID use.

Population exposure. Table 2 presents results of defined daily dose analyses for NSAIDs, using a US civilian population estimate of 232,286,000 as of July 1,

Table 4. Age and sex distributions (%) of patients using individual nonsteroidal antiinflammatory drugs*

	Sex		Age				
	M	F	0–9	10–19	20–39	40–59	60+
Fenoprofen	35	65	–	3	23	32	42
Ibuprofen	34	66	–	6	28	27	39
Indomethacin	49	51	–	2	21	32	45
Meclofenamate	36	64	–	4	18	33	44
Mefenamic acid	3	97	1	35	53	7	4
Naproxen	33	67	–	5	27	29	39
Oxyphenbutazone	50	50	–	2	33	37	28
Phenylbutazone	48	52	–	2	28	34	36
Piroxicam	32	68	–	1	10	33	56
Sulindac	34	66	–	2	19	28	51
Tolmetin	37	63	–	4	20	38	38
Zomepirac	41	59	–	7	32	35	26

* Based on data from reference no. 3.

1983 (8). The first column gives the total kilograms of each drug purchased by retail pharmacies and hospitals during 1983, and the second column displays the defined daily doses established by European researchers or derived from the official labeling. The data on DDDs/1,000 population/day indicated that there was a total of 20.54 NSAID DDDs/1,000 population/day in 1983, or enough drug quantity to provide daily treatment for over 2% of the US population.

However, this is an overestimate of actual population exposure since there seem to be considerable differences between what is prescribed in the US and the European DDDs. Prescribed daily doses in the US for ibuprofen, naproxen, sulindac, and tolmetin are all at least 50% higher than the established DDDs (Table 2). Ibuprofen is particularly discrepant, with a prescribed daily dose more than twice its defined daily dose. Prescribed daily doses are within the range of recommended doses given in the official labeling for all NSAIDs except piroxicam, which has a PDD of 22 mg and a recommended daily dose of 20 mg. Estimates of population exposure calculated with prescribed daily doses rather than defined daily doses indicate a total of 12.89 PDDs/1,000 population/day. In percentage terms, enough NSAIDs were purchased by drugstores and hospitals to treat 1.29% of the entire civilian population each day in 1983 (or almost 3 million people daily). Similarly, enough ibuprofen was available on an average day to treat about 0.3% of the population (over three-quarters of a million people).

Although the estimates based on prescribed daily doses are more accurate indicators of overall NSAID exposure in the US population, it is important to also describe usage based on defined daily doses. Since DDDs are standardized technical units of measurement that facilitate comparisons internationally, as well as on regional or local levels, analyses using the DDD methodology should always be included. Depending on the purpose of the research, any suspected discrepancies can then be investigated in more depth, as was done here using prescribed daily doses.

Concomitant use of other drugs. Table 3 presents data from the *National Disease and Therapeutic Index* on the categories of drugs that are most often used concomitantly with NSAIDs. In contrast with other data discussed in this review, only those NSAIDs classified as antiarthritics are included because it was not feasible to combine these data across categories. Antiarthritic NSAIDs were used alone about two-thirds of the time and with other drugs about one-third of the time.

Age and sex distributions. The age and sex distributions of NSAID users are displayed in Table 4. Women accounted for 60% of all *NDTI* drug mentions in 1983, and are generally more likely than men to use NSAIDs as well. Only indomethacin, oxyphenbutazone, and phenylbutazone approached equal use by men and women. Mefenamic acid was used almost exclusively by women. NSAIDs were almost never used by children under 10 years of age, and except for mefenamic acid, the percentage of NSAIDs used by children aged 10–19 years was low. Eighty-eight percent of mefenamic acid mentions were for patients aged 10–39 years. Use of zomepirac and oxyphenbutazone peaked in the 40–59 age group and decreased among patients 60 years or older, whereas the percent-

Table 5. Diagnoses for diseases of bones and organs of movement (DBOM) associated with nonsteroidal antiinflammatory drug "mentions"*

	% of specific diagnoses				
Drug	Arthritis NOS	Osteoarthritis	Rheumatoid arthritis	Bursitis	% of all DBOM
Fenoprofen	13	16	6	6	59
Ibuprofen	11	14	3	7	49
Indomethacin	13	13	5	11	57
Meclofenamate	13	19	6	8	61
Mefenamic acid	–	–	–	–	–
Naproxen	11	17	7	8	56
Oxyphenbutazone	4	5	1	23	43
Phenylbutazone	5	4	–	22	47
Piroxicam	23	27	10	5	78
Sulindac	17	22	7	10	71
Tolmetin	14	20	7	11	67
Zomepirac	–	5	1	4	17

* Based on data from reference no. 3. NOS = not otherwise specified.

Table 6. Diagnoses associated with 10% or more of drug "mentions" for any nonsteroidal antiinflammatory drugs*

	% of all associated diagnoses				
Drug	DBOM	Sprains/ strains	Surgical aftercare	Gout	Dysmenorrhea
Fenoprofen	59	12	5	–	1
Ibuprofen	49	10	5	1	6
Indomethacin	57	6	4	10	–
Meclofenamate	61	8	3	–	2
Mefenamic acid	–	1	2	–	59
Naproxen	56	9	4	1	7
Oxyphenbutazone	43	8	4	6	–
Phenylbutazone	47	10	4	7	–
Piroxicam	78	3	3	1	–
Sulindac	71	7	4	2	–
Tolmetin	67	13	3	–	–
Zomepirac	17	16	19	–	3

* Based on data from reference no. 3. DBOM = diseases of bones and organs of movement.

ages were comparable in these 2 age groups for tolmetin and phenylbutazone. The percentage use for the other NSAIDs increased with age.

Diagnosis profiles. Age and sex distributions will frequently vary with different uses of a drug, and Tables 5 and 6 present *NDTI* data on diagnoses (categorized in the *International Classification of Disease,* or *ICD7* [7]) associated with each NSAID. All specific diagnoses that accounted for at least 10% of the total diagnoses associated with any NSAID are included in the 2 tables.

As might be expected, NSAIDs are used largely for the *ICD7* class "diseases of bones and organs of movement." As indicated in Table 5, arthritis not otherwise specified (NOS), osteoarthritis, rheumatoid arthritis, and bursitis were the most frequently mentioned specific diagnoses within the broader diagnosis class. Oxyphenbutazone and phenylbutazone were less likely to be used for arthritic conditions and more likely to be used for bursitis, while most of the other NSAIDs were more likely to be used for arthritic conditions. The entire diagnosis class accounted for practically none of the use of mefenamic acid and for only 17% of all diagnoses associated with the use of zomepirac.

Table 6 provides a broader diagnostic profile and shows the conditions for which mefenamic acid and zomepirac are most often used. Dysmenorrhea accounted for 59% of the diagnoses associated with the use of mefenamic acid, whereas sprains, strains, and surgical aftercare represented over one-third of diagnoses associated with zomepirac. Diagnoses commonly associated with zomepirac usage that do not appear in Table 6 were mainly those included in the general diagnostic classes of "accidents and poisonings" (e.g., fractures, contusions, lacerations) and "symptoms and senility" (e.g., back pain, headache, chest pain).

Table 7. Drug therapy prescribed for arthritis patients*

Drug category	% of all arthritis patient visits
No drug therapy	15
Nonsteroidal antiiflammatory drugs	55
Ibuprofen	11
Naproxen	11
Piroxicam	10
Sulindac	7
Indomethacin	7
Fenoprofen	3
Tolmetin	3
Meclofenamate	3
Zomepirac	1
Phenylbutazone	1
Oxyphenbutazone	1
Mefenamic acid	–
Aspirin, APC, etc.	12
Plain corticoids (oral)	6
Plain corticoids (injectable)	5
Codeine and combination analgesics (oral)	5
Propoxyphenes	4
Other over-the-counter analgesics	3
Gold therapy	3

* Includes ICD7 (7) diagnoses of acute pyogenic arthritis, acute nonpyogenic arthritis, rheumatoid arthritis, spondylitis ankylopoietica, osteoarthritis, spondylitis osteoarthritis, arthritis not otherwise specified, and other specified arthritis. Based on data from reference no. 3. APC = acetylsalicylic acid, phenacetin, and caffeine.

Drug treatment for arthritis. The *National Disease and Therapeutic Index* estimated that there were 29 million visits by patients for the broad diagnosis of arthritis in 1983. Four specific diagnoses represented 96% of this total: osteoarthritis (40%), arthritis NOS

(29%), rheumatoid arthritis (18%), and spondylitis osteoarthritis (9%). About 55% of the total number of visits involved prescription NSAID therapy. Only 15% of the patients were not given some type of drug therapy. Percentages for individual NSAIDs and other drug categories are presented in Table 7.

DISCUSSION

Utilization patterns are fairly similar for 8 of the 12 NSAIDs. They are basically used to treat arthritic conditions in older patients. Mefenamic acid differs strikingly; almost 60% of its use was for treatment of dysmenorrhea, and it was virtually never used in the treatment of arthritis. Women accounted for 97% of the use of mefenamic acid and 88% of its use was in the 10–39-year age group.

Zomepirac, phenylbutazone, and oxyphenbutazone also differ from the other NSAIDs and are similar to one another and to mefenamic acid in several ways. They were less likely to be used for treatment of elderly patients and more likely to be used to treat acute conditions. The proportion of new prescriptions was higher and the average prescription size was lower for these drugs compared with other NSAIDs. The percentage of use for arthritis was relatively low for all 3 drugs. Bursitis was the specific diagnosis most frequently associated with both phenylbutazone and oxyphenbutazone, and surgical aftercare was the main diagnosis for which zomepirac was used. A high proportion of zomepirac was also used for various pain symptoms and accidents.

As a class, the NSAIDs are among the most widely used drugs in current practice. In 1983, enough NSAIDs were available to treat almost 3 million people daily. Their use has nearly tripled over the past 10 years and continues to grow. This particular market appears to be an elastic one: with few exceptions, each new product introduced expands the market rather than detracting from the existing products. The unavailability of zomepirac in the latter part of 1983 was not compensated for by an increase in the use of other NSAIDs (probably because zomepirac had a different diagnosis/use pattern). Whether the market will continue to expand with introduction of new NSAIDs remains to be seen.

REFERENCES

1. National Prescription Audit. Ambler, Pennsylvania, IMS America, Ltd., 1983
2. The US Pharmaceutical Market–Drugstore and Hospital Purchases. Ambler, Pennsylvania, IMS America, Ltd., 1983
3. National Disease and Therapeutic Index. Ambler, Pennsylvania, IMS America, Ltd., 1983
4. Bergman U, Grimsson A, Wahba AHW, Westerholm B, editors: Studies in Drug Utilization. Copenhagen, World Health Organization Regional Office for Europe, 1979
5. Nordic Council on Medicines: Nordic Statistics on Medicine. Part II. Uppsala, Nordic Council on Medicines, 1982
6. Kennedy DL, Forbes MB, Baum C, Jones JK: Antibiotic use in U.S. hospitals in 1981. Am J Hosp Pharm 40:797–801, 1983
7. World Health Organization: Manual of the International Classification of Disease, Injuries, and Causes of Death. Geneva, World Health Organization, 1957
8. Estimates of the population of the United States July 1, 1981 to 1983. United States Bureau of the Census. Advance Report. Population estimates and projections, Series P-25, No. 944, January 1984

APPLICATION, TO JAPANESE PATIENTS, OF THE 1982 AMERICAN RHEUMATISM ASSOCIATION REVISED CRITERIA FOR THE CLASSIFICATION OF SYSTEMIC LUPUS ERYTHEMATOSUS

RYUICHI YOKOHARI and TOKUGORO TSUNEMATSU

The 1982 American Rheumatism Association revised criteria for the classification of systemic lupus erythematosus were tested on Japanese patients. Sensitivity and specificity data were comparable with those presented in the development of the revised criteria by the American Rheumatism Association. Complement determinations were evaluated for their ability to improve the criteria for the diagnosis of early systemic lupus erythematosus.

The 1982 American Rheumatism Association (ARA) revised criteria for the classification of systemic lupus erythematosus (SLE) (1) were applied to Japanese patients. This study evaluated the revised criteria in the context of 2 questions: How effective are the revised criteria when tested against a patient population outside the United States? How much do the sensitivity and specificity of the revised criteria depend on the point in the course of the patient's illness at which they are applied?

METHODS

The Research Committee for Autoimmune Diseases of the Ministry of Health and Welfare of Japan obtained the SLE criteria study protocol, instructions, and data recording form which were used in the development of the revised criteria. The protocol, instructions, and data form were translated into Japanese, slightly modified, and distributed in September 1983 to 29 investigators throughout Japan, who were members of the Committee. The modifications included selecting as controls, if possible, patients with progressive systemic sclerosis (PSS), polymyositis or dermatomyositis (PM/DM), or Sjögren's syndrome (SS), as well as rheumatoid arthritis (RA). Patients with mixed connective tissue disease or overlap syndromes were excluded. Each investigator was requested to submit report forms on 10 consecutive patients with unequivocal SLE observed during a period of active disease and forms on 10 control patients by December 1983. The diagnosis of the patients' disease was made using each participant's own criteria, except that patients with RA were diagnosed as having definite or classic disease, using the ARA criteria (2).

The forms noted the presence or absence of each variable at any time during followup, as well as at the initial evaluation. The collected data from 285 patients with SLE and 272 control patients were processed by a microcomputer (NEC PC-8801); accuracy was ensured by checking original forms against computer data printouts and, when necessary, checking outlying information against original data at the home institution. The data were analyzed with programs written by Inforex Company Ltd., Japan, tabulating the frequencies of each variable and of each of the revised criteria, as well as the 1971 ARA preliminary criteria (3) in the patient groups. The difference was regarded as statistically significant when P was <0.01, by chi-square analysis.

RESULTS

Table 1 shows the distribution of patients from whom data were obtained in this study. The mean age at disease onset was 27.2 ± 10.0 years in SLE patients and 40.4 ± 13.3 years in the control group. The mean age at study entry was 33.1 ± 10.6 years in SLE patients and 47.2 ± 13.3 years in the control group.

From the Research Committee for Autoimmune Diseases, the Ministry of Health and Welfare of Japan, Tokyo.

Supported by a research grant from the Japanese Ministry of Health and Welfare.

Ryuichi Yokohari, MD, PhD: Head, Division of Collagen Diseases, National Medical Center, Tokyo; Tokugoro Tsunematsu, MD, PhD: Professor, Third Department of Internal Medicine, Shimane Medical University and Chairman of the Research Committee for Autoimmune Diseases.

Address reprint requests to Ryuichi Yokohari, 1-21-1 Toyama, Shinjuku-ku, Tokyo 162, Japan.

Submitted for publication August 17, 1984; accepted in revised form February 8, 1985.

Table 1. Patient population

	Male	Female	Total
Systemic lupus erythematosus patients	17	268	285
Control patients			
Progressive systemic sclerosis	11	77	88
Rheumatoid arthritis	13	84	97
Polymyositis/dermatomyositis	11	34	45
Sjögren's syndrome	0	24	24
Others*	10	8	18
Total	62	495	557

* Others included 4 patients with polyarteritis nodosa, 4 with generalized morphea, 3 with Behçet's disease, 3 with aortitis, 2 with allergic granulomatous angiitis, 1 with Wegener's granulomatosis, and 1 with ankylosing spondylitis.

The mean duration of disease was 7.8 ± 8.7 years in SLE patients and 8.9 ± 9.3 years in the control group. The period of time from disease onset to the first visit was comparable in the 2 groups.

Every variable tested, except Raynaud's phenomenon and focal neurologic disorder, occurred with significantly different frequency in SLE patients versus controls (Table 2).

When our data were compared with data presented in the analysis of the revised criteria (1), the prevalence of various manifestations was found to be similar for Japanese and American patients, with statistically significant differences in the frequencies of malar rash, Raynaud's phenomenon, nonerosive arthritis, pleurisy, leukopenia, and DNA antibody, as indicated in Table 3.

When the revised criteria were tested on the Japanese patients with the above-mentioned disease features, sensitivity was 97% and specificity against the control group was 89%. When the 1971 preliminary criteria (3) were used, sensitivity was 92% and specificity 94%. A similar analysis was performed on the

Table 2. Frequency of manifestations in Japanese patients

	Systemic lupus erythematosus patients	Control patients
Malar rash	219/285 (77)*	8/272 (3)
Discoid lupus	78/285 (27)	4/272 (1)
Alopecia	157/285 (55)	17/272 (6)
Photosensitivity	129/284 (45)	8/271 (3)
Oral ulcers	70/285 (25)	16/271 (6)
Raynaud's phenomenon	135/284 (48)	108/271 (40)
Arthritis		
Nonerosive	228/285 (80)	106/272 (39)
Erosive	3/285 (1)	84/272 (31)
Proteinuria		
>0.5 gm/day	151/280 (54)	15/263 (6)
>3.5 gm/day	78/281 (28)	3/271 (1)
>3+	123/277 (44)	12/267 (4)
Granular casts	147/278 (53)	23/271 (8)
Dementia	4/285 (1)	1/272
Seizures	27/285 (9)	1/272
Coma	17/285 (6)	0/272
Psychosis	41/285 (14)	3/272 (1)
Focal neurologic disorder	31/285 (11)	22/271 (8)
Pleurisy	51/284 (18)	14/270 (5)
Pericarditis	45/284 (16)	11/269 (4)
Hemolytic anemia	45/278 (16)	12/269 (4)
Leukopenia	191/285 (67)	36/271 (13)
Lymphopenia	195/279 (70)	79/270 (29)
Thrombocytopenia	68/282 (24)	12/269 (4)
Lupus erythematosus cells	161/267 (60)	10/200 (5)
Antinuclear antibody	281/285 (99)	133/255 (52)
DNA antibody	244/272 (90)	54/219 (25)
Sm antibody	49/183 (27)	4/166 (2)
False-positive serologic test for syphilis	52/267 (19)	5/223 (2)
C3	208/255 (82)	40/215 (19)
C4	178/240 (74)	42/203 (21)
CH50	208/244 (85)	53/214 (25)
Abnormal renal biopsy findings	90/99 (91)	3/17 (18)
Abnormal skin biopsy findings	37/50 (74)	6/36 (17)

* Numbers in parentheses = percentages.

Table 3. Comparison of frequency of manifestations in the Japanese patient group versus the American Rheumatism Association (ARA) patient group*

	Systemic lupus erythematosus patients		Control group	
Criterion	Japanese (n = 285)	ARA (n = 177)	Japanese (n = 272)	ARA (n = 162)
Malar rash	219/285 (77)	101/177 (57)	8/272 (3)	6/162 (4)
Raynaud's phenomenon	135/284 (48)	51/176 (28)	108/271 (40)	30/162 (19)
Arthritis, nonerosive	228/285 (80)	152/177 (86)	106/272 (39)	102/162 (63)
Pleurisy	51/284 (18)	92/177 (52)	14/270 (5)	18/162 (11)
Leukopenia	191/285 (67)	82/177 (46)	36/271 (13)	17/161 (11)
DNA antibody	244/272 (90)	113/168 (67)	54/219 (25)	7/91 (8)

* Only frequencies with significant difference are shown. Numbers in parentheses = percentages.

data obtained at the initial evaluation. The revised criteria were 89% sensitive and 96% specific, while the preliminary criteria were 78% sensitive and 98% specific. These results revealed that the revised criteria show better sensitivity than the preliminary criteria at any point in the patient's illness (Table 4). The most important contributory item to sensitivity of the revised criteria was the fluorescent antinuclear antibody (FANA) test, since its exclusion resulted in a loss of sensitivity of up to 89% at any time during followup and up to 74% at the time of initial evaluation. Exclusion of other items such as DNA antibody, Sm antibody, or lymphopenia did not significantly reduce sensitivity.

Using the revised criteria, there were 29 false-positive patients, including all but 2 of the 15 false-positive patients identified using the preliminary criteria. These 29 patients consisted of 12 patients with PSS, 8 with RA, 3 with DM, 5 with SS, and 1 with Wegener's granulomatosis (Table 5). Of these patients, 7 with PSS, 2 with RA, 1 with DM, and 3 with SS were also false-positive by the preliminary criteria, as illustrated in Figure 1. These results seemed to indicate a lower specificity for the revised criteria than for the preliminary criteria. However, a statistically significant difference in specificity was not obtained between the 2 criteria sets ($0.05 > P > 0.01$). Using the revised criteria, false-positive patients, when compared with true-negative patients, had significantly higher frequencies of the following elements: photosensitivity, oral ulcers, cellular casts, psychosis, peripheral neuropathy, pleurisy, leukopenia, lymphopenia, thrombocytopenia, LE cells, FANA, DNA antibody, Sm antibody, CH50, and C4 (Table 6).

Thirty-six patients with SLE did not fulfill the revised criteria at the initial evaluation. They had lower frequencies of malar rash, photosensitivity, nonerosive arthritis, profuse proteinuria, cellular casts, leukopenia, lymphopenia, LE cells, FANA, and DNA antibody when compared with the patients who fulfilled the revised criteria at the time of initial evaluation, as seen in Table 7. Eighteen of them had low levels of either C3, C4, or CH50. If hypocomplementemia was used as an additional criterion, sensitivity increased to 93% with a reduction in specificity by 2%.

Table 4. Comparison of sensitivity and specificity of the 1971 and 1982 American Rheumatism Association (ARA) criteria for the classification of systemic lupus erythematosus in the Japanese patient group versus the ARA patient group

	% sensitivity*		% specificity	
	Japanese patients	ARA patients	Japanese patients	ARA patients
1971	92 (78)	88	94 (98)	95
1982	97 (89)	95	89 (96)	96

* Numbers in parentheses = percentage at the initial evaluation.

Table 5. Number of revised criteria fulfilled by patient group*

No. of criteria	SLE	PSS	RA	PM/DM	SS	Controls (combined)
0	0	8	23	10	2	46
1	0	21	37	12	7	87
2	1	26	19	11	3	63
3	7	21	10	8	7	47
4	25	9†	7†	2†	3†	22†‡
5	51	3†	0	1†	2†	6†
6	70	0	1†	0	0	1†
7	68	0	0	0	0	0
8	39	0	0	0	0	0
9	17	0	0	0	0	0
10	7	0	0	0	0	0
11	0	0	0	0	0	0
Total	285	88	97	45	24	272

* SLE = systemic lupus erythematosus; PSS = progressive systemic sclerosis; RA = rheumatoid arthritis; PM/DM = polymyositis/dermatomyositis; SS = Sjögren's syndrome.
† False-positive patients.
‡ Includes 1 patient with Wegener's granulomatosis.

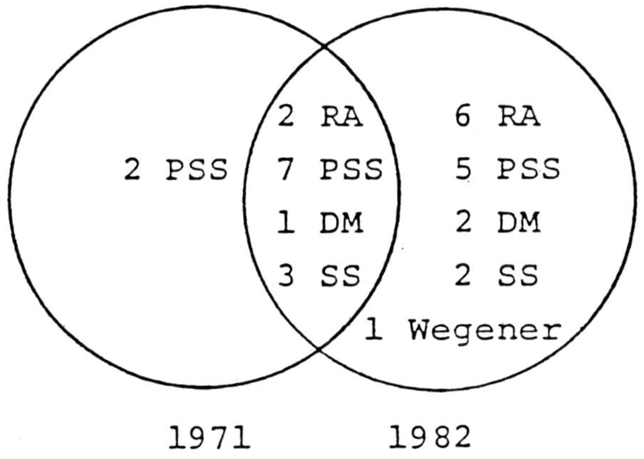

Figure 1. Distribution of patients classified as false-positive by the 1971 American Rheumatism Association (ARA) preliminary criteria for systemic lupus erythematosus and by the 1982 ARA revised criteria. RA = rheumatoid arthritis; PSS = progressive systemic sclerosis; DM = dermatomyositis; SS = Sjögren's syndrome; Wegener = Wegener's granulomatosis.

DISCUSSION

Japanese patients under consideration in this study show somewhat different disease features than patients in the United States. There were higher frequencies of malar rash and leukopenia in SLE patients and lower frequencies of nonerosive arthritis in the control group. There also were higher frequencies of Raynaud's phenomenon and DNA antibody and a lower frequency of pleurisy in both SLE patients and the control group. When tested on these patient groups, the 1982 revised criteria revealed a significantly higher sensitivity than the 1971 preliminary criteria, with a slight, but not significant, decrease in specificity. We did not try to apply a different set of criteria for Japanese patients, since the sensitivity of the revised criteria was sufficiently high, and significantly higher sensitivity could not be expected. Among items which were added to the revised criteria, FANA was found

Table 6. Frequency of manifestations in false-positive patients and true-negative patients using the 1982 American Rheumatism Association revised criteria for systemic lupus erythematosus

	False-positive	True-negative	Chi-square
Malar rash	3/29 (10)*	5/243 (2)	3.67
Discoid lupus	1/29 (3)	3/243 (1)	0.01
Alopecia	5/29 (17)	12/243 (5)	4.76†
Photosensitivity	4/27 (15)	4/244 (2)	10.49‡
Oral ulcers	7/29 (24)	9/242 (4)	19.44‡
Raynaud's phenomenon	16/29 (55)	92/242 (38)	3.19
Arthritis, nonerosive	16/28 (57)	90/244 (37)	4.33†
Proteinuria			
>0.5 gm/day	3/26 (12)	12/237 (5)	0.82
>3.5 gm/day	1/28 (4)	2/243 (1)	0.13
>3+	1/26 (4)	11/241 (5)	0.11
Cellular casts	8/29 (28)	15/242 (6)	15.25‡
Seizure	1/29 (3)	0/243 (0)	1.63
Coma	0/29 (0)	0/243 (0)	
Psychosis	3/29 (10)	0/243 (0)	16.82‡
Focal neurologic disorder	7/29 (24)	15/242 (6)	11.17‡
Pleurisy	7/28 (25)	7/242 (3)	24.95‡
Pericarditis	3/28 (11)	8/241 (3)	1.87
Hemolytic anemia	4/28 (14)	8/241 (3)	4.74†
Leukopenia	10/29 (34)	26/242 (11)	12.67‡
Lymphopenia	20/29 (69)	59/241 (24)	24.75‡
Thrombocytopenia	8/29 (28)	4/240 (2)	34.93‡
Lupus erythematosus cells	8/27 (30)	2/173 (1)	34.09‡
Fluorescent antinuclear antibody	25/29 (86)	108/226 (48)	13.70‡
DNA antibody	17/26 (65)	37/193 (19)	26.34‡
Sm antibody	3/19 (16)	1/147 (1)	16.33‡
False-positive serologic test for syphilis	1/26 (4)	4/197 (2)	0.01
C3	9/24 (38)	31/191 (16)	6.37§
C4	10/22 (45)	32/181 (18)	9.22‡
CH50	12/22 (55)	41/192 (21)	11.67‡

* Numbers in parentheses = percentages.
† $P < 0.05$.
‡ $P < 0.01$.
§ $P < 0.02$.

Table 7. Frequency of manifestations in false-negative patients and true-positive patients using the 1982 American Rheumatism Association revised criteria for systemic lupus erythematosus at the time of initial evaluation

	False-positive	True-negative	Chi-square
Malar rash	10/36 (28)*	186/248 (75)	32.78†
Discoid lupus	4/34 (12)	56/242 (23)	1.65
Alopecia	10/36 (28)	117/243 (48)	5.25‡
Photosensitivity	5/33 (16)	107/238 (45)	8.39†
Oral ulcers	2/36 (6)	51/242 (21)	3.94§
Raynaud's phenomenon	12/33 (36)	110/246 (45)	0.82
Arthritis, nonerosive	15/35 (43)	197/247 (80)	22.37†
Proteinuria			
>0.5 gm/day	6/33 (18)	102/230 (44)	8.16†
>3.5 gm/day	4/33 (12)	47/238 (20)	0.66†
>3+	4/31 (13)	84/225 (37)	6.17‡
Cellular casts	4/32 (13)	90/240 (38)	6.74†
Seizure	0/36 (0)	13/248 (5)	0.96
Coma	0/36 (0)	8/247 (3)	0.31
Psychosis	0/36 (0)	20/249 (8)	2.00
Focal neurologic disorder	4/36 (11)	17/245 (7)	0.30
Pleurisy	0/36 (0)	31/243 (13)	3.96§
Pericarditis	0/35 (0)	25/243 (10)	2.80
Hemolytic anemia	2/34 (6)	32/237 (14)	0.96
Leukopenia	11/35 (31)	143/244 (59)	9.14†
Lymphopenia	11/32 (34)	136/226 (60)	7.61†
Thrombocytopenia	8/33 (24)	43/240 (18)	0.76
Lupus erythematosus cells	10/28 (36)	135/216 (63)	7.38†
Fluorescent antinuclear antibody	21/29 (72)	230/241 (95)	20.97†
DNA antibody	13/27 (48)	178/215 (83)	17.31†
Sm antibody	3/13 (23)	33/112 (29)	0.02
False-positive serologic test for syphilis	3/27 (11)	44/220 (20)	0.72
C3	13/24 (54)	131/180 (73)	3.53
C4	10/16 (63)	101/152 (66)	0.10
CH50	11/20 (55)	147/188 (78)	5.32§

* Numbers in parentheses = percentages.
† $P < 0.01$.
‡ $P < 0.02$.
§ $P < 0.05$.

to contribute most to an increase in sensitivity. A similar result was reported by Levin et al (4).

The specificity of the revised criteria in this study was slightly lower than that presented in the development of the revised criteria (89 versus 96%), although the difference was not significant ($0.05 > P > 0.01$). This may be because of different distributions of the control patients. In the ARA study (1), when the revised criteria were tested against the combined PSS and PM/DM patients on whom data had been collected by the Subcommittee for Scleroderma Criteria of the ARA, specificity was 89%. In our study also, specificity against PSS or SS was relatively low (86 and 79%, respectively) in comparison with that against RA (93%). Inclusion of connective tissue diseases other than RA in the control group probably reduced the specificity of the revised criteria to some extent. False-positive patients in this study had significantly higher frequencies of abnormal urinary, hematologic, and immunologic findings than did true-negative patients. It seems likely that laboratory findings contained in the revised criteria had the effect of lowering specificity. In order to improve specificity, it may be necessary to weight the criteria, as proposed by Clough et al (5).

Thirty-six patients with SLE did not fulfill the revised criteria at the time of initial evaluation. They had lower frequencies in many characteristic manifestations of SLE, compared with those who fulfilled the revised criteria at the time of initial evaluation. Hence, early classification of SLE is difficult. Half of the false-negative patients at the time of initial evaluation were already hypocomplementemic. Using hypocomplementemia as an additional criterion, 15 patients fulfilled 4 of the criteria, and sensitivity increased from 89% to 93%. In developing the revised criteria, the ARA

Subcommittee was unable to improve the accuracy of the criteria by using any combination of serum complement determinations either as a separate criterion or by including those determinations with one of the other combined variables. The same was also true in this study, when the data obtained at any time over the course of followup were analyzed. However, at the initial evaluation, hypocomplementemia appeared to assist in the process of classifying SLE.

Complement determinations have been widely used as one of the tools for monitoring disease activity in SLE, especially in lupus nephritis. Weinstein et al (6) showed a high predictive value of high DNA binding and low C3 levels for the diagnosis of SLE. Hypocomplementemia should be reevaluated for its ability to improve sensitivity of the criteria at the first evaluation, when the disease manifestations are not fully developed.

ACKNOWLEDGMENTS

The authors are grateful to Dr. Eng M. Tan for his cooperation, and thank Shinichi Aotsuka and Makiko Kinoshita for their valuable assistance.

REFERENCES

1. Tan EM, Cohen AS, Fries JF, Masi AT, McShane DJ, Rothfield NF, Schaller JG, Talal N, Winchester RJ: The 1982 revised criteria for the classification of systemic lupus erythematosus. Arthritis Rheum 25:1271–1277, 1982
2. Ropes MW, Bennett GA, Cobb S, Jacox R, Jessar RA: 1958 revision of diagnostic criteria for rheumatoid arthritis. Bull Rheum Dis 9:175–176, 1958
3. Cohen AS, Reynolds WE, Franklin EC, Kulka JP, Ropes MW, Shulman LE, Wallace SL: Preliminary criteria for the classification of systemic lupus erythematosus. Bull Rheum Dis 21:643–648, 1971
4. Levin RE, Weinstein A, Peterson M, Testa MA, Rothfield NF: A comparison of the sensitivity of the 1971 and 1982 American Rheumatism Association criteria for the classification of systemic lupus erythematosus. Arthritis Rheum 27:530–538, 1984
5. Clough JD, Elrazak M, Calabrese LH, Valenzuela R, Braun WB, William GW: Weighted criteria for the diagnosis of systemic lupus erythematosus. Arch Intern Med 144:281–285, 1984
6. Weinstein A, Bordwell B, Stone B, Tibbetts C, Rothfield NF: Antibodies to native DNA and serum complement (C3) levels: application to diagnosis and classification of systemic lupus erythematosus. Am J Med 74:206–216, 1983

BRIEF REPORT

JUVENILE PROGRESSIVE SYSTEMIC SCLEROSIS: CLINICAL AND SEROLOGIC FINDINGS

MARÍA E. SUÁREZ-ALMAZOR, LUIS J. CATOGGIO, JOSÉ A. MALDONADO-COCCO, RUBÉN CUTTICA, and OSVALDO GARCÍA-MORTEO

Progressive systemic sclerosis (PSS) is a rare disease among children. The largest series of patients whose disease onset occurred before the age of 16 years were reported by Hanson in 1976 (1) and Cassidy et al in 1977 (2). In both reports, clinical features of juvenile PSS appeared to be similar to those described in adult-onset disease. Although cardiac and pulmonary involvement have been extensively studied in adult patients with PSS, they have been rarely described in children with this disease. Using conventional methods of immunofluorescence, antinuclear antibodies (ANA) are detected with similar frequency in adults and in children with PSS (1,2). However, the frequency and clinical significance of the more recently described antibodies considered to be highly specific for PSS, e.g., antinucleolar, anticentromere (ACA) (3), and anti–Scl-70 (4), have not been determined in the juvenile form of the disease. In this report we describe the clinical features in 5 children with PSS, with emphasis on the cardiovascular involvement and serologic findings.

From the Section of Rheumatology, Department of Medicine, Instituto Nacional de Rehabilitación, and the Laboratory, Centro Médico San Luis, Buenos Aires, Argentina.

María E. Suárez-Almazor, MD: Fellow in Rheumatology, Instituto Nacional de Rehabilitación; Luis J. Catoggio, MD: Physician in Charge, Rheumatology Section, Hospital Italiano de Buenos Aires and Laboratory, Centro Médico San Luis; José A. Maldonado-Cocco, MD: Chief, Section of Rheumatology, Department of Medicine, Instituto Nacional de Rehabilitación; Rubén Cuttica, MD: Staff Physician, Hospital de Niños "Dr. Pedro de Elizalde," Buenos Aires; Osvaldo García-Morteo, MD: Associate Professor of Medicine, Universidad de Buenos Aires and Head, Department of Medicine, Instituto Nacional de Rehabilitación.

Address reprint requests to José A. Maldonado-Cocco, MD, Sección Reumatología, Instituto Nacional de Rehabilitación, Echeverría 955, 1428 Buenos Aires, Argentina.

Submitted for publication June 11, 1984; accepted in revised form January 3, 1985.

PATIENTS AND METHODS

Five children with juvenile PSS (4 girls and 1 boy) were studied over a 2-year period. In all patients, disease began before age 16 years; all patients fulfilled American Rheumatism Association criteria for the diagnosis of PSS (5). In addition to the usual clinical and laboratory evaluations, the following studies were performed: barium swallow radiographs of the esophagus, resting electrocardiogram (EKG), exercise EKG (treadmill), 24-hour ambulatory EKG (Holter), echocardiogram (M mode), spirometry, and arterial blood gas analysis with the patient at rest, breathing room air.

Antinuclear antibodies were detected by indirect immunofluorescence using mouse liver and HEp-2 cells as substrates (6). Antibodies to Scl-70, Sm, Ro (SS-A), La (SS-B), and nuclear RNP (nRNP) were investigated by the Ouchterlony double immunodiffusion technique with 0.6% agarose (6). Human spleen extract was used as a source of Ro (7), calf thymus extract for La, nRNP, and Sm (8), and rabbit thymus extract for Scl-70 (6). Rheumatoid factors were investigated by the latex fixation test.

RESULTS

Clinical manifestations. Four of the 5 patients studied had diffuse scleroderma, and 1 had incomplete CREST syndrome (calcinosis, Raynaud's phenomenon, esophageal dysmotility, sclerodactyly, telangiectasias), with Raynaud's phenomenon, sclerodactyly, and telangiectasias (Table 1). In all cases, initial signs and symptoms were Raynaud's phenomenon and skin tightening on the hands; these occurred either simulta-

Table 1. Clinical manifestations in 5 children with progressive systemic sclerosis (PSS)

Patient	Type of PSS	Sex	Age at onset (years)	Disease duration (years)	Presenting signs/ symptoms	Pitting scars	Hypo/ hyper-pigmentation	Telangi-ectasias	Muscle weakness	Arthritis	Abnormal esophageal motility	Digital tuft resorption	Calcinosis
1	Diffuse	M	10	2	Raynaud's, skin tightening, knee arthritis	Yes	Yes	Face, hands	Yes	Yes	Yes	No	Yes
2	Diffuse	F	10	3	Raynaud's, skin tightening	Yes	Yes	No	Yes	No	Yes	Yes	No
3	Diffuse	F	9	2.5	Raynaud's, skin tightening	Yes	No	No	No	No	No	No	No
4	Diffuse	F	8	1.5	Raynaud's, skin tightening, arthralgia	Yes	Yes	No	No	No	No	No	No
5	RST*	F	10	8	Raynaud's, skin tightening, telangiectasias	Yes	No	Face, hands, trunk	Yes	No	No	Yes	No

* Raynaud's phenomenon, sclerodactyly, telangietasias.

neously or less than 1 year apart. Other clinical features are shown in Table 1. Three children developed proximal muscular weakness; the electromyographic pattern was compatible with myositis in 2 of them. Only 1 patient had mild elevation of creatine kinase and aldolase. All patients showed joint contractures in various degrees, mainly in the hands and elbows. Although 2 patients had radiologic evidence of esophageal hypomotility, only 1 of them had transient dysphagia. Digital tuft resorption was observed in the 2 children who had the longest disease duration. Nasal septal perforation was observed in 1 patient. None had intestinal symptoms or evidence of renal disease.

Cardiopulmonary findings. Patient 1 had pulmonary hypertension, heart enlargement, congestive heart failure, and peaked P waves on the EKG (Table 2). Cardiac catheterization showed a pulmonary artery pressure of 80/40 mm Hg (mean 56 mm Hg). During catheterization, immersion of the patient's hands in cold water produced Raynaud's phenomenon, with a simultaneous increase of 5 mm Hg in diastolic pulmonary pressure. The child died of refractory heart failure 2 years after disease onset; autopsy was not performed.

None of the other patients showed clinically significant cardiovascular disease (Table 2). Although

Table 2. Cardiopulmonary findings in 5 children with progressive systemic sclerosis*

Patient	Clinical features	Cardiac catheterization	Resting EKG	Exercise EKG	Holter EKG	Echocardiogram	Chest radiograph	FVC (spirometry)	Arterial blood gases
1	Pulmonary hypertension, congestive heart failure, died	LV 105/0–8 mm Hg, LA 11 mm Hg, RA 10 mm Hg, RV 80/0 mm Hg, PA 80/40 (56) mm Hg	Right ventricle hypertrophy	NT	Normal	Pericardial effusion, pericardial and endocardial thickening, RV enlargement	Cardiomegaly	52%	PO_2 59 mm Hg
2	Crackling rales	NT	Normal	Normal response	Normal	Pericardial effusion	Bibasilar linear densities	37%	NT
3	None	NT	Normal	Normal response	Isolated supraventricular arrhythmia (2/hour)	Normal	Normal	60%	PO_2 82 mm Hg
4	None	NT	IRBB	Normal response	Normal	Normal	Normal	68%	Normal
5	None	NT	Normal	Normal response	Normal	Normal	Normal	73%	NT

* EKG = electrocardiogram; FVC = forced vital capacity; LV = left ventricle; LA = left atrium; RA = right atrium; RV = right ventricle; PA = pulmonary artery; NT = not tested; IRBB = incomplete right bundle branch block.

only 1 (patient 2) had clinical and radiologic features of pulmonary fibrosis, spirometric evaluation showed varying degrees of restrictive ventilatory incapacity in all patients. Hypoxemia was observed in 2 of 3 patients (patient 1, 59 mm Hg; patient 3, 82 mm Hg).

Serologic findings. By immunofluorescence with mouse liver as substrate, 2 patients showed ANA. However, when HEp-2 cells were used, all 5 sera had positive ANA with a nucleolar pattern (Table 3). In 2 sera, no other nuclear or cytoplasmic staining was observed, but 1 of them had anti-Ro antibodies shown by immunodiffusion. In the remaining 3 patients, the nucleolar pattern was accompanied by a diffuse grainy staining of the nucleus with chromosomal staining. Anti–Scl-70 antibodies were present in 2 of them. All patients were seronegative for rheumatoid factor.

Table 3. Serologic findings in 5 children with progressive systemic sclerosis

Patient	Antinuclear antibodies (mouse liver)	Antinuclear antibodies (HEp-2)	Anticentromere antibodies	Anti–Scl-70	Other antibodies*
1	Negative	4+ nucleolar	Negative	Negative	Negative
2	1:500, homogeneous	3+ nucleolar, 2+ DG†	Negative	Positive	Negative
3	Negative	2+ nucleolar, 1+ DG	Negative	Negative	Negative
4	Negative	3+ nucleolar, 2+ DG	Negative	Positive	Negative
5	1:500, nucleolar speckled	4+ nucleolar	Negative	Negative	Anti-Ro

* Anti-Ro, anti-La, anti–nuclear RNP, anti-Sm.
† DG = diffuse grainy.

DISCUSSION

Reports of PSS in children have not been frequent. There have been occasional reports on small numbers of children, and some of these series included patients with localized scleroderma (9,10). Hanson (1) and Cassidy et al (2), respectively, described 13 and 15 juvenile patients with PSS; clinical features of disease appeared to be the same as in adults. In most cases, initial manifestations were Raynaud's phenomenon and cutaneous induration of the hands. These features were also observed in our juvenile patients.

Although cardiovascular abnormalities, including pulmonary hypertension, have been adequately studied in adults (11–13), their prevalence and characteristics in children are unknown. To our knowledge, only 1 juvenile patient with scleroderma and pulmonary hypertension has been described (14). As in that case, our patient died a few months after the onset of pulmonary hypertension, showing the severe, rapid course of this complication. It has been previously suggested that pulmonary vessels are susceptible to cold-induced vasospasm (15), and in our patient with pulmonary hypertension, immersion of his hands in cold water produced Raynaud's phenomenon and a simultaneous increase in diastolic pulmonary pressure.

Although without clinical significance, 3 other patients showed some cardiologic abnormalities. It is of interest that despite the short disease duration and absence of prominent clinical or radiologic findings of pulmonary fibrosis in 4 of the patients, they all showed varying degrees of restrictive ventilatory incapacity. As in adults, the children with more severe visceral disease were those with more extensive cutaneous involvement.

To our knowledge, there are no reports regarding the recently described antibodies characteristic of scleroderma in the juvenile form of systemic disease. Although only 2 of our 5 patients had ANA on mouse liver substrate, all of them showed nuclear staining when monolayer cell cultures (HEp-2) were used. As has been previously shown, this is due to the higher sensitivity of the latter substrate (16). All patients had antinucleolar antibodies using HEp-2 cells, including the 3 patients with negative ANA on mouse liver substrate. This pattern is considered to be highly characteristic of PSS, and a recent report stated that patients with these antibodies had more severe disease (17). However, with the increasing use of highly sensitive substrates, their true clinical significance remains to be determined.

No ACA were found in our patients; this is consistent with previous data, since 4 of the 5 patients had diffuse disease and ACA is highly characteristic of the CREST variant (6,16,17). Two patients had anti–Scl-70 antibodies; both had diffuse disease and 1 of them had severe pulmonary fibrosis. It is of interest to note that this antibody has been associated with disease that is more systemic (6,16), in particular, with lung involvement (6).

In summary, cardiopulmonary findings were frequent in these children with PSS and were similar to those observed in adult-onset systemic sclerosis. Serologic findings known to be characteristic of PSS in adults were also found in children with this disease and appear to have similar clinical implications.

Acknowledgments. We wish to thank Drs. Jorge Yabkowski and Maria Romanelli for referring 2 patients and for their criticism of an earlier draft of this manuscript. We would also like to thank Drs. Ricardo Gené and Horacio Casabé for performing some of the cardiovascular studies.

REFERENCES

1. Hanson V: Dermatomyositis, scleroderma and polyarteritis nodosa. Clin Rheum Dis 2:455–464, 1976
2. Cassidy JT, Sullivan DB, Dabich L, Petty RE: Scleroderma in children. Arthritis Rheum (suppl) 20:351–354, 1977
3. Moroi Y, Peebles C, Fritzler M, Steigerwald J, Tan EM: Autoantibody to centromere (kinetochore) in scleroderma sera. Proc Natl Acad Sci USA 77:1627–1631, 1980
4. Douvas AS, Achten M, Tan EM: Identification of a nuclear protein (Scl-70) as a unique target of human antinuclear antibodies in scleroderma. J Biol Chem 254:10514–10522, 1979
5. Subcommittee for Scleroderma Criteria of the American Rheumatism Association Diagnostic and Therapeutic Criteria Committee: Preliminary criteria for the classification of systemic sclerosis (scleroderma). Arthritis Rheum 23:581–590, 1980
6. Catoggio LJ, Bernstein RM, Black CM, Hughes GRV, Maddison PJ: Serological markers in progressive systemic sclerosis: clinical correlations. Ann Rheum Dis 42:23–27, 1983
7. Clark G, Reichlin M, Tomasi TB: Characterization of a soluble cytoplasmic antigen reactive with sera from patients with systemic lupus erythematosus. J Immunol 102:117–122, 1969
8. Mattioli M, Reichlin M: Heterogeneity of RNA protein antigens reactive with sera of patients with systemic lupus erythematosus: description of a cytoplasmic nonribosomal antigen. Arthritis Rheum 17:421–429, 1974
9. Ansell BM, Nasseh GA, Bywaters EGL: Scleroderma in childhood. Ann Rheum Dis 35:189–197, 1976
10. Stogmann W, Sandhofer M, Fritz J: Immunological studies in childhood scleroderma. Eur J Pediatr 124:223–230, 1977
11. Clements PJ, Furst DE, Cabeen W, Tashkin D, Paulus HE, Roberts N: The relationship of arrhythmias and conduction disturbances to other manifestations of cardiopulmonary disease in progressive systemic sclerosis. Am J Med 71:38–46, 1981
12. Roberts NK, Cabeen WR, Moss J, Clements PJ, Furst DE: The prevalence of conduction defects and cardiac arrhythmias in progressive systemic sclerosis. Ann Intern Med 94:38–40, 1981
13. Ungerer RG, Tashkin DP, Furst D, Clements PJ, Gong H, Bein M, Smith JW, Roberts N, Cabeen W: Prevalence and clinical correlates of pulmonary arterial hypertension in progressive systemic sclerosis. Am J Med 75:65–74, 1983
14. Kass H, Hanson V, Patrick M: Scleroderma in childhood. J Pediatr 68:243–256, 1966
15. Naslund MJ, Pearson TA, Ritter JM: A documented episode of pulmonary vasoconstriction in systemic sclerosis. Johns Hopkins Med J 148:78–80, 1981
16. Tan EM, Rodnan GP, Garcia I, Moroi Y, Fritzler MJ, Peebles C: Diversity of antinuclear antibodies in progressive systemic sclerosis: anti-centromere antibody and its relationship to CREST syndrome. Arthritis Rheum 23:617–625, 1980
17. McCarty GA, Rice JR, Bembe ML, Barada FA Jr: Anticentromere antibody: clinical correlations and association with favorable prognosis in patients with scleroderma variants. Arthritis Rheum 26:1–7, 1983

BRIEF REPORT

PROTECTIVE EFFECT OF POLIOMYELITIS ON PSORIATIC ARTHRITIS

STEVEN R. WEINER, LAWRENCE W. BASSETT, and RONALD P. REICHMAN

Neurologic lesions resulting in paralysis of an extremity have been reported to spare that extremity clinically and radiographically, when the patient subsequently develops rheumatoid arthritis (1–9), tophaceous gout (10), or osteoarthritis (11–16). The same phenomenon has been reported in animals with adjuvant arthritis (8). The reports cited involved women 3 times more commonly than men. The mean age of the patients in previously cited reports was 54 (range 12–76) (1–16). The time from onset of neurologic lesion to onset of arthritis in these patients was 8 months to 70 years (1–16). The majority of rheumatoid arthritis patients were seropositive, and nodule formation was absent in the neurologically involved extremities in 70% (1–10). Nerve lesions and hemiplegia occurring after the onset of rheumatoid arthritis may also have a protective effect on the involved extremity in terms of the inflammatory arthropathy (9,17). To our knowledge, this is the first report of paralysis sparing an extremity from psoriatic polyarthritis.

Case report. A 72-year-old right-handed man was evaluated for psoriatic arthritis. At the age of 30 months he had been afflicted with polio, which left him with a totally nonfunctional left arm. The patient had worked as a golf caddy for over 30 years and complained of pain, stiffness, and loss of function in his right hand over the last 10 years. The onset of joint pain was in 1971 and initially involved the first and fifth fingers of his right hand. One year later, a classic psoriatic rash blossomed over his trunk, extensor surfaces of the extremities, face, and buttocks. The rash was diagnosed clinically and by skin biopsy as psoriasis and has persisted to date despite treatment. The arthritis has also persisted for 12 years, with pain, swelling, and stiffness of the right hand and wrist, right shoulder, spine, knees, ankles, and feet.

The patient was otherwise in good health except for well-controlled essential hypertension. On physical examination, his skin showed erythematous scaly plaques with some satellite lesions in the axilla, groin, scalp, umbilicus, intergluteal folds, and on the extensor surfaces of the knees. There was no pitting of the nails. Motion in the left arm was limited to a slight shoulder shrug and finger extension if no resistance was applied. Marked wasting was noted in the muscles of the left arm.

The musculoskeletal examination revealed a Z deformity of the right thumb, no motion (frozen) across the third, fourth, and fifth distal interphalangeal joints, and swelling and tenderness in the first carpometacarpal joint and all proximal interphalangeal and metacarpophalangeal joints of the right hand. The right trapeziometacarpal joint was fixed in 15° of abduction and approximately 10° of radial extension. The right wrist was swollen, tender, and limited to 5° of flexion and 10° of extension. The right elbow had a full range

From the Department of Radiology, University of California, Los Angeles Medical Center and the Department of Medicine, Olive View Medical Center, Van Nuys, California.

Steven R. Weiner, MD: Chief of Rheumatology, Olive View Medical Center and Assistant Professor of Medicine, UCLA School of Medicine; Lawrence W. Bassett, MD: Associate Professor of Radiology, UCLA School of Medicine; Ronald D. Reichman, MD: Assistant Clinical Professor, UCLA/Cedars-Sinai Medical Center.

Address reprint requests to Lawrence W. Bassett, MD, UCLA Medical Center—CHS, Department of Radiology, B2-240, 10833 Le Conte Avenue, Los Angeles, CA 90024.

Submitted for publication September 14, 1984; accepted in revised form January 14, 1985.

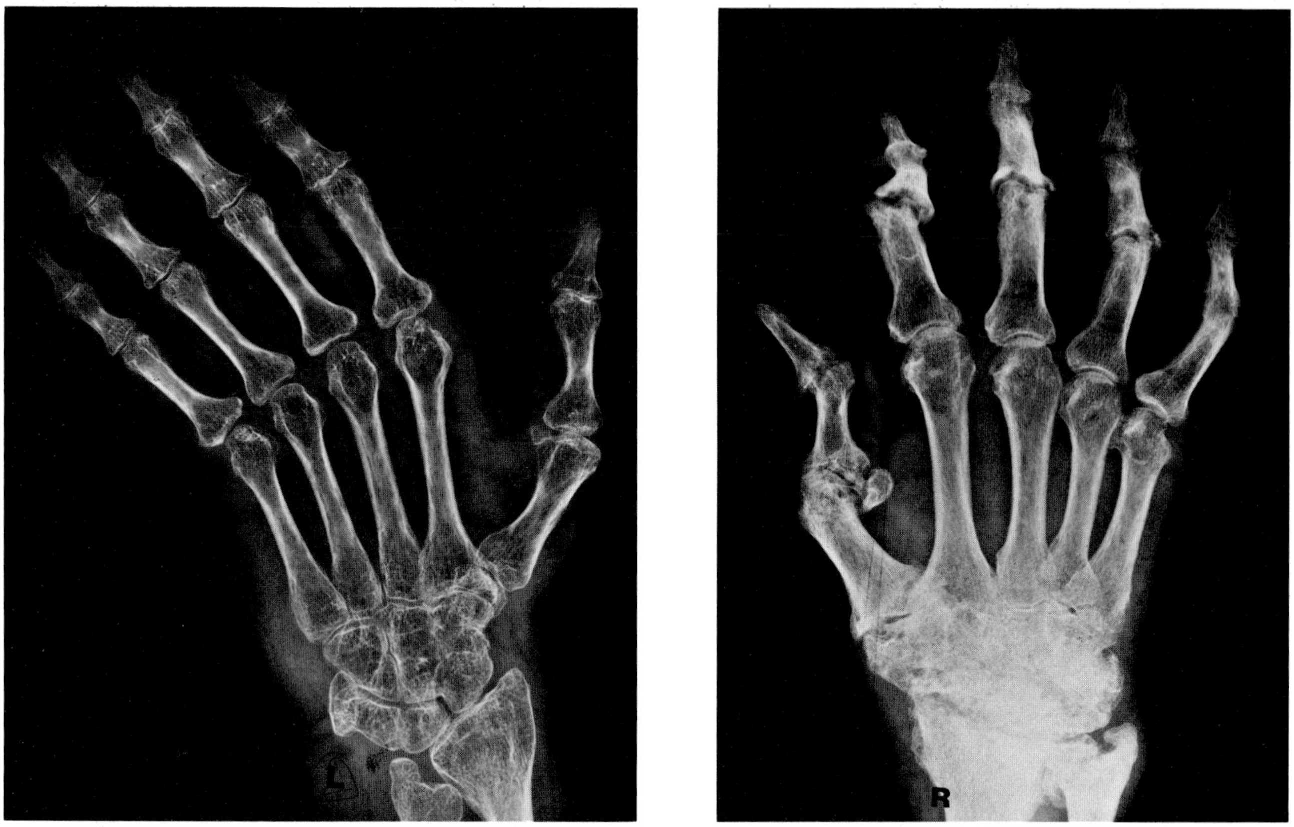

A B

Figure 1. Hand radiographs of a 71-year-old man with a 12-year history of psoriasis and joint pain, whose left arm and hand have been nonfunctional since he was afflicted with polio at age 30 months. **A,** Anteroposterior view of the left hand. Bones and cartilage are atrophic. There is ulnar deviation of the phalanges and partial carpal ankylosis; however, there is no evidence of active inflammatory joint disease. **B,** Anteroposterior view of the right hand, showing severe psoriatic arthritis. There is destruction and/or fusion of the carpal and interphalangeal joints. Joint destruction is accompanied by proliferative bone formation at the radioulnar joint, bases of several phalanges, and the sesamoid bone of the first interphalangeal joint. Bone density is preserved despite extensive joint disease.

of motion although the joint was tender to palpation; the left was a flail elbow. The right shoulder was limited to 30° of active and passive abduction, with rotation and flexion also limited. Both knees and all toes of both feet were warm and tender with small effusions. Both ankles were swollen, and the heels were tender to compression.

Laboratory studies revealed a Westergren erythrocyte sedimentation rate of 13 mm/hour, a normal complete blood count, negative rheumatoid factor by latex fixation, and negative HLA–B27.

Radiographs of the hands are shown in Figure 1. The left hand and wrist showed sparing of the joints, with no evidence of active arthritis. Films of the right hand and wrist revealed severe psoriatic arthritis. Other radiographs demonstrated bilateral calcaneal spurs, erosions in the interphalangeal joint of the right fourth toe, and fusion of the first, third, fourth, and fifth interphalangeal joints of the left foot with erosion of the third. The sacroiliac joints were sclerotic, and the cervical and lumbar spine had anterior osteophytes. The third and fourth cervical spinous processes were fused posteriorly.

Discussion. The association of a prior neurologic lesion, either upper or lower motor neuron, with sparing of an extremity from the effects of subsequent rheumatoid arthritis, osteoarthritis, tophaceous gout, or adjuvant arthritis has been previously reported in 134 patients (1–16) (Table 1). The phenomenon has been attributed to a protective effect of the neural lesion or to a reduction of motion (although not necessarily all motion or weight-bearing) (1,4–6,11).

Table 1. Sparing of extremities from rheumatoid arthritis (RA), tophaceous gout (TG), osteoarthritis (OA), and psoriatic arthritis (PA) due to prior neurologic/traumatic lesion

Reference	Type of arthritis	Type of lesion (n)*	No. of cases
Thompson and Bywaters (1)	RA	Meningioma (1), CVA (2), neurovascular lues (1)	4
Yaghmai et al (2)	RA	Cerebral palsy	1
Hammoudeh et al (3)	RA	Traumatic ulnar and radial neuropathy	1
Glick (4)	RA	Poliomyelitis (12), encephalitis (1)	13
Bland and Eddy (5)	RA	CVA	1
Ueno et al (6)	RA	Poliomyelitis	1
Jacqueline (7)	RA	CVA	1
Courtright and Kuzell (8)	RA	Laceration of flexor tendon	1
Velayos and Cohen (9)	RA	CVA	1
Glynn and Clayton (10)	TG	CVA	1
Winter (11)	OA	CVA	1
Hench (12)	OA	Infantile paralysis	1
Coste and Forestier (13)	OA	CVA	2
Stecher and Karnosh (14)	OA	CVA, laceration of median nerve	2
Forestier (15)	OA	CVA	1
Glyn et al (16)	OA	Poliomyelitis	100
Thompson and Bywaters (1)	OA	Erb's palsy	1
Present report	PA	Poliomyelitis	1

* CVA = cerebrovascular accident (thrombotic, embolic, or bleed).

This effect has been used to justify rest therapy for these disorders. Studies of rest therapy for rheumatoid arthritis support the hypothesis that immobilization has a protective and beneficial effect (18–21).

The protective effect of immobilization can also be seen with animal studies of osteoarthritis, using the model of anterior cruciate ligament resection in dogs and iodoacetate intraarticular injection in guinea pigs (22,23). While prolonged immobilization in animals results in cartilage atrophy, there is no loss of the integrity of the articular surface, no fibrillation, no augmentation of proteoglycan synthesis, no osteophyte formation, and no increased extractability of matrix proteoglycans (22,23).

In the human model, researchers disagree as to whether limb immobilization occurring after the onset of rheumatoid arthritis, tophaceous gout, or osteoarthritis can prevent further arthritis progression (15,17,19). This case of psoriatic arthritis contributes a different perspective in that the pathologic and immunogenetic findings in psoriatic arthritis are distinct from those of rheumatoid arthritis or osteoarthritis (24,25), and adds support to the hypothesis that the protective effects of immobilization and/or neural lesions apply to inflammation of articular structures in general, and not just in rheumatoid arthritis or osteoarthritis.

REFERENCES

1. Thompson M, Bywaters EGL: Unilateral rheumatoid arthritis following hemiplegia. Ann Rheum Dis 21:370–377, 1962
2. Yaghmai I, Rooholamini SM, Faunce HF: Unilateral rheumatoid arthritis: protective effect of neurologic deficits. AJR 128:299–301, 1977
3. Hammoudeh M, Khan MA, Kushner I: Unilateral rheumatoid arthritis (letter). Arthritis Rheum 24:1218, 1981
4. Glick EN: Asymmetrical rheumatoid arthritis after poliomyelitis. Br Med J 3:26–28, 1967
5. Bland JH, Eddy WM: Hemiplegia and rheumatoid hemiarthritis. Arthritis Rheum 11:72–80, 1968
6. Ueno Y, Sawada K, Imura H: Protective effect of neural lesion on rheumatoid arthritis (letter). Arthritis Rheum 26:118, 1983
7. Jacqueline F: Un cas de polyarthrite evolutive a localisations contro-d'une hemiplegie. Rev Rhum Mal Osteoartic 20:323–324, 1953
8. Courtright LJ, Kuzell WC: Sparing effect of neurological deficit and trauma on the course of adjuvant arthritis in the rat. Ann Rheum Dis 24:360–367, 1965
9. Velayos EE, Cohen BS: The effect of stroke on well-established rheumatoid arthritis. Md State Med J 21:38–42, 1972
10. Glynn JJ, Clayton ML: Sparing effect of hemiplegia on tophaceous gout. Ann Rheum Dis 35:534–535, 1976
11. Winter S: Unilateral Heberden's nodes in a case of hemiplegia. NY State Med J 52:349–350, 1952

12. Hench PC: Heberden's nodes: heredity in hypertrophic arthritis of the finger joints. JAMA 115:2024–2025, 1940
13. Coste F, Forestier J: Hemiplegie et nodosites d'Heberden controlaterales. Bull Soc Med Hop Paris 51:772–775, 1935
14. Stecher RM, Karnosh LJ: Heberden's nodes: the effect of nerve injury upon the formation of degenerative joint disease of the fingers. Am J Med Sci 213:184–191, 1947
15. Forestier J: Rheumatism d'Heberden chez une hemiplegique lesions articulaires limitées au côte sane. Rev Neurol 63:442–448, 1935
16. Glyn JH, Sutherland I, Walker GF, Young HC: Low incidence of osteoarthritis in hip and knee after anterior poliomyelitis: a late review. Br Med J 2:739–742, 1966
17. Smith RD: Effect of hemiparesis on rheumatoid arthritis (letter). Arthritis Rheum 22:1419–1420, 1979
18. Alexander GJM, Hortas C, Bacon PA: Bedrest, activity and the inflammation of rheumatoid arthritis. Br J Rheumatol 22:134–140, 1983
19. Partridge REH, Duthie JJR: Controlled trial of the effect of complete immobilization of the joints in rheumatoid arthritis. Ann Rheum Dis 22:91–99, 1963
20. Smith RD, Polley HF: Rest therapy for rheumatoid arthritis. Mayo Clin Proc 53:141–145, 1978
21. Gault SJ, Spyker JM: Beneficial effect of immobilization of joints in rheumatoid and related arthritides: a splint study using sequential analysis. Arthritis Rheum 12:34–44, 1969
22. Palmoski MJ, Brandt KD: Immobilization of the knee prevents osteoarthritis after anterior cruciate ligament transection. Arthritis Rheum 25:1201–1208, 1982
23. Williams JM, Brandt KD: Immobilization ameliorates chemically induced articular cartilage damage. Arthritis Rheum 27:208–216, 1984
24. Moll JHM: The clinical spectrum of psoriatic arthritis. Clin Orthop 143:66–75, 1979
25. Kammer GM, Soter NA, Gibson DJ, Schur PH: Psoriatic arthritis: a clinical, immunologic and HLA study of 100 patients. Semin Arthritis Rheum 9:75–97, 1979

BRIEF REPORT

ALLOPURINOL HYPERSENSITIVITY IN A PATIENT WITH SEVERE, CHRONIC, TOPHACEOUS GOUT

ELLA WEBSTER and RICHARD S. PANUSH

We report our experience managing a patient with severe, chronic, tophaceous gout and allopurinol hypersensitivity. Our patient was successfully desensitized to allopurinol and also benefited from extensive removal of tophi as well as amputation of tophaceous digits. We are aware of 2 previous case reports of desensitization to allopurinol in patients with associated hypersensitivity (1,2). This experience illustrates possible approaches to an unusual and seemingly hopeless clinical situation.

Case report. The patient, a 61-year-old white man, has a history of gout dating back to 1944. Within 5 years of that time he developed tophi over his ankles, knees, wrists, elbows, and shoulders. Despite therapy with allopurinol, probenecid, colchicine, and occasionally prednisone, he had acute attacks every 2–3 months and in 1973 was forced to retire from his job as a postal carrier.

While being treated with allopurinol, the patient developed a pruritic, erythematous, maculopapular rash of the face, trunk, and extremities; the allopurinol was discontinued with apparent resolution of the rash. The rash recurred following re-challenge with allopurinol. Biopsies were not performed. He was then treated with colchicine, probenecid (1.5–2 gm/day), and indomethacin. His serum uric acid level ranged from 10.0–10.9 mg/dl. In May 1980, with poorly controlled, recurrent episodes of gouty arthritis superimposed on chronic, draining tophi, the patient was admitted for desensitization and retrial of allopurinol under close observation, and for surgical drainage and debridement of tophi.

Physical examination results were notable for a confluent, erythematous, maculopapular rash with some scaling and excoriation, diffuse swelling of both wrists, elbows, knees, ankles, and multiple metacarpophalangeal and proximal interphalangeal joints, and ulcerated, draining tophi over the elbows, hands, wrists, knees, and ankles (Figures 1 and 2). Laboratory findings included blood urea nitrogen (BUN) 18 mg/dl, serum creatinine 1.2 mg/dl, serum uric acid 11.5 mg/dl, erythrocyte sedimentation rate 12 mm/hour, normal SMAC profile and complete blood count with differential, 24-hour urinary uric acid 304 mg, and creatinine clearance 44 cc/minute.

He was initially treated with sulfinpyrazone (400 mg/day) and indomethacin (150 mg/day), but his BUN rose to 28 mg/dl and serum creatinine to 1.7 mg/dl, while serum uric acid was 9.7 mg/dl. Indomethacin dosage was then decreased to 25 mg twice a day, sulfinpyrazone was discontinued, bicarbonate was begun, and fluid intake increased. His creatinine clearance improved to 77 cc/minute, and 24-hour urinary uric acid level rose to 1,008 mg.

From the Division of Clinical Immunology, Department of Medicine, College of Medicine, University of Florida and the Clinical Immunology Section, Medical and Research Services, Veterans Administration Medical Center, Gainesville, Florida.

Supported by grants from the Veterans Administration and the Florida Chapter of the Arthritis Foundation.

Ella Webster, MD: Postdoctoral Fellow, Division of Clinical Immunology, Department of Medicine, College of Medicine, University of Florida; Richard S. Panush, MD: Associate Professor of Medicine and Immunology and Medical Microbiology, Chief, Division of Clinical Immunology, Department of Medicine, College of Medicine, University of Florida, and Chief, Clinical Immunology Section, Veterans Administration Medical Center, Gainesville.

Address reprint requests to Richard S. Panush, MD, Division of Clinical Immunology, Department of Medicine, Box J-277, JHMHC, University of Florida, Gainesville, FL 32610.

Submitted for publication August 27, 1984; accepted in revised form January 17, 1985.

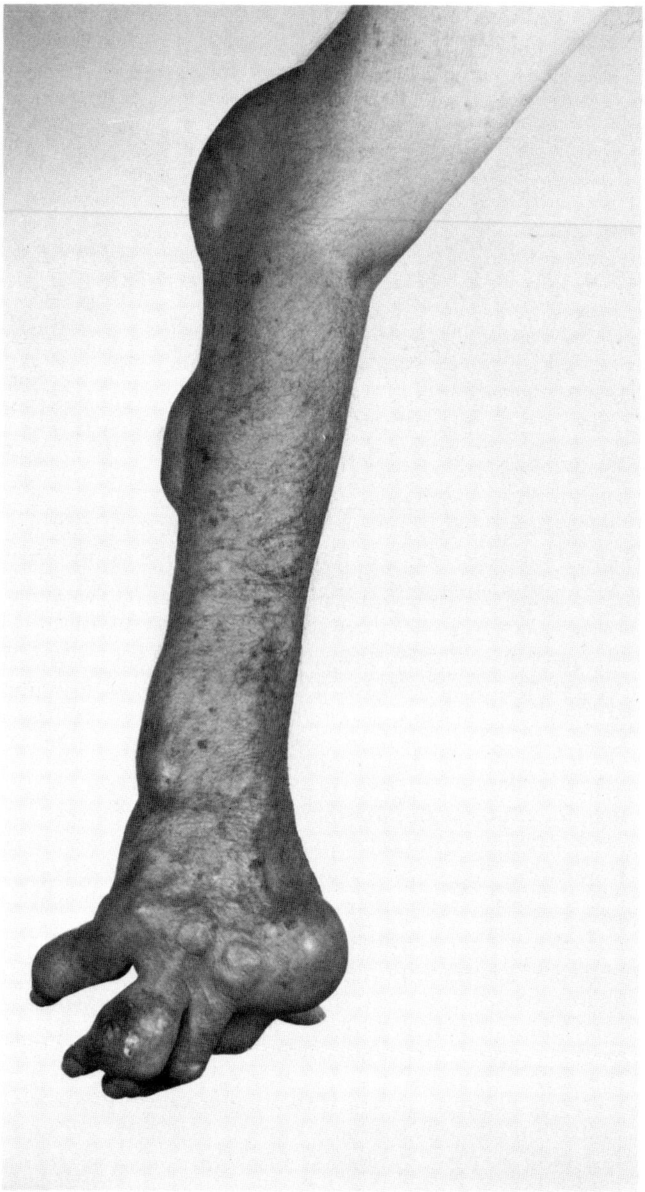

Figure 1. Gouty involvement of the patient's right arm.

On June 24, 1980, allopurinol desensitization was initiated as shown in Table 1. The patient tolerated desensitization without complication, receiving gradually increasing doses of oral solution and then tablets of allopurinol. There was an initial increase in his serum creatinine; this improved with continued hydration and alkalinization of his urine. Serum uric acid decreased from a peak of 11.5 mg/dl while he was in the hospital to 8.5 mg/dl at discharge.

The patient was subsequently transferred to the orthopedic surgery service where he underwent resection of ulcerating tophi on both index fingers and excision of tophi from the right elbow, right prepatellar bursa, left great toe, left ankle, and left Achilles tendon. He had an uneventful recovery and continued on a regimen of allopurinol 300 mg/day, colchicine 0.6 mg twice a day, and indomethacin.

Discussion. Allopurinol is now commonly used for treatment of certain patients with hyperuricemia and gout. Adverse reactions include fever, pruritis, gastrointestinal distress, diarrhea (3,4), toxic epidermal necrolysis, interstitial nephritis, renal insufficiency (5), granulomatous hepatitis (6), and vasculitis (7). Reports estimate that up to 10% of patients given allopurinol will have minor adverse reactions (3,4), particularly cutaneous reactions (8,9) which could limit use of this drug.

Allopurinol is particularly important for therapy of patients with tophaceous gout and/or gouty nephritis. Drug hypersensitivity, as occurred in our patient, would seriously limit the ability to manage such patients. Our patient had severe, debilitating, tophaceous gout which benefited from amputation of digits and excision of ulcerated, draining lesions. He may have also had some underlying renal insufficiency,

Table 1. Allopurinol desensitization regimen

Day	Dosage of allopurinol (mg)
1	0.008
2	0.016
3	0.024
4	0.032
5	0.040
6	0.048
7	0.056
8	0.064
9	0.072
10	0.080
11	0.160
12	0.320
13	0.480
14	0.640
15	0.800
16	0.960
17	1.120
18	1.280
19	1.600
20	2.000
21	2.560
22	5.120
23	10.240
24	20.000
25	50.000
26	75.000
27	100.000
28	150.000
29	200.000
30	300.000

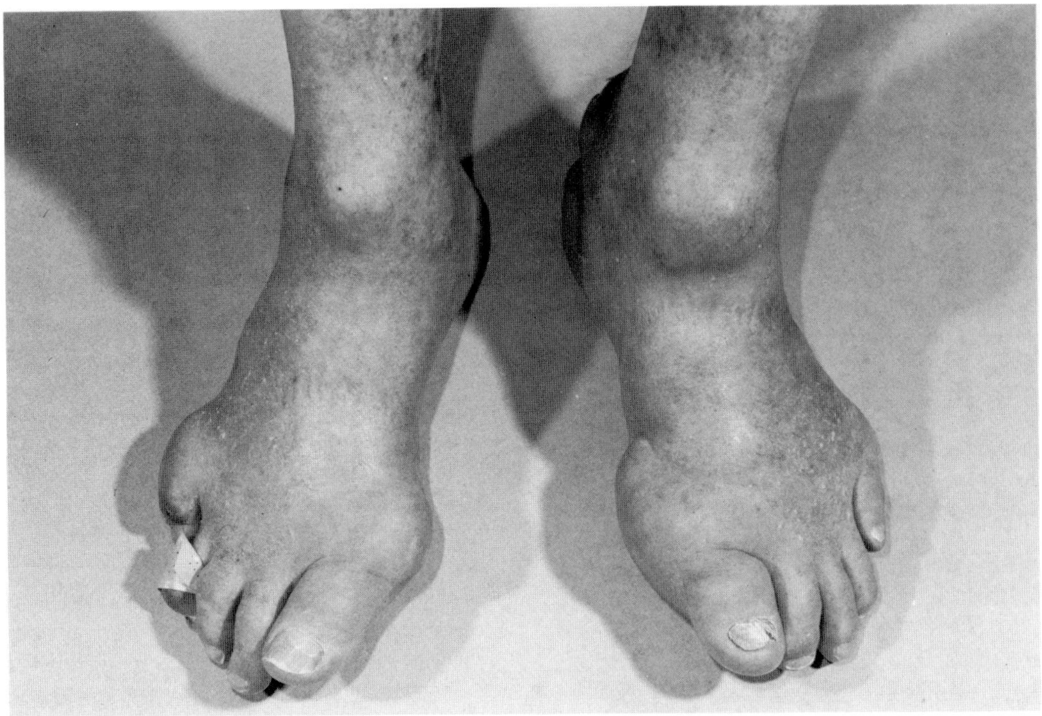

Figure 2. Gouty involvement of the patient's feet.

possibly related to his tophaceous gout. He did well with both desensitization and operative procedures and is now managed in a conventional manner with adequate control of joint discomfort and serum urate level.

Our experience, which supports that of others, indicates that cautious desensitization of patients with cutaneous hypersensitivity to allopurinol is both feasible and clinically useful.

Acknowledgments. The authors appreciate the assistance of Barbara Gibbs in preparing the manuscript and the helpful advice of Drs. Selden Longley and N. Lawrence Edwards.

REFERENCES

1. Meyrier A: Desensitization in a patient with chronic renal failure and severe allergy to allopurinol (letter). Br Med J 2:458, 1976
2. Fam AC, Paton TW, Chaiton A: Reinstitution of allopurinol therapy for gouty arthritis after cutaneous reactions. Can Med Assoc J 123:128–129, 1980
3. Rundles RW, Metz EN, Silberman HR: Allopurinol in the treatment of gout. Ann Intern Med 64:229–258, 1966
4. Gutman AB: Hyperuricemia and its management. Drug Ther 5:29–39, 1971
5. Yong JL, Boswell RB, Nies AS: Severe allopurinol hypersensitivity (association with thiazide and prior renal compromise). Arch Intern Med 134:553–558, 1974
6. Simmons F, Feldman B, Gerety D: Granulomatous hepatitis in a patient receiving allopurinol. Gastroenterology 62:101–104, 1972
7. Jarzofski J, Ferry J, Wombolt D, Fitch DM, Fegan JD: Vasculitis with allopurinol therapy. Am Heart J 79:116–121, 1970
8. Frisch JM, Lovatt GE, Sproit ARM, Turmer R: The adverse reaction profile of allopurinol, Frontiers of Internal Medicine, 1974. Edited by SH Blondheim. Basel, Karger, 1975, pp 412–419
9. Boston Collaborative Drug Surveillance Program, Boston University Medical Center: Excess ampicillin rashes associated with allopurinol or hyperuricemia. N Engl J Med 286:505–507, 1972

BRIEF REPORT

ORAL GOLD THERAPY IN A PATIENT WITH RHEUMATOID ARTHRITIS AND PREEXISTING UREMIA

WINFRIED GRANINGER, GERALD SEIDL, JOSEF KOVARIK, WULF PINGGERA, and JOSEF S. SMOLEN

The use of slow-acting, disease-modifying drugs is a well-established and effective therapy for rheumatoid arthritis. Aside from immunosuppressive agents, gold salts, D-penicillamine (DP), and hydroxychloroquine are most frequently used for this purpose (1). Administration of these drugs, however, may be accompanied by severe side effects.

Although not commonly observed, rheumatoid arthritis (RA) can occasionally occur in patients with azotemia due to some unrelated, underlying disease. In such patients, use of gold salts or DP may be dangerous. Patients with mild impairment of renal function may run the risk of further deterioration; moreover, in such patients as well as in those requiring long-term hemodialysis, accumulation and increased incidence of non-nephrologic side effects could occur, since these drugs, as well as hydroxychloroquine, are excreted primarily by the kidney (2–4).

Recently, an oral gold compound, auranofin, has been developed (5). In contrast to parenteral gold preparations, it is excreted primarily via the feces (6) and should therefore be especially useful in patients with impaired kidney function. In this report we present the results of auranofin therapy in a uremic patient with rheumatoid arthritis.

From the Second Department of Internal Medicine, University of Vienna, Vienna, Austria.

Winfried Graninger, MD: Fellow, Rheumatology Section; Gerald Seidl, MD: Assistant Professor of Radiology, Radiology Section; Josef Kovarik, MD: Assistant Professor of Medicine, Nephrology Section; Wulf Pinggera, MD: Professor of Medicine, Nephrology Section; Josef S. Smolen, MD: Associate Professor of Medicine, Rheumatology Section.

Address reprint requests to Dr. Josef S. Smolen, Second Department of Internal Medicine, University of Vienna, A-1090 Vienna, Garnisongasse 13, Austria.

Submitted for publication September 4, 1984; accepted in revised form January 14, 1985.

Case report. A 50-year-old man was referred to our outpatient rheumatology department in September 1983 because of continuing arthralgias. History-taking revealed that the patient's right arm had been amputated in 1962 as a consequence of an accident. In 1971 hemodialysis was initiated because of end-stage glomerulonephritis. Bilateral nephrectomy had been performed in 1972. Renal transplantations in 1975 and 1978 were unsuccessful. In 1981, the patient underwent parathyroidectomy because of secondary hyperparathyroidism. Since then he received 1,25-dihydroxycholecalciferol substitution therapy.

In the fall of 1981, the patient had surgery for carpal tunnel syndrome. Since approximately November 1981 he had noted tenderness and pain upon motion in his wrist joint as well as several metacarpophalangeal (MCP) joints and proximal interphalangeal (PIP) joints. There was also intermittent swelling of these joints.

Since no improvement was attained with analgesic drugs, clinical, radiologic, and laboratory investigations were performed in April 1982. At that time, his erythrocyte sedimentation rate (ESR) was 52 mm/hour, serum creatinine was 8.6 mg/dl (normal $\leq$1.4), blood urea nitrogen was 65 mg/dl (normal $\leq$20), alkaline phosphatase was 396 units/liter (normal $\leq$170) with the elevation solely due to the liver and not bone isoenzyme, in the presence of known cholecystolithiasis; uric acid, calcium, and phosphate levels were within normal limits. Hematocrit level was 23%; leukocytes, differential count, and thrombocytes were within the normal range. Total protein was 6.7 gm/dl with 48% albumin (normal ≥52%) and 25.1% gamma globulins (normal ≤21%).

IgM was elevated to 240 mg/dl (normal ≤180); IgG and IgA were within normal limits. Rheumatoid factor was negative, but the antinuclear antibody (ANA) titer was 1:640. However, no DNA binding could be seen by Farr assay, and no antibodies to the ANA subsets Ro, La, Sm, RNP, or Scl-70 could be demonstrated (kindly performed by Dr. E. Penner, University of Vienna). A C1q binding test for circulating immune complexes produced negative results.

Radiologic assessment of the patient's hand revealed juxtaarticular demineralization and several erosions and areas of cystic destruction (Figure 1), findings not seen on a previous radiograph obtained in 1979. There was no evidence of subperiosteal resorption characteristic of secondary hyperparathyroidism (7,8).

When the patient was seen by the rheumatologists in September 1983, he complained of morning stiffness of 60 minutes duration and pain upon motion in his wrist joint and several finger joints. Tenderness and swelling were noted at his wrist joint, second through fourth MCP joints, and second and fourth PIP joints. Tenderness and mild swelling were found at his right shoulder joint, and a mild effusion and tenderness were noted at his knee joints. Positive Tinel's sign and Phalen's maneuver indicated relapse of carpal tunnel syndrome.

Radiologic reassessment of his hand revealed changes similar to those found in 1982. A deep erosion was found in the humeral head; the bony structures of the knee joints appeared normal.

ESR was 70 mm/hour; other routine laboratory results were essentially similar to those obtained in 1982. Rheumatoid factor was still negative; ANA titer was 1:320.

Based on clinical, laboratory, and radiologic examinations, the patient was diagnosed as having definite, seronegative rheumatoid arthritis.

The patient was initially treated with nonsteroidal antiinflammatory drugs (diclofenac, 75–150 mg/day), but experienced only slight relief. With 8 mg of methylprednisolone/day he was somewhat more comfortable, but any attempt to reduce this dosage led to an increase in pain. Therefore, we decided to begin oral gold therapy, and the patient received auranofin in a reduced dosage of 3 mg/day, beginning at the end of December 1983.

Within 2 months, morning stiffness decreased to ≤15 minutes per day, and the methylprednisolone dosage could be gradually tapered to 4 mg every other day. By the end of June 1984, the patient's clinical rheumatologic status was stable with no or very brief morning stiffness, occasional mild swelling, and only occasional, minimal tenderness in the affected joints. Radiographic reassessment of his hand revealed no progression of disease. Laboratory reassessment showed an ESR of 25 mm/hour with otherwise unchanged parameters; however, ANA was negative at that time.

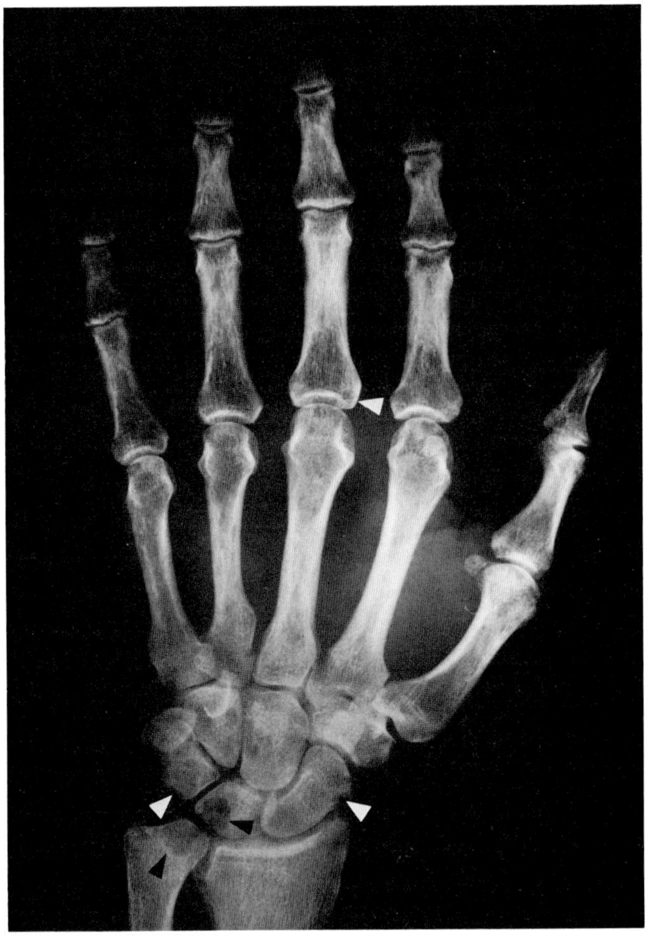

Figure 1. Radiograph of the left hand of the patient (who had lost his right arm in a traffic accident) taken in 1982, 6 months after the onset of arthritis symptoms. Erosions and cystic lesions can be seen at several carpal bones, the distal end of the ulna, and the third metacarpophalangeal joint (**arrowheads**).

With regard to potential side effects of gold therapy, clinical and laboratory examinations performed every 2–4 weeks since initiation of auranofin treatment did not reveal any abnormality, and subjectively, the patient tolerated the drug very well. During the initial phase of auranofin application, serum gold levels (kindly tested by Smith, Kline and French, Germany, by atomic absorption spectrophotometry using a modification of the method of Schattenkirchner [9]) rose progressively, reaching a level of 585 ng/ml after 8 weeks and 850 ng/ml after 5 months, when medication was reduced to 3 mg every other day. When the dialysate fluid was examined, gold could not be detected. The assay employed has a sensitivity of 50 ng/ml. This indicates that with hemodialysis, gold from auranofin is either nondialyzable or dialyzable only in very low amounts.

Discussion. The presence of rheumatoid arthritis in a patient with preexisting uremia is uncommon. Treatment of such patients requires special considerations, since the risk:benefit ratio naturally is much higher compared with that in patients who have normal kidney function. This is particularly true if renally excreted drugs are employed. Thus, although gold sodium thiomalate, aurothioglucose, D-penicillamine, and hydroxychloroquine are well-established treatments for rheumatoid arthritis, their application is severely limited in the context of uremia, since these compounds are predominantly renally excreted (2–4).

As described in the present report, we used auranofin, a new, primarily fecally excreted gold compound, for the treatment of a uremic patient with rheumatoid arthritis. In this patient, auranofin was effective in inducing marked clinical improvement and did not cause adverse side effects. With a reduced dosage of 3 mg/day, the serum gold level rose in the course of 5 months to a level similar to that found in patients without kidney failure who have received 6 mg/day. Thus, accumulation of gold apparently occurred in this patient, indicating that normally it is renally excreted to a certain extent. This is in accordance with previous observations of 20–50% renal excretion of absorbed auranofin (10). In contrast, parenteral gold preparations are primarily (70%) renally excreted (11). Finally, gold from auranofin could not be dialyzed in significant amounts by hemodialysis; this indicates that similar to parenteral gold preparations which can be removed only by peritoneal dialysis (12), auranofin gold is mainly protein-bound.

We believe that more patients similar to the one described will have to be studied in order to fully determine potential hazards of auranofin therapy in uremic patients; however, from the observations reported here we conclude that auranofin, albeit in a reduced dosage, may be the remission-inducing drug of choice in patients with rheumatoid arthritis and impaired kidney function.

REFERENCES

1. Bunch TW, O'Duffy JD: Disease modifying drugs for progressive rheumatoid arthritis. Mayo Clin Proc 55:161–169, 1980
2. Krusius FE, Markkanen A, Deltola P: Plasma levels and urinary excretion of gold during routine treatment of rheumatoid arthritis. Ann Rheum Dis 29:232–235, 1979
3. Aposhian HU: Biochemical and pharmacological properties of the metal-binding agent penicillamine. Fed Proc (suppl) 20:10, 1961
4. Fabre J, de Freudenreich J, Druckert A, Pitton JS, Rudhardt M, Virieux C: Influence of renal insufficiency on the excretion of chloroquine, phenobarbital, phenothiazines and metacyline. Helv Med Acta 33:307–316, 1966
5. Berglof FE, Gerlof K, Walz DT: Auranofin: a new oral gold compound for treatment of rheumatoid arthritis. J Rheumatol 5:68–74, 1978
6. Blodgett RC Jr: Auranofin: experience to date. Am J Med 75:86–89, 1983
7. Parfitt AM: Clinical and radiographic manifestation of renal osteodystrophy, Calcium Metabolism in Renal Failure and Nephrolithiasis. Edited by DS David. New York, John Wiley & Sons, 1977, pp 145–195
8. Lechner G, Seidl G, Urbanek A: Röntgenologische Veränderungen des Hyperparathyreoidismus, Hyperparathyreoidismus: Diagnostik und Therapie der Nebenschilddrüsenüberfunktion. Edited by A Fritsch, G Geyer. Vienna, Urban & Schwarzenberg, 1982, pp 37–48
9. Schattenkirchner M, Grobenski Z: The measurement of gold in blood and urine by atomic absorption in the treatment of rheumatoid arthritis. Atomic Absorption Newsletter 16:84–88, 1977
10. Blocka K, Furst DE, Landaw E, Dromogole S, Blomberg A, Paulus HE: Single-dose pharmacokinetics of auranofin in rheumatoid arthritis. J Rheumatol (suppl) 9:110–119, 1982
11. Gottlieb NL: Comparative pharmacokinetics of parenteral and oral gold compounds. J Rheumatol (suppl) 9:99–108, 1982
12. Combs RJ, Dentino MM, Lehrman L, Szwed J: Gold toxicity and peritoneal dialysis. Arthritis Rheum 19:936–938, 1976

In Appreciation of Nathan J. Zvaifler, MD

Editor, 1980–85

As this issue of *Arthritis and Rheumatism*—the last on which his name appears as Editor—goes to press, we take an editorial page away from Nate Zvaifler and dedicate it to him as a tribute.

The countless hours Dr. Zvaifler has devoted to his duties as Editor over the last five years have been reflected by the high quality of the articles which have appeared in *A&R*. The reduction of the manuscript acceptance rate to less than 40% is a function of two phenomena: the large number of researchers who choose *A&R* for submitting their work and the discerning eye with which Dr. Zvaifler and his associates have evaluated it.

During the period of Dr. Zvaifler's editorship, the number of pages the journal devotes to original scientific research has increased dramatically, as the yearly volumes have been expanded from 8 to 12 issues, with more pages per issue. In addition, there has been a shift in emphasis from conference proceedings to the timely publication of refereed scientific materials.

Two features introduced in *Arthritis and Rheumatism* by Dr. Zvaifler, Radiologic Vignettes and Government Affairs, reflect the broad range of interests among the members of the American Rheumatism Association and the journal's other readers. That readership over the past five years has climbed dramatically, to a point where circulation is now over 8,000, in 80 countries. By increasing the size of *A&R*'s Editorial Board, Dr. Zvaifler has expanded the involvement of ARA members, to the journal's benefit as well as their own.

With Dr. Zvaifler's editorship came computerization of the *A&R* editorial office. For her able and creative handling of that and the many other office functions, we thank Henri Albert, Dr. Zvaifler's Assistant Editor for the past three years. Much gratitude is also owed to the Editorial Board, and especially to Dr. Zvaifler and his Associate Editors—Drs. Wayne H. Akeson, Michael A. Becker, Harry G. Bluestein, F. Richard Convery, James W. Hollingsworth, Donald L. Resnick, and Michael H. Weisman.

As Bill Koopman assumes the role of Editor, the Zvaifler stamp will remain imprinted upon *A&R*. We look forward to the continued growth of the journal as it serves the rheumatology community in the years ahead.

Jane Diamond
Managing Editor

Irving H. Fox, MD
Chair, Committee for the Publication of A&R

Introducing the New Editor: William J. Koopman, MD

It has been the privilege of some Presidents of the American Rheumatism Association to introduce an incoming Editor of our prestigious publication, *Arthritis and Rheumatism*. This year it is my pleasure to introduce Dr. William J. Koopman who, on July 1, 1985, will become the sixth Editor of *Arthritis and Rheumatism*.

Bill Koopman inherits a tradition of excellence and responsibility which is in some ways awesome to behold. Under the superb guidance of its previous Editors—William S. Clark, Daniel J. McCarty, Charles L. Christian, J. Claude Bennett, and the most recent Editor, Nathan J. Zvaifler—*Arthritis and Rheumatism* has been recognized as the world's premier journal in the discipline of rheumatology. It is a journal which is a valuable reference not only for clinicians, but also for biochemists, immunologists, and molecular biologists. Many students of history recognize that this kind of excellence in any endeavor occurs sequentially and takes time to develop and mature. The success of the journal has been fostered and promoted by its Editors, the Editorial Board and staff, and by its scholarly contributors.

A search committee chaired by one of our elder statesmen, Dr. Morris Ziff, selected Bill Koopman to succeed Nate Zvaifler as the Editor. Bill Koopman has inherited some noble bloodlines. He is in an academic institution where his department chairman, Dr. J. Claude Bennett, was an illustrious previous Editor of *Arthritis and Rheumatism*. Bill Koopman is Director of the Division of Clinical Immunology and Rheumatology of the Department of Medicine at the University of Alabama at Birmingham. He graduated summa cum laude from Washington and Jefferson College with a BA and magna cum laude from Harvard University with an MD. His academic experiences have been at outstanding institutions which have included Harvard University, where he worked and published on mediators of inflammation in immediate hypersensitivity. Following this, he was at the National Institutes of Health, where he studied lymphokines and immunoregulation, before joining the University of Alabama, where he is now working on rheumatoid factors—their synthesis, localization, and role in pathogenic mechanisms. In 1982 he was the recipient of the prestigious Carol Nachman Prize for outstanding research in rheumatology.

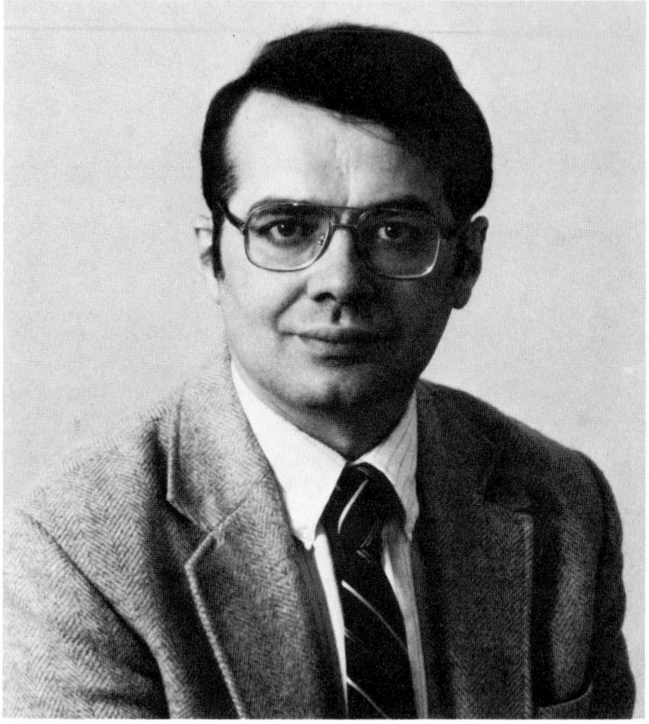

William J. Koopman, MD

The ARA can feel secure in knowing that the journal is in the hands of Bill Koopman and his Associate Editors in Birmingham. Under his stewardship, we look forward to an unbroken continuum of this tradition of excellence.

Eng M. Tan, MD
President, 1984–85
American Rheumatism Association

LETTERS

Evaluation of the 1982 American Rheumatism Association revised criteria for the classification of systemic lupus erythematosus

To The Editor:

The sensitivity of the 1971 preliminary criteria for the classification of systemic lupus erythematosus (SLE) was 90% according to Cohen et al (1), who assembled those criteria. This high degree of sensitivity was not found by other investigators (2–6). The 1982 revised criteria proposed by Tan et al (7) showed a 96% sensitivity among their patients.

In a recent work, Levin et al (8) compared the 1971 and the 1982 American Rheumatism Association (ARA) criteria in 156 of their patients and found 88% sensitivity with the 1971 preliminary criteria and 91% with the 1982 revised criteria. The increased sensitivity was attributed to the addition of the fluorescent antinuclear antibody (FANA) test as a criterion, whereas lowering the value required for fulfilling the proteinuria criterion did not affect sensitivity.

We compared the 2 criteria as did Levin et al (8). In 135 of our SLE patients, we found 81% sensitivity using the 1971 preliminary criteria and 90% with the 1982 revised criteria. In our group of patients, the improvement in sensitivity was 9%. This improvement was due to the decrease in the level of proteinuria to fulfill that criterion in 4% of the patients, to the addition of the anti–native DNA criterion in 2% of the patients, and to the inclusion of FANA in 9%.

The elimination of alopecia and Raynaud's phenomenon as criteria, the selection of cellular casts as an alternative to proteinuria, and the use of the false-positive reaction for syphilis as an alternative to LE cells (not as a separate criterion) did not change the overall sensitivity. Although we observed a decrease in the total number of the criteria present in our patients, the total number was never fewer than the necessary 4 criteria. The gain in sensitivity with the 1982 ARA criteria was higher in our patients (9%) than it was in the patients of Levin and coworkers (3%) (8). This gain is essentially due to the addition of FANA as a criterion.

F. Davatchi, MD
Shariati Hospital
C. Chams, MD
Razi Hospital
M. Akbarian, MD
Shariati Hospital
Tehran Medical School
Teheran, Iran

1. Cohen AS, Reynolds WE, Franklin EC, Kulka JP, Ropes MW, Shulman LE, Wallace SL: Preliminary criteria for the classification of systemic lupus erythematosus. Bull Rheum Dis 21:643–648, 1971
2. Davatchi F, Chams C, Atarian H, Baygan F, Akbarian M: Systemic lupus erythematosus in Iran. "R" 13:129–135, 1983
3. Davis P, Atkins BC, Josse RG, Hughes GRV: Criteria for the classification of SLE. Br Med J 3:88–89, 1973
4. Estes D, Christian CL: The natural history of systemic lupus erythematosus by prospective analysis. Medicine (Baltimore) 50:85–95, 1971
5. Fries JF, Siegel RC: Testing the preliminary criteria for classification of SLE. Ann Rheum Dis 32:171–177, 1973
6. Trimble RB, Townes AS, Robinson H, Kaplan SB, Chandler RW, Hanissian AS, Masi AT: Preliminary criteria for the classification of systemic lupus erythematosus: evaluation in early diagnosed SLE and rheumatoid arthritis. Arthritis Rheum 17: 184–188, 1974
7. Tan EM, Cohen AS, Fries JF, Masi AT, McShane DJ, Rothfield NF, Schaller JG, Talal N, Winchester RJ: The 1982 revised criteria for the classification of systemic lupus erythematosus. Arthritis Rheum 25:1271–1277, 1982
8. Levin RE, Weinstein A, Peterson M, Testa MA, Rothfield NF: A comparison of the sensitivity of the 1971 and 1982 American Rheumatism Association criteria for the classification of systemic lupus erythematosus. Arthritis Rheum 27:530–538, 1984

Autoantibodies in Argentine patients with systemic sclerosis (scleroderma)

To the Editor:

Data from studies of progressive systemic sclerosis (PSS) patients, conducted in North America (1–4) and Europe (5–7), appear to confirm the specificity and clinical implications of the presence of anticentromere antibodies (ACA) and anti–Scl-70 antibodies in this disease. The presence of ACA is highly characteristic of CREST (calcinosis, Raynaud's phenomenon, esophageal dysmotility, sclerodactyly, telangiectasias) and identifies patients with less severe disease (1–6). Anti–Scl-70, however, is associated with more systemic involvement (1,6). The prevalence of pulmonary fibrosis in these patients, a finding first described by investigators in Great Britain (6), has recently been confirmed in a large series of PSS patients from the United States (8). Information obtained on PSS patients in other parts of the world, however, is still lacking. We therefore undertook to examine the frequency and clinical significance of ACA and anti–Scl-70 antibodies, as well as other autoantibodies in 16 Argentine PSS patients whom we have been following prospectively since 1983.

Antinuclear antibodies were detected by indirect immunofluorescence using HEp-2 cells; we sought, in particular, the nucleolar and centromere patterns. Antibodies to soluble cellular antigens, including Ro (SS-A), La (SS-B), nRNP, Sm, and Scl-70, were investigated by immunodiffusion in 0.6% agarose (6). Statistical analysis was performed using the chi-square test with Yates' correction.

Clinical and serologic data obtained on our patients

Table 1. Clinical and serologic characteristics of 16 Argentine patients with progressive systemic sclerosis

Characteristic*	Diffuse (n = 9)	CREST (n = 7)†	P‡
Mean age (range)	39 (17–59)	53 (23–71)	
Disease duration, median years (range)	3 (2–16)	13 (10–30)	
Calcinosis, n (%)	–	6 (86)	<0.01
Raynaud's phenomenon, n (%)	8 (89)	6 (86)	
Sclerodactyly, n (%)	–	5 (71)	<0.02
Acrosclerosis, n (%)	–	2 (28)	
Telangiectasia, n (%)	1 (11)	5 (71)	
Esophageal involvement, n (%)	7 (78)	1 (14)	<0.05
Pulmonary involvement, n (%)	3 (33)	2 (28)	
Cardiac involvement, n (%)	–	1 (14)	
Renal involvement, n (%)	1 (11)	–	
Arthritis, n (%)	5 (55)	2 (28)	
Myositis, n (%)	1 (11)	–	
Antinucleolar antibodies, n (%)	5 (55)	1 (14)	
Anticentromere antibodies, n (%)	–	5 (71)	<0.02
Anti–Scl-70 antibodies, n (%)	4 (44)	1 (14)	

* Esophageal involvement defined as an abnormal result on barium swallow fluoroscopy with the patient in the supine position. Pulmonary involvement defined as bibasilar fibrosis on chest radiographic examination. Cardiac involvement defined as conduction abnormalities or heart failure in the absence of other causes. Renal involvement defined as proteinuria >0.5 gm/24 hours, creatinine clearance <60 ml/minute, abnormal sediment, or rapidly progressing hypertension. Two patients had both antinucleolar and anti–Scl-70 antibodies.

† CREST = calcinosis, Raynaud's phenomenon, esophageal dysmotility, sclerodactyly, telangiectasias.

‡ *P* value calculated using chi-square analysis with Yates' correction.

are shown in Table 1. The 16 patients, of whom 12 were women, were of various ethnic backgrounds, including Spanish, Italian, Arabic, Russian, and Polish; 1 was descended from local aborigines. All patients fulfilled the American Rheumatism Association preliminary criteria for PSS (9), with the exception of 1 patient who had calcinosis, sclerodactyly, and telangiectasias. Nine patients had diffuse disease, and 7 patients had the CREST variant. Two patients with acrosclerosis were included in the latter group.

The frequency of antinucleolar (37%) and anti–Scl-70 (31%) antibodies in the whole group and of ACA (71%) in the CREST patients is similar to that previously reported (1–6). Fourteen of the 16 patients had at least 1 of these antibodies. Table 2 further compares these patients according to the presence or absence of ANA and anti–Scl-70.

ACA occurred only in CREST patients and was associated with prolonged disease duration (median 14 years versus 5 years for ANA negative patients), limited scleroderma ($P < 0.05$), and, aside from lung disease, less systemic involvement. Four of 5 patients with anti–Scl-70 antibodies had diffuse PSS. Disease duration among these patients was shorter (median 6 years versus 10 years for anti–Scl-70 negative patients), and overall, they had more systemic involvement, including lung disease (60% versus 18% for patients without anti–Scl-70, $P > 0.05$). Antinucleolar antibodies occurred mainly in patients with diffuse scleroderma,

Table 2. Comparison of relevant clinical characteristics of 16 Argentine patients, according to the presence or absence of ACA and anti–Scl-70 antibodies*

Characteristic	ACA+ (n = 5)	ACA− (n = 11)	Anti–Scl-70+ (n = 5)	Anti–Scl-70− (n = 11)
Disease duration, median years (range)	14 (4–30)	5 (2–16)	6 (2–15)	10 (2–30)
Diffuse PSS, n (%)	–	9 (82)†	4 (80)	5 (45)
CREST, n (%)	5 (100)	2 (18)†	1 (20)	6 (54)
Lung involvement, n (%)	2 (40)	3 (27)	3 (60)	2 (18)‡
Esophageal involvement, n (%)	–	8 (73)†	5 (100)	3 (27)†

* ACA = anticentromere antibodies; + = positive; − = negative; PSS = progressive systemic sclerosis. See legend to Table 1 for other definitions.

† $P < 0.05$ by chi-square analysis with Yates' correction.

‡ $P > 0.05$ by chi-square analysis with Yates' correction.

but there were no apparent differences in visceral involvement. No patient had antibodies to Ro (SS-A), La (SS-B), nRNP, or Sm.

In the sera of 100 highly selected patients with connective tissue diseases (35 with PSS, 35 with systemic lupus erythematosus, 10 with mixed connective tissue disease, 12 with "early" connective tissue disease, 4 with "primary" Raynaud's, and 4 with polymyositis), referred to our laboratory, ACA occurred only in 1 patient who did not have PSS; that patient had "primary" Raynaud's. Similarly, anti–Scl-70 did not occur in any patient who did not have scleroderma. Of 24 patients with antinucleolar antibodies, 17 had systemic sclerosis. These data confirm the specificity of these antibodies, in particular, ACA and anti–Scl-70, for PSS.

In spite of the small number of patients studied, our findings support those obtained in other series demonstrating the diagnostic value of antinucleolar, anticentromere, and anti–Scl-70 antibodies and suggest that their clinical significance among patients in Argentina is similar to that among patients in other countries. Furthermore, because of the diverse ethnic backgrounds of our patients, including a patient with local aboriginal ancestors, our data suggest that these serologic abnormalities are indeed widespread.

Luis J. Catoggio, MD
Hospital Italiano de Buenos Aires and Centro Médico San Luis
Santiago Rodrigué, MD
Hugo Laborde, MD
Pedro M. Catoggio, MD
6ta Cátedra de Medicina Hospital Escuela José de San Martín
Patricia González Salas, MD
Centro Médico San Luis
Buenos Aires, Argentina

1. Tan EM, Rodnan GP, Garcia I, Moroi Y, Fritzler M, Peebles C: Diversity of antinuclear antibodies in progressive systemic sclerosis: anti-centromere antibody and its relationship to CREST syndrome. Arthritis Rheum 23:617–625, 1980
2. Fritzler MJ, Kinsella TD, Garbutt E: The CREST syndrome: a distinct serologic entity with anticentromere antibodies. Am J Med 69:520–526, 1980
3. McCarty GA, Rice JR, Bembe ML, Barada FA Jr: Anticentromere antibody: clinical correlations and association with favorable prognosis in patients with scleroderma variants. Arthritis Rheum 26:1–7, 1983
4. Steen VD, Ziegler GL, Rodnan GP, Medsger TA Jr: Clinical and laboratory associations of anticentromere antibodies in patients with progressive systemic sclerosis. Arthritis Rheum 27:125–131, 1984
5. Kallenberg CG, Pastoor GW, Wouda AA, The TH: Antinuclear antibodies in patients with Raynaud's phenomenon: clinical significance of anti-centromere antibodies. Ann Rheum Dis 41:382–387, 1982
6. Catoggio LJ, Bernstein RM, Black CM, Hughes GRV, Maddison PJ: Serological markers in progressive systemic sclerosis: clinical correlations. Ann Rheum Dis 42:23–27, 1983
7. Moutsopoulos HM, Giotaki H, Maddison PJ, Mavridis AC, Drosos AA, Skopouli FN: Antibodies to cellular antigens in Greek patients with autoimmune rheumatic diseases: anti-Ro(SSA) antibody a possible marker of penicillamine-D intolerance. Ann Rheum Dis 43:285–287, 1984
8. Powell DL, Lipinski E, Steen V, Rodnan GP, Medsger TA Jr: Clinical associations of anti-Scl 70 antibody in patients with systemic sclerosis (abstract). Arthritis Rheum (suppl) 27:S19, 1984
9. Subcommitte for Scleroderma Criteria of the American Rheumatism Association Diagnostic and Therapeutic Criteria Committee: Preliminary criteria for the classification of systemic sclerosis (scleroderma). Arthritis Rheum 23:581–590, 1980

Calcium pyrophosphate dihydrate crystal deposition in rheumatoid arthritis

To the Editor:

A recent report by Doherty et al (1) deserves comment. The authors compared "chondrocalcinosis" seen on standard knee radiographs of 100 patients who had well-defined rheumatoid arthritis (RA) with those of 135 "normal" controls who had knee radiographs taken in an emergency room for trauma. Several problems relating to this study can be enumerated.

First, the frequency of radiographically evident joint calcification (14%) in the controls, who had a mean age of 65 years, seems much too high (see Table 1). Ellman et al (2) found a 9.6% prevalence of chondrocalcinosis in a large group of patients who likewise had knee radiographs taken in an emergency room. But they correctly pointed out that this was probably a gross overestimate of the frequency in the general population, since there had obviously been symptoms referable to the knee of sufficient severity to bring the patient to the hospital. Many of these subjects may have had arthritic symptoms related to underlying crystal deposits,

Table 1. Radiologic surveys of the prevalence of chondrocalcinosis (English language)

Author (ref.)	No. of patients	No. with chondrocal-cinosis	% with chondrocal-cinosis	Mean age
Ellman et al (2)*	574	55	9.6	65
Bocher et al (3)	455	32	7	80
Hollingsworth et al (6)	142	0	0	54.9
Schmied et al (7)	61	1	0.6	61
Wilkins et al (8)†	20	3	15	65

* Films taken in emergency room.
† From the same group as studied by Doherty et al (1).

and trauma is a well-documented, common antecedent of crystal-induced arthritis.

Bocher et al (3) showed only a 7% incidence of chondrocalcinosis in a survey of a large group of subjects with an average age of 80 years. We found only a 3.2% prevalence of calcium pyrophosphate dihydrate (CPPD) crystal deposits when the menisci of 215 cadavers (mean age 72 years) were removed and examined using specimen radiography with industrial film (4). Only 7% of our cadavers had chondrocalcinosis that could conceivably have been visible on standard radiographs. This included brushite ($CaHPO_4 \cdot 2H_2O$) and apatite-type deposits. Many examples of calcified vessels supplying the outer third of the menisci were seen, however, and not systematically tabulated. When seen "on edge," as in standard knee films, these could also be called "chondrocalcinosis."

Second, the cartilage in many of the knees of Doherty's RA patients must have been thinned to an extent which would make detection of calcification within it difficult, if not impossible, since these patients had well-defined rheumatoid disease averaging 10 years in duration.

Third, as pointed out by Doherty et al in their discussion (but not in the title), chondrocalcinosis and CPPD crystal deposition are not synonymous. This alone invalidates their conclusion that CPPD deposition is less common in RA.

Fourth, 6 of the 579 patients with definite or probable CPPD crystal deposition studied by us in the past 24 years also had classic or definite RA. This approximates 1%, the accepted prevalence of RA in the general adult population.

Fifth, 26 of these 579 patients had the "pseudorheumatoid" pattern of CPPD crystal deposition. Some had even received gold therapy from rheumatologists because of synovial thickening, flexion contractures, and inflammatory-type joint fluid! Is it not possible that 7 of the 10 patients who were thought by Doherty et al to have both RA and CPPD crystal deposition had only the latter? These 7 had atypical radiologic features for RA, including exuberant osteophytosis, asymmetric erosive disease, lack of osteopenia, paucity of progressive erosive disease, and well-corticated erosions. Erosions have been described as a feature of apatite-type crystal deposition (5). An alternative interpretation of Doherty's data is that CPPD crystals can also be associated with juxtaarticular erosions and that 7 of their patients, in fact, had the pseudorheumatoid pattern associated with CPPD crystal deposition per se.

Finally, it would be of interest to know from what number of classic/definite RA cases their 10 cases of purported coincidental CPPD deposition disease were derived. One would estimate about 1,000 if 1% of subjects with CPPD crystal deposition disease have RA, as in the general population. If the prevalence is only one-fifth that of the general population, as Doherty et al suggest, then their 10 cases of "coincidental" disease must have been obtained from a population of about 5,000 patients with RA.

Although the authors of the paper in question have contributed a great deal of useful information to the subject of crystal deposition disease, the data they present in this paper should not be accepted uncritically.

Daniel J. McCarty, MD
Medical College of Wisconsin
Milwaukee, WI

1. Doherty M, Dieppe P, Watt I: Low incidence of calcium pyrophosphate dihydrate crystal deposition in rheumatoid arthritis, with modification of radiographic features in coexistent disease. Arthritis Rheum 27:1002–1009, 1984
2. Ellman MN, Brown NL, Levin B: Prevalence of knee chondrocalcinosis in hospital and clinic patients aged 50 or older. J Am Geriatr Soc 29:189–192, 1981
3. Bocher J, Mankin HJ, Berk RN, Rodnan G: Prevalence of calcified meniscal cartilage in elderly persons. N Engl J Med 272:1093–1097, 1965
4. McCarty DJ, Hogan JM, Gatter RA, Grossman M: Studies on pathological calcifications in human cartilage. I. Prevalence and types of crystal deposits in the menisci of two hundred fifteen cadavers. J Bone Joint Surg 48:309–325, 1966
5. Schumacher HR, Miller JL, Ludivico C, Jessar RA: Erosive arthritis associated with apatite crystal deposition. Arthritis Rheum 24:31–37, 1981
6. Hollingsworth P, Williams PL, Scott JT: Frequency of chondrocalcinosis of the knee in asymptomatic hyperuricemia and rheumatoid arthritis: a controlled study. Ann Rheum Dis 41:344–364, 1982
7. Schmied P, Rossum PV, Gabay R, Zahnd G: Etude radiologique sur la frequence de l'association entre la chondrocalcinose articulaire et le diabete. Schweiz Med Wochenschr 101:272–274, 1971
8. Wilkins E, Dieppe P, Maddison P, Evison G: Osteoarthritis and articular chondrocalcinosis in the elderly. Ann Rheum Dis 42: 280–284, 1983

Reply

To the Editor:

We would like to thank Professor McCarty for his interesting letter, and we appreciate having the opportunity to reply. Four of McCarty's 6 points were fully discussed in our article (1). However, taking them in order, we would like to make the following additional observations:

1. We have consistently found chondrocalcinosis in about 15% of subjects in the age group studied. This is largely due to the marked increase in incidence in subjects over the age of 65. Other European authors report similar figures (2). It may be worth exploring the possibility that the incidence varies in different groups, but we believe our figures are consistent with those in other recent surveys, and that our control group is relevant and representative.

2 and 3. We agree with these points, and highlighted them in our discussion. This was why we looked at synovial fluid crystals as well as at radiographs.

4. The incidence of rheumatoid arthritis (RA) in patients presenting with symptoms and calcium pyrophosphate dihydrate (CPPD) deposition is not relevant since it can be distorted by a variety of selection factors.

Indeed, in our own survey of symptomatic CPPD patients, we found a high incidence of atypical RA, prompting the controlled study (1).

5. We have found the "pseudo" disease subdivision unhelpful (3). Although we see polyarticular CPPD, we have not seen anyone with "pseudorheumatoid disease" in a series of over 200 patients. We, like others (4), do not accept the assertion that CPPD can cause rheumatoid-like erosions. Perhaps some of Professor McCarty's patients had modified RA! We are confident of the diagnosis of RA in the 10 cases described: as explained in the text, all fulfilled American Rheumatism Association criteria (5), all had erosive disease, and 8 had classic extraarticular features.

6. We do, indeed, see an enormous number of patients with RA. During the 5 years of recording of our cases, we have been at the only rheumatology unit serving a population of nearly 1 million. In addition, many of our patients were referred from colleagues in Bath, who are at a referral center for the southwest of England.

Professor McCarty's points are well-taken and relevant to the difficult problem of disease coincidence. It is difficult to prove positive or negative associations for a common age-related phenomenon, but we believe that our data represent the first controlled evidence concerning the relationship between CPPD and RA. The negative association is in keeping with the finding of low levels of pyrophosphate in rheumatoid synovial fluid (6).

The more important part of our paper, which we would like to stress, does not concern incidence, but the effects of the interaction. We believe it is misleading to regard pyrophosphate deposition as a disease; it is an age-related process which can be accelerated or retarded by a number of other factors, and which can interact with other pathologic conditions to induce disease. We view CPPD as a reflection of host response which is associated with a modified form of rheumatoid arthritis, just as it modifies osteoarthritis.

Michael Doherty, MD
City Hospital
Nottingham, England
Paul Dieppe, MD
Iain Watt, MD
Bristol Royal Infirmary
Bristol, England

1. Doherty M, Dieppe P, Watt I: Low incidence of calcium pyrophosphate dihydrate crystal deposition in rheumatoid arthritis, with modification of radiographic features in coexistent disease. Arthritis Rheum 27:1002–1009, 1984
2. Mitrovic D, Stankovic A, Mann J, Borda-Iriate O, Vzan M, Quntero M, Memin Y, Bard M, de Seze S, Rickewaert A: Incidence of knee-joint menisco-chondrocalcinosis at autopsy. Rev Rhum Mal Osteoartic 49:495–499, 1982
3. Dieppe PA, Alexander GJM, Jones HE, Doherty M, Scott DGI, Manhire A, Watt I: Pyrophosphate arthropathy: a clinical and radiological study of 105 cases. Ann Rheum Dis 42:371–376, 1982
4. Resnick D, Williams G, Weisman MH, Slaughter L: Rheumatoid arthritis and pseudo-rheumatoid arthritis in calcium pyrophosphate dihydrate crystal deposition disease. Radiology 140:615–621, 1980
5. Ropes MW, Bennett GA, Cobb S, Jacox R, Jessar RA: 1958 revision of diagnostic criteria for rheumatoid arthritis. Bull Rheum Dis 9:175–176, 1958
6. Micheli A, Po J, Fallett GH: Measurement of soluble pyrophosphate in plasma and synovial fluid of patients with various rheumatic diseases. Scand J Rheumatol 10:237–240, 1981

Comment on Zea-Mendoza report

To the Editor:

While the existence of the recently described, distinct clinical entity, POEMS syndrome, appears well documented (Bardwick PA, Zvaifler NJ, Gill NG, Newman D, Greenway GD, Resnick DL: Plasma cell dyscrasia with polyneuropathy, organomegaly, endocrinopathy, M-protein and skin changes: the POEMS syndrome: report on two cases and a review of the literature. Medicine [Baltimore] 59:311–322, 1980), one must exercise caution and restraint in classifying a patient with a puzzling array of symptoms and signs into this new group. The problem is illustrated by a recent case report in *Arthritis and Rheumatism* (Zea-Mendoza AC, Alonso-Ruiz A, García-Vadillo A, Moreno-Caparrós A, Beltrán-Gutierrez J: POEMS syndrome with neuroarthropathy and nodular regenerative hyperplasia of the liver. Arthritis Rheum 27:1053–1057, 1984).

The authors described a 72-year-old man with polyneuropathy, skin lesions, hepatomegaly, monoclonal gammopathy and bone marrow plasmacytosis, lytic lesions in the bones, and erosive changes (of neuropathic arthritis) in the ankles. Though biopsies of the sural nerve and liver showed no amyloid, results of a rectal biopsy were positive for amyloid deposits. Based on this constellation of symptoms, the authors arrived at the diagnosis of POEMS syndrome.

It seems likely that this patient actually had amyloidosis. Primary amyloidosis is associated with gammopathy and plasmacytosis, neuropathy, hepatomegaly, skin lesions, and erosive arthritis, such as this patient had. The authors stated that there was sufficient evidence in this case to exclude amyloidosis as the cause of the associated disorders. Though 3 biopsy specimens were negative for amyloid, the rectal biopsy showed a positive result. It seems contrary to the principle of "Ockham's razor" to postulate the existence of another, coexistent disease, in addition to the amyloidosis that this patient clearly had, to account for his syndrome. It is more likely that the 3 biopsy results that were negative for amyloid were false-negative and that the rectal biopsy result was true-positive.

John Varga, MD
Maggie Flinn, MD
Boston University Medical Center
Boston, MA

BOOK REVIEW

Antinuclear Antibodies: Contemporary Techniques and Clinical Application to Connective Tissue Disease. *Gale A. McCarty, Donald W. Valencia, Marvin J. Fritzler. New York, Oxford University Press, 1984. 95 pages. Illustrated. Indexed. $29.95.*

This book is of value to clinicians and laboratory personnel who utilize or perform antinuclear antibody (ANA) tests. It is a brief but rather comprehensive monograph combining the clinical information with the practical laboratory aspects of testing for and interpretation of specific autoantibodies of diagnostic significance in rheumatic diseases. The authors have included an extensive and up-to-date bibliography for those who wish to review specific areas in depth.

The first 2 chapters are good summaries of the clinical relevance of ANA testing. Chapter 1 briefly summarizes the clinical characteristics of patients with systemic lupus erythematosus, scleroderma, mixed connective tissue disease, rheumatoid arthritis, juvenile rheumatoid arthritis, polymyositis–dermatomyositis, and Sjögren's syndrome. It is in these disease groups that the fluorescent ANA (FANA) and specific autoantibody profiles have clinical relevance. Included are the major manifestations of the disease, the current American Rheumatism Association criteria where applicable, a brief review of the systems involved, and relevant tests, other than ANA, used in diagnosis.

Chapter 2 presents the classification of the various autoantibodies according to the biochemical characterizations of the antigens to which they bind. These include antibodies to nucleic acids (DNA and RNA), histones, and the non-histone proteins (Sm, RNP, SS-B [La], etc.). Also included are some uncommon autoantibodies, such as those to various cytoplasmic constituents, which are observed more frequently with the use of tissue culture cells.

The next 3 chapters deal with microscopy, FANA standardization and interpretation, and the use of counterimmunoelectrophoresis (CIE) to identify specific autoantibodies. I would have liked to have seen these chapters expanded to include a few more areas.

The chapter on microscopy is brief, yet includes the fundamental principles of both incidence and transmission light microscopy, the types of light sources and filters, and some suggestions for taking photomicrographs. The discussion on FANA standardization is well written, and the information can be applied to FANA testing in general. However, the section on interpretation of ANA is limited primarily to tests that use HEp-2 as the substrate. This section on standardization could well have been expanded to include a wider discussion on other substrates, primarily rodent tissues, with examples of pattern variation among them. The photographs of the various nuclear and cytoplasmic fluorescent patterns seen on the HEp-2 cells are excellent and should be helpful to individuals using this substrate.

My major criticism of this book is the use of the term "contemporary techniques" in the title, suggesting a broader discussion of the techniques used for antinuclear antibody identification than is actually presented. No discussion of anti–native DNA (anti-nDNA) tests is included. The authors include a good picture of the *Crithidia luciliae* in their photograph section, but fail to include any mention of this assay in the text. Since anti-nDNA tests are among the most important used in the laboratory, I consider this a major oversight. The only technique for the detection of extractable nuclear antigens that is included, other than FANA, is CIE. The chapter on CIE is well written and includes the authors' easy-to-follow procedure. While CIE is a useful method, the most common method, and the one which is commercially available, is double immunodiffusion. A brief discussion of double immunodiffusion and some of the problems encountered when testing for various nuclear antibodies would have been extremely helpful.

Despite the limited discussion of identification techniques other than CIE, this monograph is excellent for FANA standardization and interpretation as well as the discussion of the clinical relevance of the various autoantibodies. I highly recommend it as a valuable addition to any laboratory in which ANA tests are performed.

Carol L. Peebles, MS, MT (ASCP)
Scripps Clinic and Research Foundation
La Jolla, CA

1 9 8 5

ARTHRITIS FOUNDATION

SCIENTIFIC ABSTRACTS

ANNUAL MEETING

49TH ANNUAL MEETING

AMERICAN RHEUMATISM ASSOCIATION

★ ★ ★

20TH ANNUAL MEETING

ARTHRITIS HEALTH PROFESSIONS ASSOCIATION

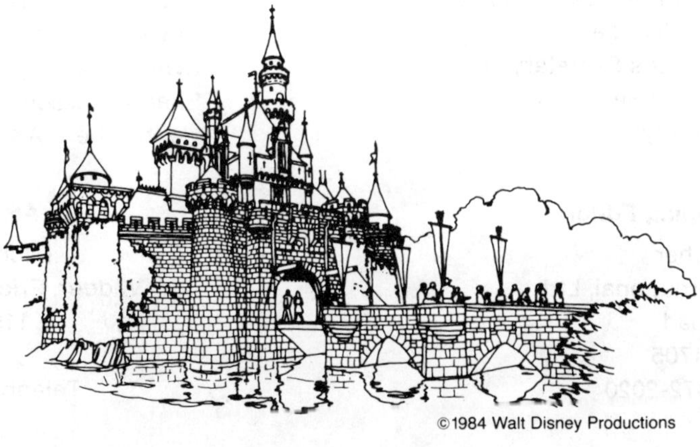

JUNE 4-8, 1985
DISNEYLAND HOTEL
ANAHEIM, CALIFORNIA

ABSTRACT VOLUME

AMERICAN RHEUMATISM ASSOCIATION

Section of the Arthritis Foundation

ARA OFFICERS 1984-85

President: Eng M. Tan, M.D.
First Vice President & President-Elect: Edward D. Harris, Jr., M.D.
Second Vice President: Michael D. Lockshin, M.D.
Secretary-Treasurer: William N. Kelley, M.D.

ARA LOCAL ARRANGEMENTS COMMITTEE

Co-Chairpersons: Dr. & Mrs. James R. Klinenberg

ARA PROGRAM COMMITTEE

Chairperson: Dennis A. Carson, M.D.

Subsection Chairpersons

A. Research Rheumatology
- Aa. Humoral Immunology: Paul H. Plotz, M.D.
- Ab. Cellular Immunology: Peter D. Lipsky, M.D.
- Ac. Inflammation: Rochelle Hirschhorn, M.D.
- Ad. Biochemistry: Donald M. Marcus, M.D.

B. Clinical Rheumatology
- Ba. Pediatrics: Earl J. Brewer, Jr., M.D.
- Bb. Rheumatoid Arthritis: J. W. Hollingsworth, M.D.
- Bc. Systemic Lupus Erythematosus: Ronald P. Messner, M.D.
- Bd. Scleroderma: James C. Steigerwald, M.D.
- Be. Osteoarthritis and Spondylitis: Irving Kushner, M.D.
- Bf. Other Rheumatic Syndromes: John T. Boyer, M.D.

C. Orthopedics
Lawrence C. Rosenberg, M.D.

D. Health Services Research
Matthew H. Liang, M.D.

ARA NATIONAL STAFF

Dallas F. Whaley, CAE, Executive Vice President

Lynn Bonfiglio, Director, Membership & Committee Affairs
Angel Fortenberry, Director, Conferences & Expositions
Jeffrey W. Haggerty, Business Manager
Gwen Brown, Membership Records Secretary
Suzanne Gould, Word Processing Secretary
Kim Turner, Department Secretary
Jane Diamond, A&R Managing Editor
Patricia Courtney, A&R Manuscript Editor
Beverly Greene, A&R Manuscript Editor
Lynne Beavers, A&R Circulation Director
Sharon Russell, A&R Assistant Editor
Henri Albert, A&R Assistant Editor (San Diego)

ARA Newsletter Managing Editor

Gerald J. Faucher
Contact Associates International, Ltd
600 Middle Road
Bayport, NY 11705
Telephone: (516) 472-2020

ARA Legal Counsel

Michael E. Reed, Esq.
Vedder, Price, Kaufman & Kammholz
115 LaSalle Street
Chicago, IL
Telephone: (312) 781-2306

ABSTRACT VOLUME PRODUCTION ASSISTANCE PROVIDED BY CONTACT ASSOCIATES

TABLE OF CONTENTS

General Information S4

ARA Tentative Meeting Schedule S6

ARA State of the Art Lecture Program S9

Henry G. Kunkel Memorial Lecture S10

ARA Scientific Workshop S10

ARA Postgraduate Clinical Seminars S11

ARA Scientific Abstracts S14

ARA Author Index S101

ARA Key Phrase Index S124

AHPA Program Committee Listing S133

AHPA Tentative Meeting Schedule S134

AHPA Abstracts S138

AHPA Author Index S153

AHPA Key Phrase Index S157

NOTE: In order to meet an early publication deadline, some of the information contained in this Abstract Volume is not complete. Corrections will be made in the final program. Any major corrections concerning the program should be forwarded to Angel Fortenberry at the ARA National Office, 1314 Spring Street, N.W., Atlanta, Georgia 30309.

ABSTRACT VOLUME

Annual Scientific Meetings

49th ANNUAL MEETING
American Rheumatism Association

20th ANNUAL MEETING
Arthritis Health Professions Association

June 4-8, 1985

ABSTRACTS OF SCIENTIFIC PRESENTATIONS

ARA Podium Presentations (175)
ARA Abstracts 1 - 175

ARA Poster Presentations (326)
ARA Abstracts A-1 - A-67
B-1 - B-56
C-1 - C-57
D-1 - D-72
E-1 - E-74

AHPA Podium Presentations (37)
AHPA Abstracts

AHPA Poster Presentations (36)
AHPA Abstracts B-22 - B-39
C-50 - C-67

AHPA Workshop/Seminar
Presentations (15)

NOTE: A separate meeting program containing all other information regarding the meeting (including the author index) will be sent to all ARA dues-paid members and registrants prior to the meeting. The information contained in this volume is subject to further corrections.

The ARA and AHPA scientific abstracts will appear only in this supplement to the April 1985 issue of ARTHRITIS & RHEUMATISM. Copies of the ARA/AHPA Abstract Volume will be available for distribution to registrants at the Annual Meeting in Anaheim.

Registration forms for the 1985 Annual Scientific Meetings of both the American Rheumatism Association and the Arthritis Health Professions Association were mailed in March from the ARA/AHPA National Office, 1314 Spring Street, N.W., Atlanta, Georgia 30309.

The registration fees for the ARA Scientific Meeting are: 125.00 (Advance) and $150.00 (On-Site) for ARA members; $150.00 and $175.00 for Non-Members; $75.00 and $100.00 for Students and Fellows.

There is a separate registration fee for the ARA State-of-the-Art Lecture Program to be held on Tuesday, June 4, 1985 (Advance $125; On-Site $150; $75 and $100 for Students and Fellows).

The registration fees for the AHPA Scientific Meeting are: $110.00 (Advance) and $130.00 (On-Site) for AHPA Members; $130.00 and $150.00 for Non-Members; $50.00 and $60.00 for Undergraduate Students.

CATEGORY I CREDIT - ARA

As an organization accredited by the Accreditation Council for Continuing Medical Education (ACCME), the Arthritis Foundation designates these activities for hour-for-hour credit in Category I of the Physician's Recognition Award of the American Medical Association.

CEU CREDITS - AHPA

CEU's are awarded on a standard of one unit per ten hours of classroom contact. The CEU is a nationally recognized unit of measure used to accumulate a standardized permanent record of an individual's participation in credit-free continuing education programs conducted under responsible, capable direction and qualified instruction.

1 9 8 5

ARTHRITIS FOUNDATION

SCIENTIFIC ANNUAL MEETING ABSTRACTS

★ ★ ★

49TH ANNUAL MEETING

AMERICAN RHEUMATISM ASSOCIATION

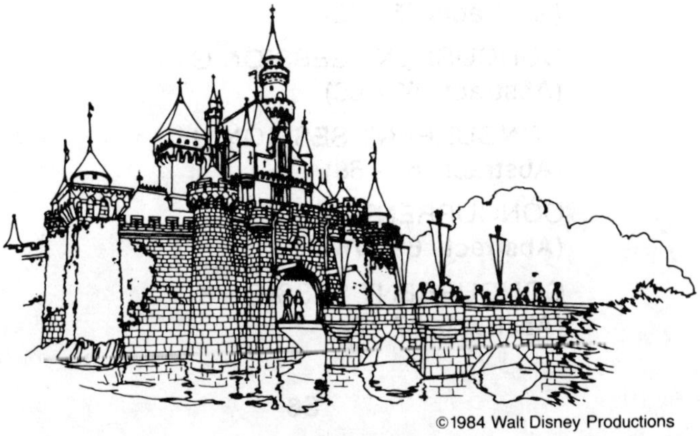

JUNE 4-8, 1985
DISNEYLAND HOTEL
ANAHEIM, CALIFORNIA

49TH ANNUAL SCIENTIFIC MEETING
Anaheim, California
June 4-8, 1985

TENTATIVE SCHEDULE

TUESDAY, JUNE 4, 1985

8:30 a.m. to 5:30 p.m.	STATE OF THE ART LECTURE PROGRAM	
6:30 p.m. to 8:00 p.m.	WELCOME RECEPTION	

WEDNESDAY, JUNE 5, 1985

7:30 a.m. to 8:30 a.m.	Continental Breakfast	Center Ballroom
8:00 a.m. to 9:30 a.m.	POSTER SESSION A (Abstracts A1 - A67)	Exhibit Hall
9:30 a.m. to 10:00 a.m.	Break	Exhibit Hall
10:00 a.m. to 11:00 a.m.	KUNKEL MEMORIAL LECTURE	Grand Ballroom
11:00 a.m. to 12:00 p.m.	PLENARY SESSION I (Abstracts 1-4)	Grand Ballroom
12:00 p.m. to 1:00 p.m.	Lunch Break	
1:00 p.m. to 3:00 p.m.	CONCURRENT SESSION A (Abstracts 5 - 12)	Center Ballroom
1:00 p.m. to 3:00 p.m.	CONCURRENT SESSION B (Abstracts 13 - 20)	South Ballroom
1:00 p.m. to 3:00 p.m.	CONCURRENT SESSION C (Abstracts 21 - 28)	North Ballroom
1:00 p.m. to 3:00 p.m.	CONCURRENT SESSION D (Abstracts 29 - 36)	Marina 3
1:00 p.m. to 3:00 p.m.	CONCURRENT SESSION E (Abstracts 37 - 44)	Marina 2
3:00 p.m. to 3:30 p.m.	Break	Exhibit Hall
3:30 p.m. to 5:30 p.m.	CONCURRENT SESSION F (Abstracts 45 - 52)	Center Ballroom
3:30 p.m. to 5:30 p.m.	CONCURRENT SESSION G (Abstracts 53 - 60)	South Ballroom
3:30 p.m. to 5:30 p.m.	CONCURRENT SESSION H (Abstracts 61 - 68)	North Ballroom
3:30 p.m. to 5:30 p.m.	CONCURRENT SESSION J (Abstracts 69 - 76)	Marina 3
3:30 p.m. to 5:30 p.m.	CONCURRENT SESSION K (Abstracts 77 - 84)	Marina 2

8:00 p.m. to 10:00 p.m.	STUDY GROUP MEETINGS:	
	Anti-Rheumatic Therapy	Marina 1
	Cartilage	Pacific
	Inflammation in Rheumatic Diseases	Serrano
	Health Services Research	Cerritos
	Non-Articular Rheumatism	Embassy East
	Orthopedics	Marina 4
	Pediatric Rheumatology	Santa Rosa
	Rehabilitative Rheumatology	Yorba
	Scleroderma	Marina 2
	SLE	Marina 3
10:00 p.m. to 11:30 p.m.	POST STUDY GROUPS RECEPTION	Grand Ballroom

THURSDAY, JUNE 6, 1985

7:30 a.m. to 8:30 a.m.	Continental Breakfast	Center Ballroom
8:00 a.m. to 9:30 a.m.	POSTER SESSION B (Abstracts B1 - B56)	Exhibit Hall
9:30 a.m. to 10:00 a.m.	Break	Exhibit Hall
10:00 a.m. to 11:00 a.m.	PLENARY SESSION II (Abstracts 85 - 87)	Grand Ballroom
11:00 a.m. to 12:00 p.m.	PRESIDENTIAL ADDRESS & BUSINESS MEETING	Grand Ballroom
12:00 p.m. to 1:00 p.m.	Lunch Break	
1:00 p.m. to 3:00 p.m.	ARA POSTGRADUATE CLINICAL SEMINAR A	North Ballroom
1:00 p.m. to 3:00 p.m.	ARA POSTGRADUATE CLINICAL SEMINAR B	South Ballroom
1:00 p.m. to 3:00 p.m.	ARA/AHPA POSTGRADUATE CLINICAL SEMINAR C	Marina 2
1:00 p.m. to 5:30 p.m.	ARA SCIENTIFIC WORKSHOP I	Marina 3
3:00 p.m. to 3:30 p.m.	Break	
3:30 p.m. to 5:30 p.m.	ARA POSTGRADUATE CLINICAL SEMINAR D	North Ballroom
3:30 p.m. to 5:30 p.m.	ARA POSTGRADUATE CLINICAL SEMINAR E	South Ballroom
3:30 p.m. to 5:30 p.m.	ARA/AHPA POSTGRADUATE CLINICAL SEMINAR F	Marina 2
6:30 p.m. to 8:00 p.m.	RECEPTION	Grand Ballroom

FRIDAY, JUNE 7, 1985

7:30 a.m. to 8:30 a.m.	Continental Breakfast	Center Ballroom
8:00 a.m. to 9:30 a.m.	POSTER SESSION C (Abstracts C1 - C57)	Exhibit Hall
9:30 a.m to 10:00 a.m.	Break	
10:00 a.m. to 12:00 p.m.	CONCURRENT SESSION L (Abstracts 88 - 95)	Center Ballroom
10:00 a.m. to 12:00 p.m.	CONCURRENT SESSION M (Abstracts 96 - 103)	South Ballroom

10:00 a.m. to 12:00 p.m.	CONCURRENT SESSION N (Abstracts 104 - 111)	North Ballroom
10:00 a.m. to 12:00 p.m.	CONCURRENT SESSION O (Abstracts 112 - 119)	Marina 3
10:00 a.m. to 12:00 p.m.	CONCURRENT SESSION P (Abstracts 120 - 127)	Marina 2
12:00 p.m. to 1:00 p.m.	Lunch	
1:00 p.m. to 2:30 p.m.	POSTER SESSION D (Abstracts D1 - D72)	Exhibit Hall
2:30 p.m. to 3:00 p.m.	Break	
3:00 p.m. to 5:00 p.m.	PLENARY SESSION III (Abstracts 128 - 135)	Grand Ballroom

SATURDAY, JUNE 8, 1985

8:00 a.m. to 9:30 a.m.	Continental Breakfast	Center Ballroom
8:00 a.m. to 9:30 a.m.	POSTER SESSION E (Abstracts E1 - E74)	Exhibit Hall
9:30 a.m. to 10:00 a.m.	Break	Exhibit Hall
10:00 a.m. to 12:00 p.m.	CONCURRENT SESSION Q (Abstracts 136 - 143)	Center Ballroom
10:00 a.m. to 12:00 p.m.	CONCURRENT SESSION R (Abstracts 144 - 151)	South Ballroom
10:00 a.m. to 12:00 p.m.	CONCURRENT SESSION S (Abstracts 152 - 159)	North Ballroom
10:00 a.m. to 12:00 p.m.	CONCURRENT SESSION T (Abstracts 160 - 167)	Marina 3
10:00 a.m. to 12:00 p.m.	CONCURRENT SESSION U (Abstracts 168 - 175)	Marina 2

AMERICAN RHEUMATISM ASSOCIATION

STATE OF THE ART LECTURE SERIES

Tuesday, June 4, 1985
8:30 AM - 5:30 PM
Disneyland Hotel
Grand Ballroom

MAGNETIC RESONANCE IMAGING IN THE RHEUMATIC DISEASES

William Martel, M.D.
University of Michigan
Ann Arbor, Michigan

MECHANICAL LOW BACK PAIN
Richard N. Stauffer, M.D.
Mayo Clinic
Rochester, Minnesota

MECHANISM OF ACTION OF GOLD
Peter E. Lipsky, M.D.
University of Texas
Dallas, Texas

SEPTIC ARTHRITIS
Don L. Goldenberg, M.D.
Boston University
Boston, Massachusetts

OSTEOPOROSIS
Bevra H. Hahn, M.D.
University of California
Los Angeles, California

MOLECULAR BIOLOGY FOR THE CLINICIAN
John D. Stobo, M.D.
University of California
San Francisco, California

KUNKEL MEMORIAL LECTURE

Wednesday, June 5, 1985
10:00 AM - 11:00 AM
Disneyland Hotel
Grand Ballroom

MURINE LUPUS - A MODEL FOR HUMAN AUTOIMMUNITY

Frank J. Dixon, M.D.
Scripps Clinic and Research Foundation
La Jolla, California

SCIENTIFIC WORKSHOP

Thursday, June 6, 1985
1:00 PM - 5:30 PM
Marina 3

VIRUSES, IMMUNITY AND RHEUMATIC DISEASES

Moderator: Michael B. A. Oldstone, M.D.

RETROVIRUS MODEL OF HUMAN ARTHRITIS: CAPRINE ARTHRITIS AND ENCEPHALITIS

Travis C. McGuire, Jr., D.V.M, Ph.D.
Washington State University, Pullman, Pennsylvania

DISEASE MECHANISMS OF HUMAN AND MURINE LYMPHOTROPIC VIRUSES

William A. Haseltine, M.D.
Harvard Medical School, Dana-Farber Cancer Institute, Boston, Massachusetts

MEDICAL IMPLICATIONS OF VIRUS INDUCED ALTERATIONS OF IMMUNE AND OTHER DIFFERENTIATED FUNCTIONS

Michael B. A. Oldstone, M.D.
Scripps Clinic and Research Foundation, La Jolla, California

MOLECULAR MIMICRY: IMPLICATIONS FOR AUTOIMMUNE DISEASE

Robert S. Fujinami, Ph.D.
Scripps Clinic and Research Foundation, La Jolla, California

ARA POSTGRADUATE CLINICAL SEMINAR A

Thursday, June 6, 1985
1:00 PM - 3:00 PM
North Ballroom

USE OF CYTOTOXIC IMMUNOSUPPRESSIVE DRUGS IN RHEUMATIC DISEASES

INTRODUCTION

Frederic C. McDuffie, M.D.
Emory University School of Medicine
Atlinua, Georgia

EFFECTS OF CYTOTOXIC DRUGS ON INFLAMMATION AND IMMUNE MECHANISMS

Peter E. Lipsky, M.D.
University of Texas Health Sciences Center
Dallas, Texas

RELATIONSHIP OF CYTOTOXIC DRUGS TO MALIGNANCY
IN RHEUMATIC AND NONRHEUMATIC CONDITIONS

Leo J. Kinlen, M.D.
University of Oxford
Oxford, England

CLINICAL USE OF CYTOTOXIC DRUGS IN RHEUMATIC DISEASE

John R. Ward, M.D.
University of Utah Medical Center
Salt Lake City, Utah

ARA POSTGRADUATE CLINICAL SEMINAR B

Thursday, June 6, 1985
1:00 PM - 3:00 PM
South Ballroom

DRGS - DOES RHEUMATOLOGY GET SUPPORTED?

THE IMPACT OF MEASURING OUTCOMES OF RHEUMATOLOGIC TREATMENT ON RHEUMATOLOGIC PRACTICE, PRESENT AND FUTURE

Matthew H. Liang, M.D., M.P.H.
Brigham and Women's Hospital
Boston, Massachusetts

THE IMPACT AND IMPLICATIONS OF CORPORATE MEDICINE IN THE MEDICAL-INDUSTRIAL COMPLEX ON THE PRESENT AND FUTURE PRACTICE OF RHEUMATOLOGY

Roy Christensen, M.D.
New Hope Pain Center, Inc.
Pasadena, California

COMPREHENSIVE AMBULATORY CARE AND RHEUMATOLOGY - A VIABLE MODEL

Robert L. Swezey, M.D.
The Arthritis and Back Pain Center
Santa Monica, California

ARA/AHPA POSTGRADUATE CLINICAL SEMINAR C

Thursday, June 6, 1985
1:00 PM - 3:00 PM
Marina 2

OSTEOARTHRITIS OF THE KNEE

Clement B. Sledge, M.D.
Brigham and Women's Hospital
Boston, Massachusetts

Jules M. Rothstein, Ph.D.
Medical College of Virginia
Richmond, Virginia

ARA POSTGRADUATE CLINICAL SEMINAR D (CORP FORUM)

Thursday, June 6, 1985
3:30 PM - 5:30 PM
North Ballroom

MEDICAL MEGATRENDS: IMPLICATIONS FOR MEDICAL PRACTICE

William J. Arnold, M.D.
Park Ridge, Illinois

REPORT BY CHAIRMAN ON CORP ACTIVITIES

Paulding Phelps, M.D.
Portland, Maine

GENERAL DISCUSSION: CONCERNS OF MEMBERS

ARA POSTGRADUATE CLINICAL SEMINAR E

Thursday, June 6, 1985
3:30 PM - 5:30 PM
South Ballroom

THE TERRIBLE TWOSOME: NSAIDs AND ULCERS

Moderator: Sanford H. Roth, M.D.
Arthritis Center, Ltd. and
St. Luke's Medical Center
Phoenix, Arizona

EVALUATION OF UNITED STATES AND FOREIGN DATA ON NSAID TOXICITY

John G. Harter, M.D.
Federal Drug Administration
Bethesda, Maryland

THE PATHOPHYSIOLOGIC BASIS OF GASTRIC ULCERS ASSOCIATED WITH ARTHRITIS THERAPY: CYTOPROTECTION AND RATIONAL PROPHYLAXIS

Sandor Szabo, M.D., Ph.D.
Harvard Medical School - Brigham and Women's Hospital
Boston, Massachusetts

GASTROENTEROLOGY ASSESSMENT OF NSAID INDUCED PEPTIC DISEASE - RECOGNIZING AND RESPONDING

Paul H. Guth, M.D.
UCLA and Wadsworth Veterans Administration Hospital
Los Angeles, California

ARA/AHPA POSTGRADUATE CLINICAL SEMINAR F

Thursday, June 6, 1985
3:30 PM - 5:30 PM
Marina 2

JUVENILE RHEUMATOID ARTHRITIS

Edith S. Shear, S.W.
Children's Hospital Medical Center
Cincinnati, Ohio

James T. Cassidy, M.D.
Creighton Health Profession Center
Omaha, Nebraska

1

D-PENICILLAMINE (D-PEN) AND HYDROXYCHLOROQUINE (HCQ) IN JUVENILE RHEUMATOID ARTHRITIS (JRA)- RESULTS OF THE DOUBLE-BLIND, PLACEBO (P) CONTROLLED TRIAL. Earl J. Brewer, Edward H. Giannini for the USA Pediatric Rheumatology Collaborative Study Group. N. Kuzmina, L. Alekseev for the USSR Cooperating Centers. Houston TX. USA. Moscow, USSR.

The purpose of the study was to evaluate the efficacy and safety of D-PEN versus P, and HCQ versus P in a group of pts with JRA who were considered candidates for slower-acting drugs. 18 pediatric rheumatology centers in the USA and USSR participated. All centers employed an identical protocol and standardized case report forms. Pts were randomized into either the D-PEN, HCQ or P group. Initial dose (in mg/kg/d) of D-PEN was 5, increased to 10 after 2 mo. HCQ was started at 3 and raised to 6. The P group received an identical number of capsules. Followup was 1 yr, with visits at 0,2,4,6,9 and 12 mo. A single NSAID was allowed; other antirheumatic drugs were not permitted.

162 pts (54 D-PEN, 57 HCQ, 51 P) were randomized. 87% had polyarticular, 7% pauciarticular, and 6% systemic JRA. There were no significant inter-group differences (by Dunnett's Method) in any demographic, articular,or hematologic variables at randomization.

Results: 159 pts completed at least 2 mo of therapy and were considered for efficacy. According to the physician's global assessment, 54% of the D-PEN, 61% of the HCQ, and 47% of the P pts were classified as "better" or "much better" at their final visit. Significant clinical improvement (defined as >=25%) in the number of joints with active arthritis occurred in 54% of the D-PEN, 55% of the HCQ, and 52% of the P pts. Change in the number of active joints averaged -2.2 for D-PEN, -4.9 for HCQ, and -4.2 for P. The proportion of pts in whom the ESR returned to nl did not differ significantly among the groups. Adversity was rare and usually attributable to the NSAID. Nephrotic syndrome developed in a pt receiving D-PEN and tolmetin. By 12 mo 20% had dropped from the D-PEN, 19% from HCQ, and 33% from P. Inefficacy drops were highest in the HCQ group, followed by D-PEN and then P.

These data suggest that, in combination with NSAID, neither D-PEN nor HCQ offer a significant advantage over P in the treatment of JRA. A large proportion of pts considered candidates for SAARDS improve dramatically on NSAID alone. Further data analysis may identify sub-groups of pts who are more likely to respond to D-PEN or HCQ than to P.

2

CLONING OF A HUMAN RHEUMATOID FACTOR (RF) IMMUNOGLOBULIN LIGHT CHAIN GENE ASSOCIATED WITH A MAJOR CROSS-REACTIVE IDIOTYPE (CRI). Frank Jirik, Joe Sorge, Sherman Fong, PoJen Chen, Robert Goldfien, John Curd and Dennis Carson, Scripps Clinic and Research Foundation, La Jolla, CA 92037. Joy Heitzmann, Salk Institute, La Jolla, CA 92037.

A fundamental question in immunology concerns the genetic and molecular basis for autoantibody synthesis. Whether germ-line genes encode autoantibodies, or whether they arise through somatic mutation of Ig genes, is not known. To analyze these questions directly requires monoclonal sources of autoantibody-secreting cells and specific DNA probes. Cells from a patient with chronic lymphocytic leukemia (CLL) associated with high titers of monoclonal IgM-RF were characterized by: 1) *in vitro* RF production by freshly explanted CLL lymphocytes; 2) continual secretion of RF by 17/24 human-human hybridomas derived from the CLL cells; 3) the presence of a major CRI on the RF light chains, that is shared by 70% of monoclonal human RFs. The CLL cells were used to generate a genomic library in the phage vector EMBL3. Kappa joining- and variable-region DNA probes permitted the isolation of a recombinant phage containing the single light chain gene rearrangement. Southern blotting revealed identity in restriction fragment size of the rearranged light chain gene in the patients B lymphocytes, the RF-secreting hybridomas, and the isolated recombinant clone. The cloned gene (and its sequence) will provide specific probes to enable: a) isolation of the corresponding germline V-region gene; b) delineation of the size of the gene family encoding RF-light chains; c) direct examination of genes utilized by RF in autoimmune disease.

3

THE ARTHROPATHY OF ADULT HUMAN PARVOVIRUS INFECTION. Anthony D. Woolf, +Diana G. White, °Philip P. Mortimer, °Bernard J. Cohen, David R. Blake and Paul A. Bacon. RNHRD Bath, +PHL Bath, °CPHL London, England.

Patients presenting in 1979/80 with early synovitis have been entered into a prospective clinical, serological and radiological study. All were first reviewed within 3 months of onset of joint symptoms, many within 2 weeks. Sera were examined for evidence of a variety of possible infective causes. These included human parvovirus (HPV)-specific IgM, IgG, and HPV antigen. HPV has been associated with erythema infectiosum (EI) which may be accompanied by arthropathy in adults.

HPV-specific IgM was found in 19 of 153 patients' sera, 12 with high levels, falling in the 11 available follow-up sera, with a rise in HPV-specific IgG in 9. HPV antigen was not detected. Other infective causes were identified in 6 additional cases. The 19 cases of HPV infection were all female, aged 18-58 years (median 38 years) and the arthropathy was characterised by an acute onset, symmetrical, peripheral polyarthritis, usually commencing in hands or knees. This became widespread within 1-2 days and improved within 1-2 weeks, but arthralgia and occasionally synovitis has persisted for 2 months to at least 5 years, median 6 months, either continuously (11 cases) or intermittently (6 cases). 13 patients described prodromal features, rash in 4 but only typical of EI in 1. Immune complexes by either ACA, C1q binding or platelet aggregation were detected at low levels in 9 cases and synovial biopsy in 1 case at 2 weeks was non-specific.

Thus, HPV arthropathy is a clinical entity distinct from that in adults with EI. It was a common identifiable cause of synovitis and can have a persistent but mild course.

4

REGULATION OF THE ALTERNATIVE PATHWAY OF T CELL ACTIVATION BY ANTI-T3 MONOCLONAL ANTIBODY. David A. Fox, Stuart F. Schlossman and Ellis L. Reinherz, Dana-Farber Cancer Inst., Harvard Medical School, Boston, MA.

Recent studies have delineated a novel, alternative pathway of human T cell activation that is mediated by triggering of the 50KD T11 sheep erythrocyte binding protein on the T cell surface. Monoclonal antibodies anti-$T11_2$ and anti-$T11_3$, directed at distinct epitopes of the T11 molecule, induce mature T cells to proliferate and to express their functional programs, in a manner independent of specific antigen or accessory cells. When thymocytes are stimulated by anti-T11 antibodies, interleukin 2 (IL-2) receptors are expressed on cells in both T3+ and T3- populations. In the present studies we have found that a non-mitogenic anti-T3 antibody, which binds to a component of the T3-Ti antigen/MHC receptor complex, blocks subsequent activation of both peripheral blood T cells and T3+ thymocytes via the T11 pathway. Although anti-T3 led to modulation of the T3 antigen from the T cell surface, neither expression of T11 nor the ability to expose the activation-related $T11_3$ epitope were affected. However, cells treated first with anti-T3 and subsequently cultured with anti-$T11_2$ and anti-$T11_3$ could not generate IL-2 receptors or produce optimal amounts of IL-2. In contrast, blockade or modulation of the T11 molecule by non-mitogenic anti-$T11_1$ antibodies did not inhibit subsequent activation of T cells via the T3-Ti antigen receptor complex. These results suggest that a regulatory interaction between antigen-triggered and antigen-unrelated pathways of T cell activation may be important during both thymic T cell ontogeny and activation of mature T cells. Given the central role of T lymphocytes in the pathogenesis of diseases such as rheumatoid arthritis, an understanding of pathways of T cell activation may lead to insights into the immunologic basis of such conditions.

5

LIVER HISTOLOGY IN RHEUMATOID ARTHRITIS BEFORE AND AFTER PROLONGED METHOTREXATE THERAPY. AP Koo, AH Mackenzie, RJ Tuthill, JR Leatherman, Cleveland Clinic Foundation, Cleveland, OH 44106, USA.

Methotrexate (MTX) therapy for rheumatoid arthritis (RA) has become widespread. A liver biopsy study of patients (pt) taking MTX for a longer duration was done to follow a prior study*. 107 pt (73 female, 34 male) with classical or definite RA underwent liver biopsy. 25 pt were biopsied prior to oral MTX therapy (pre-MTX). 82 biopsied pt had received MTX for a minimum of 2 years: mean dose 7.9 mg/week (range 2.5-12.5). mean total MTX dose 3092 mg (range 727-8400), and mean duration 91 months (range 27-202). 100 (93%) pt were RA stage II or more. 88% were seropositive, and 46% had ANA. MTX pt had significantly worse disease, but were of similar age. Most pt (72%) took MTX once weekly. BIOPSIES: The overall degree of fatty change, fibrosis, anisonucleosis, cell necrosis, and inflammatory activity were analyzed histologically, and assigned a final grade 1-4. FINDINGS: All pre-MTX pt received Grade 1 or 2, in addition to 77 (94%) pt on MTX. Four pt in MTX group received a Grade 3 (dose range 727-4752): mild bridging fibrosis (Grade 3) occurred in 4 (4.9%) pt on MTX. Grade 3 overall fibrosis was seen in only 1 pt; the rest had less. No pt received a Grade 4. There was no significant correlation between histopathology and age of pt, duration of RA, total amount of MTX, duration of MTX use, or maximum dose of MTX (mg/kg/week). CONCLUSION: This study revealed minimal histologic hepatotoxicity of MTX given for RA. The low weekly dose may minimize toxicity. The liver toxicity of MTX appears clinically acceptable even for very prolonged therapy.

*J Rheumatol, I (Suppl.1): 73, 1974.

6

FOOD-INDUCED (ALLERGIC) ARTHRITIS. I. RHEUMATOID ARTHRITIS EXACERBATED BY MILK. R. S. Panush, R. M. Stroud, E. M. Webster, L. P. Endo, J. Nauman. University of Florida and VAMC, Gainesville, FL 32610.

Suggestive, but largely unproven, observations have associated RA with environmental antigens, including foods. We studied a patient with RA in a prospective, blinded, controlled fashion to determine whether symptoms were associated with food sensitivities. This 52 year-old, white female, with 11 yrs of class I, stage I, active RA, had symptomatic exacerbations allegedly associated with meat, milk, and beans. We observed increased symptoms following an unblinded food challenge. She was then studied in our CRC. On her normal diet for 6 d, she averaged 30 min AM stiffness, 9 tender and 3 swollen joint scores, 87% subjective and 89% examiner assessments (100% = best possible). While fasting (3 d) or on Vivonex (2 d), we noted no AM stiffness, 1 tender and 0 swollen joint scores, and assessments of 100% ($p<0.05$ vs. normal diet). She was then nourished with Vivonex for 33 d without difficulty and challenged in a blinded fashion at meal times with lyophyllized foods in opaque capsules. 4 milk challenges (equivalent to $\geq$8 oz per meal) produced up to 30 min AM stiffness, 14 tender and 4 swollen joint scores, 85% subjective and 80% objective assessments ($p<0.05$ vs. fasting-Vivonex), peaking 24-48 hrs post-challenge. Placebo and other foods (lettuce and carrot) were without effect. Immunologic studies indicated both delayed and immediate cutaneous reactivity to milk, no ↑IgE anti-milk, marked ↑IgG4 anti-milk, milk antigen-containing CICs, and cellular milk sensitivity. These observations associate symptomatic exacerbation of RA with milk in this instance and suggest new insights as to the pathogenesis of inflammatory joint disease and its therapeutic control.

7

CHRYSIASIS: THE ROLE OF SUN EXPOSURE IN THE HYPERPIGMENTATION SECONDARY TO GOLD THERAPY. P.A. Leonard, Farhad Moatamed and John R. Ward. University of Utah, Salt Lake City, UT 84132

Chrysiasis is a striking pigmentation of the sun-exposed skin seen in patients receiving high doses of gold therapy. To investigate the role of sun exposure in chrysiasis, we studied the skin biopsies of non-sun exposed and sun exposed-skin in 3 groups of patients with rheumatoid arthritis: I) the chrysiasis group consisted of 4 patients with clinically apparent chrysiasis. (Total gold dose equals 4.8-24 grams). II) The "high dose control" group consisted of 3 patients without apparent skin pigmentation. (Total gold dose 4.4-5.9 grams). III) The "low dose control" group consisted of 3 patients without pigmentation. (Total gold dose 0.35-.550 grams). The mean melanin (MEL) score for each group (number of basal epithelial cells per high power field containing melanin) and the mean concentration of gold in the dermis (ng/mg of tissue) quantified by atomic absorption for each group in the sun exposed (EXP) and non-exposed (NON) are shown in the table below.

	EXP: Gp I	GP II	Gp III	NON: Gp I	Gp II	Gp III
MEL score	19.2	13.9	3.2	3.5	3.3	.7
Au ng/mg tissue	374.6	138.0	0	119.0	36.8	0

Tansmission electron microscopy showed electron-dense deposits in the macrophages (primarily melanophores) in the dermis. X-ray dispersive analysis identified these as gold. Our results suggest that the deposition of gold in the dermis stimulates melanin production and that the melanin itself may have an important role in the hyperpigmentation of chrysiasis. In addition, there appears to be a preferential uptake of gold induced by sun exposure.

8

LOW-DOSE CYTOTOXIC DRUG COMBINATION THERAPY IN INTRACTABLE RHEUMATOID ARTHRITIS: Butler, D., Tiliakos, N. Atlanta, Georgia.

The efficacy, in intractable RA, of a combination therapy of an alkylating and an antimetabolite agent with hydroxychloroquine (HCQ), was studied and compared to single cytotoxic agent, as well as, to conventional treatment. 18 patients with intractable RA were randomized in 3 therapeutic schemes over a 6-month period. A) Methotrexate 5mg/wk, cyclophosphamide 25mg/d, HCQ 400mg/d. B) MTX 10mg/wk. C) Continuation of the non-immunosuppressive remittive agents. As intractable was characterized the RA of ARA class III, associated with persistent activity unremitted by gold or D-pen. The joint counts and swellings, the AM stiffness, the physician and patient global assessments improved significantly, in 3-4 wks in groups A and B, and the grip strength in A. The erosive osseous changes recorticated radiographically in 4 out of 5 (gr. A), while new erosions appeared in gr. B and C. The sed. rates decreased by 10-20% in gr. B and by 80-100% in gr. A. In gr. A the hypergammaglobinemia and thrombocytosis decreased by 25% and the rheumatoid factors became negative in 2. Treatment interruption occurred in gr. A by preference (I) and stomatitis (I), and in gr. B by severe anorexia and wt loss (3). Severe rebound activity followed 1 month after the discontinuation of treatment (I) in gr.A. In conclusion, low-dose cytotoxic combined treatment was not only efficacious and associated with recortication of the erosions, but was also relatively free of serious adverse effects.

9

CLINICAL UTILITY OF ACOUSTIC ARTHROGRAPHY AND TENDONOGRAPHY. I. Jon Russell, M.D., Ph.D., The University of Texas Health Science Center at San Antonio, San Antonio, TX 78284.

Clinicians have long been aware of joint crepitance and tendon popping but there has been little systematic effort to document such "sounds" or to identify the anatomic basis for them. In the present study, a sensitive electronic stethoscope transducer with fidelity characteristics of ± 3 decibels in the 30-500 Hertz frequency range was secured to periarticular skin in a standardized manner. Sounds produced by flexion and extension of normal or rheumatic arthritic joints (acoustic arthrography) were recorded, stored in digital form, computer edited and printed graphically with an integrated system from Andries Tek, Inc., Austin, TX. Simultaneous video recording of joint motion allowed synchronization of mechanical and acoustic events. Flexion of rheumatoid knees (RA) exhibited higher (300 vs 150 Hertz) peak sound frequencies with approximately twice the sound intensity as did the knees of age and sex-matched normal (NL) controls. Similarly interesting differences were seen with shoulder, wrist and tendon (acoustic tendonography) motion. It is proposed that available instrumentation can accelerate the construction of a musculoskeletal acoustic database similar to that which required over 100 years to develop for cardiac and pulmonary ausculation.

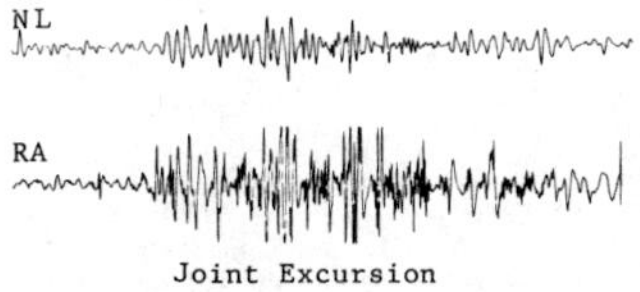

Joint Excursion

10

DANA TOTAL SHOULDER REPLACEMENT: 1-7 YEAR RESULTS. Harlan C. Amstutz, Riyaz Jinnah, Teresa Dalseth. UCLA, Los Angeles, CA 90024.

Between 1976 and 1984, 51 total shoulder replacements were performed at UCLA. The DANA shoulder replacement (formerly known as the UCLA total shoulder) was used in all patients. This system provides four sizes of humeral components with matching glenoid components. In addition, "hooded" glenoid components are available in patients with irreparable or absent rotator cuffs. The diagnosis for which this operation was performed was OA in 16; RA in 16; post trauma in 10; failed hemireplacement in 4; ON in 3; other in 2. Followup ranges from 6 months to 7 years (mean 28 mos.). Each patient was evaluated according to the UCLA 10 point joint replacement scale. All diagnostic categories had good pain relief with pain improving from 3.1 to 8.2. Function improved from 3.1 to 6.6 with 17 patients having a rating below 6. Flexion improved from 63° to 92°; abduction from 55° to 83° and external rotation from 19° to 40°. Eight patients had internal rotation contractures preop vs. none postop. Taking only the rheumatoid patients, pain improved from 2.6 to 8.2 and function from 2.8 to 6.1. Complications include 4 re-operations, 1 for removal of painful wires, 1 for a loose glenoid component with a fractured acromion and 2 for instability. Both the unstable shoulders were revised by a hooded component and are presently doing well.

These results show that total shoulder replacement provides excellent pain relief. Function and ROM were diagnosis-dependent with best results in OA and AVN. In the rheumatoid patient, where cuff pathology is common, the hooded component provides extra stability without undue restraint.

11

RADIOGRAPHIC FINDINGS AND EVALUATION OF SKELETAL CHANGES IN PATIENTS WITH RHEUMATOID ARTHRITIS TREATED WITH ETODOLAC AND ASPIRIN.
Alex Norman, Adam Greenspan. Hospital for Joint Diseases-Orthopedic Institute, New York, NY 10003; Ginette Jacob, Shawki Salem, Marie Sanda, and John F. Mullane. Ayerst Laboratories, New York, NY 10017.

It was reported that treatment with etodolac, a new nonsteroidal anti-inflammatory agent, has a potential to reverse the skeletal changes associated with Freund's adjuvant arthritis in rats. Based on this observation, a clinical study investigating the effect of etodolac on skeletal changes associated with rheumatoid arthritis was undertaken. In this double-blind, parallel group study, the skeletal changes were analyzed by evaluation of the pre-treatment and post-treatment radiographs of hands and wrists of patients with active rheumatoid arthritis. Of 178 patients included in this analysis, 99 received etodolac (mean dose 296 mg/day) and 79 received aspirin (mean dose 4.4 g/day) for a period of 6 to 12 months. The treatment groups were comparable in their demographics, RA history, concomitant use of disease modifying antirheumatic drugs, and length of treatment with the study drug. The results, based on the differences in the osseous defects (OD) and joint space narrowing (JSN) pre-treatment and post-treatment scores, indicate that the changes observed in the etodolac treated patients (mean change in OD 0.60 ± 0.35, JSN 0.37 ± 0.42) are significantly ($p < 0.01$) different from those seen in the aspirin treated group (OD 2.64 ± 0.61, JSN 2.38 ± 0.68). In conclusion, in comparison with aspirin treatment, etodolac therapy appears to retard the radiographic progression of rheumatoid arthritis.

12

IS LARGE BOWEL FUNCTION ALTERED IN RHEUMATOID ARTHRITIS?
P.J.Rooney, R.T.Jenkins, R.L.Goodacre, K.Smith, and G.Coates
From the Departments of Medicine, Pathology, Radiology and Nuclear Medicine, McMaster University, Hamilton, Ontario, Canada, L8N 3Z5.

^{51}Cr EDTA has been used as a probe of intestinal macro-molecular permeability. Increased urinary excretion of this probe has been demonstrated in patients with inflammatory large bowel disease.(IBD). That this occurs in the large bowel itself is suggested by our observations that rectal administration of ^{51}Cr EDTA in patients with IBD results in urinary excretion of approximately 40%/Day of the total dose. The normal excretion of an oral dose ranges from 2.65-2.59%/Day and this increases in patients with total or subtotal ulcerative colitis to a median value of 4.59%/Day. A similar increase in excretion of an oral dose of ^{51}Cr EDTA has been observed in rheumatoid arthritis (RA). This has been attributed to the use of non steroidal anti inflammatory drugs (NSAID's). This agrees with our observation that a two fold increase in bowel permeability occurs in normal subjects after 48 hrs. of naproxen 500 mg. bid po. This effect is lost 10 days after ingestion ceases. To investigate the possibility that this effect of NSAID's is due to their causation of large bowel inflammation 6 patient volunteers with classical or definite RA who had no symptoms of bowel abnormality and who were ingesting NSAID's were submitted to ^{111}Indium WBC scans of the abdomen. Of these patients 4/6 showed an increased uptake of ^{111}Indium over the caecum and ascending colon. Of these 4 patients, 3 underwent ^{51}Cr EDTA absorption studies within 48 hours. 2 were significantly elevated. It is not known whether the abnormalities on ^{111}Indium scanning and ^{51}Cr EDTA excretion reflect the same pathology nor if there is any morphological abnormality of the large bowel. Studies to answer these questions are under way.

13

SUPPRESSIVE STEROID TREATMENT OF TEMPORAL ARTERITIS.

L.A. Healey. The Mason Clinic, Seattle, WA 98111.

It is well recognized that temporal arteritis responds well to steroid treatment, but questions persist as to the appropriate dose and duration of treatment necessary to suppress the inflammation. Sixty-six patients with biopsy-proven temporal arteritis have been followed for 5 to 20 years (median 6.5 years). No patient treated with at least 50 mg of prednisone daily for 1 month had a subsequent flare of arteritis. This daily dose was gradually tapered. Rises in the erythrocyte sedimentation rate (to as high as 90 mm/hr) were occasionally noted in patients on low-dose maintenance therapy. These were not accompanied by symptoms, the steroid dose was not increased, and the sedimentation rates gradually returned to normal. On this steroid schedule, 2 patients developed osteoporosis and vertebral collapse, and 1 patient had avascular necrosis of both hips and one shoulder.

Some patients had a symptomatic response to smaller doses, but their course was not so predictable if the steroid dose were less than 50 mg daily or continued for a shorter period. Three patients treated with less steroid subsequently lost vision, and in two others, biopsy showed persistence of inflammation in the temporal artery.

Conclusion: Predisone in a dose of 50 mg daily for 1 month has proven to be effective in suppressing the inflammation of temporal arteritis. No patient so treated subsequently lost vision or had other symptoms of cranial arteritis. Late rises in the sedimentation rate, unaccompanied by symptoms, do not require steroid treatment.

14

PRIMARY ANGIITIS OF THE CENTRAL NERVOUS SYSTEM (PACNS); A REPORT OF SEVEN NEW CASES AND A PROPOSAL FOR DIAGNOSTIC CRITERIA. Mallek JA, Calabrese LH. Cleveland Clinic Foundation, Cleveland, Ohio 44106

PACNS is an infrequently reported and poorly understood disorder. Few large series have been reported and antemortem pathologic material has been infrequently obtained which may explain the lack of a unified clinical picture. We have identified seven new cases of PACNS and have combined them with 39 cases previously reported. Based upon these data we have proposed diagnostic criteria and have examined the results of therapy in the combined series. The requirement for a definite diagnosis is a positive pathologic specimen of CNS tissue or a characteristic angiogram. In addition, a number of conditions or circumstances must have been excluded including: evidence of vasculitis outside the CNS, diseases associated with systemic vasculitis, herpes zoster opthalmicus, or lymphoma. Arteriography was characteristic in 19 of 29 cases (six present series) for an overall sensitivity of 66%. A biopsy of CNS tissue was positive in 10 of 13 (two present series) for a sensitivity of 77%. The overall mortality was 61% in the combined series. In those patients receiving no treatment only 1 of 21 survived while in those treated with corticosteroids alone 5 of 15 survived. Combination therapy with corticosteroids and cytotoxic agents resulted in no deaths among these 10 patients although three were left with substantial neurologic impairment. Angiographic resolution was noted in one of our patients treated with combination therapy. It appears that prompt diagnosis and aggressive treatment has a favorable effect on the outcome in PACNS.

15

FACTOR VIII ANTIGEN IN TAKAYASU'S ARTERITIS (TA) J.E. Richardson, M. Grady, M. Glynn, E.C. Keystone. Department of Medicine, University of Toronto, Toronto, Canada.

TA is an inflammatory disorder affecting predominantly large elastic arteries, in which the adjacent endothelium may be affected causing cell injury. Endothelial cell damage results in release of factor VIII antigen (VIII:Ag) which may be reflected by an increased serum concentration of VIII:Ag. We measured VIII:Ag in the serum of 19 patients with TA and 15 normal controls.

The mean (±SD) VIII:Ag concentration was increased in TA (195±131%) versus controls (106±44%) with P<0.02. This elevation did not correlate with an increased ESR. The mean VIII:Ag concentration in patients with a normal ESR (231±172%) did not differ significantly from patients with an increased ESR (179±88%). Nine angiograms were done in 8 patients who had simultaneous serum VIII:Ag concentrations performed. In the 5 angiograms that demonstrated deterioration the mean VIII:Ag concentration was 295±147% and in 4 stable angiograms it was 84±31% this difference was significant (P<0.05). Serial VIII:Ag serum concentrations were performed in 7 patients in whom disease activity could be accurately assessed. In the 3 patients with persistently active disease VIII:Ag was elevated on initial measurement (360±85%) and remained elevated (400±140%). In the 4 patients whose disease became clinically quiescent VIII:Ag decreased (240±144% initially, 130±47% at follow-up), although this trend was not significant.

The data show that the serum factor VIII:Ag concentration is elevated in TA and that it may be a useful marker of progressive vessel involvement.

16

DIAGNOSTIC STRATEGIES IN POLYARTERITIS NODOSA (PAN): A DECISION ANALYTIC APPROACH. Daniel A. Albert and Marc D. Silverstein, Univ. Chicago, Chicago, IL 60637.

A strategy for diagnostic evaluation using a computer derived sequence of available tests based on their sensitivity and specificity (Arth. Rheum. 27 S87) was extended to include morbidity, mortality and dollar cost. The sequence of tests was ordered by accuracy and invasiveness. For individuals without clinically localizing findings, initial angiography is followed by testicular biopsy (for males), blind muscle and needle kidney biopsy. The sequence is preceded by muscle or nerve biopsy if a site is symptomatic. The strategy has a 90% sensitivity and 91% specificity for patients without localizing symptoms. For patients without a symptomatic site, at a prevalence of 50% and a male/female ratio of 9/1, the positive and negative predictive value of the strategy is approximately 90% with a cost of $5906 per case diagnosed. As prevalence decreases to 10% the positive predictive value decreases to 53% whereas the negative predictive value increases to 99%, and the cost per case diagnosed rises to $36,929. For patients with localizing muscle or nerve involvement the sensitivity is 96% and 97% respectively, and the specificity is 88%. The strategy improves with increasing sensitivity of angiography reaching sensitivity of 95% if angiography is 80% sensitive, and similar findings are noted for testicular biopsy. As the proportion of males declines the sensitivity of the strategy decreases without affecting specificity. The strategy is also affected by the specificity of angiography; thus "over-reading" angiographic abnormalities will lead to a false diagnosis of PAN in up to 1 in 5 tested patients if 10% of angiograms in patients without PAN are read as vasculitis. This is an effective diagnostic strategy, however it is sensitive to the accuracy of angiographic evaluation.

17

CRYOGLOBULINEMIA AND HEPATITIS B SURFACE MARKERS IN RAYNAUD'S DISEASE

Horowitz J., Klien, M., Sukenik, S. Beer-Sheva, Israel and Birmingham, Alabama, USA.

Twenty patients with Raynaud's disease were examined for cryoglobulins. Mixed IgG and IgM cryoglobulinemia was found in 11 patients (132 mg/l to 556 mg/l). One patient has monoclonal IgMκ and 10 patients had polyclonal cryoglobulinemia. Hepatitis B surface markers were found in the serum of 8 cryoglobulinemic patients (6 ab, and 2 ag). The cryoprecipitates of 10 of the 11 patients contained hepatitis B surface markers (8 ab, 2 ab and ag.). Although the clinical picture of both patients with and without cryoglobulinemia was identical, there were demographic and some laboratory differences between the groups. All patients with cryoglobulinemia were females and all but one was of North African origin. Six patients with cryoglobulinemia had elevated ESR, 9 had rheumatoid factor and 2 decreased serum C_3 and C_4. Of the 9 patients without cryoglobulinemia, 5 were males, none was of North African origin and none had abnormal laboratory values. During 5 years follow up only one of the cryoglobulinemic patients developed the typical clinical picture of mixed cryoglobulinemia. The other patients continued to exhibit only Raynaud's phenomenon. This study indicate that in populations with high prevalance of hepatitis B markers such as North African jews (prevalence of 4.5% ag and 42% ab) mixed cryoglobulinemia should be considered as an important etiologic factor of Raynaud's disease. In these patients cryoglobulinemia can present only as Raynaud's phenomenon without the other manifestations of this syndrome. This study, also adds further confirmation for the association between hepatitis B infection and essential mixed cryoglobulinemia.

18

TRANSDERMALLY ADMINISTERED PROSTAGLANDIN E_2 ANALOGUE, (CL 115, 347 - CYANAMID) FOR RAYNAUD'S PHENOMENON - A CONTROLLED, DOUBLE-BLIND TRIAL

Y.B.Kassam, E.M.Grace, W.F.Kean, W.W.Buchanan, P.Tugwell, G.Norman, W.S.Beattie, McMaster University, Hamilton, Ont. Canada, L8N 3Z5

The effectiveness of a prostaglandin E_2 analogue (PGE_2), CL 115, 347 (Cyanamid), administered transdermally, was evaluated in a 10 week double-blind placebo controlled study in 36 patients with Raynaud's including 32-idiopathic, 1-MCTD, 2-CREST and 1-Occupational. After 2 weeks of baseline measurements, eligible patients were randomised into the active treatment/placebo group for a period of 4 weeks with a post treatment follow-up of 4 weeks. The following variables were documented a) frequency, duration and severity of attacks from a daily diary, b) at each weekly visit, overall severity of Raynaud's was determined using 10 cm visual analog scales.

PGE_2 significantly shortened the duration of Raynaud's attacks, (P<0.02). Despite falling temperatures, PGE_2 group had less frequent and milder episodes. A cumulative score (using number of attacks, duration and severity) of changes from baseline was calculated. (range -9 to +9) (Table).

Study Week	3	4	5	6
Outside Temp (^{o}C)	3.8	-2.2	-5.4	-7.6
Placebo	1.38	1.52	0.94	2.4
Active	0.07	-1.6	-0.2	-0.06
P	NS	<0.025	NS	<0.025

Side effects were mild and infrequent except for local erythema (Active - 73%, Placebo - 12%)

These results show that PGE_2 ointment is effective, well tolerated and provides a non-invasive method of prostaglandin administration for the treatment of Raynaud's phenomenon.

19

C4 DEFICIENCY: C4 METABOLIC AND INHERITANCE STUDIES IN A KINDRED WITH AN UNUSUAL VARIANT (C4D-V). J.Wisnieski, M.Nathanson, G.Naff, CWRU, Cleve., OH 44106; A.E.Davis, C.A.Alper, Harvard Univ., Boston, MA 02115

We recently described a kindred with C4D-V. Unlike usual C4D, deficiency in this kindred was partial, was not caused by null genes at C4 loci, and showed no HLA linkage. C4D-V in 7/14 persons at risk in 2 generations suggested dominant transmission (JCI,74,1509,1984). We here report on the mechanism and inheritance of C4D-V in this kindred. C4a levels were assayed by RIA (Upjohn) and were normal in healthy C4D-V members. C4 metabolism was studied by IV injection of 5 μCi of ^{125}I-C4; EDTA plasma aliquots were collected for 7 days from 4 normal family and 3 healthy C4D-V members, 3 controls and 1 vasculitis patient. The % radioactivity remaining in each aliquot was measured, and C4 fractional catabolic rate (FCR) was calculated for each subject from a 3-exponential model of plasma radioactivity disappearance. C4 synthetic rate (SR) was calculated from the FCR, weight, plasma volume and C4 level. Extravascular/plasma (E/P) ratio was also determined. FCR and E/P were normal in all 3 test groups; however, SR was decreased in C4D-V members vs. normal members and controls ($p<.005$, t-test). Group means are shown.

	FCR (%/hr)	SR (mg/kg/hr)	E/P ratio
Controls (3)	2.1	0.23	0.60
Nl. members (4)	2.0	0.18	0.49
C4D-V members (3)	2.0	0.06	0.56
Vasculitis pt.	4.7	0.13	0.39

C4 was low (<10 mg/dl) in a previously untested member and in 2 of 4 third generation children. To date, 10/19 members at risk have C4D-V, (♂=6, ♀=4). In conclusion, C4D-V members of this kindred are hyposynthetic for C4, even though their genome contains intact C4 structural genes. Analysis of 3 generations shows autosomal dominant inheritance.

20

MAGNETIC RESONANCE IMAGING (MRI) AS A DIAGNOSTIC TOOL IN ISCHEMIC NECROSIS OF THE FEMORAL HEAD IN PATIENTS RECEIVING GLUCOCORTICOIDS (GC). K. Kalunian, B. Hahn, and L. Bassett. UCLA, Los Angeles, CA 90024.

Preliminary observations at our institution suggested that MRI had better sensitivity and specificity for ischemic necrosis of bone (INB) in femoral heads than did standard x-ray or scanning techniques. Therefore, 7 patients receiving GC therapy for various disorders who had recently developed new hip pain received a) standard radiographs of both hips, b) technetium diphosphonate (TcDP) bone scans, c) technetium sulfur colloid (TcSC) scans, and d) MRI of the pelvis and hips. Identical studies were performed in 5 patients with no history of GC therapy but recent onset of new hip pain.

In the patients receiving GC, INB was proven to exist in 8 of 14 femoral heads by a) Stage II or greater radiographic changes either initially or in follow-up, and/or b) INB on biopsy of the femoral head(s). There was no evidence of INB initially or on follow-up in the 10 control hips. In the 8 hips where INB was present, only 3 were associated with abnormal x-rays initially or on follow-up, 4 had positive TcDP scans, 1 had a positive TcSC scan, and all had positive MRI. In the 10 control hips, 2 had positive TcDP scans and all other tests including MRI were negative.

By chi square testing, MRI was significantly more sensitive than each of the other techniques at $p<.05$ or better. Overall, 10 of 32 observations using non-MRI techniques were positive for INB when it was present, versus 8 of 8 observations by MRI ($\chi^2=12.2$, p .02). In this small study, MRI seemed to be specific for INB. MRI was significantly more sensitive in GC treated patients than routine techniques in detecting INB of the femoral heads, including Stage I disease (6 of 8).

21

ENHANCED OXIDATIVE METABOLISM OF NEUTROPHILS IN PATIENTS WITH PROGRESSIVE SYSTEMIC SCLEROSIS (PSS). Peter J. Maddison, Christina Maslen, Anthony D. Woolf and Nicolas D. Hall. Bath, England.

Oxygen-derived free radicals released from phagocytic cells could be implicated in certain features of PSS including damage to vascular endothelium, depressed activity of serum protease inhibitors and increased frequency of chromosome breakage. Accordingly, oxidative metabolism, determined as hydrogen peroxide and HPETE production, has been assessed in neutrophils from 16 patients with PSS, 15 patients with RA, 8 patients with peripheral vascular disease and 16 healthy volunteers. Measurements were made on unstimulated cells and following incubation with heat-aggregated IgG (HAGG) or with the chemotactic peptide FMLP.

Unstimulated cells from PSS patients produced significantly more hydrogen peroxide than those of any other group ($p < 0.05$). Following stimulation with HAGG, neutrophils from PSS patients generated significantly more HPETE than the control groups ($p < 0.005$). In contrast, the response to FMLP was the same in all 4 groups. In view of these results, the expression of Fc (IgG) receptors on PSS and healthy neutrophils was determined by EA rosette formation. Cells from PSS patients showed significantly greater rosette formation than did controls due to increased number or avidity of Fc receptors. A strong correlation was found between Fc receptor expression and HPETE formation in response to HAGG (r=0.85, n=9).

These results suggest that peripheral blood neutrophils in PSS patients are in an activated state, secreting significant amounts of hydrogen peroxide. This could be an important factor in causing endothelial cell damage and subsequent vascular involvement in this disease.

22

Immune Complexes in Bronchoalveolar Lavage Fluid of Patients with Systemic Sclerosis (Scleroderma). R.M. Silver, J.F. Metcalf and E.C. LeRoy, Medical University of South Carolina, Charleston.

Analysis of bronchoalveolar lavage (BAL) fluid from patients with systemic sclerosis has revealed neutrophilic alveolitis and elevated IgG in approximately 50% of cases, similar to what has been found in idiopathic pulmonary fibrosis (IPF). Immune complexes (IC) are believed to play an important role in the pathogenesis of IPF. This study was undertaken to determine whether IC might play a role in the alveolitis of scleroderma lung disease. A solid phase Clq enzyme immunoassay was used to study IC in sera and BAL fluids. Sera were available on 23/24 patients and 32 healthy controls; BAL fluids were available on 21/24 patients and 7/32 healthy controls. IC were detected in the sera of 6/23 (26%) patients and 0/32 controls ($p < 0.01$). All six patients with serum IC had increased neutrophils (5/6) or lymphocytes (1/6) in BAL fluid. Of the 12 patients with a normal BAL cell differential, 0/12 had serum IC detected ($p < 0.02$). IC were detected in the BAL fluids of 13/21 (62%) patients and 1/7 (14%) controls. Patients with IC in BAL fluid had increased BAL inflammatory cells (7) or a normal BAL cell differential (6).

The presence of IC in over 50% of scleroderma BAL fluids suggests that IC may play a role in the pathogenesis of scleroderma lung disease. The concentration of IC in BAL fluid (ug AHGG equiv/mg albumin) was 35x that of scleroderma serum, suggesting that serum IC are selectively deposited in the lung or that IC formed in the lung may, in some cases, appear in the serum.

23

BRONCHOALVEOLAR LAVAGE (BAL) EOSINOPHILIA IN SCLERODERMA (PSS) LUNG DISEASE. R.R. Greene, D.R. Suarez, O.P. Sharma, M.M. Glovsky, D.A. Horwitz, and R.C. Kitridou. LAC/USC Med. Center, Los Angeles 90033.

Four of 16 patients with PSS had lavage eosinophilia (EO), 12.3±4.8, vs. 0.5±0.3 in the remaining 12. The 4 with EO had shorter disease duration (1.2±0.3 vs. 5.7±1.7) and greater disease activity by clinical and laboratory parameters: arthritis, 2/4 vs 4/12; tendinitis, 2/4 vs. 3/12; vascular lesions, 2/4 vs. 2/12; myositis, 1/4 vs. 1/12; low complement, 2/4 vs. 1/12; and elevated cryoglobulins, 4/4 vs. 6/11. An activity index, derived from the above clinical and laboratory parameters in addition to skin involvement, correlated with lavage EO (r=0.65). Patients with BAL EO tended to have more dyspnea and chest x-ray changes.

Studies of lavage fluid C3a and C4a in 7 patients failed to show evidence of complement activation.

In two patients with 6-12 month sequential studies, reduction in BAL EO accompanied increases in pulmonary function, while on methylprednisolone and D-penicillamine:

Patient	Eo%	Residual Vol.	DLCO
1 A	21	47	36
1 B	5	50	48
1 C	3	105	ND
1 D	18	56	ND
2 A	20	76	46
2 B	6	105	63

We suggest that alveolar eosinophils correlate with lung involvement and PSS activity in general, and may be pathogenetically important in PSS alveolitis. To date we have no evidence for complement participation in the genesis of the pulmonary lesion.

24

TOMOGRAPHIC THALLIUM-201 MYOCARDIAL PERFUSION SCINTIGRAMS AFTER MAXIMAL CORONARY ARTERY VASODILATION WITH INTRAVENOUS DIPYRIDAMOLE IN PRIMARY SCLERODERMA MYOCARDIAL DISEASE (PSMD). André Kahan, Bernard Amor, Charles J. Menkès, Jean Y. Devaux, Jean M. Foult, and Jean C. Roucayrol. Hôpital Cochin, 75674 Paris Cedex 14, France.

Recent studies using exercise and redistribution thallium scans have demonstrated abnormalities of myocardial perfusion in patients (pts) with progressive systemic sclerosis. To investigate the potential effects of vasodilator drugs on these perfusion defects, we studied 15 pts with PSMD with thallium-201 (Tl) myocardial single photon emission computed tomography at rest, and after intravenous dipyridamole (DPD, 0.14 mg/kg/min for 4 min). The left myocardium was divided into 9 segments. Tracer activity was visually graded in 5 steps (2 ; 1.5 ; 1 ; 0.5 ; 0 ; 2 = normal perfusion, 0 = no tracer activity) by 3 independent observers. Scores for each segment were averaged. Tl defects (D) were defined as mean scores of less than 1.5. After DPD, a variation greater than 0.5 in a given segment was interpreted as an improved or aggravated defect. At rest, all 15 pts had diffuse D ; 99 D were found in a total of 135 segments. After DPD, 43 D were improved, 48 unchanged, and 8 aggravated ; global defect score was improved in 8 pts, unchanged in 5, and worsened in 2. The DPD-induced aggravation in 8 D is consistent with irreversible damage of the myocardium. In contrast, the major observation in this study is the DPD-induced improvement in 43 defects. Eight of 9 pts had normal coronary arteriography.

We conclude that in PSMD thallium defects can be improved after coronary arteriolar vasodilation in approximately half of the cases. These findings suggest that some vasodilator drugs may be beneficial in the treatment of patients with PSMD.

25

INCREASED NOREPINEPHRINE TURNOVER IN RAYNAUD'S SYNDROME.

M Hooper, JJ Condemi, and JL Izzo, Jr. Univ. of Roch., Rochester, NY 14642.

We have evaluated the activity of the sympathetic nervous system in 13 patients with Raynaud's Syndrome (RS) (6 with 1°RS and 7 with RS 2° to SLE or scleroderma) who were compared to age and sex-matched controls. Under carefully controlled conditions, we measured basal catecholamines as well as the norepinephrine (NE) metabolites, dihydroxyphenyl glycol (DHPG) and NE-sulfate. We then performed steady state NE infusions in order to calculate the turnover rate of NE in RS and controls.

Basal plasma NE was elevated in 1°RS (441±113 vs. 219±16 pg/ml in controls, p<.05) but not in 2°RS (258±49 vs. 211±12 pg/ml in controls). Epinephrine (E) levels were identical among the groups, so these differences probably were not due to stress. The metabolic clearance rate of NE (rate of NE infusion ÷ steady state - basal plasma NE) was elevated in both 1°RS (92±17 vs. 51±5ml/min/kg, in p<0.05) and 2°RS (89±13 vs. 61±5ml/min/kg, controls p<0.05). The plasma appearance rate of NE (basal NE x NE metabolic clearance rate) was elevated in both groups of RS patients (35±11 vs. 13±1 ng/min/kg in controls, p<0.01). Levels of the intraneuronally (monoamine oxidase) derived metabolite DHPG were normal in 1°RS (1100±110), 2°RS (1160±142), and controls (1120±68 pg/ml). Levels of the extraneuronally derived metabolite, NE-S, were higher in 1°RS (1120±240) compared to 2°RS or controls (760±260 and 610±113 pg/ml, p<0.1) in keeping with the higher basal plasma NE concentrations and increased NE turnover in the 1°RS group.

Thus, 3 lines of indirect evidence (elevated basal plasma NE, NE-S levels, and NE appearance rate) support the conclusion that NE release and therefore sympathetic nervous activity are increased in RS. 1° RS appears to have the most exaggerated increase in NE turnover while 2°RS is intermediate between 1°RS and normals.

26

KETANSERIN RELIEVES BUT DOES NOT PREVENT COLD-INDUCED VASOCONSTRICTION IN PRIMARY RAYNAUD'S PHENOMENON.

J.R.Seibold and C.A.Terregino, UMDNJ-Rutgers Medical School, New Brunswick, NJ.

In a double-blind placebo crossover trial, we studied the influence of time of administration of intravenous(IV) ketanserin(K), a selective serotonin$_2$ receptor antagonist, on digital artery response to cold challenge in primary Raynaud's phenomenon(1°RP). 4 women, ages 23-28 with 7-18 yr histories of RP, no clinical evidence of connective tissue disease, Class I nailfold capillaroscopy, absent serum antinuclear and anticentromere antibodies and normal levels of plasma β-thromboglobulin and platelet factor 4, were monitored by serial digital strain gauge plethysmography during controlled cycles of hand warming and cooling.

Following 2cc of IV 0.9% saline, plethysmographic evidence of loss of digital flow occurred at finger temperature 27.5°C ± 3.7(N=8). IV K (10 mg), if administered prior to cold challenge, did not improve the ability to maintain digital flow during cold challenge nor alter the finger temperature at which loss of digital flow occurred(27.0°C ± 5.0, N=4). However, K administered at the time of loss of digital artery flow caused a prompt increase in digital flow and finger temperature in all 4 subjects.

The present data suggest that serotonin is an important element in maintenance of vasospasm in 1°RP but that other factors(? adrenergic) are involved in initiation of a RP episode. "Local fault" is hypothesized to represent the effect of intermittent local platelet activation. Mechanical interaction of platelets with constricted vasculature, altered platelet reactivity and/or vascular responsiveness to platelet-derived mediators at lower temperatures are possible participating factors.

27

NIFEDIPINE MAY BE HARMFUL IN THE TREATMENT OF RAYNAUD'S PHENOMENON SECONDARY TO SYSTEMIC SCLEROSIS - RESULTS OF A DOUBLE BLIND STUDY.

G. Lindsey, R.G. McCullough J. Seaman, R. Hawkins, J. Weil, and J. Steigerwald, Univ. Colorado Health Sci. Ctr., Denver CO

We have conducted a double-blind cross-over trial of nifedipine versus placebo for secondary Raynaud's among 18 of our scleroderma patients (pts.). Each was given placebo or nifedipine (20 mg t.i.d.) for four weeks and then crossed over after a one week wash-out period. The trial was conducted during the coldest months. Each pt. kept a daily diary recording the number, length and quality of each attack of Raynaud's. Serial whole hand plethysmography (measuring total volume change) with simultaneous mean blood pressure measurement was performed on each patient prior to the study and after each treatment period. These measurements allow us to determine blood flow as well as peripheral vascular resistance.

Five pts. noted a subjective clinical response while on nifedipine while 3 improved on the placebo. No patient reported an absolute cessation of Raynaud's attacks, nor did any patient report worsening. Four patients dropped out before completion of the study because of side effects (2 with unremitting headache, one with ankle edema and one with dizziness).

Objective measurement at 35°C and 25°C revealed a decrease in blood flow in 90% of patients on nifedipine when compared to controls or placebo (p=.01). Measurement of the resistance at these temperatures revealed an increase in resistance in > 95% of patients while on nifedipine when compared to controls or placebo, p < .01. Blood presure was essentially unchanged.

We conclude that nifedipine does not appear to be useful in the treatment of the Raynaud's phenomenon seen in scleroderma pts. and may indeed be harmful if the decreased peripheral blood flow and increased resistance were to be sustained.

28

THE PROGNOSTIC VALUE OF BLOOD EOSINOPHILIA AND ANTI-ssDNA ANTIBODIES IN LINEAR SCLERODERMA

V. Falanga, TA Medsger, Jr., and M. Reichlin, Departments of Dermatology and Medicine, University of Pittsburgh, Pittsburgh, PA, and Department of Medicine, University of Oklahoma, Oklahoma City, OK.

We evaluated 53 patients with linear scleroderma for the presence of ANAs, anti-ssDNA antibodies, hypergammaglobulinemia, rheumatoid factor, and blood eosinophilia (> 300 cells/mm^3). The disease was defined as inactive if no clinical progression had occurred for at least 6 months. The patients were separated into those with 1 linear lesion and those with 2 or more lesions. None of the patients have developed internal organ involvement in a follow up period of 2-14 years.

Blood eosinophilia was present in 50% of patients and was more common during active disease (p<0.05). Elevated IgG was present in 42% and rheumatoid factor in 25% of patients. Elevated IgG was more common in patients with impaired joint motion (p< 0.05). ANAs were present in 33% of patients using a mouse substrate and in 43% on Hep-2 cells. The nuclear immunofluorescence pattern was homogeneous in 55%, nucleolar in 35%, and fine speckled in 10%. High levels of anti-ssDNA antibodies were found to correlate with both disease activity (p< 0.05) and number of lesions (p< 0.05). Negative reactions with Crithidia substrate were observed in all patients. Discordance in the immunofluorescence patterns and the presence of anti-ssDNA antibodies suggests that at least 3 separate antibody systems are present in the sera of patients with linear scleroderma: ssDNA antibodies and ANAs with homogeneous and nucleolar pattern. We conclude that the presence of blood eosinophilia and the level of anti-ssDNA antibodies are useful tests in both the diagnosis and prognosis in patients with linear scleroderma.

29

TRANSMEMBRANE SIGNALLING BY THE T CELL ANTIGEN RECEPTOR.

John Imboden & John Stobo. Howard Hughes Medical Institute and University of California, San Francisco, Ca. 94143.

We have shown that the antigen receptor on the human T cell line, Jurkat, initiates activation by increasing cytoplasmic free calcium ($[Ca^{2+}]_i$). The ability of this cell-surface receptor to transmit a signal leading to lymphokine production is critically linked to its ability to increase $[Ca^{2+}]_i$. When extracellular Ca^{2+} is depleted to <60 nM with 10 mM EGTA, a monoclonal antibody to the antigen-receptor heterodimer still increases $[Ca^{2+}]_i$, demonstrating that the receptor causes release of Ca^{2+} from intracellular stores. In Jurkat cells loaded with ^{3}H-inositol, perturbation of the antigen receptor or its associated structures, T3, (but not other cell-surface determinants) generates significant increases in ^{3}H-inositol trisphosphate (IP_3) as well as the other ^{3}H-inositol phosphates. Purified IP_3 (0.1 to 1 uM) releases Ca^{2+} from saponin-permeabilized Jurkat cells, indicating that this compound can mobilize intracellular Ca^{2+} in Jurkat. Pretreatment of Jurkat with either cholera or pertussis toxin (toxins known to affect GTP-binding proteins) abolishes both receptor-mediated increases in IP_3 and in $[Ca^{2+}]_i$. These receptor functions are not blocked by either forskolin or 8 bromocyclic AMP and thus are not influenced by toxin-induced changes in cAMP. These results indicate that the T cell antigen receptor is linked to a phosphodiesterase that generates IP_3 from its parent phospholipid. In turn, IP_3 releases Ca^{2+} from intracellular stores and is responsible for the increase in $[Ca^{2+}]_i$ that initiates activation. The studies with toxins suggest that a GTP-binding protein couples the antigen receptor to this phosphodiesterase in a fashion analogous to the coupling of the beta-adrenergic receptor to adenylate cyclase by Gs.

30

INTERLEUKIN 2 (IL-2) UPREGULATES IL-2 RECEPTOR GENE TRANSCRIPTION

Joel M. Depper, Warren J. Leonard, Cynthia Drogula, Martin Krönke, Thomas A. Waldmann, and Warner C. Greene. NCI, NIH, Bethesda, MD.

The early rise and subsequent fall in IL-2 receptor number following lymphocyte activation suggests that IL-2 receptor expression contributes to the regulation of T lymphocyte immune responses. We now demonstrate that IL-2 alone may upregulate IL-2 receptor gene expression in cultured PHA lymphoblasts which have lost >90% of their surface receptors for IL-2. Purified Jurkat or recombinant IL-2 increased cell surface IL-2 receptors 2-5 fold as measured by the binding of radiolabeled anti-Tac antibody. Increased expression was maximal after 12 hours, and did not represent the mobilization of cryptic, preformed receptors to the cell surface, as it was inhibited by actinomycin D or cycloheximide. Moreover, maximal increases in both IL-2 receptor number and cell proliferation were mediated by IL-2 concentrations which selectively interact with the high affinity class of IL-2 receptors. Using an IL-2 receptor cDNA probe, IL-2 receptor mRNA levels were increased 7-fold after IL-2 incubation in Northern blotting experiments. IL-2 also induced increases in the levels of mRNA encoding the lymphocyte activation antigens c-myc and the transferrin receptor, but did not increase mRNA for the beta chain of the T cell antigen receptor. We performed nuclear transcription experiments to demonstrate that the increased mRNA accumulation did not reflect changes in RNA transport or processing. Nuclei isolated from IL-2 incubated cells demonstrated a 2-3 fold increase in IL-2 receptor gene transcription. Thus, IL-2 may regulate IL-2 dependent immune responses, at least in part, by affecting the transcription rate of the IL-2 receptor gene.

31

5-AZACYTIDINE DE-DIFFERENTIATES MATURE T CELLS. Bruce Richardson, Larry Kahn, E.J. Lovett and Jerry Hudson. University of Michigan, Ann Arbor, MI 48109.

Human thymocytes simultaneously express surface molecules identified by the monoclonal antibodies OKT6, OKT8, and OKT4. During maturation, thymocyte interactions with thymic stromal major histocompatability complex (MHC) determinants and thymic hormones result in thymocyte proliferation, suppression of T6 expression, and suppression of either the T4 or T8 determinants. Mature T cells leaving the thymus express either T4 or T8, and can recognize self MHC determinants but also require antigen (Ag) to induce proliferation. To study the role of DNA methylation in the regulation of these events, cloned human T4+ and T8+ tetanus toxoid (TT) reactive T cells were treated with 5-azacytidine (5-azaC), a nucleoside analog which inhibits methylation of newly synthesized DNA. Cloned T8+ TT reactive T cells treated with 5-azaC subsequently express T4 and T8, but not T6, and physically bind macrophages (MØ), but do not proliferate to MØ plus TT. In contrast, T4+ TT reactive T cells treated with 5-azaC remain T4+ T8- T6-, but acquire the ability to proliferate in response to Class II MHC determinants on autologous MØ without TT. Another inhibitor of DNA synthesis which does not affect DNA methylation, hydroxyurea, failed to induce these changes. These results demonstrate that 5-azaC induces T4 expression on T8+ cells and allows T4+ cells to proliferate to MØ without Ag. This indicates that expression of these altered phenotypes and functions, which are observed in thymocytes, may be suppressed by DNA methylation in mature T cells (NIADDKD 1R23AI21454-1).

32

DEVELOPMENT OF NOVEL MONOCLONAL ANTIBODIES AGAINST HUMAN IMMUNOREGULATORY T CELL SUBSETS. C. Morimoto, N.L. Letvin and S.F. Schlossman, Dana-Farber Cancer Institute and Harvard Medical School, Boston, MA 02115

To further dissect the heterogeneity of T cell subsets, we have developed two monoclonal antibodies, anti-2H4 and anti-4B4 which define the functionally unique human T cell subsets. Anti-2H4 antibody was reactive with approximately 42% of unfractionated T cells, 41% of T4+ inducer cells and 54% of T8+ cytotoxic/suppressor cells. This antibody subdivided peripheral blood T4+ cells into two functionally distinct populations. T4+2H4+ proliferates well to Con A stimulation, but poorly to soluble antigen stimulation and provides poor help to B cells for PWM-driven Ig synthesis. T4+2H4- subset proliferates poorly upon stimulation with Con A but well on exposure to soluble antigen and provides a good helper signal for PWM-driven Ig synthesis. Moreover, this antibody defines the subset of T4+ cells which is the inducer of T8 suppressor cells in a PWM Ig synthesis system. In contrast, anti-4B4 antibody defines the subset which proliferates well on exposure to soluble antigen and provides a good helper signal for PWM-driven Ig synthesis. Furthermore, phenotypic and functional studies suggest that anti-4B4 antibody defines the human helper inducer subset (T4+4B4+/H.I.) of lymphocytes which is the reciprocal of that defined by anti-2H4 (suppressor inducer subset, T4+2H4+/S.I.). Moreover, these antibodies are functionally distinct from those previously reported as TQ1 and Leu 8. These monoclonal antibodies should prove an important tool for dissection of the immune dysregulation seen in autoimmune diseases such as SLE.

33

HUMAN MONOCYTES AND U937 CELLS BEAR TWO DISTINCT Fc RECEPTORS FOR IgG (FcγR): EVIDENCE FROM AFFINITY PURIFICATION AND SUPPORT OF T-CELL MITOGENESIS. RJ Looney, GN Abraham, and CL Anderson. Univ. of Rochester, Rochester, NY 14642.

Despite observations that murine macrophages bear two or more FcγR, human monocytes and the human monocyte line (U937) are thought to bear only one FcγR, a 72 Kd sialoglycoprotein (p72) with high affinity (Ka = 10^8-10^9 M^{-1}) for human (h) IgG1 & IgG3 & for murine (m) IgG2a. Two lines of evidence suggest that these human mononuclear phagocytes bear a second type of FcγR. First, two molecules (p72 and p40) were specifically purified by ligand-affinity with Sepharose-hIgG from detergent lysates of ^{125}I-U937 & from most (4/5) ^{125}I-monocyte preparations (p72 always appeared as a strong band whereas p40 was variable and was absent in one monocyte preparation). Only p40 was recovered from Daudi cells, a human B cell line. A goat antibody raised against p72 and p40 of U937, after adsorption with Daudi, did not precipitate p40 from U937, suggesting that p40 of U937 and Daudi are similar. Second, stimulation of human T cell mitogenesis by an IgG2a anti-T3(OKT3) is mediated by monocytes from 100% of healthy people, whereas mitogenisis by mIgG1 anti-T3(Leu 4) is mediated by monocytes from 80% of normals (responders=R). About 20% of individuals (nonresponder=NR) show little or no mitogenesis with mIgG1 anti-T3. Mitomycin-treated U937 or Daudi added to monocyte-depleted lymphocytes mediated Leu 4 T cell mitogenesis but only U937 mediated OKT3 mitogenesis. Thus Daudi and U937 both bear p40 and mediate FcR activity which is missing from NR monocytes. Our working hypothesis is that U937 and R monocytes bear two types of FcγR, p72 and p40. The smaller receptor, p40, is altered or missing on NR monoctyes, but is present on Daudi cells.

34

INTERFERON-γ INDUCES THE EXPRESSION OF HLA-D REGION DETERMINANTS AND THE CAPACITY TO PRESENT ANTIGEN BY ENDOTHELIAL CELLS AND FIBROBLASTS. Thomas D. Geppert and Peter E. Lipsky. UTHSCD, Southwestern Medical School, Dallas, TX.

Endothelial cells (EC) and fibroblasts (FB) express class II major histocompatibility complex (MHC) encoded gene products (HLA-D) at inflammatory sites. It is felt that these normally HLA-D(-) cells are induced to express these determinants by gamma interferon (IFN-γ), a product of activated T cells. The ability of EC and FB to accomplish HLA-D restricted functions once induced by IFN-γ to express MHC antigens in vitro was therefore examined. HLA-D expression was assessed by staining with various specific monoclonal antibodies and analysis on the fluorescence activated cell sorter. IFN-γ induced HLA-DR expression on nearly 100% of each cell type at similar densities. Highly purified peripheral blood T4 cells were used as responders for functional analysis of HLA-D restricted activity. Neither control EC nor FB stimulated allogeneic T4 cell DNA synthesis. In contrast, both IFN-γ treated EC and FB stimulated the mixed lymphocyte reaction (MLR), although EC were markedly more effective. Moreover, IFN-γ stimulated but not control FB were capable of processing and presenting the soluble antigens tetanus toxoid and SK-SD to syngeneic T4 cells, albeit markedly less efficiently than monocytes. Antigen presentation by IFN-γ stimulated FB was blocked by monoclonal antibodies directed at HLA-DR determinants and required that the HLA-D region of the responding T cell and the IFN-γ stimulated FB be identical. These data suggest that both HLA-D (+) EC and FB found at inflamatory sites are capable of functioning as fully effective antigen presenting cells.

35

BINDING OF HUMAN RECOMBINANT INTERFERON GAMMA (rIFN) TO ITS RECEPTOR ON HUMAN MONOCYTES AND U937 AND HL60 CELL LINES. D.S. Finbloom, D. Hoover, Walter Reed Army Institute of Research, Washington, DC 20307 and L. Wahl, NIH, Bethesda, MD 20205

Interferon-gamma induces many effector functions in macrophages presumably through binding to cell surface receptors. This report demonstrates that IFN-gamma interacts with a specific receptor on human monocytes. rIFN (Genentech) was radioiodinated using Bolton-Hunter reagent to a specific activity of 203 Ci/mmol. ^{125}I-rIFN bound in a specific and saturable manner. Saturation of binding sites occurred at 10^{-9}M (300 U/ml); there were 4000 specific binding sites per cell for both monocytes and the cell lines. Highly purified lymphocyte-derived IFN-gamma and rIFN both competed for binding sites with ^{125}I-rIFN. Binding of the ligand reached maximal levels within 30min at 4^oC and 10min at 37^oC. The foward rate constant (k_1) at 4^oC was about $9 \times 10^5 M^{-1} sec^{-1}$ for each cell type studied. The dissociation rate constant (k_{-1}) (derived from data generated by measuring the loss of ^{125}I-rIFN from cells at 4^oC in the presence of excess unlabeled IFN) was about 1×10^{-4} sec^{-1} for each cell type. The K_a calculated from these constants was $9 \times 10^9 M^{-1}$. There was no inhibition of binding of the ^{125}I-rIFN by rIFN-alpha or rIFN-beta. 90% of the rIFN bound at 4^oC could be released into the media by exposure of cells to pH3 for 5min. SDS-PAGE analysis of acid-released rIFN revealed it to be monomeric. These studies demonstrate that rIFN binds in a specific and saturable manner and with high affinity to a receptor on human monocytes and monocytic cell lines. Neither rIFN-alpha nor rIFN-beta effectively competes for the binding site on these cells. There was no evidence for dimeric binding of the rIFN.

36

DENDRITIC CELLS IN RHEUMATOID SYNOVIAL FLUIDS. Nathan J. Zvaifler, Ralph M. Steinman, and Gilla Kaplan. UCSD, San Diego CA 92103, and Rockefeller University, New York NY 10021.

Blood dendritic cells (DC) are potent accessory cells for T cell replication. Synovial membrane contains stellate-appearing cells but DC have not been identified in joint effusions. Irradiated synovial fluid mononuclear cells (SFM) from RA patients stimulated mixed leukocyte reactions 3 to 5 times better than DC-enriched blood cells. Complement (C') lysis of macrophages treated with monoclonal antibodies increased rather than decreased SFM accessory function, while anti-DR treatment abrogated mitogenic capacity. A cocktail of anti-T, anti-B, anti-macrophage antibodies plus C' eliminates 85-95% of SFM but T-cell stimulation by the residual population increased 4-8 fold. 60-80% of the remaining viable cells are spiny, dendritic-appearing cells which stain for DR, DQ, and the 3Cbi receptor but not with monoclonal anti-macrophage antibodies (63D3, 3C10). Transmission electron microscopy of SFM show macrophages whose cytoplasm contains large endocytic vacuoles filled with cellular debris. In contrast, cells remaining after antibody cocktail plus C' resemble blood DC, i.e., an irregular nucleus rimmed with thick heterochromatin and a cytoplasm with many mitochondria, but few lysosomes or endocytic vacuoles. Birbeck granules were absent. At higher magnification the perinuclear zones showed a well-developed smooth reticulum made up of short tubular profiles with electron dense content, as seen in interdigitating cells and large bundles of intermediate filaments sweeping around the nucleus.

RA effusions contain 5-10 times more DC than blood. These cells may be important in perpetuating the joint inflammation characteristic of this disease.

37

IDIOTYPIC ANALYSIS OF HUMAN RHEUMATOID FACTORS (RF) BY ANTIBODIES TO SYNTHETIC HYPERVARIABLE-REGION PEPTIDES. Pojen P. Chen, Richard A. Houghten, Sherman Fong, Frank Jirik, Robert Goldfien, John H. Vaughan and Dennis A. Carson. Scripps Clinic and Research Foundation, La Jolla, CA 92037. Fernando Goni and Blas Frangione, New York University Medical Center, New York, NY 10016.

Previously, we induced anti-idiotypic antibodies against two synthetic peptides (PSH3 and PSL2) corresponding to the hypervariable regions (i.e. complementarity-determining regions, CDR) of human RF molecules. The antibodies to the second CDR of the RF-Sie light chain (anti-PSL2) reacted with light chains from 10 out of 12 monoclonal human IgM RFs. We have now analyzed five additional anti-idiotypic antibodies against peptides corresponding to the 3rd CDR of Sie light chain (PSL3), the 2nd and the 3rd CDRs of RF-Pom heavy chain (PPH2 and PPH3), and the 2nd and the 3rd CDRs of RF-Wol heavy chain (PWH2 and PWH3). As analyzed by Western blotting, both anti-PSL3 and anti-PSL2 reacted with 11 of 16 (70%) monoclonal IgM-RFs. In contrast, all five anti-idiotypes induced by the heavy chain-peptides reacted only with their corresponding proteins, i.e. Sie, Pom and Wol respectively. These results show that the majority of human RFs share two cross-reactive idiotypes (CRI), and that both CRI are on the light chains. Since the peptide-induced anti-idiotypes recognize mainly the primary structures (i.e. the amino acid sequences), they in essence identify phenotypic markers of the corresponding variable region genes. Thus, the majority of human IgM-RF probably employ only a single variable-region gene for light chains, but a large number of genes for heavy chains. The data suggest a central role for conserved light chains for the RF autoantibody activity.

38

ANTI-IDIOTYPIC ANTIBODIES DISTINGUISH RHEUMATOID FACTORS (RF) FROM PATIENTS WITH RHEUMATOID ARTHRITIS (RA) AND SEROPOSITIVE ADULTS. Sherman Fong, Timothy A. Gilbertson, Pojen P. Chen, Robert I. Fox, John H. Vaughan and Dennis A. Carson. Scripps Clinic and Research Foundation, La Jolla, CA 92037.

The structural features of RF autoantibodies from patients with RA, Primary Sjogren's Syndrome (1°SS) and normal elderly subjects were defined with two types of anti-idiotypic antibodies: 1) monoclonal antibody (MoAb) 17.109, prepared against intact IgM RF Sie, which recognizes a cross-reactive idiotype of the kappa light chains of monoclonal RFs, and 2) rabbit antibodies prepared against synthetic peptides corresponding to the 2nd and 3rd complementarity-determining regions (CDR) of Sie light chains. By inhibition studies, MoAb 17.109 reacted with only $4.6 \pm 5.9\%$ of serum IgM RF from RA patients, as opposed to $42.8 \pm 9.8\%$ of RF from 1°SS and $28\% \pm 8.5\%$ of RF from elderly subjects. By immunoblot analysis, antibodies against both the 2nd and 3rd CDR bound efficiently to every affinity-purified 17.109 idiotype positive serum Ig and RF paraproteins. Further characterization of affinity purified RF from RA patients revealed that they reacted strongly with antibodies to the 2nd CDR. These data show that serum RFs from elderly subjects and patients with 1°SS have structurally similar light chains to RF paraproteins, and most likely are the products of a single V-Kappa gene or gene family. By comparison, the RFs from RA patients are much more diverse, but probably derive from somatic variants of the same V-kappa gene(s). The factors that cause somatic diversification of light chains gene(s) may be crucial to the pathogenesis of seropositive RA.

39

SPECIFICITY ANALYSIS OF A MONOCLONAL ANTI-Sm ANTIBODY. David S. Pisetsky, Cynthia Klatt, and Michael O'Donnell. Durham VA Hospital, Durham, NC 27705.

MRL mice are unique among the murine models of systemic lupus erythematosus in their expression of antibodies to the Sm antigen. To investigate the mechanisms of this novel response, the specificity and idiotypic determinants of a monoclonal anti-Sm antibody were studied. 2G7 is an IgG2aK monoclonal product derived from fusion of MRL-lpr/lpr mouse spleen cells using the 653 myeloma line. Its specificity for Sm antigen was demonstrated using an ELISA with affinity-purified Sm as well as precipitation of radiolabeled RNAs. An anti-idiotypic antiserum was prepared in a rabbit and used to assess the presence of crossreactive 2G7 idiotypic determinants by direct and inhibition ELISAs. Interestingly, 2G7 demonstrated at least two idiotypic determinants, both of which were also expressed by monoclonal anti-DNA antibodies. Crossreactivity with an independently derived anti-Sm monoclonal was also found. To define the basis of this crossreactivity, 2G7 was tested for anti-DNA activity. By an ELISA with single-stranded DNA, 2G7 bound DNA with specificity for certain synthetic homopolymers by inhibition studies. The activity was present moreover in each one of a series of recloned 2G7 lines but was not present in two other monoclonal anti-Sm antibodies. These results suggest that polyspecificity of anti-DNA antibodies may extend to the Sm antigen, and that some anti-Sm antibodies arise from anti-DNA antibody families.

40

THE EXPRESSION IN SLE OF AN IDIOTYPE COMMON TO DNA-BINDING AND NON-BINDING MONOCLONAL ANTIBODIES PRODUCED BY NORMAL HUMAN LYMPHOID CELLS. Ewa Cairns, David A. Bell, University of Western Ontario, London, Ontario, Canada, N6A 3K7.

We previously reported on the production of monoclonal anti-DNA auto-antibodies derived from normal human tonsillar lymphoid cells, which in common with SLE bind to different nucleic acid antigens. We now report on studies designed to determine whether these normal anti-DNA autoantibodies also share idiotypes (id) with SLE anti-DNA antibodies.

Rabbit antiserum vs one normally derived monoclonal anti-DNA antibody (4.6.3) was used for id analysis, after absorption with pooled normal human IgM and IgG to render it specific for 4.6.3. id. Anti-4.6.3 recognized an antigen binding site region of the id since the binding of monoclonal 4.6.3. anti-DNA antibody to DNA could be inhibited with anti-id. Anti-4.6.3 also bound 7/22 (31.8%) other monoclonal anti-DNA antibodies from the same fusion, but it did not interfere with the antigen recognition by these antibodies. Anti-4.6.3 also bound 21/69 (30.4%) anti-DNA negative IgM and/or IgG-containing hybridoma supernatants. The common 4.6.3 id present on these normal monoclonal antibodies was also present in 18/23 (72%) SLE sera, and 4/25 (16%) of normal serum studied to date.

Therefore anti-DNA antibodies bind to nucleic acid antigens characteristic of SLE anti-DNA antibodies, and the id of these normal and SLE antibodies share common structural determinants. Such common cross-reactive idiotypes in SLE and normals imply common germ line Ig genes, and suggest that the difference between SLE and normals lies in the expression of these genes.

41

ANTI-IDIOTYPES (A-ID) DIRECTED AGAINST ANTI-DOUBLE STRANDED DNA (DS-DNA) IDIOTYPES IN SERA OF FAMILIES OF LUPUS PATIENTS. N.I. Abdou, R. Suenaga, M. Evans, and M. Aultman. Kansas Univ. Med. Ctr., Kansas City, KS 66103.

We have shown that spontaneous a-Id regulate anti-ds-DNA Id in lupus sera and are associated with disease remission (J Clin Invest 67:1297). We searched for a-Id in 39 unaffected family members of 8 lupus families. Controls were normals (n=15) without personal or family history of lupus. Serial dilutions of family members or normals sera were tested for binding to lupus anti-ds-DNA $F(ab')_2$ fragments (framework binding), to lupus non-anti-DNA $F(ab')_2$, using a sensitive Elisa assay. Blocking of the binding of anti-ds-DNA to DNA by the family members sera or normal sera (antigen binding site) were also tested. Antigen specificity of the binding was tested by using anti-tetanus toxoid (TT) obtained from the lupus patient. Compared to normal controls, family members sera of 6 families had significantly higher binding to $F(ab')_2$ anti-ds-DNA (2SD). The isotype of anti-Id was IgG. Majority of sera that bound to $F(ab')_2$ anti-DNA blocked the binding of the latter to ds-DNA. Within each family, the binding to $F(ab')_2$, anti-ds-DNA was higher than to $F(ab')_2$ non-anti-ds-DNA. Blocking of binding of the lupus patient anti-TT to TT by the family members sera was insignificant when compared to the blocking of anti-DNA binding to DNA. Anti-Id play a role in regulating levels of anti-DNA in family members. Whether the acquisition of anti-Id in families is dependent on environmental exposure or genetic make-up or both remains to be seen.

42

IN VITRO EXPRESSION OF NUCLEAR ANTIGENS ON MONOCYTE CELL SURFACES. Brian L. Kotzin, Ronald E. Arndt, R. Joseph Massoni, V. Michael Holers, and William P. Arend. VA Med Ctr and Univ of Colorado, Denver, CO 80220.

We reported recently that after normal human blood mononuclear leukocytes are cultured for 24 hours, a subpopulation of viable monocytes bear surface antigens recognized by several monoclonal anti-histone and anti-DNA antibodies. These monoclonal antibodies were used with indirect immunofluorescence and FACS analysis to further study the mechanism of in vitro expression of surface nuclear antigens.

The appearance of histone- and DNA-positive monocytes was inhibited by 0.25 ug/ml cycloheximide in the 24 hr culture ($38.7 \pm 3.2\%$ without cycloheximide vs $2.6 \pm 0.6\%$ with, N=7). Cycloheximide did not reduce the amount of nuclear material found in the 24 hr culture supernatants. To examine whether monocyte surface nuclear material was passively adsorbed, freshly isolated cells were incubated with 24 hr-old supernatants. Less than a 1% increase in nuclear antigen positive monocytes was detected (N=9). Monocytes cultured in media with <0.01 ng/ml bacterial lipopolysaccharide (LPS) failed to show a marked increase in cell surface nuclear antigens after 24 hr in culture. The addition of LPS led to a dose-dependent appearance of cell surface nuclear material ($30.1 \pm 1.9\%$ positive cells with 2 ng/ml LPS vs $7.2 \pm 1.8\%$ without, N=9). The effect of LPS on stimulating the appearance of nuclear antigens on the monocyte surface was not associated with higher levels of nuclear material in the cell supernatants.

In summary, the appearance of nuclear antigens on the monocyte cell surface during 24 hr culture requires protein synthesis and cell activation. The surface nuclear material appears not to be secondary to passive adsorption but may be endogenously synthesized and selectively placed on the cell surface. Monocytes activated in vivo may also express surface nuclear antigens, and be involved in the production or damage of specific antinuclear antibodies in autoimmune diseases.

43

GENETICALLY ENGINEERED MONOCLONAL ANTIBODIES. S.H.Pincus, C.E. Carmack, and J.R. Ward. University of Utah School of Medicine, Salt Lake City, UT 84132

The therapeutic potential of monoclonal antibodies may be limited by the development of immune complex disease in recipients. Using recombinant DNA techniques, it may be possible to construct antibodies that avoid immune complex formation and deposition, and at the same time retain the desired biological effects. The heavy-chain constant-region would be a logical place to start.

We have produced a series of monoclonal antibodies to the synthetic polypeptide antigen poly-(Tyr, Glu)-Ala--Lys, designated TGAL. One hybridoma, T17, secreting mu, kappa antibody was subjected to treatment with anti-mu antibody and complement. Variant cells were selected. One of these, called T17.2, secretes kappa chains but has lost the heavy chain genes. This cell served as the recipient for DNA mediated gene transfer. Recombinant DNA plasmids were constructed containing a cloned anti-TGAL heavy chain variable region gene, a murine mu gene, and the gene transfer vector pSV-neo. These were introduced into target cells with DEAE-dextran. Using the appropriate plasmids, as many as 60% of the transfected cells secreted anti-TGAL antibody. Thirteen cell lines with different rates of secretion of the reconstituted antibody were cloned. The antibody products have been characterized with regard to idiotype, fine specificity, and molecular weight. Relative rates of heavy and light chain production have been compared to copy number of inserted genes.

This experiment demonstrates the feasibility of attaching heavy chain constant region genes to hybridoma derived variable region genes, and obtaining the expression of appropriate antibodies.

44

MOLECULAR NATURE OF AUTOANTIBODY-REACTIVE T CELL MEMBRANE ACTIVATION ANTIGENS IN SYSTEMIC LUPUS ERYTHEMATOSUS. Seiji Minota, Barry Myones, and John B. Winfield. UNC, Chapel Hill, NC, 27514.

Anti-lymphocyte antibodies of various specificities appear to be fundamentally important with respect to T cell dysfunction in systemic lupus erythematosus (SLE). The present experiments were designed to provide information concerning the molecular nature of T cell activation determinants to which a novel type of autoantibody inhibiting antigen-induced T cell proliferation is directed. Nonidet P-40 lysates of unstimulated and mitogen-activated T cells were electrophoresed under reducing conditions on sodium dodecyl sulfate polyacrylamide gels and examined for IgG antibody reactivity following Western blotting using immunoperoxidase staining techniques. Excluding the ~60-65 kD IgG Fc receptor, 7 of 14 membrane glycoproteins, identified by binding to lentil lectin, exhibited specific staining with antibodies from a group of 15 patients with SLE. Of special interest were several ~50-55 kD proteins localized exclusively to activated T cells, which reacted widely with SLE sera inhibiting tetanus toxoid-induced T cell proliferation in vitro. While co-migrating with Tac, preliminary data from immunoprecipitation experiments suggest that these proteins were distinct from the interleukin-2 receptor. Two SLE antibody-reactive proteins (~70 kD and ~120 kD) were demonstrable on both resting and activated cells, and 3 (~80 kD, ~95 kD and ~105 kD) were demonstrable only on activated cells. Antibodies to Ia antigen were not detected.

These experiments identify several distinct T cell activation antigens reactive with IgG anti-lymphocyte antibodies in SLE. The most interesting ~50-55 kD molecules may be of functional relevence in antigen-induced T cell responses.

45

CATABOLIN SYNTHESIS BY OSTEOARTHRITIC (OA) PERIPHERAL BLOOD MONONUCLEAR CELLS (MNC): IN VIVO AND IN VITRO EFFECTS OF PIROXICAM. Jerome H. Herman and Evelyn V. Hess. University of Cincinnati Medical Center, Cincinnati, OH 45267.

Catabolins are products of monocyte/T-cell interaction and synovium which induce the synthesis and release of proteinases from chondrocytes. Their importance in the pathophysiology of OA is unknown. In the current study, catabolins were generated in 72 hr cultures of isopyknic gradient derived MNC of 12 OA patients both following a 72 hr NSAID washout and one month of 20 mg daily piroxicam. Matched controls were studied in parallel. MNC were cultured with and without PHA and a therapeutic level of piroxicam (5 μg/ml) or drug added post-culture to determine effect on catabolin activity. Catabolin was assessed by release of $^{35}SO_4$-labelled proteoglycans from cartilage.

Spontaneous catabolin release was detected more frequently in OA than control subjects (83 vs 50%). Quantity of label release was also significantly greater (9 ± 1.9% vs 3.4 ± 0.6%). Levels were higher in patients having moderate to severe (n=7, 13.7 ± 1.4% release) vs mild disease (n=5, 3.7 ± 1.8%). PHA enhanced catabolin synthesis in 75% of controls but in only 3 OA patients having mild disease. Lectin induced DNA synthesis was comparable in groups.

Oral piroxicam had no effect on catabolin production. However, drug used in vitro blocked spontaneously released activity in 90% of OA assays and had an inhibitory effect on both the synthesis and activity of PHA-induced catabolin. Thus increased spontaneous production of catabolin occurs in OA which correlates with extent of disease. Piroxicam can modulate its production and/or activity.

46

RUNNING AND OSTEOARTHRITIS: A CONTROLLED STUDY. N. Lane, D. Bloch, H. Jones, P. Wood, & J.F. Fries, Stanford University, Stanford, CA 94305

Thirty million Americans now run, a change that may influence the incidence and severity of osteoarthritis. Stanford Arthritis Center has begun a prospective, 5-year longitudinal controlled study. This report introduces the study design and presents initial cross-sectional data on runners and matched controls.

The "Over-50 Runners Club" provided access to enroll 550 running enthusiasts (9,983 average total miles) and the Lipid Research Project access to a 450 member community sample. Cases and controls were matched for age, sex, years of schooling, and occupation, but unselected for exercise, injuries, calcium intake, family history, and other variables. Forty-one runners and paired matched controls formed an intensive study group who underwent rheumatological examination, and x-rays of hands, spine and knees. CAT scan of L1 for bone mineralization was obtained in 40 subjects. Runners had more mineral content (130 vs 106) ($p < .01$) in L1. They also showed more apparent sclerosis and somewhat more spur formation in blindly-read weight-bearing knee and spine films, but not in hand films. Importantly, there were no significant differences in joint-space narrowing between runners and non-runners. Runners weighed less (146 vs 160 lbs.), reported better overall health, and had less disability. Both groups had similar family history of arthritis, calcium intake, and sports history. Because of the multiple comparisons involved, these findings suggest but do not prove a hypothesis that relates running to increased radiologically apparent sclerosis and new bone formation, but not to loss of cartilage, crepitation, pain, or dysfunction of the joints; e.g., clinical osteoarthritis. A prospective study is now in progress to confirm or deny this hypothesis.

47

ATLANTO-AXIAL (C1-C2) FACET JOINT OSTEOARTHRITIS (OA) WITH AND WITHOUT NON-REDUCIBLE ROTATIONAL HEAD TILT (NRRHT). J. T. Halla, Abilene, TX 79601; S. Fallahi, University of AL in Birmingham, 35294; and J. G. Hardin, University of South AL, Mobile, 36617.

OA of the C1-C2 facet joints has received little scientific attention and this study was designed to define its frequency and clinical expressions. Of 600 consecutive patients with OA, 16 (2.6%) had symptomatic C1-C2 facet joint involvement. Mean age of these 16 patients was 76.6 years and 13 were women; peripheral OA varied from monarticular to polyarticular and symptoms had been present from 6 months to 30 years. At the initial evaluation all but 1 complained of neck pain (severe in 3, moderate in 10 and mild in 2); occipital pain was interpreted as headache in 8 and 6 also had posterior auricular pain. All had audible crepitus on head rotation and 5 had palpable crepitus. All had suboccipital trigger points, usually more tender on the side of the greatest roentgenographic involvement. Head position was abnormal in 9 (NRRHT in 4 and reversible head tilt in 5) and all had limited rotation, usually to the side of greatest roentgenographic involvement. Routine cervical spine roentgenograms demonstrated mild to moderate subaxial OA in 9. Tomography showed C1-C2 facet joint OA with normal atlanto-occipital joints in all patients; C1-C2 OA was bilateral in 7; 6 had predominantly unilateral lateral mass collapse (LMC); and 6 had subluxations (lateral in 6; rotatory in 4), usually with LMC. NRRHT due to predominantly unilateral collapse of the C1-C2 lateral masses has been reported by us in patients with inflammatory arthropathies (ARTHRITIS RHEUM 25:1316-1324, 1982) (ARCH INTERN MED 143:471-474, 1983); apparently it may also result from OA. C1-C2 facet joint OA seems to be relatively common and may produce a clinical picture which differs from that of the subaxial disease.

48

BILATERAL HIP AND KNEE ARTHROPLASTY: LONG TERM RESULTS. J. David Grauer, M.D., Andrea Cracchiolo, III, M.D., Gerald A. M. Finerman, M.D. UCLA Medical Center, Division of Orthopaedic Surgery, Los Angeles, CA 90024

Twenty-five patients underwent bilateral hip and knee replacement in the ten year period from 1973 to 1982. Twenty-two patients were evaluated and the data recorded on the UCLA hip and knee forms. Index diagnosis was rheumatoid arthritis (14), juvenile rheumatoid arthritis (4), ankylosing spondylitis (2), and osteoarthritis (2). The age at surgery ranged from 16 to 81, with a mean of 53.

At mean 6.8 year follow-up (2.5-11.8 years), pain relief was obtained but functional results were disappointing. Based upon the UCLA rating scale of 1-10, with 1 being the worst and 10 the best score, pain improved from 3.8 to 8.4 (occasional and slight), function from 3.2 to 4.2 (independent, limited housework), and walking from 3.7 to 5.2 (one support, less than 2 blocks). Thirteen patients were walking further and using less walking supports, while nine patients were unchanged or worse. Ability to climb stairs and arise from a chair was only improved in six patients. Two patients ultimately underwent bilateral girdlestone procedures, two underwent knee arthrodesis, and an additional seven joints required revision. Other complications included femoral fracture (1), tibial fracture (1), wound infection (2), dislocation (1), nerve palsy (1), and trochanteric nonunion (1). Average hospital stay was 80 days per patient.

These results confirm that our major goal of pain relief was achieved, but functional improvement was limited. There were a significant number of complications in this patient population.

49

REITER'S SYNDROME AND THE ACQUIRED IMMUNE DEFICIENCY SYNDROME.
H. Fischer, G. Solomon, R. Enlow, R. Winchester. Hospital for Joint Diseases, New York, NY 10003

The profound but selective immune deficiency underlying the acquired immune deficiency syndrome (AIDS) affords an opportunity to evaluate whether the immunologic mechanisms in Reiter's Syndrome (RS) were dependent on the integrity of the immunoregulatory circuits that are compromised in the AIDS patient. Over a three year period 9 individuals were identified with RS and AIDS (5) or the AIDS related complex (4) (AIDSRC) of lymphadenopathy, weight loss, anergy and decreased helper cells. There were 7 male homosexuals, 1 female I.V. drug abuser and 1 male without known risk factors. All had an asymmetric polyarticular inflammatory arthritis. Other clinical features included HLA B27 positivity (6), enthesopathy (8), urethritis (6), conjunctivitis (6), sacroiliitis (6), chronic diarrhea (8) and post enteritic onset (2). In 4 patients (2 AIDS, 2 AIDSRC) the immune deficiency preceded RS by 5-18 months while in 5 patients (3 AIDS, 2 AIDSRC) RS preceded the immune deficiency by 1-34 months (17 years in 1 patient). No change in the characteristics of the arthritis was noted when AIDS or AIDSRC developed. Four patients had particularly severe and extensive disease. One patient with AIDSRC received Imuran and had an overall deterioration of health. Shortly after beginning Methotrexate (MTX) in two patients one developed fatal Pneumocystis and the other Kaposi's Sarcoma which regressed upon cessation of MTX. In summary, in RS occurring in AIDS the immune deficiency did not prevent or attenuate the arthritis. In some instances the arthritis proved particularly difficult to treat and immunosupressives were tried. These agents, however, should be used with extreme caution in patients with RS at risk for AIDS.

50

THE ONSET, EVOLUTION AND FINAL STAGES OF JUVENILE ANKYLOSING SPONDYLITIS (JAS) ARE DIFFERENT FROM THOSE OF ADULT ANKYLOSING SPONDYLITIS (AAS). Javier Jiménez and Gregorio Mintz, Hospital General, Centro Médico Nacional, México City. México.

We compared 22 patients with JAS (onset before 15 years) with 22 matched AAS (onset after 17 years) followed for 20 years. Both groups are comparable in male/female ratio and in B27+/- ratio. The differences found were: at onset, 55% of JAS had fever against 5% of AAS ($p < 0.001$), only 9% of JAS had clinical or radiographic sacroiliitis compared to 100% of AAS ($p < 0.001$), 32% of JAS had leukocytosis against 9% of AAS ($p < 0.05$), 95% of JAS had knee arthritis compared with 50% AAS ($p < 0.001$) and ankles were involved in 68% of JAS and 32% of AAS ($p < 0.03$). The evolution of disease was episodic in 91% of JAS and in 32% of AAS ($p < 0.001$) and the final radiological stage after 20 years of disease was: sacroiliitis only in 55% of JAS against 5% of AAS ($p < 0.001$) and "bamboo" spine or ankylosis of sacroiliac joints in 36% of JAS and 82 of AAS ($p < 0.001$). Uveitis, hip involvement or arthroplasty and invalidity are similar in both groups.

We conclude that JAS has more differences with AAS in onset, evolution of disease and late radiologic findings than has been heretofore recognized.

51

CROSS-REACTIVITY BETWEEN YERSINIA ENTEROCOLITICA AND HLA-B27 IN REACTIVE ARTHRITIS. D. H. KONO, M. OGASAWARA, H. PRINCE, M. S. PARK, A. TOIVANEN, AND D. T. Y. YU. UCLA, Los Angeles, CA 90024; American Red Cross, Los Angeles, CA 90006; University Turku, Turku, Finland.

Possible mimicry between bacteria and HLA-B27 has been identified with allo- and monoclonal anti-HLA-B27 antibodies. We used a different approach to assess this possibility. Monoclonal antibodies were generated against an arthritis-causing bacteria, *Yersinia enterocolitica* 0:3. One monoclonal antibody was found to cross-react with HLA-B27 positive lymphoblastoid cell lines using complement dependent microcytotoxicity. Testing of 53 cell lines and several mutated cell lines that had the loss of different HLA molecules showed that this antibody reacted primarily with all HLA-B27 and a few HLA-B7 cells. The anti-*Yersinia* reactivity could be decreased following absorption of the monoclonal antibody by HLA-B27 positive, but not HLA-B27 negative cell lines.

This antigenic mimicry would be of clinical significance if cross-reactive antibodies could also be detected in the sera of arthritis patients or in patients who have been infected with *Yersinia*. Three methods were used to test for anti-HLA-B27 antibodies in sera: 1) complement dependent microcytotoxicity, 2) FACS analysis, and 3) competitive inhibition to the binding of a radio-labelled anti-B27 monoclonal antibody. Sera from ankylosing spondylitis, Reiter's syndrome, and *Yersinia*-infected patients were tested. Multiple cell lines and peripheral blood cells were used. No anti-HLA-B27 antibodies could be detected.

In conclusion, cross-reactivity between HLA-B27 antigens and bacteria is a very likely possibility. However, it is unlikely for this to induce arthritis through an antibody-dependent reaction.

52

THE VALUE OF CT SCAN IN THE EVALUATION OF INFLAMMATORY BACK PAIN. G. S. Alarcón, G.V. Ball, W.D. Blackburn, J.J. Vitek, B.O. Barger, and R.T. Acton. University of Alabama at Birmingham, B'ham., AL. 35294

Early diagnosis of inflammatory back disease (IBD) is difficult. Neither the history, physical exam, conventional radiographs, nor radionucleide scanning of the sacroiliac (SI) joints, nor B27 typing can accurately predict the occurrence of sacroiliitis or IBD.

The purpose of the present work was to study in a systematic way individuals selected because of histories suggesting IBD. Twenty-three males (M) were identified and evaluated by questionnaire, physical examination, pelvic and lumbosacral spine radiographs, radionucleide scanning of the SI joints, CT of the lumbar spine and the SI joints, and B27 typing. Only one of the 23 patients studied had sacroiliitis as evidenced by conventional radiographs. Twenty of the 23 had CT abnormalities falling into the following categories: proliferative facet joints (PFJ): 7, bulging disc (BD): 15, spina bifida occulta (SB): 4, spondylolisthesis (SL): 1, and non-diagnostic SI joint abnormalities (ASI) (asymmetry, irregularity and haziness): 12.

In view of these findings we evaluated a group of 23 M without back pain who had been identified as controls (C) for our immunogenetics studies. They were comparable to the pts in age, occupation, lumbar spine mobility and B27 positivity. Only 3 had normal CT; the remaining 20 had CT abnormalities as follows: PFJ:13, BD: 11, SL 1, SB 1; ASI 11, and 1 each with spinal stenosis and spondylolysis. Our studies suggest that: 1) CT scanning of the lumbar spine and SI joints fails to distinguish between individuals with and without back pain. 2) The predictive value of an abnormal CT for either the development of a spondyloarthropathy or mechanical back pain remains to be determined.

53

SEVERE OCULAR DISEASE IN SYSTEMIC LUPUS ERYTHEMATOSUS: OCULAR AND SYSTEMIC MANIFESTATIONS. DA Jabs, GG Heiner, and MB Stevens. Johns Hopkins University, Baltimore, MD.

The major ophthalmic manifestations of systemic lupus erythematosus (SLE) are: 1) mucocutaneous involvement of the lids; 2) secondary Sjögren's syndrome; 3) retinopathy and; 4) optic neuropathy. Retinopathy, occurring in 3 to 28% of patients with SLE, is the most common manifestation and generally consists of cotton wool spots, with or without intraretinal hemorrhages, and microvascular abnormalities. A less common, but visually devastating, retinal vaso-occlusive disease has been described. At the Rheumatic Disease Unit of the Johns Hopkins Medical Institutions, we have seen 12 patients with either a severe vaso-occlusive retinopathy (9 patients) or an optic neuropathy (3 patients). The severe retinal vaso-occlusive lesions included arterial occlusion, extensive peripheral non-perfusion of the retina, secondary neovascularization, and vitreous hemorrhage. Visual outcome was often poor with 39% of the involved eyes having a final visual acuity of 20/200 or worse. Two systemic clinical features correlated with the presence of severe ocular disease. Nine of these 12 patients (75%) had central nervous system (CNS) lupus, compared to a prevalence of 40% in our overall patient population (p=0.02). Serositis, present in 7 of 12 patients (58%), was statistically more common in patients with severe ocular disease than in our overall population (11%, p=0.0001). The most common central nervous system lesion seen in patients with severe ocular disease was an organic brain syndrome. Retinal vasculitis in SLE should be considered a marker for CNS lupus in most instances and probably reflects the small vessel disease present in both the retina and CNS.

54

EVOKED POTENTIALS (EPs): A sensitive test for CNS-SLE. L.M.Billingsley, G.D.Yannakakis, M.B.Stevens. The Johns Hopkins University School of Medicine, Baltimore, Maryland 21205.

The diagnosis of central nervous system lupus (CNS-SLE) is primarily clinical since sensitive laboratory indices are lacking. It is our purpose here to determine the usefulness of evoked potentials (EPs) as an indicator of CNS involvement in SLE.

Fifteen patients with CNS-SLE were studied, 14 fulfilling ARA criteria for SLE, and the exception the only patient without multilevel neurologic disease who had recurrent transverse myelitis, ANA(+) and L.E. cells. Visual (V), auditory (A) and somato sensory (SS) EPs were performed in patients independent of neurologic assessments and were coded blindly before analysis. Laboratory studies showed:

Patients	EEG	CT	CSF	EPs
No. abnormal / No. studied	9/13	7/14	7/15	14/15
(% abnormal)	(69%)	(50%)	(47%)	(93%)

EP abnormalities included: A in 4/15 (27%), SS in 6/14 (43%) and V in 12/14 (86%). Both V and SS abnormalities occurred in 5; V and A, in 3. In 13 patients (87%) the neurologic lesion clinically correlated with EP abnormalities, but 5 patients had abnormal visual EPs without symptoms/signs. Of seven controls, minimally abnormal EPs were noted in 2 (A1;V1). In the single CNS-SLE patient with normal EPs initially, abnormal EPs (SS and V) were noted on repeat one month later.

These data support the usefulness of EPs as a sensitive measure of CNS involvement in SLE (more sensitive than conventional testing) with capability not only of detecting occult CNS lesions but also localizing anatomic pathways involved.

55

IMPROVED IDENTIFICATION OF FOCAL BRAIN LESIONS IN CEREBRAL LUPUS BY MAGNETIC RESONANCE IMAGING.

W. Joseph McCune, Anne M. MacGuire, Alex M. Aisen. University of Michigan, Ann Arbor, MI 48109.

We studied 28 acute neuropsychiatric events in 25 patients with > 4 ARA lupus criteria, employing a Diasonics 3.5 kilogauss magnetic resonance (MR) scanner. Events were classified as: Group 1: onset of focal deficits detectable on neurologic examination (9 patients), Group II: seizures (5 patients), Group III: exclusively nonlocalizing neurologic events (13 patients) including organic brain syndromes, psychosis, headaches, movement disorders. Focal abnormalities were detected in brain substance by MR in 8/9 (89%) Group I scans, 4/5 (80%) Group II scans, but only 1/13 Group III scans. Thus, compared with Group III, focal lesions were more common in Group I ($p<0.01$) and Group II ($p<0.05$). Patients with localized lesions or seizures were more likely to have focal abnormalities by MR (12/14 (86%) scans) than x-ray computerized tomography (3/8 (38%) scans ($p < 0.05$)).

MR showed predominately gray matter lesions in 4 patients, large predominately white matter lesions in 2 patients and single or multiple >1 cm white matter lesions in 5 patients. Gray matter lesions in two patients (seizure 1, aphasia 1), which were initially visible by MR but not CT, resolved on subsequent MR scans within 2 and 3 weeks.

Thus, MR showed good correlation with clinical findings of focal neurologic deficits or seizures, and was more sensitive than CT. Two "transient" gray matter lesions were identified, which may represent a distinct subset of localized brain lesions in lupus.

56

CEREBROSPINAL FLUID BETA$_2$-MICROGLOBULIN IN CENTRAL NERVOUS SYSTEM LUPUS ERYTHEMATOSUS.

Steven J. Golombek and Steven K. Magid. The Hospital for Special Surgery-Cornell University Medical College, New York, NY 10021.

Beta$_2$-microglobulin (B2m) is a low molecular weight protein found on the surface of lymphocytes and other cells. Elevated levels are seen in the serum and synovial fluid in SLE patients.

Fifty-six samples of cerebrospinal fluid (CSF) from 36 lupus patients and 14 samples from 14 patients without inflammatory neurologic diseases were retrospectively studied. There was a significant elevation of CSF B$_2$m in the 32 samples from patients with active CNS lupus (mean ±SE 2.60±0.29mg/L) as compared to both the 24 samples from those lupus patients without active CNS disease (1.20±0.18, $P<0.001$) and controls (1.01±0.35, $P<0.001$). Levels were elevated in 18/32(56%) samples from patients with CNS lupus, 3/24(12%) samples from patients without CNS lupus and 0/14 (0%) controls. There was only weak correlation of the CSF B2m level and either CSF pleocytosis ($r=0.46, P<0.05$) or protein concentration ($r=0.51, P<0.05$). No correlation was seen between the CSF B$_2$m level and either renal function or peripheral activity in the lupus patients. It is concluded that CSF B$_2$m levels are useful and specific in distinguishing patients with active disease from those without.

57

CORRELATION OF IDIOTYPE EXPRESSION WITH DISEASE ACTIVITY IN SYSTEMIC LUPUS ERYTHEMATOSUS.

Lucille P. Frank and Betty Diamond. Albert Einstein College of Medicine, Bronx, New York 10461.

Three murine monoclonal anti-idiotypic antibodies directed against different framework determinants on human anti-DNA antibodies were evaluated for their usefulness in determining activity of systemic lupus. Idiotype titers were measured by RIA in serum samples from over twenty patients who were examined over months to years encompassing periods of clinical exacerbation and remission. In over two-thirds of patients, titers of one or more of the idiotypes associated with anti-DNA antibodies were significantly elevated compared to normal controls even during periods of clinical remission. However, changes in expression of idiotype often correlated with clinical flares and remissions. In several cases titer of one or more idiotype provided a more consistent reflection of disease activity than anti-DNA or complement levels. Isoelectric focussing of serum samples in patients in whom idiotype titer correlates with clinical activity demonstrates that during periods of disease exacerbation there is a specific increase in idiotype expression in the cationic bands suggesting that charge is an important factor in anti-DNA activity.

These data suggest that determinations of idiotype expression may be a useful adjunct in assessing disease activity and may reflect alterations in immunologic regulation that are often not detected by measuring anti-DNA or complement levels.

58

LUPUS CRISIS: C3a desarg AND LIPOXYGENASE PRODUCTS APPEAR IN PLASMA.

H.M. Belmont, R. Ludewig, S. Kimmel, G. Weissmann and S. Abramson. NYU Medical Center, New York, NY

Complement is activated at sites of immune complex deposition in active SLE. To determine whether activated complement components are released into the circulation of such patients, we have measured C3a desarg (C3a) and C5a desarg (C5a) by radioimmunoassay. Mean C3a for ten normals was 101.3 ± 16.7 (ng/ml ±S.E.M.). Mean C3a for 9 patients with lupus crisis (group I; 3 or more organ systems involved) was 446.0 ± 61.4 ($p<0.0001$). In 22 moderately active SLE patients (group II; 1-2 organ involvement) plasma C3a was 164.0 ± 9.2, above control ($p<0.001$) but less than group I patients ($p<0.01$). Levels of total C3 (immunodiffusion) did not correlate with C3a. C5a levels in groups I and II were 2.9 ± 0.7 and 2.0 ± 0.4 ng/ml respectively, versus 1.4 ± 0.5 in normals (data did not attain significance). In group I patients there was a positive correlation between levels of C3a and C5a ($r=0.59$). Since platelets and neutrophils could be stimulated by circulating C3a/C5a, products of these cells were sought in patient plasma. Lipid material was extracted (chloroform:methanol and ether) and analyzed by reverse-phase HPLC. In plasma from 3 of 9 patients peaks absorbing at O.D. 235 nm were detected which co-eluted with standard 12-HETE. Two of these 3 plasmas also yielded material which co-eluted with reference 15-HETE. These peaks, probably monohydroxy acids derived from activated platelets and neutrophils respectively, were not detected in 10 normal and 7 febrile controls. We conclude not only that the elevation in plasma of C3a/C5a and the appearance of lipoxygenase products represent novel probes of the inflammatory process in SLE, but that serial measurements of C3a may prove useful in the clinical assessment of these patients.

59

A MODEL FOR IMMUNE COMPLEX DISEASE IN SLE: BIPARTITE Fc RECEPTOR AND COMPLEMENT-DEPENDENT DYSFUNCTION.

Robert P. Kimberly, New York, NY 10021; Nancy L. Meryhew, Ronald P. Messner and Olaf A. Runquist, Minneapolis, MN 55435.

Recent data have implicated both Fc receptor (FcR) and complement (C) mechanisms in the handling of immune complexes (IC). To explore the possible roles of FcR-mediated and C-dependent clearance mechanisms in SLE, we analyzed clearance rate data from 32 SLE pts and 49 controls for the four rate constants regulating mononuclear phagocyte system (MPS) clearance. We also constructed a model for the pathogenesis of IC disease utilizing these constants and concurrent data for circulating IC (CIC), C and anti-DNA antibodies. CIC were measured by Raji and Clq binding assays, C by total hemolytic complement, anti-DNA by the Farr technique and MPS function by clearance of opsonized RBC. Results indicate that:

1. Fc-mediated splenic clearance and C-associated hepatic phagocytosis were lower for all SLE ($p<.001$ and $p<.05$, respectively) with the largest defects in the active renal subgroup ($p<.0001$ and $p<.001$).
2. As predicted by the disease model, the correlation between disease activity and impaired Fc clearance was poor in normocomplementemic pts ($r=.025$; $p>.10$) but was high in hypocomplementemic pts ($r=.77$; $p<.001$).
3. As predicted by the model, with increasing [CIC] handled by Fc mechanisms (high [anti-DNA]/[CH50] ratio) and increasingly impaired Fc clearance, disease activity was higher; ie, the correlation of the product of the anti-DNA/CH50 ratio and Fc clearance with activity score gave an $r=0.86$, $p<.001$.

The model suggests a bipartite mechanism for handling immune complexes. Fc clearance, with a slower kinetic rate than C mechanisms, may be most important in the context of C-mediated dysfunction. Active renal disease occurs with dysfunction in both mechanisms.

60

FAMILIAL AGGREGATION (FA) OF SYSTEMIC LUPUS ERYTHEMATOSUS (SLE).

M.C.Hochberg, P.Florsheim, J.Scott, The Johns Hopkins Medical Institutions, Baltimore, and F.C.Arnett, University of Texas, Houston.

A genetic predisposition to SLE is supported by 1)familial occurrence in 10-12% of cases, 2)greater concordance in mono- than dizygotic twins, and 3)association with HLA-DR and other genetic markers. A case-control study was performed to determine whether SLE exhibits FA and what host/disease-related factors are associated with this phenomenon.

Seventy-seven patients with SLE and their age and race-matched 'associate' controls were interviewed. Detailed family pedigrees were constructed and the occurrence of SLE and 19 other autoimmune diseases (AID) in first-degree relatives (FDR) was determined. Medical records of persons reported to have SLE were reviewed to validate diagnosis.

Eight(10.4%) of the cases had a total of 9 FDR with SLE, while only 1(1.3%) of the controls had a single FDR with SLE ($RR=8, P=.0337$). The cases and controls had a total of 541 and 540 FDR, respectively. Thus, the prevalence of SLE in FDR of cases was 16.6 per 1000 compared to 1.8 per 1000 among FDR of controls.

Four(17.4%) of 23 black compared to 3(5.7%) of 52 white cases had affected FDR ($RR=3.4, P=.124$). Of 45 cases with age at diagnosis ≤ 30 years, 7(15.6%) had affected FDR compared to only 1(3.1%) of 32 with age ≥ 31 years ($RR=5.7, P=.08$). There were no associations of any HLA-DR or C4A phenotype with FA in either racial group.

There was no evidence of FA of other AID in SLE; 15 SLE cases had 21 FDR with other AID compared to 13 controls with 16 affected FDR.

These data confirm the occurrence of FA in SLE. In addition, they suggest that FA may be more common in blacks and among probands with age at diagnosis ≤ 30 years. Further studies are needed to identify other markers for the genetic predisposition in families with SLE.

61

THE INFLUENCE ON HEALING OF TREATMENT WITH ASPIRIN AND PREDNISONE VS ASPIRIN ALONE IN AN ANIMAL MODEL OF CORONARY ARTERITIS. Albert R. Katz, Vladamir Mahnovski, Thomas J. A. Lehman. Childrens Hospital of Los Angeles, California 90027.

Coronary arteritis and myocarditis which histologically resemble the lesions in Kawaskai's Disease were induced in 60 C57Bl/6 mice by intraperiotneal injection of Lactobacillus casei cell wall fragments. Beginning 3 weeks after injection 20 mice were treated with aspirin 100 mg/kg/day plus prednisone 2 mg/kg/day and 20 were treated with the aspirin alone; 20 control mice were untreated. All mice were sacrificed 8 weeks after injection.

Aspirin and prednisone treated mice exhibited more frequent, severe luminal narrowing of the coronary arteries (CA) (83% vs 57%; ≥ 50% narrowing), more frequent aneurysm formation (20% vs 10%), and more frequent thrombosis (20% vs 0%) than did aspirin only treated mice. These differences were accompanied by histologic differences in the healing process. Aspirin and prednisone treated mice exhibited smooth muscle hyperplasia in the CA media, marked intimal proliferation and focal areas of myocardial fibrosis and necrosis. Aspirin only treated mice exhibited less intimal proliferation, but marked fibrosis in both the media and adventitia without medial muscular hypertrophy, and no myocardial fibrosis or necrosis. Compared to the treated mice, the control group exhibited more frequent aneurysms and thrombosis, as well as more severe myocardial fibrosis and necrosis. These data support the present use of aspirin alone in preference to aspirin and prednisone for Kawasaki's Disease, but in our animal model neither treatment could be termed adequate since the fibrous scarring in the aspirin only group would be expected to result in CA stenosis and delayed myocardial infarction.

62

LYMPHOCYTE SUBSET ABNORMALITIES IN CHILDREN WITH ACTIVE JUVENILE RHEUMATOID ARTHRITIS (JRA). K.S. Barron, D.E. Lewis, E.J. Brewer, W.T. Shearer. Baylor College of Medicine, Houston, Texas 77030.

Previous studies have shown that the majority of patients with active JRA have cytotoxic anti-T cell antibodies. It has been postulated that these antibodies may be involved in the selective depletion of suppressor-inducer T cells. The present investigation was designed to determine if JRA patients did indeed have abnormalities in lymphocyte subset number as well as function. Lymphocytes from 12 children with active JRA and 7 normal controls were evaluated. We found that patients with active JRA can be divided into 2 subsets: those with normal numbers of B cells and those with increased number of B cells, both absolute number and %, as reflected by both B4 and Ia staining. Patients with elevated numbers of B cells also had decreased % of T3 cells (pan-T cells), however the absolute number was normal, reflecting the absolute lymphocytosis. In contrast to previous reports, the number and % of T4 (helper T cells) was normal in both JRA subsets, however the % of cells with both T4 and Leu8 antigens (found to be inducers of suppression) was significantly decreased in the subset of JRA patients with elevated B cells.

	% B4+*	% Ia+	% T3+	% T4+	% T4+,Leu8+	% T8+
JRA ↑ B (n=5)	30±4**	37±3**	40±2**	30±2	13±1**	18±2
JRA nl B (n=7)	6±2	22±3	52±4	34±3	23±4	25±2
Control (n=7)	5±1	15±4	52±4	36±3	26±4	24±2

* % positive ± SEM; ** p < .04 compared to JRA normal B and controls.

These data provide direct evidence for the contention that the T4+,Leu8+ subpopulation containing suppressor-inducer T cells is reduced in a subset of active JRA patients.

63

OUTCOME OF CHILDREN WITH POST-STREPTOCOCCAL REACTIVE DISEASE NOT TREATED WITH ANTIBIOTIC PROPHYLAXIS. Carmen L. De Cunto, Earl J. Brewer, Edward H. Giannini, Donald A. Person. Baylor College of Medicine, Texas Children's Hospital, Houston, TX 77030.

Patients with evidence of Group A Beta hemolytic streptococcal infection and articular disease who do not fulfill the modified Jones criteria for a diagnosis of acute rheumatic fever (ARF) have been termed post-streptococcal reactive arthritis/arthralgia (PSRA). We reviewed the outcome of 9 PSRA patients who were seen at our institution between 1978 and 1984. There were 5 girls and 4 boys with an average age of 9 yrs (range 4-17). Six children were white, 2 hispanic and 1 black. During the initial episode 4 had polyarthralgia, 3 polyarthritis, and 2 pauciarthritis. Large joints were involved in 9/9. Hand involvement was seen in 1/9, fever 4/9, and elevated ESR 6/9. The chest x-ray was normal in 8/8, 8/9 had a normal EKG, and 7/7 had a normal ECHO. A recent strep infection was documented as follows:

Patient	1	2	3	4	5	6	7	8	9	
ASO	+	+	+	-	-	+	+	+	+	
streptozyme	nd	+	nd	nd	nd	nd	+	+	+	(-)=nl or neg
anti-hyaluronidase	nd	+	+	-	-	+	+	+	nd	(+)=abnl or pos
anti-DNAase	+	+	+	nd	nd	+	+	+	+	(nd)=not done
throat culture	nd	-	nd	+	+	-	-	-	+	

All pts were treated with aspirin for short periods, and all received 10 days of penicillin. Following this, none were treated with prophylactic antibiotic therapy. After the initial episode, the children were followed for an average of 14 mo (range 6-27). One pt developed ARF with valvulitis 18 mo of the initial episode, 2 pts had recurrent episodes of arthritis and streptococcal infection without carditis and 1 pt had an isolated episode of arthritis within 4 mo.

In conclusion we have shown that some patients who have reactive arthritis/arthralgia with proven streptococcal infection, but who do not fulfil the Jones criteria for a diagnosis of ARF, can and do develop subsequent rheumatic heart disease or recurrent episodes of arthritis. These observations suggest that a larger, prospective study needs to be done to assess whether prophylactic antibiotic therapy should be prescribed for all PSRA patients.

64

LONG TERM FOLLOW-UP OF TOTAL HIP REPLACEMENT IN JUVENILE RHEUMATOID ARTHRITIS. Paul F. Lachiewicz, Bernie L. McCaskill, Allan E. Inglis, C. S. Ranawat and Byron D. Rosenstein. UNC School of Medicine, Chapel Hill, NC 27514

From 1971 to 1980, 45 patients with juvenile rheumatoid arthritis had 82 conventional total hip replacements (THR's) at the Hospital for Special Surgery and North Carolina Memorial Hospital (UNC - Chapel Hill). Thirty-four patients with 62 THR's returned for examination and radiographs. There were 27 females and 7 males. The average age at surgery was 26 years (range 14-49 years). Twenty-seven patients with 49 hips were 30 years of age or less at the time of the procedure. The average follow-up was 6 years (range 2-11), with 36 hips having 5 to 11 year follow-up. The hips were rated according to the HSS hip rating system. The clinical results were: 30 hips excellent, 19 good, 9 fair and 4 poor. There were no early or late deep infections. One patient developed severe heterotopic ossification with ankylosis of both hips postoperatively. Two patients have required revision: one for acetabular loosening six years postoperatively, and one for a broken stem ten years postoperatively. Radiographic review demonstrated progressive radiolucencies or migration of 25% of the acetabular components and 8% of the femoral components. The frequency of acetabular migration or progressive radiolucencies was related to the position of the component in the true acetabulum. These results represent a somewhat more optimistic view of conventional total hip replacement in young patients than other published reports. This is likely related to the lower average weight and decreased activity level of these patients with juvenile rheumatoid arthritis.

65

THE PROGNOSTIC SIGNIFICANCE OF ANTIBODIES DIRECTED AGAINST CARDIOLIPIN IN CHILDREN WITH SYSTEMIC LUPUS ERYTHEMATOSUS (SLE). Deborah K. McCurdy and Thomas J. A. Lehman. Childrens Hospital of Los Angeles, California, 90027.

Antibodies directed against cardiolipin (ACA) have been associated with thrombosis, thrombocytopenia, and cerebral vascular disease in adult patients with SLE. To determine whether ACA were of prognostic significance in children with SLE, we measured ACA by an ELISA technique in the initial serum specimen from 85 children with SLE. The medical records of these patients were reviewed for abnormalities of platelets, PT, PTT, and the presence of circulating anticoagulants; and clinical complications including thrombocytopenia, thrombosis, aseptic necrosis, CNS or renal disease, and patient outcome. Sera from 36/85 (42%) of the children contained ACA. Of the 36 patients with ACA 12 are dead, 9 have continuing active disease, 4 are in remission and 5 are lost to followup. In contrast of the 49 children with SLE who did not have ACA in their initial serum specimen 3 have died, 20 are in remission, 20 have continuing active disease and 6 are lost to followup ($p < .0001$). In addition to correlating with an unfavorable overall outcome ACA correlated with renal disease (nephrotic syndrome, renal failure, or nephritis) ($p < .02$), and an abnormal PTT ($p < .03$). However, there was no correlation with thrombocytopenia, bleeding diathesis, thrombotic episodes, aseptic necrosis, or CNS disease.

These findings suggest that ACA at the time of diagnosis identify a subset of children with SLE who are at increased risk of continuing active disease and a poor outcome, irrespective of the presence of renal or CNS disease.

66

AUTOIMMUNITY TO ARTICULAR ANTIGENS IN JUVENILE RHEUMATOID ARTHRITIS. CG Ragsdale, FC Garbrecht, SL Bowyer, RE Petty, PF Cirenza, and DB Sullivan Departments of Pediatrics, Ann Arbor, MI, and Vancouver, BC.

We studied 100 children with JRA, 46 controls and 25 patients with osteoarticular syndromes (OAS) to determine whether immune reactivity correlated with onset, course, or outcome.

Cell-mediated immunity to native type II collagen (NIIC) and proteoglycan monomer (PM) was measured by assaying for leukocyte inhibitory factor. Autoantibodies to NIIC and PM were measured using enzyme-linked immunosorbent assays. Results were analyzed using Fisher's exact test.

In the LIF assay, JRA patients were more reactive than controls to NIIC and PM, but their reactivity did not differ from that of patients with noninflammatory OAS. In the occurrence of antibodies to NIIC JRA patients differed from both controls and OAS patients. Antibodies to PM were found only in 2 JRA patients.

	NIIC		PM	
# Pos/n	CMI	ab	CMI	ab
Control	8/46	1/31	2/46	0/30
JRA	51/99+	23/86+	23/100*	2/64
OAS	18/25+	0/20	5/24	0/12

Different from control Pc*<0.05, +<0.001

In controls CMI to collagen was associated with HLA-DR4 positivity ($p<0.01$). CMI in JRA did not correlate with onset, course, outcome, ANA, RF, or HLA type. Humoral immunity to NIIC, however, was associated with the occurrence of erosive arthritis ($p<0.001$).

CMI to articular antigens may be of pathogenetic significance in arthritis but it is not associated with clinical or genetic factors in JRA. The presence of antibodies to NIIC may be of greater importance in signaling poor outcome in this disease.

67

NUCLEOLAR ANTI-HISTONES (H) ANTIBODIES (Ab) IN JUVENILE DERMATOMYOSITIS. Carlos M. Arroyave, Lauren M. Pachman, Kenneth C. Rich, Murray Passo, Jeffrey L. Kaine, Charles H. Spencer, Robert W. Nickeson, Jr. Northwestern University Medical School, Children's Memorial Hospital, Department of Pediatrics, Chicago; and Departments of Pediatrics, Indiana University Medical Center, Indianapolis; Washington University School of Medicine, St. Louis; Louisiana State University Medical Center, New Orleans; University of Oklahoma Health Science Center, Oklahoma City.

Ten positive antinuclear antibody (ANA) sera from JDMS patients obtained within 4 months of disease onset were examined by indirect immunofluorescence (IF), radial immunodiffusion, hemagglutination, and enzyme immunoassays for the specificity of the Ab. Antihistones Ab was identified by IF using HEp-2HCl washed slides and confirmed by histones reconstitution. No sera had Ab to Sm, RNP, SS-A, SS-B, DNA, and Scl 70. Seven of ten showed the presence of IgG, IgA-H, and three IgM-H antinuclear Ab. All patients with anti-H Ab were reconstituted with H2b and H3 and three with H2a; after reconstitution, the initial IF homogeneous-speckled pattern changed to speckled nucleolar in 5/7 H-positive sera. In vitro complement fixation with HEp-2-1 reconstituted slides and JDMS sera showed that C1q but not C3 and C4 fixed this immune complex. We concluded that JDMS sera with positive ANA has more than one Ab and the H Ab may account for a portion of the Abs, and immune complexes formed in the presence of JDMS-H sera fixed C1q only.

Supported in part by a grant from Illinois Capter of the Arthritis Foundation and the Marlene Apfelbaum Foundation.

68

Heterogeneous Composition of Highly Frequent Dw14 Specificities in Children With Seropositive Juvenile Rheumatoid Arthritis. Jorg Goronzy, Kornelia Weyand, and C. Garrison Fathman.

Seropositive juvenile arthritis (JRA) has been reported to be highly associated with the HLA-D type DR4. By cellular typing, a high proportion of the diseased children were heterozygous for Dw4 and Dw14 which is a rare combination in the normal population. To analyze the HLA-D region in patients with JRA, we generated alloreactive human T cell clones against a lymphoblastoid cell line of a JRA patient, which expressed the Dw4/Dw14 heterozygosity. The specificities of the clones were characterized on a panel of well defined homozygous typing lines. A group of clones, the specificities of which could be clearly assigned to Dw14, were tested on a series of JRA patients. Although the individual T cell clones seemed to be specific for Dw14, we found at least five different recognition patterns in the group of the JRA children. But all children tested, even if they were Dw14 negative by conventional typing, were seen by at least two of the Dw14 specific T cell clones. The antigenic sites recognized by different Dw14 reactive clones can be further differentiated by target inhibition studies. Only some of the clones can be blocked by monoclonal anti-DR antibodies.

We conclude that the MLR defined specificity Dw14 is a hetergeneous composition of different determinants. In HLA-D region molecules of children with seropositive JRA, the individual Dw14 determinants are not necessarily linked but are expressed in very high frequencies.

69

DIMINISHED EXPRESSION AND REARRANGEMENT OF T-CELL RECEPTOR GENES IN MRL/MP-LPR/LPR (lpr) MICE. Janet Evans, Jeffrey Frelinger, James Allison, Robert Eisenberg, and Philip Cohen. UNC, Chapel Hill, NC 27514 and UT, Smithville, TX 78957.

The hyperplastic cells which accumulate in lpr mice are of uncertain lineage. Because they may serve to stimulate autoreactive B cells, we examined their T-cell receptor gene configuration and their expression of T-cell receptors.

DNA from 2 and 5 month old lpr and MRL/Mp-+/+ (+/+) was digested with the restriction enzymes Eco RI, Bam HI, Pvu II, or Hind III, electrophoresed through 0.8% agarose, blotted onto nitrocellulose, and hybridized with p86T5, a probe for the J region of the T-cell receptor β chain. The lpr lymph node and spleen β chain DNA was in germline configuration, without additional bands. In +/+, by comparison, the germline bands were reduced in intensity, suggesting substantial polyclonal rearrangement.

T-cell receptor expression was determined by surface radioiodination, detergent lysis, immunoprecipitation with antiserum (8177) to the T-helper receptor, and resolution by diagonal SDS-PAGE. Receptor expression was markedly diminished in 5 month old lpr lymph node cells compared to young lpr and +/+ controls of both ages.

The data indicate that the hyperplastic cells in lpr lymphoid tissue are not monoclonal or oligoclonal T cells. Their T-cell receptor DNA appears to be mostly in germline configuration, but the data do not rule out some degree of polyclonal rearrangement. The dilution with age of receptor-positive cells also suggests that the infiltrating cells are not typical T-helper cells. Thus, their contribution, if any, to humoral autoimmunity is likely to involve a mechanism other than antigen-specific help.

70

T CELL CLONES FROM ATUOIMMUNE MICE HAVE DUAL REACTIVITY FOR SELF AND NUCLEIC ACID. M. Fischbach, D. Infante, and N. Talal. University of Texas Health Science Center and Audie Murphy V A Hospital, San Antonio Tx 78284.

We have prepared T cell clones from MRL/lpr and C57Bl/6/lpr mice, murine models of human systemic lupus erythematosus. Clones reactive with an autoantigen,polyriboadenylic acid(poly A), present on all messenger RNA, were obtained by culturing immunized T cells in a standard cyclic fashion using antigen stimulation followed by rest. Clones were obtained by limiting dilution selecting T cells from wells plated at<0.3 cells/well. All clones have been in culture for >8 mos. They display typical helper phenotype, but in addition possess the unusual lpr associated markers 14D10 and 9F3. Clones obtained from mice immunized with poly A had dual specificities, reacting to both antigen presenting cells(APC) as well as poly A. Stimulation indexes were 30 and 60 respectively. Both responses were inhibited by specific monoclonal anti-Ia antibodies. The reactivity to the APCs was due to surface Ia antigens. The use of recombinant inbred lines usggested that these antigens mapped to the I-A MHC subregion. There was no reactivity to xenoproteins from serum since these reactions occurred in synthetic serum free media. The nucleic acid response was specific for poly A. There was no reactivity to poly dA, double or single stranded RNA or DNA. Poly A polymers ranging in size from 2 to 276 adenine residues gave equal reactivity. Thus, the binding specificities are very similar to those for anti-poly A antibodies.

These studies demonstrate dual reactivity by a single T cell clone to both poly A and Ia antigens of APCs. They suggest a possible naturally occurring mechanism linking autologous recognition with poly A reactivity.

71

ANALYSIS OF AUTOREACTIVE T CELL LINES FROM MRL MICE. Philip L. Cohen, Rebecca Rapoport, Robert A. Eisenberg. University of North Carolina, Chapel Hill, NC 27514

In an effort to characterize further the role of T cells in the autoimmune disease of MRL/Mp-lpr/lpr (lpr) mice, continuous cell lines were established from spleen and lymph nodes using EL-4 lymphoma supernatants as a source of T cell growth factor(s). Five lines were derived from lpr spleen and lymph nodes, and an equal number from MRL/Mp-+/+ (+/+). All of the lines lost their alloreactivity after a short time in culture. Surprisingly, every line manifested marked proliferation in response to autologous irradiated spleen cells. This response was restricted to I-A^k, as it was blocked with monoclonal anti-I-A^k antibodies, and as B10.A(4R) accessory cells were stimulatory while B10.A(3R) were not. There was no difference in the degree of stimulation from lpr accessory cells compared to those from +/+ or other H-2^k mice. The T cell lines bore Thy 1, Ly 1, L3T4, and 7D4 (interleukin 2 receptor), but lacked Ly 2 and surface Ig. They proliferated in response to both conventional and recombinant DNA-derived interleukin 2. When co-cultured with Ia-identical B cells, the T cell lines provoked B cell division and antibody production. The latter was most marked when lpr B cells were used. The results indicate that lpr lymphoid tissue contains functional T cells reactive to autologous Ia molecules and capable of inducing B cell activation. Such cells may be of importance in inducing hypergammaglobulinemia and autoantibody production in these SLE mice.

72

T CELL ANTIGEN RECEPTOR STUDIES ON AUTOIMMUNE-PRONE MICE BEARING THE LPR GENE. Howard Dang and Norman Talal. University of Texas Health Science Center and Audie L. Murphy VA Hospital, San Antonio, Tx 78284.

Mice bearing the lpr gene locus spontaneously develop a lupus-like syndrome and massive lymphadenopathy. Moreover, T cells from these mice demonstrate an inability to respond to antigen in vitro when primed in vivo. The proliferation of an aberrant Lyt-1^+, L3T4^- T cell population is associated with the occurrence of autoimmunity and antigen unresponsiveness.

In order to define this aberrant T cell population, we have studied the nature of their antigen receptor. Using a monoclonal anti-allotypic T cell receptor antibody, KJ16, we have found that the KJ16 allotype is present on the same number of T cells from lpr mice when compared to their normal congenics (15-20% of the total T cell population). Biochemical studies of the lpr antigen receptor were performed by using diagonal sodium dodecylsulfate-polyacrylamide gel electrophoresis (SDS-PAGE) analysis of ^{125}I cell surface labeled T cells. Gels suggested that the α and β chains of the receptor from lpr T cells has a lighter molecular weight compared to the α and β chains from normal T cells. These results suggest that the T cell antigen receptor may be aberrant in lpr mice. This result could explain their inability to respond to antigen and to manifest normal immunologic reactivity.

73

ENHANCEMENT OF IgG ANTI-DS DNA RESPONSES BY ANTIGEN AND T CELL HELP IN MURINE LUPUS. D. Ando, E. Sercarz, and B. Hahn UCLA Los Angeles, CA 90024

T cell requirements for the hyperactive B cells of NZB/W mice to produce pathogenic DNA antibodies are controversial. For the first time direct measurements have been made of IgG anti-ds DNA antibody forming cells (D-AFC) and cellular interactions controlling them. B/W spleen cells were cultured in a modified Mishell-Dutton system and D-AFC were measured by the ELISPOT method. In old B/W females with nephritis mean ds D-AFC in whole spleen cultures was 89/culture. This response increased with added antigen: the mean ds D-AFC with 1ng/ml of ds DNA was 189 per culture(p<.01).In contrast old females without nephritis had a mean baseline response of 15/culture;the response did not change after addition of ds-DNA from 0.8ng to 100μg/ml.Purified B cells($3x10^6$) from mice with and without nephritis when added to nylon wool purified T cells($3x10^6$) from mice with nephritis showed an increase in ds D-AFC from 14 to 64/culture(p<.001).T cells from mice without nephritis did not augment D-AFC. Splenic T cells were subjected to cycles of cultures with DNA and irradiated antigen presenting cells to enhance DNA T helper populations. Addition of small numbers ($2x10^5$) of these cells to B cells($3x10^6$) showed an incremental increase in dsD-AFC from 59 to 115/culture(p<.001). There was no parallel increase in ssD-AFC. In summary D-AFC from nephritic mice were amplified by addition of antigen; D-AFC from non nephritic mice were not. There are T helper cell (Th) populations in the spleens of nephritic B/W mice which augment production of IgG antibodies to ds DNA. B cells from both nephritic and non nephritic mice were responsive to this Th. Cloning of these cells are in progress.

74

STUDIES OF AUTOIMMUNE B CELL DEFECTS IN CONTINUOUS DNP SPECIFIC B CELL LINES. Michael S. Brooks and Marlene Aldo-Benson. Indiana University, Indianapolis, IN 46223

Resistance to tolerance induction in autoimmune mice has been described, but it is unclear whether this is due to an inherent B cell defect or to abnormal regulation by T cells. We developed continuous cell lines of dinitrophenyl (DNP) specific B cells from BALB/c mice and from NZB X NZW F1 hybrid (BWF_1) mice which we used to study abnormalities in autoimmune B cells. These cell lines have less than 1% staining with anti thy 1.2, 0% cytotoxicity with anti thymocyte sera, and 0% esterase staining. Both BALB/c and BWF_1 cell cultures required the addition of supernatant from El-4 lymphoma (El-4 SUP) and irradiated rat thymus filler cells (FC) in order to produce an immune response upon stimulus with the antigen DNP-Ficoll. Thus, requirements for antigen stimulation in BWF_1 cells are similar to those of normal B cells. To study tolerance we incubated cell line B cells for 48 hrs with DNP conjugated to murine IgG_{2a} (DNP-MGG), removed the DNP-MGG and cultured the cells with DNP-Ficoll, El-4 SUP, & FC. BALB/c B cells were made tolerant, but BWF_1 cells were not tolerant.

Cell line	Plaque Forming Cells/10^6 Cells (± SE) DNP-MGG	DNP-Ficoll	P	% Suppression
BWF_1-41	159,708 (15,581)	71,983 (19,989)	-	0
BWF_1-21	98,296 (9,510)	106,536 (49,169)	.25	7.8
BALB/c-H_7	64,426 (15,500)	197,594 (32,442)	.05	67.4
BALB/c-C_9	8,412 (2,541)	86,380 (19,743)	.01	90.3

This data indicates that resistance to tolerance in BWF_1 mice is associated with an inherent defect in the B cells.

75

FUNCTIONAL STUDIES OF T-CELL SUBSETS OF THE LPR AUTOIMMUNE MOUSE. R. Budd, J.-C. Cerottini, H.R. MacDonald, Epalinges, Switzerland and J.-L. Davignon, S. Izui, Geneva, Switzerland.

The homozygous lpr mouse develops a thymus-dependent age-related autoimmune disease consisting of vasculitis, arthritis, and immune-complex glomerulonephritis, associated with a massive lymphadenopathy. Phenotypic analysis of adult lpr/lpr lymph nodes (LN) demonstrates accumulation of a dull Lyt-1+, Thy-1+ population which expresses neither Lyt-2 nor L3T4 (i.e. L2-4-). Previous functional studies have examined only the total lpr/lpr lymphoid population which includes Lyt-2+ and L3T4+ cells. Using a method of complement lysis with anti-Lyt-2 mAb, 31 M (IgM) and a new anti-L3T4 mAb, RL 172.4 (IgM), we have purified the L2-4- subset. This population comprises on average 80% of adult C57 lpr/lpr lymph node (LN) T cells. These cells are not actively cycling by Propidium Iodide staining which correlates with their lack of receptors for Interleukin-2 (IL-2) using PC61, a mAb to the mouse IL-2 receptor, and by an ^{3}H IL-2 binding assay. In limiting dilution analysis the L2-4- subset displays an antiallogeneic CTL-precursor frequency of only 1/36,086 compared to total lpr/lpr LN of 1/1012, an lpr/lpr Lyt-2+ enriched population of 1/145, and normal C57 LN of 1/194. IL-2 production with Con A + PMA by the L2-4- population was 1/20 that of total lpr/lpr LN population and 1/64 that of normal LN. Similarly, no interferon- production was detected by the L2-4- subset under these conditions. Thus, the major cell subset of the adult lpr/lpr LN appears to be a noncycling cell with very limited potential for antigenic stimulation or lymphokine production.

76

ABROGATION OF COLLAGEN ARTHRITIS AND MODULATION OF DELAYED TYPE HYPERSENSITIVITY (DTH) BY A TYPE II COLLAGEN REACTIVE T CELL LINE. Ernest Brahn and David E. Trentham. Harvard Medical School and Brigham and Women's Hospital, Boston, MA 02115.

Lymph node cells (LNC) were isolated from inbred Lou-MN rats that had been immunized 10 days earlier with type II collagen emulsified in incomplete Freund's adjuvant. These LNC were cultured with native type II collagen for 3 days. The antigen-responsive lymphoblasts were separated by discontinuous gradient centrifugation and selectively expanded by periodic stimulation with antigen plus irradiated syngeneic accessory cells. In thymidine incorporation assays, the line cells proliferated in response to native and denatured type II collagen but not to type I collagen, PPD, or ovalbumin. The passive transfer of line cells to naive recipients induced DTH, as measured by a radiometric ear index, but no IgG antibodies by ELISA to collagen.

Additional rats were injected intravenously with 2.5 to 10 x 10^7 line cells 2 weeks prior to immunization with type II collagen. None of 5 recipient rats developed arthritis compared to 7 of 10 controls that were immunized without prior cell transfer (p<0.05). Four weeks after immunization, the cell line recipients had significantly lower DTH to collagen (1.6±0.2 vs 3.1±0.5, respectively, p<0.02). Serum IgG antibody titers to collagen, as determined immediately prior to the expected onset of arthritis (9 days post immunization), were similar in both groups ($-\log_2$ 10.0±0 vs 9.7±0.7, respectively). These findings demonstrate protection from arthritis afforded by T cell line transfer and suggest that the phenomenon results from down-regulation of the recipients' cellular immunity to collagen.

77

LYMPHOKINE-ENHANCED NEUTROPHIL (PMN) ACTIVATION BY COMPLEMENT. Kwan, L., Weisbart, R.H., Chan G., Gasson, J., & Golde, D.W. VAMC, Sepulveda, CA 91343, and UCLA, Los Angeles, CA 90024.

Complement attracts neutrophils to sites of tissue injury and initiates neutrophil oxidative metabolism. Our laboratory recently showed that a single 22,000 M.W. T-cell-derived lymphokine in natural and recombinant form induced precursor cells to differentiate to neutrophils and macrophages (colony-stimulating activity, or GM-CSF), inhibited the motility of mature neutrophils (NIF-T activity), and primed neutrophils for activation of oxidative metabolism in response to the bacterial chemoattractant, f-MLP (NAF activity). In the present study, we determined whether the lymphokine (GM-CSF) also regulated neutrophil oxidative metabolism in response to serum complement. Superoxide anion production was measured as superoxide dismutase-inhibitable cytochrome C reduction. In six separate experiments natural GM-CSF produced by a human T lymphoblast cell line increased superoxide anion production in response to zymosan-treated serum (activated complement) from an average (mean±SEM) of 10±2 nmol-/min/10^6PMN to 24±4 nmol/min/10^6PMN measured over 1 minute. In ten separate experiments, recombinant GM-CSF increased superoxide anion production in response to complement from an average of 18±2 nmol-/min/10^6PMN to 34±2 nmol/min/10^6PMN measured over 1 minute. In contrast, GM-CSF did not enhance oxidative metabolism of neutrophils in response to zymosan alone or phorbol myristate acetate (PMA). These results suggest that GM-CSF may be a natural regulator of neutrophil inflammatory responses induced by serum complement. This finding may be of pathophysiologic significance in some immune-mediated inflammatory diseases.

78

A NEW FUNCTION FOR ADENOSINE: PROTECTION OF VASCULAR ENDOTHELIAL CELLS AGAINST NEUTROPHIL MEDIATED INJURY. BN Cronstein, RI Levin, J Belanoff, G Weissmann and R Hirschhorn. Dept. of Medicine, New York University Medical Center, NY, NY.

Stimulated neutrophils (PMN) generate oxygen metabolites which are toxic to endothelial cells (EC) in vitro. Adenosine and its analogues, acting at specific receptors on PMN inhibit release of these toxic oxygen species. To determine whether adenosine prevents damage to EC induced by PMN, we studied the effects of 2-chloroadenosine (ClAdo), a poorly metabolized but potent adenosine analogue, on two measures of EC viability: % adherent cells and ^{51}Cr release after incubation for 90 minutes with PMN stimulated with the chemoattractant F-Met-Leu-Phe. Whereas unstimulated PMN did not alter the percentage of EC adherent after incubation, stimulated PMN decreased the percentage of adherent cells by 29±8% (S.D., n=3, p<0.03 vs. unstimulated PMN). The loss of adherent cells was not due to detachment of EC since no EC appeared in the supernatant medium. Addition of ClAdo (10uM) before stimulation of PMN resulted in a 79% inhibition of EC loss induced by PMN (6% vs. 29%). Activated PMN caused a three-fold increase in release of ^{51}Cr from EC (46±15% vs. 14±3% release, stimulated vs. unstimulated PMN, respectively, p<0.02, n=3). ClAdo (10uM) also almost completely abolished the increased ^{51}Cr release caused by stimulated PMN reducing it to 19±6% (p<0.04 vs. stimulated PMN). The data indicate that engagement of adenosine receptors prevents cell death caused by activated PMN in this in vitro model of acute vascular damage. Thus, adenosine, which is specifically released by damaged vascular cells, is a potent anti-inflammatory agent which protects vascular endothelium from further damage by the formed elements of the blood.

79

LOW DENSITY LIPOPROTEIN (LDL) MAY MODULATE INFLAMMATION BY HINDRANCE OF CELLULAR INTERACTION WITH PARTICULATES. R. Terkeltaub, J. Martin, L. Curtiss, M. Ginsberg. Scripps Clinic, La Jolla, CA 92037

We recently observed that LDL is a major inhibitor of neutrophil (PMN) oxidative and lytic responses to urate crystals (UC). The level of LDL in synovial fluid is highly variable and could thus regulate PMN inflammatory responses. We have therefore defined LDL's mechanism of action. LDL (40μg/ml) markedly inhibited PMN chemiluminescence (CL) induced by UC and latex beads (LB) but not by aggregated IgG or soluble agents including phorbol esters. LDL binding to UC, but not to LB, was greatly reduced by extensive acetylation of apolipoprotein B lysine residues. Acetylated LDL lost inhibitory activity for UC-induced CL but retained its effect on LB-induced CL. Thus LDL must be bound to a surface to express this activity. LDL effects were not cell-specific. LDL profoundly suppressed the platelet secretory response to silica and UC in a stimulus-specific manner. As LDL also progressively abrogated apparent PMN phagocytosis of UC we hypothesized interference with initial crystal-cell association by LDL. To test this, we measured LDL effects on early physical platelet-UC interaction using a differential low speed centrifugation assay under nonlytic, nonaggregating incubation conditions (4°C,5mM EDTA). Up to 97% of the cells sedimented (30xg, 5 min) in the presence of UC; only 35.2% in their absence. LDL blunted platelet-UC association and was 10-100 fold more inhibitory than acetylated LDL or lipoprotein-depleted plasma. These data suggest that the binding of LDL to particulates renders them less capable of stimulating phagocytic and secretory cells. Variability in concentration of intrasynovial LDL may help to explain differences in opsonic capacity of inflammatory joint fluids for certain particulates.

80

ACQUISITION OF STIMULUS RESPONSE COUPLING OF GRANULOCYTES AT A DEFINED STAGE OF MATURATION. J. Buyon, S. Seremetis, V. Sloan and R. Winchester. Hospital for Joint Diseases, New York, NY 10003.

The maturational stage at which cells of the granulocyte lineage acquire the ability to generate a respiratory burst and degranulate in response to various stimuli was studied by fractionating peripheral blood from patients with chronic myelogenous leukemia or blood from normal bone marrow on a Percoll gradient. The phenotypes of the cells in fractions of different densities were characterized by Wright's stained cytocentrifuged preparations and by monoclonal antibodies to Ia antigens (DR and DQ), U_{26} (GP120) and PMN_1 antigen. Cytochalasin B treated cells were evaluated for superoxide anion generation (O_2-) in response to stimulation by FMLP (10^{-7}M) or PMA (1ug/ml) and betaglucuronidase release in response to FMLP. Analysis of the low density fractions primarily consisting of blasts and promyelocytes with the phenotype Ia^+ 56%, $U_{26}{}^+$ 50%, $PMN_1{}^+$ 18%, revealed that FMLP induced O_2^- was 3% of the response of mature granulocytes separated by buffy coat dextran sedimentation, and 5% after PMA. In contrast, in fractions containing cells with the phenotype $Ia^-U_{26}{}^-PMN_1{}^+$ 95%, and consisting of 60% granulocytes with fully mature morphology, the values for O_2^- were 98% of the mature FMLP response and 100% of the PMA response. In the fractions of intermediate density, O_2^- after stimulation by either FMLP or PMA was directly proportional to the number of $Ia^-U_{26}{}^-PMN_1{}^+$ cells. In accordance with these findings diminished release of betaglucuronidase was observed in the less dense fractions with greater percentages of Ia^+, $U26^+$ cells. Similar studies of normal bone marrow gave comparable results. These data suggest that oxidative metabolism and degranulation are differentiated functions associated with the expression of certain surface molecules.

81

SUPPRESSIVE EFFECTS OF COLCHICINE ON NEUTROPHIL CHEMOTAXIS IN VITRO AND MIGRATION IN VIVO ARE INDEPENDENT OF ITS EFFECT ON MICROTUBULES.

Yi-Han Chang and Annie T.A. Fong. UCLA, Los Angeles, CA 90024

Effect of drugs on chemotaxis (measured by Boyden chamber technique) of rabbit peripheral blood polymorphonuclear leukocytes(PMN) was determined by preincubating the cells in the presence of each drug at concentrations from 10^{-9} to 10^{-5}M for 90 minutes at 37°C. Chemotaxis directed toward serum-derived chemotactic factors (zymosan-activated serum, ZAS) was clearly suppressed by colchicine at concentrations as low as $1x10^{-8}$M (37.5±0.7%), whereas that toward cell-derived chemotactic factor(CCF), or that toward synthetic chemotactic peptide (FMLP) was not affected at 1000 times the concentration ($1x10^{-5}$M). The selective effects suggests that colchicine may affect initial steps rather than the final common pathway of the chemotactic response. The low effective concentration, the rapid suppressive action and the selectivity further suggest that the suppression of chemotaxis by colchicine may not involve its binding to cytoplasmic tubulin. This conclusion is supported by the finding that oncodazole, a more potent inhibitor of microtubule polymerization which competitively inhibits colchicine binding to tubulin, failed to affect ZAS-induced chemotaxis at $1x10^{-5}$M. Effects similar to that on chemotaxis were observed for PMN migration in vivo. A non-leukopenic dose of colchicine (0.2mg/kg), oncodazole (0.14mg/kg) or placebo was administered i.v. to rabbits followed by an injection of a chemotactic solution into a preformed ear pouch. The number of PMN's present in the ear pouch was determined at 5.0 hours after the injection of chemotactic solution. Colchicine treatment brought about a suppressions of PMN migration induced by ZAS or by Na urate crystals (MSU) (54.1±7.3%, 73.1±5.8%), but not that induced by CCF. Administration of oncodazole had no effect on MSU-induced PMN migration.

82

HUMAN RHEUMATOID SYNOVIAL MACROPHAGES INDUCE ANGIOGENESIS. Alisa E. Koch, S. Joseph Leibovich, Peter J. Polverini. Northwestern University Chicago, Ill., 60611.

The rheumatoid synovial pannus is an aggressive, invasive, fibrovascular proliferative lesion, neovascularization playing a crucial role in its development. We have investigated whether macrophages isolated from fresh rheumatoid synovia produce an angiogenic factor. Macrophages were isolated from fresh rheumatoid synovial tissue by enzymatic digestion. The cell suspension was centrifuged through isopycnic continuous Percoll density gradients and fractionated into five fractions (F1-F5). The percentage of macrophages in each fraction was determined using histochemical and functional markers. F_2, F_3, and F_4 (densities 0.98-1.042 g/ml, 1.042-1.062 g/ml, and 1.062-1.082 g/ml, respectively) contained the bulk of the macrophages (1-19%, 6-29% and 1-32% respectively). Macrophages were purified by adherence to fibronectin-coated collagen gels. Several cell types adhered to the gels. Non-macrophage cells were removed by trypsinization. 95% pure macrophages were obtained by dissolving the gels with collagenase. Macrophages from each fraction were tested in rat corneas for their ability to induce neovascularization. F_2 and F_4 were inactive while F_3 induced angiogenesis in 13 of 13 corneas tested. Cultured rheumatoid synovial fibroblastic cells did not induce a neovascular response in 11 of 12 corneas tested. Thus, within the rheumatoid synovium there is a heterogeneous population of macrophages, some of which induce angiogenesis and some of which do not. While rheumatoid fibroblastic synovial cells do not possess angiogenic activity, synovial macrophages are potent inducers of neovascularization. Macrophages may play a key role in the induction of neovascularization in rheumatoid arthritis.

83

FLARE UP OF ANTIGEN INDUCED ARTHRITIS AFTER CHALLENGE WITH ORAL ANTIGEN WB van den Berg, JW Lens, LBA van de Putte, Dept of Rheumatology University Hospital, St Radboud, 6525 GA Nijmegen, The Netherlands.

Intravenous injection of methylated bovine serum albumin (mBSA) in mice with unilateral chronic mBSA induced arthritis causes a flare up of the smouldering arthritis without affecting the contralateral noninflamed knee joint[1]. We examined whether orally administered antigen can also provoke such a flare up reaction. C57Bl mice were immunized with mBSA in Freunds complete adjuvant and unilateral arthritis was induced at day 21 by intraarticular injection of 60 ug mBSA. At day 56 groups of mice received oral doses ranging from 1-60 mg mBSA, and flare up of arthritis was quantitated by ^{99m}Tc uptake of the knee joints. With an oral dose of 20 mg mBSA nearly all mice (8/9) showed a flare up, but with lower doses the response was more variable (11/16 with 10 mg and 3/11 with 5 mg). The flare up reached a maximum within 6 hours and lasted for at least 2 days. Using ^{125}I-mBSA (20 mg), 5-10% of the administered label was found in the blood between 1 and 6 hrs. Only 0.1% of the label was proteinbound and less than 10% of the protein could be specifically precipitated, indicating that the amount of circulating antigen was at any event less than 200 ng. Knee joints dissected at 3 hr. after challenge, contained an amount of radiolabel equivalent to 1 ug protein (probably less than 100 ng mBSA). Local intraarticular injection of mBSA revealed that a dose of 1 ug is needed to induce inflammation in the contralateral nonarthritic joint whereas a dose of 10 ng suffices to provoke a clear flare up of the smouldering arthritis. Our data indicate that passage of tiny amounts of antigen through the gastrointestinal mucosa may play a role in exacerbation (and perpetuation) of arthritis. [1] Lens, Clin.Exp.Imm. (1984) 55, 287.

84

ELECTRICAL CHARGE OF AN ANTIGEN DETERMINES ITS LOCALIZATION IN THE JOINT Wim B. van den Berg, Levinus B.A. van de Putte Dept of Rheumatology University Hospital, St Radboud, 6525 GA Nijmegen, The Netherlands

Intraarticular injection of cationic bovine serum albumin(BSA) induces a chronic arthritis in immune mice, whereas the negatively charged native BSA fails to cause a protracted joint inflammation[1]. We examined the role of antigenic charge as a determinant of antigen retention and exact localization within the knee joint. Immune and nonimmune mice received an intraarticular injection of either radiolabeled native BSA (^{125}I-BSA) or charge modified BSA rendered cationic(pI 8.5) by amidation (aBSA), and autoradiographs were prepared of whole joint sections. Native BSA shows no affinity for negatively charged joint structures and in nonimmune mice the antigen was hardly detectable after day 1. In immune mice antibody mediated retention of BSA was found in the ligaments and fibrous cartilage structures of the joint,but appeared to be absent at the hyaline cartilage. The amount retained is restricted both by the antibody titer and by the presence of loose enough joint tissues to permit in situ immune complex(IC) formation. In contrast,large amounts of the cationic aBSA were retained at all collagenous structures of the joint, in particular at the highly negatively charged cartilage. The most striking observation was the deep penetration of aBSA in the dense hyaline cartilage. This was found both in immune mice,in the presence of joint inflammation,as well as in nonimmune mice. In addition to deep penetration,clear surface labeling was found in immune mice,and immunofluorescence on IgG and C_3 made clear that this pattern represents IC formation. Large parts of the joint surface consist of hyaline cartilage and due to its charge mediated penetration and excellent retention large amounts of cationic antigens may be retained to provide long lasting antigen supply to sustain inflammation. [1]van den Berg J. Clin. Invest.(1984) 74 1850

85

IMPACT OF DIAGNOSIS-RELATED GROUP (DRG)-BASED REIMBURSEMENT FOR RHEUMATIC DISEASES IN A TEACHING HOSPITAL. RM Hartley, MH Liang, KE Cullen. Depts. of Medicine and Rheumatology/Immunology and Multipurpose Arthritis Center, Brigham & Women's Hospital, Boston, MA 02115.

The impact of Medicare's DRG-based reimbursement system is examined for 734 rheumatology inpatients admitted to a teaching hospital during 1982 and 1983. The analysis accounted for "outliers" as defined by Medicare and distinguished costs from charges.

The mean costs for patients, excluding length of stay outliers, in DRGs 240 and 241 were $4450.54 and $3174.74, resulting in net revenues of $1126 and $1794 per patient, respectively. The difference between DRGs in cost is significant ($p < 0.001$), indicating that DRGs identify two different groups of patients. Excluding outliers, the coefficients of variation in costs for DRGs 240 and 241 were 72% and 80%, which were average for DRGs at our hospital. Mean total charge per patient was different for groups defined by their primary rheumatological diagnosis in DRG 240 but not DRG 241. For the largest groups in DRGs 240 and 241, rheumatoid arthritis and systemic lupus erythematosus, the charges per patient did not differ, but SLE patients received more technology-intensive care.

The mean cost of outliers in DRG 240 was $34,515 and $23,622 for DRG 241, resulting in an average loss of $18,400 and $16,500, respectively. Outliers accounted for 34.5% and 21.8% of the DRGs' total costs, respectively, but only 6.4% and 3.6% of the total number of patients.

Under current DRG reimbursement rules, costs of care for rheumatology patients would be adequately reimbursed in our hospital. Losses on outliers would be offset by inliers if Medicare adjustments for capital and medical education continue.

86

ADMINISTRATION OF ANTI-T CELL ANTIBODIES RETARDS MURINE LUPUS IN BXSB MICE. David Wofsy. VAMC and UCSF, San Francisco, CA 94121.

Murine lupus in BXSB mice is associated with monocyte proliferation, polyclonal B cell activation, and impaired T cell function, but the relationship among these abnormalities and their significance are unknown. To examine the pathogenetic role of T cells in BXSB mice, we specifically depleted T cells using rat IgG2b monoclonal antibodies (MAb) to either Thy-1.2 (on all T cells) or L3T4 (on "helper" T cells). Treatment with anti-Thy-1.2 (6 mg i.v.) at age 3 months produced a sustained 40-50% reduction in circulating T cells for 6 months. Treatment prevented monocytosis, reduced anti-DNA Ab by >75%, and significantly retarded renal disease, but it did not prolong life. Rat IgG2b MAb to Thy-1.2 elicits host Ab to rat Ig, and repeated injection caused anaphylaxis in BXSB mice. In contrast, rat IgG2b MAb to L3T4 did not elicit Ab to rat Ig. We therefore were able to treat BXSB mice weekly with anti-L3T4 (2 mg i.p.) from age 3 to 12 mo. Treatment reduced L3T4+ cells by 70-80%. It also significantly reduced monocytosis, anti-DNA Ab levels, renal disease, and mortality:

Treatment	Monocytes/mm^3 (8 mo)	Anti-DNA Titer (8 mo)	BUN (mg/dl) (8 mo)	Mortality (10 mo)
saline	5270 ± 1760	1:200 ×÷ 1.2	24.8 ± 3.9	70%
anti-L3T4	610 ± 200	1:60 ×÷ 1.2	15.5 ± 1.2	20%
rat IgG	(died from anaphylaxis/serum sickness			100%

These findings establish that monocytosis and autoimmunity in BXSB mice are T-cell dependent. They extend our previous observation that MAb to L3T4 retards autoimmunity in NZB/NZW mice. L3T4 is homologous to T4 in humans. Our finding that MAb to L3T4 is effective in two murine models for SLE suggests that MAb to T4 may be effective in humans with SLE.

87

POLYARTHRITIS, NEUTROPENIA, AND CIRCULATING LARGE GRANULAR LYMPHOCYTES: SUBSET OF FELTY'S SYNDROME. W.J. Wallis, T.J. Loughran, Jr., M.E. Kadin, E.A. Clark, G.A. Starkebaum. University of Washington, Seattle, WA 98195, USA.

We have identified five patients with polyarthritis, splenomegaly and neutropenia who had markedly increased numbers of circulating large granular lymphocytes (LGL) with the phenotype of immature natural killer (NK) cells. LGL comprised 61 ± 14% (S.D.) of peripheral blood mononuclear cells. All five had recurrent infections with fevers during episodes of profound neutropenia. Three had simultaneous onset of neutropenia and polyarthritis (prominent at wrists and hands) of less than 2 years duration, one had chronic polyarthralgias 15 yrs., and one had chronic erosive polyarthritis 20 yrs. Anti-neutrophil IgG, ANA's, rheumatoid factor activity and immune complexes (Ciq binding activity) were detected in the sera of all patients. Bone marrow biopsies from four revealed a maturation arrest at the myelocyte stage with lymphoid infiltrates. NK- like cells were defined by characteristic morphology on peripheral blood smear (large "activated" lymphocytes with prominent azurophilic granules) and the following reactivity pattern with monoclonal antibodies: OKT3 +, OKT8 +, HNK-1 +, OKT4-, OKM1-. Studies with two-color FACS confirmed that this panel of surface markers was shared on LGL. Most cells were also HLA-Dr+. Peripheral blood mononuclear cells exhibited little NK activity (mean 6% of normal controls) in assays with K562 target cells. Clonal cytogenetic changes (trisomy 14) were observed in mononuclear cells from the spleen and peripheral blood of one patient supporting the diagnosis of LGL leukemia. Synovial biopsy did not reveal leukemic infiltrates. Increased LGL with the phenotype of immature NK cells may reflect a reactive or neoplastic process. These cells may play a role, as yet undefined, in the pathogenesis of neutropenia, humoral immunologic disturbances and synovitis in a subset of patients with Felty's Syndrome.

88

SENSITIVITY TO CHANGE OF HEALTH STATUS MEASURES IN A CLINICAL TRIAL OF AURANOFIN IN RA. The Auranofin Cooperating Group.

We tested the sensitivity of a battery of Health Status measures in a 6 month multi-center randomized clinical trial of Auranofin vs Placebo in 311 patients. Independent assessors, trained centrally, administered questionnaires selected to assess various dimensions of the disease. Four distinct dimensions were identified and represented by 4 composite scores. Changes in these scores were expressed as % of baseline standard deviations. The Auranofin group improved significantly more than the Placebo group in all 4 dimensions.

DIMENSION	CHANGE IN COMPOSITE SCORES(%) AURANOFIN	PLACEBO	P VALUE
Physical	34.5	15.7	0.003
Functional	29.2	4.9	0.001
Pain	74.1	49.7	0.026
Global	50.0	26.8	0.006

Physical score included: tender/swollen joints, AM stiffness, grip & 50 ft walk. Functional score included the Health assessment questionnaire (HAQ), the Index of Wellbeing (IWB) and the Keitel. The pain score included the McGill pain questionnaire, a 10 cm line and a categorical scale. The Global score consisted of measures of disease status and Global Health. Pairwise correlations between composite scores ranged from 0.45 to 0.67 indicating that these represent different dimensions of the impact of RA. The NIMH depression scale and the RAND Health Perception scale did not differ between the 2 groups. These results indicate that several Health Status measures are sensitive to clinical changes and support their use in clinical trials. These results also show that auranofin effectively improves several dimensions of RA.

89

DO RA PATIENTS IN HEALTH MAINTENANCE ORGANIZATIONS HAVE WORSE OUTCOMES OF CARE THAN THOSE IN FEE-FOR-SERVICE? Edward Yelin, Martin Shearn and Wallace Epstein. UCSF, San Francisco, CA 94117.

The purpose of this project is to determine if, after an average of 18 months of follow-up, persons with RA in health maintenance organizations (HMOs) differ from those in fee-for-service (FFS) in the amount of care received and in outcomes. We reported last year that 626 RA pts. in FFS did not differ from 186 in HMOs in their baseline (1982) measures of severity of disease as reported by rheumatologists, or in pt. report of symptoms, rates of hospitalization, length-of-stay per admission, or rates of joint replacement surgery. We re-interviewed 92% of these RA pts. (95% of HMO pts., 91% of FFS) in 1984. After adjusting for differences in patient report of sex, race, marital status, education, age, baseline functional score (HAQ), # of comorbid conditions, health insurance, overall health status, # of painful, swollen, or stiff joints, and in MD report of # of joints with erosions, sed rate, rheumatoid factor, we could find no significant difference ($p > .05$ by t test) between HMO and FFS pts. in: # of visits to MDs for RA (13.8 HMO, 13.6 FFS); # of visits to MDs for all reasons (16.35 HMO, 16.16 FFS); # of hospital stays for RA (.25 HMO, .19 FFS); hospital days per capita (1.43 HMO, 1.37 FFS); or length-of-stay in days (7.1 HMO, 6.83 FFS). After similar adjustment, HMO and FFS pts. with RA did not differ in these outcome measures: 1984 HAQ score (1.18 HMO, 1.19 FFS); change in HAQ score from baseline (.14 HMO, .15 FFS); % of pts. stating their RA had worsened (45% HMO, 51% FFS). After adjustment including baseline status, HMO pts. stated that their 1984 overall health status was better than FFS pts. (1-4 scale, 4=poor) (2.45 HMO, 2.60 FFS). HMO pts.' overall health status improved from baseline (-.09 in 1-4 scale), whereas FFS pts.' worsened (.05). We conclude that RA pts. in HMOs have similar use of medical care and at least as good outcomes over almost two years of follow-up as FFS pts.

90

EFFECTS OF VARYING PHYSICAL THERAPY INTENSITY ON OUTCOMES IN TOTAL JOINT ARTHROPLASTY. MH Liang, KE Cullen, MG Larson, JA Schwartz, C Robb-Nicholson, AH Fossel, Multipurpose Arthritis Center, Brigham & Women's Hospital, Boston, MA 02115.

Between 1973 and 1981 the amount of physical therapy (PT) for patients following total joint arthroplasty was successively reduced because of fiscal pressure. Patients and staff perceived that the reduction impaired quality of care and surgical outcomes. To evaluate this, a retrospective analysis of the surgical results during four periods of varying PT intensity was performed.

Two hundred patients treated under four periods of different PT intensity were randomly chosen. The patients were similar in age (66 years), sex (71% female), diagnosis (68% osteoarthritis, 32% rheumatoid arthritis), and joints replaced (51% hips, 49% knees). The patients received significantly different average hours of PT during their hospital stays ($p=0.00025$), 52.4 hours, 46.4 hours, 41.2 hours and 37.9 hours.

There were no statistically significant differences in outcome as measured by length of hospital stay (26.2 days), functional outcome, or numbers of surgical complications and manipulations. During one period patients had an increased number of medical complications judged unrelated to reduced PT. The statistical power of the study to detect a 5-day length of stay difference between one or more groups was 50%. Perceived loss of quality with decreased PT may be more apparent than real and may be due to loss of emotional support rather than to significant differences in physical outcome.

91

SYNOVIAL FLUID ANALYSIS IN HOSPITAL LABORATORIES. Peter Hasselbacher, Gerald T. O'Connor, Nancy A. Tehan. University of Louisville, Louisville KY, and Dartmouth Medical School, Hanover NH.

We sent a questionnaire to all hospitals in NH and VT to determine the frequency and methods of synovial fluid(SF) analysis. To cooperating labs we sent "unknown" SFs for specific studies.42 of 54 labs responded. The median number of SF studied was 3/mo. The panel of tests in a "routine" SF analysis varied widely. The majority regularly performed WBC and RBC counts. Other tests, as WBC differential, viscosity, mucin clot, glucose, protein, complement, enzymes, or antibody studies were done with widely different frequencies (from always to never). More than half the labs performed a gram stain and cultures on all SF. 26% of labs used an electronic cell counter. 4 labs were diluting SF in acetic or other acid to perform cell counts. Of 38 sets of test fluids, 26 were returned. In one fluid, only 4 labs identified the frequent CPPD crystals (3 urate,5 undefined,13 none). In a 2nd fluid containing innumerable urate crystals, 20 labs reported urate (1 CPPD, 3 undefined,1 none). A 3rd fluid contained both urate and CPPD crystals:a single lab identified both (18 urate only, 1 CPPD only, 3 undefined,3 none). A 4th fluid contained no crystals and only 1 lab saw CPPD. Average WBC count from this SF was 6683 ± 1192mm/3 (max=12,000. min=2467). There was even wider variation in RBC and differential counts. Our survey demonstrated a clear lack of general guidelines for routine SF analysis. Many unnecessary, cost-ineffective, archaic, or inaccurate tests were performed. The majority of hospital labs were inadequate in performing crystal identification. Those components of the SF analysis which are truly useful must be identified, and unnecessary testing eliminated if SF analysis is to be recommended as a cost-effective procedure.

92

A DISABILITY ADJUSTED MEDICARE CAPITATION PAYMENT FOR RHEUMATOID ARTHRITIS. M. Nevitt, E. Yelin, C. Henke, W. Epstein. UCSF, San Francisco, CA 94117

Capitation payments to prepaid health plans (PHP) must reflect the potentially high medical costs of RA if Medicare beneficiaries with RA are to have access to prepaid health care. Age/sex adjustments now used by Medicare do not capture these high costs. We have performed annual utilization surveys in a panel of 822 persons with RA (derived from a random sample of N. Calif. rheumatologists), accumulating 1581 person years of observation. Crude hospital admissions (HAd) in this sample are 4 to 5 times greater than the average for all members of U.S. PHPs. Our sample had 215 ± 16 RA HAds/1000/yr., 1,565 ± 145 RA hospital days (HD)/1000/yr. and 261 ± 24 non-RA HAds/1000/yr. Comparing RA pts. in the 1st with those in the 4th quartile of baseline Health Assessment Questionnaire (HAQ) disability scores, we found a 500% increase in subsequent RA HAds, a 600% increase in RA HDs and a 300% increase in non-RA HAds. RA HDs, but not RA HAds, increased slightly with age, while non-RA HAds increased sharply with age.

	RA HAd/1000	RA HD/1000	non-RA HAd/1000
HAQ 1st quart	77 ± 21	505 ± 134	116 ± 25
" 2nd "	119 ± 25	530 ± 200	292 ± 43
" 3rd "	231 ± 39	1,446 ± 310	290 ± 63
" 4th "	395 ± 59	3,108 ± 597	341 ± 54

We performed ANOVA on HAd and HD measures using 10 age/sex strata and 4 HAQ disability strata. Non-RA HAd ($p<.05$), but not RA HAd or RA HD, differed by age/sex. RA HAd ($p<.01$), RA HD ($p<.01$) and non-RA HAd ($p<.05$) differed by HAQ. Variance in RA HAd and HD explained by HAQ was 4X that explained by age/sex. HAQ explained more variance in non-RA HAd than a general functional status measure. In addition to its clinical applications, HAQ disability score is a good predictor of hospital use in RA pts. and could be added to age/sex to adjust capitation payments of RA pts. for health risk.

93

EXPERIMENTAL EVIDENCE THAT CHANGES IN PSYCHOLOGICAL FACTORS ARE ASSOCIATED WITH CHANGES IN ARTHRITIS PAIN. Kate Lorig, Stanford Shoor, Halsted R. Holman, Stanford University, Stanford, CA 94305.

Psychological factors have long been thought to influence arthritis pain. However, there has been little experimental evidence in arthritis patients that psychological factors could be changed or that such changes would be associated with changes in pain. On the other hand, self-care activities such as arthritis specific exercise, relaxation and walking are generally believed to assist in alleviating arthritis pain.

To test these beliefs, 140 arthritics were randomized to take the 12-hour, lay-taught Arthritis Self-Management (ASM) course or to control status. Comparing treated subjects to controls after 4 months, pain was reduced ($p<.01$). Self-care activities, exercise, relaxation and walking increased ($p<.01$) and psychological status (a combined scale of coping, pain self-efficacy, satisfaction with treatment, and treatment expectancy) improved ($p<.01$).

Tests of association were performed on the treated subjects. Utilizing multilinear regression, controlling for baseline pain, age, sex, education, and type of arthritis, the expected association between changes in self-care activities and changes in pain was not significant (R=0.08). However, the association between changes in pain and changes in psychological status was significant (R=-.42) ($p<.05$).

Thus, psychological factors impacted by patient education appear to correlate better with changes in pain than do more commonly measured self-care behaviors. The unidentified features of the ASM course which enhanced psychological status with an associated reduction in pain are being explored.

94

FUNCTIONAL STATUS ASSESSMENT: DEVELOPMENT AND APPLICATION OF HEALTH STATUS PROFILES. Robert F. Meenan, Jennifer J. Anderson, Lewis E. Kazis. Boston University Multipurpose Arthritis Center, Boston, MA.

Although the clinical relevance of functional status assessments is conceptually clear, the method for depicting this information in a scientific fashion that is clinically useful is questionable. This study describes the development and reliability testing of a format for the presentation of health status information to clinicians in the treatment of patients with rheumatoid arthritis (RA). Health Status Profiles (HSP) are generated using the Arthritis Impact Measurement Scales (AIMS), a reliable and valid instrument, which estimates physical disability, psychological status and pain. HSP's are single page summary formatted reports for expressing functional assessments contained in the AIMS instrument.

Ten prototypical patients were selected for representativeness and uniqueness from an extensive RA patient population using both graphics and cluster analysis. HSP's were generated, one for each patient. One hundred and two clinicians responded to a mailing that asked for the ranking of the 10 profiles in order of decreasing health status. The coefficient of concordance was .784 indicating the relative reliability of HSP's. Two clusters of the profile rankings revealed a cluster loading on physical function, while the other stressed psychological and pain status.

HSP's communicate functional assessments in a reliable fashion, a prerequisite if this format is to have clinical utility. Clinicians also weigh their assessments by emphasizing different components of health status. These findings support the more widespread use of HSP's in clinical practice.

95

THE IMPACT OF CHILDHOOD RHEUMATOLOGICAL DISEASE ON THE FAMILY. Marie C. McCormick, Balu H. Athreya, Margaret M. Stemmler. Children's Seashore House, Atlantic City, NJ 08404, and University of Pennsylvania School of Medicine, Philadelphia, PA, USA, 19104.

Rheumatological conditions in children are often associated with limitations in activities of daily living, psychological problems secondary to chronic illness and increased use of health services. This report examines the health status and health care utilization of 138 children with various rheumatic diseases (the majority with juvenile rheumatoid arthritis), and assesses the impact on the children's families. The data was obtained by a telephone survey using a questionnaire covering sociodemographic characteristics; acute and chronic health problems and associated health care use; limitation of daily activities of health; parental perception of child's health; and impact of the child's health problem on the family using the Stein and Riessman Scale (impact scale).

In spite of the chronic medical condition, most children (71%) were perceived to be healthy by the parents. However, 42% were limited in two or more activities of daily living. High scores on impact scale were correlated at a statistically significant level with limitation of activities and not with the diagnosis. Other variables associated with greater family impact score were lower educational attainment of the mother, male child, number of hospitalizations, family income less than $10,000 and number of doctor visits.

These results suggest that chronic rheumatic disease presents a particular strain for families with modest resources in the face of increased need for nursing care. In assessing the effects of chronic illness on children and their families, special attention should be paid to the effect of the child's functioning in the home and to the financial impact, as well as to the clinical symptoms and the diagnosis.

96

ADULT-ONSET STILL'S DISEASE (AOSD); DISEASE COURSE AND HLA ASSOCIATIONS. J.M.G.W. Wouters, P. Reekers, L.B.A. Van de Putte and Cooperating Centres. University Hospital, 6500 HB Nijmegen. The Netherlands.

Twenty-nine patients with definite and 13 patients with probable AOSD from 15 rheumatologic centres were studied to determine disease course and possible HLA associations.

Diagnosis of AOSD was based on the ARA criteria for systemic JRA. Twenty-five patients were female. Mean age of disease onset was 28 years (range 16-65 years). Mean follow-up after onset was 54 months (range 12-168 months). The main clinical and laboratory features of the 42 patients were: fever in 42, arthritis in 42, typical rash in 34, splenomegaly in 14, pericarditis in 9, neutrophilic leucocytosis in 41 and hepatic dysfunction in 33.

Sixteen patients had persistent disease with continuous disease activity for at least one year. On X-ray examination 26 patients showed evidence for joint destructions. In 15 patients at least one root joint was impaired. Between patients with and without persistent disease, patients with and without joint destructions and patients with and without involvement of the root joints no statistical differences were found for sex, age at onset, follow-up and the main clinical and laboratory features. The frequency of DR4 was increased in the total group of 42 patients (35%,p=0.03) and the 29 patients with definite AOSD (41%, p=0.02) as compared to healthy controls (20%). None of the patients was positive for DR1 and only one was positive for Bw35. The frequency of DRw6 was increased in the patients with involvement of at least one root joint (40%,p=0.03)as compared to patients without involvement of these joints(11%).These results suggest that AOSD is associated with DR4 and that DRw6 may be an unfavourable prognostic marker in this disorder

97

ADULT-ONSET STILL'S DISEASE: CLINICAL COURSE AND LONG-TERM OUTCOME.

J.J. Cush, T.A. Medsger, Jr., W.C. Christy, D.C. Herbert, L.A. Cooperstein, University of Pittsburgh, Pittsburgh, PA, 15261

We have reviewed the long-term natural history and functional outcome in 21 patients with adult-onset Still's disease first evaluated during 1971-1981. There were 12 men and 9 women with a median onset age of 21 years and a median disease duration of 11.6 years (range 3-40) at the time of reevaluation in 1984. Patients were classified into four clinical patterns 4 had monocyclic systemic (MS), 2 polycyclic systemic (PS), 10 chronic articular (CA) and 5 a mixed pattern of chronic articular-polysystemic disease (CA-PS). MS patients had either no arthritis or oligoarthritis at onset, an oligoarticular course requiring little or no therapy at followup, and all remained in ARA functional class I or II. In contrast, CA and CA-PS patients generally had a polyarticular onset and course, more frequently developed carpal bony ankylosis (10/15) and because ARA class II or III (14/15). Five individuals had a history of a childhood illness consistent with an episode of JRA and all had CA or CA-PS involvement. Three patients, all with chronic articular disease, required bilateral total hip replacement, and 10 of 15 CA patients continue to receive maintenance NSAID, corticosteroid and/or remittive agent therapy for persistent inflammatory and/or secondary osteoarthritis.

In nearly all instances, systemic features were controlled only after the addition of corticosteroid therapy. There were two deaths, one sudden and unexplained and the other secondary to pulmonary tuberculosis during corticosteroid therapy. We conclude that adult-onset Still's disease, especially the chronic articular type, may pursue a rheumatoid-like course with disabling polyarthritis.

98

SEROLOGIC CROSS-REACTIVITY BETWEEN LYME DISEASE SPIROCHETE AND TREPONEMA PALLIDUM IN INDIRECT IMMUNOFLUORESCENT ASSAY.

P.E. Lavoie, M.D., A.J. Wilson, M.D., Pacific Presbyterian Medical Center, San Francisco, CA. 94115 and R.S. Lane, Ph.D., Univ. of Calif., Berkeley, CA. 94720.

Patients with syphilis have been previously shown to also react serologically to the Lyme Disease Spirochete (LDS) (Borrelia burgdorferi). We investigated this cross-reactivity using control reagents and substrates. Fluorescein isothiocyanate labelled anti-LDS conjugate prepared in rabbits (1:5 dilution) was applied to T. pallidum substrate in the FTA test and the reaction was compared with the usual 1+ and 4+ controls. FTA control serum at dilutions of 1:5 (4+) and 1:640 (1+) was applied to LDS substrate. Results were as follows:

FTA control serum 1:5 with LDS	= 4+ reaction
FTA control serum 1:640 with LDS	= 1+ reaction
Anti-LDS conjugate with FTA substrate	= 3+ reaction

Also we studied fresh serum from a former Lyme Disease patient (A) and from a patient with active Acrodermatitis Chronica Atrophicans and previous Lyme Disease (B). Serologic testing in these patients showed:

(A) LDS titer 1:128 FTA 1+
(B) LDS titer 1:512 FTA 3+

There appears to be substantial immunologic cross-reactivity between T. pallidum and B. burgdorferi by the IFA method. These findings argue against the widely held concept of high specificity of the FTA test for syphilis. This should raise the consideration of antecedent Lyme Disease in patients with a positive FTA who lack a syphilis history.

99

ANTICARDIOLIPIN ANTIBODIES DETECTED IN THE SERA OF PATIENTS WITH LYME DISEASE: RELATIONSHIP TO NEUROLOGICAL FEATURES.

Charles Mackworth-Young, Nigel Harris, Azzudin Gharavi, Allen C. Steere, Stephen E. Malawista, and Graham Hughes. Royal Postgraduate Medical School, London W12, UK, and Yale University School of Medicine, New Haven, CT 06510.

Lyme disease is a spirochaete-related disorder, the clinical features of which may include a rash, widespread neuropathy, and arthritis. Conventional tests for syphilis, such as the VDRL, are usually negative. These employ cardiolipin as a ligand, but are not as sensitive in detecting anticardiolipin antibodies (ACA) as solid-phase radioimmunoassays (RIA). In view of the fact that raised levels of ACA's detected by the latter method are associated with neurological disease in SLE we were interested in determining with a solidphase RIA whether patients with Lyme disease also have elevated levels of these antibodies.

Twenty-five patients with active Lyme disease were studied: four with erythema chronicum migrans only, seven with arthritis and fourteen with neurological disease. VDRL tests were negative in all of them. Seven patients (28%) had raised levels of ACA's (IgM class). Three were weakly positive in the assay (defined as values between 2.76 and 5SD above the mean of the normal controls), and consisted of one patient from each group. Four were strongly positive (range 5.4 to 9.9SD): all of these had neurological features. There was no correlation between the degree of anticardiolipin activity and specific antibody titres against the Lyme spirochaete as measured by indirect immunofluorescence.

These results demonstrate that anticardiolipin activity may be raised in roughly a quarter of patients with active Lyme disease, and suggest that in some individuals there may, as in SLE, be a relationship between elevated levels of ACA's and the presence or development of neurological disease.

100

PALINDROMIC RHEUMATISM LEADING TO PERSISTENT, EROSIVE, ASYMMETRIC SYNOVITIS IN CYSTIC FIBROSIS.

Perry Rush, Wellesley Hospital, and Dan Wilmot, John Lee, Henry Levinson and Abraham Shore, Hospital for Sick Children, Toronto, Canada

We describe 12 cystic fibrosis (CF) patients, 7 females and 5 males, with arthritis unrelated to hypertrophic osteoarthropathy. The average age was 23 years with an average duration of symptoms of 7 years.

10/12 patients presented with recurrent episodic attacks of a debilitating, asymmetric, non-nodular, effusive, non-erosive, synovitis involving large and small joints above and below the waist in a classic palindromic pattern. Involvement was polyarticular in 5, pauciarticular in 4 and monoarticular in one patient. Three of these 10 patients, one of whom became latex positive, progressed to a persistent synovitis requiring chronic therapy with anti-inflammatory agents. Two developed cartilage loss and erosions.

2/12 patients had no previous history of palindromic attacks and presented with a latex positive, non-nodular, effusive, erosive, asymmetric, polyarthritis involving large and small joints above and below the waist.

All patients had negative anti-nuclear factors, normal complements and normal uric acid levels. Immunoglobulins were normal or diffusely elevated. Joint involvement was unrelated to severity of the chest disease or any medication.

A subgroup of CF patients with palindromic rhematism develop persistent, asymmetric, erosive disease. In all, 5/12 patients with CF arthritis had erosions and 4 of these 5 had a positive latex. CF arthritis may not be benign as has been previously reported.

101

MUSCULOSKELETAL DISEASE AND CONTROL OF SERUM CALCIUM AND PHOSPHATE IN CHRONIC HEMODIALYSIS PATIENTS.

J.H. Uhl, D.R. Maxwell, and S.L. Myers. Indianapolis Veterans Administration Medical Center and Indiana University, Indianapolis, IN 46223.

A high prevalence of musculoskeletal symptoms has been observed in chronic hemodialysis patients. We tested the hypothesis that these symptoms are related to loss of serum calcium and phosphate homeostasis. Fifty chronic hemodialysis patients were entered, on the basis of mean serum [calcium] x [phosphate] product (CaP) during the previous year, into 2 study groups: "controlled" (C), n=25; or "uncontrolled" (UC), n=25. Initially, 20 patients were interviewed and examined by a single blinded observer, 12 from Group C (mean age, 54.4 years; mean duration of treatment, 58 months; mean CaP=34.4) and 8 from Group UC (mean age, 51.6 years; mean duration of treatment, 39 months; mean CaP=71.0). Periarticular tenderness overlying tendons, tendinous insertions, or bursae was noted in 7 of 12 C patients and in 7 of 8 UC patients. Joint or bursal effusions were seen in 3 UC patients but not in any C patients. Normal joint examinations were recorded for 5 C patients but only one UC patient. There was a positive correlation between the patient's subjective assessment of severity of joint disease and CaP ($r=.74$; $p<.001$), and also between the number of painful joints and CaP ($r=.56$; $p<.01$). Two chronic effusions (one knee, one olecranon bursa) from UC patients contained non-birefringent material which stained with Alizarin red S, and are being further evaluated by electron microscopy. These data suggest that hemodialysis patients with poor control of CaP more frequently have symptoms of joint pain, and have a higher incidence of synovitis and periarticular tenderness than patients whose CaP is well controlled.

102

MONOSODIUM URATE CRYSTALS (MSUC) IN KNEE JOINTS OF ASYMPTOMATIC PATIENTS WITH NONTOPHACEOUS GOUT.

John S. Bomalaski, G. Lluberas, H.R. Schumacher. U. of Penn., VAMC, Med. Coll. Penn., Philadelphia, PA 19104

Rheumatologists often see patients with clinical diagnoses of non-tophaceous gout in whom synovial fluid (SF) has not been examined for MSUC. Some consider that the diagnosis of gout can only be made by documenting MSUC in SF. MSUC may be documented by examination of SF from asymptomatic metatarsophalangeal joints. Aspiration of knee joints is easier and would hopefully provide more SF for examination while maintaining the sensitivity of toe joint aspiration. MSUC have been reported in asymptomatic knees in tophaceous gout. We attempted to aspirate knee SF from 26 asymptomatic patients with nontophaceous gout in whom SF MSUC had previously been documented in at least one joint, not necessarily the knee. SF was obtained from 41/43 (95%) knees and MSUC were documented in 22/41 (54%) joints and 16/25 (64%) patients in whom SF was obtained. The presence of MSUC was not related to patient age, duration of gout, duration since the last attack of gout, alcohol abuse, hypertension, congestive heart failure, obesity, diabetes mellitus, treatment with allopurinol, concurrent serum uric acid (SUA) nor serum creatinine. Fifty percent of patients with and without MSUC had a SUA <7.1 mg/dl. A SF bulge sign was present in 6 patients and MSUC were present in 5/6 (83%) knee SF. Six patients had MSUC in one knee SF but not the other. Intracellular MSUC were seen in 70% of the positive samples. The SF WBC and volume of fluid aspirated were not different in the MSUC positive and negative groups. Knee joint aspiration is a sensitive method for demonstrating MSUC in non-tophaceous gout. Also, the implications of persistent MSUC despite normalization of SUA need to be determined.

103

TRANSITIONAL URATE CRYSTALS: A FACTOR IN GOUTY ARTHRITIS? Peter A. Simkin and Richard S. Benedict. U. of Wa., Seattle, Washington 98195.

Apparent crystal-negative effusions are sometimes seen in the early course of acute gouty arthritis. Also, newly-prepared urate crystals become less phlogistic after heating in vitro. A plausible explanation for these phenomena lies in the tendency for some solutes to precipitate first as highly hydrated structures which then evolve into more stable, less hydrated crystals. Polyhydrated urate salts could be intensely phlogistic yet invisible in polarized light. We examined this hypothesis after finding only needle-shaped, non-birefringent, intracellular objects up to 15 microns long in a gouty synovial fluid.

A supersaturated urate solution (500 mg/dl) was prepared in 0.1 N NaOH at 90°, allowed to cool, neutralized to pH 7.2 with HCl, and incubated at 37°. Serial observations of this solution revealed rod-like structures which appeared after 60 minutes and became birefringent over 24 hours. This transition sometimes occurred uniformly, but more often progressed from individual foci within the crystal. The non-birefringent urate crystals were avidly ingested by isolated normal PMNs on incubation in vitro.

For 25 years, monosodium urate monohydrate has been accepted as "the gout culprit" because its presence is recognized as a pathognomonic sign of gout. It now seems likely, however, that one or more polyhydrated, transitional form(s) of urate may also participate in the acute inflammatory process. Such crystals may be missed by observers using conventional polarizing microscopes.

104

CELL MEDIATED CYTOTOXICITY TO AUTOLOGOUS MUSCLE CULTURES IN POLYMYOSITIS. Ilan Bank, Armand Miranda, and Leonard Chess. College of Physicians & Surgeons, Columbia Univ., New York, NY 10032.

Several studies have suggested that peripheral blood mononuclear cells (PBMC) from patients with polymyositis and dermatomyositis (PM/DM) are cytotoxic to xenogeneic and allogeneic embryonally-derived muscle cultures. We report on the cytotoxicity of PBMC and their subsets to autologous and allogeneic muscle cultures derived from diagnostic biopsies. Dissociated muscle biopsy specimens from patients were cultured in vitro, transferred to microtiter plates and allowed to differentiate to multinucleated muscle cells. Lymphocyte cytotoxicity of cultured muscle cells was measured in an 8 hour, ^{51}Cr release assay. Cytotoxicity by unfractionated PBMC was detected in all patients. Isolated T cells from PM/DM patients were specifically cytotoxic to autologous but not allogeneic muscle cultures. In contrast, normal T cells were not specifically cytotoxic. Non-T cells from both PM/DM patients and normal controls were cytotoxic to both autologous and allogeneic muscle cultures. These results demonstrate for the first time that patients with PM/DM contain T cells capable of specifically killing autologous muscle cells. The non-T cell myocytotoxicity observed in patients with PM/DM was also prominent in normal controls and therefore has no apparent disease specificity. The recent findings of T cells in the inflammatory infiltrate in muscle biopsies from these patients suggest that the in vitro killing of autologous muscle by T cells may have pathogenetic relevance.

105

FUNCTIONAL HETEROGENEITY OF HUMAN ANTIGEN-PRESENTING CELLS (APC): PRESENTATION OF SOLUBLE ANTIGEN BUT NOT SELF Ia BY MONOCYTES. José Moreno and P.E. Lipsky. Univ of TX Health Science Center, Southwestern Medical School, Dallas, Texas 75235.

APC are necessary for the activation of T cells by soluble antigens. The autologous mixed lymphocyte reaction (AMLR) describes the proliferative response of T cells to autologous non-T cells in the absence of exogenous antigen. Both types of responses involve the recognition of self HLA-D region-encoded determinants on the APC. A number of cells including monocytes (Mϕ) and dendritic cells among others have been claimed to function as APC and to stimulate the AMLR. In order to address this issue, Mϕ were purified from peripheral blood adherent cells (AC) with the use of the Mϕ-specific monoclonal antibodies (Mab) 63D3, 3C10 and 61D3 and the fluorescence activated cell sorter. Responder populations consisted of autologous T4 cells that were extensively depleted of potential APC. Both Mϕ-Mab(+) and (-)AC effectively presented the recall antigens SK-SD and tetanus toxoid to T cells with as few as 500 cells supporting such responses. In contrast, only Mϕ-Mab(-)AC were effective stimulators of the AMLR. In no instance did Mϕ-Mab(+)AC stimulate the AMLR. This could not be explained by the release of inhibitory factors by Mϕ. Moreover, there were no significant differences in surface expression and density of HLA-DR and DQ-encoded determinants between Mϕ-Mab(+) and (-)AC populations. These results indicate that Mϕ are effective APC for soluble antigens but lack the ability to stimulate the AMLR. The dissociation between soluble antigen presentation and the AMLR suggests that the AMLR is not a prerequisite for succesful antigen presentation.

106

IMMUNOBIOLOGICAL FUNCTIONS OF ARTICULAR CHONDROCYTES. Moti L. Tiku, Shirley Liu, Marius Teodorescu, and John L. Skosey. University of Illinois College of Medicine, Chicago, IL 60612

Ia antigen expression on articular chondrocytes (CH) has been demonstrated in normal and diseased human cartilage, but immunological functions of these cells have not yet been studied. We therefore initiated studies to investigate the ability of enzyme dissociated CH to present antigen, and to induce allogenic and autologous mixed lymphocyte reactions. For antigen presentation, adult rabbits were immunized in front foot pads with ovalbumin (OVA) in complete Freund's adjuvant. Four to six weeks later draining lymph node cells (LNC) were obtained. CH were obtained by overnight collagenase, deoxyribonuclease and hyaluronidase digestion of cartilage from both ends of femurs and the proximal ends of tibias. Antigen presenting cells from spleen were used as positive controls. LNC or nylon wool purified T cells were cultured with OVA pulsed or nonpulsed and mitomycin C treated CH and spleen cells. LNC proliferation was measured by ^{3}H-thymidine uptake. Both CH and spleen cells showed antigen presenting activity. LNC proliferation in response to antigen pulsed CH or spleen cells was inhibited by 2c4a monoclonal anti-rabbit Ia antibodies. When T cells were purified first by Sephadex G10 and later by nylon wool, the proliferative response of these cells to the immunogen (OVA) was absolutely dependent on antigen presenting cells. Again CH under these strict experimental conditions presented antigen to T cells. In addition, CH were able to induce allogenic and autologous mixed reaction resulting in lymphocyte proliferation. These experiments establish the presence of Ia antigen associated functional properties of normal articular chondrocytes. The knowledge gained from this study may have significance in the understanding of the pathogenesis of immune arthritis.

107

THE REGULATORY PROPERTIES OF THE THIRD MONONUCLEAR POPULATION ON LYMPHOCYTE PROLIFERATION AND IMMUNOGLOBULIN SYNTHESIS. W. Abo, A.C. Bakke and D.A. Horwitz. USC School of Medicine, Los Angeles, California 90033.

The objective of this study was to define non-T/non-B lymphocytes with the capacity to regulate immunoglobulin production and to compare properties of these cells with typical OKT8 suppressor cells. Lymphocytes (PBL) were stained with a pan T (Leu 1) and a Pan B (B1) cell monoclonal antibody and the non-reactive cells were isolated with the FACS. This fraction contained all lymphocytes reacting with Leu 11, and OKM1, an antibody recognizing the C3bi receptor. Most also displayed azurophilic granules. We report that a cell subset with high density Fc receptors for IgG (FcR) labelled by Leu 11 has the capacity to suppress pokeweed mitogen-induced proliferation and Ig synthesis. Immune complexes (IC) were required to induce Leu 1/B1 negative cells to suppress proliferation, but not Ig production. Exposure of these cells to recombinant (r)-IL-2, r-Interferon α, but not r-Interferon γ markedly enhanced the suppressive activities. Leu 1/B1 negative cells were more radioresistant than OKT8+ cells. Treatment of non-T/non-B cells with Leu 11 and complement completely abolished suppression. Although Leu 11+ cells are the effectors of NK activity, we were able to disassociate suppression from killing. Kinetic studies revealed that Leu 11+ cells exerted maximum effects during the first 24 hours of culture and trypsinization of these cells abolished NK, but not suppression. Leu 11+ cells are markedly reduced in active SLE, a finding that may in part account for unregulated Immunoglobulin production.

108

MECHANISM OF ACTION OF GLUCOCORTICOIDS: INHIBITION OF T CELL PROLIFERATION IS REVERSED BY LEUKOTRIENE B4. J.S. Goodwin and D. Atluru. University of New Mexico School of Medicine, Albuquerque, N.M. 87131.

The mechanism whereby glucocorticosteroids are immunosuppressive is unknown. One potential mechanism of action of these compounds is by inhibition of arachidonic acid metabolism. If the immunosuppressive effect of hydrocortisone is indeed secondary to inhibition of arachidonic acid metabolism, then one should be able to mimick the effect of hydrocortisone with nonspecific lipoxygenase-cyclooxygenase inhibitors, and one should be able to reverse the effect of hydrocortisone by adding one or more specific arachidonic acid metabolites back to the assay. Phytohemagglutinin (PHA)-stimulated lymphocytes produce ∿ 10^{-9}M leukotriene B4 (LTB4), a 5-lipoxygenase product of arachidonic acid. Concentrations of hydrocortisone (10^{-5} to 10^{-6}M) that caused > 80% inhibition of 3H thymidine incorporation into PHA-stimulated lymphocytes also inhibited production of LTB4 by those lymphocytes by > 90%. In addition, inhibition of lymphocyte proliferation by hydrocortisone was mimicked by nonspecific lipoxygenase inhibitors (BW755, NDGA, nafazatrom) and also by a specific 5-lipoxygenase inhibitor (AA861), but not by specific cyclooxygenase inhibitors. The inhibition of lymphocyte proliferation by either hydrocortisone or by the 5-lipoxygenase inhibitor was totally reversed by LTB4 in low concentrations (10^{-8} to 10^{-12}M), but not by other arachidonic acid metabolites, including PGE2, LTC4, 5-HETE, 12-HETE and 15-HETE (means of 10 experiments: PHA 21,204; PHA + 10^{-5}M hydrocortisone, 5,930; PHA + 10^{-10}M LTB4, 18,408; PHA + hydrocortisone + LTB4, 20,840). Thus, glucocorticosteroids may inhibit lymphocyte proliferation by inhibiting endogenous LTB4 production.

109

FIBROBLAST-MODULATING LYMPHOKINES DERIVED FROM HUMAN T CELL HYBRIDOMAS Robert O. Endres, Arnold E. Postlethwaite and Andrew H. Kang, Memphis, TN.

Human T lymphocyte hybridomas have been produced in an effort to study T cell derived factors that influence fibroblast function. The hybridomas were produced by polyethylene glycol mediated fusion of 6-thioguanine resistant mutants of the human T cell leukemia lines CEM and HSB-2 with phytohemagglutinin stimulated peripheral blood mononuclear cells. All but one of the hybridomas tested were Leu 2^- and weakly Leu 3+, indicating they are derived from T cells of the helper/inducer subset. Serum-free supernates from some hybridomas (unstimulated) exhibited latent chemotactic activity for fibroblasts. Chemotactic activity was evident only after incubation of the supernates with an extract of sonicated monocytes, which is not chemotactic by itself. When concentrated supernates were chromatographed on Sephadex G-200 and incubated with sonicated monocyte extract, a major peak of latent fibroblast chemotactic activity was found eluting just behind IgG. Hybridoma supernates have also been found that either stimulate or inhibit fibroblast production of hyaluronic acid. The molecular weight of the inhibitor is approximately 55kd, and the stimulator exhibited three peaks of activity at 200kd, 65kd and 16kd as estimated by Sephadex G-200 chromatography. Other activities found in some hybridoma supernates include both stimulation and inhibition of fibroblast collagen synthesis and collagenase release. These human T cell hybridomas should serve as useful tools for the biochemical characterization of fibroblast-modulating lymphokines. This work was supported by USPHS Grant AM-26034, research funds from the Veterans Administration, and the Arthritis Foundation.

110

B CELL ACTIVATION BY CLONED ALLOSPECIFIC HUMAN HELPER T CELLS. S. M. Friedman, A. Green, A. R. Lewison, M. K. Crow, and A. B. Gottlieb. Hospital for Special Surgery and Rockefeller University, New York, NY 10021.

In the mouse, B cell activation and autoantibody production during graft-versus host disease (GVHD) is mediated by abnormal cooperation across major histocompatibility disparities between alloreactive donor T helper cells (T_h) and recipient B cells. To extend the GVHD model to man, we have generated a number of interleukin-2 dependent alloreactive T_h clones. These clones proliferate specifically to allogeneic stimulator cells bearing a particular DR antigen (e.g. clone A-7 is DR 3 reactive while A-57 is DR 2 responsive). Coculture of x-irradiated T_h cells with allogeneic B cells bearing the relevant DR antigen results in B cell activation as assessed by both proliferation and differentiation into immunoglobulin secreting cells (ISC). In some studies, B cell subsets were isolated with respect to cell density and expression of the 4F2 activation antigen. We found that after antigen specific activation, T_h cells can "recruit" a proliferative and ISC response by in vivo activated B cells regardless of their DR type. In contrast, effective activation of resting B cells requires direct MHC restricted interaction of T_h and B cell surface DR antigens. These data define two pathways of human T_h-B cell interaction and should prove useful for studying resting B cell activation in normals and patients with autoimmune disease.

111

Adult and Juvenile Rheumatoid Arthritis Patients Share HLA-Class II Antigens Defined by Alloreactive T Cell Clones. C. M. Weyand, J. J. Goronzy, C. G. Fathman.

To compare Class II antigens in patients with juvenile and adult rheumatoid arthritis,we generated a panel of alloreactive T cell clones.T lymphocytes were primarily stimulated against a lymphoblastoid line of a JRA patient typed DR4,Dw4/Dw14,an HLA type which has been described to be strongly associated with seropositive rheumatoid arthritis in children.We selected a couple of clones which were specific for Dw14 specificities present in a very high frequency in a group of JRA patients.Tested on 25 adult seropositive rheumatoid patients,at least one Dw14 specificity could be identified in most of the patients.Two of the clones which gave an identical reactivity for the Dw14 homozygous typing lines and the Dw4/Dw14 heterozygous JRA patients recognized antigenic sites expressed by two different subgroups of adult patients.With the exception of one patient which was recognized by both clones,the two different determinants seen by the two Dw14 reactive clones are mutually exclusive.On the basis of target inhibition studies with monoclonal antibodies,the two antigenic structures can be clearly differentiated, too.Thus,the specificity Dw14 defined by conventional typing is composed of different determinants.Frequently,adult rheumatoid patients share Dw14 determinants with the clinically identical group of seropositive juvenile patients.The minority of adults not seen by any of the different Dw14 specific clones included patients which failed to respond to conventional therapy and underwent treatment with total lymphoid irradiation.The results suggest that the Dw14 specificities as defined by alloreactive T cell clones can be used to subdivide adult rheumatoid patients into clinical relevant subgroups.

112

IDENTIFICATION AND MOLECULAR CLONING OF CENP-B, A HUMAN CENTROMERE PROTEIN RECOGNIZED BY ALL HUMAN ANTICENTROMERE ANTIBODIES (ACA). William C. Earnshaw, Kevin F. Sullivan, William Saunders, Don W. Cleveland, Johns Hopkins University, Baltimore, MD 21205, and Naomi F. Rothfield, Univ. of Conn., Farmington, CT 06032.

Sera was studied from a patient prior to and after the appearance of ACA. At the time ACA appeared, the sera was found to simultaneously acquire antibodies recognizing 3 chromosomal proteins (M_r=17, 80, and 140kD). Antibodies binding to each protein were affinity purified from preparative immunoblots made from isolated human HeLa chromosomes. Indirect immunofluorescence using the purified antibody revealed that the 3 antigens are localized to the centromere and have therefore been designated CENP-A (17kD), CENP-B(80kD), and CENP-C(140kD).

Sera containing ACA were used to clone cDNAs encoding the CENP antigens by the expression vector method. One clone (in lamda phage gt11) apparently corresponds to CENP-B, since affinity purified anti-CENP-B binds to the cloned fusion protein synthesized in E. coli. This antigen, CENP-B, is recognized by all ACA positive sera from 39 patients and is not recognized by ACA negative sera from patients with Raynaud's syndrome and similar connective tissue diseases or from 25 normal age, sex, race matched normal controls. All ACA positive patients have Raynaud's syndrome plus a connective tissue disease or Raynaud's disease.

The identification and molecular cloning of the human centromere protein, CENP-B (80kD) will allow for future studies on the pathophysiologic significance of ACA in human diseases.

113

CYTOSKELETAL BINDING OF MONOCLONAL ANTI-DNA ANTIBODIES DERIVED FROM NORMAL HUMAN LYMPHOID CELLS. Ewa Cairns, Ronald Komar and David A. Bell. University of Western Ontario, London, Ontario, Canada, N6A 3K7.

Recent reports have indicated a high frequency of anti-vimentin serum antibodies in SLE. We have examined the ability of monoclonal IgM anti-DNA antibodies derived from normal human lymphoid cells to bind to cellular constituents by immunofluorescence, using the human epithelial cell line HEP-2 as substrate. Hybridoma supernatants (HS) from 10 different clones were studied. 4/10 gave a strong fibrillar cytoplasmic staining resembling cytoskeletal staining (CS), 1/10 showed strong nuclear staining only, 3/10 showed weak nucleolar staining only and 2/10 showed no staining. HS showing CS were either polyspecific for various nucleic acid antigens (ssDNA, DNA, poly (dA-dT), poly dG.poly dC, RNA, cardiolipin), relatively restricted (poly dG.poly dC, RNA, cardiolipin), or monospecific (cardiolipin only). Negative HS or the parent cell line GM 4672 (used for fusion) were negative. CS staining identical to HS was also seen with 2 different mouse monoclonal anti-vimentin antibodies. Inhibition of CS was accomplished in 3/4 HS by pre-absorption of HS with cardiolipin and/or ssDNA, or by pre-incubationof the HEP-2 cells with the mouse monoclonal anti-vimentin antibody.

Therefore some normal human monoclonal anti-DNA antibodies bind to CS, probably vimentin. Lack of any known structural homology of vimentin or other CS components with nucleic acid antigens or cardiolipin suggests that configurational determinants or charge on these different molecules may account for their common binding and hence may also account for the presence of anti-vimentin autoantibodies in SLE serum.

114

MYOSITIS SERA RECOGNIZE ALANYL-tRNA SYNTHETASE AND TRANSFER RNA INDEPENDENTLY: IMPLICATIONS FOR AUTOIMMUNITY.
MB Mathews, RM Bernstein, CC Bunn, Cold Spring Harbor Laboratory, New York and Hammersmith Hospital, London.

In contrast to SLE, where antinuclear antibodies are general, autoantibodies in polymyositis and dermatomyositis are frequently directed at cytoplasmic components. These are often associated with transfer RNA. Jo-1, the commonest specificity, is found in 30% of myositis cases, especially those with interstitial lung disease (70%). The antigen is histidyl-tRNA synthetase. Another charging enzyme, threonyl-tRNA synthetase, is the target in the less frequent PL-7 system.

Five examples of a third system, PL-12, have now been studied. The sera precipitate a protein of M.Wt. 110,000 which appears to be alanyl-tRNA synthetase, based on the ability of PL-12 IgG to block tRNA charging with alanine. PL-12 antibodies, unlike Jo-1 and PL-7 antibodies, also bind deproteinized tRNA. Removal of anti-tRNA antibody by preabsorption with immobilized tRNA leaves the anti-protein antibody fully active. Surprisingly, tRNA was not associated with the protein antigen precipitated by the preabsorbed IgG.

We conclude that the PL-12 specificity consists of separate antibodies to naked tRNA and to alanyl-tRNA synthetase. This implies that (i) antibodies are generated against both components of a macromolecular complex; and (ii) one antibody might be an anti-idiotype to the other. Experimental tests of this hypothesis will be discussed.

115

ASSOCIATION OF NOVEL PROTEIN ANTIGENS REACTIVE WITH IgG-ANTINUCLEOLAR ANTIBODIES AND DIFFUSE SCLERODERMA. G. Reimer, K.M. Rose* and E.M. Tan. Scripps Clinic and Research Foundation, La Jolla, Ca. 92037 and *University of Texas, Houston, Texas 77225.

Immunofluorescent (IF) antinucleolar IgG antibodies (ANoA) were present in 14 (16%) of 89 scleroderma sera. We have analyzed the macromolecular nature of the ANoA reactive antigens by using Protein A facilitated immunoprecipitation followed by SDS-polyacrylamide gel electrophoresis.

The polypeptides immunoprecipitated from ^{35}S-labeled HeLa-cell extracts by ANoA could be divided into two distinct groups. Scleroderma sera with speckled nucleolar staining (n=3) precipitated 9 polypeptides with molecular weights (MW) from 190 to 12.5K (=Scl-A). The same 9 polypeptides were immunoprecipitated by anti-RNA polymerase I antibodies from a rabbit which was immunized with purified enzyme. This rabbit serum also showed the same speckled nucleolar pattern by IF staining. These findings strongly suggest that RNA polymerase I is the target of anti-Scl-A autoantibodies. A second group of ANoA with a homogeneous nucleolar IF pattern (n=7) precipitated 7 polypeptides with MW from 100 to 20K (= Scl-B). The 78K polypeptide was phosphorylated. The Scl-A and Scl-B proteins were not associated with RNA as shown by ^{32}P-RNA analysis of the phenol-extracted immunoprecipitates in 7M urea 8% polyacrylamide gels. Deproteinized RNA was not a target of the antinucleolar sera investigated.

Anti-Scl-A and anti-Scl-B antibodies were only detected in antinucleolar scleroderma sera and found to be associated with diffuse scleroderma.

116

IDENTIFICATION OF THE RIBOSOMAL PROTEIN ANTIGENS IN SYSTEMIC LUPUS ERYTHEMATOSUS (SLE). K. B. Elkon, C. L. Foster, A. P. Parnassa. Hospital for Special Surgery, New York, NY.

Antinuclear antibodies are regarded as the hallmark of SLE whereas autoantibodies to cytoplasmic constituents have received far less attention. Antiribosomal antibodies (ARA) have been reported to occur in 1-70% of patients with SLE and the question as to whether the RNA or protein moieties are antigenic is also controversial. To precisely define the specificity of ARA, dog and rat ribosomes were isolated by homogenization, differential centrifugation and discontinuous sucrose density ultracentrifugation. Ribosomes and their subunits were analyzed by fractionation on a 15-30% sucrose gradient and by composite gel electrophoresis. The molecular weight and charge characteristics of the ribosomal antigens were determined by one- and two-dimensional gel electrophoresis followed by Western blotting. CM cellulose chromatography and NH_4Cl ethanol extraction studies were also performed.

ARA reacted with ribosomal proteins of approximately 38 (major) and 18/19 (minor) Kd from the large subunit. The antigens were acidic and were distinguishable from the other soluble major antigens Ro, La, Sm, RNP and Jo-1. The protein antigens were identified as Po, P1 and P2 on the basis of their size and charge and behavior on CM cellulose and NH_4Cl-ethanol. These proteins function in the elongation step of protein translation. The selective production of antibodies to these 3 (of 80 ribosomal proteins) may be relevant to the genesis of autoantibodies in SLE.

117

HISTONE EPITOPES BINDING ANTIBODIES FROM DRUG-INDUCED AND IDIOPATHIC SYSTEMIC LUPUS ERYTHEMATOSUS. J. GOHILL, M.J. FRITZLER, Calgary, CANADA, C. CRANE-ROBINSON, Portsmouth, ENGLAND.

We studied the epitopes on histones reacting with drug-induced lupus (DIL) and systemic lupus erythematosus (SLE) sera. Core histone limit peptides were produced by treating chicken erythrocyte nuclei with 25U/ml trypsin for 25 min at 37°C, extracted with 0.2M sulfuric acid and separated by HPLC. Four polypeptides purified in this manner were identified as amino acids 12-118 of H2A, 21-125 of H2B, 27-129 of H3 and 20-102 of H4. Thus, trypsin cleavage removed the amino (N) terminus of all core histones and the carboxyl (C) terminus of H2A and H3. The sera of 10 DIL, SLE and controls were tested by ELISA using intact and limit peptides. The results are average OD at 405 nm:

	Intact Histone				Limit Peptides			
	H2A	H2B	H3	H4	H2A	H2B	H3	H4
SLE	.98	1.26	.93	.85	.28	.29	.33	.23
DIL	.97	1.29	.55	.47	.23	.49	.16	.16
CONTROL	.12	.20	.11	.14	.10	.11	.07	.18

9/10 SLE and 9/10 DIL sera showed highest reactivity with intact histones while reactivity with limit peptides was near control values. This suggested that the antigenic epitope reacting with most DIL and SLE sera was in the N and/or the C terminus of histone cleaved by trypsin. This was confirmed by chemically and enzymatically prepared peptides that contained the C and N terminus and testing them for reactivity by ELISA and immunoblotting and finding that 9/10 sera from each group reacted with the N and/or C terminus. Therefore the epitope of histones reacting with both groups of sera are found in the C and/or the N terminus and the reactivity of DIL antibodies with these epitopes are no less restricted than those from SLE.

118

CROSS-REACTIVITY OF MONOCLONAL NZB ANTI-MOUSE ERYTHROCYTE ANTIBODIES WITH NON-ERYTHROCYTE AUTOANTIGENS. Barry S. Handwerger, Nancy L. Meryhew, James M. Peterson, Kenji Tani, John B. Harley, Dennis A. Gastineau and Ronald P. Messner. Mayo Clinic, Rochester, MN, University of Minnesota, Minneapolis, MN and Oklahoma Medical Research Foundation, Oklahoma City, OK.

NZB mice develop a lupus-like illness characterized primarily by autoimmune hemolytic anemia (AIHA). As previously reported, we have produced a panel of monoclonal NZB anti-mouse erythrocyte antibodies (mono-aRBC) which recognize several distinct epitopes present on intact mRBC and differ in their ability to mediate AIHA in BALB/c mice and to fix complement from several animal species. To further characterize the specificity of these mono-aRBC, three mono-aRBC were affinity purified and tested for cross-reactivity with several non-RBC autoantigens. Mono-aRBC # 20, 114 and 245 all reacted with cardiolipin in a solid phase ELISA assay. Furthermore, cardiolipin but not phosphytidylglycerol or phosphytidylethanolamine, inhibited the binding of the antibodies to mRBC in an indirect RIA. Mono-aRBC # 20 and 114 had strong and # 245 mild lupus anti-coagulant activity, measured by prolongation of the recalcified platelet-rich plasma clot time. Mono-aRBC #20, but not #114 or 245, reacted strongly with several different preparations of affinity-purified nuclear RNP (Sm). None of the mono-aRBC had anti-lymphocyte, anti-thymocyte or anti-DNA activity or gave a positive FANA with mouse liver substrate. These data demonstrate that NZB mono-aRBC cross-react with several non-RBC autoantigens, and support the concept that the autoantibody repertoire in SLE may be less complex than previously appreciated.

119

AN IDIOTYPIC INTERACTION BETWEEN RHEUMATOID FACTOR AND ANTI-PEPTIDOGLYCAN ANTIBODIES? Peter M. Johnson, Kia-Kien Phua, and Helen B. Evans. Dept. of Immunology, University of Liverpool, UK.

There is known to be an association between bacterial (notably streptococcal) infections and RF production. Furthermore, IgG antibodies reactive with Gram-positive bacterial cell wall peptidoglycan-polysaccharide (PG-PS) polymer are found at elevated levels in human RA. We have investigated the relationship between RF and anti-PG-PS antibody by repeated immunization of groups of Balb/c mice with separate sterile affinity-purified polyclonal RF preparations from five high-titre seropositive RA sera. In all cases, there was a substantial anti-PG-PS antibody response detectable by both immunodiffusion and ELISA against Str. pyogenes PG-PS. This antibody could be absorbed by excess PG-PS or RF, but not by isolated human non-RF IgG or IgM preparations. Groups of mice similarly immunized with non-RF IgG (n=3) or IgM (n=2) preparations produced no significant anti-PG-PS response compared with pre-immune sera (p>0.05), unlike RF-immunized animals (p<0.001). All immunogens lacked detectable PG-PS. Thus, anti-PG-PS antibody may be produced by RF immunization (in the absence of PG-PS), and it appears that RF carries the internal image of a streptococcal PG-PS epitope.

This work suggests some idiotypic complementarity between RF and anti-PG-PS antibodies, and that RF cross-reacts both with an anti-PG-PS idiotype as well as an IgG-Fc isotypic determinant. Thus, RF may react as an immunoregulatory auto-anti-idiotype against certain anti-bacterial antibodies, and uncontrolled RF production would represent an imbalance in this system.

120

EXPRESSION DEFECTS OF MUTANT HUMAN ADENOSINE DEAMINASE. PETER E. DADDONA, Ann Arbor, STEWART H. ORKIN, Boston, WILLIAM N. KELLEY, Ann Arbor.

A severe deficiency of adenosine deaminase (ADA) is associated with an autosomal recessive form of severe combined immunodeficiency disease, while subjects with partial enzyme activity are immunocompetent. To further our understanding of this enzyme deficiency, specific ADA mRNA levels and rates of protein turnover were determined in cells from subjects with partial ADA deficiency and enzyme expression of cloned human ADA cDNA was assessed. Genetic expression of ADA in cultured B lymphoblast cell lines from 4 partially (5-50% activity) ADA deficient subjects showed normal to 2-fold normal ADA mRNA levels (Northern blot). Among these cell lines enzyme synthesis varied from 165% to 15% of normal. ADA degradation rates were 1.5 to almost 3 times faster than normal, consistent with the complete absence of the enzyme in patient erythrocytes. From these analyzes apparent abnormalities in mRNA regulation, translation and protein degradation can be identified to explain the steady state enzyme level expressed in these partially ADA deficient cell lines. Cloned normal human ADA cDNA inserted into an SV_{40} based expression vector was shown to generate human ADA activity in monkey kidney (COS) host cells (7-fold over host). An unexpected finding was the identification of another normal human ADA cDNA construct which failed to produce human ADA activity or immunoreactive protein upon transfection. DNA sequence analysis revealed a single nucleotide substitution within this clone that altered the predicted sequence of ADA protein at amino acid 50. This mutation, caused by a cloning artifact, defines one critical region of the human ADA protein.

Thus, our studies define transcriptional, translational and post-translational defects in partial ADA deficiency and identify a point mutation in ADA cDNA which mimics the phenotype expressed in severe ADA deficiency.

121

UI RNP SECONDARY STRUCTURE DETERMINED BY LOCALIZATION OF ANTIGENIC SITES. Paul F. Agris, Andra Boak, Shirley Kovacs, and Theodore Munns, University of Missouri, Columbia, MO. 65211 and Washington University, St. Louis. 63110.

UI RNP has been shown to be involved in mRNA processing by its removal from in vitro processing systems with addition of the autoimmune antibodies RNP or Sm. We had previously shown that the two antigenic determinants for these antibodies are conferred by different peptides and are both part of the UI RNP complex. We had also shown the structural relationship between nucleotides 40-90, of the 165 nucleotide UI RNA, and the protein antigenic determinant for RNP antibody. Others demonstrated the localization of the Sm determinant at the 3' terminal nucleotide sequence. We have now defined by two independent methods the structural positions of these antigenic determinants relative to each other and two other structural positions. A newly recognized autoimmune antibody, Me, defines the third locale; and antibody directed against m^7G defines the fourth position, that of the 5'-cap of UI RNA within the complex. This approach has demonstrated the closeness of the Me and Sm peptides at the 3'-terminus of the RNA with each other and the 5'-cap, and the distance of the RNP determinant. A two dimensional picture of UI RNA and UI RNP peptides results. (Supported by NIH AM 20305)

122

A MOLECULAR SURVEY OF HPRT DEFICIENCY. BEVERLY J. DAVIDSON, THOMAS D. PALELLA, JAMES M. WILSON, PETER E. DADDONA, TIMOTHY O'TOOLE, WILLIAM N. KELLEY, Ann Arbor.

Virtually complete deficiency of hypoxanthine phosphoribosyltransferase (HPRT) results in the Lesch-Nyhan syndrome. Partial deficiency of HPRT results in gout. We have previously sequenced the normal enzyme and documented the amino acid substitution in four mutant forms of the enzyme. We have undertaken a molecular genetic survey of cell lines derived from HPRT-deficient patients in order to define specific mutations for which protein sequencing is impractical or impossible. Lymphoblasts derived from 17 patients deficient in HPRT (9 with the Lesch-Nyhan syndrome; 8 with partial HPRT deficiency) were studied. Restriction mapping employing the Southern blot technique has been performed with several common restriction enzymes (Pst I, Bgl II, Bam HI, Hpa II and Eco RI). No abnormal restriction patterns were found. Northern blot analysis of mRNA derived from these cell lines were used to determine the molecular size and relative concentrations of message. Three cell lines had no detectable HPRT mRNA. In the remaining cell lines, all but one exhibited normal molecular size (1.6 Kb); the exception had a molecular weight of 1.8 Kb. Relative concentrations of mRNA ranged from slightly diminished in 3, normal in 11 and increased in 3. To more completely define the molecular abnormality, we have generated a cDNA library derived from mRNA obtained from one patient's cultured B-lymphoblasts. From this library, a mutant HPRT cDNA was cloned. This cDNA is 1200 base pairs in length and has restriction maps with Hae III, Hinc II and Hind III identical to normal HPRT-cDNA. This approach provides a direct method for defining the mutation in all $mRNA^+$ $HPRT^-$ subjects. From this survey we conclude that analysis of mutant HPRT at the DNA and mRNA level provides a powerful tool to define specific mutations.

123

A NEW MOLECULAR DEFECT ASSOCIATED WITH HEREDITARY AMYLOIDOSIS. M Benson and FE Dwulet, VAMC and Indiana University, Indianapolis, Indiana 46223

Familial amyloidotic polyneuropathy (FAP) type II (Indiana-Swiss) differs from FAP type I by its association with carpal tunnel syndrome, prominent cardiomyopathy and lack of significant renal amyloidosis. Recently it has been shown that both FAP type I and type II are associated with depressed serum prealbumin levels but only in FAP type II are retinol binding protein (RBP) levels also depressed. These differences suggest different molecular defects in plasma prealbumin which is the subunit protein for all dominant hereditary amyloids described to date. To identify this presumed molecular defect the amino acid sequence of FAP type II amyloid protein was determined.

Amyloid fibrils were isolated from cardiac tissue of a 61 yr. old man with FAP type II. Reduction and alkylation in 6M guanidine and fractionation on Sepharose CL6B gave several retarded peaks; the smallest having a molecular weight of 14,000. Sequence analysis of tryptic peptides of this protein proved its homology with prealbumin but revealed both threonine and glycine at position 49 of the 127 amino acid residue molecule. A search for glycine at position 49 in plasma prealbumin of patients in this family, however, failed to show any glycine at this position. Complete sequencing of both the amyloid subunit protein and plasma prealbumin revealed a significant amount of prealbumin with a serine substitution for isoleucine at position 84 of the molecule. This substitution has not been reported before. It is hypothesized that this region of the molecule is involved in the binding of RBP and can explain the variations in plasma RBP levels that distinguish FAP type II from type I. In addition, this amino acid substitution may be the inherited factor that determines FAP type II fibril formation.

124

IMMUNOHISTOCHEMICAL ANALYSIS OF CARTILAGE PROTEOGLYCAN MONOMER IN EXPERIMENTAL OSTEOARTHRITIS. Roland W. Moskowitz and Thomas F. Kresina. Case Western Reserve University, Cleveland, OH 44106.

Monoclonal antibodies specific for unique epitopes on proteoglycan (PG) molecules were utilized to analyze cartilage PG structure in experimental osteoarthritis (OA).

Methods. Femoral/tibial cartilage sections from nonoperated, 6-wk sham operated, and 6-wk partial meniscectomy rabbits were separately incubated with fluorescein-conjugated normal mouse IgG, and monoclonal antibodies 2G2, 2E9, and 6C9. The monoclonals were generated on fusion of splenic cells from rabbit xiphoid process PG monomer (A1D1D1). PG epitope specificity was determined utilizing competitive inhibition of DEAE cellulose-resolved tryptic PG fragments with A1D1D1 in solid phase radioimmunoassay, and uronic acid and amino acid analysis of tryptic fragments. 2G2 recognizes a recurrent eiptope on native PG; 2E9 a private single native protein epitope; and 6C9 a recurring epitope on denatured (50°C, 30 min) PG monomer.

Results. In normal and sham-operated animals, 2G2 and 2E9 stain cellular/pericellular (C/PC) and matrix (M) areas; 6C9 stains only C/PC. Augmented C/P and M staining of femoral (but not tibial) OA cartilage occurred with 2G2 and 6C9; increased 2E9 stain was seen in C/P regions.

Conclusions. Monoclonal antibodies allow study of PG localization in normal and OA cartilage. Quantitative and qualitative differences in staining patterns were observed; these differences seen in OA may represent a switch to a new PG gene product, or unmasking of PG epitopes. [AM30134 (NIH), AM20618 (NIH), and Revco Arth Res Ctr.]

125

BIOCHEMICAL PURIFICATION OF PROLIFERATING CELL NUCLEAR ANTIGEN (PCNA) AND ITS USE IN AN ELISA ASSAY. T.S. LIEU, R.D. SONTHEIMER and E.M. TAN. Depts. of Dermatology, UTHSCD, Dallas, Tx and Scripps Research Institute, La Jolla, Ca.

Autoantibodies to PCNA can be detected by immunodiffusion in 5% of systemic lupus erythematosus sera. Since the biochemical characteristics of this soluble nuclear antigen found only in rapidly dividing cells have not been fully determined, we devised a simple scheme to purify PCNA from rabbit thymus extract. The antigenic activity of PCNA was separated from U1-RNP and Sm activities by sequential ammonium sulfate precipitation. The U1-RNP and Sm antigenic activities were precipitated in the 33-60% saturated ammonium sulfate fraction whereas PCNA activity remained in the supernatant. The 60-80% saturated ammonium sulfate fraction of rabbit thymus extract contained both SS-B/La and PCNA antigenic activities. In polybuffer ion exchange column chromatography, the SS-B/La antigenic activity was eluted by 0.1 M and 0.2 M NaCl whereas PCNA activity was recovered in the 0.5M and 1M NaCl eluate. In SDS gel electrophoresis, the 0.5M NaCl eluate contained one major 35,000 molecular weight component and two minor bands with molecular weights of 70,000 and 19,000. The result of Western Blot analysis indicated that all of the PCNA antigenic activity was contained in the 35,000 molecular weight component. The isoelectric point of PCNA was found to be 4.88 as determined by electrofocusing in polyacrylamide gel. In an enzyme linked immunoabsorbent assay (ELISA) the purified PCNA antigen reacted with immunodiffusion defined monospecific anti-PCNA sera but not with monospecific anti-Sm, anti-SS-A/Ro, anti-SS-B/La, anti-U1-RNP or normal serum.

126

REGULATION OF COLLAGEN FIBRIL FORMATION. Raul Fleischmajer, Jerome S. Perlish, Bjorn Olsen, Rupert Timpl. Mount Sinai School of Medicine, New York, NY 10029; Rutgers Medical School, Piscataway, NJ 08854; Max Planck Inst. fur Biochemie, Munich, West Germany.

Collagen is synthesized in a precursor form known as procollagen with extension propeptides at the amino and carboxy ends. "In vivo" and "in vitro" studies suggested that the amino propeptide (AP) and carboxy propeptide (CP) may regulate collagen fibril diameter. Human skin from embryos (18-24 weeks old) and adults were studied by immunofluorescence and immunoelectron microscopy and by Western immunoblotting with purified antibodies against the AP of type I and type III procollagens. These antibodies derive from calf procollagens and cross-react with human collagens. The AP of type I procollagen was found in embryonic skin in fibrils up to 35 nm but was absent in adult skin consisting mainly of fibrils 50-100 nm in diameter. The AP of type III procollagen was found in both young (20-30 nm) and mature (40-50 nm) collagen fibrils. Immunoblotting confirmed the presence of the AP of type I procollagen in embryonic skin. However, the AP of type III procollagen was present in both embryonic and adult skin. Ten day old chick embryo tibia were studied by immunoelectron microscopy with antibodies directed against the AP and CP of type I procollagen. These antibodies were prepared from chick tendons incubated in organ culture. In the periostium, thin fibrils about 20 nm labeled with the AP while thick fibrils 60-80 nm labeled with the CP. Type II collagen did not label. This study gives further support to the hypothesis that the AP and CP participate in collagen fibrillogenesis and may regulate fibril diameter in the extracellular matrix.

127

CARBOHYDRATE HETEROGENEITY OF FIBRONECTINS: IDENTIFICATION OF PLASMA AND SYNOVIAL FORMS BY LECTIN BINDING. S.E.Carsons, B.B. Lavietes, H.S. Diamond, E. Berkowitz. Long Island Jewish Hospital, SUNY Stony Brook, New Hyde Park, N.Y. 11042.

Glycosylation of fibronectin (Fn) affects the protease resistance and solubility properties of the molecule. Fibronectins isolated from different tissues have been shown to have specific oligosaccharide side chain composition. We have compared Fns isolated from human plasma (PFn), rheumatoid synovial fluid (SFFn), and medium of primary rheumatoid synoviocytes (SCFn) by western blotting with labeled lectins and biochemical analysis after hydrolysis to determine differences in carbohydrate composition.

PFn and SFFn both contain 3% neutral hexose; and both show moderate binding to Con A, consistent with the presence of mannose containing biantennary N-asparagine linked side chains. In contrast, while SFFn reacts strongly with WGA, PFn binds weakly. Fn isolated from cultured synoviocytes has a lectin-binding pattern similar to SFFn. Chymotryptic cleavage shows that after release, the carbohydrate rich gelatin-binding domains of SFFn and PFn react equally with WGA and that the site of differential reactivity is located on the Fn C-terminal fragment.

Differences in sialic acid content were also seen among the Fn species. PFn contains 6 mol/monomer; SFFn, 2 mol/monomer and SCFn, no detectable sialic acid.

Carbohydrate analysis reveals major differences between PFn and SFFn. The sugar composition of RASFFn more closely resembles that of SCFn than that of PFn providing further evidence for the synovial origin of SFFn. Differences in Fn glycosylation may affect the protease sensitivity and function of Fn in the inflamed joint.

128

HLA-DP (SB) ANTIGENS IN PAUCIARTICULAR JRA WITH IRIDOCYCLITIS. R. W. Hoffman, S. Shaw, L. Francis, R.A. Petersen, L.T. Chylack, D.N. Glass. Immunology Branch, NIH, Bethesda, MD 20205, Children's Hospital Medical Center and Brigham and Women's Hospital, Boston, MA 02115

A form of early-onset pauciarticular JRA with chronic iridocyclitis has been shown to be associated with the HLA antigens HLA-DR5, DRw8, Bw35, Bw44, Cw4. We have typed thirty North American Caucasian patients (29 female, 1 male) by primed lymphocyte typing (PLT) for HLA-DPw (SB) 1-6, the most centromeric of the HLA-D region polymorphisms. We found that there was an increased frequency of DPw2 antigen in patients (20/30, 67%; $p<0.036$, RR=2.1) compared to controls (67/210, 32%). Furthermore a T cell clone was identified whose reactivity was closely related to DPw2 but was even more closely associated with the disease (25/30 patients react with the clone) than with the two DPw2-specific PLT bulk T cell populations.

Previous studies have identified pauciarticular JRA "high risk" haplotypes Cw4/Bw35/DR5, Cw4/Bw44/DR5 and DRw8. The increase in DPw2 frequency in patients appears not to be due to its linkage disequilibrium with these haplotypes since: 1) in the patients there was no positive association between DRw8 or DR5 and DPw2, 2) there was no increased frequency of DPw2 among the DR5 positive controls.

This is the first report of a rheumatic disease associated with a HLA-DP region polymorphism. These results suggest that the DPw2 antigen may be a new marker of a HLA-linked disease susceptibility gene. Family studies are in progress to establish the genetics of the HLA-DP in these patients.

129

IMMUNOGLOBULIN VARIABLE REGION GENE ARRANGEMENTS IN ANTI-NUCLEAR ANTIBODIES. S.H.Pincus, F.M.Ebling, B.H.Hahn, D.S.Pisetsky, and J.R. Ward, University of Utah, Salt Lake City, UT 84132, University of Calif. Los Angeles, CA 90024, and Durham VA Hospital,Durham NC 27705.

We have used Southern DNA hybridization to study immunoglobulin variable (V)-region gene arrangements in 19 hybridoma cell lines secreting monoclonal anti-nuclear antibodies. Data from such analyses are informative regarding the V and joining (J) genes that encode the antibody combining site.

Antibodies analyzed were specific for single stranded DNA, double stranded DNA, and Sm antigen, and derive from the following mouse strains: MRL/lpr, BXSB, and NZB/NZW F1. DNA was extracted from the cell lines and cut with a restriction enzyme, either EcoRI or HindIII. It was size separated and blotted onto a solid support. The DNA was hybridized with radiolabelled kappa or heavy chain J-gene probes. Heavy chain analysis reveals several common arrangements in different hybridomas. The similarity of these arrangements was confirmed using both enzymes. The most common arrangement seen among anti-DNA hybridomas has the V-region genes on an EcoRI fragment of 4.4-5.2 Kb, and a 15Kb HindIII fragment. This probably represents the use of the same V-gene with different J-genes. All antibodies expressing the public idiotype BWds1 use this arrangement. However, some anti-DNA antibodies use a distinctly different gene arrangement, implying the use of different V-genes. Surprisingly, the anti-Sm antibodies seem to use arrangements similar to those used by the majority of the anti-DNA antibodies. These results suggest that the same or similar heavy chain V and J-genes encode many spontaneously arising anti-nuclear antibodies.

130

SELECTIVE INHIBITION OF EXCESSIVE PROGRESSIVE SYSTEMIC SCLEROSIS (PSS) FIBROBLAST COLLAGEN SYNTHESIS BY RECOMBINANT γ-INTERFERON (rec. γ-IFN). Sergio A. Jimenez, Bruce Freundlich and Joel Rosenbloom. Univ. of Pennsylvania, Philadelphia, Pennsylvania, 19104

Excessive deposition of collagen in the skin and various internal organs is a characteristic feature of PSS and is responsible for many of the clinical manifestations of the disease. Increased collagen synthesis by PSS fibroblasts appears to be the most likely mechanism responsible for this abnormality. At present there is no adequate therapy to control the progressive fibrotic process in PSS. It has recently been shown that rec. γ-IFN is a potent and selective inhibitor of collagen synthesis by normal human dermal fibroblasts. The inhibition of fibroblast collagen synthesis by rec. γ-IFN was apparently due to a decrease in specific collagen mRNA levels as determined employing Type I collagen cDNA probes. The present study was performed to determine if rec. γ-IFN could similarly modulate the excessive collagen biosynthesis characteristic of PSS fibroblasts. For this purpose the effect of various concentrations of rec. γ-IFN on collagen production by confluent cultures of PSS dermal fibroblasts was examined employing biosynthetic methods. Five cell lines obtained from patients with early onset, rapidly progressive systemic disease were studied. All PSS cell lines exhibited increased collagen production ranging from 60 to 160% when compared to control cells. Rec. γ-IFN caused marked inhibition of collagen production in each of the PSS cell lines tested in a dose dependent manner. These effects were selective for collagen since the synthesis of non-collagenous proteins was not significantly affected. The results indicate that rec. γ-IFN can modulate the excessive collagen biosynthesis characteristic of PSS fibroblasts and may have a place as a possible therapeutic agent for this incurable disease.

131

CHILDHOOD LYME ARTHRITIS: EXPERIENCE IN AN ENDEMIC AREA. A.H. Eichenfield, D.P. Goldsmith, F.X. Loeb, A.H. Ross, B.H. Athreya. Children's Seashore House; St. Chris. Hosp. Child., Philadelphia, PA; SUNY-Stony Brook, NY.

Arthritis following erythema chronicum migrans (ECM) is part of a well described illness which may also affect the nervous and cardiovascular systems. In the absence of a history of rash, cardiac or neurologic disease, however, identification of Lyme disease may be difficult. We report 25 children with oligoarticular arthritis seen between 8/83 and 12/84 with Lyme disease documented by immunofluorescent (IFA) and ELISA assays.

There were 16 boys and 9 girls (M:F 1.8:1), ages 2-15 years. Thirteen children (52%) had no history of ECM or other rash. Thirteen had fevers as high as 105°F up to 2 months before onset of arthritis. Twelve recalled definite tick bites and all live in deer tick-infested areas.

Ten children (40%), of whom 7 had no history of rash, were hospitalized for presumed septic arthritis (knee-9, hip-1). Another 7 patients had less acute, recurrent episodes. Four children carried diagnoses of pauciarticular JRA for as long as 3 years. Two children suffered Bell's palsy 2 months before onset of arthritis.

All patients showed antibodies to the Lyme spirochete by IFA with IgG titers from 1:128 to >1:2048. In 19, IgM titers ranged from 1:16 to 1:256. ELISA was positive in 11/11 patients. In 12 patients, synovial fluid WBC counts ranged from 180 to 97,700/mm^3 (>65% polymorphs). ESR was elevated in 16 cases (range 6-171 mm/hr). ANA was transiently positive in 5 children in titers as high as 1:320. One child had a low-titer RF; 3/10 patients had elevated serum IgM; 1/5 had an IgM cryoglobulin.

In endemic areas Lyme disease is now being recognized as a more common cause of oligoarticular arthritis. Its initial presentation may be confused with acute septic arthritis or recurrent pauciarticular JRA, particularly when there is no characteristic rash.

132

DIFFERENTIAL IN VIVO BINDING OF SPECIFIC LUPUS SERA IN HUMAN SKIN. LA Lee, WL Weston, JO Stevens, GG Krueger, M Emam, DA Norris. Univ. of Colorado, Denver, CO 80262, and Univ. of Utah, Salt Lake City, UT 84112.

Antibodies to the SSA/Ro antigen are found in 80% and 98% of patients, respectively, with subacute cutaneous lupus (SCLE) and neonatal lupus (NLE). Though SSA antigen has been demonstrated in and on keratinocytes, it is not known if antibodies to SSA are directly related to the diseases. We have shown in an animal model, the nude mouse with grafted human skin, that intravenous (IV) injection of anti-SSA serum results in granular deposits of IgG in human skin at the dermal-epidermal (D-E) junction and on basal keratinocytes, and that this deposition is augmented by ultraviolet light (UVL). To determine if IgG binding to basal keratinocytes is specific for certain lupus sera in this model, we compared anti-SSA specific sera from 3 SCLE/NLE patients to sera from 5 SLE patients without skin disease who had comparable titers of autoantibodies, either to native DNA (nDNA) or to Sm. Animals received 0.3cc serum IV and biopsies were taken 24 hours later. In all 10 animals injected with anti-SSA sera, there was granular IgG on basal keratinocytes in the graft. In none of the 7 animals injected with anti-SSA negative SLE sera was there deposition of IgG at the epidermis or D-E junction, even after a minimal erythema dose (MED) of UVL.

We conclude that there is specific binding of anti-SSA antibodies to SSA antigen in situ: (1) IgG from anti-SSA sera was found in human skin, which contains SSA antigen, but not in mouse skin, which does not; (2) binding of IgG to skin did not occur with anti-nDNA or -Sm SLE sera, even after UVL. The IgG deposition with anti-SSA sera occurs on the basal keratinocyte, where cellular injury is seen in histologic exam of lupus lesions, and the pattern of deposition in the animal model reproduces the pattern observed in SCLE and NLE patients' lesions. Specific antibody binding in situ to basal keratinocytes may be directly related to the development of SCLE and NLE lesions.

133

MAGNETIC RESONANCE IMAGING (MRI) AS A DIAGNOSTIC TOOL IN ISCHEMIC NECROSIS OF THE FEMORAL HEAD IN PATIENTS RECEIVING GLUCOCORTICOIDS (GC). K. Kalunian, B. Hahn, and L. Bassett, UCLA, Los Angeles, CA 90024

Preliminary observations at our institution suggested that MRI had better sensitivity and specificity for ischemic necrosis of bone (INB) in femoral heads than did standard x-ray or scanning techniques. Therefore, 7 patients receiving GC therapy for various disorders who had recently developed new hip pain received a) standard radiographs of both hips, b) technetium diphosphonate (TcDP) bone scans, c) technetium sulfur colloid (TcSC) scans, and d) MRI of the pelvis and hips. Identical studies were done in 5 patients with no history of GC therapy but recent onset of new hip pain.

In the patients receiving GC, INB was proven to exist in 8 of 14 femoral heads by a) Stage II or greater radiographic changes either initially or in follow-up, and/or b) INB on biopsy of the femoral head(s). There was no evidence of INB initially or on follow-up in the 10 control hips. In the 8 hips where INB was present, only 3 were associated with abnormal x-rays initially or on follow-up, 4 had positive TcDP scans, 1 had a positive TcSC scan, and all had positive MRI. In the 10 control hips, 2 had positive TcDP scans and all other tests including MRI were negative.

By chi square testing, MRI was significantly more sensitive than each of the other techniques at p .05 or better. Overally, 10 of 32 observations using non-MRI techniques were positive for INB when it was present, versus 8 of 8 observations by MRI(χ^2=12.2, p .02). In this small study, MRI seemed to be specific for INB.

MRI was significantly more sensitive in GC treated patients than routine techniques in detecting INB of the femoral heads, including those with Stage I x-rays(6 of the 8).

134

PERIPHERAL INFLAMMATORY VASCULAR DISEASE (IVD) IN SJOGREN'S SYNDROME (SS): ASSOCIATION WITH NERVOUS SYSTEM COMPLICATIONS. RODOLFO MOLINA, THOMAS T. PROVOST, ELAINE L. ALEXANDER. Johns Hopkins Medical Institutions, Baltimore, MD.

Two histopathologic types of peripheral inflammatory vascular disease (IVD) have been described in SS: neutrophilic (NIVD) and mononuclear (MIVD). 50 SS patients with and 50 without biopsy documented IVD were examined for nervous system disease (NSD). A total of 54 biopsies were performed (skin 46, muscle 4, peripheral nerve 4). Histopathologically, 30 patients had NIVD and 20 MIVD. Cutaneous manifestations included purpura, chronic urticaria, or erythematous lesions and were identical for both types of IVD. 33 (66%) SS patients with IVD had NSD [peripheral (PNS) or central (CNS)] unattributable to other causes, in contrast to 10 (20%) SS patents without IVD (p = 0.0026). CNS disease occurred in 24 patients (brain 21, spinal cord 5) and were often multifocal and recurrent over time. PNS disease occurred in 28 patients: peripheral neuropathy 17, carpal tunnel syndrome 10, cranial neuropathy 3, autonomic neuropathy 2. Patients with IVD of both types were at equal risk for the development of NSD [NIVD, 17/30 (57%); MIVD 16/20 (80%)]. Retrospective analysis of the therapeutic response to corticosteroid therapy showed improvement or stabilization of cutaneous IVD in 23 of 37 (63%) and CNS disease in 13 of 24 (54%) patients. The concomitant presence of peripheral IVD and active NSD and their response to therapy suggest that, at least in a subset of SS patients, IVD may play a role in the immunopathogenesis of NSD. Furthermore, the observations that both histopathologic types of IVD can give rise to similar cutaneous vasculitic lesions and are associated with serious NSD implicates MIVD, as well as the well recognized NIVD (leukocytoclastic vasculitis), in the pathogenesis of vascular damage.

135

FACTORS RESPONSIBLE FOR FORMATION OF SYNOVIAL-LIKE MEMBRANE AFTER TOTAL HIP REPLACEMENT (THR); ITS ROLE IN PROSTHESIS LOOSENING. Steven R. Goldring, Murali Jasty, Merrilee Roelke, Carolyn M. Rourke, and William H. Harris. Department of Medicine and Orthopaedic Surgery, Harvard Medical School, Massachusetts General Hospital, and the New England Deaconess Hospital, Boston, MA 02114.

We previously reported that the tissue obtained from the bone cement interface (BCT) from loosened THRs is organized into a synovial-like membrane. Conditioned medium from this tissue releases high levels of PGE_2 and induces bone resorption in vitro. To investigate mechanisms responsible for the synovial transformation, we compared the histological features of the BCT in revision THR in which one component was fixed and the other loosened (22 fixed and 106 loosened). In membranes from loosened components, in addition to the synovial-like membrane, the tissue was heavily infiltrated with particulate methylmethacrylate (MM) or polyethylene (PE) associated with a giant cell/histiocyte reaction. Tissue from THRs using only PE or MM in the initial implant, was similar suggesting that either PE or MM in particulate form could induce inflammatory responses. In contrast to the membranes from loosened components, no synovial-like lining was present in tissue associated with rigidly fixed components. The membrane was predominantly fibrous with rare histiocytes without particulate PE or MM. Mean levels of PGE_2 released from tissue cultured from loosened components were 3x greater than that from non-loosened [mean PGE_2, loose = 62.5 ng/ml (range 17.7 - 136.0) and mean, non-loose = 20.5 (range 2.7 - 58.3)]. Synovial-like transformation does not occur in the absence of loosening. Release of particulate MM or PE wear debris are likely important in the pathogenesis of the bone resorption which accompanies loosening.

136

LONG-TERM OUTCOME IN TOTAL LYMPHOID IRRADIATION (TLI) AND IMMUNOSUPPRESSIVE (IS) DRUG TREATED PATIENTS WITH INTRACTABLE RHEUMATOID ARTHRITIS (RA). Y. Sherrer, D. Bloch, & J. Fries, Stanford University, Stanford, CA 94305

Outcomes were compared between consecutive patients who had received either TLI or IS for the treatment of intractable RA. At our center there were 33 standard TLI recipients and 32 IS recipients between 1972 and 1983. Patients received these treatments if they had severe disease and had failed standard therapy. Average follow-up from the start of therapy was 2.7 years for TLI and 5.9 years for IS.

	Initial [Avg. ±SE(n)]		Follow-Up (proportion with outcome)		
	TLI	IS		TLI	IS
Age	53±2 (33)	50±2 (32)	Deaths	4/33	2/30
Duration	13±1 (33)	11±2 (32)	Leukopenia	9/33	3/28
ESR	59±7 (23)	57±6 (15)	Infectious Hosp.	10/32	1/25
PCV	36±.9(32)	38±.9(21)	Herpes	7/32	0/25
Log latex	3.1±.2(31)	3.1±.2(10)			

Average disability (HAQ) was 2.1 for both TLI and the IS group in follow-up. TLI patients were older and had greater average disease duration and severity. Thirteen TLI patients had no prior IS therapy; their average disability at follow-up was 2.1 as well. Definite infections requiring hospitalizations were more common after TLI. 22 of 33 TLI and 12 of 18 IS recipients required additional remittive therapy or high dose steroids. There has been only one possible infectious death in our TLI group after 80 patient years of follow-up. Continuing long-term follow-up of these cohorts will help establish relative efficacy and toxicity.

137

CYCLOSPORINE IN RHEUMATOID ARTHRITIS. Maxime Dougados, Bernard Amor. Paris. FRANCE.

The efficacy and the tolerance of cyclosporine (CyA) in severe rheumatoid arthritis (R.A.) were evaluated in 2 open trials. Statistical analysis was performed upon the changes in the clinical statues. The first trial : 6 patients (pts) used CyA 8.5 mg/kg/day. Clinical statement improved at day 15 with a reduction of morning stiffness (-100± 72 mns p<0.02), number of swollen joints (-2.0±1.9 p<0.05), Ritchie Index (I.) (-6.8±3.0 p<0.01), sedimentation rate (-17.0±13.3 mms p< 0.05). The second trial (12 pts) used CyA 5 mg/kg/day. Clinical statement was not modified at day 15 but improved at day 30 and overall at day 60 with a reduction of morning stiffness (-48.6±56.4 mns p<0.02) pain (-15.6±16.0 mms p<0.01), number of swollen joints (-3.2±3.5 p<0.02), Lee I. (-4.5±2.4 p<0.001), proximal interphalangeal circumference (-12.3±10.1 mms p<0.01). Five pts dropped out of the first trial : one death at the 3th month from myocardial infarction ; thrombocytopenia at the 3th month (1 pt) ; hypertension and temporary renal insufficiency at the 2th month (1 pt) ; fatigue and weight loss at the 2th month (1 pt), hypertension at the 2th month (1 pt). Two pts dropped out of the second trial : thrombocytopenia at the 3th month (1 pt), dyspepsia (1 pt). Other side effects occured in these trials (dyspepsia, hirsutism, gengivitis, paresthesias, tremor) but were less frequent and severe in the second trial. No side effect occured in 4 pts in the second trial. The mean maintenance daily dose of CyA at day 60 was 7.8±2.1 mg/kg in the first trial and 5.5±2.6 mg/kg in the second. These data suggest that : 1) CyA is an effective treatment of R.A. 2) the drug efficiency onset seems to be dose related. 3) side effects are frequent, might be severe and seem also to be dose related.

138

TOXICITY TO METHOTREXATE (MTX) IN RHEUMATOID ARTHRITIS (RA): CLINICAL AND HLA STUDIES. G.S. Alarcón, J.M. Guyton, R.T. Acton, B.O. Barger, and W.J. Koopman. University of Alabama at Birmingham, B'ham., AL 35294.

Only in the last few years has MTX become an acceptable form of remittive treatment in RA pts who had either failed or developed toxicity to other agents. Its toxic potential, however, has been less emphasized. We have thus reviewed the experience with MTX in the treatment of RA in a tertiary care facility. Seventy-two RA pts (classical or definite RA by ARA criteria) had been treated with pulse weekly po MTX (range dose 2.5-12.5 mg) with a mean follow-up of 1 year (range 1 mo - 3 yrs). Mean age 57.1 y, 66.6%F and 87.5% caucasians (C). Patients were divided into those who did not develop toxicity (NT) (n=19; 26.4%) and those who developed toxicity (n=53;73.6%). Minor toxicity (oral ulcers, transient ↑ in liver enzymes, nausea, vomiting) were present in 46 pts (63.8%), whereas major toxicities (MT) (severe infection, cytopenia, progressive respiratory failure) were present in 7 (9.7%)(2 deaths). Patients with MT differed from those with NT in a shorter disease duration (9.1 ± 2.6 y vs 15.2 ± 7.9 y; P<0.05), increased frequency of extraarticular manifestations (85.7% vs 57.9, P<0.05) and a shorter follow-up (0.56 y vs 1.05 y; P<0.05). Previous toxicity to either gold salts or d-penicillamine did not predict a toxic response to MTX. HLA- A, B, and DR data were available in 29 of 63 C. No significant differences in the distribution of HLA-A or B antigens was found, but DRW 53 was found to be significantly decreased in the NT as compared to those developing a toxic reaction (P=0.006, Relative Risk=0.06). Our study emphasizes: 1) the relatively high frequency of toxicity to MTX, 2) the need for close follow-up to anticipate and/or detect major complications, and 3) the possible protective effect of DR53 in RA pts receiving MTX.

139

RHEUMATOID SYNOVIAL MEMBRANE PRODUCTION OF IMMUNOGLOBULINS AND RHEUMATOID FACTORS IS NOT SUPPRESSED BY LYMPHOID IRRADIATION.

John Hanly, Jaythoon Hassan, Alex Whelan, Con Feighery, Barry Bresnihan
St. Vincent's Hospital and St. James's Hospital, Dublin, Ireland.

Synovial membrane (SM) production of rheumatoid factors (RFs) is believed to be important in the pathogenesis of rheumatoid arthritis (RA). Irradiation of lymph nodes has a measurable effect on intractable rheumatoid synovitis. This study investigated the effect of lymphoid irradiation on SM production of immunoglobulins (Igs) and RFs. Ten patients with intractable RA received 2000 rad to the mantle and inverted Y fields. SM production of Igs and RFs was calculated from a diffusion line based on the linear relationship between the synovial fluid to serum ratios of three proteins, transferrin, caeruloplasmin and alpha 2 macroglobulin, and the log of their molecular weights. IgM, IgG and IgA RFs were measured by ELISA. Before treatment the mean SM production of IgM was 94 iu/ml, and of IgM RF was 97 iu/ml. Up to one year after treatment there was a significant improvement in six of seven standard clinical parameters. However, there was no change in SM production of IgM (112 iu/ml) or IgM RF (86 iu/ml). Similarly, SM production of other Igs and RFs was not suppressed. In addition, in vitro production of IgM RF by blood mononuclear cells, and serum and SF concentrations of Igs and RFs showed no significant change. In conclusion, clinical improvement following lymphoid irradiation was not associated with any measurable effect on Ig or RF production.

140

PULSE METHOTREXATE (MTX) THERAPY FOR INTRACTABLE RHEUMATOID CUTANEOUS ULCERS (RCU) Tiliakos, N. Atlanta, Georgia.

Cutaneous vasculitic ulcers in RA by being associated with widespread vasculitis and intractability, carry appreciable morbidity. Various treatments have been used with unpredictable results and serious complications. In this study, we report our experience with weekly low-dose pulse MTX therapy for intractable RCU. Intractability was defined as failure of RCU healing, despite adequate trial of D-pen, immunosuppressives and local surgical care, including skin-grafting. Our material included 14 successive RCU of 20-14 months duration which were located in legs (11), elbows (2), and sacrum (1) and had repeatedly been debrided, skin-grafted, and treated with antibiotics, St, D-pen, AZ, or CTX, unsuccessfully. The diagnosis of RCU was made by the presence of deep ulcers, in association with either histologic evidence of vasculitis (4pts) or hypocomplementemia with mononeuritis (1pt). The patients had chronic seropositive, nodular RA with interstitial lung disease. Two had SS. Resistant RCU superinfections were developed in 3 pts. Two of them had the immunosuppressive drugs withheld, and, subsequently underwent amputations. (Controls of the standard treatment). The remaining patients were started on MTX at 12-hr-intervals for 3 successive doses, totaling 10-15mg/wk. The synovitis and morning stiffness improved by 60%. ESR and C3-C4 were normalized. The RCU and adjacent leukocytoclastic vasculitic lesions, including one superinfected with pseudomonas, healed completely within 45-100 days. No adverse reactions occurred. In conclusion, low-dose MTX is quite efficacious in treating intractable RCU.

141

HEPATIC HISTOLOGY FOLLOWING PROLONGED TREATMENT OF RHEUMATOID ARTHRITIS WITH BOLUS METHOTREXATE. Julio Aponte, Mary Petrelli.
CASE WESTERN RESERVE UNIVERSITY, FAIRVIEW GENERAL, CLEVELAND METROPOLITAN GENERAL HOSPITALS, Cleveland, OH 44111.

The potential hepatotoxicity of Methotrexate (MTX) has been a source of concern. We are following a large number of Rheumatoid Arthritis (RA) patients who have been taking MTX for extended periods (Clin Res 30:803A, 1982). We investigated liver histopathology in RA patients treated for over ten years with MTX. Patients received 5-15 mg. of MTX administered as a single oral dose (bolus) once a week. All patients were advised not to drink more than 30 cc. of ethanol daily. Of 23 such patients, 20 agreed to a liver biopsy. Minimal cumulative MTX dose was 4,690 mg.

Liver sections stained with H & E and Masson trichrome were graded in a blind manner among other biopsies performed in a clinical setting. None of the biopsies showed cirrhosis. All showed variable degrees of anisonucleosis but only 4 were graded more than 2+. 7/20 showed no other abnormalities. In the remainder, histopathologic changes were mild and included; 5 with hepatic steatosis, 2 with portal fibrosis (1 with steatosis), 2 with non-specific triaditis, 2 with Kupffer cell hyperplasia, 1 with chronic persistent, 1 with non-specific reactive, and 2 with granulomatous hepatitis.

Duration and severity of disease, total cumulative dose, weekly MTX dose, and use of other drugs did not correlate with the degree of hepatocellular changes.

This study indicates that substantial hepatotoxicity must be rare in RA patients treated for extended periods with bolus MTX therapy, and that routine liver biopsies are not necessary in the management of these patients.

142

MALIGNANCY IN CYCLOPHOSPHAMIDE-TREATED RHEUMATOID ARTHRITIS PATIENTS: A LONG-TERM FOLLOWUP STUDY. Gary L. Baker, Leslie E. Kahl, Thomas A. Medsger, Jr., Bertrand L. Stolzer, Carl H. Eisenbeis, Jr., Amrit K. Agarwal. University of Pittsburgh and St.Margaret Memorial Hospital, Pittsburgh, PA 15261

The use of cyclophosphamide (CY) in the treatment of rheumatoid arthritis (RA) is limited by serious side effects, including the potential for malignancy. From 1968-1973, 113 RA patients from one private rheumatology practice were treated with CY after conventional remittive agents had failed. We have completed long-term followup (mean 143 months) on a representative 56 of these patients (CY-RA), as well as 56 RA controls not treated with CY (NCY-RA) matched for age, sex, disease duration, and ARA functional class. Sixteen malignancies developed in 15 (27%) CY-RA patients compared to 7 in 7 (13%) NCY-RA patients ($p < 0.05$). Cancer was found more frequently in both CY-RA and NCY-RA males (40% and 27%, respectively) than in females (22% and 7%). In the CY-RA group 10 (67%) patients had tumors diagnosed 9 or more years after starting CY, whereas in the NCY-RA group the timing of the tumors was more random. CY-RA cancer patients received a mean total dose of 64.8g CY over a mean of 37.3 months, whereas CY-RA patients without cancer received 50.4g over 31.6 months. The only 4 bladder carcinomas occurred in CY-RA patients after 9 years, and after greater mean CY dose and duration compared with all other CY tumor patients. Alcohol use appeared to be more frequent among CY-RA cancer patients than among all other study groups.

We conclude that: 1) RA patients treated with cyclophosphamide have a two-fold increased frequency of malignancy on long-term followup compared with matched controls; and 2) these patients appear to be at high risk for the development of bladder carcinoma.

143

ELBOW SYNOVECTOMY IN RHEUMATOID ARTHRITIS, Clayton Patchett, Box 337, Beaumont, Ca.92223, Don Ferlic, Mack Clayton, 2005 Franklin, Denver,Co. 80205.

The purpose of this study was to evaluate the long-term results of elbow synovectomies in patients with rheumatoid arthritis. 57 elbows in 46 patients were followed for up to 20 years after undergoing elbow synovectomy. Follow up averaged 86 months. Excellent, improved and poor categories were established and x-rays were classified. On follow up 77% of the elbows were found to be either excellent or improved. While only 23% of the elbows showed poor results. Elbows followed for less than 10 years and those for more than 10 years (47%) showed similiar results. No major complications were noted and post operative loss of motion was not generally a problem. Patients who underwent additional radial head replacement had results similiar to patients who did not. Optimal results were noted in patients who failed conservative treatment and had early stage x-ray changes. Less satisfactory results were associated with pre-operative advance x-ray changes; post operative x-ray progression and Juvenile Rheumatoid Arthritis. Early reports of Total elbow replacements have shown poor results. However, elbow synovectomy is a straight forward procedure with minimal risks. Synovectomy of the elbow is not a staging procedure to gain time before an arthroplasty is performed, but rather it is a definitive procedure with 77% of the patients being helped on follow up. The Authors feel that Synovectomy of the elbow may be one of the best synovectomies in RA based on the long term results of this study.

144

CROSS-REACTIVITY OF RO/SSA AND IMMUNOGLOBULIN G. Mark J. Mamula, Owen F. Fox, and John B. Harley. Univ. of Oklahoma and the Arthritis and Immunology Program of the Okla. Med. Res. Fnd., Oklahoma City.

Anti-Ro/SSA precipitating antibody has been demonstrated in approximately 30% of SLE patients, 60% of patients with subacute cutaneous lupus erythematosus and 40% of Sjögrens syndrome patients. Of all patients with anti-Ro/SSA precipitins, 70% have rheumatoid factor. Data from this study is consistent with IgG and the Ro/SSA particle sharing antigenic specificities which has implications for the basis of their clinical association.

Precipitating heteroimmune anti-Ro/SSA serum has been obtained from a Ro/SSA immunized rabbit host. By enzyme-linked immunosorbent assay (ELISA) for anti-Ro/SSA, the anti-Ro/SSA activity of this rabbit serum is inhibited up to 60% by preincubation with either human or bovine IgG and by greater than 95% by purified Ro/SSA. Conversely, the anti-IgG activity may be inhibited 75% by prior incubation with purified Ro/SSA and 98% by IgG. Applying the rabbit anti-Ro/SSA serum to bovine and human IgG immunoadsorbent columns removed greater than 90% of the anti-Ro/SSA activity. Further, the eluates from these IgG adsorbents demonstrate anti-Ro/SSA binding in both ELISA and Western blots. Similar experiments have been performed with human autoimmune anti-Ro/SSA serum. Bovine IgG inhibits 60% of the human anti-Ro/SSA activity in the ELISA. IgG adsorption removes autoimmune anti-Ro/SSA binding in the anti-Ro/SSA ELISA and Western blots. This relationship must be specific for the Ro/SSA antigen and IgG since antibodies against other autoantigens such as La/SSB show no cross-reactivity with IgG. These observations suggest that an intimate association exists between rheumatoid factor and anti-Ro/SSA in autoimmune disease.

145

INTERACTION OF DNA WITH CONNECTIVE TISSUE MATRIX PROTEINS REVEALS PREFERENTIAL BINDING TO TYPE V COLLAGEN. Steffen Gay, Michele J. Losman, William J. Koopman, and Edward J. Miller. UAB Medical Center, Birmingham, AL 35294.

A particular affinity of glomerular basement membrane and collagen for DNA has been proposed as a possible basis for local formation of DNA-anti-DNA complexes in SLE (J. Exp. Med. 144:428, 1976). Since these studies utilized only uncharacterized glomerular structures and type I and III collagens, we have evaluated the affinity of DNA for several highly purified matrix components. The latter include the structural components of basement membranes, type IV collagen and the glycoprotein laminin, as well as the other interstitial collagen types.

All of the components were isolated by established procedures (Meth. Enzymol. 82A:33, 1982). DNA-binding studies were performed with ^{125}I-DNA and purified connective tissue components immobilized on disposable Immulon™ Strips or in solution.

Essentially no binding could be detected with type I, II, III, IV, and VI collagens and their denaturation products or to laminin or BSA. Significant binding to native type V collagen was observed in which case approximately 20% of the added radioactivity was bound. Inhibition was complete by adding 0.5 µg of unlabeled DNA, or preincubation of 1.25 ng ^{125}I-DNA with 600 ng of type V collagen.

The results demonstrate that under physiological conditions, DNA has a much higher, conformation-dependent affinity for type V collagen than for the other collagens, laminin, or their denatured components. Type V collagen, which is largely found in pericellular matrices, is an intercalated component of the mesangial matrix and may be the specific "receptor" for DNA and its immune complexes in glomerular lesions of SLE.

146

CROSSREACTIVITY OF HUMAN AND MURINE ANTI-DNA ANTIBODIES WITH HEPARAN SULPHATE

Peter Faaber, Jo H.M. Berden, Truus P.M. Rijke, Levinus B.A. van de Putte and Peter J.A. Capel
Departments of Nephrology and Rheumatology, St.Radboud Hospital, University of Nijmegen, The Netherlands

In sera of SLE patients (n=63) and MRL/1 mice (n=10) antibodies are present reacting with heparan sulphate, the major glycosaminoglycan of the glomerular basement membrane. The anti-heparan sulphate titer in these sera was significantly correlated with the anti-DNA titer as determined by the ELISA technique with DNA or heparan sulphate as coated antigen. That the antibody binding to heparan sulphate was caused by crossreactive binding of anti-DNA antibodies, was substantiated along two different lines of evidence. First, we could demonstrate that DNA could completely inhibit the binding of SLE sera to heparan sulphate, whereas on the other hand the binding of these sera to DNA could be inhibited by heparan sulphate. The dosages of both antigens to achieve 50% inhibition were identical. Second, two murine monoclonal anti-DNA antibodies showed binding to heparan sulphate comparable to DNA. Antibodies eluted from human and murine kidneys with diffuse proliferative SLE glomerulonephritis showed a similar binding in vitro with heparan sulphate as with DNA. The binding of these eluted antibodies to heparan sulphate could also be inhibited by DNA. Heparan sulphate is present in the glomerular basement membrane in a discrete granular pattern. Direct binding of anti-DNA antibodies to this compound may therefore occur in SLE and might play a role in the initiation of glomerular damage.

147

FACILITATION OF THE B TO Z TRANSITION OF SYNTHETIC DNA BY HYDRALAZINE OR PROCAINAMIDE: A POSSIBLE MECHANISM FOR DRUG INDUCED LUPUS. T.J. Thomas and Ronald P. Messner, University of Minnesota, Minneapolis, MN 55455.

Recent reports indicate that left-handed Z-DNA is more immunogenic than the native right-handed B-form and that antibodies specific for Z-DNA occur in SLE. Equilibrium between B and Z forms of DNA is influenced by the frequency of alternating guanine (G)-cytosine (C) sequences, cations, and substituents attached to the polymer. DNA isolated from SLE immune complexes has a high G-C content. We questioned whether lupus-inducing drugs may act by inducing or stabilizing the Z form of DNA. The effect of hydralazine and procainamide on the salt-induced B to Z transition of poly(dG-me^{5}dC), poly(dG-me^{5}dC) was determined using circular dichroism and ultraviolet spectroscopy. The concentration of NaCl required to induce the midpoint of the B to Z transition was reduced from 0.8 to 0.5M by both drugs at a DNA phosphate to drug ratio (P/D) of 40. Similarly, the rate of the B to Z transition of the synthetic-polymer in the presence of 1M NaCl was increased in the presence of these drugs. At low ionic concentrations (0.1M NaCl), high concentrations of hydralazine induced aggregation of poly(dG-me^{5}dC) . poly(dG-me^{5}dC). Aggregation of synthetic and natural DNA by hydralazine was concentration dependent and was confirmed by quasi-elastic laser light scattering.

Thus, two drugs known to induce lupus can facilitate the B to Z transition of DNA. Induction or stabilization of the more immunogenic Z form of DNA by drugs or other agents may be important in the pathogenesis of some cases of lupus.

148

ANTIGUANOSINE ANTIBODIES IN DRUG-INDUCED SLE. Yee, W., Weisbart, R.H., Colburn, K.K., Wong, S., Kacena, A., Johnson, J., Heng, M., & Boucek, R. VAMC, Sepulveda, CA 91343 and Loma Linda University, Loma Linda, CA 92354.

Antinuclear antibodies are present in the majority of patients receiving procainamide and hydralazine irrespective of SLE symptoms, suggesting that only certain specificites are pathogenic. We described the association of IgG antiguanosine antibodies with idiopathic SLE, and recently found these antibodies in patients with drug-induced SLE as well. In order to determine whether IgG antiguanosine antibodies were associated with SLE symptoms, we compared their levels in the sera of asymptomatic and symptomatic patients taking procainamide and hydralazine. IgG antibodies to guanosine (G), cytidine (C), thymidine (T), and adenosine (A), conjugated to human serum albumin, and IgG antibodies to single-stranded DNA (ssDNA) were simultaneously measured by ELISA in 50 asymptomatic patients receiving procainamide or hydralazine and in 21 patients with drug-induced SLE manifested by arthralgias, arthritis, pleuritis, pericarditis, leukopenia, or thrombocytopenia. Elevated levels of antiguanosine antibodies were present in 86% of symptomatic patients but in only 2% of asymptomatic patients. Anti-ssDNA antibodies were present in 81% of symptomatic patients, but they were also present in 32% of asymptomatic patients. In contrast to antiguanosine antibodies, antibodies to C & A did not correlate with symptoms. Antibodies to T were present in 33% of symptomatic patients (all with anti-G antibodies), and in only 2% of asymptomatic patients. These results indicate that IgG antiguanosine antibodies are strongly associated with drug-induced SLE.

149

IgG ANTICARDIOLIPIN ANTIBODY (ACAG): POSSIBLE PREDICTOR FOR THROMBOSIS, THROMBOCYTOPENIA, AND RECURRENT ABORTION.
EN HARRIS, JKH CHAN, RA ASHERSON, AE GHARAVI, GRV HUGHES.

We have previously reported an association between the presence of ACAG, determined by solid phase radioimmunoassay, and thrombosis, thrombocytopenia and recurrent abortion in patients with SLE and other autoimmune disorders. We since have investigated 100 patients to determine whether the degree of ACAG elevation (measured as standard deviations (S.D.) above mean normal control level) correlated with frequency of these complications.

Patients were classified as 0, 1, 2, 3 according to whether they experienced 0, 1, 2, 3 of the events, arterial or venous thrombosis, thrombocytopenia, and recurrent abortions. Logarithms of the (ACAG + 1) values were taken to get approximately constant variance. Analysis of variance showed a significant increase in ACAG levels with increasing number of events ($p < 0.001$), Table 1 below.

NUMBER OF EVENTS	NUMBER OF PATIENTS	MEAN ACAG LEVEL (S.D.)
0	30	1.8
1	38	3.5
2	22	5.9
3	10	11.2

As a method of determining the most descriminating level of ACAG for each event, the value that best separated patients with or without the event was taken. These values were for arterial and venous thrombosis (≥5 S.D.); thrombocytopenia (≥7 S.D.) and recurrent abortion (≥5 S.D.).

ACAG determinations may identify patients with autoimmune disorders prone to thrombosis, thrombocytopenia, and/or recurrent abortion. Therapy to lower these antibodies in affected patients may be beneficial.

150

CORRELATION STUDY BETWEEN PROLACTIN AND ANDROGENS IN MALE PATIENTS WITH SYSTEMIC LUPUS ERYTHEMATOSUS (SLE).
C. Lavalle, E. Loyo, R. Paniagua, J.A. Bermudez, J. Herrera A. Graef, R. Navarrete, D. González-Bárcenas, A. Fraga.
Hospital de Especialidades C.M. La Raza y Unidad de Investigación Biomédica, C.M.N., I.M.S.S., Mexico City, Mexico.

We studied the hypothalamic-pituitary-gonadal-axis in 8 male (ARA) SLE patients. Five were untreated, none had liver, renal or thyroid diseases. Eight matched healthy men were used as controls. Serum samples were taken before and after I.V. administration of 25 µg of LH-RH. Hormones were determined by RIA. Serum testosterone (T) and dihydrotestosterone (DHT) resting values were lower in SLE (1004 ± 168 Vs 2227 ± 260 and 267 ± 42 Vs 327 ± 27 pg/ml; $p < 0.01$ and $p < 0.02$). Serum estradiol levels were lower ($p < 0.01$) and estrone higher ($p < 0.05$) in SLE. Serum LH resting values were higher in SLE ($p < 0.02$). Serum prolactin (PRL) resting values were higher in SLE (16.99 ± 3.07 Vs 4.32 ± 0.52 ng/ml; $p < 0.01$). Inverse correlation was observed between PRL and T levels ($p < 0.05$). After LH-RH stimulation T and DHT levels remained below and PRL significantly higher. The high PRL male in SLE is a novel finding which explains the low T and DHT serum levels by interfering the convertion of androstendione to T and T to active DHT. PRL plays a role in immunocompetence and could be an important factor in autoimmunity.

151

ANTI-CARDIOLIPIN ANTIBODY, PLACENTAL INSUFFICIENCY AND FETAL DEATH IN SLE PREGNANCIES. M. Lockshin, S. Goei, T. Qamar, L. Jovanovic, M. Druzin, M. Magid The Hospital for Special Surgery and The New York Hospital, New York, N.Y. 10021

Placental insufficiency, defined by abnormal non-stress tests (NST) and/or fetal death, complicated 9 of 21 prospectively studied pregnancies in patients with SLE. Pregnancies with placental insufficiency had increased frequency and quantity of antibody to cardiolipin (9/9 positive [mean 209.8 units]) measured by ELISA assay, compared to pregnancies without placental insufficiency (0/12 positive [mean 25.5 units, $p<0.01$]). SLE patients with placental insufficiency had subnormal levels of human chorionic gonadotrophin (HCG) and beta-HCG and more frequent history but not simultaneous presence of lupus anticoagulant (4/9 complicated vs 0/12 uncomplicated pregnancies, $p<0.05$), as well as statistically indeterminate trends toward more frequent thrombocytopenia (5/9 vs 1/12) and history of prior fetal death (3/9 vs 0/12). Features which did not identify placental insufficiency pregnancies included: clinical lupus activity (excluding thrombocytopenia), VDRL, anti-DNA antibody, anti-Ro antibody, C3, C4, CH50, plasma prolactin, or sex of the child. Placentas of affected pregnancies were small and showed histologic evidence of only minor vasculopathy.

Placental insufficiency can be predicted in lupus pregnancy; antibody to cardiolipin is the most sensitive marker and may be of pathogenic significance. (Supported in part by AM 32929 and by a Summer Student Grant from the New York Chapter of the Arthritis Foundation.)

152

PRIMARY SJÖGREN'S SYNDROME (SS) WITH CENTRAL NERVOUS SYSTEM DYSFUNCTION (CNS-SS) MIMICKING MULTIPLE SCLEROSIS (MS). ELAINE L. ALEXANDER, KENNETH L. MALINOW, JANE E. LEJEWSKI, THOMAS T. PROVOST, GARRETT E. ALEXANDER, Johns Hopkins Medical Institutions, Baltimore, MD

Since our initial report of CNS-SS, we have seen over 50 SS patients with CNS disease, unattributable to other causes, a subset of whom closely resemble patients with MS. We report the clinical and neurologic features of 20 primary SS patients in whom MS was initially considered the most likely diagnosis by at least one neurologist. All patients were symptomatic for the sicca complex with KCS, a positive minor salivary gland biopsy or both. The mean age at onset of CNS disease was 38 yrs, while the diagnosis of SS was 42 yrs. All patients had multifocal CNS events [brain (20), spinal cord (17)] over time with a relapsing/remitting pattern in 18 and chronic progressive course in 4. A mean of 4.7 CNS events occurred per person (range 2 to 12). Evoked response testing was abnormal in 15 of 18 patients tested (VER'S, 10/17; BAER'S, 8/15; SSER'S 5/11). No patient had plaques on enhanced CT scan. The following CSF studies were abnormal: [total protein (6), IgG (5), IgG/total protein ratio (5), IgG index (10), oligoclonal bands (OCB's) (16), myelin basic protein (2), mononuclear pleocytosis with lymphocytes and lymphoblastoid cells (9)]. Distinguishing features from MS, subtle and usually previously unrecognized, included peripheral neuropathy (10), vasculitis (8), and serologic abnormalities (13). 13 of 14 patients treated with cortico-steroids responded clinically with a concomitant decrease in IgG index, OCB's, and cell count. Since primary SS is a common CTD and approximately 25% of patients at our institution have CNS disease, CNS-SS should be considered in the differential diagnosis of patients presenting with an MS-like symptom complex.

153

RELATIONSHIP OF TEAR LYSOZYME LEVELS TO THE OCULAR SYNPTOMS AND SAINING TESTS IN PATIENTS WITH SJÖGREN'S SYNDROME. Yoshinari Takasaki,Juntendo University,Tokyo, Minoru Tanaka, Tastuko Ueda, Shinichi Yoshino, Takeshi Tojo, Shoji Miyawaki, Kimihiro Miyagawa, Mistuyoshi Nakajima, Yuichi Shiokawa,Bromhexine for Sjögren's syndrome research group,Tokyo,Japan.

Eighty-eight patients with Sjögren's syndrome(SS) who met diagnostic criteria of the Ministry of Health and Welfare of Japan were studied to know the relationship between lysozyme concentration in tears and,ocular symptoms and staining tests. The tears of patients were collected by the standard filter strip for the Schirmer test to measure lysozyme concetration. The severity of ocular synptoms(dry feeling, forein body sensation and pain) was evaluated, and divided into four grades. Fluorescein and Rose bengal tests were performed and their results were also divided into four grades from - to +++.

The lysozyme concentrations in patients with SS were significantly lower($P<0.05$) than those in 19 healthy controls(53.9 ± 35.2 µg/ml versus 146.0 ± 98.9 µg/ml, respectively). Patients with the lower lysozyme concentrations had the severer synptoms and they were significantly correlated irrespective of the types of synptoms($P<0.05$-$P<0.01$). The grades of both ocular staining tests were also significantly related with lysozyme concentrations, and patients with the more advanced changes in ocular tests showed the lower lysozyme concentrations($P<0.01$).

At the same time, the effectsof bromhexine(36mg/day) on lysozyme concentration in tears were studied by means of double blind comparision trial(DBT) with placebos for 8 weeks. In the present DBT, bromhexine was found to increase the tear lysozyme concentration significantly, whereas placebo did not cause any changes in the concentration.

These results suggest that the tear lysozyme level is a useful clinical marker and bromhexine may increase its level in patients with SS.

154

TREATMENT OF THE CUTANEOUS CALCINOSIS OF DERMATOMYOSITIS OR SCLERODERMA WITH LOW DOSE WARFARIN: RESULTS OF A DOUBLE-BLIND STUDY. Robert G. Berger, Nortin M. Hadler. University of North Carolina, Chapel Hill, NC 27514

Patients with calcinosis universalis secondary to dermatomyositis or scleroderma have increased levels of the calcium binding amino acid, gamma carboxy glutamic acid, in involved tissue and urine. The enzyme that effects gamma carboxylation of glutamic acid is warfarin sensitive. In a previous Phase I study, 3/4 patients treated with 1 mg of warfarin daily had decreases in the size of calcinotic lesions. We now report on a double-blind comparison of low dose warfarin versus placebo in 8 patients with calcinosis universalis.

Patients were randomized to receive 1 mg of warfarin daily or a placebo. No changes were made in other medications. Progression of existing calcinosis and appearance of new areas of activity was assessed before treatment and at six month intervals by clinical exam, plane radiology of involved areas, and qualitative and quantitative 99m TC diphosphonate whole body nuclear scans. One patient (on warfarin) was dropped from the study because of noncompliance.

During the 18 months of the study, no patient in either group developed new areas of calcium deposition. However, in 2/3 patients taking warfarin compared with 0/4 of control patients, the number and size of existing lesions decreased.

We conclude: 1) The natural history of calcium deposition in calcinosis universalis is a slow or intermittent process. 2) Low dose warfarin can be used safely in the treatment of calcinosis universalis. 3) While not definitive, these results suggest benefits.

155

RISK OF MALIGNANCY IN POLYMYOSITIS/DERMATOMYOSITIS. Sharad Lakhanpal, Thomas W. Bunch, Lee J. Melton, III, and Duane M. Ilstrup. Mayo Clinic, Rochester, MN 55905.

Numerous reports have suggested an association between polymyositis/dermatomyositis (P/D) and malignancy. Most of these lack specific diagnostic criteria for P/D and none have a comparably evaluated control population. To investigate the validity of this association, we identified all patients with a biopsy diagnosis of P/D seen from 1965 to 1974. The other criteria for diagnosis included proximal muscle weakness, elevated muscle enzymes, EMG changes and a characteristic skin rash. All patients below the age of 18 years were excluded as were those with other associated connective tissue disease or muscular dystrophy. For each case, a chronologically matched control was selected of the same age, sex, race and from the same geographic area of residence. The records of all cases and controls were reviewed and followed up to death or October 1984.

Based on above criteria, 115 patients were included in the study. There were 40 men and 75 women with an age range of 18 to 81 years (mean 52 years). Because of matching, controls had an identical distribution. Of the 115 patients, 65 had P and 50 D. Overall, more P/D patients had malignancy than controls but the difference was not statistically significant ($P>0.5$). Likewise, there was no significant difference in the proportion of P patients with malignancy as compared to D patients. When patients were separated into groups based on geographic area of residence, it was seen that the slight excess of malignancies in the P/D patients was confined to the most distant referrals and can be explained by referral bias. We did not find a significant association between P/D and malignancy.

156

RELAPSING POLYCHONDRITIS AND HEMATOPOIETIC DISEASE IN 11 PATIENTS. J. McGill, C. Michet, J. Goldberg, L. Pedell and L. McAdam. William Beaumont Hospital, Royal Oak, MI 48067, Marshfield Clinic, Marshfield, WI 54449 and Mayo Clinic, Rochester, MN 55901.

Relapsing polychondritis (RP) is an uncommon disorder that may present at any age. It has been associated with many other diseases, most of them autoimmune. This report presents the unusual occurrence of RP in older patients who had hematopoietic disorders diagnosed concurrently.

Eleven patients from four institutions were studied. RP was diagnosed in nine men and two women between the ages of 50 and 86 years, average age of 68.3 years. All of the patients were anemic at presentation, six had an increased MCV. Peripheral WBC was variable. Normal WBC (3 pts), leukocytosis (3 pts), leukopenia (2 pts), early forms (7 pts), eosinophilia (1 pt) and monocytosis (1 pt) were observed. Three patients had thrombocytopenia. Ten patients had bone marrow examinations within 1 year of onset of RP and all demonstrated myelodysplastic syndrome. Of these ten patients, 3 developed leukemia (2 myelomonocytic, 1 CGL) and expired at 5-15 months. Three patients have failing marrows and require transfusions. Three patients have died of other causes and 1 has a stable anemia. One patient (without an initial BM exam) died at 7 mo. of diffuse histiocytic lymphoma.

An extensive review of the literature disclosed one documented case of a 46-year-old male with RP and Hodgkin's disease. We are reporting eleven patients who developed relapsing polychondritis at an older age and were found to have myelodysplasia or lymphoma simultaneously. This is a new finding and should prompt further investigation of patients with RP and abnormal peripheral smears.

157

JAW CLAUDICATION IN PRIMARY SYSTEMIC AMYLOIDOSIS (AL).
Morie A. Gertz, Robert A. Kyle, W. Leroy Griffing and Gene G. Hunder. Mayo Clinic, Rochester, MN. 55905.

Amyloid deposits in the temporal artery were observed more than 40 years ago but the presence of vascular ischemic symptoms in patients with amyloidosis has been poorly recognized. From January 1, 1970, through December 31, 1980, we saw 22 patients who had typical jaw claudication with biopsy proved primary amyloidosis. This number constituted nine percent of the total group of 229 amyloid patients seen over this period. In none was vasculitis documented to be a contributing cause of the claudication. However, two patients were misdiagnosed initially as temporal arteritis and polymyalgia rheumatica and treated with corticosteroids which resulted in significant drug toxicity. Subsequent temporal artery biopsy revealed extensive luminal and interstitial amyloid deposits in both. There was an association between jaw claudication and other ischemic vascular symptoms in that calf claudication was present in five and arm claudication was present in four at the time the jaw pain became evident. Carpal tunnel syndrome present in nine was also seen in the 22 patients with a higher incidence than expected. This subset of systemic amyloidosis patients had a median survival of 42 months, compared to a median survival of 12 months for the entire group seen with amyloidosis in this time period. The improved survivorship presumably results from more extensive vascular amyloid deposition with less interstitial amyloid infiltration of other viscera. Vascular symptoms related to amyloidosis are not rare and amyloidosis should be considered in the differential diagnosis of patients with jaw claudication. Appropriate staining of temporal artery biopsy specimens can yield the correct diagnosis in such cases.

158

A DOUBLE BLIND STUDY OF AMITRIPTYLINE VERSUS PLACEBO IN PATIENTS WITH PRIMARY FIBROSITIS.
Simon Carette, Laval University, Quebec City, P.Q. Glenn A. McCain, David A. Bell, UWO, London, Ont., Adel G. Fam, University of Toronto, Ont. Canada.

Seventy patients with primary fibrositis satisfying Smythe's criteria were randomized into a 9 week double-blind trial comparing amitriptyline 50 mg (A) to placebo (P). Patients were evaluated at baseline and weeks 5 and 9 for duration of morning stiffness, pain severity (analogue scale) and myalgic scores (determination of fibrositic point tenderness by dolorimeter). Other parameters of efficacy included evaluation of sleep quality by questionnaire and patient (PGA) and physician's (PhGA) global assessments. Fifty-nine patients (27 A, 32 P) completed the trial.

Patients on A improved significantly in their morning stiffness and analogue scores of pain at 5 and 9 weeks as compared to baseline, whereas no changes were noted in these parameters in the P group. Myalgic scores did not improve significantly in either of the treatment groups.

When compared to the P group, the A group improved significantly at 5 weeks with regards only to sleep, PGA and PhGA. This improvement however was not significantly different from the P group at 9 weeks for the last two parameters. A summary of these results is shown in the table:

	Percentage of patients improved					
	SLEEP		PGA		PhGA	
Weeks	5	9	5	9	5	9
A	69	70	77	70	70	66
P	34	40	43	50	37	43
p value (X^2)	.008	.02	.008	.11	.01	.07

This study shows some therapeutic benefit of amitriptyline over placebo in patients with primary fibrositis. It also shows that an unusually high proportion of patients with this condition improved with placebo.

159

A RANDOMIZED CLINICAL TRIAL OF NAPROXEN (N) AND AMITRYPTILENE (AM) IN PRIMARY FIBROMYALGIA.
Hal Dinerman, David Felson, Don Goldenberg. Boston University Arthritis Center, Boston, MA 02118.

Patients with fibromyalgia are often treated with tricyclic antidepressants for the sleep disorder and with nonsteroidal agents for the pain. Nonetheless, neither medicine has been studied in a controlled fashion. We conducted a six week placebo-controlled double blind randomized clinical trial using a 2x2 factorial design with four treatment groups: group 1 received 500mg naproxen (N) twice daily and 25mg amitryptilene (AM) at night; group 2 N and placebo AM; group 3 AM and placebo N; and group 4 double placebo. A power analysis suggested a study size of 32 was needed to show the efficacy of a single agent but was not necessarily sufficient to demonstrate differences between the four treatment groups. Outcome measures evaluated at study onset, 2, 4, and 6 weeks included patient global assessment, pain and sleep (all on 1-10 analog scales), physician global assessment and trigger point score. 40 patients with primary fibromyalgia entered; five distributed across treatment groups dropped out early because of side effects.

Results for 35 patients showed N treated patients had less pain ($p=.05$) but no significant improvement in other measures. AM treated patients had improvement in patient global assessment ($p < .01$) and pain ($p < .01$), findings not explained by concomitant N use. AM treated patients also had a nonsignificant trend toward improved sleep. Group 1 patients did best, with better global response ($p=.02$) and pain relief ($p=.02$) than other treatment groups combined.

Combined N and AM are effective in treating primary fibromyalgia. The efficacy of AM may confirm the hypothesis that fibromyalgia is due to a sleep disorder. More patients are being entered into the study to evaluate differences between individual therapeutic regimens.

160

CLEARANCE OF MODEL DNA anti-DNA IMMUNE COMPLEXES IN MICE.
W.Emlen and G.Burdick Pacific Medical Center/University of Washington, Seattle, WA.

DNA/anti-DNA immune complexes are important in the pathogenesis of SLE, but the clearance and organ localization of these complexes is not well studied. We have examined the clearance, in mice, of DNA/anti-DNA complexes made at varying degrees of antibody excess, both before and after DNAse digestion of immune complexes.

Immune complexes (IC) were made by incubating IgG from a patient with SLE with sonicated calf thymus ^{125}I dsDNA (300 bp) at 37° overnight. ICs were injected directly into mice, or digested with DNAse to remove exposed DNA (DNA not covered by antibody) prior to injection. Blood samples were removed at varying intervals after injection and ammonium sulfate precipitable radioactivity remaining in the serum was measured. In some animals, IC remaining in serum were analyzed on a 3-12% polyacrylamide gradient gel.

ICs formed in antigen excess or in moderate antibody excess, but in which some DNA is exposed (not covered with IgG) were cleared rapidly like DNA alone. Clearance of these complexes was slowed by concurrent administration of excess cold DNA, confirming that clearance of these complexes was mediated by antigen in the IC. If, however, exposed DNA was removed by prior digestion with DNAse, IC were cleared more slowly than DNA, at rates proportional to the number of IgG molecules contained in the complex. Analysis of IC size on gradient gels showed that ICs containing 1-4 IgGs persisted in the circulation, whereas ICs containing more than 4 IgGs were cleared rapidly by the liver. These data suggest that large complexes containing multiple IgGs, and ICs containing exposed DNA are cleared rapidly. However, smaller complexes containing no exposed DNA can persist in circulation and may therefore be important in the pathogenesis of SLE.

161

DEGRADATION OF SMALL COVALENTLY CROSS-LINKED POLYMERS OF HUMAN IgG1 BY HUMAN MONOCYTES.
R.W. Strickland, D.S. Finbloom, Walter Reed AMC, Washington, DC 20307, and L.M. Wahl, NIH, Bethesda, MD 20205.

Soluble immune complexes (IC) are implicated in the pathogenesis of several human diseases. Large IC are rapidly removed by the mononuclear phagocyte system; their phlogistic potential is therefore limited. Small IC are cleared poorly from the blood of animals and are known to fix complement. Since no probe exists for study of interactions of soluble IC with monocytes in vivo, we have studied endocytosis of small oligomers of IgG by peripheral blood monocytes in vitro. Dimers and oligomers (mostly trimers and tetramers) were prepared by crosslinking myeloma-derived IgG1 with dimethylsuberimidate and separated by gel filtration. About $2x10^5$ and $7x10^4$ IgG molecules/cell of oligomer and dimer were bound, respectively. Monocytes, purified by gradient centrifugation and counterflow centrifugal elutriation, were incubated at 4°C for 16 hrs with dimer or oligomer, washed, and then incubated for up to 5 hrs at 37°C for degradation to occur. Radioactivity not precipitated by acid represented degraded IgG molecules. At 5 hr of incubation, $3x10^4$ IgG molecules of oligomer were degraded per cell (the equivalent of 14% of those oligomers initially bound to the cell). In contrast, of the dimers only $2.5x10^3$ IgG molecules per cell were degraded (3% of the dimers initially bound to the cell). These results show that: (1) five-fold less dimers than oligomers were degraded when expressed as a percent of that initially bound. (2) since less dimers than oligomers bind to the cell, the number of molecules degraded per hr is 1/12 that of the oligomers, and (3) the degree of multivalency of the IC markedly alters its fate.

162

ROLE OF COMPLEMENT RECEPTOR (CR_1) IN THE PATHOGENESIS OF SLE AND OTHER DISORDERS ASSOCIATED WITH COMPLEMENT ACTIVATION II: CORRELATION WITH DISEASE ACTIVITY.
W. J. Yount, G. D. Ross, J. B. Winfield. UNC, Chapel Hill, NC 27514, C. J. Parker, Duke, Durham, NC, and R. Taylor, UVA, Charlottesville, VA.

CR_1, C3c, C3d, C3g, C4d and IgG were quantified on erythrocytes (E) with monoclonal antibodies labeled with ^{125}I. Significantly lower CR_1/E, and higher C3d, C3g, C4d and IgG/E were found in SLE, primary Sjogren's Syndrome, serum sickness, and a variety of autoimmune hemolytic disorders vs. normals and disease controls. Significant differences also were documented in a blinded comparison of active vs. inactive SLE and in serial studies of individual SLE patients. In in vitro kinetic analyses of these phenomena using normal E, maximum binding of cold agglutinins or well-characterized ds DNA/anti-DNA immune complexes (IC) and activated complement fragments was noted within 5 minutes, with only residual C3d and C3g present after 60-120 minutes. No change in levels of CR_1/E was noted, even when maximal levels of IgG, C3d and C3g were present on E. Incubation of sensitized E with an excess of peripheral blood leukocytes produced no diminution in CR_1/E suggesting that if CR_1 is "stripped" from cells, this process probably does not occur in peripheral blood. Binding of IC to E could be blocked by a polyclonal antibody to CR_1. These studies provide further support for the hypothesis that IC rapidly bind to E, that levels of CR1/E are decreased in active disease, perhaps by "stripping" in the liver, leaving a population of E with diminished CR_1 and increased C3 fragments and IgG.

163

IMMUNOLOGICAL IDENTIFICATION OF A COMPONENT IN IMMUNE COMPLEXES ISOLATED FROM RHEUMATOID ARTHRITIS SERUM. Stewart G. Greisman, Patricia B. Redecha and Charles L. Christian. Hospital for Special Surgery, New York, NY 10021.

Antisera raised against isolated immune complexes (IC) have proved useful probes in analyzing the constituents of IC. IC were isolated from serum by polyethylene glycol precipitation followed by competitive binding to protein A-bearing Staphylococci. Eluants from the Staphylococci were analyzed by SDS-polyacrylamide gel electrophoresis and then, by a Western blot technique, transferred to nitrocellulose paper. The paper was subsequently overlaid with selected antisera and developed with radiolabeled protein A, followed by autoradiography. IC were isolated from rheumatoid arthritis (RA) and other diseases and probed with various antisera raised in rabbits, including several raised against IC isolated from a patient with Lactobacillus casei endocarditis and IC from synovial fluid of a RA patient. Six to 10 common bands appeared in the IC of all isolates overlaid with these antisera. However, RA IC (12 of 16 isolates) showed a band at 60,000 daltons which was not seen in IC from systemic lupus erythematosus, hepatitis B-associated polyarteritis, juvenile rheumatoid arthritis or normals. In addition, this 60,000 dalton band was not demonstrated by an overlay with an antiserum raised in rabbits against normal human serum.

These results suggest that certain IC isolated from RA patients may contain a distinct component not present in IC isolated from patients with other rheumatic diseases.

164

ANTIBODY TO BamHI-K FRAGMENT OF EPSTEIN-BARR VIRUS NUCLEAR ANTIGEN (EBNA) IN RHEUMATOID ARTHRITIS. T.M.Wright, A.L.Scott, G.Milman and M.C.Hochberg. The Johns Hopkins Medical Institutions, Baltimore.

Patients with rheumatoid arthritis(RA) have antibodies which react with a nuclear antigen derived from Epstein-Barr virus(EBV) infected cells(RANA). Recent studies suggest that RANA may be identical to EBNA, although anti-RANA and anti-EBNA activities commonly differ, and elevated anti-EBNA titers have not consistently been demonstrated in RA.

A fragment of EBV DNA encoding the carboxy-terminal third of EBNA (BamHI-K) was inserted into E.coli via a high expression plasmid. The EBNA polypeptide segment thus produced was purified by sequential chromatography on phosphocellulose and hydroxylapatite columns. This 28K polypeptide was used as the antigen in an ELISA to detect IgG-anti-EBNA antibody in sera from 88 normal controls and 83 RA patients.

Anti-EBNA antibody was present in 82% of controls and 100% of RA patients($P<.001$). Of the RA patients, 51(61%) had anti-EBNA titers that were > 2 standard deviations above the mean of controls. Among these 51 patients, there was a suggestion of milder disease activity as reflected by a lower mean painful/tender joint count and score (17.8 vs 25.8, P=.024; 22.5 vs 32.8, P=.046). There were no differences in mean age, sex or race ratio, duration of disease, functional class, geometric mean titer of antinuclear antibodies or rheumatoid factor or frequency of any HLA-DR, MB or C4A and C4B phenotype between these 51 and the remaining 32 RA patients.

These data demonstrate that anti-EBNA antibodies occur in all RA patients and that a majority have significantly elevated titers when compared to normals. There were no associations of any HLA or C4 phenotype with anti-EBNA production. Serial measurements are needed to examine the relationship between anti-EBNA titers and disease activity.

165

RHEUMATOID ARTHRITIS SYNOVIAL MEMBRANES CONTAIN A 62 KD PROTEIN THAT SHARES AN ANTIGENIC EPITOPE WITH THE EBV ENCODED ANTIGEN EBNA. Robert Fox, Gary Rhodes, Dennis Carson, John Vaughan. Scripps Clinic and Research Foundation, La Jolla, CA 92037. Janos Luka and Gary Pearson, Georgetown University, Washington D.C., 20007.

Recent studies have shown that the Epstein-Barr virus (EBV) encoded antigen EBNA contains repetitive (gly-ala) sequences and that similar repetitive sequences also are expressed by EBV genome negative cell lines (Luka et al.,J.Virol 52:833,1984). We have used a monoclonal antibody (MoAb P135) that reacts with a cross reactive antigenic determinant on EBNA (a 70-85 KD molecule) and on a 62 KD molecule found in EBV negative cell lines to show that: a) synovial membrane lining cells from 10/11 RA patients exhibited strong reactivity when frozen tissue sections were examined using immunoperoxidase techniques; b) only rare synovial lining cells were stained in biopsies from osteoarthritis or psoriatic arthritis patients; and c) no staining of RA or control synovial biopsies was noted with anti-CMV, anti-HSV or anti-HuTLV antibodies. Analysis of tissue extracts from RA synovium by SDS gel electrophoresis and immunoblotting showed that the reactive molecule was 62 KD, similar to the normal cellular protein and smaller than the EBNA molecule. Normal lymph node tissues contained a small but detectable amount of the 62 KD antigen on immunoblotting even though these tissues were not reactive in immunoperoxidase assays. Taken together, these results suggest that RA synovial membranes contain a relatively high concentration of the 62 KD protein that shares an antigenic epitope with EBNA. The chronic inflammatory response in RA synovial membrane may result from an immune response against this cross reactive epitope.

166

EFFECTS OF ANTI-L3T4 ANTIBODY ON THE DEVELOPMENT OF MURINE COLLAGEN INDUCED ARTHRITIS (CIA). Gerald E. Ranges, Subramaniam Sriram and Sheldon M. Cooper, University of Vermont, Burlington, VT 05405

Immunization of DBA/1 mice with bovine type II collagen results in a severe inflammatory arthritis (CIA) which has features that are similar to rheumatoid arthritis. Using this model, we tested the effect of in vivo administration of the monoclonal antibody GK1.5 on the development of CIA. GK1.5 recognizes a non-polymorphic determinant on the L3T4 antigen of murine T lymphocytes that is analogous to the human OKT4/Leu3 antigen present on the helper T cell subset. GK1.5 blocks all class II MHC antigen restricted functions of T cells in vitro. Three groups of mice (n=10) were immunized with native type II collagen on day 0 and boosted on day 32. Mice in Group A were treated with 100 μg GK1.5 on day -1, +1 and every two weeks thereafter until day 46. Group B mice were treated with 100 μg GK1.5 on day 28 and day 42. By day 28 a vigorous immune response to collagen is already present. Group C did not receive GK1.5. On day 52 each limb of each animal was scored for the presence and severity of arthritis on a scale from 0 to 4. Group C showed a 90% incidence of CIA with an average score of 4.9. Group A showed a 10% incidence with an average score of 1.0 and in Group B a 50% incidence and average score of 4.1 was observed. Cell sorter analysis of lymph node cells following GK1.5 treatment showed a >95% decrease in L3T4+ cells at 3 days and a 50% decrease at 14 days. These data indicate a pivotal role for L3T4+ T cells in the development of CIA and confirm the therapeutic possibility of using monoclonal antibodies to deplete specific T cell subsets.

167

SUPPRESSION OF B CELL IMMUNE RESPONSE ANTIGEN EXPRESSION BY CORTICOSTEROIDS. Gregory Dennis, Fred D. Finkleman and James J. Mond. Walter Reed Army Medical Center, Washington, D.C.; Uniformed Services University of the Health Sciences, Bethesda, Maryland.

The immune response-associated (Ia) antigens encoded in the I-region of the major histocompatibility complex in mice are analogous to the HLA-Dr antigens in humans and play an important role in influencing immune responsiveness. The quantitative variation in expression of B cell surface Ia that is induced by corticosteroids in vivo and in vitro was studied by flow microfluorometry after staining of murine splenic cells with fluorescein labeled anti-Ia antibodies. Intravenous injection of 40 mcg of dexamethasone resulted in a 35-40% reduction in the expression of Ia which occurred within 3 hours, reached its maximum suppressive effect (75% suppression) within 6 hours and by 12 hours was beginning to return towards baseline levels. The suppressive effect of dexamethasone on B cell surface Ia was dose dependent with respect to the length of time required to reach maximal suppression and to the magnitude of Ia suppression attained. In addition, B cell surface Ia was reduced after injection of dexamethasone into athymic (nude) mice, as well as after in vitro incubation of purified B cells with dexamethasone. However, when B cells were activated in vivo by injection of anti-δ antibodies, dexamethasone was significantly less effective in suppressing the expression of Ia suggesting that its maximum effect on B cell Ia was exerted on resting and not activated B cells. Since B cell surface Ia has been shown to play a critical role in antigen presentation and in influencing B cell- T cell interactions, the suppression of Ia on B cells by corticosteroids may be an important mechanism whereby corticosteroids influence antibody producing pathways in the normal or autoimmune state.

168

EVIDENCE FOR MULTIPLE ARTHRITOGENIC AND IMMUNOGENIC EPITOPES ON TYPE II COLLAGEN MOLECULES. P.H. Wooley+, H.S. Luthra+, M.M. Griffiths*, J.M. Stuart#, A. Huse+ and C.S. David+. +Mayo Clinic, Rochester, MN 55905, *Univ. UT, Salt Lake City, UT 84132 and #Univ. TN, Memphis, TN 38163.

Type II collagen obtained from chick (CII), bovine (BII), deer (DII), rat (RII), human (HII) and porcine (PII) sources was tested for the ability to cause collagen-induced arthritis (CIA) in 14 independent haplotype and 12 recombinant haplotype mouse strains congenic to the C57/B10 background. $H\text{-}2^q$ haplotype mice (B10.Q and B10.G) developed a high CIA incidence injected with CII, BII, DII, RII, or HII, but were resistant to disease using PII. B10.RIII mice ($H\text{-}2^r$) only developed CIA using BII, DII or PII. Analysis of the recombinant haplotypes demonstrated CIA susceptibility was associated with the $I\text{-}A^q$ subregion using CII, BII, or RII, but exceptions to this genetic restriction were observed using DII. The regulation of susceptibility to CIA by both collagen species source and immunoregulatory genes indicate the presence of at least 2 arthritogenic epitopes, one restricted to CII, RII and HII, and the other restricted to PII. Variations in the optimum arthritogenic doses between $H\text{-}2^q$ and $H\text{-}2^r$ strains suggest both epitopes may be expressed on BII and DII, in different concentrations. $H\text{-}2^q$ haplotype strains were consistent high antibody responders to all type II collagens, including PII, with high interspecies cross-reactivity. B10.RIII only produced high antibody responses to BII, DII and PII; antibody levels to CII were intermediate and did not crossreact strongly. Analysis of the antibody response in CIA resistant strains suggested the presence of at least 3 other species restricted antigenic epitopes, capable of inducing an immune response to type II collagen which did not result in CIA.

169

MACROPHAGE ACTIVATION BY SEROTONIN (5-HT) IS AFFECTED BY INTERFERON γ (IFNγ) CONCENTRATION AND IS INHIBITED BY 5-HT RECEPTOR ANTAGONISTS. E.M. Sternberg, J. Trial, C.W. Parker. Howard Hughes Medical Institute and Washington University School of Medicine, St. Louis, Mo. 63110

In previous studies we have shown that 5-HT decreases the percent of mouse bone marrow macrophages expressing Ia and augments phagocytosis in cultures grown in supernatants from Concanavalin A treated spleen cells (Con A sup). Since IFNγ is one lymphokine present in Con A sups and has been shown to induce Ia and augment phagocytosis, we have now examined the effect of 5-HT on IFNγ induced Ia expression and phagocytosis. After 48 hours, increasing concentrations, from 1 U to 100 U, of E. Coli-derived recombinant DNA murine IFNγ (Genentech) increased both the percent of cells phagocytosing >21 latex particles (from 7% to 55%) and the percent of cells expressing Ia (from 34% to 95%). Control cultures contained 10% cells phagocytosing >21 particles per cell, and 1% to 10% Ia positive cells. At low but not high IFNγ concentrations, 5-HT induced a 3 to 5 fold increase in the percent of cells phagocytosing >21 particles, and decreased the percent of Ia positive cells by 60% compared to IFNγ alone. In Con A sup treated cultures, the 5-HT receptor antagonists spiperone and ketanserin antagonized both the phagocytosis enhancing and Ia inhibiting effects of 5-HT. These data suggest that the macrophage-activating effect of 5-HT is affected by IFNγ concentration and the state of activation of the macrophage, and may be mediated by a specific 5-HT surface receptor.

170

REGULATION OF SUSCEPTIBILITY TO TYPE II COLLAGEN-INDUCED ARTHRITIS (CIA) BY GENES MAPPING EXTERIOR TO THE MAJOR HISTOCOMPATIBILITY COMPLEX (H-2) IN MICE. P.H. Wooley, H.S. Luthra, A. Huse and C.S. David. Immunology and Rheumatology Depts., Mayo Clinic, Rochester, MN 55905.

Susceptibility to CIA has been shown to be associated with the $H\text{-}2^q$ and $H\text{-}2^r$ haplotypes in mice congenic to the C57/B10 background. B10.Q mice are susceptible to chick type II collagen (CII), and resistant to porcine type II collagen (PII), while B10.RIII mice are resistant to CII CIA but susceptible to PII CIA. Inbred strains now indicate non-MHC gene involvement, since DBA/1J ($H\text{-}2^q$) was susceptible to both CII and PII, while SWR/J ($H\text{-}2^q$) and RIII/J ($H\text{-}2^r$) were resistant to both collagens. F_1 analysis of (resistant x susceptible) strains with homozygous H-2 genes demonstrated that resistance to arthritis was a dominant trait: (SWR/J x B10.Q)F_1 was resistant to CII CIA and (RIII/J x B10.RIII)F_1 was resistant to PII CIA. Gene complementation analysis [(resistant H-2, susceptible background x (susceptible H-2, resistant background)]F_1 indicated that the CIA resistance trait was multigenic or showed incomplete penetrance, since the CIA was influenced by the species source of type II collagen. (SWR/J x B10.RIII)F_1 was resistant to CII CIA, but susceptible with a moderate frequency to PII CIA. Backcross analysis implicated multiple gene involvement, since [SWR/J x (SWR/J x B10.RIII)] yielded either $H\text{-}2^{q/q}$ haplotype mice resistant to both CII and PII, or $H\text{-}2^{q/r}$ mice susceptible to both collagen species with a low CIA frequency. Mice phenotypically $H\text{-}2^{r/q}$ from the [B10.RIII x (SWR/J x B10.RIII)] cross were resistant to CII and susceptible to PII, but $H\text{-}2^{r/r}$ offspring were able to overcome the MHC regulation and develop CII CIA with a low frequency.

171

PHOSPHOLIPID (PL) METABOLISM IN MONONUCLEAR PHAGOCYTES (MNP) FROM PATIENTS WITH RHEUMATOID ARTHRITIS (RA). John S. Bomalaski, Michael Clark, Robert B. Zurier. Univ. of Penn. and Smith Kline & French Labs., Philadelphia, PA 19104

Macrophages (MØ) found in RA synovium likely derive from peripheral blood monocytes (PBM). PBM allowed to mature in culture for 12 days (M-MØ) were incubated for 2 hr with radiolabeled linoleic (LA) and arachidonic acids (AA). Cells (M-MØ) from RA patients take up significantly more LA and AA than M-MØ from normal controls. Distribution of fatty acid (FA) incorporated into PL was determined by thin layer chromatography (TLC). Incorporation of LA into phosphatidylcholine (PC) was restricted in RA M-MØ ($p<0.05$ vs controls; N=6). Stimulation of M-MØ with calcium ionophore A23187 or zymosan resulted in striking and preferential hydrolysis of LA from PC in RA M-MØ (65% reduction of labeled LA in PC) compared to controls (7% reduction). However, hydrolysis of AA after M-MØ stimulation was similar in RA and control cells. To further investigate these differences we examined phospholipase A_2 (PLA_2) and phospholipase C (PLC) activity in PBM from RA patients and controls. Cell free sonicates were incubated with radiolabeled PL and reactants were separated by TLC. Enzyme activity is expressed per 10^{-5} mol substrate hydrolyzed/mg protein/min. No significant differences in PLA_2 activity were noted. However, an increase in PLC activity was seen in RA cells against 2-linoleyl PC (8.6 ± 0.4 RA vs 2.2 ± 0.4 normal; $p<0.05$; N=9) and against 2-linoleyl phosphatidylinositol (0.6 ± 0.1 RA vs 0.26 ± 0.13 normal; $p<0.05$; N=9). These studies suggest that FA and PL metabolism is altered in MNP from RA patients. Changes in distribution and availability of eicosanoid precursors may affect profoundly cell function and inflammatory responses.

172

ELEVATED FIBROBLAST INORGANIC PYROPHOSPHATE (PPi) AND ECTO-NUCLEOSIDE PYROPHOSPHOHYDROLASE (ENP) IN CALCIUM PYROPHOSPHATE DIHYDRATE (CPPD) CRYSTAL DEPOSITION DISEASE. LM Ryan, RL Wortmann, BJ Karas, DJ McCarty. Medical College of Wisconsin, Milwaukee, WI. 53226.

Elevated cellular PPi levels have been reported in cells from members of a French kindred with CPPD deposition (Lust et al, Science 214: 809, 1981); and elevated ENP (which generates PPi in the reaction NTP → NMP + PPi) activity was observed in extracts of cartilage containing CPPD crystals (Tenenbaum et al, Arthritis Rheum 24:492, 1981). We measured intracellular PPi and ENP activity in cultured skin fibroblasts from 44 donors: CPPD-familial (11), CPPD-sporadic (13), osteoarthritis (OA) (13), normal (N) (7).

{PPi} was elevated in both CPPD-sporadic ($p<0.05$ Wilcoxon's rank sum) and CPPD-familial ($p<0.01$) fibroblasts compared to OA or N. ENP activity was elevated in CPPD-sporadic ($p<0.01$), but not CPPD-familial. Other ectoenzyme activities (5'nucleotidase and pyrophosphatase) in CPPD donor cells were not different from OA or N. When all 44 donors were combined, {PPi} correlated with ENP ($p<0.01$, Spearman's rank correlate).

Elevated PPi levels in skin fibroblasts may serve as a biochemical marker for some patients with familial or sporadic CPPD deposition disease; ENP activity may further separate sporadic and familial disease types. Expression of these abnormalities in nonarticular cells lends support to the postulate of a generalized metabolic defect(s) accompanying CPPD crystal deposition in joints (Lust et al).

173

IMMUNE INTERFERON SUPPRESSES LEVELS OF PROCOLLAGEN mRNA AND TYPE II COLLAGEN SYNTHESIS IN HUMAN CHONDROCYTES. Mary B. Goldring, Linda J. Sandell, Mary L. Stephenson, Edward P. Amento, and Stephen M. Krane. Harvard Med. School, MGH, Boston, MA 02114, Rush-Presbyterian St. Luke's Medical Center, Chicago, IL 60612.

After chondrocytes are cultured they begin to synthesize types I and III collagens as well as type II. In this study, we have examined some controls of collagen synthesis by cultured human chondrocytes. Proteins in medium from cells pulsed with [^{3}H]proline were analyzed by SDS-PAGE before and after pepsinization at 4°C. Adult articular chondrocytes synthesized type II collagen >> I and III during weeks 1-3 in culture and I and III > II after first subculture. Costal chondrocytes (from a 3-year-old) synthesized ∿ no α2(I) chains until after week 1 and type II >> I even after weeks of culture. Previous studies showed that immune interferon (IFN-γ) inhibits synthesis of types I and III collagens by human skin and synovial fibroblasts. We found here that recombinant IFN-γ (0.1 to 100 U/ml) inhibited synthesis of type II as well as types I and III collagens by chondrocytes; levels of procollagen mRNAs were decreased (dot blot hybridization with cDNA probes for α1[I], α2[I], α1[II] and α1[III] procollagen chains). Human leukocyte interferon-α (10 to 1000 U/ml) had no effect on collagen synthesis or on the levels of procollagen mRNAs. In articular chondrocytes or synovial fibroblasts, levels of α2(I) mRNA were disproportionately high [α1(I)/α2(I) < 1.0] vs. costal chondrocytes or dermal fibroblasts [α1(I)/α2(I) ∿2]. IFN-γ suppressed the levels of all α1 mRNAs > α2(I)mRNA in all types of cell. The lymphokine IFN-γ could, therefore, have a role in suppressing matrix synthesis in inflammatory joint disease and other conditions.

174

CALCIUM PYROPHOSPHATE CRYSTAL DEPOSITION IN PURIFIED MENISCUS COLLAGEN GELS. Neil S. Mandel and Gretchen S. Mandel. Medical College of Wisconsin, Veterans Administration Medical Center, Milwaukee, WI 53193.

Calcium pyrophosphate dihydrate crystal (CPPD) growth in cartilage was modeled using gels composed of purified porcine meniscus collagen. Gels were prepared such that CPPD crystal growth would occur at or near physiological ionic levels established by ionic diffusion gradients. The gels were incubated at 37° C and harvested over a 6 month period. The crystals were identified by x-ray diffraction, the [Ca] determined by atomic absorption and the [PPi] by enzyme assay.

Amorphous calcium pyrophosphate (a-CaPPi) formed after 2 days at the Ca/PPi ionic interface. Within 2 weeks, a-CaPPi formed throughout the tube, inducing the [Ca] and [PPi] to fall to physiological levels. At 3 to 4 months, most of the a-CaPPi had disappeared leaving a clear gel which contained large clumps of the two crystal dimorphs observed in vivo, triclinic (t) and monoclinic (m) CPPD. In contrast to previous studies using denatured collagen (biologic gelatin), gels composed of native-type collagen did not yield any other crystalline calcium pyrophosphates observed in vivo, particularly orthorhombic calcium pyrophosphate tetrahydrate or any mixed Ca/Na PPi salts. Further, the growth morphology of the t-CPPD crystals formed in the native-type collagen gels paralleled in vivo observations of large prismatic crystals compared to the needles observed in denatured collagen gels.

175

A CHONDROITIN SULFATE PROTEOGLYCAN FROM HUMAN NEUTROPHILS

K.S. ROSTAND, W.D. BLACKBURN, L. HECK, Birmingham, AL 35294

Purified human neutrophils were labelled *in vitro* with ^{35}S-sulfate. Incorporation of $^{35}SO_4$ into macromolecules increased up to 24h; radioactivity was 80-90% cell associated, was totally digested by chondroitinase AC, and eluted from DEAE-Sephacel at 0.6M NaCl. Treatment of the cell associated sulfated molecules with alkaline borohydride shifted their elution position on molecular sieve chromatography from K_{AV} = 0.45 to K_{AV} = 0.82. Subcellular distribution of incorporated radioactivity was analyzed by fractionation on Percoll gradients. Gradient fractions were assayed for elastase, cathepsin G, lactoferrin, myeloperoxidase, lysozyme, alkaline phosphatase, and radioactivity. Only 1% of the radioactivity was localized to the azurophilic granules; the specific granule (SP) and plasma membrane (PM) fractions contained 32% and 65%, respectively. SDS-PAGE (5-15%) of SP and PM fractions labelled with ^{35}S-Sulfate and 3H-leucine revealed multiple (8-10) Coomassie staining bands; fewer (5-6) radiolabelled components were seen. A broad diffuse band, M_R>200,000, was a component of both SP and PM fractions, was Coomassie positive and radiolabelled, and was the only band labelled by $^{35}SO_4$ alone. Chromatography of solubilized SP and PM components on DEAE-Sephacel produced a broad peak of $^{35}SO_4$-labelled material eluting at 0.6M NaCl. Our data suggest that mature human neutrophils synthesize a condroitin sulfate proteoglycan that resides in at least two subcullular compartments.

A1

INHIBITION OF HUMAN MONOCYTE COLLAGENASE PRODUCTION BY ANTI-RHEUMATIC AGENTS. Akihide Ohta, James S. Louie and Jouni Uitto. Harbor-UCLA Medical Center, Torrance, CA 90509

Previously, human peripheral blood monocytes have been shown to synthesize and secrete collagenase in short term culture (Arthritis Rheum. 27:1397, 1984). In this study, we have tested the effects of various anti-rheumatic agents on monocyte collagenase production in vitro. Peripheral blood mononuclear cells, isolated by Ficoll-Hypaque density gradient centrifugation, were placed in 24-well microtiter plates, 10^6 cells/well. The cells were allowed to adhere for 2 hrs and the non-adherent cells were removed by washing. The adherent cells, consisting predominantly of monocyte-macrophages as determined by non-specific esterase staining, were incubated in serum-free DMEM for 48 hrs at 37°C. Aliquots of the media were assayed for collagenase activity in the presence of 10 mM Ca^{2+} with [^{3}H]proline-labeled type I collagen as substrate. The cultured cells spontaneously produced small but detectable amounts of active collagenase and the production could be markedly increased by incubation with 20 µg/ml of Con-A. The Con-A-induced production of collagen was inhibited in a dose dependent manner by three anti-rheumatic agents, 1)gold sodium thiomalate (GST), 2)Auranofin (AF), and 3)indomethacin (IM). GST inhibited the collagenase production by 32 and 62% in 30 and 300 µg/ml concentrations, respectively (mean of 3 separate experiments). AF showed a 68% inhibition in concentrations ≥ 0.5 µg/ml. 10^{-4} M IM inhibited the enzyme production by 54%. The results indicate that anti-rheumatic agents inhibit the collagenase production by monocyte-macrophages in vitro, and such inhibition may contribute to the clinical efficacy of these compounds in vivo.

A2

INCREASED COLLAGEN BIOSYNTHESIS AND INCREASED EXPRESSION OF TYPE I AND TYPE III COLLAGEN GENES IN TIGHT SKIN (TSK) MOUSE FIBROBLASTS. Sergio A. Jimenez, Charlene Williams, Jeanne Myers and Reza I. Bashey. University of Pennsylvania, Philadelphia, PA 19104

The TSK mouse mutant strain displays connective tissue abnormalities similar to those present in patients with scleroderma (PSS) and is therefore a useful model to study the pathogenesis of uncontrolled fibrosis in PSS. To examine the mechanisms responsible for these alterations, normal and TSK mouse dermal fibroblasts cell lines were established and studies of collagen biosynthesis and regulation were performed. Identical secondary cultures of 5 normal and 5 TSK fibroblasts were incubated in media containing 10% FCS and 50 µg/ml ascorbic acid and after labeling with [14 C]-proline for 72 h the amount of newly synthesized collagen was determined. The results showed that TSK dermal fibroblasts produced significantly greater amounts of collagen than normal fibroblasts ($118 \pm 28.3 \times 10^{-2}$ dpm/µg DNA vs $53.7 \pm 21.9 \times 10^{-2}$ dpm/µg DNA; $p < 0.004$). Subsequently, the expression of three collagen genes in normal and TSK fibroblasts was analyzed by Northern blot hybridization of polyadenylated RNA to the human cDNA clones α12, Hf 32 and RJ 5 which are specific probes for transcripts of α1(I), α 2(I) and α1(III) collagen chains, respectively. It was found that the TSK fibroblasts consistently displayed increased levels (up to five-fold) of all three collagen transcripts examined. The results demonstrate that TSK fibroblasts produce excessive amounts of collagen in culture which is accompanied by a dramatic increase in the level of expression of collagen-specific mRNAs. These findings suggest that a similar increase in the level of expression of collagen genes may be responsible for the collagen overproduction characteristic of PSS.

A3

A NEW PROTEOGLYCAN COMPONENT OF THE HLA CLASS I COMPLEX. Joel Schiffenbauer* and Benjamin D. Schwartz. Wash. Univ. Med. School, and the Howard Hughes Med. Inst., St. Louis.

The HLA class I molecules act as target antigens on allogeneic cells and restrict T cell mediated killing directed against viral antigens. These molecules consist of a 45,000d chain associated with β_2 microglobulin. We have recently discovered that these molecules are associated with a high molecular weight sulfated component. This sulfated material was tested for the three characteristics of a proteoglycan (PG): 1) polyanionicity, 2) linkage of SO_4 to a large non-protein moiety and 3) sensitivity to enzymes specific for a PG. Class I molecules were isolated from $^{35}SO_4$ labeled Swei cells, and immunoprecipitated with various anti-class I antibodies. The $^{35}SO_4$-labeled associated class I molecule were solubilized in 8M urea and incubated with DEAE Sephacel under conditions in which proteoglycans, but not proteins or glycoproteins would bind. 91% of the class I-associated $^{35}SO_4$ labeled material bound to the column confirming its polyanionicity. Pronase digestion of the sulfated component resulted in a product which was excluded by Biogel P10, suggesting that the sulfated moiety was of large molecular weight. Finally, the SO_4 labeled component was treated with chondroitinase AC. The released material migrated with a chondroitin 4-sulfate standard. Therefore, the SO_4-labeled component associated with class I molecules meets the three criteria of a proteoglycan. The finding of a proteoglycan associated with the class I molecules and the known role of proteoglycans in cell-cell interactions suggests that the class I associated proteoglycan may have a role in immunologically important events.

A4

MOLECULAR EVENTS ASSOCIATED WITH INTERLEUKIN-1 INDUCTION OF SYNOVIAL CELL PLASMINOGEN ACTIVATOR. Eugene Mochan, Joanne Uhl and *Robert Newton. UMDNJ-SOM, Camden, NJ, 08103 and *E.I. duPont de Nemours & Co., Glenolden, PA., USA 19036.

We previously presented evidence (J. Rheum. 11:123, 1984; JAOA 84: 216, 1984) that the mononuclear cell product, interleukin-1 (IL-1), stimulates human synovial cell plasminogen activator (PA) production and that PA, via its proteolytic conversion of plasminogen to plasmin, might participate in cartilage destruction associated with rheumatoid arthritis (RA). In the present study, we have examined the mechanistic features associated with IL-1 stimulation of human synovial cell PA. Employing purified human peripheral blood mononuclear cell IL-1, we have found that IL-1 stimulates both intracellular and extracellular PA production in a dose dependent manner at a 50% maximum stimulation level comparable to that seen with enhancement of mouse thymocyte proliferation. This IL-1 stimulation caused increased levels of synovial cell PA, as detected by immunoperoxidase staining, and was prevented by cycloheximide and actinomycin D, and therefore, appears to involve de novo protein synthesis. The molecular weight of the induced synovial cell PA was ∼55,000 and thus resembles one of the forms of PA found in our earlier studies to be elevated in RA synovial fluids. The cyclooxygenase inhibitor, indomethacin ($IC_{50} = 2.5\mu M$), inhibited the IL-1 induction of PA and simultaneous addition of Prostaglandin E_2 (PGE_2) partially prevented this inhibition. On the other hand, addition of the phosphodiesterase inhibitor, theophylline, or dibutyryl c-AMP caused an approximate 2-fold enhancement of the IL-1 induction of PA. These results suggest that the IL-1 induction of synovial cell PA occurs via generation of endogenous PGE_2 and c-AMP.

A5

STRUCTURAL STUDIES ON B LYMPHOCYTE CYTOSKELETAL PROTEINS. Fiona Hunter, Jianyun Dong, Ajit Bhown, and J. Claude Bennett. UAB, Birmingham, AL 35294.

The proteins comprising the cytoskeleton of erythrocytes have been well characterized. Recent studies in other laboratories have indicated that a molecule (fodrin) which is structurally and immunologically related to erythrocyte spectrin is present in some non-erythroid cells. We have found that affinity purified rabbit antibodies to human erythrocyte spectrin give a positive immunofluorescence pattern with human (Daudi, Raji, LBW-46 and PBL) and murine (38C-13) lymphocytes. The cytoplasmic staining reveals a diffuse pattern which is different from that observed with affinity purified rabbit antibodies to actin, tubulin and IgM. Surface staining is negative. Omission of the primary antibody, normal rabbit serum and affinity purified rabbit anti-myosin are the negative controls. Immunoblot analysis of human erythrocyte ghost proteins separated by SDS gels and probed with the affinity purified rabbit antibodies to erythrocyte spectrin show reactivity with polypeptides of 220kD and 240kD as expected. Similarly polypeptides of 240kD and 270kD were found in the LBW-46 cell line when reacted with the same purified antibodies. In both cases some reactivity with a 45kD molecule was observed. Gel filtration chromatographic techniques have been developed to purify the spectrin-like molecule from extracts of lymphocyte cell lines. SDS gel analysis of the purified material yeilds proteins of 240kD and 270kD with additional aggregates of higher molecular weight. These studies are being pursued to gain an understanding of the structure of the lymphocyte cytoskeleton and its interaction with membrane receptors.

A6

BIOCHEMICAL AND IMMUNOLOGICAL DIFFERENTIATION OF HUMAN NEUTROPHIL COLLAGENASE AND HUMAN SKIN COLLAGENASE. Karen A. Hasty, George P. Stricklin, Margaret S. Hibbs, Jerome M. Seyer and Andrew H. Kang, Memphis, TN 38104.

Increased collagenase activity in acute and chronic inflammation plays a major role in in vivo degradation of native collagen and is the irreversible step in articular destruction. The presence of polymorphonuclear cells (PMN) during inflammatory processes underscores the necessity for further information about the role of PMN collagenase in disruptive alterations of the collagen framework. Since, classically, all mammalian collagenases are metalloproteases that cleave interstitial collagens approximately 3/4 of the distance from the NH_2-terminus, present analyses of tissues fail to differentiate the cellular origin of the collagenase. We have purified human neutrophil collagenase (HNC) and compared this enzyme to purified human skin collagenase (HSKC) biochemically with respect to the peptide bond cleaved in native collagen and immunologically for crossreactivity. HNC degrades Type I collagen between residues 775 and 776 of the α1(I) chain, as does HSKC. However, immunological comparisons showed each enzyme to contain unique and shared epitopes. Polyclonal antibody to HNC was inhibited 50% with HSKC in competitive inhibition ELISA confirming that some structural domains are conserved while others are unique to HNC. Paradoxically, polyclonal antibody to HSKC was not significantly inhibited by HNC, evidence of unique immunodominant epitope(s) of HSKC. Therefore, HNC and HSKC, although similar to each other in the precise site of substrate cleavage, differ in immunologically defined structural domains.

A7

MODULATION OF CELL PROLIFERATION BY HYALURONATE: RELEVANCE TO RHEUMATOID ARTHRITIS. R.L. Goldberg, J.-W. Hwang and B.P. Toole Tufts University School of Medicine, Boston, MA 02111

Synovial cell proliferation and decreases in the concentration and molecular weight (mol. wt.) of hyaluronate (HA) in the synovial fluid are characteristics of rheumatoid arthritis. We tested the effect of various concentrations and mol. wts. of HA, similar to those found in normal and diseased synovial fluid (0.3-2.9 mg/ml), on proliferation of cultured cells using radioactive thymidine incorporation into DNA and cell counts. Cells grown for 24 h in the presence of high mol. wt. HA (greater than 2,000,000 as determined by gel filtration) exhibited a dose dependent decrease in thymidine incorporation. A decrease of 50% occurred for rabbit synovial cells at 0.5 mg/ml of this HA, for 3T3 cells at 0.1 mg/ml, and for SV-3T3 cells at 0.7 mg/ml. Thymidine incorporation was inhibited by 90% in cultures of rabbit synovial cells grown in the presence of 1 mg/ml high mol. wt. HA for 24 or 48 h and cell number was inhibited by 50%. Incorporation of radioactive amino acids into cellular protein in these cultures was not affected. Lower mol. wt. HA (10,000-500,000) was not as effective an inhibitor; at 0.5 mg/ml, rabbit synovial cells were inhibited by only 20%, 3T3 by 15% and SV-3T3 had an increased incorporation of 45%. Also, with low concentrations of the lower mol. wt. HA (0.1 mg/ml) there was an increase of 30% in thymidine incorporation for rabbit synovial and 3T3 cells. Thus the alterations of HA in the synovial fluid of patients with rheumatoid arthritis may set a more favorable environment for synovial cell proliferation and disease progression. (Supported by NIH grant DE05838 to BPT and National Arthritis Foundation fellowship to RLG.)

A8

LIPOXYGENASE PATHWAY METABOLISM OF ARACHIDONIC ACID BY HUMAN SYNOVIAL CELLS IN CULTURE. Kathleen Gans, *Eugene Mochan, Debbie Cipriano, *Joanne Uhl, Robert Newton, & Neil Ackerman, E.I. duPont de Nemours & Co., Wilmington, DE., 19898 & *UMDNJ-SOM, Camden, NJ., 08103.

Cyclooxygenase metabolites of arachidonic acid (20:4) are synthesized by human synovial cells and may play a role in synovial joint destruction. Klickstein et al (J. Clin. Invest. 66: 1166, 1980) have detected 5-hydroxyeicosatetraenoic acid (5-HETE) and leukotriene B_4 (LTB_4) in human rheumatoid synovial fluid, but the source of these products was not identified. Others (BBA 753:257, 1983) did not detect production of lipoxygenase (LO) products by cultured rabbit synovial cells. In the current study, release of LO products from human synovial cells was investigated. Concentrations of various 20:4 metabolites were determined by radioimmunoassay (RIA). Human synovial cells from patients with rheumatoid or osteoarthritis were grown in primary monolayer culture. No macrophages were observed in the cultures used (5-8 passages). The 20:4 metabolites, PGE_2, 5-HETE, 12-HETE, LTB_4 and LTC_4 were detected following a 3 hour incubation in Eagles MEM. Using a purified human mononuclear cell interleukin-1 (IL-1), no stimulation in release of LO products was observed under conditions (3 hr, 37°c) that gave a 5-fold stimulation in PGE_2 release. These results demonstrate that cultured human synovial cells release LO products as well as PGE_2 and suggest that IL-1 predominately influences the cyclooxygenase pathway.

A9

ABNORMAL DNA REPAIR IN UNAFFECTED FAMILY MEMBERS OF RHEUMATOID ARTHRITIS PROBANDS, MAY BE AN ACQUIRED DEFECT. C. Bernard Colaco, G. Harris, P.D. Lawley, P.M. Lydyard and I.M. Roitt. The Middlesex Hospital, Immunology Department, Tottenham Street, London W1, UK.

A previous report of defective repair of a potent pre-mutagenic lesion 0^6-methylguanine (MeGua) in peripheral blood lymphocytes (PBLs) from patients with rheumatoid arthritis (RA) and SLE, might suggest that reduced expression of the necessary repair enzyme activity has a role in the development of auto-immunity (1).

We have studied 17 RA pedigrees to examine any putative hereditary or environmental influences in the expression of this enzyme.

Test PBLs are exposed to [^{14}C]N-methyl-N-nitrosourea (MNU) for one hr, followed by DNA extraction, acid hydrolysis and HPLC of free bases, and measurement of 0^6MeGua/7MeGua as a ratio, to assess relative proficiency of repair of 0^6MeGua. In a comparison with 32 healthy controls, 10/17 RA probands were found to be relatively deficient in DNA repair (p<0.005), but so also were 11/32 1° and 2° relatives (p<0.01) and 6/13 spouses (p<0.025). Interestingly a significant correlation between levels of 0^6MeGua repair in PBLs of each RA proband and their respective spouse (n=13, r=0.81, p<0.001) and also their respective 1° and 2° relatives (n=32, r=0.57, p<0.001) would suggest an environmental influence on the expression of this methyltransferase enzyme, but a hereditary component cannot yet be excluded.

Ref

(1) Defective repair of 0^6-methylguanine in auto-immune diseases. G. Harris et al. Lancet ii, 952, 1982.

A10

C1q AND RHP LEVELS AS DEFINITIVE BIOLOGICAL MARKERS FOR ACTIVE RHEUMATOID ARTHRITIS. CHARLES HURWITZ, CARMEN L. ROSANO AND NOUROLLAH PARHAMI. ALBANY, NEW YORK.

We have previously shown that serum levels of unbound C1q are elevated in active adult rheumatoid arthritis (RA) uncomplicated by vasculitis. We now report that all sera of such patients thus far examined contain a specific protein (RHP) which is absent from, or present in undetectable amounts in normal sera or sera from patients with other arthritides.

RHP is not rheumatoid factor, an immunoglobulin, the chondroitin-4-sulfate C1q inhibitor, or an acute phase reactant. It has a M.W. of 135 K, a pI of 5.1-5.3, and it inhibits those functions of C1q dependent on the exposed region to which C1r·C1s binds to form C1.

These findings suggest that both elevated C1q serum levels and the presence of detectable levels of RHP may serve not only as unambiguous biological markers for diagnosis of active RA but also as objective measures of changes in disease states since we have observed marked increases in serum levels of C1q and of RHP in a patient in remission one month before his disease flared.

The finding that RHP inhibits physiological functions of unbound C1q, such as its hemolytic action, binding of C1r·C1s, and binding to fibronectin, suggests that elevated serum levels of RHP and of unbound C1q may play roles in the immunopathogenesis of RA; since subsets of B lymphocytes, macrophages, and neutrophils contain specific receptor sites for unbound C1q. Unbound C1q has been shown to activate neutrophil metabolism.

A11

THE PREVALENCE OF SJOGREN'S SYNDROME (SS) IN PATIENTS WITH SYSTEMIC LUPUS ERYTHEMATOSUS (SLE) WHO HAVE ANTI-SS-A ANTIBODIES. **S.G. West, P.A. Andersen. Fitzsimons Army Medical Center, Denver CO 80045.**

The frequency of SS in SLE patients with anti-SS-A(Ro) antibodies is debated. The present study found 2i of 78 (27%) SLE patients to have antibodies against SS-A. These 21 patients were evaluated by clinical, serologic, genetic, radiographic, and pathologic criteria for the presence of SS.

Seventeen of these 21 patients had antibodies against SS-A without having antibodies against SS-B(La). Ten of these 17 patients had SS documented by lip biopsy while the other 7 had negative lip biopsies.

These 10 lip biopsy positive patients had the following positive results: sicca - 8; Schirmer's - 7; rose bengal - 4; parotid scan - 6; polyclonal gammopathy(PG) - 3; positive rheumatoid factor(+RF) - 2; and anti-RANA antibodies - 0. Nine of the 10 were HLA DR 3 positive.

The 7 lip biopsy negative patients had the following positive results: sicca - 3; Schirmer's - 2; rose bengal - 1; parotid scan - 1; PG - 3; +RF - 1; and anti-RANA antibodies - 0. One of the 7 was HLA DR 3 positive.

Four of the 21 patients had antibodies against both SS-A and SS-B. Three of the 4 had lip biopsies positive for SS. The 3 lip biopsy positive patients had the following positive results: sicca - 2; Schirmer's - 2; rose bengal - 1; parotid scan - 3; PG - 1; +RF - 3; and anti-RANA antibodies - 1. All 4 patients were HLA DR 3 positive.

Ten patients were randomly selected from the 57 patients who did not have antibodies against SS-A. Two of these 10 patients had SS documented by lip biopsy while the other 8 had negative lip biopsies. The 2 lip biopsy positive patients had the following positive results: sicca - 2; Schirmer's - 2; rose bengal - 1; parotid scan - 1; PG - 1; +RF - 1; anti-RANA antibodies - 1 and both had antibodies against SL antigen. One of the 2 was HLA DR 3 positive. The 8 lip biopsy negative patients had the following positive results: sicca - 3; Schirmer's - 1; rose bengal - 0; parotid scan - 0; PG - 2; +RF - 2.

These data suggest that HLA DR 3 positive, anti-SS-A positive SLE patients have an increased incidence of SS compared to HLA DR 3 negative, anti-SS-A positive SLE patients ($p<.01$) and compared to SLE patients without anti-SS-A ($p<.01$).

A12

SERUM LYMPHOCYTOTOXINS AND NEUROCOGNITIVE FUNCTION IN SYSTEMIC LUPUS ERYTHEMATOSUS (SLE). Aidan A. Long, Ramona Carbotte, Susan D. Denburg, Peter Temesvari, Dharam Singal and Judah A. Denburg, McMaster University, Hamilton, Ont. L8N 3Z5, CANADA.

Brain cross reactive serum lymphocytotoxic antibodies (LCA) have been associated with neuropsychiatric involvement in SLE (NP-SLE) but clearcut demonstration of their role has been hampered by lack of a standardized approach to the clinical classification of NP-SLE. We have investigated the relationships among LCA, detected by microcytotoxicity assay against panel lymphocytes, and simultaneous clinical and neurocognitive assessments in 26 patients with SLE. Previous correlations of LCA with overt neuropsychiatric events have been reported (Temesvari et al., Clin Immunol Immunopathol 28:243, 1983). LCA were present in 11/26 patients, of whom 6 had active NP-SLE and 5 had a history of NP-SLE assessed by a standardized clinical rating. 11/11 exhibited impaired neurocognitive function, using a standardized reproducible battery of tests, compared to 7/15 who were LCA negative ($p<0.05$). None of the 9 patients who had normal neurocognitive function had LCA. Furthermore, in the 22 patients whose serum was simultaneously examined for antineuronal antibodies (by a mixed hemadsorption assay against cell lines in culture) a positive correlation was found between the presence of these antibodies and LCA. These results provide further evidence that brain cross-reactive LCA are associated with NP-SLE. Moreover, utilizing neurocognitive status as a diagnostic criterion, the association is stronger, suggesting the biological importance of LCA in relation to brain dysfunction.

A13

DANAZOL IN SYSTEMIC LUPUS ERYTHEMATOSUS : A TWO YEARS PROSPECTIVE CONTROLLED TRIAL IN FOURTY FEMALE PATIENTS. Maxime Dougados, Bernard Amor, Chantal Job-Deslandre, Charles-Joël Menkès. Paris. FRANCE.

Since sex hormones seem to influence the natural course of systemic lupus erythematosus (S.L.E.) with a deleterious effect of estrogens and a protective effect of androgens, it seemed interesting to study danazol (D) as baseline treatment of S.L.E. Fourty female patients (pts) with mild disease and on low corticosteroid (C.S) dosage (less than 20 mg prednisone daily) were randomly allocated to either of two groups. The first group received D. 400 mg daily together with C.S. while the second only C.S. Patients crossed over after one year and then received the alternate treatment. Thirteen pts withdrew from the study because of pregnancies while taking C.S. alone (3 pts) and of side effects while taking D (10 pts) : skin rash (4 pts), amenorrhoea badly psychologically accepted (3 pts), hepatitis (1 pt), dyspepsia (1 pt), depressive syndrome (1 pt). The results were combined with respect to treatment modality : patients taking D. (groupe D+) or not (group D-). Statistical analysis was performed upon the clinical and biological changes after one year period follow up and demonstrated in groupe D+ a reduction of C.S. daily dosage (-5.2±4.7 mg V.S.+1.1±6.7 in group D-, p<0.01) and number of flarings (1 V.S. 15 in group D-, p<0.001) ; an increase in haemoglobin level (+1.1±1.1 gr/100 ml V.S. 0.8±1.0 in group D-, p<0.001), platelet count (+65.3±59.0 x 10^3/mm3 V.S. 10.3±48.7 in group D-p<0.01) and in C4 level (+9.4±9.0 mg/l V.S. -1.1±6.7 in group D- p<0.01). These data suggest the beneficial effect of D. in female S.L.E. and therefore that hormonomodulation of human lupus is possible.

A14

EVIDENCE THAT ANTI-RO/SSA MAY BE INVOLVED IN THE GENESIS OF CONGENITAL COMPLETE HEART BLOCK. John B. Harley, Jeffrey L. Kaine, Owen F. Fox, Morris Reichlin, Barry Gruber. Univ. of Okla. and Okla. Med. Res. Fnd., Oklahoma City; Wash. Univ., St. Louis; and State Univ. of New York, Stony Brook.

Anti-Ro/SSA precipitating antibodies have been closely associated with congenital complete heart block. The mechanism of congenital complete heart block pathogenesis is unknown. We, therefore, conducted a study of a pedigree with twins and of cardiac tissue using a sensitive solid phase immunosorbent assay for anti-Ro/SSA. The affected neonate, his fraternal HLA-identical unaffected twin, and his mother all had anti-Ro/SSA precipitating antibody in an immunodiffusion assay. The proband, however, had less than 10% of the anti-Ro/SSA binding activity in the immunosorbent assay that was present in either the twin sister or the mother. Meanwhile, the proband and his twin had identical titers in a fluorescent antinuclear antibody assay using a mouse kidney substrate. Purified Ro/SSA blocked the immunosorbent anti-Ro/SSA binding activity, but not the antinuclear antibody activity. In separate experiments, the immunosorbent assay was modified to measure Ro/SSA in extracts. Adult and fetal cardiac extract contained a similar level of Ro/SSA demonstrating that cardiac tissue contains Ro/SSA antigen activity. These findings demonstrate that this autoantigen is present in cardiac tissue and show that anti-Ro/SSA is specifically reduced in the serum of a child with congenital complete heart block. These observations are consistent with models of complete congenital heart block which require the participation of anti-Ro/SSA in the immunopathogenesis of congenital complete heart block.

A15

DYSLIPOPROTEINEMIA IN SYSTEMIC LUPUS ERYTHEMATOSUS. **W. Ettinger, D.Applebaum-Bowden, F. Wigley, A. Goldberg, and W. Hazzard, Gerontology Research Center and Johns Hopkins University, Baltimore, MD 21205.**

Recent evidence suggests that patients with systemic lupus erythematosus (SLE) develop premature atherosclerosis. Since dyslipoproteinemia is a major cause of atherosclerosis we measured triglycerides (TG), total cholesterol (C), high density lipoprotein C (HDL-C), HDL-C subclasses (HDL_2-C, HDL_3-C), low density lipoprotein C (LDL-C) and apoprotein AI (ApoAI) in 36 females with SLE and age matched female controls (CT). The mean ±SE values (mg/dl) were:

	TG	C	HDL-C	HDL_2-C	HDL_3-C	LDL-C	ApoAI	
SLE	175.6*	220.5**	53.6	9.5*	44.0*	132.4	135.2	
	±17.5	±10.5	±3.1	±1.6	±2.5	±8.1	±11.6	*p<.001
CT	81.7	186.7	53.7	23.7	33.7	127.6	135.7	**p<.01
	±6.8	±6.6	±2.4	±1.1	±1.3	±9.2	±8.9	

TG, C and HDL_3-C were higher and HDL_2-C lower in SLE subjects than in controls. Despite similar mean values for HDL-C and LDL-C, 7 SLE subjects had LDL-C values above the Lipid Research Clinics 95th percentile level as compared to 1 control (p<.005) while 7 others had HDL-C values below the 5th percentile compared to 1 control (p<.005). In the SLE subjects corticosteroid dose correlated with TG (r=0.38), C (r=0.44), HDL-C (r=0.47) and HDL_3-C (r=0.41) but not HDL_2-C. HDL_2-C was inversely correlated with TG (r=-0.38) in SLE subjects but not controls. Thus, dyslipoproteinemia is common in SLE and consists of hypertriglyceridemia, hypercholesterolemia, low HDL_2-C and in a sub-group of patients, low HDL-C. These lipoprotein abnormalities may explain why SLE patients develop premature atherosclerosis.

A16

PLASMAPHERESIS IN LUPUS NEPHRITIS: A CONTROLLED STUDY. PRELIMINARY RESULTS. Daniel J Wallace, Dennis Goldfinger, James R Klinenberg, Cedars-Sinai Med Ctr, Los Angeles, CA 90048.

Patients with aggressive lupus nephritis are usually managed with prednisone, and if this intervention is not satisfactory, immunosuppressive therapy is added. To date, we have studied 20 patients who have active nephritis despite adequate courses of treatment with both prednisone and immunosuppressive agents in an ongoing study. In addition to continuing the above treatment (C group), 13 of the patients also underwent 12 plasmaphereses over 4 weeks (P group) in an effort to see if this approach could improve the poor prognosis attributed to this subset. 19 of the 20 patients (95%) were women with nephrotic syndrome. The mean age at study entry was 36 with a mean disease duration of 5 years. 14 of the 18 patients biopsied had Class IV (diffuse proliferative) lesions, 3 Class III (focal proliferative) and 1 Class V (membranous). Concurrent immunosuppressive therapy included cyclophosphamide 13, azathioprine 6, and chlorambucil 1. 12 patients had received prior pulse medrol. In a mean 19 month follow-up, one patient in each group died and one in each group was dialyzed.

P patients had a greater mean decrement in blood pressure, weight, steroid dose, 24 hour urine protein, anti DNA and serum creatinine than C patients. They also had a greater rise in serum albumin and C3 levels. Preliminary evidence reveals that at 19 months, P patients had less active renal disease but similar life table curves.

A17

A NOVEL HIGH MOLECULAR DNA FRAGMENT IN CRYOPRECIPITATES FROM SYSTEMIC LUPUS ERYTHEMATOSUS. Carmen E. Contreras, Manuel Rieber, Ornella Melijson and Nicolás E. Bianco. WHO Collaborative Center for Clinical Immunology and IVIC, Caracas, Venezuela.

Cryoprecipitates from 3 groups of patients with Systemic Lupus Erythematosus (SLE): group A (high serum levels of anti DNA, circulating immune complexes (CIC) and cryoprecipitate protein content), group B(high levels of CIC only) and group C (all 3 parameters within normal limits), were investigated for the presence of DNA fragments.Cryoprecipitates from non SLE patients and young healthy individuals were included as controls. DNAs were obtained by pretreatment of cryoprecipitates with proteinase k and extracted by phenol-chloroform, ethanol method. Size and nature of DNAs were achieved by ethidium bromide agarose gel electrophoresis and enzymatic treatments with DNAseI and restriction enzyme Eco RI. Our results showed a consistent 9.7 kbp DNA fragment, detected in cryoprecipitates from control groups and from SLE groups B and C patients.In contrast in SLE group A cryoprecipitates, in addition to the 9.7kbp DNA,a unique high molecular weight (17.5kbp) DNA and 3 minor DNA fragments(1.77-2.24kbp; 1775- 975 bp and<975bp) were demonstrated . All DNA fragments from the selected patients groups and normal donors were susceptible to DNAseI treatment. Furthermore, all fragments with the exception of 9.7 kbp fragment, were digested by the Eco RI enzyme suggesting their double stranded nature.Contrary to previous reports,our results suggest the presence of a novel high molecular weight DNA fragment in the cryoprecipitates of active SLE patients. The origen and significance of these DNAs needs further elucidation.

A18

LONG TERM USE OF METHOTREXATE (MTX) IN INFLAMMATORY ARTHRITIS: CLINICAL AND X-RAY EVALUATION. Larry Boh, Art Schuna, Michael Pitterle, Elaine Adams, and Walter Sundstrom. UW and VA, Madison, WI 53705.

We prospectively evaluated the clinical efficacy of MTX in the management of inflammatory arthritis. MTX 12.9±5.05mg was administered once weekly to 57 patients,(27 males,30 females) for 11.86±9.7 months. All patients failed or developed toxicity to gold, penicillamine, and hydroxychloroquine. Mean patient age was 61. Disease duration was 10.8 yr (range 1-26). Forty-nine patients had RA (39 sero +) 6 had psoriatic arthritis, 2 MCTD. Prednisone was used in 85%,(mean=5.6mg/d), NSAIDs in 72% of patients.

Clinical Parameters Demonstrating Significant Improvement

month	0	6	12	18	24
Joint Count	15.5±7.3	10.2±6.3*	8.2±5.9*	7.4±3.3*	7.9±4.3*
A.M. Stiffness	6.1±8.5	2.0±4.1	0.7±0.9*	3.8±7.3	1.0±1.6
Pain Scale	6.65±2.6	4.4±1.6*	4.3±1.9*	4.2±1.6*	3.5±1.7*
Activity Scale	6.7±2.4	3.9±1.6*	4.3±1.9*	4.3±1.5*	3.8±1.5*

*p<0.05

Grip strength,fatigue,ring size,hgb,hct,ESR,platelets,SGOT,SGPT showed no significant change. A reduction in Prednisone dose was observed at 6,12,18,24 months but was not statistically significant. Elevated transaminase was the most frequent toxicity observed. No toxicity was observed after 18 months. MTX was discontinued in 7 patients (3 toxicity,4 lack of efficacy).

A total of 24 new erosions were observed in 30 patients followed for 1 year,incidence 0.8 erosions/patient year. Additional x-ray data will be presented. MTX is an effective therapy with an acceptable risk-benefit ratio for patients who have failed or developed toxicities from traditional remission-inducing agents.

A19

SEGREGATION AND LINKAGE STUDIES ON SEROPOSITIVE RHEUMATOID ARTHRITIS. B. Barger, G.S. Alarcón, R.C.P. Go, W.J. Koopman, R.T. Acton, University of Alabama at Birmingham, Birmingham, AlaLama 35294

Segregation and linkage analyses were conducted as a means of assessing the mode of inheritance in white patients with rheumatoid arthritis (RA). The relationship between HLA and rheumatoid factor (RF) pro duction was also examined. HLA haplotypes and RF seropositivity were determined on all available members of 14 multiply-affected and 15 simplex families. Each family member who reported symptoms of RA was clinically examined. Analysis of haplotype sharing between 10 affected -sib pairs showed 10/10 shared at least one haplotype, with 3/10 sharing both haplotypes. Haplotypes assorted randomly among unaffected sibs in both the multiply-affected and simplex families.

Linkage analysis was performed on 11 families, using a penetrance of 36% and recombination rates from 0.0 to 0.4. No linkage with HLA was found. In addition, the association of RF with HLA was assessed and no association of linkage was found.

The segregation data on 151 white families identified through a proband with RA indicated that the frequency of clinically confirmed RA among first degree relatives was 6.0%. An age of onset segregation model will be used to test for existence of major gene(s) or genetic heterogeneity. These results will be used to further define the linkage analyses reported here.

A20

PERSONALITY AND STRESS IN RHEUMATOID AND OSTEOARTHRITIS. Neal Latman, School of Pharmacy, SWOSU, Weatherford, OK 73096.

In the last 50 years, many investigators have implicated personality and stress in the onset and development of rheumatoid arthrits (RA). The purpose of this study was to determine if; a.) people with RA have different personality characteristics than people with osteoarthritis (OA), b.) onset of RA is associated with more life stress than onset of OA, and c.) any personality differences that were found are the result of the chronic disease process. The 16 Personality Factor Questionaire and a life stress measure was administered to 128 RAs and 77 OAs. The RAs had an average of 51 (+/- 4.8 S.E.) Life Change Units compared to 33 (+/- 4.7 S.E.) for the OAs. ($P < 0.01$) The RAs also exhibited a different personality pattern on 11 on the 16 primary personality factors and 2 of the 4 second order personality factors ($P < 0.005$). A lack of correlation between duration of RA and personality factor scores implied that the personality differences were present at onset and not the result of the chronic disease process. Although this study found distinct differences in personality and stress at disease onset between the matched groups of RA and OA, the differences are more complex than had previously been reported and do not exhibit a normal frequency distribution.

A21

AN ANALYSIS OF HEMATURIA IN RHEUMATOID PATIENTS ON GOLD AND D-PENICILLAMINE THERAPY. Patrice A. Leonard, Stephen R. Bienz, Daniel O. Clegg, and John R. Ward. University of Utah School of Medicine, Salt Lake City, UT 84143

A membranous nephropathy presenting as proteinuria is the most common manifestation of renal toxicity from gold and D-penicillamine therapy for rheumatoid arthritis. Hematuria is considered a less commonly encountered manifestation of nephrotoxicity from these drugs; however, its incidence and relationship to treatment have not been well defined. We reviewed the stored data on urinalyses from two multicenter controlled randomized trials, one comparing gold sodium thiomalate (GST), auranofin and placebo, the other comparing moderate dose D-penicillamine, low-dose D-penicillamine and placebo. We define hematuria as 3 or more red blood cells per high power field found in 3 or more of the weekly urinalyses in the gold trial or the bi-monthly urinalyses in the D-penicillamine trial. Of the 225 patients in the D-penicillamine trial, 29% of the 52 patients on placebo, 35% of the 87 patients on 125 mg/day of D-penicillamine and 28% of the 86 patients on 500 mg of D-penicillamine had recurrent hematuria. Of the 161 patients in the GST/auranofin trial, 35% of the 43 placebo-treated patients, 35% of the 54 GST-treated patients and 29% of the 64 auranofin-treated patients had hematuria. There were no statistical differences between treatment groups in either trial. Further analysis showed that menstruating females did not account for the majority of patients with hematuria. These findings suggest that the traditionally held belief that gold and D-penicillamine cause hematuria should be reconsidered.

A22

ANKLE ORTHOSIS FOR RHEUMATOID DISEASE. L. Gerber, G. Hunt, National Institutes of Health, Bethesda, Md. S. Hurwitz, G. W. University Hospital, Washington, D. C.

Five patients with rheumatoid arthritis, moderate-to-severe ankle pain, abnormal gait characteristics and decrease in function were provided an ankle orthosis in an attempt to improve these parameters. The orthosis was designed to immobilize the subtalar joint, partially immobilize the tibiotalar joint, but permit articulation at the midfoot and forefoot. All patients had failed to obtain adequate relief using local injections, other types of orthotics or gait aids.

Patients received careful evaluation of the foot, including: gait parameters as measured by Stride Analyzer®, range of motion of hindfoot, x-rays, subjective pain assessment, and activity level.

All patients were comfortably fit with a custom made orthotic, made in an office setting by the physiotherapist in 2 hours. The orthotic enclosed the heel, extended over the maleoli, limiting only hindfoot motion.

All patients had restricted subtalar motions and radiographic changes in the subtalar joint primarily. Stride length increased an average of 12%, and velocity increased an average of 11M/min in all patients with the orthotic. All patients had severe pain on ambulating without the orthotic and 4 experienced minimal or no pain when ambulating with the orthotic. Five patients required gait aids prior to using the orthosis, and 4 ambulate without aids while using the orthosis. Five patients resumed activities previously abandoned.

An orthosis that controls hindfoot motion is effective in reducing pain and increasing functional activity. The orthotic should be considered for patients who have not responded to conventional ankle-foot orthotics who have primarily subtalar joint disease.

A23

A CONTROLLED TRIAL OF AURANOFIN AND PLACEBO IN RHEUMATOID ARTHRITIS(RA). The Auranofin Cooperating Group.

A six month multi-center, prospective, randomized, double blind study comparing Auranofin (AU) with Placebo (P) was conducted in patients with definite and classical RA taking stable doses of NSAIDS. 311 patients entered the trial, 275 remained on coded medication. Baseline characteristics were similar in both groups. At 6 months, the AU group showed a significant improvement in clinical ($p=0.003$), functional ($p=0.001$), pain ($p=0.026$) and global scores ($p=0.006$). Mean changes in selected components of the clinical score are illustrated below:

	P:Mean Change ± SE	AU:Mean Change ± SE	p
Tender joints	-4.5 ± 0.9	-7.3 ± 0.9	0.01
Swollen joints	-3.6 ± 0.6	-5.5 ± 0.7	0.01
Morning stiffness	-12.3 ± 13.4	-28.3 ± 12.0	0.09

Diarrhea or loose stools occurred in 60% of AU patients and 19% of P patients. Coded medication was discontinued in 48 patients(15%)as follows:

	Auranofin (N=158)		Control (N=153)		Total (N=311)	
	#	%	#	%	#	%
Adverse effects	16	10.1	6	3.9	22	7.1
Lack of efficacy	6	3.8	6	3.9	12	3.9
Other	9	5.7	5	3.3	14	4.5

Adverse effects which required discontinuation included: P group: diarrhea 1, rash 2, oral ulcers 1, headache 1, elevated liver enzymes 1. AU: diarrhea 7, rash 2, thrombocytopenia 2, proteinuria 1, forgetfulness 1, gastritis 1, tachycardia 1, irritability 1. All were reversible on cessation of therapy. These results demonstrate that 6 months of Auranofin therapy is safe and more effective than Placebo in controlling RA.

A24

CLINICAL SIGNIFICANCE OF ANTI-SSA (Ro) IN RHEUMATOID ARTHRITIS. Gilles Boire and Henri-A. Ménard. Rheumatic Diseases Unit, Faculty of Medicine, University of Sherbrooke, Sherbrooke, Québec, Canada, J1H 5N4.

Anti-SSA has been found in SLE (notably the sub-acute and neonatal form) and Sjogren's syndrome (SS) but no specific association with RA has been reported. Reviewing the charts of 30 anti-SSA positive patients seen in the last year, we made the following observations:

Antibody to	No (%)	SLE	RA	SS	CTD
SSA	9(30)	0	7(78)	1	1
SSA/dsDNA	7(23)	7	3*	0	0
SSA/SSB	5(17)	0	1	2	2
SSA/RNP/others**	8(27)	3	0	2	3
SSA/PM-1	1(3)	0	0	0	1
TOTAL	30(100)	10(33)	11(37)*	5(17)	7(23)

(*) Satisfy both the ARA criteria for SLE and RA and are also included under SLE. (**) Sm 1, SSB 5, unidentified 1, none 1.

Hence: 1- anti-SSA is frequently (70%) found with other nuclear auto-antibodies in which case almost 50% are SLE. 2- When anti-SSA is found alone, the most common diagnosis is RA (78%). 3- These RA patients (3 with SS) have generally an unfavorable clinical course, do not respond well to remitting drugs and require steroid or immunosuppressive therapy. Furthermore, vasculitis, liver abnormalities, neutropenia and circulating immune complexes are prominent. 4- Three patients with classical sero-positive RA developped clinical and serological features of SLE. Our study suggests that an isolated anti-SSA identifies a sub-group of severe RA.

A25

PROGRESSIVE ANKYLOSIS IN THE MOUSE: A MURINE MODEL OF ANKYLOSING SPONDYLITIS. Maren L Mahowald and Joel Taurog. Minneapolis VA Medical Center and Univ of Minn Medical School, Minneapolis, MN 55417

Progressive Ankylosis (ANK) in the mouse was described as a recessive skeletal mutation by Sweet and Green (1981). This report concluded that ANK/ANK mice had: "calcification of cartilage and tissues adjacent to joints, proliferation of joint cells and tissues; and degeneration in tendons and ligaments of joints." We have studied 32 litters from 4 heterozygous breeder pairs. Abnormalities occurred in 23/106 (22%) of males and 18/87 (21%) of females and included: decreased grasp and cling by forepaw digits at wk 3-4 and hindpaws at wk 5; decreased flex/ext of wrists at wk 5, elbows wk 7, ankles wk9; dec mobility of cervial spine and a stiff thorax by wk5 and a crouched posture with thoracic kyphosis by wk 6. By wk 8 digits were hyperextended and wrists and ankles so stiff that gait was markedly abnormal. Animals were unable to cling to a wire grid, unable to keep heads above water while swimming and unable to eat food from overhead cage covers. Brief swelling without erythema was occasionally found in digits. Several females developed crusting vaginal excrescences and several males developed striking balanitis. No eye inflammation was found, affected animals were smaller than unaffected littermates and by mo 4 fur was scruffy.

Histologic changes at 1 mo included synovial proliferation, synovial fluid contained a few mononuclear cells and a few PMNS in subsynovium. At 3 mo there was striking joint destruction by hyperplastic synovial pannus eroding cartilage and producing ankylosis as well as extensive periosteal new bone. Clinical features of this murine model resemble human ankylosing spondylitis. The histopathologic and genetic features remain to be investigated.

A26

PROSTAGLANDIN E (PGE) GENERATION BY MONOCYTES FROM SYSTEMIC LUPUS ERYTHEMATOSUS (SLE) PATIENTS. Bruce Freundlich, Barbara R. Shoback and Robert B. Zurier. University of Pennsylvania, Philadelphia, PA 19104

The disease process in murine SLE models responds in a positive fashion to treatment with exogenous PGE. The metabolism of PGE was therefore studied in human SLE peripheral blood monocytes, the major secretor of PGE among mononuclear cells. Monocytes with low platelet contamination from 13 patients were compared to those from matched controls. One x 10^6 cells/well were incubated in 24 well plastic plates from 1 to 14 hr with or without Con A. Overnight viability was >95% and plating frequencies were comparable among SLE patients vs normals. At 18 hr there was maximum production of PGE in both groups of donors as measured by radioimmunoassay: means 18.2 ng/ml (SLE) and 22.2 ng/ml (nl). SLE monocytes produced less PGE than normals after Con A stimulation 27.2 ng/ml vs 54.1 ng/ml ($p < 0.05$). Patients were divisible into: good producers, 18 hr mean 30.2 ng/ml (N=7) and low producers, 6.1 ng/ml (N=6). Low producers had a poor PGE response to Con A and tended to have more active disease and were off prednisone. Good producers had inactive disease. Two patients who were low producers with active disease were placed on prednisone and upon restudy became good producers with diminished disease activity. In one of these patients a similar rise in monocyte production of $PGF_{2\alpha}$, 6-Keto $PGF_{1\alpha}$ and LTC_4 was noted after the institution of prednisone. Since PGE has been implicated in suppressor responses these results may be relevant to the abnormal immunosuppression often seen in SLE patients.

A27

AN INHIBITOR OF SUPEROXIDE (O_2^-) GENERATION AND PHAGOCYTOSIS IN SYNOVIAL FLUID OF GOUT AND PSEUDOGOUT PATIENTS. Alejandro Alvarellos, Isaias Spilberg. V.A. Medical Center and Washington U. St Louis, MO 63106.

An explanation for the self-limited nature of the acute attacks of crystal-induced arthritis postulates the appearance of an inhibitor of phagocytosis in the synovial fluid (SF) during the later phases of the process. To test the above, SF from patients with gout (G), pseudogout (PG), RA and DJD were assessed for their inhibitory properties on PMN fluorescent latex beads phagocytosis and FMLP induced O_2^- generation by the cytochrome C assay. In the O_2^- experiments, cells were preincubated in medium or 1/10 SF for 30' and then exposed to 10^{-7} FMLP for 10'. Phagocytosis assays were performed preincubating cells with medium or 1/10 SF for 30', fluorescent latex beads added and incubated for 1 hr. Intracellular beads were then counted with a fluorescent microscope. Results are expressed as % of inhibition of O_2^- generation and latex beads phagocytosis by PMN exposed to SF. Cells incubated with G SF had a 30.8%±7.7 inhibition of O_2^- generation ($p<.001$) and 45.1%±16.7 decrease of phagocytosis ($p<.001$). Sequential SF samples from a patient with acute gout showed an increasing O_2^- inhibition: 1st day: 18.3%; 2nd day: 23.3%; 4th day: 42.5%; 5th day: 54.1%. PG SF showed a 21.9%±5.6 inhibition of O_2^- generation ($p<.05$) and a 22.8%±8.1 decrease in phagocytosis ($p<.05$). RA and DJD SF showed no significant inhibition of O_2^- generation or phagocytosis. Treatment of SF with hyaluronidase or heat did not affect the results. HPLC analysis of G SF showed the bulk of inhibitory activity present in a peak with a MW @ 15K. These results suggest that an inhibitor(s) of O_2^- generation and phagocytosis by PMN is present in the SF of patients with G and PG but is not seen in RA or DJD.

A28

OXY RADICAL DEGRADATION OF HYALURONIC ACID (HA) BY NEUTROPHILS (PMNs). Robert A. Greenwald and Susan A. Moak Long Island Jewish-Hillside Medical Center, New Hyde Park, NY 11042.

Oxygen radicals are the probable mediators of HA degradation *in vivo*. This reaction has been studied in the xanthine oxidase (XO) system, but is not well documented for PMNs, the probable source of radicals in inflamed joints. PMNs stimulated with PMA reproducibly decreased the viscosity of HA (40% at 60 min, 65% at 90 min). When XO and PMN systems were calibrated to identical maximal superoxide fluxes, the magnitude of the XO effect exceeded that of PMNs and had an earlier onset of action. For a given superoxide flux, prolonged incubation time enhanced the degree of PMN degradation but not that due to XO. However, both systems showed identical behavior when dose response inhibition curves were done with SOD or catalase, and their requirements for exogenous ferric ion were identical as well. Physical disruption of HA by PMNs was demonstrated by altered chromatographic profiles on Sepharose CL-2B (PMN degraded material shifting from V_o to V_t) and by loss of intrinsic viscosity from 1770 ml/gm down to 750 in sequential steps as a function of incubation time. PMN lysates or supernatants from stimulated cells had no effect on HA. PMA was the only PMN stimulus that caused HA degradation; neither concanavalin A nor FMLP, when used at equal or greater superoxide generating fluxes, affected HA. PMNs, containing no enzyme capable of degrading HA, do so by generating superoxide, which exerts its effect by secondary generation of hydroxyl radical; generation of the latter is a function of concomitant H_2O_2 production. Stimuli *in vivo* which do not yield the latter will not result in loss of synovial fluid viscosity.

A29

EXCESSIVE PRODUCTION OF AND RESPONSE TO B CELL GROWTH FACTOR (BCGF) BY CELLS FROM PATIENTS WITH SYSTEMIC LUPUS ERYTHEMATOSUS (SLE). Jorge Alcocer-Varela, Erasmo Martínez-Cordero and Donato Alarcón-Segovia. Instituto Nacional de la Nutrición. México 14000, D.F. MEXICO.

B-cell hyperactivity in SLE may be due to decreased suppressor cell function, increased helper-cell function or direct lymphokine action. We therefore studied the production of and the response to BCGF by peripheral blood cells from 18 untreated SLE patients (10 active, 8 in remission).

T cells from SLE patients with active disease but not those from patients in remission (table) released significanly more BCGF activity than those of controls whether stimulated with PHA ($p<.0025$) or by autologous mixed lymphocyte reaction (AMLR) ($p<.01$) as determined by the 3TdR incorporation by normal purified Staph aureous Cowan I-activated B cells.

SLE	(n)	PRODUCTION, CPMx10^{-3} PHA	PRODUCTION, CPMx10^{-3} AMLR	RESPONSE, CPMx10^{-3}
ACTIVE	(10)	11.8 ± 2.7	4.9 ± 0.3	17.0 ± 4
INACTIVE	(8)	4.2 ± 0.9	2.7 ± 0.5	5.4 ± 0.6
CONTROLS	(13)	4.0 ± 0.6	2.9 ± 0.2	4.4 ± 1.1

The proliferative response of purified SLE B-cells to BCGF from a cloned T cell was increased in patients with active disease ($p<.001$) but not in patients in remission.

Because most T cell functions remain abnormal despite disease remission the increased production of BCGF may be a determining factor in switching on the production of autoantibodies upon activation of SLE.

A30

SPECIFICALLY DECREASED SUPPRESSION OF IgM-RHEUMATOID FACTOR (RF) SYNTHESIS BY OKT8(+) CELLS IN RHEUMATOID ARTHRITIS (RA). N. Olsen and H.E.Jasin. University of Texas Health Science Center, Southwestern Medical School, Dallas Texas 75235

Circulating B cell precursors specific for IgM-RF are present in normal (N) subjects, but spontaneous production of RF occurs only in RA. The regulatory role of RF-specific suppressor T cells was studied in pokeweed mitogen-stimulated in vitro cultures. Increasing numbers of purified N or RA T8 cells were added to allogeneic normal B + T4 cell mixtures. RA-T8 cells were observed to be consistently less effective than N-T8 cells in suppressing normal IgM and IgM-RF synthesis. At several cell concentrations, twice as many RA-T8 cells were required to achieve levels of suppression comparable to normals. An autologous preculture system was then used to probe for RF-specific suppressor precursors. T cells from N or RA donors were precultured with or without 10 ug/ml heat aggregated IgG (HAG) for 4 days, then panned for T8(+) cells which were added to fresh autologous B + T4 cells. At T8:T4=1, mean suppression of baseline RF synthesis was 48±10% for 7 N donors and only 12±4% for 7 RA donors (p=0.010). Suppression of total IgM was comparable in both groups (36%,30%) indicating a defect in generation of RF-specific suppression in the RA precultures. Addition of HAG to the preculture increased RF suppression in RA from 12 to 48% (p=0.006). Specificity for suppression of RF was indicated by a decrease in the RF/M ratio from 2.1 in RA control cultures to 0.9 in HAG cultures (p=0.035) while corresponding ratios in normals increased (0.8 to 1.4; p=0.041). The data suggest that OKT8-mediated suppression of RF synthesis is decreased in RA but can be specifically induced in vitro by IgG complexes.

A31

ANTIGEN-INDUCED ACCELERATION OF SURFACE Ig TURNOVER AND IgD LOSS ON ANTIGEN-BINDING B CELLS DEPENDS ON INTERACTION WITH MATURE T CELLS. R.F. Ashman and B.J. Noel. University of Iowa and VA Medical Center, Iowa City, IA 52242.

We are determining which early and intermediate events in the response of antigen-binding B cells to a T-dependent antigen (sheep erythrocytes) require T help. Nonimmune sheep erythrocyte antigen-binding spleen B cells (ABC) from Balb/c nu/nu mice resemble those of nu/+ and +/+ mice in surface IgM and IgD expression and turnover rate. But 5 days after in vivo immunization: 1) The proportion of ABC expressing surface IgD declined in +/+ mice (87% decreased to 47%) and in nu/+ mice (90% to 43%), but not in nu/nu mice (96% to 93%). 2) Recovery of antigen-binding occurred by 2 hr after pronase treatment in +/+ ABC (19% of initial ABC count increased to 62%) and in nu/+ ABC (15% to 44%) but not in nu/nu ABC (12% to 18%). 3) When spleen cells were incubated 2.5 hr in 100 µg/ml cycloheximide to prevent receptor replacement, uncompensated receptor shedding reduced ABC by 79% in +/+ mice and by 84% in nu/+ mice, but only by 6% in nu/nu mice. Thus, although the ABC in nonimmune nu/nu mice appear normal in their surface Ig turnover, day 5 immune nu/nu ABC fail to undergo the normal antigen-induced acceleration of surface Ig shedding and replacement with reduced expression of surface IgD, suggesting that these activation events require interaction with mature T cells. Indeed, when nu/+ T cells were transferred intravenously to nu/nu littermates 1 day before immunization, pronase-treated day 5 ABC were then able to recover to 30-60% of their initial ABC count in 2 hr and also shed receptors rapidly, like +/+ and nu/+ ABC.

A32

MECHANISM RESPONSIBLE FOR ABNORMAL CONTROL OF EPSTEIN-BARR VIRUS(EBV) IN RHEUMATOID ARTHRITIS (RA). Martin Lotz, Constantine D. Tsoukas, Dennis A. Carson and John H. Vaughan. Scripps Clinic and Research Foundation, La Jolla, CA 92037.

After in vitro infection of peripheral blood mononuclear cells with Epstein Barr virus, RA T lymphocytes are deficient in IL-2 and IFNγ production. This defect could be restored by monocyte depletion of the cultured cells. The mechanism of this monocyte effect does not involve prostaglandins, oxygen radicals or soluble immune response suppressor substances, as judged by the failure of indomethacin, 2-mercaptoethanol, or catalase to neutralize it. EBV infection of RA lymphocytes induces both IL-1 and an inhibitor of IL-1. The latter was found in all RA cultures examined for it. The balance of simultaneously present IL-1 and IL-1 inhibitor determined the levels of detectable IL-1 activity, and this correlated with the levels of IL-2 and IFNγ.

In contrast to the deficiency in T cell response to EBV infection, the response to stimulation with OKT_3 is normal as measured by proliferation and IL-2 and IFNγ release. Thus, these in vitro studies on RA lymphocytes indicate that antigenic stimulation with EBV, in contrast to the normal OKT_3 mitogen response, induces inhibition of IL-1 with subsequent defects in IL-2 and IFNγ. This may be the basis for the previously reported defect of RA lymphocytes in regulating EBV infection of B cells.

A33

CHARACTERIZATION OF LEU 2+ SUPPRESSORS OF INTERLEUKIN 2 PRODUCTION IN SLE M. Linker-Israeli, F.P. Quismorio, B. Uddis, L.Balisi and D.A. Horwitz. USC School of Medicine, Los Angeles, CA 90033.

Previously we have reported that Interleukin-2 production by peripheral blood mononuclear cells (PBM) from patients with SLE is impaired and that removal of OKT8+ cells reversed this defect. Our objective was to define the phenotype of the suppressor cells and to determine the effect of irradiation on these cells. PBM from SLE patients and healthy controls were labeled with Leu 2 or double labeled with this antibody and Leu 7, anti-Ia, or with an anti- C3bi receptor (OKM1 or Leu 15). Various populations were removed with the FACS, the remaining cells were stimulated with Phytohemagglutinin for 48 hours and the supernatants tested for IL-2 activity. As reported before, removal of all Leu 2+ cells markedly elevated IL-2 in SLE (from 11.4 u/ml to 68.0 u/ml). Removal of Leu 2+/Leu 7+ cells increased values to 39.0 u/ml and depletion of Leu 2+/Ia+ cells increased values even further to 64.0 u/ml. In 3 of 5 studies removal of Leu 2+/Leu 7- or of Leu 2+/ Ia- cells did not elevate IL-2 production. However, removal of Leu 2+/C3bi R+ cells did increase IL-2 values in these donors. The Leu 2+ suppressor cells were radiosensitive. Irradiation of PBM enhanced IL-2 to levels comparable to depletion of Leu 2+ cells. Irradiation of PBM depleted of Leu 2+/Leu 7+ cells or Leu 2+/Ia+ cells also increased IL-2 values indicating more than one subset of radiosensitive suppressor cells. These studies provide further evidence that the low IL-2 production in SLE is the result of excessive suppression and that several lymphocyte subsets, including some which differ from typical T cells, are responsible for this in vitro defect.

A34

MONONUCLEAR CELLS FROM PATIENTS WITH POLYMYOSITIS INHIBIT CALCIUM BINDING BY SARCOPLASMIC RETICULUM. Apostolos E. Kalovidouris. VAMC/Indiana University Medical Center. Indianapolis, IN 46202

Mononuclear cell infiltration is a key pathologic feature of polymyositis (PM). In this study the effect of supernatants from peripheral blood mononuclear cells (PBMC) of PM patients exposed to autologous muscle on calcium binding by sarcoplasmic reticulum (SR) membrane was investigated. PBMC isolated from 10 patients with PM and from 8 patients with neuromuscular complaints but without myositis were incubated with various dilutions of autologous muscle homogenates (w/v ranging from 1:180 to 1:4800) in RPMI with 5% AB serum for 5 days. Proliferative responses of PBMC were measured by ^{3}H-thymidine incorporation into DNA. SR membranes were derived from rat muscle. Ca^{2+} binding was measured by a millipore filter technique at 23°C in a medium containing 0.1M KCl-30mM histidine, pH 6.8, 5mM $MgCl_2$, 0.1mM $^{45}CaCl_2$, 2mM ATP, 300µg SR protein and supernatants from PBMC dialyzed against the assay medium.

After incubation with autologous muscle, PBMC from 7 out of 10 patients with PM showed proliferative responses with stimulation indices ranging from 3 to 14. Supernatants from muscle-stimulated PBMC from 6 of these patients produced inhibition of ATP-dependent Ca^{2+} binding by SR ranging from 25% to 59% (mean 45 ± 12). Neither proliferative responses nor inhibition of Ca^{2+} binding by SR membrane was observed in PBMC and supernatants of controls.

These results suggest that mononuclear cells in PM are sensitized to autologous muscle and release soluble factors which inhibit the function of SR muscle membrane, the key regulator of muscle contraction.

A35

DIFFERENCES IN T LYMPHOCYTE ION CHANNEL EXPRESSION IN NORMAL AND AUTOIMMUNE MICE. M. Fischbach, T.E. DeCoursey, K.G. Chandy, N. Talal S. Gupta, and M.D. Cahalan. University of Texas Health Science Center and Audie Murphy VA Hospital, San Antonio,TX 78284 and University of California, Irvine, CA 92717.

MRL/lpr mice are a model for human systemic lupus erythematosus. Massive lymphadenopathy is the hallmark of these mice with the predominate cell in lymph node and spleen being weakly expressive of the $Lyt1^+2^-$ phenotype, but also displaying unusual combinations of other T cell and B cell markers. These T cells are functionally abnormal failing to respond to a number of different immunological stimuli including mitogens, presented antigens, and self-Ia.

We investigated the mechanism underlying this T cell abnormality by studying expression of ion channels in T cells of MRL/lpr mice and their normal +/+ congenic controls. Utilizing the gigaohm seal voltage clamp technique, the predominant ion channel in the mouse T cell is a potassium (K) selective channel. $Lyt1^+$ cells had 20 times more K channels than $Lyt1^+$ +/+ T cells. The +/+ T cells expressed 2 types of K channels, N and L, which differ both in kinetics of channel gating and in their sensitivity of the K channel blocker tetraethylammonium (TEA). Half-blockage of K currents by TEA occurred at less than 100uM in lpr T cells(L-type channels) while in +/+ T cells expressing mainly N-type channels, half-blockage by TEA was 10mM. TEA inhibited mitogenesis at concentrations high enough to block the type-N channels, suggesting that the type-N but not the type-L channels may be required for T cell activation. Lpr T cells express predominately type-L channels. This abnormal expression of K channels may explain the unresponsiveness of lpr T cells.

A36

LEFT VENTRICULAR DYSFUNCTION IN ANKYLOSING SPONDYLITIS (AS). DH Goddard, L Shapiro*, RE Moore*, R. Canepa-Anson°, DG Gibson* and DA Brewerton. Departments of Rheumatology & Cardiology°, Westminster Hospital and Department of Cardiology*, Brompton Hospital, London, UK.

Cardiac function has been studied in 30 men with definite AS selected for having relatively mild symptoms and restriction of spinal movement, with minimal or no deformity. Group I (age 20-40, n=15) included 9 with mild symptoms requiring no treatment and 6 taking NSAID's. Group II (age 41-65, n=15) included 6 with mild spinal restriction, 8 with moderate to severe restriction, and 1 taking NSAID's. None had cardiac abnormalities on clinical assessment, chest x-ray or ECG, apart from 1 man with minor ST segment changes.

On digitised echocardiography all 30 patients had a prolonged interval from minimum dimension to mitral valve opening (MD-MVO). When compared with 30 age-matched controls, $p<0.001$ (Mann-Whitney U test). In Group I the range was 40-100 msec (mean 64) compared with controls 5-15 msec (mean 7.5). In Group II the range was 27-73 msec (mean 50) compared with controls 5-20 msec (mean 10). This abnormality was not related to age, disease activity, deformity, or treatment, and it was present in athletically fit young men with little or no discomfort. Isovolaemic relaxation was also prolonged in 4 men in each group. One patient had unsuspected aortic root dilatation without reflux.

This abnormality of LV relaxation suggests myocardial abnormality (but not amyloid). It does not reflect disease of coronary arteries, valves, or conducting tissues. The pathological explanation and possible clinical significance of this finding require extensive investigation.

A37

ROLE OF FACTOR B SS PHENOTYPE IN THE DEVELOPMENT OF ANKYLOSING SPONDYLITIS IN MEXICAN SUBJECTS. Julio Granados, Donato Alarcón-Segovia, Graciela Ibáñez de Kasep, Carlos Abud-Mendoza, Erasmo Martínez-Cordero and Adrián García-Soto. Instituto Nacional de la Nutrición. México D.F. México.

Because not all ankylosing spondylitis (AS) patients are HLA-B27 positive, it is felt that this marker may not be the only one involved. We addressed this question by studying factor B polymorphism thas is coded within the major histocompatibility complex and has 12 electrophoretically distinctallele products. In a sample of 200 Mexican healthy individuals the frequency of these alleles was found to be in Hardy Weinberg equilibrium. This equilibrium was lost, however, in a sample of 36 mexican patients with AS. Of them 33 had the SS phenotype, none had S1 or F1 alleles and only one had the FF phenotype.
Interestingly, two of the 4 women in this group had phenotypes other than SS (one FF, one FS).
Eight of the AS patients were HLA-B27 negative and all but one had factor B SS phenotype. The exception was the female with FS phenotype. The difference between patients and the 200 controls (n=70 with phenotypes other than SS) was significant at the p<0.01 level (X^2 with Yates correction).
Our findings suggest, at least in this ethnic group, the role of 3 predisposing factors to the development of overt AS: HLA-B27 positivity, factor B SS phenotype, and maleness. The interactions among them and their combined role in other ethnic groups seem to merit further study.

A38

DISCORDANCE BETWEEN HLA B27 AND ANKYLOSING SPONDYLITIS (AS) - A FAMILY INVESTIGATION. D. Gladman, M. Urowitz, K. Anhorn, H. Mervart. The Wellesley and Women's College Hospitals, Toronto.

Thirty five members in 4 generations of a family were evaluated clinically for the presence of AS. Clinical assessment, in addition to eliciting history and physical findings of back and sacroiliac involvement and assessment of peripheral joints, included radiological examination of the back and sacroiliac joints in all family members age 18 and over. Twelve members, including the propositus, 7 siblings, the parents and maternal grandparents, were HLA typed using 9th International Workshop antisera, including monoclonal antisera to HLA B27. HLA typing for HLA A, B, C, DR and MT antigens were performed on all members, using Canadian Red Cross tissue typing trays. Lymphocytes were separated from peripheral blood by centrifugation over hypaque ficoll gradients. B lymphocytes were further purified by passage over nylon wool columns. The NIH microcytotoxicity test was used.

The propositus and 4 of 5 male sibs demonstrated AS. A sister had evidence of sacroiliitis but did not fulfill criteria for AS. Three of the members with AS shared the B27 containing haplotype (A32, B27, CW2, DR6, MT1, 2), inherited from the mother. The remaining 3 individuals, 2 with AS and one with sacroiliitis lacked B27 but shared the other maternal haplotype (A2, B61, CW2, DR6, MT1, 2). Three other individuals with the B27 containing haplotype did not show evidence of either sacroliitis or AS. Monoclonal antibodies confirmed the B27 typing with alloantisera but did not discern between patients with or without spondylitis. The lack of association of known HLA antigens with disease expression in this family suggests that some, as yet unknown, genetic and/or environmental influence may be necessary for disease expression in Ankylosing Spondylitis.

A39

STUDIES OF MONOCYTE PHAGOCYTIC FUNCTION IN ANKYLOSING SPONDYLITIS. Stanley P. Ballou, Muhammad A. Khan, Irving Kushner. Case Western Reserve University/Cleve. Metro. General Hospital, Cleveland, OH 44109.

Recent evidence has suggested that neutrophil chemotaxis is increased in B27(+) patients with ankylosing spondylitis (AS). To further explore phagocytic cell function in spondylitic diseases, we evaluated the phagocytic activity of adherent peripheral blood mononuclear cells (monocytes) from 10 patients with spondylitic diseases (6-AS; 4-Reiter's syndrome) off treatment at the time of study. Fc receptor-mediated phagocytic activity of monocyte monolayers was assessed in serum-free buffer using opsonized sheep red blood cells (SRBC). In these patients the percent phagocytic cells (PPC, 91 ± 3%) and the phagocytic index (PI = number of SRBC ingested per monocyte, 2.8 ± 0.3) were significantly increased compared to 8 normal individuals: PPC = 82 ± 9%, p <0.01; PI = 2.1 ± 0.4, p <0.001. In contrast, nonspecific phagocytic activity (latex beads) was similar in 7 patients (PPC = 93%) and 5 normals (PPC = 95%). In the spondylitis patients both PPC and PI were significantly correlated with serum levels of CRP (p < 0.05) but not with levels of immune complexes (C_1q binding) or plasma fibronectin. We also assessed the effect of serum on phagocytosis. In the presence of normal serum, phagocytic activity was depressed using both normal (PPC = 51, PI = 1.09) and patient (PPC = 49, PI = .98) monocytes. In comparison, phagocytosis in AS serum appeared less depressed: normal monocytes: PPC = 63, PI = 1.59; patient monocytes: PPC = 62, PI = 1.34. The differences, however, did not attain significance. These findings indicate that monocyte Fc receptor-mediated phagocytosis is increased in patients with active spondylitic diseases. Further studies are underway to determine whether serum factors in such individuals may enhance monocyte phagocytosis.

A40

PROTECTION BY CORTICOSTEROIDS AGAINST CHEMICALLY INDUCED ARTICULAR CARTILAGE DAMAGE AND OSTEOPHYTE FORMATION. James M. Williams, Rush Medical School, Chicago, IL and Kenneth D. Brandt, Indiana University Medical Center, Indianapolis IN 46223

Although corticosteroids have been shown to cause articular cartilage degeneration, studies of experimentally-induced osteoarthritis indicate that under certain conditions they may protect against cartilage damage and osteophyte formation. We herein examine the in vivo effect of triamcinolone hexacetonide (TH) on the degeneration of articular cartilage which occurs following intraarticular injection of sodium iodoacetate (IA) into the normal guinea pig knee.

Three weeks after a single injection of IA (3 mg/kg), ipsilateral femoral condylar cartilage exhibited fibrillation, loss of staining with Safranin-O, depletion of chondrocytes, and prominent osteophytes. In striking contrast, when TH (0.40 mg/kg) was injected into the ipsilateral knee 24 hours after the intraarticular injection of IA, fibrillation was noted in only one of six samples, osteophytes were much less prominent, pericellular staining with Safranin-O persisted, and cell loss was less extensive. Knees of animals which received only 1/10 as much intraarticular TH (0.04 mg/kg) after the IA injection also exhibited marked reduction in size and extent of osteophytes. However, fibrillation, loss of Safranin-O staining and chondrocyte depletion were as severe as in animals injected with IA but not treated with steroid. No apparent morphologic or histochemical changes were observed after intraarticular injection of the steroid alone. Thus, TH produced a dose-dependent marked protective effect in this model of chemically-induced articular cartilage damage.

A41

THE NON-PROGRESSIVE NATURE OF OSTEOARTHRITIS OF THE KNEE (OAK). David Kaplan, Downstate Medical Center, Brooklyn, NY; Roy Altman, U. Miami, Miami, FL; William Murphy, Washington U., St. Louis, MO.

A recent report (J.Rheum. 10:282, 1983) suggests that by the 7th decade the signs and symptoms of OAK no longer show increasing severity with age. Data on 139 pts. with the clinical diagnosis of OAK collected by the ARA Osteoarthritis Criteria Subcommittee were reviewed. The following were scored for severity: knee Xrays (read blindly) for osteophytes, sclerosis, joint narrowing and cysts (range 0-36), signs (range 0-6) and symptoms (range 0-23). Results were as follows:

AGE	≤ 50	51-60	61-65	66-70	71-80	81+
(n)	(18)	(39)	(31)	(21)	(26)	(4)
Symptoms	7.56	8.95	8.98	9.90	9.69	14.40
Signs	1.83	2.08	2.81	2.14	2.96	4.25
Xray	3.22	5.05	6.58	7.90	6.77	7.00
TOTAL	12.61	16.08	18.35	19.95	19.04	25.25

Dur. of Sx	1 yr	2 yrs	3-6yrs	7-10yrs	11-15yrs	16+yrs
(n)	(10)	(15)	(33)	(26)	(31)	(24)
Symptoms	9.30	8.60	8.64	9.35	9.87	9.29
Signs	2.00	2.47	2.21	2.54	2.71	2.50
Xray	3.00	5.40	6.48	5.46	6.58	6.58
TOTAL	14.30	16.47	17.33	17.35	19.16	18.38

We conclude that OAK is a disease beginning in middle age (mean age of onset of symptoms: 51.6yrs) and shows little evidence of progression after the seventh decade or after 1-2 years of symptoms.

A42

A HUMAN MONOCLONAL AUTOANTIBODY REACTIVE WITH DNA, AN EXTRACTABLE NUCLEAR ANTIGEN, AND NUCLEOLI. Nicholas Chiorazzi and Westley H. Reeves. The Rockefeller University, New York, N.Y. 10021.

The immortalization of autoantibody producing B lymphocytes has proven to be a powerful tool for analyzing autoantibodies and the autoantigens bound by these antibodies. Recently human-human B cell hybridomas were constructed using mitogen-stimulated B cells from a patient with SLE and an HGPRTase-deficient EBV-transformed human cell line (0467). This fusion resulted in 97 growth positive wells, of which 36 secreted human monoclonal antibody reactive with DNA. One of these DNA-reactive monoclonal antibodies also bound to nucleoli in a HEp-2 fluorescent antinuclear antibody assay. This nucleolar staining could be completely eradicated by pretreatment with RNase but was unaffected by DNase, suggesting that the antigenic determinant resided on a ribonucleoprotein. ELISA studies demonstrated that this antibody bound to a highly charged eluate of rabbit thymus extract implying that at least a portion of the antigen-monoclonal antibody interaction was charge related. Antigen binding assays using antigens which spanned a wide isoelectric range confirmed this impression. SDS-PAGE analysis of internally labeled K562 cells using this monoclonal antibody revealed two bands in the 16-20kD range which were clearly different from those immunoprecipitated by sera containing known autoantibody specificities including Sm, RNP, Ro, and La. A similar protein doublet was precipitated from the radiolabeled cell extract using the original patient's serum. Thus, an autoantibody producing clone from the patient was immortalized and its secreted human monoclonal antibody may define a novel autoantigen.

A43

DE NOVO STIMULATION OF ANTIBODY TO SS-B/La IN NORMAL MICE BY ACTIVE IMMUNIZATION. E.K.L. Chan, A.M. Francoeur and E.M. Tan. Scripps Clinic and Research Foundation, La Jolla, CA.

Anti-SS-B autoantibodies are found in sera from patients with SLE and Sjogren's syndrome. However, these antibodies have not been demonstrated in autoimmune strains of mice. This report describes the induction of anti-SS-B antibodies in normal mice by active immunization. Balb/c mice were injected ip. with either affinity-purified SS-B from calf thymus extract (CTE) in Complete Freund's adjuvant (bi-weekly) or washed beads from immunoprecipitation of CTE, human anti-SS-B sera, and Protein A-Sepharose (weekly). Within 3 months after the initial injection, anti-SS-B antibodies could be detected in sera from both groups of mice using ELISA, Western blotting (WB) and ^{32}P immunoprecipitation of HeLa cell extracts. ELISA activity of mouse sera could be inhibited by human anti-SS-B. WB showed reactivities to SS-B polypeptides from CTE, Rabbit thymus and HeLa. These mouse sera precipitated both precursors of 5S RNA and tRNAs and the 48K SS-B phosphoprotein, a pattern of reactivity similar to human anti-SS-B sera. This documented the successful induction of antibodies to SS-B in normal mice and will be a useful model to study autoimmune and pathogenic mechanisms of this autoantigen-antibody system.

A44

NO EVIDENCE OF CROSSREACTING ANTI-HLA-B27 ANTIBODIES IN SERA OF PATIENTS WITH ENTERIC GRAM NEGATIVE BACTERIAL INFECTIONS. D. Cavender and M. Ziff. Univ Texas Health Science Center at Dallas, TX 75235.

Enteric infections with certain gram-negative bacteria (GnB) may initiate spondyloarthropathy in HLA-B27$^+$ individuals. Studies with rabbit antisera, human HLA typing sera and murine monoclonal antibodies have suggested that serological crossreactivity may exist between the B27 molecule and one or more antigens of GnB. To determine whether patients with these infections actually form such crossreactive antibodies, sera from patients with culture-proven and/or firm serological and clinical evidence of infection with *Shigella flexneri* (n=3), *Campylobacter jejuni* (n=31), *Yersinia enterocolitica* (n=26), or *Salmonella typhi* (n=6) were tested for anti-B27 antibodies by a dye-exclusion microcytotoxicity assay using an EBV-transformed B27$^+$ lymphoblastoid cell line and three of its B27$^-$ variants as control cells. Two commercially available lots of monospecific anti-B27 sera were used as positive serum controls. These sera routinely killed >90% of the B27$^+$ cells at 1:8 dilution but <10% of the B27$^-$ variant cells; in addition, the cytotoxicity could be removed by adsorption with the B27$^+$ cells but not with B27$^-$ cells. None of the 66 patient sera tested, including 9 from patients who had developed arthritis following *Yersinia* infection, contained detectable anti-B27 antibodies. However, all of 54 of the 66 sera tested to date contained antibacterial antibodies as measured by agglutination and/or an avidin-biotin immunoperoxidase ELISA method. Attempts to inhibit the cytotoxicity of the positive anti-B27 sera with GnB antigens have also been unsuccessful. These results do not support the hypothesis that B27 crossreactive antibodies are involved in the etiology of the B27-associated spondyloarthropathies.

A45

SERUM ANTIBODIES TO CARDIAC CONDUCTING TISSUE IN RHEUMATIC DISEASES. William R. Caruso, Maria de Guzman, Francisco P. Quismorio, Jr. USC School of Medicine, Los Angeles, California.

Cardiac abnormalities including conduction defects constitute a common manifestation of rheumatic diseases such as RA, SLE and PSS. Circulating antibodies to cardiac conducting tissue (anti-CCT) have been recently described in RA (Clin Exp Immunol 53:336, 1983) and these abs. were found to be more prevalent in RA pts. with right bundle branch block. We examined some of the immunological properties of the anti-CCT ab. in RA and studied the occurrence of the ab. in other rheumatic disorders .

Anti-CCT ab. was tested by an indirect immunofluorescent test using bovine ventricular septum as substrate. The ab. reacted with Purkinje fibers but not with myocardial, skeletal or smooth muscle fibers. Rabbit ab. to human collagen Type I as well as ab. to skin keratin did not bind Purkinje fibers. Anti-mitochondrial ab. in primary biliary cirrhosis sera reacted with the fibers but in a different pattern. Anti-CCT abs. were found in 39/86 (45.3%) of RA pts. and in 3/42 (7.1%) of healthy controls (p=0.001). In contrast, ab. prevalence was not increased in SLE 3/34 (8.6%), PSS 5/23 (21.7%), MCTD (17.4%) or in seronegative spondyarthritides 0/8. Anti-CCT ab. in RA was predominantly IgG, while IgM and IgA abs. were rarely found. The ab. did not fix human C' in vitro. The frequency of EKG abnormalities was similar in RA pts. with anti-CCT (5/19, 26.3%) and RA pts. without the ab. (6/19, 31.6%). The ab. in RA did not correlate with presence of ANA.

Circulating anti-CCT ab. is a serological characteristic of RA but not of other systemic rheumatic diseases which often can also manifest clinically with cardiac conduction abnormalities.

A46

AN IMMUNOGENETIC STUDY OF 22 PATIENTS WITH SCLERODERMA : RAISED HLA DR3 AND C4AQO ALLELES

Carol M.Black, R.S.Pereira, D.Briggs*, K.I.Welsh*
Rheumatology Dept.,West Middlesex University Hospital,Middx.TW7 6AF
*Tissue Typing Dept.,Guy's Hospital, St Thomas Street, London SE1 9RT

Family typing allowed full HLA-A,B,C,DR haplotype assignments in 22 patients with systemic sclerosis. 3/22 patients were male. 12/22 patients were DR3 (P<0.01) and 8 of these also carried HLA B8 on the same haplotype. Complement allotyping (C2,C4,Bf) allowed definitive assignment of QO alleles in 15 families. All with the HLA B8,DR3 haplotype have null alleles at C4A. 3/4 of the DR3+ that were not B8 also carried C4AQO alleles, and overall 12/21 patients were C4AQO (P=0.002). Incidence of C4BQO and other complement alleles was normal. C3 allotyping (chromosome 19) showed no deviation from the expected frequency. A similar high incidence of null alleles at the C4A complement locus has been shown in systemic lupus erythematosus (1).

A previous population study has shown an increased incidence of DR5 and DR3 (2). The lower incidence of DR5 in this family study reflects the increased severity of disease in these patients, DR5 being associated with the CREST form of disease.

(1) Fielder AHL, Walport MJ, Batchelor JR et al.1983, Br Med J 286:425
(2) Black CM, Welsh KI, Maddison PJ et al.1984, Br J Rheumatol 23:267

A47

PROPYLTHIOURACIL-INDUCED IMMUNE-MEDIATED DISEASE. DA Aucoin, RG Lahita, SM Krator, ME Peterson, DE Drayer, , AI Hurvitz, and MM Reidenberg, Depts Pharmacology and Medicine, Cornell Univ Medical College and The Rockefeller University, N.Y., N.Y.

Over 50% of cats given propylthiouracil(PTU), 150 mg/d, develop severe lethargy, anorexia, lymphadenopathy, Coombs' positive hemolytic anemia and antinuclear antibodies (ANA) within 6 weeks. Four cats redeveloped disease when rechallenged with 150 mg/d of PTU within 4 weeks; however, when rechallenged with 12.5 mg/d of PTU for 10 weeks, recurrence of disease or ANA did not develop indicating a dose response relationship for disease induction. To identify the protein to which the ANA was directed, ANA positive serum was tested for binding specificity toward ssDNA, dsDNA and 3 histone fractions using ELISA methodology. Antibodies toward RNP and Sm were tested by hemagglutination. All tests were negative. This serum was immunoprecipitated with S-35 methionine in vitro labelled soluble cellular protein from a K526 cell line using rabbit anti-cat IgG bound to Sepharose. The IP was electrophoresed under reduced conditions on a 15% SDS-PAG and fluorographed. Non-labeled histones were run concurrently on the same gel and detected by Coummassie blue staining. Fluorography revealed a 12,000 MW protein from cat sera with ANA titers >1:80 that differed from any of the 5 histone fractions.
We conclude that there is a dose-response relationship for PTU-induced immune-mediated disease in cats. This suggests that a pharmacologic effect of PTU is required for disease induction rather than PTU simply functioning as a hapten. Preliminary results indicate that the ANA is directed against a nuclear protein which, unlike other drug-induced ANA's, does not appear to be a monomeric histone fraction.

A48

THERAPY OF REFRACTORY PAGET'S DISEASE OF BONE WITH SYNTHETIC HUMAN CALCITONIN (SHC). Roy D. Altman and Barbara Collins. Miami VAMC and University of Miami, Miami, FL 33101.

SHC was administered as 0.5 mg subcutaneously daily to 11 patients who had failed or become refractory to Synthetic Salmon Calcitonin, disodium etidronate (EHDP), or the combination of both.

Assessments included general status, a 4 point pain scale, (0-3), and serum alkaline phosphatase (AP).

Patients were 71±6 years old upon entry, 10 men, 1 woman, and have been followed for 15±13 months (range 4-42 mo). Nine (90%) felt improved. Two discontinued the program after 1 month. Pain assessment changed from 2.4±.7 to 0.8±.7 (P=.029 Wilcoxan Signed Rank). Although symptomatically better, patient #6 had no change in serum chemistries. The Alkaline Phosphatase decreased significantly by 3 months (P=.03) and 6 months (P=.03). The pain and AP response is reflected in Table 1:

TABLE 1: SERUM ALKALINE PHOSPHATASE (TIME IN MONTHS)

	INITIAL	3	6	12	18	24	30	36
VALUE XN*	18.5	12.9	12.0	5.6	7.7	4.3	6.0	6.0
±SD	15.5	8.5	10.4	3.5	5.7	1.5	1.4	2.8

*XN = multiple of the upper limits of normal.

Patient #5 had further improvement in clinical status and suppression of AP by the addition of EHDP. Patient #4 had previously received transient benefit from Mithramycin.

Adverse reactions included nausea (4), mild diarrhea (2), mild abdominal cramps (1), facial flush (1), and rhinorrhea and headache (1). Most were transient and required no change in regimen. Nausea in Patient #2 required reducing SHC to 0.5 mg for 3 months. Rhinorrhea and headache caused discontinuation in patient #11.

SHC was clinically and chemically effective in 8 of 11 patients with severe Paget's disease refractory to their prior therapies. The response to EHDP plus SHC was additive in a patient who had become refractory to EHDP previously.

A49

CLASSIFICATION PARAMETERS FOR OSTEOARTHRITIS (OA) OF THE KNEE: INTERIM REPORT. ARA Osteoarthritis Diagnostic and Therapeutic Criteria Subcommittee. Chairman, Roy D. Altman.

A prospective trial was designed to evaluate combinations of clinical parameters (para) that might exceed the sensitivity and specificity of an x-ray alone the classification of knee OA. The study included 130 patients with idiopathic OA and 107 controls with non-osteoarthritic painful conditions of the knee.

Diagnoses were established by each center coordinator and verified by 3 independent chart reviews. Clinical OA was distinguished from asymptomatic OA by the presence of pain. The committee first selected 13 para by "Delphi" technique felt to be both sensitive and specific. These were included in 24 historical, 16 physical, 12 laboratory and 28 x-ray para obtained on each subject. X-rays were interpreted by each center coordinator and then blindly by a musculoskeletal radiologist.

The following para were identified following data analysis (ARAMIS): (Format: para, %OA/%control), **Clinical:** age >40 years 96/60; knee stiffness <30 minutes 69/50; crepitus on active motion 85/46; absence of palpable effusion 63/35; absence of palpable warmth 84/46; bony enlargement 56/10; bony (without synovial) tenderness 63/26; **Laboratory:** OA synovial fluid (clear, viscous, or WBC <2,000) 100/50; ESR <40 mm/hr 86/45; latex fixation <1:40 titer 82/30. **X-ray:** osteophytes 92/23.

Criteria for classification were divided into groups: Group 1: (Clinical) knee pain with 4/7 **clinical** para, sensitivity 84%, specificity 72%; Group 2: (Clinical and laboratory) knee pain with 5/10 **clinical** and **laboratory** para, sensitivity 88%, specificity 82%; Group 3: (Clinical and x-ray) knee pain and 2 of 3 **clinical:** (age >40 yr, stiff <30 min, crepitus) and **x-ray:** (osteophytes), sensitivity 90%, specificity 91%.

The development of such criteria is expected to help differentiate OA from other diseases for the purpose of uniform reporting of OA in clinical/epidemiologic studies.

A50

RELAPSING POLYCHONDRITIS (RP) AND CHRONIC REFRACTORY ANEMIA (CRA).
J.C.Piette, M.A.Prince-Zucchelli, S.Herson, C.J.Menkes, P.J.Weiller, M.Mongin, P.Godeau. Hôpital de la Pitié - 75013 Paris; Hôpital Cochin, 75014 Paris; Hôpital La Timone, 13005 Marseille - FRANCE.

Hematologic findings in RP are thought to be unremarkable except for moderate "anemia of chronic disorders" and mild leukocytosis during flares. In our series of 55 patients with RP, 7 patients developed CRA. RP preceded CRA in 3; both diseases were diagnosed simultaneously in 4.

All patients were males. Their age at onset ranged from 45 to 87 (mean: 70). All fulfilled Mac Adam's criteria for RP (Medicine 55: 193-215, 1976). Main symptoms were: auricular chondritis (n=7), respiratory tract chondritis (n=7), nasal chondritis (n=5), ocular inflammation (n=7) and polyarthritis (n=5). High dose of corticosteroids were required in all patients for control of RP.

Anemia was normochromic, macrocytic (mean MCV: 112 fl), aregenerative, chronic and severe, requiring transfusions in 6 patients. A marked leukopenia and/or thrombocytopenia were present in 5 patients. Bone marrow studies showed excessive (n=5) or normal (n=2) cellularity. Maturation was quantitatively and qualitatively abnormal in most patients, without any leukemic change. Myelofibrosis was absent. Prussian blue staining revealed no major iron overload. In 3 patients, kinetic studies suggested a primary bone marrow defect. Usual causes of CRA could be ruled out. No patient had recieved dapsone or cytotoxic drugs prior to the onset of CRA. Treatments of CRA were ineffective. Conclusion: CRA is not uncommun in RP, especially in elderly male patients. Further studies are needed to understand its mechanism.

A51

ACEBUTOLOL-INDUCED LUPUS (AIL).
J.C.Piette, P.Bourgeois, S.Herson, S.Etienne, M.F.Kahn and P.Godeau. Hôpital de la Pitié, 75013 - Hôpital Bichat 75018 Paris - FRANCE.

Eleven patients treated with acebutolol, a beta-blocking agent widely used in France, developed a lupus-like syndrome. There were 8 females and 3 males. Their age ranged from 35 to 84 (mean: 57). Prior to acebutolol treatment, Raynaud's phenomenon was present in two patients, Sjögren's syndrome in one, and another patient had a past history of idiopathic thrombocytopenic purpura. In all patients but one, acebutolol was introduced for hypertension. AIL appeared after 4 to 36 months of treatment (mean: 13). The daily dose of acebutolol was 400 to 2400 mg (mean: 800).

AIL main symptoms were: polyarthritis/arthralgias (n=10), fever (n=5), myalgias (n=3), pericarditis (n=3), pleuropulmonary involvement (n=3), relapse of thrombocytopenic purpura (n=1) and arterial thrombosis (n=1). Renal and neurologic involvement were not encountered. High titers of ANA were present in all patients, anti-DNA were negative (n=8) or weakly positive (n=3), complement levels were normal (n=8) or slightly decreased (n=3).

In all patients, AIL clinical symptoms resolved within weeks after acebutolol withdrawal, whereas ANA disappearance was slower. Corticosteroid treatment was required in 3 patients only. One patient died from cardiac tamponade after incidental readministration of acebutolol.

Conclusions: 1)- A lupus-like syndrome may occur during acebutolol treatment. 2)- Further studies are needed to evaluate the safety of acebutolol in patients with prior immunological abnormalities.

A52

MONONUCLEAR CELL PROFILES IN MUSCLE BIOPSIES FROM PATIENTS WITH POLYMYOSITIS AND CHILDHOOD DERMATOMYOSITIS. Laurie C. Miller and Alfred F. Michael. University of Minnesota, Minneapolis, MN. 55455

Quantitative profiles of mononuclear cell subsets were assessed in muscle biopsy tissues from 5 patients with polymyositis, 8 children with dermatomyositis and 4 normal individuals. Tissue sections were stained with monoclonal antibodies directed against the OKT11, OKT3, OKT4, OKT8, BA1, OKM1, and LEU7 determinants on inflammatory cells, and counterstained with ethidium bromide. All cells were counted, and positive cells for each antibody expressed as a percentage. A significant difference was found in the number of cells positive for the OKT11 marker, with 3.3% positive in childhood dermatomyositis biopsies and 9.2% positive in polymyositis biopsies ($p < .05$). Positive cells were also found in normal biopsies. Significant differences in labelling patterns were found between normal biopsies and dermatomyositis biopsies using antibodies to OKT8, BA1, and OKM1 ($p = .05, <.05, <.01$). The same antibodies demonstrated significant differences between polymyositis and normal biopsies (all $p < .01$). The T4:T8 ratios were not significantly different in the two patient groups.

The significant difference in the number of cells bearing the OKT11 marker in childhood dermatomyositis and polymyositis may support the notion that different pathogenetic mechanisms are involved. This study also demonstrates the importance of using quantitative methods and normal controls in assessing patterns of inflammatory cell infiltration in tissue sections.

A53

SUCRALFATE THERAPY IN NONSTEROIDAL ANTI-INFLAMMATORY DRUG-INDUCED GASTRITIS. J.R. Caldwell, S.H. Roth, W.H. Marsh, M.D. Heller, W.C. Wu, E.L. Semble. Gainesville, FL 32605; Phoenix, AZ; Lynnfield, MA; Charleston, SC; Winston-Salem, NC.

PURPOSE: A multicenter double-blind study comparing the efficacy of sucralfate (SCR) versus placebo (P) in the therapy of nonsteroidal anti-inflammatory drug (NSAID0-induced gastritis.
METHODS: 120 patients (pts) with symptoms of NSAID-induced gastritis underwent pandendoscopy. Pts received SCR 1g. qid or P qid for 4 weeks. Treatment for the 46 pts with lesions was randomized separately from symptomatic pts without lesions. NSAID dosage continued unchanged from prestudy dosage. Changes in endoscopic lesion grade (0,1,2,3,4,5; 0=normal mucosa, 5=multiple ulcers) and symptoms scores were measured.
RESULTS: SCR produced greater improvement in both gastric lesion healing and symptom scores than P.

No. of pts	Mean changes in lesion scores			
	Improved	Same	Worse	Lesion grade
SCR (N=23)	14	7	2	-1.130 P< 0.01
P (N=23)	11	5	7	-0.435
SYMPTOMS SCORE MEAN CHANGES:		Frequency		Intensity
SCR (N=61)		-27.06		-58.90 P< 0.05
P (N=59)		-14.15		-32.25

CONCLUSION: A significant difference in favor of SCR in treating drug-induced GI damage/symptoms is evident. Results are consistent with recent pharmacologic evidence of SCR stimulation of prostaglandin mediated mucosal responses (cytoprotection). Continuing research in the area is warranted as SCR represents a means of managing NSAID-induced gastritis while continuing NSAID therapy.

A54

OLIGOCLONAL BANDS IN SJOGREN'S SYNDROME. Douglas R. Hough, Roger W. Strickland, David M. Lewis, and Gary L. Klipple. Walter Reed Army Medical Center, Washington, D.C. 20307-5001.

The clinical significance of oligoclonal bands in the sera of patients with Sjogren's Syndrome (SS) is not known. Although a prior study by Moutsopoulos et al. (J.Immunol. 130:2663-5, 1983) reported monoclonal bands in the sera of 66% of 1° SS patients; most had extraglandular disease.

38 patients with sicca symptoms were evaluated with a record review, history, examination, Schirmer and rose bengal testing. Lip biopsies were obtained in 31. An extensive serologic evaluation and high resolution protein electrophoresis (HREP) using Helena plates were performed on sera from each patient. Oligoclonal bands were identified with immunofixation.

SS patients fulfilled 2 of 3 criteria: (1) lip biopsy focus score >1; (2) confirmed keratoconjunctivitis sicca (KCS); and (3) a connective tissue disease or positive SSA and/or SSB antibodies. Three patient groups resulted: 14 had 1° SS, 10 had 2° SS, and 14 had a "sicca-like" syndrome satisfying less than 2 criteria. 3 patients with 1° SS had a positive lip biopsy and SSA or SSB antibodies, but had no evidence of KCS. 6/14 with 1° SS had extraglandular disease.

HREP was abnormal in 16/24 with SS compared to 4/14 with the "sicca-like" syndrome. Oligoclonal bands were detected in 50% of 1° SS patients with extraglandular disease (3/6) and 1 patient with 2° SS. Oligoclonal bands in 1° SS patients seem to correlate with a subpopulation having associated extraglandular disease such as interstitial pulmonary fibrosis, autoimmune thyroiditis, lymphadenopathy, and neutropenia.

A55

DESTRUCTIVE ARTHROPATHIES OF LARGE JOINTS IN PATIENTS ON LONG TERM HEMODIALYSIS (HD). T. Bardin, D. Kuntz, Hôpital Lariboisière, Paris, T. Drueke, J. Zingraff, Hôpital Necker, Paris, M.C. Voisin, Hôpital H. Mondor, Créteil - FRANCE.

Rheumatic disorders are increasingly recognized as potentially severe complications of long term HD treatment. We report the occurrence of destructive arthropathies of large joints of the limbs in 6 patients (5 females, 1 male) aged 52-66, who had been on HD for an average of 123 months (range 80-180). Affected joints were shoulders (5), hips (4), and knees (3). X rays showed rapid and severe narrowing of the articular space, usually associated with subchondral radiolucent cysts and/or erosions without osteophytosis. Disability appeared rapidly and 2 prosthetic replacements of the hip and one of the knee were performed. Small joints of the hands were affected in 3 patients ; destructive spondylarthropathies were seen in 5 (Arthr. Rheum., 1984, 27, 369-375).

The pathophysiology of these disorders is uncertain. Only 3 patients had an history of secondary hyperparathyroidism, 2 of whom had undergone successfull parathyroidectomy. Serum aluminum level was elevated in all patients ; 2 had suffered from Al osteomalacia and 1 from Al encephalopathy. Apatite crystals were found by transmission electron microscopy (TEM) in a meniscus from the operated knee. Periarticular calcifications were seen in X rays of 6 other affected joints. Finally, massive amyloid deposits were identified by congo red staining and TEM in synovium and capsula of the 2 replaced hips.

Destructive arthropathies may be a major source of disability in patients on long term HD. This study shows that they are frequently associated with apatite deposition and dialysis amyloidosis. The pathophysiology of these rheumatic disorders needs further investigation.

A56

HIGH PREVALENCE OF REITER'S SYNDROME (RS) IN THE INUIT (ESKIMO) POPULATION OF GREENLAND. T. Bardin, M. Lathrop, C. Enel, F. Becker-Christensen Hôpital Lariboisière, U. Paris 7, FRANCE and Egedesminde Hospital, Greenland.

A clinical and epidemiological survey of post-veneral RS was undertaken in the Egedesminde (EGM) and Jakobshavn (JAK) regions of west Greenland as high frequencies of HLA-B27 (approximating 25 %) and veneral disease had been reported. In 1983, the regions had respectively 3055 and 3799 inhabitants. Complete medical records on all inhabitants, centralized in the two district hospitals, were reviewed. Potential patients were given a medical examination during a field study. Diagnosis was made following the proposed ARA criteria (Arthr. Rheum., 1981, 24, 844). Gonococcal arthritis was eliminated on favorable response to penicillin. X-rays were taken for diagnosis of ankylosing spondylitis (AS).

51 patients (50 males, 1 female) were found to have a definite history of Reiter's syndrome. The prevalence was 1.08 % in EGM and 0.34 % in JAK in the general population, and 1.96 % and 0.68 % respectively in the group over 40. The mean age of onset was 27.3 with a mean follow-up of 10.9 years (range 0-39). Ocular involvement occurred in 66 % of patients (including uveitis in 47 %, balanitis in 18 %, keratoderma blennorrhagica in 10 %. Recurrences of arthritis occurred in 74 % and 85 % of patients with a follow-up exceeding 5 and 10 years respectively, 50 % of the attacks being oligoarticular. 11 patients had a definite bilateral sacroiliitis, 8 of whom met the NY criteria for AS. 29 % of RS patients had one or more close relative affected.

Our work shows a very high prevalence of RS in an Inuit population, and confirms the chronicity of the disease in an epidemiological study benefiting from complete follow-up due to stability of the population and centralization of medical care.

A57

ALIZARIN RED STAINING OF SYNOVIAL FLUID (SF). SIMILAR RESULTS IN OSTEOARTHRITIS (OA) AND RHEUMATOID ARTHRITIS (RA). T. Bardin, B. Bucki, A. Dryll, J. Lansaman, A. Ryckewaert, Hôpital Lariboisière, Paris - FRANCE

Alizarin red staining has been proposed as a sensible test to detect calcium compounds, including apatite crystals, in SF. We report our results in a series of 230 unselected SF. Results were graded as negative, + positive (rare stained clumps), ++ positive (stained clumps in over 50 % of low power field), and +++ positive (stained clumps in every low power field). 29 SF were also processed for transmission electron microscopy (TEM). X rays of the aspirated joint and precise clinical data were obtained for 199 patients.

Intra and inter observer variations in the graduation of Alizarin red staining results were negligible. By TEM, no apatite crystal was found in 20 negative or + to ++ positive SF ; 5 +++ positive SF contained apatite crystals whereas 4 other +++ positive SF contained only CPPD crystals. 10 % of 230 SF were +++ positive, including 2 SF from "Milwaukee shoulders", 6 (16 %) of 38 RA SF, 5 (14 %) of 35 OA SF, and 11 (52 %) of 21 SF containing CPPD crystals by polarizing light microscopy. In the 3 latter categories positivity did not correlate with SF cellularity but was strongly associated with the extent of joint deterioration as assessed by X-rays. No positive result was found in patients with other diseases, including 25 patients with internal derangement of the knee, 11 with gout and 21 with seronegative spondylarthropathies.

Our results confirm that Alizarin red S staining is a valid technique to detect apatite or small CPPD crystals in SF, provided that only strongly positive results are taken into accounts. The incidence of strong positives we found in RA and OA are similar, suggesting non specific association of the presence of calcium compounds in SF with cartilage and/or subchondral bone deterioration.

A58

LUPUS BAND TEST AND ANTINUCLEAR ANTIBODIES IN FIBROMYALGIA. HAL DINERMAN, DAVID T. FELSON, DON L. GOLDENBERG, JAMES SOLOMON, Boston University School of Medicine, Boston, MA 02118.

A recent study (A&R 27:1174, 1984) found immunoglobulin deposition of IgG at the DEJ of normal forearm skin in 76% of 25 patients with fibromyalgia (Fib). We performed skin biopsies on 36 patients who all met the clinical criteria for the diagnosis of Fib. A control group of 11 patients with systemic lupus erythematosus (SLE) also had skin biopsies obtained during the course of their disease. All biopsies in both groups were taken from uninvolved forearm skin on the extensor surface. The results were as follows:

	No.	IgG	IgM	C'	IC Ig
SLE	11	9	10	4	
Fib	36	4	1	0	11

Thus, 12% of patients with Fib had Ig deposition at the dermal-epidermal junction (DEJ) characteristic of a positive lupus band test, whereas 100% of patients with SLE had a positive lupus band test. 30% of patients with Fib had intercellular (IC) deposits of Ig in the dermis, but the significance of this is not yet clear. 6 of the 36 patients with Fib had a positive ANA in low titer on at least 1 occasion, including 2 of the 4 patients with a positive lupus band test. However, none of these patients went on to develop an autoimmune disorder at a mean follow-up of 4 years.

We conclude that identification of immunoflourescence at the DEJ is not present in a large percentage of patients with Fib and is not a useful marker in helping to diagnose Fib.

A59

DISCREPANCIES IN SYNOVIAL FLUID (SF) ANALYSIS RESULTS FROM FOUR LABORATORIES. M.S. Sieck, M.S. Rothfuss, G.M. Clayburne, D.F. Baumgarten, B. Paralapiano, J. Kant, and H.R. Schumacher. VAMC and U of PA, Philadelphia, PA 19104.

There are no established standards for quality control in SF analysis. In order to learn how frequently discrepancies occur, 30 specimens were immediately separated into aliquots for 4 labs. Lab A was a specialized rheumatology lab, B and C were clinical labs in university associated hospitals and D was a commercial lab. The results obtained from labs B, C, and D were compared to those from A. In 20 reports there was a discrepancy of > 50% in the leukocyte (WBC) count. In 6 cases the error was much more and large enough to affect diagnosis and treatment. All 4 labs counted WBCs manually. Labs A and D used 0.3% saline as diluent, B used NSS and C used buffered ammonium oxalate. In 10 reports there was a discrepancy of > 50% in the WBC differential. D reported only the percent of neutrophils present and did not differentiate mononuclear cells. Although lab B did a full differential, only neutrophils and lymphocytes were ever reported. One lab reported 85% eosinophils not found by any other lab. Multiple fat droplets were apparently counted as WBC by lab C and were correctly identified by only lab A. In 7 reports there were discrepancies in the crystal identification with urates or CPPD either missed or erroneously identified by one or more labs. Errors in crystal identification would have resulted in inappropriate, potentially dangerous treatments.

Differing WBC counts may well be due to delays in performance as well as technical problems. Discrepancies in crystal identification may be due in part to lack of reference standards for comparison. Standardization of procedures and quality control should be strongly considered for labs doing SF analysis.

A60

PRIMARY SJÖGREN'S SYNDROME (SS) AND ACTIVE CNS DISEASE (CNS-SS) EVIDENCE FOR INTRATHECAL IgG SYNTHESIS AND LYMPHOID CELLS WITHIN THE CEREBROSPINAL FLUID (CSF). Elaine L. Alexander, Jane E. Lijewski, and Garrett E. Alexander. Johns Hopkins Medical Institutions, Baltimore, MD 21205.

The present study was designed to examine CSF immunoglobulin and cellular abnormalities in primary SS patients in whom the diagnosis of an additional connective tissue disease had been rigorously excluded were studied. CSF from 30 patients with active CNS-SS (SS_A) was examined and the results contrasted with those of 20 SS patients without CNS involvement (SS_{IA}) and 20 patients with systemic lupus erythematosus and active CNS disease (SLE_A). The following CSF determinations were elevated significantly in the SS_A, as opposed to the SS_{IA} group: total protein concentration, IgG concentration, IgG to total protein ratio, and IgG/albumin index. Agarose gel electrophoresis was abnormal, with one or more bands, in 25 of 29 (87%) SS_A patients, but in only 3 of 18 (17%) SS_{IA} patients. Similar, but less striking CSF abnormalities were seen in a subset of SLE_A patients. Fifteen (50%) SS_A patients had transient mild to moderate CSF pleocytosis, while only one (5%) SS_{IA} patient had similar findings. Cytology was abnormal in 18 (60%) SS_A patients with plasma cells, lymphocytes, and large mononuclear cells which resembled lymphoblastoid cells or activated lymphocytes. Similar cytologic findings were not observed in SS_{IA} or SLE. Thus, CSF analyses demonstrated the presence of immunocompetent lymphoid cells and evidence for the intrathecal synthesis of IgG in patients with active, but not inactive, CNS-SS. With corticosteroid therapy, elevated IgG indices, oligoclonal bands, and pleocytosis tended to normalize. CSF abnormalities serve as markers to monitor disease activity and response to therapy and suggest an immune-mediated pathogenesis for CNS-SS.

A61

HYPOCOMPLEMENTEMIC URTICARIAL VASCULITIS SYNDROME (HUVS): STUDIES ON C1q BINDING BY HUVS IgG. J. Wisnieski, G. Naff, CWRU, Cleve., OH 44106

HUVS is a rare vasculitis syndrome. Although "SLE-like," its relationship to SLE is problematic. Characteristically, serum or IgG from HUVS patients precipitates C1q in agarose immunodiffusion (ID). HUVS IgG is polyclonal, does not contain antibody to C1q, and binds C1q via its Fc fragment, suggesting that HUVS IgG may be part of a low mol wt (~7S) immune complex (IC) (J Immunol, 121, 613, 1978). We report here evidence that HUVS IgG is not part of an IC but is functionally abnormal. IgG was isolated by DEAE-Affigel blue chromatography (IgG Fx). When necessary, IgG Fx was further purified by affinity chromatography. Affinity purified IgG contained no polyaggregates, since both HUVS IgG and normal IgG eluted as a single, identical peak (K_{av}=.25) by Sephacryl-300 chromatography. C1q binding and precipitation by IgG Fx (1000 mg/dl) was studied in 1% gels at low ionic strength (.05μ) with decreased well size (10 μl) and increased C1q (80 mg/dl). These modifications allowed detection of precipitation in 12-24 hrs, maximal at 48-72 hrs vs 5 days by previous methods. Under these conditions, only HUVS IgG Fx precipitated C1q; normal control and 20 SLE IgG Fx's and HUVS heavy chains did not. Purified IgG was studied at physiologic ionic strength (.15μ) and pH (7.4) by a modified ^{125}I-C1q binding method. Cpm bound by normal IgG were equal to background (1-2%); in contrast, HUVS IgG bound 10-15% of added cpm. By SDS-PAGE, no difference in mol wt was found between HUVS light or heavy chains and normal controls. In 11% gels run under dissociative, non-reducing conditions, no low mol wt species (0-20,000 daltons) was found on staining with Coommassie blue, silver, or PAS stains. In conclusion, HUVS IgG and its chains have normal molecular weights; HUVS IgG is monomeric and does not appear to be part of an immune complex. Unlike normal IgG, it binds C1q under physiologic ionic strength and pH.

A62

CORRELATION OF ANGIOGRAPHIC ABNORMALITIES WITH DISEASE SEVERITY IN POLYARTERITIS NODOSA. Edward A. Ewald, and W. Joseph McCune. University of Michigan, Ann Arbor, Michigan 48109.

We evaluated angiograms of patients with polyarteritis nodosa (PAN) as well as the associated clinical and laboratory features. All patients had visceral angiograms and either biopsy or angiographic proof of PAN. Severe disease was defined as CNS PAN, renal failure requiring dialysis, gangrene of fingers or toes, cardiomyopathy, bowel infarction, hepatic failure, or hepatic infarction.

Angiograms were abnormal in 16 of 26 (62%) patients. Aneurysms were found in 15 of 26 (58%) patients, in 3 of 22 (14%) mesenteric circulations, 5 of 21 (24%) celiac circulations and in 14 of 26 (54%) renal circulations. An abnormal angiogram was found in 11 of 12 (92%) patients with clinically severe disease and in 6 of 14 (43%) patients without severe disease ($p < .01$). Clinical features were similar in aneurysm and non-aneurysm patients except for severe hypertension which was present in 10 of 15 (67%) aneurysm patients and in 3 of 11 (27%) non-aneurysm patients ($p < .05$). Hepatitis B surface antigen was found in 4 of 8 (50%) aneurysm patients and in 0 of 9 (0%) non-aneurysm patients ($p < .05$). An abnormal celiac angiogram was present in 6 of 9 (67%) patients with clinical hepatic involvement but in only 1 of 12 (8%) without hepatic involvement ($p < .01$).

The presence of aneurysms was associated with severe hypertension, hepatitis B surface antigenemia and clinically severe disease. Angiography may therefore identify a subset of patients with more severe involvement and may be of value in management decisions.

A63

FAMILIAL SLE - PRESENCE OF A CROSSREACTIVE IDIOTYPE IN HEALTHY FAMILY MEMBERS
Halpern, R., Davidson, A., Lazo, A., Lahita, R., Solomon, G., Diamond, B. Albert Einstein College of Medicine, Bronx, New York

Sera of 27 members of 3 human kindreds with familial systemic lupus erythematosus (SLE) were examined for expression of a crossreactive idiotype present on anti-DNA antibodies (aDNA ab) of SLE patients.

By radioimmunoassay serum samples from 7/8 SLE patients and 14/19 family members had high titered reactivity with the anti-idiotype, 3I. Isoelectric focussing and Western blot analysis of 3I reactive bands revealed either a pattern of bands present at pH5-7, or additional bands present at pH7-8.5. Cationic bands were found to correlate with the presence of aDNA ab indicating that immunoglobulin charge may be a factor in determining specificity for DNA. Millipore filter analysis revealed aDNA ab in sera of 4/8 SLE patients and 2/19 unaffected family members. In 2 additional SLE patients and 2 additional family members aDNA ab were revealed when sera were analyzed under conditions that dissociate immune complexes.

This study indicates that expression of an idiotype associated with aDNA ab is significantly increased in healthy relatives of SLE patients and usually occurs in the absence of aDNA activity. Investigation of the differences between idiotype positive antibodies which bind DNA and those which do not may lead to elucidation of the molecular basis for pathogenic autoantibody production.

A64

ANTIBODIES TO BOVINE CASEIN IN HUMAN SLE AND NZB/W MICE. R. I. Carr and D. Tilley, Dalhousie University, Halifax, N.S., Canada, B3H 1V9

We have found a significant increase in antibodies to bovine casein in patients with SLE. 25 ng of ^{125}I-casein in 100 ul was added to 100 ul of a 1:10 diln of sera from 47 SLE patients and 25 age and sex matched normal controls. 200 ul of 20% Polyethylene Glycol 6000 (PEG 6000) was added, the tubes vortexed, and incubated overnight at 4°C. They were then centrifuged, decanted, the precipitates washed with 1 ml of 10% PEG 6000, and then counted. The following results were obtained:

Sera	Mean Binding ± S.D.	
Normal Controls	20.5 ± 9.2	
SLE	42.5 ± 15.5	p<0.01

Since ingestion is the presumed route of exposure to casein in the patients, and since oral antigen exposure normally results in orally induced tolerance in experimental animals, we wondered if the increased casein antibody in SLE might represent a failure of oral tolerance to casein.

We examined this possibility in 4 month old NZB/W and BDF$_1$ female mice. The mice were fed casein by i.g. tube and immunized 7 days later. On day 21 they were boosted and bled on day 28. Antibodies were assessed by titering the sera in the assay above and the results expressed as ug of antigen bound per ml of undiluted serum (ABC_{33}).

Strain	Saline Fed	Protein Fed	
BDF$_1$	9.5 ± 2.4	3.2 ± 1.5	p<0.01
NZB/W	13.3 ± 8.0	21.5 ± 14.2	p>0.05

Thus, although the normal mice were tolerized by casein presented orally, the B/W mice were not and indeed may have been primed. Thus the increase in antibody seen in human SLE may reflect a similar failure of orally inducible tolerance in this disease.

A65

COST-EFFECTIVENESS (CE) OF TOTAL JOINT ARTHROPLASTY (TJA) IN OSTEOARTHRITIS (OA). MH Liang, KE Cullen, MG Larson, MS Thompson, JA Schwartz, AH Fossel, WN Roberts, CB Sledge. Multipurpose Arthritis Center, Brigham & Women's Hospital, Boston, MA 02115.

Although TJA is a major advance in the treatment of patients with OA, its cost-effectiveness has been questioned. We report the 6-month results in a study of the costs and benefits of TJA in unselected patients with OA.

Consecutive OA patients 50 to 80 years of age, with no prior upper extremity arthroplasty and no cognitive deficits were enrolled in a one-year prospective study. Health status was measured by the Index of Well Being (BUIWB), costs of services for arthritis by interview and validated against billing records.

The sample had 18 males and 27 females (mean age 66.4). A third were full or part-time employed, a third were retired and 20% were unemployed because of OA and 13% were unemployed for other reasons. Preoperatively, substantial pain, activity limitation and impaired global health were reported.

Six months after TJA, significant improvements were seen in global health (mean BUIWB change=0.087,$p < 0.0001$) and in functional status (mean BUMPS change=0.063,$p < 0.001$). The average cost for the six months prior to TJA was $933. The average 6-month cost after TJA was $22,730 per patient due almost entirely to costs of surgery.

For all patients, the CE ratio was 0.4 with large CE differentials associated with initial health status. The highest CE ratios were observed in 10 patients who had poorest health initially. TJA is more cost-effective for patients with the most to gain and "ineffective" for those with better preoperative health status.

A66

MURINE RECOMBINANT INTERLEUKIN 1 (rIL-1) INDUCES THE PRODUCTION OF COLLAGENASE AND PROSTAGLANDIN E_2 BY RHEUMATOID SYNOVIAL CELLS AS WELL AS STIMULATES THE PROLIFERATION OF MURINE THYMOCYTES.
C. Fiedler-Nagy, C. Batula-Bernardo, R. Semionow, and A.S. Stern. Hoffmann-La Roche, Inc., Nutley, N.J. 07110.

The monokine, interleukin 1 (IL-1) has previously been shown to functionally activate a variety of cell types including thymocytes and rheumatoid synovial cells. However, the question whether these effects result from the action of a single peptide has so far not been conclusively answered. The cDNA for murine IL-1 has recently been cloned and expressed in *E. coli* (Lomedico et al., Nature 312, p. 458, 1984). The rIL-1 was extracted from protein-containing inclusion bodies found within the *E. coli* expressing the lymphokine and purified by size-exclusion chromatography. The purified peptide stimulated the proliferation of murine thymocytes and was found to be endotoxin free by the Limulus Amebocyte Lysate test. When incubated with human rheumatoid synovial cells, the rIL-1 induced the production of collagenase and PGE_2 in a dose-dependent manner at concentrations slightly above those required for thymocyte proliferation. The biological activity of the rIL-1 was completely abolished when the peptide was heated at 90° for 30 min. Several retinoids including retinol, retinal, trans-retinoic acid, 13-cis-retinoic acid and Ro 10-9359 inhibited the rIL-1-induced production of collagenase but not PGE_2 by synovial cells at 1×10^{-6}M. These results are in agreement with previously published observations using IL-1 preparations at various stages of purity and conclusively confirm that a single peptide can induce thymocyte proliferation and stimulate the production of collagenase and PGE_2 by rheumatoid synovial cells.

A67

SPECIFIC SUPPRESSION OF ANTI-DNA PRODUCTION IN VITRO. M.R. Liebling, C. Wong, and J. Radosevich. Harbor-UCLA Medical Center, Torrance, CA.

Peripheral blood mononuclear cells (PBMC) from SLE patients produce measurable quantities of IgG antibodies to DNA (a-DNA) and tetanus toxoid (a-tet) as assessed by sensitive and specific radioimmunoassays. In an attempt to induce specific suppression of a-DNA production in vitro, antigen specific T-suppressor (Ts) cells were generated by incubating $5x10^6$ normal human T-cells and 5% monocytes (T+M) with calf thymus DNA (0-100 ug/ml) in 2 ml of RPMI 1640, 10% fetal calf serum, 25mM HEPES and antibiotics. After 5 days, of culture in this media, the T+M cells were washed thoroughly and a population enhanced for Ts cells was obtained by "panning" for OKT8+ cells using a negative selection technique (Benveniste E. et al, J Clin Immunol 3:166, 1983). These DNA educated, normal human, Ts cells were then co-cultured with $2x10^6$ SLE PBMC in the absence of DNA. The ratio of normal Ts cells to SLE B cells in these co-cultures was varied from 0.1:1 to 1:1. After 8 days, the co-culture supernatants were assessed for a-DNA and a-tet. In three separate experiments, specific suppression ranging from 57±2% to 87±4% was obtained employing this system. This suppression could be eliminated by irradiating the normal T-cells prior to co-culture and was not attributable to antigen transfer. Moreover, when SLE T-cells were educated with DNA in this manner and then co-cultured with either autologous or allogeneic SLE PBMC, no specific suppression of a-DNA was detected. We conclude that: 1) Ts cells specific for a-DNA can be generated from normal T+M cells after incubation with DNA, 2) these cells act across HLA-DR barriers and, 3) SLE patients appear to have a defect in their ability to generate Ts cells specific for a-DNA.

A68

RADIONUCLIDE JOINT-BONE SCANNING IN CHILDREN WITH RHEUMATIC COMPLAINTS. M. Moore, W. Moore, E. Giannini, E. Brewer, S.Long, R.Sonnemaker, D.Person. Baylor College of Medicine, Texas Children's Hospital, Houston, TX 77030

Radionuclide scanning is a useful diagnostic modality in the evaluation of adults with connective tissue disorders. Scanning in childhood rheumatic disorders has been less extensively studied, and the indications for scans are not well established. The purpose of this study was to identify the clinical characteristics of children with rheumatic complaints in whom scans proved most useful.

We reviewed the medical records and scans of all children who presented to the Pediatric Rheumatology Service over a 3 yr period (160 scans). The scans were interpreted independently by 3 nuclear medicine physicians who were unaware of the original interpretation. All children underwent radionuclide scanning using Tc-99 labeled phosphate complexes. The scan interpretations were identical to the original in 151 cases (94.3%).

The mean age was 7.6 years. By history, arthralgia occurred in 136 pts, fever in 50, and joint swelling in 50. On clinical exam, 137 joints had active arthritis; 57 had only pain on motion. Final diagnoses were varied: 34 pts had definite or probable JRA, 32 had arthralgia alone, 22 other connective tissue disorders, 10 infection, 4 tumors, 68 other.

There were 172 active areas by radionuclide scanning. In 57 joints with arthralgia alone, the scan identified 13 areas of activity not clinically apparent. The amount of agreement between scan results and clinical impression varied, depending on the joint being evaluated. Of 92 children without active arthritis on exam, 29 (32%) had abnl scans. Elevated ESR, young age, clinically active joint disease, abnl radiograph, patient diagnosis, and the presence of arthritis at any point were all associated with radionuclide scan abnormalities (p<.001; Chi square). There was no association of scan results with fever, duration of symptoms, condition at follow-up, arthralgia,WBC, hemoglobin, ANA, immunoglobulin levels or complement levels.

In conclusion, when arthralgia alone is present, a scan may confirm the presence of synovitis or other abnormalities. When arthritis is clinically present, the scan often confirms synovitis. Further, the scan is frequently useful in identifying areas of active arthritis not clinically apparent.

B1

EPIDEMIOLOGY OF SYSTEMIC-ONSET JRA. Carol B. Lindsley, University of Kansas Medical Center, Kansas City, KS 66103.

As there is no known cause or triggering factor in JRA, it would be expected that disease onset would be equally distributed over the warm and cold months of the year. Furthermore, we would expect an equal number of cases to be distributed across the four seasons of the year as well as across the twelve months of the year.

A review of all new patients with systemic-onset JRA seen at a university-based pediatric arthritis center over the past ten years revealed a significant difference existed between the number of observed cases falling into each category and the expected distribution.

	Expected Frequency	Observed Frequency		Expected Frequency	Observed Frequency
Warm Months	14	26	Winter	7	0
Cold Months	14	2	Spring	7	9
			Summer	7	8
			Fall	7	11

Chi-square tests of the above, observed-frequency distributions demonstrated that both were significantly different from the expected frequency distributions, based on chance. The chi-square values and consequent p values were respectively:

20.57, df=1, p <.001
10.00, df=3, p <.02

Additionally, a test of the distribution across the twelve months of the year was found to be significantly different from chance (p<.001).

These data suggest that regional or national data collection on seasonal patterns of disease onset in this subtype of JRA may be indicated.

B2

CHARACTERISTICS OF RESPONDERS (R) AND NON-RESPONDERS (NR) TO SLOWER-ACTING ANTIRHEUMATIC DRUGS (SAARDS) IN JUVENILE RHEUMATOID ARTHRITIS (JRA). Edward H. Giannini, Earl J. Brewer, Baylor College of Med, Texas Children's Hosp. Houston,TX 77030.

A double-blind, parallel, randomized, placebo (P) controlled, 12 mo, multi-centered, trial of d-penicillamine (D-PEN) and hydroxychloroquine (HCQ) was conducted in 162 pts with JRA. No statistically significant inter-group differences in response variables were detected. Despite these findings, there may be a select sub-group of pts who have a higher likelihood of response to SAARDS than to P. The purpose of this paper is to describe and compare the clinical and demographic characteristics of those pts who responded favorably versus those who did not respond to D-PEN, HCQ, or P. Pts were classified as R if they met at least 3 of the following 5 criteria at the final visit: 25% or more improvement in 1) the total no. of joints with active arthritis, 2) severity score, or 3) duration of AM stiffness; 4) classification as 'better' or 'much better' on the global assessment by the physician or 5) by the parent. Results: 159 pts completed at least 8 weeks of therapy and were considered for efficacy analysis. 62% of the D-PEN, 67% of the HCQ, and 60% of the P pts responded favorably. The median values of selected variables for the R and NR at randomization are shown in the table.

	D-PEN		HCQ		P	
Median values at randomization	R	NR	R	NR	R	NR
total number of active joints	12	21	14	23	13	16
total severity score	48	78	33	66	36	42
duration of AM stiffness (min)	30	50	25	10	15	15
erythrocyte sed rate (mm/hr)	27	18.5	17	27	21.5	16.5
age at rndzation (yrs)	10.2	10.5	10.0	10.4	8.0	10.6
duration of disease at rndzation (yrs)	2.0	2.3	1.8	4.3	2.1	2.5

From these and other data we conclude that pts with less articular involvement are more likely to respond favorably to SAARD + NSAID medication. However, this relationship is seen also in the placebo + NSAID group, perhaps indicating the response seen is attributable to NSAID alone. The amount of elevation of the ESR, the age of the pt, and the duration of disease at initiation of therapy do not appear to be associated with a higher likelihood of response.

B3

ASSESSMENT OF PHYSICAL WORK CAPACITY (PWC) IN JUVENILE RHEUMATOID ARTHRITIS (JRA) PATIENTS. Manuela S. Jasso, Elizabeth J. Protas, Edward H. Giannini, Earl J. Brewer, Texas Children's Hospital, Texas Woman's University, Baylor College Med. Houston 77030.

The rate of oxygen (O2) consumption while performing incremental exercise tests has become the standard method for assessing PWC. The usefulness of this method in determining PWC among patients with JRA has not been described previously. The objectives of this pilot study were; 1) to determine the feasibility of using such exercise testing to establish PWC in JRA, and 2) to describe quantitatively the relationship between PWC and the severity of articular involvement using regression analysis. Subjects were 9 JRA pts aged 8 to 11 yrs (mean=10.4). The total number of joints with active arthritis averaged 18.5 (range 1-46; median=15): severity scores averaged 64 (range 1-241; median=40). Each pt was tested on a bicycle ergometer using increasing workloads of 30, 60, 90, 120, and 150 watts. Workloads were increased stepwise every 2 min until the child could no longer pedal at a constant rate. An open-circuit method and a Gould 9000 IV Cardiopulmonary Exercise Lab were used to analyze expired gases.

Results of regression analysis showed that there was a positive correlation between O2 consumption and the number of active jts and the severity scores. There was a strong inverse correlation between disease severity and the workload that the pt was able to complete (table).

	active joints		severity score	
	N	r value	N	r value
O2 consumed at 30 watts	9	.43	9	.62
O2 consumed at 90 watts	7	.49	7	.40
highest workload completed	9	-.60	9	-.72

No adverse reactions were reported during or after testing.

We conclude graded exercise testing is an objective method of quantitatively assessing the effect of JRA articular disease severity on the cardiopulmonary system and may also be useful in measuring the response to treatment. A larger study is necessary to establish, with greater certainty, the extent and strength of the relationship between disease severity and PWC in pts with JRA.

B4

THE FREQUENCY OF ANTINUCLEAR ANTIBODY (ANA) IN CHILDREN USING MOUSE KIDNEY (MK) AND HUMAN EPITHELIAL CELLS (HEp-2). CM Arroyave, LM Pachman, M Giambrone, KC Rich, J Merphuyan. Northwestern University Medical School, Children's Memorial Hospital, Chicago, IL 60614.

The frequency of positives and the screening dilution of sera for ANAs has not been rigorously established in the pediatric population. The purpose of this study was to determine the frequency of ANA in non-rheumatic, non-allergic, non-infected children without malignancy undergoing surgery. The records were reviewed for the presence of abnormal CBC, ESR, and medical history. Serum from 251 children (age range 4 mos. to 16 yrs.) were tested for IgG ANAs by 3 different investigators using indirect immunofluorescence and two commercially available substrates, MK and HEp-2, at 3 dilutions by 3 different investigators. Five sera (2.4%) were positive:

SUBSTRATE	DILUTION OF SERA	# POSITIVE	% POSITIVE	TOTAL%+
MK	1:5	2	0.8	
	1:10	1	0.4	
	1:20	0	0	1.2
HEP_2	1:10	4	1.6	
	1:20	2	0.8	
	1:40	0	0	2.4

The IF pattern observed was speckled in 4/5 and homogeneous in 1/5. Only 1 was positive on both substrates. In contrast, 10/10 newly diagnosed children with definite (ARA criteria) SLE were positive at a dilution of 1:80 or greater on both substrates.

This is the first large scale study of pediatric sera using two commonly available substrates. We conclude that ANA is rare in this pediatric population. Supported in part by a grant from the SLE Society of Illinois and the Children's Mem. Hosp. Res. Foundation.

B5

SPECKLED PATTERN ANTINUCLEAR ANTIBODIES IN JUVENILE RHEUMATOID ARTHRITIS. Thomas G. Osborn, Terry L. Moore. St. Louis University School of Medicine, St. Louis, MO 63104.

In a previous investigation, antinuclear antibodies (ANA) were determined in 217 juvenile rheumatoid arthritis (JRA) patients by indirect immunofluorescence (IF) using HEp-2 cells as substrate. Significant ANA titers (≥ 1:40) were detected in 131 (60%) of these children. The speckled pattern of IF was found most commonly (72%).

Sera from 20 children found to have the highest titer speckled-pattern ANA were further investigated. Enzyme sensitivity of the antigens was determined by treating HEp-2 slides with deoxyribonuclease I (DNase I) 100 µg/ml in 0.01 M phosphate-buffered saline (PBS), pH 7.4 containing 3 mM $MgCl_2$ for 60 minutes at 37° C; ribonuclease A (RNase A) 100 µg/ml in PBS for 60 minutes at 37° C, and trypsin 3 µg/ml in PBS for 30 minutes at 25° C. HEp-2 substrates were also treated with 0.1 N HCl for 30 minutes at 25° C.

There was no significant change in ANA titer in the 20 patients when the HEp-2 cell substrate was treated with DNase I. However, sera were found to have at least an eight-fold drop in ANA titer when the HEp-2 cells were treated with trypsin. All sera were also found to have at least a four-fold drop in ANA titer when the substrate was treated with RNase A. There was no drop in titer when the cells were treated with 0.1 N HCl.

These findings suggest the antigen, to which the speckled ANA of these patients with JRA is directed, may be a tightly bound nuclear protein or nuclear ribonucleic acid.

B6

ABNORMAL SUPPRESSOR CELL FUNCTION AND CYCLIC AMP RESPONSE IN JUVENILE ARTHRITIS. E.Silverman, Hospital for Sick Children, Toronto, Canada, C.Somma, M.Khan, K.Melmon, E.G.Engleman. Stanford University, Stanford, Ca. 94305

We have previously shown that Leu 2+,9.3- T cells contain the precursors of Con-A and histamine-inducible suppressor cells. In addition, isolated Leu 2+,9.3- cells have a 2-7x↑ in cyclic AMP (cAMP) after histamine (his.) and isoproterenol (iso.) stimulation. Peripheral blood from 24 patients (pts.) with various forms of Juvenile Arthritis (JA) and 9 pediatric controls was separated on Ficoll-Hypaque and then divided into T and non-T cells by rosetting. T cells were then "panned" sequentially using anti-Leu 3 and 9.3 antibodies. Isolated Leu 2+,9.3- cells were pretreated with his. or Con-A, irradiated and tested for their ability to suppress the proliferative response of autologous Leu 3+ cells. In some experiments the intracellular cAMP response to iso. and his. was measured.

All controls and 11/24 JA pts. had normal Con-A and his.-inducible suppressor cells and 6/6 tested had a normal cAMP response to his. and iso. In 6/24 JA pts. there was minimal his. but normal Con-A-inducible suppressor cell function and in 2/2 pts. there was no cAMP response to his. but a normal response to iso. In 7/24 JA pts., both Con-A and his.-inducible suppressor cell function was abnormal and in 2/2 pts. there was no cAMP response to iso. and his. No JA pt. had decreased Con-A but normal his.-inducible suppressor cell function.

We have identified 2 groups of JA pts. with abnormal suppressor cell function. One has abnormal Con-A and his.-inducible suppressor cells with absent cAMP response to both iso. and his. while the other has an isolated defect in his.-inducible suppressor cell function with an absent cAMP response to his. and not to iso. Abnormal immunoregulation in JA may be related to a failure of an appropriate suppressor cell cAMP response.

B7

IMMUNE COMPLEXES (IC) IN THE SERUM AND CARDIAC TISSUE OF CHILDREN WITH KAWASAKI'S SYNDROME (KS).

B Herold, LM Pachman, AT Davis, ST Shulman, CM Arroyave, M Hang, J Robb, J Schaller, B Beckwith. Northwestern University Medical School, Children's Memorial Hospital, Department of Pediatrics, Chicago, IL 60614; Scripps Clinic, LaJolla, CA 92037; and University of Washington, Seattle, WA 98105.

To evaluate the role of IC in the pathogenesis of KS, we studied autopsy specimens from 6 children who died with cardiac complications of KS for IC, and sera from 10 children with active KS for the presence of cryoprecipitates (cryos) and soluble IC (S-IC). All ten sera contained S-IC by C1q binding and cryos were present in 7/10. The immunoglobulin (Ig) within the cryos consisted primarily of IgG and IgM. In limited serial studies, the concentration of protein within the cryos diminished in parallel with clinical improvement.

In 6 children who died with cardiac complications of KS, IgG and IgM were deposited in the coronary vessel wall in a granular pattern suggestive of IC ($p<.05$, $p<.01$). and IgM was present more frequently within myocardium when compared to age/date of death matched controls ($p<.05$).

We conclude: 1) soluble IC and cryos were present in serum of most KS children 2) the Ig within cryos consists predominantly of IgG and IgM; 3) the concentration of the cryos tends to parallel the clinical activity; 4) IC are seen in cardiac tissue of children who die from cardiac sequelae of KS and are found most frequently within coronary vessel walls, the major site of pathologic damage; and 5) these IC may be pathogenically related to coronary artery disease in KS.

B8

THE ROLE OF EPSTEIN BARR VIRUS IN JUVENILE ARTHRITIS.

Leonard D. Stein Sasson Lavi, Chaim Roifman, Bonnie Cameron, Ronald Laxer and Erwin Gelfand. Division of Immunology/Rheumatology. The Hospital for Sick Children, Toronto, Canada M5G 1X8.

Epstein-Barr virus (EBV) is a ubiquitous Herpes virus with lymphotrophic properties. EBV causes infectious mononucleosis and is associated with other diseases. Investigations suggest that the natural immune response to EBV infection is cytotoxicity and/or suppression of the early outgrowth of EBV infected B lymphocytes, and maintenance of long-term immune surveillance. Virtually all adult Rheumatoid Arthritis (RA) patients reported have had serologic evidence of EBV infection. Recent studies of RA patients have demonstrated a defect in the suppressor T lymphocyte system's ability to suppress EBV infected cells and have hypothesized a pathogenic role in RA. Prior to examining whether a similar EBV related immune defect exists in patients with juvenile arthritis (JA) we assessed the EBV immune status of these patients. Serologic studies of early antigen (EA) and viral capsid antigen (VCA) were performed on 41 JA patients. VCA and EA titers were negative in 38% of patients. Fifty-eight percent of pauci-articular, 28% of polyarticular and 20% of systemic onset subgroups were negative for both EA and VCA titers. Two rheumatoid factor positive patients were VCA positive. No patient had EA positive and VCA negative titers. In contrast to adult RA these studies suggest that EBV infection has not occurred in a large proportion of patients with JA, making it unlikely that an EBV specific T suppressor defect is integrally related to the pathogenesis of JA.

B9

ANTIBODIES TO PEPTIDOGLYCAN (PG) IN JUVENILE ONSET ANKYLOSING SPONDYLITIS (JAS) AND PAUCIARTICULAR ONSET JUVENILE ARTHRITIS ASSOCIATED WITH CHRONIC IRIDOCYCLITIS (CI).

Ruben Burgos-Vargas, Arthur Howard* and Barbara M. Ansell*. Hospital General de Mexico, S.S.A., Mexico 06726 and *Clinical Research Centre, Northwick Park Hospital, Harrow, Middlesex, HA1 3UJ.

PG is a heteropolymer of glycan chains cross linked through short peptides present in the cell wall of all bacteria. Its biological activities, including the adjuvant arthritis induced in rats, depend on a complex formed with residual pentose polysaccharide (GSP). The sera of both seropositive and seronegative rheumatoid arthritis and juvenile arthritis patients contain high level of antibodies to PG-GSP. Using an indirect enzyme linked immunosorbent assay antibodies of the IgG class to Streptococcus pyogenes group A PG-GSP were measured in the sera of 37 patients with JAS, 22 with CI and 20 healthy children. Mean antibody activity, measured in arbitrary units, was 184 in the JAS and 250 in the CI (p N.S.). The results in both groups differed from those found in healthy children ($p < 0.001$ and $p < 0.01$ respectively). This suggests either a possible role of bacterial cell wall products in the pathogenesis of these diseases or a state of immune reactivity to PG-GSP in these children.

B10

A RELATION BETWEEN SPONTANEOUS PRODUCTION OF RHEUMATOID FACTOR AND SUBSETS OF MONONUCLEAR CELLS IN PATIENTS WITH RHEUMATOID ARTHRITIS.

Sarah B. Clarkson, Roger D. Rossen and Donald M. Marcus. Baylor College of Medicine, Houston, TX 77030

Mononuclear cells (MNC) from the blood of many patients with seropositive rheumatoid arthritis (RA) spontaneously secrete rheumatoid factor (RF) in vitro. The objective of this study is to analyze the relationship between spontaneous production of IgM and RF, disease activity and subsets of MNCs. Although equal amounts of IgM were secreted by unstimulated MNCs from normal individuals and RA patients, RF production was detected only in RA patients (17/25, 68%). Patients with active disease secreted higher levels of RF (6.2 ± 5.2 ng/100 ul) than inactive patients (3.0 ± 1.2 ng/100 ul) ($p<0.05$). Patients who spontaneously secreted RF (RF-SP) differed from RF non-producers (RF-NP) in the proportions of their MNC subsets. The RF-SP patients had statistically significant fewer T3+, T4+ and more Mo2+ cells than normals, and fewer T4+, Ia+ and Mo2+ cells than RF-NP patients.

Number of positive cells (mm^3)

	T3	T4	T8	Ia1	B1	Mo2
RF-SP	787	501*	312	542**	143	418**
RF-NP	955	708	369	678	118	497

*p<0.01 **p<0.05

These data provide the first evidence that spontaneous secretion of RF by blood MNCs of RA patients is correlated with an alteration in MNC subsets. A decrease in the number and/or function of T4+ cells that induce suppressor cells may be responsible for the spontaneous secretion of RF.

B11

COLLAGEN-INDUCED ARTHRITIS IN RATS: REACTIVITY OF ANTICOLLAGEN ANTIBODIES WITH THE RENATURED CYANOGEN BROMIDE (CB) PEPTIDES OF TYPE II COLLAGEN.

M.A. CREMER, K. TERATO, A.S. TOWNES, and A.H. KANG. Veterans Administration Medical Center and University of Tennessee Center for the Health Sciences, Memphis, TN 38104, USA.

Rats immunized with native (N) BII collagen develop a brisk antibody response to N-BII and inflammatory arthritis. To determine which regions of N-BII contained antibody epitopes, we cleaved BII with CB, isolated peptides CB6, CB8, CB10, CB11, and CB12, renatured them by stepwise cooling, and confirmed their renaturation by viscometry or optical rotation studies. Reactivity of CB-peptides with IgG was determined by ELISA using sera collected serially on days 9, 15, 30, 75 from arthritic rats immunized with N-BII. Absorbance values were greatest for CB11, CB10 and CB8; intermediate for CB12; and, least for CB6. Sera obtained on day 30 from nonarthritic rats showed a similar pattern of reactivity but lower values for each CB-peptide. Other studies showed little IgG cross-reactivity between the different CB-peptides, but good cross-reactivity with the corresponding CB peptide prepared from either rat or chick type II collagen. The conformation dependency of epitopes was measured by inhibition studies. Microtiter wells were coated with renatured or denatured (D) CB-peptide and reacted with pooled serum (day 15). N-BII or D-BII were added as inhibitors. Reactivity to renatured peptides CB10 and CB11 was inhibited best with N-BII; denatured CB10 and CB11, inhibited best with D-BII. CB8 and CB12 reactivity was inhibited well with N-BII or D-BII irrespective of CB-peptide conformation. These findings show that N-BII immunization induces antibodies that react with several different epitopes present on the N-BII molecule.

B12

ANTIBODIES TO snRNPS AND scRNPS: DETECTION WITH UNLABELED CELL EXTRACTS.

M.Forman, J.A.Hardin, T.Mimori, and C.Gelpi. Yale University School of Medicine, New Haven, CT 06510.

Patients with rheumatic diseases produce a broad range of autoantibodies that bind specific protein components of different ribonucleoprotein (RNP) particles. Immunoprecipitation of extracts of ^{32}P labeled HeLa cells provides a highly sensitive and precise approach for characterizing these antibodies. However, this assay is complicated by the need for ^{32}P labeled substrate. Our aim has been to find a way to perform this assay that avoids the use of radioisotopes.

We adhered patient antibodies to protein A-sepharose particles and used them to immunoprecipitate extracts of unlabeled HeLa cells. Immunoprecipitated RNA molecules were recovered with phenol and resolved in urea-acrylamide gels. The gels were then stained with silver stain or ethidium bromide.

Both stains readily demonstrated patterns of small RNA molecules characteristic of immunoprecipitates based on antibodies to (U1)RNP, Sm, Ro, La, Th, U3, ribosomes, tRNAs, and several unidentified RNAs. In comparison with immunodiffusion, silver stained gels were 1000x as sensitive for detecting anti-(U1)RNP, 64x as sensitive for anti-Sm, 4x as sensitive for anti-Ro, and equally as sensitive for detecting anti-La antibodies. Accuracy was also improved. For example, we found that sera which immunoprecipitate only the Th RNA give false positive results for anti-La antibodies in immunodiffusion (the Th RNA is a single species of the La RNAs).

We conclude that most antibodies to ribonucleoproteins can be precisely characterized with the gel staining methods described here, even without specific standard control reference sera. They are sufficiently simple to be performed in most clinical laboratories.

B13

IMMUNOLOGIC EVIDENCE FOR HOMOLOGIES BETWEEN IMMUNOGLOBULINS AND THREE NUCLEAR ANTIGENS: Sm, nRNP AND Scl-70. Angeline S. Douvas, Robin A. Dyleski and Martin A. Turman. USC, Los Angeles 90033 and U. of Colorado Denver 80262.

Three RNA-associated polypeptides, P13, P30 and P26 react with anti-Sm and anti-nRNP antibodies. The single polypeptide Scl-70 and its phosphorylated form pScl-70 react with autoantibodies occurring in scleroderma. We have demonstrated that all four nuclear proteins cross-react with anti-immunoglobulin (Ig) antibodies, and also bind to protein A independently of any interactions with human antibodies. Binding of I^{125}-protein A to the P13,P30,P26-ribonucleoprotein (RNP) particle was demonstrated by solid phase radioimmunoassay (RIA). Also, it was possible to adsorb P13 and P30 out of solution using protein A-Sepharose, and to demonstrate direct binding of protein A to P13 by electroblotting (Western blots). Control proteins of similar size and charge did not bind to protein A in any of these experiments. I^{125}-protein A bound to detergent-denatured Scl-70 in electroblots, although native unphosphorylated Scl-70 showed little affinity for protein A in RIAs or on Sepharose beads. In contrast, pScl-70 bound avidly and quantitatively to protein A Sepharose suggesting that conformational changes may be needed to maximally expose binding sites on Scl-70. Direct binding of anti-Fc and anti-F(ab') anti- bodies to P13, P30 and P26 was demonstrated by electroblotting. These antibodies also bound to the P13,P30,P26-RNP particle and to Scl-70 in RIAs. The above observations suggest that Ig homologous sites on nuclear protein antigens may be central to the mechanisms which cause these molecules to react with autoantibodies in rheumatic diseases.

B14

IMMUNOGLOBULIN CLASS SPECIFICITY OF ANTI-HISTONES ANTIBODIES (AHA). Stamatia Gockel and Walter L. Binder, Behring Diagnostics, La Jolla, CA, 92037.

We have detected IgM class anti-histone antibodies (AHA) using a solid phase enzyme linked immunoassay (ELISA) in 41 of 60 (68%) ANA positive sera, 18 of 45 (40%) sera from old people (age >65) and 32 of 50 (64%) "general health screen" participants. The IgM antibodies found in the 18 older persons were further examined to determine their reactivity towards different histone subclasses. While most of the sera showed antibody activity towards all histone subclasses, 3 of 18 demonstrated elevated reactivity towards H_3 and 1 reacted mainly with H_{2a}-H_{2b}.

Antibodies of the IgG class appear to be more specific and were detected in 27 of 60 (45%) ANA positive sera, 1 of 48 (2%) sera from old people and in only 6 of 109 (5.5%) of "general health screen" participants. Of the 27 ANA and AHA positive sera, 21 were of homogenous pattern, 4 gave a speckled pattern and 2 were anti-centromere positive. All ANA positive sera had a titer of $\geq$1:80 on HEp-2.

These studies demonstrate that, IgM class AHA are widespread and are the main AHA found in old people and in the normal population. These antibodies are probably "transporteur" or physiologic auto-antibodies as described by Grabar and as such may have no pathological significance. IgG class antibodies on the other hand are more disease specific with a very low incidence in the random and older normal population.

In all future studies of histone antibodies factors to be carefully considered should include conjugate specificity as well as patient population and age.

B15

CHARACTERIZATION OF ANTI-Ki AUTOANTIGENS. P.T. Gompper, A.M. Francoeur, C.L. Peebles and E.M. Tan. Scripps Clinic and Research Foundation, La Jolla, Ca.

Anti-Ki autoantibodies occur in approximately 10% of patients with SLE, often in association with anti-Sm autoantibodies. Clinically, anti-Ki antibody is suspected to be associated with arthritis, pericarditis and pulmonary hypertension. Immunofluorescent staining of HeLa and HEp-2 cells with anti-Ki sera showed a predominant diffuse speckled nuclear and nucleolar pattern. Two autoantigens were identified, Ki-1 (MW 86,000d) and Ki-2 (MW 66,000d) by immunoprecipitation and immunoblotting. The antisera formed two groups separable by reaction in immunoblots. Some antisera reacted with both Ki-antigens while others reacted much more strongly with Ki-2 than Ki-1. The antigens did not appear to be phosphorylated, nor were they found associated with DNA or RNA. The Ki antigens were purified by affinity chromatography and SDS-PAGE. The amino acid composition of both proteins was determined and proved very similar. Anti-Ki antibodies were antigen-affinity purified by two separate technologies and found to cross-react with both Ki antigens, suggesting a shared epitope. A primary *in vitro* translation product was detected for Ki-2 antigen but not for Ki-1 suggesting the possibility that the latter may be a post-translational modification of Ki-2.

The ability to define more precisely the molecular nature of the Ki antigen/s would help to classify this antigen-antibody system and to relate it to clinical syndromes.

B16

SOLID PHASE-IMMUNE COMPLEX (SP-IC) BINDING OF C1q, AND FIBRONECTIN (FN) BINDING TO SP-C1q. Cynthia Gustafson, John J. Weiss, Frank R. Schmid, Ruth A. Entwistle, Azalia Kang, and Byron Anderson. Northwestern U. Medical School, Chicago, IL 60611.

FN may play a role in the metabolism of ICs by binding to the C1q component of the complement system possibly facilitating IC clearance and/or the localization of ICs in tissues containing FN (e.g., synovial and other joint tissues). Therefore, the stoichiometric and kinetic parameters of C1q binding to SP-IC ± FN were investigated. Two antigens of Di-N-acetylchitobiose coupled to a poly-lysine-glutamic acid copolymer (DNAC-poly-LG) and methotrexate coupled to bovine serum albumin (MTX-BSA), were adsorbed to the polystyrene tube SP. Rabbit polyclonal antibodies specific for the haptenic groups DNAC and MTX, respectively, were added and the bound antibodies titered using an enzyme-linked immunoassay. Radiolabeled (^{125}I) C1q was then added and percent binding determined under varying conditions.

At saturating concentrations of antibody bound to antigen, 22-25% ^{125}I-C1q was bound at 1.5 nM concentration and saturation of C1q binding sites achieved at concentration of 39 nM C1q. Competition of ^{125}I-C1q and unlabeled C1q binding to the SP-IC yielded a dissociation equilibrium constant (Kd) of 2 X 10^{-13}M. ^{125}I-FN bound to varying concentrations of SP-adsorbed C1q was shown to be dependent on ionic strength of the buffer system. The stoichiometry was approximately 1:1 (FN:C1q) and Scatchard analyses yielded two Kds of 1 and 10nM FN concentrations. The binding curves suggested that the interaction was avidity-dependent in that each molecule of FN forms more than one interaction with one or more C1q molecules. These conditions for FN binding to C1q could prevail *in vivo* and permit a role for FN in IC mediated inflammation. (Supported by PHS grant #AI-18317).

B17

IMMUNOCHEMICAL PROFILES OF IgA IN SERUM AND SYNOVIAL FLUID OF REITER'S SYNDROME (RS). R.D. Inman, M.E.A. Johnson, M.H. Klein. University of Toronto, Toronto, Ontario, Canada M5T 2S8.

Alteration in IgA level in RS has been of interest since it may reflect an immune response to a mucosaly acquired bacterial antigen which is serving as a provocative stimulus for RS in an immunogenetically susceptible host. Determination of immunoglobulin levels revealed elevated levels of IgA, in the presence of normal IgG and IgM levels, in 8/17 RS. Elevated IgA was seen more commonly with antecedent gastrointestinal infection (5/5 post-GI RS) than with antecedent genitourinary infection (2/7 post-GU RS). To resolve whether the elevated IgA levels might reflect the presence of IgA immune complexes, serum (S) and synovial fluid (SF) were subjected to sucrose density gradient (15-45%) ultracentrifugation, and density patterns of IgA determined by an IgA ELISA. The predominant pattern of IgA was 7s for S and 11s for SF: (i) of 12 S, 7 were primarily 7s IgA, 5 were both 11s and 7s, none was primarily 11s IgA; (ii) of 8 SF, none was predominantly 7s IgA, 4 were both 11s and 7s, 4 were 11s IgA. That the 11s IgA represented polymeric IgA was supported by the following: (i) the 11s IgA corresponded to the buoyant density on ultracentrifugation of a control dimeric IgA, (ii) ultracentrifugation at pH 2.8 did not lead to dissociation of the 11s IgA, (iii) radiolabelled secretory component bound exclusively to the 11s fraction, (iv) IgA rheumatoid factor (measured by an ELISA) was absent from both S and SF. J chain synthesis and polymerizing enzyme activity have recently been shown to be early markers of B cell activation. The polymeric IgA in RS may be a manifestation of local B cell activation within SF.

B18

CHARACTERIZATION AND CELL SURFACE REACTIVITY OF MONOCLONAL ANTI-DNA ANTIBODIES. Ruthann Kibler, James L. Parsons and Theresa A. Banks. U. of AZ. and Southwestern Clinic and Research Inst., Tucson, AZ 85724.

Spleen cells from female New Zealand Black/White autoimmune mice (age 4-7 months)were fused with SP2/0-Ag14 myeloma cells. An enzyme-linked immunosorbent assay with double stranded DNA as the antigen was used to detect those hybridomas specifically secreting monoclonal anti-DNA antibodies. From three separate fusions, a total of six anti-DNA secreting hybridomas were selected. These secreted the following immunoglobulin isotypes: 3-$\mu\kappa$, 2-$\gamma_{2a}\kappa$, and 1-$\gamma_1\kappa$. Additional characterization of these anti-DNA antibodies revealed that all of the μ isotypes yielded a peripheral staining pattern in the anti-nuclear-antibody test whereas the γ isotypes all demonstrated a homogeneous staining pattern. The six antibodies also displayed different reactivities against various nucleosides, denatured DNA and sonicated DNA.

A Rose Bengal binding assay was used to demonstrate that the anti-DNA antibodies adhered to the surface of various lymphoid cell lines. This could be explained by several mechanisms. Recent reports indicate that lymphoid and myeloid cell surfaces possess DNA receptors and that exogenous DNA can be processed by certain cells with these receptors (Biochem.Biophys.Res.Comm. 122:1034, 1984;Western Regional ARA abstract 19, 1984). The monoclonal anti-DNA antibodies could be adhering to this exogenous DNA. Consequently, it is possible to speculate that the presence of high titers of anti-DNA antibodies and the subsequent formation of immune complexes in systemic lupus erythematosus is due to a defective processing of DNA after its binding to cell surface receptors. A second alternative for binding of anti-DNA antibodies is that they actually recognize DNA or a "DNA-like" antigen inherent to the surface of lymphoid cells.

B19

MONOCLONAL ANTI-Z DNA AUTOANTIBODIES FROM MRL/1 MICE. W.J. KOOPMAN, M.J. LOSMAN, H.R. BERGEN, J.E. LARSON, T.R. O'CONNOR, and R.D. WELLS, UNIVERSITY OF ALABAMA SCHOOL OF MEDICINE, BIRMINGHAM, ALABAMA 35294.

Antibodies specific for the left-handed (Z) conformation of DNA have been previously identified in the sera of the spontaneously autoimmune murine strain MRL lpr/lpr; however, the fine specificity of these antibodies has not been delineated. To this end, we rescued B cells from MRL lpr/lpr spleens secreting antibodies against Z DNA $[Br\text{-}poly(dG\text{-}dC)]_2$ using hybridization techniques and examined the binding specificity of these IgMκ monoclonal products (Za, Ze and Zi) using solid phase ELISA and fluid phase immunoprecipitation assays. Antibody Za bound strongly to $[Br\text{-}poly(dG\text{-}dC)]_2$ and to a slightly lesser extent to $[poly(dG\text{-}5BrdC)]_2$ but not to B DNA (pBR322), denatured calf thymus DNA, the B form of $[poly(dG\text{-}dC)]_2$, $[poly(dG\text{-}dC)]_2$ brominated at 0.2M NaCl or to 2 other preparations of left-handed DNA, $[poly(dG\text{-}5MeC)]_2$ and $[poly(dG\text{-}thiodC)]_2$. In contrast, protein Ze bound to both $[Br\text{-}poly(dG\text{-}dC)]_2$ and denatured calf thymus DNA but not to B DNA (native calf thymus DNA, $[poly(dG\text{-}dC)]_2$) or to the other three left-handed forms of DNA tested. Antibody Zi exhibited similar binding specificity as Za but with lower avidity for $[Br\text{-}poly(dG\text{-}dC)]_2$.

Our results indicate that MRL lpr/lpr mice elaborate specific anti-Z DNA antibodies and suggest that these autoantibodies may be useful probes for analyzing fine structural heterogeneity of Z DNA.

B20

CLONED SCLERODERMA FIBROBLASTS EXPRESS A UNIFORM HIGH-SYNTHETIC PHENOTYPE. ROBERT BUCKINGHAM, THERESA WHITESIDE, Pittsburgh, PA.

Progressive systemic sclerosis (PSS, scleroderma) is characterized by fibrosis and extensive accumulation of connective tissues in the skin and internal organs. The mechanisms responsible for these changes are unknown, and both "activation" and "selection" of dermal fibroblasts (DF) with a high-synthetic phenotype may play a role in the pathogenesis. We established and studied DF clones from normal and PSS skin to compare their synthetic and proliferative characteristics. Limiting dilution assay (LDA) was used to determine frequencies of cloning in the microcultures of DF plated at 2, 1 and 0.5 cells/well. The clones derived from single cells were expanded in vitro and studied in passages C-E for growth (cell numbers, ^{3}H-thymidine incorporation) and synthesis of glycosaminoglycan (GAG) and collagenase-sensitive protein (CSP). Each clone inoculated at $20X10^3$ cells/well was fed on days 2 and 4, pulsed with ^{3}H-glucosamine or ^{3}H-proline and harvested 12 hours later. The cloning efficiency determined in 4 experiments by a statistical method of Taswell was similar for normal and PSS DF (35-50%, $p < 0.05$). Normal fibroblast clones (NFC) had heterogeneous phenotypes, while PSS clones (PSS-FC) were much less heterogeneous:

NORMAL CLONES No. of Clones	GAG cpm $x10^{-3}/10^6$ fibroblasts	CSP	PSS CLONES No. of Clones	GAG cpm $x10^{-3}/10^6$ fibroblasts	CSP
2	300 - 550	500 - 1,000	9	300 - 915	300 - 1,000
7	170 - 275	160 - 140	1	240	220
6	46 - 150	90 - 140	1	0	82

Clones were tested in passages C or D on day 4 of culture. Culture wells were assayed in triplicates. A representative experiment.

PSS-FC were also more uniform than NFC in cell growth kinetics and retained their characteristic growth and synthetic phenotypes in culture from passage C to F. Our experiments indicate that, unlike normal skin, skin of scleroderma patients is composed of DF which synthesize uniformly large quantities of GAG and CSP and which retain this synthetic phenotype throughout many generations in culture.

B21

α-INTERFERON RELEASE AFTER STIMULATION OF NORMAL LYMPHOCYTES WITH SLE ANTI-LYMPHOCYTE ANTIBODY. Francisco Ramirez and Ralph C. Williams, Jr. UNM, Albuquerque, NM 87131.

Several previous studies have shown that heterologous rabbit antilymphocyte antisera or mouse monoclonal anti-T-cell reagents such as OKT3 produced stimulation of interferon production by cultured normal human lymphocytes. Accordingly, anti-lymphocyte antibody obtained from SLE serum either by heat elution from normal lymphocytes preincubated with SLE serum at 4°C or from euglobulin preparations was incubated with normal peripheral blood mononuclear cells (PBMC) for periods of 3-7 days. This treatment resulted in production by PBMC of striking elevations of interferon (IFN) as measured by vaccinia virus plaque inhibition assay. This IFN activity was neutralized by anti-alpha interferon antiserum and showed acid lability. Antilymphocyte antibody present largely in IgM fractions of SLE serum was measured in parallel by microcytotoxicity and showed a direct correlation with ability of the same preparations to induce acid labile αIFN after culture with normal PBMC. Control eluates from PBMC using normal sera or euglobulins from normal sera produced no detectable IFN activity in cultured lymphocyte supernatants. These findings may help to explain the presence of acid labile αIFN in the serum of patients with SLE. They also indicated that anti-lymphocyte antibody from SLE serum is capable of inducing production of acid labile αIFN by normal PBMC.

B22

DNA INTERNALISATION - A FUNCTIONAL ROLE FOR THE DNA RECEPTOR. J. Peller, M. Merritt & R.M. Bennett. Oregon Health Sciences University Portland, Oregon 97201

Monocytes, T cells, B cells and neutrophils bind DNA in a saturable manner with a Kd of 10^{-9} M; a single species of cell surface binding molecule, M.W. 30,000, has been described (BBRS, 122:1034-1039, 1984). The stoichiometry suggests a ligand-receptor union, but a functional role has not hitherto been described. DNA binding/internalisation studies were performed using lambda phage ^{3}H DNA (nick translation) incubated with human monocytes and neutrophils (37°C, $7x10^6$ cells, HBSS). Timed aliquots of cells were washed x2 with 0.1 M glycine buffer, pH 3.0, (to remove surface DNA), and solubilised pellets were treated with 10% TCA. Internalisation of DNA occurred over a 36 hour period; evidence for receptor mediated endocytosis was provided by competitive inhibition by excess cold DNA, and abrogation of internalisation by omitting Ca++ (receptor mediated DNA binding is Ca++ dependent). Adding cold DNA after exposure to ^{3}H DNA enhanced internalisation in a manner indicative of "up regulation". Both monocytes and neutrophils maximally internalised $2.4x10^6$ DNA molecules per cell after 36 hours of incubation, whereas their surface binding capacity was only $2x10^3$ molecules - suggesting receptor recycling. Internalised DNA is degraded to oligo-nucleotides (<12 b.p.), but the quantitative results are inconsistent. Direct visualisation of internalisation was obtained by using a probe of biotinylated DNA and indirect immunofluorescence (goat anti-biotin and FITC anti-goat). At 37° C surface redistribution and capping of DNA occurred over a 3 hour course with a 90% internalisation at 18 hours. These results indicate that DNA internalisation may be a receptor mediated process, and it is hypothesized that this is a major functional role for the DNA receptor. These findings may have some relevance in regard to DNA processing and the clearance of free DNA and DNA-anti DNA immune complexes in patients with SLE.

B23

TWO DISTINCT IgG Fc RECEPTORS ON A HUMAN MONOCYTE LINE (U937): DIFFERENCES IN BINDING OF MURINE IgG SUBCLASSES. Douglas H. Jones and Clark L. Anderson. University of Rochester, Rochester, NY 14642.

Although murine (m) macrophages have been shown to bear 3 distinct Fc Receptors (FcR) for IgG, only one FcR, a 72,000 d sialoglycoprotein with high affinity for monomeric IgG, has been described on human (h) monocytes and U937 cells. Studies of receptor-specific binding of radioiodinated murine IgG subclasses to U937 cells at low ionic strength (employed to enhance low affinity interactions) indicate the presence of a second class of IgG FcRs on these cells. We found, first, that the amount of cell-bound heat aggregated (agg) mIgG2b and mIgG1 increased 5-fold as the ionic strength of the medium was decreased from 0.150 μ to 0.050 μ, whereas the amount of cell-bound monomeric mIgG2a and hIgG1 was unaltered at $1.5\text{-}3 \times 10^4$ molecules/cell. Second, receptor-specific binding at low ionic strength of agg mIgG2b was completely inhibited by agg hIgG (I50 = 25 μg/ml) and agg mIgG2b (I50 = 25 μg/ml) but was not inhibited by monomeric mIgG2a (20%Inh at 1000 μg/ml) or hIgG1 (0%Inh at 180 μg/ml). On the other hand, the binding of monomeric mIgG2a was inhibited by agg mIgG2b 65-fold less efficiently than by monomeric mIgG2a or hIgG1 consistent with a minor contamination of the agg mIgG2b preparation with mIgG2a. Third, in three experiments trypsinization of U937 cells resulted in a 32% mean decrease in the amount of monomeric mIgG2a bound to the cells whereas agg mIgG2b binding was increased 8% over untrypsinized cells. These studies suggest that U937 cells bear two distinct FcRs for IgG. One, previously well described, shows high affinity for monomeric hIgG1 or mIgG2a and is relatively trypsin sensitive. The other shows low affinity for agg mIgG2b, agg mIgG1 and agg hIgG and is trypsin resistant. The resemblance of these two FcRs to the murine macrophage FcRs for IgG2a and IgG2b/1, respectively, is striking.

B24

EFFECT OF AURANOFIN ON MACROPHAGE ACCESSORY CELL FUNCTION. JaNahn Scalapino and Barry S. Handwerger, Mayo Clinic, Rochester, MN

Previous studies have demonstrated that auranofin (AF) diminishes macrophage (MØ) accessory cell function in mitogen- and antigen-stimulated proliferation assays. To define the mechanism(s) responsible for this defect, we separated mononuclear cells from normal volunteers by plastic adherence into MØ-enriched fractions and non-adherent peripheral blood lymphocytes (PBL). MØ were treated for 1 hr with AF (0-0.5 μg/ml) and washed thoroughly. PBL were further depleted of adherent cells by incubation on nylon wool, then recombined with treated or untreated MØ and stimulated with Con A for 72 hrs. A dose-related decrement in Con A-induced PBL proliferation (^{3}H-TdR incorporation) was observed in the presence of AF-treated MØ, which could be completely restored by the addition of untreated MØ. The defect was not due to decreased IL 1 production, as 1) addition to culture of affinity-purified IL 1 (0.5-50 U/ml) only minimally enhanced proliferation, and 2) AF-pretreatment of purified MØ resulted in augmented (rather than decreased) lipopolysaccharide-stimulated IL 1 production, measured in a sensitive LBRM/HT-2 cell assay. The AF effect could not be attributed to diminished cell-cell contact, since MØ-PBL cluster formation was not appreciably altered by AF pretreatment of MØ. These data suggest that the effect of AF on MØ accessory cell function is not due to diminished IL 1 production or decreased MØ-lymphocyte contact. Accessory cell function is known to be influenced by Ia (HLA-DR) expression. AF treatment of MØ resulted in a measurable decrease in HLA-DR expression as determined by quantitative FACS analysis. The functional significance of the AF effect on MØ expression of HLA-DR remains to be determined.

B25

CONCANAVALIN-A MEDIATED PHAGOCYTOSIS: AN Fc-RECEPTOR RELATED FUNCTION.

Jane E. Salmon, Robert P. Kimberly, Allan Gibofsky, Nancy Tappe and Marilena Fotino. Hospital for Special Surgery and the New York Blood Center, New York, NY 10021.

We have previously demonstrated a specific decrease in Fc-receptor (FcR)-mediated phagocytosis of IgG sensitized erythrocytes (EA) as compared to phagocytosis of neuraminidase-treated erythrocytes (an Fc-independent probe) in disease-free individuals with the HLA allotypes DR2, DR3 or DQw1 which are seen with increased frequency in SLE. The specificity of this immunogenetically-associated alteration was studied in further detail by examining blood monocyte ingestion of Concanavalin A-treated erythrocytes (EConA) in 66 disease-free Caucasian adults. Phagocytosis of EConA was decreased in those groups in which decreased FcR-mediated phagocytosis has been shown: DR2+ (mean $\pm$ S.D.:2.89 $\pm$ 0.79, EConA phagocytosed/monocyte/hr, $p<0.01$); DR3 + (3.31 $\pm$ 1.64, $p<0.05$); and DQw1+/DR2- (3.45 $\pm$ 0.57, $p<0.025$) as compared to all others (4.16 $\pm$ 1.52). To investigate the relationship between Con A-mediated phagocytosis and FcR-mediated phagocytosis, ingestion of EConA, EA and zymosan was studied in monocytes which were adherent to coverslips coated with aggregated-IgG (Agg) or IgG-free fetal calf serum (FCS). Modulation of FcR from the surface of monocytes following adherence to Agg resulted in decreased ingestion of both EConA and EA, as compared to FCS controls (% phagocytosis: 6 $\pm$ 5 vs 70 $\pm$ 9 and 8 $\pm$ 8 vs 72 $\pm$ 12, respectively). No change in phagocytosis of zymosan was observed (79 $\pm$ 9 vs 93 $\pm$ 7). These results suggest that 1) FcR participates in Con A-mediated phagocytosis and that 2) since Con A binds mannose, FcR may have an oligosaccharide(s) with exposed mannose. Other Con A-mediated effects might involve participation of the FcR via crosslinking of such mannose-containing residues.

B26

PROLIFERATION OF NORMAL "RESTING" HUMAN T CELLS IS INDUCED BY INTERLEUKIN 2 IN THE ABSENCE OF OTHER KNOWN STIMULI.

Sharad Lakhanpal, Nick J. Gonchoroff, Jerry A. Katzmann and Barry S. Handwerger. Mayo Clinic, Rochester, MN 55905.

Defects in IL 2 production and responsiveness have been reported in SLE and RA. Further characterization of the biological properties of IL 2 should enhance our understanding of immune mechanisms in these diseases. IL 2 is known to stimulate the progression of activated T cells from G_1 through the rest of the cell cycle. We have demonstrated that addition of purified recombinant, human IL 2 to fresh normal human peripheral blood mononuclear cells (PBM), which were IL 2 receptor (Tac)-negative by FACS analysis, stimulated marked proliferation of the PBM. Proliferation peaked at days 7-9, was equivalent in magnitude to the maximal PHA response and was inhibited by anti-IL 2 receptor (anti-Tac) antibodies added at day 0. Significant proliferation was seen with IL 2 doses as low as 1 unit/ml (110 fM) and was maximal at 40-400 units/ml. IL 2-induced proliferation was also observed with PBM obtained from umbilical cord blood. Monocyte (MØ) depletion of PBM resulted in a marked reduction of IL 2 response which could be restored by addition of MØ to the cultures. The proliferating cells were shown by two color FACS analysis to be primarily Leu 1+ and Leu 4+ cells (both Leu 3+ and Leu 2+ subsets), but some Leu 1- and Leu 4- cells also responded. The proliferative cells were negative for markers present on B cells (B1,B2,B4), MØ (Mo2, 63D3) and NK cells (Leu 7 and Leu 11). These data demonstrate that IL 2 at femtomolar concentrations induces marked, MØ augmentable, proliferation of normal, "resting" (Tac-negative) Leu 1+ and Leu 4+ human T cells and a population of Leu 1- and Leu 4- cells which lacks B cell, MØ and NK cell markers.

B27

JUVENILE ARTHRITIS IS ASSOCIATED WITH THE NEW HLA ANTIGEN DRw52.5,6,8.

Linda K Myers, Edward J Ball, Chester W Fink and Peter Stastny. Depts of Int. Med. and Pediatrics, The University of Texas Health Science Center at Dallas, Texas 75235

Previous studies of HLA antigens in juvenile arthritis (JA) have shown that patients with pauciarticular onset and those with rheumatoid-factor-negative polyarticular onset have increased frequencies of the antigens DR5, DRw6, DRw8 and DRw52. Heterozygous phenotypes such as DR5-DRw8 were however, not associated with increased risk, suggesting that a single mechanism might explain the association with each of the antigens. One possibility was that the main HLA association was with a determinant shared by the individual specificities. Analysis of recently-typed patients showed that DR5, DRw6 or DRw8 were found in 44/59 compared to 62/140 in controls (X^2=14.1). Chi square values for DR5 (5.0), DRw6 (12.9), DRw8 (1.3) and for DRw52 (12.2), were all lower. While DRw52 is known to include virtually all individuals positive for either DR3, DR5, DRw6 or DRw8, the pattern in JA appeared to lack the DR3 component. Two typing sera appeared to recognize such a specificity associated with DR5, DRw6, and DRw8. Absorptions substantiated the fact that a single specificity was recognized and lysostrip experiments showed that cytotoxicity was inhibited by anti-DRw52-like monoclonal antibodies I-LR2, 7.3.19.1 and MCS7. In addition, three alloreactive T cell clones were generated which recognized a similar antigen shared by DR5, DRw6 and DRw8 cells. The proliferative responses of these T cell lines were inhibited by addition of murine monoclonal antibodies reacting with DRw52-like antigens. Thus, DRw52.5,6,8 appears to be a separate HLA antigen which may have a strong association with susceptibility for development of juvenile arthritis.

B28

EFFECT OF NONSTEROIDAL ANTIINFLAMMATORY DRUGS ON ARTICULAR CARTILAGE.

Calvin R. Brown, Giles G. Bole, Jeanne M. Riddle, University of Michigan, Ann Arbor, MI 48109

Male guinea pigs were used to assess the effects of three drugs on normal and experimental osteoarthritis induced by gluteal myectomy and infrapatellar tendotomy. Normal and osteoarthritic animals were fed oral solutions of salicylate (100 mg/kg), ibuprofen (25 mg/kg), and sulindac (5 mg/kg) to produce serum values comparable to human levels. After dosing orally for one week, animals were given intraperitoneal $^{35}SO_4^{=}$ 24 hours before sacrifice. Cartilage from femoral heads, tibial condyles and tibial plateaus was removed, water content measured and radioactivity in proteoglycans determined. Normal guinea pigs untreated or treated with salicylate, ibuprofen or sulindac demonstrated similar values for $^{35}SO_4^{=}$ incorporation in cartilage proteoglycan (10-11 dpm x 10^3/uM uronic acid). Twelve to fourteen week postoperative osteoarthritic animals had an average 15% increase in $^{35}SO_4^{=}$ incorporation in knee proteoglycans and 80% depression in hip proteoglycans over unoperated controls. These values were unaffected by drug treatment. Cartilage water content in both normal and osteoarthritic animals was depressed by 25±1.2% in ibuprofen, but not salicylate or sulindac treated groups. By scanning electron microscopy osteoarthritic animals appear to show a progressive change in cartilage matrix from surface to enchondral plate. The extent of these changes did not appear to be affected by treatment with nonsteroidal antiinflammatory drugs. There was no affect from treatment with oral nonsteroidal drugs on proteoglycan synthesis, but ibuprofen altered cartilage water content without other observed ultrastructural changes in cartilage matrix integrity.

B29

STIMULATION OF HUMAN CHONDROCYTES BY GROWTH FACTORS.

M.L. Jurisson and C.W. Castor. University of MI, Ann Arbor, MI 48109.

It has been suggested that chondrocytes are hypermetabolic and actively engaged in repair of damaged cartilage in osteoarthritis (OA). We sought to ascertain the responsiveness of chondrocytes to circulating or locally derived mediators as possible regulators of this behavior. In human OA chondrocyte cultures we demonstrated stimulation of glycosaminoglycan synthesis by naturally occurring growth factors. Increased synthesis of hyaluronic acid (HA) and sulfated glycosaminoglycans (S-GAG) was demonstrated by incorporation of ^{14}C-glucosamine and $^{35}SO_4$ respectively into CPC precipitable material in tissue culture supernatants. Gel filtration (Sephacryl S-500) showed two peaks, the larger peak, a proteoglycan monomer, consisted nearly entirely of chondroitin-4/6 sulfate, whereas the smaller peak also contained substantial amounts of dermatan sulfate.

Addition of Interleukin-1, CTAP-III, insulin, or an extract of osteoarthritic synovial cells to chondrocyte cultures enhanced ^{14}C-glucosamine and $^{35}SO_4$ incorporation, suggesting increased HA and S-GAG synthesis. Interleukin-1, in nanogram amounts, stimulated much greater synthesis of ^{14}C-HA than ^{35}S-GAG. Half-maximal response to CTAP-III occurred at a concentration of 0.5 μg/ml. It can be concluded that human OA chondrocytes are metabolically active in culture and that their production of proteoglycan monomer, S-GAG chain, and HA may be increased by naturally occurring growth factors.

B30

LEUKOTRIENE PRODUCTION BY HUMAN SYNOVIAL MEMBRANE.

J.A. Kopicky, S.P. Peters, D.W. Lennox, F.M. Wigley. The Johns Hopkins Medical Institutions, Baltimore, MD 21224

Leukotrienes (LT) have been demonstrated to be mediators of immediate hypersensitivity reactions and inflammation. Although LTB_4 has been measured in inflammatory synovial fluid, the role of the synovial membrane (SM) in the production of LT, especially sulfidopeptide LT, has not been studied. SM obtained at arthroplasty in 10 patients {5 osteoarthritis (OA), 4 rheumatoid arthritis (RA), 1 chondromatosis} was dissected into fragments which were incubated for 18 hours in DMEM with 10% fetal calf serum, then washed and incubated in DMEM with 0.2% lactalbumin for 4 hours either with or without the calcium ionophore A23187. Media was extracted (chloroform:ethanol:formic acid) and subjected to high performance liquid chromatography. Aliquots that migrated with standard LTC, LTD and LTE were analyzed by radio-immunoassay with the following results, expressed as mean ± SEM:

	LEUKOTRIENE (ng/g wet tissue)		
	C	D	E
Control	12.3±3.6	10.7±4.3	39.1±14.3
A23187(10um)	15.7±4.1	20.4±7.4	242.1±93.3

LTC, LTD and LTE were all detectable. LTE production was significantly increased by inophore stimulation over control values ($p<0.05$). There was no significant difference in LT synthesis between OA and RA synovium. The stimulated synovial chondromatosis demonstrated a 22 fold rise in LTE over baseline. We conclude that SM has the capacity to synthesize and metabolize LT and that these mediators may play a significant role in acute and chronic synovitis.

B31

Adenosine Deaminase and Purine Nucleoside Phosphorylase Activities in the Acquired Immunodeficiency Syndrome. Edwin Mejías, and Rosa Lluberes. Veterans Administration Hospital, San Juan, P.R. 00936

Deficiencies of the purine catabolic enzymes adenosine deaminase (ADA) and purine nucleoside phosphorylase (PNP) have been described in severe combined immunodeficiency disease and selective T-cell immunodeficiency disease respectively. The recently described acquired immuno deficiency syndrome (AIDS) resembles the immunologic alterations observed in children with a congenital deficiency of PNP.

In an attempt to further investigate immunologic alterations in AIDS, erythrocyte and lymphocyte ADA and PNP activities were measured by highly sensitive radiochemical methods in 6 patients with AIDS and 26 controls. Our results are as follows: 1. Erythrocyte ADA activity for controls was 0.66 nmol/min/mg protein and 0.80 nmol/min/mg protein in AIDS. 2. Lymphocyte ADA activity in controls and AIDS were 6.86 nmol/min/mg protein and 5.57 nmol/min/mg protein respectively. 3. Lymphocyte PNP in controls was 5892 ± 501 nmol/hr/mg protein and AIDS 2740 ± 865 nmol/hr/mg protein ($p<0.0025$). 4. Erythrocyte PNP activity in controls and AIDS were 2680 ± 190 and 1618 ± 137 nmol/hr/mg protein respectively ($p<0.0005$). PNP activity in three patients with AIDS was reduced to 56% in the spleen and 65% in lymph nodes of the activity as compared to 8 controls.

From our studies we conclude that: 1. Abnormalities in purine catabolic enzymes should be included among the alterations in AIDS. 2. It is unlikely that the decreased PNP activity in AIDS is causally related to the syndrome, nevertheless this may be a facilitating factor in perpetuating the abnormal T-cell dysfunction in this entity.

B32

SYNOVIAL FLUID NUCLEOTIDE PYROPHOSPHOHYDROLASE LEVELS IN BASIC CALCIUM PHOSPHATE DEPOSITION ARTHROPATHY. JW Rachow, LM Ryan, PB Halverson. Medical College of Wisconsin, Milwaukee, WI. 53226.

We recently reported that synovial fluids (SF) containing calcium pyrophosphate dihydrate (CPPD) crystals exhibited elevated ATP pyrophosphohydrolase activity compared to fluids from patients with primary osteoarthritis (OA), rheumatoid arthritis (RA), and gout. We subsequently found that the enzyme responsible for this activity is a non-specific nucleotide pyrophosphohydrolase (NPPH) which generates inorganic pyrophosphate from nucleoside triphosphates. In addition to generating PPi, NPPH promotes matrix vesicle induced formation of basic calcium phosphate (BCP) crystals, which frequently occur in joint fluids containing CPPD crystals. We sought to determine whether NPPH activity was elevated in fluids containing BCP crystals with or without CPPD crystals.

We studied SF from 73 patients with a variety of arthropathies: 3 gout, 8 RA, 17 OA, 14 CPPD deposition, 21 BCP deposition, and 10 CPPD+BCP deposition. NPPH activity was measured as production of p-nitrophenol from p-nitrophenyl thymidine monophosphate at pH 7.3 and 37°C.

Activity in OA was 1571±810 (mean ± SD) pmol/hr/mg protein. This was lower than CPPD deposition (2070±730, $p < 0.05$, independent samples t-test), BCP deposition 2240±810, $p < 0.014$) and BCP+CPPD deposition (2550±960, $p < 0.02$). The lowest activities were observed in gout (765±50) and RA (1230±370).

We conclude that elevated SF NPPH activity may be a marker for CPPD and BCP crystal deposition in joints. Whether it plays a role in pathologic articular mineralization is still speculative.

B33

SUPPRESSION OF ACTIVE COLLAGENASE FROM CALCIFIED LAPINE SYNOVIUM BY ARTEPARON. Paul B. Halverson, Herman S. Cheung, Daniel J. McCarty, Medical College of Wisconsin, Milwaukee, Wisconsin 53226.

Arteparon (ART) is a polysulfated mucopolysaccharide with inhibitory activity against a variety of proteinases in vitro. ART has also been shown to retard progression of arthritis in a lapine meniscectomy model of osteoarthritis (Howell et al Arthritis Rheum 27:S41, 1984). The mechanism of action is unknown. We have studied the effect of ART on collagenase production from calcified lapine synovium cultured ex vivo.

Calciphylaxis was induced in New Zealand white rabbits by oral administration of cholecalciferal 600,000 units and on the following day intra-articular injection of 8μmoles $FeCl_2$ in phosphate buffered saline. Approximately 3 weeks later, calcified synovium was collected, washed, minced, and cultured in DMEM with 10% lactoalbumin hydrolysate. ART 10^{-3}M was added to 2 samples. Media was changed daily and was assayed for active and total collagenase. One unit of collagenase = 1μg collagen digested/ml/min.

Collagenase (u/mg tissue)	Day 1	Day 2	Day 3
Total	4.56	6.91	32.74
Active	0	.01	2.40
Active + ART	0	.52	5.35

Total collagenase was not affected by addition of ART. By day 3 cultures with ART have less than one half the active collagenase of cultures without ART. There was no further suppression of active collagenase by ART 10^{-3}M. Conclusion: Calcified lapine synovium produces active collagenase by day 2 of organ culture. ART significantly suppresses generation of active collagenase without decreasing total collagenase. ART may inhibit the activation process of collagenase.

B34

QUANTITATIVE SOLID PHASE FLUORESCENCE IMMUNOASSAY (FIAX) OF RHEUMATOID FACTOR (RF) AND C-REACTIVE PROTEIN (CRP) IN RHEUMATOID ARTHRITIS (RA). G.W. Cannon, M.J. Egger, J.R. Ward, L.J. Blonquist. University of Utah, Salt Lake City, UT 84132.

FIAX is a semi-automated solid pnase fluorescence immunoassay metnod for detection and quantitation of RF and CRP in international units/ml (IU/ml) over a continuous range. RF was measured in 150 patients with active RA. RF measured by latex agglutination (LA) methods in two fold dilution titer (1:20-1:40,960) correlated significantly witn FIAX ($r=.8689$, $p <.001$). A positive RF was detected by both FIAX and LA in 141 patients, by FIAX only in 1 patient, by LA only in 1 patient and neither FIAX or LA in 7 patients.

RF LA titer	Negative	1:20	1:40	1:80	1:160	1:320	>1:320
RF FIAX (IU/ml)	11±1.8	19±10	25±20	33±16	48±27	111±57	840±377
Patients (N)	8	5	6	6	13	14	98

CRP and Westergren erythrocyte sedimentation (ESR) were measured in 151 patients. CRP measured by FIAX and nephelometric methods (NM) correlated significantly with each otner ($r=.9412$ $p <.001$) and witn ESR (data below). An elevated CRP (>.8 IU/ml) was detected by botn FIAX and NM in 120 patients, FIAX only in 10 patients, NM only in 2 patients, and neitner FIAX or NM in 19 patients.

ESR (mm/hr)	1-20	21-30	>31	r (CRP vs ESR)	p
CRP (NM) (IU/ml)	1.43±1.62	2.86±1.91	4.61±3.24	.5451	<.001
CRP (FIAX) (IU/ml)	1.50±2.05	3.20±2.15	5.87±4.50	.5970	<.001
Patients (N)	26	23	102		

In RA patients tne FIAX method of measuring RF and CRP appears similar to LA and NM metnods for measuring these parameters. Tne CRP measured by botn FIAX and NM metnods correlated significantly witn ESR.

B35

CHLOROQUINE RETINOPATHY: EARLY DIAGNOSIS AND PROGNOSIS. Michael Easterbrook. University of Toronto, Toronto, Ontario, Canada, M5S 2T5.

Elaborate testing with dark adaptation, retinal light threshhold testing fluorescein angiography and automated perimetry are time-consuming, expensive and difficult to perform in many arthritic patients taking chloroquine or hydroxychloroquine. Chloroquine retinopathy may be present with normal vision, normal colour vision and a normal fundus appearance. There is therefore need for a simple, self-administered test that would alert patients and ophthalmologists to the possibility of early chloroquine retinopathy. 23 patients initially diagnosed with the Amsler grid have been investigated. This simple visual field test may be performed in a few seconds with excellent correlation to more difficult and time-consuming visual field testing by static and kinetic perimetry. Not only is the correlation with traditional forms of visual field testing excellent; Amsler grid testing by the patient may preceed visual field defects found by static and kinetic perimetry.

These patients have been followed for 6 months to 5 years. The natural history of these patients so diagnosed will be discussed. Patients with early bilateral chloroquine retinopathy with relative scotomas, normal colour vision, electroretinograms, electrooculograms and fluorescein angiography have not progressed. Patients presenting with absolute scotomas, abnormal colour vision, and abnormal fluorescein angiography progress in 50% of cases.

B36

ONE YEAR EXPERIENCE IN PATIENTS TREATED WITH AURANOFIN FOLLOWING COMPLETION OF A TRIAL COMPARING AURANOFIN, GOLD SODIUM THIOMALATE AND PLACEBO. Stephen L. Dahl and H. James Williams for tne Cooperative Systematic Studies of Rheumatic Diseases, Salt Lake City UT 84132.

One hundred thirty-seven patients who completed a 22 week parallel, controlled trial comparing placebo (P), auranofin (AUR) and gold sodium thiomalate (GST) entered a one year open-label study. Patients were treated witn 3 mg AUR twice daily. Background anti-inflammatory therapy was modified as needed at the discretion of the investigator. Of those who enrolled into tnis study, 41 nad received placebo during the controlled trial, 49 nad received AUR, and 47 nad received GST. Eighty patients were still receiving AUR after 52 weeks. Twenty-two patients (54%) who transferred from P to AUR completed 52 weeks of treatment. There were no statistically significant improvements in joint counts for pain/tenderness or for swelling. Thirty-seven patients (76%) who continued AUR during the open label study completed 52 weeks. For tnese patients there was no apparent additional improvement during AUR therapy. Twenty-one (45%) of patients who switched from GST to AUR completed 52 weeks of treatment. For those patients evidence suggests that AUR could sustain the initial response achieved by GST.

Thirteen patients were withdrawn for adverse effects of which 8 occurred in patients previously treated with GST. Tnirty-four patients were withdrawn for lack of acceptable therapeutic response and the numbers were similar among tne groups when stratified by previous treatment. Thus AUR appears capable of sustaining an initial response to GST but continued improvement is not apparent with increased duration of AUR therapy.

B37

Immunohistologic Evaluation of the Synovium in Intractable Rheumatoid Arthritis (RA). H. Gaston, N. Lane, R. Warnke, D. Schurman, S. Strober.

This study was designed to evaluate the initial appearance of the rheumatoid synovium in 15 patients who have classical or definite RA with active joint disease which was not controlled with NSAID's gold salts and penicillamine.

Multiple knee synovial biopsies were obtained by arthroscopy and evaluated using conventional and immunohistological techniques. Lymphocyte function studies and measurements of autoantibodies in the serum and synovial fluid were performed concurrently. Synovial biopsies showed marked heterogeneity in histological appearances. In particular, there was a wide variation in both synovial hypertrophy and lymphocytic infiltration. Some biopsies were characterized by infiltration with T lymphocytes (9 biopsies), while in others lymphocyte infiltration was rare (6 biopsies). In general, biopsies with heavy lymphocytic infiltration also showed marked synovial proliferation. Lymphocytic proliferation in response to soluble antigens was evaluated in 12 patients. 8 patients showed significant responses to tetanus toxoid (S.I. >5 mean 20±14) while 4 were unresponsive. There was no correlation between the degree of lymphocytic infiltration of the synovium and a failure to respond to soluble antigens. All synovial fluids had a high titer of rheumatoid factor (RF) regardless of the intensity of lymphocytic infiltrate. Thus, the majority of patients with intractable RA had a T cell infiltrate in the synovium as well as RF in the joint fluid.

B38

SALICYLATE OTOTOXICITY IN PATIENTS WITH RHEUMATOID ARTHRITIS (RA) - A CONTROLLED STUDY. James T. Halla and Joe G. Hardin. Abilene, TX 79601 and Univ. of South AL, Mobile 36617.

To assess the significance of symptoms suggestive of salicylate ototoxicity, 135 consecutive patients with RA who were presumably taking salicylates regularly and 182 normal subjects who were not taking any anti-inflammatory drugs (controls-C) were studied. The symptoms of tinnitus (T) and subjective hearing loss (SHL) were elicited and analyzed by structured interview and serum salicylate (SS) levels were measured in all of the RA patients. Each group was divided into four subgroups on the basis of symptoms: (1) those with both T and SHL, (2) those with T alone, (3) those with SHL alone and (4) those with neither. The RA and C groups did not differ significantly with regard to symptoms; 21% of the RA and 13% of the C subjects were in subgroup (1), 11% and 12% in subgroup (2), 10% and 15% in (3) and 58% and 60% in (4). Within the RA group, SS levels were >19.6mg/dl in 38% of subgroup (1), 33% of (2), 77% (13 patients) of (3) and 35% of (4); there was no significant difference between subgroups (1) and (4). Audiometric responses were measured in 28 of the RA patients. All 10 in subgroup (1) had a mild-severe sensorineural hearing loss, while only about half of the subjects in the other subgroups had such a defect. All 3 patients with SS levels >30mg/dl had an abnormal audiometric response, but mean SS levels did not differ significantly between subgroups (1) (23mg/dl) and (4) (21mg/dl).

Symptoms suggestive of salicylate ototoxicity seem to occur no more frequently in RA patients taking salicylates than in normal individuals taking no anti-inflammatory drugs; when these symptoms occur in patients at risk for ototoxicity they correlate poorly with SS levels within or below the usual therapeutic range and both correlate poorly with audiometric responses.

B39

BRONCHOALVEOLAR LAVAGE IN PATIENTS WITH RHEUMATOID ARTHRITIS. G. Ho, Jr. B. Zimmermann, S. Davis, and A. Erickson. Veterans Administration Medical Center and Brown University, Providence, RI 02908.

Twenty-five randomly selected patients (pts) with definite or classical rheumatoid arthritis (RA) underwent bronchoalveolar lavage (BAL) to investigate interstitial lung disease (ILD) associated with RA. The population consisted of 23 men and 2 women with a mean age of 57 yrs (range 29-76). The average duration of RA was 14 yrs (range 1-40). All were Steinbrocker's functional grade II or III and 76% were positive for rheumatoid factor (RF). Based on the results of the differential cell counts of recovered BAL fluid, the pts were separated into two groups: Gp I, those with abnormal lavage results defined as neutrophils (PMNs) > 5% (n=3) and/or lymphocytes ≥ 10% (n=7), and Gp II, those with normal lavage results who had percentages of PMNs and lymphocytes below these limits.

	Group I (n = 8)	Group II (n = 17)
"velcro" rales present	3/8 (38%)	6/17 (35%)
chest x-ray showing ILD	2/8 (25%)	5/17 (29%)
abnormal PFTs*	3/8 (38%)	3/16 (19%)
current remittive drugs**	4/8 (50%)	15/17 (88%)

Gp I and Gp II pts did not differ in mean age, disease severity or duration, RF positivity, or mean total cell number from BAL. Both groups contained similar proportions of pts with clinical evidence of ILD. Remittive drugs appear to be associated with a lower incidence of BAL abnormalities. Our data show that 1/3 of randomly selected RA pts have abnormal BAL results and support previous reports of increased proportion of lymphocytes among BAL cells from RA pts.

* 2 or more of TLC, FRC, or DLco < 80% or single parameter < 65% of predicted. ** gold, penicillamine, methotrexate, or hydroxychloroquine.

B40

ANTI-GALACTOSYL IgG ANTIBODY (aGAL AB) LEVELS IN RHEUMATOID ARTHRITIS PATIENTS (RA). CORRELATION WITH THE SPLENIC UPTAKE (SU) OF HEAT-DAMAGED RED BLOOD CELLS (HD-RBC). MG MALAISE, JB FOIDART, PR MAHIEU and P FRANCHIMONT. State University of Liege, Liege, Belgium.

Recently, an unique natural aGAL IgG AB was described on thalassemic RBC and subsequently characterized in normal human sera (Galili et al; Blood, 1983; J Exp Med, 1984). 99Tc-labeled HD-RBC mainly accumulate into the spleen by unknown mechanisms. Testing the hypothesis that HD-RBC clearance is mediated at least by splenic Fc-receptors, we measured in the same subjects the SU of HD-RBC and aGAL AB titers, whose role in the clearance of thalassemic or senescent RBC has been suggested. The aGAL AB titers were then measured by passive hemaglutination using rabbit RBC and by RIA using affinity-purified 125I- aGAL AB and desialylated orosomucoid-coated plates in 20 controls (C) and in 31 NSAIDs- or low doses steroid-treated RA whose HD-RBC SU was simultaneously explored as previously described (Malaise et al, J Rheum, 1985). Anti-GAL AB levels were also tested in 4 AIDS. In C, aGAL AB ranged from 1:20 to 1:80 and iterative tests showed no significant variations; all AIDS had titers of 1:1 and titers of RA ranged from 1:20 to 1:320 (19.4 % out of C titers). A prior incubation of sera with melibiose inhibited the aGAL AB activity while that with aIgG-, aIgA- or aIgM-coated immunobeads confirmed the main IgG nature of the aGAL activity. In C, mean SU (+/- 1 SD) was 31.6 +/- 3.5 % and iterative tests showed a variation coefficient of 6.7 %. In RA, mean SU was 28.2 +/- 7.6 % and 32 % of RA showed defective values, i.e. < 24.6 %. A direct positive linear correlation was noted between aGAL AB and SU (R = .67; P < .01) in RA that did not belong to the normal range for both parameters (14/31 = 45 %). In vitro experiments using labeled protein A showed a higher binding of affinity purified aGAL AB onto human autologous HD-RBC than onto the corresponding untreated RBC. Lastly, the Fc-mediated rosetting capacities of C human monocytes were inhibited by the aGAL AB. In conclusions: 1) Abnormal aGAL AB titers in AIDS and RA reflect an overall alteration of humoral immune response; 2) HD-RBC can bind to aGAL AB and be cleared at least by splenic Fc-receptors in RA.

B41

HLA-DR2 AND DR3 ASSOCIATE WITH TWO DISTINCT ANTI-Ro(SS-A)/La(SS-B) SUBGROUPS MARKING AGE AT DIAGNOSIS IN SYSTEMIC LUPUS ERYTHEMATOSUS(SLE). M.C.Hochberg, R.E.Boyd, P.H.Howard, R.H.McLean, W.B.Bias, T.T.Provost, F.C. Arnett and M.B.Stevens. Johns Hopkins University, Baltimore, Md.

In a search for more homogeneous serologic-genetic subsets of SLE, we examined relationships between the anti-Ro/La antibody responses and HLA antigens, as well as age at diagnosis, in 147 patients with SLE.

Among 111 whites, three groups were defined based on anti-Ro/La antibody status; their HLA-DR frequencies are listed below.

	Group	No	DR2(%)	DR3(%)
I	Anti-Ro alone	24	75.0	41.7
II	Anti-Ro & La	13	30.8	76.9
III	Neither	74	36.5	23.0

Group I had a significantly higher frequency of DR2 than both GroupII(P=.01) and III(P=.001), while Group II had a significantly higher frequency of DR3 than both Group I(P=.04) and III(P=.0003). There were no differences in the frequency of DR2 between Groups II and III or DR3 between Groups I and III. DR2+ Group I patients had a younger mean age at diagnosis than DR3+ Group II patients (30.2 vs 45.1 years, P=.006).

In addition, 63 of the whites were studied for HLA-linked C4A and C4B phenotypes. The 27 with a C4A null(Q0) allele had an older mean age at diagnosis (40.6 vs 31.4 years, P=.008) and higher frequency of DR3 (67% vs 17%, P=.00006) than the 36 without the C4AQ0 allele. There were no associations of C4AQ0 with anti-Ro or anti-La antibody status.

Among the 36 blacks, no HLA associations were apparent for SLE overall, and no serologic-genetic age-related subgroups were identified.

These data suggest that age at diagnosis of SLE in whites may reflect different immunogenetic risk factors which mediate distinctive auto-antibody responses.

B42

EVIDENCE FOR RIGHT CEREBRAL LATERALITY IN PATIENTS WITH SYSTEMIC LUPUS ERYTHEMATOSUS AND THEIR MALE RELATIVES. Robert G. Lahita, New York, N. Y. and Norman Geschwind Boston, Mass.

The reasons for the female predominance of SLE may have its origin in early life. Disordered estradiol and testosterone metabolism in human SLE has been reported and murine work has indicated that sex steroids are important to the disease. New evidence, based on tests for handedness, suggest that a greater incidence of right cerebral laterality and learning disability exists in patients with SLE and their family members in comparison to controls. An increase in left handedness and ambidexterity was found in a group of 93 SLE patients (Laterality quotient 61.6 vs 73.0 for 507 normal controls). Moreover 12% of SLE patients had some form of learning disability rangeing from dyslexia to stuttering. Such findings were exaggerated in two male Klinefelter patients with SLE. Sons and brothers of patients with SLE had a higher incidence of learning disability. 5.1% of SLE patients tested reported one or more first degree male relatives with dyslexia (nl=0.8%:n=507) whereas 5.8% of patients reported one or more members who stuttered. In families where multiple cases of SLE were reported up to 22% of relatives were learning disabled. Such findings suggest a hormone effect on the developing brains of both SLE patients and their first degree male relatives. A specific antibody effect cannot be ruled out during brain development.

B43

LIPOPROTEIN HANDLING BY ABNORMAL MACROPHAGES OF AUTOIMMUNE MRL/LPR+ LUPUS-LIKE MICE. Prem C. Chatpar, Robert P. Kimberly, Domenick J. Falcone and Charles L. Christian. Hospital for Special Surgery, New York, NY 10021.

Since macrophages play a central role in the development of atherosclerosis and SLE is associated with an increased incidence of coronary artery disease, we examined macrophage handling of lipoproteins in lupus-like mice. Low density lipoprotein (LDL) handling by peritoneal macrophages (PM) was studied by the incorporation of 14-C-oleate into cholestryl-esters (CE). Adherent resting PM were incubated overnight in media. PM were pulse labeled with 14-C-oleate in the presence of acetyl -LDL (ALDL) for 6 hrs at 37°C in DMEM with 20% FCS. Oleate incorporation via the acylCoA:cholesterol acyltransferase enzyme (ACAT) was measured as cholesteryl 14-C-oleate after organic extraction of the cell layer and radiometric thin layer chromatography. Results indicate that ALDL is metabolized and re-esterified at a rate 4-10 times faster than LDL. Mean values for ALDL stimulated 14-C-oleate incorporation (nmoles/mg of cell protein) is shown below:

Added ALDL	NIH Swiss	MRL/lpr+
0 ug	0.7	1.5
25 ug	2.6	7.8
50 ug	2.6	18.7

The basis of increased accumulation of cholesteryl esters by macrophages from autoimmune mice may represent defective receptor handling, altered metabolic rates or the abnormal elimination of the cholesteryl esters from the macrophage. The resultant increased macrophage associated cholesterol leads to a foam cell which may play a role in accelerated atherogenesis in murine SLE.

B44

DIRECT MEASUREMENT OF PLASMA IC3b-NEOANTIGEN LEVEL IN LUPUS NEPHRITIS BY RADIOIMMUNOASSAY. N. Negoro*, T. Inoue*, M. Okamura*, K. Amatsu*, J.G. Curd and Y. Kanayama*. Scripps Clinic and Research Foundation, La Jolla, CA. * Osaka City University Medical School, Osaka, Japan.

Using monoclonal antibody specific for C3dg and iC3b(i-C3b-neoantigen), we have developed a solid phase radioimmunoassay for measurement of plasma iC3b-neoantigen(iC3b-NEO) without pretreatment of plasma with polyethyleneglycol. Plasma iC3b-NEO level in normal subjects (n=38) was 10.0±5.2 ug/ml (iC3b equivalent). Plasma iC3b-NEO level in 26 lupus patients was highly elevated to 201±52 ug/ml, and the values in almost all (25/26) patients were abnormally high. In 26 patients with untreated lupus nephritis, plasma iC3b-NEO level correlated well with renal histologic activity index (rS=0.60,p<0.01). Plasma iC3b-NEO level in patients with diffuse proliferative lupus nephritis (WHO classification, type IV) was significantly higher than in other types of lupus nephritis (p<0.01). Although the plasma iC3b-NEO level decreased promptly after corticosteroid treatment it remained in abnormal level in some patients whose C3 level had normalized.

iC3b-NEO assay, C1q-binding assay and anti-C3 assay for immune complexes were done simultaneously after sucrose density gradient ultracentrifugation and applied to some lupus plasma. A 3-5S peak and a much greater 7-11S peak were found by iC3b-NEO assay. Almost identical 7-11S peak was found by both C1q-binding and anti-C3 assay.

B45

ABNORMAL FINDINGS IN MAGNETIC RESONANCE IMAGING IN PATIENTS WITH ACTIVE CENTRAL NERVOUS SYSTEM LUPUS ERYTHEMATOSUS. Douglas C. Conaway, Gary DeFilipp, Steven N. Berney, and Charles D. Tourtellotte. Temple University, Philadelphia, PA 19140.

Magnetic resonance imaging (MRI) is a new diagnostic technique in which anatomic images are generated by recording the response of atomic nuclei in a magnetic field. We have compared the usefulness of MRI and computed tomography (CT) in studying the central nervous system (CNS) in 17 patients with lupus erythematosus (LE). All patients had active LE at the time of the study and met 1982 ARA revised criteria for diagnosis. Patients were subgrouped according to activity of CNS disease. CT showed an abnormality in only one patient (basal ganglia calcifications in a patient with inactive CNS disease). In contrast, MRI showed definite abnormalities in all three patients with focal neurologic presentation of active CNS LE; these abnormalities were in areas of the brain where a lesion might cause the focal neurologic signs. MRI showed no abnormalities in patients without past CNS disease (6), in patients with inactive CNS disease (3), in patients with recurring seizure disorders (3), and in patients with diffuse neuropsychiatric presentations of active CNS LE (2). We believe MRI is more useful than CT in evaluating a subgroup of patients with active CNS disease and focal neurologic presentations.

B46

ANTINEURONAL ANTIBODIES AND NEUROCOGNITIVE FUNCTION IN SYSTEMIC LUPUS ERYTHEMATOSUS (SLE). Judah A. Denburg, Susan D. Denburg, Ramona M. Carbotte, Angela How, Peter Dent and S.-K. Liao. McMaster University, Hamilton, Ont. L8N 3Z5, CANADA.

The pathogenesis of neuropsychiatric lupus (NP-SLE) is unclear, but may involve vasculitis or antibodies against nervous system tissue, or both. A major difficulty in determining the significance of antineuronal antibodies in NP-SLE has been lack of consistent clinical diagnostic approaches. We have therefore prospectively evaluated the relationship between IgG antineuronal antibodies as measured by a mixed hemadsorption binding assay to neuroblastoma cell lines, and a standardized, clinical classification of NP-SLE or a sensitive, reproducible neuropsychological assessment of brain function in SLE patients. Frequency of serum IgG binding to neuroblastoma lines was significantly higher in 53 patients with active or inactive NP-SLE (30%) than in 36 without NP-SLE (11%) or in 77 controls (12%), in accordance with our earlier findings (Arthr. Rheum., in press), but this constituted neither a specific nor a sensitive test for NP-SLE. Antibody-positivity was found in 8/25 (32%) NP-SLE patients with diffuse disease, and in 1/16 (6%) with focal NP-SLE ($p<0.05$). When serum IgG neuroblastoma binding was related to neurocognitive status in all SLE patients, it was found that 14/16 (88%) antibody-positive subjects were impaired, compared to 32/55 (58%) antibody-negative subjects ($p<0.02$). Fourteen of 46 (30%) neurocognitively impaired SLE patients were antibody-positive, compared to only 2/25 (8%) unimpaired subjects ($p<0.02$). These observations indicate that antineuronal antibodies are specifically related to brain dysfunction, and stress the biological importance of clinical or subclinical neurocognitive impairment in SLE.

B47

ASSOCIATION OF MIGRAINE HEADACHE (MH) AND RAYNAUD'S PHENOMENON (RP) IN SYSTEMIC LUPUS ERYTHEMATOSUS (SLE). Wesly T. Mizutani, Maria Hutchinson and Francisco P. Quismorio, Jr., USC School of Medicine, Los Angeles, CA.

RP is more prevalent in subjects with MH than in non-migranous controls. Both RP and MH are frequently seen in pts. with variant angina pectoris. These observations have raised the possibility that these disorders represent expressions of a generalized vasospastic disorder. We studied the occurrence of MH and RP in SLE and correlated them with clinical and serological features.

79 SLE pts. (76 females), ages ranging 19-73 (mean - 38 yrs.) and 46 healthy controls (43 females), ages ranging 21-60 (mean = 36 yrs.) were studied. Each subject answered standardized questionnaires pertaining to MH and RP (New Engl J Med 30:763, 1981). Affirmative answers were assigned points and the diagnoses of RP and MH were based on the total score.

MH and RP were more prevalent in SLE than in controls (62% vs. 24%; 49% vs. 8.7% respectively). More importantly, RP was more common in SLE pts. with MH (60%) than those without MH (25%). SLE pts. with both MH and RP tended to have more frequently digital gangrene due to vasculitis, hemolytic anema and anti-RNP ab. The attacks of MH were not temporally related to RP episodes in SLE pts. with both symptoms. Kidney, central nervous system, cardiac, pulmonary, skin involvement, cryoglobulins, anti-DNA, anti-SSa, anti-ribonucleoprotein and anti-Sm abs. were not associated with the presence of MH or RP, either singly or both.

Our study indicates that MH and RP in SLE may be related to a common vasospastic phenomenon, occurring in different vascular beds, influenced and precipitated by different factors.

B48

CREATININE CLEARANCE OVERESTIMATES GLOMERULAR FILTRATION RATE IN LUPUS NEPHROPATHY. Michelle Petri, Gregory Fitz, Quinn Whiting-O'Keefe, Anthony Sebastian, and David Hellmann. UCSF, San Francisco, CA, 94143.

To determine the degree to which creatinine clearance (Ccr) overestimates the true glomerular filtration rate (GFR), as represented by inulin clearance (Cin) and iothalamate clearance (Cio), we determined the Ccr, Cin and Cio in 15 patients with lupus nephropathy (LN). LN was defined as the presence of serum creatinine > 1.5, Ccr < 80cc/min, proteinuria (2+ by dipstick or > 600mg/24hr) or hematuria, excluding other known causes of renal disease. Cin and Cio were determined using intravenous bolus and infusion of inulin and iothalamate, with six 30-minute urine collections. The ratio Ccr/Cin (mean 1.5, range 1.0-2.1) was greater than 1.2 ($p < 0.00005$). The ratio of Ccr/Cin was > 1.3 in 12/.5 patients and > 1.5 in 7/15 patients. A prospectively hypot .esized four variable linear regression model that included serum potassium (K^+), Ccr, proteinuria, and an index of lupus activity accounted for 47% of the variation in Ccr/Cin. K^+ alone accounted for 37% of the variation and was the only significant single variable predictor of an increased ratio of Ccr/Cin ($p < 0.02$). In addition, a stepwise linear regression model selected high serum K^+ as the strongest predictor of an increased ratio of Ccr/Cin among 41 clinical, serologic, and renal parameters. The predictive value of K^+ was not accounted for by the use of diuretics. Cio, which can be more readily adapted to outpatient use, correlates highly with Cin (r = 0.99; mean Cio/Cin = 1.1). Use of creatinine or Ccr as an indicator of GFR may be misleading, since Ccr overestimates GFR in the majority of patients with LN.

B49

ENDOCYTOSIS IS REQUIRED FOR MITOGENESIS INDUCED BY CALCIUM CONTAINING CRYSTALS. A Borkowf, HS Cheung, DJ McCarty. Medical College of Wisconsin, Milwaukee, WI. 53226

Mitogenesis is induced in cultured fibroblasts by calcium containing crystals. Although cell-crystal contact is required for mitogenesis, the role of crystal endocytosis is unclear. Synthetic crystals, uniformly labelled with ^{45}Ca, were added to cultured, synchronized confluent human foreskin fibroblasts. After 24 hrs, cultures were pulsed with ^{3}H thymidine for 1 hr. Cells were washed with 10 mM EDTA to remove surface crystals. Fractions were collected after centrifugation at 500 X g for 15 min on a preformed Percoll (1.07 gm/ml) density gradient. Control cells without crystals were similarly separated. Incorporation of ^{3}H thymidine and/or ^{45}Ca in a representative experiment was as follows: (X ± SEM; n=4)

	^{45}Ca HA (100 μg/ml)		Control
Fractions	^{45}Ca cpm	^{3}H thymidine cpm	^{3}H thymidine cpm
1.(bottom)	6509 ± 838	7772 ± 237	46 ± 8
2.	6001 ± 172	12706 ± 358	328 ± 10
3.	2670 ± 152	8797 ± 1391	508 ± 37
4/5.	543 ± 38	2624 ± 159	509 ± 92
6/7.	397 ± 19	3324 ± 253	822 ± 129
8.	804 ± 14	4382 ± 149	2419 ± 194
9.(top)	1564 ± .03	8243 ± 439	5680 ± 125

When ^{45}Ca HA crystals alone were placed on the gradient, most cpms were found in fraction 1. These data show that crystal endocytosis and thymidine uptake are coincident phenomena in cultured fibroblasts. These findings may relate to synovial cell hyperplasia associated with calcium crystals.

B50

FURTHER CHARACTERIZATION OF GROWTH FACTORS FROM HUMAN URINE (CTAP-U). A.R. Cabral, D.A. Walz, and C.W. Castor. University of MI, Ann Arbor, MI 48109, Wayne State University, Detroit, MI 48201.

As reported earlier, connective tissue activating peptide(s) from human urine (CTAP-U) is a potent stimulator of glycosaminoglycan and DNA formation in human synovial, dermal, cartilage and muscle connective tissue cells and does not compete for epidermal growth factor receptor. Here we describe two CTAP-U species of differing molecular weight and provide data supporting their possible relatedness.

Albumin-free, concentrated human urine subjected to preparative isoelectric focusing and gel filtration chromatography yielded two equally potent bioactive growth factors localized in anionic (pH 4-5) zones. Two single band fractions of 28-29 kd and 16-17 kd (reduced and non-reduced SDS-PAGE) were isolated.

Rabbit antisera raised against each CTAP-U molecular weight species react (double immunodiffusion and Western blot) with both antigens. Anti-CTAP-U antibodies also react strongly with extracts of human kidney and heart; extracts of liver, lung, spleen, muscle, bladder, normal human plasma and joint fluids were negative.

These data suggest that human urine contains at least two anionic growth factors with similar antigenic determinants and biologic activity. Amino acid composition and sequence studies (in progress) may clarify the structural relationship of these materials. The present data suggest that heart and kidney may be sources of these materials; their role in health and disease states remains to be determined.

B51

MITOGENIC ACTIVITY OF HYDROXYAPATITE: REQUIREMENT FOR SOMATOMEDIN C. HS Cheung, JJ Van Wyk, W Russell and DJ McCarty. Medical College of Wisconsin, Milwaukee, WI 53226 and University of North Carolina, Chapel Hill, NC 27514.

Synovial hyperplasia is associated with hydroxyapatite (HA) or calcium pyrophosphate dihydrate crystal deposition. These and other crystals containing calcium stimulated mitosis of cultured human skin fibroblasts or synovial cells. Serum derived from platelet-poor plasma (SP) from a hypopituitary patient was depleted of somatomedin C (SmC) by affinity chromatography. HA crystals were tested for mitogenic effect in the presence of SP, SmC and monoclonal antibodies against SmC (A-SmC). Values expressed as % of control (1% SP) uptake of ^{3}H thymidine (n-4). Normal serum (NS) and platelet-derived growth factor (PDGF) were also tested.

Protein(%)	Addition	CPM(X±SE)	Protein(%)	Addition	CPM(±SEM)
SP(1)	None	100± 3	SP(1)	ASmC(40ng/ml)	75± 5
SP(1)	SmC(40ng/ml)	170± 7	SP(1)	ASmC(40ng/ml) +HA (50μg/ml)	151± 3
SP(1)	HA (50 μg/ml)	241± 5			
SP(1)	SmC(40ng/ml) HA(50 μg/ml)	598±15	SP(1)	ASmC(40ng/ml) +PDGF(15ng/ml)	141± 7
SP(1)	SmC(40ng/ml)+ HA(100 μg/ml)	640±20	SP(1)	ASmC(40ng/ml) +HA(50μg/ml) +SmC(40ng/ml)	388±19
SP(1)	PDGF(15ng/ml)	252±14			
			NS(1)	None	145± 6
SP(1)	PDGF(15ng/ml) +SmC(40ng/ml)	652±22	NS(10)	None	655±24

HA (and probably other calcium-containing crystals) act as a growth factor like PDGF and require somatomedin C for full mitogenic activity.

B52

OPPOSING IMMUNOREGULATORY PROPERTIES OF D-PENICILLAMINE. N.D. Staite, R.P. Messner, D.C. Zoschke, Univ. of Minnesota, Minneapolis, MN 55455.

The proliferative response of human mononuclear cells (PBMC) to mitogens is profoundly suppressed by the addition of D-penicillamine (D-PEN) and copper (Cu). Suppression can be reversed with catalase implicating the involvement of H_2O_2. Our studies have quantitated H_2O_2 production from D Pen reacted with physiological amounts of Cu and have examined whether this is relevant to the action of the drug in vivo.

H_2O_2 production was measured by a colorimetric assay involving the oxidation of phenol red. After 5 mins maximum H_2O_2 production (4.9 ± 0·24 nmoles) was observed at 250 ug/ml D-PEN and 30 μM $CuSO_4$; a concentration of Cu commonly found in RA serum. Kinetic studies show that, using 30 μM Cu, the concentration of D-PEN giving maximal H_2O_2 production increases with time and H_2O_2 levels plateau after 10 mins of incubation. To simulate physiological conditions D-PEN was reacted with 30 μM Cu and ceruloplasmin (Cp). During incubations of up to 15 mins H_2O_2 production was lower with Cp-Cu compared with Cu alone suggesting that only free Cu ions can oxidise D-PEN.

H_2O_2 production by D-PEN decreases at higher concentrations of the drug suggesting that D-PEN also scavenges H_2O_2. When added to H_2O_2 in the absence of Cu, D-PEN rapidly diminishes H_2O_2 levels in a concentration dependent manner. Scavenging by D-PEN was also seen in the presence of 5g/dL human serum albumin. Importantly, using physiological concentrations of H_2O_2, D-PEN completely reverses H_2O_2-mediated suppression of Con-A stimulated PBMC proliferation.

Our results show that D-PEN may have two opposing effects. A suppressive action mediated by H_2O_2 production in the presence of available copper and a direct H_2O_2 scavenging action that could protect lymphocytes at inflammatory sites from oxidative damage.

B53

MIGRATION OF POLYMORPHONUCLEAR LEUKOCYTES ACROSS CULTURED MONOLAYERS OF ENDOTHELIAL CELLS. Martha B. Furie, Ada J. Huang, Beth L. Naprstek, and Samuel C. Silverstein. College of Physicians and Surgeons of Columbia University, New York, NY 10032.

A critical early event in inflammation is passage of circulating polymorphonuclear leukocytes (PMNs) across vessel walls. Monolayers of bovine microvascular endothelial cells (ECs) cultured on connective tissue derived from human amnion were used for the in vitro study of the mechanisms that control PMN extravasation. Purified human PMNs placed above EC-amnion cultures migrated across the endothelial monolayers and into the amniotic tissue in response to gradients of the chemoattractant formyl-methionylleucylphenylalanine. The process of PMN migration across the EC-amnion cultures, as revealed by transmission electron microscopy, closely resembled PMN extravasation observed in vivo by other investigators. Endothelial cells from human umbilical vein also were cultured to confluence on amnion; the rate and extent of PMN migration across the human ECs were similar to those observed using the bovine ECs. PMN migration across bovine EC monolayers was unaffected by the following treatments: a) removal of plasminogen from the serum used in the assay; b) acid treatment of the serum to inactivate protease inhibitors; c) addition of purified human plasminogen to physiologic levels; and d) addition of antibodies to urokinase, which is the major type of plasminogen activator secreted by stimulated PMNs. Therefore, it appears that plasminogen activator is not used by PMNs to aid in their transendothelial migration. Migration was also unaffected by a variety of protease inhibitors, including leupeptin, antipain, α_1-antitrypsin, soybean trypsin inhibitor, and p-nitrophenyl p'-guanidinobenzoate.

B54

DRUG PROTECTION OF SERUM AND TISSUE ANTIPROTEINASE FROM OXIDATIVE INACTIVATION AND PREVENTION OF CARTILAGE PROTEOGLYCAN DEGRADATION. John L. Skosey, Donald C. Chow, Charalampos Arsenis, and Klaus Kuettner. University of Illinois College of Medicine and Rush Medical College, Chicago, IL 60612.

Results of previous studies demonstrated that D-penicillamine (PSH), gold compounds and other drugs used in the treatment of rheumatoid arthritis (RA) retarded inactivation of serum antiproteinases by oxygen radicals ($[O_x]$). We have suggested that preservation of antiproteinases by these drugs could result in decreased tissue destruction by enzymes secreted by inflammatory mediator cells. Studies on the interaction of these factors in cartilage proteoglycan (PG) degradation have now been initiated. Rabbits were injected with $Na_2{}^{35}SO_4$ and radiolabeled articular cartilage removed and boiled, minced and stored frozen until used. Supernatant fluids from human peripheral blood neutrophils (N) stimulated with opsonized zymosan contained enzymes which promoted cartilage PG degradation. This was inhibited by fresh serum. The ability of serum exposed to $[O_x]$ generated by stimulated N was diminished. PSH, 10^{-5}-10^{-3} M, protected serum antiproteinase from inactivation by $[O_x]$ and preserved its ability to inhibit cartilage PG degradation. Anti-invasion factor (AIF) from bovine cartilage has antiproteinase (anti-elastase) activity, which was diminished after it was pre-incubated with an $[O_x]$-generating system (acetaldehyde-xanthine oxidase). The antiproteinase activity of AIF was protected from oxidative inactivation by PSH, 10^{-4}-10^{-3} M. The ability of AIF to protect cartilage from enzymatic attack in inflammation may be impaired by the action of $[O_x]$. Drugs with antioxidant activity may protect AIF and other antiproteinases from oxidative damage and, subsequently, cartilage from enzyme mediated inflammatory tissue damage.

B55

DECREASED CHEMOTACTIC FUNCTION AND C5a RECEPTOR EXPRESSION OF SYNOVIAL FLUID MONONUCLEAR CELLS (MNC) IN INFLAMMATORY ARTHRITIS.

Ildy M. Katona, Kiyoshi Ohura, Dennis E. Chenoweth, Ronald L. Wilder, and Sharon M. Wahl. USUHS, NMRI, and NIH, Bethesda, MD 20814, VA Medical Center, San Diego, CA 92161.

Inflammatory arthritis is characterized by the accumulation of leukocytes in the synovial fluid and tissues. Increased concentrations of complement components and the chemotactic response of certain MNC might provide a mechanism for the cell accumulation at these sites. In the present study, normal peripheral blood (PB) MNC and synovial fluid MNC from patients with inflammatory arthritis were isolated by Ficoll-Paque gradients. These cells were then incubated with saturating concentrations of fluorochrome labelled phenotype specific markers and the chemotactic ligands, C5a and f-met-leu-phe (fMLP) followed by single or dual parameter cell sorter analysis.

The percentage of synovial fluid T and B lymphocytes was variable, but monocytes were the predominant synovial cell type. Whereas receptors for C5a and fMLP were coexpressed on the majority of $OKMI^+$ PBMNC, the majority of synovial monocytes were $fMLP^+$, but lacked C5a receptors. The synovial cell chemotactic response for C5a was greatly decreased compared to PBMNC, consistent with their C5a receptor expression. However, synovial cell chemotaxis toward fMLP and fMLP receptor expression were comparable to PBMNC. These results indicate that 1) the chemoattractant receptor phenotype of synovial fluid monocytes is different than that of the PB monocytes or that 2) C5a-induced chemotaxis of monocytes toward the inflammatory site occurred in vivo and the C5a receptor-ligand interaction resulted in decreased free C5a receptor expression.

B56

LOW MOLECULAR WEIGHT RHEUMATOID FACTOR - A SEROLOGICAL MARKER IN SYSTEMIC LUPUS ERYTHEMATOSUS.

Roberta J. Jacobs and Morris Reichlin. Okla. Med. Res. Fdn., Oklahoma City, OK 73104.

The antibody excess anti-C3 assay (J. Immunol. 130:2775, 1983) is a quantitative assay for measuring C3-bearing immune complexes (IC). In this assay, all C3 and C3-bearing material is precipitated from plasma with rabbit antisera to C3. Precipitated IC are then quantitated by uptake of $F(ab')_2$ ^{125}I-anti-human IgG. This assay effectively discriminates between clinically active systemic lupus erythematosus (SLE) (70% positive, 16/23) and clinically inactive SLE (22% positive, 4/18). In contrast, with the same samples, the Clq binding assay showed 19% and 6% positivity, respectively, and neither population was significantly different from the normal.

In the anti-C3 assay, the formation of C3-anti-C3 precipitates provides a reactant for any rheumatoid factor (RF) present in the patient sample and this RF is subsequently detected by the uptake of ^{125}I-anti-IgG. This can be eliminated by using $F(ab')_2$ anti-C3 to form C3-anti-C3 precipitates. Thus, the difference in reactivity observed with non-digested and $F(ab')_2$ anti-C3 was used to assess the RF content in the most reactive of these samples. In ten of eleven samples, >66% of the reactivity was due to RF. Using this same technique after density gradient centrifugation of these samples, the RF was found to be almost exclusively low molecular weight (7S-18S), strongly suggesting that it was IgG RF. These results indicate that low molecular weight RF is a better serological marker of clinical activity in SLE than the measurement of IC and emphasize the need to reexamine the role of RF in the pathogenesis of this autoimmune disease.

C1

SOMATOSENSORY EVOKED POTENTIALS IN THE EVALUATION OF THE UNSTABLE RHEUMATOID SPINE. Paul F. Lachiewicz, Richard Shoenfeldt and Allen E. Inglis. UNC School of Medicine, Chapel Hill, NC 27514.

Median nerve somatosensory evoked potentials (SEP) were prospectively performed in 24 consecutive patients with rheumatoid arthritis who had symptomatic cervical spine instability. Eighteen patients had C1-C2 instability: in ten, the subluxation was completely reducible, and in eight, the subluxation was irreducible, with or without superior migration of the odontoid process. Four patients had superior migration alone, and two had subaxial subluxation alone. Abnormal SEP's were found in seven of the twenty-four patients overall. However, 58% of those patients with irreducible atlanto-axial subluxation and/or superior migration of the dens demonstrated abnormal SEP conduction latencies. Rheumatoid patients with these radiographic abnormalities may be at a higher risk for the development of myelopathy. Seven patients underwent successful surgical stabilization for the relief of pain. SEP examinations should be performed in rheumatoid patients with symptomatic cervical spine instability.

C2

PATHOPHYSIOLOGY OF CARPAL TUNNEL SYNDROME: ELECTRO-THERMOGRAPHIC ASSESSMENT. B.M. Rothschild, J. Fisherowitz, J. Reiss, E. Prostic, B. Abrams and R.A. Carlson, Menorah Medical Center and University of Kansas School of Medicine and University of Missouri, Kansas City, Missouri, 64110.

A double-blind controlled trial was conducted of thermographic perturbations as a function of symptoms, clinical signs and electrophysiologic evidence of carpal tunnel syndrome. Two basic thermographic patterns were noted: Baseline thenar hypothermia and stress (Phalen test)-induced hypothermia. Thermographic evidence of thenar hypothermia correlated with electrophysiologic evidence of carpal tunnel syndrome ($p = 0.042$). The presence of nocturnal symptoms correlated equally with electrophysiologic abnormalities ($p = 0.032$) and thermography findings ($p = 0.033$). Electrophysiologic abnormalities were not correlated with presence or absence of a Tinel or Phalen sign. The presence of Tinel sign correlated with thenar hypothermia ($p=0.010$) while the presence of either Tinel or Phalen sign correlated with a positive stress thermogram ($p=0.009$ and 0.038), respectively. The presence of both Tinel and Phalen signs correlated even more strongly with thermographic findings ($p = 0.0004$). Although compression-induced alteration in sympathetic activity could be considered as partial explanation of thermographic perturbations in carpal tunnel syndrome, an equally plausible consideration is decreased metabolic activity of those muscles with median nerve innervation, which compose the thenar eminence. Compression, sufficient to affect those nerve fibers responsible for baseline muscle tone, may explain the correlation of thermographic changes with the Tinel and Phalen tests. The specificity of stress thermography for a positive Tinel or Phalen sign was, respectively, 100% and 96%. This study demonstrates the efficacy of thermography for assessment of carpal tunnel syndrome.

C3

COMPUTED TOMOGRAPHY WITH MULTIPLANAR REFORMATION AND THREE-DIMENSIONAL IMAGE ANALYSIS IN THE PREOPERATIVE EVALUATION OF ISCHEMIC NECROSIS OF THE FEMORAL HEAD. David J. Sartoris, MD, Donald Resnick, MD, David Gershuni, MD, Marvin Meyers, MD.

In order to extend the potential utility of CT, we have applied multiplanar reformation and three-dimensional image reconstruction to the analysis of the ischemic femoral head.

Patients with varying degrees of infarction and/or collapse of the femoral head were studied. CT image data were acquired on a Technicare 2060 Scanner using 2mm contiguous sectioning. Multiplanar reformation and three-dimensional processing were performed on a Contour Medical Systems Cemax 1000. Based upon CT data and three-dimensional contouring, plastic models of the femoral heads were constructed preoperatively and compared with resected specimens in patients undergoing subsequent total hip replacement.

As judged by both radiologists and orthopedic surgeons, multiplanar reformation and three-dimensional analysis were felt to contribute valuable preoperative information regarding extent of infarction and degree of subchondral bone collapse in each instance. Plastic models were found to represent actual head configurations with reasonable accuracy. The ability to completely remove the obscuring influence of adjacent soft tissue and acetabular bone, and the capability of displaying three-dimensional sections through the femoral head were additional advantages of the technique.

Based upon our limited experience, we feel that CT combined with multiplanar reformation and three-dimensional analysis is the optimal preoperative means for evaluating ischemic necrosis of the femoral head.

C4

HIP RESURFACING - PROGNOSTIC DETERMINANTS FOR DURABILITY: A TEN YEAR EXPERIENCE WITH 584 CASES. Harlan C. Amstutz, Fred Dorey. UCLA, Los Angeles, CA 90024.

Despite an initial world-wide enthusiasm for surface replacement of the hip, most designs have been abandoned. From 1975 to 1984, 584 acrylic fixed THARIES resurfacing implants have a 1 to 10 year follow-up. Results have been studied by survivorship analysis and have compared favorably to conventional hip replacements in patients under 40, those with osteoarthritis and congenital dysplasia of the hip. The overall observed failure rate is 12%. The most common mode of failure has been acetabular loosening which can lead to absorption of the femoral neck and loosening. The most adverse prognostic factors are youth and a high activity level. An experienced surgeon and rheumatoid arthritis are favorable prognostic factors. When age was eliminated, bone stock deficiency of osteonecrosis and dysplasia was not significant. Despite our failures, the clinical results have been sufficiently promising to try to achieve the goals of preservation of femoral stock. Its primary other advantages include a stable hip, a low sepsis (1 in 600), less blood loss. The resurfacing concept seems ideal for biologic ingrowth into a porous substrate. Preliminary clinical trials in 50 patients have shown a promise of improved durability with 2 years followup.

C5

TIDAL KNEE LAVAGE IN PATIENTS WITH CHRONIC PAIN DUE TO OSTEOARTHRITIS OF THE KNEE. WJ Arnold, SE Mather, N. Mostello and J. Tongue, Park Ridge Il and Portland, ORE.

Seventeen patients (pts) [aver. age 68 yrs (range 48-87 yrs), 15F/2M] with chronic pain associated with clinical and radiographic (x-ray Stage I 3 pts; Stage II 3 pts; Stage III 4 pts; Stage IV 10 pts) evidence for osteoarthritis (OA) of the knee underwent 20 tidal knee lavages (TKL) instead of arthroscopic surgery or more extensive surgical procedures. The average duration of knee pain prior to lavage was 7.5 yrs (range 5-30 yrs). All had failed to respond to more than one NSAID and physical therapy and 17/20 had received an intra-articular glucocorticoid injection. TKL was carried out with a total of 1000 ml of normal saline instilled and withdrawn via a spring-loaded 30 ml syringe through an 11 gauge Veres needle. All procedures were performed as an outpatient using 0.25% Bupivicaine intra-articular anesthesia. At an average of 5.3 mos (range 1-9 mos) following the procedure, a subjective clinical outcome score (SCOS) was determined for the treated knee. Ten/20 procedures resulted in a good/excellent (G/E) SCOS and 10/20 in a Fair/Poor (F/P) SCOS. A G/E SCOS was found in 2/3 pts with x-ray Stage I, 3/3 with Stage II, 3/4 with Stage III but only 2/10 with Stage IV. None of the 10 pts with a G/E SCOS have required further surgical therapy. However 5/10 pts with a F/P SCOS have subsequently undergone more extensive surgical procedures. Our observations suggest that TKL may produce relief of chronic pain in pts with OA of the knee resistant to standard nonsurgical therapy. Particularly in pts who are candidates for arthroscopic surgery, TKL alone can produce relief from chronic pain thereby avoiding or delaying the arthroscopic procedure.

C6

THE FOOT IN JUVENILE RHEUMATOID ARTHRITIS (JRA). John J. Calabro, Aldo Vincent Londino, Jr, Caroline Eyvazzadeh, Saint Vincent Hospital, Worcester, MA 01604

Unlike the hand, there has been relatively little attention focused on the foot in JRA. Yet, these joints are affected in almost all of JRA patients and are occasionally the major source of disability. Clinically, foot problems include pain, stiffness, loss of function, and deformity. Consequently, because of the frequent need for orthotic or other supportive measures as well as surgical intervention, the orthopedic surgeon should be familiar with the spectrum of foot problems induced by JRA.

Of 100 patients with JRA, 62 girls and 38 boys, consecutive referrals to a pediatric rheumatology clinic, now observed prospectively for 25 years, the foot was involved in 46%. Foot synovitis occurred in 6 of 20 with systemic JRA, in 26 of 48 with polyarticular disease, and in 14 of 32 with pauciarticular JRA.

In polyarticular JRA, the hallmark of foot involvement was generalized and symmetrical metatarsophalangeal (MTP) joint involvement, unlike pauciarticular disease where heel pain or swelling of a single proximal, distal, or MTP joint predominated. In systemic JRA, both generalized and lcoalized synovitis were observed.

Continuing MTP inflammation promoted contractures of supporting tendons and ligaments, resulting in progressive hallux valgus, hammer or cockup toes, subluxation of MTP joint,spreadfoot, and fibular deviation. Progressive heel involvement resulted in cavus deformity from apophyseal overgrowth. As a consequence of vasculitis, painful leg ulcerations and permanent foot drop occurred in one patient.

C7

The Histology Of The Bone-Cement Interface In Failed Total Hip Arthroplasty. N.A. Johanson, P.G. Bullough, Philip D. Wilson, Jr., Eduardo A. Salvati, Chitranjan S. Ranawat. The Hospital For Special Surgery, New York, N.Y.

The purpose of this study was to examine the histological features of the bone cement interface in clinically loosened, noninfected total hip arthroplasties, with attention toward possible pathophysiological mechanisms of loosening.

Twenty-five patients who had undergone revision total hip replacements for aseptic loosening from July through December 1983 were studied. Thirty membranes taken from the bone-cement interface of the acetabular and/or femoral components were studied, using routine histological sections. The membranes were oriented by the operating surgeon as to the side of the membrane facing the cement mantle of the prosthesis and the side facing bone.

On Microscopic examination, histiocytosis, fibrosis and necrosis were present on every specimen. Histiocytic proliferation was seen primarily on the cement side of the membrane, but this reaction was seen to a lesser degree in the mid-substance and bone side as well. Other prominent features included evidence of acrylic cement particles of varying size distributed throughout the membrane, particles of high-density polyethylene and fragments of necrotic trabecular bone.

This study demonstrated histologically two different modes of failure. Cement failure was suggested by the high frequency of particulate acrylic cement seen grossly and microscopically in the membranes. Bone Failure was suggested by bone detritus throughout the membranes of 88% of the patients. These findings, in combination with the prominence of histiocytosis in these specimens, suggest that clinical failure may be dependent on cement particle size, immunogenicity and bone debris.

C8

DEFORMING ARTHRITIS IN SYSTEMIC LUPUS ERYTHEMATOSUS (SLE). POSSIBLE ROLE OF RHEUMATOID FACTOR AND DISTINGUISHING FEATURES FROM THOSE OF RHEUMATOID ARTHRITIS (RA). Carlos Abud-Mendoza, Donato Alarcón-Segovia, Jorge Alcocer-Varela, Victor De los Reyes, Jorge Hernández-Ortíz, Antonio Iglesias-Gamarra and Efraín Díaz-Jouanen. Instituto Nacional de la Nutrición. México 14000, D.F. MEXICO.

The arthropathy of SLE may cause deformity. Of 858 patients with SLE (ARA criteria) 41 had deforming arthritis (DA). Their clinical characteristics were compared with those of 60 randomly picked SLE patients without deforming arthritis who turned out to be of similar age and disease duration. SLE patients with DA were found to have higher frequency of symptomatic Sjögren's syndrome ($p<.05$), rheumatoid factor ($p<.001$) and lymphopenia ($p<.05$). Conversely, they had lower frequency of malar rash ($p<.005$), photosensitivity ($p<.01$), and renal involvement than SLE patients without DA. Other clinical and serologic findings were similar.

Three observers compared hand X-rays from the 41 SLE patients with DA to those of 40 patients with classic or definite RA and found them to have more frequent ulnar deviation($p<.05$), swan neck deformity ($p<.005$) and MCP (2,3,4 & 5) subluxation ($p<.005$) but less frequent carpal ($p<.001$) and styloid ($p<.005$) erosions, and decreased carpometacarpal space ($p<.005$).

Our findings may indicate a role of rheumatoid factor in the pathogenesis of DA in SLE and show that this DA of SLE is distinguishable from that of RA.

C9

ENZYME-LINKED-IMMUNOSORBENT-ASSAY FOR ANTI-SM ANTIBODY USING "FREE SM" AS AN ANTIGEN. Yoshinari Takasaki, Akira Kodama, Keiji Mastumoto, Hiroshi Hashimoto, Shunichi Hirose. Juntendo University, Tokyo, 113 Japan.

Buchanan, et al., reported that there were two molecular species of the Sm antigen and one was reactive with both anti-U1-RNP and Sm antibodies, the other reacted only with anti-Sm antibody. The later was called "free Sm"(Clin.exp.Immunol.,51,8,1983). In this report, free Sm was purified, and using this antigen, enzyme-linked-immunosorbent-assay(ELISA) for anti-Sm antibody in various rheumatic diseases was studied.

Sm antigen from calf thymus extract was purified using ammonium sulfate precipitation and Sephadex G200 gel filtration. anti-Sm reacted with elution fractions, both molecular weight of about 200K and 88K, but anti-U1-RNP reacted only with 200K elution fraction on G200 column. 88K eluate (free Sm) was further purified by anti-Sm affinity chromatogaphy. The purified free Sm gave two major bands with molecular weight of 70K and 12-13K on SDS-polyacrylamide gel electrophoresis. Using free Sm as an antigen source(2.5μg/ml), ELISA was performed and this preparation was devoid of nuclear antigens U1-RNP, SS-A, SS-B, Scl-70, Jo-1 and PCNA. But all sera with precipitating antibodies to Sm by immunodiffusion gave reactions(normal range OD 405 0.153 ± 0.132 estimated by 30 normal controls). Of 115 patients with systemic lupus erythematosus(SLE), 30 with mixed connective tissue disease(MCTD), 42 with scleroderma(SD), 59 with rheumatoid arthritis, 23 with polymyositis, 6 with Sjogren's syndrome, 19.4% of SLE, 6.9% of MCTD and 2.6% of SD had anti-Sm antibodies. But only 13.9% of SLE showed anti-Sm precipitin in immunodiffusion. Of 30 SLE with IgG anti-Sm antibodies, 8 sera had IgM anti-Sm and 4 sera had IgA anti-Sm. These results suggest that ELISA using free Sm is sensitive and specific for anti-Sm antibody and may help to know the relationship of immunoglobulin class to clinical features in patients with SLE.

C10

ASSOCIATION OF ANTISPERM ANTIBODIES WITH LUPUS ERYTHEMATOSUS. Morris Reichlin and Gilbert G. Haas, Jr. Oklahoma Medical Research Foundation and Departments of Medicine and Ob/Gyn., Oklahoma University Health Sciences Center, Oklahoma City, OK 73104

Unselected patients with systemic lupus erythematosus (SLE) were studied for serum IgG antisperm antibodies with a radiolabelled antiglobulin assay. Of 25 patients tested, 10 (40%) were positive for antisperm antibodies; less than 1% of normal fertile controls have antisperm antibody. About 1% of infertile persons have antisperm antibody. In the SLE sera, 12 had anti-DNA while 13 sera did not have anti-DNA. Interestingly, 8 of 12 anti-DNA positive sera contained antibody to sperm while only 2 of 13 anti-DNA negative sera contained antisperm antibody. They were present with equal frequency in males and females (40%). Serial studies of individual patients revealed that when anti-DNA titers fell, antisperm antibody titers also fell. Thus both antibodies were present in clinically active patients and were absent or much diminished in clinically inactive patients. Absorption of anti-DNA positive sera with DNA dramatically lowered anti-DNA titers but did not affect antisperm antibody titers.

Thus, antisperm antibodies were temporally associated with anti-DNA antibody but were independent of and differentiated from this specificity by the absorption experiments. Electron microscopic localization by the ferritin technique revealed the antisperm antibody attachment site to be the sperm plasma membrane over the acrosomal region of the sperm. Antisperm antibodies like anti-DNA seem to be a marker for active disease. Their possible role in infertility remains to be evaluated.

C11

C1s-C1 INHIBITOR COMPLEX (C1s-Inh): IMPROVED SPECIFICITY FOR DISEASE ACTIVITY IN PREGNANT AND NOT PREGNANT SLE PATIENTS. M. Lockshin, P. Harpel, T. Qamar, M. Druzin, The Hospital for Special Surgery and The New York Hospital, New York, N.Y. 10021.

To study persistent hypocomplementemia in pregnant SLE patients and to validate a new measure of complement activation rate, C1s-Inh, we studied serial CH50, C3, C4 (clinical complement) and C1s-Inh in 24 pregnant and 33 not pregnant women with SLE. At first measurement, C1s-Inh varied inversely with CH50 and C4 in both patient groups but it correlated poorly with C3. Judged by an independent clinical activity index, first assay of C1s-Inh correctly identified 74% (19/24) pregnant and 76% (25/33) not pregnant patients, compared to 67% and 85% for clinical complement measures (n.s.). C1s-Inh gave 12% false positive results compared to 48% for clinical complement ($p < 0.05$). C1s-Inh gave 31% false negative results compared to 0% for clinical complement ($p<0.05$). In serial studies all measures of complement improved with corticosteroid therapy in not pregnant patients but in pregnant patients C1s-Inh alone improved while clinical complement remained abnormal until the end of the pregnancy. Three pregnant but 0 not pregnant patients had worsening of C1s-Inh despite therapy and despite stability of (abnormal) clinical complement.

We conclude that C1s-Inh is a more specific though less sensitive assay for clinical lupus activity than are clinical complement measures, that clinical complement frequently remains depressed throughout pregnancy, and that C1s-Inh may be the preferred assay for examining the complement system in pregnant SLE patients. (Supported in part by AM 32929).

C12

AUTOANTIBODIES TO SOLUBLE INTRACELLULAR PROTEINS IN THE CEREBROSPINAL FLUID OF LUPUS PATIENTS. S. J. Golombek, K. B. Elkon, Hospital for Special Surgery, New York, NY.

Increased immunoglobulin levels and antineuronal antibodies are found in the cerebrospinal fluid (CSF) of lupus patients. In this study the CSF from 25 lupus patients and 9 controls was evaluated for the presence of autoantibodies by the dot blot nitrocellulose method. 9/15 with definite central nervous system involvement (CNS^+) and 3/10 patients without CNS involvement (CNS^-) had a positive test. CSF autoantibodies were confirmed to be present by indirect immunofluorescence (11/14 patients positive, 5/11 speckled pattern) and by Western blotting. Western blotting of dog spleen and human B-cell extracts revealed IgG autoantibodies to proteins ranging in molecular weight from 18,000 to 68,000 daltons. CSF autoantibodies reflected serum specificity and included antibodies to SM, RNP, and La. No autoantibodies were present in the controls.

As determined by the CSF/serum albumin levels, CSF autoantibodies occurred in patients without disruption of the blood brain barrier. An elevated IgG index (CSF/serum IgG) (CSF/serum albumin) indicated local CNS production of IgG in some patients. It is concluded that IgG autoantibodies to intracellular proteins are present in the CSF of approximately 60% of CNS^+ lupus patients and have similar specificities to antibodies produced in the serum. The relationship of the antibodies to disease expression remains to be determined.

C13

AN HYPOTHESIS FOR DIFFERENCES IN THE OCCURRENCE OF AUTOANTIBODIES AGAINST EXTRACTABLE ANTIGENS. K.K. Gaither, O.F. Fox, M. Reichlin and J.B. Harley. Univ. of Oklahoma and the Okla. Med. Res. Fdn., Oklahoma City.

In systemic lupus erythematosus (SLE), autoantibodies to Ro/SSA and La/SSB tend to occur together while anti-Sm is associated with anti-nRNP. The basis for these relationships is not known. Sensitivity of autoantibody detection using purified autoantigen preparations and solid phase immunosorbent assay techniques is greatly enhanced compared to immunodiffusion assays. Consequently, we have been able to detect low levels of anti-Ro/SSA in 7 of 40 normal control sera (17.5%) and anti-La/SSB in 3 of the 40 (7.5%). These binding activities have been inhibited in competition assays by purified Ro/SSA or La/SSB, respectively, and can also be demonstrated by Western blotting. Binding activity is found in the $F(ab')_2$ fragment of IgG and thus cannot be attributed to non-specific Fc binding. Two of 7 anti-Ro/SSA normal donors displayed additional serologic abnormalities. One had low levels of anti-La/SSB. The other normal was HLA B8, DR3 positive and had low titer antinuclear antibody, anti-ssDNA, a false-positive VDRL and, previously, a low titer rheumatoid factor. It is possible that this normal individual is at risk to develop autoimmune disease. None of the 40 normal sera bound the purified nRNP and Sm preparation. The finding that anti-Ro/SSA commonly occurs at low levels in the normal population while anti-nRNP(Sm) does not (p = 0.007, Fisher's Exact Test) would be consistent with different mechanisms of autoantibody generation being responsible for their presence in SLE. Anti-Ro/SSA and anti-La/SSB may occur in SLE by enhancing the production of antibody already present while the production of anti-nRNP or anti-Sm may require a primary autoimmune response.

C14

TEMPORAL SHIFT FROM Sm TO RNP ANTIGEN RECOGNITION BY SERA FROM PATIENTS WITH SYSTEMIC LUPUS ERYTHEMATOSUS (SLE). David E. Fisher, Westley H. Reeves, Rosanne Wisniewolski, and Robert G. Lahita. Rockefeller University, New York, NY 10021.

The relative amounts of Sm and RNP antibodies in serial sera from patients with SLE were examined by pulse-labeling of snRNP proteins, competition experiments and analysis of immunoprecipitated snRNA. Immunoprecipitation and SDS-PAGE of snRNP proteins pulse-labeled with ^{35}S-methionine, revealed distinct patterns of antigen recognition using anti-RNP sera (A and C proteins), and anti-Sm sera (A, B, B', C, D, E, F, and G proteins). Two patients were identified whose sera initially displayed the anti-Sm pattern of recognition which evolved over time to the anti-RNP pattern. A competition assay using biochemically separated snRNP particles confirmed the evolution from a predominantly anti-Sm response to a predominantly anti-RNP response in the sera. Analysis of ^{32}P-labeled snRNAs immunoprecipitated by serial sera also indicated a decrease in the relative intensities of U2, U4, U5, and U6 RNAs with little change in the intensity of U1 by autoradiography. By all three techniques, the relative amount of anti-Sm antibodies decreased markedly over time, while anti-RNP antibodies remained relatively constant. Anti-Sm reactivity never completely disappeared from the sera, however. These studies demonstrate a temporal shift from Sm to RNP antigen recognition in sera of certain SLE patients.

C15

SELECTIVE EFFECTS OF PLASMAPHERESIS ON SERUM ANTINUCLEAR ANTIBODIES IN MAN. Keith K. Colburn, Satian Pooprasert, Judy A. Johnson, Department of Medicine, Pettis Memorial Veterans Administration Medical Center, Loma Linda, CA 92354; and Richard H. Weisbart, Department of Medicine, UCLA-San Fernando Valley, Veterans Administration Medical Center, Sepulveda, CA 91343.

Plasmapheresis has been used therapeutically in some patients with systemic lupus erythematosus (SLE) with reports of improvement in clinical symptoms. The mechanisms for its clinical efficacy are unknown but include the nonspecific removal of immunoglobulins and immune complexes. It is also possible, however, that plasmapheresis specifically affects immune regulation by facilitating the clearance of autoantibodies or preventing their production. We decided, therefore, to determine whether plasmapheresis has a selective effect on auto-immune responses. To do this we studied the effects of plasmapheresis on plasma levels of IgG antinuclear antibodies in six patients with SLE. Antibodies were measured to the nuclear antigens single stranded DNA (ss-DNA) and the nucleoside, guanosine. These autoantibodies were compared with IgG antibody levels to microbial antigens. IgG antibodies were measured by an enzyme linked immunosorbent assay (ELISA). Daily plasmapheresis treatments for 2-4 days resulted in a 24% reduction in total plasma IgG (p<0.05) and a 5% decrease in the mean IgG antibody levels to streptococcal antigens and pneumococcal and influenza viral vaccine antigens. In contrast IgG antibodies to ss-DNA and the nucleoside, guanosine, were reduced 43% (p<0.017) and 50% (p<0.007) respectively. The reduction of antibodies to both ss-DNA and guanosine were significantly greater than the reduction of antibodies to the combined microbial antigens (p<0.0002) and the reduction of total plasma IgG (p<0.04). The clinical symptoms of all the patients subjectively improved with plasmapheresis while drug therapy remained unchanged. These data suggest that plasmapheresis selectively lowered plasma levels of antinuclear antibodies in patients with SLE. In addition to its non-specific effects, plasmapheresis may selectively facilitate the clearance of antinuclear antibodies or inhibit their production. These effects may contribute to the clinical efficacy of plasmapheresis in SLE.

C16

CYCLOSPORIN A: A POTENTIAL DISEASE MODIFYING DRUG IN RHEUMATOID ARTHRITIS (RA). R Madhok, H Capell. Centre for Rheumatic Diseases, Glasgow Royal Infirmary, Glasgow, Scotland.

The immunopharmacological profile of Cyclosporin A (CSA) suggests that it is a potential disease modifying drug (DMD) in RA. Its toxicity and efficacy is being evaluated in a long-term open study of 20 patients with active RA (CSA dose 5mg/kg). Patients are seen at 2 weekly intervals to determine toxicity and 6 weekly assessments of benefit (pain score, functional ability, articular index and morning stiffness) are made by an independent observer.

Preliminary results are presented:

Toxicity: No patient has been withdrawn because of toxicity. A dose dependent but reversible decline in renal function was noted in 16 patients; hirsutium in 2 and tremor in one.

Efficacy: All 4 clinical indices showed improvement at week 6 (n = 18), week 12 (n = 14) and week 18 (n = 11). ESR at 18 weeks was significantly reduced; no change in rheumatoid factor, immunoglobulins or T-helper/T-suppressor was noted. Updated results of 6 to 12 month follow up will be presented.

Our preliminary results indicate that CSA appears to have a DMD effect. To date reversible renal dysfunction has been the major side effect observed.

C17

A LONG-TERM PROSPECTIVE STUDY OF METHOTREXATE (MTX) IN RHEUMATOID ARTHRITIS (RA). Joel M. Kremer, M.D., Albany Medical College, Albany, N.Y.

29 patients (pts.) with active RA who had previously failed on hydroxychloroquine, gold and penicillamine entered a prospective study of the safety and efficacy of MTX. 52 liver biopsies have been performed including 29 baseline, 16 at 2 years (yrs.) (mean total dosage [T.D.] MTX -1.46g), 6 at 3 yrs. (mean T.D.-2.01g), and 1 at 4 yrs. (T.D.-2.5g). There have been 2 dropouts; one for a MTX pneumonitis which resolved and one from a death from an unrelated cause. The mean duration of therapy of the 27 pts. still active is 25.1 months. Pts. ingested a mean dose of 12.4mg of weekly oral MTX.

Number of tender joints decreased from a mean of 14.4 to 7.7(p=<.001). Swollen joints decreased from a mean of 18.3 to 11.1 (p=<.001), and AM stiffness decreased from a mean of 157.4 minutes to 50.4 (p=<.001). Mean prednisone dosage in 18 pts. decreased from 8.22mg to 3.0mg (p=<.01). Sequential radiographs demonstrated lack of progression of disease in 8 of 8 pts. examined, and healing of erosions were noted in 3 of 8 pts. Sequential liver biopsies showed little change from baseline. 2 pts. progressed from mild to moderate fatty infiltration at the 2 yr. biopsy and neither of these pts. showed progression in their 3 yr. biopsy.

26 pts. (90%) reported an adverse effect (A.E.) of MTX at some time during the course of the study although most were mild. 13 pts. (48%) reported a moderate A.E. at some time. 10 pts. had A.E.s become tolerable after a decrease in weekly MTX dosage.

MTX is an effective drug in active RA which has failed other regimens. A.E.s usually respond to an adjustment of dosage. No hepatotoxicity was demonstrated in limited numbers of pts. after 2 and 3 yrs. of therapy when follow-up biopsies were compared to baseline.

C18

CLINICAL EFFECT OF THERAPEUTIC NON-ACETYLATED SALICYLATE (TRILISATE) PLUS NAPROXEN IN RHEUMATOID ARTHRITIS (RA). D. Furst, K. Blocka, S. Cassell, E. Harris, J. Hirschberg, N. Josephson, R. Trimble, and A. Lachenbruch. University of Iowa, Iowa City, IA 52242.

Previous studies using combinations of non-steroidal drugs to treat RA have yielded conflicting results. We used Trilisate at therapeutic serum salicylate concentrations (150-300 mg/l) and naproxen (1500 mg qd) in a randomized, double-blind, placebo-controlled cross-over (1 month per arm) study of full-dose Trilisate (FD-TRIL), full-dose Naproxen (FD-NAP), full-dose both (FD-BOTH) and half-dose both (½-BOTH) to examine their additive or synergistic efficacy/toxicity in treating RA. We used standard measures of disease activity, and high-pressure liquid chromatography to measure plasma drug concentrations. This analysis concerns the 43 patients who completed the study; 41 dropouts were equally distributed among the four groups. FD-BOTH was statistically superior to all other treatments for 8 of 11 variables including joint tenderness count, activity of daily living scale and patient pain visual analog scales. FD-BOTH was better than FD-TRIL or ½-BOTH for 7 of 11 variables and to FD-NAP for 4 of 11 variables. FD-TRIL, FD-NAP and ½-BOTH were clinically equal and more effective than placebo. Tinnitus was more common when TRIL was used (28-30 complaints) than when only NAP was used (13 complaints). GI complaints were equally common for all regimens. FD-BOTH, altho statistically superior to FD-TRIL or FD-NAP, showed neither synergy nor a pharmacologically defined additive effect versus NAP or TRIL alone. On the other hand, no increased toxicity was easily discernible for FD-BOTH versus any of the other active drug regimens.

C19

RANDOMIZED DOUBLE-BLIND CROSSOVER TRIAL OF LOW-DOSE METHOTREXATE (MTX) FOR RHEUMATOID ARTHRITIS (RA).
M.E. Weinblatt, J.S. Coblyn, D.A. Fox, P.A. Fraser, D.E. Holdsworth, D.N. Glass, and D.E. Trentham, Harvard Medical School, Brigham and Women's Hospital, Beth Israel Hospital, and Dana Farber Cancer Institute, Boston, MA 02115.

Thirty-five patients with active RA entered a 24 week double-blind crossover trial comparing oral low-dose "pulse" MTX (2.5-5 mg q12h for 3 doses weekly) to placebo. All had failed gold and 80%, penicillamine. At 12 weeks (crossover), the MTX group, versus the placebo group, exhibited significant ($p<0.01$) improvement in the number of painful or tender joints, duration of morning stiffness, and overall investigator and patient assessment scores; a significant ($p<0.05$) decrease also occurred in the number of swollen joints and 50-foot walking time. All variables, as well as the sedimentation rate, showed significant ($p<0.01$) improvement at 24 weeks in the patients crossed over to MTX. All patients that responded to MTX in the first period flared on placebo. A significantly ($p<0.03$) increased frequency of HLA-DR2 occurred in the 8 patients that had the most substantial response to MTX. Adverse reactions during MTX therapy included transaminase elevation resolving with temporary drug interruption (21%), nausea (18%), diarrhea (12%), alopecia (6%), oral ulcers (6%), and a superficial skin infection (6%). One withdrew from the trial because of drug toxicity (diarrhea). Rheumatoid factor and immune complex levels, as well as blood lymphocyte subsets and thymidine incorporation responses to mitogens and antigens, did not change significantly on MTX. Although the mechanism of action is unknown, this trial provides evidence of the short-term efficacy of MTX in patients with refractory RA.

C20

SCANNING ELECTRON MICROSCOPIC EVALUATION OF THE ARTHRITIS OF MRL MICE.
F.X. O'Sullivan, F. Denys, W.J. Koopman, S. Gay. University of Alabama School of Medicine, Birmingham, Alabama 35294.

We have previously shown that the spontaneously occurring arthritis in knees of MRL/1 mice is characterized by proliferation of synovial cells and early destruction of bone and cartilage in the absence of a significant inflammatory response. Detailed light microscopic studies have shown that tissue destruction is closely associated with the presence of proliferating synovial cells in the same focal area. We have examined the articular surfaces of MRL knee joints to further explore the correlation between synovial cell proliferation and tissue destruction.

Disarticulated knee joints from 9 MRL/1 and 6 MRL/n mice, aged 4-33 weeks were examined by scanning electron microscopy. Two types of lesions involving articular cartilage of MRL/1 mice were detected. The first consisted of areas of articular cartilage covered by tightly adherent non-confluent monolayers of stellate-shaped cells with intertwining cytoplasmic processes. The integrity of the underlying cartilage matrix was disrupted, with exposure of collagen fibers. The second lesion consisted of well-circumscribed, dense sheets of amorphous cells loosely attached to the underlying collagen matrix, which had similarly been denuded. Occasional mononuclear-appearing cells were attached singly and in clusters to membrane fragments. Similar lesions were not seen in MRL/n knee joints. In areas without overlying cell layers the articular cartilage had either a smooth, fine fibrillar, or gently pockmarked appearance; features that have all been described in normal mammalian articular cartilage.

These lesions likely consist of proliferating synovial cells and support previous observations in arthritic MRL mice of joint destruction closely associated with the presence of proliferating synovial cells.

C21

IMPACT OF SPECIFIC THERAPY UPON RHEUMATOID ARTHRITIS (RA).
J. F. Fries, P. Spitz, & D. Bloch, Stanford University, Stanford CA 94305

An observational study of 889 consecutive drug starts among 580 patients of 13 commonly used drugs in patients with definite or classical RA from five geographically dispersed sites was carried out, using outcome assessment methodology. Patients were studied by protocol at six month intervals using a validated outcome questionnaire (HAQ) with endpoints of disability, pain, patient global assessment, drug costs, laboratory costs, and number of physician visits. Controls were both historical (the patient's previous status), and concurrent (other drug starts in the same cohort).

Striking effects upon these patient outcome measures were limited to use of intramuscular gold, pencillamine (DPA), and methotrexate (MTX), the three "disease-modifying" drugs studied. Gold resulted in highly significant reductions in disability ($p < .005$) and in pain ($p < .001$) after an average period of nine months. DPA and MTX showed similar trends in decreasing pain; MTX also decreased disability. Gold showed marked effects upon patient global assessment ($p < .005$). On the other hand, the number of doctor visits nearly doubled with gold and MTX, drug costs increased strikingly with gold ($p < .005$), and laboratory costs increased markedly with all three of these drugs, tripling on gold therapy ($p < .001$). In contrast, relatively minor differences in outcomes between the non-steroidal anti-inflammatory agents were difficult to interpret with certainty.

Outcome assessment methodology introduced in this study confirms disease impacts predicted from experimental studies and extends those observations to new outcomes such as disability and cost. These methods are sensitive and permit approaches to longer-term studies of a full range of disease outcome measures.

C22

ASSESSMENT OF RADIOLOGIC PROGRESSION IN RHEUMATOID ARTHRITIS (RA): A RANDOMIZED CONTROLLED TRIAL.
J.F. Fries, J. Sharp, D.A. Bloch, D.J. McShane, G. Bluhm, D. Forrester, P. Gofton, C. Weissman, H. Genant, S. Richman, F. Wolfe, P. Spitz. Stanford University & associated institutions of the Beaver Creek Conference Study Group

Radiologic progression is a definitive endpoint for assessment of RA progression; progression must be assessed optimally to have efficient, reliable, and valid results from clinical trials. The Beaver Creek Conference convened established investigators to work toward consensus by means of a randomized controlled trial of alternative reading methods. Twenty-four pairs of RA hand films in random sequence were read twice by eight observers--by erosion counting, weighted erosion counting, global assessment, and joint space narrowing. Films were scored by comprehensive (34 joints) and selective (18 joints) techniques, giving a total of eight methods for direct comparison. Satisfactory (.74-.88) correlation coefficients were obtained for both first and second readings for all methods. Simultaneous reading of paired films (in unknown sequence) was more reliable than reading separated in time. Smaller numbers of joints assessed (18) gave reliability similar to larger numbers (34). Statistically, ranked data was superior to raw data. Both erosion and joint space narrowing assessments are required. There was some increase in precision with weighted erosion counts. Readers with previous experience in reading for clinical trials scored better than those without such experience. Reliability and validity are greatly enhanced by use of 3 or more readers. The power requirements of a study are dramatically influenced by use of optimal reading techniques, which can reduce the required number of patients (and the cost) of a study by more than one-half.

C23

STRUCTURAL REQUIREMENTS FOR CHEMOTACTIC ACTIVITY OF LEUKOTRIENE B_4 LTB_4.
S.T. Hoffstein. R.M. Manzi. K.A. Razgaitis*. P.E. Bender* and J. Gleason*. Departments of Immunology and Medicinal Chemistry. Smith Kline and French Laboratories. Philadelphia. PA 19101.

LtB_4 (5S. 12R dihydroxy-6. 14-cis-8. 10-trans-eicosatetraenoic acid) is an extremely potent chemotaxin. We examined the structural requirements for chemotactic activity using synthetic LtB_4. several of its isomers. and two analogs. nor- and homo- LtB_4. Dose response curves for neutrophil chemotaxis to these compounds were obtained using a modified Boyden chamber. The mean distance cells moved into the filter was determined after 30 min. Peak chemotactic activity of LtB_4 was at 10^{-7}M. At higher concentrations. chemotactic activity was decreased. The shape of the dose response curve was similar to that with FMLP except that maximum chemotaxis to LtB_4 was consistently greater than chemotaxis to FMLP. A mixture of epimers at C-5 and C-12 shifted the response curve to the right and lowered maximum activity to that induced by 10^{-6}M LTB_4. Increasing or decreasing the chain by one carbon between the first OH and the COOH also shifted the curve to the right but maximal activity was comparable to the LtB_4 maximum. Changing the Δ^6 double bond from cis to trans had a greater effect. Activity was only detectable at high concentrations and maximum activity achieved was less than 50% that of LtB_4. Each of the compounds was capable of desensitizing neutrophils to LtB_4-induced aggregation. suggesting that they were acting at the same receptor. Thus the chain length between carboxyl and C-5 hydroxyl groups. the C-5 and C-12 absolute stereochemistry and the stereochemistry of the Δ^6 double bond are all important structural features for chemotactic activity with 6 stereochemistry apparently having the greatest contribution.

C24

COXSACKIEVIRUS B 1-INDUCED MURINE POLYMYOSITIS REQUIRES ACTIVE MUSCLE INFECTION BY LIVE VIRUS TO INITIATE DISEASE.
Steven R. Ytterberg, Minneapolis VAMC, Univ. of Minnesota, Minneapolis, MN 55417.

A myopathic strain of Coxsackievirus B1 (CVB 1) has been shown to induce in mice a syndrome resembling human polymyositis (PM). These studies were undertaken to determine whether persistent myositis requires initial viral infection of muscle to results from a primary immune response to viral antigens. Neonatal CD-1 Swiss mice were inoculated ip with varying doses of live CVB 1 (LV) or uv-killed virus (KV). LV produced dose-dependent mortality (LD_{50}=500 pfu), while survival of KV mice was comparable to controls. Clinically, proximal hindquarter weakness developed in most surviving LV mice but not in KV mice. Histologic changes in LV animals included initial extensive muscle necrosis, followed by regeneration and diffuse inflammation, and later focal inflammation, fatty replacement and calcification. Muscle from KV animals was normal. Infectious virus was recovered from LV mice for up to 14 days, with a peak titer of 10^7 pfu/gm muscle. No infectious virus could be recovered from KV mice, confirming the complete inactivation of this preparation. Neither repeated daily ip injections of high doses of KV, comparable to virus loads in LV mice, nor direct im injection of KV produced clinical or histologic evidence of myositis. These data demonstrate that live CVB 1, able to replicate in vivo and produce muscle necrosis, is required for the induction of murine PM, and that the disease does not develop as a result of simple exposure to viral antigens in the absence of infection. The possibility that a subsequent immune response, induced by the primary infection, is involved in the persistent inflammatory process is being investigated.

C25

SUSCEPTIBILITY OF MONONUCLEAR (MNC) AND LYMPHOBLASTOID CELLS TO HYDROGEN PEROXIDE. Nigel D. Staite Ronald P. Messner, David C. Zoschke, University of Minnesota, Minneapolis, MN 55454.

Activated phagocytes release H_2O_2 at sites of inflammation. Evidence of lipid peroxidation can be found in rheumatoid synovial fluid and the immunosuppressive action of D penicillamine may involve H_2O_2 formation. Thus H_2O_2 may play an important role in the pathogenesis of RA. We have examined the quantities of H_2O_2 that cause oxidative cytotoxicity, whether lymphocyte populations could differ in their susceptibility to H_2O_2 mediated damage and have compared these to the quantities of H_2O_2 that inhibit cellular proliferation.

50% oxidative cytotoxicity of MNC, measured by fluorescein diacetate (FDA), was seen after a 1hr exposure to 350 nmoles $H_2O_2/10^5$ cells. Six lymphoblastoid cell lines, RPMI 1788 (B), Raji (B), IM-9 (B), Daudi (B), CCRF-CEM (T) and MOLT-3 (T) were studied as examples of T and B-lymphocytes. Less than 30% cytotoxicity was seen in all cell lines with up to 512 nmoles $H_2O_2/10^5$ cells. 50% cytotoxicity was seen between 750 and 1500 nmoles of H_2O_2 in all but the MOLT-3 and Daudi cell lines, which were highly resistant to H_2O_2 mediated killing. In contrast to cytotoxicity studies, Con-A induced proliferation of MNC at 3 days was inhibited by 50% after a 1hr exposure to 2 - 3 nmoles H_2O_2 /10^5 cells.

Our studies reveal marked differences in susceptibility to H_2O_2 mediated oxidative cytotoxicity between MNC and lymphoblastoid cell lines and among the cell lines themselves. In addition, 100 fold less H_2O_2 is required to inhibit Con-A induced proliferation of MNC compared to that which causes immediate cytotoxicity. Thus by influencing functional aspects of discreet lymphocyte populations, small quantities of H_2O_2 may play an important role in the immunoregulation of RA.

C26

MONONUCLEAR CELL FACTOR INDUCES SECRETION OF SYNOVIAL MAST CELLS. Barry Gruber, Mary Haak-Frendscho, and Allen P. Kaplan. SUNY Stony Brook, N.Y. 11794

Numerous reports have documented mast cell hyperplasia in rheumatoid joints and suggest a role for these cells in contributing to the pathogenesis of proliferative synovitis. The activation of synovial mast cells has been studied following enzymatic digestion and dispersal of synovial cells. We have previously shown these mast cells to be responsive to specific antigens, anti-IgE, compound 48/80, and calcium ionophore. Histologic analysis of 40 synovium indicate that mast cells may reside at the periphery of lymphoid aggregates in the subsynovial layer. Mononuclear cells obtained during apheresis were cultured in the presence of Streptokinase/Streptodornase and the conditioned media contained a factor capable of releasing histamine (HRF) from human basophils. The partially purified HRF has a molecular weight of 32,000 by gel filtration and two isoelectric forms were found (pH 6.9 and 7.5 - 8.4) by chromatofocusing and isoelectric focusing in gels. SDS gel electrophoresis and radioautography of iodinated gel filtered material revealed a band at molecular weight 30,000 coincident with histamine releasing activity. Synovial cells obtained from 9 separate rheumatoid joints were then exposed to HRF for 30 mins. at 37°C and a significant histamine release (mean 24.8%, SEM ± 7.9) was detected. Preliminary studies also suggest the presence of HRF in rheumatoid synovial fluid. Interactions between synovial mononuclear cells and mast cells may be important in the pathogenesis of erosions and joint destruction in rheumatoid arthritis. The activation of mast cells by HRF may represent one such mechanism.

C27

PHENOTYPE AND CHARACTERISTICS OF STELLATE-SHAPED SYNOVIAL CELLS DERIVED FROM MRL/1 MICE. R.E. Gay, F. Denys, F.X. O'Sullivan, W.J. Koopman, H. Nagase, E.D. Harris, Jr., S. Gay. UAB Medical Center, Birmingham, AL and Rutgers Medical School, New Brunswick, NJ.

Previous observations in our laboratory have revealed that the proliferating synovial lining in the arthropathy of MRL/1 mice consists of distinct types of cells: round, non-spreading cells of the $MØ^+$ lineage, typical Ia^- $MØ^-$ fibroblasts and polymorphic stellate-shaped cells with a more or less dendritic appearance. We have examined the phenotype and characteristics of the latter cells in more detail.

Knee joints of 13 to 20 week old MRL/1 mice were opened and the menisci were dissected away in such a manner that proliferating synovial living cells remained attached. Under these conditions the synovial cells obtained, which were composed of less than 20% of fibroblasts and no inflammatory cells, were cultured and subsequently cloned in MEM containing 10% FCS in plastic dishes coated with a native collagenous matrix consisting of cartilage-derived type II and bone-derived type I collagen. These cells were examined by LM, IF, TEM and SEM.

15-25% of the primary culture displayed a polymorphic, stellate or slightly dendritic appearance. The stellate-shaped cells appeared transformed based on the frequent presence of large, pale double nuclei with little condensed chromatin, several enlarged nucleoli, highly developed rough endoplasmic reticulum and numerous small primary lysosomes. SEM revealed loss of the culture matrix at the sites of cell attachment. Synovial collagenase-specific antibodies labeled the cytoplasm and vesicles present within the long cellular processes.

The large, stellate, transformed appearing cell type is defined as being primarily responsible for the erosion and degradation of the collagenous matrix of cartilage and bone.

C28

FENRETINIDE [N-(4-HYDROXYPHENYL) RETINAMIDE; (4-HPR)] AS AN EFFECTIVE INHIBITOR OF ADJUVANT ARTHRITIS IN THE LEWIS FEMALE RAT. Carol Fisher and Francis Persico. Department of Biological Research, McNeil Pharmaceutical, Spring House, PA 19477-0776.

Brinckerhoff et al. (Science, 221: 756, 1983) demonstrated that 13-*cis*-retinoic acid was active in adjuvant arthritis, and Haraoui et al. (A&R, 27: S68, 1984) reported activity with 4-HPR in a model of streptococcal cell wall-induced arthritis in rats. Therefore, we tested 4-HPR for its capacity to inhibit adjuvant arthritis.

4-HPR (25-200 mg/kg/day p.o.), administered at the time of induction of adjuvant disease by intraplantar injection of *Mycobacterium butyricum*, and daily thereafter for 21 days, produced significant dose-dependent inhibition of the inflammatory response (quantitated as edema by plethsmography in a mercury bath) in the non-injected, contralateral paw. Statistically significant, dose-dependent inhibition of both the primary (acute) and secondary responses were also observed in the ipsilateral, injected paw. In other experiments, 4-HPR (25-200 mg/kg/day) was administered beginning 11 days after the induction of arthritis and continued for 16 additional days. Statistically significant dose-related inhibition of the edema was noted. Treatment of adjuvant arthritic rats with fully established disease (e.g. starting dosing 18 or 28 days after induction) resulted in amelioration of inflammation that was accompanied by a reversal of the bony changes that are associated with this chronic condition.

Thus, orally administered 4-HPR is capable of significantly reducing the inflammation and bony changes associated with developing and established adjuvant arthritis in the rat.

C29

A NEW METHOD MEASURING IgG ANTIBODY FORMING CELLS TO DNA (D-AFC) CORRELATES BETTER IN MURINE LUPUS WITH CLINICAL NEPHRITIS THAN MEASUREMENT OF CIRCULATING ANTIBODIES. D.Ando,F.Ebling,and B. Hahn, UCLA Los Angeles, CA 90024.

Detection of Ig ds D-AFC has been difficult using previous techniques such as the Jerne plaque assay. We developed an ELISPOT method in which ds or ss DNA is coated on to microtiter plates, murine spleen cells are cultured in the wells for 4 hours and the imprints of the cells secreting specific antibodies are developed with enzyme linked anti-IgG or Igm and agarose-substrate. Spots representing AFC are counted visually. Advantages include direct visualization of IgG AFC, no requirement for complement fixation and availability of standard reagents. Specificity of IgG AFC for DNA was shown by significant dose dependent competitive inhibition by ds and ss-DNA but not by Poly AU. A study of 16 NZB/W F_1 females showed a significant increase in IgG D-AFC with age: mean AFC per 10^5 splenocytes for dsDNA-17 at ages 10-29 weeks versus 48 at ages 30-40 weeks($p<.01$):for ssDNA-28vs.70($p<.05$). There were significant linear correlations between measurements of ds and ss D-AFC and a) age in weeks(R=0.68,0.57),b) rising BUN(R=0.83,0.78), and increasing proteinuria(R=0.78,0.77). In contrast although linear correlations with circulating ds and ssDNA antibodies and age were significant (R=0.54,0.66,$p<.05$) correlations with BUN and proteinuria were not (R's<0.34). D-AFC secreted predominantly IgM up to 18 weeks of age:IgG ds and ssD-AFC predominated thereafter. This is the first report of the ELISPOT method for use in measuring IgG D-AFC. In addition to its simplicity, the method yields results which correlate better with clinical parameters of nephritis than do standard measurements of circulating antibodies.

C30

CHARACTERIZATION OF INTERLEUKIN-2 (IL-2) SYNTHESIS IN SJOGREN'S SYNDROME USING ANTIBODIES AGAINST CHEMICALLY SYNTHESIZED PEPTIDES OF IL-2. Robert Fox, Argyrios Theofilopoulos, and Amnon Altman. Scripps Clinic and Research Foundation, La Jolla, CA 92037.

Abnormalities in interleukin-2 (IL-2) production previously have been reported in several autoimmune diseases. However, these studies utilized peripheral blood lymphocytes (PBL) and such abnormalities may not be present in the inflammatory site lymphocytes. Therefore, we studied patients with primary Sjogren's syndrome (SS, keratoconjunctivitis sicca) where PBL of 8/24 patients had markedly decreased IL-2 production. However, salivary gland lymphocytes (SGL) from these patients all had normal IL-2 production. To directly detect cells producing IL-2, we immunized rabbits with chemically synthesized peptides corresponding to amino acids 1-12 (peptide 81, p81) or 59-72 (peptide 84, p84) of human IL-2 and used immobilized peptides to prepare affinity purified antisera (PNAS:81,2176,1984). We found that: a) prior to mitogen stimulation, <1% of normal PBL or SS PBL were reactive; b) after mitogen stimulation, >40% of normal or SS PBL were reactive and the staining was blocked by pre-incubation of the antisera with the appropriate peptide; c) prior to mitogen stimulation, reactive cells were found among SGL (3.4 ± 1.4%) and normal LN (2.5 ± 1.5%); after mitogen stimulation, >50% of T-cells were reactive. These results emphasize that alterations of IL-2 production found in PBL in autoimmune diseases may not occur in the inflammatory site lymphocytes. Further, specific antisera against IL-2 peptides can provide new probes to understand the regulatory interactions that occur *in vitro* and to detect lymphocytes producing IL-2 *in situ*.

C31

LECTINS AND THE FC RECEPTOR: AFFINITY ISOLATED FC-GAMMA RECEPTOR BINDS CONCANAVALIN A. Robert P. Kimberly, Patricia Redecha, Theresa M. Prendergast and Stewart Greisman. Hospital for Special Surgery, New York, NY 10021.

The phagocytosis of Concanavalin A-treated erythrocytes by blood monocytes can be inhibited by the down-modulation of surface Fc-gamma receptors via adherence of monocytes to IgG-aggregate coated surfaces. To test the prediction that the Fc-gamma receptor contains an oligosaccharide(s) with terminal mannose residue(s), we have isolated Fc-gamma receptors by affinity chromatography and have demonstrated concanavalin A binding by Western blot analysis. Blood monocytes, separated by Ficoll-hypaque centrifugation and purified by adherence to plastic, were lysed in nonionic detergent in the presence of a protease inhibitor cocktail. Binding of putative receptor to DEAE-purified human IgG, immobilized on Sepharose beads, was carried out at 4°C by overnight incubation of ultracentrifuged lysate supernatant with beads. After extensive washing, the IgG-binding material was harvested by SDS or pH elution and dialyzed extensively against distilled water. SDS-PAGE and silver stain analysis of lyophilized receptor material showed predominantly two bands of approximately 51 and 68 kilodaltons. Electrophoretic transfer of PAGE'd proteins to nitrocellulose and overlay with iodinated tetravalent Concanavalin A demonstrated several bands of reactivity. Two bands were coincident with the putative Fc-gamma receptor evident on silver stain; several other bands of Con A reactivity were also seen.

These data suggest that the Fc-gamma receptor contains an oligosaccharide with a terminal mannose. Accordingly, binding to and cross-linking of Fc receptors may provide one mechanism for the effects of Concanavalin A.

C32

MECHANISM RESPONSIBLE FOR ABNORMAL CONTROL OF EPSTEIN-BARR VIRUS(EBV) IN RHEUMATOID ARTHRITIS (RA). Martin Lotz, Constantine D. Tsoukas, Dennis A. Carson and John H. Vaughan. Scripps Clinic and Research Foundation, La Jolla, CA 92037.

After in vitro infection of peripheral blood mononuclear cells with Epstein Barr virus, RA T lymphocytes are deficient in IL-2 and IFN γ production. This defect could be restored by monocyte depletion of the cultured cells. The mechanism of this monocyte effect does not involve prostaglandins, oxygen radicals or soluble immune response suppressor substances, as judged by the failure of indomethacin, 2-mercaptoethanol, or catalase to neutralize it. EBV infection of RA lymphocytes induces both, IL-1 and an inhibitor of IL-1. The latter was found in all RA cultures examined for it. The balance of simultaneously present IL-1 and IL-1 inhibitor determined the levels of detectable IL-1 activity, and this correlated with the levels of IL-2 and IFN γ.

In contrast to the deficiency in T cell response to EBV infection, the response to stimulation with OKT_3 is normal as measured by proliferation, IL-2 and IL-2 and IFN γ release. Thus, these in vitro studies on RA lymphocytes indicate that antigenic stimulation with EBV, in contrast to the normal OKT_3 mitogen response, induces inhibition of IL-1 with subsequent defects in IL-2 and IFN γ. This may be the basis for the previously reported defect of RA lymphocytes in regulating EBV infection of B cells.

C33

MODULATION OF SPONTANEOUS IMMUNOGLOBULIN PRODUCTION BY NATURAL KILLER CELLS IN RHEUMATOID ARTHRITIS. Zair Tovar, Richard Pope, Norman Talal. The University of Texas Health Science Center and Audie Murphy V.A. Hospital, San Antonio, TX 78284.

Mononuclear cells (MNC) from the synovial fluid (SF) of patients with rheumatoid arthritis (RA) spontaneously produce immunoglobulin (Ig). Natural killer (NK) cells down regulate Ig production both in vivo and in vitro. NK activity in the rheumatoid joint is present but reduced. We examined the ability of residual NK cells (Leu11b+) to modulate the spontaneous production of Ig in RA peripheral blood (PB) and SF. MNC were isolated from normal PB and RA PB and SF, and treated with complement (C') alone or anti-Leu 11b plus C'. After 7 days in culture, the cells were harvested and analyzed for NK activity employing the cell line K-562. The supernatants were frozen for later quantitation of Ig. As expected, the spontaneous production of IgG was greater in RA SF (1368±682 ng/ml/5x10^6 cells) than in RA(845±356 ng/ml) or normal (568±108 ng/ml) PB. The baseline NK activity was significantly ($p<0.05$) lower in RA SF (14.5±3.7%) than RA(40±5.9%) or normal (59.5±4.7%) PB. Treatment with anti-Leu 11b and C' resulted in reduced NK activity: from 14.5±3.7% to 9.7±2.4% in RA SF, from 40±5.9% to 3.9±1.7% in RA PB and from 59.5±4.7% to 13.1±2.7% in normal PB. Treatment with anti-Leu 11b resulted in a significant increase of IgG production in RA SF (from 1368±682 ng/ml to 2549±1531 ng/ml) as well as in RA PB (from 845± 356 ng/ml to 1125±410 ng/ml) and normal PB (from 568±108 ng/ml to 625±97 ng/ml. Lysis of NK cells with anti-Leu 11b plus C' also resulted in a significant ($P<0.01$) increase of IgM production in the SF (from 375±165 ng/ml to 984±460 ng/ml). We conclude that the residual SF Leu $11b^+$ (NK) cells modulate the ongoing synthesis of both IgG and IgM in the rheumatoid joint.

C34

RESTORATION OF THE IMMUNOGLOBULIN SECRETING CELL RESPONSE OF MONONUCLEAR CELLS TO POKEWEED MITOGEN BY INTERLEUKIN-1 AND INTERLEUKIN-2 IN SYSTEMIC LUPUS ERYTHEMATOSUS. L. Bidulo, R.J. DeHoratius, C. Monihan, Hahnemann University School of Medicine, Philadelphia, PA.; A.I. Levinson, University of Pennsylvania School of Medicine, Philadelphia, PA.

Despite polyclonal in vivo activation of peripheral blood mononuclear cells (PBM) and the resultant increased spontaneous immunoglobulin secreting cell (IgSC) number in patients with systemic lupus erythematosus (SLE), PBM from SLE patients demonstrate an impaired in vitro IgSC response to pokeweed mitogen(PWM). The role of interleukin-1 (IL-1) and Interleukin-2 (IL-2) in enhancing the deficient PWM induced IgSC response was studied. PBM from 14 patients with active SLE were incubated with PWM alone and in combination with IL-1, IL-2, and IL-1 + IL-2 in a 6 day culture and IgSC responses were then measured using a modified reverse hemolytic plaque assay (RHPA). The combination of IL-1 + IL-2 provided significant enhancement of the mean PWM induced IgSC response ($p < 0.01$) but had no effect on the PWM induced response of PBM obtained from 12 normal subjects. Neither IL-1 alone nor IL-2 alone fully reconstituted the PWM induced IgSC response of SLE PBM. An augmentation index was also performed for each manipulation. Again, only the combination of both IL-1 + IL-2 provided significant enhancement of the baseline PWM induced IgSC response ($p < 0.05$). This study supports the hypothesis that both IL-1 and IL-2 may be deficient in patients with active SLE as evidenced by the requirement for both interleukins for optimal enhancement of the IgSC response. Depressed lymphokine levels may be one important aspect in accounting for the multifactorial causes of disordered immunoregulation characteristic of SLE.

C35

IMMUNOGLOBULIN SECRETING CELL (IgSC) RESPONSE TO EPSTEIN BARR VIRUS(EBV) IN SYSTEMIC LUPUS ERYTHEMATOSUS (SLE) PATIENTS. B.Matteucci, R.J.DeHoratius, C.Monihan, Hahnemann University School of Medicine, Philadelphia, Pa. 19102.

Patients with SLE manifest the paradoxical combination of increased in vivo polyclonal activation of peripheral blood mononuclear cells (PBM) with impaired in vitro response to mitogens such as pokeweed mitogen (PWM). As we have shown previously, this impaired in vitro response is correctable by addition of lymphokines. In order to further delineate the intrinsic immune defects in mitogen responses in SLE, we have utilized EBV, a purely B cell polyclonal activator as an inducer of IgSC since it is unclear where the defects occur in SLE patients. The use of this mitogen would obviate the problems associated with the T cell dependent PWM system. PBM from 37 patients with active SLE and 24 controls were incubated with EBV-containing supernatant derived from a B95-8 lymphoblastoid cell line in 8 day cultures. The same sample population was also stimulated with PWM in 6 day cultures. IgSC responses were then measured using the modified reverse hemolytic plaque assay. The SLE patients had a mean IgSC response of 5169/10^6 plaque forming cells while the controls had 5435/10^6 plaque forming cells in response to EBV. In contrast the SLE patients had 13,464/10^6 plaque forming cells while controls had 27,219/10^6 plaque forming cells in response to PWM ($p<.001$). Our results demonstrate no significant difference in IgSC response to EBV between patients and controls while there is a significant difference to PWM. We conclude that B cell function in SLE patients in response to a polyclonal T cell independent stimulant is normal. The abnormal responses noted in T cell dependent systems may reflect abnormal function of T cells and/or macrophages.

C36

C3b (CR1) AND C3d (CR2) RECEPTOR EXPRESSION ON B LYMPHOCYTES IN SYSTEMIC LUPUS ERYTHEMATOSUS (SLE) AND RHEUMATOID ARTHRITIS (RA). J.G. Wilson, W.D. Ratnoff, P.H. Schur, and D.T. Fearon. Boston MA

Patients with SLE have inherited and acquired deficiencies of CR1 on erythrocytes (E). We have now assessed B cells of these patients for the expression of CR1 and CR2 to determine whether receptor abnormalities occur on a cell type more critically involved in immune reactions. Peripheral blood lymphocytes from SLE and RA patients and from normal individuals were stained with XRITC-anti-B1 to identify B cells and either FITC-anti-CR1 or FITC-anti-CR2 and analyzed by two-color flow cytometry. The average mean fluorescent channel of CR1-staining for B1-positive cells of 9 RA patients and 12 SLE patients was 85 ±5% (SEM; $p <0.01$) and 54 ±6% ($p <0.001$) that of B cells from normal persons. CR1 expression on B cells from 6 active SLE patients (47 ±10% of normal) was slightly less ($p >0.2$) than that of 6 inactive patients (61 ±6%). When the B cells were assessed for CR2 expression, the average mean fluorescence of cells from RA and SLE patients was 87 ±3% ($p <0.05$) and 56 ±7% ($p <0.001$) that of normal B cells. CR2 expression on B cells from 4 active SLE patients (42 ±6%) was approximately half ($p <0.01$) that of 4 inactive patients (70 ±6%). These deficiencies of CR1 and CR2, which are more marked in SLE than in RA patients and are caused at least in part by pathologic processes associated with active disease, may alter B cell function or may indicate that these cells have already been altered by interaction with C3-bearing immune complexes.

C37

JOINT CONTRACTURES AND NODULES AS PRESENTING MANIFESTATIONS OF JUVENILE SCLERODERMA. Donald P. Goldsmith, Masoud Shamaszedeh, Robert G. Sanford, Charles D. Tourtellotte. Temple Univ. Sch. Med., St. Christopher's Hospital for Children, Philadelphia, PA 19133

Current ARA diagnostic criteria for scleroderma are derived primarily from adults and may not be wholly adaptable to children. Childhood onset scleroderma unlike adult disease is more often characterized by localized morphea or linear lesions, and up to 10% of children with localized scleroderma initially present with arthritis. In our experience, more diffuse juvenile scleroderma may also have a similar articular presentation.

We follow 5 children (ages 7 to 15; 3 females, 2 males), all referred to us as probable polyarticular JRA because of multiple joint contractures and subcutaneous nodules. Four now have biopsy proven proximal skin changes of scleroderma which developed from 6 months to 4 years after recognition of joint involvement.

None have typical CREST syndrome although 1 has calcinosis and sclerodactyly; 1 has Raynaud's phenomenon; and 1 has esophageal dysfunction and sclerodactyly. Joints commonly involved are elbows, wrists, small joints of the hands, and hips; none have active synovitis. Although clinical weakness is minimal myositis is documented in 2; none have myocarditis. Pulmonary functions are abnormal in 2 of 4. Nodule biopsy in 3 of 4 revealed rheumatoid nodules in 2 and fibrotic nodules in 1. Two developed positive nucleolar pattern ANA (1:640, 1:10, 240); 1 has positive RF (1:1280); none have anti-DNA, Sm, RNP, anticentromere or SCL-70 antibodies. We feel that all children who present with gradual evolution of multiple painless joint contractures require careful observation for the development of skin changes suggestive of scleroderma.

C38

EARLY HISTOLOGIC AND RADIONUCLIDE SCAN CHANGES IN CHILDREN WITH REFLEX SYMPATHETIC DYSTROPHY SYNDROME (RSDS). Robert Nickeson, Earl Brewer, Donald Person. University of Oklahoma, Oklahoma City, OK 73126, Baylor College of Medicine, Houston, TX 77025.

No previous reports of RSDS in children have documented histologic changes in the involved tissues. Clinical findings in children with RSDS may differ from the typical pattern in adults. A group of seven children with typical RSDS were studied for evidence of altered immunity, and with technitium pyrophosphate scintigrams. Three patients also agreed to undergo biopsy of skin, muscle, and nerve of the involved region of their legs.

One patient had decreased serum IgA and depressed serum C3 and C4 during an acute episode of RSDS. Otherwise serologic studies in the patients were normal.

Scintigrams immediately post-injection consistently showed decreased perfusion of the affected areas. Delayed scans showed regional decreased bone uptake in the symptomatic region. No child had increased uptake around involved joints. All of the patients studied had initial scans performed within 14 months of onset of symptoms.

Abnormal capillary morphology was present in each of the three children biopsied. Electron micrographs showed endothelial swelling and basement membrane thickening and reduplication. Muscle tissue in one patient had endomesial IgG deposits with patchy fiber atrophy and degeneration suggesting ischemic injury.

We believe the initial symptoms in childhood RSDS are due to vascular insufficiency as documented by scintigraphy. The cause of this ischemia, probably at the capillary level, is unclear. Our patients were studied early in the course of their disorder prior to developing osteoporosis from disuse.

C39

HIDDEN 19S IgM RHEUMATOID FACTOR IN ADULTS WITH JUVENILE RHEUMATOID ARTHRITIS ONSET. James C. Speiser, Terry L. Moore, Thomas G. Osborn, Robert W. Dorner, Jack Zuckner. St. Louis University School of Medicine, St. Louis, MO 63104.

Hidden 19S IgM rheumatoid factors (RF), i.e., 19S IgM RF detected in the IgM-containing fraction of serum after separation by acid-gel filtration, were found in 68% of children with seronegative juvenile rheumatoid arthritis (JRA) by the complement-dependent hemolytic assay (HA).

In the present study, 48 adult patients with JRA onset (<16 years of age) were evaluated in adulthood ($\geq$17 years of age) for the presence of hidden 19S IgM RF. There were 6 men and 42 women with a median age of onset of 9.4 years. The average age of the patients when studied was 25.3 years with a mean duration of disease of 16.5 years. Thirty-seven patients had polyarticular-onset (7 positive for 19S IgM RF in the serum), 9 pauciarticular-, and 2 systemic-onset disease. The sera were subjected to acid-gel filtration on a Sephadex G-200 column and the IgM-containing fraction concentrated to the original serum by vacuum dialysis. The IgM fraction was heat inactivated at 56°C for 30 min, absorbed with washed sheep red blood cells for 90 min at 37°C, and then assayed for 19S IgM RF by the HA. Hidden 19S IgM RF (titers > 1:16) were found in 32 patients (67%) and correlated well with fluctuations in disease activity. Overall, in 88 serum samples evaluated in the 48 patients, disease activity correlated with IgM hidden RF titers in 55/88 (62%).

These results indicate that seronegative JRA-onset patients continue to have significant titers of hidden 19S IgM RF in their sera into early adulthood.

C40

NAILFOLD CAPILLARY AND ENDOTHELIAL CELL PRODUCT ABNORMALITIES IN JUVENILE DERMATOMYOSITIS (JDMS). W.A. Price, H.R. Maricq, J. Lazarchick and R.M. Silver, Medical University of South Carolina, Charleston

JDMS is a multisystem rheumatic disorder of unknown etiology which primarily affects small blood vessels of muscle and skin. Previous reports have demonstrated characteristic morphologic abnormalities in nailfold capillaries and abnormalities of coagulation parameters including factor VIII-related antigen (VIII:Ag), an endothelial cell product. This study attempts to correlate capillary abnormalities with coagulation studies using children with other rheumatic diseases as controls. In vivo capillary microscopy and coagulation studies were performed on 3 groups of patients: 5 with JDMS and 1 with JPMS; 12 with JRA; and 4 with SLE.

Abnormal capillaries by in vivo capillary microscopy were seen in 5/5 JDMS, 0/1 JPMS, 0/4 SLE, and 0/12 JRA. Abnormal results of VIII:Ag and fibronectin (FN) (endothelial cell products) assays are as follows:

	VIII:Ag	FN
JDMS	2/5	2/5
JRA	2/11	1/11
SLE	4/4	0/4

Mean PT, PTT, fibrinogen, fibrin-split products, FVIII procoagulant activity, plasminogen and β-thromboglobulin did not show differences for JDMS as compared with JRA or SLE. Thrombocytosis was noted only in JRA (3/12) and thrombocytopenia only in SLE (1/4).

Our results show that nailfold capillary changes in JDMS are accompanied by abnormalities in serum levels of endothelial cell products but that patients with SLE, JRA and JPMS may have similar abnormalities without changes in capillary morphology.

C41

19S IgM RHEUMATOID FACTOR-7S IgG RHEUMATOID FACTOR IMMUNE COMPLEXES ISOLATED IN SERUM OF PATIENTS WITH JUVENILE RHEUMATOID ARTHRITIS. Terry L. Moore, Thomas G. Osborn, Patricia L. Haber, Courtney R. Johnson, Robert W. Dorner. St. Louis University School of Medicine, St. Louis, MO 63104.

Serum from 25 children with juvenile rheumatoid arthritis (JRA), 6 polyarticular-onset seropositive (poly+), 12 polyarticular-onset, seronegative (poly-), and 7 pauciarticular-onset (pauci), were subjected to affinity chromatography (F[ab']$_2$ fragments of goat IgG anti-human IgM antibody) [αHIgM] to assay for immune complexes (IC). Material retained by the column was eluted sequentially by 1M NH_3 and 0.1M glycine-HCL buffer, pH 3.0. Isolated fractions were assayed by ELISA for 19S IgM rheumatoid factors (RF) and 7S IgG RF and by immunodiffusion for associated IgG. The fractions were further analyzed by preparative isoelectric focusing (IEF).

Isolation of the IC-like material eluted from the αHIgM column revealed IgG, 19S IgM RF in 5 patients, and IgG RF in 4 of the 5 in the NH_3-eluted fraction. These patients were all poly+. Significant 19S IgM RF titers plus IgG were also detected in 16 patients in the glycine-HCl eluate (5 poly+, 7 poly-, and 4 pauci). 7S IgG RF were also demonstrated in 7 patients glycine-HCl eluate (the same 5 poly+ and 2 poly-).

Analysis by preparative IEF of the IgM and IgG RF positive NH_3 and glycine-HCl eluates showed IgM RF throughout the pH range, but the highest quantity of IgM RF was in bands in the pH range 4.5-5.0, along with the IgG RF when present.

These studies demonstrate (1) IC containing 19S IgM-IgG and 19S IgM RF-7S IgG RF can be detected by ELISA in JRA patient's serum; and, (2) most of 19S IgM RF and IgG RF when present are in the pH band 4.5-5.0 by preparative IEF.

C42

JUVENILE PSORIATIC ARTHRITIS (JPSA) - CLINICAL ANALYSIS AND HLA ANTIGENS. M.L. Ganczarczyk, D. Gladman, A. Shore. Women's College and The Wellesley Hospitals, Toronto, Canada, M4Y 1J3.

JPSA is an uncommon arthritis of childhood. Our aim was to further define it in terms of clinical and laboratory analysis and compare it to adult PSA seen in our centre (presented at ARA meeting, June 1984). 17 patients with JPSA were evaluated according to a standard protocol, including a complete history, physical examination, radiologic and laboratory testing with HLA typing for A, B, C, D antigens.

Female to male ratio was 1.4:1. The mean age of onset of arthritis was 12 years with Psoriasis (PS) preceding arthritis in 11/17 of patients. A family history of PS was present in 13/17 of patients and PSA in 3/17. The most common presentation was that of gradual onset of poly- or oligoarthritis with or without axial involvement (7/17). Simultaneous flare of skin and joints was seen in 7/17. The disease appeared rather benign, with the majority of patients in Functional Class II at the time of assessment. Nail involvement of PS was common (14/17). None of the patients showed other extraarticular features.

There appeared to be a trend towards increased frequency of B17, BW38, CW6, DR1, and DR7, compared to healthy controls. No increase in B8 or B27 was seen in contrast to the previous report (Annals of CRMCC Vol. 17, #3, 1981). DR locus association was seen when none was observed in adult PSA. The results also differed from those reported for subgroups of juvenile arthritis (DR4-polyarticular group, B27, DR5 and DR8 pauci articular and DR5 alone - systemic) (A&R Vol. 26, Jan. 1983).

Based on clinical evaluation confirming previous reports and unique HLA typing - JPSA appears to be an entity separate from adult PSA and subgroups of JA.

C43

CHARACTERISTICS OF HLA B27 POSITIVE (B27+), ANTINUCLEAR ANTIBODY POSITIVE (ANA+) CHILDREN WITH ARTHRITIS. Alan M. Rosenberg. University of Saskatchewan, Saskatoon, Canada, S7N OXO.

Typically HLA B27 associated arthropathies are not associated with positive tests for antinuclear antibodies. Tabulated below are the features of 6 children (<16 years old) with chronic arthritis who are both B27+ and ANA+ (titer ≥1:80; HEp-2 cell substrate).

Patient	Sex	Race	Onset Age	Total # of Joints	Enthes-itis	Sacro-iliitis	Other Features
1	F	I*	10	8	yes	yes	Nodules, RF¶
2	M	I/C†	14	3	yes	yes	
3	F	C†	10	2	yes	yes	No IgA, Crohn's
4	F	I	3	18			
5	F	I	10	30			
6	F	I/C	4	19			

*I=Native Indian,†I/C=Mixed Race,†C=Caucasian,¶RF=Rheumatoid Factor

In the table below the group of 6 B27+, ANA+ children is compared to a group of 15 B27+ children without antinuclear antibodies (ANA-).

	Sex (F:M)	Race (I:C:I/C)	Onset Age (yr) (Mean ± 1SD)	Total Number of Joints (Mean ± 1SD)
ANA+, B27+	5:1	3:1:2	8.5 ± 3.8	13.3 ± 10.0
ANA-, B27+	2:13	4:11:0	12.4 ± 2.6	4.0 ± 2.2

When compared to B27+, ANA- children with arthritis, B27+, ANA+ children are more frequently females (χ^2=6.56,p=.01), have a younger onset age (t=2.59,p=.009) and have more joints involved (t=3.26,p=.002). Thus, in several notable respects B27+, ANA+ children are distinguishable from B27+, ANA- children and may represent a distinctive subset of chronic childhood arthritis. Co-existant features of more than one disease (cases 1 and 3) may be more common in B27+,ANA+ children.

C44

THE RELATIONSHIP BETWEEN OCULAR AND ARTICULAR DISEASE ACTIVITY IN CHILDREN WITH JUVENILE RHEUMATOID ARTHRITIS (JRA) AND ASSOCIATED UVEITIS. Alan M. Rosenberg, Kiem G. Oen. Universities of Saskatchewan and Manitoba, Saskatoon and Winnipeg, Canada.

To establish if activity of arthritis in children with JRA correlates with activity of anterior uveitis (U) we reviewed the onset patterns of 34 children with JRA (ARA criteria) and associated U. The subsequent courses of 20 of these children whose follow-up was sufficiently detailed are also described. In 21 children the onset of U followed the onset of arthritis by 1 to 6 years (mean 1.6 yrs). In 10 children U was first noted at the time of joint onset. In 3 children presenting with band keratopathy, synechiae and cataracts, the diagnosis of U antedated joint manifestations by .5 to 1 year. Eleven of 20 patients who had had regular follow-up had a remitting/relapsing (r/r) articular course; in 5 of these eye activity was also r/r, 3 had a single episode of U and in 3 others U was unremitting. Of 5 patients with a single episode of arthritis, 3 had r/r U and 2 had unremitting U. Of 4 patients with unremitting arthritis 2 had unremitting U and 2 had r/r U. Thus, in 13 of 20 patients (65%) the pattern of eye and joint activity differed. Together the 20 patients were seen 181 times. At 55 visits both articular and ocular inflammation were present. At 33 visits neither eye nor joint inflammation was present. At 45 visits U was active and joints inactive and at 48 visits U was inactive and joints active. Thus, at 51% of visits U and arthritis activity were discordent. In 20 instances coincident remission of both eye and joint activity was followed by relapse of eye and/or joint activity. In 7 such cases articular and ocular flare occurred simultaneously. Joint flare was not associated with U relapse in 6 cases and eye relapse was unassociated with joint flare in 7. Thus, in JRA, the course of U usually differs from that of arthritis.

C45

COMPLEMENT FIXATION BY INTERMEDIATE SIZED DNA/ANTI-DNA COMPLEXES C. Horgan, G. Burdick and W. Emlen Univ. of Washington, Seattle WA

The pathogenic potential of DNA/anti-DNA immune complexes (IC) may depend in part on IC size. Large complement fixing IC incorporate C3b and bind rapidly and stabily to C3b receptors on red blood cells (RBC); these IC are then cleared by the liver. Small IC do not activate complement (C) and may therefore be innocuous. IC which are intermediate in size may activate C and incorporate C3b but may be too small for stable binding to RBC, and thereby escape clearance via the RBC pathway. The purpose of this study is to investigate the ability of these intermediate sized IC to fix complement.

IC were prepared with ^{125}I-DNA(300bp) and IgG from SLE sera, then treated with DNAse to generate stable nuclease resistant IC. The size of the IC and the # of IgG antibodies (Ab) /DNA in the IC were estimated by sucrose gradient ultracentrifugation and polyacrylamide gel electrophoresis (PAGE). The size of the DNA was measured by PAGE after the IgG was digested with Proteinase K. Incorporation of C3b was measured by precipitation of the IC with monoclonal Ab to C3d(which also bound C3b) after the IC had been incubated with normal human C. Binding of the IC to RBC was also measured after incubation of the IC with C. Prior to DNAse digestion, IC formed over a wide range of Ab/DNA ratios were able to both incorporate C3b and bind to RBC. After DNAse digestion, IC did not bind to RBC, and only IC prepared at high Ab excess incorporated C3b. Thus, a population of IC can fix C, yet escape RBC-mediated clearance. DNAse digested IC containing 1 or 2 IgG/protected DNA fragment (35-70bp) did not incorporate C3b or bind to RBC. Larger DNAse digested IC did incorporate C3b, but could not bind to RBC. Because these IC do not bind to RBC, they may be able to persist in the circulation and yet still activate C, and thereby ellicit pathogenic effects.

C46

IMMUNOGLOBULIN AND COMPLEMENT DEPOSITION IN CARTILAGE IN EXPERIMENTAL OSTEOARTHRITIS. Roland W. Moskowitz and Thomas F. Kresina. Case Western Reserve University, Cleveland, OH 44106.

Immune responses may play a role in osteoarthritis (OA) responses, and may differentiate 1° and 2° OA. Cartilage deposition of immunoglobulins and complement in experimental OA is presented.

Methods. OA was induced in NZW female rabbits by partial meniscectomy (PM), and in vitro studies performed on nonoperated, 6 wk sham-operated and 6 wk PM animals. Medial/lateral femoral/tibial cartilage, and prepatellar synovium were separately studied for direct immunofluorescence with fluorescein-conjugated goat IgG, and with goat anti-rabbit IgM, IgG and C_3.

Results. Nonoperated and sham-operated animals revealed negative staining patterns. Cellular/pericellular (C/P), matrix (M) and surface (S) staining (grade 0-4) in the PM cartilages are shown (table).

	αIgM			αIgG			αC_3		
	C/P	M	S	C/P	M	S	C/P	M	S
Med femur	0	0	2+	0	3+	2+	0	0	3+
Lat femur	0	0	0	1+	1+	2+	3+	0	0
Med tibia	2+	2+	0	0	0	3+	0	0	2+
Lat tibia	0	0	0	2+	0	2+	1+	0	2+

Uniform deposition of IgG and C_3 in parallel was most striking at the joint surface. Contralateral knees were negative. Augmented synovial staining was seen only with αIgG.

Conclusions. IgG/C_3 deposition occurs in secondary OA, likely associated with secondary synovitis. Immune complexes may contribute to OA pathology. [AM30134 (NIH), and Revco Arth Res Ctr.]

C47

DISSOCIATION OF RHEUMATOID FACTOR (Id)-ANTIGEN COMPLEXES BY ANTIIdS. J.L. Nelson, F. Nardella, M. Mannik. U. of Wa., Seattle, WA 98195.

Rabbits were immunized with two IgG RFs F(ab')$_2$ and one IgM RF. Each rabbit antiserum was adsorbed over normal human serum and normal F(ab')$_2$ columns. A liquid phase radioimmunoassay (RIA) was used to detect RF(Id)-antiId binding. Rabbit antiIds bound their own Ids and did not bind normal IgG, normal F(ab')$_2$, Fc, or a monoclonal IgM. Normal rabbit F(ab')$_2$ did not bind to the RFs. Unexpectedly, each of the three Id-antiId interactions was not inhibited by the appropriate antigen, IgG, when added up to 100 times the amount of Id. Partial inhibition was observed only when a molar excess of antigen to Id of 24,000 to 1 was added. In marked contrast to the first experiments, relatively small amounts of antiIds were able to inhibit the binding of their respective RFs to solid phase IgG. Next the percent of RFs bound to solid phase IgG was determined, and then antiIds were added. The antiIds to the IgG RFs readily dissociated their Ids from solid phase IgG. IgM RF was not dissociated by its antiId, and this difference is most likely attributable to the known greater affinity of IgM RF than of IgG RF for solid phase IgG.

The experimental observations described can be explained by a relatively greater affinity of antiId for Id than Id for antigen, and serve to underscore the importance of considering relative affinities in Id-antiId and Id-antigen interactions. These findings indicate that both the specificity and affinity of antiIds to Ids should be considered in the manipulation of the immune response by antiId.

C48

ANTIBODIES TO CARTILAGE COMPONENTS IN RHEUMATOID ARTHRITIS (RA). S. Larrian Johnston, Janet L. Johnson, Lorne A. Runge, and Paul E. Phillips, SUNY-Upstate Medical Center, Syracuse, N.Y.

Humoral antibodies to cartilage may contribute to chronicity in RA. In a matched control study, we examined antibodies to various cartilage components using ELISA. Guanidine-HCl extracts of bovine nasal cartilage were separated into proteoglycan fraction A_1 and matrix protein fraction A_4 by associative CsCl density gradients; collagen was prepared by limited pepsin digestion on previously extracted cartilage. Although several RA sera had markedly elevated anti-collagen antibodies, mean antibody levels were not significantly elevated in the RA group compared to matched controls. However, RA sera did have significantly elevated mean antibody levels for fractions A_1 and A_4. Matrix protein fraction A_4 was the most reactive with mean absorbance values of 0.830 for RA and 0.440 for non-RA (p < .001). Fraction A_4 contained 8 major proteins with a molecular weight range of 12-135 kd by SDS-PAGE and two electrophoretically distinct low buoyant density proteoglycans. Subfractions of A_4, prepared on a second associative CsCl density gradient with an overall lighter density, resulted in a proteoglycan fraction $A_{4.1}$ and a proteoglycan-free fraction $A_{4.6}$. Fraction $A_{4.1}$ also contained two proteins of 57 and 66 kd, and fraction $A_{4.6}$ contained six major protein bands with a molecular weight range of 13-66 kd. RA sera previously shown to possess high antibody levels to fraction A_4 were found to react well in ELISA with proteoglycan-free subfraction $A_{4.6}$, but not at all with proteoglycan subfraction $A_{4.1}$. Western blot analysis following SDS-PAGE revealed that these sera were reacting with three protein components of molecular weights 13, 48 and 57 kd. The data suggest that antibodies to these matrix proteins may be involved in perpetuating RA.

C49

GENETIC REGULATION OF THE IMMUNE RESPONSE TO CHICK TYPE II COLLAGEN IN MICE. P.H. Wooley, H.S. Luthra, A. Huse and C.S. David. Immunology and Rheumatology Depts., Mayo Clinic, Rochester, MN 55905.

The humoral immune response to chick type II collagen was assessed in 13 independent haplotype mouse strains congenic to C57/B10, to investigate the significance of the antibody response in the development of collagen-induced arthritis (CIA. Mice were injected with 25 μg of chick collagen, i.d., and ELISA assays were carried out to measure the antibody response after 28 days. High antibody responses were detected in the CIA susceptible strains B10.Q and B10.G. The predominant isotype observed was IgG2b, with high levels of IgG2a, and intermediate levels of IgG1 and IgM present. Anti-collagen antibodies from B10.Q and B10.G mice inhibited (>60%) the binding of antibody extracted from the joints of arthritic B10.Q mice (JE-Ab), and crossreacted with a high degree with 4 of 6 collagen species tested. High anti-collagen antibody responses were also observed in B10.D2, B10.P and B10.F mice. The predominant isotype was IgG2b, with intermediate levels of IgG2a, IgG3 and IgM present. None of these antisera showed >25% inhibition of JE-Ab, and only B10.P anti-collagen antibodies showed crossreactivity with other collagen species. Intermediate antibody responses were detected in B10, B10.RIII, B10.M and B10.PL mice. The predominant isotype was IgG2b, with IgG2a, IgG1 and IgG3 low or absent. Inhibition of JE-Ab >50% was observed in B10.PL antisera, but none of the strains crossreacted highly with other collagen species. The remaining strains produced low antibody responses to type II collagen. Isotyping of JE-Ab indicated the presence of IgG2a and IgG2b. These results suggest that both specificity and isotype of the anti-collagen antibody response may be important in the development of CIA.

C50

UNMASKING OF CYTOPLASMIC FLUORESCENCE OF ANTI-JO-1 BY PURIFICATION OF ANTIBODY. Ira N. Targoff and Morris Reichlin. V.A. Med. Ctr., Dept. of Med., OU Health Sci. Ctr., and Okla. Med. Res. Fdn., Oklahoma City, OK 73104.

Most antibodies recognized by immunodiffusion (ID) of serum with tissue extracts also react in indirect immunofluorescence (IIF) to give a characteristic pattern. IIF is generally a quantitatively more sensitive technique than ID. We have observed 6/23 sera with anti-Jo-1 by ID that are negative by IIF. Although anti-Jo-1 should give a cytoplasmic pattern since anti-Jo-1 is a cytoplasmic enzyme, this pattern was seen in only 7/23 sera. The cytoplasmic staining was more common with very high ELISA values, seen in 4 of the 6 sera with the highest ELISA readings, although a perfect correlation was not seen. Specific antibody was isolated from two IIF negative anti-Jo sera with good ELISA activity by acid treatment of immune precipitates. When redissolved in the same volume as the original serum from which it was purified, specific antibody stained cytoplasm at 1/8 and 1/16 dilutions, respectively, while neither whole serum had cytoplasmic staining at 1/5. Thus, the lack of IIF activity is not due to antigenic deficiency of the substrate. If an activity unit is defined as the activity giving the weakest definite staining, specific antibody was >66- and >114-fold increased over the respective sera in activity per mg IgG. Whole IgG isolated from both sera was positive with 9- and 7-fold increases in activity per mg IgG over the whole sera. A serum with anti-Mi-2 and high titer nuclear fluorescence had twice the activity/mg of whole IgG isolated from that serum, an effect opposite to that seen with anti-Jo sera. Thus, there appears to be a factor in whole serum from Jo patients interfering with IIF.

C51

OCCURRENCE OF MONOMERIC IgA RF IN RHEUMATOID ARTHRITIS (RA). R.E. Schrohenloher and W.J. Koopman. University of Alabama School of Medicine, Birmingham, AL 35294.

IgA RF has been shown to be present in many RA sera and synovial fluids (SF). Where characterized, it was almost exclusively polymeric although total IgA was predominantly monomeric. Using a monoclonal IgA RF paraprotein, we recently demonstrated that monomeric IgA RF (mIgA RF) can escape detection by previously described RIAs, but its binding activity can be markedly enhanced by the presence of a hybridoma anti-human α-chain antibody. Monomeric and polymeric IgA fractions from 37 RA sera containing IgA RF were obtained by gel chromatography or density gradient ultracentrifugation in acidic buffer and examined for the presence of IgA RF by RIA in the presence and absence of the hybridoma antibody. Quantities were estimated by comparison to isolated monoclonal mIgA RF and pIgA RF proteins. mIgA RF was detected in 29 (78%) of the sera at levels ranging from 1-516 μg/ml (representing 5-88% of the IgA RF recovered) and did not correlate (P>0.05) with pIgA RF or serum IgA. Moreover, the ratio of mIgA RF to pIgA RF did not correlate with the serum IgA RF as measured by the conventional RIA. pIgA RF was recovered from all the sera. mIgA RF was also found in all of 10 SF examined. Levels ranged from 3-43 μg/ml and represented 9-39% of the recovered IgA RF. Neither form of IgA RF was detected in normal serum analyzed under the same conditions. Thus, previous studies may have underestimated the occurrence of mIgA RF in RA. Further, the highly variable proportions of monomer and polymer suggest that distinct regulatory pathways govern expression of these two molecular forms of IgA RF.

C52

IDENTIFICATION OF ANTI-RIBOSOMAL AUTOANTIGENS. C.L. Peebles, A.M. Francoeur, E.M. Tan and J.C. Lee*, Scripps Clinic and Research Foundation, La Jolla, Ca., *University of Texas, San Antonio, Texas.

Certain patients with connective tissue disease synthesize autoantibodies to components of the ribosome. Immunoprecipitations and immunoblots with selected anti-ribosomal RNP sera were used to identify three autoantigens, rRNP-1, rRNP-2 and rRNP-3. The antigens were found to be phosphoproteins, having approximate molecular weights of 38,000d, 16,000d and 15,000d. Occasionally another antigen of molecular weight 30,000d was also detected. The human sera reacted with similar proteins present in a number of eukaryotic species but not with prokaryotic antigens.

Immunoblotting with purified proteins and specific antisera was used to identify the rRNP-2 and rRNP-3 autoantigens. These correspond to the acidic phosphoproteins associated with the large ribosomal subunit called A1/A2 (yeast), P1/P2 (rat), and eL7/eL12 in other eukaryotes. Similarly, the rRNP-1 antigen was identified as a 38,000d non-acidic, large ribosomal subunit-associated phosphoprotein.

The molecular identity of ribosomal autoantigens have now been defined. The presence of different groups of anti-ribosomal sera with distinct reactivities would have to be considered in previous reports associating anti-rRNP with renal disease.

C53

CHARACTERIZATION OF THE DNA-BINDING AUTOANTIGEN KU. Tsuneyo Mimori, John A. Hardin and Joan A. Steitz. Yale University, New Haven, CT 06510.

Certain patients with rheumatic disorders develop autoantibodies that recognize an acidic nuclear protein antigen termed Ku, which we have identified as DNA-binding protein doublet of 70KDa and 80KDa (J. Clin. Invest., 68:611, 1981). Our aim is to elucidate a mechanism of interaction between Ku and DNA and to understand the biological function of the Ku proteins.

In the present studies, Ku proteins were purified from HeLa cell extract using anti-Ku immunoaffinity column chromatography. Binding of Ku to DNA was examined in the filter assay using a single ^{32}P-DNA fragment derived from HeLa cell DNA with EcoRI endonuclease (300bp, labeled at 3' of 5' end). These studies demonstrated that double stranded (ds) DNA bound Ku with much greater affinity than did single stranded (ss) DNA; that Ku dissociated from dsDNA at ionic strength greater than 0.35M NaCl; and that Ku binding to the DNA fragment was not inhibited in the presence of superhelical closed circular DNA (from plasmid pBR322) but was inhibited when the latter DNA was denatured or cleaved with appropriate restriction endonucleases.

The Ku-binding site on DNA was investigated by foot-print analysis. The end-labeled ^{32}P-DNA probe (with or without bound Ku proteins) was partially digested with DNase I and residual fragments were analyzed electrophoretically. Bound Ku protected only the free end-portions of both strands of the dsDNA probe.

Thus, the Ku proteins bind specifically to free ends of dsDNA and, to a lesser extent, ssDNA. These findings suggest that the Ku antigen plays a role in DNA metabolic events such as replication or repair.

C54

THE COMPLEMENT MEDIATED BINDING OF ANTIBODY(AB)/dsDNA IMMUNE COMPLEXES (IC) TO NON-PRIMATE PLATELETS. G.A. Kujala and R.P. Taylor, University of Virginia School of Medicine, Charlottesville, VA.

We studied the in vivo and in vitro binding of Ab/^{3}H-dsPM2 DNA and Ab/^{125}I-dsDNA IC to rabbit and guinea pig cellular blood components. SLE plasma was the Ab source. In the in vivo experiments the IC were injected intravenously into the animals, and shortly thereafter blood samples anti-coagulated in EDTA were obtained. Binding was determined by pelleting the cells and the fraction of radiolabeled IC bound to the cells was measured. The binding for these two non-primates was very similar, was almost entirely due to platelets and required homologous, intact complement. Maximal binding of the ^{3}H-DNA was >90% in vivo and in parallel in vitro experiments. Binding in vitro was 60% to 65% in mixtures of cells containing approximately 100,000 platelets per microliter, whether dilutions of a) citrated whole blood, b) recombined platelets, neutrophils and mononuclear cells, or c) platelets alone were used. Furthermore, no appreciable binding was observed when neutrophils, mononuclear cells or erythrocytes were used alone at normal blood concentrations. The in vivo binding reaction occurred quite rapidly (less than one minute for 90% binding) and over 60% of the cell bound counts were removed from the circulation in less than 5 minutes. These observations suggest that relatively large, complement-fixing IC are bound to non-primate platelets in vivo. Thus, animal models of immune complex mediated diseases will have to take into account the role of platelet (in non-primates) and erythrocyte (in primates) binding in the clearance of complement fixing IC from the circulation.

C55

METHOTREXATE IS SAFE AND EFFECTIVE IN THE LONG TERM MANAGEMENT OF RHEUMATOID ARTHRITIS.

Arthur Weinstein, Sally Marlowe, Joseph Korn, and Faripour Farouhar. U Conn Health Center, Farmington, CT 06032.

We have reported the short term benefit of low dose methotrexate (MTX) in 21 patients (pts) with classical rheumatoid arthritis (RA). These pts have been reevaluated to analyze the effectiveness and toxocity of MTX after an additional 2.5 yrs.

15/21 pts (71%) have continued on MTX for 20-67 (mean 42) mos. Cumulative MTX dose was 2021mg (range:915-3705). Clinical assessment at the first (I) and most recent (II) evaluations are noted below:

	PreMTX	I(11 mos)	II(42 mos)
# tender/swollen jts	22/15	13/7*	6/4**
grip strength (mm)	82	123*	136**
AM stiffness (hrs)	8.2	3.4*	0.4
sed rate (mm/hr)	68	43*	33

* I vs Pre: $p<0.006$, ** II vs I: $p<0.02$

3/21 (14%) achieved a complete clinical remission (ARA criteria) and 9/21 (43%) had an excellent response. AM stiffness disappeared in 8/15 pts and the sed rate normalized in 9/15.

Mild nausea and stomatitis were common (10/18). MTX was discontinued in 6 pts because of clinical hepatitis, planned pregnancy, fear of toxicity, noncompliance, nausea and vomiting, nausea and transaminase increase. Elevated transaminases occurred in 10/21 pts. Liver biopsies in 17 pts at cumulative MTX dose of 1950 mg (range:915-3125) revealed mild to moderate steatosis and moderate to marked variation in nuclear size. These changes did not correlate with the occurrence of abnormal transaminases. Mild fibrosis was seen in 6 biopsies but severe fibrosis or cirrhosis was not present. MTX is effective and reasonably safe for the long term treatment of RA.

C56

PILOT STUDY OF GRADED EXERCISE TESTING OF ARTHRITIS PATIENTS.

T.E. Dreisinger, M.A. Minor, R.R. Webel, R.B. Whiting, D.R. Kay, University of Missouri-Columbia Multipurpose Arthritis Center, Columbia, MO. 65212

Prescribed rest and range of motion exercise are considered fundamental in the basic management of many types of arthritis, but rest and lack of appropriate physical activity decreases functional capacity. We developed conditioning exercise protocols for AP to test the hypothesis that deconditioning is a component of arthritis disability. Testing of this hypothesis required a pilot study to answer 3 questions: 1) Can AP successfully perform graded exercise tests (GXT); 2) will pain limit GXT performance, and 3) can AP exercise at sufficiently high levels to potentially increase functional capacity? Seven AP (diagnosis RA (4), OA (2), MCTD (1); weight bearing joint involvement (7); functional class II (6), III (1); XRay Stage 2 (5), 3 (2)) were given a standardized GXT (Naughton Protocol, motor driven treadmill) to their subjective maximum performance. Table describes subjects age at pretest; preconditioning maximal treadmill level ($Level_{max}$); oxygen uptake (VO_{2max}L/min); minute ventilation (VE_{max} L/min); heart rate (HR_{max}), and metabolic equivalent (MET_{max}).

	AGE_{yrs}	$LEVEL_{max}$	VO_{2max}	VE_{max}	HR_{max}	MET_{max}
Mean±SD	57±20	2.8±2	1.05±.22	26±6	151±17	4.4±1
Range	34-82	0-6	.820-1.400	18-35	123-170	3.7-6.5

HR_{max} was within 90% of the age predicted maximal HR for an able bodied population. VO_{2max} and $Level_{max}$ confirmed AP's poor fitness levels. VE_{max} was within normal ranges for exercise performed. All of the patients terminated the test because of subjective fatigue and not pain. We conclude that arthritis patients can tolerate GXT's, their performance is limited by deconditioning and not pain and they can exercise at levels sufficient to potentially increase their cardio-respiratory capacity. This testing protocol is in use to measure the efficacy of conditioning exercise protocols.

D1

LUNG INVOLVEMENT IN SYSTEMIC LUPUS ERYTHEMATOSUS AND AUTOANTIBODIES.

Shigeko Inokuma, Shigeru Takafuji, Haruhito Sugiyama, Keiko Miyahara, Tokyo Metropolitan Komagome Hospital, and Yukio Matsumura, Matsumura Clinic and Research Inst. for Asthma and Immunological Diseases, Tokyo.

Lung involvement in systemic lupus erythematosus(SLE) and autoantibodies were studied in 49 patients with SLE diagnosed with revised ARA criteria. They were 4 males and 45 females, 44.1 ± 12.7 years of age. The duration of the disease was 9.3 ± 7.3 years, and 42 of them had been treated with corticosteroids.

Lung involvements were evaluated carefully by clinical symptoms, x-ray examinations, and pulmonary function tests. Interstitial pneumonitis was recognized in 8 cases, pleural effusion was seen in 5 cases, and pulmonary vascular disease was suspected in 3 cases. Pulmonary diseases not caused by SLE (bacterial pneumonia, tuberculosis, and lung congestion) were excluded.

Number of positive cases/number tested in autoantibody exams were ANA 49/49, LE-test 11/49, anti-dsDNA 20/47, RNP 14/40, Sm 4/36, SS-A 12/40, SS-B 2/40, RF 12/46. Positive LE, dsDNA, Sm, SS-B, or RF had no relation to lung involvement. However, among 14 patients with positive RNP, 5 had pneumonitis, 2 had pleuritis, and 3 had pulmonary vascular disease. The incidence of lung involvement in RNP-positive patients(10/14, 71.4%) was significantly higher than that in RNP-negative patients(4/22, 15.3%) ($p < 0.01$). Among 12 patients with SS-A, 6 had pneumonitis and 1 had pleuritis. The incidence of pulmonary involvement in SS-A positive patients(7/12, 58.3%) was also significantly higher than that in SS-A negative patients(7/28, 25%) ($p < 0.05$). All 4 patients with both RNP and SS-A were suffering from pneumonitis.

Anti-RNP and SS-A antibodies might be some risk factors or correlating factors for lung involvement in SLE.

D2

NON-PRECIPITATING ANTI-Sm ANTIBODIES AND ANTIBODY ISOTYPES IN CONNECTIVE TISSUE DISEASES.

J. T. Tesar, D. Axelrod, J. Armstrong, and P. Wheeler. Walter Reed Army Medical Center, Washington, D.C. 20307

A sensitive immunoassay was used for quantitation of anti-Sm antibody (Ab) and its isotypes in 174 pts with various connective tissue diseases and 106 controls. A highly purified Sm antigen (Ag) (2 ug/ml) was used to coat micro-titer plates using Engvall's ELISA method. The Ag was devoid of immune reactivity with 14 monospecific reference sera against known nuclear and cytoplasmic Ag-s (including RNP). The homogeneity of the Sm antigen was also proven by immunoblotting, after electrophoretic separation. All sera were also examined for precipitating anti-Sm Ab-s using immunodiffusion in agarose. Most of control sera contained no anti-Sm Ab-s. 15 normal subjects (14%) had low titer Ab-s (≤1/320 ELISA). Although non-precipitating IgG anti-Sm AB-s (≥1/640) were found mainly in SLE pts (21/87=24%) they were also present in scleroderma (4/20) and RA (4/42) pts. 14% of SLE pts had precipitating anti-Sm Ab-s which were not present in any of the other rheumatic diseases including 18 scleroderma, 5 polymyositis, 42 RA and 8 vasculitis. 14 SLE pts had IgM and/or IgA anti-Sm isotypes. Statistical analysis revealed no association of Sm-Ab-s with CNS, renal or hematological involvement in 87 SLE pts. We conclude that in SLE there was no correlation between anti-Sm-Ab-s and presence of renal or CNS involvement; that non-precipitating Sm-Ab-s occur also in scleroderma and RA and finally that low level anti-Sm-Ab-s may be present in normal pts.

D3

ASSOCIATION BETWEEN SYSTEMIC LUPUS ERYTHEMATOSUS (SLE) AND T4 EPITOPE PHENOTYPE.

William Stohl and Joyce Z. Singer. The Rockefeller University, New York, NY 10021, and The State University of New York at Downstate, Brooklyn, NY 11203.

A heterogeneity in expression of the T4 epitope (as detected by staining with monoclonal antibody OKT4) on T helper cells is found in Blacks (but not in Whites) giving rise to three distinct T4 epitope phenotypes: intact; intermediate (heterozygote); and deficient. Inasmuch as the prevalence of SLE is 3- to 4-fold greater in Blacks than in Whites, 346 Blacks (112 SLE; 101 normals; 133 non-rheumatologic diseases) were screened for T4 epitope expression to correlate phenotype with development of SLE. A trend toward the preferential expression of the intermediate and deficient phenotypes in SLE compared to normals and disease controls was noted, although this did not achieve statistical significance. However, in individuals of Jamaican ancestry a significant correlation between development of SLE and expression of the T4 epitope-intermediate or deficient phenotype was demonstrated ($P < 0.025$), whereas non-Jamaican individuals demonstrated no such correlation. In the nine Jamaican SLE patients with the intermediate or deficient phenotype, central nervous system (CNS) disease and lymphadenopathy each was manifest in six patients whereas they were each manifest in only two of the seven Jamaican SLE patients with the intact phenotype. We suggest that the T4 epitope-intermediate or deficient phenotype may be an identifying factor in the development of SLE. CNS disease and lymphadenopathy may also correlate with T4 epitope phenotype. However, other factors must also be playing a role since the correlation between T4 epitope phenotype and development of SLE could be demonstrated in the Jamaican population but not in non-Jamaicans.

D4

RELATIONSHIP BETWEEN CIRCULATING ANTI RO/SSA ANTIBODY (a-Ro) LEVELS AND SKIN DISEASE ACTIVITY IN SUBACUTE CUTANEOUS LUPUS ERYTHEMATOSUS (SCLE).

Purcell SM, Lieu TS, Davis BM and Sontheimer RD, Derm Depts. UTHSCD, Dallas, Tx 75235 and Wilford Hall USAF, San Antonio, Tx 78236

If a-Ro plays a pathogenetic role in the development of SCLE skin lesions as has been suggested by some workers, one might expect a positive correlation between a-Ro levels and skin disease activity in SCLE. To investigate this possibility we have examined the relationship between a-Ro levels and skin disease activity in 12 SCLE patients whom we had examined and collected blood from on at least three separate occasions. A-Ro levels were determined in 80 serum specimens by double immunodiffusion using Wil-2 cell extract as the antigen source. 9/12 (75%) of the patients had detectable a-Ro levels. 3/12 had no detectable a-Ro in spite of multiple exacerbations of skin disease activity. 8/12 (67%) had fluctuations in a-Ro levels during the course of the study. Seven of these 8 patients showed a rising titer after the onset of skin disease activity. Four of these 7 patients showed a ≥2 titer increase in a-Ro. The preliminary results of a more sensitive ELISA assay using biochemically purified Ro/SS-A antigen also suggest that in most patients IgG a-Ro antibody levels tend to rise as skin disease activity abates. These preliminary results suggest that there is no significant increase in a-Ro immunodiffusion titers prior to or coincident with flares of skin disease activity in SCLE patients. These findings argue somewhat against the possibility that free a-Ro is directly mediating cutaneous injury in SCLE, but do suggest that elevations of a-Ro levels in these patients might result from increased antigen load released during cutaneous tissue injury.

D5

NEURONAL ANTIBODIES (NA) IN NEUROPSYCHIATRIC SYSTEMIC LUPUS ERYTHEMATOSUS (NP-SLE) PROBABLY ACCESS THE CENTRAL NERVOUS SYSTEM THROUGH A DAMAGED BLOOD-BRAIN BARRIER.

Marta Kelly, William Swanston, Jack Gauldie, Peter B. Dent, Shuen-Kuei Liao and Judah A. Denburg. McMaster University, Hamilton, Ont. L8N 3Z5, CANADA.

It is not clear whether NA, when found in patients with NP-SLE, gain access to the central nervous system through a damaged blood-brain barrier or are locally produced therein. We have measured CSF/serum albumin and IgG ratios, CSF oligoclonal bands and/or paired CSF/serum specific IgG binding activity to neuroblastoma cell lines by mixed hemadsorption assay in 14 patients with SLE and 67 controls with inflammatory, infectious, vascular, neoplastic or traumatic neurological and/or psychiatric conditions. Four of 14 SLE CSFs contained NA, and all 4 also had serum NA; 4 additional SLE patient sera were positive for NA without CSF positivity and 3 of these had abnormal CSF/serum albumin ratios. None of 14 SLE CSFs had abnormal IgG ratios or oligoclonal bands. None of 24 control CSFs tested were positive for NA; 19/67 showed abnormal albumin ratios, 19/67 had evidence of local CSF IgG production, 15/67 had oligoclonal bands, and 6/67 had both increased albumin and IgG ratios. We conclude that NA, as measured by our IgG binding assay, are specific for SLE and most likely enter the CSF through a damaged blood-brain barrier. Such findings could explain the variable expression of clinically overt NP-SLE in serum NA-positive individuals.

D6

SSA ANTIBODIES: INFLUENCE ON PREGNANCY OUTCOME IN WOMEN WITH SYSTEMIC LUPUS ERYTHEMATOSUS (SLE).

Rosalind Ramsey-Goldman, David Hom, J. S. Deng, Gayle Casterline Ziegler, Leslie E. Kahl, Virginia D. Steen, Ronald E. LaPorte, Thomas A. Medsger, Jr., University of Pittsburgh, Pittsburgh, PA 15261

Congenital complete heart block (CHB) occurs in infants of some women with SLE who have serum SSA antibodies. Other adverse pregnancy outcomes in these patients have not been ascertained. We studied pregnancy outcome in 83 women with SLE seen from 1979-1984 (24 SSA positive and 59 SSA negative). Fertility was reduced in SSA vs no-SSA patients (0.08 pregnancies per year menstruating vs 0.11, p=0.097), but the proportion never pregnant was similar. There were no significant differences in the rates of miscarriage (Mc), prematurity (Pr), stillbirth (Sb), neonatal complications (Nc) or maternal lupus or non-lupus complications. Adverse outcomes did not differ according to race, age at lupus onset or diagnosis, or timing of pregnancy in relation to SLE onset.

SLE Patients	Total Pregnancies	Fetal Outcomes				
		Mc	Pr	Sb	Nc	
SSA (N=24)	42	4(10%)	5(12%)	0	6*(14%)	*3CHB
no-SSA (N=59)	126	21(17%)	12(9%)	5(4%)	13(10%)	

CHB occurred exclusively in infants of anti-SSA mothers. Only one of the 45 pregnancies of women symptomatic from lupus resulted in a CHB baby, compared with 2/123 pregnancies in initially asymptomatic women. We therefore estimate an approximate 1:40 risk of CHB in all women with definite or probably SLE, and considering these results and reports in the literature, a higher risk in those with SSA antibody.

D7

APPLICATION OF A NEW ELISA ASSAY FOR THE MEASUREMENT OF ANTI-HISTONE ANTIBODIES. Alan Epstein, Mark Greenberg, Peter Barland and Seymour Halbert. Montefiore Medical Center/Albert Einstein College of Medicine, Bronx, NY 10467.

Antibodies reactive with nuclear histones have been identified in SLE, rheumatoid arthritis, drug-induced lupus erythematosus (DILE), and in asymptomatic patients with drug-induced antinuclear antibodies (DANA). The clinical method most commonly employed to detect these antibodies is a tedious indirect immunofluorescence assay (IF), in which acid extracted mouse kidney sections are reconstituted with histone fraction 2A. We have developed a new technique in which unfractionated nuclear histones (UH) are covalently bonded to plastic discs and employed in an ELISA system for the measurement of anti-histone antibodies (AHAb). There is significant quantitative agreement between the ELISA and IF assays ($r=0.470$, $p < 0.01$), thus validating the new technique. Further, when applied to patients in clinically defined categories the diagnostic value of this technique is apparent (Table).

Group	#	%+	mean*	S.D.*
Control	24	0%	8.2	4.4
DILE	20	100%	323	393
DANA	18	22%	17.8	17.5
SLE	60	42%	32.2	65.7
RA (RF+)	20	15%	13.3	8.0

*Standardized O.D. units

The ELISA assay using discs coated with UH is a rapid, reliable method for the measurement of AHAb which correlates with the presently used IF assay. The results can help differentiate between patients with DILE and DANA ($p < 0.01$). Although AHAb are demonstrable in patients with SLE they are present in lower amounts than in patients with DILE ($p<0.01$) and have no association with disease activity.

D8

CLINICAL AND LABORATORY FEATURES ASSOCIATED WITH ANTI CARDIOLIPIN ANTIBODIES IN NON-SLE PATIENTS,
Asherson RA, Chan JKH, HarrisEN, Gharavi AE, Hughes GRV.

From: The Rheumatology Unit, The Royal Postgraduate Medical School of London, The Hammersmith Hospital, London, ENGLAND.

A strong association between thromboses(arterial and venous) thrombocytopenia , recurrent abortions and the "lupus anticoagulant"in SLE patients has been demonstrated. Recently a strong correlation between anticardiolipin antibodies and the "lupus anticoagulant" has been shown by our Department.
Seventeen patients, not fulfilling the ARA criteria for a diagnosis of SLE are presented, all of whom had elevated levels of IgGAnticardiolipin antibodies and who manifested the same associations as the SLE group. They had been diagnosed clinically as "Lupus-like", "Variant" Lupus or unspecified autoimmune disorders.
14/17 had arterial or venous occlusions. The seven with arterial thrombi had cerebral(6) and mesenteric(1) involvement. TIA's occurred in 2. DVT's(often multiple)were seen in 7 and superficial phlebitis in 3.
8/14 females had multiple abortions(>2). Migraines and livedo were common while polyserositis, renal involvement and polyarthritis were rare.
CNS manifestations such as epilepsy/chorea were not uncommon.
IgG antibodies to cardiolipin were present in all and false positive VDRL's were demonstrated in 8/14 tested, DNA bindings has always been negative but ENA's were positive in six. Ten were ANA +ve and seven ANA -ve.
Thrombocytopenia was present in 8/17.
Prospective studies are currently in progress in order to determine if the patients in this group are in fact "pre- lupus" or whether they represent a specific subset of the autoimmune spectrum.

D9

WHICH IS THE ACTIVE COMPONENT OF SULPHASALAZINE IN RHEUMATOID ARTHRITIS? T Pullar, J A Hunter, H A Capell. Centre for Rheumatic Diseases, Glasgow Royal Infirmary and Gartnavel General Hospital, Glasgow.

Sulphasalazine (SASP) has been shown to be an active second-line drug in the treatment of rheumatoid arthritis (RA). SASP is split in the large bowel to sulphapyridine (SP) and 5-aminosalicylic acid (5ASA). We have evaluated these two compounds separately in an attempt to identify the active moiety of SASP and to try to separate toxic from beneficial effects.

Sixty patients with active RA were randomly allocated to SP 2g/day or 5ASA (Asacol) 1.2g/day. At 24 weeks 21 patients remained on 5ASA and 17 on SP. Inefficacy was the most common reason for discontinuation of treatment in the 5-ASA group while most patients stopping SP did so because of side-effects (nausea, vomiting, rash). The patients who continued SP showed significant improvement in both laboratory and clinical parameters of inflammation (Wilcoxon) whereas only articular index improved significantly in the 5ASA group and haemoglobin fell significantly. There was a greater improvement in ESR, articular index and grip strength in the SP patients compared with the 5ASA group (Mann-Whitney). This implies that SP has a second-line action in RA, whereas any beneficial action of 5ASA would appear to be a first-line effect. The toxicity profile of SP is similar to SASP and it is doubtful whether its use would confer additional benefit. However, the ability of an antibiotic to 'modify' RA may indirectly throw some light on the aetiopathogenesis of RA.

D10

ESTIMATION OF THE RELATIVE AFFINITY OF 19S IgM RHEUMATOID FACTOR SECRETED BY RHEUMATOID SYNOVIAL CELLS FOR HUMAN IMMUNOGLOBULIN G SUBCLASSES. Dick L. Robbins, Jeffrey Skilling, William F. Benisek, UCD, Davis, CA 95616, Richard Wistar, Jr., Naval Medical Research Center, Bethesda, MD 20814.

19S IgM rheumatoid factors (RF) in rheumatoid arthritis (RA) are polyclonal autoantibodies directed at antigenic determinants on the Fc piece of IgG molecules. Serum RF demonstrate a heterogeneity of specificities for determinants on IgG Fc. For example, many serum RF have greater specificity for rabbit than for human IgG and the affinity for human IgG is low with an association constant of 10^4 to 10^5 liters/mole. Serum RF also has specificity for human IgG subclasses 1, 2, and 4, but little or none for IgG3. However, the plaque forming cell assay (PFC) allows determination of specificity and affinity characteristics of antibody molecules produced at a given time by a given cell. RF detected in a rheumatoid synovial cell (RSC) RF-PFC have greater specificity for human IgG and subclass IgG3 relative to autologous serum RF.

The purpose of this study was to extend previous observations of RSC RF specificities and to estimate the relative affinities of RSC RF for human IgG subclasses. This was done by calculation of fractional RF expression in the RSC RF-PFC following inhibition by IgG subclasses. In particular, the diameters of individual plaques from each assay were measured and the cubes of the diameters were summed to give a quantity proportional to total plaque volume, which is expressed as percent of the control. This provides a more valid estimate of relative RF affinity than does inhibition of RSC RF-PFC number. The greatest specificity and highest relative affinity of RSC RF was for human IgG and for subclass IgG3.

D11

ULTRASTRUCTURAL PATHOLOGY OF MUSCLE IN RHEUMATOID ARTHRITIS (RA) AND LUPUS ERYTHEMATOSUS(SLE). M.L. Russell, D. Friesen, W.M. Hanna, Women's College Hospital, University of Toronto, Toronto, Canada.

Weakness and myalgia are common complaints in RA and SLE, although the reason for this is usually unclear, especially in the absence of contiguous joint disease. Light microscopy of muscle is usually unimpressive and often normal. No systematic ultrastructural studies have been done.

We have examined quadriceps biopsies from 16 RA and 15 SLE patients unselected for muscle symptoms. Seven RA and 4 SLE patients had myalgia and/or weakness. Symptoms appeared unrelated to drug therapy or joint disease, and in only 1 RA were muscle enzymes elevated. Light microscopy was normal, specifically showing no vasculitis.

Ultrastructural abnormalities found included lymphocytic infiltrates, degeneration/necrosis, fibre atrophy and disarray, and microvascular basement membrane changes. Milder non-specific changes included increased glycogen and mitochondria, and myelin bodies due to chloroquine.

Quantitation of the number of abnormal muscle sections/biopsy revealed that overall RA and SLE patients had more pathologic changes than controls, and that symptomatic patients had more frequent and more severe changes (table below).

	% Abnormal Sections		
	Weak	Strong	Controls
RA	54%	26%	17%
SLE	56%	28%	17%

It appears that muscle fibre abnormalities are not uncommon in RA and SLE. While non-specific, the degree and severity of pathologic change appears to correlate with clinical symptomatology.

D12

LIVER BIOPSIES IN PATIENTS ON LOW DOSE PULSE METHOTREXATE (MTX) FOR THE TREATMENT OF RHEUMATOID ARTHRITIS. R. F. Willkens, D. O. Clegg, J. R. Ward, C. R. Marks, M. L. Greene, K. G. Tolman, G. J. Roth, C. G. Jackson, P. A. Leonard. University of Washington, Washington.

The emphasis by dermatologists of the potential hepatoxicity of MTX which can be recognized consistently only by a tissue examination mandated such an evaluation of rheumatoid patients treated with low dose pulse therapy. Consequently 59 patients treated intermittent low dose pulse regimens were biopsied. Cumulative dose of MTX ranged from 792 to 4000 mgm and duration of therapy was in excess of 2 years in the majority of patients. Biopsies were graded on a scale of I - IV depending upon the presence and extent of inflammatory and/or cellular infiltration, fibrosis, or cirrhosis.

Twenty-seven patients showed essentially no abnormality; 17 showed mild fatty and cellular infiltration; 13 showed more extensive change with mild fibrosis. No biopsy was graded category IV or cirrhosis. Histologic findings did not correlate with dose, duration of administration, or with liver function test abnormalities, although patients in category III A had one or more abnormal liver function tests. The most consistent correlation with histopathology was alcohol use.

In summary, only two of 59 patients on low dose pulse MTX demonstrated sufficient change to consider discontinuing MTX therapy after two years or approximately 1.5 gms of MTX.

D13

PULMONARY ABNORMALITIES IN ADULT-ONSET STILL'S DISEASE (AOSD).

Orrin M.Troum, John G. Mohler, Michael N. Koss and Francisco P. Quismorio, Jr., USC School of Medicine, Los Angeles, CA. 90033

Pleurisy, cough and lung infiltrates occur as pulmonary manifestations of AOSD. These symptoms are acute, transitory and respond to steroid therapy. An AOSD pt. with persistent and progressive interstitial lung fibrosis was recently reported (Ann. Rheum. Dis. 42:452, 1984). To determine whether chronic lung disease occurs frequently in AOSD, we studied 12 pts. followed for 1 to 18 yrs. (mean = 6 yrs.) for respiratory symptoms. Chest x-rays and pulmonary function tests (PFT) were performed. There were 7 females and 5 males with ages from 19 to 55 yrs. (mean = 37.5 yrs.). The pts. had arthritis, high intermittent fevers, typical skin rash, leucocytosis, adenopathy, liver dysfunction and negative tests for rheumatoid factors, anti-DNA and anti-ENA abs. None had evidence of infection or malignancy.

Nine pts. had respiratory involvement: pleurisy in 7, with pleural effusion in 3, lung infiltrates in 3, cough in 4 and shortness of breath in 4. None had clubbing. X-ray changes consisting of pleural effusion, parenchymal infiltrate, plate-like atelectasis and elevated diaphragm were found in 9 pts. Lung biopsy in one pt. showed acute alveolitis. Lung symptoms were acute and occured during disease exacerbation and responded to anti-inflammatory agents. PFT showed changes of restrictive lung disease including decreased DLCO and total lung capacity in 7 of 8 pts.

Our study shows that acute as well as chronic pulmonary functional abnormalities constitute a common clinical feature of AOSD. Evidence for restrictive lung disease should be sought for in pts. with AOSD.

D14

SERIAL Clq LEVELS IN RELATION TO THE DISEASE SUBSETS OF RA BASED ON JOINT DAMAGE.

T. Ochi, R. Iwase, K. Yonemasu, M. Matsukawa, M. Yoneda, H. Owaki and K. Ono. Osaka University Medical School, Osaka 553, Japan.

We reported that serum Clq levels in patients with RA had a prognostic value in tissue damage indicated by the number of joints with erosion (NJE) (Arthritis Rheum. 1984 No.8). We have advanced studies to make clearer the relationship between Clq levels and the suspected disease subsets of RA based on NJE.

Using the NJE from 68 joints throughout the whole body as an index, a population study was done statistically involving patients who had had RA for 10 yrs or more. Three groups, each showing Poisson's distribution, were found. Mean NJE of each were 10.8 (1st group; Less Erosive Subset,LES), 32.4 (2nd group; More Erosive Subset,MES) and 52.5 (3rd group; Mutilating Disease,MUD),respectively. These 3 groups were suspected to be disease subsets of RA based on the extent of joint damage.

In each of the 3 groups, we measured the following: (1) the mean incidence of joint involvement at the disease period of 10 yrs or more (2) retrospective yearly profile of Clq level change. Results were as follows: LES; (1) wrist 72%, MPJ 25%, others<15%. (2) Clq levels remained constantly below 250μg/ml for the whole disease period. After 7 yrs of RA, they began to decrease to normal level (Mean;137μg/ml). MES; (1) DIP a few %, hip 56%, others>70%. (2) For the first 7 yrs of RA, Clq levels remained constantly above 250μg/ml. After 7 yrs, Clq levels began to decrease and after about 20 yrs, the levels were, in many cases, almost normal. MUD; (1) DIP 60%, others>90%.(2) similar to MES.

To summarize, (I) 3 disease subsets of RA could be found statistically based on the extent of joint damage. (II) Clq level could be a good indicator to discriminate LES from MES or MUD for the first 7 yrs of RA.

D15

STUDIES ON THE MECHANISM OF PIROXICAM INHIBITION OF THE ACTIVITY OF ANABOLINS PRODUCED BY RHEUMATOID (RA) SYNOVIUM.

Jerome H. Herman, Alan M. Appel, and Evelyn V. Hess. University of Cincinnati Medical Center, Cincinnati, OH 45267.

Anabolins are products of T lymphocytes and pathologic synovium which modulate chondrocyte proteoglycan and collagen synthesis. It was previously shown (Arthritis Rheum 27:S81, 1984) that piroxicam used in vitro in a therapeutic concentration of 5 μg/ml had an inhibitory effect on both the synthesis and activity of anabolins produced by RA synovium. The current study evaluates mechanisms responsible for this inhibition of activity.

Six day RA synovial membrane organ cultures were established. Anabolin was assayed in synovium conditioned media (SCM) by assessing its effect on glycosaminoglycan (GAG) synthesis in 72 hr articular cartilage cultures. Anabolins suppressing GAG synthesis were produced by each of 3 synovial specimens (mean suppression 73.5 ± 1.1%). Post-culture addition of piroxicam to SCM significantly blocked this effect (mean suppression 24.2 ± 5.3%).

Anabolins were partially purified by anion exchange and Sephacryl S200 chromatography. Chondrocytes preincubated with piroxicam overnight and washed free of drug were less responsive to anabolin than cells unexposed to drug (7.1 ± 4.1 vs 28.1 ± 3% suppression GAG synthesis, n=2). Drug did not effect chondrocyte viability. Preincubating anabolin with piroxicam followed by drug removal by extensive dialysis reduced the anabolin effect (15.4 ± 2.4 vs 39.3 ± 1.6% suppression, n=2). Thus piroxicam has been shown to modulate anabolin activity at a chondrocyte level (potential effect on cell receptor vs cell metabolism) as well as by direct binding to anabolin.

D16

RELEASE OF SUPEROXIDE ANION (O_2^-) AND HYDROGEN PEROXIDE (H_2O_2) FROM NEUTROPHILS BY IMMUNE COMPLEXES CANNOT BE INHIBITED BY ENGAGEMENT OF ADENOSINE RECEPTORS.

BN Cronstein, SM Kubersky, G Weissmann and R Hirschhorn. Dept. of Med., NYU Med. Ctr., New York, NY 10016.

Adenosine and its analogues, acting at specific surface receptors, inhibit generation by neutrophils (PMN) of toxic oxygen metabolites provoked by soluble stimuli (e.g. chemoattractants such as F-Met-Leu-Phe and C5a, concanavalin A, and ionophore A23187). To determine whether engagement of adenosine receptors also inhibits the generation of oxygen metabolites by cells exposed to particles, we studied the effects of 2-chloroadenosine (ClAdo), a potent adenosine receptor agonist, on O_2^- and H_2O_2 generation by PMN challenged by serum treated zymosan particles (STZ), latex particles, or immune complexes (BSA-antiBSA). ClAdo (10uM) inhibited O_2^- and H_2O_2 generation by PMN stimulated by STZ (57±8% and 50±12% inhibition, n=6, p<0.001, for O_2^- and H_2O_2 generation, respectively). ClAdo (10uM) also inhibited H_2O_2 generation stimulated by latex particles (69±11% inhibition, n=4, p<0.008). Therefore, engagement of adenosine receptors inhibited O_2^- and H_2O_2 generation in response to STZ and latex particles. In direct contrast, when cells were exposed to BSA-antiBSA, ClAdo (10uM) inhibited O_2^- generation by a trivial amount (16±5% inhibition, n=6, p<0.02). Nor was generation of H_2O_2 in response to immune complexes affected by ClAdo. Neither BSA nor IgG alone interfered with ClAdo inhibition of O_2^- generation induced by F-Met-Leu-Phe. These data indicate that while adenosine and its analogues inhibit PMN responses to most ligands, they have no effect on activation of PMN via F_c receptors. Thus, adenosine receptors permit PMN to respond selectively to inflammatory signals at their surface.

D17

NEUTROPHIL PRODUCTION OF AN INTERLEUKIN I INHIBITOR.

Katherine Tiku, John L. Skosey, and Moti L. Tiku. University of Illinois College of Medicine, Chicago, IL 60612

Recently Liao et al. (J. Exp. Med. 159: 126, 1984) have identified a specific inhibitor of interleukin I (IL-1) in the urine of febrile patients. The cellular source of this inhibitor is not known. During our previous studies on neutrophil derived thymocyte activating factor, i.e., interleukin I, we observed that when neutrophils were cocultured with macrophages in the presence of zymosan there was inhibition of macrophage IL-1 activity. We initiated the present studies to investigate if neutrophils produced an inhibitor of IL-1. Supernatants collected from 18 hour zymosan stimulated or unstimulated purified human neutrophils were tested for their ability to inhibit human monocyte derived IL-1 activity. The assay consisted of C_3H/HeJ thymocyte proliferation. Supernatants obtained from stimulated (S-sup) and unstimulated (US-sup) neutrophils inhibited IL-1 derived thymocyte proliferation in a dose response manner. At 15% concentration of supernatants, US-sup caused 51% inhibition while S-sup produced 77% suppression of thymocyte ^{3}H-thymidine incorporation in the presence of 1 μg/ml phytohaemagglutinin. The factor was non-dialyzable. The inhibition was evident even when macrophage IL-1 and neutrophil supernatants were preincubated at 37°C for 1 hour before being tested in IL-1 assay. These studies suggest that neutrophils may be a source of an inhibitor of IL-1 and production of this inhibitor is enhanced by zymosan stimulation. Our previous studies indicated that neutrophils produce an IL-1 like factor. In addition these cells may be producing an inhibitor of IL-1 which is involved in negative regulation of IL-1 action. These findings may explain the presence of an inhibitor to IL-1 in the urine of febrile patients, since neutrophils are involved in the biology of acute febrile reaction.

D18

INDOMETHACIN AUGMENTS LEUKOTRIENE PRODUCTION DURING ACUTE ANAPHYLAXIS.

Dwight R. Robinson, K.J. Bloch, C. Melvin, E. Hayes, E. Lowenstein, M. Skoskiewicz, G. Castorena, J. Moss, F. Michelassi, and W.M. Zapol. Massachusetts General Hospital, Boston, MA 02114.

Cyclooxygenase (CO) inhibition by nonsteroidal anti-inflammatory drugs (NSAID) appears to account for their major toxic and therapeutic effects, but shunting of the metabolism of arachidonic acid by NSAIDS to lipoxygenase products, including leukotrienes (LT), could contribute undesirable effects. We have examined the effects of indomethacin (indo) on eicosanoid production during acute anaphylaxis in sheep. Sheep were sensitized with ascaris suum extract (ASE) subcutaneously 2 weeks before the experiment, and anaphylaxis was induced by intravenous ASE after general anesthesia. Mean levels of thromboxane B_2 and the prostacyclin metabolite, 6 keto $PGF_{1\alpha}$, in arterial plasma, measured by radioimmunoassay (RIA), increased 7-fold and >10-fold, respectively, after challenge of 4 sensitized sheep, whereas changes in mean levels of these mediators in 4 indo-treated sensitized sheep and 4 non-immunized controls did not change significantly. Levels of sulfidopeptide (SP) LTs were not detectable in plasma by RIA, but in pulmonary lymph there was a >5-fold increase in SPLT to a maximum of 35 ng/ml (as LTE_4) after challenge of indo-treated sheep whereas no change was seen in sensitized sheep or in controls. Reverse phase HPLC analyses of lymph demonstrated that all of the SPLT was present as LTE_4. Therefore, cyclooxygenase blockade results in marked augmentation of SPLT formation in vivo. These changes in arachidonic acid metabolism could contribute to certain toxic effects of NSAIDS such as bronchospasm and impaired renal function. Augmentation of LT formation by NSAIDs could also blunt the therapeutic efficacy of these agents.

D19

EFFECT OF JOINT MOTION ON EXPERIMENTAL CALCIUM PYROPHOSPHATE (CPPD) CRYSTAL-INDUCED ARTHRITIS. A.G. Fam, H.R. Schumacher, G. Clayburne, T. Villanueva, D. Baker, S. Jimenez. VAMC and U of PA. Phila., PA 19104.

Exercise has been shown to exacerbate acute urate crystal-induced inflammation in canine joints (A&R 15,609,1972). The influence of joint motion on chronic experimental articular inflammation has received less study. We now describe the effects of exercise and immobilization on acute and chronic CPPD crystal-induced arthritis in lapine joints.

Ten NZ white rabbits received a single 10 mg CPPD injection into each knee. L knees were cast-immobilized, R knees were either free at cage activity(5), or passively moved from 60° to 120° every 20"x5 hrs using a modified human elbowmobile continuous passive motion machine (5). Controls included 9 non-injected (-inj) rabbits casted and exercised as above. Six other rabbits received repeated knee injections of 10 mg CPPD q5d x 4; L knees cast-immobilized; R knees free at cage activity.

Synovial fluid (SF) WBCs were higher in the acute CPPD-inj exercised knees compared to immobilized joints ($\bar{x}$ difference 36,025/mm^3,p=0.05) but only equivocally so in the chronic. SF prostaglandin E_2 activity showed no consistent change. Synovitis histologic scores were greater in acute and chronic CPPD-inj exercised compared to immobilized knees ($p < 0.001$). Inj & non-inj knees immobilized for 24 d showed significant loss of cartilage safraninophilia and chondrocyte disarray. Non-immobilized joints with or without repeated CPPD inj showed no such changes; longer experiments are pending. Results of proteoglycan synthesis ($^{35}SO_4$ incorporation) and content (uronic acid) are being analyzed.

Active and passive joint motion have an enhancing effect on both acute and chronic CPPD-induced inflammation. Chronic CPPD-induced synovitis did not affect cartilage Safranin-O staining in non-immobilized joints over 24 days.

D20

LIPOSOME-INDUCED SYNOVITIS IN RABBITS. S.J. Choi, H.R. Schumacher, G. Clayburne, and M.S. Rothfuss. U of PA. and VAMC Phila., PA 19104.

Several reports have described patients with acute or chronic arthritis with intracellular (IC) birefringent lipid spherulites in joint fluids and suggested that these liposome-like particles might have induced the inflammation. Since there was no proof of phlogistic potential for such spherulites, we have studied whether liposomes injected into rabbit joints can induce acute or chronic inflammation.

Liposomes were prepared by Vortex mixing of phosphatidylcholine, dicetyl phosphate and cholesterol at molar ratios of 7:2:1 in 0.145M K_2HPO_4 under sterile conditions. Nine rabbits had right knees (RK) injected with 0.5 ml liposomes; left knees (LK) as controls received only 0.5 ml K_2HPO_4. At 6 hours (hrs) and 2,4 and 6 days (d) after injection, synovial fluids (SF) and membranes (SM) were examined by polarized, light and electron microscopy (EM). At 6 hrs, RKs showed leukocyte counts (WBC) of 11,600-90,400/mm^3 (mean 58,450/mm^3) with 94-99% polymorphonuclear cells (PMN); LKs had WBC of 1,300-19,900 (mean 12,650) with 68-96% PMN. At 2 d, 1 RK had 35,500 WBC with 48% synovial lining cells (SLC) and 39% lymphocytes (lymph); the LK showed only 750 WBC. At 4 d, 1 RK had 3,500 WBC with 77% lymph and 10% SLC; the LK had 450 WBC. At 6 d, the RK had 1,650 WBC with 68% lymph and 22% SLC; the LK showed 850 WBC. Liposomes seen as birefringent Maltese crosses or vesicles were mostly extracellular at 6 hrs and almost all IC at 2 d; there were still IC liposomes at 4 and 6 d. EM of SFs at 6 hrs showed membranous arrays of liposomal material in PMN vacuoles and adhering to cell surfaces. Histology of SMs showed many PMN in RKs and much fewer in LKs at 6 hrs. At 2 d, RK showed subacute and chronic inflammation, while the LK was normal.

Liposomes can induce either acute or chronic synovitis; this supports a phlogistic role for similar spherulites found in some patients.

D21

CHARACTERIZATION OF AN INTERLEUKIN-I INHIBITOR DERIVED FROM HUMAN SYNOVIAL FLUID. Jacob A. Aelion, Robert O. Endres and Arnold E. Postlethwaite. UTCHS, VAMC, Memphis, TN 38163.

Interleukin-1 (IL-1) is a macrophage derived mediator whose properties suggest that it could be an important mediator in arthritis. An IL-1 like factor has previously been isolated from human joint effusions and inflamed synovium. We observed the presence of an IL-1 inhibitor in synovial fluid collected from routine knee arthrocentesis in 75% (9/12) of rheumatoid and 70% (7/10) of osteoarthritic patients. The inhibitor suppresses both human and guinea-pig IL-1 activity as measured by the standard murine thymocyte proliferation assay but has no cytotoxic effect on thymocytes. It does not suppress interleukin-2(IL-2) activity as measured by an IL-2 dependent T-cell growth assay. The molecular weight of the inhibitor activity is heterogenous (250-60Kd), however, the maximal inhibitory activity consistently elutes in advance of IgG on Sephadex G-200. The presence of the inhibitor is not restricted to joint cavities. The inhibitor was also isolated from normal guinea-pig saline peritoneal washouts (30/30), 90% (9/10) of human cirrhotic ascitic fluids and is a constituent of normal human serum. The data suggest that an IL-1 inhibitor is present in synovial and other body fluids and may play an important role in controlling and modulating the biological effects of IL-1 in vivo.

D22

DO PEOPLE WITH ARTHRITIS LACK COMMITMENT TO WORK? Edward Yelin and Wallace Epstein. UCSF, San Francisco, CA 94117.

We analyzed the 1978 Social Security Survey of Disability and Work (SDA) to determine if: 1) persons with arthritis (ARTH) differ from those with other chronic conditions in commitment to work; and 2) persons with ARTH had different rates of work disability (cessation of work after onset of illness) when controlling for commitment to work, health and functional status, demographics, and physical and social characteristics of jobs (JOB). 6,405 individuals in the SDA had 1+ chronic conditions causing activity limitation. Of these, 4,002 (76%), had 1+ forms of ARTH. We first regressed each of 7 commitment to work variables (vars) on the absence(0)/presence(1) of ARTH, 6 health vars, 10 demographic vars, and 12 job vars. The 7 vars include two measures of satisfaction with work, four measures of alienation from work, and one measure of eligibility for disability programs one could receive if one left work. After controlling for health, demographic, and job vars, persons with ARTH did not have significantly less commitment to work ($p>.05$ by t-test) on any of the seven measures. We then regressed current work disability status (0=disabled, 1=working) on absence/presence of ARTH, as well as health, demographic, job vars and each commitment to work var. In each case, persons with ARTH were significantly more likely to be working than those with other chronic conditions, all other vars held constant. For example, after controlling for health, demographic, job vars and extent of boredom on job, persons with ARTH were 7% more likely to be working. We conclude that persons with ARTH have at least the same commitment to work as those with other conditions and, net of health, demographic, job vars and commitment to work, they are no more likely to stop working in the presence of illness.

D23

RELATIONSHIP BETWEEN HAND RADIOGRAPHS AND FUNCTIONAL HEALTH STATUS IN RHEUMATOID ARTHRITIS. M.G. Regan-Smith, G.T. O'Connor, C.K. Kwoh, L. Brown, E.M. Olmstead. Dartmouth-Hitchcock Medical Center, Hanover, NH 03756

A cross sectional study was conducted to assess if there was a significant correlation between the functional health status of individuals with rheumatoid arthritis(RA) and changes in their hand radiographs. Of 179 patients with classical or definite RA and no significant comorbidity 38 (22%) had radiographs of the hands taken within six months. Radiographic changes were classified according to the Steinbrocker criteria. All patients completed the Arthritis Impact Measurement Scales (AIMS) questionnaire and both the patients and the physicians rated the patient's physical functioning using a simple global index of physical health status. Correlations between radiograph stage, physician and patient ratings, and AIMS scores were calculated.

Radiograph Stage versus:	Rs*	p	
AIMS (physical score)	-.1000	.550	*Spearman's
Physician Rating	.0928	.579	rank order
Patient Rating	.0169	.920	correlation

There was poor correlation between the hand radiograph Steinbrocker stage and the AIMS score and the patient's or physician's rating of physical functioning. We conclude that RA patients' hand radiograph stage is not well correlated with either the patients' or the physicians' rating of the patient's functional health status or the AIMS, a comprehensive and well-validated health status indicator. We believe that this finding calls into question the clinical utility of using routine hand radiographs as a marker of functional health status in RA patients.

D24

CONCORDANCE BETWEEN CLINICIANS' AND PATIENTS' ASSESSMENT OF PHYSICAL AND MENTAL HEALTH STATUS. G.T.O'Connor, C.K. Kwoh, M.G. Regan-Smith, E.M. Olmstead, L.Brown, J.Burnett, R. Hochman, K.King, G.J. Morgan. Dartmouth-Hitchcock Medical Center, Hanover, NH 03756.

We examined the degree of concordance between clinicians' and patients' assessment of physical and mental health status in 176 consecutive eligible outpatients with definite or classical RA and no significant co-morbidity. The clinician and patient independently rated the patient's physical and mental functioning on similar four-category ordinal scales based on the Steinbrocker criteria. The percent agreement for physical disability was 60% and for mental disability it was 73%. The weighted Kappa statistic, an index of concordance that corrects for chance-related agreement, was .38 for physical disability and .31 for mental disability. These results show a low level of agreement between clinicians and patients in their rating of physical and mental disability. At all levels of mental disability and at high levels of physical disability, the patients' self-ratings indicated greater impairment as compared to the clinicians' ratings. In contrast, at low levels of physical disability, the clinicians' ratings indicated greater impairment as compared to the patients' self ratings.

We conclude: 1) Clinicians and patients with RA often disagree in their assessment of physical and mental health status; 2) This disagreement will differ in magnitude and direction depending on the specific type of disability (physical vs. mental) and on the level of disability present; 3) These disagreements may compromise the validity of studies using health status measures to assess therapeutic success or failure and 4) These disagreements need to be recognized and resolved when managing individual patients.

D25

COST-UTILITY ANALYSIS OF MANAGEMENT STRATEGIES FOR ASYMPTOMATIC HYPERURICEMIA IN A GERIATRIC POPULATION. C. J. Shamess, McMaster University, Hamilton.

Asymptomatic hyperuricemia predisposes to nephrolithiasis and gout but treatment is often withheld because acute events are rare and hypouricemic therapy may be toxic. This study compares the economic consequences of management methods from a societal viewpoint in the context of a specific medical center situated in Ontario, Canada. Mathematical models based on decreasing exponential functions of the form e^{-kt} were devised to simulate the following strategies in an asymptomatic hyperuricemic male geriatric population subject to ongoing mortality: I. No Rx until an acute event. Rx acute event only (No subsequent hypouricemic Rx); II. No Rx until an acute event. Rx acute event. Give subsequent lifetime hypouricemic Rx; III. Lifetime hypouricemic Rx from ascertainment. Costs are measured in 1983 Canadian dollars and consequences in quality-adjusted life years, both discounted to present value. Using fully allocated prices prevailing at the medical center, the OHIP (Medicare) fee schedule and the OHIP drug benefit formulary, several treatment scenarios were costed. Utilities were determined from a multiattribute model. Utility-cost ratios and incremental utility-cost ratios revealed that Strategy I was most efficient and Strategy III least so. Because of the inherent uncertainty of the data, a rigorous sensitivity analysis incorporating conditions least and most favorable to prophylaxis was undertaken. The strategies consistently retained their relative ranks, suggesting that, in an asymptomatic male hyperuricemic population, Strategy I is most efficient, while Strategy II is next best.

D26

RHEUMATOLOGISTS' MANAGEMENT PRACTICES IN "PURE" POLYMYALGIA RHEUMATICA: RISK-BENEFIT CONSIDERATIONS USING A DECISION ANALYTICAL MODEL. Rowland W. Chang, Theodore M. Pass, Emily Wen, Northwestern University Medical School, Chicago, IL 60611

A decision analysis of PMR management practices using published data suggested that in patients with PMR without cranial signs or symptoms ("pure" PMR), empiric treatment with high dose steriods was rarely warranted and the decision to do a temporal artery biopsy depended on risk-benefit considerations related to treatment toxicity and prevention of blindness (Med Decis Making 3:459-475, 1983). Recognizing that data in the literature may not represent the experience of clinicians, 392 adult rheumatologists sampled from the 1983 ARA Membership Directory were asked by mail to estimate probabilities of uncertain events which could occur in PMR and to indicate which management strategy they preferred in treating a patient with "pure" PMR. 204 (52%) of the initial sample responded to the questionnaire. Of the respondents, 73% favored empiric treatment with low dose steriods (Strategy A); 23% favored a temporal artery biopsy as the initial management step, treating positive biopsy patients with high dose steriods and negative biopsy patients with low dose steriods (Strategy B); 2% favored empiric treatment with high dose steriods (Strategy C) and 2% favored other non-specified strategies. A computer program which incorporated the original decision analytical model and Monte Carlo simulation was utilized to calculate expected occurrences of blindness (B) and of severe medication side effects (SE) and ranges of acceptable risk-benefit ratios (R-BR) for Strategies A, B, and C while taking into consideration the variability of the probability estimates. Mean outcomes for a typical analysis of 100 Monte Carlo simulations were:

Strategy	B(/10,000 cases)	SE(/10,000 cases)	R-BR(cases of severe toxicity /case of blindness averted)
A	231	500	< 1
B	64	670	1 to 24
C	0	2200	> 24

Again it appears that Strategy C is rarely warranted. The stability of these estimated outcomes given the variability of the probability estimates will be discussed.

D27

PLASMA PLASMINOGEN ACTIVATOR IN SYSTEMIC SCLEROSIS. E. Godín-Ostro, M. Mitrane, I. Heller, H.C. Kim, J.R. Seibold. UMDNJ-Rutgers Medical School, New Brunswick, N.J.

Plasminogen activator (PA) is an endothelial-derived protease important in endogenous fibrinolysis and in angiogenesis. We measured plasma PA levels by ELISA technique with goat antihuman tissue-type PA immunoglobulin in 50 samples from 36 patients with systemic sclerosis (SS) and 28 normal controls. Plasma was drawn from an antecubital vein without tourniquet and after at least 10 minutes of rest. Correlations of results of plasma PA assay were sought with extensive clinical and laboratory data compiled on these patients.

Levels of plasma PA in ng/ul were higher in SS patients (mean 8.06 ± 2.59) than in controls (6.98 ± 1.82) (P<0.05, paired t test). However only 7 (14%) of 50 SS patients had plasma PA>10.62 (mean + 2SD of normals). Patients with generalized SS (N=24) had higher levels (8.62 ± 3.03) than those with limited SS (7.54 ± 2.01, N=26) but this difference was not significant. Results in patients with early SS (<3y disease duration) (8.08 ± 2.52, N=31) were comparable to those with late SS (8.02 ± 2.75, N=19). SS patients with severe interstitial lung disease (x-ray fibrosis, D_LCO<50% predicted) had plasma PA elevations (10.61 ± 2.55, N=8) significantly higher than all SS patients (P<0.02). Plasma PA levels did not identify other patterns of visceral involvement including renal, gastro-intestinal, myocardial and sicca syndrome, nor did they identify digital ulcerations or correlate with severity of Raynaud's phenomenon or measures of in vivo platelet activation.

Our results are further evidence of endothelial damage in SS. Further study is required to gauge the utility of serial measurements in determining disease activity and/or response to therapy.

D28

COAGULATION STUDIES DURING COLD STIMULATION IN SYSTEMIC SCLEROSIS. Rafael G. Grau, Brenda L. Monson and Alfonse T. Masi. Univ. of Illinois, Peoria, IL 61656

In vivo release of factor VIII-related antigen (fVIII:rAg) after cold stimulation of patients with systemic sclerosis (SS) has been suggested to represent cold induced endothelial cell injury (Ann Intern Med 1981; 94:428). We report the effect of local cold stimulation on coagulation and endothelial cells, the latter as reflected by fVIII:rAg release. Six patients with SS and 6 age and sex matched controls were studied. The following assays were done on venous blood from the arm to receive the cold stimulation, before, during and 15 minutes after a 5 minute immersion into water at 15°C: fibrinopeptide A (FPA), fibrin(ogen) degradation products, fibrinogen, platelet aggregates (PA), platelet factor 4, β-thromboglobulin and fVIII:rAg.

Prior to the cold stimulation, only FPA levels (mean ± SD) of SS patients reached statistical significance when compared to control values (4.66 ± 2.01 ng/ml vs 2.25 ± 0.83 ng/ml, P<0.05). During cold stimulation, fVIII:rAg levels were significantly elevated as compared to control levels (133 ± 20% vs 95 ± 16%, P<0.04). Similar results were obtained with platelet aggregate levels (18 ± 7% vs 6 ± 4%, P<0.01). Post stimulation values of fVIII:rAg and PA did not reach statistical significance. These preliminary results support the hypothesis that cold stimulation induces platelet aggregation and injury to endothelial cells in SS patients.

D29

SPECIFICITY AND CLINICAL CORRELATIONS OF PROXIMAL NAILFOLD BIOPSIES IN CONNECTIVE TISSUE DISEASE. E.V.Lally, R.K.Scher, D.W.K.Tom, H.A.Bogaars. Brown University Program in Medicine, Providence, RI

In vivo capillary microscopy (IVCM) of the proximal nailfold (PNF) may provide diagnostic and prognostic data in patients (pts) with early connective tissue disease (CTD). Abnormalities on IVCM have been shown to correlate with histopathologic changes in biopsied specimens from the PNF. Thompson found characteristic PAS+ deposits in the cuticles of 14 of 15 pts with CTD or Raynaud's phenomenon only (RPO) but in none of 9 controls (Arthritis Rheum 27:97, 1984). In order to assess the specificity of these deposits for CTD, we performed biopsies of the PNF in 10 pts with CTD (4 CREST, 3 PSS, 1 dermatomyositis (DM), 2 undifferentiated CTD), 4 pts with RPO and 6 pts with non-CTD. Deposits in the cuticle were graded arbitrarily on a scale of 0-3+ according to the amount of material deposited. Eosinophilic, PAS+ material was found in 9 of 10 pts with CTD, 3 of 4 pts with RPO and 4 of 6 pts with non-CTD. Heavy deposits (2+,3+) were noted in 4 of 4 pts with CREST, 2 of 3 pts with PSS, 1 pt with DM, 1 pt with RPO and 2 pts with non-CTD. Heavy deposits were found in 6 of 7 pts with CTD and RP but in only 2 of 7 pts with RPO or CTD without RP. Eight of 8 pts with heavy deposits but only 2 of 9 pts with light deposits (1+) or no deposits had abnormal IVCM. The amount of PAS+ deposition correlated in general with the severity of capillary changes on IVCM. In pts with CTD, the presence or histologic grade of PAS+ deposits did not correlate with duration of symptoms, severity of the underlying disease or specific visceral organ involvement.

We conclude that the presence of PAS+ material in the PNF is not specific for CTD. The amount of PAS+ material correlates with the severity of IVCM patterns. The combination of heavy deposits and characteristic IVCM appears to be associated with RP secondary to CTD.

D30

RENAL VASCULAR HISTOLOGY AND MORPHOMETRY IN SYSTEMIC SCLEROSIS SUBSETS: A CASE-CONTROL AUTOPSY STUDY. David C. Trostle, Carlos D. Bedetti, Virginia Steen, Radwan Al-Sabbagh, Thomas A. Medsger, Jr., University of Pittsburgh, Pittsburgh, PA 15262

To examine the spectrum of renal vascular changes in systemic sclerosis (SS) we studied autopsy specimens in 9 CREST syndrome (CS) patients, 17 diffuse scleroderma (DS) patients and 9 additional DS patients with "renal crisis". Each patient had an age, race and sex-matched control. Light microscopic evaluation and morphometric measurements using a Zeiss image analyzer were completed on 4-16 (mean 9) arteries per patient. The vessels were arbitrarily divided by diameter: small (< 200μ), medium (200-325μ) and large (> 325μ) and the ratio of the intimal to medial areas (Ai/Am) and the percent luminal occlusion were determined (Virchows Arch A Path Anat Histol 385:351-359, 1980). For all sized arteries except medium and large vessels in CREST patients, the mean Ai/Am ratio was significantly greater in cases than controls in all SS subsets (p< 0.05). The small sized arteries of CS patients (p< 0.05) and small and medium sized vessels in both DS groups (p<0.01) had significantly increased luminal occlusion compared to controls. The Ai/Am ratio and the percent luminal occlusion were significantly greater in DS than CS in the small and medium sized arteries (p<0.05). The majority of non-renal DS and CS patients had moderate fibroelastic, sclerotic intimal thickening. Elastic lamina reduplication was more prevalent in SS patients without renal crisis and was correlated with disease duration in CS.

We conclude that many CS and DS patients without overt kidney disease have pathologic abnormalities of the renal arteries. Each variant has a different propensity to affect the vessels.

D31

GROWTH ASSESSMENT OF DERMAL FIBROBLASTS FROM TIGHT-SKINNED MICE.

Thomas G. Osborn, Nancy E. Bauer, Terry L. Moore. St. Louis University School of Medicine, St. Louis, MO 63104.

The tight-skinned (TSK) mouse has an autosomally dominant single gene different from the normal C57 mouse. The result of this single gene mutation is a marked proliferation of connective tissue components in its skin, lung, heart, fascia, and bone.

Previous studies have shown the TSK mouse to have an increase in its skin thickness, weight, collagen (hydroxyproline) content, and glycosaminoglycan content.

Light microscopy has revealed the thickened dermis is more cellular than normal. The vast majority of these cells are spindle-shaped, basophilic stained, and appear to be fibroblasts.

Fibroblasts cultured from newborn TSK and normal mouse dermis were obtained by sharp scalpel dissection and trypsin treatment. These cells were subsequently grown in parallel replicate 24-well plates. Following trypsin treatment cell viability was determined by trypan blue exclusion. Growth was assessed by counting live and dead cells at 24 hour intervals for 10 days.

Identical growth curves for living cells were found for TSK and normal mouse fibroblasts. Doubling time was 76 hours for both during the exponential growth phase. Total non-viable cell counts were the same for TSK and normal mice at each time.

These findings suggest the abundance of connective tissue in the skin of the TSK mouse is not due to an accelerated growth of this animal's fibroblasts.

D32

SIGNIFICANCE OF ANTICENTROMERE ANTIBODY IN IDIOPATHIC RAYNAUD'S SYNDROME.

J. Sarkozi, A.A.M. Bookman, P. Lee, E.C. Keystone, University of Toronto, Toronto, Canada, M.J. Fritzler, University of Calgary, Calgary, Canada.

Fifty-eight patients with idiopathic Raynaud's syndrome (IRS) followed prospectively on a standard protocol between November 1981 to June 1984 had serum analyzed for the presence of anticentromere antibody (ACA) using indirect immunofluorescence techniques on HEp-2 cell lines. Eighteen patients (31%) were ACA positive (ACA+), 17 with ACA titres $\geq 1/320$. Forty were ACA negative (ACA-).

The ACA+ and ACA- groups were comparable in age, sex distribution, duration of IRS, incidence of digital pits and ulcers, pulp atrophy, sclerodactyly, pulmonary function or esophageal motility abnormalities, rheumatoid factor, cryoglobulins, and low C3.

The ACA+ group demonstrated significantly more frequent digital telangiectases ($p<0.02$), digital edema ($p<0.001$), elevated immunoglobulins ($p<0.05$), and low C4 ($p<0.05$).

Photoplethysmography (PPG) on maximally vasodilated digits revealed significantly diminished digital blood flow (DBF) in the ACA+ group ($p<0.05$) using wave form analysis. Capillary microscopy revealed significantly increased avascularity ($p<0.001$) and number of dilated loops ($p<0.001$) in the ACA+ group. Giant loops were seen only in the ACA+ group ($p<0.01$).

We conclude that the presence of ACA in IRS is associated with greater impairment of DBF, and more profound capillary abnormalities than ACA- patients. Clinical findings in the ACA+ group are suggestive of a transition to connective tissue disease, with features of the CREST syndrome.

D33

MARKERS OF PROGRESSION TO SYSTEMIC ILLNESS IN RAYNAUD PHENOMENON (RP).

O.Fitzgerald, and E.V. Hess, University of Cincinnati Medical Center, Cincinnati, OH 45267, and C.Spencer-Green, Dartmouth-Hitchcock Medical Center, Hanover, NH 03756.

While RP is the most common presenting feature in systemic sclerosis (SS), markers in RP patients that predict eventual development of connective tissue disease (CTD) are unknown. To attempt to identify early markers of disease progression, we prospectively followed 58 patients (48F:10M, median age 35.2 years) who presented with either RP alone (37) or RP plus minor laboratory abnormalities but no definable CTD (21). At follow-up (mean 2.7 years), 11 patients had developed a definable CTD (3 SS, 8 CREST-like syndrome), and 23 patients remain free of identifiable disease other than RP. An additional 24 patients have clinical or laboratory abnormalities without defined disease including 7 with ANA+ (2RNP+, 1 SS-A+), 2 anticentromere antibody+, 1 SS-A+, and 14 patients with esophageal dysmotility who also had ANA+ (3), restrictive lung disease (2) or SS-A+ (2). At entry 9 patients had abnormal nailfold capillary pattern (NCP). During the period of observation, 2 of these 9 developed SS, 4 CREST syndrome and 2 digital ulceration (1 ANA+, 1 esophageal dysmotility). Only 1 patient has not evolved. Of the 11 patients who developed a definable CTD during the study period, all but 1 black patient whose capillaries could not be visualized had an abnormal NCP either at entry or during the follow-up period. In this study approximately 20% of all patients studied evolved to SS or CREST syndrome, 40% have nondiagnostic clinical or laboratory findings and 40% have RP only. Abnormal NCP is a sensitive and specific marker for progression to systemic illness in RP.

D34

IL-2 PRODUCTION BY PERIPHERAL MONONUCLEAR CELLS (PBM) FROM PATIENTS WITH DIFFUSE SCLERODERMA (PSS) IS ENHANCED AND IS HIGHLY CORRELATED WITH EXTENT OF SKIN INVOLVEMENT.

E. C. Keystone, A. Shore, S. Jaglal, M. Ramsden, P. Lee, D. Gladman, The Wellesley Hospital, Toronto, Ont. M4Y 1J3

Since augmented fibroblast proliferation may be pathogenetically important in PSS and IL-1 has been shown to regulate this proliferation, we studied Il-1 and Il-2 generation by peripheral blood adherence cell selected monocytes (AC) and PBM respectively from 17 patients with PSS, 14 patients with Psoriatic Arthritis (PsA) and 13 age and sex matched normals. Cells from each subject were cultured for IL-1 and IL-2 at the same time using optimal conditions previously established for normals. Supernatants from AC were assayed for IL-1 using the mouse thymocyte assay and supernatants from PBM were assayed for IL-2 using IL-2 dependent T cell proliferation. Supernatants were always assayed using six serial two-fold dilutions. Results were analyzed by using probit analysis to compare resulting test curves with those from a constant IL-1 and IL-2 standard and are expressed as units activity ± SE.

	IL-1	IL-2
PSS	77±17	52±9 †
PsA	80±16	24±4
Normal	69±14	29±4 † p<.01

Although isolated AC from PSS secrete normal amounts of IL-1, PBM from PSS generate excessive amounts of IL-2. Elevated IL-2 levels were seen almost exclusively in PSS patients with diffuse skin involvement (85 units ± 12) compared with those with limited involvement (33 units ± 5) ($p<0.01$). There was a highly significant correlation between the extent of skin involvement and the amount of IL-2 generated (Spearman Rank Correlation Coefficient $r=0.78, p=0.001$).

D35

SUPPRESSION OF ANTIGEN-SPECIFIC INTERLEUKIN-2 (IL-2) PRODUCTION BY MRL/MpJ-lpr/lpr and MRL/MpJ-+/+ LYMPH NODE CELLS.

S.J. Naides, B. Benacerraf and M.-S. Sy, Harvard Medical School, Boston, Massachusetts 02115

The MRL/MpJ-lpr/lpr (MRL-l) mouse strain develops a lupus-like autoimmune disease characterized by a massive lymphoproliferation of an abnormal "dull" Lyt 1^+, 2^- lymphocyte. By 5-6 months of age ("old"), MRL-l spleen and lymph node cells neither produce IL-2 in response to mitogen or antigen, nor respond to exogenous IL-2. Mice of the MRL/MpJ-+/+ (MRL-+) strain develop both a milder disease and the IL-2 defect at a later age than the MRL-l mouse. In order to determine if the failure to produce IL-2 is due to the presence of suppressor cells in MRL-l mice, naive MRL-l or MRL-+ lymph node cells (LN) were cocultured for 24 hours with LN from young MRL-+ mice primed to the hapten trinitrobenzene sulfonate (TNBS). Cultures included irradiated TNBS modified naive MRL-+ spleen cells as stimulators. Coculture of "old" MRL-l LN with an equal number of primed MRL-+ LN resulted in suppression of IL-2 production by 54-57% compared to control cultures. Coculture of 2-3 month old MRL-l LN resulted in 20-45% suppression. Coculture of naive MRL-+ LN resulted in suppression comparable to age matched MRL-l cells. However, coculture of H-2 syngeneic C3H/HeJ LN failed to suppress at all ages tested. Negative selection with anti-Lyt 1.2, but not anti-Thy 1.2 or Lyt 2.1, and complement partially but significantly reversed suppression by MRL-l cells. Anti-Lyt 1.2 selection had no effect on suppression by MRL-+ LN. Of interest, intravenous transfer of "old" MRL-l LN into primed MRL-+ mice markedly suppressed hapten-specific IL-2 responses tested seven days later. Transfer of young MRL-l or "old" MRL-+ LN, or "old" MRL-l or MRL-+ spleen cells had no effect. Thus, lymph node cells from mice of the MRL background contain cell(s) capable of suppressing antigen-specific IL-2 responses *in vitro*. *In vivo* expression of suppressor cell function may play a role in the development of both the IL-2 defect and disease expression.

D36

EVIDENCE FOR EXPRESSION OF ENDOGENOUS RETROVIRUS PROTEINS ON THE SURFACE OF PRECURSOR OR REGULATORY CELLS DURING B CELL DIFFERENTIATION.

T. Pincus and B. Alberto, Vanderbilt University, Nashville, TN.

Retrovirus proteins are expressed during B cell differentiation in cultures of mouse spleen cells exposed to bacterial lipopolysaccharide (LPS). After 4 days in culture, approximately 40% of living mononuclear cells express cytoplasmic mu chains, while 2-15% express cytoplasmic retrovirus proteins. Almost all cells which express retrovirus proteins also express mu chains. Addition of anti-mu antibodies to these cultures results not only in suppression of mu chain expression, as noted previously by others, but also in suppression of retrovirus proteins, despite enhanced cellular proliferation. Addition of antibodies to retrovirus proteins also results in suppression of cytoplasmic retrovirus proteins and mu chains. However, retrovirus antisera are suppressive of these proteins by suppressing cell proliferation and viable cells recovery. Suppression by retrovirus antisera involves primarily IgG, rather than other serum proteins, and is greatest using antisera to whole virus or envelope glycoproteins, rather than to internal structural proteins. Retrovirus proteins and mu chains do not co-cap on the cell surface, and therefore reciprocal inhibition by antisera to these proteins is not explained for the basis of physical interactions at the cell surface. These data indicate interactions between mu chains and retrovirus proteins at two stages of B cell differentiation: a) activation of the retrovirus genome occurs concomitant with mu chain expression; b) retrovirus proteins are expressed on the surface of a precursor or regulatory cell, rendering B cell differentiation suppressible by retrovirus antisera.

D37

ACCESSORY CELLS (AC) IN RHEUMATOID SYNOVIAL TISSUE AND FLUID. David M. Spalding and Marianne Egan. University of Alabama at Birmingham. Birmingham, AL 35294.

We have examined AC activity of populations from rheumatoid synovial fluid and Dispase[R] digested synovial tissue which have been separated on the basis of adherence and bouyant density (ρ). Oxidative mitogenesis, which assesses incorporation of ^{3}HTdR by periodate treated human T cells, was used to detect accessory cell activity. In synovial fluid essentially all AC activity was detected in non-adherent populations with $\rho<1.078$. Studies with synovial tissue cells from three patients using populations separated by density on discontinuous BSA gradients were next performed: example - 5 x 10^5 periodate treated T cells co-cultured with 25 x 10^3 non-adherent synovial cells of $\rho<1.063$, $\rho=1.068\rightarrow1.063$, $\rho=1.078\rightarrow1.068$, $\rho>1.078$ or adherent cells showed ^{3}HTdR incorporation of 20729, 6348, 4148, 4248 and 3570 CPM respectively. Dose response curves with graded number of cells from each fraction demonstrated an 8-12 fold enrichment for accessory activity in the lowest density cells ($\rho<1.063$). Simultaneous examination of cell preparations by phase contrast microscopy showed a cell type morphologically resembling mouse spleen dendritic cells predominantly in the $\rho<1.063$ population and totally absent from the high density ($\rho>1.078$) population. Ia^+ cells were detected in all fractions and constituted 25-56% of the cells but only the lowest density fractions ($\rho<1.068$) contained a large, intensely Ia staining cell type with cytoplasmic veils. These data suggest that AC are present in rheumatoid synovium and that AC activity correlates best with the presence of a very low density cell with morphologic features and an Ia staining pattern compatible with dendritic cells. These DC in rheumatoid synovia resemble those previously described in peripheral blood but lack an adherent phase.

D38

DIFFERENT EFFECTS OF CALCIUM IONOPHORE AND PHORBOL MYRISTATE ACETATE ON IMMATURE AND MATURE T CELL PROLIFERATION. C. Sandborg, M. Berman, B. Andrews, G. Friou, B. Calabia. Univ. Calif. Irvine, Irvine, CA 92717.

The effects of calcium ionophore(A23187) and phorbol myristate acetate(PMA) on mouse thymocytes and human lymphocytes were studied. A23187(.25uM) was used for its effects on increasing intracellular Ca^{2+} and PMA(2.5ng/ml) for its ability to activate protein kinase C. PMA alone was mitogenic for both human lymphocytes depleted of macrophages by adherence and human T cells purified by E rosettes, however, A23187 was mitogenic only for the macrophage depleted whole lymphocyte fraction. This mitogenic effect of PMA was enhanced by IL-1 or PHA and to a lesser degree by IL-2. IL-1, PMA+A23187 and IL-1+A23187 resulted in only minimal proliferation (2X background). In contrast, only the combination of PMA and A23187 led to thymocyte proliferation, whereas either one alone had no effect. PMA with lug/ml PHA also induced marked proliferation as did purified IL-1 with A23187 though to a lesser extent. The combinations PMA+IL-1, IL-2+PMA, IL-2+A23187, or PHA +A23187 did not lead to thymocyte proliferation. Serum-free medium+ transferrin did not support proliferation with either IL-1+PHA or PMA+ A23187. PMA+A23187 had no direct effect on an IL-2 dependent T cell line(CTLL), but stimulated large amounts of IL-2 to be produced by thymocytes. Neither PMA nor A23187 alone stimulated IL-2 production in thymocytes. An inhibitor(MW 50-100K) of IL-1 and IL-2 activity markedly inhibited the action of PMA+A23187 on thymocytes. The suppressive activity of this inhibitor was reversed by large amounts of IL-2 in the IL-2 assay, suggesting its site of action is inhibition of IL-2/receptor interaction. These results suggest that 2 signals are required to stimulate IL-2 production and IL-2 receptor expression in immature T cells, whereas more mature T cells may require only 1 signal.

D39

HIGH LEVELS OF IN VITRO IgM-RHEUMATOID FACTOR (RF) SYNTHESIS BY BLOOD MONONUCLEAR CELLS CORRELATE WITH HLA-DR4 IN NORMAL INDIVIDUALS. N. Olsen, P. Stastny, H.E.Jasin. University of Texas Health Science Center Southwestern Medical School, Dallas Texas 75235

The HLA-DR4 histocompatibility type is correlated with seropositive but not seronegative rheumatoid arthritis. The possibility that the DR4 haplotype is associated with in vitro IgM-RF synthesis was investigated in 35 normal subjects using cultures containing 50,000 B cells, 50,000 T cells and pokeweed mitogen. When total T cells were used, there was no significant difference in IgM-RF synthesis between DR4(+) and DR4(-) donors. However, when the T population was depleted of OKT8(+) suppressor cells, significant differences emerged. For 13 DR4(+) donors, mean IgM-RF synthesis was 13.6±3.6 ng and 22 DR4(-) donors had a corresponding mean of 5.3±1.4 ng (p=0.0167). Moreover, 6 of 8 high responders (HR; RF>12.0 ng) were DR4(+) while only 7 of 27 low responders (LR;RF<12.0 ng) were DR4(+) (p=0.035). The DR4(+) group also produced higher levels of total IgM (25.2 μg/ml) than the DR4(-) group (14.1 μg/ml; p=0.025). However, relative specificity for RF was shown by the mean RF/M ratio of 1.03 for DR4(+) HR compared to 0.40 for DR4(-) LR (p=0.026). There was no significant difference between the number of circulating B cells between HR (6.9±0.6%) and LR (8.1±1.2%). Mixing experiments with B and T8-depleted populations demonstrated that high responses were associated with HR B cells and not HR T cells. The data indicate that a subset of DR4(+) normal individuals have an expansion of the RF-specific B cell precursor population which may facilitate RF synthesis. Environmental factors may than act to trigger clinical disease in a genetically susceptible individual.

D40

INHIBITION BY CYCLOSPORIN A (CSA) OF GROUP A STREPTOCOCCAL CELL WALL (SCW)-INDUCED ARTHRITIS AND HEPATIC GRANULOMAS IN RATS. DE Yocum*, JB Allen, SM Wahl, GB Calandra, and RL Wilder. NIH, Bethesda, MD 20205.

The effects of CsA, an inhibitor of T helper/inducer lymphocyte activation, on the development of SCW-induced arthritis and hepatic granulomas in LEW/N female rats were investigated. Continuous daily treatment with CsA (25 mg/kg/day) beginning 24 hours prior to or up to 13 days after SCW administration and continued to 6 weeks, significantly inhibited the chronic, proliferative, erosive synovitis(p 0.05). Chronic arthritic indices(AI, range 0-16) at 42 days were as follows (Mean ± SEM):

	SCW only	SCW + CSA from day: -1 to 42	7 to 42	13 to 42
AI	9.7 ± 0.6	2.4 ± 0.7	1.5 ± 0.4	3.5 ± 0.8

In contrast, treatment only during the acute phase (day -1 to 12) of the arthritis did not inhibit the development of the chronic disease. When CsA was stopped at 6 weeks, its effect was maintained for at least another 5 weeks (AI=1.2 ± 0.3), demonstrating long term benefit without continued administration of the drug. Histologic examination of the joints demonstrated significantly less synovial proliferation and bone erosion in the CsA treated animals. Similar inhibition of the SCW-induced hepatic granuloma formation was observed. These data provide additional evidence for an important role of the T helper/inducer lymphocyte in this experimental model and suggest that CsA may be a useful probe in defining molecular and cellular processes involved in chronic erosive synovitis.

D41

NATURALLY OCCURRING POLYCLONAL B CELL ACTIVATOR OF NORMAL AND AUTO-ANTIBODY RESPONSES. David A. Bell, Michael J. Atkinson and Sharwan K. Singhal. UWO, London, Ontario, Canada, N6A 5A5.

We have previously reported on the immunogenicity of LMW DNA (~160 BP) molecules in normal and preautoimmune mice. These protein free DNA molecules could be readily obtained from thymocyte cell free supernatant (S/N) cultures and their immunogenic effects were specific for DNA. We now report on the presence of a naturally occurring polyclonal B cell activator (sPBA) isolated from autoimmune and some normal mouse spleen cell culture S/N. This S/N when separated from a relatively LMW inhibitor we have previously termed SIF (<10,000 daltons) is mitogenic for spleen cells and was observed to have a direct mitogenic effect on T cell, macrophage depleted spleen cells, and bone marrow cells, but not thymocytes. sPBA lacks properties associated with Il-1 or Il-2 or endotoxin. sPBA can stimulate polyclonal antibody responses in vitro in the presence or absence of added antigen in addition to significantly augmenting anti-DNA antibody responses in vitro in normals or in vivo in preautoimmune B/W mice. sPBA is able to augment IgG as well as IgM anti-DNA antibody responses in vitro. Physical-chemical studies suggest that sPBA is a protein-DNA complex of 120,000-180,000 daltons with properties of nucleosomes. The DNA moiety of the active material behaves in a manner identical in ethidium bromide stain gels to the LMW immunogenic DNA previously described. The protein (histone?) moiety of sPBA, lacking in LMW DNA may be responsible for its property of polyclonally activating B cells.

This naturally occurring molecule may play an important role as an endogenous polyclonal B cell activator in autoimmune susceptible mice.

D42

STAPHYLOCOCCUS AUREUS COWAN I IS A POTENT STIMULUS OF IgM RHEUMATOID FACTOR PRODUCTION. Leslie Tar, Ciro Carafa, and Arnold I. Levinson. University of Pennsylvania and Veterans Administration Medical Center, Philadelphia, PA 19104.

Polyclonal B cell activation may result in the production of rheumatoid factor (RF). Staphylococci and their cell wall components are polyclonal B cell activators (PBA) of potential clinical significance but it is not known how often or how prominently they elicit RF production. We studied IgMRF production of peripheral blood mononuclear cells (PBM) stimulated in vitro with protein A containing S. aureus Cowan I (SAC), protein A negative S. aureus Wood strain (Sansorbin) or PWM, a standard PBA. We cultured PBM from 8 healthy volunteers for 7 days with varying concentrations of these agents and measured IgMRF, total IgM and IgG responses in culture supernatants by ELISA. We observed greater IgMRF responses in cultures stimulated by SAC (17.4ng/ml ± 6, mean ± SEM) than by Sansorbin (0.9ng/ml ± 0.4, p < 0.025) or by PWM (1.9ng/ml ± 0.6, p < 0.025). We observed IgMRF production (>2.5ng/ml) in cultures of a) 8/8 subjects stimulated with SAC, b) only 1/8 subjects stimulated with Sansorbin and c) 4/8 subjects stimulated with PWM. All 3 agents induced significant polyclonal IgG and IgM responses and the higher magnitude and frequency of SAC induced IgMRF responses were not due to more prominent total IgM responses to this agent. SAC is a powerful stimulus of RF production and this property may relate to its protein A content. It should prove useful in exploring the activation of precursors of RF secreting cells which are likely present in most healthy individuals.

D43

DIFFERENTIAL EXPRESSION OF IgG3 and IgG4 ANTI-Fab ANTIBODIES IN RHEUMATOID ARTHRITIS.

J.E. Persselin and R.H. Stevens, UCLA School of Medicine, Los Angeles, CA 90024

We have found most serum anti-Fab antibodies (aFABA) in rheumatoid arthritis (RA) to be acidic IgG molecules which show clonal restriction and circulate as immune complexes. The acidic nature of these aFABA suggested their being minor subclasses as most IgG molecules are alkaline. Twenty RA, 10 normal, and 10 systemic lupus erythematosus (SLE) sera were chromatofocused (CF) over a pH of 8 to 5, and the distribution of IgG aFABA subclasses were quantitated by ELISA using monoclonal antisera. Acidic IgG4 and IgG3 aFABA comprised the majority of IgG aFABA in 15/20 of the RA sera. Although IgG3 and IgG4 aFABA also predominated in the normal and SLE populations, the levels were lower in both normal (p .001) and SLE (p .001) sera. When aFABA levels were elevated in normal sera, they tended to be IgG4, whereas elevated aFABA in SLE tended to be IgG3. Urea treatment of sera and preparative isolation of aFABA by CF prior to ELISA were necessary for maximum detection of all IgG aFABA subclasses.

Anti-Fab antibody clonotypic and IgG aFABA subclass analyses were also performed on serial samples of serum obtained from individual RA patients over 1 to 60 week periods of time. The aFABA clonotypes and IgG3 and IgG4 aFABA levels in several RA sera showed temporal changes, in some cases in as little as 1 week. Furthermore, changes in IgG3 and IgG4 aFABA levels tended to be inversely correlated.

These data indicate that most aFABA in human sera are comprised of minor IgG subclasses, with elevated levels of IgG3 and IgG4 aFABA in RA. When elevated, aFABA tend to be IgG4 in normal individuals and IgG3 in SLE patients. Additionally, aFABA expression appears to be a dynamic process. This suggests: 1) a possible role for the minor subclasses of IgG in the regulation of immune responses, 2) variable abberant aFABA expression in autoimmune disorders, and 3) differential IgG3 and IgG4 aFABA expression in RA may reflect alterations in disease activity and/or therapeutic intervention.

D44

RHEUMATOID FACTOR IDIOTYPE CROSS-REACTIVITY IN RHEUMATOID ARTHRITIS PATIENT SERA.

J. L. Nelson, F.A. Nardella, M. Mannik. U. of Wa. Seattle, WA 98195.

Idiotypic cross-reactivity with each of 3 rheumatoid factors (RFs) was evaluated testing a panel of sera from patients with rheumatoid arthritis (RA). Rabbits were immunized with the $F(ab')_2$ of two IgG RFs and one IgM RF. Rabbit antisera were adsorbed over normal human serum and normal $F(ab')_2$ columns. A liquid phase radioimmunoassay (RIA) was used to detect RF (Id) antiId binding. Each rabbit antiId bound its own Id and did not bind normal IgG, normal $F(ab')_2$, Fc, or a monoclonal IgM. Normal rabbit $F(ab')_2$ did not bind to the RFs. The amount of normal IgG present in the serum samples did not inhibit the Id-antiId interactions. Therefore, whole serum could be used to test for cross-reactivity to the RF Ids. A panel of 42-51 RA sera and another of normal sera were tested in each of three Id-antiId systems. No serum caused complete inhibition of an Id-antiId interaction, however, partial inhibition by some RA sera was observed with 13 of 51 and 3 of 49 in the IgG RF systems, and 21 of 42 in the IgM RF system. This partial inhibition of RA sera was not striking, since 1 µl or less of autologous serum caused 50% inhibition in each assay, whereas even 150 µl of each of the RA sera caused less than 50% inhibition. These inhibition studies suggest that private idiotypes are prominant on IgG RFs as recognized by polyclonal xenogenic antisera.

D45

SELECTIVITY OF ANTINUCLEAR ANTIBODY PRODUCTION IN MURINE LUPUS.

Brian L. Kotzin, Henry N. Claman, Ronald E. Arndt, Joseph P. Portanova. V.A. Medical Center and University of Colorado, Denver, CO 80220.

Anti-histone antibodies (AHA) and anti-ssDNA antibodies are produced in high levels in SLE and in murine models of lupus. To study the selectivity of this production, we measured serum levels of these autoantibodies, antibodies to different self and heterologous non-nuclear antigens, and total Ig levels.

IgM AHA and anti-DNA antibodies were elevated at 3-4 months of age in NZB/NZW mice compared to non-autoimmune mice. However, because of a general increase in IgM levels, there was little evidence for selective production at this young age. From ~4-7 months of age, there was a dramatic increase in IgG (but not IgM) AHA and anti-DNA antibodies (>500 and >200 fold, N=30) while total IgG levels increased by less than 2 fold. (C57BL/6 x DBA/2) F_1 mice injected with DBA/2 lymphoid cells develop chronic graft vs host disease (GVH) and very high serum levels of IgG AHA and anti-DNA, as well as lupus-like disease. During GVH, these autoantibodies increased 20-200 fold, while antibodies to a variety of other mouse proteins and total IgG levels did not increase. Spleen cells from GVH mice spontaneously produced antibodies to histones but not to mouse fibrinogen, hemoglobin, or transferrin. In contrast, lipopolysaccharide-stimulated normal F_1 cells produced antibodies to histones and equivalent amounts to the other antigens, indicating that B cells with all specificities were present.

These data as well as preliminary studies in MRL mice indicate that antinuclear antibody production in murine lupus is selective and not solely due to generalized B cell activation, and emphasize the likely importance of antigen-specific cellular interactions with certain forms of self-antigens.

D46

DECREASED CR1 IN SYSTEMIC LUPUS ERYTHEMATOSUS: ACQUIRED OR INHERITED?

Asad Zoma, Elizabeth Holme, Anne Fyfe and Keith Whaley. University Departments of Pathology and Medicine, University of Glasgow, Scotland.

Clearing of antigen-antibody complexes (IC) is partly facilitated by its interaction with receptors for C3b (CR1), the activated third component of complement. Wilson et al (1) recently reported decreased numbers of erythrocyte CR1 in patients with systemic lupus erythematosus (SLE). Our study was undertaken to further elucidate the distribution of CR1 and its relationship to disease activity in SLE. Erythrocyte CR1 was measured using ^{125}I-labelled $F(ab')_2$ anti-CR1. The mean numbers of receptor sites were 380 (range 332-5871) and 229 (range 0-4500) in 46 normal subjects and 19 SLE patients respectively. The distribution of receptor site numbers in both normals and SLE patients was distinctly unimodal. From our study we conclude that the reduced numbers of CR1 in SLE is an acquired abnormality for the following reasons: 1) Family studies do not support the notion that low numbers of CR1 in SLE patients are inherited. 2) Levels of CR1 are lower in patients with active rather than inactive SLE.

It therefore appears that reduced numbers of CR1 are a consequence rather than a cause of SLE. The observation that CR1 numbers are also reduced in other immune complex diseases such as rheumatoid arthritis lends support to this argument.

1. Wilson, JG et al. N Engl J Med 1982; 16: 981-86.

D47

KINETIC STUDIES OF THE CLEARANCE OF ANTIBODY(AB)/RADIOLABELED dsDNA IMMUNE COMPLEXES (IC) FROM RABBIT CIRCULATION.

R.P. Taylor, G.A. Kujala, J. Edberg and J.S. Davis, IV, Univ. of VA. Charlottesville,VA.

When Ab/dsDNA IC containing high MW PM2 dsDNA and 7S IgG Ab are injected into the circulation of rabbits, >90% of the input counts are rapidly cleared in a single exponential process (t 1/2=80 seconds). If the dsDNA is of lower MW (LMW-dsDNA, 100,000 to 500,000 Daltons), 75% of the input counts are cleared in a slower exponential process (t 1/2=140 seconds) and the majority of the residual radiolabeled DNA circulates for periods of >15 minutes, and remains insoluble in 5% trichloroacetic acid (TCA). Farr assays confirmed the DNA was Ab bound. If the Ab is reduced and alkylated (R/A 7S IgG) to inhibit complement fixation, t 1/2 for clearance of the IC with LMW-dsDNA increases to 270 seconds for 60% of the input counts. Most of the residual DNA persisting in the circulation remains insoluble in 5% TCA. If the IC are prepared with R/A 7S IgG Ab, LMW-dsDNA, and Rheumatoid Factor, 75% of the input counts are cleared in a rapid exponential process (t 1/2=75 seconds). If normal human IgG is used in place of anti-dsDNA, >75% of the input counts are cleared in a rapid process (t 1/2=60 seconds) for LMW-dsDNA, and only a small amount of the residual radiolabelled DNA remains insoluble in 5% TCA. These results suggest that IC may persist in the circulation of non-primates for extended periods if our proposed platelet mediated IC clearance mechanism is compromised. The results in this animal model system should have significant parallel implications for the erythrocyte IC clearance mechanism in human IC mediated diseases such as SLE.

D48

ANTI-IDIOTYPIC (ID) ANTIBODIES TO ANTI-DR IN PATIENTS WITH RHEUMATOID ARTHRITIS (RA).

Susan M. Savage, Robert P. Searles, Gary M. Troup, and James S. Goodwin. Lovelace Medical Foundation and University of New Mexico School of Medicine, Albuquerque, NM, 87108.

We have previously reported that RA patients have anti-DR antibodies (Arth.Rheum. 26:486,1983). These antibodies could be antigenic by virtue of the hypervariable region causing the production of anti-id antibodies. Therefore, RA sera were examined for potential anti-id antibodies to anti-DR. Anti-id were identified using an ELISA method with murine monoclonal anti-DR-coated plates incubated serially with either normal or RA sera and peroxidase goat anti-human Fc. Significant binding of 5/14 (36%) RA sera (O.D.=.200±.060) (Mean±SD) to anti-DR was found compared to 0/44 normals (O.D.=.030±010) (P<.01). No binding was found to the following monoclonal antibodies: anti-cytochrome c, anti-breast tumor antigen, anti-M5 (monocyte) or anti-OKT8 (suppressor). However, RA sera also showed binding to anti-Leu 3a (helper/inducer). Differential specificity of anti-id in RA sera for anti-DR was demonstrated by competitive inhibition studies using monoclonal anti-DR and anti-Leu3a. Moreover, anti-id were entirely absorbed by monoclonal anti-DR but not anti-Leu3a or anti-OKT8.

In addition, anti-DR antibodies were determined in RA sera by ELISA method as per cent inhibition by RA sera of peroxidase goat anti-mouse IgG binding to murine monoclonal anti-DR-coated plates. The results show anti-DR antibodies correlated with the simultaneous presence of anti-id antibodies in 4 of the 5 anti-id-positive RA patients. We conclude that some RA patients have anti-id-like antibodies potentially involved in immunoregulation of anti-DR antibodies.

D49

PURIFICATION AND N-TERMINAL AMINO ACID SEQUENCE OF PROLIFERATING CELL NUCLEAR ANTIGEN (PCNA). K. Ogata, Y. Ogata, R.M. Nakamura and E.M. Tan. Scripps Clinic and Research Foundation, La Jolla, Ca.

PCNA is a nuclear protein related to cell proliferation and blast transformation and is also known as cyclin. Autoantibody to PCNA occurs in 3% of patients with lupus.

PCNA was extracted from rabbit thymus acetone powder in PBS, pH 7.2. This extract was fractionated with ammonium sulfate and purified by DEAE-Sephacel, HPLC ion exchange, and HPLC gel filtration column chromatography. PCNA was concentrated more than 1,400 times and was analyzed by SDS-PAGE and immunoblotting. SDS-PAGE showed that a 36K protein was selectively isolated and this protein was identified as PCNA by the immunoblotting. Other previously identified nuclear antigens, Sm, U1-RNP, SS-A/Ro, SS-B/La, histones and DNA were not present in this preparation. Purified PCNA was electrophoretically eluted from SDS gel slices of the 36K protein and analyzed, and has the following N-terminal amino acid sequence:

1 2 3 4 5 6 7 8 9 10 11 12 13 14 15 16 17
Met-Phe-Glu-Ala-Arg-Leu-Val-Gln-Gly-( )-Ile-Leu-Lys-Lys-Val-Leu-Glu-
18 19 20 21 22 23 24 25 26
Ala-Leu-Lys-Asp-Leu-Ile-Asn-Glu-Ala-

The amino acid sequence of PCNA/cyclin was found to be unique and showed little sequence homology with existent proteins in nationwide computer databanks. The current information will be useful in designing experiments such as gene cloning and other studies to determine its function in regulating cell proliferation and transformation.

D50

ANTINUCLEAR ANTIBODIES IN THE FAMILIES OF PATIENTS WITH SYSTEMIC SCLEROSIS R.S.Pereira, P.J.Maddison, and U.K. Scleroderma Study Group. West Middlesex Hospital (Isleworth), Royal National Hospital for Rheumatic Diseases (Bath), Northwick Park Hospital (Harrow), Hope Hospital (Salford), and Leeds General Infirmary (Leeds), U.K.

The families of 60 patients with progressive systemic sclerosis were examined clinically and serum samples from each subject were tested for anti-nuclear antibodies(ANA) by immunofluorescence on HEp-2 cells and for precipitating antibodies to soluble cellular antigens including Scl-70.

Of 272 blood relatives, 57(21%) had ANA (41 speckled, 5 nucleolar, 7 both, 2 centromere, 2 homogeneous); 28(10%) had precipitins (2 anti-Ro+anti-La, 1 anti-nRNP,remainder unidentified). Family members tended to share ANA patterns. Of 36 spouses, 9 (25%) had ANA (8 speckled, 1 centromere) and 2 showed (unidentified) precipitins. This compares with an incidence of ANA and precipitins in a control population of 10% and 1% respectively. Seven patients (two of whom were related), but no other relatives, had antibodies to Scl-70 antigen. Antibodies were more common in female than male relatives (particularly in mothers and daughters of probands). 27 of the 57 family members with ANA had clinical features of connective tissue disease; the remainder were asymptomatic.

The presence of genetic factors influencing auto-immunity is suggested by the incidence of auto-antibodies in first degree relatives; however, similar observations in spouses indicates that environmental factors may also have a role in these immune abnormalities.

D51

PREFERENTIAL BINDING OF SLE ANTIBODIES TO LOW MOLECULAR WEIGHT DNA AND Z-DNA. M. R. Liebling, T. Schulte, and J.S. Louie, Harbor-UCLA Medical Center, Torrance, California.

Antibodies directed against DNA are a hallmark of systemic lupus erythematosus (SLE). The reactivity of these antibodies with endogenous and exogenous DNA was compared. DNA was obtained from dividing SLE peripheral blood mononuclear cells and separated into low (L) and high (H) molecular weight fractions by sucrose density centrifugation. Calf thymus was used as the source of exogenous DNA (CT-DNA). Employing a solid phase radioimmunoassay, SLE sera (24) uniformly displayed greater binding to L-DNA (5738 ± 535 CPM) than to H-DNA (1660 ± 79 CPM) or CT-DNA (1515 ± 130 CPM). p<0.001. This binding was not related to the quantities of DNA fixed to the solid phase. Moreover, normal sera (4) failed to show significant binding to any DNA.

Because L-DNA has a high content of guanine-cytosine residues, the specificity of antibodies in SLE sera (10) was examined with the following artificial polynucleotides: 1) poly dG-dC, 2) poly dG-me^{5}dC (Z-DNA), 3) poly dAdT, 4) poly G, and 5) poly C. The predominant binding was directed against Z-DNA or poly dG-dC, in quantities similar to the binding to L-DNA (Table). These observations can be linked by the hypothesis that the SLE antibodies to endogenous L-DNA are directed against poly dG-dC determinants in a Z conformation. Preliminary inhibition studies support this hypothesis.

Table. Binding of SLE Sera[a] to Polynucleotides

	L-DNA	Z-DNA	dG-dC	dA-dT	poly G	poly C
CPM	30.469	29.682	31.708	12.232	11.382	10.936
± SE	2.466	2.559	3.491	655	693	733

a - all sera (10) diluted 1:10.000

D52

PROSPECTIVE STUDY OF TREATMENT IN POLYARTERITIS NODOSA (PAN). Aileen M. Dillon, Doyt L. Conn, Stephen D. Armstrong, Duane M. Ilstrup. Mayo Clinic, Rochester, MN 55905.

21 patients with active PAN were randomized to receive Prednisone (T1) or Prednisone plus Cyclophosphamide (T2), and studied prospectively to determine clinical indicators of outcome and the effect of treatment. Cyclophosphamide dose was initially 2 mg/kg/day and Prednisone was 60 mg/day in divided doses. Twelve randomized to T1, 9 to T2.

There were 14 males, 7 females, mean age 63.7 yrs (range 35-78). The duration from onset of symptoms to diagnosis was 0.5-12 mo ($\bar{m}$ 4.6). The followup was 2-48 mo ($\bar{m}$ 24.6). Five deaths occurred, 3 on T1, 2 on T2. All occurred early, 2.0-7.5 mo ($\bar{m}$ 4.4) - 2 due to vasculitis, 2 superimposed infection, 1 unknown.

The mean followup on those alive was 31 mo. Of 9 remaining on T1, 8 are in remission - 5 off Prednisone and 3 on <10 mg/day. One failed to respond, but improved on T2. Of the 7 remaining on T2, 4 are off therapy and 1 is controlled on low doses. Cyclophosphamide was stopped for side effects in 2 - aphthous stomatitis and leukopenia in 1, and hemorrhagic cystitis in 1; both are now in remission. Projected two year survival was 75% for T1, 78% T2, and 76% overall.

Visceral angiograms were performed on 15; 4 were normal, 6 showed extensive involvement and 5 mild-moderate involvement. The type and number of organs involved clinically and by angiography, initial Hb <9 gm/dl, creatinine >2 gm/dl, proteinuria or hematuria >grade 2, low serum complement or abnormal liver function tests did not affect outcome.

In this small number of patients, we were unable to detect different outcomes in the two treatment groups.

D53

INFLAMMATORY ARTHRITIS ASSOCIATED WITH FOLLICULAR OCCLUSION. J.M. Lipstate, W.D. Blackburn, J.M. Guyton, and G.S. Alarcón. University of Alabama at Birmingham, Birmingham, AL 35294.

Six patients are described with inflammatory arthritis and one or more features of the follicular occlusion (FO) triad of hidradenitis suppurativa (HS), acne congoblata (AC), or dissecting cellulitis of the scalp (DCS). All patients are black, 4 females and 2 males, varying in age from 16 to 54. Skin disease and arthritis appeared concurrently in 3 patients, skin lesions preceded arthritis in 2 patients by 3 and 14 years, and arthritis anteceded skin lesions by 6 years in 1 patient. All patients had HS, additionally, 2 patients had AC, 1 patient had DCS, and a fourth iritis and pyoderma gangrenosum. Five patients had peripheral arthritis most commonly involving the ankle, wrist, knee, PIP, MCP, and MTP joints. Half of the patients had axial involvement with radiographic evidence of spondyloarthropathy. All had elevated erythrocyte sedimentation rates and negative rheumatoid factor, whereas antinuclear antibody test was negative in 5 patients screened. Four patients were anemic and 3 had a mild leukocytosis. Inflammatory synovial fluid was found in 2 of 3 patients, and a synovial biopsy performed on 1 patient demonstrated synovial hyperplasia with acute and chronic inflammatory infiltrates. The cases reported here and by Rosner et al. (Ann. Intern Med. 97:520, 1982) further suggest an association between an inflammatory arthritis and FO. A large number of these patients seem to develop evidence of a spondyloarthropathy. A study to determine the frequency of arthritis in patients with FO is currently underway.

D54

THE CLINICAL SIGNIFICANCE OF GIANT CELLS IN TEMPORAL ARTERITIS. C. Michael Franklin, James L. Perruquet, Peter Cera, Thomas M. Harrington, and Dennis Torretti. Geisinger Medical Center, Danville, Pennsylvania 17822.

The clinical significance of the presence of giant cells on temporal artery biopsy in temporal arteritis remains uncertain. In an effort to define any differences between patients with giant cell arteritis and temporal arteritis without giant cells, we reviewed the clinical course of all patients with biopsy proven temporal arteritis from 1976-1983. Fifty-three patients with biopsy proven temporal arteritis were evaluated. All temporal artery biopsies were re-examined and resectioned by a single pathologist. Six biopsies previously negative for giant cells were found to have giant cells. Following reclassification, there were 35 patients in the giant cell positive (GCP) group and 18 in the giant cell negative (GCN) group. There was no difference in age, sex distribution, ESR, laboratory features, initial steroid dose, the number of patients in whom prednisone was discontinued, the number of relapses while on therapy, or the number of recurrences between the two groups. The duration of symptoms prior to diagnosis appeared longer in the GCP group (11.5 ± 5.8 weeks vs. 6.3 ± 4.2 weeks, p=.18), but the difference did not achieve statistical significance. Clinical manifestations were strikingly similar in both groups except for visual loss. In the GCP group 8/35 (22.8%) became blind while only 1/17 (5.9%) became blind in the GCN group (p=.11). The duration of symptoms prior to diagnosis was similar in patients with blindness and those without blindness (10.4 ± 5.2 weeks vs. 9.6 ± 2.5 weeks).

Although the differences are not statistically significant, the data suggest an increased incidence of visual loss in patients with giant cells on biopsy.

D55

COLD AIR INHALATION AFFECTS DIFFUSING CAPACITY (DL_{CO}) IN PATIENTS WITH RAYNAUD'S PHENOMENON (RP). JJ Condemi, MA Bauer, and MJ Utell, Univ. of Roch., Rochester, NY 14642.

Patients with RP experience spasm in vascular systems other than the extremities with exposure to cold stimuli. To determine if patients with RP develop vasospasm in the pulmonary vasculature, we studied changes in DL_{CO} and airway reactivity after cold air inhalation (in 28 subjects). Nine healthy subjects were controls, 8 subjects had secondary Raynaud's and 11 had primary Raynaud's (1°R). All subjects were non-smokers and denied any history of asthma or allergies. Cold air challenge (-12±2°C) was performed at 3 successive rates, for 4 min each, of isocapnic ventilation (V_E): resting V_E, V_E=30L/min and V_E=60L/min. We measured before and immediately after each cold air exposure FVC, FEV_1, specific airway conductance (SGaw) and functional residual capacity. DL_{CO} was measured at baseline and only following the final (V_E=60 L/min) cold air exposure. Following the maximun cold air inhalation (V_E60L/min) there was no significant difference in airway reactivity in the 1°R group compared to controls as determined by FEV_1(-2.7±3.1(SD)% vs. -0.7±2.6%, p=NS) or SGaw (-14±21% vs. 1±16%, p=NS). In contrast, cold air inhalation caused a significant reduction of DL_{CO} only in the 1°R group as shown below (DL_{CO} expressed as ml/min/mm Hg, mean± SD):

	Baseline	Post Cold Air	%Change
Control	25.0±4.8	26.9±5.0	+7.6*
Primary Raynaud's	24.1±3.8	22.8±4.1	-5.4*
Secondary Raynaud's	18.5±2.4	18.0±2.4	-2.7

*Difference from baseline significant at: p<0.05

These data suggest that cold air inhalation in patients with 1°R may produce vasospasm of the pulmonary vasculature to account for the reduction in DL_{CO} and support prior findings that some patients with Raynaud's have a systemic abnormality of the vasoregulatory mechanism.

D56

EFFECTS OF INJECTABLE CORTICOSTEROIDS ON EXTRA-ARTICULAR SOFT TISSUES OF THE EXTREMITIES: A RABBIT MODEL. Robert G. Trapp, James J. Hill, Che Su, Nat Mody. Southern Illinois University School of Medicine, Springfield , IL. 62708.

Complications from soft-tissue corticosteroid (CS) injection therapy are well recognized. We have studied the local tissue effects of three CS preparations injected into musculotendinous junctions of the rabbit. One relatively soluble CS, Dexamethasone Phosphate (DP), and two relatively insoluble CS's, Prednisolone Tebutate (PT) and Triamcinalone Hexacetonide (TH), were used either alone or mixed in the syringe with Lidocaine (L). Injections of saline, L and the vehicle of one CS were controls. Tissue samples from the injection sites were studied 1, 3, 7 and 28 days after injection. White deposits were observed in 39% and 78% of the sites injected with PT and TH respectively, but no deposits were seen at control or DP sites. The former two percentages are significantly greater than the latter two (p <0.0070). Spectrophotometric analysis of tissues taken at days 7 and 28 detected CS in 19 of 40 sites injected with PT and TH but in 0 of 11 DP injected sites (p = 0.0039). Inflammatory cellular infiltrates were most common at day 3. Light microscopy revealed that late inflammation at day 28 occurred more often with PT and TH (7/21) than with DP (0/8) (p = 0.0008). Insoluble CS's were more commonly associated with inflammation when injected without L (p = 0.0184). Muscle necrosis and calcium deposits occurred more commonly with the relatively insoluble CS's and no calcium deposits were seen when the CS was mixed with L(p = 0.0038). These findings suggest that several soft tissue changes occur at the site of CS injection. These may depend in part on the type of CS preparation and its method of administration. Further study of this model is warranted.

D57

COMPARISON OF BARIUM AND TECHNETIUM ESOPHOGRAMS AS SCREENING TESTS FOR ESOPHAGEAL MOTILITY IN RAYNAUD PHENOMENON (RP). O. FitzGerald, G. Bongiovanni, G. Merhar, M. Ulloa-Fernandez, E.V. Hess, G. Spencer-Green. University of Cincinnati Medical Center, Cincinnati, OH 45267, USA.

Barium esophogram (Bar-E) is routinely used as a screening evaluation for esophageal dysmotility in patients with RP, although technetium esophogram (Tch-E) may be a more sensitive test and result in less radiation exposure. To compare the relative sensitivity and specificity of the two methods, we performed both tests in 40 patients with RP who were being evaluated for an underlying connective tissue disease (CTD). Sixteen patients had abnormal Bar-E and 13 abnormal Tch-E, but discordance between the two techniques was noted in 13 patients (Table).

	Normal Technetium(27)	Abnormal Technetium(13)
Normal Barium (24)	19	5
Abnormal Barium (16)	8	8

Because of the high level of discordance, 8 patients to date have been further evaluated by esophageal manometry (EM). Of 3 patients with normal Bar-E and abnormal Tch-E, 2 had normal and 1 abnormal EM. Of 2 patients with abnormal Bar-E and normal Tch-E, 1 had normal and 1 abnormal EM. Two of 3 patients with concordant esophogram results also gave similar results on EM. Esophageal dysmotility is an important marker in establishing visceral involvement in early CTD. This study suggests that there is 30% discordance in results of Bar-E and Tch-E and that abnormal results on either test should be confirmed by esophageal manometry.

D58

THE NATURAL HISTORY OF FIBROMYALGIA (FIB). David Felson, Hal Dinerman, Don Goldenberg. Boston University Arthritis Center, Boston, MA 02118.

The natural history of fibromyalgia (FIB) was studied in 39 patients with primary FIB seen consecutively by one rheumatologist. A survey instrument validated to ensure that it accurately reflected patients' assessment of illness activity was administered in 11/83 and again in 11/84. All patients were being seen in clinic in 11/83 and mean duration of follow-up at that time was 13.7 months (range 1-84). At survey 2 (S2) 38 of 39 patients were assessed; 10 either no longer received formal medical care or received care elsewhere.

At both surveys all patients had persistent FIB symptoms. At S2: 27/38 (71%) had moderate or severe pain from their FIB, while only 2, both of whom no longer saw a physician, had no pain or stiffness. 15/38 (39%) felt fair or poor with respect to FIB symptoms, although 71% stated that symptoms had improved since diagnosis. Sleep difficulties were present in 87%, albeit improved since diagnosis in two-thirds. All patients took medicines to control symptoms either regularly (31 patients) or on a PRN basis (7). Of 9 patients doing well with respect to all symptoms, six took sleeping medicines regularly and only one rarely need any medicine. Of 29 still followed, persistent symptoms and tender points on exam corroborated survey findings. At S2, there were no differences between those no longer followed and those still seen. The following variables were not predictive of patient status at S2: patient age and sex, history of psychiatric illness, symptom duration prior to diagnosis, and severity of illness at diagnosis (as measured by trigger point score and number of tender areas). Status at survey 1 correlated with S2 status (p=.05).

We conclude that patients with FIB tend to have persistent symptoms that require therapy for at least two years after diagnosis.

D59

DOES RUNNING LEAD TO DEGENERATIVE JOINT DISEASE? R. Panush, N. L. Edwards, S. Longley, J. Caldwell, R. Yonker, E. Webster, J. Nauman, H. Pettersson, J. Stork, C. Schmidt. Univ FL, Gainesville, Florida.

In recent years increased interest in physical fitness has resulted in millions of people of all ages undertaking exercise programs, usually running. However little information is available regarding the long-term effects, if any, of running on the musculoskeletal system. We therefore determined whether there was an increased prevalence of degenerative joint disease (DJD) among runners. 22 male runners and 18 male non-runners completed a detailed health and running questionnaire, underwent physical examinations, and x-ray evaluations of hips, knees, ankles, and feet. Examinations and x-ray interpretations were carried out in a "blinded" fashion. Runners averaged 53 yrs of age (range 46-74), 5'11" height (5'9"-6'3"), 164 lbs weight (141-220), compared with 60 yrs (50-74), 5'10" height (5'8"-6'4"), and 171 lbs (150-210) for non-runners. Running subjects (including 54% marathoners) ran an average of 28 miles per week (range 20-50) for 11½ years (5-27). 54% of runners had experienced knee pain and/or swelling, which was statistically comparable with 33% of non-runners. Examinations revealed 77% of both runners and non-runners had knee crepitation. Other musculoskeletal evaluations were similar for running and non-running subjects. Radiologic examinations also showed no notable differences among groups. 1 runner had degenerative changes of the hip and another of knees (9% prevalence), while 3 control subjects had knee DJD (17% prevalence). We do not find an increased prevalence of DJD among our runners. Our observations suggest, within the limits of our study, that long-duration, high-mileage running need not lead to premature DJD of the lower extremities.

D60

SEPTIC ARTHRITIS DUE TO GROUP G STREPTOCOCCUS IS ASSOCIATED WITH ABNORMALITIES OF THE GASTROINTESTINAL AND GENITOURINARY TRACT. Robert W. Ike and Thomas J. Schnitzer. University of Michigan, Ann Arbor, MI 48109

Septic arthritis due to group G Streptococcus is uncommon with only twenty-five cases having been reported to date. A cluster of cases of arthritis due to this organism at our hospital prompted a review of the institutional experience over the past five years. Six episodes occurring in four patients were identified. Each episode presented as an acute monoarthritis (knee-4, shoulder-1, wrist-1). Three patients had underlying joint disease (OA, RA, and SLE). Significantly, all patients had an underlying abnormality of the GI tract (asymptomatic carcinoma of the colon; enterocutaneous fistula complicating diverticulitis; Barrett's esophagus, gastric ulcer, and tubular adenoma of the colon in the same patient) or GU tract (neurogenic bladder with vesicostomy). Response to adequate therapy was slow with sterile effusions persisting after bacteriologic cure in half the episodes. Septic arthritis recurred in 2 patients 1 month and 34 months following the initial episode; GI/GU abnormalities had not been corrected in either patient.

Thus, the universal occurrence of GI and GU tract abnormalities in our series suggests that a search for such abnormalities should be undertaken in any patient with group G streptococcal arthritis when the source of the organism is not evident.

D61

POLYARTHRITIS IN POLYARTERITIS NODOSA (PAN). C.M. Ziminski, T.M. Zizic, M.B. Stevens. The Johns Hopkins University School of Medicine, Baltimore, Md. 21205.

Neither the pattern nor prevalence of arthritis in classical polyarteritis (PAN) has been firmly established in the literature. In view of the gravity of this systemic illness, it is not surprising that little attention has been focused on its articular component. A recent patient presented with such dominant polyarthritis as to delay the diagnosis of polyarteritis. This experience prompted our retrospective study.

Patients admitted to our Rheumatic Disease Unit 1971-1983 were selected for review only on the basis of certainty of diagnosis with histologic and/or angiographic confirmation of medium-sized vessel arteritis. Patients with a clinical diagnosis alone, or with variants of polyarteritis were specifically excluded.

Of 19 patients with PAN, nine (47%) had polyarthritis; and in four of these nine, it was the dominant presenting feature. The arthritis was migratory, symmetrical and non-deforming with both small (67%) and large (77%) joint involvement. The pattern of arthritis was strikingly polyarticular with $\geq$ 5 joints involved in seven (77%) and $\geq$ 10 joints in four (44%). Articular involvement occurred early and uniformly by the time of diagnosis. In addition to those with frank polyarthritis, four (21%) had arthralgias alone involving fewer and predominantly large, lower extremity joints.

There were no demographic or clinico-laboratory features of PAN which correlated significantly with the presence of arthritis, although those four patients with dominant polyarthritis tended to be younger, with mean age at onset 28 years.

Thus, polyarthritis is a frequent, prominent, and often presenting manifestation of PAN.

D62

CARTILAGE METAPLASIA INDUCED IN VITRO BY RHEUMATOID SYNOVIUM. B.B.Lavietes, S.E. Carsons, B.J. Diamond, H.S. Diamond, R.S. Laskin. Depts. of Medicine and Orthopaedic Surgery, Long Island Jewish -Hillside Medical Center, New Hyde Park, NY USA 11042

Freshly extirpated rheumatoid synovium and rheumatoid synovial cells maintained in tissue culture were co-cultured with cylindrical plugs of normal pig cartilage removed from articular surfaces with a cork borer (4.8 mm diameter). All cultures were maintained in Dulbecco's modified Eagle's medium with 10% human serum and antibiotics.

Under these conditions, cartilage cultured alone maintained its morphology over 3 weeks in culture. Some outgrowth of fibroblastic cells from basal endochondral bone surface was seen, but it did not extend beyond the proliferative zone. In co-culture with pieces of synovium, this outgrowth extended around and completely enveloped cartilage and synovium. At the articular surface in contact with synovium, proteoglycan was lost (toluidine blue stain), and matrix was replaced by dense deposits of fibrillar collagen (van Gieson stain). The interior of the cartilage retained its normal morphology. A transition zone was seen between unaffected cartilage and the fibrous area; this zone showed loss of metachromasia with toluidine blue, breakdown of lacunae, and appearance of small fibrils. These changes were not seen with passaged rheumatoid cells alone (up to 5×10^4 cells/well) but could be induced by addition of monocyte supernatant medium. Addition of media from primary cultures of synovium that had effected cartilage metaplasia produced some transitional areas at the articular surface suggesting initiation of the process.

These results suggest the effects of rheumatoid synovium on other tissues of the joint are not an inherent property of synovial cells but rather the result of complex interactions between monocytes and cells of cartilage, bone, and synovium. The co-cultures provide a system in which to study these interactions. (Supported by grants from NIH and Arthritis Foundation, New York chapter)

D63

WESTERN BLOTTING ANALYSIS OF CHLAMYDIA TRACHOMATIS (Ct) AND YERSINIA ENTEROCOLITICA (Ye) ANTIGENS IN REITER'S SYNDROME. R.D. Inman, M.E.A. Johnson, B. Chiu, M. Petric, J.A. Falk. University of Toronto, Toronto, Ontario, Canada, M5T 2S8.

Reiter's syndrome (RS) occurs in immunogenetically susceptible hosts following gastrointestinal (GI) or genitourinary (GU) infections by a relatively narrow spectrum of pathogens, suggesting that these organisms may have certain antigenic determinants in common. Anti-Ct antibodies were detected by microimmunofluorescence in 15/17 RS patients (8/8 post-GU, 3/4 post-GI), 5/10 B27-positive reactive arthritis (ReA) patients (1/2 post-GU, 4/8 post-GI), 8/10 B27-negative nonspecific urethritis (NSU) patients, 4/7 B27-positive normals, 0/9 B27-negative normals. Anti-Ye antibodies were detected by microagglutination in 5/12 RS patients (2/5 post-GU, 3/4 post-GI), and 3/5 ReA (all post-GI). 2 post-Salmonella ReA patients were negative for anti-Ct and anti-Ye antibodies. Western blotting analysis was performed in which antigens derived from Ye (serotypes 0:3, 0:8, 5:27), Ct (sero-type L_2) and S.enteritidis were electrophoresed, transferred to nitrocellulose, reacted with serum and synovial fluid and detected by radiolabelled Protein A. Post-GI RS showed preferential reactivity to Ye or Salmonella antigens, with anti-chlamydial reactivity confined primarily to the major outer membrane protein (MOMP) of Ct, with molecular weight of 40,000 daltons. Post-GU RS sera reacted with several Ct antigens in addition to MOMP, most commonly 60,000 and 62,000 daltons in molecular weight. Concurrent reactivity with Ye and S.enteritidis was seen in some, but not all, post-GU RS. No single cross-reacting antigen links this group of microorganisms despite their shared propensity to induce RS and ReA in susceptible hosts.

D64

DECREASED SUPPRESSIVE B CELL FACTOR ACTIVITY IN RHEUMATOID ARTHRITIS: CORRELATIONS WITH RHEUMATOID FACTOR PLAQUE-FORMING CELLS AND DISEASE ACTIVITY. Edward J. Pisko, Randal E. White, Susan L. Foster and Robert A. Turner. Bowman Gray School of Medicine, Winston-Salem, NC 27103.

We have described a 32,000 molecular weight lymphokine, suppressive B cell factor (SBF), that is produced by human OKB7 positive B lymphocytes after stimulation with heat-aggregated IgG (HAIgG), a model for immune complexes (IC). To assess IC mediated feedback suppression in rheumatoid arthritis (RA), we evaluated the ability of SBF from patients with RA and normal controls to suppress the pokeweed mitogen (PWM)-induced rheumatoid factor plaque-forming cell (RF-PFC) response of normal peripheral blood mononuclear leukocytes (PBL).

The PBL from patients with RA produced decreased SBF activity following HAIgG stimulation. Patients with RA on only non-steroidal anti-inflammatory drugs (NSAID) had the poorest ability to generate SBF activity while RA patients on immunosuppressive drugs and NSAID were comparable to age-matched controls. Pretreatment of PBL from patients with RA with trypsin and DNase did not affect the production of SBF activity. Suppressive activity correlated inversely with the number of spontaneously occurring RF-PFC in patients and normal controls ($r = .45$, $p \leq .01$). RA disease activity, as measured by erythrocyte sedimentation rate and joint count, was shown to inversely correlate ($r = .56$, $p \leq .02$ and $r = .67$, $p \leq .01$, respectively) with SBF activity. We conclude that RA patients produce decreased SBF. The decreased in vitro responsiveness of PBL to HAIgG in patients with RA does not appear to be due to IC coating or exogenous proteins. This study supports a defect in IC stimulated B cell suppressor activity in RA leading to further IC formation. This defect may be involved in the pathogenesis and chronicity of RA.

D65

DNA BINDING TO THE COLLAGEN-LIKE SEGMENT OF C1Q. Alan M. Rosenberg, Patricia A. Prokopchuk. University of Saskatchewan, Saskatoon, Canada.

This study was undertaken to determine if DNA, which is known to bind to collagen, also binds to the collagen-like segment of Clq (CLS). Purified human Clq, isolated by IgG-Sepharose 4B affinity chromatography, was pepsin digested and applied to a Sephadex G-200 column. CLS eluted with the void volume. Six sera with antibodies to denatured (ss-) DNA (as determined by an enzyme linked immunoassay {ELISA}) and 6 sera with antibodies to native (ds-) DNA (radioimmunoassay) were employed in an ELISA to detect CLS bound ss- or dsDNA. Twelve sera without such antibodies served as controls. The ELISA methodology included: 1. coating with 50 µg/ml CLS or phosphate-buffered saline (PBS)(4^0C×16 hr) 2. addition of 50 µg/ml ssDNA or dsDNA (<2% S1-nuclease sensitive) or PBS (37^0 C×30 min) 3. addition of sera in duplicate (1:10)(37^0C×30 min) 4. detection of antibody binding by employing an anti-IgG alkaline phosphatase/phosphate substrate system. The results follow:

Wells Coated with	CLS	CLS	CLS	PBS	PBS
ssDNA Added:	yes	no	no	yes	no
dsDNA Added:	no	yes	no	no	yes
Sera with Antibody to					
ssDNA ($\bar{X}$±1SD)(n=6)	.41±.10*		.18±.02	.16±.01	
dsDNA ($\bar{X}$±1SD)(n=6)		.73±.12	.17±.02		.15±.01
Normal Sera ($\bar{X}$±1SD)(n=12)	.18±.02	.19±.02	.18±.02	.15±.02	.16±.01

* Values represent the Mean ($\bar{X}$) O.D.(405nm)±1 Standard Deviation (SD)

These results indicate that ss- and dsDNA bind to CLS. CLS, altered in conformation by interaction of Clq with Cl activators, is the binding site for Clr and then $C\bar{1}r_2C\bar{1}s_2$. Thus, molecules such as DNA, which may bind to CLS, could be factors important in modulating Cl activation.

D66

RADIOIMMUNOASSAY OF CIRCULATING INTERFERONα IN HUMAN PLASMA. MEASUREMENT OF INTERFERONα-LIKE SUBSTANCE IN HEALTHY INDIVIDUALS & VARIOUS RHEUMATIC DISEASE PATIENTS. Shunichi Shiozawa, Kazuo Chihara, Kazuko Shiozawa, Shinichi Shimizu, Takuo Fujita, Hakuo Ikegami, Shunsaku Koyama, and Masashi Kurimoto. Kobe Univ.,Kobe,& Hayashibara Biochem. Lab., Okayama, Japan

Radioimmunoassay for human circulating interferonα(IFNα) was developed using IFNα from human leukemic BALL-1 cell line. Antibody was made by immunizing rabbit with IFNα. Lactoperoxidase was used for radiolabelling. The assay paralleled with bioactivity & did not cross-react with IFNβ, IFNγ, or ACTH. Dilution curve of plasma completely paralleled with the standard curve. IFNα-like substance (IFNα-LS) was extractable and and concentrated from plasma either by silisic acid or anti-IFNα affinity method. Extracted sample of plasma showed identical dilution to the standard IFNα. Circulating IFNα-LS in healthy individuals at the age 25 to 40 was 0.207+0.055ng/ml in male(n=49) and 0.172+0.076ng/ml in female(n=32). Plasma IFNα-LS decreased gradually with ageing. In rheumatoid arthritis(n=39),plasma IFNα-LS was below 0.07ng/ml,whereas it was not decreased in rheumatoid patients with vasculitis. IFNα-LS was high in active SLE,while it was low in inactive SLE with prednisolone(n=56). Plasma IFNα-LS was also decreased in Sjøgren's syndrome. Decreased plasma IFNα-LS may have pathogenetic importance in relation to defective natural killer cell activities. By gel chromatography, plasma IFNα-LS eluted in the same position as standard IFNα, however,the position indicated smaller molecular weight.Incubation of standard IFNα with plasma showed gradual shift of IFNα to the smaller peak on Sephadex G-75, suggesting a possibility of tryptic digestion of IFNα. Treatment of plasma with enzyme inhibitors abrogated the shift, however, plasma IFNα-LS remained small in size.PlasmaIFNα-LS may be presentin a fragmented form.

D67

INTRAOSSEOUS PRESSURE AND OUTFLOW RESISTANCE IN STEROID TREATED RABBITS. C. McAllister, P.A. Simkin. U. of Wa., Seattle, WA 98195.

Intraosseous hypertension and increased resistance to injected saline are recognized features of osteonecrosis in man. To quantify these variables in an accepted animal model, we studied both bones of the hip in control (C) and steroid-treated (T) NZW rabbits. Surgical exposure of the femoral head and acetabulum allowed transchondral insertion of needles to a depth of 3-5 mm. Outflow resistance (mm Hgxmlxmin^{-1}) and baseline pressure (mm Hg) were determined from regression analysis of intraosseous pressures at successive flow rates.

	9 days	3 weeks	5 weeks	7 weeks
Femoral Head Resistance ($\bar{x}$±SE (n))				
C	32±2(2)	61±25(2)	32±5(4)	33±9(2)
T	263±112(4)	8332±4299(4)	619±224(5)	100±7(4)
Acetubular Resistance				
C	24±2(2)	26±1(3)	63±6(2)	---
T	124±30(4)	533±260(4)	326±67(5)	282±81(4)
Femoral Head Pressure (mmHg)				
C	9±1(2)	16±5(2)	15±3(4)	7±1(2)
T	36±4(4)	49±13(4)	72±27(5)	25±6(4)
Acetubular Pressure				
C	10±3(2)	6±3(3)	12±0(2)	---
T	25±4(4)	33±9(4)	19±7(5)	16±10(4)

Both baseline pressure and outflow resistance rose significantly within 9 days of starting steriods, peaked between 3 and 5 weeks, and fell thereafter. Similar, though attenuated, changes were found in the acetabulum. Quantitiatve determinations of these properties may be helpful in clinical as well as experimental osteonecrosis.

D68

ROTATOR CUFF TENDINITIS: COMPARISON OF LOCAL CORTICOSTEROID INJECTIONS VERSUS NONSTEROIDAL THERAPY. Richard H. White, Dana M. Paull, Kenneth W. Fleming Univ. of CA., Davis, Sacramento, CA. 95817.

Local injection of corticosteroid (S) has not been rigorously compared to nonsteroidal therapy in the treatment of rotator cuff tendinitis. We compared subacromial bursa injection of 40 mg of triamcinolone acetonide versus indomethacin (I), 100 mg/day PO, in a 6 week, prospective, double-blind, double-dummy study of 40 patients with impingment symptoms for less than 12 weeks who could abduct above 90° after bursal injection of 3 ml of 1% lidocaine. All patients received a placebo or (S) injection in an opaque syringe, (I) or placebo capsules, and instructions for home physical therapy, with repeat injection and medication refill after 3 weeks if necessary. Initial demographics, physical findings and pain scores were similar.

Using a 0-3 point scale for severity of pain and motion deficit, at 6 weeks: 8/20 pts. receiving (I) had minimal pain and good motion, 2/20 had some improvement, 5/20 had continued pain and decreased motion, and 5/20 had were lost. In comparison, in the (S) group: 6/20 did well, 3/20 improved, 6/20 did poorly and 5/20 were lost.

Changes in measured variables (±SD) for the 30 pts. followed were:

Variable	I (n = 15)	S (n = 15)
Δ Initial Arc of Pain (abduction)	+ 41 ± 48	+ 46 ± 41
Δ Highest Arc of abduction	+ 16 ± 45	+ 30 ± 37
Δ Pain Score (0 - 18)	- 5.5 ± 8.3	- 4.3 ± 5.2
Δ Overall severity score (0 - 3)	- 1.1 ± 1.2	- 1.0 ± 1.1

If the trend continued we would need 70 patients in each group to detect a significant difference favoring (S) using the highest arc parameter with a power of 95%. We conclude that, clinically, there is little difference between (I) and injection of (S).

D69

ROTATOR CUFF TENDINITIS: CORRELATION OF CLINICAL FEATURES AND RADIOGRAPHIC FINDINGS WITH RESPONSE TO THERAPY. Richard H. White, David C. Hardy, Dana M. Paull, Univ. of CA., Davis, Sacramento, CA 95817 and Travis AFB, Fairfield, CA 94535

In a study comparing the efficacy of subacromial injection(s) of corticosteroid vs. oral indomethacin, clinical efficacy was nearly identical. We correlated the clinical response after 6 weeks therapy with either agent with clinical and radiographic parameters in 30 patients. Combining pain and motion scores, 14/30 patients had an excellent response, 5/30 a fair response, and 11/30 a poor response.

The mean age of excellent and fair responders (Grp 1), 52±13 years (±SD), was significantly less than the poor responders (Grp 2), 65±10 years. History of work related use or trauma of the shoulder was noted in 11/19 in Grp 1 vs. 1/11 in Grp 2 ($p < 0.05$). Similarly, a precipitating event such as lifting or falling was noted in 11/19 Grp 1 patients vs. 3/11 in Grp 2 ($p < 0.05$). In Grp 1, 7/19 had prior episodes of shoulder pain vs. 5/11 in Grp 2 (NS). Onset of symptoms was 3.4±3.0 weeks prior to therapy in Grp 1 vs. 6.8±2.7 in Grp 2 (p=0.08).

Twenty-seven of the 30 patients had shoulder x-rays evaluated blindly by a bone radiologist. Using a 0-3 point scoring system for subacromial spurs, degenerative changes in the humeral head and inferior acromioclavicular joint spurs (total 0-9 points), the mean total score for Grp 1 was 2.8±2.0 vs. 3.3±2.0 in Grp 2 (NS). Small calcium deposits were noted in 9/19 in Grp 1 versus 3/11 in Grp 2 (NS).

We conclude: Patients with rotator cuff tendinitis who have a favorable short-term response to conservative treatment tend to be younger and give a history of shoulder use and/or trauma; radiographic findings and the short-term response to therapy do not correlate.

D70

NONSTEROIDAL ANTI-INFLAMMATORY DRUGS (NSAIDS): EFFECTS ON NEUTROPHIL (PMN) ACTIVATION MEDIATED NOT BY CYCLOOXYGENASE INHIBITION BUT BY AN EFFECT ON ADENYLATE CYCLASE (AC). S. Abramson, R. Ludewig, H. Korchak and G. Weissmann. NYU Med. Center, New York, NY.

NSAIDS, including sodium salicylate (NaS), a poor cyclooxygenase inhibitor, inhibit activation of PMN (cells with little cyclooxygenase activity). To investigate this inhibition we tested the effect of aspirin (3mM), NaS (3mM), indomethacin (indo, 30µM) and piroxicam (50µM) on the rise in cyclic AMP (cAMP) induced by the chemoattractant f-met-leu-phe (FMLP). Following stimulation of PMN by FMLP(10^{-7}M) cAMP rose from 5.3 pmoles to 12.4 at 15 sec. and 7.9 at 120 sec. Preincubation of PMN with each of the NSAIDS potentiated the FMLP-induced rise in cAMP; e.g.,NaS increased cAMP at 15 sec. to 18.6 ($p<0.01$); at 120 sec. to 12.7 ($p<0.05$). To test whether NSAID inhibition of PMN depended on AC we utilized 9-(tetrahydro-2-furyl) adenine (THFA), an inhibitor of AC. Indo (30 µM) reduced FMLP-induced lysozyme release (LR) from PMN to 75.9%, superoxide generation (O_2-) to 55.9%, and aggregation to 66.6% of control (all $p<0.01$). THFA (100uM) reversed this inhibition by indo, whereas THFA alone had no effect on cell function: When cells were preincubated with both THFA and indo, FMLP-induced LR was restored to 100% ($p<0.03$), O_2- increased to 70.3% ($p<0.01$), and aggregation increased to 75.8% ($p<0.02$) of control. THFA similarly reduced the effects of indo on cAMP: preincubation of PMN with indo (30µM) increased FMLP-induced cAMP (15 sec.) to 15.4 (greater than control, $p<0.05$). However, preincubation with both THFA and indo before FMLP reduced cAMP to 12.6 ($p<0.05$). Studies indicate that NSAIDS inhibit PMN function not by cyclooxygenase inhibition (NaS) but by influencing membrane events linked to the activation of adenylate cyclase.

D71

EFFECT OF INCREASING DOSE OF METHOTREXATE IN PATIENTS WITH RHEUMATOID ARTHRITIS. H. James Williams for the Cooperative Systematic Studies of Rheumatic Diseases, Salt Lake City, UT 84132

One hundred eighty-nine patients were studied in a prospective, controlled, double-blind multicenter trial comparing methotrexate (MTX) and placebo. Patients taking MTX were significantly improved in all clinical and laboratory variables examined compared to placebo. Patients were begun on 7.5 mg MTX weekly given in tnree divided doses 12 nours apart. Patients who were not responding by the physician's assessment at 6 weeks nad the dosage of MTX doubled to 15 mg/week. Comparison of patients who completed tne trial indicates that response to MTX occurs early. Doubling tne dose in unresponsive patients recruited only a few more responders and degree of response was more modest (see table).

Median improvement in selected variables

	Maximum weekly dosage	
Variable	7.5 mg (N=19)	15 mg (N=38)
Morning stiffness (min)	150	83
Joint pain/tenderness count	19	8*
Joint pain/tenderness score	27	14*
Joint swelling count	10	6*
Joint swelling score	17	10*
Erythrocyte sed. rate (mm/hr)	37	22*

* p <.05

Toxicity was similar to both doses. Patients generally respond to MTX witnin tne first 6 weeks of tnerapy and 7.5 mg MTX per week appears to be an appropriate dose.

D72

PRE "EROSIVE" DEFECTS IN THE SUBCHONDRAL PLATE (SCP) OF NONARTHRITIC METACARPAL HEADS (MCH). James Leisen, Howard Duncan, Jeanne Riddle, Wayne Pitchford. Henry Ford Hospital, Detroit, MI 48202.

Radiographic erosions and cysts of the MCH are commonly seen in rheumatoid arthritis (RA). The earliest erosions are known to occur on the radiovolar aspect. Histologic studies have also shown that rheumatoid pannus may disseminate through perforations in the SCP. To further explore these findings, we examined the topography of the SCP from the MCH's of nonarthritic cadavers by scanning electron microscopy (SEM).

Cadaver hands were examined by standard and Brewerton radiographs. No defects in the SCP, including cysts, were seen. The second and third MCH (N=16) were removed, macerated and the articular surface of the SCP surveyed by SEM. We observed perforations of the SCP. The holes ranged in diameter from 100 to 290 microns (avg. 180) or about 10-20 times the size of the calcified chondrocyte lacunae. These holes penetrated into the marrow space through the thin SCP. Holes were found in greatest number on the radial condyle where they were distributed in an oval shaped pattern across this surface.

From our study, we conclude that perforations of the SCP are a normal anatomical feature of the MCH primarily in the condylar areas. Furthermore, we suggest that coalescence of these perforations might possibly give rise to the dot dash or Bywaters lesions seen in early RA. The location of these holes might also explain why erosions in RA are first seen on the radiovolar aspect of the MCH.

E1

Splenic Dysfunction in SLE: Correlation with Serum IgM Level
Wendell Wilson, Rajendra Marwah, Julian Foreman, Hugh McGrath and Myriam Perez, LSU Medical Center, New Orleans, Louisiana 70112

We assessed the relationship between serum IgM level and splenic function in SLE because previous studies using particulate tracers suggested that splenic dysfunction occurs in SLE, and other studies have reported that low serum IgM levels occur in subjects following surgical splenectomy for trauma. Splenic phagocyte function was quantitated by giving 5 millicuries of 99m Tc sulfur colloid intravenously; 30 minutes later, the ratio of splenic to hepatic intensity of uptake of the colloid (S/L ratio) was quantitated by computer scintigraphy. Patients (n = 15, 14 females, age 19-75 mean 35 years) were classified by the revised ARA criteria, and were outpatients with normal hepatic function, and with duration of SLE from 2 to 14 years mean 6.3 years.

S/L ratio was correlated with serum IgM level $r = 0.75$, $p < 0.005$, but not with IgG nor IgA level. Patients with the lowest IgM levels (64, 60, 52 and 40 mg per 100 ml) had abnormal or borderline S:L ratio (0.40:1, 0.33:1, 0.50:1, and 0.59:1 respectively). S:L ratio (normal range 0.53 to 1.45) was low in 5/15 patients. S:L ratio or IgM level were not related to the following: features or duration of SLE, prednisone, immuran or plaquenil therapy, anti n-DNA, C_3, C_4, immune complexes, HLADR3 or DR7. Our findings are consistent with the known role of the spleen in IgM production, and indicate that splenic dysfunction may cause the relative paucity of IgM autoantibodies previously observed in SLE. Also, splenic phagocytosis, as well as IgM antibody have roles in the early immune responses to bacteremia and may therefore be implicated in severe infection , now a leading cause of death in SLE.

E2

CLINICAL CHARACTERISTICS OF PATIENTS WITH ANTIBODIES TO PROLIFERATING CELL NUCLEAR ANTIGEN. Yoshinari Takasaki, Noriko Ohata, Mistuhiko Yasuma, Hiroshi Hashimoto, Shunichi Hirose. Juntendo University, Tokyo, 113 Japan.

In 1978, Miyachi et al reported that an autoantibody which was reactive with a nuclear antigen in proliferating cell(PCNA) had been demonstrated in a small percentage of patients with systemic lupus erythematosus (SLE)(J. Immunol,121,2228). In this report, we studied the frequency of anti-PCNA antibody in various rheumatic diseases and the clinical features of patients with anti-PCNA.

569 patients with various rheumatic diseases were tested for anti-PCNA antibodies by standard immunodiffusion. Anti-PCNA antibodies were detected only in patients with SLE and its incidence was 2.1%(7 Out of328). The clinical and serological features of 7 patients with anti-PCNA were studied and the frequencies of thrombocytopenia(66.7%) and seizure(44.9 %) in those patients were significantly higher compared with 293 SLE patients without anti-PCNA($P<0.005$, $P<0.05$, respectively). The relationship between those clinical features and anti-PCNA was further studied longitudinally(0.5-8 years,mean 5.6). Thrombocytopenia was observed in parallel with the elevation of titer of anti-PCNA in 3 out of 4 patients . On the contrary, seizure was not observed with the relation to appearance nor elevated titer of anti-PCNA. All seven patients with anti-PCNA had renal involuvement and 2 of them were diagnosed as nephrotic syndrome, and one with DPGN lacked anti-DNA antibody. In those patients, the elevation of anti-PCNA titer was observed preceding to the dvelopment of protenuria and the titer of anti-PCNA was decreased by the treatment with corticosteroid therapy.

Those results suggest that anti-PCNA antibody is a useful clinical marker for SLE related to thrombocytopenia and renal involvement and its production is sensitive to corticosteroid therapy.

E3

THE "EUTHYROID SICK SYNDROME" IN SYSTEMIC LUPUS ERYTHEMATOSUS.
Frederick W. Miller, Gerald F. Moore, and Alfred D. Steinberg, Arthritis and Rheumatism Branch, NIADDK, Bethesda, MD. 20205

Patients (pts) with systemic nonthyroidal diseases have altered thyroid hormone metabolism resulting in depressed T_3, low to normal (nl) T_4, elevated reverse T_3 (rT_3) and nl TSH values, known as the "euthyroid sick syndrome." The extent of underlying disease activity often correlates with the decrease in T_3 and elevation of rT_3. We studied 119 data sets ($\leq$ 3/pt) consisting of 58 routine laboratory tests and concurrent TSH, T_4, T_3, and rT_3 values from 65 hospitalized pts with systemic lupus erythematosus (SLE) without known thyroid disease, in order to determine the incidence of this syndrome and correlations among these tests.

This data was divided into four groups on the basis of thyroid function tests:(1) 34 data sets (29%) included nl T_4 and TSH but low T_3 values, consistent with the "euthyroid sick syndrome";(2) 26 (22%) had a nl T_3 and T_4 but high TSH;(3) 17 (14%) had high TSH and low T_3 and T_4 levels consistent with the laboratory diagnosis of hypothyroidism; and (4) only 42 sets (35%) had nl T_3, T_4, and TSH values. The "euthyroid sick" group had the highest rT_3 levels, and in this group selected laboratory indicators of disease activity significantly ($p<.05$) correlated with T_3 and rT_3 but not with T_4 or TSH levels: T_3 correlated positively with albumin and hematocrit and negatively with creatinine, BUN, uric acid, ESR, gammaglobulin, IgG, IgA, and anti-DNA titers; while rT_3 correlated positively with creatinine, phosphate, and amylase.

These data suggest that the "euthyroid sick syndrome" is the most common cause of thyroid function test abnormalities in pts with SLE without clinical evidence of thyroid disease, and that the extent of decrease of T_3 and elevation of rT_3 correlate with many laboratory parameters of systemic disease activity.

E4

RELATIONSHIP BETWEEN ANTI-CARDIOLIPIN ANTIBODIES AND DISEASE ACTIVITY AND DISEASE SUBSETS IN SLE.
David A. Isenberg , Carol Dudeney and Bernie Colaco°. Departments of Rheumatology, UCH and The Middlesex° Hospitals, London

As part of a prospective study 42 SLE patients were examined on 4 or more occasions between August 1983 and August 1984. At each clinic attendance a wide range of clinical and serological features were noted and compared with IgG and IgM anti-cardiolipin antibody levels measured by a sensitive RIA. These antibody levels were shown to distinguish inactive/mild disease activity from moderate/severe activity ($p=0.025$, Mann-Whitney U test) in the group overall, with even greater discriminant function in patients with marked dermatological and pleural/pericardial involvement. Further, persistently raised IgM (but not IgG) anti-cardiolipin antibody levels were found to be associated with a history of spontaneous abortion and/or thrombosis and with cerebral disease ($p<0.05$, Fisher's exact test) though not with thrombocytopenia. These results indicate the clinical utility of measuring anti-cardiolipin antibodies in SLE.

E5

ANTI-LA/SSB AND LA/SSB ANALYSIS WITH A MONOCLONAL ANTIBODY. John B. Harley, Myra O. Rosario, Hajime Yamagata, Owen F. Fox, Eugen Koren. Univ. of Oklahoma and Okla. Med. Res. Fnd., Oklahoma City.

Purified bovine La/SSB was used to immunize a Balb/C mouse from which anti-La/SSB producing hybridoma cell lines were detected and cloned. Of these La 1, a γ_1 kappa antibody, was chosen for careful characterization. La/SSB containing extracts from a bovine source, but not from a human or rabbit source, inhibited the reactivity of La 1 in an anti-La/SSB solid phase assay. La 1 was positive in an antinuclear antibody flourescent assay on a bovine substrate with a fluorescent pattern identical to the speckled nuclear pattern produced by a selected anti-La/SSB containing human serum. The antinuclear antibody fluorescence of both La 1 and the anti-La/SSB containing serum was inhibited by purified La/SSB. The La 1 antibody, unlike the human anti-La/SSB containing serum, had negative antinuclear antibody fluorescence when human, rabbit, or mouse cell lines were used as substrates. Both solid phase assays using a purified La/SSB peptide preparation and Western blotting demonstrated that La 1 bound the larger 41 Kd La/SSB peptide but not the 29 Kd La/SSB peptide. An anti-La/SSB solid phase assay was established using La 1 and bovine La/SSB containing extracts from which Ro/SSA had been removed. This assay was more than 10-fold more sensitive than an analogous solid phase assay using purified La/SSB and 1000-fold more sensitive than immunodiffusion for anti-La/SSB binding activity. Beyond confirming that some normal sera contained anti-La/SSB, results from this assay demonstrated that nearly all anti-Ro/SSA containing sera also contained some La/SSB binding activity.

E6

FAMILIAL SYSTEMIC LUPUS ERYTHEMATOSUS(SLE): FURTHER EVIDENCE FOR ASSOCIATION WITH AN EXTENDED HAPLOTYPE ON THE 6TH CHROMOSOME, INCLUDING C4A*QO. J. Verrier Jones, E. Jones, S.J. Forsyth, R.I. Carr, J.M. MacSween, S. Eastwood, Division of Rheumatology, Department of Medicine, Dalhousie University, Halifax, Nova Scotia, B3H 3J5, Canada, V. Skanes, Memorial University, St. John's, Newfoundland, M. Reichlin, Oklahoma Medical Research Foundation, Oklahoma City, Oklahoma, U.S.A.

SLE is associated with the HLA antigens HLA-DR2 and DR3, and with the null alleles of C4 (C4AQO, C4BQO). Antibodies to the Ro/SSA antigen are increased in individuals positive for DR3. There are no published reports of antibodies to Ro/SSA and La/SSB in patients with C4 half null alleles. We report a family from Prince Edward Island, Canada, in which two sisters from a sibship of 14 have SLE. 27 members of the family have been tested for ANA, antibodies to Ro/SSA, La/SSB, Sm, and nRNP, and typed for HLA-A, B, C, and DR, C4 and Bf. The affected sisters have the following genotype: HLA-DR3, C4AQO, C4B1, BfS, HLA-B8, HLA-C7, HLA-A1/HLA-DR8, C4AQO, C4B1, BfS, HLA-B8, HLA-C7, HLA-A1. One has antibodies to Ro/La and nRNP, the other to nRNP. In Generations II and III, two of four unaffected antibody producers share an HLA haplotype with the affected sisters, and are half null heterozygotes for C4AQO: one produces antibodies to nRNP, one to Ro and nRNP. Of the two remaining antibody producers, one has antibodies to nRNP, and normal alleles for C4A, (A3/A3) and is homozygous for DR4, while the other has a positive ANA, but no antibodies in the Ro/La/nRNP system. This family thus confirms the association between SLE and homozygosity for the C4AQO, and between C4AQO and the extended haplotype C4B1, BfS, HLA-B8, HLA-A1. The haplotype also includes HLA-C7. On one chromosome, this family shows the characteristic HLA-DR3, while on the other, this is replaced by HLA-DR8.

E7

ARTERIAL OCCLUSIONS ASSOCIATED WITH ANTIBODIES TO CARDIOLIFIN

Asherson RA *, Harris EN*, Gharavi AE*, Derksen RHWM[+], Kater L[+], Lendrum R**, Bird G**, Hughes GRV*.
From: The Rheumatology Unit, The Royal Postgraduate Medical School of London, England
+The University Hospital, Utrecht, The Netherlands.
**The Newcastle General Hospital, Newcastle Upon Tyne, England.

It has long been recognised that venous thromboses, often multiple, have been associated with the "lupus anticoagulant". Recently a strong correlation has been found with the presence of antibodies to cardiolipin. This association has led to a search for these antibodies in arterial occlusions and a strong association with cerebral infarction in S.L.E. has already been documented. We have recently seen several patients with large vessel arterial occlusions suffering from S.L.E., "lupus -like" or other autoimmune disorders who have demonstrated these antibodies. We wish to document 11 such patients, six of whom suffered major arterial occlusions leading to gangrene of the extremities (with amputation of digits or limbs in three). Two presented with bowel infarctions necessitating partial colectomy, two (both males) developed myocardial infarctions in early 20's and one who demonstrated an "aortic arch syndrome"

Histological examination of the vessels examined in four of the patients (two with gangrene and two with mesenteric infarctions) did not reveal any evidence of vasculitis or atheromatous disease.

We suggest that these antibodies are implicated in the pathogenesis of the arterial occlusions in these patients.

E8

SAFETY PROFILE OF SULPHASALAZINE IN RHEUMATOID ARTHRITIS. H A Capell, T Pullar, J A Hunter. Centre for Rheumatic Diseases, Royal Infirmary and Gartnavel General Hospital, Glasgow.

Recent controlled studies have established a role for sulphasalazine (SASP) as a second-line drug in the treatment of rheumatoid arthritis (RA). Since it is possible that toxicity will be different in RA patients compared to those with inflammatory bowel disease close attention needs to be paid to the safety profile of SASP.

158 patients with RA have been treated with SASP (50 1.5g/day; 108 3g/day). 107 (68%) of these patients remained on treatment for 6 months and this group showed significant improvement in clinical and laboratory indices of inflammation (Wilcoxon). Of the 51 (32%) of patients who discontinued SASP 7 (4%) did so because of leucopenia (in 2 cases $< 0.5 \times 10^9/l$ polymorphs). This occurred in the first 12 weeks of therapy and reversed in all cases on withdrawal of SASP. 4 (3%) developed a rash and 21 (13%) stopped because of nausea. Other patients suffering upper GIT symptoms responded to dose adjustment or a brief course of prochlorperazine. Patients who were elderly (> 65) or slow acetylators had a significantly greater incidence of upper GI side effects. Unusual adverse reactions included oral ulceration, hepatitis, acute dyspnoea, dizziness and drowsiness. 5 patients (3%) found SASP ineffective.

Thus while SASP is a useful second-line agent in RA it has a range of side effects similar to gold and penicillamine. Close haematological monitoring is essential particularly in the first 12 weeks of therapy. Prolonged follow up will be needed to determine the long term safety profile.

E9

MICROWAVE RADIOMETRY. A NEW TECHNIQUE FOR ASSESSMENT OF INFLAMMATORY JOINT DISEASE. S Fraser, D Land and R D Sturrock. Centre for Rheumatic Diseases, Royal Infirmary and Department of Physics, University of Glasgow.

Microwave radiometry is a technique measuring microwave emission from sites of inflammation. Microwaves have a wavelength of approximately 10 cms and can penetrate clinically useful depths of up to 4 cms directly measuring tissue thermal radiation.

A microwave detector was used to study joint inflammation in rheumatoid arthritis (RA) patients compared with normal controls. Fifty two knee joints were evaluated clinically for pain, inflammation and range of movement. Laboratory parameters measured included haemoglobin and erythrocyte sedimentation rate (ESR). The microwave emission from each knee was measured and a microwave radiometry index (MRI) calculated for each individual. There was a significant difference between the median MRI of the RA and control groups (2.07) (1.06) and a correlation with ESR ($p < 0.001$) and pain index ($p < 0.001$) was found. The technique was found to be quick, simple to use at the bedside and reproducible and has potential as an objective method for measuring changes in joint inflammation.

E10

MEASUREMENT OF GOLD EFFECTIVENESS: A PROSPECTIVE STUDY. F. Wolfe, M. Cathey, S. Kleinheksel, University of Kansas, Wichita, Ks 67206, P. Spitz, Stanford University, Palo Alto, Ca 94305.

Although gold is a widely used treatment for rheumatoid arthritis (RA), there is little information concerning the length of time gold remains effective, nor quantitative data as to the degree of its effectiveness. To investigate this aspect of gold therapy (GT) we used the Disability Index (DI) of the Stanford Health Assessment Questionnaire (HAQ), an outcome index that worsens (increases) with duration of disease. The HAQ DI computes a 0-3 score from patient self-assessment of 6 ADL activities. We administered this instrument to 69 RA patients at the onset of GT, and at 3-6 month intervals during a 2 to 4 year follow-up. Predicted DIs for each patient were calculated from regression equations derived from 426 gold treated patients, utilizing disease duration and age as independent variables. Gold treated patients had a sharp fall in the DI from pretreatment levels (DI=1.18) and predicted levels (mean DI=1.2) which was maximum at 3 to 6 months of treatment (DI=0.93 - 0.95), and returned to baseline levels at 12 months. Differences between pretreatment and/or predicted DIs were significant ($p<0.05$) at 3 and 6 months of therapy, but not thereafter. Patients completing at least six months of treatment or identified as gold responders had similar temporal patterns of response. The reduction in DI from baseline and/or predicted levels can be expressed as Disability Days (ΔDI x days), and provides a method to express quantitatively the benefit of GT. In this cohort a reduction of 52 disability days occurred during the first 12 months of follow-up. Our data suggest that measureable, clinically significant improvement in function follows gold administration, but is not sustained beyond 12 months.

E11

SURVIVAL IN RHEUMATOID VASCULITIS. Randall S. Vollertsen, Doyt L. Conn, Duane M. Ilstrup, Raymond E. Kazmar, and Joel C. Silverfield, Mayo Clinic, Rochester, MN 55905.

We reviewed survival in 52 patients who had definite rheumatoid arthritis (ARA criteria) and clinical vasculitis which was diagnosed between 1/1/75 and 12/31/80. We defined vasculitis as the presence of classical skin lesions or mononeuritis multiplex or a positive tissue specimen. We measured survival by the Kaplan-Meier method, using age and sex matched upper Middle Western controls. We examined individual clinical findings to determine which were associated with decreased survival ($p\leq0.05$).

Twenty patients died. We observed the others for 57.0 $\pm$ 24.8 months, (mean $\pm$ standard deviation). Manifestations of vasculitis included skin ulcers (28 patients), purpura and petechia (17), gangrene and infarctions other than leg ulcers (13), mononeuritis multiplex (22), and positive tissue specimens (24 of 26 patients). The positive tissue specimens were from skin (17 patients), nerve (5), and other tissues (2).

We found significantly decreased survival at 6 months (91.2% vs 98.9%, patient vs controls) through 6 years (57.6% vs 88.7%) after diagnosis. Even those patients who survived for three years continued to demonstrate significantly decreased survival over the subsequent three years (74.7% vs 94.7%).

The two clinical factors which were most significantly associated with decreased survival were increased age at diagnosis of vasculitis and cytotoxic-immunosuppressive therapy before diagnosis of vasculitis.

E12

TOTAL HEMOLYTIC COMPLEMENT ASSAY IN RHEUMATOID ARTHRITIS: INTERFERENCE BY RHEUMATOID FACTOR AND RELATIONSHIP TO DISEASE ACTIVITY. Sharad Lakhanpal and Doyt L.Conn. Mayo Clinic, Rochester, MN 55905.

Total complement levels (CH50) are reported to be prognostically useful in the evaluation of rheumatoid arthritis (RA). We observed that CH50 could not be measured in some patients with RA because their sera agglutinated the sensitized sheep erythrocytes (SSE) that are used for complement assay. We evaluated disease severity in these patients. An age and sex matched group of RA patients seen during the same period of time, whose sera did not agglutinate SSE, served as controls.

There were 33 patients in the study group and 35 in the control. The mean ages were 64.9 years and 75 years, M:F ratio was 9:24 and 7:28 and mean duration of RA was 11.5 years and 14.6 years, in the two groups, respectively. C'3 and C'4 levels were normal in the 23 study patients evaluated. Significant differences were seen in the numbers of patients in the two groups with vasculitis (13 and 1), subcutaneous nodules (23 and 11), keratoconjunctivitis sicca (4 and 0), complicating infections (11 and 2), Felty's syndrome (6 and 0), pulmonary involvement (14 and 2), leukopenia (6 and 1), antinuclear antibody (22 and 7), rheumatoid factor (RF) (33 and 19), hypergammaglobulinemia (15 and 8) and erosive arthritis (17 and 6).

Patients in the study group had higher RF titers which presumably was responsible for agglutination of SSE. CH50 levels were measurable in 5 of the study patients some time either before or after the period during which they agglutinated the SSE. Their RF titers were lower at these times.

The sera of some RA patients agglutinates SSE when tested for CH50. These patients have higher RF titers and more severe rheumatoid disease.

E13

MODULATING EFFECTS OF HYPERURICEMIA ON RHEUMATOID DISEASE ACTIVITY. Carlos A.Agudelo,Winston-Salem,Armin Good,Ann Arbor, Chris Wise, Robert Turner and Edward Pisko, Bowman Gray School of Medicine,Winston-Salem,NC 27103.

The negative association between gout and rheumatoid arthritis (RA) is well accepted. In vitro studies have described hyperuricemic suppression of rheumatoid factor production. In this study, we provide in vivo evidence for the immunosuppressive effects of hyperuricemia by showing flares of RA disease activity during hypouricemic therapy. We describe 3 male patients who first presented with gouty arthritis. Pertinent findings included acute arthritis with podagra (3/3),monosodium urate crystals (MSU) in inflammatory synovial fluids (2/2), hyperuricemia (3/3), and self limited attack with improvement after colchicine therapy (3/3). While on hypouricemic therapy, these 3 patients developed classic RA (2) and a symmetric seronegative polyarthritis (1). Findings included a symmetrical inflammatory arthritis (3/3), high titer rheumatoid factor (2/3), inflammatory synovial fluid with repeatedly negative MSU crystals (3/3), erosive x-ray changes (3/3), subcutaneous nodules (2/3), rheumatoid synovial biopsy (2/2). Serum uric acid levels were repeatedly normal during active RA. Hypouricemic therapy has been discontinued with gradual return to hyperuricemic levels and concomitant objective improvement in their RA process with no other changes in their treatment. This study provides further evidence that hyperuricemia modulates the clinical expression of inflammation in some RA patients.

E14

MICROVASCULAR PRESSURES IN NORMAL CANINE JOINTS. Peter A. Simkin and Richard S. Benedict. U. of Wa., Seattle, WA 98195.

Net water exchange between plasma (p) and synovial fluid (sf) reflects the interaction of opposing hydrostatic (HP) and oncotic (OP) pressures. Proximal filtration is driven by relatively high arteriolar pressure, whereas distal reabsorption occurs at the lower intravascular pressure of the venules. At the point of transition from net filtration to net reabsorption, all forces are in balance and the "mean microvascular pressure" may be calculated from the equation: $HP_{sf}+OP_{p}-OP_{sf} = HP_{p}$. We measured these forces (in mm Hg) in the shoulders, wrists and knees of 10 normal, recumbent, live dogs aged 2-10 years:

	HP_{sf}	OP_{p}	OP_{sf}	HP_{p}
Shoulder	-2.8 ± 1.7(SE)	20.5 ± 0.5	8.0 ± 0.6	9.7 ± 1.7
Wrist	1.3 ± 2.5	20.5 ± 0.5	$6.2\pm0.8^{\circ}$	$15.7\pm2.4^{\circ}$
Knee	$-4.5\pm1.1^{\circ}$	20.5 ± 0.5	$7.9\pm0.7^{+}$	$7.9\pm1.0^{+}$

$^{\circ} = p < 0.05$, $+ = p < 0.001$ (by paired t)

Subatmospheric pressures were found regularly in canine knees and shoulders but rarely in wrists. Conversely, the oncotic pressure of sf was consistently lowest in the wrist. These factors combine to implicate a low pressure microvascular bed in the knee in contrast to a relatively high pressure bed in the wrist. We also found a strong, positive correlation between the age of each dog and the mean oncotic pressure of its sf (r=0.93, p<0.001).

These findings establish highly significant differences in normal microvascular function between joints and between individual dogs. Such physiological variation may prove to be an important determinant of synovial susceptibility to specific rheumatic diseases.

E15

STUDIES OF CELLULAR SOURCE OF PROINFLAMMATORY ENZYME PHOSPHOLIPASE A_2 IN RHEUMATOID SYNOVIAL FLUID. Peter Vadas, Waldemar Pruzanski, John Kim, Helene Jacobs and Ewa Stefanski. University of Toronto, Canada. M4Y 1J3.

High phospholipase A_2 (PLA_2) was found in rheumatoid synovial fluids (SF). PLA_2, a Ca^{++}-requiring lipolytic protein, MW 12,000, is both vasoactive and proinflammatory, implicating it in the propagation of inflammation in RA. The source of PLA_2 in SF has not yet been identified. Since FMLP-stimulated rabbit PMN's release PLA_2 (Lanni and Becker, Am. J. Path. 113:90,83) we compared intracellular PLA_2 and FMLP-induced PLA_2 release from rabbit peritoneal exudate cells (PEC) and rheumatoid SF cells, as well as PLA_2 in peripheral blood (PB) leukocytes in rabbit and man. Cells were purified from at least 3 donors, sonicated and assayed for PLA_2 activity. Sonicates of unstimulated human PB leukocytes had negligible intracellular PLA_2 (20-38 Units/5 X 10^6 cells). Rabbit buffy coat cells had 15-fold higher intracellular PLA_2 activity than human buffy coat cells (294 vs 20 Units/5 X 10^6 cells). This confirms and extends previously reported high PLA_2 in rabbit PEC. Treatment of PEC with FMLP caused rapid release of lysosomal PLA_2 (141 vs 49 in controls). However, SF cells which exhibit high PLA_2, did not release it in response to FMLP. Human PB PMN's incubated in rheumatoid SF with high PLA_2 showed increased membrane-associated PLA_2. Our study has shown a species difference between rabbit and man in both the intracellular content and FMLP-stimulated extracellular PLA_2 release. The fact that human SF PMN's as well as PB PMN's incubated with SF exhibit comparable PLA_2 levels, may mean that these cells acquire PLA_2 passively and are not a significant source of SF PLA_2. SF PLA_2 may originate from inflamed synovium. Studies are now in progress to determine the cellular source of SF PLA_2 using immunofluorescent-labeled anti-PLA_2 antibodies. Supported by the Arthritis Society.

E16

Clq BINDING ASSAY: MECHANISM AND APPLICATION TO SEROPOSITIVE RHEUMATOID ARTHRITIS. Roberta J. Jacobs and Raman Mocharla. Okla. Med. Res. Fndn., Oklahoma City, OK 73104.

The mechanism of the Clq binding assay (ClqBA) was examined using ^{131}I-heat aggregated IgG (HAIgG) as an immune complex (IC) model. No difference in the amount of ^{131}I-HAIgG precipitated by 2.5% polyethylene glycol (PEG) was observed in the absence or presence of varying concentrations of ^{125}I-Clq, indicating that crosslinking of IC by Clq does not lead to increased precipitation by PEG. Instead, the amount of ^{131}I-HAIgG precipitated was strictly a function of its concentration.

The incidence of positivity with ClqBA in clinically active SLE was 19% (4/21) compared to 96% (27/28) in seropositive rheumatoid arthritis, a disease not thought mediated systemically by IC. The correlation between ClqBA reactivity and rheumatoid factor (RF) titer (latex agglutination) was not significant (r = 0.28), p > 0.1). By density gradient centrifugation, ClqBA reactivity was found in low (7-11S) and intermediate (11-18S) molecular weight (MW) fractions, suggesting that reactive material was not IgM RF nor complement activating IC. Results with the antibody excess anti-C3 assay for IC (J. Immunol. 130:2775, 1983) showed an absence of low MW C3-bearing immunoglobulin and the presence of low MW RF in these samples. This, along with a strong correlation between ClqBA and anti-C3 assay reactivity in unfractionated sera (r = 0.59, $p \leq .001$), suggest that intermediate complexes of IgG RF may be the ClqBA reactive material in seropositive rheumatoid arthritis.

E17

EXPERIMENTAL AUTOIMMUNE MYOCARDITIS (EAM) IN THE GUINEA PIG. Stephen M. Campbell, Jeffrey D. Hosenpud, Mark V. Hart, and Nelson S. Niles. Oregon Health Sciences University, Portland, OR 97201.

We have produced EAM in the guinea pig (GP) by immunizing (IZ) animals to heterologous heart protein, Freund's adjuvant, and pertussis vaccine. Eleven to 15 weeks following onset of immunization, in vivo hemodynamic pressures, cardiac outputs, blood volume (BV), in vitro pressure-volume relationships, collagen content, histology, serology, and lymphocyte transformation studies were performed on control and IZ GPs. There were no differences in heart rate, aortic pressure, cardiac outputs, or stroke volumes between groups. LVEDP was increased in IZ GPs, as was mean RA pressure. Blood volume was markedly increased. LV weight was increased, as was LV volume as assessed by PV relationships. Collagen content was also increased, and histology revealed inflammation, myocyte necrosis, and fibroblast proliferation. Antibody to GP heart antigen was detected in IZ GPs by hemagglutination and solid-phase radioimmunoassays. IZ GPs also demonstrated increased lymphocyte transformation to GP heart antigen.

These results show that an inflammatory myocarditis can be produced by immunization, that this can be monitored by in vivo hemodynamic measurements, and that immunological mechanisms may play a role. EAM in GPs may be a useful model to study immune mediated myocardial injury in rheumatic and other diseases.

E18

Effects of cationic catalase and superoxide dismutase on experimental arthritis.

J. Schalkwijk, W.B. van den Berg, L.B.A. van de Putte, L.A.B. Joosten and L. van den Bersselaar.
Dept. Rheumatology, St.Radboudhospital, Geert Grooteplein Zuid 8, 6500 HB Nijmegen, the Netherlands.

Several enzymes were made cationic by coupling to polylysine or shielding of anionic sites. These enzymes, all having an isoelectric point higher than 8.5 exhibited an excellent retention in articular structures when injected in mouse knee joints. Autoradiography and histochemistry show that cationic forms of catalase, superoxide dismutase and horseradish peroxidase are firmly retained by negatively charged tissues such as cartilage and synovium. The halflife of these enzymes in the joint is thus significantly extended compared to the native enzymes. It was found that injection of cationic catalase or peroxidase induced a marked suppression of the inflammatory response in two types of experimental arthritis, as measured by ^{99m}Tc-uptake and ^{125}I-albumin leakage. Native catalase and peroxidase were less or not at all effective. Cationic superoxide dismutase or cationic proteins in general did not suppress inflammation. These data suggest that elimination of hydrogen peroxide contributes to the suppression of the inflammatory response.

E19

ANTINUCLEOLAR ANTIBODIES (ANoA): Sucheelar Panicheewa, C.E. Harmon. University of Colorado Health Sciences Center, Denver, Colorado

ANoA have been reported in 8.3% of patients (pts) suspected clinically of having a rheumatic syndrome with scleroderma the most frequently associated disease. We first studied the sera of 570 consecutive pts. with a known or suspected rheumatic disease by the indirect immunofluorescence technique (IF) to determine the frequency of ANoA positivity on 2 different substrates, mouse kidney (MK) and HEp-2 cells.

The sera of 15/570 (2.6%) pts. demonstrated ANoA on MK while 28/570 (4.9%) had ANoA when HEp-2 cells were used as the substrate. Differences in ANoA positivity were apparent when various commercially available HEp-2 substrates were used. Compared to our best substrate (Antibodies, Inc.), ANoA positivity in the 28 sera varied from 29 to 86% on 5 other HEp-2 substrates. There were 3 distinct patterns of nucleolar IF: homogeneous (H), clumpy (C), and discrete speckles (DS). The most common diagnosis was lupus.

We next examined 101 MK-ANoA positive sera on our most reliable HEp-2 substrate. Of the 101, 91 were also ANoA positive on HEp-2 with 3 distinct No IF patterns observed: 63 H, 20 C, and 8 DS. Clinical information was available in 50 pts. Irrespective of pattern, the most common diagnoses were SLE and scleroderma, 18% each, and Raynaud's (14%). SLE, scleroderma and Raynaud's were associated with H-No IF while SLE was rarely associated with clumpy or DS No IF.

This study demonstrates that: 1) ANoA are uncommon in unselected sera although use of a cell line substrate nearly doubles the rate of positivity, 2) the proper HEp-2 substrate is critical in the detection of ANoA, 3) SLE, scleroderma and Raynaud's are the most frequently associated diseases with ANoA, 4) there are 3 distinct No IF patterns which may be associated with different rheumatic diseases.

E20

IMPOTENCE IN SCLERODERMA. NS Nowlin, JE Brick, DJ Weaver, DA Wilson, HL Judd, and HE Carlson. VA Medical Center and University of Missouri-Columbia, Columbia, MO 65201, and UCLA, Los Angeles, CA 90024.

Impotence has been reported in patients with scleroderma (PSS); however, both the incidence and the etiology remain unclear. Sexual function was evaluated in 10 male PSS patients in our rheumatology clinic. Ten age-matched male patients with rheumatoid arthritis were also studied. Serum levels of testosterone (TEST), prolactin (PRL), estradiol (E_2), follicle stimulating hormone (FSH), luteinizing hormone (LH), and thyroxine (T_4) were measured; penile and leg blood flow was evaluated using the Doppler technique. Of the 10 PSS patients (aged 35-69) interviewed, 5 reported complete impotence, 3 had impaired potency, and 2 had normal sexual function. Of the 10 RA patients (aged 34-67), none was impotent, 3 had impaired potency, and 7 had normal sexual function. TEST, PRL, E_2 and T_4 were normal in all patients. FSH and LH were elevated in some patients, but there were no significant differences between the PSS and RA groups. The results of the penile blood pressure studies are shown below. Two PSS patients also had evidence of large vessel disease in the legs.

	PSS Impotent	PSS Partially Potent	PSS Potent	RA Partially Potent	RA Potent
# Abnormal	3	1			
# Intermediate	2		1		
# Normal	0	2	1	3	4

Impotence is more common in our PSS patients (50%) than in age-matched patients with a different chronic disease. Our results indicate that impotence in scleroderma appears to be due principally to vascular insufficiency, perhaps reflecting small-vessel involvement by PSS.

E21

CONTINUOUS ESOPHAGEAL pH MONITORING IN SCLERODERMA. W Ravich, F Wigley, R Wilson, W Ettinger Jr., R Johannes, and T Hendrix. Divisions of Gastroenterology and Rheumatology. The Johns Hopkins Medical Institutions. Baltimore, MD. 21205.

Gastroesophageal reflux disease is common in scleroderma. It has been assumed that the severity of esophageal involvement, as defined by manometric examination, correlates with the severity of reflux. We examine this assumption by comparing the results of esophageal manometry (EM) with continuous pH monitoring (CpHM).

METHODS. 9 patients with systemic sclerosis (6 diffuse, 3 CREST, 1 overlap syndrome) were evaluated. EM was performed using a multilumen catheter perfused by a low compliance pump. Lower esophageal sphincter pressure (LESP) was defined as the average of end-expiratory pressure during a single slow pull-through. The results were scored on a scale of 0 to 5, with 0 being normal and 5, aperistalsis and very low (≤5 mmHg) LESP. CpHM was performed using a portable instrument developed at Johns Hopkins. CpHM began prior to the dinner and extended through the night. The % time with esophageal pH ≤4 was calculated for a 4-hr postprandial(PP) and an 8-hr supine(sleep) period as a measure of reflux severity. Scattergrams followed by linear regression analysis of the results of EM scoring and of LESP separately against 4-hr PP and 8-hr supine reflux were used. The Fisher's Exact test was used to look for significant differences between subgroups.

RESULTS. 7 of 9 patients had EM scores of 4 or 5 representing severe degrees of esophageal involvement. All patients had abnormal CpHM, however a dissociation of reflux severity during the PP and supine periods was common.

	4-hr PP	8-hr supine
mean % reflux (range)	10.1(0-20.6)	14.2(0-48.2)

No significant correlation was noted between either EM score or LESP and either CpHM period.

CONCLUSIONS. The results of esophageal manometry do not correlate well with reflux severity as measured by CpHM. This suggests that other factors than those measured by EM are involved in the production of reflux. CpHM provides a more direct measure of reflux severity than does EM.

E22

D-PENICILLAMINE TOXICITY IN SYSTEMIC SCLEROSIS. Virginia D. Steen, Sandra Blair, Thomas A. Medsger, Jr., University of Pittsburgh, Pittsburgh, PA 15261

We have evaluated D-penicillamine (DPA) toxicity in 259 systemic sclerosis (SS) patients treated since 1972. Eighty-four percent had diffuse scleroderma. Their mean age was 46 years and their median disease duration was 2.1 years. The average daily dose of DPA was 635mg given for a mean of 1.8 years.

The proportion of SS patients with DPA side effects was 47%, similar to the 60% found in 10 published series of 1219 rheumatoid arthritis (RA) patients. Toxicities included: rash 15% SS vs. 19% RA; proteinuria 8% vs. 11%; gastrointestinal (GI) symptoms 8% vs. 13%; dysgeusia 3% vs. 13%; oral ulcers 3% vs. 8%; thrombocytopenia 3% vs. 5%; and neutropenia 2% vs. 3%. Four episodes each of myasthenia gravis and pemphigus occurred in our patients; both are rarely reported in RA. GI symptoms due to DPA were more prevalent in patients with underlying SS esophageal involvement with dysphagia. HLA-DR3 was more frequent in DPA treated patients with proteinuria (4/11 or 36%) than in those without this complication (23/118 or 19%). All four myasthenia gravis patients had HLA-DR5.

Drug withdrawal due to toxicity was necessary in 30% SS and 33% RA patients from the literature. Fifty-four of our SS patients (21%) discontinued DPA for non-toxicity reasons and 126 (49%) remain on DPA for a mean of 2 years. Although DPA is a toxic drug with a high frequency of adverse effects, it can be used safely in systemic sclerosis. The autoimmune disorders pemphigus and myasthenia gravis may occur more commonly in SS compared to RA.

E23

ALPHA-2 ADRENERGIC RECEPTORS IN PATIENTS WITH MCTD. J. Peller, E. Keenan, G. Gabor, J. Porter and R.M. Bennett. Oregon Health Sciences University, Portland, Oregon 97201.

Raynaud's phenomenon (RP) is a frequent occurence in MCTD and is due to both organic vascular disease and vasospasm. In this study an attempt has been made to dissect out these 2 variables with particular attention to platelet $\alpha 2$ receptors. Eight patients with MCTD and RP had upper limb angiography, digital plethysmography and $\alpha 2$ receptor studies; they were compared to 14 normal healthy subjects and 22 patients with spastic RP. Platelet $\alpha 2$ receptors were quantitated in membrane fractions (200µg of protein) incubated (25°C, 20 min) with ^{3}H-dihydroergocryptine (0.5 to 25 nM, 23 Ci/m mol); unlabelled phentolamine (100 µM) was run in parallel to establish specific binding; bound ligand was separated from free ligand by filtration.

All 8 patients with MCTD and RP had abnormal digital plethysmography and angiography as evidenced by occlusion of 43/80 digital arteries and 4/8 ulnar arteries - these findings are indicative of significant organic vascular disease. The $\alpha 2$ receptor capacity in the 14 normal control was 78±8 fm/mg (mean ±SEM) of membrane protein; the 8 patients with MCTD had values of 168.7, 84.2, 263.4, 79.4, 93.3, 77.5, 444.8 and 97.3. Three of these values are >2 S.D. above the mean value for controls and compare to values seen in purely spastic RP (192±15 fm/mg). The 2 MCTD patients with the greatest $\alpha 2$ receptor capacity had a Kd one order greater than the other MCTD patients and controls - 1.9×10^{-8} and 2.5×10^{-8} M versus a mean Kd of 2.3×10^{-9} M (MCTD) and a mean Kd of 5×10^{-9} M (controls). These findings indicate a high prevalence of organic vascular disease in patients with MCTD, but also point to a subgroup of patients with a pattern of increased $\alpha 2$ receptor capacity, as is seen in patients with purely spastic RP. Whether these changes in platelet receptors are mimicked by similar changes in vascular smooth muscle may be a fruitful area of future research with implications for treatment.

E24

DIGITAL VASCULAR ASSESSMENT OF PATIENTS WITH RAYNAUD'S PHENOMENON (RP). Peter Lee, Jeff Sarkozi, Edward C. Keystone, and Arthur A. Bookman. The Wellesley Hospital, Toronto, ON M4Y 1J3.

Capillary microscopy*, measurement of digital blood pressure (BP), photoplethysmography (PPG) and evaluation of digital arterial circulation by doppler ultrasonic tracing were carried out in 30 patients with systemic sclerosis (PSS) (mean age 43.4 ± 15.0 yrs, disease duration 2.0 ± 3.4 yrs), 56 with RP (mean age 41.3 ± 12.6 yrs, duration RP 7.0 ± 9.2 yrs; 16 primary and 40 with undifferentiated connective tissue disease:UDCT) and 20 normal controls (mean age 35.3 ± 9.0 yrs).

Results (All means ± SD)

	*No. enlarged capillary loops(ECL)	*Avascular score (AS)
Controls	0.1 ± 0.1	0
RP:	3.3 ± 4.5	0.3 ± 0.4
Primary	1.2 ± 1.6	0.1 ± 0.2
UDCT	4.1 ± 5.0	0.4 ± 0.4
PSS	12.0 ± 7.4	1.6 ± 0.8

	PPG Index	Digital/Brachial BP	Doppler Index
Controls	2.5 ± 3.8	0.95 ± 0.10	70.3 ± 6.7
RP	7.6 ± 6.0	0.76 ± 0.14	65.3 ± 11.8
PSS	15.3 ± 7.1	0.56 ± 0.26	47.9 ± 16.6

Differences between controls, RP and PSS were all highly significant ($P < 0.005$) except Doppler between normals and RP ($p < 0.05$). Differences between primary RP and UDCT were only significant in mean ECL and AS (both $p < 0.025$). ECL was measurement with greatest sensitivity (100%), specificity (81%) and positive predictive value (90%) for secondary RP. Doppler was least sensitive (67%); digital BP and PPG were least specific (62.5%).

E25

ELECTRON MICROSCOPIC STUDY OF RHEUMATOID SYNOVIAL VASCULATURE: INTIMATE RELATIONSHIP BETWEEN TALL ENDOTHELIUM AND LYMPHOID AGGREGATES.
T. Iguchi, H. Ishikawa, K. Hirohata, and M. Ziff. UTHSCD, Dallas, TX 75235, and Kobe University School of Medicine, Kobe, Japan.

Rheumatoid (RA) synovial membranes with well-developed mononuclear cell infiltrates have areas of lymphoid aggregation and areas containing lymphocytes, plasma cells and macrophages (transitional areas). To determine whether there was a relation between the composition of the cellular infiltrates and the structure of the neighboring blood vessels, we examined the features of the vessels in infiltrated areas in relation to the cellular composition of the surrounding infiltrates. In view of the role of tall endothelium in lymphocyte emigration from post capillary venules of lymph node, the "tallness" of the EC was quantitated by measurement of the ratio of the height of the cell to its base (H/B). The vessels of 20 RA synovia varied between 7 and 70μ in outer diameter, and the height of EC of between 0.8-8.3μ. H/B showed a strong correlation with the number (τ=0.91, $p<0.001$) and per cent (τ=0.94, $p<0.0001$) of lymphocytes around the vessel, i.e. the denser the aggregation, the taller the endothelium. In contrast, H/B showed a negative correlation with per cent plasma cells (τ=-0.76, $p<0.0002$) and per cent macrophages (τ=-0.83, $p<0.0001$), i.e. EC were flatter in the antibody-producing transitional areas of the synovium. Such correlations were not found for capillaries or for the vessels of the interstitial areas. These observations indicate that the formation of lymphoid aggregates in RA synovium occurs around vessels with tall endothelium, as in normal lymphoid tissue. In contrast, EC in antibody-producing areas are by comparison significantly decreased in height. These findings suggest that the pattern of synovial cellular infiltration may be intimately related to the structure of neighboring blood vessels.

E26

CA ANTAGONISTS INHIBIT PERIPHERAL BLOOD MONONUCLEAR CELL PROLIFERATION. SB Kramer & R Hirschhorn. Dept. of Med., NYU Med. Ctr, NYC

Calcium (Ca^{++}) fluxes have been reported to be essential for activation of peripheral blood mononuclear cells (PBM). Three classes of Ca^{++} antagonists, represented by nifedipine (Nf), verapamil (Vp) and diltiazem (Dl), have all been shown to block the flow of Ca^{++} through voltage-sensitive Ca^{++} channels. The effects of the different drugs appear to be mediated via different but allosterically linked sites. We therefore tested the effect of these three structurally different classes of Ca^{++} antagonists on PBM proliferation induced by PHA and allogeneic cells (MLR) as well as spontaneous proliferation. All three classes of Ca^{++} antagonists inhibited PHA induced, MLR and spontaneous PBM proliferation in a dose dependent fashion. The IC_{50}'s for PHA induced proliferation for Vp, Nf and Dl were 34, 80, and 191uM respectively. The dose response curves for Vp and Dl were parallel, while that for Nf was distinctly different (slope=-3.2±0.3 and -2.8±0.3 vs -1.4±0.3, respectively, $p<0.01$). Nicardipine, a Ca^{++} antagonist in the same class as Nf, demonstrated a curve identical to that of Nf (IC_{50}=87±6uM and slope = -1.3±0.2, $p<0.01$). Chelation of extracellular Ca^{++} by EGTA abolishes PBM proliferation in response to PHA and MLR. The effect of EGTA can be overcome by increasing extracellular Ca^{++}. In contrast, increasing extracellular Ca^{++} did not reverse the inhibition of proliferation induced by Nf, Vp and Dl, which have been reported to block $^{45}Ca^{++}$ influx into lymphocytes. These data are still consistent with a requirement for Ca^{++} for PBM proliferation since not all effects of Ca^{++} antagonists can be reversed by excess Ca^{++} in other systems. The data also indicate that, as in cells with voltage-sensitive Ca^{++} channels, Dl and Vp interact at a site on PBM different from that for Nf.

E27

SYSTEMIC LUPUS ERYTHEMATOSUS (SLE) ANTIBODY REACTIVITY WITH VLA-LIKE MEMBRANE PROTEINS ON LYMPHOCYTE AND NEURONAL CELLS. Ken D. Pischel, Harry G. Bluestein, and Virgil L. Woods, Jr. University of California, San Diego; San Diego CA 92103.

Systemic lupus erythematosus (SLE) sera frequently contain many antibodies, including ones reactive with lymphocyte and neuronal cell surface antigens. These antibodies may be important in the pathogenesis of SLE immunologic abnormalities and lupus neuropsychiatric disease. By reacting SLE serum with intact normal T cells and subsequent immunoprecipitation, we have previously shown some SLE sera react with discrete surface proteins of heterogeneous molecular weights, including frequent reactivity with chains of 150 kd mass. Now we examine those sera for cross reactivity between lymphocytes and neurons. Several SLE sera react with similar-sized molecules from both T lymphocytes and neuronal cells. These precipitated molecules have been shown by electrophoresis to be different in molecular weight from T200, CR1, OKT9, and OKM1. The molecular weight of these molecules most closely resembles that of VLA glycoproteins precipitated by the monoclonal antibody A-1A5 (M. Hemler et al; J. Immunol. 131:334, 1983). VLA molecules have been reported to be present on long-term mitogen or alloantigen activated T cells and a subset of other cells. VLA molecules were demonstrated to be present on neuronal cells by immunoprecipitation with monoclonal antibody A-1A5 of iodinated SK-N-SH neuronal cells and coelectrophoresis with A-1A5 immunoprecipitated lymphocyte VLA. Rabbit anti-PBL immunoprecipitates prepared from neuronal cells contained VLA-like molecules as predominant bands. Thus VLA-like molecules represent major cross-reactive surface antigens between lymphocytes and neuronal cells and may contribute significantly to the lymphocyte-neuronal cross reactivity of SLE sera.

E28

PRODUCTION OF THE GLYCOSAMINOGLYCAN (GAG)-STIMULATORY FACTOR BY CLONED, IN VITRO-ACTIVATED HUMAN T LYMPHOCYTES. Min Tsao, Adriana Zeevi, Theresa Whiteside, Pittsburgh, PA.

Supernatants of mitogen-activated mononuclear cells (MNC) contain a factor which stimulates up to 15-fold the synthesis of glycosaminoglycan (GAG) by cultured normal dermal fibroblasts (DF). We have previously shown that the production of the GAG-stimulatory factor by MNC, T lymphocytes and T-cell subsets depends on the presence of monocytes. To demonstrate that the GAG-stimulatory factor is a product of T lymphocytes, we cloned normal T lymphocytes that were activated in mixed lymphocyte culture. Selected alloreactive T cell clones were activated with irradiated stimulator cells (PBL or B cell line) and the supernatants collected after 72h. The GAG activity was determined by adding aliquots of supernatants to confluent DF for 72h. ^{3}H-glucosamine was added for the last 24h. of culture and the newly-synthesized GAG determined. Representative results are shown below.

CLONE	STIMULATOR	CPM GAG*
HA6	-	13 ± 1
HA6	PBL	50 ± 4
HA18	-	21 ± 1
HA18	PBL	104 ± 13
-	PBL	17 ± 2
Medium (Neg. cont.)		24 ± 2
MNC + Con A (Pos cont)		235 ± 16

CLONE	STIMULATOR	CPM GAG*
310	-	6 ± 1
310	BLCL	73 ± 6
-	BLCL	9 ± 2
Medium (Neg. cont.)		7 ± 2
MNC + Con A (Pos cont)		32 ± 1

*cpm GAG x $10^{-3}/10^6$ cells

Only supernatants from alloactivated T cell clones contained GAG stimulatory factor, whereas supernatants from non-stimulated T cell clones or irradiated PBL and BLCL had no activity. Our results suggest that activated T cells release factors that modulate synthetic activities of dermal fibroblasts in vitro.

E29

ABNORMAL EXPRESSION OF SURFACE IMMUNOGLOBULIN ON TOLERANT ANTIGEN-BINDING CELLS. Richard D. Brasington, Mary Morton, Cynthia Baumgartner, Jan Reichard-Brown, Beth J. Noel, and Robert F. Ashman. University of Iowa, Iowa City, IA 52242.

Temporary B cell tolerance to the trinitrophenyl (TNP) hapten can be produced in BDF_1 mice by intraperitoneal injection of trinitrobenzene sulfonic acid (TNBS). Antigen-binding cells (ABC's) specific to TNP, measured as TNP donkey erythrocyte rosettes, are found in tolerant mice as well as in immune mice. We have studied the surface immunoglobulin isotype profile of these TNP-binding lymphocytes (TNP-ABC) in 4 groups of animals: nonimmune, immune, tolerant, and tolerant-challenged. Immune mice received intravenous TNP sheep erythrocytes (TNP-SRC), whereas tolerant-challenged mice received TNP-SRC and TNBS on day 0. TNP-ABC for mice immunized with TNP-SRC exhibit increased expression of surface IgG and decreased expression of surface IgD, compared to the ABC from nonimmune mice. Tolerant mice have a higher proportion of ABC with surface IgG, and a lower proportion with surface IgD, than nonimmune mice. Tolerant-challenged mice have a lower proportion of ABC with surface IgG, and a higher proportion with surface IgD, than immune mice. Thus, B cell tolerance in this model entails an attenuation of the surface Ig isotype switch (loss of IgD and gain of IgG) on ABC seen in the normal immune response. For most TNP-ABC, tolerogen exposure prevents the switch in surface isotypes normally induced by exposure to TNP antigen, i.e., the tolerance lesion precedes the surface isotype switch. However, a minority of the TNP-ABC appear to switch surface isotypes in response to the tolerogen itself.

E30

DEXAMETHASONE (DEX) INCREASES BINDING OF RECOMBINANT HUMAN INTERFERON-GAMMA (rIFN) TO HUMAN MONOCYTES. R.W. Strickland and D.S. Finbloom, Walter Reed Army Medical Center, Washington, DC 20307, and L.M. Wahl, NIH, Bethesda, MD 20205.

Interferon-gamma modulates many monocyte effector functions, including enhancement of IgG Fc receptors (FcR) on monocytes. This may be important in those autoimmune diseases where a defect in Fc receptor-mediated clearance of immune complexes exists. Exposure of monocytes to rIFN in the presence of DEX results in even greater binding of IgG to the cell than with monocytes exposed to rIFN alone. One possible mechanism for this DEX-induced enhancement may be increased rIFN receptors on the monocytes. This was examined by measuring binding of ^{125}I-rIFN (Genentech Inc.) to human monocytes. Monocytes, obtained by leukapheresis, were purified by Ficoll-Paque gradient centrifugation and counterflow centrifugal elutriation. Following exposure to DEX for 18 hr at 37°C, monocytes were incubated for 1hr at 4°C with 200-300 units/ml ^{125}I-rIFN. Cells were separated from media by centrifugation through phthalate oils. Non-specific binding was 5% or less. The number of rIFN molecules binding to DEX-treated cells was increased 60%. The effect of DEX was apparent at the lowest dose of DEX tested, 25 nM, and maximal at the higher doses tested, 200-400 nM. Similar studies using the human promyelocytic cell line HL-60 showed no increase in rIFN binding following exposure to DEX. These results suggest that effects of DEX on the rIFN-enhancement of FcR may be due to increased receptor number for rIFN on human monocytes; the lack of effect in HL-60 cells may be due to their undifferentiated state.

E31

FURTHER ANALYSIS OF THE NK-LIKE CELLS IN RHEUMATOID SYNOVIAL FLUID.
R.M. Silver, Medical University of South Carolina, Charleston.

We have previously shown that cytotoxic lymphocytes (L) in rheumatoid synovial fluid differ from natural killer (NK) cells in peripheral blood by their lack of Fc receptors for IgG (FcR-) and by their cytotoxicity toward cell targets normally resistant to short-term NK lysis. In the following experiments, the phenotype of rheumatoid peripheral blood (PB) NK cells and synovial fluid (SF) NK-like cells were compared using the monoclonal antibody, anti-Leu-11. Paired PBL and SFL were incubated with anti-Leu-11 with or without complement (C'), and the remaining viable cells were tested at various effector:target (E:T) ratios for cytotoxicity against the NK target K562 in a 4h ^{51}Cr release assay. Pre-treatment of PBL with anti-Leu-11 + C' eliminated virtually all cytotoxicity toward K562, but similar treatment of SFL had little effect:

	% specific ^{51}Cr release ± SD			
	PBL (n=15)		SFL (n=7)	
E:T	Leu-11	Leu-11 + C'	Leu-11	Leu-11 + C'
100:1	53±21	5±4	45±14	35±17

PBL NK activity could still be significantly reduced by anti-Leu-11 + C' after short-term incubation of PBL with heat aggregated IgG (AHGG) or autologous SF or mitomycin-treated SFL.

From these data the following conclusions can be drawn: (1)most rheumatoid PBL NK cells express Leu-11, but most rheumatoid SFL NK-like cells do not express Leu-11, yet another example of disparity of phenotype and function of RA SFL; (2)the lack of reactivity of anti-Leu-11 with RA SFL NK-like cells (FcR-) supports the conclusion that anti-Leu-11 is directed against the FcR on NK cells; (3)reactivity of anti-Leu-11 with PBL pre-treated with AHGG suggests that the FcR is re-expressed or that anti-Leu-11 competes successfully with AHGG for the FcR.

E32

ELEVATED B CELL SURFACE IgM TO IgD RATIO IN NZB MICE: ROLE OF MEMBRANE ASSOCIATED SECRETORY IgM. Eliot A. Goldings, Dorothy Yuan. University of Texas Health Science Center, Dallas, Tx 75235.

Previous measurements of total B cell surface immunoglobulin (Ig) have revealed an abnormally high ratio of IgM to IgD in adult NZB mice. In this study we have investigated whether the high μ/δ ratio is due to the presence of an abnormally large proportion of plasmablasts with the surface Ig phenotype of activated B lymphocytes. Spleen cells from 8-12 wk old female autoimmune NZB/BINJ and control DBA/2J and B6D2F1/J mice were separated by percoll density gradient centrifugation. The degree of polyclonal B cell activation in each fraction was assessed by determining the number of immunoglobulin secreting cells (ISC) in a reverse hemolytic plaque assay. An abnormally increased number of ISC in NZB mice (2,637±236/10^6 vs 783 ±307/10^6 spleen cells in control strains) was localized to the low density fraction, containing approximately 1/3 of the total number of NZB B cells, whereas the high density fractions in both NZB and control strains contained similar numbers of ISC (389±67/10^6 vs 233±49/10^6 respectively). Correspondingly, the μ/δ ratio of cell surface Ig of the high density cells in the NZB mice (0.9) was much lower than that of unfractionated cells (4.2). Polyacrylamide gel electrophoretic analysis of ^{125}I-labeled surface IgM of the latter cells revealed the presence of a high level of μ chain with the molecular size of secreted IgM. Incubation of these iodinated NZB lymphocytes for 2 hrs allowed the secretion of this μ species in the form of 19s IgM and resulted in membrane μ/δ ratios (1.2) that were similar to those of cells in the high density fraction and akin to resting B lymphocytes (0.5 to 1.0). These results indicate that a major determinant of the increased μ/δ ratio in NZB spleen cells is secreted IgM which becomes transiently membrane-associated.

E33

ENHANCEMENT OF IMMUNOGLOBULIN (Ig) SYNTHESIS BY HUMAN LARGE GRANULAR LYMPHOCYTES (LGL). Martin A. Rodriguez, Isaac Blanca, Miren L. Baroja, Isaac Abadi, and Nicolas Bianco . Centro Nacional de Enfermedades Reumaticas and Centro Nacional de Inmunologia Clinica. Hospital Universitario de Caracas. Caracas, Venezuela.

It has been recently reported that LGL can suppress Ig synthesis. We examined the effect of this cell population on spontaneous and mitogen stimulated IgG synthesis by B cells from healthy donors. Peripheral blood mononuclear cells (PBMC) were separated into B and T populations. LGL (purity > 90%) were obtained after fractionation of nylon non-adherent cells on percoll gradients followed by E-rosetting at 29 C. In some experiments LGL or T cells were preincubated with media or interferon gamma (IFN) for 18 hr at 37 C . Supernatants from cell cultures were tested for IgG levels by ELISA. Both fractions increased spontaneous IgG synthesis: B = 1488 ± 488; B+LGL (5 x 10^4) = 2280 ± 569; B+T (5 x 10^4) = 2138 ± 579 ng/ml (n=6, $p < 0.03$). In contrast, in the presence of T cells fresh LGL failed to enhance IgG production by unstimulated or PWM activated cultures. Unlike fresh cells, low numbers (1x10^3 - 1x10^3) of preincubated LGL enhanced PWM induced IgG synthesis regardless of the presence of T cells. This effect was even stronger after preincubation with IFN (50 to 1000 IU): PBMC 3479 ± 1206, PBMC+LGL-media 5483 ± 1794, PBMC+LGL-IFN (50 IU) 5279 ± 2206, PBMC+LGL-IFN (100 IU) 7698 ± 2844 and PBMC+LGL-IFN (1000 IU) 9564 ± 5654 ng/ml (n=4)(added LGL 1x10^3). We conclude that fresh LGL from healthy donors can enhance spontaneous IgG synthesis by autologous B lymphocytes in the absence of T cells. Preincubation of LGL with media or IFN increased their helper effect regardless of the presence of T cells. Our results support a promoting rather than an inhibitory effect of LGL on IgG synthesis.

E34

ABNORMAL REGULATION OF IMMUNOGLOBULIN (Ig) AND RHEUMATOID FACTOR (RF) SYNTHESIS IN PATIENTS WITH PRIMARY SJOGREN'S SYNDROME (SS). Martin A. Rodriguez, Miren L. Baroja, and Isaac Abadi . Centro Nacional de Enfermedades Reumaticas. Caracas, Venezuela.

Primary SS patients show high serum levels of RF, antinuclear antibodies and circulating immune complexes. The mechanisms underlying this abnormal humoral response were examined in a group of untreated patients. Unstimulated or PWM activated blood lymphocytes cultures were tested for IgG, IgM and IgM-RF production by ELISA. Suppressor T cell activity was abrogated by 2000 rads treatment. OKT8(+) suppressor cells were depleted by a panning technique. As compared to controls (n=17), patients' B cells (n=10) spontaneously produced higher amounts of IgG (923 ± 208 vs 247 ± 32 ng/ml), IgM (363 ± 119 vs 40 ± 15 ng/ml), and IgM-RF (16± 10 vs 1 ± 0.09 ng/ml) ($p < 0.01$). PWM stimulated IgM-RF production was higher in patients (34 ± 15 ng/ml) compared to controls (2 ± 0.3 ng/ml) ($p < 0.05$). T cell irradiation enhanced IgG and IgM production in PWM-driven B+T cocultures from healthy donors. In contrast, this maneuver caused a significant increase in IgG (247 ± 68 %, $p< 0.01$) but not IgM (184 ± 72 %, ns) or IgM-RF (182 ± 56 %, ns) synthesis in cultures from patients. OKT8(+) cell depletion led to a significant increase of IgG production in cultures from controls (1957 ± 833 v.s. 4404 ± 1359 ng/ml, n=7, $p < 0.05$), but not in cultures from SS patients (2678 ± 1263 v.s. 2921 ± 1312 ng/ml, n=6, n.s.). Our results suggest that SS patients have: 1. in vivo hyperactivation of B cells; 2. a selective decrease in radiosensitive T cell suppressor activity for IgM and IgM-RF production; and 3. a competent radiosensitive suppressor function for IgG synthesis which is not fully identified by the OKT8 monoclonal antibody.

E35

MODULATION OF ANTI-DNA PRODUCTION BY DNA:ANTI-DNA IMMUNE COMPLEXES. JD Clough, SA Frank, LH Calabrese, DM Getzy. Cleveland Clinic Foundation, Cleveland, OH 44106.

T cells are known to exert important modulating effects on antibody production, including help, suppression, and control of the IgM-IgG switch. We investigated the effects of incubation of isolated T cells with DNA:anti-DNA immune complexes, prepared in various Ag:Ab ratios, on their ability to modulate specific anti-DNA production and polyclonal Ig production in vitro. T cells isolated by E-rosette sedimentation were preincubated with IC made from calf thymus DNA and immunoabsorbent-purified human anti-DNA in Ag:Ab ratios of 50:1, 10:1, 5:1, and 2.5:1 (wt:wt). After washing, these cells were cocultured with autologous B cells isolated by affinity chromatography (anti-Fab) with 1:50 PWM for 7 days. Supernates were assayed for polyclonal IgM and IgG as well as specific DNA-binding IgM and IgG by solid-phase RIA. There was a directly proportional relationship of the DNA-binding fractions of both IgM (r=.99) and IgG (r=.94) to log[Ag:Ab ratio] of the IC used for preincubation. Furthermore, there was a directly proportional relationship of IgM:IgG ratio within the DNA-binding fraction to log[Ag:Ab ratio] (r=.98). These findings suggest that as T cells are exposed to IC with progressively decreasing Ag:Ab ratio there is a shift from primarily IgM to IgG antibody production as well as a tendency to terminate the response. With autologous cell combinations this is accompanied by only minimal effects on total Ig production and, thus, appears to be specific for the Ag:Ab system in the IC used for preincubation.

E36

UNUSUAL METACARPOPHALANGEAL ARTHROPATHY. WV Williams, TS Hoyt, R Cope, WD Gaunt, TA Pressly, SE Walker. Dept. of Medicine and Radiology, University of Missouri, Columbia, MO 65212.

Degenerative-like arthropathy affecting the metacarpophalangeal (MCP) joints with relative sparing of proximal and distal interphalangeal joints has been described in chondrocalcinosis (CPPD) and hemochromatosis (HC). Eight males aged 51-72 years with MCP arthropathy mimicking CPPD/HC were evaluated with complete history, physical examination, occupational history, detailed hand examination; radiographs of hands, feet, shoulders, lumbar spine, pelvis, knees; joint scans (Tc-PYP); Fe, IBC, ferritin levels; median and ulnar nerve conduction velocities.

The results showed no evidence of CPPD/HC in any patients. Six samples of joint fluid or tissue (5 from 2 patients) were negative by x-ray crystallography. All patients were manual laborers involved in heavy hand use for 30 years or more. Two patients fulfilled clinical criteria for definite rheumatoid arthritis and 2 had asymptomatic decreases in median nerve conduction velocity. An underlying cause other than occupation was not found in 4 patients. The 2nd and/or 3rd MCP joints were involved radiologically in all cases (7/8 bilateral), with Tc-PYP scan positive in 7/8 (5/8 bilateral). Seven of 8 patients were symptomatic at these joints and physical findings included soft tissue swelling (8/8), bony spurs (7/8), tenderness (6/8) and decreased range of motion (6/8). The hand radiographs were reviewed blinded by a radologist intermixed with 22 age, sex, and occupation matched controls. He correctly identified 7/8 as having arthropathy similar to CPPD/HC; 3 new cases were detected. We conclude MCP arthropathy similar to CPPD/HC can be seen without these disorders, mild rheumatoid arthritis and neuropathy can be associated with this radiographic appearance, and an occupational predisposition can be identified.

E37

ARE WOMEN RELATIVELY PROTECTED FROM DEVELOPING ANKYLOSING SPONDYLITIS? S van der Linden, H Valkenburg, A Cats and MA Khan, Universities of Leiden and Rotterdam (The Netherlands) and Case Western Reserve University/Cleveland Metropolitan General Hospital, Cleveland, Ohio.

Ankylosing Spondylitis (AS) is less often diagnosed in females than in males (1 : 3.5), although HLA-B27 distribution is equal in the two sexes. One reason could be a clinically more benign and slow course in females. In radiological surveys, however, the prevalence of AS according to the New York criteria is about the same in both sexes. (To fulfill the New York criteria bilateral sacroiliitis (SI) grade 2 or unilateral grade 3-4 has to be present).

Our family study (Arth Rheum 26:S18,1983) enabled us to evaluate whether borderline SI occurs more often in females, which would suggest some relative protection of females from developing clinical manifestations of AS. Each of 5 observers read twice the pelvic films of 19 B27(-) male, 22 B27(-) female, 24 B27(+) male and 35 B27(+) female relatives of 20 B27(+) AS probands. All readings were done independently and without knowledge of the clinical status and the HLA data. Borderline SI (unilateral grade 2; the contralateral joint showing grade 0 or 1) not fulfilling the New York criteria was seen in 1.1% of the readings of the B27(-) males versus 2.3% readings of the B27(-) females (p value is not significant), and in 1.7% of the readings of the B27(+) males versus 5.4% readings of the B27(+) females ($p < 0.05$).

These findings indicate that borderline SI occurs more frequently in females than males and suggest a shift towards a relatively milder form of AS in females.

E38

An Immunohistological analysis of the synovial membrane in Ankylosing Spondylitis.

*O. Duke, S. Hobbs, L.W. Poulter,
*G.S. Panayi
*Depts. of Medicine and Rheumatology
Guy's Hospital, and Dept. of Immunology,
Royal Free Hospital, London).

We have examined the immunohistology of the synovial membrane (SM) from 6 patients with ankylosing spondylitis (AS) in an attempt to define the cellular interactions and microenvironment occuring in the SM in this disease. Furthermore, we wished to examine the possible differences between AS SM and the SM of other inflammatory arthropathies which maybe of pathogenetic and diagnostic significance.

Monoclonal antibodies to T lymphocyte subsets (OKT4 and OKT8), macrophages (RFD1), B lymphocytes (RFB4 and RFB6), and HLA-DR antigens (directed against monomorphic determinants) were used in the standard immunoperoxidase test performed on frozen 6 μ sections of AS SM.

The results show that no qualitative differences exist between the immunohistological appearances of either rheumatoid arthritis (RA) or AS SM in terms of HLA-DR antigen expression or T cell subset distribution and that a similar microenvironment to that seen in RA SM is observed in the AS SM.

E39

TREATMENT OF OSTEOARTHRITIS OF THE HAND WITH LOW POWER INFRARED LASER, Micha Abeles, Sally Marlowe, Fran Ingenito, University of Connecticut Health Center.

The potential efficacy of low power infrared laser therapy in osteoarthritis (OA) of the joints of the hand was investigated in a randomized double blind study of 20 patients. A Gallium Aluminum Sulfate Laser (physio-technology - Chicago) was used with direct appication of the laser probe to the joint (wavelength 904 mm, pulse rate 1000 Hz at 60 sec/point). The study consisted of 9 laser or sham treatments over 3 weeks. All patients had a pre-study evaluation including hand x-rays and serologic testing. The first C-MC joint was involved in 3 patients and the rest had PIP or DIP joint involvement. Evaluation consisted of a pain analogue scale, grip testing, and the use of the McGill-Melzack pain questionnaire (MMQ).

Statistical analysis showed the experimental group to have a statistically significant decrease of pain (p= .05) on the MMQ in the immediate post treatment and at one month followup periods. Improvement in the other parameters occurred in the laser treated group but did not reach statistical significance.

Although a small number of patients were used in this preliminary study, the results are encouraging and suggest the need for continuing investigation of laser therapy for treatment of OA of the hands.

E40

PATHOLOGY OF EARLY HIP DISEASE IN FEMALE ANKYLOSING SPONDYLITIS. Amrit K. Agarwal, Howard E. Reidbord, Carl H. Eisenbeis, Jr., Burton H. Pollock. St. Margaret Memorial Hospital, Pittsburgh, PA 15215

Various investigators have emphasized the difficulty in studying the histopathology of Ankylosing Spondylitis (AS), especially in the early stages of the disease. The histopathology of a diarthrodial joint in AS is usually described as indistinguishable from that seen in Rheumatoid Arthritis. Changes more characteristic of AS have also been described, and these include a less intense inflammatory infiltrate, less prominent hypertrophy of synoviocytes, reduced proliferation of fibroblasts, more fresh hemorrhage and increased synovial fibrosis in the later stages.

It has recently been postulated that occasionally a unique focal lesion consisting of subchondral vascular proliferation with osteoclastic activity unrelated to pannus formation, contributes significantly to cartilage destruction in AS. The present study examines in detail the histopathology of the hip joint of four female patients with clinically limited and early AS. Their ages ranged from 28 to 51 years. The average duration of hip disease was 4 years. HLA B27 was present in all. Latex test for rheumatoid factor was negative in all. Two patients had bilateral sacroiliitis and one of these was the lone patient with peripheral joint involvement. One had unilateral sacroiliitis. None had thoraco-lumbar spine involvement.

Along with the expected modest degrees of inflammation in surface synovium, intensive vascular proliferation and osteoclastic activity was observed in the subchondral areas of all four hips. These subchondral changes, unrelated to surface pannus, have not been described in clinically early RA.

E41

THE ARTHROPATHY OF WILSON'S DISEASE: EVALUATION FOR A CALCIUM CRYSTAL ETIOLOGY. Kathleen Menerey, Wendy Eider, George Brewer, Armin E. Good, Gregory Irvine, H. Ralph Schumacher, Ethan M. Braunstein, and Irving H. Fox. The University of Michigan, Ann Arbor, Michigan 48109.

Wilson's disease is associated with an osteoarthritis involving the back and large joints. The purpose of this study was to determine if Wilson's disease arthropathy is caused by Calcium Pyrophosphate Dihydrate (CPPD) crystals. Twenty-two patients with Wilson's disease were evaluated with history, physical examination, radiographs, and arthroscopy with cartilage and synovial biopsy in four patients. Patients ranged in age from 19 to 54 years (mean 30). Seventeen of twenty-two patients had findings consistent with a premature osteoarthritis involving in descending order of frequency knees, shoulders, ankles, lumbo-sacral spine, metacarpophalangeals, feet, wrists, hips, and neck. Symptoms consisted primarily of pain and stiffness in affected joints with associated physical findings of tenderness on motion and crepitations with no effusions. Disability was mild. Radiologic findings included spur formation with hyperostosis (11 patients), subchondral cysts (8 patients), joint space narrowing (5 patients) and chondrocalcinosis (3 patients). There was no correlation between severity of neurologic involvement and severity of arthropathy. There were no crystals by preliminary light and electron microscopic studies, but degeneration of chrondrocytes was present in two out of four patients.

These data confirm the existence of a mild premature osteoarthritis in 17 patients and chondrocalcinosis in 3 patients, but at present there is no evidence of CPPD crystals in pathologic studies.

E42

SYNOVIAL FLUID (SF) AND SYNOVIAL MEMBRANE (SM) STUDIES OF ARTHRITIS ASSOCIATED WITH HIDRADENITIS SUPPURATIVA (HS), ACNE CONGOBLATA (AC) AND ACNE FULMINANS (AF). A.J. Reginato, J.S. Bomalaski, L. Guzman, C.R. O'Connor, and M. Sieck. Cooper Med. Ctr., Camden, NJ, Univ. of Pa. and VAMC, Philadelphia, PA 19104.

Pathological studies of articular tissue and SF are needed to characterize the arthritis (AR) associated with the related skin diseases HS, AC and AF. We report 6 patients who presented with seronegative AR and HS (4), AC (1) and AF (1). Patterns of AR in HS included: chronic recurrent asymmetrical erosive AR of hands, knees, ankles, midtarsal joints and destructive toe changes (2), recurrent knee AR and chronic wrist synovitis (1) and asymmetrical nonerosive polyarthritis (1). One pt. presented with sacroiliac joint involvement and increased density of the ilium. SF from 2 pts. was clear with normal viscosity and 800 - 1000 WBC/mm^3 with 80% mononuclear cells. Light and electron microscopy of SM revealed synovial lining cell proliferation, hypervascularization and abundant diffuse and perivascular plasma cell infiltrates. Two pts. also had pyoderma gangrenosum and 1 had keratitis and microabscesses at venipuncture sites. The pt. with AC had symmetrical poly-AR and erosive spondylo-AR with increased bone density of the cervical spine and ilium and destructive toe changes. The pt. with AF had migratory poly-AR followed by ankle AR associated with new bone formation and a large erosion on the fibula. SF from a knee and ankle were both clear with poor viscosity and cell counts ranged from 2400-5400 WBC/mm^3 with 20-50% polymorphonuclear cells. Fibrotic synovium showed sparce mononuclear cell infiltrates and eroded bone and cartilage. AR associated with HS, AC and AF may mimic other destructive or erosive arthropathies. However, SF is only mildly hypercellular and SM shows only mild signs of chronic inflammation with invasion of bone and cartilage.

E43

PALEOPATHOLOGY OF ANKYLOSING SPONDYLITIS AND DIFFUSE IDIOPATHIC SKELETAL HYPEROSTOSIS. Bruce M. Rothschild, Menorah Medical Ctr and Kansas University School of Medicine, Kansas City,MO, 64110.

Serendipitous observation of ceratopsian cervical spine fusion in the British Museum stimulated a variety of site visits to determine the uniqueness of the observation. Similar cervical pathology was documented, not only in both major species of the propositus but, also in other members of the Ceratopsia family of dinosaurs. As this group is characterized by rostral overgrowth and massive skulls, it is proposed that cervical fusion played a protective role, facilitating support of the heavy skull. This cervical fusion not only involved the centrum but also affected the posterior elements of the first three or four cervical vertebrae. Further evidence for a protective role of cervical fusion is noted in the pre-Miocene mole, Mesoscalops, which apparently used its head as a "battering ram" in digging. Such fusion can easily be distinguished from the isolated fusion of caudal vertebrae noted in Diplodoccus and Apatosaurus. Absence of apophyseal joint fusion and the nature of the fusion in the latter two species of Sauropod dinosaurs is more in keeping with a diagnosis of Diffuse Idiopathic Skeletal Hyperostosis (DISH). The site of occurrence of "DISH" in Sauropods is at a highly stressed spinal region. While it may represent a response to trauma, the absence of apophyseal joint damage suggests a protective role, distributing the stress over a wider region of spine. Classical changes of DISH were also noted in two Miocene Mysticetes, Pelocetus and Thinocetus. The extent of spinal calcification in the latter actually led to the species designation, arthritus.

E44

ENDOGENOUS AND NEWLY SYNTHESIZED PROTEOGLYCAN (PGs) IN HUMAN OSTEOARTHRITIC (OA) CARTILAGE. Johanne Martel-Pelletier, Jean-Pierre Pelletier, Jean-Marie Cloutier and Charles J. Malemud, University of Montréal, Montréal, Québec, Canada and Case Western Reserve University, Cleveland, Ohio, U.S.A.

One of the chemical changes that occur early in the OA cartilage is a quantitative diminution in the amount of PGs. It is not known, however, whether this PG defect is related to the decrease in the synthesis of the newly synthesized PG or to the modification of its structure.

In the present investigation, we have examined and compared the structure and the aggregation properties of both endogenous and newly synthesized PGs within the human OA cartilage.

Cartilage specimens were obtained from the tibial plateaus of 7 OA patients. The PGs were radio-labeled with $^{35}SO_4$, extracted in 4 M GuHCl, isolated by a density gradient and analysed on a column chromatography. Our results showed that the PG measured either by uronic acid or by $^{35}SO_4$, was mostly found in the A_1 fraction. The amount of the newly synthesized PGs ($^{35}SO_4$) was significantly higher ($p<0.05$) than the amount of endogenous PG. Conversely, in the higher bouyancy fractions, a significant decrease ($p<0.05$) of the newly synthesized PG was found over that of the endogenous macromolecules. Furthermore, the analysis of the A_1 fraction indicates that the $^{35}SO_4$-PGs are to a large extent, aggregated to hyaluronic acid. On the Sepharose CL2B, the average partition coefficient of the newly synthesized PG was smaller (Kav=0.25) than the endogenous uronic acid containing macromolecules (Kav=0.33). This result indicates that for the endogenous PGs, there could be a reduction in the size of the chondroitin sulfate-rich region.

Supported by MRC Canada and NIH # AG02205.

E45

DEGRADATIVE CHANGES IN HUMAN ARTICULAR CARTILAGE INDUCED BY CHEMOTHERAPEUTIC AGENTS. Johanne Martel-Pelletier and Jean-Pierre Pelletier, University of Montréal, Montréal, Québec, Canada.

Chemotherapeutic agents are therapeutically valuable in treating autoimmune diseases such as inflammatory arthritis. However, their effect on the articular cartilage matrix has not yet been studied. In the present investigation, we evaluated the effects of chemotherapeutic drugs on the articular cartilage by 1) an electron microscopy analysis and 2) a biochemical analysis.

The tibial plateaus of 13 patients, treated with chemotherapeutic agents for malignant tumors, were used. Control specimens, obtained from post-mortem patients were used for comparison. The histological and ultrastructural studies showed that the degenerative and the repair processes were both present simultaneously. The degenerative changes included: alterations in the cells, a decrease in the Safranin-O staining at the superficial layer and around the midlayer chondrocytes, and a collagen fiber disruption in the perilacunar area. A repair process was characterized by an increase in the number of chondrocytes. In the deep layer, some of the chondrocytes showed more intense perilacunar metachromasia staining. Abnormal biochemical values were found. They were associated with a significant increase in: 1) the DNA content (1.5X, $p<0.05$); 2) the total neutral collagenolytic enzyme ($p<0.01$) and metalloproteoglycan-degrading enzyme ($p<0.01$) activities and 3) the active form of the neutral collagenolytic enzyme ($p<0.05$). The uronic acid content of the cartilage of treated patients was decreased compared to that content found in the controls, but the difference did not reach a significant level.

The results of this study indicate that chemotherapeutic agents can induce cartilage changes, which are similar in many ways to those found in early osteoarthrosis. Supported by MRC Canada.

E46

IN VIVO AND IN VITRO EVIDENCE OF A ROLE FOR COMPLEMENT C5 IN TYPE II COLLAGEN-INDUCED ARTHRITIS. William C. Watson, Alexander S. Townes, Peggy S. Brown, James A. Pitcock. VAMC & UTCHS, Memphis, TN 38104; Paul H. Wooley, Mayo Clinic, Rochester, MN 55905.

Passive transfer studies have demonstrated that IgG autoantibody to type II collagen (CII), the major protein of joint cartilage, will initiate arthritis in normal rodents. A recent report (Mayo Clinic Proc 59:737, 1984) described the passive transfer of arthritis to mice by injection of anti-CII antibody isolated from the serum of a patient with rheumatoid arthritis (RA). Complement activation appears to be an integral part of the humoral mechanism, since complement depletion inhibits the development of arthritis after active or passive immunization in rodents. We designed studies to further define the role of complement in CII-induced arthritis. In vivo studies utilized passive transfer techniques with affinity purified rat anti-CII IgG in C5 complete B10.D2/new line and C5 deficient B10.D2/old line mice. Based upon clinical and histological analyses, C5 complete mice were found to be susceptible (75% incidence), while C5 deficient mice were resistant (0% incidence) to the induction of arthritis by a single I.V. injection of 9mg antibody. In vitro studies utilizing an RIA for C5a demonstrated that both rat anti-CII IgG and mouse anti-CII IgG2a activated C5 to C5a when bound to mouse cartilage in vitro. A CII-Sepharose purified fraction from the serum of the above RA patient activated C5 to C5a when bound to human cartilage in vitro. These studies support an important role for complement C5 in the initiation of arthritis by autoantibody to joint cartilage CII and provide additional evidence of a pathogenic potential for human autoantibodies to CII.

E47

CHARGING INHIBITION AS A MEASURE OF ANTI-JO-1. Ira N. Targoff and Morris Reichlin. V.A. Med. Ctr., Dept. of Med., OU Health Sci. Ctr. and Okla. Med. Res. Fdn., Oklahoma City, OK 73104

Antibody to Jo-1 is a marker of polymyositis and of interstitial lung disease in myositis. Jo-1 antigen is histidyl-tRNA synthetase (HtS) and anti-Jo-1 has been shown to inhibit the charging of $tRNA^{His}$. We have studied the use of this inhibitory activity as an assay for Jo-1 antibody in patient serum. When the enzyme is limiting, the charging reaction is a measure of HtS activity. Before the source of HtS (liver extract) is added to start the reaction, it is incubated with a dilution of serum. A 1/50 dilution in the final reaction mixture is used for screening. All nine normal sera caused some inhibition of charging activity, averaging 35% (65% original activity remained). Cohn fraction II caused no inhibition. Twenty-three myositis sera with anti-Jo-1 by immunodiffusion (ID+) and 14 myositis sera negative for anti-Jo-1 by ID (ID-) were tested. Addition of 22 of the ID+ sera resulted in 80-99% inhibition of activity expected with normal serum (66% with serum 23). 13 ID- sera caused <32% inhibition (observed activity = 68-186% of activity seen with addition of normal serum) while the last (1 of 3 that had small elevations on ELISA) inhibited 64%. The charging inhibitory ability (CI) of 24 anti-Jo-1 ID+ sera was quantitated by determining the dilution resulting in 50% inhibition (from a plot of serum dilution vs charging activity). This value was plotted against optical density of the respective serum by ELISA using affinity purified Jo-1 as antigen. A good overall linear correlation (r = .83) was seen. A subset appeared to have more CI for the amount of ELISA activity. Thus, CI can be used to detect and quantitate anti-Jo-1. CI is more sensitive and quantitative than ID. Unlike ELISA, it does not require antigen purification.

E48

THE INFLUENCE OF Y^{aa} ON B6-lpr ANTI-DNA RESPONSES. David S. Pisetsky, Cynthia Klatt, and John B. Roths. Durham VA Hospital, Durham, NC and The Jackson Laboratory, Bar Harbor, ME 04609.

To define genetic interactions in murine SLE, anti-DNA levels were assessed in B6-lpr mice expressing the Y^{aa} autoimmune accelerator gene derived from the BXSB strain. Subclass specific ELISAs were used to measure both total IgG and IgM immunoglobulins as well as anti-DNA specific responses. Male B6-lpr, Y+ mice showed only slight increases in IgG anti-DNA levels in comparison to B6-+/+ controls while female B6-lpr mice had significantly elevated anti-DNA levels in comparison to sex-matched controls. In contrast, B6-lpr, Y^{aa} mice had markedly elevated anti-DNA responses which exceeded levels of both male and female lpr mice. lpr homozygotes with or without lpr failed to show an increase in IgM anti-DNA responses, however. For B6-lpr, Y^{aa} mice increases in IgG anti-DNA levels were disproportionately elevated in comparison to total IgG. These results indicate that lpr and Y^{aa} can act synergistically to promote anti-DNA production and that the impaired anti-DNA response of B6-lpr male mice does not preclude a significant response to another genetically determined mechanism of autoimmunity. The disproportionate increase in anti-DNA levels further suggests that B cells producing anti-DNA may be preferentially expressed during the polyclonal B cell activation of murine autoimmunity.

E49

HUMORAL SENSITIVITY TO NATIVE COLLAGEN TYPES I-VI IN THE ARTHRITIS OF MRL/1 MICE. Steffen Gay, Frank X. O'Sullivan, William J. Koopman. UAB Medical Center, Birmingham, AL 35294.

The presence of immune reactivity to collagen in patients with RA as well as recent interest in the type II collagen-induced arthritis model have suggested a role for autoimmunity to collagen as a major disease mechanism. However, data concerning the occurrence of antibodies (ab) against the different types of collagen during a spontaneously occurring, histologically well-defined arthritis have been lacking.

Sera from 48 MRL/1 mice with spontaneously occurring hindlimb arthritis aged 5 to 25 weeks were obtained. 18 mice were bled at consecutive 4 week intervals. Sera were tested for auto-ab against collagens utilizing highly purified native collagen types I-VI (Meth. Enzymol. 82A:33, 1982) immobilized by coating disposable Immulon^{TM} strips.

Significant levels of circulating ab against native collagen types I, III, and VI could not be detected in any age group. Ab against type II were found in low levels in 9-10 week-old mice, with a moderate elevation at 13-15 weeks and a subsequent decline at >19 weeks. Ab against type IV collagen were detected in slightly elevated levels with a maximum at 9-10 weeks. Most strikingly, ab against type V were markedly elevated after 19 weeks. The data show there is a moderate rise in type II collagen ab levels as cartilage destruction progresses. The presence of type IV collagen ab suggests glomerular lesions. The occurrence of high levels of ab against type V collagen, largely found in the pericellular matrix of smooth muscle cells, is associated with the late stage of disease characterized by histologically documented vasculitis. The results suggest that ab to collagen occur as a consequence of tissue destruction and evidence for a pathogenetic role of ab in MRL/1 arthritis is lacking.

E50

IgA RHEUMATOID FACTOR (RF) ACTIVITY IN B6 AND B6-lpr/lpr MICE. Robert W. Warren and Denise M. Sailstad. UNC, Chapel Hill, NC 27514.

RFs are not limited to autoimmune diseases; RF quantity and/or specificity may determine pathogenic potential. We have previously shown that IgM RFs occur spontaneously in autoimmune B6-lpr/lpr and aged normal B6 (+/+) mice, and are inducible in young normal B6 mice with chronic mitogenic (LPS) or antigenic (KLH) stimulation. The specificity of IgM RFs in the B6-lpr/lpr female appears unique.

Significant IgA RF (anti-mouse IgG) activity was found in normal B6 sera by ELISA, but titers increased only 2-4 fold from 2 to 18 mo of age. Though chronic LPS and KLH immunization induced high IgM RF titers, IgA RF titers did not rise. While 2 mo lpr/lpr IgA RF titers were not different from +/+, 9 mo female and male lpr/lpr titers exceeded matched +/+ controls by 10.8 and 3.0 fold, respectively.

IgA RF specificity was assessed by direct binding to heterologous IgGs (het IgG) and by ELISA inhibition assays. While both +/+ and lpr/lpr sera bound rabbit and human IgG, only 6-9 mo female lpr/lpr sera bound goat and bovine IgG significantly. Spontaneous +/+ IgM RFs had shown no binding to het IgGs. In general, IgA binding to these het IgGs was clearly inhibitable by mouse IgG (and vice versa), suggesting significant +/+ and lpr/lpr IgA RF cross-species IgG reactivity. Unlike IgM RFs which showed a binding preference by inhibition for mouse IgG_1, both 2 mo +/+ and lpr/lpr IgA RFs showed strong preferences for IgG_{2a} and IgG_{2b}.

In sum, RF immunoregulation is complex; these studies show that the lpr gene influences IgA RF production, and also suggest differences in IgA RF quantity and specificity from simultaneously occurring IgM RFs in normal B6 and autoimmune B6-lpr/lpr mice.

E51

AUTOANTIBODY TO MICROFILAMENT (MF) ANCHORING SITES. J.L. Senécal, F. Joyal and A. Roussin. University of Montréal School of Medicine, Montréal, QC, Canada H2L 4K8.

Actin MF are a major component of the eucaryotic cytoskeleton (CY). In cultured cells MF are organized in cytoplasmic bundles which, in order to exert a contractile force during motility, are anchored to the plasma membrane within cell-to-substratum focal adhesion sites.

Sera from patients with connective tissue diseases (CTD) have been studied by indirect immunofluorescence for anti-CY antibodies (Ab). PTK2 cells, a rat kangaroo kidney epithelial line with a well characterized CY, were permeabilized and fixed with 0.005% digitonin in 2% paraformaldehyde (5 min., 37°C) and used as substrate. One serum contained a high titer Ab which decorated elongated cytoplasmic patches. These were more numerous along the leading edge of cell growth and were of a morphology similar to that reported for adhesion sites. Other CY structures were not labeled. With double staining, using first the index serum followed by incubation with fluoresceine anti-human IgG and rhodamine phalloidin (a highly specific actin binding drug derived from the mushroom Amanita phalloides; Wulf et al, PNAS 76:4498,1979), the sites decorated by this serum were localized at the ends of MF. These observations suggest that this unique Ab is directed to MF anchoring sites (MFAS).

This serum was from a patient with Raynaud's phenomenon (RP) and sclerodactyly and did not contain other autoAb specificities. One year serial studies revealed persistence of anti-MFAS. Anti-MFAS was not detected in sera from 20 normals, 18 RP, 15 undifferentiated CTD, 20 scleroderma and 20 systemic lupus patients or on routine ANA substrates.

Anti-MFAS may be a useful probe to further explore MF and cell motility. (Supported by the Medical Research Council of Canada)

E52

ANTI-KU ANTIBODIES IN AMERICAN PATIENTS WITH SLE: DETECTION WITH ELISA, IMMUNOBLOTTING AND IMMUNODIFFUSION ASSAYS. M.Nakamura, T.Mimori, and J. A.Hardin. Yale University School of Medicine, New Haven, CT 06510

Anti-Ku antibodies have been found by immunodiffusion in Japanese patients with polymyositis/scleroderma overlap syndrome and rarely SLE (less than 1%) J.Clin.Invest.68:611,1981. We have now used more sensitive methods to search for anti-Ku in American patients with SLE.

The antigenic 70 and 80 kDa Ku proteins were purified from HeLa cell extracts using anti-Ku immunoaffinity chromatography. When tested in overloaded acrylamide gels, the eluted antigen consisted only of the Ku proteins along with a trace contaminant of 43 kDa (likely to be actin). This antigen was used to develop assays based on ELISA and immunoblotting techniques. Our results with these assays (I.D.=immunodiffusion; I.B.=immunoblot assay) are shown in the Table.

		Patients Positive		
	Pts.studied	I.D.	I.B.	ELISA
SLE	60	2(3%)	3(5%)	21(35%)
Other rheumatic diseases	51	0	0	0
Normal controls	29	0	0	0

The two sera positive in immunodiffusion were among the three positive by immunoblotting and the latter were among the 21 positive by ELISA. When studied by immunoblotting, seven of the 21 patients positive by ELISA exhibited weak binding to various non-Ku components within the antigen preparation that were not visible in overloaded gels stained with coommassie blue.

We conclude that anti-Ku antibodies occur in at least 5% of patients with SLE. Contaminants in immunoaffinity purified antigen preparations may lead to unreliable results in ELISA assays for anti-Ku as well as other autoantibodies.

E53

AUTOANTIBODIES IN MURINE GRAFT VERSUS HOST (GVH) DISEASE. K.M. Pollard, E.K.L. Chan, R.L. Rubin and E.M. Tan. Scripps Clinic and Research Foundation, La Jolla, CA. 92037

Lupus-like GVH disease was induced in male 10 week old C57BL/10 x DBA/2 F1 mice by the intravenous injection of spleen and thymus cells (2:1) from 10 week old male DBA/2 mice. GVH mice were bled at two week intervals one month after injection and tested for autoantibody. Using HEp-2 cells as substrate, antibody to nuclear antigens (ANA) were found by immunofluorescence. ELISA showed that ANA consisted, in part, of antibody to histones and DNA. The titer and frequency of ANA was found to correlate with the number of cells injected. In order to determine the spectrum of ANA in GVH disease mice were reinjected with optimum cell numbers (120×10^6 cells), and the splenocytes from two mice with the higher titer ANA were fused to the mouse myeloma P3x63Ag8.653. Hybridomas were tested for ANA by immunofluorescence and ELISA. Sixty-eight clones were found which secreted ANA. Of these 59 percent produced antibody to DNA or histones and 41 percent antibody which gave a variety of nuclear immunofluorescence patterns. These included the nuclear staining patterns of speckled, homogeneous, nuclear matrix, mitotic spindle apparatus and nucleolar. The fine antigenic specificity of these hybridomas remains to be determined. The maneuver of a booster injection of DBA/2 cells (GVHx2) appears to enhance the yield of autoantibody producing cells. This study indicates that GVH disease provides an excellent source of splenocytes for the production of ANA-producing hybridomas.

E54

PURIFICATION OF Jo-1 ANTIGEN (HISTIDINE-tRNA LIGASE) AND AN ENZYME-LINKED IMMUNOSORBENT ASSAY FOR QUANTITATION OF ANTI-Jo-1 ANTIBODY. Frederick W. Miller, Tapas Biswas, Yutaka Takagaki, Paul H. Plotz NIH, Bethesda, MD; and Morris Reichlin, OMRF, Oklahoma City, OK.

The Jo-1 antigen to which antibodies are directed in adult patients with myositis is the enzyme histidine-tRNA ligase (EC 6.1.1.21). We have biochemically purified this enzyme from HeLa cells and mouse liver over 1100-fold by a rapid two step method using Blue Sepharose batch affinity chromatography followed by diethylaminoethyl ion-exchange high performance liquid chromotography (HPLC). The purified HeLa and mouse liver enzymes comigrate as dimers with an apparent molecular size of 120 kD by size exclusion HPLC. Immunoblotting experiments, using anti-Jo-1 sera, show the antigen, whether from HeLa or liver, to be a single 50 kD protein by denaturing sodium dodecyl sulfate gel electrophoresis run under fully reducing conditions, confirming previous findings.

We have developed an enzyme-linked immunosorbent assay (ELISA) using purified HeLa antigen and affinity-purified, peroxidase-conjuated IgG $F(ab')_2$ fragments from goat anti-human IgG. By this assay sera diluted 1:30 from anti-Jo-1 positive patients (n=7) gave significantly (p<.0001) greater readings (0.087 ± 0.014 OD_{492nm} [mean ± SD]) than sera from anti-Jo-1 negative patients with SLE (0.010 ± 0.0049 OD_{492nm}, n=7), and normal sera (-0.0026 ± 0.010 OD_{492nm}, n=15). Significant titers of both IgG and IgM anti-Jo-1 antibodies were detected in all positive patients, and all positive sera cross-reacted with mouse liver enzyme in the ELISA.

This ELISA should allow for the rapid screening of sera, serial quantitation of antibody titers, and a better understanding of the clinical and pathogenetic significance of anti-Jo-1 antibodies.

E55

A MUSCULOSKELETAL SYNDROME ASSOCIATED WITH MITRAL VALVE PROLAPSE (MVP). Harry Spiera, Frederick Swerdlow and Jose Meller. Mount Sinai School of Medicine, New York, N.Y. 10029.

We have seen a number of patients with documented MVP who experienced the relatively acute onset of severe aching muscle pain. In contrast to the classic fibrositis syndrome, the pain was more prominent in the extremities than in the axial skeleton. Extensive investigation including ESR, ANA, rheumatoid factor, CPK, aldolase, electrodiagnostic studies and muscle biopsies were consistently unrevealing.

Subsequently, 11 patients who presented with the identical clinical syndrome but who lacked the classic mid-systolic click or murmur were prospectively evaluated by echocardiography. 10 had evidence of MVP. All but one of these patients were young women ranging in age from 14 to 45. Most patients were not obviously psychoneurotic and led normal lives prior to the onset of this syndrome. None of these patients improved symptomatically with either NSAID's or analgesics. 13 patients received steroid therapy without significant improvement. 30% of the patients had some alleviation of their symptoms coincident with the use of beta blockers.

The constellation of a relatively acute myalgic syndrome with a negative work-up for other etiologies, the discovery of MVP prospectively, and the occasional response to beta blockers suggests an association between MVP and this myalgic syndrome which warrants further investigation.

E56

TAKAYASU'S ARTERITIS (TA) J.E. Richardson, E.C. Keystone. Department of Medicine, University of Toronto, Toronto, Canada.

Since 1970, 23 patients (18 caucasian) with TA were seen by Toronto area rheumatologists and followed an average of 4.7 yrs. The onset of symptoms occurred at a mean age of 28 with frequently a long delay before diagnosis (mean 16.3 mo.). The patients presented most commonly with a pulse deficit (11) or cerebrovascular event (6). Most of the patients had an elevated ESR (20/23), however, 2 patients had persistently normal ESRs despite angiographic evidence of progressive disease. All 20 patients with clinical evidence of aortic arch involvement had abnormal arch angiograms, as did 1 patient with a normal clinical exam. Abdominal vessel involvement was common (16/17 tested) and often the only clinical evidence of its presence was an epigastric bruit. All patients were treated with prednisone (mean dose 47 mg.) and in 21 that were followed more than 6 months, the response to treatment was variable. 3 patients, initially untreated, developed progressive vessel involvement but stabilized with subsequent treatment. Of 13 patients who initially responded with normalization of the ESR, and stable or improved pulses, 9 received a further course(s) of prednisone for angiographic deterioration and/or a elevated ESR. An additional 8 patients had a poor initial response because of persistent inflammatory symptoms or worsening angiograms. There was a poor correlation between clinical improvement or stabilization and follow-up angiograms. Of 6 improved pulses, the angiograms improved in only 2, suggesting that improvement was due to the development of collaterals. Despite stable pulses in 12 patients, angiograms revealed both deterioration (4) and improvement (3). This study shows that serial angiograms are often necessary for evaluation of TA as the clinical assessment may be misleading and the response to treatment variable.

E57

THE ARTHRITIS OF BRUCELLOSIS (Br): IMMUNOGENETIC STUDIES. G.S. Alarcón, E. Gotuzzo, T.S. Bocanegra, M.O. Castañeda, A. Calvo, J. Guerra, C. Carrillo, S.A. Hinostroza, I. Rolando, H. Hernandez, R.C.P. Go, R.T. Acton, B.O. Barger, and L.R. Espinoza. Universidad Peruana Cayetano Heredia, Lima 1, Perú, University of Alabama at Birmingham, B'ham., AL. 35294 and University of South Florida, Tampa,Florida 33612.

During the last 15 years 498 Br pts have been seen by us. Of these 498 pts, 180 or 36.1% had a form of arthritis (BrA): sacroiliitis, spondylitis, peripheral arthritis, mixed arthritis, or periarthritis. The pathogenesis of BrA is poorly understood. In some instances it is clear cut infections with brucella recovered from the affected joint if synovial fluid is adequately cultured (Ruiz-Castañeda biphasic medium). Other cases, regardless of the articular form are likely to be reactive but the clinical distinction between both may not be readily apparent. The genetic predisposition for the occurrence of BrA had previously been postulated but not conclusively proved. The present study attempts to further define the predisposing genetic factors for the occurrence of BrA. To do so we studied: (1) a group of 14 pts with BrA (spondylitis) in whom B27 and B7-CREG specificities were tested. The frequency of these antigens in these pts was similar to that found in a local control population. 2)Eight families for a total of 62 individuals in whom more than 1 member had Br ($\bar{x}$: 3.1/family) and at least 1 had BrA. Sib-pair analysis (15 pairs) and inspection of the family trees failed to reveal any distortion in the distribution of the haplotypes among affected family members. Our studies suggest that: 1) other HLA antigens native to our population and yet to be determined may be the predisposing factor(s) in BrA and/or 2) other non-genetic factors may play an important role in its development.

E58

THE VALUE OF VON WILLEBRAND'S FACTOR RELATED ANTIGEN IN DERMAL VASCULITIS. S.R. Nuslnow, T.S. Zimmerman and J.G. Curd. Scripps Clinic and Research Foundation, La Jolla, CA.

The purpose of this study was to evaluate von Willebrand's factor related antigen (vWF:Ag) in patients presenting with dermal vasculitis (palpable purpura, erythema nodosum, nodular vasculitis, and/or urticarial vasculitis). The plasma concentration of vWF:Ag was measured by quantitative immunoelectrophoresis, and is expressed as a percent of pooled normal human plasma (normal 100%±50%). Of 50 patients with vasculitis studied, 13 patients presenting with a dermal vasculitis were identified. The latter had a mean vWF:Ag concentration of 191±67% (range 90-270). 8 of 13 patients have been followed prospectively for a period of 1 month to 5 years. The concentration of vWF:Ag measured in serial samples from these patients was never greater than 300%. vWF:Ag levels greater than 300% were associated with a medium or large vessel vasculitis. Clinically, the patients with a dermal vasculitis and low vWF:Ag did well, and the vasculitis did not progress to involve larger blood vessels. The results of this study indicate that a patient presenting with dermal vasculitis and concentration of vWF:Ag less than 300%, has a good prognosis and low probability that the disease will progress to involve larger blood vessels.

E59

OUTCOME IN COGAN'S SYNDROME. Randall S. Vollertsen, Thomas J. McDonald, and Brian R. Younge, Mayo Clinic, Rochester, MN 55905.

We reviewed 78 cases of Cogan's syndrome -- (nonsyphilitic interstitial keratitis and audiovestibular symptoms) -- including 18 from our institution to identify the clinical characteristics which were significantly associated ($p \leq 0.05$) with serious outcomes, and to evaluate treatment. The median duration of observation was 22 months.

Serious outcomes occurred in 49 of 78 patients and included blindness (6 patients), deafness (34), aortic insufficiency (11), and vasculitis (12). We could not obtain appropriate data to analyze death. Of these, vasculitis and aortic insufficiency were significantly associated with one another.

A longer duration of observation correlated with blindness. Deafness was more likely if there was initial audiovestibular involvement, weight loss, or cardiac findings other than aortic insufficiency (systolic murmur, cardiomegaly, dysrhythmia). Weight loss, abdominal discomfort, the absence of vertigo, tinnitus, and nystagmus, an elevated erythrocyte sedimentation rate, anemia, and neutrophilia were more common in those with aortic insufficiency.

Vasculitis was significantly associated with weight loss, fever, arthritis, arthralgias and myalgias, peripheral neuropathy, psychological symptoms, subcutaneous nodules, splenomegaly, lymphadenopathy, chest findings, abdominal discomfort, and an abnormal urinalysis. An elevated erythrocyte sedimentation rate, leukocytosis, lymphopenia, thrombocytosis, and anemia were more common in vasculitis patients.

Glucocorticosteroids are helpful, although patients who are deaf when therapy is begun are unlikely to regain hearing. Aortic valve replacement and arterial bypass grafting are useful in selected cases.

E60

A SURVEY OF MUSCULOSKELETAL PROBLEMS ENCOUNTERED IN HIGH LEVEL MUSICIANS. Caldron P, Calabrese L, Lederman R, Clough J, Stulberg B, Bergfeld J. Cleveland Clinic Foundation, Cleveland, Ohio 44106

The requirement of rapid controlled repetitive musculoskeletal (MS) activity by high level musicians suggests they mey be a population at risk for a variety of occupational injuries, yet aside from pianists, little information exists in the medical literature. To evaluate the occurrence and types of occupational injuries, aside from pianists, little information exists in the medical literature. To evaluate the occurrence and variety of MS problems acquired through playing musical instruments, 250 high level musicians (woodwinds excluded) completed a detailed questionnaire. Group I (n=92) had MS problems severe enough to seek medical care (36.8%) Group II (n=55) reported problems without a physician diagnosis (20.2%). Group III (n=103) reported no MS problems (40%). 30% of Group I as opposed to 4% of Group II and 2% of Group III reported some income loss resulting from musically related injuries. Group I reported a median practice time lost due to injury of 5 weeks which was significantly greater than Groups II and III ($p<0.0001$). Female musicians were more likely to report injuries ($p=.002$), and to seek medical care. No significant age difference was found between those who did and did not report injuries. The most common injuries reported were tendinitis, muscle spasm, and nerve impingements. The percussionists, violinists/violists, pianists and harpists were more likely to report injuries than bassists, cellists, organists or guitarists (p=ns). We submit that musicians commonly seek physician care for MS problems which may result in loss of professional income and practice time. Detailed studies of these injuries are needed to clarify pathogenesis, treatment and prevention.

E61

IMMUNOLOGICAL STUDIES OF SKIN AND CIRCULATING AUTOANTIBODIES IN PRIMARY FIBROSITIS SYNDROME. Xavier J. Caro, Francisco P. Quismorio, Jr. Northridge Hospital Medical Center-UCLA School of Medicine, and USC School of Medicine, Los Angeles, Ca.

We have previously reported the presence of granular IgG deposits at the dermal-epidermal junction (DEJ) of clinically normal skin in Primary Fibrositis Syndrome (PFS). Here we attempted to characterize the nature of these deposits, compared them to SLE skin deposits and tested PFS sera for autoantibodies. Twenty PFS patients (16 female), mean age 44 years(28-71 yrs), and 22 healthy controls(17 females), mean age 44 years(27-62 yrs), were studied. The prevalence of ten different organ and non-organ specific autoantibodies tested for by indirect immunofluorescence(IF)using rat tissue substrates, was not different in the two groups. The number of subjects with at least one autoantibody was similar in PFS (9/20) and controls (6/22). Ab to basement membrane zone(BMZ), intercellular antigen, and basal cell antigens were negative when tested against monkey esophagus and human skin. IF staining of IgG at the DEJ was blocked by unlabeled anti-IgG but not by PBS or anti IgM. DEJ Ig deposits in 4 PFS and 2 SLE patients were partially eluted after incubation with 0.2M citrate buffer (pH 3.2)but not with 2M NaCl, 0.01M glycine buffer (pH 11) or PBS. IgG deposits in PFS did not fix C3 or C1q when skin sections were reacted with fresh human sera. Neither PFS or SLE skin bound fluorescein-labeled pemphigoid anti-BMZ Ab. Although these data do not show autoimmunity to skin and other antigens to be a feature of PFS they do suggest an immunologically related process, resembling that seen with immune complexes, occurring at the DEJ in this disorder. The lack of skin staining with anti-BMZ Ab and exogenous C' may be due to the absence of BMZ antigens, local inhibitory factors, and/or a non-C' fixing IgG subclass at the DEJ.

E62

CENTRAL NERVOUS SYSTEM VASCULITIS. R. Yonker, E. Webster, N. L. Edwards, S. Longley, R. S. Panush. University of Florida and VAMC Gainesville, FL 32610

We are frequently requested to evaluate complex patients for possible vasculitis of the central nervous system (CNS). To provide a perspective of possibly helpful clinical and laboratory features, diagnostic studies, therapies, and outcome, we reviewed our experience with 17 patients encountered during 1977-1983. Patients with and without CNS vasculitis had generally comparable clinical features (diffuse or focal neurologic deficits, rheumatic complaints) and laboratory findings (leukocytosis, elevated ESR, proteinuria, negative RF, negative ANA, normocomplementemia, absent cyroglobulinemia or circulating immune complexes, and abnormal CSF). Positve diagnoses in 5 patients were based on angiography (granulomatous angiitis, amphetamine abuse angiitis), brain biopsy (granulomatous angiitis), sinus/kidney biopsy (Wegener's granulomatosis), and clinical criteria (Behcet's disease). CNS vasculitis was excluded in the other 12 patients by negative angiography (6/6), negative biopsy (3/3), and CT findings of thrombotic CVA, ventricular dilatation, and/or atrophy (7/7). Vasculitis has not developed in these 12 patients during follow-up. Patients with CNS vasculitis were treated with steroids (2/5), immunosuppressives (1/5), or observation (3/5). Three patients recovered and 2 died. Our observations indicate that CNS vasculitis is uncommon, is difficult to appreciate clinically, and requires an aggressive diagnostic approach to confirm or exclude the diagnosis. Such an approach may identify patients for whom early use of steroids or cytotoxic drugs may be beneficial.

E63

CAUSES OF DEATH IN RELAPSING POLYCHONDRITIS (RP). J.C.Piette, S.Herson, C.Chapelon, I.Bourgault, O.Bletry, B.Wechsler and P.Godeau. Hôpital de la Pitié, 75013 Paris. - FRANCE.

Because of the lack of epidemiologic data concerning mortality in RP, we reviewed 60 cases of dead patients: 11 from our personal series and 49 from the literature. The average duration of RP before death was 4.8 yr. The ratio female/male (I) and the age at onset of RP (45 yr.) were identical among dead and alive patients. Patients were divided into three categories according to the cause of death:

- Death directly related to RP (34 patients):
  - + airway collapse or obstruction: 19 patients (group I);
  - + RP related cardiovascular involvement: 13 patients (group II);
  - + renal failure: 2 patients.
- Death related to treatment complications: 7 patients.
- Death unrelated to RP: neoplasia (5 patients), miscellaneous (9 patients), or unknown (5 patients).

Symptoms of respiratory tract chondritis were present during the first year following onset of RP in 17 out of 19 group I patients. The ratio female/male was 3.7 in group I and 0.3 in group II ($p < .005$). This result can be explained in part by the higher prevalence of respiratory tract involvement in female (64%) than in male (45%) either dead or alive. The average duration of RP before death was significantly higher in group II than in group I (8.2 vs. 3.7 yr, $p < .05$), because of the late occurence of arterial aneurysms in the course of RP.

Conclusion: The leading causes of death in RP are respiratory tract and cardiovascular involvement. The former occurs mainly in women while the latter is more often encountered in men.

E64

HYPERMOBILITY - THE MISSING LINK TO FIBROSITIS. John A. Goldman. Northside and St. Joseph's Hospitals, Atlanta, GA 30342

One hundred six patients with the diagnosis of fibrositis were examined for the presence of hypermobility. Fibrositis was diagnosed as chronic pain, multiple tender points, a positive trapezius roll sign, poor sleep pattern, normal laboratory studies and no other identifiable disease. Hypermobility was identified by the following: (1) Passive opposition of the thumb to the forearm, (2) Passive hyperextension of the fingers beyond 90 degrees, (3) Active hyperextension of the elbow >10 degrees, (4) Active hyperextension of the knees>10 degrees, and (5) Ability to place palms on the floor without bending the knees. The ages ranged from 24 to 78 years with an average of 44 years. 103 were women. 62 (58%) had one, 36 (34%) had two and 21 (20%) had three or more areas of ligamentous laxity. Hypermobility due to another disorder was not found in these patients. The results showed that hypermobile patients had less sleep disturbance and more often responded to exercise. Both groups had similar fatigue, morning stiffness and responsiveness to tricyclics. This looseness suggests there may be a structural difference in the tissue of a subset of patients who develop fibrositis. Caro suggested the dermal epidermal junction of fibrositis patients allows the diffusion of non-immunoglobulin protein into it suggesting increased vascular permeability. (Arthritis Rheum 27: S76, 1984). It is possible that looseness of the tissue predisposes to the events that lead to the development of clinical fibrositis. Since most of the patients were sedentary at the time of diagnosis, the hypermobility subgroup of fibrositis may represent a clinical syndrome due to deconditioning. Finding clinical hypermobility may be a useful diagnostic and management clue in the treatment of patients with fibrositis.

E65

TREATMENT OF PSORIATIC ARTHRITIS WITH HYDROXYCHLOROQUINE: FAVORABLE RESPONSE BUT INCREASED DERMATOLOGIC TOXICITY. John L. Juozevicius and Richard I. Rynes, Albany Medical College, Albany, N.Y.

Because some investigators believe that potential, severe dermatologic reactions preclude the use of hydroxychloroquine (HCQ) in treating psoriatic arthritis (PSA), we reviewed the course of all patients in our practice treated with HCQ for PSA. Fifteen patients treated with HCQ, 200 mg p.o. b.i.d., were compared to an age and sex-matched control group with rheumatoid arthritis (RA).

Among PSA patients, 6/15 had at least a 50% improvement in articular index with 4 having decreased morning stiffness and 2 able to taper concommitant prednisone. Three PSA patients failed to improve. The other 6 developed dermatologic reactions within 8 to 70 days of drug institution. Two of these had a moderate flare of psoriasis, one associated with an erythematous pruritic drug eruption without exfoliation. Another had a mild psoriatic flare limited to the scalp. The fourth patient had an urticarial rash, the fifth generalized erythema and edema involving the hands and face. The final patient originally had gastrointestinal intolerance with his first course of HCQ. A leukocytoclastic vasculitis developed within 10 days of restarting HCQ 6 months later. All dermatologic reactions subsided within 2 weeks of stopping the drug. No patient required systemic steroids or hospitalization to manage toxicity. Among RA controls 11 improved and 4 had no response to HCQ. No side effects were noted.

We conclude that HCQ is effective in treating PSA; however, dermatologic toxicity is frequent. Patients with PSA treated with HCQ should be carefully monitored for dermatologic toxicity during the first 3 months of HCQ treatment.

E66

ANALYSIS OF IMMUNE COMPLEXES (IC) IN RHEUMATOID ARTHRITIS (RA) FOR EPSTEIN-BARR VIRUS (EBV) ANTIGENS. R.D. Inman, B.A. Chiu. University of Toronto, Toronto, Ontario, Canada M5T 2S8.

The present study was undertaken to assess the role of EBV antigens in IC formation in serum and synovial fluid of patients with RA. IC were isolated from synovial fluids of RA and non-RA arthritides by differential polyethylene glycol precipitation and competitive binding to Staphylococcal Protein A. Anti-IC antisera, raised in rabbits by immunization with the isolated IC, were examined for reactivity with specific viral antigens. Pre-immune sera were negative for antiviral antibodies, but anti-IC antisera were positive for anti-viral capsid antigen (VCA) of EBV by microimmunofluorescence (mean titer 1:512) and by ELISA. This was seen in antisera raised against IC of both RA and non-RA synovial fluids. Anti-IC antisera were negative for reactivity against EB nuclear antigen (EBNA), rubella, cytomegalovirus, and herpesvirus. Reactivity against EBV early antigen (EA) was seen in some antisera. The anti-VCA reactivity of the rabbit anti-IC antisera was completely removed by absorption against human IgG, regardless of the presence or absence of anti-VCA antibodies in that IgG. Thus there was no evidence for idiotype/anti-idiotype interactions. Evidence supporting shared determinants of VCA and IgG derived from ELISA studies in which (1) Fc fragment of IgG specifically inhibited the binding of a monoclonal anti-VCA antibody to VCA (2) monoclonal anti-VCA effectively competed with anti-IgG for binding to solid phase Fc fragment. These results demonstrate certain cross-reactivity of VCA and IgG Fc fragment but do not support the notion of complexed EBV antigens contributing to IC in RA synovial fluid.

E67

IMPAIRED PHAGOCYTOSIS BY YOUNG AUTOIMMUNE MURINE SPLENOCYTES. Louis T. Merriam and Robert P. Kimberly. Hospital for Special Surgery, New York, NY 10021.

Defective clearance of both model immune complexes and IgG opsonized erythrocytes has been demonstrated in MRL/lpr mice. To examine whether the basis for this defect parallels the dissociation of Fc receptor-ligand binding and internalization in SLE, we studied the Fc-mediated binding and endocytosis by adherent splenocytes obtained from normal NIH-Swiss mice and autoimmune MRL/lpr mice. Spleens, harvested within 1 minute of sacrifice, were teased apart in media with .004% CaCl2 and 200 units/ml collagenase. After adherence to glass coverslips and subsequent washing, cells were incubated with IgG sensitized sheep erythrocytes (SRBC). To assess ligand binding nonadherent SRBC were washed away; to assess phagocytosis all external SRBC were lyzed with an NH4Cl buffer.

The mean number of bound SRBC per phagocytic cell was significantly higher than normals for both young (mean age: 7 wks) and old (mean age: 19 wks) MRL mice (1.63 vs 1.17 for young, $p<.05$; 1.49 vs 0.91 for old, $p<.05$). The mean number of internalized SRBC was higher than age-matched normals for old MRL (2.34 vs 1.49; $p<.05$), but not for young MRLs (1.87 vs 1.54; $p>.10$) despite increased ligand binding. Fractional phagocytosis (fraction of total SRBC bound that were phagocytosed) was significantly lower in young as compared to old MRLs (.535 vs .612; $p<.01$).

Phagocytic splenocytes from MRL mice show increased Fc ligand binding. Unlike older mice, young MRL do not show a proportionate increase in phagocytosis suggesting an internalization defect similar to SLE. Such decreased internalization predating major disease expression may contribute to the immune complex manifestations of autoimmune disease.

E68

DIFFUSE IDIOPATHIC SKELETAL HYPEROSTOSIS (DISH) AND RETINOL METABOLISM. M. Abiteboul-Clinical Research, LERS-SYNTHELABO, Paris 75013 ; M. Sarrabay, B. Mazières, J. Arlet-CHR Rangueil, Toulouse 31400. FRANCE.

In animal and in man high doses of retinol and retinoids cause spinal and peripheral hyperostosis very similar to DISH. These considerations prompted us to explore retinol metabolism in DISH patients.

In 34 DISH patients and 12 control patients the concentration of retinol in serum (normal 0.3 - 0.7 mg/l) was measured by HPLC. β-carotene was measured by absorption spectrophotometry (n=0.50 - 0.90 mg/l), retinol binding protein (RBP) and prealbumin by radial immunodiffusion (respectively n=37-56 mg/l, 100-400 mg/l). In DISH patients, retinolemia was abnormal and significantly higher ($p<0.05$) than in controls after a 12-hour fast (0.74 $\pm$ 0.19 vs 0.59 $\pm$ 0.13), and 5 hours after ingestion of retinol 50.000 IU (0.77 $\pm$ 0.17 vs 0.60 $\pm$ 0.13). Intra subject comparison of T0 and T5-retinol levels yielded significantly different values in the DISH group ($p<0.05$) in contrast with the control group. A similar difference was seen in RBP (higher in DISH patients). β-carotene was similar in both groups.

In conclusion, retinolemia was significantly higher in the DISH group, and rose abnormally 5 hours after an oral administration of retinol (50.000 IU). These findings suggest that abnormal retinol metabolism might be involved in DISH lesions.

E69

IDENTIFICATION OF A NEUTRAL METALLOPROTEINASE SECRETED BY HUMAN MACROPHAGES WHICH DEGRADES GELATIN AND NATIVE TYPE V COLLAGEN. Margaret S. Hibbs, John R. Hoidal and Andrew H. Kang, Memphis, TN 38104.

Monocyte-macrophages are a frequent component of chronic inflammatory processes such as rheumatoid arthritis where they may secrete proteinases which participate in cartilage destruction. A neutral proteinase which degrades gelatin was detected in culture media of human macrophages. The proteinase was maximally detected after 3-5 days of culture and continued to be secreted in the media for 2 weeks. The activity was predominantly found in the culture media and its secretion could be blocked by the presence of cycloheximide. The proteinase could be isolated by affinity chromatography on gelatin sepharose. It was found to be inhibited by metalloproteinase inhibitors, to consist of a major component of approximately 92 kDa and to degrade native type V collagen. This component shows immunologic cross-reactivity with a polyclonal antisera to neutrophil gelatinase. Thus both neutrophils and monocytes are capable of elaborating proteinases which may participate in articular destruction by virtue of their ability to act synergistically with interstitial collagenase as well as their ability to degrade native type V collagen.

E70

SERUM KERATAN SULFATE (KS) CONCENTRATIONS ARE LOWER IN CHILDREN WITH JUVENILE RHEUMATOID ARTHRITIS (JRA) THAN IN CHILDREN WITHOUT RHEUMATIC DISEASE. LM Pachman, ME Lenz, B Caterson, J Goletz, J Jacobitz, KE Kuettner, and EJMA Thonar. Dept. of Pediatrics, Northwestern Univ. Med. Schl., Children's Mem. Hosp., and Dept. of Biochemistry, Rush Presbyterian-St. Luke's Med. Ctr. Chicago, IL 60614.

Sera from over 100 children without rheumatic disease were tested by ELISA assay using a monoclonal antibody (1/20/5/-D-4) directed against KS which is primarily derived from cartilage proteoglycans (PG). The assay accurately quantitates as little as 5 ng KS/ml and documents that human sera contains significant levels of KS, present as single chains bearing litle or no protein. The mean levels of KS were calculated for the different age groups (0-20 yrs) and compared with those from over 50 children with JRA. During the first few years of life, there is a gradual rise in KS values in non-JRA sera (0-1 yrs: 352 ng/ml $\pm$ 84, n=12; 2-4 yrs: 445 ng/ml $\pm$ 115, n=17; 5-8 yrs: 554 ng/ml $\pm$ 112, n=26; 9-12 yrs: 558 $\pm$ 152 ng/ml, n=27) becoming fairly constant between the ages of 5-12. In the 13-15 year group, there is a dramatic decrease in the KS levels, 374 ng/ml $\pm$ 176, n=18, which remains constant in the 16-20 yr olds (331 ng/ml $\pm$ 138, n=17) and in older adults. When sera from patients with JRA are compared to nonrheumatic sera, there is a marked decrease in KS in the 5-12 year age group, (419 ng/ml $\pm$ 100, n=24, $p<.001$). We conclude that: 1) KS levels show a gradual increase in early childhood and a rapid drop in the 13-15 yr age range, when turnover of cartilage PG may be increased, and 2) the low levels of KS in JRA may reflect an alteration of metabolism of cartilage PG.

Supported by NIH Grant# 1 P60 AM-30692-01A1 and McGaw Medical Center Interinstitutional Research Funds.

E71

DIFFERENTIAL EFFECT OF BIOMECHANICAL STRESS ON ARTICULAR CARTILAGE AND SYNOVIUM FROM INDIVIDUAL JOINTS. Christiane L. Arsever, Giles G. Bole, Patricia Taylor. University of Michigan, Ann Arbor, MI 48109.

This study further describes changes in articular cartilage proteoglycan (PG) metabolism from an experimental model of osteoarthritis (OA). Previous studies have described this non-invasive model in guinea pigs that produces progressive histologic and biochemical changes consistent with OA. These studies have also shown that co-culturing cartilage with synovium using the Fell-Jubb system induces greater $^{35}SO_4^{=}$-PG release into spent media than culturing cartilage alone. After *in vivo* administration of $^{35}SO_4^{=}$, pairs of animals (control and experimental) were sacrificed simultaneously 4-20 wks postoperatively. Articular cartilage from the femoral head (FH), tibial plateau (TP), and femoral condyles (FC) and synovial tissue from both the hip and knee were removed from each animal. Cultures using the Fell-Jubb system were set up as follows: experimental cartilage (EC) alone, control cartilage (CC) alone, EC + experimental synovium (ES), EC + control synovium (CS), CC + CS, CC + ES, CS alone, and ES alone. $^{35}SO_4^{=}$-PG release for EC + ES was greater than EC + CS from the rt hind limb at 4 wks, but EC + CS was greater than EC + ES at 20 wks. The left unoperated side showed greater $^{35}SO_4^{=}$-PG release of EC + CS at 20 wks postoperatively. At 4 wks $^{35}SO_4^{=}$-PG release from CC + ES was greater than CC + CS in the rt FC and TP (knee) as compared to 20 wks; while on the left side this combination showed greater $^{35}SO_4^{=}$-PG release from the femoral head. Co-culturing with freeze/thawed synovium did not eliminate the synovial tissue stimulation of $^{35}SO_4^{=}$-PG release. There appears to be a series of metabolic interactions between the synovium and articular cartilage which is dependent upon changes in joint biomechanics and the stage of OA development in individual joints.

E72

LUMBAR SPINE SURGERY IN THE ELDERLY By: Alexander E. Brodsky, M.D. and Peter L.R. Wood, F.R.C.S.; St. Luke's Episcopal Hospital, Houston, Texas 77030.

Back and leg pain due to degenerative disease in the lumbar spine in the elderly does not always respond to conservative measures. Many practitioners are reluctant to consider surgery because of the patient's age. Surgery for degenerative conditions of the lumbar spine was performed in 154 patients over the age of 60, between 1960 and 1979. 32 of the patients were over 70. Patients with prior lumbar surgery, infectious, or neoplastic diseases of the spine were omitted from the study. 78 patients (51%) had spinal stenosis and disc herniations. 13 patients (8%) had spinal stenosis without disc herniation, and 62 patients (41%) had disc herniation without stenosis. 11 patients had intermittent neurogenic claudication; otherwise symptoms were similar to those in younger people. 18 (22%) had extruded disc fragments. Adequate follow up was secured in 139 patients. 102 patients (74%) with no symptoms or minimal symptoms were rated excellent. 15 patients (11%) had partial relief of symptoms but required no medication and 21 (15%) were considered poor due to subjective complaints. There were two late post operative deaths in high risk patients, one with cirrhosis and the other with coronary artery disease; both were in unremitting pain and both were cleared medically. 7 of 10 patients rated as "poor" had second operations and obtained good results. With proper preoperative preparation and good anesthesia, lumbar spine surgery should not be denied to the elderly because of age. The results are similar to that observed in younger patients. The major obstacle to improving results were because of persistent subjective complaints without objective findings.

E73

RHEUMATOID FACTOR ISOTYPES FOLLOWING IMMUNIZATION. Peter R. Levine and David Axelrod. Walter Reed Army Medical Center, Washington, D.C. 20307.

Multiple prophylactic immunizations have been reported to be a cause of serum rheumatoid factor (RF) positivity. We examined this phenomenon using an enzyme-linked immunosorbent assay (ELISA) for IgM, IgG and IgA RF isotypes, and a standard sheep-cell agglutination test (SCAT).

Serum was obtained from 422 healthy military recruits (296 male, 126 female) prior to and four weeks after immunization with polyvalent meningococcal, influenza, and oral polio vaccines, and tetanus and diphtheria adsorbed toxins. All specimens were assayed in triplicate for IgM, IgG and IgA RF by ELISA. Post-immunization sera from subjects demonstrating a significant increase in IgM RF by ELISA were also assayed with a commercially-available SCAT.

Mean pre-immunization values for RF were IgG 48 International Units (IU), IgA 64 IU, IgM 72 IU. Significant increases in IgM occurred in 22% of subjects, increases in IgA in 13%, and increases in IgG in 6% post-immunization. Mean post-immunization values for subjects with significant increases were IgG 1246 IU, IgA 2960 IU, and IgM 1468 IU. No post-immunization serum from a subject with a significant increase in IgM RF by ELISA was positive by SCAT.

Multiple immunizations may cause an increase in RF as detected by ELISA in a significant minority of subjects 4 weeks post-immunization. However, this immunization regimen was not associated with a positive RF as measured by a routinely available assay.

E74

COMPARATIVE SPECIFICITIES OF SERUM AND SYNOVIAL CELL 19S IgM RHEUMATOID FACTORS IN RHEUMATOID ARTHRITIS. Dick L. Robbins, UCD, Davis, CA 95616, Richard Wistar, Jr., Naval Medical Research Center, Bethesda, MD 20814.

Rheumatoid factor (RF) may play a critical role in sustaining the inflammatory events leading to tissue damage in rheumatoid arthritis (RA). However, many serum RF's have greater specificity for rabbit IgG than for human IgG, thus raising unresolved questions regarding RF's pathogenicity in RA. Serum RF also has specificity for human IgG subclasses 1, 2 and 4, but little, if any, for IgG3. The synovium is central to the pathology of RA: thus RF made there may be of greater pathogenic importance than is the serum RF. We examined the specificity of 19S IgM RF in a RF plaque forming cell assay (RF-PFC) using RA synovial cells (RSC). The following observations were made: 1) RSC produced greater numbers of RF-PFC/10^6 cells than did RA peripheral blood mononuclear cells (PBM); 2) RSC RF-PFC had greater specificity for human than for rabbit IgG compared to autologous serum RF; 3) RSC RF had significantly greater specificity for human IgG3 relative to autologous serum RF. This was in contrast to the finding that RSC RF and autologous serum RF had the same relative specificities for polyclonal human IgG, and monoclonal subclasses, IgG1, IgG2, and IgG4. Thus, the specificity of a significant portion of the RF synthesized by RSC differed from serum RF.

ARA AUTHOR INDEX

ABADI,I., E34,E33
Caracas
ABDOU,N.I.,MD, PhD 41
Kansas City,KS
ABELES,M.,MD E39
Farmington,CT
ABITEBOUL,M.J.,MD E68
Paris
ABO,W.,MD, PhD 107
Los Angeles,CA
ABRAHAM,G.N.,MD 33
Rochester,NY
ABRAMS,B.,MD C2
Kansas City,KS
ABRAMSON,S.,MD D70, 58
New York,NY
ABUD-MENDOZA,C.,MD C8,A37
Mexico City
ACKERMAN,N.,PhD A8
Wilmington,DE
ACTON,R.T., E57,A19,52,138
Birmingham,AL
ADAMS,E.,MD A18
Chicago,IL
AELION,J.A.,MD D21
Memphis,TN
AGARWAL,A.K.,MD 142,E40
Pittsburgh,PA
AGRIS,P.F.,PhD 121
Columbia,MO
AGUDELO,C.A.,MD E13
Winston-Salem,NC
AISEN,A.M.,MD 55
Ann Arbor,MI
AL-SABBAGH,R., D30
Pittsburgh,PA
ALARCON,G.S.,MD, MPH A19,138,52,E57,D53
Birmingham,AL
ALARCON-SEGOVIA,D., C8,A29,A37
Mexico City
ALBERT,D.A.,MD 16
Chicago,IL
ALCOCER-VARELA,J.,MD A29,C8
Mexico City
ALDO-BENSON,M.,MD 74
Indianapolis,IN
ALEKSEEV,L.,MD 1
Moscow
ALEXANDER,E.L.,MD, PhD 134,A60,152
Baltimore,MD
ALEXANDER,G.E., 152,A60
Baltimore,MD
ALLEN,J., D40
Bethesda,MD
ALLISON,J.,PhD 69
Smithville,TX
ALPER,C.A.,MD 19
Boston,MA
ALTMAN,A.,PhD C30
La Jolla,CA
ALTMAN,R.D.,MD A49,A48,A41
Miami,FL
ALVARELLOS,A.,MD A27
St. Louis,MO
AMATSU, K., MD B44
Osaka, Japan
AMENTO,E.P.,MD 173
Boston,MA
AMOR,B.,MD 137,24,A13
Paris
AMSTUTZ,H.C.,MD C4,10
Los Angeles,CA
ANDERSON,B., B16
Chicago,IL
ANDERSON,C.L.,MD 33,B23
Rochester,NY
ANDERSON,J.J., 94
Boston,MA
ANDERSON,P.A.,MD A11
Aurora,CO
ANDO,D.,MD 73,C29
Los Angeles,CA
ANDREWS,B.,MD D38
Irvine,CA
ANHORN,K., A38
Toronto,ON
ANSELL,B.,CBE,MD D50,B9
Isleworth
ANSELL,B.M., B9
Harrow
APONTE,C.,MD 141
Cleveland,OH
APPEL,A.M.,PhD D15
Cincinnati,OH
APPLEBAUM-BOWDEN,D.,PhD A15
Baltimore,MD
AREND,W.P.,MD 42
Denver,CO
ARLET,J.,MD E68
Toulouse
ARMSTRONG,J.,BS D2
Washington,DC
ARMSTRONG,S.D.,MD D52
Springfield,MD
ARNDT,R.E.,BS 42,D45
Denver,CO
ARNETT,F.C.,MD B41,60
Houston, TX
ARNOLD,W.J.,MD C5
Park Ridge,IL
ARROYAVE,C., B7
Chicago,IL
ARROYAVE,C.M.,MD, PhD B4,67,B7
Chicago,IL
ARSENIS,C.,PhD B54
Chicago,IL

ARSEVER,C.L., ... E71
Ann Arbor,MI
ASHERSON,R.A.,MB,ChB,FCP E7,D8
London
ASHMAN,R.F., ... E29,A31
Iowa City,IA
ATHREYA,B.H.,MD 131,95
Philadelphia,PA
ATKINSON,M.J., ... D41
London,ON
ATLURU,D., ... 108
Albuquerque,NM
AUCOIN,D.,DVM A47
New York,NY
AULTMAN,M.,PhD 41
Kansas City,KS
AXELROD,D.,MD D2,E73
Washington,DC
BACON,P.,MD, FRCP D50,3
Birmingham,UK
BAKER,D.G.,MD D19
Philadelphia,PA
BAKER,G.L.,MD 142
Pittsburgh,PA
BAKKE,A.C.,PhD 107
Los Angeles,CA
BALESTRIERI,G., ... 149
Brescia,Italy
BALISI,L.,BS A33
Los Angeles,CA
BALL,E.J.,PhD B27
Dallas,TX
BALL,G.V., ... 52
Birmingham,AL
BALLOU,S.P.,MD A39
Cleveland,OH
BANK,I.,MD 104
New York,NY
BANKS,T.A.,MS B18
Tucson,AZ
BARDIN,T.,MD A57,A56,A55
Paris
BARGER,B.O.,PhD 138,A19,52,E57
Birmingham,AL
BARLAND,P., ... D7
Bronx,NY
BAROJA,M.L., ... E33,E34
Caracas
BARRON,K.,MD 62
Houston,TX
BASHEY,R.I.,PhD A2
Philadelphia,PA
BASSETT,L.W.,MD 20,133
Los Angeles,CA
BATULA-BERNARDO,C.,BS A66
Nutley,NJ
BAUER,M.A.,MD D55
Rochester,NY
BAUER,N.E.,BA D31
St. Louis,MO
BAUMGARTEN,D.F., ... A59
Philadelphia,PA
BAUMGARTNER,C., ... E29
Iowa City,IA
BEATTIE,W.,MD, PhD 18
Hamilton,ON
BECKER-CHRISTENS,F.,MD A56
Egedesminde,Greenland
BECKWITH,B., ... B7
Seattle,WA
BEDETTI,C.D., ... D30
Pittsburgh,PA
BELANOFF,J., ... 78
New York,NY
BELL,D.A.,MD,FRCP(C) 158,D41,40,113
London,ON
BELMONT,H.,MD 58
New York,NY
BENACERRAF,B.,MD D35
Boston,MA
BENDER,P., ... C23
Philadelphia,PA
BENEDICT,R.S.,BS 103,E14
Seattle,WA
BENISEK,W.,PhD D10
Davis,CA
BENNETT,J.,MD A5
Birmingham,AL
BENNETT,R.M.,MD B22,E23
Portland,OR
BENSON,M.D.,MD 123
Indianapolis,IN
BERDEN,J.M.,MD 146
Nijmegen,The Netherlands
BERGEN,H., ... B19
Birmingham,AL
BERGER,R.G.,MD 154
Chapel Hill,NC
BERGFELD,J.A.,MD E60
Cleveland,OH
BERKOWITZ,E.,BA 127
Stony Brook,NY
BERMAN,M.,PhD D38
Irvine,CA
BERMUDEZ,J., ... 150
Mexico City
BERNEY,S.N.,MD B45
Philadelphia,PA
BERNSTEIN,R.M.,MD 114
London
BHOWN,A.S.,PhD A5
Birmingham,AL
BIANCO,N., ... A17,E33
Caracas
BIAS,W.B., ... B41
Baltimore,MD
BIDULO,L.,MD C34
Chapel Hill,NC
BIENZ,S.R., ... A21
Salt Lake City,UT
BILLINGSLEY,L.M.,MD 54
Baltimore,MD
BINDER,W.L., ... B14
La Jolla,CA
BIRD,G., ... E7
Newcastle Upon Tyne
BISWAS,T., ... E54
Bethesda,MD

BLACK,C.M.,MD, MRCP A46,D50
Isleworth,UK
BLACKBURN,W.D.,MD D53,52,175
Birmingham,AL
BLAIR,S., ... E22
Pittsburgh,PA
BLAKE,D.R.,MRCP 3
Birmingham,UK
BLANCA,I., ... E33
Caracas
BLESILA,A.,MS D36
Nashville,TN
BLETRY,O.,MD E63
Paris
BLOCH,D.,PhD 46,136,C21,C22,A49
Stanford,CA
BLOCH,K.J., ... D18
Boston,MA
BLOCKA,K.,MD C18
Saskatoon,SA
BLONQUIST,L.,BS B34
Salt Lake City,UT
BLUESTEIN,H.G.,MD E27
San Diego,CA
BLUHM,G., ... C22
Stanford,CA
BOAK,A.,PhD 121
Houston,TX
BOCANEGRA,T.S., ... E57
Birmingham,AL
BOGAARS,H.A.,MD D29
Providence,RI
BOH,L.,MS, RPh A18
Madison,WI
BOIRE,G.,MD, BSc A24
Sherbrooke,PQ
BOLE,G.G.,MD B28,A49,E71
Ann Arbor,MI
BOMALASKI,J.S.,MD 171,102,E42
Philadelphia,PA
BOMBARDIER,C.,MD A23,88
Toronto,ON
BONGIOVANNI,G.,MD D57
Cincinnati,OH
BOOKMAN,A.A.,MD D32,E24
Toronto,ON
BORKOWF,A.,PhD B49
Milwaukee,WI
BOUCEK,R., ... 148
Loma Linda,CA
BOURGAULT,I.,MD E63
Paris
BOURGEOIS,P.,MD A51
Paris
BOWYER,S.L.,MD 66
Ann Arbor,MI
BOYD,R.E., ... B41
Baltimore,MD
BRAHN,E.,MD 76
Boston,MA
BRANDT,K.D.,MD A40,A49
Indianapolis,IN
BRASINGTON,R.D.,MD E29
Iowa City,IA
BRAUNSTEIN,E.,MD E41
Ann Arbor,MI
BRESNIHAN,B., ... 139
Dublin,Ireland
BREWER,E.J.,MD 1,62,63,B2,B3,C38
Houston,TX
BREWER,G.,MD E41
Ann Arbor,MI
BREWERTON,D.,MD, FRCP A36
London,UK
BRICK,J.E.,MD E20
Morgantown,WV
BRIGGS,D.,BSc A46
London,UK
BRODSKY,A.E.,MD E72
Houston,TX
BROOKS,M.S.,MD 74
Indianapolis,IN
BROWN,L.J.,MD D24,D23
Hanover,NH
BROWN,P.S., ... E46
Memphis,TN
BROWN, JR,C.R.,MD B28
Ann Arbor,MI
BUCHANAN,W.,MD,FRCP(C) 18
Hamilton,ON
BUCKI,B.,MD A57
Paris
BUCKINGHAM,R.B.,MD B20
Pittsburgh,PA
BUDD,R.C.,MD 75
Epalinges,Switzerland
BULLOUGH,P.G.,MD C7
New York,NY
BUNCH,T.W.,MD 155
Rochester,MN
BUNN,C.,MI 114
London
BURDICK,G., ... 160,C45
Seattle,WA
BURGOS-VARGAS,R.,MD B9
Mexico City
BURNETT,J.B.,MD D24
Hanover,NH
BUTLER,D.E.,MD 8
Decatur,GA
BUYON,J.,MD 80
New York,NY
CABRAL,A.R.,MD B50
Ann Arbor,MI
CAHALAN,M.D.,PhD A35
Irvine,CA
CAIRNS,E.,MSc 113,40
London,ON
CALABIA,B.,BS D38
Irvine,CA
CALABRESE,L.H.,DO E35,E60,14
Cleveland,OH
CALABRO,J.J.,MD C6
Worcester,MA
CALANDRA,G., ... D40
Bethesda,MD
CALDRON,P.,DO E60
Evanston,IL
CALDWELL,J.R.,MD A53,D59
Gainesville,FL

CALVO,A., ... E57
Lima,Peru
CAMERON,B.,MD B8
Toronto,ON
CAMPBELL,S.M.,MD........ E17
Portland,OR
CANEPA-ANSON,R.,MRCP A36
London,UK
CANNON,G.W.,MD B34
Salt Lake City,UT
CAPEL,P.A.,PhD........ 146
Nijmegen,The Netherlands
CAPELL,H.,MBChB,MRCP E8,D9,C16
Glasgow
CARAFA,C.,MD D42
Philadelphia,PA
CARBOTTE,R.M.,........ A12,B46
Hamilton,ON
CARETTE,S.,MD,FRCP(C) 158
Quebec,PQ
CARLSON,H.E., ... E20
Columbia,MO
CARLSON,R., ... C2
Kansas City,MO
CARMACK,C.,........ 43
Salt Lake City,UT
CARO,X.J.,MD E61
Northridge,CA
CARR,R.I.,MD, PhD........ E6,A64
Halifax,NS
CARRILLO,C.,........ E57
Lima, Peru
CARSON,D.A.,MD 2,37,C32,165,38
La Jolla,CA
CARSONS,S.E.,MD D62,127
New Hyde Park,NY
CARUSO,W.R.,MD........ A45
Los Angeles,CA
CASSELL,S.L.,MD C18
Eugene,OR
CASTANEDA,M., ... E57
Lima, Peru
CASTOR,C.,MD B29,B50
Ann Arbor,MI
CASTORENA,G., ... D18
Boston,MA
CATERSON,B.,........ E70
Chicago,IL
CATHEY,M.,BSN E10
Kansas City,KS
CATS,A.,MD E37
Leiden,The Netherlands
CAVENDER,D.E.,PhD........ A44
Dallas,TX
CERA,P.,........ D54
Danville,PA
CEROTTINI,J.,MD........ 75
Epalinges,Switzerland
CHAN,E.L.,PhD........ E53
La Jolla,CA
CHAN,E.L.,PhD........ A43
La Jolla,CA
CHAN,G., ... 77
Sepulveda,CA
CHAN,J.H.,........ D8
London
CHANDY,K.,MD, PhD A35
Irvine,CA
CHANG,R.W.,MD, MPH D26
Chicago,IL
CHANG,Y.,PhD, PhD 81
Los Angeles,CA
CHAPELON,C.,MD E63
Paris
CHATPAR,P.C.,MD B43
New York,NY
CHEN,P.P.,PhD........ 3,38,37
La Jolla,CA
CHENOWETH,D.E.,MD, PhD B55
San Diego,CA
CHESS,L.,MD 104
New York,NY
CHEUNG,H.S.,PhD B51,B33,B49
Milwaukee,WI
CHIHARA,K.,........ D66
Kobe
CHIORAZZI,N.,MD A42
New York,NY
CHIU,B.,PhD D63,E66
Toronto,ON
CHOI,S.,MD D20
Philadelphia,PA
CHOW,D.C.,MS B54
Chicago,IL
CHRISTIAN,C.L., ... B43,163
New York,NY
CHRISTY,W.C.,MD 97
Pittsburgh,PA
CHYLACK, JR,L.T.,MD........ 128
Boston,MD
CIPRIANO,D.,BS A8
Wilmington,DE
CIRENZA,P.F., ... 66
Ann Arbor,MI
CLAMAN,H.N.,MD D45
Denver,CO
CLARK,E.A., ... 87
Seattle,WA
CLARK,M., ... 171
Philadelphia,PA
CLARKSON,S.B.,MD........ B10
New York,NY
CLAYBURNE,G., ... A59,D19,D20
Philadelphia,PA
CLAYTON,M., ... 143
Denver,CO
CLEGG,D.O.,MD D12,A21
Salt Lake City,UT
CLEVELAND,D.W.,PhD 112
Baltimore,MD
CLOUGH,J.D.,MD E35,E60
Cleveland,OH
CLOUTIER,J.,MD........ E44
Montreal,PQ
COATES,G.,MBBS........ 12
Hamilton,ON
COBLYN,J.S.,MD C19
Boston,MA

COHEN,B.J.,PhD ... 3
London,UK
COHEN,P.L.,MD ... 71,69
Chapel Hill,NC
COLACO,C.B.,BSC,MBChB ... A9,E4
London
COLBURN,K.K.,MD ... 148,C15
Loma Linda,CA
COLLINS,B.,ARNP ... A48
Miami,FL
CONAWAY,D.C.,MD ... B45
Philadelphia,PA
CONDEMI,J.J.,MD ... 25,D55
Rochester,MN
CONN,D.L.,MD ... D52,E11,E12
Rochester,MN
CONTRERAS,C.E.,MSc ... A17
Caracas
COOKE,D.V.,MB, BCHIR ... A49
Kingston,ON
COOPER,S.M., ... 166
Burlington,VT
COOPERSTEIN,L.A.,MD ... 97
Pittsburgh,PA
COPE,R.,MD ... E36
Columbia,MO
CRACCHIOLO, III,A.,MD ... 48
Los Angeles,CA
CRANE-ROBINSON,C.,PhD ... 117
Portsmouth,UK
CREMER,M.A.,MD ... B11
Memphis,TN
CRONSTEIN,B.N.,MD ... D16,78
New York,NY
CROW,M., ... 110
New York,NY
CULLEN,K.E.,MEd ... A65,85,90
Boston,MA
CURD,J.,MD ... 2,E58
La Jolla,CA
CURTISS,L., ... 79
La Jolla,CA
CUSH,J.J.,MD ... 97
Dallas,TX
DADDONA,P.E.,PhD ... 122,120
Ann Arbor,MI
DAHL,S.L.,PharmD ... B36
Salt Lake City,UT
DALSETH,T., ... 10
Los Angeles,CA
DANG,H.,PhD ... 72
San Antonio,TX
DAVID,C.S., ... 170,168,C49
Rochester,MN
DAVIDSON,A., ... A63
New York,NY
DAVIDSON,B.J.,MD ... 122
Ann Arbor,MI
DAVIGNON,J.,PhD ... 75
Geneva
DAVIS,A., ... B7
Chicago,IL
DAVIS,B.M.,MD ... D4
Lackland AFB,TX
DAVIS,S.,MD ... B39
Providence,RI
DAVIS III,A.E.,MD ... 19
Boston,MA
DAVIS IV,J.,MD ... D47
Charlottesville,VA
DE CUNTO,C.L.,MD ... 63
Houston,TX
DE FILIPP,G.,MD ... B45
Philadelphia,PA
DE GUZMAN,M.,MD ... A45
Los Angeles,CA
DE KASEP,G.I., ... A37
Mexico City
DE LOS REYES,V., ... C8
Mexico City
DECOURSEY,T.E.,PhD ... A35
Irvine,CA
DENBURG,J.,MD,FRCP(C) ... A12,B46,D5
Hamilton,ON
DENBURG,S.D., ... A12,B46
Hamilton,ON
DENG,J.,PhD ... D6
Pittsburgh,PA
DENNIS,G.J.,MD ... 167
Washington,DC
DENT,P.B., ... D5,B46
Hamilton,ON
DENYS,F., ... C27,C20
Birmingham,AL
DEPPER,J.M.,MD ... 30
Bethesda,MD
DERKSEN,R., ... E7
Utrecht,The Netherlands
DEVAUX,J.Y., ... 24
Paris
DIAMOND,B., ... A63
New York,NY
DIAMOND,B.J.,BA ... D62
New Hyde Park,NY
DIAMOND,B.A.,MD ... 57
Bronx,NY
DIAMOND,H.S.,MD ... D62,127
New Hyde Park,NY
DIAZ-JOUANEN,E., ... C8
Mexico City
DILLON,A.M.,MB,BCh,BAO ... D52
Rochester,MN
DINERMAN,H.,MD ... A58,D58,159
Boston,MA
DONG,J.,MD ... A5
Birmingham,AL
DOREY,F., ... C4
Los Angeles,CA
DORNER,R.W.,PhD ... C39,C41
St. Louis,MO
DOUGADOS,M.,MD ... 137,A13
Paris
DOUVAS,A.S.,PhD ... B13
Los Angeles,CA
DRAYER,D., ... A47
New York,NY
DREISINGER,T.E.,PhD ... C56
Columbia, MO

DROGULA,C., ... 30
Bethesda,MD
DRUEKE,T.,MD ... A55
Paris
DRUZIN,M.,MB ... C11,151
New York,NY
DRYLL,A.,MD ... A57
Paris
DUDENEY,C.,BSc ... E4
London
DUKE,O.,MRCP ... E38
London
DUNCAN,H.,MD ... D72
Detroit,MI
DWULET,F.E.,PhD ... 123
Indianapolis,IN
DYLESKI,R.A.,BA ... B13
Los Angeles,CA
DeHORATIUS,R.J.,MD ... C34,C35
Philadelphia,PA
EARNSHAW,W.C.,PhD ... 112
Baltimore,MD
EASTERBROOK,M.,MD,FRCP(C) ... B35
Toronto,ON
EASTWOOD,S.,BSc ... E6
Halifax,NS
EBLING,F.,PhD ... 129,C29
Los Angeles,CA
EDBERG,J., ... D47
Charlottesville,VA
EDWARDS,N.,MD ... D59,E62
Gainesville,FL
EGAN,M.,PhD ... D37
Birmingham,AL
EGGER,M.,PhD ... B34
Salt Lake City,UT
EICHENFIELD,A.H.,MD ... 131
Philadelphia,PA
EIDER,W.,MD ... E41
Ann Arbor,MI
EISENBEIS, JR,C.H.,MD ... E40,142
Pittsburgh,PA
EISENBERG,R.,MD ... 69,71
Chapel Hill,NC
ELKON,K.B., ... C12,116
New York,NY
EMAM,M., ... 132
Salt Lake City,UT
EMLEN,W.,MD ... C45,160
Seattle,WA
ENDO,L.P.,MD ... 6
Gainesville,FL
ENDRES,R.O., ... D21,109
Memphis,TN
ENEL,C.,PhD ... A56
Aguamassalik
ENGLEMAN,E.G.,MD ... B6
Stanford,CA
ENLOW,R.,MD ... 49
New York,NY
ENTWISTLE,R.A.,MS ... B16
Chicago,IL
EPSTEIN,A.L.,MD ... D7
Bronx,NY
EPSTEIN,W.V.,MD ... D22,92,89
San Francisco,CA
ERICKSON,A.,MD ... B39
Providence,RI
ESPINOZA,L.R., ... E57
Tampa,FL
ETIENNE,S.,MD ... A51
Paris
ETTINGER, JR,W.,MD ... A15,E21
Baltimore,MD
EVANS,J.,BS ... 69
Chapel Hill,NC
EVANS,M.,BA ... 41
Kansas City,KS
EWALD,E.A.,MD ... A62
Ann Arbor,MI
EYVAZZADEH,C.,MD ... C6
Worcester,MA
FAABER,P.,PhD ... 146
Nijmegen,The Netherlands
FALANGA,V.,MD ... 28
Pittsburgh,PA
FALCONE,D.J., ... B43
New York,NY
FALK,J.,BSc ... D63
Toronto,ON
FALLAHI,S.,MD ... 47
Birmingham,AL
FAM,A.G.,MD, FRCP ... D19,158
Toronto,ON
FATHMAN,C.,MD ... 68,111
Stanford,CA
FEARON,D.T.,MD ... C36
Boston,MA
FEIGHERY,C., ... 139
Dublin
FELSON,D.,MD, MPH ... 159,A58,D58
Boston,MA
FERLIC,D., ... 143
Denver,CO
FIEDLER-NAGY,C.,PhD ... A66
Nutley,NJ
FINBLOOM,D.S.,MD ... E30,35,161
Washington,DC
FINERMAN,G.M.,MD ... 48
Los Angeles,CA
FINK,C.W.,MD ... B27
Dallas,TX
FINKLEMAN,F.D.,MD ... 167
Bethesda,MD
FISCHBACH,M.,MD ... A35,70
San Antonio,TX
FISCHER,H.D.,MD ... 49
New York,NY
FISHER,D.E.,PhD ... C14
New York,NY
FISHER,M.C.,BA, ASCP ... C28
Spring House,PA
FISHEROWITZ,J.,RPT ... C2
Kansas City,KS
FITZ,G.,MD ... B48
San Francisco,CA
FITZGERALD,O.,MB, MRCP ... D33,D57
Cincinnati,OH

FLEISCHMAJER,R.,MD 126
New York,NY
FLEMING,K.W.,MD D68
Sacramento,CA
FLORSHEIM,P., ... 60
Baltimore,MD
FOIDART,J., ... B40
Liege,Belgium
FONG,A.A., ... 81
Los Angeles,CA
FONG,S.,PhD 2,38,37
La Jolla,CA
FOREMAN,J.B.,MD E1
New Orleans,LA
FORMAN,M.S., ... B12
New Haven,CT
FORRESTER,D., ... C22
Stanford,CA
FORSYTH,S.J.,BSc E6
Halifax,NS
FOSSEL,A.H., ... A65,90
Boston,MA
FOSTER,C., ... 116
New York,NY
FOSTER,S.L.,MA D64
Winston-Salem,NC
FOTINO,M., ... B25
New York,NY
FOULT,J.M., ... 24
Paris
FOX,D.A.,MD 4,C19
Boston,MA
FOX,I.H.,MD E41
Ann Arbor,MI
FOX,O.F.,PhD 144,C13,A14,E5
Oklahoma City,OK
FOX,R.I.,MD, PhD 165,38,C30
La Jolla,CA
FRANCHIMONT,P., ... B40
Liege,Belgium
FRANCOEUR,A.,PhD B15,A43,C52
La Jolla,CA
FRANGIONE,B.,MD, PhD 37
New York,NY
FRANK,L.P.,MD 57
Bronx,NY
FRANK,S.A.,BS E35
Cleveland,OH
FRANKLIN,C.,MD D54
Danville,PA
FRASER,P.A.,MD C19
Boston,MA
FRASER,S.M.,MBChB,MRCP E9
Glasgow
FRELINGER,J.,PhD 69
Chapel Hill,NC
FREUNDLICH,B.,MD 130,A26
Philadelphia,PA
FRIEDMAN,S.M.,MD 110
New York,NY
FRIES,J.F.,MD C22,C21,46,136
Stanford,CA
FRIESEN,D., ... D11
Toronto,ON
FRIOU,G.,MD D38
Irvine,CA
FRITZLER,M.J.,MD,FRCP(C) D32,117
Calgary,AL
FUJITA,T., ... D66
Kobe,Japan
FURIE,M.B.,PhD B53
New York,NY
FURST,D.E.,MD C18
Iowa City,IA
FYFE,A.,BSc D46
Glasgow
GABOR,G., ... E23
Portland,OR
GAITHER,K.K.,BS C13
Oklahoma City,OK
GANCZARCZYK,M.,MD C42
Toronto,ON
GANS,K.R.,PhD A8
Wilmington,DE
GARBRECHT,F.C.,MD 66
Vancouver,BC
GARCIA-SOTO,A., ... A37
Mexico City
GASSON,J., ... 77
Sepulveda,CA
GASTINEAU,D.A., ... 118
Rochester,MN
GASTON,J.H.,MD, PhD B37
Stanford,CA
GAULDIE,J., ... D5
Hamilton,ON
GAUNT,W.D.,MD E36
Columbia,MO
GAY,R.E.,MD C27
Birmingham,AL
GAY,S.,MD 145,C20,C27,E49
Birmingham,AL
GELFAND,E.,MD B8
Toronto,ON
GELPI,C., ... B12
New Haven,CT
GENANT,H., ... C22
Stanford,CA
GEPPERT,T.D.,MD 34
Dallas,TX
GERBER,L.H.,MD A22
Bethesda,MD
GERTZ,M.A.,MD 157
Rochester,MN
GESCHWIND,N., ... B42
Boston,MA
GETZY,D.M., ... E35
Cleveland,OH
GHARAVI,A., ... E7
Newcastle Upon Tyne,UK
GHARAVI,A.,MD, MSc 99,149,D8
London,UK
GIAMBRONE,M., ... B4
Chicago,IL
GIANNINI,E.H.,DrPH 63,B2,B3,1
Houston,TX
GIBOFSKY,A.,MD B25
New York,NY

GIBSON,D.,MD, FRCP A36
London
GILBERTSON,T.A., ... 38
La Jolla,CA
GINSBERG,M., ... 79
La Jolla,CA
GLADMAN,D.D.,MD,FRCP(C) A38,C42,D34
Toronto,ON
GLASS,D.N.,MD 128,C19
Boston,MD
GLEASON,J., ... C23
Philadelphia,PA
GLOVSKY,M.,MD 23
Los Angeles,CA
GLYNN,M.X.,MD 15
Toronto,ON
GO,R.P., ... A19,E57
Birmingham,AL
GOCKEL,S.,MS B14
La Jolla,CA
GODDARD,D.,MD, MRCP A36
Philadelphia,PA
GODEAU,P.,MD A50,A51,E63
Paris
GODIN-OSTRO,E.,MD D27
New Brunswick,NJ
GOEI,S., ... 151
New York,NY
GOFTON,P., ... C22
Stanford,CA
GOHILL,J.,BSc 117
Calgary,AL
GOLDBERG,A.,MD A15
Baltimore,MD
GOLDBERG,J.,MD 156
Marshfield,WI
GOLDBERG,R.L.,PhD A7
Boston,MA
GOLDE,D., ... 77
Sepulveda,CA
GOLDENBERG,D.L.,MD 159,A58,D58
Boston,MA
GOLDFIEN,R.,MD 2,37
La Jolla,CA
GOLDFINGER,D., ... A16
Los Angeles,CA
GOLDINGS,E.A.,MD E32
Dallas,TX
GOLDMAN,J.A.,MD E64
Atlanta,GA
GOLDRING,M.B.,PhD 173
Boston,MA
GOLDRING,S.R.,MD 135
Boston,MA
GOLDSMITH,D.P.,MD C37,131
Philadelphia,PA
GOLETZ,J., ... E70
Chicago,IL
GOLOMBEK,S.J.,MD 56,C12
New York,NY
GOMPPER,P.,BS B15
La Jolla,CA
GONCHOROFF,N.J., ... B26
Rochester,MN
GONI,F.,PhD 37
New York,NY
GONZALEZBARCENAS,D., ... 150
Mexico City
GOOD,A.E.,MD E13,E41
Ann Arbor,MI
GOODACRE,R.,MB,FRCP(C) 12
Hamilton,ON
GOODWIN,J.S.,MD 108,D48
Albuquerque,NM
GORONZY,J.J.,MD 68,111
Stanford,CA
GOTTLIEB,A., ... 110
New York,NY
GOTUZZO,E., ... E57
Birmingham,AL
GRACE,E.,RN, MHSc 18
Hamilton,ON
GRADY,M., ... 15
Toronto,ON
GRAEF,A., ... 150
Mexico City
GRANADOS,J.,MD A37
Mexico City
GRAU,R.G.,MD D28
San Antonio,TX
GRAUER,J.,MD 48
Los Angeles,CA
GREEN,A., ... 110
New York,NY
GREENBERG,M., ... D7
Bronx,NY
GREENE,M.L.,MD D12
Seattle,WA
GREENE,R.R.,MD 23
Los Angeles,CA
GREENE,W.C., ... 30
Bethesda,MD
GREENWALD,R.A.,MD A49,A28
New Hyde Park,NY
GREISMAN,S.G.,MD 163,C31
New York,NY
GRIFFING,W.,MD 157
Rochester,MN
GRIFFITHS,M.M., ... 168
Salt Lake City,UT
GRUBER,B.,MD A14,C26
Stony Brook,NY
GUERRA,J., ... E57
Lima,Peru
GUPTA,S.,MD A35
Irvine,CA
GUSTAFSON,C.J.,MD B16
Chicago,IL
GUYTON,J.M., ... D53,138
Birmingham,AL
GUZMAN,L.,MD E42
Santiago,Chile
HAAK-FRENDSCHO,M., ... C26
Stony Brook,NY
HAAS, JR,G.G., ... C10
Oklahoma City,OK
HABER,P.L.,MD C41
St. Louis,MO

HADLER,N.M., ... 154
Chapel Hill,NC
HAHN,B.,MD ... 129
Los Angeles,CA
HAHN,B.H.,MD ... 129,133,20,73,C29
Los Angeles,CA
HALBERT,S., ... D7
Bronx,NY
HALL,N.D.,MA, PhD ... 21
Bath,UK
HALLA,J.T.,MD ... 47,B38
Abilene,TX
HALPERN,R.,PhD ... A63
New York,NY
HALVERSON,P.B.,MD ... B32,B33
Milwaukee,WI
HANDWERGER,B.S.,MD ... B24,118,B26
Rochester,NY
HANG,M., ... B7
La Jolla,CA
HANLY,J.,MB, MRCPI ... 139
Dublin
HANNA,W.M.,MBBCh,FRCP ... D11
Toronto,ON
HARDIN,J.G.,MD ... 47,B38
Mobile,AL
HARDIN,J.A.,MD ... B12,C53,E52
New Haven,CT
HARDY,D.C.,MD ... D69
Fairfield,CA
HARLEY,J.B.,MD, PhD ... 144,C13,118,A14,E5
Oklahoma City,OK
HARMON,C., ... E19
Denver,CO
HARPEL,P.C.,MD ... C11
New York,NY
HARRINGTON,T.M., ... D54
Danville,PA
HARRIS,E.N.,MD ... D8,E7.149,99
London,UK
HARRIS,E.,MD ... C18
Whittier,CA
HARRIS,G.,MD ... A9
London
HARRIS,W.H.,MD ... 135
Boston,MA
HARRIS, JR,E.D.,MD ... C27
New Brunswick,NJ
HART,M.V., ... E17
Portland,OR
HARTLEY,R.M.,MD ... 85
Boston,MA
HASHIMOTO,H.,MD ... E2,C9
Tokyo
HASSAN,J., ... 139
Dublin
HASSELBACHER,P.,MD ... 91
Louisville,KY
HASTY,K.A.,PhD ... A6
Memphis,TN
HAYES,E., ... D18
Boston,MA
HAZZARD,W.R.,MD ... A15
Baltimore,MD
HEALEY,L.,MD ... 13
Seattle,WA
HECK,L.,MD ... 175
Birmingham,AL
HEINER,G.G.,MD ... 53
Baltimore,MD
HEITZMANN,J.,PhD ... 2
La Jolla,CA
HELLER,I.,MS ... D27
New Brunswick,NJ
HELLER,M., ... A53
Charleston,SC
HELLMANN,D.,MD ... B48
San Francisco,CA
HENDRIX,T.,MD ... E21
Baltimore,MD
HENG,M., ... 148
Sepulveda,CA
HENKE,C.J.,PhD ... 92
San Francisco,CA
HERBERT,D.L.,MBBS ... 97
Pittsburgh,PA
HERMAN,J.H.,MD ... D15,45
Cincinnati,OH
HERNANDEZ,H., ... E57
Lima
HERNANDEZ-ORTIZ,J., ... C8
Mexico City
HEROLD,B.,MD ... B7
Chicago,IL
HERRERA,J., ... 150
Mexico City
HERSON,G.,MD ... A51,E63
Paris
HERSON,S., ... A50
Paris
HESS,E.V.,MD ... 45,D57,D15,D33
Cincinnati,OH
HIBBS,M.S.,MD ... E69,A6
Memphis,TN
HILL,J.J.,MD ... D56
Springfield,IL
HINOSTROZA,S.A., ... E57
Lima,Peru
HIROHATA,K., ... E25
Kobe,Japan
HIROSE,S., ... C9,E2
Tokyo
HIRSCHBERG,J.M.,MD ... C18
Rancho Mirage,CA
HIRSCHHORN,R.,MD ... D16,E26,78
New York,NY
HO, JR,G.,MD ... B39
Providence,RI
HOBBS,S., ... E38
London,UK
HOCHBERG,M.C.,MD, MPH ... 60,164,A49,B41
Baltimore,MD
HOCHMAN,R.,MD ... D24
Sayre,PA
HOFFMAN,R.W.,DO ... 128
Bethesda,MD
HOFFSTEIN,S.T.,PhD ... C23
Philadelphia,PA

HOIDAL,J.R., ... E69
Memphis,TN
HOLDWORTH,D.E.,MD C19
Boston,MA
HOLERS,V.,MD 42
St. Louis,MO
HOLMAN,H.R., ... 93
Stanford,CA
HOLME,E.,MSc D46
Glasgow
HOM,D., ... D6
Pittsburgh,PA
HOOPER,M.M.,MD 25
Rochester,NY
HOOVER,D., ... 35
Washington,DC
HORGAN,C.J.,PhD C45
Seattle,WA
HOROWITZ,J.,MD 17
Birmingham,AL
HORWITZ,D.A.,MD 23,107,A33
Los Angeles,CA
HOSENPUD,J.D., ... E17
Portland,OR
HOUGH,D.R.,MD A54
Washington,DC
HOUGHTEN,R.A.,PhD 37
La Jolla,CA
HOW,A., ... B46
Hamilton,ON
HOWARD,A.,MSc B9
Harrow,UK
HOWARD,P.H., ... B41
Baltimore,MD
HOWELL,D.S.,MD A49
Miami,FL
HOYT,T.S.,MD E36
Columbia,MO
HUANG,A.J.,MD B53
New York,NY
HUDSON,J.,PhD 31
Ann Arbor,MI
HUGHES,G.V., ... 149,99,D8,E7
London,UK
HUNDER,G.G.,MD 157
Rochester,MN
HUNT,G.C., ... A22
Bethesda,MD
HUNTER,F.,PhD A5
Birmingham,AL
HUNTER,J.,MBChB,MRCP D9,E8
Glasgow
HURVITZ,A., ... A47
New York,NY
HURWITZ,C.,PhD A10
Albany,NY
HURWITZ,S., ... A22
Washington,DC
HUSE,A., ... C49,170,168
Rochester,MN
HUTCHINSON,M.,BS B47
Los Angeles,CA
HWANG,J.,BS A7
Boston,MA
IGLESIAS-GAMARRA,A., ... C8
Mexico City
IGUCHI,T.,MD E25
Dallas,TX
IKE,R.W.,MD D60
Ann Arbor,MI
IKEGAMI,H., ... D66
Kobe,Japan
ILSTRUP,D.M., ... D52,E11,155
Rochester,MN
IMBODEN, JR,J.B.,MD 29
San Francisco,CA
INFANTE,D.,MS 70
San Antonio,TX
INGENITO,F., ... E39
Farmington,CT
INGLIS,A.E.,MD 64,C1
New York,NY
INMAN,R.D.,MD D63,E66,B17
Toronto,ON
INOKUMA,S.,MD D1
Tokyo
IRVINE,G.,MD E41
Ann Arbor,MI
ISENBERG,D.A.,MD, MRCP E4
London,UK
ISHIKAWA,H.,MD E25
Kobe,Japan
IWASE,R.,MD D14
Osaka
IZUI,S.,PhD 75
Geneva
IZZO, JR,J.L.,MD 25
Rochester,NY
JABS,D.A.,MD 53
Baltimore,MD
JACKSON,C.G.,MD D12
Salt Lake City,UT
JACOB,G.,MD 11
New York,NY
JACOBITZ,J., ... E70
Chicago,IL
JACOBS,H., ... E15
Toronto,ON
JACOBS,R.J.,PhD B56,E16
Oklahoma City,OK
JAGLAL,S.,BSc D34
Toronto,ON
JASIN,H., ... D39,A30
Dallas,TX
JASSO,M.S.,LPT B3
Houston,TX
JASTY,M.,MD 135
Boston,MA
JAYSON,M.V.,MD, FRCP D50
Salford,UK
JENKINS,R.,PhD 12
Hamilton,ON
JIMENEZ,J.,MD 50,50
Mexico City
JIMENEZ,S.A.,MD 130,A2,D19
Philadelphia,PA
JINNAH,R., ... 10
Los Angeles,CA

JIRIK,F.R.,MD 2,37
La Jolla,CA
JOB-DESLANDRE,C.,MD A13
Paris
JOHANNES,R.,MD E21
Baltimore,MD
JOHANSON,N.A.,MD C7
New York,NY
JOHNSON,C.R.,MD C41
St. Louis,MO
JOHNSON,J., ... C48
Syracuse,NY
JOHNSON,J.A., ... 148,C15
Loma Linda,CA
JOHNSON,M.,MSc B17,D63
Toronto,ON
JOHNSON,P.M.,PhD,MRCP 119
Liverpool,UK
JOHNSTON,S.,PhD C48
Syracuse,NY
JONES,D.H.,MD B23
Rochester,NY
JONES,E.,MB,MRCP E6
Halifax,NS
JONES,H., ... 46
Stanford,CA
JONES,J.V.,BM,FRCP(C) E6
Halifax,NS
JOOSTEN,L., ... E18
Nijmegen,The Netherlands
JOSEPHSON,N.,MD C18
Des Moines,IA
JOVANOVIC,L.,MD 151
New York,NY
JOYAL,F.,MD,FRCP(C) E51
Montreal,PQ
JUDD,H.L.,MD E20
Los Angeles,CA
JUOZEVICIUS,J.L.,MD E65
Albany,NY
JURISSON,M.L.,MD B29
Ann Arbor,MI
KACENA,A., ... 148
Sepulveda,CA
KADIN,M.E., ... 87
Boston,MA
KAHAN,A.,MD 24
Paris
KAHL,L.E.,MD D6,142
Pittsburgh,PA
KAHN,L.,MS 31
Ann Arbor,MI
KAHN,M.F.,MD A51
Paris
KAINE,J.L., ... 67,A14
Chicago,IL
KALOVIDOURIS,A.E.,MD A34
Indianapolis,IN
KALUNIAN,K.C.,MD 20,133
Los Angeles,CA
KANG,A.H., ... A6,B11,109,E69
Memphis,TN
KANG,A.,BS B16
Chicago,IL
KANT,J.,MD, PhD A59
Philadelphia,PA
KANTOR,S.,MD A47
New York,NY
KAPLAN,A.P., ... C26
Stony Brook,NY
KAPLAN,D.,MD A41,A49
Brooklyn,NY
KAPLAN,G., ... 36
New York,NY
KARAS,B., ... 172
Milwaukee,WI
KASSAM,Y.B.,MBChB,FRCP 18
Hamilton,ON
KATER,L., ... E7
Utrecht,The Netherlands
KATONA,I.M.,MD B55
Bethesda,MD
KATZ,A.R.,MD 61
Los Angeles,CA
KATZMANN,J.A., ... B26
Rochester,MN
KAZIS,L.E., ... 94
Boston,MA
KAZMAR,R.E.,MD E11
Olympia Fields,IL
KEAN,W.,MD,FRCP(C) 18
Hamilton,ON
KEENAN,E., ... E23
Portland,OR
KELLEY,W.N.,MD 122,120
Ann Arbor,MI
KELLY,M.,BSc, MD D5
Hamilton,ON
KEYSTONE,E.C.,MD, FRCP 15,D32,E24,D34,E56
Toronto,ON
KHAN,M.,PhD B6
Stanford,CA
KHAN,M.A.,MD E37,A39
Cleveland,OH
KIBLER,R.,PhD B18
Tucson,AZ
KIM,H.C.,MD D27
New Brunswick,NJ
KIM,J., ... E15
Toronto,ON
KIMBERLY,R.P.,MD E67,C31,59,B25,B43
New York,NY
KING,K.,ARNP D24
Belmont,MA
KITRIDOU,R.C.,MD 23
Los Angeles,CA
KLATT,C., ... 39,E48
Durham,NC
KLEIN,M.,MD B17
Toronto,ON
KLEIN,M., ... 17
Birmingham,AL
KLEINHEKSEL,S.,OTR E10
Kansas City,KS
KLINENBERG,J.R.,MD A16
Los Angeles,CA
KLIPPLE,G.,MD A54
Washington,DC

KOCH,A.,MD ... 82
Chicago,IL
KODAMA,A., ... C9
Tokyo
KOMAR,R.,MSc ... 113
London,ON
KONO,D.H.,MD ... 51
Los Angeles,CA
KOO,A.P.,MD ... 5
Cleveland,OH
KOOPMAN,W.J.,MD ... E49,A49,145,C51,B19,C27,C20,A19
138
Birmingham,AL
KOPICKY,J.A.,MD ... B30
Baltimore,MD
KORCHAK,H., ... D70
New York,NY
KOREN,E.,PhD ... E5
Oklahoma City,OK
KOSS,M.,MD ... D13
Los Angeles,CA
KOTZIN,B.L.,MD ... D45,42
Denver,CO
KOVACS,S.,PhD ... 121
Columbia,MO
KOYAMA,S., ... D66
Kobe
KRAMER,S.B.,MD ... E26
New York,NY
KRANE,S.M.,MD ... 173
Boston,MA
KRATOR, S.M.,MD ... A47
New York,NY
KREMER,J.M.,MD ... C17
Albany,NY
KRESINA,T.F.,PhD ... C46,124
Cleveland,OH
KRONKE,M., ... 30
Bethesda,MD
KRUEGER,G.G.,MD ... 132
Salt Lake City,UT
KUBERSKY,S.M., ... D16
New York,NY
KUETTNER,K.,PhD ... B54,E70
Chicago,IL
KUJALA,G.A.,MD ... C54,D47
Charlottesville,VA
KUNTZ,D.,MD ... A55
Paris
KURIMOTO,M., ... D66
Kobe
KURSŪNOGLU,S.,MD ... C3
San Diego,CA
KUSHNER,I.,MD ... A39
Cleveland,OH
KUZMINA,N.,MD ... 1
Moscow
KWAN,L.,MD ... 77
Sepulveda,CA
KWOH,C.,MD ... D23,D24
New Haven,CT
KYLE,R.A.,MD ... 157
Rochester,MN
LACHENBRUCH,A.P.,PhD ... C18
Iowa City,IA
LACHIEWICZ,P.F.,MD ... C1,64
Chapel Hill,NC
LAFFERTY,C.,MD ... C3
San Diego,CA
LAHITA,R.G.,MD ... C14,B42,A63,A47
New York,NY
LAKHANPAL,S.,MB,BS,MD ... B26,155,E12
Rochester,MN
LALLY,E.V.,MD ... D29
Providence,RI
LAND,D.V.,BSc, PhD ... E9
Glasgow
LANE,N.E.,MD ... 46,B37
Stanford,CA
LANE,R.S.,PhD ... 98
Berkeley,CA
LANSAMAN,J.,MT ... A57
Paris
LaPORTE,R.E.,PhD ... D6
Pittsburgh, PA
LARSON,J., ... B19
Birmingham,AL
LARSON,M.G.,DSc ... 90,A65
Boston,MA
LASKIN,R.S.,MD ... D62
New Hyde Park,NY
LATHROP,M.,PhD ... A56
Paris
LATMAN,N.S.,PhD ... A20
Weatherford,OK
LAVALLE,C.,MD ... 150
Mexico City
LAVI,S.,MD ... B8
Toronto,ON
LAVIETES,B.,PhD ... 127,D62
Stony Brook,NY
LAVOIE,P.E.,MD ... 98
San Francisco,CA
LAWLEY,P.,PhD ... A9
London
LAXER,R.,MD ... B8
Toronto,ON
LAZARCHICK,J.,MD ... C40
Charleston,SC
LAZO,A., ... A63
New York,NY
LEATHERMAN,J.R.,BS ... 5
Cleveland,OH
LEDERMAN,R.J.,MD ... E60
Cleveland,OH
LEE,J.,MD,FRCP(C) ... 100
Toronto,ON
LEE,J.,PhD ... C52
San Antonio,TX
LEE,L.,MD ... 132
Denver,CO
LEE,P.,MD,FRCP(C) ... D32,E24,D34
Toronto,ON
LEHMAN,T.A.,MD ... 61,64
Los Angeles,CA
LEIBOVICH,S.J.,PhD ... 82
Chicago,IL
LEISEN,J.,MD ... D72
Detroit,MI

LEJEWSKI,J.E., ... 152
Baltimore,MD
LENDRUM,R., ... E7
Newcastle Upon Tyne
LENNOX,D.W.,MD B30
Baltimore,MD
LENS,J.,PhD 83
Nijmegen,The Netherlands
LENZ,M., ... E70
Chicago,IL
LEONARD,P.A.,MD A21,D12,7
Salt Lake City,UT
LEONARD,W.J., ... 30
Bethesda,MD
LeRoy,E.C.,MD 22
Charleston, SC
LETVIN,N.L.,MD 32
Boston,MA
LEVIN,R.I., ... 78
New York,NY
LEVINE,P.R.,MD E73
Washington,DC
LEVINSON,A.I.,MD D42,C34
Philadelphia,PA
LEVISON,H.,MD,FRCP(C) 100
Toronto,ON
LEWIS,D.M.,DDS A54
Washington,DC
LEWIS,D.E.,PhD 62
Houston,TX
LEWISON,A., ... 110
New York,NY
LIANG,M.H.,MD, MPH 90,A65,85
Boston,MA
LIAO,S., ... D5,B46
Hamilton,ON
LIEBLING,M.R.,MD D51,A67
Torrance,CA
LIEU,T.,PhD 125,D4
Dallas,TX
LIJEWSKI,J.E.,BS, MT A60
Baltimore,MD
LINDSEY,G.T.,MD 27
Denver,CO
LINDSLEY,C.B.,MD B1
Kansas City,KS
LINKER-ISRAELI,M.,PhD A33
Los Angeles,CA
LIPSKY,P.E.,MD 105,34
Dallas,TX
LIPSTATE,J.M.,MD D53
Birmingham,AL
LIU,S.,BS 106
Chicago,IL
LLUBERAS,G.,MD 102
Philadelphia,PA
LLUBERES,R., ... B31
San Juan,PR
LOCKSHIN,M.,MD C11,151
New York,NY
LOEB,F.X.,MD 131
Philadelphia,PA
LONDINO, JR,A.V.,MD C6
Worcester,MA
LONG,A.A.,MB, MRCPI A12
Hamilton,ON
LONGLEY,S.,MD D59,E62
Gainesville,FL
LOONEY,R.J.,MD 33
Rochester,NY
LORIG,K.R.,RN, DrPH 93
Stanford,CA
LOSMAN,M.J.,PhD 145,B19
Birmingham,AL
LOTZ,M.,MD C32
La Jolla,CA
LOUGHRAN,T.J., ... 87
Seattle,WA
LOUIE,J.S.,MD A1,D51
Torrance,CA
LOVETT, III,E.J.,PhD 31
Scarborough,ME
LOWENSTEIN,E., ... D18
Boston,MA
LOYO,E., ... 150
Mexico City
LUDEWIG,R., ... 58,D70
New York,NY
LUKA,J.,PhD 165
Washington,DC
LUTHRA,H.S., ... 170,168,C49
Rochester,MN
LYDYARD,P.,PhD A9
London
MACKWORTH-YOUNG,C.G.,MRCP 99
Boston,MA
MACSWEEN,J.,MD,FRCP(C) E6
Halifax,NS
MADDISON,P.J.,MD, MRCP D50,21
Bath,UK
MADHOK,R.,MBChB,MRCP C16
Glasgow
MAGID,M.,MD 151
New York,NY
MAGID,S.K.,MD 56
New York,NY
MAHIEU,P., ... B40
Liege,Belgium
MAHNOVSKI,V.,MD 61
Los Angeles,CA
MAHOWALD,M.L.,MD A25
Minneapolis,MN
MALAISE,M.,MD B40
Liege,Belgium
MALAWISTA,S.E.,MD 99
New Haven,CT
MALEMUD,C.J.,PhD E44
Cleveland,OH
MALINOW,K.L., ... 152
Baltimore,MD
MALLEK,J.A.,MD 14
Cleveland,OH
MAMULA,M.J.,MS 144
Oklahoma City,OK
MANDEL,G.S., ... 174
Wood,WI
MANKIN,H.J.,MD A49
Boston,MA

MANNIK,M.,MD D44,C47
Seattle,WA
MANZI,R., ... C23
Philadelphia,PA
MARCUS,D.M.,MD B10
Houston,TX
MARICQ,H.R.,MD C40
Charleston,SC
MARKS,C.R.,RN D12
Seattle,WA
MARLOWE,S., ... E39
Farmington,CT
MARSH,W., ... A53
Lynnfield,MA
MARTEL-PELLETIER,J.,PhD E45,E44
Montreal,PQ
MARTIN,J., ... 79
La Jolla,CA
MARTINEZ-CORDERO,E., ... A29,A37
Mexico City
MARWAH,R.,MD E1
El Paso,TX
MASI,A.T.,MD, DRPH D28
Peoria,IL
MASLEN,C.,BPharm,MPS 21
Bath,UK
MASSONI,R.,BS 42
Denver,CO
MASTUMOTO,K., ... C9
Tokyo
MATHER,S.E., ... C5
Chicago,IL
MATHEWS,M.B.,PhD 114
Cold Spring Harbor,NY
MATSUKAWA,M.,MD D14
Osaka
MATSUMURA,Y.,MD D1
Tokyo
MATTEUCCI,B.M.,MD C35
Philadelphia,PA
MATTREY,R.,MD E72
San Diego,CA
MAXWELL,D.R.,MD 101
Indianapolis,IN
MAZIERES,B.,MD E68
Paris
MEDSGER, JR,T.A.,MD 97,D30,E22,28,142,A49
Pittsburgh,PA
MEENAN,R.F.,MD A49,94
Boston,MA
MEJIAS,E.,MD B31
San Juan,PR
MELIJSON,O., ... A17
Caracas
MELLER,J.,MD E55
New York,NY
MELMON,K.,MD B6
Stanford,CA
MELTON III,L.J.,MD 155
Rochester,MN
MELVIN,C., ... D18
Boston,MA
MENARD,H.A.,MD A24
Sherbrooke,PQ
MENEREY,K.A.,MD E41
Ann Arbor,MI
MENKES,C.J., ... 24,A13,A50
Paris
MERHAR,G.,MD D57
Cincinnati,OH
MERPHUYAN,J., ... B4
Chicago,IL
MERRIAM,L.T., ... E67
New York,NY
MERRITT,M.,BS B22
Portland,OR
MERVANT,H., ... A38
Toronto,ON
MERYHEW,N.L., ... 118,59
Rochester,MN
MESSNER,R.P.,MD 118,147,59,C25,B52
Rochester,MN
METCALF,J.F.,MD 22
Charleston,SC
MICHAEL,A.F., ... A52
Minneapolis,MN
MICHELASSI,F., ... D18
Boston,MA
MICHET,C.,MD 156
Rochester,MN
MIKKELSEN,W.M.,MD A49
Ann Arbor,MI
MILLER,E.J.,PhD 145
Birmingham,AL
MILLER,F.W.,MD, PhD E54,E3
Bethesda,MD
MILLER,L.C.,MD A52
Minneapolis,MN
MILMAN,G., ... 164
Baltimore,MD
MIMORI,T.,MD C53,B12,E52
New Haven,CT
MINOTA,S.,MD 44
Chapel Hill,NC
MIRANDA,A.,PhD 104
New York,NY
MITRANE,M.,MD D27
New Brunswick,NJ
MIYAGAWA,K., ... 153
Tokyo
MIYAHARA,K.,MD D1
Tokyo
MIYAWAKI,S., ... 153
Tokyo
MIZUTANI,W.,MD B47
Los Angeles,CA
MOAK,S.A., ... A28
New Hyde Park,NY
MOATAMED,F., ... 7
Salt Lake City,UT
MOCHAN,E.,PhD, DO A4,A8
Camden,NJ
MOCHARLA,R.,PhD E16
Ardmore,OK
MODY,N.J.,MD D56
Springfield,IL
MOHLER,J.G.,MD D13
Los Angeles,CA

MOLINA,R., ... 134
Baltimore,MD
MOND,J.J.,MD 167
Bethesda,MD
MONGIN,M., ... A50
Paris
MONIHAN,C., ... C35,C34
Philadelphia,PA
MONSON,B.L., ... D28
Peoria,IL
MOORE,G.F., ... E3
Bethesda,MD
MOORE,R.,MD A36
London
MOORE,T.L.,MD B5,C39,D31
St. Louis,MO
MOORE,T.,MD C41
St. Louis,MO
MOORE,W.,MD 65
Housotn,TX
MORENO-RODRIGUEZ,J.,MD 105
Dallas,TX
MORGAN, JR,G.,MD D24
Hanover,NH
MORIMOTO,C.,MD 32
Boston,MA
MORTIMER,P.P.,MD 3
London
MORTON,M., ... E29
Iowa City,IA
MOSKOWITZ,R.W.,MD A49,124,C46
Cleveland,OH
MOSS,J., ... D18
Boston,MA
MOSTELLO,N.,RN C5
Park Ridge,IL
MULLANE,J.,MD 11
New York,NY
MUNNS,T.,PhD 121
St. Louis,MO
MURPHY,W.A.,MD A49
St. Louis,MO
MYERS,J.,PhD A2
Philadelphia,PA
MYERS,L.K.,MD B27
Dallas,TX
MYERS,S.L.,MD 101
Indianapolis,IN
MYONES,B.,MD 44
Chapel Hill,NC
MacDONALD,H.,PhD 75
Epalinges, Switzerland
MacGUIRE,A.M.,MD 55
Ann Arbor,MI
MacKENZIE,A.H.,MD 5
Cleveland,OH
McADAM,L.P.,MD 156
Thousand Oaks,CA
McALLISTER,C.M.,BS D67
Seattle,WA
McCAIN,G.A.,MD,FRCP(C) 158
London,ON
McCARTY,D.J.,MD B33,B49,B51,172
Milwaukee,WI
McCASKILL,B.L.,MD 64
Dallas,TX
McCORMICK,M.C.,MD, ScD 95
Philadelphia,PA
McCULLOUGH,R.G.,RN 27
Denver,CO
McCUNE,W.,MD A62,55
Ann Arbor,MI
McCURDY,D.K.,MD 64
Los Angeles,CA
McDONALD,T.J.,MD E59
Rochester,MN
McGILL,J.,MD 156
Royal Oak,MI
McGRATH,H.,MD E1
New Orleans,LA
McLEAN,R.H., ... B41
Baltimore,MD
McSHANE,D.J.,MD A49,C22
Palo Alto,CA
NAFF,G.B.,MD A61,19
Cleveland,OH
NAGASE,H., ... C27
New Brunswick,NJ
NAIDES,S.J.,MD D35
Boston,MA
NAKAJIMA,M., ... 153
Tokyo
NAKAMURA,M.C.,BA E52
New Haven,CT
NAKAMURA,R.M.,MD D49
La Jolla,CA
NAPRSTEK,B.L.,BA B53
New York,NY
NARDELLA,F.A.,MD D44,C47
Seattle,WA
NATHANSON,M.,PhD 19
Cleveland,OH
NAUMAN,J.,BSN 6,D59
Gainesville,FL
NAVARRETE,R., ... 150
Mexico City
NELSON,J.,MD C47,D44
Seattle,WA
NEVITT,M.C.,PhD 92
San Francisco,CA
NEWTON,R.,PhD A4,A8
Glenolden,PA
NICKESON,R.,MD C38
Oklahoma City,OK
NICKESON, JR,R.W., ... 67
Chicago,IL
NILES,N.S., ... E17
Portland,OR
NOEL,B.J., ... E29,A31
Iowa City,IA
NORMAN,A.,MD 11
New York,NY
NORMAN,G., ... 18
Hamilton,ON
NORRIS,D.A.,MD 132
Denver,CO
NOWLIN,N.S.,MD E20
Columbia,MO

NUSINOW,S.R.,MD E58
La Jolla,CA
O'CONNOR,C.R.,MD E42
Camden,NJ
O'CONNOR,G.T.,PhD D23,D24,91
Hanover,NH
O'CONNOR,M., ... 162
Syracuse,NY
O'CONNOR,T., ... B19
Birmingham,AL
O'DONNELL,M., ... 39
Durham,NC
O'SULLIVAN,F.X.,MD E49,C27,C20
Birmingham,AL
O'TOOLE,T., ... 122
Ann Arbor,MI
OCHI,T.,MD D14
Osaka
OEN,K.G.,MD C44
Winnipeg,MA
OGATA,K.,PhD D49
La Jolla,CA
OGATA,Y.M.,DVM D49
La Jolla,CA
OHATA,N.,MD E2
Tokyo
OHTA,A.,MD A1
Torrance,CA
OHURA,K.,DDS, PhD B55
Bethesda,MD
OLMSTEAD,E.M.,BA D23,D24
Hanover,NH
OLSEN,B.,MD, PhD 126
Piscataway,NJ
OLSEN,N.J.,MD A30,D39
Dallas,TX
ONO,K., MD D14
Osaka
ORKIN,S.H., ... 120
Boston,MA
OSBORN,T.G.,MD B5,C39,C41,D31
St. Louis,MO
OWAKI,H.,MD D14
Osaka
PACHMAN,L.M.,MD 67,E70,B4,B7
Chicago,IL
PALELLA,T.D.,MD 122
Ann Arbor,MI
PANAYI,G., ... E38
London
PANIAGUA,R., ... 150
Mexico City
PANICHEEWA,S.,MD E19
Denver,CO
PANUSH,R.S.,MD D59,E62,6
Gainesville,FL
PARALAPIANO,B., ... A59
Philadelphia,PA
PARHAMI,N.,MD, FACP A10
Albany,NY
PARK,M.,PhD 51
Los Angeles,CA
PARKER,C.W.,MD 169
St. Louis,MO
PARNASSA,A., ... 116
New York,NY
PARSONS,J.L.,MD B18
Tucson,AZ
PASS,T.M.,PhD D26
Newton,MA
PASSO,M., ... 67
Chicago,IL
PATCHETT,C.E.,MD 143
Beaumont,CA
PATE,D., ... C3
San Diego,CA
PAULL,D.M.,MD D69,D68
Sacramento,CA
PEARSON,G.,PhD 165
Washington,DC
PEDELL,L.,MD 156
Royal Oak,MI
PEEBLES,C.L.,MS B15,C52
La Jolla,CA
PELLER,J.,MD E23,B22
Portland,OR
PELLETIER,J.,MD E45,E44
Montreal,PQ
PEREIRA,R.,MB, PhD A46,D50
Isleworth
PEREZ,M.,MD E1
New Orleans,LA
PERLISH,J.S.,PhD 126
New York,NY
PERRUQUET,J.L., ... D54
Danville,PA
PERSICO,F.J.,PhD C28
Spring House,PA
PERSON,D.A.,MD 63,C38
Houston,TX
PERSSELIN,J.,MD D43
Los Angeles,CA
PETERS,S.P.,MD, PhD B30
Baltimore,MD
PETERSEN,R.,MD 128
Boston,MD
PETERSON,J.M., ... 118
Rochester,MN
PETERSON,M., ... A47
New York,NY
PETRELLI,M.,MD 141
Cleveland,OH
PETRI,M.A.,MD B48
San Francisco,CA
PETRIC,M.,PhD D63
Toronto,ON
PETTERSSON,H.,MD D59
Gainesville,FL
PETTY,R.E.,MD 66
Vancouver,BC
PHILLIPS,P.E.,MD C48
Syracuse,NY
PIETTE,J.,MD E63,A50,A51
Paris
PINCUS,S.H.,MD 129,43
Salt Lake City,UT
PINCUS,T.,MD D36
Nashville,TN

PISCHEL,K.D.,MD, PhD E27
San Diego,CA
PISETSKY,D.S.,MD, PhD 39,E48,129
Durham,NC
PISKO,E.J.,MD D64,E13
Winston-Salem,NC
PITCHFORD,W., ... D72
Detroit,MI
PITCOCK,J.A.,MD E46
Memphis,TN
PITTERLE,M.,MS, RPh A18
Madison,WI
PLOTZ,P.H.,MD E54
Bethesda,MD
POLLARD,K.M.,PhD E53
La Jolla,CA
POLLOCK,B.H.,MD E40
Pittsburgh,PA
POLVERINI,P.J.,DDS,DMSc 82
Chicago,IL
POOPRASERT,S., ... C15
Loma Linda,CA
POPE,R.,MD C33
San Antonio,TX
PORTANOVA,J.P.,PhD D45
Denver,CO
PORTER,J., ... E23
Portland,OR
POSTLETHWAITE,A.E.,MD 109,D21
Memphis,TN
POULTER,L., ... E38
London
PRENDERGAST,T., ... C31
New York,NY
PRESSLEY,T.A.,MD E36
Columbia,MO
PRICE,W.A.,BS C40
Charleston,SC
PRINCE,H.,PhD 51
Los Angeles,CA
PRINCE-ZUCCHELLI,M., ... A50
Paris
PROKOPCHUK,P.A.,BSc D65
Saskatoon,SA
PROSTIC,E.,MD C2
Kansas City,KS
PROTAS,E.J.,LPT, PhD B3
Houston,TX
PROVOST,T.T., ... 134,152,B41
Baltimore,MD
PRUZANSKI,W., ... E15
Toronto,ON
PULLAR,T.,MBChB,MRCP E8,D9
Glasgow
PURCELL,S.M.,DO D4
Lackland AFB,TX
QAMAR,T.,BS C11,151
New York,NY
QUISMORIO, JR,F.P.,MD E61,A33,B47,D13,A45
Los Angeles,CA
RACHOW,J.,MD, PhD B32
Milwaukee,WI
RADOSEVICH,J., ... A67
Torrance,CA
RAGSDALE,C.G.,MD 66
Ann Arbor,MI
RAMIREZ,F.,MD B21
Albuquerque,NM
RAMSDEN,P.,MD,FRCP(C) D34
Toronto,ON
RAMSEY-GOLDMAN,R.,MD D6
Pittsburgh,PA
RANAWAT,C.S.,MD C7,64
New York,NY
RANGES,G.E.,PhD 166
Burlington,VT
RAPOPORT,R., ... 71
Chapel Hill,NC
RATNOFF,W.D.,MD C36
Boston,MA
RAVICH,W.,MD E21
Baltimore,MD
RAZGAITIS,K., ... C23
Philadelphia,PA
REDECHA,P.B.,BS 163,C31
New York,NY
REEKERS,P.,PhD 96
Nijmegen,The Netherlands
REEVES,W.H., ... A42,C14
New York,NY
REGAN-SMITH,M.G.,MD D23,D24
Hanover,NH
REGINATO,A.J.,MD E42
Camden,NJ
REICHARD-BROWN,J., ... E29
Iowa City,IA
REICHLIN,M.,MD E47,28,C10,C50,A14,C13,E6,B56,E54
Oklahoma City,OK
REIDBORD,H.E.,MD E40
Pittsburgh,PA
REIDENBERG,M., ... A47
New York,NY
REIMER,G.,MD 115
La Jolla,CA
REINHERZ,E.L.,MD 4
Boston,MD
REISS,J.,MD C2
Kansas City,KS
RESNICK,D.,MD E72,C3
San Diego,CA
RHODES,G.,PhD 165
La Jolla,CA
RICH,K.C., ... 67,B4
Chicago,IL
RICHARDSON,B.C.,MD, PhD 31
Ann Arbor,MI
RICHARDSON,J.E.,MD E56,15
Toronto,ON
RICHMAN,S., ... C22
Stanford,CA
RIDDLE,J.,PhD D72
Detroit,MI
RIDDLE,J.M.,PhD B28
Ann Arbor,MI
RIEBER,M., ... A17
Caracas
RIJKE,T.M., ... 146
Nijmegen,The Netherlands

ROBB,J., ... B7
Seattle,WA
ROBB-NICHOLSON,C.,MD 90
Boston,MD
ROBBINS,D.,MD E74,D10
Davis,CA
ROBERTS,W.,MD A65
Boston,MA
ROBINSON,D.R.,MD D18
Boston,MA
RODRIGUEZ,M.A.,MD E34,E33
Caracas
ROEKLE,M., ... 135
Boston,MA
ROIFMAN,C.,MD B8
Toronto,ON
ROITT,I.,FRS A9
London
ROLANDO,I., ... E57
Lima,Peru
ROONEY,P.J.,MD,FRCP 12
Hamilton,ON
ROSANO,C.L.,MS A10
Albany,NY
ROSARIO,M.O.,PhD E5
Oklahoma City,OK
ROSE,K.M.,PhD 115
Houston,TX
ROSENBERG,A.M.,MD C44,C43,D65
Saskatoon,SA
ROSENBLOOM,J.,MD, PhD 130
Philadelphia,PA
ROSENSTEIN,B.D.,MD 64
Chapel Hill,NC
ROSS,A.H.,MD 131
Stony Brook,NY
ROSS,G.D.,PhD 162
Chapel Hill,NC
ROSSEN,R.D.,MD B10
Houston,TX
ROSTAND,K.S.,PhD 175
Birmingham,AL
ROTH,G.J.,MD D12
Seattle,WA
ROTH,S., ... A53
Phoenix,AZ
ROTHFIELD,N.F.,MD 112
Farmington,CT
ROTHFUSS,M.S., ... A59,D20
Philadelphia,PA
ROTHS,J.B., ... E48
Bar Harbor,ME
ROTHSCHILD,B.M.,MD E43,C2
Kansas City,KS
ROUCAYROL,J.C., ... 24
Paris
ROURKE,C.M., ... 135
Boston,MA
ROUSSIN,A.,MD,FRCP(C) E51
Montreal,PQ
ROWELL,N.,MD, FRCP D50
Leeds
RUBIN,R.L.,PhD E53
La Jolla,CA
RUNGE,L.,MD C48
Syracuse,NY
RUNQUIST,O.A., ... 59
Minneapolis,MN
RUSH,P.J.,MD 100
Toronto,ON
RUSSELL,I.,MD, PhD 9
San Antonio,TX
RUSSELL,M.,MD,CM,FRCP D11
Toronto,ON
RUSSELL,W.,MD B51
Chapel Hill,NC
RYAN,L.M.,MD B32,172
Milwaukee,WI
RYCKEWAERT,A.,MD A57
Paris
RYNES,R.I.,MD E65
Albany,NY
SAILSTAD,D.M.,MSPH E50
Chapel Hill,NC
SALEM,S.,PhD 11
New York,NY
SALMON,J.,MD B25
New York,NY
SALVATI,E.A.,MD C7
New York,NY
SANDA,M.,MD 11
New York,NY
SANDBORG,C.I.,MD D38
Irvine,CA
SANDELL,L.J.,PhD 173
Chicago,IL
SANFORD,R.G.,MD C37
Harrisburg,PA
SARKOZI,J.,MD,FRCP(C) D32,E24
Mississauga,ON
SARRABAY,M.,MD E68
Paris
SARTORIS,D.J.,MD C3
San Diego,CA
SAUNDERS,W.,MS 112
Baltimore,MD
SAVAGE,S.M.,BS D48
Albuquerque,NM
SCALAPINO,J.C.,MD B24
Rochester,MN
SCHALKWIJK,J.,MSc E18
Nijmegen,The Netherlands
SCHALLER,J., ... B7
Seattle,WA
SCHER,R.K.,MD D29
Providence,RI
SCHIFFENBAUER,J.,MD A3
St. Louis,MO
SCHLOSSMAN,S.F.,MD 32,4
Boston,MA
SCHMID,F.R.,MD B16
Chicago,IL
SCHMIDT,C.,OTR D59
Gainesville,FL
SCHNITZER,T.,MD, PhD D60
Ann Arbor,MI
SCHOENFELDT,R.,MD C1
New York,NY

SCHROHENLOHER,R.E.,PhD C51
Birmingham,AL
SCHULTE,T., ... D51
Torrance,CA
SCHUMACHER,H.,MD A59,102,E41,D19,D20
Philadelphia,PA
SCHUNA,A.,MS, RPh A18
Madison,WI
SCHUR,P.H.,MD C36
Boston,MA
SCHURMAN,D.,MD B37
Stanford,CA
SCHWARTZ,B., ... A3
St. Louis,MO
SCHWARTZ,J.A.,OTR 90,A65
Boston,MA
SCOTT,A., ... 164
Baltimore,MD
SCOTT,J., ... 60
Baltimore,MD
SEAMAN,J.,MD 27
Denver,CO
SEARLES,R.P.,MD D48
Albuquerque,NM
SEBASTIAN,A.,MD B48
San Francisco,CA
SEIBOLD,J.R.,MD 26,D27
New Brunswick,NJ
SEMBLE,E., ... A53
Winston-Salem,NC
SEMIONOW,R.,BS A66
Nutley,NJ
SENECAL,J.,MD,FRCP(S) E51
Montreal,PQ
SERCARZ,E.E., ... 73
Los Angeles,CA
SEREMETIS,S.,MD 80
New York,NY
SEYER,J.M., ... A6
Memphis,TN
SHAMAZEDEH,M.,MD C37
Philadelphia,PA
SHAMESS,C.J.,MD D25
Hamilton,ON
SHAPIRO,L.,MD, MRCP A36
London
SHARMA,O.P.,MD 23
Los Angeles,CA
SHARP,J., ... C22
Stanford,CA
SHAW,S.,MD 128
Boston,MD
SHEARER,W.T.,MD 62
Houston,TX
SHEARN,M.,MD 89
Oakland,CA
SHERRER,Y.,MD 136
Stanford,CA
SHIOKAWA,Y., ... 153
Tokyo
SHIOZAWA,S.,MD, PhD D66
Kobe
SHOBACK,B.R., ... A26
Philadelphia,PA
SHOOR,S., ... 93
Stanford,CA
SHORE,A.,MD,FRCP(C) 100,D34,C42
Toronto,ON
SHULMAN,S., ... B7
Chicago,IL
SIECK,M., ... E42
Philadelphia,PA
SIECK,M.S., ... A59
Philadelphia,PA
SILVER,R.M.,MD E31,C40,22
Charleston,SC
SILVERFIELD,J.C.,MD E11
Tampa,FL
SILVERMAN,E.D.,MD B6
Toronto,ON
SILVERSTEIN,M.D., ... 16
Chicago,IL
SILVERSTEIN,S.C.,MD B53
New York,NY
SIMKIN,P.A.,MD 103,E14,D67
Seattle,WA
SINGAL,D., ... A12
Hamilton,ON
SINGER,J.Z., ... D3
New York,NY
SINGHAL,S.K., ... D41
London,ON
SKANES,V.,PhD E6
St. John's,NF
SKILLING,J.,BS D10
Davis,CA
SKOSEY,J.L.,MD, PhD 106,B54,D17
Chicago,IL
SKOSKIEWICZ,M., ... D18
Boston,MA
SLEDGE,C.B.,MD A65
Boston,MA
SLOAN,V., ... 80
New York,NY
SMITH,K.,MD 12
Hamilton,ON
SOKOLOFF,L.,MD A49
Stony Brook,NY
SOLINGER,A.M.,MD A32
Cincinnati,OH
SOLOMON,G.,MD 49,A63
New York,NY
SOLOMON,J., ... A58
Boston,MA
SOMMA,C.,MD B6
Paris
SONTHEIMER,R.D.,MD D4,125
Dallas,TX
SORGE,J.,MD 2
La Jolla,CA
SPALDING,D.M.,MD D37
Birmingham,AL
SPEISER,J.,MD C39
St. Louis,MO
SPENCER,C.H., ... 67
Chicago,IL
SPENCER-GREEN,G.,MD D33,D57
Hanover,NH

SPIERA,H.,MD ... E55
New York,NY
SPILBERG,I., ... A27
St. Louis,MO
SPITZ,P.W.,RN, MS ... E10,C21,C22
Stanford,CA
SRIRAM,S., ... 166
Burlington,VT
STAITE,N.D.,PhD ... C25,B52
Minneapolis,MN
STARKEBAUM,G.A., ... 87
Seattle,WA
STASTNY,P.,MD ... B27,D39
Dallas,TX
STEEN,V.D.,MD ... E22,D6,D30
Pittsburgh,PA
STEERE,A.C.,MD ... 99
New Haven,CT
STEFANSKI,E., ... E15
Toronto,ON
STEIGERWALD,J.C.,MD ... 27,27
Denver,CO
STEIN,L.D.,MD ... B8
Toronto,ON
STEINBERG,A.D., ... E3
Bethesda,MD
STEINMAN,R.M.,MD ... 36
New York,NY
STEITZ,J.A.,PhD ... C53
New Haven,CT
STEMMLER,M.M., ... 95
Philadelphia,PA
STEPHENSON,M.L.,PhD ... 173
Boston,MA
STERN,A.S.,PhD ... A66
Nutley,NJ
STERNBERG,E.,MD ... 169
St. Louis,MO
STEVENS,J.O.,DVM, PhD ... 132
Denver,CO
STEVENS,M.,MD ... D61,53,54,B41
Baltimore,MD
STEVENS,R.H.,MD ... D43
Los Angeles,CA
STOBO,J.D.,MD ... 29
San Francisco,CA
STOHL,W.,MD, PhD ... D3
New York,NY
STOLZER,B.L.,MD ... 142
Pittsburgh,PA
STORK,J.,MD ... D59
Gainesville,FL
STRICKLAND,R.W.,MD ... E30,161,A54
Washington,DC
STRICKLIN,G.P., ... A6
Memphis,TN
STROBER,S.,MD ... B37
Stanford,CA
STROUD,R.M.,MD ... 6
Gainesville,FL
STUART,J.M., ... 168
Memphis,TN
STULBERG,B.N.,MD ... E60
Cleveland,OH
STURROCK,R.D.,MD ... E9
Glasgow
SU,C.,PhD ... D56
Springfield,IL
SUAREZ,D.R.,MD ... 23
Los Angeles,CA
SUENAGA,R.,MD ... 41
Kansas City,KS
SUGIYAMA,H.,MD ... D1
Tokyo
SUKENIK,S., ... 17
Birmingham,AL
SULLIVAN,D.B.,MD ... 66
Ann Arbor,MI
SULLIVAN,K.F.,PhD ... 112
Baltimore,MD
SUNDSTROM,W.,MD ... A18
Madison,WI
SUTHERLAND, JR.,D.,MD ... C3
San Diego,CA
SWANSTON,W., ... D5
Hamilton,ON
SWERDLOW,F.,MD ... E55
New York,NY
SY,M.,PhD ... D35
Boston,MA
TAKAFUJI,S.,MD ... D1
Tokyo
TAKAGAKI,Y., ... E54
Bethesda,MD
TAKASAKI,Y.,MD, PhD ... 153,E2,C9
Tokyo
TALAL,N.,MD ... C33,70,A35,72
San Antonio,TX
TAN,E.M.,MD ... 125,115,B15,E53,A43,C52,D49
La Jolla,CA
TANAKA,M., ... 153
Tokyo
TANI,K., ... 118
Rochester,MN
TAPPE,N., ... B25
New York,NY
TAR,L.,MD ... D42
Philadelphia,PA
TARGOFF,I.N.,MD ... E47,C50
Oklahoma City,OK
TAUROG,J., ... A25
Minneapolis,MN
TAYLOR,P.,BA ... E71
Ann Arbor,MI
TAYLOR,R.P.,PhD ... C54,D47
Charlottesville,VA
TEHAN,N.A.,RN ... 91
Hanover,NH
TEMESVARI,P., ... A12
Budapest
TEODORESCU,M.,MD, PhD ... 106
Chicago,IL
TERATO,K., ... B11
Memphis,TN
TERKELTAUB,R.,MD ... 79
La Jolla,CA
TERREGINO,C.A.,BA ... 26
New Brunswick,NJ

TESAR,J.T.,MD D2
Washington,DC
THEOFILOPOULOS,A.,MD C30
La Jolla,CA
THOMAS,T.,PhD 147
Minneapolis,MN
THOMPSON,M.S.,PhD A65
Boston,MA
THONAR,E., ... E70
Chicago,IL
TIKU,K.,MS D17
Chicago,IL
TIKU,M.L.,MD 106,D17
Chicago,IL
TILIAKOS,N.A.,MD 8,140
Decatur,GA
TILLEY,D.,BSc A64
Halifax,NS
TIMPL,R.,PhD 126
Munich
TINCANI,A., ... 149
Brescia.Italy
TOIVANEN,A.,MD 51
Turku,Finland
TOJO,T., ... 153
Tokyo
TOLMAN,K.G.,MD D12
Salt Lake City,UT
TOM,D.K.,MD D29
Providence,RI
TONGUE,J.,MD C5
Portland,OR
TOOLE,B.P.,PhD A7
Boston,MA
TORRETTI,D., ... D54
Danville,PA
TOURTELLOTTE,C.D.,MD B45,C37
Philadelphia,PA
TOVAR,Z.,MD C33
San Antonio,TX
TOWNES,A.S.,MD E46,B11
Memphis,TN
TRAPP,R.G.,MD D56
Springfield,IL
TRENTHAM,D.E.,MD 76,C19
Boston,MA
TRIAL,J.,RESCH ASST 169
St. Louis,MO
TRIMBLE,R.B.,MD C18
Mason City,IA
TROSTLE,D.C.,MD D30
Pittsburgh,PA
TROUM,O.M.,MD D13
Los Angeles,CA
TROUP,G.M.,MD D48
Albuquerque,NM
TSAO,M.,MD E28
Pittsburgh,PA
TSOUKAS,C.,PhD C32
La Jolla,CA
TUGWELL,P.,MD,FRCP(C) 18
Hamilton,ON
TURMAN,M.A.,BA B13
Denver,CO
TURNER,R.A.,MD D64,E13
Winston-Salem,NC
TUTHILL,R.J.,MD 5
Cleveland,OH
UDIS,B., ... A33
Los Angeles,CA
UEDA,T., ... 153
Tokyo
UHL,J.,MS A4,A8
Camden,NJ
UHL, JR,J.,MD 101
Indianapolis,IN
UITTO,J.,MD, PhD A1
Torrance,CA
ULLOA-FERNANDEZ,M.,MD D57
Cincinnati,OH
UROWITZ,M.B.,MD A38
Toronto,ON
UTELL,M.J.,MD D55
Rochester,MN
VADAS,P.,MD, PhD E15
Toronto,ON
VALKENBURG,H.A.,MD E37
Rotterdam
VAN DE PUTTE,L.,MD E18,146,96,83,84
Nijmegen,The Netherlands
VAN DEN BERG,W.B.,PhD 84,83,E18
Nijmegen,The Netherlands
VAN DER LINDEN,S.,MD E37
Berne,Switzerland
VAN WYK,J.J.,MD B51
Chapel Hill,NC
VANDENBERSSELAAR,L., ... E18
Nijmegen,The Netherlands
VAUGHAN,J.H.,MD C32,37,38,165
La Jolla,CA
VILLANUEVA,T.G.,MD D19
Philadelphia,PA
VITEK,J.J., ... 52
Birmingham,AL
VOISIN,M.C.,MD A55
Creteil,France
VOLLERTSEN,R.S.,MD E59,E11
Rochester,MN
WAHL,L.M.,PhD E30,161,35
Bethesda,MD
WAHL,S.M.,PhD B55,D40
Bethesda,MD
WALDMANN,T.A., ... 30
Bethesda,MD
WALKER,S.E.,MD E36
Columbia,MO
WALLACE,D.J.,MD A16
Los Angeles,CA
WALLIS,W.,MD 87
Seattle,WA
WALZ,D.A.,PhD B50
Detroit,MI
WARD,J.R.,MD D12,A21,7,129,B34,43
Salt Lake City,UT
WARNKE,R.,MD B37
Stanford,CA
WARREN,R.W.,MD, PhD E50
Chapel Hill,NC

WATSON,W.C.,PhD ... E46
Memphis,TN
WEAVER,D.J.,MD ... E20
Columbia,MO
WEBSTER,E.,MD ... D59,E62
Gainesville,FL
WEBSTER,E.M.,MD ... 6
Gainesville,FL
WECHSLER,B.,MD ... E63
Paris
WEIL,J.,MD ... 27
Denver,CO
WEILLER,P., ... A50
Paris
WEINBLATT,M.E.,MD ... C19
Boston,MA
WEINSTEIN,A.,MD ... C55
Farmington,CT
WEISBART,R.H.,MD ... 148,C15,77
Sepulveda,CA
WEISS,J.J.,MS ... B16
Chicago,IL
WEISSMANN,G., ... 58,78,D16,D70
New York,NY
WELLS,R., ... B19
Birmingham,AL
WELSH,K.,PhD ... A46
London
WEN,E., ... D26
Evanston,IL
WEST,S.G.,MD ... A11
Aurora,CO
WESTON,W.L.,MD ... 132
Denver,CO
WEYAND,C.M.,MD ... 111
Stanford,CA
WEYAND,K., ... 68
Stanford,CA
WHALEY,K.,MD, PhD ... D46
Glasgow
WHEELER,P., ... D2
Washington,DC
WHELAN,A., ... 139
Dublin
WHITE,D.G.,MRCPath ... 3
Bath
WHITE,R.E.,MD ... D64
Winston-Salem,NC
WHITE,R.H.,MD ... D69,D68
Sacramento,CA
WHITESIDE,T.,PhD ... B20,E28
Pittsburgh,PA
WHITING-O'KEEFE,Q.,MD ... B48
San Francisco,CA
WIGLEY,F.M.,MD ... B30,A15,E21
Baltimore,MD
WILDER,R.L.,MD, PhD ... B55,D40
Bethesda,MD
WILLIAMS,C.,PhD ... A2
Philadelphia,PA
WILLIAMS,H.,MD ... D71,B36
Salt Lake City,UT
WILLIAMS,J.M.,MD ... A40
Indianapolis,IN
WILLIAMS,W.V.,MD ... E36
Columbia,MO
WILLIAMS, JR,R.C., ... B21
Albuquerque,NM
WILLKENS,R.F.,MD ... D12
Seattle,WA
WILMOT,D.,MD,FRCP(C) ... 100
Toronto,ON
WILSON,A.J.,MD ... 98
San Francisco,CA
WILSON,D.A.,MD ... E20
Columbia,MO
WILSON,J.G.,MD ... C36
Boston,MA
WILSON,J.M.,MD ... 122
Boston,MA
WILSON,R.,MD ... E21
Baltimore,MD
WILSON,W.A.,MD ... E1
New Orleans,LA
WILSON, JR.,P.D.,MD ... C7
New York,NY
WINCHESTER,R.J.,MD ... 49,80
New York,NY
WINFIELD,J.B.,MD ... 162,44
Chapel Hill,NC
WISE,C.,MD ... E13
Winston-Salem,NC
WISNIESKI,J.J.,MD ... A61,19
Cleveland,OH
WISNIEWOLSKI,R., ... C14
New York,NY
WISTAR, JR,R.,MD, PhD ... E74,D10
Bethesda,MD
WOFSY,D.,MD ... 86
San Francisco,CA
WOLFE,F., ... C22
Stanford,CA
WOLFE,F.,MD ... E10
Wichita,KS
WONG,C., ... A67
Torrance,CA
WONG,S., ... 148
Loma Linda,CA
WOOD,P., ... 46
Stanford,CA
WOOD,P.L.,FRCS ... E72
Wrightington, UK
WOODS, JR,V.L.,MD ... E27
San Diego,CA
WOOLEY,P.H.,PhD ... E46,168,170,C49
Rochester,MN
WOOLF,A.D.,MRCP ... 3,21
Bath,UK
WORTMANN,R., ... 172
Milwaukee,WI
WOUTERS,J.W.,MD ... 96
Nijmegen,The Netherlands
WRIGHT,T.M.,MD ... 164
Baltimore,MD
WU,W., ... A53
Winston-Salem,NC
YAMAGATA,H.,MD ... E5
Oklahoma City,OK

YANNAKAKIS,G.D.,MD 54
Towson,MD
YASUMA,M.,MD E2
Tokyo
YEE,W.,MD 148
Sepulveda,CA
YELIN,E.H.,PhD D22,92,89
San Francisco,CA
YOCUM,D.E.,MD D40
Bethesda,MD
YONEDA,M.,MD D14
Osaka
YONEMASU,K.,MD D14
Osaka
YONKER,R.,DO D59
Gainesville,FL
YONKER,R.A.,DO E62
Gainesville,FL
YOSHINO,S., ... 153
Tokyo
YOUNGE,B.R.,MD E59
Rochester,MN
YOUNT,W.J.,MD 162
Chapel Hill,NC
YTTERBERG,S.R.,MD C24
Minneapolis,MN
YUAN,D.,PhD E32
Dallas,TX
ZAPOL,W.M., ... D18
Boston,MA
ZEEVI,A., ... E28
Pittsburgh,PA
ZIEGLER,G.C.,RN, BSN D6
Pittsburgh,PA
ZIFF,M.,MD, PhD A44,E25
Dallas,TX
ZIMINSKI,C.M.,MD D61
Baltimore,MD
ZIMMERMAN,T.,MD E58
La Jolla,CA
ZIMMERMANN, III,B.,MD B39
Providence,RI
ZINGRAFF,J.,MD A55
Paris
ZIZIC,T.M.,MD D61
Baltimore,MD
ZOMA,A.,MB, MRCP D46
Glasgow
ZOSCHKE,D.C., ... B52,C25
Minneapolis,MN
ZUCKNER,J.,MD C39
St. Louis,MO
ZURIER,R.B., ... 171,A26
Philadelphia,PA
ZVAIFLER,N.J.,MD 36
San Diego,CA

ARA KEY PHRASE INDEX

μ/α ratio in NZB mice E32
19S IgM and 7S IgG rheumatoid factors C41
1pr gene 72,E50
ANA in children B4
Ab/dsDNA immune complexes C54,D47
Abnormal B cell activation E34
Abnormal immunoglobulin IgG A61
Accessory cells in synovial tissue D37
Acebutolol induced lupus A51
Acne congoblata and arthritis E42
Acne fulminans and arthritis E42
Acoustic arthrography 9
Acoustic tendonography 9
Acquired immune deficiency syndrome 49
Activation antigens E27
Acute rheumatic fever 63
Adenosine D16,78
Adenosine deaminase 120,B31
Adenylate cyclase D70
Adjuvant arthritis C28
Adult rheumatoid arthritis 111
Adult-onset Still's disease 96,97
Alizarin red A57
Allergic arthritis 6
Alloreactive T cell clones E28
Alpha-2 receptors E23
Alternative pathway of T cell Activation 4
Alveolar eosinophilia 23
Amino and carboxy propeptide 126
Aminoacyl-tRNA synthetase 114
Amitriptyline 158
Amsler field testing B35
Amyloidosis 157,123
Amyloidosis associated with dialysis A55
Anaphylaxis D18
Androgens and SLE 150
Anemia, refractory A50
Angiogenesis 82
Angiography A62
Animal model of PSS A2
Animal model of ankylosing spondylitis A25
Animal models of coronoary arteritis 61
Ankle orthosis A22
Ankylosing spondylitis 50,A38,A39,E40,A36,E38,E43
Ankylosing spondylitis in Mexicans A37
Ankylosing spondylitis in females E37
Anti-DNA E48,149,E35,39
Anti-DNA antibodies A63,73,57,D41
Anti-DNA antigen specificity B18
Anti-DNA cell surface reactivity B18
Anti-DNA idiotypes 41,40
Anti-DNA production in vitro D51,A67
Anti-DR D48
Anti-Fab antibodies D43
Anti-Ig antibodies B13
Anti-Jo-1 antibodies C50,E47
Anti-Ki autoantigens B15
Anti-La/SSB E5
Anti-Ro/SSA A14,144,D4
Anti-SS-A antibodies A11,D6
Anti-SSA/Ro antibodies 132
Anti-Sm antibodies D2,C9,39
Anti-collagen antibodies 168
Anti-erythrocyte antibodies 118
Anti-galactosyl AB B40
Anti-histone antibodies D7,67,A47
Anti-idiotypic antibodies D48,C47,38
Anti-inflammatory drugs D18,D24
Anti-lymphocyte autoantibodies 44
Anti-rRNP C52
Anti-rheumatic agents A1
Anti-ribosomal autoantigens C52
Anti-ssDNA 28
Anti-type II collagen antibodies C49
Antiallogeneic CTL frequency analysis 75
Antibodies C10
Antibody affinities C47
Antibody binding in cutaneous lupus 132
Antibody genes 43,129
Antibody isotype and specificity C49
Antibody specificity E50
Antibody to SSA (Ro) A24
Antibody to proliferating cell nuclear E2
Anticardiolipin antibodies E7,64,99,D8,E4,151
Anticentromere antibodies (ACA) 112,D32
Antigen presentation 34
Antigen presenting cells 105
Antigen receptor 72
Antigen retention 84
Antigen specific suppressor cell A67,D51
Antigen-binding cells A31
Antigens recognized by ACA 112
Antiguanosine antibodies 148
Antilymphocyte antibodies E27,B21
Antinuclear antibodies B1,2,C15,42,A43,A47,D50,C43,B5 129,E19
Antiphospholipid antibody specificity 149
Antiproteinases B54
Antisperm C10
Apatite crystals A57
Apatite deposition disease A55
Arachidonic acid metabolism A8
Arteparon B33
Arterial occlusions E7
Arthritis impact measurement scales 94
Arthritis, juvenile rheumatoid 66
Arthritis/polyarteritis D61
Aseptic loosening of cemented prosthesis C7
Asymptomatic hyperuricemia D25
Atherogenesis B43
Atherosclerosis in SLE A15
Atlanto-axial joints 47
Auranofin B24,B36
Aranofin, clinical trials 88,A23
Aranofin, efficacy of A23
Autoantibodies B12,B19,B41,C12,C14,D45,117,C53,116, E51,A43
Autoantibodies to collagen E49
Autoantibody to nuclear antigens E53,115
Autoantibody/autoantigen A42

Autoimmune MRL-1pr/1pr mice D35
Autoimmune B cell function 74
Autoimmune antibodies (RNP and Sm) 121
Autoimmunity 86,148,70,66,72,B11,A35
Autologous mixed lymphocyte reaction 105,71
B cell activation 110,E29
B cell activation events A31
B cell differentiation D36
B cell regulation by NK cells E33
B cell tolerance E29
B lymphocytes 167,C36,A5
B to Z transition of DNA 147
B-cell growth factor, in SLE A29
Bacteria in juvenile arthritis B9
Bacterial antigens D63
Bacterial cell wall-induced arthritis 40
Bacterial cell walls in JA B9
Bacterial peptidoglycan 119
BamHI-K restriction fragment 164
Basic calcium phosphate B32
Beta-blocking agent induced disease A51
Beta 2-microglobulin 56
Bilateral hip arthroplasty 48
Bilateral knee arthroplasty 48
Biological marker for RA A10
Biopsies D12
Birefringent lipid spherulites D20
Blind reading 46
Blood eosinophilia 28
Borderline-sacroiliitis E37
Bromhexine 153
Bronchoalveolar lavage B39,23,22
Brucellosis E57
C-reactive protein B34
cDNA expression 120
C1q D65
C1q - fibronectin interactions B16
C1q binding 67,A61
C1q binding assay E16
C1q, unbound A10
C1s-C1 inhibitor complex C11
C3a desarg 58
C4 polymorphism E6
C5a and fMLP receptors B55
CNS disease 152
CNS lupus B46,A12,53,D5,54
CNS vasculitis E62
CSF D5
CSF IgG and lymphoid cells A60
CT scan 52
Calcinosis 154
Calcitonin A48
Calcium and phosphate homeostasis 101
Calcium antagonists E26
Calcium ionophore and phorbol myristate D38
Calcium pryophosphate dihydrate crystals .. A57,B32,172,174
Calcium pyrophosphate deposition disease E41
Capillary microscopy D32,C40
Cardiac abnormalities in RA A45
Cardiac tissue B7
Cardiomyopathy E17
Carpal tunnel syndrome C2
Cartilage 45,D15
Cartilage degradation B54,E45
Cartilage destruction A6
Cartilage immunology C46,124
Cartilage matrix proteins C48
Cartilage metabolism B28,E71
Cartilage metaplasia in vitro D62
Cartilage proteoglycans C48
Catabolin 45
Catecholamine 25
Cationic proteins E18
Causes of death in collagen disorders E63
Cell secretions ....]0
Cell surface nuclear antigens 42
Cellular immunology C35,C34
Cellular interactions D62
Cental nervous system E62
Central nervous system disease 134,A60,152
Central nervous system lupus C12,56,B46,A12,53,54,D5
Cerebrospinal fluid 56
Cerebrospinal fluid immunoglobulin C12
Cervical spine 47
Cervical spine instability C1
Chemotaxis 81,C23,B55
Childhood dermatomyositis C40
Childhood rheumatological disease 95
Children E70
Chloroquine retinopathy B35
Chondrocytes 173
Chondrocytes, allogenic reaction 106
Chondrocytes, antigen presentation 106
Chondrocytes, autologous mixed reaction 106
Chondroitin sulfate 175
Chrysiasis 7
Classification A49
Claudication 157
Clinical and x-ray evaluation A18
Clinical angiographic correlation E56
Clinical heterogeneity 111
Clinical sub-group of RA A24
Clinical trial 159
Clinical trial of Auranofin 88,A23
Cloned Th cells 110
Coagulation D28
Coagulation abnormalities 15
Coexistent gout and rheumatoid arthritis E13
Cogan's syndrome E59
Cold air inhalation D55
Cold stimulation D28
Collagen 126,A32,145
Collagen arthritis 76
Collagen degradation A6
Collagen gene expression in TSK A2
Collagen synthesis in TSK fibroblasts A2
Collagen synthesis in dermal fibroblasts B20
Collagen-induced arthritis B11,168,166
Collagenase B33,A1
Combination cytotoxic therapy 8
Commitment to work D22
Complement C54,77
Complement (C4) 19
Complement C5 .... E46
Complement allotypes A46
Complement assay E12
Complement fixation C45
Complement receptors C36,162
Complementarity-determining regions 37
Complete congenital heart block A14

Complications of immunosuppressive therapy 49
Computer tomography, brain B45
Computerized tomography - lupus 55
Concanavalin A C31,B25
Conduction defects in RA A45
Congenital heart block A14
Connective tissue disease E51,D29
Corticosteroid injections D56
Corticosteroids 108,167,A40
Cost-effectiveness A65
Cost-utility analysis D25
Coxsackievirus B C24
Creatinine clearance B48
Crest D29
Cross-reactivity HLA-B27 and bacteria 51
Crossreacting anti-B27 antibodies A44
Crossreactive idiotype A63
Crossreactivity 118,B13
Crossreactivity of anti-DNA antibodies 146
Cryoglobulins 17
Crystal endocytosis B49
Crystal-induced arthritis 91
Crystals A59,174
Cutaneous lupus erythematosus 132
Cutaneous ulcers 140
Cyclic AMP response B6
Cyclophosphamide 142
Cyclosporine 137
Cyclosporin A C16,D40
Cystic fibrosis arthritis 100
Cytoprotection A53
Cytoskeletal A5,113
Cytotoxic agents E45
Cytotoxicity 104
D-pencillamine nephrotoxicity A21
D-penicillamine B52
D-penicillamine, hydroxychloroquine B2,1
DANA shoulder replacement results 10
DISH E68
DNA 145,B22,D65
DNA ELISPOT C29
DNA T helper cells 73
DNA antibodies C29
DNA fragments in cryoprecipitates A17
DNA fragments in patients with SLE A17
DNA-C1q interactions D65
DNA-anti DNA 160
DNA-binding protein C53
DNA/anti-DNA complexes C45
DPA toxicity E22
Danazol A13
Decision analysis D26,16
Deconditioning E64
Decreasing exponential function model D25
Defective DNA repair A9
Defects in autoimmune B cells 74
Degenerative joint disease A49,D59
Dendritic cells 36
Dermal fibroblasts E28
Dermal vasculitis E58
Dermatologic toxicity E65
Dermatomyositis A52,155
Dexamethasone influence on monocytes E30
Diagnosis 16
Diagnosis-related groups 85
Differentiation 80
Diffuse idiopathic skeletal hperostosis E43
Digital vascular flow studies E24
Dipyridamole 24
Disability indices during gold therapy E10
Disease course 96
Disease subsets of RA D14
Doctor-patient agreement D24
Double-blind controlled trial 1
Double-blind study 154
Drug impact C21
Drug therapy B36
Drug-induced SLE 148
Drug-induced gastritis A53
Drug-induced immune mediated disease A47
Drug-induced lupus A51,D7,148
Dw 14 specificities 68
ELISA B14,E54,E52
ESR in late temporal arteritis 13
Early diagnosis 52
Early onset pauciarticular JRA 128
Early rheumatoid erosions D72
Early synovitis 3
Ecto-nucleoside pyrophosphohydrolase 172
Efficacy of Auranofin A23
Elbow synovectomy 143
Electrical charge 84
Electrophysiology C2
Endocytosis B22
Endothelial cells B53,78,E25
Endothelial cells, fibroblasts 34
Endothelial injury C40
Endothelium D27
Enzyme-linked immunosorbent assay C9,E73,D7
Epidemiology B1
Epithelial cells B4
Epstein-Barr nuclear antigen (EBNA) 164
Epstein-Barr virus 165,C32,E66,B8
Erosions C22
Eskimo A56
Esophageal motility D57
Etodolac 11
Euthyroid sick syndrome E3
Evoked potentials 54
Exacerbation of arthritis 83
Experimental CPPD crystal arthritis D19
Experimental arthritis E18,E46
Experimental model of arthritis 170
Experimental myocarditis E17
Experimental osteoarthritis E71,124
Extra-articular soft tissue injections D56
Extraglandular disease A54
FC-GAMMA receptor C31
Factor B polymorphism A37
Factor VIII 15
Familial SLE A63
Familial aggregation 60
Familial studies A19
Family impact 95
Family study A9,A38
Family study: 60 families D50
Fc receptor expression in PSS 21
Fc receptors B23,33,B25
Fell-Jubb culture sytstem E71
Felty's syndrome 87

Femoral head deformity C3
Fenretinide C28
Fibrillogenesis 126
Fibroblast cloning B20
Fibroblast glycosaminoglycan synthesis B20
Fibroblast growth D31
Fibroblasts B50,109
Fibromyalgia 158,A58
Fibronectin 127
Fibrositis E64
Fibrositis, autoantibodies in E61
Fibrositis-immunological studies of skin E61
Follicular occlusion D53
Food allergy 6
Foot involvement C6
Functional assessment 88
Functional health status D24,D23
Functional status assessment 94
GI tract D60
Gait characteristics A22
Gastroesophageal reflux disease E21
Gelatinase E69
Gene cloning 2
Gene transcription 30
Genetic analysis 170
Genetic predisposition 60
Genetics of autoimmunity E48
Giant cells D54
Glomerular lesions of SLE 145
Glucocorticoid therapy 133,20
Glycosaminoglycan (GAG) synthesis E28
Glycosaminoglycan metabolism B50
Glycosaminoglycans B29
Glycosylation 127
Gold deposition in the skin 7
Gold nephrotoxicity A21
Gold therapy: duration of benefit E10
Gold treatment C21
Gout 103,102,79
Graft versus host disease E53,D45
Gram negative bacteria A44
Granulocyte 80
Granulomatous angiitis of CNS 14
Growth factors B50,B29
Guinea pigs E17
H/2 O/2 - scavenging B52
H/2 O/2 - synthesis B52
HLA A46
HLA B27 .... C43,A38
HLA antigen DRw52.5,6,8 .... B27
HLA antigens C42,E6
HLA association 96,B41
HLA studies E57
HLA-D antigens 111
HLA-DP antigens in JRA w/ iridocyclitis 128
HLA-DR4 .... D39
HMOs versus FFS 89
HPRT deficiency 122
Health care 89
Health care utilization 95
Health status outcome 93
Health status profiles 94
Heat-damaged RBC clearance B40
Helper T lymphcytes 166
Helper/inducer subset 32
Hematuria in rheumatoid arthritis A21
Hemodialysis A55,101
Hemolytic assay C39
Heparan sulphate 146
Hepatitis B 17
Hepatotoxicity 141
Hereditary 123
Hereditary complement deficiency 19
Hidden IgM rheumatoid factor C39
Hidradenitis suppurativa D53,E42
High molecular weight DNA fragments A17
Hip resurfacing - 10 year results C4
Histamine releasing factors C26
Histones B14
Hormones and SLE 150
Hormonomudulation A13
Hospital use for rheumatoid arthritis 92
Human T cell clones 68
Human chondrocytes B29
Human class II molecules A3
Human lymphocytes D42
Human monoclonal antibody A42
Human monocyte-macrophages A1
Human monocytic cell lines 35
Human osteoarthritic cartilage E44
Human parvovirus 3
Human rheumatoid factors (RF) 37
Human synovial cells A8
Humoral antibodies in RA C48
Humoral immunity B5
Hyaluronate, molecular weight A7
Hyaluronic acid A28
Hybridomas 2,E53
Hydrogen peroxide C25
Hydroxyapatite B49,B51
Hydroxychloroquine E65
Hyperlipidemia in SLE A15
Hypermobility E64
Hyperpigmentation secondary to gold 7
Hypocomplementemic urticarial vasculitis A61
Idiotype expression 57
Idiotypic complementarity 119
Idiotypes D44
IgA B17
IgA rheumatoid factor C51
IgG 144
IgG subclasses B23
IgG3 and IgG4 subclasses D43
IgM E1
IgM to IgD ratio in NZB mice E32
Immune complex assays B56
Immune complex clearance D47,B16
Immune complex degradation by moncytes 161
Immune complex disease 59
Immune complex size C45
Immune complex-C1q-fibronectin interact B16
Immune complexes .. 162,160,22,D64,163,C46,E66,E35,B7,C41
Immune defect B8
Immune response antigens 167
Immunization E73
Immunoassay, solid phase fluorescence B34
Immunodeficiency B31
Immunofluorescence C50
Immunogenetic regulation C49
Immunogenetics of ankylosing spondylitis A37

Immunogenic molecules D41
Immunoglobulin 129,43
Immunoglobulin M D36
Immunoglobulin specific anti-histone B14
Immunoglobulin synthesis and NK cells E33
Immunoglobulin synthesis regulation E34
Immunohistologic evaluation of synovium B37
Immunohistology E38,165,C30
Immunoregulation E35
Immunosuppressive treatment 136
Immunotherapy, in collagen arthritis 76
Impotence E20
Incremental exercise test B3
Inflammation D21
Inflammatory arthritis D53,A18
Inflammatory back pain 52
Inflammatory cells 79
Inflammatory joint disease E9
Inflammatory mediators ....]0
Infrared laser E39
Inhibition A27
Inhibition of charging of +RNA E47
Inhibitor IL-1 .... D17
Inorganic pyrophosphate 172
Interferon D66,169,B21
Interferon-gamma binding by monocytes E30
Interferon-y 173,34,35
Interleukin D34
Interleukin 1 and 2 .... D38
Interleukin 2 .... C30
Interleukin 2 (IL-2) 30
Interleukin 2-induced proliferation B26
Interleukin-1 .... A4,D21,D17
Interstitial lung disease B39
Intractable 8
Intraosseous D67
Ion channels A35
Iridocyclitis C44
Ischemic necrosis C3
Ischemic necrosis of bone 20,133
JRA E70,B1
Jamaicans D3
Jo-1 antigen E54
Joint biology E14
Joint contractures C37
Joint destruction E49,C27,C20
Joint fluid A59
Joint motion D19
Joint replacement 135
Juvenile and adult spondylitis 50
Juvenile ankylosing spondylitiss 50
Juvenile arthritis B27,C43,B8,B6
Juvenile dermatomyositis 67
Juvenile psoriatic arthritis C42
Juvenile rheumatoid arthritis (JRA) 1,C44,97,62,C6,64,C39, C41,68,B2,B5,E70,B1,66
Juvenile scleroderma C37
Kawasaki syndrome B7
Keratan sulfate E70
Ketanserin 26
Ki-antigen-characterization B15
Knee A41,C5
Knee joint 102
Ku antigen C53
Ku autoantibodies E52
LPR autoimmune mouse 75
La/SSB E5
Lactobacillus casei induced disease 61
Large bowel function 12
Large granular lymphocytes E33,87
Laser E39
Learning disability B42
Length of stay 90
Lesch-Nyhan syndrome 122
Leukemic polyarthritis 87
Leukocyte extravasation B53
Leukocytes A59,E15
Leukotriene B4 .... C23
Leukotrienes B30,D18,108,A8
Linear scleroderma 28
Lipid metabolism ....]0
Lipoprotein metabolism B43
Lipoproteins and inflammation 79
Liposomes D20
Lipoxygenase products 58
Liver D12
Liver biopsies C17
Liver histopathology 5
Long-term follow-up 64
Lung involvement in SLE D1
Lupus C35,C34
Lupus - neuropsychiatric 55
Lupus anticoagulant 149
Lupus band test A58
Lupus erythematosus, brain B45
Lupus erythematosus, muscle D11
Lupus inducing drugs 147
Lupus nephropathy B48
Lyme disease 99
Lyme disease serology 98
Lyme disease without rash 131
Lymphoblastoid cells C25
Lymphocyte emigration E25
Lymphocyte proliferation E26
Lymphocyte subsets 62
Lymphocytotoxins A12
Lymphoid irradiation 139
Lymphokine production 75
Lymphokines C34,109,77,D34,A32
MCTD E23
MRL mouse strain C20
MRL-mouse C27,E49
MRL/1pr autoimmune mice E67
Macrophage 82,E69
Macrophage accessory cell function B24
Macrophage activation 169
Magnetic resonance imaging 20,133
Magnetic resonance imaging - lupus 55
Magnetic resonance imaging, brain B45
Malignancy 155,142
Management strategies D26
Measurement of gold effectiveness E10
Mechanical failure cemented total hip C7
Mechanism of T cell proliferation D38
Mechanism of action of colchicine 81
Medicare and pre-paid health plans 92
Membrane associated secretory IgM E32
Metabolic turnover studies 19
Metacarpal head D72
Metacarpophalangeal arthropathy E36

Methotrexate 141,D12,C17,C19,140,A18,138
Methotrexate dosage D71
Methotrexate therapy D71,5
Microfilament anchoring sites E51
Microtubules 81
Microvascular physiology E14
Microwave radiometry E9
Migraine headaches in SLE B47
Mitogen response 108
Mitogenesis B49
Mitogenic activity B51
Mitral valve acute myalgic syndrome E55
Model 174
Models of polymyositis C24
Modulating effects of hyperuricemia E13
Modulation of immunoglobulin production C33
Molecular cloning 122
Molecular cloning of centromere antigen 112
Monoclonal anti-DNA antibodies 113,B18
Monoclonal antibodies 40,86,32,124
Monoclonal antibodies-human response to 33
Monoclonal autoantibodies 118,39
Monocyte binding of Interferon-gamma E30
Monocyte catabolism of immune complexes 161
Monocyte degradation of IgG polymers 161
Monocytes 42,33,105,A39,B23,A26
Monocytes/macrophages 35
Mononuclear cells C25,A34
Mononuclear cells in RA B10
Mononuclear phagocyte system 59
Mononuclear phagocytes E67
Mononuclear subsets in muscle biopsies A52
Monosodium urate crystals 102
Morphometry D30
Mouse kidney B4
Multiple sclerosis 152
Murine SLE D41,B43,E48,D45,73,C29,86
Murine ankylosing spondylitis A25
Murine arthritis 83,84
Murine polymyositis C24
Murine recombinant interleukin 1 .... A66
Musically related injuries E60
Myelodysplastic syndromes 156
Myositis autoantibodies 114
N-terminal amino acid sequence D49
NSAIDS D70
NZB/W mice A64
Nailfold capillary microscopy E24
Nailfold capillary pattern D33
Naproxen C18
Naproxen and amitriptyline 159
Natural history D58
Natural killer cells C33,E31
Nephritis, lupus A16
Network regulation in SLE 41
Neurocognitive function B46
Neuronal antibodies D5,B46
Neuropathy 99
Neutrophils 77,D17,A28,175,D70,C23,D16,78
Nifedipine 27
Non-SLE D8
Non-acetylated salicylates C18
Non-erythroid spectrin A5
Non-progressive nature A41
Nonsteroidal anti-inflammatory drugs (NSAID) A53,B28,D70
Nuclear antigens 117,175
Nucleolar patterns of immunofluorescence E19
Nucleoli A42
Nucleotide pyrophosphohydrolase B32
Occupational predisposition E36
Oligoarticular arthritis in children 131
Oligoclonal bands A54
Oligosaccharide C31
Oral antigen challenge 83
Oral tolerance to casein A64
Orthopedic care C6
Osteitis deformans A48
Osteoarthritis B28,46,E41,45,A41,47,A40,A49,E39,A65,C5
Osteoarthritis pathogenesis C46
Osteonecrosis D67
Osteophytes A40
Ototoxicity B38
Outcome assessment C21
Outcome in total joint arthroplasty 90
Outcomes 89,E59
Oxidative metabolism of neutrophils 21
Oxidative mitogenesis D37
Oxygen consumption B3
Oxygen radicals B54
PCNA/cyclin D49
PGE A26
pH monitoring E21
PMN collagenase A6
PSS fibroblast collagen synthesis 130
PSS fibroblast modulation 130
Paget's disease A48
Pain 93
Paleopathology E43
Palindromic rheumatism 100
Pathology of early hip disease E40
Pediatric rheumatology 66
Pemphigus E22
Penicillin prophylaxis 63
Peptidoglycan and juvenile arthritis B9
Perflurocarbons E72
Perforations in the subchondral plate D72
Personality A20
Phagocytosis B25,A39,A27,E67
Phosphatidylinositol turnover 29
Phospholipase 171
Phospholipase A/2 .... E15
Phospholipids 171
Physical therapy 90
Physical work capacity B3
Plasmapheresis A16,C15
Plasminogen activator A4,D27
Platelets C54
Poly A 70
Polyarteritis nodosa A62,D52,16,D61
Polyarthritis D61
Polyarticular arthritis 48
Polychondritis, relapsing A50,E63
Polymorphonuclear leukocytes B53
Polymyalgia rheumatica D26
Polymyositis C50,104,A52,155,E47
Polymyositis - dermatomyositis A34
Post-streptococcal reactive arthritis 63
Pregnancy C11,151,D6
Primary CNS angiitis 14
Primary CNS vasculitis 14

Primary Sjogren's syndrome ... E34
Primary fibromyalgia ... D58,159
Primary fibrositis ... 158
Primary scleroderma myocardial disease ... 24
Production of interleukin 2 ... A33
Prognosis ... B35
Prognostic factors for hip resurfacing ... C4
Prognostic factors in SLE ... 64
Prognostic guide for joint damage in RA ... D14
Progressive ankylosis in the mouse ... A25
Prolactin and SLE ... 150
Proliferating cell ... 125
Proliferation, synovial cell ... A7
Prostaglandin E2 analogue ... 18
Prostaglandins ... 135
Protein structure ... 123
Protein turnover ... 120
Proteoglycans ... E44,175,A3
Proximal nailfold biopsy ... D29
Psoriatic arthritis ... E65
Psychological status ... 93
Psychosomatic aspects of RA ... A20
Pulmonary diffusion capacity ... D55
Purification ... D49
Purine nucleoside phosphorylase ... B31
Purkinje fiber antibody in RA ... A45
RA immunology ... E66
RF, role in deforming arthritis in SLE ... C8
RNA polymerase I ... 115
RNP ... D1
RNP autoantigen characterization ... C52
Radiographic changes ... D23
Radiographic progress ... 11
Radioimmunoassay ... D66
Radiologic progress ... C22
Radiosensitive Leu 2+ suppressor ... A33
Raynaud's ... 18,D57,B47,26,E24,27,D55,E23,D33,17,D32,25
Rc receptors reactive with leu 11 ... 107
Reactive arthritis ... 51
Receptors ... 69,B22
Receptors, IL-2 ... 30
Recombinant Y-interferon ... 130
Reflex neurovascular dystrophy ... C38
Reflex sympathetic dystrophy ... C38
Regulation of T cell ... 31
Regulation of immunoglobulin synthesis ... 107
Regulation of interleukin-2 production ... D35
Reimbursement ... 85
Reiter's syndrome ... A56,D63,B17,49
Relapsing polychondritis ... 156
Renal vessels ... D30
Responders versus non-responders ... B2
Response to treatment ... E56
Resting human T cells ... B26
Restrictive lung disease in Still's disease ... D13
Results of shoulder replacement ... 10
Retinal "vasculitis" ... 53
Retinoid ... C28
Retinol ... E68
Retinol tolerance test ... E68
Retroviruses ... D36
Rheumatoid arthritis ... 164,D48,C51,137,A9,A30,D39,C33,A24, C2,2,D64,163,C32,38,D43,141,D66,D23,D24,143,171,E74,D10, C17,136,C18,D71,C1,6,A7
Rheumatoid arthritis and SLE ... 85
Rheumatoid arthritis protein (RHP) ... A10
Rheumatoid arthritis, muscle ... D11
Rheumatoid cervical spine ... C1
Rheumatoid disease ... A22
Rheumatoid factor ... E50,D47,C51,A30,D39,D42,2,119,B10,B56 E16, E12,E73,139,B34,D44,C47,38
Rheumatoid factor specificity ... E74
Rheumatoid lung disease ... B39
Rheumatoid syndrome ... D37
Rheumatoid synovial cell ... E74
Rheumatoid synovial cell RF ... D10
Rheumatoid synovial cell collagenase ... A66
Rheumatoid synovial fluid ... E31
Rheumatoid synovial pannus ... 82
Rheumatoid synovitis and histamine ... C26
Rheumatoid synovium ... D62
Rheumatoid vasculitis ... E11
Ribonucleoproteins ... B12
Risk adjusted capitation payments ... 92
Ro/SSA ... 144
Ro/SSA nRNP ... C13
Roentgenographic study ... E36
Rotator cuff tendinitis ... D68,D69
Running ... D59,46
SB antigens and JRA ... 128
SLE ... D46,113,40,B21,B19,D6,58,E1,C11,151,A64,146
SLE disease activity ... E4
SLE disease subsets ... E4
SLE in childhood ... 64
SLE, B-cell hyperactivity in ... A29
SLE, deforming arthritis in ... C8
SLE-regulation ... 41
SS-A ... D1
SS-B/La ... A43
Sacroiliitis ... E72
Sacroiliitis in females ... E37
Salicylates ... B38
Sarcoplasmic reticulum ... A34
Scleroderma ... 115,A46,D31,E21,E20,27,D34
Scleroderma lung disease ... 22,23
Scleroderma, rheumatoid arthritis ... D2
Screening tests ... D57
Seasonal patterns ... B1
Segregation and linkage ... A19
Sensitivity of health status measures ... 88
Septic arthritis ... D60,E72
Septic arthritis and lyme disease ... 131
Seropositive rheumatoid arthritis ... E16
Serotonin ... 26,169
Serum C1q level ... D14
Sex steroids ... B42
Shoulder pain ... D68,D69
Sjogren's syndrome ... A54,153,134,A60,A11,C30,152
Skin disease activity ... D4
Skin-immunological studies in fibrositis ... E61
Sm antibodies ... C14
Sm, nRNP, Scl-70 ... B13
Small nuclear ribonucleoprotein complex ... 121
Social Security data ... D22
Soft tissue rheumatism ... 101,D56
Somatomedin C ... B51
Somatosensory evoked potentials ... C1
Specific suppression ... D51,A67
Spirochetal immune cross-reactivity ... 98
Spleen ... E1

Spondyloarthropathy A44
Staphylococcus aureus D42
Starling forces E14
Steroid-induced osteonecrosis D67
Still's disease in adults D13,96,99
Stimulus response coupling 80
Streptococcal cellwall-induced arthritis D40
Streptococcal cellwall-induced granuloma D40
Streptococcus, group G D60
Stress A20
Subacromial impingement D68,D69
Subacute cutaneous lupus erythematosus D4
Subcutaneous nodules C37
Sulphasalazine D9
Sulphasalazine, safety profile of E8
Superoxide A27,A28
Superoxide anion D16
Suppression of interleukin-2 production D35
Suppressive B cell factor D64
Suppressor T cells A30
Suppressor cell function B6
Suppressor-inducer T cells 62
Suppressor/inducer subset 32
Surface Ig turnover A31
Surface immunoglobulin E29
Survival E11
Survivorship analysis of resurfacing C4
Sympathetic nervous system 25
Synovial cells A4,C27,C20
Synovial fluid 36,127,E15,D21
Synovial fluid analysis 91
Synovial fluid lymphocyte E31
Synovial fluid mononuclear cells B55
Synovial mast cells C26
Synovial membrane B30,E25,139
Synovial tissue D15
Synovitis B30,D20,3
Synovium B33,135
Synthetic peptides 37
Systemic lupus erythematosus (SLE) .. 162,A29,E52,44,59,53,60, E27,C13,C14,54,160,A33,117,116,C36,C8,D2,147,E2, C9,A11,D3,C10 B48,E3,B56,A26,C34,C35,D46,113,40,B21, B19,D6,58,E1,C11,151, A64,146
Systemic sclerosis D50,21,D33,D30, D28,D27,E22,115,A46,D31,E21,E20,29,D34
T cell activation 29
T cell antigen receptor 29
T cell antigens 44
T cell clones B27,70
T cell hybridomas 109,A32
T cell lines, in collagen arthritis 76
T cell lymphokines C32
T cell proliferation 36
T cells 104,31,A35,69,71
T11 antigen 4
T3-Ti antigen/MHC receptor complex 4
T4 epitope phenotype D3
tDNA ligase E54
Takayasu's arteritis 15,E56
Tear lysozyme level 153
Technitium scintigraphy C38
Temporal arteritis 157,13,D54
Temporal arteritis, steroid dose in 13
Therapy 137,E59
Thermography C2
Third mononuclear population 107
Three-dimensional analysis C3
Thrombocytopenia E2
Thymic maturation 31
Thymocyte proliferation A66
Thyroid test abnormalities E3
Tidal lavage C5
Tight-skinned mice D31
Tolerance induction in autoimmune B cells 74
Tomographic thallium-201 myocardial scintigrams 24
Total hip failure C7
Total hip replacement 64
Total joint arthroplasty A65
Total lymphoid irradiation 136
Toxic oxygen metabolites E18
Toxicity 138
Toxicity of Auranofin A23
Training of laboratory technicians 91
Transdermal administration 18
Transfer RNA 114
Treatment of coronary arteritis 61
Treatment of polyarteritis nodosa D52
Type II collagen B11,168,E46
Type II collagen cDNA probes 173
Type II collagen-induced arthritis 170
Type V collagen E69
UI ribonucleoprotein complex (UI RNP) 121
Ultrastructure, muscle D11
Unbound C1q A10
Urate crystals 103
Uveitis A56,C44
Vasculitis 1
Vasculitis 134,A62,E62
Vasospactic phenomenon in SLE B47
Ventricular dysfunction A36
Viral arthropathies 3
Visceral angiography in polyarteritis D52
Visual loss D54
Von Willebrand's factor related antigen E58
Warfarin treatment 154
Western blot 163
Wilson's disease E41
Work disability in arthritis D22
Yersinia enterocolitica 51
Yersinia, chlamydia D63
Z DNA B19

1 9 8 5

ARTHRITIS FOUNDATION

SCIENTIFIC ABSTRACTS

ANNUAL MEETING

★ ★ ★

20TH ANNUAL MEETING

ARTHRITIS HEALTH PROFESSIONS ASSOCIATION

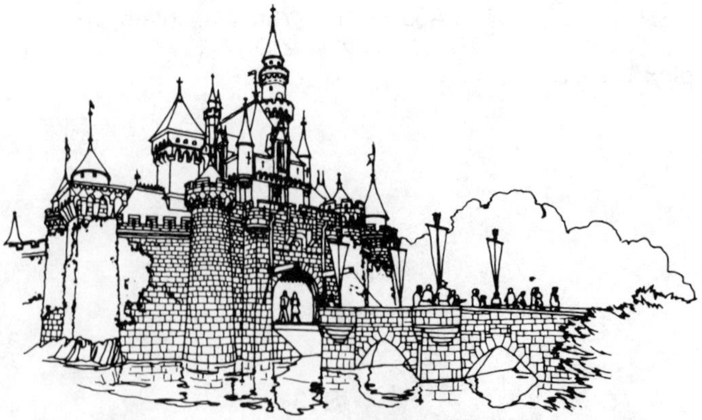

JUNE 4-8, 1985
DISNEYLAND HOTEL
ANAHEIM, CALIFORNIA

ARTHRITIS HEALTH PROFESSIONS ASSOCIATION

20th Annual Scientific Meeting
June 4-8, 1985

Disneyland Hotel
Anaheim, California

PROGRAM COMMITTEE

Cynthia A. Stabenow, OTR, Chair, *Charlottesville, Virginia*
Saralynn H. Allaire, RN, MS, *Boston, Massachusetts*
Carol Burckhardt, RN, PhD, *Portland, Oregon*
Bruce M. Clark, PT, *Vancouver, British Columbia*
Marian A. Minor, RPT, MSPH, *Columbia, Missouri*

•

REVIEW COURSE TASK FORCE

Teresa J. Brady, OTR, MA, Chair, *Minneapolis, Minnesota*
Andrew A. Guccione, RPT, MA, *Boston, Massachusetts*
Jurate A. Sakalys, RN, PhD, *Denver, Colorado*
Pamela M. Schroeder, RN, MSN, *Milwaukee, Wisconsin*
Elizabeth J. Yerxa, PhD, OTR, *Downey, California*

•

LOCAL ARRANGEMENTS COMMITTEE

Muriel MacKallor, OT, MS, *Inglewood, Califofornia*

ARTHRITIS HEALTH PROFESSIONS ASSOCIATION

20TH ANNUAL SCIENTIFIC MEETING

JUNE 4 - 8, 1985
ANAHEIM, CALIFORNIA

TENTATIVE SCHEDULE

See published program for room locations and speaker details.

TUESDAY, JUNE 4

8:30 AM - 5:00 PM	**FOUNDATIONS OF CLINICAL PRACTICE IN RHEUMATOLOGY: BEYOND MEDICAL INTERVENTION**
6:30 PM - 8:00 PM	Welcome Reception

WEDNESDAY, JUNE 5

7:30 AM - 8:30 AM	Continental Breakfast
8:30 AM - 9:45 AM	Plenary Session I **THE LEADING EDGE**
9:45 AM - 10:00 AM	Refreshment Break
10:00 AM - 11:15 AM	Plenary Session II **UNDERSTANDING OSTEOPOROSIS**
11:15 AM - 11:30 AM	Refreshment Break
11:30 AM - 12:30 AM	Concurrent Session A (Abstracts 1 - 4)
	Concurrent Session B (Abstracts 5 - 8)
	Concurrent Session C (Abstracts 9)
12:30 PM - 1:30 PM	Lunch Break
1:30 PM - 3:30 PM	Concurrent Session D **APPLICATION OF THE PRINCIPLES OF WORK CAPACITY EVALUATION TO THE PERSON WITH ARTHRITIS**
	Concurrent Session E (Abstracts 10 - 15)

3:30 PM - 4:00 PM	Refreshment Break
4:00 PM - 5:30 PM	Concurrent Session F **SOCIAL SUPPORT - RESEARCH AND APPLICABILITY TO ARTHRITIS**
	Concurrent Session G (Abstracts 16 - 20)
	Concurrent Session H (Abstract 21)
	Study Group **Multipurpose Arthritis Centers**
5:30 PM - 7:00 PM	Study Groups **Pediatrics** **Sexuality**
8:00 PM - 10:00 PM	Councils **Nursing** **Physical Therapy** **Occupational Therapy** **Social Work** **Laboratory**
10:00 PM - 11:30 PM	Study Group/Council Reception

THURSDAY, JUNE 6

6:00 AM - 8:00 AM	Run for Arthritis
7:30 AM - 8:30 AM	Continental Breakfast
8:00 AM - 9:30 AM	ARA/AHPA Poster Session B (Abstracts 22 - 39)
9:30 AM - 10:45 AM	Concurrent Session J **FIBROSITIS: A DIAGNOSTIC AND TREATMENT UPDATE**
	Concurrent Session K (Abstract 40)
	Concurrent Session L (Abstract 41)
10:45 AM - 11:00 AM	Refreshment Break
11:00 AM - 12:00 PM	Concurrent Session M **EXTRA-ARTICULAR MANIFESTATIONS IN ARTHRITIS**
	Concurrent Session N (Abstract 42)
	Concurrent Session O (Abstracts 43 - 46)
12:00 PM - 1:00 PM	Lunch Break

1:00 PM - 3:00 PM	ARA/AHPA Seminar **OSTEOARTHRITIS OF THE KNEE**
	Concurrent Session P (Abstract 47)
	Concurrent Session Q (Abstract 48)
3:00 PM - 3:30 PM	Refreshment Break
3:30 PM - 5:30 PM	ARA/AHPA Seminar **JUVENILE ARTHRITIS**
	Concurrent Session R **THE RESEARCH REVIEW: WHAT HAPPENS TO YOUR PROPOSAL AFTER YOU MAIL IT**
	Concurrent Session S (Abstract 49)
5:30 PM - 7:00 PM	Study Group **Psychosocial**
6:30 PM - 8:00 PM	Reception

FRIDAY, JUNE 7

7:30 AM - 8:30 AM	Continental Breakfast
8:00 AM - 9:30 AM	ARA/AHPA Poster Session C (Abstracts 50 - 67)
9:30 AM - 11:00 AM	Concurrent Session T **AEROBICS EXERCISE WITH ARTHRITIS: UPDATE 1985**
	Concurrent Session U (Abstract 68)
	Concurrent Session V (Abstract 69)
11:00 AM - 1:30 PM	**LUNCHEON, PRESIDENTIAL ADDRESS AND BUSINESS MEETING**
1:30 PM - 3:00 PM	Concurrent Session W **SEXUALITY WORKSHOP: SPECIFIC INTERVENTION TECHNIQUES FOR CLIENTS WITH SEXUAL PROBLEMS**
	Concurrent Session X **MICROCOMPUTERS AND THE ARTHRITIS HEALTH PROFESSIONAL: AN INTRODUCTION**
	Concurrent Session Y (Abstract 70)
	Concurrent Session Z (Abstracts 71 - 73)
3:00 PM - 3:30 PM	Refreshment Break

3:30 PM - 5:00 PM	Concurrent Session AA (Abstracts 74 - 79)
	Concurrent Session BB (Abstracts 80 - 85)
	Concurrent Session CC (Abstract 86)
5:00 PM - 6:00 PM	Study Group **Local Sections/Regional Meetings**

SATURDAY, JUNE 8

7:30 AM - 8:30 AM	Continental Breakfast
8:30 AM - 10:00 AM	Concurrent Session DD **VOCATIONAL REHABILITATION: CAN YOU ACCESS THE SYSTEM FOR YOUR PATIENT WITH ARTHRITIS**
	Concurrent Session EE (Abstract 87)
10:00 AM - 10:30 AM	Refreshment Break
10:30 AM - 12:00 PM	Concurrent Session FF **THE DEVELOPMENT AND USE OF HEALTH STATUS OUTCOME MEASURES**
	Concurrent Session GG (Abstract 88)

1

A MULTI-CENTER STUDY OF UTILIZATION AND COSTS IN RHEUMATOID ARTHRITIS. DP Lubeck, PW Spitz, JF Fries, Stanford University, Stanford; F Wolfe Wichita Arthritis Center, Wichita; D Mitchell, U. of Saskatchewan, Saskatoon Canada, SH Roth, Arthritis Center Inc., Phoenix.

The economic impact of chronic illness has important implications for medical practice and health policy. A detailed self-administered questionnaire (HAQ) was developed to determine the yearly direct and indirect costs for persons with RA, and administered to 940 subjects. This study investigates the performance of this instrument over a 2 year period (1981-82), and documents that the costs of RA can be accurately and practically measured.

Direct costs include the average annual expenditures by all patients and third party payors for: hospital care ($913 for an average stay of 2.7 days), outpatient physician costs ($206 for a mean of 8.3 visits), allied health professional visits ($71 for a mean of 2.6 visits), medications ($406), lab tests ($217), x-rays ($116), assistive devices ($24) and nontraditional therapies ($21). Annual medical costs were $2006, and other costs (transportation) ran $527 for total costs of $2553. In a multivariate analysis controlling for age ($\bar{x}$=55 years), sex (76% female), education ($\bar{x}$=13 years), and disease duration ($\bar{x}$=15 years), outpatient costs, inpatient costs and total costs were all positively related to the HAQ disability index (prob t<.01) and global health (prob t<.01), but were not associated with self-reported pain.

This instrument records costs as units of service. Dollar figures are derived by assigning the average charge in the community to each unit. Medical records were reviewed for a sample (n=66) to assess the accuracy of reported utilization. All hospitalizations are audited. Such documented cost data will be invaluable in assessing the economic gains achievable through a variety of disease interventions.

2

NURSING ASSESSMENT: A TOOL FOR PATIENT EDUCATION. Karen Cooper and Chris Lorish, Spain Rehabilitation Center, Birmingham, Alabama.

With legal ethics dictating that clients receive an adequate knowledge related to their disease and aspects of their care, it is important for health care professionals to adequately meet the educational needs of the individual.

An assessment tool was developed for staff nurses in an inpatient setting that would determine within 10 minutes a patient's reading capability, motivation to learn, physical limitations, mental status, and pain/energy level. An additional 15 minute assessment determines knowledge deficits for the client with inflammatory arthritis.

With the use of this assessment tool the primary nurse is able to develop an educational prescription for the client. A diagnostic summary is then distributed to other members of the health care team. This decreases duplication of assessment, thus speeding the educational process. If there are problem areas which will hinder the client's educational process, these are addressed by the health care team prior to beginning the educational prescription.

Upon instituting this assessment tool, nurses noted a decrease in personal frustration with educating their clients. One noted factor was an increased awareness of clients with low literary skills and methods/materials wich address those needs.

3

COMMUNITY SERVICE INFORMATION NEEDS OF PATIENTS WITH ARTHRITIS. A. L. Hull, J. Liebman, R. W. Moskowitz. Northeast Ohio Multipurpose Arthritis Center, CWRU, Cleveland, Ohio.

Information about community services is important to patients with arthritis diseases, and the need becomes critical for patients incurring significant loss of function. As part of a study to develop a community resource guide for patients with arthritis, the investigators interviewed 189 patients who were receiving treatment in several arthritis clinics in the metropolitan area. The interviews solicited information needs caused by the arthritis condition. Demographic and functional assessment questions were also asked.

A structured interview was conducted wherein each patient was asked to indicate the degree to which they had needed information about 66 potential services (e.g., public transportation, home care). The items were grouped into 3 content categories. Chronbach alpha statistics suggested that the items in each of the three groups were similar. The three item groups were labeled general information (GI), medical and personal care services (MPC) and assistive devices and equipment (ADE).

Multiple regression was used to regress each of the three need variables on eight demographic and functional assessment questions. Functional ability (FA), family income, and age were related to GI, FA and income were related to MPC, and FA and age were related to ADE. In all cases FA was positively correlated, while age and income were negative. These findings suggest that health providers and service agencies need to target service information to specific groups of patients, since younger, less affluent, and more functional patients have a more extensive need for information. Study supported by NIADDK AM 20618.

4

COMMUNITY-BASED ARTHRITIS CONTROL PROGRAM. Bonnie Denford. The Arthritis Society, Vancouver, B.C., Canada V5Z 1L7.

The Arthritis Society-B.C. Division has been operating a province-wide community-based Arthritis Control Program for 31 years. British Columbia is approximately 360,000 square miles with a population of 2,704,826. The most populated areas are in the lower third of the province with small cities and towns dispersed widely across the northern two thirds. It is a challenge to deliver consistent province-wide care for arthritis patients who live most of their lives in communities outside the large medical centres.

Servicing this population are 104 regional or community hospitals. The Arthritis Society has established a co-operative link with 45 of these hospitals located throughout the province. This link through the hospital administrator was initially established with either a Physiotherapist or Occupational Therapist. Recently Social Work and Nursing have become involved.

Accessibility to information and trained health professionals is important in the management of chronic diseases. Education in Arthritis management is initially provided by the Vancouver Centre and then the designated AHP returns to his/her community to provide services to the local patient population. Ongoing educational liaison is primarily maintained by the Vancouver Centre. In addition, clinical and further educational liaison is provided by three regionally-based Arthritis Centres. Support is provided through written material, phone consultations, on-site visits and an annual conference.

This established model for the delivery of Arthritis Allied Health Service will be discussed.

5

TRENDS IN POST-TKA TREATMENT OF PATIENTS WITH ARTHRITIS: CPM, NMES, AND CPM/NMES COMBINED. Robert Landel, Teresa Newton, Rancho Los Amigos Medical Center, Downey, California.

Early restoration of knee extension range and quadriceps strength is the key to recovery from total knee arthroplasty (TKA). Continuos passive motion (CPM) machines and neuromuscular electrical stimulation (NMES) have recently been introduced as adjuncts to conventional treatment programs and have been shown by some studies to accelerate the recovery process. A combination CPM/NMES machine is now being developed. The purpose of this study is to compare the effectiveness between a conventional treatment regimen alone and conventional regimens augmented by CPM, NMES, and CPM with NMES on gaining quadriceps strength, knee ROM, and ambulation endurance, as well as decreasing length of hospital stay in post-TKA patients with rheumatoid arthritis.

The protocol post-op TKA begins with isometric exercises, progressing to passive and active ROM exercises and ambulation. Patients are discharged when range, strength, and endurance criteria are met. The CPM protocol begins immediately post-op, increasing daily until 90 degrees of flexion is achieved. NMES programs are initiated when the patient is cleared for active exercise and continued until a F+ quadriceps contraction is achieved. The synchronized CPM/NMES program combines the above CPM and NMES protocols.

Since the CPM and NMES do not require a 1-1 patient/therapist relationship, use of these treatments can extend the hours of therapy the patient with rheumatoid arthritis receives during non-contact hours. This has the potential for improving post-op results and reducing costly hospital stays.

6

ISOKINETIC AND ISOMETRIC TRAINING IN RHEUMATOID ARTHRITIS. Jean Wessel, Vancouver,BC, Arthur Quinney, Edmonton, AB.

The purpose of this study was to compare the effects of isokinetic and isometric training of knee extension on the torque, power and work of the quadriceps muscles of women with rheumatoid arthritis (RA). Thirty-one women, aged 23 to 59, with RA were randomly assigned to one of three groups. Subjects in the two exercise groups attended 3 times weekly for 7 weeks for training of their quadriceps. The isometric group performed one maximal isometric contraction at each of three angles of the knee, while the isokinetic group performed three sets of six dynamic contractions at 180 degrees/sec. The control group received no program of exercise. Knee extension torque was tested at 5 velocities from 0 to 192 degrees/sec on a Cybex II isokinetic dynamometer. Power and work were calculated from the area under the torque curves. Both training groups improved in peak torque, and in measures of power and torque of the knee extensors. The isometric group had its greatest changes at the slow speed or isometric contractions, while the isokinetic group had improvements at faster velocities as well. It is concluded that the patient with RA can benefit from a strength training program with changes in torque, work and power of the exercised muscles. The results also suggest a trend towards specificity of training effects for the two modes of exercise employed in this study.

7

FEASIBILITY OF INPOOL AEROBIC EXERCISE FOR ARTHRITIS PATIENTS. M.A. Minor, T.E. Dreisinger, R.B. Webel, M.K. Smith, D.R. Kay. University of Missouri-Columbia Multipurpose Arthritis Center, Columbia, Missouri.

Inpool aerobic exercise is one of three exercise protocols in a controlled longitudinal study of the efficacy of physical conditioning exercise programs for people with rheumatoid or osteoarthritis. A pilot study was performed to design and evaluate an inpool protocol that would: 1) be strenuous enough to elicit heart rates within target range for conditioning, 2) be individually gradeable for duration and intensity, 3) not require swimming skills, and 4) be tolerated by the subjects. Five subjects (age 53-82) were pretested and entered into a 4 week exercise program. The aerobic component of the inpool protocol consists of ambulatory, stroking and kicking movements (with and without flotation device), and gross motor movements with partial weight bearing. For this exercise to produce a conditioning effect, it must be performed on a regular basis, strenuously enough to increase heart rates into the target range and maintain target heart rates for 20-30 minutes. Undue fatigue or exacerbration of musculoskeletal symptoms are unacceptable side effects. By the third week, subjects were able to regulate the intensity of exercise by varying the speed and type of movements performed. They achieved target heart rates and maintained activity within this training level for 25-30 minutes. All reported subjective improvement in flexibility, endurance, quality of sleep and sense of well-being. Four weeks was not long enough to produce significant changes in exercise tolerance. One subject reported increased pain and tenderness in one joint. Two subjects failed to complete the program due to scheduling conflicts. All subjects required individualized education to interpret and define sensations arising from increased activity. This study demonstrated that an inpool exercise program, performed on a regular basis, strenuously enough to produce a conditioning effect, can be safely and acceptably implemented with arthritis patients.

8

THE PHYSICAL AND PSYCHOLOGICAL EFFECTS OF A RECREATIONAL EXERCISE PROGRAM ON PERSONS WITH RHEUMATOID ARTHRITIS AND OSTEOARTHRITIS. M. Wineland, J. Zischke, G. Dennis and G. Klipple. Walter Reed Army Medical Center, Washington, D.C. and George Mason University, Fairfax, VA.

A recreational exercise program designed specifically for people with arthritis was studied for its effect on morale, depression, anxiety and functional ability in 51 adults with rheumatoid arthritis and osteoarthritis. Using a pretest-posttest control group design, subjects were randomly assigned to an experimental group which received recreational exercise and relaxation training twice a week for 12 weeks, and a control group which continued to participate in normal daily activities. Both groups kept exercise diaries throughout the study. Analysis of covariance was used to evaluate the data base which consisted of a geriatric morale scale, depression inventory, anxiety scale, disability index, observed functional test and clinical evaluation. Results on the Revised Philadelphia Geriatric Center Morale Scale, which has three subfactors, showed the experimental group had significantly higher level of total morale (p=.006), a better attitude toward their own aging (p=.012), and less agitation (p=.027) than the control group. This continuing study suggests that promoting a program of recreational exercise designed for people with arthritis might be effective in improving psychological factors that are common in chronic illnesses such as rheumatoid arthritis and osteoarthritis.

9

THE RHEUMATOLOGY NURSE PRACTITIONER. Teresa Doyle, Wayne State University, Detroit and Sally Marlowe, University of Connecticut, Farmington.

Nurse practitioners comprise a unique sub-group among arthritis health professionals, implementing practice models with great potential impact on health-care delivery to the chronically ill. The rheumatology nurse practitioner is prepared, through advanced training and a well-developed professional philosophy, to provide a wide range of services across settings to individuals and families affected by arthritis and rheumatic disease. For the most part, members of this nursing subspecialty have developed their professional roles independently and in relative isolation, each applying advanced nursing skills to the health needs of a specific rheumatology population. Nurse practitioners who specialize in rheumatology now need to identify one another, to examine critically their evolving role and to begin formulation of standards for their practice. Moreover, rheumatologists,health service administrators and the public should become acquainted with the range of services that rheumatology nurse practitioners are prepared to provide.

This roundtable session, led by two rheumatology nurse practitioners will provide partticipants with an opportunity to examine critically this developing nursing subspecialty, to identify important issues and to developsupportive networks. A brief background of the nurse practitioner movement will be presented. A model of practice will be proposed. The audience will be invited to participate in informal discussion of related experiences and concerns.

This roundtable will be presented at an intermediate level for a multidisciplinary audience; particularly nurses, nurse practitioners, physicians and health services administrators.

10

PROTEIN-CALORIE MALNUTRITION (PCM) IN RHEUMATOID ARTHRITIS (RA). G.S. Alarcón, T.L. Dunn, P. Harrell, Y. Germany, J. Wathal, and R.D. Collins, Jr. University of Alabama at Birmingham, Birmingham, Alabama 35294.

Twenty-two patients (pts) with active classic or definite RA were prospectively studied at admission to determine the incidence of PCM. A "likelihood of malnutrition" (LOM) score was calculated as previously described by R.J. Weinsier (1979), with a score of >25 being a high LOM. The eight parameters listed below were used. Sixty-eight percent of RA pts had a LOM >25 ($\bar{x}$ =51). The % of pts with abnormal values of each parameter (%patients) and the % of total points (% points) contributed by that factor are listed below. While abnormal values of albumin (Alb) and hematocrit (Hct) were common as expected, together they contributed only 23% of points. Arm muscle area (AMA) and weight per height (W/H) reflecting somatic protein and total body fat, were each of major significance. Grip strength, old age and female sex related to one or more abnormal nutritional parameters. Rheumatoid factor, ESR, functional class (FC), Ritchie index score, pinch strength, 24 hr dietary recall and evidence of xerostomia and peptic ulcer disease were similar for malnourished (MAL) and non-malnourished (NON). At a 2 yrs follow-up MAL pts did worse than NON pts as measured by worsening FC and hospitalizations directly or indirectly related to RA (p<0.05). We conclude that malnutrution per se may be a contributing factor to increased morbidity and mortality in RA.

	Serum Folate	Vit c	Skin fold	AMA	W/H	Lymphocyte	Alb	Hct
% pts	82	23	9	64	41	41	64	73
% points	14	8	2	22	21	10	12	12

11

ARTHRITIS SCREENING IN PUBLIC HEALTH CLINICS FOR OLDER ADULTS. Steven A. Mazzuca, Gloria J. Barger, Kenneth D. Brandt, Doris Wagner and Nebraska Demombery. Indiana University Arthritis Center and Marion County (Indiana) Health Department Nursing Bureau, Indianapolis.

Older adult clinics (OACs) operated by public health nurses are becoming a common source of health care for the elderly. Nurses staffing OACs need expertise in many chronic diseases--especially arthritis. The purposes of this study were to 1) assess the adequacy of arthritis screening and management in a group of municipal OACs and 2) improve screening and management by means of inservice education.

Interviews with 95 patients in 7 OACs indicated that while 64% of patients suffered joint pain or swelling and 21% experienced limited mobility, only 15-18% were screened for these problems. Therapeutic advice was offered less than 5% of the time. The 7 OACs (23 nurses) were assigned randomly to experimental (E) and control (C) conditions. E nurses received a 5-component inservice program: advanced readings, a half-day seminar, a pocket guide to arthritis screening/management, an individualized follow-up session and an Arthritis Center telephone consultation service. Content covered osteoarthritis, rheumatoid arthritis, soft tissue rheumatism and polymyalgia rheumatica. Preliminary evaluation data based on interviews with 50 patients (1/2 the anticipated patient sample) show screening for pain, swelling and mobility problems to be 25-30% more frequent in E clinics compared to control (all Fisher's Exact ps < 0.05). Also increased compared to control is E nurses' screening for morning stiffness, Raynaud's syndrome and polymyalgia rheumatica (0.01 < ps < 0.10). Continuation of these trends in the total sample will evince the capacity of multicomponent inservice programs to improve arthritis care for the elderly in public health settings.

12

A PAIN MANAGEMENT PROGRAM FOR RHEUMATOID ARTHRITIS PATIENTS F. Spilberg, F.H. Gilner, V.A. Medical Center, St. Louis, Missouri; St. Louis University, St. Louis, Missouri.

The effectiveness of a pain management treatment for rheumatoid arthritis (RA) patients was assessed employing stress inoculation training for pain and cognitive therapy for depression. Subjects were 20 male veteran outpatients, with a mean age of 55.5, who had RA for an average of 13.3 years. Ten subjects were assigned to the treatment condition and met in two groups for six sessions. The other ten subjects were assigned to a waiting list control group.

Pain perception, level of depression, and level of activity directly affected by arthritis were assessed at pretreatment and posttreatment. Pain perception was measured by the McGill Pain Questionnaire (MPQ), the Pain Rating Index, derived from the MPQ, provided qualitative data on the sensory, affective and evaluative qualities of pain perception. The Beck Depression Inventory was employed to measure level of depression and the Stanford Disability Index Questionnaire assessed level of activity.

An ANCOVA, performed for each variable, yielded results showing that the treatment had a significant effect ($p <$ .001) on the evaluative component of pain perception, lowering level of depression and increasing activity level.

Our results support the effectiveness of the outlined treatment as an intervention designed to decrease illness related stress and depression in rheumatoid arthritis patients.

13

THE USE OF LIDOCAINE WITH MYOCHRYSINE TO DECREASE POST-INJECTION DISCOMFORT. Andrea Kovalesky, Thomas J.A. Lehman, Los Angeles, David D. Sherry, Seattle.

The discomfort associated with Myochrysine injections is a chronic cause of morbidity among the rheumatic disease patients who receive them. Patients often complain of discomfort at the site of injection lasting several minutes to an hour or more. Lidocaine HCl (1%) has been added to Myochrysine in some institutions as one means of decreasing this discomfort, but its effectiveness and the appropriate dose have not been objectively determined.

In this study 8 patients received a total of 185 Myochrysine injections containing 0, 0.1, or 0.25 cc's of 1% lidocaine HCl. Patients were asked to rate their discomfort on a visual analog pain scale of 1 to 10 one minute following each of the 185 injections. The mean visual analog score reported was 4.32 following injections without lidocaine, 2.5 following injections with 0.1 cc of lidocaine, and 2.24 following injections with 0.25 cc's of lidocaine ($p < .0001$ when injections with and without lidocaine were compared). In addition, patients were asked to speculate whether lidocaine was included in their injection, based on their amount of discomfort. Patients correctly determined whether lidocaine was added to the Myochrysine 89/120 times ($p < 1 \times 10^{-6}$). No nitritoid reaction or reactions to lidocaine were seen, nor was any alteration of the effective of the Myochrysine apparent.

These data indicate that when 0.1 or 0.25 cc's of lidocaine HCl is added to Myochrysine injections most patients have a significant decrease in post-injection discomfort without an increase in adverse reactions.

14

THE RELATIONSHIP OF FAMILY DYNAMICS TO HEALTH STATUS IN RHEUMATOID ARTHRITIS. Barbara Whitmeyer, Lahey Clinic Medical Center, Boston.

Because rheumatoid arthritis (RA) effects not only the physical but also the psychosocial well being, afflicted individuals often are forced to modify numerous aspects of their lives. As with any chronic illness, these modifications have been shown to place a strain on family relationships and often lead to a breakdown of the family structure.

This study examined the relationship between the health status of the RA wife/mother and five family dynamics variables: 1) family cohesiveness; 2) conflict; 3) expressiveness; 4) functioning and 5) congruence. Fifty-three subjects completed the Arthritis Impact Measurement Scale (AIMS) and subjects and spouses completed the Family Environment Scale (FES) and the Family Functioning Index (FFI). Significant correlations were obtained for both subjects and spouses between the nine AIMS subscales and the social and psychological variables. Higher social activity scores were associated with higher family relationship scores for both subjects and their spouses, while higher depression and anxiety scores were associated with lower cohesiveness and functioning and higher conflict in subjects, and less expressiveness in spouses. Surprising, however, there were few significant relationships between the AIMS subscales measuring the physical variables and the family variables. For example, mobility and household activities were not significantly related to the family variables. The amount and intensity of pain was also not significantly related to the family variables. These findings provide direction for intervention with rheumatoid arthritic clients.

15

EFFECTIVENESS, ACCEPTABILITY AND COSTS OF THREE METHODS OF SELF-CARE EDUCATION FOR PERSONS WITH RHEUMATOID ARTHRITIS. Teresa Doyle, Marilyn Oermann, Alice Reid, Juanita Balke and Carol Zabinski, Wayne State University, Detroit.

This study examined group teaching (GT), self-instruction (SI) and one-to-one instruction (OI) for persons with rheumatoid arthritis (RA) in terms of their effects on learning and learner satisfaction. Costs of the three teaching methods were also compared.

Thirty persons with RA were assigned in order to four groups: OI, SI, GT and control. With the exception of controls, all received similar content, the only difference being the teaching method. Learning was measured by the Rheumatoid Arthritis Knowledge Inventory (RAKI), administered immediately before, immediately after and one month after the educational intervention. Satisfaction with teaching was measured with an original instrument at completion of instruction. Cost analysis took into account cost of materials and professional time spent teaching. Significance of applied statistical tests was set at 0.05.

Paired t tests indicated significant improvement in posttest over pretest RAKI scores for all three teaching groups. ANCOVA showed no significant difference in posttest scores of the three groups. Learning retention, measured by one-month RAKI scores, was not significantly different among the the three groups, per ANCOVA. All subjects indicated satisfaction with teaching; this was significanly greater for OI. Costs per subject were: $3.35 for SI, $22 for GT and $61-$91 for OI.

The results indicate that persons with RA learned and retained content equally well via three educational methods. OI was the most acceptable, albeit the most costly, method. SI was the least costly method.

16

TIMED FUNCTIONAL ASSESSMENT: RELIABILITY AND VALIDITY. Lynda McCloy. The Arthritis Society, Vancouver, B.C. and Lyn Jongbloed. University of British Columbia, Vancouver, B.C.

A unique, timed functional assessment (Robinson, H.S. et al, Canadian Journal of Occupational Therapy, 29, 4, 1962) has been examined for reliability and validity in an arthritis rehabilitation centre. The centre has extensive experience in the use of this assessment and has found 2 advantages over other functional assessments: a) objective method (timing); b) generation of patient problems for treatment plan formation.

A chart review of 100 patients was conducted to examine internal consistency, concurrent validity with A.R.A. functional scale and joint range of motion, criterion group validity and predictive validity. Content validity was examined using a survey and the nominal group technique with a panel of experts. Currently, test-retest reliability and inter-observer variability are being studied.

Early results show fairly high internal consistency (.73 alpha reliability) and moderate intercorrelation of the four sub-scales of the test. Correlation between test scores and range of movement are for the most part low (.1-.2) Mean admission and discharge scores showed significant differences when the standard deviations were examined (t-test) although a ceiling effect was noticed in the discharge scores. The survey of the panel of experts (8 O.T.'s) revealed that the functional assessment was seen to be a better measure of patient problems than treatment outcomes. However, the self-care and ambulation subscales were identified as moderately good measures of treatment outcome.

It is felt that once this review is completed, certain sections of this functional assessment will provide a useful tool for occupational therapists to use with arthritis patients in the clinical setting.

17

LONG-TERM FUNCTIONAL FOLLOW-UP OF MCP ARTHROPLASTIES. K. Patricia MacBain, Arthritis Society, Vancouver, B.C. Robert W. McGraw, University of British Columbia.

Rheumatoid arthritis often leads to reduced function in the hand. Surgical procedures aimed at improving function are frequently carried out but few studies have looked at the effectiveness of such surgery in terms of practical function over a long period of time.

Starting in 1969, two groups of patients with MCP arthroplasties have been followed by the orthopaedic surgeon who did the procedures and by an occupational therapist. A previous review was done in 1977 on 26 patients (33 hands). At this time, 12 of the same patients have been re-assessed. Seven patients (9 hands) had standard resection arthroplasties and 5 patients (6 hands) had Swanson implants. Average follow-up is 14 years for the former and 12 years for the latter.

Each patient has been functionally assessed pre-operatively and at repeated intervals after surgery; each has had at least 4 assessments. The functional assessment consists of strength tests (grip, hook, pinch, pouring, cutting) and dexterity tests (lacing, pinning, buttoning, locking, picking up coins). The orthopaedic review includes x-rays and a physical examination.

Early results have shown an initial improvement in both groups. The improvement in strength in the implant group was slower to appear but was later noted to be superior to the resection only group.

In the long term (12-14 years), of the remaining patients, a definite decline in function was recorded in both groups. There was a notable exception. Pinch strength in the index and long fingers in the implant group was maintained in the majority of patients.

18

STRETCH GLOVE EFFECTS ON HAND SYMPTOMS IN PATIENTS WITH RHEUMATOID ARTHRITIS. P. McKnight. St. Margaret Memorial Hospital, Pittsburgh, Pennsylvania.

Inflammatory synovitis of the hands is a major cause of disability in patients with rheumatoid arthritis (RA). Previous studies have shown that stretch gloves have been effective in the management of arthritis affecting the hands. In this study, two types of gloves, the Futuro and the Isotoner, were compared to determine which was more effective in the relief of hand symptoms in patients with R.A.

To date, ten out of thirty hospitalized patients, each exhibiting bilateral hand synovitis, have been studied. Each patient was randomly given one Isotoner and one Futuro glove and instructed to wear the gloves from bedtime until morning for one week. During this time, patients continued to receive routine treatments to the hands; however, air splints and steroid injections were withheld. Objective and subjective evaluations were performed on both hands before the gloves were dispensed and after one week. Objective evaluations consisted of ring size, range of motion, grip strength, and rate of finger motion. Subjective evaluations included reports of pain and morning stiffness.

Preliminary data on the ten patients was analyzed by a paired t-test to compare the effects of the hands treated with the Isotoner versus the hands treated with the Futuro. These data indicate both gloves are effective in relief of pain, stiffness and swelling and improvement of motion and strength to the .05 level. Due to the small sample size, it is unclear if one glove is more effective than the other. Data analysis from all thirty patients will be presented to determine if one glove is more effective than the other for relief of synovitis of the hands.

19

OBSERVATIONS FROM AN IN-HOME OCCUPATIONAL THERAPY PROGRAM FOR WOMEN WITH RHEUMATOID ARTHRITIS (RA). C. Rodon, M.K. Smith, M. Cadwell, D.R. Kay, University of Missouri-Columbia Multipurpose Arthritis Center, Columbia, Missouri. 65212

Occupational Therapy (OT) services traditionally offered in hospital settings restrict accessiblity, availability, and possibly relevance of care for many arthritis patients. OT services often focus on OT goals rather than patient goals. To address these problems, we implemented an individualized OT program of self-managment information delivered entirely in the patient's home. A randomized pre-post control group design with multiple observations is being used to evaluate its impact. To date, 15 women (definite RA, Functional Class 1 or 2) were invited to participate; 11 enrolled, 4 declined. For seven enrollees, their primary incentive was a desire to help others rather than expectation of personal benefit. Initial observations from this study indicate: a) working with a patient in her home provides critical information necessary for optimal OT treatment (e.g. physical setting, support systems, lifestyle, family dynamics, significant issues) (8/10); b) working in the patient's home enhanced rapport and understanding of the patient's perspectives (8/10); c) reported functional adjustment did not correlate with disease duration or severity, but appeared more related to attitude toward her disease (9/10); d) typical OT goal orientation is often discrepant with patient goals for improved function (5/5 experimental subjects); e) patients tend toward a reactive rather than a proactive approach to their arthritis (6/10); f) many patients have spontaneously made appropriate adaptations without receiving OT (8/10). In-home OT offers a unique opportunity to develop, test, and revise self-management programs with patients in their home environments. The OT services are thus relevant, individualized, and more likely to be utilized.

20

AN EFFECTIVE TOOL FOR ASSISTANCE IN DETERMINING SOCIAL SECURITY DISABILITY. Sally Bucrek and Sue Stock, Ingham Medical Center, Lansing, Michigan.

When a physician is confronted by an arthritic wage-earner who reports an inability to complete the tasks required on his/her job, the issue of disability arises. Tools for objectively measuring the degree of disability and residual functional capacity, relative to the patient's specific job requirements, have until now been unavailable.

An interdisciplinary consultation between a rheumatologist, O.T.R., and R.P.T. resulted in the development of an evaluation procedure which can be utilized to: A) determine whether a functional disability exists; B) compare functional ability to job requirements, C) recommend work place modifications to permit continued employment if appropriate, or D) verify the infeasibility of continued performance of the patient's current job. The summary of the O.T. and P.T. interview, evaluation, and recommendations are submitted for review to their physician who may add radiographic, laboratory and medical data.

This tool has been used predominantly for evaluation of rheumatoid and spondylolytic patients. Recommendations for environmental modification often permit retention of an experienced employee at a level of improved efficiency. All applications for social security disability that have been submitted with the recommendation of this evaluation have been accepted. Previously, many of these legitimate claims had been unjustly denied.

With increasing emphasis on reduced spending for disability programs this tool assists the rheumatoid patient to perform at his/her optimal functional work capacity and assists the physician in making more accurate disability judgments. A summary of social security disability requirements, specific evaluation forms and methods will be provided.

21

USING THE HEALTH CENTER OR HOSPITAL LIBRARY : A REFERENCE SEMINAR FOR ARTHRITIS HEALTH PROFESSIONALS (AHPS). L. Ray, Northeast Ohio Multipurpose Arthritis Center, Cleveland, Ohio.

AHPs come to their health center or hospital library every day for answers to clinical, educational, and research questions. They often leave with partial answers or new questions because they were unable to utilize the vast myriad of available reference services. This seminar will help AHPs to use their health center or hospital library in a more efficient and effective manner.

Participants will be able to describe how to formulate a complete and accurate reference question; identify the qualities of "factual," "bibliographic," and "verification" reference questions; identify major reference tools used in answering each type of reference question; describe the bibliographic access points and types of card catalogs; and define the purpose and procedure of responsible interlibrary loaning.

An interactive "reference interview" will be conducted to reveal to participants how to formulate better questions and to recognize the 3 types of reference questions (ie, factual, bibliographic, and verification). A lecture presentation will review major reference tools, focussing upon their formats and specific uses; how to use card catalogs; and interlibrary loan resource sharing principles. Small group exercises will provide participants an opportunity to devise reference search strategies and resource materials collection methods.

This seminar will be presented for AHPs interested in knowing more about how to use their health center or hospital library at a beginning/intermediate level.

(Supported by AM20618)

22

EFFECT OF MANUAL TRACTION ON ELBOW FLEXION CONTRACTURES IN RA. K.R. Gibson, St. Margaret Memorial Hospital, Pittsburgh.

The purpose of this presentation is to review the methodology and results of a clinical research study in which the addition of elbow joint mobilization to a standard protocol of moist heat and active exercises was evaluated with respect to its efficacy in reducing elbow flexion contractures in people with rheumatoid arthritis, compared to moist heat and active exercise alone.

Fifteen inpatients participated in the study. Both elbows of each patient had greater than a 5° flexion contracture and either Stage I or II roentgenographic changes per the American Rheumatism Association classification. On each successive patient admitted to the study, the experimental status was alternately assigned to either the right or left elbow. The fifteen control elbows received ten treatments consisting of moist heat and ten repetitions of active range of motion (AROM), while the fifteen experimental elbows received the same treatment, as well as ten repetitions of grade III elbow joint traction.

The resulting mean gain of elbow extension in the experimental group was 9.53° compared to 5.20° in the control group. A dependent t-test shows the difference to be significant at $p < .01$. There was not a significant difference between the experimental and control groups in the changes noted in the degree of flexion or in the total range of active elbow motion.

In conclusion, elbow joint traction combined with moist heat and active exercise was found to provide a significantly greater gain in elbow extension than moist heat and active exercise alone in selected patients with rheumatoid arthritis and elbow flexion contractures. Implications of these findings will be discussed.

23

SEATBELT MODIFICATIONS FOR PATIENTS WITH RHEUMATIC DISEASES. I. Harris, Arthritis Society, Vancouver. B. Gilliland and S. Whitling, University of British Columbia, Vancouver.

Mandatory seatbelt use for vehicle drivers or passengers has been enforced since October 1, 1977 in British Columbia, Canada. Persons with rheumatic diseases have sought exemption from wearing seatbelts for medical reasons. These requests for exemption prompted an investigation into the difficulties encountered when "buckling up".

A questionnaire was designed and distributed to 100 patients attending treatment at the Arthritis Society in Vancouver. Areas of difficulty in applying seatbelts were identified as 1) reach required to grip seatbelt 2) the fastening mechanism of the seatbelt 3) the releasing mechanism and 4) the pressure exerted by the seatbelt itself.

A seatbelt was designed to solve the problems identified by the questionnaire. The seatbelt modification is a universal design and therefore able to attach to any existing seatbelt. It is also easily transferable and inexpensive to produce.

24

A STRUCTURED INTERVIEW TO IDENTIFY ARTHRITIS NEED FOR SERVICE. J. Liebman, A. Hull, M. Blauner, R.W. Moskowitz. Northeast Ohio Multipurpose Arthritis Center, CWRU, Cleveland, Ohio.

Arthritis affects many aspects of day-to-day living. The needs arising out of changes in functioning and life style can be met in part by community services. To identify the needs that can be satisfied through such resources, data from actual consumers of care is required.

A structured interview was developed to inquire about arthritis patients' felt need for service, as part of a project to produce a consumer arthritis service directory. This presentation discusses the process used to formulate and administer the structured interview. The items selected for use in the questionnaire resulted from a review of current literature, interviews with patients, the concerns of health professionals, an examination of functional assessment studies, and consults with Arthritis Foundation staff about public inquiries. Demographic information and functional ability were also requested in the interview which took 45 minutes to administer each of the 189 patients receiving care in urban and suburban locations. The results of the interview indicated three groups of needs: General information (GI), medical and personal care services (MPC), and assistive devices and equipment (ADE).

The process used for identifying variables important in arthritis care facilitated the development of the structured interview. The resulting needs were later matched with known service agencies obtained from a computerized data bank of non-profit agencies and formed the basis for the consumer directory subsequently produced.

Supported by NIADDK AM 20618.

25

THE VALIDITY OF SELF-REPORTED ARTHRITIS DIAGNOSIS. Genevieve E.S. Gines, Dennis Keane, Kate Lorig, Stanford University, Stanford, CA

The National Health Survey and other studies often ask for self-reported diagnosis of arthritis. Not only are subjects asked to identify themselves as arthritics but often are asked to report their type of arthritis. In order to determine the accuracy of such self-reports, 199 subjects, recruited from the general public by public service announcements for arthritis patient education classes, were asked for a written self-diagnosis as part of the application process. This was followed within a month by a diagnosis from their physicians.

Physicians confirmed a diagnosis of arthritis in 184 (93%) of the 199 subjects (15% RA, 70% OA, 10% with other forms of arthritis, eg. ankylosing spondylitis, lupus, bursitis, and 5% with multiple forms of arthritis). Although this demonstrates a high rate of accuracy of general self-diagnosis by the subjects, their self-diagnosis for specific type of arthritis was less accurate. Eighty-nine percent correctly identified themselves as RA; 45% correctly identified themselves as OA; 33% of the non-RA, non-OA subjects correctly identified their type of arthritis; 5% of the multiple arthritics partially or completely identified their arthritis. Overall, 96 (52%) correctly identified their type of arthritis.

This study suggests that patients generally know they have arthritis but their self-reported diagnosis of specific type of arthritis is highly questionable. This error in patient self-reported diagnosis is relevant not only to the accuracy of health surveys but also to the patient's capability to manage disease. Because the various forms of arthritis each require different treatment-emphasis, knowledge of one's type of arthritis should aid patients in optimally implementing treatment programs.

26

METHODS UTILIZED BY URBAN LOW INCOME MINORITY PATIENTS TO CARE FOR THEIR ARTHRITIS. Dee Bill, Robert Rippey, Carol Pfeiffer, Micha Abeles, Maggie Jones, University of Connecticut Multipurpose Arthritis Center, Farmington.

A study of two urban low income minority (ULIM), communities was done to identify individuals with self perceived arthritis, to determine their medical diagnosis, methods of caring for their arthritis and the perceived efficacy of these methods.

ULIM individuals were identified by arthritis advocates. Individuals were examined by a rheumatologist. A social history questionnaire (SHQ) was administered orally. Of the 160 subjects, (66% Black, 34% Hispanic) 83% had a rheumatic disease. The majority of Blacks (60%) had osteoarthritis (OA), compared to 7% of the Hispanics. In contrast, the Hispanics had fibrositis (fibro) as the most prevalent diagnosis (44%) in comparison to (3%) of the Blacks. The following remedies were used at least weekly:

	Topical Ointments	ASA	Rest	Exercise	Prayer	Heat	Physician Rx Medicine
Blacks (OA)	44%	33%	31%	20%	29%	27%	27%
Hispanics (Fibro)	48%	26%	35%	28%	35%	65%	30%

In addition, 22% of the Blacks with OA used equipment (canes), and 9% used other pain medicine. None of the Hispanics with fibrositis reported using equipment, and 26% used other pain medicine. Prayer (92%), equipment (70%), and heat (33%) were reported as giving "much help" for the Blacks. Prayer (50%), heat (40%), and topical ointments (27%) were reported as giving "much help" for the Hispanics.

A spectrum of treatment modalities were utilized by the Black and Hispanic subjects. Knowledge and sensitivity of the range of modalities utilized will enhance communication and successful treatment.

27

The Effects of Hospitalization Upon the Psycho-Social and Functional Status of Rheumatoid Arthritis Patients. C. Lorish, J. Parker, S. Brown. Multi-Purpose Arthritis Center, Birmingham.

The purpose of this poster is to add to the scant published data on the effects of hospitalization upon rheumatoid arthritis patients' psycho-social and functional status. During the average 12 day stay, 123 ARA level II and III patients admitted in flared condition received comprehensive, team oriented, medical, PT and OT therapies, in addition to rest, proper nutrition, and social services.

Using the State-Trait Anxiety scale, the Beck Depression scale, the Health Locus of Control scale, the Bradburn Affect Balance scale, and the Face Test of Mood, psycho-social assessments were made upon intake, discharge, and at a clinic follow-up visit, approximately 40 days later. The Sickness Impact Profile (SIP) was used at intake and follow-up to assess the impact of the disease upon 14 discrete areas of the patient's life.

Results of the correlated t-test analysis of the psycho-social measures revealed that at discharge patients felt significantly less pain, depression, state anxiety, external control, negative mood and more energy. While there was a trend to return to the levels found at intake, significant but not as large a differences existed between intake and follow-up on these same measures. T-test analysis of the SIP scales revealed that patients' arthritis was affecting them significantly less at follow-up in the areas of sleep and rest, body care and movement, home management, mobility, social interaction, ambulation, alertness, and recreational behavior. These results suggest an important positive impact of hospitalization upon patients, although additional data is needed to determine the longevity of these gains.

28

DESCRIPTIVE CHARACTERISTICS OF FATIGUE—THE FIRST STEP TOWARD A NURSING DIAGNOSIS. A.M. Voith, J.S. Pigg, A.M. Frank, Midwest Arthritis Treatment Center, Columbia Hospital, Milwaukee WI.

Fatigue is frequently a chronic and severe problem for pts. with rheumatic diseases (RD). Nurses' involvement with RD pts. stimulated interest in fatigue as a possible nsg. diagnosis. Nsg. diagnosis is the labeling of pt. problems upon which nsg. can have an affect and is increasingly the basis of nsg. activities. Before the impact of nsg. interventions can be examined, descriptive characteristics which are the most commonly occurring cues for recognizing fatigue must be identified. This study sought to identify the descriptive characteristics of fatigue as the first step toward acceptance of this common pt. problem as a nsg. diagnosis. Recognition of fatigue as a nsg. diagnosis will increase awareness by nurses and focus appropriate care.

A questionaire was sent to a random sample of 1000 nurses representing RD, cardiac rehab, nsg. diagnosis and general nsg. asking them to rank on a 1 to 5 Likert-type scale a list of possible descriptive characteristics of fatigue compiled from literature and experience. From the 27.3% return, descriptive characteristics with a mean > 4.0 were considered critical indicators of fatigue. These included: verbalizes fatigue, inability to maintain usual activity level, poor task performance, impaired ability to concentrate, irritability and increased physical complaints.

The identification of a list of critical indicators is the first step toward acceptance of fatigue as a nsg. diagnosis. Critical indicators aid nurses in recognition, assessment and treatment of fatigue as a RD pt. problem, as well as encourage validation of the ANA/AHPA Outcome Standards of Rheumatology Nursing Practice related to fatigue.

29

NURSING DIAGNOSES IN AN ELDERLY POPULATION WITH RHEUMATIC DISEASES (RD). Diane Erlandson and Raymond E.H. Partridge, Tufts New England Medical Center, Boston, MA.

The aged, who are victims of RD are subject not only to problems resulting from their disease but also to problems related to aging.

The purpose of this study was to identify all nursing diagnoses made on patients over 65 during a 2 year period from a population being treated for RD by the staff of a Rheumatology Clinic in a university setting. (N=631). Of these 631 patients, 64 (51 female; 13 male) were being followed as primary patients of a nursing staff member. Medical diagnoses included: Rheumatoid Arthritis (N=22); Osteoarthritis (N=19); Polymyalgia Rheumatica (N=5); Lupus (N=3); Vasculitis (N=3); Myositis (N=3); and Other (N=9). Based on signs and symptoms, each patient's nursing diagnosis was documented using the nomenclature developed by the National Conference on Classification of Nursing Diagnoses. 430 diagnoses were made in all. The most commonly used diagnoses were: Alteration in Comfort, Pain (75%); Impaired Mobility (61%); Impaired Home Maintenance Management (43%); Self Care Deficit (42%); Depression (23%); Potential for Injury (22%); Knowledge deficit (22%); Disturbance in Self Concept (22%); and Anxiety (20%).

Almost one-half of the patients lived alone. There was a significantly greater incidence of problems with pain, mobility, depression and injury among those who lived alone when compared to those who did not.

Conclusion: 1) Important nursing diagnoses in the elderly with RD are Pain, Impaired Mobility, Impaired Home Management Management, and Self-care Deficit. 2) The elderly with RD who live alone appear to be at a greater risk for developing problems with pain, mobility, self-care, depression and injury.

30

NURSING ASPECTS OF INTRAVENOUS METHYLPREDNISOLONE AND INTRAVENOUS IMMUNOSUPPRESSANTS FOR RHEUMATOLOGY PATIENTS. Andrea Kovalesky, Childrens Hospital, Los Angeles and Diane Miller, Harbor-UCLA Medical Center, Torrance, California

The treatment of rheumatic diseases is becoming increasingly complex. Many medications being used on an experimental basis have significant nursing implications, including precautions in preparing and handling the medications, monitoring vital signs, care of nausea/vomiting, abnormal blood counts, alopecia, and potential for carcinogenesis and sterility. However, at present no guidelines for administering these drugs or counseling the patients who receive them are readily available to rheumatology nurses.

To determine current practice a survey was conducted of every other nurse listed in the AHPA directory regarding nursing aspects of intravenous methylprednisolone (IVMP) and intravenous cyclophosphamide (IVC) (N=174). 37% of the nurses responded, and of these, 26% had experience in administering IVMP, and 18% in administering IVC. The results showed that the majority of nurses administering these drugs (63%) had limited training in the nursing aspects of these drugs, and that a wide diversity of current practice exists. For example, 2/3's of nurses monitor vital signs every 15-20 minutes after the administration of IVMP, while 1/3 monitor vital signs only on a routine basis (every 4-8 hours).

In order to help formulate guidelines for nurses administering these drugs, all responses have been collated, and preliminary recommendations with related rationale have been extrapolated for each nursing aspect. In addition, a list of nurses with more extensive experience in experimental medications has been developed for distribution.

31

GETTING THE MESSAGE OUT: EDUCATING SCHOOL AND PUBLIC HEALTH NURSES IN THE COMMUNITY. Mary Jo Schneider, Carrie Goren Ingall, Balu H. Athreya. Pediatric Rheumatology Center, Children's Seashore House and The Children's Hospital of Philadelphia, Philadelphia.

Community outreach is an important aspect of care of children with low incidence, high impact illnesses, such as rheumatic disorders. Since school and public health nurses have more frequent contact with the children and their families, and are familiar with community resources, we developed a model to improve the skills and knowledge base of these nurses. The pediatric rheumatology nurse of a tertiary care center was instrumental in planning and implementing these educational programs.

The model designed from our experience in two outreach clinics included school and public health nurses of these counties as active members of the health care team. These nurses were expected to assess problems, make home visits, monitor progress, and identify resources for these children and their families. An educational program was introduced to help these professionals develop skills in case finding, follow-up assessment, dispelling myths, monitoring medications and therapy programs, and managing the psychosocial needs of children with rheumatic diseases. The outcome from educational sessions included improvement in referral system, fewer inappropriate referrals, and more effective communication between families, community resources, and the pediatric rheumatology center. Patient family outcome included high level of satisfaction and higher attendance rate at the outreach clinics. In the future, this model may be expanded to include community based physical and occupational therapists.

32

AN ARTHRITIS TRAINING PROGRAM FOR HOME HEALTH NURSES. S.E. Brunk, S. Wegener, C. Stabenow, A. Goodson, T. Vecchiolla, A. O'Leary, A. Thomas Doyle, University of Virginia, Charlottesville, and S. Liddle, Arthritis Foundation, Richmond, Virginia.

This paper describes a statewide educational program designed for home health nurses to increase their knowledge and skills in caring for persons having arthritis. A two day workshop was developed in cooperation with health professionals at the state university, the Arthritis Foundation, and various local health care resources. The workshop was presented to five nursing districts (n=200) of the state Health Department during the spring of 1985. Content of the program included the nature of the common rheumatic diseases, home management options, coping skills for dealing with chronic pain clients, and the range of local resources available.

The impetus for development of the workshop was three-fold. First, since the implementation of DRG's, an increase in the use of home health care services has been documented. Home health nurses are called upon to meet both competently and economically patient needs after reduced hospital stays. Second, due to the high prevalence of arthritis in the elderly, most of the population obtaining home health services, regardless of reason for referral, probably has arthritis. Third, the nurse has primary responsibility for case management, frequently without the assistance of a multidisciplinary team, particularly in rural areas.

Content areas covered were decided upon through a needs assessment of the home health nurses. The workshop uses an active learning approach of lecture/discussion and videotaped case study. An evaluation process, consisting of a pre- and post-test of both knowledge and attitudes, was conducted. The strengths and problems encountered will be presented.

This program suggests a new delivery system for disseminating information and increasing skills of home health nurses.

33

AN INSTRUCTIONAL MODEL FOR TEACHING RHEUMATOLOGY NURSING IN A BACCALAUREATE PROGRAM. Kuei-Shen Tu, University of Alabama, Birmingham, Alabama.

Greater emphasis on teaching Rheumatology Nursing in the nursing schools has been evident while the instructional strategies used may vary. It is the author's intention to present an instructional model for teaching Rheumatology nursing which has been in practice in our program. The model consists of utilization of multiple instructional strategies for facilitating student's learning. The placement of the content is in the Adult Health Nursing as a component of the concept of Mobility and Perception. The learning experience is structured based on the educational taxonomy in three phases. The initial phase of the learning experience consists of knowledge acquisition which is achieved through independent study guided by specific learning objectives. The second phase places emphasis on knowledge synthesis in a teacher guided seminar format in which students are assisted in translating the basic knowledge into a nursing process developed for a hypothetic client with rheumatoid arthritis. The final phase of the experience is achieved through clinical practice in selected clinical settings where the nursing process is carried out by the learner. The expected terminal behaviors of the students can be summarized as being able to demonstrate proficiency in the basic knowledge relevant to arthritis as a health stressor and its impact on the individual as a biological and social being, and critical skills in developing and executing the nursing process for clients experiencing the arthritic stressors.

34

PERCEPTIONS OF COMPETENCE: RHEUMATOLOGISTS VERSUS PHYSICAL THERAPISTS. C. Moncur. University of Utah, Salt Lake City, UT.

The purpose of this presentation is to describe the differences in perceptions between rheumatologists and two groups of physical therapists regarding the competencies needed for the entry level physical therapist to deliver arthritis patient care. Eighty competencies in rheumatology were identified by 288 individuals using the survey method for gathering data. The respondents were 80 rheumatologists, 108 physical therapists who were AHPs, and 100 physical therapists who were clinical educators and not AHP members. Reliability of the survey instrument was determined to be .95. Content validity was obtained from a panel of national experts in rheumatology.

Since multiple comparisons were done in this study, the Bonferroni inequality statistic was used to scale the significance level to a conservative level of .007. Nonparametric statistics were used to test for differences between groups. Levels of importance of a competency were compared for the different groups using the Kruskal-Wallis One Way ANOVA and the Mann-Whitney test for pair-wise comparisons. The Mantel-Haensel test was used to complete a test for location of standard deviations.

When comparing the three groups' responses, the data revealed that there was a significant difference in perception between these groups on 20 competencies ($p = .007$). Comparisons of standard deviations determined that each group had considerable variability in their responses on various competencies ($p = .007$).

Because of the heterogeneity of responses on these competencies, exclusion of them from a physical therapy curriculum is not warranted. Further studies should be conducted to ascertain if there are any differences between traditional and competency-based student performances.

35

PROBLEMS AND PERSPECTIVES IN MEDICAL COMPLIANCE FOR CHILDREN WITH JUVENILE RHEUMATOID ARTHRITIS (JRA) C. Ross, J. Goletz, G. Frommelt, S. Ramirez, Northwestern U. and Childrens Memorial Hospital, Chicago

The purposes of this investigation were 1) to determine the extent to which medication and exercise compliance occurs, 2) to identify factors which may increase or decrease compliance, 3) to suggest issues of importance in planning compliance education interventions.

Data, including reported medication and exercise compliance, reasons for compliance difficulty and individual responsibility for compliance, were obtained through questionnaires from 70 JRA patients and their parents. Exercise compliance was reported to be significantly lower than medication compliance ($p<.05$). In spite of provider perception that all children had some kind of exercise recommendation, nearly half reported that they had none. Reasons given for failure to comply included pain and time involved. The relationship between age and compliance was significant at the .01 level. Older children were less likely to follow recommendations. In addition, the relationship between child's age and compliance responsibility was significant, ($p<.001$). Parents were more likely to be responsible for assuring younger child compliance. For older children, the child was more often responsible.

The findings suggest that the greatest need for JRA compliance education may be for exercise with older children. Educational programs should emphasize specifity of recommendations and incentives for following recommendations. Furthermore, educational programs to increase compliance should give attention to age. Education for younger children may be aimed at the parent and child. Programs for older children may emphasize the child's responsibility and participation.

36

EVALUATION AND TREATMENT OF THE PEDIATRIC REFLEX NEUROVASCULAR DYSTROPHY PATIENT. Kathy Wotring, Joan Mehn, Carol Stengem, Childrens Hospital of Los Angeles, Los Angeles, California.

Reflex Neurovascular Dystrophy (RND), a syndrome characterized by severe pain with associated autonomic dysfunction, frequently results in serious functional impairment of the involved extremity. RND is common in adults, but considered rare in children. Since 1969, the rheumatologists and therapists here have successfully treated approximately 75 pediatric cases. The purpose of this paper is to share our methods of evaluation and treatment and to review their effectiveness in 2 representative cases.

Although often mistaken for other rheumatic diseases, typical physical and psychological characteristics have been identified that help differentiate RND. Most authorities agree that pediatric RND is less severe and disabling than adult RND, but early diagnosis and treatment are critical elements for successful and timely recovery. The main objective, breaking the pain-disability cycle, requires admission to a rehabilitation center in most cases.

A team approach is important for consistent feedback to the patient. Our team consists of a rheumatologist, psychologist, primary nurse, a physical and an occupational therapist. The team's goals and approach change as the patient progresses. The ultimate discharge goal is the patient's physical function will be normal.

An aggressive physical therapy program is essential and sensory stimulation, intensive weight bearing activities, ROM and strengthening exercises form the basis of our program. The need for drugs or surgery has been eliminated in most cases, and the patients have been discharged with normal physical function.

37

EXERCISE CARDS: A METHOD TO INCREASE COMPLIANCE AND IMPROVE ATTITUDES IN HOME EXERCISE PROGRAMS WITH THE PEDIATRIC POPULATION. C.L. Chronic and P.G. Melson, Atlanta, Emory Univ. Regional Pediatric Rheum. Center

To increase or maintain joint mobility and strength it is vital that children with juvenile rheumatoid arthritis (JRA) participate in home exercise programs. Poor compliance by the child and family in a consistent exercise routine is a frequent problem encountered by therapists and physicians. A structured program allowing children choice and variation is needed. The objective of this project was to establish a simple inexpensive format of exercise to meet that need. One effective method to increase compliance and patient involvement has been the development of individualized programs utilizing exercise cards. Instructions and photos of each exercise are placed on an index card. The child is allowed to arrange the exercise cards daily in any order he/she desires prior to beginning the program. Supplies needed for each child include index cards, photos of exercises, clear contact paper as a protective covering for the cards, file boxes or 2" steel rings for card storage. The benefits of these cards have been observed by therapists, physicians, and parents. They provide children with a method of control over their exercise program. An increase in motivation and involvement has been seen. The children are more enthusiastic about their exercise programs and regularly bring their cards to treatment sessions. Parents are comfortable with the exercise cards as it allows them to provide flexibility in their children's exercise program. Designing exercise programs utilizing an index card format has been a very effective method to increase compliance and involvement with children and their families. Cost is minimal and a definite increase in participation has been observed.

38

IPSILATERAL HIP FLEXION CONTRACTURE AS A CONSEQUENCE OF ISOLATED KNEE INVOLVEMENT IN JUVENILE ARTHRITIS: Virginia Wright and B. Cairns, Hugh MacMillan Medical Centre and A. Shore, Hospital for Sick Children, Toronto, Ontario Canada.

Children with Pauciarticular Juvenile Arthritis (PcJA) with unilateral knee synovitis and knee flexion contracture (KFC) may develope a secondary flexion contracture of the ipsilateral uninvolved hip. Prescence of an unaccomodated true leg length discrepancy (LLD) intensifies the hip flexion contracture (HFC). This report emphasises, through varied clinical presentations, the need to detect and treat early HFC in this setting. Three cases are used to highlight distinct stages of this problem. Each of the patients had PcJA with unilateral knee involvement, a LLD > 1 CM, normal hip x-rays and full painfree hip rotation. All LLD's had been accomodated only after development of the HFC. Each patient had previously received physical therapy (PT) only for their KFC.

Patient 1 presented with a 30° KFC with no measurable HFC but tight ipsilateral hip flexors on passive stretch and weaker hip extensors on this side. Patient 2 presented with a 25° KFC with a 15° ipsilateral HFC. The KFC resolved with PT, but the 15° HFC persisted. Patient 3 had a 20° KFC 6 years earlier and presented in remission with full knee extension but a persistent 20° HFC, and a fixed hyperloidosis. A gait study confirmed that movement and muscle activity about the knee joint were normal. This confirms our observations that an untreated secondary HFC may be a more persistent problem than the original KFC. In summary, secondary HFC's are a serious complication of unilateral knee involvement in PcJA requiring intensive PT intervention at the onset of disease.

39

THE MODIFIED SPHYGMOMANOMETER (MS)-A SENSITIVE TOOL FOR MEASURING MUSCLE STRENGTH IN CHILDREN: Virginia Wright, Hugh MacMillan Medical Centre and Abraham Shore, Hospital for Sick Children, Toronto, Canada.

Sequential, accurate and reproducible evaluations of muscle strength are an essential component of the clinical assessment of Juvenile Arthritis (JA) and childhood Dermatomyositis (DM). We compared a method employing MS with the conventional Oxford Grading System (OGS) as a means of quantifiying muscle strength in 5 children (3 JRA;2DM). MS muscle testing has previously been validated and used in adult Rheumatoid Arthritis (1).

MS and OGS measurements were taken twice at 3 month intervals. Muscle groups chosen corresponded with the child's disease activity. each assessment also included an active joint count, review of medications, and an evaluation of range of motion, grip strength and functional abilities. MS measurements were found to be a more sensitive indicator of the patient's changing status than OGS, grip strength or functional changes. This sensitivity was demonstrated in DM where differences in MS were the first sign of a disease flare. Decreases of muscle strength in JA, particularly at the hip, were predictors of joint involvement or worsening.

In addition, sequential MS measurements aided in the evaluation of responses to new drugs or physical therapy regimes and served as guide lines in designing and revising exercise programs. Regular monitoring added incentive to exercise compliance for both child and parent. In summary, the MS provides a sensitive objective measurement valuable in the management of JA and DM.

(1) Helena, A Goldsmith CH, Smythe, HA, J. Chron Dis. 34:353-61,1981

40

APPLICATION OF THE PRECEDE MODEL OF PLANNING A HEALTH EDUCATION PROGRAM IN THE WORKPLACE: LESSONS FROM THE BRIGHAM BACK PROGRAM. L. Daltroy, H. Eaton, L. Pallozzi, Robert B. Brigham Multipurpose Arthritis Center, Brigham and Women's Hospital, Boston.

Arthritis health professionals and physicians are increasingly involved in preventive and ameliorative programs for musculoskeletal problems in the workplace. However, many preventive programs have been based on mere provision of information and transfer of treatment-based approaches, which are unlikely to be effective.

Development of an effective program which addresses behaviors can be approached with a diagnostic and planning model developed by Green, et al. This workshop will present critical issues and planning steps, using Green's PRECEDE model, in designing an educational program for health problems in an industrial setting. A program to reduce low back injuries in the U.S. Postal Service will be used as a case study.

Participants will be able to: (1) state the steps in Green's diagnostic model for designing a health education program; (2) state the rationale for using the model in program planning; (3) describe how the model could be applied to a health problem and setting with which they are personally familiar; and (4) identify key issues influencing the design and implementation of a program to reduce low back injuries in industry.

Methods include lecture with audio-visual aids, group discussion in a seminar format, and handouts. The target audience is health care professionals interested in health education program planning for the worksite. The approach will be at the intermediate level.

41

PEDIATRIC RHEUMATOLOGY NURSING STANDARDS: UPDATE AND GOALS. SANDRA K. AMUNDSON, La Rabida Children's Hospital and Research Center, Chicago, and Diane M. Erlandson, New England Medical Center, Boston.

Pediatric rheumatology patients and their families have special needs because of the impact of a chronic unpredictable disease on normal childhood developmental processes and patterns of family functioning. Because of the relative infrequency of pediatric rheumatology disease many professionals could enhance quality of care using specific standards for pediatric practice. Nurses from several centers have proposed nursing standards appropriate to meet these needs. This roundtable will provide opportunity to review these suggested standards, which focus on pediatric rheumatology nursing and how they relate to the Outcome Standards for Rheumatology Nursing Practice (ANA and AHPA, 1983).

Six areas of outcome standards have currently been identified. These topics are to understand disease process and management; adapt effectively to disease process, realize individual potential; incorporate therapeutic measures into daily activities; performs tasks appropriate to developmental stage; and family functions effectively.

Three objectives are identified for the session: 1) Define the process being utilized to develop and validate the pediatric rheumatology nursing standards. 2) Identify how session participants may contribute to validation of the standards. 3) Provide a forum for review and critique of plans for development of the standards.

Lectures and accompanying written handouts about each topic will be followed by discussion. The content is designed for all nurses and other arthritis health professionals interested in pediatric rheumatology and the continued refinement of practice standards. This activity is supported by the H.H.S., Division of Maternal and Child Health

42

PHYSICAL THERAPY EVALUATION AND REHABILITATION PROTOCOL FOR THE POLYMYOSITIS PATIENT. Linda K. Schroeder and Edward J. Fudman. University of Michigan Hospitals, Ann Arbor, Michigan.

Physical therapy programs for the patient with polymyositis or other inflammatory muscle syndromes vary with the clinical presentation of the disease. The clinician should be aware of the indicators on which a treatment program is designed and altered. Clinical manifestations of polymyositis and current theories of the disease process will be discussed. A physical therapy rehabilitation program based on the activity of the disease will be presented. The need for coordinated team involvement will be emphasized.

This workshop will enable participants to 1) identify clinical manifestations of polymyositis, 2) develop a comprehensive rehabilitation program, 3) explain the rationale for physical therapy programs, 4) select appropriate physical therapy evaluation procedures, 5) design a physical therapy treatment program based on the activity of the disease, and 6) rcognize the importance for interdisciplinary involvement.

The workshop leaders will present information through a lecture process with audiovisual aids, handouts, and demonstration, emphasizing participatory learning.

This workshop is presented for physical therapists and all other health professionals concerned with rehabilitation needs of this population.

43

SELF-ADMINISTERED FUNCTION MEASURES: THE IMPOSSIBLE DREAM?

Jean Goeppinger, M. Anne Thomas Doyle, Marianne Murdock, Brian L. Wilcox, Susan E. Brunk. University of Virginia, Charlottesville.

Two measures of function widely used for persons with arthritis, the Health Assessment Questionnaire (HAQ) and the Arthritis Impact Measurement Scales (AIMS), are reported to be self-administerable. However, in a study comparing the two instruments in a rural population, it was found that 72% of the participants required assistance in completing the questionnaires.

Ninety subjects were tested, 30 with osteoarthritis, 30 with rheumatoid arthritis, and 30 with diabetes mellitus. All lived in rural areas. The sample had a mean age of 60.7 years, was 78% female, 12% black, and had an average of 10.5 years of formal education.

The psychometric properties of both instruments were good and closely resembled those reported elsewhere with test-retest reliabilities of r=.93 and r=.87 for the HAQ and AIMS, respectively. Differences from other reports were found in the ease of administration for both instruments. Over one third of the sample required assistance in either reading or writing the forms; one third required assistance with clarification of words and directions. Additionally, it was found that 25% of the items on the HAQ and 32% of the items on the AIMS had little or no relevance to rural persons.

These outcomes suggest that the concept of "self-administration" may need re-evaluation. Guidelines for examining this issue and its implications in other arthritis research and practice will be discussed.

44

USE OF THE ARTHRITIS IMPACT MEASUREMENTS SCALES (AIMS) FOR PATIENT EVALUATION ON AN ARTHRITIS REHABILITATION UNIT.

Cynthia A. Stabenow, Stephen T. Wegener, Amy A. O'Leary, Carolyn M. Brunner, University of Virginia Medical Center, Charlottesville, Virginia.

The measurement properties of the AIMS instrument have been investigated primarily with outpatient samples. We have administered the AIMS to a different population of respondents: RA patients (n=50) admitted to a multidisciplinary inpatient Arthritis Rehabilitation Unit (ARU). Following a patient's admission, the AIMS is used to evaluate pain, physical function, and psychological status. A comparison sample of RA outpatients (n=65) have also completed the AIMS in the clinic.

Many of our patients come from rural, medically underserved areas, and their income and education levels tend to be notably lower than those of earlier AIMS respondent samples. Our patients also appear to have more severe, disabling RA. In the first few months of data collection many patients were found to have writing or reading problems that made self-administration of the AIMS difficult or impossible. Consequently, the AIMS is now administered to our inpatients and outpatients by trained interviewers.

Descriptive statistics will be used to present the AIMS data and the demographic and disease characteristics of our respondents. Correlations between AIMS scores and demographic and disease characteristics will also be highlighted. T-test results show that the ARU patients have significantly poorer health than the outpatients on 7 of 9 AIMS scales. Thus, the AIMS may be useful for identifying patients most in need of inpatient rehabilitation. Our presentation will also show the results of discriminant analysis to determine which AIMS subscales differentiate ARU inpatients and outpatients to the greatest extent.

45

A COMPARISON OF FUNCTIONAL STATUS MEASURES IN PATIENTS WITH RHEUMATOID ARTHRITIS (RA).

M. Hambridge, Georgia State, F. Curtiss, Emory University, Atlanta, C. Hastings, B. Tack, NIH, Bethesda, R. Smith III, Atlanta, C. Wilson, Emory University, Atlanta.

There are many instruments available to AHPs for assessing functional status in patients with arthritis. The purpose of this study was to compare the Convery Arthritis Assessment Tool (CAAT) to several other functional measures for use by AHPs. Twenty-five patients with RA were seen for 6 visits at 5 week intervals. Evaluations included a subjective rating of overall functional status by the patients, the Stanford Health Assessment Questionaire (HAQ), the CAAT, an articular index (AI) and an overall functional rating by the physician.

Results were evaluated by correlating scores between instruments for each visit. Strong correlations (r .70, p.01) were found between the CAAT, the HAQ and the physician rating. Moderate correlations (r .60,p .01) were found between the CAAT and the patient self report and the AI. The relationship between the patient and physician overall ratings varied considerably.

Findings of a strong similarity between the CAAT and the HAQ suggest that a choice between the two instruments could be made on the basis of brevity and ease of use. The relationship between the patient self report and other measures raises questions about the operational definition of functional status that invite further investigation.

46

A RHEUMATOLOGY ATTITUDES INDEX (RAI): RELATION TO DEMOGRAPHIC, PERFORMANCE, QUESTIONNAIRE AND MEDICAL MEASURES IN RHEUMATOID ARTHRITIS.

L.F. Callahan and T. Pincus, Nashville, TN.

The Rheumatology Attitudes Index (RAI) consists of 15 statements, e.g., "My condition is controlling my life," for which the patient indicates one of 5 responses: "Strongly agree," "Agree," "Do not agree or disagree," "Disagree," "Strongly disagree." The Index was developed to assess patient perceptions of their capacity to control their illness, as a measure of coping with "learned helplessness" as a psychological construct. The RAI was administered to 255 rheumatoid arthritis (RA) patients, whose clinical status was also assessed with a Modified Health Assessment Questionnaire (MHAQ), regarding functional capacity in activities of daily living, joint count, and three performance tests of functional capacity--grip strength, button test and walking time. RAI scores were not significantly correlated with age, duration of disease, or sedimentation rate, but higher scores (indicating lower control) were highly associated with lower educational levels. RAI scores were significantly correlated with MHAQ scores for difficulty, dissatisfaction, and pain ($p<.001$), and at lower levels with joint count, grip strength, button test and walking time ($p<.05$). The correlations of the RAI with disease and functional measures remained significant when controlled for age, duration of disease or educational level. These data suggest that the RAI may provide a useful index for assessment of psychological status in rheumatic diseases. Self-report data in the RAI appear to be more highly correlated with self-report data regarding functional capacity, compared to data from joint count or performance tests of functional capacity.

47

THE DEVELOPMENT AND MANAGEMENT OF SELF-HELP GROUPS: A COMPARISON OF THREE MODELS.

Karen Schmid, Childrens Hospital of Orange County, Orange, California, and Christine Ellis, University of California Irvine Medical Center, Orange, California.

The continuing proliferation of self-help groups and patient clubs is evidence of both the need for and the value of such organizations. Health professionals are frequently involved in their development and management.

The purpose of this workshop is to assist the AHP in determining the skills needed in the preparation for development of a self-help group, or in the evaluation of an existing group. Three unique existing groups will be presented and compared in terms of their composition, goals, activities and roles of participants and AHP's. Groups discussed will include an arthritis group, a lupus group and a JRA parent group. Participants will gain an understanding of the concept of self-help and the need for patient groups. Further, they will learn the steps involved in assessment of a community's needs, and promoting a group designed to meet specific needs.

In addition to lecture, a videotape demonstrating group process will be viewed and discussed. Group discussion will be focused on application of this material to the participant's community and existing groups. This workshop is intended for a beginning to intermediate multidisciplinary audience, but would also be of interest to the seasoned group leader who desires consultation on the problems of a specific group.

48

NURSING RESEARCH IN RHEUMATOLOGY.

J. Sakalys, University of Colorado Health Sciences Center, Denver, CO, C. S. Burckhardt, Oregon Health Sciences University, Portland, OR, K. Lorig, Stanford Arthritis Center, Stanford, CA.

Although research conducted by nurse members of AHPA has a long and respected history, this research has been scarce and often has been conducted in isolation from nurse colleagues. As increasing numbers of nurses with research interests and credentials join AHPA, it is vital to provide this professional group with a structured opportunity to dialogue and network.

The purpose of this roundtable session, therefore, is to convene beginning and experienced nurse researchers for discussion of views, issues, concerns, state of the art, and future directions in rheumatological nursing research.

Potential outcomes of this session include increased networking among nurse researchers as well as increased scope and methodological rigor of nursing research in rheumatology.

49

INTERNATIONAL VIEWS AND ACTIVITIES OF ARTHRITIS MANAGEMENT: AHP'S (Arthritis Health Professionals) THROUGHOUT THE WORLD. Barbara Banwell, University of Michigan/Flint and Ann Arbor, and Janice Smith Pigg, Columbia Hospital, Milwaukee.

The overall goal of this workshop is to acquaint health professionals with various styles of arthritis management in countries and cultures other than the United States. Specific emphasis will be upon European countries and Australia. Information will focus upon the roles of health professionals in medication management, exercise, physical modalities, self care activities, patient education and patient/family/social issues. The activities of health professional organizations throughout the world will be discussed. The principle presenters have observed arthritis care in Europe and Australia during the past 12 months and will be prepared to share the most current issues in arthritis care throughout the world. Other professionals who have recent experience in other countries and cultures will be welcome to participate in the presentations. Attendees at the 1985 International League Against Rheumatism (ILAR) will share share impressions of those meetings. A secondary goal of the workshop will be to interest participants in the formal development of an international AHP organization and to identify individuals prepared to pursue such activities. Teaching methods will include lecture, discussion, audio-visual aids and handouts. All health professionals are welcome.

50

EXPLORING INNOVATIVE PHYSICAL THERAPY METHODS FOR YOUNG JRA CHILDREN. Margaret King, Carole Fujishige, Raquel Hicks. Pediatric Arthritis Center, Honolulu.

Experience shows that young JRA children who require regular physical therapy often find repetitious therapy sessions uninteresting. Attention span in young children is usually poor, and compliance both for attendance to PT sessions and home therapy programs is not ideal. Furthermore, a typical JRA child begins to feel "different" because he/she needs "special exercises" in a health care setting, often developing low self-esteem, ongoing anxiety, and social isolation.

In response to these determinations, PACH last year developed two group programs--the "Tiny Tots" recreational exercise group, and a swim class for young JRA children. These groups provided exercise in a casual "open air" environment utilizing a variety of age-appropriate equipment, media and music to stimulate active physical participation, and to encourage socialization among their peers.

Our groups were small, averaging 5 children ages 3½-6 years. At the beginning 4 were shy and withdrawn and 1 refused to participate. Gradually, the children met the challenge and after 12 classes, all engaged in more active participation. In the 6 post-test series, 3 children showed marked increase in gross muscle strength and coordination. Parents post-evaluation expressed satisfaction in peer interaction and positive teachers' reports.

In summary, both groups proved surprisingly beneficial. Because of salubrious weather conditions all year round, the state of Hawaii offers multiple opportunities for open-air exercise therapy to young JRA children, and it seems a worthwhile endeavor to pursue.

51

"PEDIATRIC ARTHRITIS CENTER OF HAWAII - SUPPORTING TEENS". Margery Y. Lee, Raquel V. Hicks, Pediatric Arthritis Center of Hawaii, Honolulu. (PACH).

Among our teenaged patients with rheumatic diseases, common psychosocial issues emerged. The objective of PACH's Teen Support Group was to provide supportive services to our adolescent patients using group process. Patients from ages 14 through 17 years were selected to participate in the group. A total of 8 patients expressed interest in this activity. The teens met in weekly one and a half hour sessions which was held for 8 consecutive weeks. Each session was facilitated by the social worker. All patients were given a pre and post service questionnaire. The following areas were targeted: 1) family life 2) school performance 3) peer relationships and 4) expression of feelings about their illness.

Post service results demonstrated no significant changes in patients' rating of family life, school performance or peer relationships. However, it must be noted that 7 out of 8 patients rated these targeted areas in the good to excellent category on both pre and post test questionnaires. Four patients felt they increased the expression of feelings about their illness. All patients commented that meeting and sharing with others via the support group was beneficial.

Although data analysis showed no significant changes in patients' rating of family life, school performance, and peer relationships, these were rated high prior to and after the group activity underscoring the belief that those selected patients were well-adjusted teenagers from supportive families. The important change was the increase in the expression of feelings about their illness, and it is speculated that future support groups will substantiate this finding.

52

THE DEVELOPMENT OF A J.R.A. FAMILY EDUCATION REFERENCE MANUAL. ANDREA KOVALESKY, Children's Hospital of Los Angeles, Sandra K. Amundson, La Rabida Children's Hospital and Research Center, Chicago, Michelle Boutaugh, National Office of the Arthritis Foundation, Atlanta and Nancy A. Tehan, Dartmouth-Hitchcock Medical Center, Hanover, New Hampshire.

Patient education is now recognized as a vital component of the health care plan. In rheumatology many health professionals are actively involved in developing and utilizing a wide variety of excellent patient education materials and resources. Yet sometimes there is duplication or gaps in these materials and resources, or it may be difficult for new professionals in the field to locate or obtain them. This is particularly true in pediatric rheumatology, which is a relatively new area with a number of new centers being rapidly developed on a national basis.

In an effort to provide a more comprehensive patient education program in pediatric rheumatology on a readily accessible basis to both private practitioners and multi-disciplinary centers, a nation wide pediatric rheumatology education task force was developed through the assistance of the National Office of the Arthritis Foundation. This group has been working for over a year in the collection of data through a multi-center educational needs assessment and in formulation of learning objectives with suggested interventions for implementation. The interventions have a developmental basis for the various age groups and existing resources are being incorporated as much as possible. This session is designed to share with a wide variety of rheumatology health professionals the committee's work to date, as well as be a vehicle for receiving any additional input or assistance in completing the final project (anticipated completion in 1985).

53

COMPARISON OF PAIN RATINGS BETWEEN THE JUVENILE RHEUMATOID ARTHRITIS (JRA) CHILD, THE PARENTS AND PHYSICIAN. Diane Block, Joyce Falco, J. Roger Hollister. The National Jewish Center for Respiratory and Immune Medicine, Rocky Mountain Juvenile Arthritis Center, Denver, Colorado

The purpose of this pilot study was to compare the perceptions of pain in the JRA child as rated by the child, the child's parents and the pediatric rheumatologist. The subjects are 25 JRA children from 6-16 years old and their parents. A visual analogue scale and a drawing for identification of painful joints were administered to the children privately as part of a structured interview. Simultaneously, parents completed a visual analogue scale depicting their perception of the severity of their child's pain. Additionally, the physician completed a routine joint count, recording swelling, tenderness and limitation of motion.

Correlations between the child and parent visual analogue scores, parent and physician assessment, and the child and physician ratings have revealed patterns of agreement and discrepancy. Trends of child and parental pain minimization and exaggeration were demonstrated which will be helpful in the clinical evaluation and management of children with arthritis and in future pain research.

54

IMPACT OF RHEUMATIC DISEASE ON PARENTING AND SUGGESTED MANAGEMENT STRATEGIES. S. Allaire, Boston University, Boston, P. Green, Brigham and Women's Hospital, Boston, J. Weaver, Internal Medicine Specialties, Lincoln, NE, B. Whitmeyer, Lahey Clinic, Burlington, MA.

Rheumatic diseases (RA, SLE, PSS) often occur in individuals who have or plan to have children. Disease symptoms and effects produce child care adjustments and difficulties which could be alleviated and any potential negative impact prevented. This requires recognition of common problems and application of preventive or treatment strategies. People with these diseases are seeking information from health professionals, but little exists.

This project was designed to both collect and organize existing information about disabled parenting with specific reference to rheumatic disease, and to solicit relevant new information. A literature review was conducted with information collected about problems and solutions. This information was then used to formulate an 18 item questionnaire which was administered to 20 women who have a rheumatic disease and who provide care to children. Finally child care related survey notes from a series of interviews with intact families in which the mother has RA were examined. One finding that is a potentially negative effect is maternal impatience during disease flare. Benefits were unexpectedly found also. For example, parents who cannot physically discipline tend to establish more cooperative relationships with their children.

Information from these three sources was compiled with commonalities identified. The results will assist health professionals in providing care to parents who have rheumatic diseases, and stimulate needed research on the family implications of rheumatic diseases.

55

EVALUATION OF NEW CERVICAL COLLAR. V. White, Vancouver, B.C.

An evaluation of a new cervical collar constructed from nylon tubes and soft PVC tubing has been completed. Symptomatic relief, adherence to prescribed wearing schedule and desireability of the collar's design were determined.

Twelve adult patients had been fitted with the new collar by Arthritis Centre occupational therapists. Mailed questionnaires and telephone interviews were used to obtain self-reported data.

All patients suffering from occipital headaches, neck pain (at rest or with activity) and malalignment problems reported relief or correction as a result of wearing the collar. Radiating pain to the upper extremity was relieved in two out of three cases. Neurological signs in the upper extremity were relieved in one patient but not in another.

At the time of follow-up, 46% of patients were wearing their collars some part of every day, 56% were not wearing their collars at all. Reasons given for not wearing the collar included functional limitations, uncomfortable pressure points and decline in symptoms. Weight, coolness, cosmesis and support were favourably rated design characteristics. Comfort and adaptability to a variety of activities were rated unfavourably.

In general, the collar was thought to be effective in relieving symptoms, however, specific design features need alteration to provide the comfort that is necessary for compliance.

56

WRIST WORKING SPLINT: WHAT IS IT MEANT TO DO? V. White, K.P. MacBain, The Arthritis Society, Vancouver, B.C.

The wrist working splint is commonly prescribed in the conservative management of rheumatoid arthritis patients. This study examines what health professionals expect from such a splint and how patients rate their wrist problems.

A questionnaire survey of 55 health professionals (18 doctors, 4 registered nurses, 2 social workers, 14 physiotherapists and 16 occupational therapists) showed pain with activity ranking highest among problems thought to be affected by wearing splints. Instability function and weakness followed in that order. Swelling, pain at rest, tenderness, fatigue, range of motion and deformity were thought to be affected less by the splint.

Three-quarters of patients answering questionnaires considered pain with activity to be the most serious of their wrist problems. Weakness, pain at rest and swelling were next. In general, patients expected most symptoms (except for deformity) to be somewhat relieved by splinting. The majority expected to be able to do more when wearing working splints.

The expectations which health professionals have of wrist working splints appear to satisfactorily match the actual patient problems.

A further study is planned to assess the actual effectiveness of such splints, using objective functional tests and questionnaires.

57

SPLINT USE IN RHEUMATOID ARTHRITIS. S.L. Hanneman, S.R. Weiner, Olive View Medical Center, Van Nuys, CA 91405.

A patient's views on splint use may differ from that of the occupational therapist (OT) or physician (MD). We performed a prospective study to evaluate splint use in rheumatoid arthritis (RA).

14 patients with classic RA were studied. Each was given wrist, resting and ulnar deviation splints with standard instructions and education. Followup evaluation was done at 12 months and consisted of a questionnaire, visual analogue pain scales, OT and MD assessment.

86% of patients preferred wrist splints to ulnar deviation or resting splints. 50% felt the splints made activities more awkward. 64% had difficulty sleeping with splints on. Almost all subjects (93%) recommended splints for other RA patients.

Patients were taught that splints were to be used for joint protection, reduction of inflammation andpain relief. After one year the patients felt the indications for splint use were pain (100%), joint protection (21%), and reduction of inflammation (0%). All patients noted less pain while wearing splints. Despite the belief that the splints were for pain control, NO subject consistently wore splints when in pain.

In summary, the majority of patients felt pain was the primary indication for splint use and only a minority used splints for other suggested uses. The splints did relieve pain which provided reinforcement for this indication over others. The fact that splints were not always worn for pain may relate to feeling awkward or difficulty sleeping while in splints. Wrist splints were favored because they relieved pain and left more freedom of motion.

In conclusion, patients' concern for pain and freedom of motion must be addressed before compliance and education for splint use can occur.

58

A NEW APPROACH TO SPLINTING. Angela Fairleigh, Richard E. Hannah, Vancouver, Ontario, Canada

A new approach to the contruction of splints has been developed based on nylon tubes and soft PVC tubing linked by various junctions. Custom assembly and modification is possible from written instructions, without special tools or facilities. Assembly is reversible and the components are interchangeable, permitting assembly of a wide range of splints from the same basic components.

This system has been applied in the management of arthritis for the construction of cervical collars and knee resting splints.

Coolness, increased support, fine adjustment and good cosmesis have been achieved in the collar design. For the management of knee flexion contractures in J.R.A., a lightweight splint has been developed that can be finely adjusted at each application. It can be fitted with accuracy and speed, and is consequently less alarming for the very young child.

In a survey of therapists ease of fabrication and adjustment, adequacy of support and relief of symptoms, patient compliance and device durability all scored higher than the plastazote collar. Patients generally prefer the coolness, better support and improved cosmesis of this approach to splinting.

59

ARTHRITIS EXPERIENCE AND SOCIAL SUPPORT AS PREDICTORS OF PSYCHOLOGICAL DYSFUNCTION IN RA. Perry Nicassio, Gregory Brown, Kenneth Wallston and Nancy Szydlo. Vanderbilt University.

Patients with RA differ significantly in their psychosocial adjustment and their ability to cope with this condition. The purpose of this research was to empirically identify correlates of psychological dysfunction in a survey investigation of the psychological and behavioral concomitants of RA.

The sample consisted of 347 patients, 87 males and 260 females, who had been diagnosed as having RA within the last 7½ years. Patients completed and returned by mail a questionnaire which included the assessment of the severity of arthritis experience (i.e. measures of pain, global health status and flare-ups), psychological dysfunction (i.e. measures of depression, anxiety, arthritis helplessness and a lack of general self-efficacy) and the availability, quality and extent of the social support network.

Stepwise multiple regression analysis revealed that severity of arthritis experience and social support functioned as significant, independent predictors of psychological dysfunction, accounting for greater than 57% of the variance in this index. While severity of arthritis experience was positively correlated with psychological dysfunction (r=.68), quality of social support was negatively correlated with psychological dysfunction (r=-.36). The results suggest that a strong relationship exists between degree of pain and poor health status associated with RA and psychological dysfunction in patients with more recent RA diagnoses. However, patients with effective social support may be more immune to the deleterious impact of RA, and may have a greater likelihood of achieving a more positive psychological adjustment in face of this chronic disease.

60

DO YOU KNOW WHAT PATIENTS WANT? LAY AND PROFESSIONAL PERCEPTIONS OF THE EDUCATIONAL NEEDS OF RURAL PERSONS WITH ARTHRITIS. Jean Goeppinger, M. Anne Thomas Doyle, Susan E. Brunk, Marianne Murdock, and Carolyn M. Brunner. University of Virginia, Charlottesville.

This study indicates that most arthritis health professionals do know what their patients perceive to be important educational needs. This is noteworthy as there is growing consensus about the importance of health education to informed self-care. Curricula to teach persons with arthritis about such self-care behaviors as exercise, sleep and rest, medication usage, and nutrition have been developed and widely disseminated. To our knowledge, however, these curricula have not been based on a systematic assessment of both lay and professional perceptions of specific educational needs. Since perceptions might be expected to differ because of the rigorous professional socialization of most health care providers, such an assessment is an important first step in curriculum design.

The purpose of this study was to compare the perceptions of persons with arthritis (n=52), physicians (n=77), chiropractors (n=16), physical therapists (n=34), and community workers (n=53) on the value of education about 14 self-care behaviors. The results suggest that patient-provider congruence is unexpectedly high, but that the perceptions of physical therapists differ significantly from those of physicians, patients, and community workers. These differences were in the areas of sexual behavior, medication usage, sleep and rest, energy conservation and joint protection, and nutrition and diet.

61

"BONE UP ON ARTHRITIS": AN UPDATE ON SELF-CARE EDUCATION FOR RURAL PERSONS. Jean Goeppinger, Susan E. Brunk, M. Anne Thomas Doyle. University of Virginia, Charlottesville.

Patients and health care professionals must collaborate when attempting the effective management of chronic diseases such as arthritis. Two types of educational programs have been designed to improve patients' self-care capabilities and to augment existing medical care. They are currently being tested with persons having arthritis who live in rural areas.

In the first type of program, persons with arthritis receive six audiotape/booklet sets for self-paced study in their homes. In the second type of program, persons receive the same curricular material in small groups of approximately 15 persons. The classes are taught by community members who have been identified and trained by the project staff. Both programs emphasize self-management and self-efficacy, as well as mastery of relevant content. Topics covered include exercise, pain management, and getting a good night's sleep.

These content areas were chosen from existing materials, such as Lorig's self-help curriculum, and a needs assessment conducted among patients, physicians and other health care workers living and working in rural areas. Additional considerations related to rurality, such as low literacy levels, geographic dispersion, and dependence on indigenous leadership, also guided development of the programs' content and format.

The programs are presently being implemented in eight counties of a mid-Atlantic state. Investigation is occurring to compare the efficacy of the small group and the individualized educational self-care programs as mechanisms for self-care education in rural areas.

62

CAN MICROCOMPUTER INSTRUCTION HELP OA PATIENTS. Robert Rippey, Dee Bill, John Day, Debbie Downing, Carol A. Pfeiffer, Sally Marlowe, Sara Thal, Scott Wetstone and Micha Abeles, University of Connecticut Health Center MAC, Farmington.

Purpose: In order to reach an elderly population with cost and labor effective methods, instructional computer programs for use in senior centers by persons with OA have been developed.

Computer lessons developed are: 1) facts about arthritis, 2) medication, 3) exercise, 4) sources of information and help, 5) coping, 6) relaxation, 7) joint protection, 8) communication, 9) adaptive devices. Methods of programming, production of visual material, blending text and methods of evaluating both materials and outcomes will be shown. Others have shown that older persons can and will use computers to learn more about their rheumatic disease. We have developed programs which **simplify** computer operation, **motivate** through the use of color and animation, and **emphasize** what is important through timing, pacing, contrast, and color.

Future evaluation will determine whether or not these materials can teach arthritis patients accurate information in a cost effective way.

63

ARTHRITIS SELF HELP COURSE GUIDELINES AND PROCEDURES-EASTERN PA. CHAPTER. M. Becker, D. Hicks, A. Huber, D. Small, J. Immerman, East. Pa. Chapter, Phila.

The effectiveness of the Arthritis Self Help program has been demonstrated since the initial effort of the Arthritis Foundation in 1981. Quality assurance in a community education program, such as this, is always of major concern. Coupled with inexperience of administering a new program, it became necessary to develop specific and comprehensive guidelines to assure the continuation of these efforts. Using the national guidelines as background material and addressing issues which were encountered during this rapid expansion a preliminary format was established. Progressing through a series of additions and refinements, these guidelines and procedures were achieved to assist in the implementation of the program.

The key elements of the guidelines are: organizational relationships and a co-sponsoring facility/agency agreement, a glossary, fact sheets which can stand independently, administrative procedures for both the community and leader courses, selection procedure for course leaders and an appendix containing all pertinent materials.

We have found the guidelines, thus far, to have the greatest impact on the areas of leader selection and evaluation and on the execution of administrative procedures. We anticipate the entire program will be enhanced by the ongoing use of this document.

64

EXERCISE AND PROBLEM-SOLVING EDUCATION PROGRAM FOR RHEUMATOID ARTHRITIS. S.G. Perlman, K. Connell, J. Alberti, P. Conlon, M. Mueller. Northwestern University Medical School Chicago, IL 60611.

Nine subjects with rheumatoid arthritis (functional class I,II,III) participated in a pilot study designed to examine the effects of an aerobic-like exercise/dance program coupled with an educational intervention aimed at enhancing participants' problem-solving abilities. The program was in two phases: 16-weeks (phase I) meeting two times/week (60 min. exercise and 45 min. education program), followed by an 8-week optional maintenance phase (phase II). The educational sessions, led by a medical educator, involved participants in discussion of their progress and problems, in exploring questions related to their arthritis, and in developing and testing possible solutions to personally important arthritis-related problems. Selected physiological, psychological and educational outcomes were evaluated.

Seven of the 9 participants completed Phase I; one dropped for personal reasons and 1 for medical reasons unrelated to arthritis. Of the 7 who completed Phase I, only 1 showed an increase in her articular index from pre to post; 1 showed no change; and 5 showed a significant decrease ($p < .05$). Participants were classified as internal(I;N=4) or external (E;N=3) on the basis of the Health Locus of Control. On the pretest, there was no significant difference between I's and E's on any scale of the Profile of Mood States Inventory (POMS). On the post test, I's reported significantly more vigor ($p < .05$), less depression ($p < .05$) and less anxiety and confusion (both $p < .01$) than E's. No significant differences in anger or fatigue were found. Participants' verbal reports corroborate the POMS data. All report feeling more control over their arthritis, more optimism, and more energy. Six of the 9 participants joined and completed Phase II.

This preliminary report suggests that subjects with RA are able to participate in a vigorous exercise program without adverse joint effects. In addition, the combined exercise and problem-solving education program has provided psychological benefits. Phase II data from this group as well as comparable data from additional groups will be presented.

65

DEVELOPMENT, IMPLEMENTATION AND EVALUATION OF AN EDUCATIONAL PROGRAM ON EXERCISE FOR SELECTED ARTHRITIS PATIENTS. P. Winder. San Francisco General Hospital, San Francisco.

Literature reveals that arthritis is a chronic and disabling illness. Treatment programs including exercise can help reduce disability if begun early. Non-cooperation with treatment recommendations is high.

A study was conducted of an educational program on exercise. One and one half hour sessions of individual instruction were given, including lecture, discussion, handouts and practice of specific exercises. Sixteen women and four men, sixteen of whom had osteoarthritis, participated in the study.

Data were gathered with a three-part questionnaire, exercise performance checklist and exercise diary. Measurements were taken of knowledge at pre and post test and again at six weeks using a fifteen item multiple choice test. Test-retest for reliability was done on the questionnaire with a coefficient of $r=.72$. Findings included a significant (.01) knowledge gain at posttest and at six weeks. Data were analyzed using a t test with values of 7.74 and 6.44 respectively. Sixty-five percent of the subjects were able to perform all of the exercises correctly at six week follow-up.

Correlation analyses of several variables showed no significant (.01) relationships between outcome and age, years of education, years of arthritis or level of function. A strong positive correlation was found, however, between knowledge and outcome score at six weeks ($r=.691$, $p=.01$).

It was concluded that participants significantly increased their knowledge and were able to perform the exercises correctly. Six weeks posttesting supported the fact that actual knowledge change had occurred. With a positive correlation between knowledge and outcome it was assumed that the knowledge acquired was important to the ability to perform the exercises.

More research is recommended to further test the reliability of the questionnaire and the correlation between knowledge and outcome. Also a pre/post test control group design with randomization needs to be done to increase confidence in the actual effects of the program.

66

CYBEX STRENGTH EVALUATION IN POLYMYOSITIS. Linda K. Schroeder, University of Michigan Hospitals, Ann Arbor, Michigan.

Accurate serial strength assessment of the patient with polymyositis is important in monitoring disease activity and effectiveness of the treatment program. Manual muscle testing is not adequately sensitive to note subtle differences in the 4 (holds against gravity and moderate resistance) to 5 (holds against gravity and maximum resistance) muscle strength range. Inconsistencies between clinicians frequently result. The Cybex isokinetic dynamometer has been used serially for objective strength assessment of the patient with polymyositis.

Serial Cybex strength assessment of quadriceps, hamstrings, triceps and biceps was performed at 30 degrees per second with 15 polymyositis patients. Standartized test procedures were developed to assure consistency.

Polymyositis patients were cooperative with Cybex testing. No adverse effects were identified. The Cybex test has provided accurate strength assessment in the 4 to 5 manual muscle strength range. Serial Cybex testing has yielded objective results which physicians have found useful in monitoring disease activity.

Further research is needed to determine correlates of Cybex results to laboratory indicators of disease activity.

67

COMPREHENSIVE ARTHRITIS PROGRAM. A UNIFIED TEAM APPROACH TO RECORDING PATIENTS' PROGRESS.
N. Rafferty, P. Blanner; St. Luke's Hospital, Kansas City.

To illustrate how patient information is summarized for an Arthritis Team Meeting concisely on a single page.

The Unified Arthritis Flow Sheet, detailed slides and x-rays are elements used to summarize patients' status in a weekly team meeting consisting of Nursing, OT, PT, Medical Social Work, Rheumatologist, Physiatrists, and Orthopedic Surgeon. The Unified Arthritis Flowsheet is a summary sheet which graphically displays the evaluation finding of the different disciplines.

During the weekly Arthritis Team Meeting, covering a vast amount of knowledge in a short amount of time is difficult. Utilizing visual aids to quickly summarize a patient's progress has been found to be most effective. The evaluation results from a previous hospitalization and the two evaluations from the current hospitalization are graphically displayed, thus illustrating the ongoing changes that occur in an arthritis patient.

This form of documentation and medium to convey evaluation findings from different disciplines has been utilized weekly for eight years. The entire field of rheumatology will benefit from having a concise manner to visually document arthritis patient changes.

68

RESISTANCE TO THERAPIES IN PRESCHOOL CHILDREN WITH JUVENILE RHEUMATOID ARTHRITIS (JRA): WHY AND WHAT TO DO. C. McDowell, K. Schmid, J. Driscoll, D. Barrows, C. Sandborg. Childrens Hospital of Orange County and St. Joseph Hospital, Orange, California.

Parents with young children with JRA daily face many problems related to the disease. One difficult area is encouraging their child to comply with therapeutic regimes. The purpose of this workshop is to optimize both medical care and normal development by identifying several techniques that can be used by therapists and parents to promote compliance at this difficult age. The participants will have a better understanding of normal resistance to therapy and its impact on the family. Specific techniques will be explored to help deal with this common problem.

A lecture-discussion format will be used by team members. Pediatric social worker and nurse educator will discuss resistance to therapy as a developmental phenomenon and present a variety of behavioral interventions for facilitating compliance. Pediatric physical and occupational therapists will present techniques for adapting standard therapy regimes to age-appropriate activities. Promoting the development of self-care and play skills will be specifically addressed as these are important milestones to be achieved at this age. Integration of all these techniques into a home program and lifestyle will be discussed.

This workshop is at a basic to intermediate level for health professionals directly working with and prescribing home therapies for children with JRA.

69

THE IMPACT OF RHEUMATOID ARTHRITIS ON THE HOMEMAKER Susan Reisine, Ph.D., University of Connecticut Health Center, Farmington, CT.

Research on disability associated with rheumatoid arthritis focuses largely on work disability and the ability to perform household tasks. Few studies analyze homemaking as a social role with normative obligations and privileges that go beyond household tasks and include areas such as nurturing children and maintaining an operating household. Since the prevalence of rheumatoid arthritis is much higher among women than men and since homemaking is the primary occupation of 50% of American women this, clearly, is an area of major research and clinical significance. The purpose of the proposed roundtable is to: 1) present and discuss the literature on the effects of RA on the homemaker role; 2) define the instrumental and affective aspects of the homemaker role; 3) analyze methods of operationalizing the homemaker role using a questionnaire from an on-going study on role limitations in 200 women with rheumatoid arthritis and 4) present and discuss preliminary results from this on-going study as an example of how homemaker disability is a critical but much neglected area of social functioning.

The roundtable is aimed at an intermediate level of experience in research. Both conceptual and methodological issues related to the instrumental and nurturant dimensions of the homemaker role will be discussed.

70

IMPLEMENTATION OF AN INTEGRATED OT-PT CURRICULUM IN ARTHRITIS.
Marlys Mitchell, Deborah Retzinger. University of North Carolina at Chapel Hill.

A three-year MAC funded project initiated by a rheumatologist led to the development of integrated experiences for OT and PT students. This workshop will review content of lectures, the pretest and posttest on didactic information, and the study guide for students. A project developed video tape will be viewed. Participants will address two case studies in small groups and will answer questions leading to problem solving regarding OT-PT intervention and management of the patients.

The project-developed scale, Attitudes Toward Arthritic Persons, (ATAP) will be administered to participants and discussed in the workshop.

Collaboration between OT and PT in field work placement will be described. Assessment of skills, measured by Field Work Performance Reports and questionnaires sent to field work supervisors and students, will be discussed.

Evaluation of the curriculum project used a four cell design in which it was hypothesized that experiential, instructional methods and collaborative field work experiences would be superior to didactic instruction and separate field work experiences.

This workshop will present the conceptual model of the integrated curriculum, the experiential aspects which will require participation by the attendees, and the evaluation instruments. The workshop is directed toward clinical OTs and PTs who supervise students and to educators, including rheumatologists. It will be presented at an intermediate level.

71

DOES LEARNING READINESS PREDICT LEARNING? C.S. Burckhardt, School of Nursing, Oregon Health Sciences University, Portland, OR and Peggy Raish, Denver, CO.

Assessing patient learning readiness is considered a fundamental, preliminary step in the teaching-learning process. The purpose of this research project was to determine whether variables hypothesized to measure learning readiness would predict learning in a group of adults who participated in a structured education program while hospitalized with arthritis.

Learning readiness was assessed by instruments that measured years of formal education, interest in learning specific information about arthritis, importance of health, pain, depression, anxiety, functional impairment, energy, and severity of arthritis. These instruments, along with a demographic information sheet, were administered by questionnaire format to 90 subjects ($\bar{X}$ age=55) upon admission to an inpatient arthritis unit. All subjects had a definite diagnosis of either RA or OA and participated in 3 to 5 multidisciplinary education classes. Learning was measured by posttest scores on a 10-item, knowledge test immediately after completion of the classes. Multivariate strategies were used to determine the effect of each variable on posttest scores.

The results showed a high degree of variability in the learning readiness variables scores. But, pain was the only statistically significant predictor of posttest knowledge. Specifically, recall of higher pain intensity during the past week predicted higher learning scores; whereas, higher present pain intensity predicted lower scores. These results suggest that many of the variables hypothesized to measure learning readiness may not be predictive of learning in hospitalized patients with arthritis.

72

DOES EVALUATION TELL US WHAT WE WANT TO KNOW ABOUT ARTHRITIS PATIENT "UNDERSTANDING"? DJ Holsten, SE Hazelwood, and TD TenBrink, Multipurpose Arthritis Center, University of Missouri-Columbia.

The purpose of this presentation is to raise questions and address areas of concern for arthritis professionals regarding evaluation of their verbal communication with clients. Previous investigations have shown that not all patients understand certain health-related terms commonly used in patient education. However, we have performed a study in which we found that patient understanding varies, depending upon its definition.

Twenty-nine health-related terms were selected (e.g., relieve, flare, symptom, medication, decrease, swelling, joint protection, arthritis, rest, etc.). Independent rheumatology experts reviewed the list and agreed that these terms were among those most commonly used. Twenty-three arthritis patients verbally explained each word with an open-ended response. One patient had $<50\%$ of the terms correct, six had 50-75% correct and 15$>$ than 75% correct. "Understanding" was defined to include the ability to give examples or synonyms, as well as the ability to give dictionary definitions. In contrast, other similar investigations have used multiple-choice testing methods, and found that no more than 58% of their patients understood similar terms.

Our results raise several questions: 1) Does rigorous testing actually evaluate what patients know and understand? 2) Do patients' recognize, and understand, terms that they cannot pronounce or define? 3) What levels of understanding do patients' need (e.g., to adhere to treatment)? Is recognition enough or do they need to recall and/or explain? 4) Do the instruments we use tend to measure only the highest levels of memory? These questions point out the need for further research in this area. Practitioners should be sensitive to the fact that patients do not always respond in a way which accurately reflects their level of understanding.

73

THE EVALUATION OF OUTCOMES OF ARTHRITIS EDUCATION PROGRAMS FOR LOW LITERACY PATIENTS, Robert Rippey (Moderator), Dee Bill, and Carol A. Pfeiffer, University of Connecticut Health Center MAC, Farmington, Connecticut.

Synopsis: An arthritis education program has been conducted for three years in a low income, low literacy, minority section of Hartford, CT. This program has drawn many elderly participants who have attended regularly, and expressed enthusiasm regarding benefits. However, the problems of evaluating a low literacy and culturally different community are substantial and not solved without effort.

Carol Pfeiffer will describe the initial difficulties encountered in attempting to apply conventional evaluation instruments and scales to our low literacy population. Dee Bill will describe the current program and demonstrate procedures which have been used to date in evaluating the ongoing project. These include an obstacle course, a picture test, and an oral examination. Robert Rippey will describe the evaluation plan for the next phase of the project and some newly developed evaluation ideas including pedometers, home visits, and blind rated audio recordings.

Audience participation: Responses to the following questions will be invited: 1) How do you deal with the problem of evaluating outcomes of patient education or therapy for persons with low literacy? 2) What future plans do you have for working with low literacy groups and what helpful resources can we share as a result of this symposium? 3) What would be convincing evidence that a person's life had been enhanced? How would you measure a hopeful attitude? Is hope a relevant outcome?

74

LEARNING NEEDS OF PARENTS OF CHILDREN WITH JRA: PERCEPTIONS OF PARENTS AND THEIR HEALTH CARE TEAMS. M. Boutaugh, Arthritis Foundation, Atlanta; S. Amundson, La Rabida Children's Hosp., Chicago; J. Falco, Nat'l Jewish Hosp., Denver; D. Erlandson, N. Eng. MC, Boston; A. Hull, NE Ohio MAC, Cleveland; A. Kovalesky, Children's Hosp., Los Angeles; M. Mahy, Arthritis Society, Vancouver; C. Shields, Texas Children's Hosp., Houston; N. Tehan, Dartmouth Arthritis Center, Hanover.

To determine the content of a JRA parent education program, a survey was developed, pilot tested and distributed through 12 centers with pediatric rheumatology teams (PRT). Survey recipients were asked to rate the relative importance of 38 education topics on a scale of 1 (very important) to 4 (not at all important).

Completed surveys were obtained from 300 parents and 50 PRT members. The parents and PRT agreed that most of the items were very important (mean<2). However there was wide divergence in the rank order of parents' and PRT ratings of many items, eg. joint anatomy, diet, research, stress and pain management and lab tests were ranked high by parents but relatively low by the PRT.

The items were categorized into 3 content areas: disease process (Dp), treatment (Rx) and psychosocial (Ps). Chronback alpha statistics computed for items in these groups suggested that the items in the groups are reliable. T test analyses of the group scores were used to compare the responses of the parents with the PRT. Parents rated the Dp and Rx categories as more important than did the PRT ($\alpha < .05$).

Based on these findings and other data analyses we concluded that while parents and PRT agreed on the types of topics to include in a JRA education program their perceptions of the relative importance of these items differed. When determining which topics to emphasize parent input is essential.

75

CAREER PLANNING AND ACHIEVEMENT FOR CHILDREN WITH RHEUMATIC DISEASES (RD). Edith S. Shear, Mary Gilman, Rosanne Miller and Joseph E. Levinson, University of Cincinnati, Cincinnati, Ohio.

The unpredictability and uncertainty of the RD of childhood pose a number of problems which interfere with career planning. Helping the child achieve his/her potential is further complicated by psychosocial, psychosexual and economic aspects of these diseases. Career education should begin at diagnosis and be compatible with the projected outcome. For maximum effectiveness, the child must believe his/her disease can have a serious effect on his/her career choice.

In our Center where these patients have been followed medically and continuously over long periods of time, career education and habilitation are intrinsic to the comprehensive health management program. The role of each team member, including the child, his/her family, career, health and educational professionals, is reviewed to focus interdependently on the development of competitive skills and who and what is marketable. This study discusses the career outcomes of over 200 juvenile onset RD patients at ages 18 to 33 years. Patients with nine different rheumatic diseases will be reviewed to indicate academic grade completed, current job or profession, and marital and economic status. Results indicate that these young adults limited physically or by diagnostic classification are achieving at equal or at higher levels than their peers. Appropriately prepared to think vocationally, patients whose present employability is threatened by flares learn that their jobs and equipment can be modified, and that transfer to allied or new fields is possible. We believe this report to be the most complete of its kind to date.

76

THE EFFECTIVENESS OF AN AQUANASTICS PROGRAM: A CONTROLLED STUDY. Mary Vostrejs, J. Roger Hollister, National Jewish Center for Respiratory and Immune Medicine/Rocky Mountain Juvenile Arthritis Center, Denver, CO 80206

Decreases in range of motion (ROM) experienced by children with Juvenile Rheumatoid Arthritis (JRA) have been managed with a home program of exercises. In this study we have measured the effect of a controlled warm water aerobic exercise program (Aquanastics) on ROM, and compared this program to the benefit of a free swimming period of similar duration and water temperature.

A blinded physical therapist performed goniometric measurements before and after a 45 minute program in water of 88°F. Children with JRA age 7 to 12 participated in this study. Measurements were performed on the same group of children on two separate days with the evaluating therapist being unaware of whether the children had participated in the Aquanastics program or free swimming. Only differences of ROM greater than 5° were considered for analysis because of goniometric margin of error.

Warm water exercise was beneficial in both free swimming and Aquanastics. When the children participated in the Aquanastics program, they received particular benefit over swimming in the areas of wrist extension, hamstring length, hip flexor length and low back tightness. Our preliminary results indicate the Aquanastics program produced increases in ROM more frequently and the average degree of improvement was greater than in free swimming.

Thus, warm water exercise is an effective way to increase ROM in children with JRA. The Aquanastics program is more effective on JRA problem areas than independent swimming.

77

PEDIATRIC RHEUMATOLOGY OUTREACH PROGRAM (PROP): REVIEW OF TWO YEARS EXPERIENCE. Charlotte Shields, Earl Brewer, Donald Person. Texas Children's Hospital, Houston, Texas.

The effectiveness of outreach programs in pediatric rheumatology has not been evaluated. Common goals of such programs are to provide comprehensive care in underserved areas; train local health professionals to provide continuity of care between visits; and educate health, school, and community providers to the needs of children with rheumatic diseases.

Direct care was provided by the PROP's team through coordination with local health providers at 26 day-long clinics held on a bimonthly basis in 3 outlying communities. There were a total of 227 visits by 89 patients. The number of children by diagnosis were: rheumatic complaints-36, JRA-28, hypermobility syndrome-7, dermatomyositis-4, SLE-3, miscellaneous rheumatic disease-11. Local contacts were made and persons were trained to provide followup care with telephone contact to the regional center (RC) as needed.

Local awareness of the clinics and increased knowledge about pediatric rheumatic diseases were developed by the use of local media, area physician mailings, and educational presentations. Nine presentations were made to 325 persons including physicians; house staff; and hospital, school and public health professionals. The success of these efforts was evidenced by the number of attendees and an increased number of physician referrals (from 0-4 seen at the initial clinic in each city to 11-13 by the fourth clinics) with 2 of the 3 now at capacity - 18/clinic. The referral base was 58% local physicians, 21% RC, and 21% self or agency.

The PROP can be effective in providing both service and education to outlying areas which lack a pediatric rheumatology team.

78

SUMMER CAMPS FOR CHILDREN WITH RHEUMATIC DISEASES (RD): DO THEY MAKE A DIFFERENCE? Mary E. Stefl, Trinity University, San Antonio, Edith S. Shear and Joseph E. Levinson, University of Cincinnati, Cincinnati.

Our Center annually sponsors a week long summer camping session for children with RD. Among other objectives, the camp attempts to promote participants' self-confidence and foster independence to enhance coping and disease management skills.

The effectiveness of the 1984 Camp was evaluated by obtaining measures on the Piers-Harris Self Concept (PHSC) scale and the Norwicki-Strickland Locus of Control (LOC) Scale for Children. The latter measures the degree of control a child feels he/she can exert over his/her own life, a type of independence with implications for disease management. The 9 male and 27 female campers, aged 7-20, independently completed paper-and-pencil scales both at the beginning and end of the camp week.

Initial PHSC scores were comparable to published norms (49th percentile), but LOC scores showed RD campers assume less than average self-responsibility. By the end of the camp session, significant changes were observed: self-concept was enhanced ($t=2.28$, $df=33$, $p=.029$), and LOC became more internal ($t=2.83$, $df=33$, $p=.008$), indicating greater control over life events or more independence. Greater change was noted for campers who had had previous overnight experiences away from home. In order to determine if these positive effects are sustained over time, six-month follow-up measures will be collected in January, 1985.

This study may be helpful in identifying children most likely to achieve the stated objectives for the camping experience. The results will also aid the Center staff in planning future camping experiences for children with RD.

79

SCHOOL PROBLEMS IN JUVENILE ARTHRITIS (JA). J. Taylor, M.H. Passo and J. Schade. Indiana University Multipurpose Arthritis Center, Indpls, IN.

Children with JA encounter a diversity of school problems. The purpose of this study is to compare 3 groups; parents (Pa), children (Ch), and teachers (Tr), regarding identification of JA school problems and perceived teacher responsibilities in assisting the child.

A convenience sample of 64 subjects (24 Pa, 24 Ch, 14 Tr) were surveyed using a 3 part questionnaire. Scale 1 consists of 40 school problems. Categories included physical health, ADL, peer relationships, self-concept, medication and school schedules. Scale 2 listed 28 teacher responsibilities. Scales 1 and 2 used a 5-point Likert-type scale. Part 3 solicited demographic data.

Content validity was established by submitting the questionnaire to a pediatric rheumatologist, 3 RN's, 3 Tr, and a doctoral nurse researcher. Internal consistency was determined by Cronbach's alpha. Scale 1 and 2 reliabilities were .90 and .95, respectively. Scale 1 and 2 ANOVA between Pa, Ch, and Tr were significant at p=.0002 and p=.001, respectively. Group means showed that Pa perceived problems occurring more frequently than Ch and Ch more frequently than Tr. Disease severity positively correlated with frequency of problems. Pa and Tr identified problems with physical health and ADL occurring more often; whereas Ch noted problems with peer relationships and self-concept. Ch cited major areas of concern as parental finances and developing a positive self-attitude. Pa and Tr did not acknowledge these. Sixteen of 28 teacher responsibilities were perceived significantly different between the 3 groups.

Knowing perceived problems and responsibilities, intervention can be individualized to minimize or alleviate school problems.

80

SERIAL PSYCHOLOGICAL MEASUREMENTS IN RHEUMATOID ARTHRITIS. Donna J. Hawley, Frederick Wolfe and Mary Ann Cathey, Wichita State University and University of Kansas, Wichita, Ks 67208.

Psychological status is thought to be an important component in chronic rheumatic disease. Although patients with high levels of anxiety and/or depression present difficult treatment problems, it is not clear whether psychological abnormality otherwise effects clinical status or disease outcome. To investigate the effect of psychological status we serially studied 146 patients with rheumatoid arthritis (RA) at 3 month intervals during a two year period utilizing the anxiety (ANX) and depression (DEP) scales of the Arthritis Impact Measurement Scales (AIMS). Patients with high levels (>75th percentile) of ANX (>5.0) and DEP (>3.5) were similar to those below the 75th percentile in age, sex, disease duration, rheumatoid factor positivity, ESR, joint count and grip strength at the initial evaluation, but differed in patient perceived measures: disease severity (SEV), Stanford Health Assessment Questionnaire disability index (DI), fatigue, and AM stiffness ($p<.01$). High and low DEP groups also differed in pain scores. Differences in DI, ANX and DEP persisted throughout the study period, as did SEV for depression groups, but other clinical and severity measures were similar at the final evaluation, including proportion of radiographic erosions and gold and penicillamine treatment frequency. When ANX and DEP scores were adjusted for differences in initial DI, no difference in DI could be found at any subsequent point. These data suggest that high ANX or DEP patients perceive more disability and severity than those with low scores. A high ANX or DEP score is associated with continued increases in ANX, DEP, DI and SEV, but not with more physically severe RA, or a more rapidly progressive course.

81

EXPERIMENTAL EVIDENCE THAT CHANGES IN PSYCHOLOGICAL FACTORS ARE ASSOCIATED WITH CHANGES IN ARTHRITIS PAIN. Kate Lorig, Stanford Shoor, Halsted R. Holman, Stanford University, Stanford, CA

Psychological factors have long been thought to influence arthritis pain. However, there has been little experimental evidence in arthritis patients that psychological factors could be changed or that such changes would be associated with changes in pain. On the other hand, self-care activities such as arthritis specific exercise, relaxation and walking are generally believed to assist in alleviating arthritis pain.

To test these beliefs, 140 arthritics were randomized to take the 12-hour, lay-taught Arthritis Self-Management (ASM) course or to control status. Comparing treated subjects to controls after 4 months, pain was reduced (p .01). Self-care activities, exercise, relaxation and walking increased (p .01) and psychological status (a combined scale of coping, pain self-efficacy, satisfaction with treatment, and treatment expectancy) improved (p .01).

Tests of association were performed on the treated subjects. Utilizing multilinear regression, controlling for baseline pain, age, sex, education, and type of arthritis, the expected association between changes in self-care activities and changes in pain was not significant (R=0.08). However, the association between changes in pain and changes in psychological status was significant (R=-.42) (p .05).

Thus, psychological factors impacted by patient education appear to correlate better with changes in pain than do more commonly measured self-care behaviors. The unidentified features of the ASM course which enhanced psychological status with an associated reduction in pain are being explored.

82

BELIEFS ABOUT ARTHRITIS HELD BY HEALTH PROFESSIONS TRAINEES AND UNDERGRADUATE COLLEGE STUDENTS. Marilyn K. Potts and Kenneth D. Brandt. Indiana University Arthritis Center, Indianapolis, IN 46223.

Perceptions of others about handicapped people (HP) may be a greater problem than functional limitations. This study surveys beliefs about people with arthritis (A) held by health professions trainees [physical therapy students (PTS) (n=60), nursing students (NS) (n=111), internal medicine house officers (n=63)], and undergraduate non-health professions students (n=60).

Two subscales were derived from factor analysis of a 10-item Likert-type scale: Scale N concerned the extent to which HP may lead a normal life; Scale F dealt with the emotional/physical frailty of HP. Beliefs about people with A were relatively positive on both Scales N and F [$\bar{x}$=4.9, 4.6, respectively; possible range=1.0 (low) - 6.0 (high)]. Respondents, as a whole, judged people with A to be more "normal" than those with alcoholism, blindness or mental illness ($p<.001$); comparable to those with an amputation; and less "normal" than those with epilepsy ($p<.01$). Responses to Scale F and N were similar, but people with A were viewed as more "frail" than blind people ($p<.05$). No major between-groups differences in beliefs about A were seen in the 4 student/trainee subsets, or between interns, 1st- and 2nd-yr residents. Senior PTS considered people with A to be more "normal" than junior PTS, while 1st-yr NS judged them as more "frail" than 4th-yr NS. Age and direct personal experience were not associated with beliefs about people with A, but women considered them to be more "normal" and less "frail" than did men. Since such stereotypic beliefs may have a major impact on the patient's response to treatment, educators should take these into account in designing education programs for health professions students.

83

CHANGING ARTHRITIS KNOWLEDGE AND ATTITUDES: THE EFFECT OF TEACHING. M.A. Minor, J.E. Hewett, D.E. Finan, D.R. Kay. University of Missouri-Columbia Multipurpose Arthritis Center, Columbia, Missouri.

The Arthritis Attitude Scale (AS) and Arthritis Knowledge Inventory (AKI) were used to assess arthritis attitudes and knowledge of county level personnel participating in a statewide arthritis education study. Preintervention AS and AKI scores did not differ significantly between the lay and nursing personnel in the 20 county sample. (A&R 26:4:S83). Personnel in both groups were considered competent to offer community arthritis education. A five-part educational series, Arthritis*Wise, was provided to the county offices. Office personnel were asked to report program use, but were under no obligation to use any of the materials. Program reports collected over a 15 month period show over 400 programs delivered to over 6000 participants. After this field placement period, AS and AKI were readministered (N=42). Overall group means did not show a significant increase in either AS or AKI scores at retest. To test the hypothesis that activity as a community arthritis educator favors increased arthritis knowledge and more positive attitudes, subjects were divided into two groups based on their reported use of Arthritis*Wise programs, Users (11) and Nonusers (31). Analysis with the Wilcoxson Rank Sum technique shows a highly significant increase in AS scores of Users. AKI scores of Users also increased, but not significantly. The Nonuser group did not change in either AS or AKI scores. Retrospective analysis of initial scores shows that Users and Nonusers were not significantly different on AS or AKI before the field placement period. (p values bigger than .05 are considered non-significant). Results support the hypothesis that assuming the role of arthritis educator promotes improved arthritis knowledge and attitudes in the teacher. This positive effect of active involvement should be investigated further in designing continuing education programs in rheumatology.

84

THE IMPACT OF SLE: PHYSICAL AND PSYCHOSOCIAL VARIABLES. C. Yarboro, C. Berkebile, D. Yocum, C. Hastings, K. Joyce, NIH, Bethesda.

Systemic Lupus Erythematosus (SLE) is a chronic illness that imposes many physical and psychosocial changes on the lives of affected individuals. The extent and relationship of these effects is of interest to health professionals responsible for the assessment and care of these patients.

The purpose of this study was to assess the relationship between the physical and psychosocial effects of SLE. Forty patients with SLE were asked to complete a modified Arthritis Impact Measurement Scale (AIMS), with the word "arthritis" changed to "lupus." They were also evaluated by a physician using a standardized disease Activity Index (AI) developed at NIH, which assessed for the presence of physical symptoms grouped by body system and included a physician and patient rating of overall disease activity.

Data were analyzed using the Pearson Correlation Coefficient to determine relationships between physical and psychosocial variables. The total AIMS score was significantly correlated with the total AI score (r=.40,p=.01).The total AI also correlated with the physician rating (r=.612,p=.01) and with the patient rating(r=.458,p=.01). The AIMS pain subscale correlated strongly with the total AI as well as the patient and physician ratings. Depression was not significantly correlated with any physical variable.

These results suggest that there is a relationship between the physical and psychosocial factors in SLE that needs further investigation.

85

AN EDUCATION PROGRAM FOR CLIENTS WITH SYSTEMIC LUPUS ERYTHEMATOSUS (SLE). G. Casterline-Ziegler. University of Pittsburgh, Pittsburgh, PA 15261.

Successful comprehensive rheumatic disease management requires that the client and family have knowledge of the disease process and rationale for treatment, yet little has been published which addresses the special needs of the client and family with lupus. Teaching plays an important role in the general responsibility of the arthritis health professional in helping the client to achieve independence and to assume accountability for his or her own health care. It was the purpose of this study to develop a model for lupus education and to determine the effectiveness of this program in an ambulatory care setting.

Every client seen at our Lupus Diagnostic and Treatment Center with an established diagnosis of SLE during the eight month study period was mailed a consent form and Needs Assessment Questionnaire(NAQ). Forty-four persons (53%) participated in the study and did not differ in their demographic characteristics from those declining to participate. Subjects were assigned randomly to educational intervention and control groups. There were no significant differences between the two groups when stratified for age, race, sex, education, years treated at the Center, and mean pre-test NAQ scores. Clients attending the educational sessions demonstrated significantly higher post-test scores as compared to controls immediately following the program ($p<.01$) and at four months follow-up ($p<.05$).

Health education should be an organized process which includes the identification of needs, an exchange of knowledge, and evaluation. The lupus education program has demonstrated its ability to assist the client in becoming a knowledgeable partner in his or her own health care.

86

ISSUES OF NON-COMPLIANCE CONFRONTING WOMEN IN MID-LIFE: THE PATIENT'S PERSPECTIVE. Gail E. Evans. Arthritis Foundation-Wisconsin Chapter, Milwaukee.

Women entering mid-life (ages 35-50) are beset by a variety of life changes that are further complicated by a chronic illness requiring adherence to a medical regimen. Treatment of these individuals pose special problems when issues of non-compliance are perceived differently by the professional and patient. This workshop explores the relationship between mid-life crisis, chronic illness and non-compliance as experienced by women with arthritis. Techniques for enhancing patient compliance will be addressed.

The workshop will enable arthritis health professionals to identify factors that lead to non-compliance, correlate the relationship between arthritis and mid-life crisis and provide alternative strategies that can facilitate improved compliance.

A format that incorporates lecture and experiential activities will be utilized. Participants will be asked to identify major patient compliance problems. The patient's perspective regarding non-compliance will be presented via lecture, handouts and case studies. Workshop members will role-play the case studies and methods of intervention discussed, supplemented by lecture and handouts. Workshop materials have been derived from individual counseling sessions, survey data from eight Women's Support Group series and literature review.

The workshop will be presented for all levels of a multidisciplinary audience.

87

PATHOMECHANICS OF GAIT IN THE PATIENT WITH RHEUMATOID ARTHRITIS. Claire Beekman, Lorrie Mercer, Rancho Los Amigos Medical Center. Downey.

Patients with moderate to severe RA generally present with multiple gait deviations which limit their endurance and interfere with their mobility in the community. These deviations are related to the progression of their disease process and result from joint destruction, limitations in ROM, and muscle weakness. As members of the Allied Health Profession, it is our responsibility to address these gait deviations in order to maximize function and minimize energy expenditure.

Observational gait sessions are one way of gaining information regarding patient's gait deviations. A workshop will be presented demonstrating observational gait techniques. Participants will be able to: 1) identify the 8 sub-phases of normal gait, and critical joint position and muscle activity during these sub-phases; 2) recognize common arthritic gait deviations; 3) determine the cause and penalty of each gait deviation; 4) develop a treatment program to help correct the identified gait problems.

Normal pathomechanics of gait will be presented in a lecture format. This will be followed by audience indentification of common gait deviations from film loops of an RA patient. Causes and penalties of these deviations, as well as treatment suggestions will be discussed.

The workshop will be presented primarily for physical therapists and physicians with a beginning/intermediate level of pathological gait.

88

UPDATE ON THE ROM DANCE PROGRAM: RECENT DEVELOPMENT AND RESEARCH. Diane Harlowe, St. Marys Hospital Medical Center, Madison and Julia Van Deusen, University of Wisconsin-Madison.

The purpose of this workshop is to provide an overview of the ROM Dance Program, and to present research and program developments undertaken since completion of the pilot study in 1982.

The ROM Dance is an enjoyable exercise/rest program for adults with rheumatoid arthritis. It includes two main elements: relaxation techniques to be used during regular periods of rest, and the ROM Dance Sequence. This 7 minute sequence of expressive movements is accompanied by a verse which employs images of warm water, sunshine and friendship. The ROM Dance is based on the principles of T'ai-Chi Chuan, and incorporates joint motion in all ranges usually recommended for rheumatoid arthritis. Participants will gain sufficient exposure of the program format, goals, elements and multi-media instructional materials to evaluate potential for use in their work.

A preliminary report will be presented on the current research project funded by the Arthritis Foundation. Participants will gain a general understanding of the purpose and methods used in this two-year efficacy study, and will be encouraged to discuss limitations and initial results.

Discussion will be supplemented by a video tape and printed materials. Content is appropriate for a multi-disciplinary audience at intermediate and advanced levels.

AHPA AUTHOR INDEX

ABELES,M.,MD 26,62
Farmington,CT
ALARCON,G.S.,MD, MPH 10
Birmingham,AL
ALBERTI,J.,PhD 64
Chicago,IL
ALLAIRE,S.H.,RN, MS 54
Boston,MA
AMUNDSON,S.K.,RN, MA 41,52,74
Chicago,IL
ATHREYA,B.H.,MD 31
Philadelphia,PA
BALKE,J.,BS, RN 15
Detroit,MI
BANWELL,B.A.,MA, PT 49
Flint,MI
BARGER,G.J.,RN, MS 11
Indianapolis,IN
BARROWS,D.,OTR 68
Orange,CA
BECKER,M.D.,PT 63
Philadelphia,PA
BEEKMAN,C.,MS, RPT 87
Downey,CA
BERKEBILE,C.,RN, BSN 84
Bethesda,MD
BILL,D.,MPH 26,73,62
Farmington,CT
BLANNER,P.,RPT,MS 67
Kansas City,MO
BLAUNER,M.,MS 24
Cleveland,OH
BLOCK,D.V.,MSW 53
Denver,CO
BOUTAUGH,M.L.,RN, MPH 52,74
Atlanta,GA
BRANDT,K.D.,MD 11,82
Indianapolis,IN
BREWER,E.J.,MD 77
Houston,TX
BROWN,G.,MS 59
Nashville,TN
BROWN,S.,EdD 27
Birmingham,AL
BRUNK,S.E.,RN, MSN 32,43,60,61
Charlottesville,VA
BRUNNER,C.M.,MD 60,44
Charlottesville,VA
BUCREK,S.,RPT 20
Lansing,MI
BURCKHARDT,C.S.,PhD, RN 71,48
Portland,OR
CADWELL,M.,MEd, OTR 19
Columbia,MO
CAIRNS,B.,BSc 38
Toronto,BC
CALLAHAN,L.F.,BS 46
Nashville,TN
CATHEY,M.,BSN 80
Wichita,KS
CHRONIC,C.L.,OTR 37
Atlanta,GA
COLLINS, JR.,R., ... 10
Birmingham,AL
COLON,P.,OTR 64
Chicago,IL
CONNELL,K.,MS 64
Chicago,IL
COOPER,K.R.,BSN 2
Birmingham,AL
CURTIS,F.,PT 45
Atlanta,GA
DALTROY,L.H.,DrPH 40
Boston,MA
DAY,J.,MPH 62
Farmington,CT
DENFORD,B.S.,BSR, MEd 4
Vancouver,BC
DENNIS,G.,MD 8
Washington,DC
DOMOMBERY,N.,LPN 11
Indianapolis,IN
DOWNING,D.,RPT 62
Farmington,CT
DOYLE,A.T.,MA 32
Charlottesville,VA
DOYLE,M.T.,MA 43,60,61
Charlottesville,VA
DOYLE,T.H.,MSN, RN, C 9,15
Detroit,MI
DREISINGER,T.E.,PhD 7
Columbia,MO
DRISCOLL,J.,MSN 68
Orange,CA
DUNN,T.L., ... 10
Birmingham,AL
EATON,H.,BSN 40
Boston,MA
ELLIS,C.,MSW, ACSW 47
Orange,CA
ERLANDSON,D.M.,RN, MS 41,29,74
Boston,MA
EVANS,G.E.,MS 86
Milwaukee,WI
FAIRLEIGH,A.,OT 58
Vancouver,BC
FALCO,J.,RN, BSN 74,53
Denver,CO
FINAN,D.E.,BSIE 83
Columbia,MO
FRANK,A.,RN, BSN 28
Milwaukee,WI
FRIES,J.F.,MD 1
Stanford,CA
FROMMELT,G.,BA 35
Evanston,IL
FUDMAN,E.J.,MD 42
Ann Arbor,MI
FUJISHIGE,C.M.,RN 50
Honolulu,HI

GERMANY,Y., 10
Birmingham,AL
GIBSON,K.R.,MS, PT 22
Pittsburgh,PA
GILLILAND,B., 23
Vancouver,BC
GILMAN,M.,MSW 75
Cincinnati,OH
GILNER,F.H.,.PhD 12
St. Louis,MO
GINES,G.S.,MS 25
Stanford,CA
GOEPPINGER,J.,PhD, RN 43,60,61
Charlottesville,VA
GOLETZ,J.,RN 35
Chicago,IL
GOODSON,A.S.,RN, BSN 32
Charlottesville,VA
GREEN,P.,RN, BS 54
Quincy,MA
HAMBRIDGE,M.,MCSP,DipPT 45
Atlanta,GA
HANNAH,R.E.,MSC 58
Vancouver,BC
HANNEMAN,S.L.,BSc 57
Van Nuys,CA
HARLOWE,D.,MS, OTR 88
Madison,WI
HARRELL,P., 10
Birmingham,AL
HARRIS,I.M.,BSc, OT 23
Vancouver,BC
HASTINGS,C.,RN, BSN 84,45
Bethesda,MD
HAWLEY,D.J.,MN, EdD 80
Wichita,KS
HAZELWOOD,S.E.,BS 72
Columbia,MO
HEWETT,J.E.,PhD 83
Columbia,MO
HICKS,D.,RN 63
Philadelphia,PA
HICKS,R.V.,MD 51,50
Honolulu,HI
HOLLISTER,J.,MD 76,53
Denver,CO
HOLMAN,H.R.,MD 81
Stanford,CA
HOLSTEN,D.J.,MSPH 72
Columbia,MO
HUBER,A.,BA 63
Philadelphia,PA
HULL,A.L.,PhD 3,24,74
Cleveland,OH
IMMERMAN,J.,BA 63
Philadelphia,PA
INGALL,C.G.,RN, CPNP 31
Boston,MA
JONES,M., 26
Farmington,CT
JONGBLOED,L.,BSc,MA,PhD 16
Vancouver,ON
JOYCE,K.,RN, BSN 84
Bethesda,MD
KAY,D.R.,MD 19,83,7
Columbia,MO
KEANE,D.,BA 25
Stanford,CA
KING,M.G.,MCSP, RPT 50
Honolulu,HI
KLIPPLE,G.L.,MD 8
Washington,DC
KOVALESKY,A.,RN,MSN 13,30,52,74
Los Angeles,CA
LANDEL,R.F.,MS, RPT 5
Downey,CA
LEE,M.Y.,MSW 51
Honolulu,HI
LEHMAN,T.A.,MD 13
Los Angeles,CA
LEVINSON,J.E.,MD 78,75
Cincinnati,OH
LIDDLE,S.,MS 32
Richmond,VA
LIEBMAN,J.J.,MSN 3,24
Cleveland,OH
LORIG,K.,DPH, RN 48,25
Stanford,CA
LORIG,K.R.,RN, DrPH 81
Stanford,CA
LORISH,C.D.,PhD 2,27
Birmingham,AL
LUBECK,D.P.,PhD 1
Santa Barbara,CA
MACBAIN,K.,BA 56,17
Vancouver,BC
MAHY,M.,RN 74
Vancouver,BC
MARLOWE,S.,NP 62
Farmington,CT
MARLOWE,S.M.,NP 9
Farmington,CT
MAZZUCA,S.A.,PhD 11
Indianapolis,IN
MCCLOY,L.F.,Dip P/OT 16
Vancouver,ON
MCDOWELL,C.R.,RPT 68
Orange,CA
MCGRAW,R.W.,MD, FRCS 17
Vancouver,BC
MCKNIGHT,P.T.,OTR/L 18
Pittsburgh,PA
MEHN,J.,RPT 36
Los Angeles,CA
MELSON,P.G.,RPT 37
Atlanta,GA
MERCER,L.,MS, RPT 87
Downey,CA
MILLER,D.,RN 30
Torrance,CA
MILLER,R.,MSW 75
Cincinnati,OH
MINOR,M.A.,PT, MSPH 83,7
Columbia,MO
MITCHELL,D.,MD 1
Saskatchewan,SA
MITCHELL,M.M.,PhD, OTR 70
Chapel Hill,NC
MONCUR,C.,PT, PhD 34
Salt Lake City,UT
MOSKOWITZ,R.W.,MD 24,3
Cleveland,OH

MUELLER,M.,MSN 64
Chicago,IL
MURDOCK,M.,PhD 43,60
Charlottesville,VA
NEWTON,T.L.,BS, RPT 5
Downey,CA
NICASSIO,P.M.,PhD 59
Nashville,TN
O'LEARY,A.A.,MA 32,44
Charlottesville,VA
OERMANN,M.,PhD,RN 15
Detroit,MI
PALLOZZI,L.,RPT 40
Boston,MA
PARKER,J.,RPT 27
Birmingham,AL
PARTRIDGE,R.,MD 29
Boston,MA
PASSO,M.H.,MD 79
Indianapolis,IN
PERLMAN,S.G.,MD 64
Chicago,IL
PERSON,D.A.,MD 77
Houston,TX
PFEIFFER,C.,PhD 26,62
Farmington,CT
PFEIFFER,C.A.,PhD 73
Farmington,CT
PIGG,J.S.,RN, BSN 28,49
Milwaukee,WI
PINCUS,T.,MD 46
Nashville,TN
POTTS,M.K.,MSW 82
Indianapolis,IN
QUINNEY,A.,PhD 6
Edmonton,AL
RAFFERTY,N.,OTR, BS 67
Kansas City,MO
RAISH,P.,RN,MS,ANP 71
Denver,CO
RAMIREZ,S.,BA 35
Chicago,IL
RAY,L.E.,MA, MLS 21
Cleveland,OH
REID,A.,BSN,RN 15
Detroit,MI
REISINE,S.,PhD 69
Farmington,CT
RETZINGER,D.,BS, OTR 70
Chapel Hill,NC
RIPPEY,R.,PhD 26,62,73
Farmington,CT
RODON,C.M.,MEd, OTR 19
Columbia,MO
ROSS,C.K.,ScD 35
Evanston,IL
ROTH,S.,MD 1
Phoenix,AZ
SAKALYS,J.,PhD, RN 48
Denver,CO
SANDBORG,C.,MD 68
Orange,CA
SCHADE,J.,RN 79
Indianapolis,IN
SCHMID,K.L.,MSW, LCSW 47,68
Orange,CA
SCHNEIDER,M.,RN, BSN 31
Philadelphia,PA
SCHROEDER,L.K.,PT 42,66
Ann Arbor,MI
SHEAR,E.S.,MSW 78,75
Cincinnati,OH
SHERRY,D.D.,MD 13
Seattle,WA
SHIELDS,C.D.,BSN 74,77
Houston,TX
SHOOR,S.,MD 81
Santa Clara,CA
SHORE,A.,MD, FRCP 38,39
Toronto,BC
SMALL,D.,RN, BSN 63
Phildelphia,PA
SMITH,M.K.,ADMIN.ASST 19,7
Columbia,MO
SMITH, II,R.,MD 45
Atlanta,GA
SPILBERG,F.,PhD 12
Lemay,MO
SPITZ,P.W.,RN, MA 1
Stanford,CA
STABENOW,C.A.,BS, OTR 44,32
Charlottesville,VA
STEFL,M.E.,PhD 78
San Antonio,TX
STENGEM,C.,RPT 36
Los Angeles,CA
STOCK,S.,OTR 20
Lansing,MI
SZYDLO,N.,BSW 59
Nashville,TN
TACK,B.,RN, MSN 45
Bethesda,MD
TAYLOR,J.,BSN 79
Indianapolis,IN
TEHAN,N.A.,RN, BS 52,74
Hanover,NH
TENBRINK,T.D.,PhD 72
Columbia,MO
THAL,S.,BA 62
Farmington,CT
TU,K.,MSN, CRN 33
Birmingham,AL
VAN DEUSEN,J.,PhD, OTR 88
Madison,WI
VECCHIOLLA,T.,RN, BSN 32
Chalottesville,VA
VOITH,A.,RN, BSN 28
Milwaukee,WI
VOSTREJS,M.,RPT 76
Denver,CO
WAGNER,D.,RN, MS 11
Indianapolis,IN
WALLSTON,K.,PhD 59
Nashville,TN
WATHAL,J., ... 10
Birmingham,AL
WEAVER,J.I.,RN 54
Lincoln,NE
WEBEL,R.B.,MD 7
Columbia,MO
WEGENER,S.T.,PhD 44,32
Charlottesville,VA

WEINER,S.R.,MD 57
Van Nuys,CA
WESSEL,J.,PhD 6
Vancouver,BC
WETSTONE,S.,MD 62
Farmington,CT
WHITE,V.L.,BSc, OT 55,56
Vancouver,BC
WHITLING,S., ... 23
Vancouver,BC
WHITMEYER,B.,RN, DNSc 54,14
Boston,MA
WILCOX,B.L.,PhD 43
Charlottesville, VA
WILSON,C.,MD 45
Atlanta,GA
WINDER,P.A.,RN, MS 65
San Francisco,CA
WINELAND,M.D.,RN, MSN 8
Washington,DC
WOLFE,F.,MD 1,80
Wichita,KS
WOTRING,K.D.,BS 36
Los Angeles,CA
WRIGHT,V.,BSc, PT 39,38
Toronto,ON
YARBORO,C.,RN, BSPA 84
Rockville,MD
YOCUM,D.,MD 84
Bethesda,MD
ZABINSKI,C.,BSN, RN 15
Detroit,MI
ZIEGLER,G.C.,RN, MSN 85
Pittsburgh,PA
ZISCHKE,J.,RN, MSN 8
Fairfax,VA

AHPA KEY PHRASE INDEX

Advance nursing education ... 31
Aerobic exercise ... 7
Aerobic-like exercise ... 64
Allied health ... 4
Anxiety and depression in RA ... 80
Arthritis ... 55,23
Arthritis and exercise ... 65
Arthritis costs and utilization ... 1
Arthritis experience ... 59
Arthritis groups: lupus and JRA ... 47
Arthritis knowledge ... 83
Arthritis rehabilitation ... 8
Assessing patient understanding ... 72
Assessing perceived needs ... 24
Assessment ... 17
Assessment tools ... 45
Attitudes ... 46
Attitudes about arthritis ... 83
Behavior modification for children ... 68
Beliefs about arthritis ... 82
Career achievement outcome ... 75
Career education begins at diagnosis ... 75
Cause and penalities of gait deviations ... 87
Cervical collar ... 55,58
Childhood dermatomyositis ... 39
Childhood juvenile arthritis ... 39
Children's arthritis ... 53
Community arthritis education ... 83
Community outreach clinics ... 77
Community services ... 3
Community-based arthritis program ... 4
Competence in rheumatology ... 34
Competency-based curriculum ... 34
Compliance ... 35
Computer based education ... 62
Continued enhancement ... 63
Continuous passive motion (CPM) ... 5
Coping with rheumatic disease ... 51
Cost of health care ... 15
Cybex testing ... 66
Descriptive characteristics ... 28
Developing workshops ... 32
Diagnosis ... 25
Disability evaluation ... 20
Disability on women with arthritis ... 69
Disease variables ... 84
Educational needs assessment ... 60
Effective implementation ... 63
Effects of exercise in arthritis ... 8
Effects on hand symptoms ... 18
Elderly ... 29
Elderly, older adults ... 11
Ethnic differences ... 26
Evaluation ... 73,56
Evaluation of patient knowledge ... 72
Evaluation of summer camp ... 78
Exercise ... 6,22,65
Exercise and arthritis ... 7
Exercise and relaxation ... 88
Exercise program formats ... 37
Family and rheumatoid arthritis ... 14
Family relationships ... 54
Fatigue ... 28
Function ... 17
Functional assessment ... 16
Functional measurement ... 84
Functional mobility ... 45
Functional outcome measure ... 16
Gait deviations in RA ... 87
Graphic display of team eval. findings ... 67
Group intervention with teens ... 51
Group vs. individual instruction ... 61
Guidelines and procedures ... 63
HAQ and AIMS ... 43
Health care delivery system ... 9
Health education ... 35
Health education planning ... 40
Health outcome measure ... 44
Health service utilization ... 1
Health status outcome ... 81
Hip contracture ... 38
Home health nursing ... 32
Home program compliance ... 37
Home programs ... 19
Homemaker functioning ... 69
Hospitalization effects ... 27
Illustration of patient changes ... 67
Immunosuppressants ... 30
In-pool exercise ... 7
Innovative physical therapy methods ... 50
Inpatient rehabilitation program ... 44
Instruction of rheumatology nursing ... 33
Integrated curriculum in arthritis ... 70
Integrated education & treatment service ... 4
International AHP activities ... 49
International AHP organizations ... 49
International arthritis care ... 49
JRA - Knee resting splint ... 58
JRA Patient/Family Education ... 52
JRA children under 7 years ... 50
Juvenile arthritis ... 38,79
Juvenile rheumatic disease patients ... 78,75
Juvenile rheumatoid arthritis ... 53,35,76
Knee contracture ... 38
Lay vs. professional ... 60
Learning readiness ... 71
Library, health center ... 21
Library, hospital ... 21
Lidocaine ... 13
Low back injury ... 40
Low income minority ... 26
Low literacy ... 61,73
MCP arthroplasties ... 17
Measurement of function ... 45
Measuring disability ... 69
Methylprednisolone ... 30
Mid-life experience ... 86
Modifications ... 23
Modular splinting ... 58
Motivation ... 62

Multipurpose arthritis center projects 70
Muscle testing 39
Mychorysine injections 13
Needs assessment 3,74
Neuromuscular electrical stimulation 5
Non-compliance in arthritic children 68
Non-compliance issues 86
Nurse practitioner 9
Nursing diagnoses 29
Nursing diagnosis 28
Nursing research 48
Nursing services 9
Nursing standards of care 30
Nursing students learn arthritis 33
Nutritional assessment 10
OT-PT education 70
Occupational - physical therapy 20
Occupational therapy 19
Occupational therapy assessment 16
Outreach for community professionals 31
Pain 57,81
Pain in children 53
Pain management treatment 12
Parenting 54
Patient and family education program 85
Patient education 71,74,88,73,37,62,65
Patient education methods 15
Patient service needs 3
Patient/family resources 52
Pediatric outreach programs 77
Pediatric rheumatology 74
Pediatric rheumatology outreach 77
Pediatrics 36
Physical therapy 34,36
Physical therapy evaluation 42
Physical therapy treatment 42
Play adaptations 68
Polymyositis 42,66
Post-injection discomfort 13
Preparing a needs assessment 24
Problem-solving patient education 64
Problems in elderly with arthritis 29
Professional continuing education 32
Professional education 11
Prognostic value 10
Psycho-social and functional status 27
Psychological dysfunction 59
Psychological status 81
Public health nursing 11
Quality assurance 41
Quality of care 41
Questionnaires 46
RA elbow flexion contracture 22
RA outcome and psychological status 80
Range of motion 76
Recreational exercise and arthritis 8
Recreational exercises for JRA children 50
Reference manual 52
Reference seminar 21
Reflex neurovasuclar dystrophy 36
Research 88
Rheumatic disease 54
Rheumatoid arthritis 6,10,15,18,19,57,64,71
Rheumatoid arthritis costs 1
Rheumatoid arthritis patients 12,44,27
Rheumatoid arthritis, function capacity 46
Rural population 43,60
School and public health nurses 31
School problems in juvenile arthritis 79
Seat belts 23
Self-administered measures 43
Self-care education for rural persons 61
Self-esteem/independence 78
Self-help groups 47
Self-report 25
Serial psychological measurements in RA 80
Social security disability determination 20
Social support 59
Splinting 57,55
Standards of care 41
Strength 6
Strength assessment 66
Stress and despression 12
Stretch glove 18
Structured interview development 24
Support groups: lupus and JRA 47
Systemic lupus erythematosus 85,84
Teacher responsibilities 79
Teaching strategies 33
Teen support group 51
Terminology in arthritis education 72
Tool for assessment of patient education 2
Total knee arthroplasty in RA 5
Traction 22
Treatment of gait deviations in RA 87
Unified arthritis flowsheet 67
Urban minority health care practices 26
Warm water exercise 76
Women with arthritis 86
Working splint 56
Worksite 40
Wrist 56